# Textbook of the Autoimmune Diseases

# Textbook of the Autoimmune Diseases

Edited by

**Robert G. Lahita**, M.D., Ph.D.
*Professor*
*Department of Medicine*
*The New York Medical College*
*Chief*
*Rheumatology and Connective Tissue Diseases*
*Saint Vincent's Hospital and Medical Center*
*New York, New York*

Associate Editors

**Nicholas Chiorazzi**, M.D.
*Professor*
*Department of Medicine and Pathology*
*New York University School of Medicine*
*New York, New York*
*Chief*
*Division of Rheumatology and Allergy–Clinical Immunology*
*North Shore University Hospital*
*Manhasset, New York*

**Westley H. Reeves**, M.D.
*Marcia Whitney Schott Professor of Medicine*
*Chief*
*Division of Rheumatology and Clinical Immunology*
*College of Medicine*
*University of Florida*
*Gainesville, Florida*

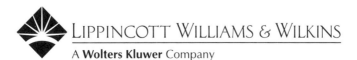
LIPPINCOTT WILLIAMS & WILKINS
A **Wolters Kluwer** Company
Philadelphia · Baltimore · New York · London
Buenos Aires · Hong Kong · Sydney · Tokyo

Acquisitions Editor: Jonathan Pine
Developmental Editor: Anne Snyder
Manufacturing Manager: Colin J. Warnock
Production Manager: Jodi Borgenicht
Production Editor: Jonathan Geffner
Cover Designer: Mark Lerner
Indexer: Kathleen Patterson
Compositor: Circle Graphics
Printer: Maple Press

© 2000 by LIPPINCOTT WILLIAMS & WILKINS
530 Walnut Street
Philadelphia, PA 19106 USA
LWW.com

Printed in the United States of America

9   8   7   6   5   4   3   2   1

**Library of Congress Cataloging-in-Publication Data**

Textbook of the autoimmune diseases / editor, Robert G. Lahita ; associate editors,
Nicholas Chiorazzi, Westley H. Reeves.
    p. ; cm.
   Includes bibliographical references and index.
   ISBN 0-7817-1505-9 (alk. paper)
   1. Autoimmune diseases. 2. Autoimmunity. I. Lahita, Robert G (Robert George),
1945- II. Chiorazzi, Nicholas. III. Reeves, Westley H.
   [DNLM: 1. Autoimmune Diseases. WD 305 T355 2000]
RC600 .T495 2000
616.97´8—dc21
                                         99-054064

To our wives and children

Terry Lahita and children Eric and Jason
Lorraine Chiorazzi and children Anne and Michael
Frances Reeves and children Lawrence and Thomas

# Contents

## Section I.  Overview

*Autoimmunity: Basic Mechanisms*

*Autoimmune Disease: Pathogenesis*

*Future Therapy of Autoimmune Disease*

# Contributing Authors

**Steven B. Abramson, M.D.**
*Professor*
*Departments of Medicine and Pathology*
*New York University School of Medicine*
*550 1st Avenue*
*New York, New York 10021*
*Chief, Department of Rheumatology*
*Hospital for Joint Diseases*
*301 East 17th Street*
*New York, New York 10003*

**Lori J. Albert, M.D.**
*Assistant Professor*
*Department of Medicine*
*University of Toronto*
*585 University Avenue*
*Toronto, Ontario M5G 2C4, Canada*
*Staff Physician*
*Department of Medicine*
*Division of Rheumatology*
*University Health Network*
*Toronto Western Hospital*
*399 Bathurst Street*
*Toronto, Ontario M5T 2S8, Canada*

**Jorge Alcocer-Varela, M.D.**
*Professor of Immunology*
*Department of Immunology*
*Instituto Nacional Nutricion*
*Vasco de Quiroga 15 Tlalpan*
*Mexico, DF 14000, Mexico*
*Chairman, Department of Immunology*
*    and Rheumatology*
*Instituto Nacional Nutricion*
*Vasco de Quiroga 15 Tlalpan*
*Mexico, DF 14000, Mexico*

**Anthony A. Amato, M.D.**
*Associate Professor*
*Department of Neurology*
*Harvard Medical School*
*Boston, Massachusetts 02115*
*Chief, Neuromuscular Division*
*Department of Neurology*
*Brigham and Women's Hospital*
*75 Francis Street*
*Boston, Massachusetts 02115*

**David E. Anderson, Ph.D.**
*Postdoctoral Fellow*
*Department of Medical Microbiology*
*    and Immunology*
*University of California, Davis School*
*    of Medicine*
*Tupper Hall, Room 3141*
*Davis, California 95616*

**Ronald A. Asherson, M.D.**
*Honorary Consultant Physician*
*Rheumatic Diseases Unit*
*Department of Medicine*
*The Groote Schuur Hospital*
*Observatory, Cape Town, South Africa 7937*

**John P. Atkinson, M.D.**
*Professor of Medicine and Molecular*
*Microbiology*
*Department of Internal Medicine*
*Division of Rheumatology*
*Washington University School of Medicine*
*Physician*
*Department of Internal Medicine*
*Barnes Jewish Hospital*
*660 South Euclid Avenue*
*St. Louis, Missouri 63110-1093*

**Daniel E. Banks, M.D.**
*N. LeRoy Lapp Professor and Chief*
*Section of Pulmonary and Critical Care Medicine*
*West Virginia University School of Medicine*
*3306 Health Sciences South*
*100 Medical Center Drive*
*Morgantown, West Virginia 26506-9166*
*Staff Physician*
*Department of Medicine*
*Ruby Memorial Hospital*
*Morgantown, West Virginia 26505*

**Richard J. Barohn, M.D.**
*Professor and Acting Chairman*
*Department of Neurology*
*The University of Texas Southwest Medical Center*
*    at Dallas*
*5323 Harry Hines Boulevard*
*Dallas, Texas 75390-8897*

**Rubens Belfort, Jr., M.D., Ph.D., M.B.A.**
*Professor and Chairman*
*Department of Ophthalmology*
*Federal University of São Paulo*
*Rua Botucatu, 822*
*04023-062 São Paulo, Brazil*
*Chief, Department of Ophthalmology*
*São Paulo Hospital*
*Rua Botucatu, 822*
*04023-062 São Paulo, Brazil*

**Robert M. Bennett, M.D.**
*Professor*
*Department of Medicine*
*Chairman, Division of Arthritis and Rheumatic*
  *Diseases*
*Department of Medicine*
*Oregon Health Sciences University*
*3181 Southwest Sam Jackson Park Road*
*Portland, Oregon 97201*

**Pierluigi E. Bigazzi, M.D.**
*Professor*
*Department of Pathology*
*University of Connecticut Health Center*
*263 Farmington Avenue*
*Farmington, Connecticut 06030*

**Warren Kline Bolton, M.D.**
*Professor*
*Department of Internal Medicine*
*Chief, Division of Nephrology*
*University of Virginia Health System*
*Box 133 Health Sciences Center*
*Charlottesville, Virginia 22908*

**D. Ware Branch, M.D.**
*Professor*
*Department of Obstetrics and Gynecology*
*The University of Utah*
*50 North Medical Drive*
*Salt Lake City, Utah 84132*

**Robin L. Brey, M.D.**
*Associate Professor*
*Department of Medicine*
*Division of Neurology*
*The University of Texas Health Science Center*
  *at San Antonio*
*7703 Floyd Curl Drive*
*San Antonio, Texas 78284-7883*

**Ricard Cervera, M.D., Ph.D.**
*Associate Professor*
*Department of Medicine*
*University of Barcelona*
*Villarroel, 170*
*08036 Barcelona, Catalonia, Spain*
*Senior Specialist*
*Systemic Autoimmune Diseases Unit*
*Hospital Clínic*
*Villarroel, 170*
*08036 Barcelona, Catalonia, Spain*

**Nicholas Chiorazzi, M.D.**
*Professor*
*Departments of Medicine and Pathology*
*New York University School of Medicine*
*550 1st Avenue*
*New York, New York 10021*
*Chief, Division of Rheumatology and*
  *Allergy–Clinical Immunology*
*Department of Medicine*
*North Shore University Hospital*
*350 Community Drive*
*Manhasset, New York 11030*

**Philip L. Cohen, M.D.**
*Professor*
*Department of Medicine*
*The University of Pennsylvania*
*421 Curie Boulevard*
*Philadelphia, Pennsylvania 19104-6100*
*Attending Physician*
*Philadelphia Veterans Affairs*
*38th Street and Woodland Avenue*
*Philadelphia, Pennsylvania 19103*

**P. K. Coyle, M.D.**
*Professor of Neurology*
*Director, Stony Brook Multiple Sclerosis*
  *Comprehensive Care Center*
*Department of Neurology*
*State University of New York at Stony Brook*
*Attending Neurologist*
*Health Sciences Center, T12*
*School of Medicine*
*Stony Brook, New York 11794-8121*

**Mary K. Crow, M.D.**
*Professor*
*Department of Medicine*
*Weill Medical College of Cornell University*
*Attending Physician*
*Department of Medicine*
*Hospital for Special Surgery*
*535 East 70th Street*
*New York, New York 10021*

**Marta Lucia Cuellar, M.D.**
*Assistant Professor*
*Department of Medicine*
*Section of Rheumatology*
*Tulane University School of Medicine*
*1430 Tulane Avenue, SL 46*
*New Orleans, Louisiana 70112*
*Department of Medicine*
*Tulane University Hospital and Clinic*
*1415 Tulane Avenue*
*New Orleans, Louisiana 70112*

**David I. Daikh, M.D., Ph.D.**
*Assistant Professor*
*Department of Medicine*
*University of California, San Francisco*
*505 Parnassus Avenue*
*San Francisco, California 94143*
*Attending Rheumatologist*
*Department of Medicine*
*Rheumatology Section*
*Veterans Administration Medical Center*
*4150 Clement Street*
*San Francisco, California 94121*

**Harish P. G. Dave, M.D.**
*Associate Professor*
*Division of Hematology–Oncology*
*George Washington University*
*2150 Pennsylvania Avenue Northwest*
*Washington, DC 20037*
*Assistant Chief, Hematology Section*
*Chief, Laboratory of Molecular Hematology*
*Veterans Affairs Medical Center*
*50 Irving Street Northwest*
*Washington, DC 20422*

**Kevin A. Davies, M.D.**
*Senior Lecturer*
*Rheumatology Section*
*Division of Medicine*
*Imperial College School of Medicine*
*London W12 0NN, United Kingdom*
*Clinical Director of Medicine*
*Directorate of Medicine*
*Hammersmith Hospital*
*Du Cane Road*
*London W12 0NN, United Kingdom*

**Luis A. Diaz, M.D.**
*Professor and Chairman*
*Department of Dermatology*
*University of North Carolina at Chapel Hill*
*3100 Thurston Building*
*CB #7287*
*Chapel Hill, North Carolina 27599*

**Luis R. Espinoza, M.D.**
*Professor and Chief*
*Department of Medicine*
*Section of Rheumatology*
*Louisiana State University School of Medicine*
*1542 Tulane Avenue*
*New Orleans, Louisiana 70112-2822*

**Janet A. Fairley, M.D.**
*Professor*
*Department of Dermatology*
*Medical College of Wisconsin*
*8701 Watertown Plank Road*
*Milwaukee, Wisconsin 53226*
*Section Chief*
*Department of Dermatology*
*Zablocki VA Medical Center*
*1000 National Avenue*
*Milwaukee, Wisconsin 53226*

**Manish J. Gharia, M.D.**
*Resident Physician*
*Department of Dermatology*
*Medical College of Wisconsin*
*9200 West Wisconsin Avenue*
*Milwaukee, Wisconsin 53226*
*Resident Physician*
*Department of Dermatology*
*Froedtert Memorial Lutheran Hospital*
*9200 West Wisconsin Avenue*
*Milwaukee, Wisconsin 53226*

**Allan Gibofsky, M.D.**
*Professor of Medicine and Public Health*
*Weill Medical College of Cornell University*
*Attending Physician*
*Department of Rheumatology*
*Hospital for Special Surgery*
*535 East 70th Street*
*New York, New York 10021*

**George J. Giudice, Ph.D.**
*Professor*
*Departments of Dermatology and Biochemistry*
*Medical College of Wisconsin*
*8701 Watertown Plank Road*
*MFRC Room 4070*
*Milwaukee, Wisconsin 53226*

**Jörg J. Goronzy, M.D.**
*Professor of Medicine and Immunology*
*Department of Medicine*
*Division of Rheumatology*
*Mayo Clinic and Foundation*
*200 First Street Southwest*
*Rochester, Minnesota 55905*

**Peter K. Gregersen, M.D.**
*Professor*
*Departments of Medicine and Pathology*
*New York University School of Medicine*
*401 East 30th Street*
*New York, New York 10016*
*Chief, Division of Biology and Human Genetics*
*North Shore University Hospital*
*350 Community Drive*
*Manhasset, New York 11030*

**David A. Hafler, M.D.**
*Breakstone Professor*
*Department of Neurology (Neuroscience)*
*Harvard Medical School*
*77 Avenue Louis Pasteur*
*Boston, Massachusetts 02115*
*Director, Laboratory for Molecular Immunology*
*Center for Neurologic Diseases*
*Brigham and Women's Hospital*
*77 Avenue Louis Pasteur*
*Boston, Massachusetts 02115*

**Harry H. Hatasaka, M.D.**
*Associate Clinical Professor*
*Department of Obstetrics and Gynecology*
*The University of Utah*
*Medical Director*
*Department of Reproductive Endocrinology*
*Utah Center for Reproductive Medicine*
*University of Utah School of Medicine*
*50 North Medical Drive*
*Salt Lake City, Utah 84132*

**Kevan C. Herold, M.D.**
*Associate Professor*
*Department of Medicine*
*Columbia University College of Physicians*
  *and Surgeons*
*Associate Attending Physician*
*Columbia Presbyterian Medical Center*
*1150 St. Nicholas Avenue*
*New York, New York 10032*

**Richard D. Huhn, M.D.**
*Associate Professor*
*Coriell Institute for Medical Research*
*401 Haddon Avenue*
*Camden, New Jersey 08103*

**Anna Huttenlocher, M.D.**
*Assistant Professor*
*Departments of Pediatrics and Pharmacology*
*University of Wisconsin*
*3780 Medical Sciences Center*
*1300 University Avenue*
*Madison, Wisconsin 53706-1532*
*Assistant Professor/Attending*
*Department of Pediatrics*
*University of Wisconsin*
*600 Highland Avenue*
*Madison, Wisconsin 53792*

**Robert D. Inman, M.D.**
*Professor*
*Department of Medicine and Immunology*
*University of Toronto*
*585 University Avenue*
*Toronto, Ontario M5G 2C4, Canada*
*Director, Arthritis Center of Excellence*
*University Health Network*
*Toronto Western Hospital*
*399 Bathurst Street*
*Toronto, Ontario M5T 2S8, Canada*

**Suresh Kerwar, Ph.D.**
*Director*
*CV Therapeutics*
*3172 Porter Drive*
*Palo Alto, California 94304*

**Robert G. Lahita, M.D., Ph.D.**
*Professor*
*Department of Medicine*
*The New York Medical College*
*Valhalla, New York 10595*
*Chief, Department of Rheumatology*
*Saint Vincent's Hospital and Medical Center*
*153 West 11th Street*
*New York, New York 10011*

**Robert S. Lebovics, M.D.**
*Clinical Associate Professor*
*Department of Otolaryngology*
*Mt. Sinai School of Medicine*
*1 Gustave Levy Place*
*New York, New York 10027*
*Chief, Otolaryngology*
*Department of Surgery*
*Cabrini Hospital and Medical Center*
*219 East 19th Street*
*New York, New York 10003*

**Mong-Shang Lin, Ph.D.**
*Assistant Professor*
*Department of Dermatology*
*University of North Carolina at Chapel Hill*
*3100 Thurston Building*
*C.B. #7287*
*Chapel Hill, North Carolina 27599*

**M. Kathryn Liszewski, B.A.**
*Research Scientist*
*Department of Medicine*
*Division of Rheumatology*
*Washington University School of Medicine*
*660 South Euclid Avenue, Box 8045*
*St. Louis, Missouri 63110*

**Zhi Liu, Ph.D.**
*Assistant Professor*
*Department of Dermatology*
*Medical College of Wisconsin*
*8701 Watertown Plank Road*
*Milwaukee, Wisconsin 53226*

**Robert W. McMurray, M.D.**
*Associate Professor*
*Department of Medicine*
*University of Mississippi Medical Center*
*2500 North State Street*
*Jackson, Mississippi 39216-4505*
*Staff Rheumatologist*
*Department of Medicine*
*G. V. (Sonny) Montgomery Veterans*
*    Affairs Hospital*
*1500 East Woodrow Wilson*
*Jackson, Mississippi 39216*

**Amy J. Miga, B.S.**
*Department of Microbiology*
*Dartmouth Medical School*
*One Medical Center Drive*
*Lebanon, New Hampshire 03756*

**Stanley J. Naides, M.D.**
*Thomas B. Hallowell Professor of Medicine*
*Professor of Microbiology and Immunology*
*Head, Section of Rheumatology*
*Department of Medicine*
*Pennsylvania State College of Medicine*
*Milton S. Hershey Medical Center*
*M.C. H038, P.O. Box 850*
*500 University Drive*
*Hershey, Pennsylvania 17033*

**Randolph J. Noelle, Ph.D.**
*Professor*
*Department of Microbiology*
*Dartmouth Medical School*
*One Medical Center Drive*
*Lebanon, New Hampshire 03756*

**Robert L. Ochs, Ph.D.**
*Senior Staff Scientist*
*Precision Therapeutics*
*3636 Boulevard of the Allies*
*Pittsburgh, Pennsylvania 15213*

**C. Lowell Parsons, M.D.**
*Professor*
*Department of Surgery*
*Division of Urology*
*University of California, San Diego*
*200 West Arbor Drive*
*San Diego, California 92103*

**Edward Penner, M.D.**
*Internal Medicine Clinic IV*
*University of Vienna*
*Waehringer Guertel 18-20*
*A-1090 Vienna, Austria*

**Westley H. Reeves, M.D.**
*Marcia Whitney Schott Professor of Medicine*
*Department of Medicine*
*Chief, Division of Rheumatology*
*University of Florida*
*College of Medicine*
*P.O. Box 100221*
*Gainesville, Florida 32610-0221*

**Walter Reinisch, M.D.**
*Department of Gastroenterology and Hepatology*
*Internal Medicine Clinic IV*
*University of Vienna*
*Waehringer Guertel 18-20*
*A-1090 Vienna, Austria*

**Hanno B. Richards, M.D.**
*Assistant Professor*
*Department of Medicine*
*Division of Rheumatology and Clinical Immunology*
*University of Florida*
*1600 Southwest Archer Road*
*P.O. Box 100221*
*Gainesville, Florida 32610*

**Lisa G. Rider, M.D.**
*Staff Scientist and Medical Officer*
*Laboratory of Molecular*
*  and Developmental Immunology*
*Division of Monoclonal Antibodies*
*Center for Biologics Evaluation and Research*
*U.S. Food and Drug Administration*
*Building 29B, Room 2G11, HFM-561*
*8800 Rockville Pike*
*Bethesda, Maryland 20892*

**Luiz Vicente Rizzo, M.D., Ph.D.**
*Professor*
*Department of Immunology*
*Institute of Biomedical Science*
*University of São Paulo*
*Av. Prof. Lineu Prestes, 1730*
*São Paulo, Brazil 05508-900*
*Scientific Director*
*Division of Allergy and Clincal Immunology*
*Hospital Das Clínicas*
*University of São Paolo*
*São Paolo, Brazil 05403-000*

**Michael Robson, B.A., M.R.C.P.**
*Research Fellow*
*Division of Medicine*
*Imperial College School of Medicine*
*Hammersmith Hospital*
*Du Cane Road*
*London W12 ONN, United Kingdom*

**Noel R. Rose, M.D., Ph.D.**
*Professor*
*Department of Pathology and of Molecular*
  *Microbiology and Immunology*
*The Johns Hopkins University*
*615 North Wolfe Street*
*Baltimore, Maryland 21205*
*Physician, Active Staff*
*Department of Medicine*
*The Johns Hopkins Hospital*
*600 North Wolfe Street*
*Baltimore, Maryland 21205*

**Anthony S. Russell, M.A., M.B., B.Chir.**
*Professor*
*Department of Medicine*
*University of Alberta*
*562 Heritage Medical Research Centre*
*Edmonton, Alberta, Canada T6G 2S2*

**David H. Sarne, M.D.**
*Associate Professor*
*Department of Medicine*
*University of Illinois at Chicago*
*1819 West Polk Street*
*Chicago, Illinois 60612*
*Attending*
*Department of Medicine*
*University of Illinois at Chicago Medical Center*
*1740 West Taylor Street*
*Chicago, Illinois 60612*

**Minoru Satoh, M.D.**
*Research Associate Professor*
*Department of Medicine*
*University of Florida*
*1600 Southwest Archer Road*
*P.O. Box 100221*
*Gainesville, Florida 32610-0221*

**Peter H. Schur, M.D.**
*Professor*
*Department of Medicine*
*Harvard Medical School*
*25 Shattuck Street*
*Boston, Massachusetts 02115*
*Professor*
*Department of Medicine*
*Division of Rheumatology, Immunology, and Allergy*
*Brigham and Women's Hospital*
*75 Francis Street*
*Boston, Massachusetts 02115*

**Margaret D. Smith, M.D.**
*Assistant Professor*
*Department of Medicine*
*New York Medical College*
*Program Director*
*Department of Rheumatology*
*St. Vincent's Hospital and*
  *Medical Center of New York*
*153 West 11th Street*
*New York, New York 10011*

**V. Bala Subramanian, M.D.**
*Instructor*
*Department of Medicine*
*Division of Rheumatology*
*Washington University School of Medicine*
*660 South Euclid Avenue*
*Box 8045*
*St. Louis, Missouri 63110*
*Assistant Physician*
*Barnes–Jewish Hospital*
*One Barnes–Jewish Hospital Plaza*
*St. Louis, Missouri 63110*

**Ira N. Targoff, M.D.**
*Associate Professor*
*Department of Medicine*
*University of Oklahoma*
*920 Stanton L. Young Boulevard*
*Oklahoma City, Oklahoma 73104*
*Oklahoma Medical Research Foundation*
*825 Northeast 13th Street*
*Oklahoma City, Oklahoma 73104*
*Department of Medicine*
*Veterans Affairs Medical Center*
*921 Northeast 13th Street*
*Oklahoma City, Oklahoma 73104*

**David O. Taylor, M.D.**
*Associate Professor*
*Department of Medicine*
*Division of Cardiology*
*University of Utah Health Sciences Center*
*50 North Medical Drive*
*Salt Lake City, Utah 84132*

**Sanjeev Trehan, M.D.**
*Assistant Professor of Medicine*
*Department of Internal Medicine*
*Division of Cardiology*
*University of Utah*
*50 North Medical Drive*
*Salt Lake City, Utah 84132*
*Attending Physician*
*Division of Cardiology*
*University Hospital*
*50 North Medical Drive*
*Salt Lake City, Utah 84132*

**David E. Trentham, M.D.**
*Associate Professor*
*Department of Medicine*
*Harvard Medical School*
*25 Shadduck Street*
*Boston, Massachusetts 02115*
*Physician*
*Department of Medicine*
*Beth Israel Deaconess Medical Center*
*110 Francis Street*
*Boston, Massachusetts 02215*

**Kenneth S. K. Tung, M.D.**
*Professor of Pathology and Microbiology*
*Department of Pathology*
*University of Virginia Health Sciences Center*
*Box 214, Old Medical School, Room 4888*
*Charlottesville, Virginia 22908*

**Jan H. Vaile, B.Med.(Hons), M.S.**
*Clinical Lecturer*
*Faculty of Medicine*
*University of Sydney*
*Sydney, New South Wales 2006, Australia*
*Staff Specialist*
*Department of Rheumatology*
*Royal Prince Alfred Hospital*
*Missenden Road*
*Camperdown, New South Wales 2050, Australia*

**Xavier Valencia, M.D.**
*Division of Rheumatology and Immunology*
*Harvard Medical School*
*Brigham and Women's Hospital*
*Smith Building*
*One Jimmy Fund Way*
*Boston, Massachusetts 02115*

**Kumar Visvanathan, M.D., Ph.D.**
*Research Associate*
*Laboratory of Clinical Microbiology*
  *and Immunology*
*Physician*
*Rockefeller University Hospital*
*The Rockefeller University*
*1230 York Avenue*
*New York, New York 10021*

**Rhonda R. Voskuhl, M.D.**
*Assistant Professor*
*Department of Neurology*
*University of California, Los Angeles*
*710 Westwood Plaza*
*Los Angeles, California 90095*

**Mark J. Walport, Ph.D.**
*Chairman and Head*
*Division of Medicine*
*Imperial College School of Medicine, Technology,*
  *and Medicine*
*Hammersmith Campus*
*Du Cane Road*
*London W1 ONN, United Kingdom*
*Professor of Medicine*
*Consultant*
*Department of Rheumatology*
*Hammersmith Hospital*
*Du Cane Road*
*London W12ONN, United Kingdom*

**Józefa Węsierska-Gądek, Ph.D.**
*Associate Professor and Head*
*Cell Cycle Regulation*
*Institute of Tumorbiology—Cancer Research*
*8a Borschkegasse*
*A-1090 Vienna, Austria*

**Cornelia M. Weyand, M.D., Ph.D.**
*Professor of Medicine and Immunology*
*Department of Medicine*
*Division of Rheumatology*
*Mayo Clinic and Foundation*
*Guggenheim Building 401*
*200 First Street Southwest*
*Rochester, Minnesota 55905*

**David Wofsy, M.D.**
*Professor*
*Departments of Medicine and Microbiology/*
  *Immunology*
*University of California, San Francisco*
*4150 Clement Street (111R)*
*San Francisco, California 94121*
*Chief, Rheumatology Section*
*Department of Medicine*
*Rheumatology Section*
*Veterans Administration Medical Center (111R)*
*4150 Clement Street*
*San Francisco, California 94121*

**John B. Zabriskie, M.D.**
*Associate Professor*
*Head, Laboratory of Clinical Microbiology*
  *and Immunology*
*Senior Physician*
*Rockefeller University Hospital*
*The Rockefeller University*
*1230 York Avenue*
*New York, New York 10021*

**Xi-Xue Zhao, M.D., Ph.D.**
*Associate Scientist*
*POC.KIT Corporation*
*73 Galaxy Boulevard*
*Toronto, Ontario M9W 5T4, Canada*

# Foreword

It is difficult to say whether the end of an old century is more dramatic than the inauguration of a new century, but there is no doubt that the opening of the twenty-first century brings with it promises of innovations in the medical sciences that were undreamed of at the start of the twentieth century. These prospects sweep across the entire scope of medicine, from pediatrics to geriatrics, and from surgery to psychiatry. They arose from a century-long saga of fundamental research in biochemistry and genetics, which culminated in the modern era of molecular biology and such clinical advances as vaccination, diagnostic radiology, blood transfusion, antibiotics, and organ transplantation. These and many other landmarks of progress have irreversibly changed medical practice from guesswork to precise knowledge of the cause, prevention, and cure of numerous previously fatal or disabling diseases. Indeed, the ever-increasing population of healthy elderly in the modern industrialized world is a phenomenon that Thomas Malthus could not envision at the end of the eighteenth century in his *Essay on Population.*

Even so, many medical problems remain unsolved. Among these are diseases mediated by elements of the immune system, whether they are antibodies or cytotoxic T cells, and whether the inciting antigen is from an exogenous or endogenous source. Some of these disorders seem to be part of the costs of industrialization and economic inequality; asthma is an example of the health burden of pollution and poverty. Others, such as rheumatoid arthritis and Type I diabetes, arise primarily from a complex set of germline genes, which—unlike pollution and poverty—are inescapable once they have been inherited. These disease-permissive genes cannot be exclusive causes, however, because the concordance of a particular autoimmune disease—type 1 diabetes, for example—in identical twins is not even close to one hundred percent. It is ironic that the causes of so many immune-mediated diseases remain behind a veil of ignorance given the triumphant advances in fundamental immunology, which have shown us the gears and springs of the immune system in exquisite detail. The yawning gap between our knowledge of the organization of the immune system—down to the atomic level—and our ignorance as to why the patient with systemic lupus erythematosus is sick is symptomatic of the chasm between the reductionism of molecular biology and the essentially holistic problem of disease.

At the beginning of the twentieth century, knowledge of the properties of the immune system underwent a seismic shift. Before then, immunity was considered only in the light of a beneficial defense against infectious diseases. In 1881, Louis Pasteur demonstrated the protection of sheep against anthrax by immunization with an attenuated strain of the bacillus. In 1890, Behring and Kitasato found that serum from patients convalescing from diphtheria protected others against the infection. These events provided strong evidence for the emerging germ theory of disease. They also revealed the fundamental attribute of the immune system: a safeguard against infection.

In 1902, however, the possibility that immunity could be harmful was raised by Richet and Portier, who described the phenomenon of anaphylaxis. In rapid succession, Clemens von Pirquet discovered the mechanism of serum sickness and coined the term *allergy* (1903); Maurice Arthus described local anaphylaxis (1903); and Donath and Landsteiner reported the first autoimmune disease in man, paroxysmal cold hemoglobinuria (1904). If we include Robert Koch's discovery, in 1891, of the tuberculin reaction, then the basic elements of immunopathology were discovered within a mere thirteen-year period using simple technical means, and, with the exception of Karl Landsteiner, by investigators who were not professional immunologists but physiologists and physicians.

Autoimmunity was the most contentious aspect of the new science of immunology. In 1901, Paul Ehrlich, one of the founders of immunology and a Nobel Laureate (1908) propounded his dictum of *honor autotoxious*, which evolved from his studies of isoantibodies in goats. Unfortunately, *honor autotoxicus* was misunderstood as a claim that autoantibodies could not exist, when what Ehrlich really meant was that the body has ways of preventing them from developing and causing harm. Indeed, rather than deny the possibility of autoantibodies, Ehrlich proposed that the pathogenic effects of autoantibodies were blocked by corresponding

xix

autoantibodies—what today would be called antiidiotypes. So great was Ehrlich's influence that fifty years after *honor autotoxious*, Ernest Witebsky delayed for three years publication of the discovery of autoantibodies against thyroglobulin in his rabbit model of experimental thyroiditis while he looked for an error in the experiments.

A turning point in reversing the negative attitude about autoimmunity and autoimmune diseases was the demonstration in 1959 of autoimmune hemolytic anemia in the New Zealand Black mouse. The description of a spontaneous autoimmune disease in an animal loosened the stranglehold of the naysayers on studies of autoimmunity—if it happened in mice, why not in humans? By 1965, general acceptance of the reality of autoimmune diseases prompted the first international congress on autoimmunity, sponsored by the New York Academy of Sciences.

A key factor in the evolution of ideas about autoimmunity was McFarlane Burnet's theory of clonal selection, one of the earliest attempts to understand the cellular basis of immunity. Burnet was struck by evidence that exposure to an antigen in utero rendered an animal incapable of responding to that antigen after birth. This phenomenon, of which there were several examples during the 1950s, led Burnet to the ideas of immunological tolerance and the immunological self. Burnet held that one of the main functions of the immune system is to differentiate between self and nonself, and added that when this distinction breaks down the result is autoimmunity. It seems appropriate, at the beginning of this millennium, to abandon such anthropomorphic terms as "self" and "nonself." Immunology is riddled with references to human attributes for descriptions of biological phenomena ("see," "recognize," "tolerate," and "defend" are other examples). These substitutes are valuable as shorthand, and especially useful in disguising ignorance, but it is time to abandon the verbal and conceptual distinction between "self" and "nonself," because it is beyond doubt that the immense universe of receptor-binding properties of normal T cells and B cells includes the capacity to accommodate epitopes on autoantigens. The profound implications of this fact are far more useful today than any artificial distinction between self and nonself.

We now have an abundance of animal models of autoimmune diseases, but each of them has to be understood in the context of the corresponding human disease. Inbred strains of mice in which type 1 diabetes, systemic lupus erythematosus, or autoimmune hemolytic anemia develop are invaluable as long as we acknowledge that these animals are, in a way, case reports. They may depend on a single mutant gene, and often display a predictable clinical course and uniform lesions. None of them shows the extraordinary and unpredictable variations of multigenic human autoimmune diseases. We also have at our disposal exquisitely refined methods of studying T cells, B cells, antigen-presenting cells, and the lesions of autoimmune diseases, both in animal models and humans. The power of these methods places a high price on new ideas, hypotheses, and concepts about autoimmune diseases. The question is no longer how to do it, but what to do.

The enormous progress made in studies of autoimmunity and autoimmune diseases during the past century warrants a textbook devoted entirely to the field. The publication of this book marks a new beginning for investigators of autoimmunity and physicians who care for patients with autoimmune diseases. There is every reason to believe that the numerous lessons learned at the laboratory bench will be applied with increasing frequency and effectiveness to the treatment, and perhaps cure of autoimmune diseases. The induction of anergy to pathogenic autoantigens has already been achieved in patients, and many equally exciting therapeutic advances growing out of knowledge of regulatory and pathogenic cytokines are expected. Indeed, it is more than possible that such therapeutic advances will lead the way to defining the causes of autoimmune diseases, a necessary step if we are to devise the means of preventing them. The original meaning of "gamut" was the first note in the scale of medieval music; later, it came to mean all the notes of the musical scale. This book covers the gamut of autoimmune diseases—all the elements that will serve to transform the present cacophony into a coherent euphony.

*Robert S. Schwartz, M.D.*
*Deputy Editor*
*New England Journal of*
*Medicine*

# Preface

Autoimmunity cuts across many scientific disciplines and clinical specialties. A single idea drives this book: that physicians and scientists should have access, in one place, to authoritative and up-to-date information on the myriad autoimmune diseases. We hope that this text will provide a broad understanding of auto-immunity in disparate systems.

While this is not the only book dealing with autoimmunity and autoimmune diseases, it is unique in its breadth of coverage of the topic. Although these diseases usually are considered to fall within the realm of rheumatology or allergy, autoimmune processes can affect virtually any organ system. We have assembled a group of outstanding clinicians and scientists to provide different perspectives on the autoimmune processes affecting various organs. This "bench-to-bedside" approach continues a tradition followed at the Rockefeller University Hospital long before the phrase became fashionable. We intend to explain the clinical presentations of autoimmune disease in the context of new advances in basic immunology and immunopathology.

Although the immunology may at times seem complex to a nonimmunologist, understanding the immune mechanisms will provide the clinician with valuable insight into the diagnosis and treatment of patients with autoimmune diseases. Conversely, an appreciation of the various autoimmune syndromes is of considerable importance to scientists investigating disease pathogenesis. In the era of managed care, the practice of medicine increasingly has become disengaged from the basic science that is its foundation. This text represents an effort to reverse this unfortunate trend.

It should be recognized that immunology is a broad and rapidly changing field. While every effort has been made to be comprehensive, inevitably there have been omissions. The reader also will find some duplication within the book. This is purposeful and permits the reader to weigh opposing viewpoints. We have not avoided controversy but have attempted to provide a balanced perspective on such topics as the role of autoimmunity in individuals with silicone implants or fibromyalgia. Besides serving as an authoritative source of information about diseases generally accepted to be autoimmune in origin, the text will serve as a starting point for the reader trying to understand disorders that are not certain to be autoimmune-mediated.

*Robert G. Lahita, M.D., Ph.D.*
*Nicholas Chiorazzi, M.D.*
*Westley H. Reeves, M.D.*

# Acknowledgments

We would like to thank our Developmental Editor, Anne Snyder, for her hard work and dedication. This book would not be possible without her work and effort. We would also like to thank Ruth Weinberg for getting the book started and our Lippincott Williams & Wilkins Acquisitions Editor, Jonathan Pine, for bringing the book to final fruition.

# Textbook of the Autoimmune Diseases

# SECTION I

# Overview

*Textbook of the Autoimmune Diseases,*
Edited by R. G. Lahita, N. Chiorazzi, and W. H. Reeves,
Lippincott Williams & Wilkins, Philadelphia © 2000.

# CHAPTER 1

# Overview of the Immune System

Philip L. Cohen

The immune system protects against infection by recognizing microorganisms and disposing of them, by limiting the growth of certain neoplasms, and by eliminating senescent cells and macromolecules. To accomplish these tasks, it must reliably distinguish between self and nonself molecules. Disorders in this process may lead to pathologic autoimmunity. Clinical pathology may also arise from immune reactivity to exogenous antigens, producing allergic and other types of hypersensitivity. Immune recognition may occur through the action of complement proteins or through nonspecific receptors (i.e., nonspecific or innate immunity), or it may proceed through the engagement of the highly specific receptors on T and B lymphocytes (i.e., specific immunity).

## NONSPECIFIC IMMUNITY

Although lacking the exquisite specificity of the T-cell and B-cell receptors, natural killer (NK) cells, neutrophils, eosinophils, basophils, mast cells, and mononuclear phagocytes nonetheless have specific receptors that enable them to focus their potent effects on appropriate targets (1,2). So essential is the *mononuclear phagocyte system* (3) that its genetic absence or severe malfunction apparently constitutes a nonviable state. Blood monocytes represent newly formed mononuclear phagocytes in transit to more permanent resting sites in tissues. Different names have been given to the mononuclear phagocytes depending on the organs in which they are found (e.g., tingible bodies, fixed macrophages, histiocytes, Kupffer cells). Their variable appearance in tissues and their ability to take on different forms such as giant cells when involved in inflammatory processes belie their common origin. Tissue macrophages have the exceedingly important task of recognizing, engulfing, and disposing of the many apoptotic cells arising from senescence and injury (4). Recognition of dying cells depends on CD36/vitronectin

receptor, CD14, phosphatidyl serine receptors, and probably other mechanisms.

Macrophages must remain ready to undergo activation in response to T-cell–derived cytokines when infection is encountered. They are capable of undergoing remarkable enlargement, an increased metabolic rate, and increased phagocytic and pinocytic activity in response to cytokines, and they can secrete their own proinflammatory cytokines such as interleukin-1 (IL-1), interleukin-6 (IL-6), and tumor necrosis factor-$\alpha$ (5). Their generation of reactive oxygen products, nitric oxide, and important antimicrobial enzymes such as myeloperoxidase is vastly increased under conditions of T-cell activation and constitutes a crucial defense against intracellular organisms (6). Once ingested, most bacteria and viruses are killed through the formation of phagolysosomes by the merger of phagocytic vesicles with lysosomes (7). Enzymes, acidity, and toxic small molecules such as hydrogen peroxide and molecular oxygen bring about the death of most organisms and their subsequent degradation to simple molecules. Those that evade destruction through their waxy coats or other protective mechanisms are held in check, sometimes for years, and remain intracellular and latent. The role of the macrophages in the presentation of antigen to T cells through intracellular peptide association with nascent class II molecules has been de-emphasized in favor of dendritic cells, but macrophages probably do play a role in presenting peptide antigens to T lymphocytes.

*Mast cells* are pharmacologically active cells capable of receptor-mediated rapid release of agents stored in granules (e.g., histamine, heparin, heparan sulfate) and of synthesizing prostaglandins and leukotrienes. All of these substances have powerful effects on vascular permeability and on the recruitment of inflammatory cells. Mast cells are widely distributed, and there are some differences in the biology of those that line the respiratory tract and those in the intestine. Triggering of both types of mast cells may take place through their IgE receptors, through C3a and C5a receptors, or through direct interaction of certain agents with cell-membrane signaling pathways (8).

P. L. Cohen: Department of Medicine, University of Pennsylvania School of Medicine, Philadelphia, Pennsylvania 19103; Philadelphia VA Medical Center, Philadelphia, Pennsylvania 19103.

The *complement system* (9) serves a key role in host defense through activation of C3 by nonself surfaces, leading to the deposition of C3b and C3d on foreign particles. CR1, CR2, and CR3 receptors on neutrophils and macrophages enable these cells to bind to and phagocytose coated particles and constitute a crucial limb of host defense (Chapter 10). Other components of the complement system regulate its overall activation and affect opsonization and recruitment of additional inflammatory cells. The importance of C3 and its receptors in antimicrobial defense is clear: people born with defects in this system suffer severe and repeated pyogenic infections.

The *interferons* (α and β) are a family of macrophage-derived molecules with potent antiviral and proinflammatory activity (10). They induce class I and class II major histocompatibility complex (MHC) expression in addition to direct antiviral activity. Interferon-γ is produced by CD4 T lymphocytes and NK cells and has several key functions in addition to its antiviral properties. It is a key regulator of the $T_H1/T_H2$ polarization of cytokine responses, a concept discussed more fully later. It is itself a key $T_H1$ cytokine, and it promotes its own further production and that of other $T_H1$ cytokines while suppressing the production of $T_H2$ cytokines (11).

A variety of cytokines participate in nonspecific response to microbial stimuli, notably bacterial endotoxins. The immune system is remarkably sensitive to the effects of endotoxins, which are mediated in part through specific cell receptors (e.g., CD14) (12) and in part through the activation of the complement, kallikrein, and coagulation pathways. An array of vascular and inflammatory events ensues after local exposure to endotoxin; if sufficient endotoxin enters the circulation, vascular collapse, intravascular coagulation, fever, myocardial suppression, and diffuse capillary leakage due to massive cytokine production can be lethal.

An important defense against altered cells, especially tumor cells, is provided by NK cells. Like cytotoxic T lymphocytes, they possess large granules containing enzymes (granzymes) that induce apoptosis when injected into target cells, and they can mediate death of Fas (CD95)–bearing targets through the action of Fas ligand. Unlike cytotoxic T cells, their receptor lacks exquisite specificity and rather relies on the ability to detect abnormally low expression of class I MHC molecules, such as may be the case for a tumor or a cell infected by certain viruses (13).

## SPECIFIC IMMUNITY

Specificity and memory are the hallmarks of T-cell and B-cell immunity, the highly evolved and interdependent systems of antimicrobial and antitumor defense in higher vertebrates. T and B lymphocytes generate their receptors through the combined permutative effects of the use of multiple gene segments, which are rearranged and annealed to each other (Fig. 1.1). For B cells, somatic mutation plays an important additional role in creating remarkable diversity, providing a repertoire in which cells of nearly any specificity exist and are available for clonal expansion to provide cellular or humoral immunity against innumerable protein, lipid, and nucleic acid antigens (14). Unlike their nonspecific leukocyte counterparts, T and B lymphocytes undergo a complex process of differentiation involving prereceptors (for T cells) and a surrogate receptor for the light chain of the B cell.

### T Cells in the Immune Response

The thymus provides a site for the positive selection of desirable T cells and for the negative selection (by apoptosis) of T cells with harmful autoreactive receptors or with neutral nonuseful receptors. So stringent is thymic selection that only a few percent of T-cell precursors arriving from the marrow eventually exit the thymus as mature T cells (15).

The specificity of T cells is a property of their recognition of the molecules of the MHC (see Chapter 4). The T-cell receptor, a two-chain, cell-bound, immunoglobulin-like molecule, binds peptide fragments of protein antigens embedded in specific pockets of the α chain of class I MHC molecules or the β chain of class II molecules (16). T cells can be broadly divided into those recognizing class I–associated peptides (these usually also express the CD8 molecule, which in-

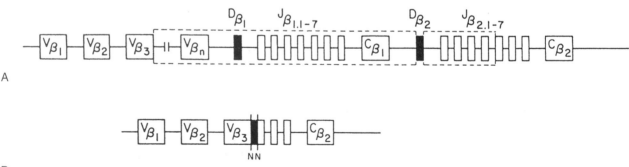

**FIG. 1.1.** Organization and rearrangement of the genes for the β chain of the human T-cell receptor. **A:** Germline configuration. **B:** Possible somatic rearrangement that uses the $V_\beta3$ gene, $D_\beta2$ element, $J_\beta2.5$ element, and $C_\beta2$ constant region gene. Portions of DNA *(dashed boxes)* in **A** are deleted during the process of somatic rearrangement to produce the complete T-cell receptor gene shown in **B**. The N regions marked are short sequences of nucleotides added at the junctions between the variable region and the D region and between the D and J regions.

creases the avidity of the class I interaction) and those recognizing class II–associated peptides (17). Class II–reactive T cells express CD4, which enhances signalling by virtue of its interaction with class II. The specificity of the T-cell receptor is derived from both of its chains; most T cells express αβ receptors, but a significant minority express the γδ receptor, which may be of special importance in the skin, gut, and female reproductive tract. The β chain encoded by certain $V_β$ genes can bind to superantigens, proteins that bind to regions shared by all members of a $V_β$ gene family, and consequently stimulate significant fractions of the T-cell repertoire (18). Because many of these superantigens are of microbial origin, this broad T-cell stimulation has important consequences.

T-cell receptors are located adjacent to the CD3 complex, a group of proteins with cytoplasmic tails that mediate T-cell activation after T-cell receptor cross-linking. Activation involves a series of kinases and results in signals for cellular proliferation and for the production of certain cytokines, particularly IL-2. The activation of T cells requires presentation of appropriate antigens and interaction between costimulatory molecules (19). The CD28 receptor on T cells interacts with B7.1 or B7.2 on T cells, and this interaction appears necessary for the CD3-mediated events described previously. The CTLA-4 molecule may also interact with B7.1 and B7.2, and transmit a negative signal that competes with the CD28-mediated positive signal.

Activated CD4 T cells can be thought of as executive cells, whose function is to influence the behavior of other cells, principally through the secretion of cytokines. CD4 T cells can be roughly divided into $T_H1$ cells, which secrete cytokines associated mainly with cell mediated immunity (e.g., IL-2, interferon-γ, IL-12, IL-18), and $T_H2$ cells, whose products mostly promote humoral immunity and allergy (e.g., IL-4, IL-5, IL-10, IL-13) (20).

In contrast to CD4 T cells, CD8 T cells recognize peptides associated with class I MHC molecules and are capable (like NK cells) of bringing about the death of their target cells (21). This they accomplish by expression of CD95L (FasL), which oligomerizes CD95 (Fas), which is likely to be present on activated cells harboring viruses or other intracellular parasites and induces rapid apoptosis, or by extrusion of perforins, proteins that form membrane channels resulting in increased electrolyte permeability and activate granzymes, provoking the apoptosis cascade. The destruction of class I MHC–bearing cells by T cells is crucial to the control of viral infections. The generation of specific CD8-bearing cytotoxic T lymphocytes requires CD4 helper T cells, probably as a source of IL-2 and other cytokines.

Specialization into CD4- or CD8-bearing cells occurs in the thymus after acquisition of the T-cell receptor. An important population of T cells matures extrathymically, perhaps representing as much as 50% of the total number of T cells. Most of this process takes place in intestinal lymphoid tissue, where most CD8-bearing intestinal T cells can be distinguished from those that mature in the thymus by their ex-

pression of two CD8 α chains instead of the CD8 αβ dimer expressed on thymus-derived CD8 cells.

A key feature of T cells is their recognition of peptide fragments of antigen that become associated with MHC molecules through the process of antigen presentation. For class I MHC molecules, peptides are generated from proteins already within the cell (and generally of microbial origin) through the proteasome, a particulate complex of proteolytic enzymes, and gain entry to the endoplasmic reticulum through transporter proteins. Seven to nine amino acid fragments of proteins are brought together with MHC molecules and intercalate into the peptide-binding groove of the third hypervariable region of the MHC alpha chain. Complete, peptide-bearing MHC molecules are exported to the cell surface associated with the $β_2$-microglobulin.

Some T cells recognize lipid-like antigens, such as lipoteichoic acid, presented by CD1, a molecule with structural homology to classic MHC antigens. These cells, which are predominantly CD4⁻CD8⁻ and express the γδ receptor, may be important in defense against mycobacteria and related pathogens.

## B Cells and Antibody Production

B lymphocytes are the source of circulating immunoglobulins: IgG, IgM, IgA, and IgE. IgD exists only in minute quantities in serum and functions primarily as a surface receptor. Antibodies consist of at least two identical heavy (H) chains and two identical light (L) chains (22) (Fig. 1.2). IgM exists as a pentamer of this $H_2L_2$ structure, and IgA usually exists as a dimer. Antibodies may bind to a wide variety of molecules, ranging from organic ring structures to proteins to

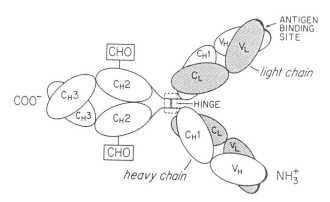

**FIG. 1.2.** Structure of an IgG molecule. Two identical heavy chains and two identical light chains are joined together by noncovalent and disulfide interactions. Additional disulfide bonds may exist between the $C_H1$ domain of the heavy chain and the $C_L$ domain of the light chain. The hinge regions between the $C_H2$ and the $C_H1$ domains are cross-linked by several disulfide bonds. Carbohydrate (CHO) is bound to the $C_H2$ domain. Antibodies of other isotypes have similar structures, although they may have different placement of disulfide bonds and carbohydrates and may be complexed into multimers of the basic $H_2L_2$ subunit.

polysaccharides and even to nucleic acids. The specificity of binding results from unique amino acid sequences in the amino termini of the heavy and light chains. These are encoded by the genetic recombination of a single $V_H$ or $V_L$ gene from a large number, with deletion of the intervening variable region (V) genes to a constant region (C) gene (this may be for one of the isotypes of IgG or for the other immunoglobulins or may be for the κ and λ chain constant region). For heavy chain genes, there is recombination with an additional D element, which further adds to the diversity of the final sequence (Fig. 1.3).

Added to the many recombinatorial possibilities of gene rearrangement is somatic mutation of the variable regions of mature antibody genes. This process is discussed more fully in Chapter 20. A B cell may rearrange only a single complete antibody gene; the inability to generate more than one antibody per B cell has been called *allelic exclusion,* and it is the basis of the clonal selection model of antibody production. Antibody responses arise from the clonal expansion of specific antibody-forming B cells through the interaction of antigen with their surface receptors. A B cell ordinarily uses IgM and IgD antibodies as its receptors but is capable of switching heavy-chain genes once engaged in an immune response. This process requires further genetic recombination. Antibody responses to newly encountered exogenous antigens generally begin with IgM antibody, followed in 7 to 10 days by IgG. The avidity (binding strength) of the IgG increases

with time, especially if the antigen is persistent or is administered again. Antibody responses to antigens to which antibody has previously been made result in more rapid and higher avidity responses, generally by IgG. This enhanced response is known as the *anamnestic response*, which results from the availability of memory B cells that persist from the initial responding clones. Immunologic memory is a key property of the specific immune system and may last for decades.

There are important roles for antibody in the serum, where it may neutralize toxins, opsonize particulate antigens, and recruit the complement system; and on mucosal surfaces. IgA is actively secreted into all regions of the gut and into the female genital tract, and it is of considerable importance in protecting these mucosal areas from infection.

IgE differs from all of the other immunoglobulin classes in that the bulk of this antibody is bound to mast cells by high-affinity receptors for its Fc region. Each mast cell expresses a representative sample of the IgE repertoire on its surface. If there are sufficient antigen molecules to cross-link sufficient receptors, mast cell degranulation and mediator synthesis occur, resulting in release of the potent pharmacologic mediators of immediate hypersensitivity. Depending on the location of the activated mast cell, local vascular permeability, inflammation, or bronchospasm may result.

T cells play a crucial role in promoting and regulating B-cell antibody production. Most antibody responses require collaboration between T and B cells, with direct T-B contact-

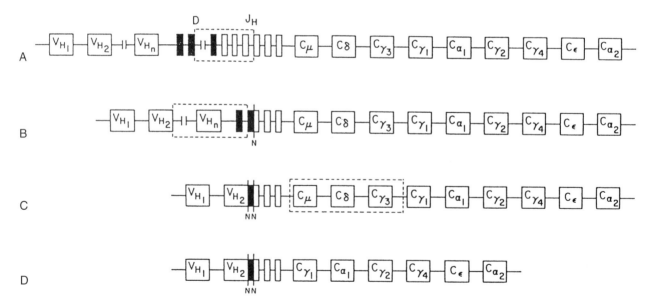

**FIG. 1.3.** Genetic organization and rearrangement of immunoglobulin heavy chain genes. This portion of chromosome 14 contains the immunoglobulin heavy chain variable region and constant region genes. **A:** Genomic organization found in all cells except committed B cells. **B:** Initial rearrangement produces the D-J joining, which results from deletion of the DNA *(dashed box)* shown in **A**. The junction between D and J regions includes additional nucleotides, constituting an N region. **C:** The next step in rearrangement is a V-D-J joining, which results from deletion of the DNA *(dashed box)* shown in **B**. A B cell expressing the rearranged gene shown in **C** may express IgM with the $V_H2$ variable region. **D:** Such a B cell could then undergo an isotype switch by deleting the DNA *(dashed box)* shown in **C** to express IgG1 with the same $V_H2$ variable region.

mediated (cognate) T-cell help facilitated by the interaction of T-cell CD40 ligand (CD154) with B-cell CD40 (23). T cells also supply critical cytokines that influence B-cell differentiation. In particular, the cytokines supplied by $T_H2$ helper T cells promote (human) IgG3, IgG4, and IgE production (24), whereas $T_H1$ cytokines promote (human) IgG1 production. T-T interactions further control the humoral immune response. Some antibody responses, principally of the IgM class, are relatively independent of T cells. Such responses are generally elicited by repeating polysaccharide antigens such as those found in certain bacterial capsules (25). Antibodies have a finite circulating half-life, depending on class, and their production is further controlled by feedback downregulation of several types, notably by antibody itself through Fc receptors on B cells.

Most B cells reside in marrow, lymph nodes, and spleen. An important B-cell subset, called B1 cells (26), primarily populates the peritoneal cavity and is responsible for a different repertoire of antibodies, primarily against commonly encountered bacterial antigens such as phosphatidylcholine. They also produce low-avidity autoantibodies, such as antierythrocyte and rheumatoid factors. Unlike conventional, or B2, cells somatic mutation of antibody genes does not occur among these cells.

### Antigen Presentation to CD4 T cells

CD4 and CD8 T cells bear receptors that recognize peptide fragments of antigen embedded in MHC molecules. For CD4 T cells, B cells are an important antigen-presenting cell population. Because of their specific surface immunoglobulin, they efficiently bind antigens. Protein antigens are engulfed to form a phagolysosome, in which degradation to peptides occurs with the help of proteolytic enzymes (27). Transport to the endoplasmic reticulum puts peptides in proximity with nascent class II MHC antigens, which are bound to the Ii (invariant) chain before binding to antigen peptides. Class II–peptide complexes are exported to the surface, where they are available for T-cell receptor binding and activation of specific T cells.

Dendritic cells, another bone marrow–derived population, have an important role in presentation of peptide antigens, probably mostly in splenic follicles. These cells express a high density of class II MHC antigens and are the most efficient antigen-presenting cells known.

### Immunologic Memory

One of the remarkable features of the immune response is the generation of more rapid, more vigorous, and higher-affinity antibody or T cells on secondary exposure to antigen. This is caused by the existence of memory T and B lymphocytes, small but vital populations that undergo rapid clonal expansion on recognition of antigen (28). Memory T cells bear the surface marker CD44 (in mice) and are $CD45RA^-CD45RO^+$ in humans. Autoantibody responses,

which involve chronic T-cell and B-cell stimulation, presumably recruit such memory cells.

### Tolerance

Specific unresponsiveness of T or B lymphocytes to antigens is known as tolerance. This process may occur by elimination of reactive lymphocytes by their inactivation, or it may be a result of the initial absence of reactive T and B lymphocytes (i.e., clonal ignorance) (29). The maintenance of self-tolerance is a high priority of the immune system. For T lymphocytes, the thymus serves as the locale where newly generated T cells with high-avidity receptors for self–MHC antigens plus peptides are eliminated through apoptosis. Further elimination of self-reactive T cells occurs in peripheral lymphoid organs and may involve deletion or inactivation of autoreactive T cells. A parallel situation exists for B lymphocytes, which undergo negative selection in marrow and fetal liver at early stages in their development and which are also subject to deletion or inactivation in the periphery.

### Regulation of the Immune Response

The characteristic waning of immune responses reflects several levels of control. The diminished presence of antigen resulting from immune clearance or from the resolution of an infection leads to a reduction in immunogenic stimulation. Antibody itself has a potent negative-feedback effect on further antibody production, mediated chiefly through Fc receptors on B lymphocytes. An important level of control comes from regulatory cytokines, particularly IL-10, which exert a negative action on further B-cell antibody production. Anti-idiotypic antibody, directed against antibody or T-cell variable region epitopes, may also play an important role in downregulating immune responses.

### Immune Injury

Injury by the immune system has historically been referred to as hypersensitivity. Hypersensitivity reactions typically arise in response to agents that themselves are not intrinsically harmful (30).

### *Type I: Anaphylactic Hypersensitivity*

Also known as immediate hypersensitivity reactions, anaphylactic reactivity is caused by the release of pharmacologic mediators stored in mast cell granules, which can result in formidable vascular effects in minutes. Mast cell degranulation is triggered by cross-linking of IgE, an immunoglobulin isotype that is primarily bound to mast cells through a unique Fc receptor; by interaction with the "anaphylatoxins" C3a and C5a; by some isotypes of IgG (notably IgG4); and by a variety of environmental agents, drugs, and chemicals. (The poorly understood cutaneous basophil hypersensitivity, or

Jones-Mote reaction, represents an analogous phenomenon precipitated by T-cell factors that bind to mast cells.) Antigens that can bind to two or more molecules of surface IgE cause a series of rapid events in the inositol triphosphate pathway, resulting in increased intracellular calcium and activation of protein kinase C. There is release of histamine, heparin, eosinophil, and neutrophil chemotactic factors, and platelet-activating factor (all stored in granules) and the synthesis and release of leukotrienes $B_4$, $C_4$, and $D_4$; prostaglandins; cytokines; and thromboxanes. These agents have potent pharmacologic effects. The most calamitous reaction is caused by degranulation of massive numbers of mast cells, causing systemic anaphylaxis.

Local anaphylaxis is manifested as allergic rhinitis, urticaria (hives), and bronchial asthma. Allergic rhinitis and bronchial asthma are precipitated by the inhalation of airborne allergens, such as pollen or dust, which trigger vasoactive mediator release in the nasal mucosa, conjunctivae, or bronchi. Urticarial reactions are usually caused by food allergens, but in many cases a cause cannot be identified. Only a minority of the population is prone to develop such allergic reactions. These atopic individuals have higher levels of circulating IgE (upward of 12 μg/mL, compared with 0.3 μg/mL in normal subjects) and have nearly all of their mast cell Fcε receptors occupied (compared with 20% to 50% in normal subjects). Atopy is genetically determined and usually results in broad reactivity against many allergens. Its survival advantage is unclear.

Allergic reactions have a late-phase component in addition to the immediate phase caused by the release of preformed mediates. The late-phase response is caused by the synthesis of prostaglandins and leukotrienes (products of arachidonic acid metabolism) and typically occurs about 6 hours after exposure, peaking at 12 hours. It is probably more significant for bronchial asthma than the immediate response.

### Type II: Antibody-Mediated Cytotoxic Hypersensitivity

In type II injury, antibody reactive to host cells causes injury. The antibody may be of self-origin (as in autoimmune diseases or certain drug reactions); it may have been infused (as in a blood transfusion); or it may have reached a fetus by crossing the placenta.

Immune injury may occur by four possible mechanisms: antibody-dependent cellular cytotoxicity; phagocytosis by Fc-receptor expressing cells; phagocytosis by C3b-receptor expressing cells (after C3 fixation); and lysis through activation of the entire complement cascade. Certain drugs have the capacity to elicit immune responses as haptens, with self-protein acting as carrier. Cell-bound drug becomes the target of drug-specific antibody, causing injury to the cell. Penicillin and other drugs can cause this form of hypersensitivity.

### Type III: Immune Complex–Mediated Hypersensitivity

Depending on the nature and valence of the antigen and on the relative amounts of antibody and antigen, antibody-antigen immune complexes can be large and insoluble. Their deposition in tissues can lead to many different pathologic conditions because of the ability of antibody to fix complement and initiate inflammation. In serum sickness, antigens elicit an antibody response and, at a particular antigen-antibody ratio, complexes deposit in tissues causing arthritis, glomerulonephritis, and rash. The antigen need not be foreign serum and is most commonly drugs, particularly antibiotics administered for long periods in large amounts.

### Damage From Antineutrophil Cytoplasmic Antibody

Certain types of renal and vascular injury have been recognized in the past decade to occur in association with antibody to neutrophil cytoplasmic antigens (ANCAs). Perinuclear (P-ANCAs) antibodies are usually directed against myeloperoxidase and cytoplasmic antibodies (C-ANCAs) antibodies are specific for a serine protease. ANCAs are thought to mediate damage by cross-linking small amounts of surface-bound antigen and triggering neutrophil release of toxic mediators. The pathogenic mechanism remains to be fully worked out, but the antibodies have considerable diagnostic value in certain forms of vasculitis (particularly Wegener's granulomatosis) and pauci-immune glomerulonephritis (31).

### Antiphospholipid Antibody–Associated Disease

Systemic lupus and related disorders can be associated with antibody to phospholipids, such as cardiolipin. The actual antigen recognized is controversial, but it may require the serum protein $β_2$-glycoprotein I. Paradoxically, the antibodies prolong *in vitro* coagulation (hence the term *lupus anticoagulant*) but are associated with thrombosis and thromboembolism *in vivo* and with recurrent fetal loss due to placental insufficiency (32).

### Type IV: Delayed-Type Hypersensitivity

The "delay" in delayed-type hypersensitivity (DTH) comes from the 24- to 48-hour latent period before the appearance of local redness and swelling and distinguishes DTH from the immediate (or nearly immediate) local reactions mediated by IgE. The tuberculin reaction, a paradigm of DTH, depends on specific immune T cells that patrol the body and localize to the site of injected antigen. They secrete cytokines that inhibit the migration of wandering macrophages (e.g., macrophage migration-inhibition factor) and other cytokines that call forth additional T cells and activate the T cells that are present (33). The result is a gradual accumulation of large numbers of "round cells," which are mostly activated macrophages. The end result is an inflammatory lesion known as a granuloma, which is centered on the invading organism or antigen and walls it off and destroys or inactivates it. Granulomas can be short lived, or they can be chronic, lasting many years.

# REFERENCES

1. Mahoney JA, Gordon S. Macrophage receptors and innate immunity. *Biochemist* 1998;20:12–16.
2. Ravetch JV. Fc receptors. *Curr Opin Immunol* 1997;9:121–125.
3. Van Furth R. *Mononuclear phagocytes: biology of monocytes and macrophages.* Dordrect, Netherlands: Kluwer, 1998.
4. Ren Y, Savill J. Apoptosis: the importance of being eaten. *Cell Death Differ* 1998;5:563–568.
5. Beelen RHJ. The macrophage: basic and clinical aspects. *Immunobiology* 1996;195:401–664.
6. MacMicking J, Xie Q, Nathan C. Nitric oxide and macrophage function. *Annu Rev Immunol* 1997;15:323–350.
7. Karnovsky MC, Bolis L. *Phagocytosis—past and future.* New York: Academic Press, 1982.
8. Marone G, Casolaro V, Patella V, et al. Molecular and cellular biology of mast cells and basophils. *Int Arch Allergy Immunol* 1997;144: 207–217.
9. Prodinger WM, Wuerzner R, Erdei A, et al. Complement. In: Paul WE, ed. *Fundamental immunology,* 4th ed. Philadelphia: Lippincott–Raven Publishers, 1999:967–995.
10. Hayes MP, Zoon KC. Production and action of interferons: new insights into molecular mechanisms of gene regulation and expression. *Prog Drug Res* 1994;43:239–270.
11. Bradley LM, Dalton DK, Croft M. A direct role for IFN-gamma in regulation of $T_H1$ cell development. *J Immunol* 1996;157:1350–1358.
12. Fenton MJ, Golenbock DT. LPS-binding proteins and receptors. *J Leukoc Biol* 1998;64:25–32.
13. Yokoyama WM. Natural killer cell receptors. *Curr Opin Immunol* 1998;10:298–305.
14. Manser T, Tumas-Brundage KM, Casson LP, et al. The roles of antibody variable region hypermutation and selection in the development of the memory B-cell compartment. *Immunol Rev* 1998;162:183–196.
15. Laufer TM, Glimcher LH, Lo D. Using thymus anatomy to dissect T-cell repertoire selection. *Semin Immunol* 1999;11:65–70.
16. Davis MM, Chien Y. T-cell antigen receptors. In: Paul WE, ed. *Fundamental immunology,* 4th ed. Philadelphia: Lippincott–Raven Publishers, 1999:341–366.
17. Chan S, Correia-Neves M, Benoist C, et al. CD4/CD8 lineage commitment: matching fate with competence. *Immunol Rev* 1999;165:195–207.
18. Florquin S, Aaderling L. Superantigens: a tool to give new insights into cellular immunity. *Res Immunol* 1997;148:373–386.
19. McAdam AJ, Schweitzer AN, Sharpe AH. The role of B7 co-stimulation in activation and differentiation of CD4+ and CD8+ T cells. *Immunol Rev* 1999;165:231–247.
20. Mosmann TR, Sad S. The expanding universe of T-cell subsets: Th1, Th2, and more. *Immunol Today* 1996;17:138–146.
21. Henkart P. CTL effector functions. *Semin Immunol* 1997;9:85–86.
22. Frazer JK, Capra JD. *Immunoglobulins: structure and function.* In: Paul WE, ed. *Fundamental immunology,* 4th ed. Philadelphia: Lippincott–Raven Publishers, 1999:37–74.
23. Lederman S, Cleary AM, Yellin MJ, et al. The central role of the CD40-ligand and CD40 pathway in T-lymphocyte–mediated differentiation of B lymphocytes. *Curr Opin Hematol* 1996;3:77–86.
24. Pene J, Rousset F, Briere F, et al. IgE production by normal human lymphocytes is induced by interleukin 4 and suppressed by interferons gamma and alpha and prostaglandin $E_2$. *Proc Natl Acad Sci USA* 1988;85:6880–6884.
25. Mond JJ, Vos Q, Lees A, et al. T-cell–independent antigens. *Curr Opin Immunol* 1995;7:349–354.
26. Hardy RR, Hayakawa K. CD5 B cells, a fetal B-cell lineage. *Adv Immunol* 1994;55:297–339.
27. Robertson M. Antigen presentation. *Curr Biol* 1998;8:R829–R831.
28. Swain SL, Croft M, Dubey C, et al. From naive 1997 to memory cells. *Immunol Rev* 1996;150:143–147.
29. Goodnow CC. Balancing immunity, autoimmunity, and self-tolerance. *Ann N Y Acad Sci* 1997;815:55–66.
30. Kay AB. Concepts of hypersensitivity. In: Kay AB, ed. *Allergy and allergic diseases.* Oxford: Blackwell Sciences, 1997:23–25.
31. Ewert BH, Jennette JC, Falk RJ. The pathogenetic role of ANCA. *Am J Kidney Dis* 1991;18:188–195.
32. Roubey RA. Immunology of the anti-phospholipid syndrome. *Arthritis Rheum* 1996;39:1444–1454.
33. Kalish RS, Ashkenase PW. Molecular mechanisms of CD8+ T cell–mediated delayed-type hypersensitivity: implications for allergies, asthma, and autoimmunity. *J Allergy Clin Immunol* 1999;103:192–199.

*Textbook of the Autoimmune Diseases,*
Edited by R. G. Lahita, N. Chiorazzi, and W. H. Reeves,
Lippincott Williams & Wilkins, Philadelphia © 2000.

CHAPTER 2

# Antibodies

Nicholas Chiorazzi

## STRUCTURE OF ANTIBODIES

Antibodies are complex glycoprotein molecules that are members of the immunoglobulin (Ig) superfamily. This family includes other immunologically important molecules such as the T-cell antigen receptor, the T-cell and B-cell receptor signal-transducing molecules, the major histocompatibility complex (MHC) molecules, several cytokine receptors, Fc receptors, and various inhibitory receptors (1,2).

The members of this superfamily share a structural feature that characterizes their shapes as glycoproteins. This distinctive feature is a series of peptide segments that fold into globular shapes held together by intrachain disulfide bonds. These characteristic repeating units are called Ig domains (Fig. 2.1).

In the case of antibodies, the repeating Ig domains are approximately 110 amino acids long (3) and are contained within two separate polypeptide chains that differ primarily in length and mass (4). For these reasons, the two chains are called the Ig heavy (H) and light (L) chains. Like the Ig domains that characterize these chains, the H and L chains are held together by disulfide linkages, although in this instance they are interchain in nature (5). Figure 2.2 illustrates the predicted three-dimensional shape of a secreted human IgG antibody molecule.

A final level of complexity is introduced by differences in the degree of amino acid sequence similarity between the Ig domains present at the amino-terminal portions of the H and L chains compared with those at the more distal and carboxyl-terminal portions of the two chains. When the structures of many different antibody molecules are examined, it becomes clear that the amino-terminal portions of each chain are much more variable in amino acid sequence than those further down in the molecule. The amino-terminal domains of each H and L chain comprise the *variable domain* of the

N. Chiorazzi: Departments of Medicine and Pathology, New York University School of Medicine, New York, New York 10016; Department of Medicine, Division of Rheumatology and Allergy–Clinical Immunology, North Shore University Hospital, Manhasset, New York 11030.

antibody molecule. In contrast, the amino acid sequences of the domains of the remainder of the molecule are more similar among different classes of antibody molecules, and these domains therefore comprise the *constant domains* of the antibody molecule (Fig. 2.2).

The constant domains of antibody molecules can be segregated into five classes of H chains and two classes of L chains that determine the isotypes of antibody molecules. These include IgM (μ H chain), IgD (δ H chain), IgG (γ H chain), IgA (α H chain), IgE (ε H chain), and the κ and λ L chains. The five H chain isotypes differ somewhat in their domain composition. Whereas IgM and IgE contain four constant domains, IgD, IgG, and IgA contain three.

The first constant domains are separated from the others by a relatively flexible region that varies in length among the isotypes (6,7). This area is called the *hinge region.* Because of the structural differences in the length and composition of the hinge region among the various isotypes, the various Ig classes differ in their abilities to accommodate antigenic epitopes separated by differing distances in space. IgG3 and IgD are especially flexible because of their long hinge regions (8,9). Table 2.1 lists some of the general characteristics of these five classes of antibody molecules (10).

Within the variable domain of the H and L chain, there are three regions that are the most diverse in their amino acid sequence (11). These regions come together when the antibody molecule folds into its three-dimensional shape and form a "pocket" into which antigen rests (12). The hypervariable regions of the variable domain that make contact with antigen are called the *complementarity-determining regions* (CDR). There are three CDRs for the H chain (HCDR1, HCDR2, and HCDR3) and three for the L chain (LCDR1, LCDR2, and LCDR3). In most instances, all of the CDRs contribute to the binding of antigen.

An antigen-binding pocket cannot encompass an entire macromolecule. In most instances, units of only 6 to 8 amino acids can adequately fit into an antigen-binding site (13). These units are called *epitopes.* Large protein molecules of the size expressed by foreign organisms or by autoantigens

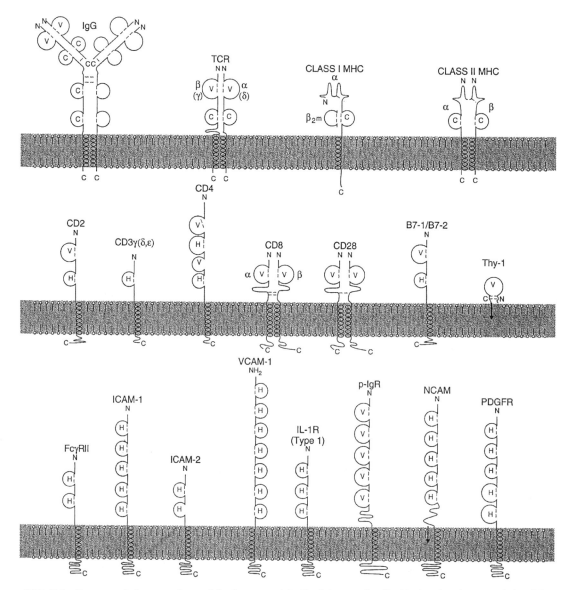

**FIG. 2.1.** Representative members of the immunoglobulin (Ig) superfamily. Notice the characteristic globular domains in each protein created by intrachain disulfide bonds. The amino acid sequences of these domains within an individual protein can be much more variable than the others (marked with V) or similar to the others (marked with C to indicate constant). (From Hunkapiller T, Hood L. Diversity of the immunoglobulin gene superfamily. *Adv Immunol* 1989;44:1–63, with permission.)

are usually composed of many epitopes, which can be bound by distinct antibody combining sites on separate antibodies.

The interaction of the variable domains of the H and L chains with antigen is noncovalent, consisting of relatively weak protein-protein interactions mediated by various physicochemical forces. Because the antigen-antibody binding reaction is noncovalent, the association between the two molecules is continually being formed and dissociated, resulting in a state of dynamic equilibrium. The measurement of the "strength" of this equilibrium reaction is the *affinity* of a given antibody for an antigen.

Because the interaction between the antigen-binding pocket of an antibody molecule and an antigen is noncovalent and dynamic, it is possible for several different antigens to fit into and occupy a given antigen-binding site, although not simultaneously. The "specificity" of an individual antibody molecule for antigen is relative and is a function of the strengths of the equilibrium reaction (affinity) of a given antibody for a series of antigens. Certain antigens fit into an individual antigen-binding site more tightly (avidly) than others; however, several may be able to occupy the site with various degrees of affinity. This concept is important for understanding some of the cross-reactivities of antibodies and possibly some of their autoreactivities.

The antigen-binding sites of antibody molecules accommodate antigens in their characteristic three-dimensional shape (i.e., as they occur in nature). This allows an antibody molecule to bind a foreign antigen when it enters the body.

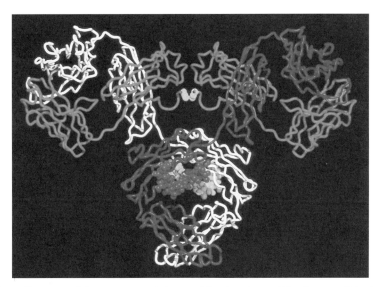

**FIG. 2.2.** Ribbon diagram of the x-ray crystallographic structure of the human (Mcg) IgG1 immuno-globulin. One of the heavy chains is represented in magenta and the other in white. Both light chains are in blue. The carbohydrate moieties in the Fc region are denoted as green and orange space-filling spheres. Each heavy chain is folded into four immunoglobulin domains and each light chain into two domains. The antigen-binding sites are positioned at the tips of each arm of the Y-shaped structure and are composed of the CDR1, CDR2, and CDR3 loops of the variable portion of the heavy chain and the CDR1, CDR2, and CDR3 loops of the variable portion of the light chain. (Courtesy of Drs. A. Edmundson and P. Rams-land, Oklahoma Medical Research Foundation, Oklahoma City, OK.) See color plate 1.

**TABLE 2.1.** *General characteristics of immunoglobulins of the various classes*

| Property | IgM | IgD | IgG | IgA | IgE |
|---|---|---|---|---|---|
| Molecular form | Pentamer, hexamer | Monomer | Monomer | Monomer, dimer | Monomer |
| Number of C region domains | 4 | 3 | 3 | 3 | 4 |
| Tailpiece | + | − | − | + | − |
| Accessory chains | J chain, SC | None | None | J chain, SC | None |
| Subclasses | None | None | G1, G2, G3, G4 | A1, A2 | None |
| Molecular weight | 950 kd, 1150 kd | 175 kd | 150 kd | 160 kd, 400kd | 190 kd |
| Carbohydrate content (%) | 10 | 9 | 3 | 7 | 13 |
| Percentage of total serum Ig | 5–10% | 0.3% | 75–85% | 7–15% | 0.02% |
| Average adult free serum level (mg/ml) | 0.7–1.7 | 0.04 | 9.5–12.5 | 1.5–2.6 | 0.0003 |
| Synthesis rate (mg/kg/d) | 7 | 0.4 | 33 | 65 | 0.016 |
| Serum half-life (d) | 5 | 3 | 23 | 6 | 2.5 |
| Antibody valence | 10, 12 | 2 | 2 | 2, 4 | 2 |
| Bacterial lysis | + | ? | + | +++ | ? |
| Placental transfer | − | − | + | − | − |
| Mast cell/basophil binding | − | − | − | − | + |
| Macrophage binding | − | − | + | + | − |
| Classic complement activation | ++ | − | + | − | − |
| Alternate complement activation | − | + | + | A1+, A2- | − |
| Other biological properties | Primary antibody responses; secretory immunoglobulin | Unknown; useful as a B-cell marker | Hallmark of secondary immune responses | Main secretory immunoglobulin | Allergic and antiparasite responses |

Adapted from Frazer JK, Capra JD. Immunoglobulins: structure and function. In: Paul W, ed. *Fundamental immunology,* 4th ed. Philadelphia: Lippincott Williams & Wilkins, 1999, with permission.

The antigen-binding sites of antibody molecules accommodate antigens without the need for the antigen to be associated with another molecule. This is different for T-cell receptors that react with antigens in a linear, denatured, and "processed" conformation and in association with major histocompatibility molecules (14).

## ANTIBODIES AS SIGNALING RECEPTORS ON B CELLS

As can be surmised from their characteristic structural features, antibody molecules have evolved to recognize and interact with antigen and then to lead to effector functions to eliminate these foreign molecules. The CDRs of the H and L chains that reside in the variable domains of antibody molecules permit the *recognition phase* of an antibody-mediated immune response. In contrast, the major characteristic features of antibody molecules that allow for the *reaction phase* of variable domain recognition reside in the constant domains of the H chain.

The antibody molecules that are integral components of the surface membrane of a B lymphocyte initiate the recognition and reaction phases of antibody-mediated immune responses. Each B lymphocyte that is created *de novo* in the bone marrow synthesizes an IgM antibody whose antigen-binding pocket is unique. These antibody molecules, each with its own unique antigenic specificity, are inserted into the surface membrane of the B cell and act as the B cell's recognition unit for its outside world (15).

Mature B cells that have exited the bone marrow display on their surface membranes IgM and IgD antibody (16) molecules that contain identical, unique antigen-binding pockets (17). These antibody molecules and their unique antigenic specificity allow the B cell to "know" when it has encountered the type of foreign stimulus to which it has been pre-programmed to respond. The occupation of the surface bound antibody receptor molecules by antigen is the critical event that marks the recognition phase of the B-cell response and sets in motion the reaction phase.

However, because even unique antigen-binding sites are not completely restricted to only one antigen, the affinity of the interaction between the antigen and the receptor becomes of critical importance. In general, those interactions with antigens whose shapes are most complementary to the antigen binding pocket (and consequently have higher affinity) are more likely to result in a positive reaction by the B cell. This contrasts with the interactions with antigens whose shapes are less complementary to the antigen binding pocket and consequently have lower affinity for the receptor. The latter interactions may lead to negative or tolerization signals (see Chapter 7).

The functional consequence (positive versus negative reaction) of antigen binding to surface membrane antibody molecules depends on the state of development of the B cell. High-affinity interactions between the antigen-binding receptor and antigen that take place during the early stages of B-cell development in the bone marrow probably lead to tolerization or cell death (16), whereas such interactions that take place in the periphery lead to cellular activation.

Because the purpose of this chapter is to discuss the production of antibodies as effector molecules in the reaction phase of an antibody-mediated immune response, only those interactions between antigen and membrane-bound antibody molecules that result in positive signals to the B cell are considered. These signals result in cellular interactions that lead to cell expansion or cell maturation to antibody producing plasma cells.

When the surface-bound antibody molecules on B cells encounter an antigen with adequate and appropriate affinity, a signal is transduced to the inside of the B lymphocyte indicating that it should initiate its effector programs (18). For the B cell, there are two major types of effector programs initiated by surface antibody-antigen interactions. The first is designed to cause B-cell proliferation to increase cell numbers and then to differentiate these B cells into plasma cells to produce the antibody that neutralizes or eliminates the foreign antigen. The second program is designed to internalize the antigen and to digest it into fragments that can be used to elicit the help of T cells in carrying out the first effector program (19). B cells elicit this help by placing digested antigenic fragments on their surfaces in association with MHC molecules. These antigen-MHC fragments are recognized by specific T cells, causing them to exercise their effector programs, one of which is to provide costimulatory signals to the B cell in the forms of contact-mediated and soluble cytokine-mediated help.

The initiation of the proliferation and differentiation and the antigen-presenting programs of B cells require that several conditions be satisfied by the interaction between the membrane-bound antibody molecule and the antigen (20). The interaction with antigen must engage several antibody molecules simultaneously, thereby causing cross-linking of several receptors. This cross-linking phenomenon induces motion of the grouped antibody receptors within the B cell's surface membrane. This motion causes a similar effect on a protein that surrounds the antibody molecule in the B-cell membrane and is noncovalently associated with it. This protein, called CD79, is composed of two chains of different composition (CD79a and CD79b) that are held together by disulfide linkages (21–23). It is through the CD79 molecule that B-cell signal transduction and activation occurs and through which the proliferation and differentiation and the antigen-presenting programs are triggered. The actual intracellular mechanisms induced by signal transduction through the surface antibody/CD79 complex are beyond the scope of this discussion but can be reviewed elsewhere (18,20).

Antigens differ in their need and capacity to elicit T-cell help for B cells. They therefore can be classified as T-cell–independent antigens or T-cell–dependent antigens (Fig. 2.3). Structurally, T-cell–independent antigens usually are multimeric molecules that display repeating antigenic epitopes in long linear arrays. These arrays of epitopes can effectively

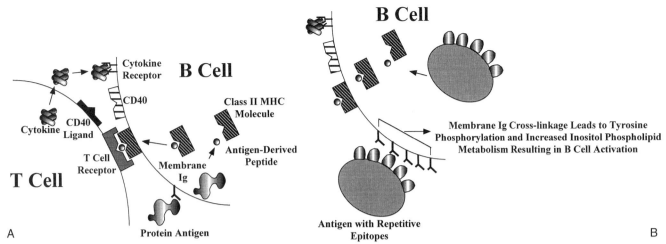

**FIG. 2.3.** Two types of B-cell activation. **A**: Cognate interactions between T cells and B cells. A resting B cell can bind a foreign protein antigen by its surface membrane immunoglobulin receptor and internalize it by endocytosis. After degradation of the foreign protein, some of its peptides are complexed with class II major histocompatibility complex (MHC) molecules and reexpressed on the cell surface. These peptide–MHC II complexes are then recognized by specific T cells. The recognition event induces expression of CD40 ligand, which interacts with CD40 on the B cell and promotes B-cell activation and expression of other costimulatory molecules such as B7.1 and B7.2, which interact with CD28 on the T cell. **B**: T-cell–independent B-cell activation. A resting B cell can bind an antigen with many repetitive epitopes, which causes extensive cross-linking of the surface membrane immunoglobulin receptor and stimulates biochemical signals of cellular activation. It does not appear that CD40 ligand–CD40 interactions are directly involved in this form of B-cell activation. (From Paul WW, ed. *Fundamental immunology,* 4th ed. New York: Lippincott–Raven, 1999:5, with permission.)

cross-link multiple surface membrane antibody molecules and thereby induce B-cell activation. T-cell–independent antigens cannot be processed into fragments that can be presented to T cells in association with MHC molecules. Examples of T-cell–independent antigens include polysaccharides (e.g., pneumococcal polysaccharide), nucleic acids, and glycolipids. The primary antibody responses to vesicular stomatitis virus, hepatitis B, and polyomavirus appear to be T-cell–independent mechanisms (24–26). The antibody responses induced by T-cell–independent antigens are usually different than those induced by T-cell–dependent antigens. They are primarily of the IgM isotype and the affinity of these antibodies does not change appreciably over time.

B cells stimulated by T-cell–dependent antigens are able to elicit other signals that aid in their proliferation and differentiation program. The signals needed to promote this type of B-cell differentiation result from a dynamic interplay between the B cell and the T cell (27,28). This interplay involves a series of cell interaction molecules and cytokines that are upregulated and downregulated in a coordinated manner on the basis of each preceding cellular communication. Dominant interacting pairs include CD40 and CD40 ligand, B7.1 and B7.2 with CD28, and others (Fig. 2.3). The details of the cell-contact and soluble cytokine signals that promote this T-cell–dependent type of B-cell maturation are described in Chapter 13.

As a consequence of these antigen-initiated interactions, some of these B cells undergo new DNA gene rearrangements (30) that allow them to produce antibodies with a wide isotype display (IgG, IgA, and IgM [31]) and that undergo the affinity maturation and immune memory responses. These antibodies are more effective in providing long-lasting and effective protection.

Because the recognition phase and the reaction phase of immune responses depend on the unique specificity of an individual B-cell clone, it is necessary for the immune system to be able to generate as many unique antigen binding sites as there are foreign antigens. Otherwise, there would be "holes" in the antigen recognition and reaction phases of the immune reaction leading to potentially disastrous consequences.

As explained in Chapter 1, much of this diversity in antigen recognition is generated at the time of the "birth" of an individual B-cell clone in the bone marrow. This diversity is the consequence of the rearrangement of different $V_H$, D, and $J_H$ segments for the H chain and of different $V_L$ and $J_L$ segments for the L chain. Additional diversity is introduced by enzymatic activities that add or subtract nucleotides, apparently randomly, at the junctions between the rearranging segments. These "combinatorial" and "junctional" mechanisms create the antigen binding sites for B cells that have never interacted with foreign antigen (i.e., "naive" or "virgin" B cells).

However, the immune system has evolved another mechanism that allows these naive B cells to react more avidly with even more diverse antigenic shapes. This is a mechanism that goes into operation after the mature B cell has left the bone marrow and has interacted with its foreign antigen in the periphery (32). This mechanism occurs in B cells after they have homed to lymphoid follicles within lymphoid organs (e.g., spleen, lymph nodes, tonsils). When an antigen-activated B cell enters a lymphoid follicle, it takes up residence in a specialized structure called a *germinal center.* Germinal centers are assembled and disassembled continuously in healthy individuals. These assembly-disassembly processes occur as a consequence of local interactions within the spleen or lymph node between the B and T cells that have been activated by the foreign antigen and by other cells presumably of the reticuloendothelial system such as follicular dendritic cells.

The purpose of assembling a germinal center is to allow the individual B-cell clone that has been stimulated by foreign antigen to generate a broader, and hopefully more protective, scope of antigen binding possibilities. This is done by a series of events that allow the B-cell clone to expand enormously in number and to develop mutations in the gene segments that encode the variable domains of the H and L chains (Fig. 2.4). These mutations alter the antigen binding site of the many progeny of the original B-cell clone.

Mutations in the variable region genes generate new and more diverse sets of receptors. However, these mutations and the changes in structure that they effect are built on the template of a receptor that originally had sufficient affinity for the foreign antigen to activate the B cell to start the germinal center diversification process. The variable domains of the B cells expressing these mutations can become more reactive or less reactive with the original foreign antigen.

Operationally, only a small number of these mutations increase affinity for the original antigen. Those B cells that have generated receptors for the original foreign antigen with similar or even greater affinity are preserved, whereas the B cells that have generated receptors for the original antigen that have lower affinities die by apoptosis (i.e., programmed cell death) (Fig. 2.4). When this germinal center reaction process works effectively, the immune system has an ongoing opportunity to develop new clones of B cells at the time of foreign antigen exposure to help react to and eliminate the antigen (32).

The germinal center reaction is potentially dangerous. Because this process generates mutations randomly, it is likely that some mutations result in B cells with receptors that react with significant affinity with autoantigens. This requires the immune system to have a protective mechanism to eliminate or silence the B cells that develop receptors for autoantigens. This process of peripheral tolerance safeguards us from the enormous danger inherent in the germinal center reaction process. These tolerance mechanisms are discussed in Chapter 7. Figure 2.4 illustrates in a diagrammatic fashion the events that occur to these B cells as they migrate through the different areas of a germinal center (33).

## ANTIBODIES AS SOLUBLE EFFECTOR MOLECULES

Although IgM and IgD represent the major cell-bound antibody classes of mature B cells, their secreted serum levels represent relatively minor portions of the available antibodies (Table 2.1). IgM is the antibody secreted in primary immune reactions and usually is of lower affinity for antigen than IgG or IgA antibodies, because many IgM-producing B cells have not gone through the germinal center reaction and developed Ig V gene mutations that lead to affinity maturation. In the serum, IgM antibodies exist primarily as pentamers or hexamers. IgM antibodies appear to carry out their major protective roles in conjunction with the complement system. After interaction with antigen, these pentameric antibodies are especially efficient activators of the complement cascade through C1q binding (34). IgM, like IgA and possibly like IgD, can serve as a protective antibody at mucosal surfaces and in breast milk, because it can also be transported through epithelial cells by the polyIg receptor.

In contrast, IgD does not appear to be able to engage the complement system in the inflammatory cascade. However, IgD molecules are enriched in breast tissue and milk, suggesting an effector function that has not yet been extensively studied (35).

IgG represents about 75% of antibodies in the circulation of adults. It is also the most plentiful in the lymph and the cerebrospinal fluid. IgG exists as four subclasses that differ in their constant domains, and these differences often translate into relatively unique functional differences. For instance, like IgM, IgG antibodies can initiate the complement cascade by permitting the binding of C1q to a constant domain. However, the various IgG subclasses vary in their abilities to initiate the complement cascade (IgG3 > IgG1 > IgG2 > IgG4) (36,37). This interaction occurs only after IgG has bound soluble or cell-surface antigen.

IgG molecules can also promote opsonization (38), antibody-dependent cellular cytotoxicity (ADCC) (39), and transplacental transport (40) by engaging receptors on various cell surfaces called Fcγ receptors (FcγR) (41,42). Table 2.2 lists some of the biologic properties of these receptors. Opsonization is the process whereby cell-associated IgG facilitates phagocytosis of an antibody-bound target cell or organism by mononuclear phagocytes. ADCC can be mediated by a series of cellular effector populations (i.e., NK cells and mononuclear phagocytes), all of which are enhanced in their cytolytic capability by the presence of IgG bound to the target. The IgG subclasses vary in their abilities to initiate and promote ADCC (IgG1 > IgG3 > IgG2 and IgG4).

IgA is the major antibody found in external secretions such as tears, saliva, and breast milk. Like IgG, IgA antibodies can be of different subclasses (e.g., IgA1 and A2). IgA also can exist in several molecular forms ranging from monomers (most common in the serum) to dimers and trimers. Serum IgA is mainly of the A1 subclass. Secretory IgA, found at most mucosal surfaces, is composed exclusively of dimers of IgA2 (held together by the J chain) in association with the secretory piece. Secretory piece allows mucosal transport and protects the IgA molecule from degradation by enzymes contained in external secretions and milk. Because of its unique

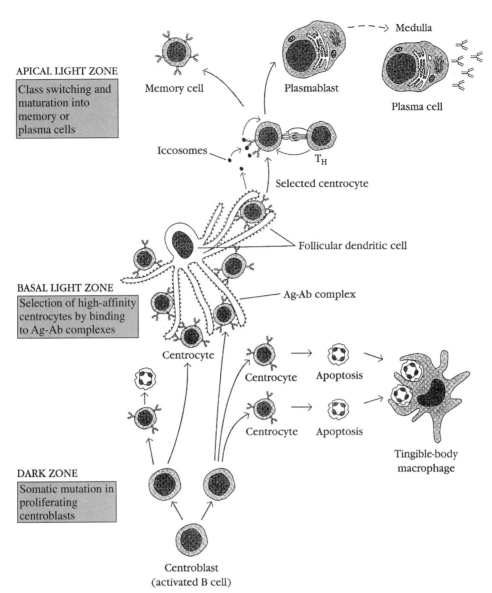

**FIG. 2.4.** Cellular events within the secondary follicles of peripheral lymph nodes. Activated B cells (centroblasts) lose surface membrane immunoglobulin receptor expression and undergo extensive proliferation and somatic mutation in the dark zone of the germinal center. After exiting the dark zone, these B cells reexpress a mutated surface immunoglobulin receptor. If the specificity of this new receptor is complementary to the antigens displayed on the surface of follicular dendritic cells in the basal light zone, the B cells are temporarily rescued from programmed cell death. However, if the specificity of the new receptor does not have adequate complementarity and affinity for the antigens displayed on the follicular dendritic cells, the B cells cannot avert programmed cell death. The B cells that have bound, internalized, and presented antigenic fragments on their major histocompatibility complex class II molecules receive a permanent rescue signal from antigen-specific T cells in the apical light zone. These B cells then enter the memory pool and are available for restimulation in the future or can differentiate into plasma cells and secrete their modified immunoglobulin. (From Kuby J, ed. *Immunology,* 2nd ed. New York: WH Freeman, 1994:341, with permission.)

molecular properties and its location at mucosal surfaces, IgA along with IgM acts as the major protective antibody barrier to invasion by infectious organisms at these sites (43).

IgE is the antibody present in the lowest amounts in the serum, primarily because it binds to the FcγRI on mast cells and basophils and eosinophils with extremely high affinity, thereby effectively removing it from the circulation (44,45).

Nevertheless, cell-bound IgE is an extremely potent effector antibody because it uses the vasodilatory and inflammatory capabilities of mast cells, basophils, and eosinophils to produce its effects. Although many of these effects are salutary (especially in the setting of helminthic and other parasitic infections), IgE is responsible for the annoying and sometimes life-threatening consequences of allergic reactions.

**TABLE 2.2.** *Human Fc receptors*

| Type | Cellular expression | Ig Fc bound with highest affinity | Effector function |
|------|--------------------|-----------------------------------|-------------------|
| FcγRI (CD64) | Constitutively on mononuclear phagocytes; induced by IFN-γ on neutrophils | IgG1 and IgG3 >IgG4; no affinity for IgG2 | Phagocytosis and ADCC |
| FcγRIIA (CD32) | Neutrophils and macrophages and megakaryocytes | IgG1 and IgG3 | Phagocytosis |
| FcγRIIB (CD32) | B lymphocytes | IgG1 and IgG3 | B-cell inhibition |
| FcγRIIIA (CD16) | Mononuclear phagocytes and NK cells | IgG1 and IgG3 | ADCC |
| FcγRIIIB (CD16) | Neutrophils (GPI-linked) | IgG1 and IgG3 | Phagocytosis and ADCC |
| FcεRI | Mast cells, basophils, eosinophils, and Langerhans cells | IgE | Immediate hypersensitivity |
| FcεRII (CD16) | B lymphocytes | IgE | B-cell regulation |

ADCC, antibody-dependent cellular cytotoxicity; GPI, glycosylphosphatidyl inositol; IFN, interferon; NK, natural killer.

# REFERENCES

1. Williams AF, Barclay AN. The immunoglobulin superfamily—domains for cell surface recognition. *Annu Rev Immunol* 1988;6:381–405.
2. Hunkapiller T, Hood L. Diversity of the immunoglobulin superfamily. *Adv Immunol* 1989;44:1–63.
3. Hill RL, Delaney R, Fellows RE, Lebovitz HE. The evolutionary origins of the immunoglobulins. *Proc Natl Acad Sci USA* 1966;56:1762–1769.
4. Fleischman JB, Porter RR, Press E. The arrangement of the peptide chains in γ-globulin. *Biochem J* 1963;88:220–228.
5. Amzel LM, Poljak RJ. Three dimensional structure of immunoglobulins. *Annu Rev Biochem* 1979;48:961–997.
6. Schumaker VN, Phillips ML, Hansen DC. Dynamic aspects of antibody structure. Mol Immunol 1991;28:1347–1360.
7. Wade RH, Tavequ JC, Lamy JN. Concerning the axial flexibility of the Fab regions of IgG. *J Mol Biol* 1989;206:349–356.
8. Dangl JL, Wensel TG, Morrison SL, et al. Segmental flexibility and complement fixation of genetically engineered chimeric human, rabbit and mouse antibodies. *EMBO J* 1988;7:1989–1994.
9. Nezlin R. Internal movements in immunoglobulin molecules. *Adv Immunol* 1990;48:1–40.
10. Paul WW, ed. *Fundamental immunology*, 4th ed. New York: Lippincott–Raven Publishers, 1999:60.
11. Wu TT, Kabat EA. An analysis of the sequences of the variable regions of Bence Jones proteins and myeloma light chains and their implications for antibody complementarity. *J Exp Med* 1970;132:211–250.
12. Hasemann C, Capra JD. Mutational analysis of arsenate binding by a CRIA⁺ antibody. *J Biol Chem* 1991;266:7626–7632.
13. Padlan EA. Anatomy of the antibody molecule. *Mol Immunol* 1994;31:169–217.
14. Germain RN. MHC-dependent antigen processing and peptide presentation: providing ligands for T lymphocyte activation. *Cell* 1994;76:287–299
15. Rajewsky K. Clonal selection and learning in the antibody system. *Nature* 1996;381:751–758.
16. Forster I, Vieira P, Rajewsky K. Flow cytometric analysis of cell proliferation dynamics in the B cell compartment of the mouse. *Int Immunol* 1989;1:321–331.
17. Fu SM, Winchester RJ, Kunkel HG. Similar idiotypic specificity for the membrane IgD and IgM of human B lymphocytes. *J Immunol* 1975;114:250–254.
18. DeFranco AL. Transmembrane signaling by antigen receptors of B and T lymphocytes. *Curr Opin Cell Biol* 1995;7:163–175
19. Lanzavecchia A. Receptor-mediated antigen uptake and its effect on antigen presentation to class II restricted T lymphocytes. *Annu Rev Immunol* 1990;8:773–793.
20. Kurosaki T. Molecular mechanisms in B cell antigen receptor signaling. *Curr Opin Immunol* 1997;9:309–318.
21. Reth M. Antigen receptors on B lymphocytes. *Annu Rev Immunol* 1992;10:97–121.
22. Hashimoto S, Chiorazzi N, Gregersen PK. The complete sequence of the human CD79b (Ig-β/B29) gene: identification of a conserved exon/intron organization, immunoglobulin-like regulatory regions, and allelic polymorphism. *Immunogenetics* 1994;40:145–149.
23. Hashimoto S, Gregersen PK, Chiorazzi N. Chromosomal location, structure, and allelic polymorphisms of the human CD79a (Ig-α/mb1) gene. *Immunogenetics* 1994;40:287–295.
24. Bachmann M, Hengartner H, Zinkernagel R. T helper cell–independent neutralizing B cell response against vesicular stomatitis virus: role of antigen patterns in B cell induction. *Eur J Immunol* 1995;25:3445–3451.
25. Milich D, McLachlan A. The nucleocapsid of hepatitis B virus is both a T cell–independent and a T cell–dependent antigen. *Science* 1986;234:1398–1401.
26. Szomolanyi-Tsuda E, Welsh RM. T cell–independent antibody-mediated clearance of polyoma virus in T cell–deficient mice. *J Exp Med* 1996;183:403–411.
27. Noelle RJ, Snow EC. Cognate interactions between helper T cells and B cells. *Immunol Today* 1990;11:361–368.
28. Clark EA, Ledbetter JA. How B and T cells talk to each other. *Nature* 1994;367:425–428.
29. Paul WW, ed. *Fundamental immunology,* 4th ed. New York: Lippincott-Raven, 1999:5.
30. Harriman W, Volk H, Defranoux N, Wabl M. Immunoglobulin class switch recombinations. *Annu Rev Immunol* 1993;11:361–384.
31. Wabl MR, Forni L, Loor F. Switch in immunoglobulin class production observed in single clones of committed lymphocytes. *Science* 1978;199:1078–1080.
32. MacLennan ICM. Germinal centers. *Annu Rev Immunol* 1994;12:117–139.
33. Kuby J, ed. *Immunology,* 2nd ed. New York: WH Freeman, 1994:341.
34. Wright JF, Shulman MJ, Isenman DE, Painter RH. C1 binding by mouse IgM. *J Biol Chem* 1990;265:10506–10513.
35. Litwin SD, Zehr BD, Insel RA. Selective concentration of IgD class-specific antibodies in human milk. *Clin Exp Immunol* 1990;80:263–267.
36. Papadea C, Check IJ. Human IgG and IgG subclasses: biochemical, genetic, and clinical aspects. *Crit Rev Clin Lab Sci* 1989;27:27–58.
37. Brekke OH, Michaelsen TE, Sandlie I. The structural requirements for complement activation by IgG: does it hinge on the hinge? *Immunol Today* 1995;16:85–90.
38. Indik ZK, Park JG, Hunter S, Schreiber AD. Structure/function relationships of Fcγ receptors in phagocytosis. *Semin Immunol* 1995;7:45–54.
39. Unkeless JC. Function and heterogeneity of human Fc receptors for IgG. *J Clin Invest* 1989;83:355–361.
40. Saji F, Koyama M, Matsuzaki N. Current topic: human placental Fc receptors. *Placenta* 1994;15:453–466.
41. Kimberly RP, Salmon JE, Edberg JC. Receptors for IgG. *Arthritis Rheum* 1995;38:306–314.
42. Ravetch JV, Kinet J-P. Fc receptors. *Annu Rev Immunol* 1991;9:457–492.
43. Mestecky J, McGee JR. Immunoglobulin A: molecular and cellular interactions involved in IgA biosynthesis and immune response. *Adv Immunol* 1987;40:153–245.
44. Helm B, Marsh D, Vercelli D, et al. The mast cell binding site on human immunoglobulin E. *Nature* 1988;331:180–183.
45. Metzger H. The receptor with high affinity for IgE. *Immunol Rev* 1992;125:37–48.

Textbook of the Autoimmune Diseases,
Edited by R. G. Lahita, N. Chiorazzi, and W. H. Reeves,
Lippincott Williams & Wilkins, Philadelphia © 2000.

# CHAPTER 3

# Superantigens

## Mary K. Crow

The observations that eventually led to the definition of superantigens came from two lines of investigation. First, it became clear in the 1970s that toxins from certain bacteria had the capacity to induce lymphocyte proliferation *in vitro* (1–3). Although it was possible that some of this response could be attributable to antigen-specific recall responses, the stimulation in many cases had more of a mitogenic character, in that the proliferative response was rapid and of high magnitude. The second body of data was accumulated during the 1970s from studies of murine mixed cell cultures (4,5). Vigorous proliferative responses were observed by T cells of one mouse strain when cultured with B lymphocytes of a different but major histocompatibility complex (MHC)–identical mouse strain. The reaction was attributed to minor lymphocyte–stimulating (Mls) antigens—inherited antigens (not MHC encoded) that induce a mixed lymphocyte reaction between MHC-identical mouse strains, although the molecular characteristics of those antigens were not defined. These disparate phenomena came together when investigators in the Kappler and Marrack laboratories found that bacterial proteins could stimulate the proliferation of a subset of T cells based on restricted reactivity with the β chains encoded by some T-cell receptor (TCR) variable gene families (6–8). Moreover, in studies of murine T-cell repertoires, these investigators and others found that subpopulations of T cells, defined by their expression of particular TCR $V_\beta$ gene families, were deleted in mice expressing the Mls antigens (9–13). Bacterial proteins and molecules expressed on the surface of B cells of certain mouse strains have a similar property—the capacity to interact with T cells based on their expression of a particular TCR β chain. This rule contrasts with the one that governs recognition by T cells of peptide antigens, in which an antigenic peptide bound to MHC class I or II antigens interacts with the antigen-binding region of a TCR, comprising amino acids predominantly encoded by segments of the

variable (V), joining, and diversity regions of the β chain genes and variable and joining regions of the α chain genes. Molecules that activated subsets of T cells based on reactivity with TCR encoded by particular TCR $V_\beta$ gene families were called *superantigens* (6). This descriptor reflects their broader T-cell specificity and the more vigorous proliferative response that they elicit compared with classic protein antigens.

Although the similar functional properties of certain bacterial products and Mls antigens were clear, the molecular basis of these superantigenic effects only began to be understood when the expression of Mls antigens was tied to the presence in those mouse strains of an endogenous retrovirus, encoded by the mouse mammary tumor virus (MMTV) (14–22). It was found that the 3′ long terminal repeat (3′LTR) region of MMTV encoded a protein with superantigenic properties. The T-cell proliferative responses elicited by superantigens represent responses of the immune system to products of a subset of infectious organisms, whether derived from bacteria or virus.

The abundant data derived from *in vitro* and *in vivo* studies during the past 10 years have contributed to the current definition of a superantigen:

1. A superantigen is a potent inducer of a strong immune response. It activates 5% to 30% of T lymphocytes and acts at femtomolar concentrations (8,23).
2. A superantigen has sites for binding to two immune system receptors: the β chain of the TCR and α or β chain of MHC class II molecules (8,24–33) (Fig. 3.1).
3. A superantigen does not require intracellular processing by an antigen-presenting cell (APC) and is not restricted to a particular MHC class II allele (8,24–27).

## MOLECULAR STRUCTURE AND PROPERTIES OF SUPERANTIGENS

Bacterial superantigens are small, nonglycosylated proteins that are usually of 22 to 30 kd. They are translated as proteins with an amino-terminal signal peptide that is enzymatically

---

M. K. Crow: Department of Medicine, Weill Medical College of Cornell University, New York, New York 10021; Department of Medicine, Hospital for Special Surgery, New York, New York 10021.

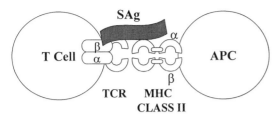

**FIG. 3.1.** Superantigens physically link the MHC class II molecule and the T-cell receptor β chain.

cleaved, yielding a mature protein with immunomodulatory activity. The typical bacterial superantigen has two domains; one domain has a beta "grasp" structure, and the other domain has a folded structure, similar to that found in immunoglobulin-binding molecules, such as protein A or protein G. The two domains may have come together through a recombination event (28–33). The structure of viral superantigen is less well defined. Although the amino acid sequences of some viral superantigens are known, these have not been crystallized (15,20,21,34). The bacterial superantigens are secreted as soluble products from the microbe of origin, and viral superantigens are synthesized by the infected host cell using RNA transcripts derived from the virus. There is little information regarding the mechanisms and manner in which these viral superantigens arrive at the host cell surface after their translation into protein, but like bacterial superantigens, it is presumed that they are coexpressed with MHC class II molecules.

Bacterial superantigens are highly stable molecules, maintaining their function over a wide range of pH values (2.5 to 11) and at temperatures up to 60°C. They bind multiple alleles of MHC class II antigens from various species. Although most superantigens bind most MHC molecules, there is relative preference of some superantigens for certain class II allelic products (35). For example, DR4 Dw10 binds staphylococcal enterotoxin B (SEB) and not toxic shock syndrome toxin-1 (TSST-1), and DR7 binds TSST-1 but not SEB. A similar observation has been made for viral superantigens, with I-E class II products preferentially bound by superantigens compared with certain I-A products. The successful crystallization of several superantigen molecules bound to class II has elucidated the likely basis for some of these differences (32,33) (Fig. 3.2).

Certain superantigens bind exclusively to the nonpolymorphic regions of class II, and others have some interaction with the part of DR that binds to antigenic peptide. In the latter case, the binding of different peptides to MHC class II β chain may confer an altered conformation and modulation of binding of the superantigen. The segment of TCR $V_\beta$ that recognizes the superantigen is somewhat variable, depending on the superantigen molecule. Although early data suggested that superantigen bound to hypervariable region 4, encompassing amino acids 70 through 74 (between complementarity-determining regions [CDR] 2 and 3) of TCR $V_\beta$ (28), later data support a unique binding pattern for each superantigen,

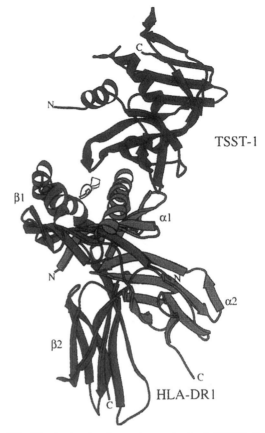

**FIG. 3.2.** The toxic shock syndrome toxin-1 (TSST-1) complex. The TSST-1 molecule interacts with the α1 domain of HLA-DR1 and about one half of the peptide binding groove. (From Kim J, Urban RG, Strominger JL, et al. Crystallographic structure of toxin shock syndrome toxin-1 complexed with a human class II major histocompatibility molecule, HLA-DR1. *Science* 1994;266:1870, with permission.)

with some also having binding contacts with the junctional CDR3 region that contacts antigenic peptide (36). The binding of superantigen to TCR is weak, but binding to class II is strong. The functional implications of these properties are that superantigen must first bind to MHC. If that operation is successfully accomplished, binding to TCR may follow. Each superantigen, whether bacterial or viral, has a distinct pattern of reactivity with TCR β gene products (Table 3.1). These patterns probably reflect the structural basis of their binding to TCR.

## MICROBIAL ORGANISMS THAT PRODUCE SUPERANTIGENS

### Bacteria

#### Gram-Positive Bacteria

Microbial superantigens produced by gram-positive bacteria have been classified on the basis of the clinical syndromes they produce and their serologic reactivity with antibody reagents (7,8). The pyrogenic toxin superantigens include the

**TABLE 3.1.** *Superantigens produced by human pathogens*

| Microbial source | Superantigen | T-cell receptor $V_\beta$ preference |
|---|---|---|
| *Staphylococcus aureus*<br>Enterotoxins | SEA | $V_\beta$1.1, 5.3, 6.3, 6.4, 6.9, 7.3, 7.4, 9.1, 18 |
| | SEE | $V_\beta$8.1, 5.1, 6.3, 6.4, 6.9, 18 |
| | SED | $V_\beta$5, 12 |
| | SEB | $V_\beta$3, 12, 13.2, 14, 15, 17, 20 |
| | SEC1 | $V_\beta$3, 12, 13.2, 14, 15, 17, 20 |
| | SEC2 | $V_\beta$12, 13.1, 13.2, 14, 15, 17, 20 |
| | SEC3 | $V_\beta$12, 13.1, 13.2, 14, 15, 17, 20 |
| | TSST-1 | $V_\beta$2 |
| *Staphylococcus aureus*<br>Exofoliative toxins | ETA | $V_\beta$2 |
| | ETB | |
| *Streptococcus pyogenes*<br>Exotoxins | SPEA | $V_\beta$2, 4, 8, 12, 14, 15 |
| | SPEB | $V_\beta$2, 8 |
| | SPEC | $V_\beta$1, 2, 5.1, 10, 15 |
| | SPEF (mitogenic factor) | $V_\beta$2, 4, 8, 15, 19 |
| | SSA | $V_\beta$1, 3, 15 |
| | M protein | $V_\beta$2, 4, 8 |
| Gram-negative toxins | | |
|   *Yersinia enterocolitica* | NK | |
|   *Yersinia pseudotuberculosis* | NK | |
| Viral superantigens | | |
|   EBV (human herpesvirus 4) | NK | $V_\beta$13 |
|   CMV (human herpesvirus 5) | NK | $V_\beta$12 |
|   HIV | Nef | NK |
|   Rabiesvirus | N protein | $V_\beta$8 |
|   Human spumavirus | Bel | |
|   HERV-K | IDDMK$_{1,2}$22 | $V_\beta$7 |
| Parasite | | |
|   *Toxoplasma gondii* | NK | $V_\beta$5 (in mice) |

CMV, cytomegalovirus; EBV, Epstein–Barr virus; ET, exofoliative toxin; HERV, human endogenous retrovirus; NK, not known; SE, staphylococcal enterotoxin; SPE, streptococcal toxins; SSA, streptococcal scarlet fever toxin; TSST-1, toxic shock syndrome toxin-1.

staphylococcal enterotoxins and TSST. Of the *Staphylococcus aureus*–derived toxins, SEA and SEE are most similar in amino acid sequence (92.2% similarity), and SEB, SEC1, SEC2, and SEC3 are also quite homologous (50% to 66%). Some of the *S. aureus*–derived superantigens (i.e., SEA, SEE, SEC2, and SED) have a zinc-binding motif that contributes to interaction with MHC class II, and others do not. Not all *S. aureus* bacteria produce superantigens. Some make multiple superantigens; some produce none. For example, superantigens are not made by coagulase-negative staphylococci, and expression of SEB and TSST-1 by a given *S. aureus* is mutually exclusive. The transcriptional regulation of all of the staphylococcal superantigens is unknown, but in the case of TSST-1, its gene *(tst)* is in a large DNA insert in the bacteria's chromosome. Transcription is under the control of an accessory gene regulator, staphylococcal accessory regulator, and an extracellular protein regulator. A distinct subset of staphylococcal superantigens, the staphylococcal exfoliative toxins, produce scalded skin syndrome and have distinct TCR $V_\beta$ specificities.

Superantigen products of *Streptococcus pyogenes* include the streptococcal scarlet fever toxins SPEA, SPEB, SPEC, SPEF, and SSA. SPEA and SSA are highly homologous (37). As is the case with the staphylococcal superantigens, some streptococcal organisms produce superantigens, and some do not. The streptococcal M proteins that make up part of the bacterial surface coat have the properties of superantigens, although some investigators debate that claim (38–40).

### Gram-Negative Bacteria

Gram-negative superantigens probably are less prevalent and less well studied than the staphylococcal and streptococcal superantigens. *Yersinia enterocolitica* and *Yersinia pseudotuberculosis* produce superantigens (42,43). No superantigens have been attributed to some of the most common gram-negative bacteria, such as *Escherichia coli*. It may be that some of the immunomodulatory activities mediated by superantigens, particularly the potent induction of cytokines, can also be produced by lipopolysaccharide, the important immunostimulatory product of gram-negative bacteria. However, the synergy between superantigens and lipopolysaccharide in some systems supports a functional role for the nonoverlapping properties of these two classes of microbial products.

## Mycoplasmal Organisms

Some of the first superantigens to be described were found in the supernatants of cultured mycoplasmal organisms. The best studied of these products is the *Mycoplasma arthritidis* mitogen (MAM) (44–50). MAM has specificity for human $V_\beta 17$ T cells, and MAM also binds to a high-molecular-weight molecule that may be an immunoglobulin. The amino acid sequence of MAM has been determined (50). Although its overall sequence is not similar to that of other known microbial products, several short stretches of amino acids are strikingly homologous to the superantigens encoded by the MMTV retrovirus. Although MAM is not known to be a human pathogen, the capacity of MAM to promote human B-cell differentiation *in vitro* (47) and *in vivo* (48) and produce inflammatory arthritis in a murine system (49) has supported a potential role for superantigens in induction or perpetuation of autoimmunity.

## Viruses

### Retroviral Superantigens

The Mls products that trigger T-cell activation in mixed-cell cultures containing lymphocytes from two murine strains are encoded by the MMTV retrovirus. Although there is evidence that other retroviruses also encode superantigens (34,51–54), most experimental data are derived from work on MMTV (55). MMTV is a B-type RNA retrovirus that is transmitted from mother to offspring in the mother's milk. The integrated MMTV is under control of glucocorticoid or progesterone hormones, resulting in increased viral transcription during pregnancy. For successful completion of the retroviral life cycle, the host immune system is required (56–58). Gut B cells become infected when newborns drink the mother's infected milk. The capacity of MMTV superantigen products to stimulate T-cell proliferation facilitates infection of those T cells by the virus; the virus infects only actively dividing cells. T-cell activation by superantigens promotes expansion of the T cells that can be infected with virus and leads to B-cell activation, augmenting the level of infection in those cells. Certain mouse strains (e.g., C57BL) are less susceptible than others to infection through milk. One resistance gene was mapped to the MHC; C57BL mice do not have the I-E gene, through which the MMTV superantigen product is presented to T cells (59). Mice deficient in CD40 ligand (CD40L), an important helper T-cell molecule that mediates cognate help for B-cell activation, do not become infected with MMTV (60), possibly because of insufficient induction of costimulatory molecules on CD40+ B cells or because CD40 ligation is needed for viral superantigen expression (Fig. 3.3).

MMTV may be sequestered in lymphoid cells until puberty. At that time, when epithelial cells of the mammary gland undergo proliferative expansion, those cells may become competent for infection by MMTV. MMTV can cause breast tumors when integrated near host protooncogenes (61).

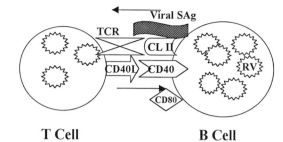

**FIG. 3.3.** Potential role of CD40 ligand (CD40L) and CD40 interactions in retrovirus infection. Studies using CD40L knockout mice indicate that CD40L is required for efficient infection of the host immune system by a retrovirus. CD40 ligation by CD40L may trigger expression of viral superantigens on the B-cell surface, induce expression of B-cell surface costimulatory molecules (e.g., CD80) that help to amplify T-cell expansion and infection, augment production of infective viral particles by B cells, or have other effects that promote retroviral infection and amplification of immune system activity.

In view of the dependence of MMTV on the immune system for expression of its infectious potential, it is not surprising that T-cell–deficient thymectomized and nude mice are relatively resistant to tumor induction by MMTV. Endogenous forms of the virus that are stable in the germline, having been introduced from the infectious virus, can encode proteins but cannot produce infectious virus particles. An approach devised by evolution to avoid MMTV-triggered mammary tumors is the transmission in the germline of MMTV retroviral sequences that can encode a superantigen (15,16, 18,19,21,22). The superantigen is encoded in the 3'LTR of the retroviral genome, a region that also encodes the env and pol proteins. The predicted superantigen protein is a type II transmembrane protein, with the carboxyl-terminal amino acids exposed to the extracellular space and sequence variability in that region correlating with TCR $V_\beta$ specificity. Different endogenous forms of MMTV (Mtv) show different tissue specificities, with Mtv-7 and Mtv-9 preferentially expressed in lymphoid cells (55). This differential expression may be caused by small differences in transcription factor binding sites in promoter regions of the endogenous viruses. Dissemination of a superantigen gene through generations of mice can eliminate MMTV and tumors. Activation-induced cell death of T cells mediated by the endogenous viral superantigens can lead to deletion of the TCR $V_\beta$ expressing subset for which the superantigen is specific, resulting in failure to recognize virus on later infection and freedom from tumor development. Inheritance of an endogenous MMTV would confer a survival advantage, because the host would be less likely to become productively infected and develop tumors.

In view of the extensive data documenting functional properties of endogenous retroviral gene products in the murine system, it seemed likely that comparable endogenous viral sequences would also inhabit the human genome. Full-length copies of several classes of endogenous retroviruses in human DNA are documented, and transcription and translation of proteins encoded by these viral parasites are well established (34,62,63). One of these classes of human endogenous retroviruses (HERV) has been shown to encode a superantigen that is expressed by human leukocytes and preferentially activates $V_\beta 7$ T cells (34). This sequence, called IDDMK$_{1,2}$22, is highly related to the HERV-K family, with overall sequence homology to murine MMTV. The superantigen protein is encoded by the env region of the genomic sequence but shows no sequence similarity to the MMTV superantigen that is encoded by the more 3′LTR of that retrovirus. In an effort to identify additional human endogenous superantigen mRNAs, polymerase chain reaction (PCR) primers that identify the MMTV open reading frame (ORF) have been used to amplify similar sequences from human cells (64). Three human sequences were identified: one that is unique, one that is related to a previously described human endogenous retroviral sequence, and one that is similar to a human autoantigen with histone-binding properties expressed in testes and sperm. Further study is needed to determine whether these intriguing mRNAs encode proteins with superantigen properties.

Whether the human immunodeficiency virus (HIV) encodes a superantigen has been a topic of considerable interest (53,54,65,66). A 3′ORF is found in the HIV nef sequence that encodes a protein that induces T-cell proliferation (53). However, the T cells activated by nef do not show specificity based on TCR $V_\beta$ expression.

### Rabies Virus Superantigen

Rabies virus is an enveloped virus of the Rhabdoviridae family that bears a negative-stranded RNA genome. The nucleocapsid is composed of three internal proteins (N, NS, and L), along with the viral RNA (67). The N protein has superantigen activity, because it binds MHC class II, induces proliferation of $V_\beta 8$ human T cells, and causes deletion of some T-cell subsets (67–69). The intact nucleocapsid can trigger T-cell–dependent IgG production and has weak T-cell mitogenic activity. The rabies virus N protein may also act as a B-cell superantigen, because it binds to IgG. It appears that superantigen helps to promote rabies infection in mice, because animals without the proper T cells ($V_\beta 6$) are not susceptible to infection. Additional evidence for a role for rabies superantigen is that neutralization of superantigen with antirabies N protein antibody confers resistance to infection.

### Cytomegalovirus

Data from patients with cytomegalovirus (CMV) and HIV infections who show preferential infection of $V_\beta 12$ T cells with HIV suggest that a CMV-encoded superantigen is responsible for T-cell activation and facilitation of HIV infection (70). However, no superantigen has been purified from CMV-infected cells, and it is not known what part of a CMV genome may encode such a protein.

### Epstein–Barr Virus

Epstein–Barr virus (EBV) has been implicated as a superantigen-producing virus. Culture of lymphoblastoid cell lines with the tumor promoter phorbol myristate acetate (PMA) augments the capacity of those cells to stimulate T-cell proliferation, with $V_\beta 13$ T cells preferentially activated (71). This T-cell stimulation is HLA-DR–dependent but not restricted to particular haplotypes, a feature of superantigens. At least one of the known effects of PMA is induction of the viral lytic cycle and upregulation of viral transcription. These PMA-induced effects may depend on transcription of an EBV-encoded protein, or alternatively, it is possible that EBV transactivates a normal B-cell gene, such as an endogenous retroviral sequence. An EBV superantigen may activate T cells to promote helper T-cell–dependent B-cell activation and survival of latently infected resting B cells (71), a scenario similar to the one that occurs with MMTV in mice. In that case, the superantigen promotes viral persistence.

### Parasites

The parasite *Toxoplasma gondii* codes for a murine $V_\beta 5$-specific superantigen (72). Susceptibility to toxoplasmosis in mice is linked to the presence of $V_\beta 5$ T cells in the T-cell repertoire, and survival is improved in mice lacking those superantigen target cells.

## EVOLUTIONARY ORIGIN OF SUPERANTIGENS

With growing understanding of the molecular features and functional properties of bacterial and viral superantigens, it is hard to escape the conclusion that the genetic material that encodes superantigens has played an important role in the course of evolution and the maintenance of balanced survival among organisms. The endogenous forms of MMTV were probably derived from an infectious retrovirus propagated in the environment, and it is likely that human endogenous retroviral sequences have a similar source. Many bacterial superantigen gene sequences originated in bacteriophage genes, also derived from viral genetic material (73,74). Bacterial and viral superantigens may represent an important evolutionary stimulus for the extensive polymorphism in MHC, TCR, and to a lesser extent, immunoglobulin molecules.

Why are superantigen genes maintained? Their products must provide an advantage to the microorganism and host. In the case of the microbe, viral superantigens activate compartments of the immune system that promote their propagation. Bacterial superantigens divert immune system activity or induce inflammation and tissue damage sufficiently long that the microbe can replicate and spread. For the host, endogenous retroviruses that encode superantigens may mold the immune repertoire by deleting or anergizing subpopulations of cells to avoid sequestration of oncogenic viruses. Superantigens may also have an adjuvant function, magnifying the immune response to a microbe. As with most modifiers of immune function, superantigens can be good or bad for the host, depending on the magnitude and quality of the immune response generated.

## IMMUNOLOGIC PROPERTIES OF SUPERANTIGENS

Superantigen effects on T cells parallel the range of responses that follow traditional activation of T cells after ligation of TCRs by antigenic peptide–MHC complexes. However, the quality of the T-cell response is more rapid and of greater magnitude, based on the relatively high proportion (5% to 30%) of the T-cell repertoire targeted by the superantigen (8). Depending on the concentration and avidity for MHC class II and TCR molecules, superantigen can induce partial T-cell activation, demonstrated as expression of cell-surface interaction molecules such as CD40L or FAS ligand, or full T-cell activation, including production of cytokines such as interleukin-2 (IL-2), tumor necrosis factor-$\alpha$ (TNF-$\alpha$), or interferon-$\gamma$; expression of cytokine receptors; and proliferation (1,3,6,8,9). As can occur with TCR activation by antigenic peptide, some conditions favor induction of T-cell anergy or deletion by superantigen. For example, in the thymus, superantigens tend to delete the reacting T-cell population, and in the periphery, systemic exposure to superantigen in the absence of costimulatory signals can anergize the T cells. When the inflammatory environment generates adequate

costimulatory signals, the superantigen often results in a massive expansion of the specific superantigen-reactive T cells, followed by activation-induced cell death and relative depletion of those cells later in the response. When administered concurrently with or subsequent to immunization with a weak antigen, a superantigen can augment the immune response to that antigen.

Depending on the properties of the superantigen and the context in which it interacts with the T-cell receptor, including the presence of costimulatory molecules and cytokines, the effector functions generated may differ. Massive cytokine secretion and proliferation by T cells is often a consequence of stimulation by SE (6,75), whereas less vigorous T-cell proliferation but effective T-cell help for B-cell activation and differentiation results from much lower concentrations of the SE or, typically, on stimulation with MAM (45,47,49,76,77). In addition to the functional outcomes of TCR ligation by superantigen, the unique capacity of superantigen to form a "bridge" between TCR $\beta$ chain and MHC class II molecule permits directional targeting of T-cell surface and cytokine signals to the interacting MHC class II–positive cell (45,47,76,78) (Fig. 4). When the bridge ties together helper T cell and B cell, the consequences are often increased expression of B-cell surface costimulatory molecules and the cell death molecule FAS, B-cell proliferation, and B-cell maturation, including immunoglobulin class switching to mature isotypes. When the superantigen bridge forms

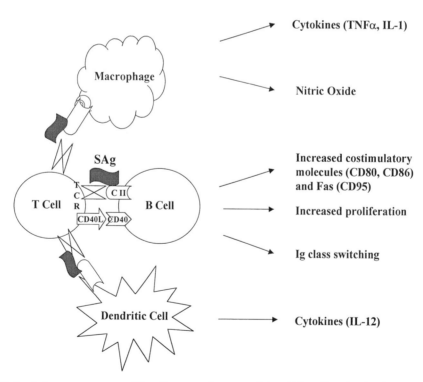

**FIG. 3.4.** Potential consequences of B-cell, macrophage, and dendritic cell activation by a superantigen bridge. By virtue of their capacity to link MHC class II molecules and T-cell receptors, superantigens direct helper T cell signals to B cells, macrophages, dendritic cells, and other MHC class II–positive target cells, leading to target cell activation.

between cytotoxic cells and MHC class II–positive cells, death of the target cell may be promoted. T cell–macrophage or T cell–dendritic cell interaction mediated by a superantigen bridge may trigger activation of those cells with cytokine secretion and nitric oxide release.

In addition to their capacity to activate T cells and mediate MHC class II target cell activation through a superantigen bridge with the T cell, superantigens can transduce activating signals directly by virtue of their fairly high-affinity binding to MHC class II molecules (79,80). In this way, macrophages, B cells, and cells that can be induced to express MHC class II molecules under inflammatory conditions can be stimulated to secrete cytokines, even without T-cell help. The cytokines, particularly IL-1 and TNF-α, produced by macrophages by direct activation by superantigen or through the superantigen bridge are responsible for much of the toxicity and pyrogenicity that are important clinical effects of infection with superantigen-producing bacteria. Superantigens are also synergistic with lipopolysaccharide, promoting greater cytokine secretion and inhibition of liver phagocyte function and contributing to increased susceptibility to endotoxin shock.

A comprehensive picture of the effects of superantigens *in vivo* comes from a study of the geography of the response to immunization of mice with MMTV (81). The architecture of the lymph nodes from such mice is in many ways comparable to that of mice immunized with a typical protein antigen. In the case of this retrovirus, immunization resulted in an initial infection of B cells with expression of superantigens on the B-cell surface. Migration of those B cells to lymph nodes was followed by T-cell activation and expansion, with a high proportion of those T cells expressing the relevant $V_\beta 6$ gene product. A role for interdigitating dendritic cells in this T-cell activation was suggested by the expression of the superantigen product and the MMTV envelope protein on those cells. T-cell activation was rapidly followed by B-cell activation and expansion in the intramedullary cords of the lymph node, with subsequent migration of those B cells to germinal centers, further expansion, and immunoglobulin production, including antibodies specific for the MMTV envelope protein. Although MMTV infection in the study resulted in deletion of $V_\beta 6$ T cells in the peripheral immune system, those cells persisted for at least 100 days in the lymph node. The important role of the MMTV superantigen in this *in vivo* immune response was documented by the near absence of a response to immunization in mice expressing a related endogenous retrovirus, resulting in elimination of $V_\beta 6$ T cells from the T-cell repertoire. This study documents the capacity of retrovirus-encoded superantigen to induce an immune response that includes activation and expansion of a large proportion of T cells expressing the appropriate TCR $V_\beta$ gene product, expansion of the B cells infected with the virus, and production of antibodies that are specific for viral gene products. It did not describe an induction of autoreactive T cells or B cells in the setting of immunization with MMTV, but the spectrum of T and B cells activated suggests the potential for such lymphocyte activation in the presence of sufficient self antigen.

## ROLES OF SUPERANTIGENS IN HUMAN DISEASE

### Pyrogenic and Toxic Shock Syndromes

The prototype human disease mediated by superantigens is TSS (82). A sometimes lethal condition characterized by fever and systemic manifestations of shock, the clinical picture of TSS is similar to that mediated by gram-negative endotoxin. In the case of TSS and related syndromes, however, the toxins are derived from gram-positive bacteria and have the properties of superantigens. TSST-1 is a *S. aureus*–derived pyrogenic toxin that is highly potent; 3 to 5 µg can lead to shock. TSST-1 causes all menstrual cases and 50% of nonmenstrual cases of TSS; 25% of TSS cases are mediated by SEB or SEC superantigen (83). $V_\beta 2$ T cells are increased during the acute phase of TSS and TNF-α, IL-2, and interferon-γ are released by lymphocytes and macrophages. A similar syndrome can be triggered by infection with group A streptococci. In either case, the result is capillary leak, hypotension, and fever. The clinical presentation and management of TSS are reviewed later in this chapter.

### Food Poisoning

Staphylococcal enterotoxins are an important cause of acute gastrointestinal illness, manifested by vomiting and diarrhea. SEB and SEC1 are among the superantigens that induce this syndrome after ingestion of *S. aureus*–contaminated food.

### Exfoliative Skin Diseases

Two *S. aureus*–derived superantigens, ETA and ETB, can produce sloughing of skin. This mechanism is involved in toxic epidermal necrolysis, staphylococcal scarlatiniform rash, and bullous impetigo, terms that describe a bullous rash in the setting of *S. aureus* infection.

### *Streptococcus pyogenes*–Related Disorders

Impetigo, erysipelas, scarlet fever, necrotizing fasciitis, pharyngitis, acute rheumatic fever, post-streptococcal glomerulonephritis, and streptococcal TSS are clinical disorders associated with infection with various streptococcal bacteria (84). The role of streptococcal superantigen in each of these conditions is not well characterized, but it is likely that those toxins play a role in at least some of these disorders. In the case of rashes associated with streptococcal infections, prior exposure to group A streptococci can predispose to a hypersensitivity reaction based on superantigenicity of the infecting bacteria. The rash itself may be caused by cytokine release after T-cell activation. The *S. pyogenes* superantigens include SPEA, SPEB, SPEC, SSA (related by protein sequence to SEB, SEC1, and SEC3), and mitogenic factor (now called streptococcal pyrogenic exotoxin F [SPEF]).

## Kawasaki Disease

Kawasaki disease is an acute inflammatory syndrome that is most often diagnosed in children. The syndrome was first described in 1967 by Kawasaki, who called the illness mucocutaneous lymph node syndrome, based on the prominent maculopapular erythematous rash over trunk and extremities, oral mucosal erythema with "strawberry tongue," and marked cervical lymphadenopathy (85). Additional characteristic clinical manifestations include fever and conjunctival injection. The syndrome is often accompanied by arthritis and arthalgias, aseptic meningitis, and most significantly, carditis and coronary arteritis (86). The acute phase of the disease, lasting 1 to 2 weeks, is followed by a subacute phase, with desquamation of the skin at the site of the rash and, in some cases, development of peripheral gangrene or coronary artery aneurysms. Unlike TSS, Kawasaki disease is rarely accompanied by shock or renal failure. The disorder can resolve without further complications, but cases with the more severe manifestations can have significant long-term morbidity.

Kawasaki disease is not obviously an autoimmune disease, because no characteristic autoantibodies have been described nor have autoantigen-reactive T cells been implicated. However, good support has been provided for an etiologic role for superantigens (87). Expanded populations of $V_\beta 2$, $V_\beta 6.5$, and $V_\beta 8$ T cells have been found early in the disease (87,88). Moreover, staphylococcal (TSST-1) and streptococcal (SPEC) superantigens have been implicated by studies showing that many Kawasaki disease patients have been infected with *S. aureus* bacteria that produce a superantigen capable of activating $V_\beta 2$ T cells or have antibodies to SPEC. $V_\beta 2$ T cells have also been detected in coronary arteries and in the myocardium in patients with Kawasaki disease. Despite these observations, a role for superantigen in the pathogenesis of Kawasaki disease is not firmly established, because some groups have failed to find $V_\beta$-restricted T-cell populations. Treatment with intravenous immunoglobulin containing antibodies reactive with bacterial toxins along with aspirin has proven efficacious.

## Infectious Mononucleosis

Infectious mononucleosis is a subacute systemic disease, characterized by lymphadenopathy and with hepatitis and its sequelae, that is associated with lymphoproliferation of T cells. EBV is the causative agent. Indirect evidence for an EBV-encoded superantigen has been presented (71,89). An activation antigen, CD69, is preferentially expressed on $V_\beta 13$ T cells in cultures with EBV-transformed B-cell lines that had been activated to undergo lytic cell cycle amplification. This T-cell activation is HLA-DR dependent.

## Atopic Dermatitis

Atopic dermatitis is a recurrent pruritic inflammatory skin disease most commonly seen in patients with type I hyper-sensitivity reactions. It has been suggested that *S. aureus* can contribute to atopic dermatitis (90). *S. aureus* organisms that secrete superantigen toxins have been isolated from more than 50% of patients with the disorder, and more than 50% of patients have antibody to *S. aureus* superantigen.

## Human Immunodeficiency Virus Disease

A murine disease with clinical features similar to acquired immunodeficiency syndrome (AIDS) has served as a model for retrovirus-induced immunodeficiency syndromes. Murine acquired immunodeficiency syndrome (MAIDS) is initiated by infection with a defective retrovirus, the murine leukemia virus, that is only able to generate one gene product, the p60 gag protein. The immunologic disease in these mice requires T cells and MHC class II–positive B cells, and the early phase of the disease is characterized by expansion of $V_\beta 5$ T cells (51). In contrast to *in vivo* exposure to superantigen in other systems, the T cells in MAIDS mice are not deleted. A relatively weak interaction between the putative retroviral superantigen and the TCR on $V_\beta 5$ T cells has been described and may explain the failure of those cells to undergo extensive activation-induced cell death (91).

Superantigens have been sought in human HIV disease (53,65,66,70). HIV encodes a protein, nef, that binds directly to HLA-DR and stimulates T-cell proliferation and cytokine production. It is not clear whether those T cells are activated in a TCR-specific manner. Like the MMTV superantigen, nef is encoded in the 3'ORF of the HIV genome. A soluble form of another HIV protein, gp160, may represent a superantigen, as it selectively activates $V_\beta 3$, $V_\beta 12$, $V_\beta 14$, and $V_\beta 15$ T cells.

## Diagnosis and Treatment of the Prototype Superantigen-Mediated Disease: Toxic Shock Syndrome

TSS is the human disease for which a pathogenic role for superantigen is best documented and that serves as a model for study of superantigen-mediated disease mechanisms and for diagnosis and treatment. TSS associated with staphylococcal infection was first described in the late 1970s, followed by the well-publicized series of cases associated with tampon use (92). In the 1990s, attention shifted to the more lethal TSS associated with highly invasive streptococcal infection (93,94). Although the increase in diagnoses of TSS is in part attributable to improved awareness among patients and physicians, there has also been an important shift in the virulence of those bacteria that has conferred a more significant pathogenic potential. A subtype of the M1 strain of group A streptococci has become dominant in some regions, and it has been suggested that increased production of certain virulence factors, including superantigens, may be a feature of this subtype (95).

With the understanding that tampons could serve as a reservoir of TSST-producing staphylococcal bacteria, the epidemiology of TSS has expanded to include children and adults with any source of *Staphylococcus* infection, although menstruating woman still represent the population at highest risk (92). The clinical presentation of TSS is characterized by high fever, generalized malaise and myalgias, headache, rash, and hypotension. In contrast to TSS mediated by streptococcal toxins, skin and mucous membrane involvement is typical of staphylococcal TSS. An erythematous rash over the trunk and extremities, erythema and swelling of the palms and soles, and erythema of the mucous membranes and conjunctivae are common. This rash usually progresses and desquamates several weeks after the onset of the illness. The symptoms of shock can be severe, resulting in hypoperfusion of kidneys, liver, and central nervous system, progressing to organ failure and occasionally to respiratory distress syndrome. Laboratory features of staphylococcal TSS include leukocytosis with many early band forms (very early in the course of the illness) or lymphopenia (later in the course), thrombocytopenia, and the laboratory correlates of hypoperfusion and organ damage. Disseminated intravascular coagulation can also develop. Antibodies to TSST-1 are not detected or of lower titer in patients with TSS than in healthy control subjects, suggesting that the absence of immunity to the toxin may be a risk factor for TSS (92).

TSS associated with group A streptococcal infection can manifest even more dramatically and with more lethal results. Although the basic research studies that link the clinical syndrome to superantigens are less complete for the patients with streptococcal infection compared with staphylococcal TSS, the streptococcal syndrome is also likely to be mediated by the immunologic effects of a superantigen, in this case SPEA or SPEB. Stevens wrote an excellent review that provides a comprehensive picture of the epidemiology and clinical features of streptococcal TSS (94). The estimated prevalence is 1 to 5 cases per 100,000 persons in the general population, with a mortality rate of 30% to 70%, and like staphylococcal cases, all age groups can be affected. The infecting streptococci must gain entry to the body, usually through the skin, but in many cases entry may not require breaking of the skin and may follow relatively minor trauma or bruising. Although generally similar to the clinical presentation of TSS associated with staphylococci, TSS in the setting of streptococcal infection is characterized by deep pain at the locus of infection, which may precede any physical sign of infection or inflammation. The tissue at the site of pain often progresses to necrotizing fasciitis or myositis, or the infection may be localized to the pelvis or abdomen. Unlike staphylococcal TSS, rash occurs only in about 10% of cases. Fever, generalized flulike symptoms, confusion, and soft tissue pain are often followed by shock and organ failure, including renal failure and adult respiratory distress syndrome. In addition to the laboratory abnormalities described previously, patients with streptococcal TSS with deep soft tissue infection often have very high creatine kinase levels, reflecting muscle necrosis. The rapidity of progression of this destructive illness must be emphasized, because even in the hospital setting, death can occur less than 24 hours after presentation.

In view of the galloping course of the illness, diagnosis of TSS must be based on acute awareness of the possible diagnosis by the physician. Formal diagnosis is based on isolation of group A streptococci from a normally sterile site, hypotension, and multiorgan involvement. In addition to microbial cultures and standard laboratory tests, the specific detection of superantigen genes using PCR enzyme immunoassays is being developed by several groups (96) and may at some point be an option. Treatment cannot wait for the results of such diagnostic studies.

The management of TSS, whether caused by staphylococcal or streptococcal infection, is based on rapid initiation of antimicrobial therapy along with fluid replacement and appropriate cardiovascular and respiratory support. Stevens reviews the advantages of clindamycin, based on its capacity to inhibit toxin and M protein synthesis by streptococci and TNF-$\alpha$ synthesis by monocytes (94). If a defined locus of infection can be identified, drainage and removal of foreign bodies is required. Particularly in the case of streptococcal TSS, necrotizing fasciitis or other deep foci of infection may be present and require debridement or other major surgery. Intravenous dexamethasone has been used in some patients, and intravenous immunoglobulin therapy has been tried and been successful in some cases, a rationale being the neutralization of bacterial toxin by antisuperantigen antibodies in the IgG preparation (97). Additional approaches under investigation include the administration of pentoxifylline, an agent that inhibits release of cytokines triggered by lipopolysaccharide or superantigen (98), and hemofiltration to attempt to remove inflammatory mediators (99).

## ROLES OF SUPERANTIGENS IN AUTOIMMUNE DISEASE

### Potential Mechanisms of Superantigen-Mediated Autoimmune Disease

Consideration of potential mechanisms of induction of autoimmunity have traditionally focused on mechanisms of "breaking tolerance." A dominant function of the immune system is discriminating "self" from "other." The extensive apoptosis that occurs in the thymus, particularly early in ontogeny, underlies the deletion of T cells with self-reactivity. Similarly, deletion of B cells interacting with high affinity with self antigens through surface immunoglobulin receptors skews the B-cell repertoire toward reactivity with foreign antigens and away from self-reactivity. With regard to B cells, this winnowing mechanism is imperfect; the machinery of somatic mutation drives altered antigenic reactivity of mature B cells and the antibodies they produce. With the key regulatory role for maintenance of self-tolerance falling to the T cell, whose antigen receptor genes do not undergo somatic mutation, a firm belief in a requirement for strict maintenance of T-cell tolerance to self antigens persisted among immunologists, although this view has softened recently. Elucidation of the role of relative affinity and valency between antigenic peptide–MHC complex and the TCR in the deletion, anergy, and activation of T cells has contributed to understanding T-cell repertoire development as a continuum (100). Self antigens with high affinity for TCR probably lead to deletion of those T cells, but self antigens with lower affinity or low valency may permit persistence of self-reactive T cells in a partially activated or ignorant state. The hypothetical presence of T cells with self-reactivity based on affinity models is supported by documentation of autoreactive T cells in normal individuals (101). Unlike the traditional view of strict tolerance to self as the normal situation, current views allow for the persistence of potentially autoreactive T cells in the peripheral T-cell repertoire.

The presence of T cells with low affinity TCR specific for self antigens is unlikely to present a problem for the host under typical circumstances. Self antigens seem to coexist with those T cells capable of response. Only when the context of presentation of those self antigens shifts is the threshold for activation of self-reactive T cells met. This scenario may apply when tissue damage leads to augmented innate immune system activation and increased expression of co-stimulatory molecules or in situations of unusually high concentrations of self antigens, as may occur with extensive burn trauma or apoptotic responses (102).

The exception to these requirements for activation of self-reactive T cells is presented by superantigen. In view of the capacity for superantigens to activate any T cells expressing the appropriate TCR $V_\beta$ gene product, the affinity of the TCR for its cognate antigen is less of a consideration. The threshold for activation of those autoreactive T cells is readily met when activation is through superantigen-TCR interaction rather than through antigenic peptide–TCR interaction. Activation of a high proportion of T cells, without regard for their antigenic specificity, represents the most important potential scenario through which superantigens may trigger autoimmunity (Table 3.2 and Fig. 3.5).

There are many potential consequences of superantigen-mediated activation of T cells. Cytokines are secreted with the potential to nonspecifically expand immune and inflammatory activity. "Non-specific" cell-surface interaction molecules are likely to be expressed. The most important of these is CD40L, the expression of which follows activation of CD4-positive (CD4+) helper T cells through their TCRs (103). CD40L expression, induced by microbial superantigens, has the potential to bind CD40 on target cells, including B cells, macrophages, dendritic cells, and activated endothelial cells and fibroblasts. Ligation of B-cell CD40 mediates B-cell proliferation, immunoglobulin class switch-

ing, and increased expression of costimulatory molecules and cytokines by the B cell. When the B-cell surface immunoglobulin receptor is coordinately ligated by antigen, CD40-activated B cells express their full potential to mature into antibody secreting cells. In the case of macrophages and dendritic cells, CD40 ligation induces secretion of cytokines, such as IL-12, and increased capacity, as in the case of dendritic cells, to promote generation of specific cytotoxic lymphocytes.

An important mechanism of superantigen action is the capacity of superantigen to form a bridge between superantigen-activated T cell and a superantigen-bound B cell (45,78) (Figs. 3.4 and 3.5). This mechanism uses superantigen as a glue to bring together T and B cells, and it mediates activation signals to T and B cells, which results in B-cell activation through MHC class II molecules, CD40, and cytokines. Because multivalent self antigens with the capacity to provide strong cross-linking of surface immunoglobulins are those most available to the B cell, full maturation of autoreactive B cells would be favored over maturation of B cells reactive to usually unavailable foreign antigens. Studies have suggested that a relatively high concentration of superantigen might favor a dominant T-cell activation response, with secretion of toxic cytokines, over the superantigen-mediated T-cell–dependent B-cell activation scenario, with the dominant activation of humoral immunity and autoantibody production (47). The staphylococcal superantigens SEB and TSST-1 are highly potent and favor T-cell activation and cytokine production. Only at very low concentrations do those superantigens mediate immunoglobulin secretion in *in vitro* studies. In contrast, MAM, a less potent superantigen, is a weak T-cell mitogen and a more effective inducer of B-cell activation and immunoglobulin secretion (47). The *in vivo* studies of the immune response to MMTV referred to earlier support T-cell and B-cell expansion and B production of antibody (81), more similar to the *in vitro* effects of MAM than those of the staphylococcal superantigens. It is likely that there is a continuum of responses to bacterial and viral superantigens that range from low-level T-cell–dependent B-cell activation and differentiation, to modest T-cell activation accompanied by B-cell differentiation, to dominant T-cell activation and cytokine secretion, and to vigorous T-cell activation with important T-cell apoptosis through activation-induced cell death (Fig. 3.6).

Although T-cell activation by superantigens provides the most powerful mechanism for activation of autoreactive specificities, the direct binding of superantigen to MHC class II molecules on B cells has been shown to induce B-cell activation in some systems (79). Moreover, some bacterial products, such as the SE, staphylococcal protein A, and HIV gp120, bind to the protein products of certain immunoglobulin heavy-chain gene families through a mechanism that parallels their binding to the products of TCR $V_\beta$ gene families (104,105). An endogenous molecule, protein Fv, is a sialoprotein that preferentially binds to IgM expressing $V_H3$ and $V_H6$ heavy chains. Data indicate that only a subset of

**TABLE 3.2.** *Potential role for superantigens in autoimmune disease*

1. Initiate autoimmune disease by expanding populations of T cells containing self-antigen specificities
2. Induce autoimmune disease after subthreshold activation of the immune system by self antigens
3. Reactivate a quiescent autoimmune disease

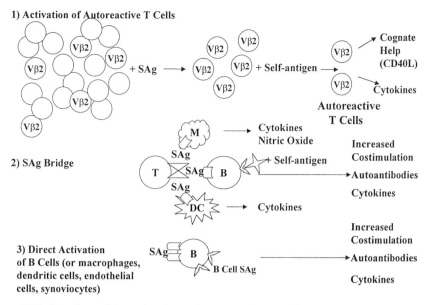

**FIG. 3.5.** Potential mechanisms of superantigen-mediated autoimmunity.

immunoglobulin gene products can be bound and ligated by superantigens. Among these, the most prominent is the $V_H3$ heavy-chain gene family (104). As in the case of T cells, cross-linking of the B-cell antigen receptor by B-cell superantigen can transduce an activation signal, leading to B-cell proliferation and differentiation or rescuing the B-cell from the consequence of other signals that would otherwise result in B-cell apoptosis. B-cell superantigen may also promote the secretion of antibodies with the properties of rheumatoid factor. Rheumatoid factors, immunoglobulins with specificity for the Fc fragment of IgG, are enriched in the $V_H3$ heavy

chain and therefore may be preferentially generated by B-cell superantigen.

APCs, expressing high surface levels of MHC class II antigens with superantigen-binding properties, are also potential targets for superantigens (79). Cytokines, including TNF-$\alpha$, are secreted by superantigen-activated macrophages, and these cytokines, along with nitric oxide released by the activated APCs, can contribute to tissue damage in settings such as inflammatory arthritis. Although APC activation through superantigen binding to MHC class II molecules could hypothetically alter the processing of self antigens to

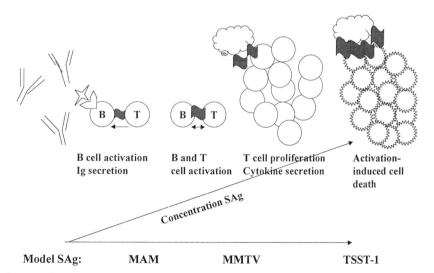

**FIG. 3.6.** Superantigens mediate a continuum of immune responses, depending on the binding characteristics of the superantigen and its concentration. *Mycoplasma arthritidis* mitogen (MAM) and very low concentrations of staphylococcal superantigen favor B-cell activation and immunoglobulin secretion. Higher concentrations of staphylococcal enterotoxin (SE) favor T-cell proliferation, cytokine secretion, and activation-induced cell death. Mouse mammary tumor virus (MMTV), based on *in vivo* data, can mediate a wide spectrum of immune effects.

expose cryptic epitopes, there are no data available that support such a mechanism.

## Exacerbation of Autoimmune Disease by Superantigens

Beyond the hypothetical mechanisms that implicate superantigens in the initiation of autoimmune disease, preexisting autoimmunity may be worsened or retriggered by exposure to superantigens, a mechanism that is strongly supported by studies using animal models and has been suggested in human diseases such as Sezary syndrome, in which TSST-1 may perpetuate cutaneous inflammation associated with T-cell lymphoma (106). Among the data related to inflammatory arthritis are those for experimental murine models in which TSST-1 reactivates or exacerbates streptococcal cell wall arthritis and MAM exacerbates collagen-induced arthritis (48,107). Superantigens also may augment a subclinical autoimmune process to a degree that it is clinically apparent and important. Mice that receive a dose of collagen inadequate to induce arthritis develop the disease after injection of MAM. The capacity of superantigens to exacerbate rather than initiate autoimmune disease is further supported by data for the rodent multiple sclerosis model, experimental autoimmune encephalomyelitis (EAE). Superantigens have been administered to mice before or after the initiation of EAE (108–110). Injection of SEB, a superantigen specific for the $V_\beta 8$ T cells that are enriched among pathogenic T cells, protects animals from induction of EAE by myelin basic protein (MBP). In contrast to the outcome of administering SEB before the onset of EAE, once EAE is established, SEB was shown to reactivate the disease or induce EAE in animals that remained asymptomatic after sensitization with MBP. Different results were obtained in experiments using the nonobese diabetic (NOD) murine model, for which it was found that superantigens can alleviate disease if administered after the onset of diabetes (111). The complex results of administering superantigens in murine models of inflammatory arthritis, diabetes, and multiple sclerosis illustrate the importance of timing, dose of superantigens, and the *in vivo* setting to the outcome of these interventions.

In studies of lupus, T cells bearing $V_\beta 8$ TCR are enriched among the pathogenic T cells in the spontaneous MRL/lpr model, and administration of SEB to those mice resulted in decreased autoantibody production and decreased renal disease (112). SEB, reactive with $V_\beta 8$ T cells, may be acting to delete T cells activated *in vivo* and playing a pathogenic role. Taken together, these animal data strongly suggest that, regardless of the potential role of superantigens in triggering autoimmune disease, those mediators have the capacity to modulate ongoing disease, negatively or favorably.

## Evidence for Superantigens in Autoimmune Diseases

Examples of autoimmune diseases that are associated with microorganisms are well known. Acute rheumatic fever

follows infection with certain streptococcal species, hepatitis B has been linked to polyarteritis nodosa, and hepatitis C infection is associated with mixed cryoglobulinemia. Reactive inflammatory arthritides or Reiter's syndrome can follow enteric or genitourinary infection with *Yersinia, Salmonella,* or *Shigella* organisms. Although no superantigen has been definitively shown to induce autoimmunity, suggestive data have been reported for several autoimmune disorders. Studies using murine models provide strong support for a role for superantigens in exacerbating or retriggering preexisting autoimmune disease. Discussion begins with a review of the data supporting a role for superantigens in the autoimmune disease that is the prototype for a molecular mimicry mechanism, acute rheumatic fever.

### Rheumatic Fever

In contrast to the more traditional view that antibodies reactive with streptococcal proteins cross-react with host muscle proteins, the superantigen hypothesis proposes a more important role for T cells in rheumatic fever pathogenesis. Antibodies that react with various heart antigens are present in patients with rheumatic fever, but these antibodies do not correlate with disease activity and do not efficiently transfer disease to recipient animals. However, infiltration of cardiac tissue with CD4$^+$ T cells supports a role for T cells. Characterization of specificity of T cells eluted from cardiac tissue of rheumatic heart disease patients has shown reactivity with several antigens from streptococci. Among these antigens is the M protein (39,40,113). M protein stimulation of T-cell responses has been shown in cord blood lymphocytes, suggesting that priming by the streptococcal bacteria is not required to elicit these proliferative responses. Response to pep-M5, an M protein peptide from a streptococcal subtype, requires accessory cells and MHC class II expression on the APC, but it is not restricted to particular MHC haplotypes. Pep-M5 preferentially activates $V_\beta 2$, $V_\beta 4$, and $V_\beta 8$ T cells, with the T-cell CDR3 regions showing diversity, consistent with a superantigen response. Other M proteins, including M6, M18, M19, and M24, also have characteristics of superantigens, but each stimulates a different panel of TCR $V_\beta$ gene products. Although the superantigen activity of M protein is controversial (41), a documented superantigen, SPEC, is made by many rheumatogenic strains of streptococci and has been associated with predisposition to cardiotoxicity. However, the pathogenic connection of SPEC to rheumatic fever has not been established.

### Rheumatoid Arthritis

Human rheumatoid arthritis has been intensively studied with an eye toward detection of signs of a role for superantigens. The approach taken by most investigators has been to characterize the TCR expressed on T cells in the rheumatoid joint or the TCR mRNA extracted from those T cells. The premise has been that skewing of the T-cell repertoire at the site of disease, with certain TCR $V_\beta$ gene products overrepresented, could be consistent with a superantigen driving the joint inflammation. A heterogeneous collection of CDR3 amino acid sequences would be consistent with superantigen drive. However, a restricted representation of CDR3 sequences may suggest that, although only certain TCR $V_\beta$ gene families dominate in the joint, those TCRs are enriched in β chains that are likely to have been selected by antigenic peptides. That argument is strengthened when similar amino acids comprise the CDR3 antigen-binding segment, while the nucleotides that encode those amino acids differ. Such a picture suggests a selection for capacity to bind a particular antigenic peptide. The data are abundant and subject to various interpretations, but a conservative evaluation could fairly conclude that the expression of TCR $V_\beta$ gene families is generally restricted in rheumatoid arthritis joint T cells. Many studies have found a striking prevalence of $V_\beta 3$, $V_\beta 14$, and/or $V_\beta 17$ T cells (114–117). At first glance, these data might be thought to support the presence of a superantigen in the rheumatoid joint, particularly because of the heterogeneous representation of TCR $V_\beta$ gene products in the peripheral T-cell repertoire found in many studies. However, further analysis of TCR sequences across the CDR3 segment has shown that those T cells are "oligoclonal." Certain TCR sequences are repeatedly represented. This picture suggests "antigen drive," with a subset of antigenic peptides selecting and expanding certain T cells that have a good fit for that antigenic peptide in their antigen binding region, the CDR3. Although none of these data provides a definitive answer to whether superantigens are involved in the immune system inflammation in the rheumatoid joint, a possible interpretation is that a superantigen may initially select or expand a subset of the T-cell repertoire, based on TCR $V_\beta$ expression, and that a joint antigen or set of antigens further expands those T cells at the site of disease. However, studies of the T-cell response to protein antigens have documented the preferential selection of certain TCR $V_\beta$ gene products by peptide antigens presented in the traditional MHC-restricted manner (118). A comparable TCR profile may be generated by peptide antigen or by superantigen drive, followed by further selection by self antigens.

Another mechanism by which superantigens may play a role in rheumatoid arthritis pathogenesis is the activation of synoviocytes from rheumatoid tissue by T cells and a superantigen bridge. This interaction could work in both directions, with activation of superantigen-reactive T cells. The capacity of superantigen to induce TNF-α production and secretion in rheumatic fever was discussed previously. Superantigens may mediate or exacerbate inflammatory arthritis by any number of the mechanisms described, but definitive evidence of a role for superantigens in human rheumatoid arthritis has not been presented, and a place for superantigens in the pathogenesis of that disease remains speculative.

### Insulin-Dependent Diabetes Mellitus

Destruction of the pancreatic islet cells after lymphocytic infiltration underlies insulin-dependent diabetes mellitus (IDDM). Data from patients with diabetes and studies using the NOD murine model of spontaneous diabetes have provided some of the most intriguing support for the role of viral superantigens in the pathogenesis of autoimmune diseases (34,119,120).

Human data include the observation of expanded T cells expressing $V_\beta 7$ TCR in pathologic specimens from two patients who died early in the course of IDDM (34,119). Sequencing of those TCRs showed diversity in the CDR3 junctional regions, suggesting that there was unlikely to have been strong selection by antigenic peptide. The alternative possibility, that a superantigen with preference for $V_\beta 7$ T cells was an etiologic factor, was proposed. Detailed study of the tissues of those two patients has culminated in the detection of a full-length HERV that encodes a superantigen with specificity for $V_\beta 7$ T cells. This virus of the HERV-K family, called $IDDMK_{1,2}22$, was detected in supernatants from short-term cultures of pancreatic islet cells of the two IDDM patients. Identical or highly similar sequences were also detected in plasma of 10 patients with recent-onset IDDM but not from the plasma of nondiabetic controls. The endogenous retroviral activity was relatively enriched in leukocytes compared with islet cells, based on assay of reverse transcriptase activity in spleen and pancreas preparations. This retrovirus encodes a superantigen from its env region, as MHC class II–positive transfectants expressing the N-terminal part of the envelope protein of $IDDMK_{1,2}22$ stimulated $V_\beta 7$ T cells. In contrast to the interpretation of that study, a subsequent report suggested that expression of this HERV is not a requirement for induction of IDDM (120). Conrad's work has generated considerable controversy. This series of studies lent substantial support to the proposal that humans can generate proteins encoded by endogenous retroviral sequences harbored in all human genomes and that those proteins include some with the immunologic properties of superantigens. As suggested by the many TCR sequences generated from patients with rheumatoid arthritis, in which evidence supports TCR $V_\beta$ restriction and junctional CDR3 diversity, Conrad's data led to a model of IDDM pathogenesis in which an endogenous superantigen expands a large subset of T cells, based on their expression of $V_\beta 7$, and among those activated T cells are those with specificity for self antigens expressed in the pancreas. However, there is the possibility that the retroviral superantigen is expressed in response to inflammation rather than being a primary trigger. Studies of retroviral gene sequences expressed by mammalian cells have been plagued by technical difficulties. Nevertheless, although the data presented for IDDM require confirmation by other groups, this study begins a new chapter in the investigation of a role for the superantigen products of HERVs in human autoimmune diseases.

In the NOD mouse model, there are parallel observations of restricted expression of TCR $V_\beta 3$ and $V_\beta 7$ subsets, although only before the onset of clinical diabetes (119). The restricted T cells are present in peri-islet infiltrates, and T cells are more heterogeneous by the time islets are damaged. The T cells found in these early peri-islet lesions are particularly enriched in $V_\beta 3$ T cells, which is of interest because most $V_\beta 3$ cells should be deleted in the NOD strain that expresses an endogenous Mtv superantigen. These results suggest the possibility that animals that have less efficient deletion of superantigen-reactive T cells during development may be predisposed to stimulation of the remaining cells expressing that $V_\beta$ gene product later on. These human and murine data provide some support for superantigen effects early in the disease, followed by later diversification of the response or subsequent superimposed selection by antigenic peptides. Some studies have found that superantigens can alleviate disease if administered after the onset of diabetes (110). A possible explanation for these findings is that in the presence of an endogenous superantigen or pancreatic self antigen, exogenously administered superantigen provides a sufficiently strong TCR stimulus to delete the T cells preactivated *in vivo* in the pancreas.

### Multiple Sclerosis

As in rheumatoid arthritis, much effort has been devoted to characterization of the T cells that infiltrate the central nervous system in multiple sclerosis, an inflammatory disease that damages the myelin sheaths of nerves, and in the closest murine model, EAE. In human multiple sclerosis, $V_\beta 5.2$ T cells are enriched in the plaques of patient brains (121), although no specific superantigen has been implicated as a trigger in this disease.

Administration of superantigen to mice suggests that T cells that have already been activated *in vivo* may be resistant to deletion or anergy on exposure to superantigens in this system. Reactivation of disease by superantigens may also drive "determinant spreading" of the autoantibody response to a broader range of epitopes of MBP than the one that initiates the autoimmune response.

### Psoriasis

Psoriasis is an inflammatory skin disease characterized by scaling plaques, particularly at sites disposed to infection with microorganisms, and psoriatic arthritis is associated with a destructive form of inflammatory arthritis. For many years, keratinocytes were the focus of investigation of the pathology of psoriasis. T cells have been increasingly implicated in that disease, as supported by therapeutic trials in which T cells have been eliminated with anti-CD3 monoclonal antibodies or toxin-coupled IL-2. These therapies have often resulted in amelioration of disease. Support for a pathogenic role for superantigens in psoriasis is only suggestive (122–124). The keratinocytes are MHC class II positive in psoriatic skin and have been shown to have stimulatory capacity for autologous T cells. As in rheumatoid arthritis, expansions of T-cell subsets expressing restricted TCR $V_\beta$ gene products have been described in guttate psoriasis. $V_\beta 2$ and $V_\beta 5.1$ T cells have been found and have diversity in the CDR3 junctional regions, as documented by sequencing studies. This pattern is consistent with a superantigen driving the expansion of the lesional T cells. Moreover, in guttate psoriasis, increased titers of antistreptococcal antibodies have been observed, and some of those antibodies also react with keratinocyte antigens (125). The strains of streptococcus that have been associated with guttate psoriasis make SPEC superantigen.

### Systemic Lupus Erythematosus

The prototype systemic autoimmune disease, systemic lupus erythematosus (SLE), is characterized by generalized immune system activation and hypergammaglobulinemia. Among many specificities of autoantibodies that are secreted in patients with SLE are those reactive with nucleic acids and nucleic acid binding proteins. No compelling support for an etiopathogenic role for superantigen in SLE has as been presented, despite the attractive hypotheses that would implicate such a mechanism. The superantigen bridge model mimics the polyclonal T-cell help for B-cell activation that mediates the murine parent → F1 model of graft-versus-host disease, in which parental T cells recognize the allogeneic MHC class II allele on recipient B cells, resulting in production of autoantibodies specific for self antigens that provide a strong crosslinking signal to those B cells (78,126). Moreover, the strong 9 : 1 female predominance and frequent onset of SLE after puberty suggests a scenario much like the one that occurs in mice infected with MMTV. At the time of mouse puberty, hormone response elements in the regulator regions of incorporated retroviral genomes promote transcription of those retroviral genes, probably including superantigen. However, even in murine models of spontaneous SLE, there is no clear evidence for involvement of retroviral or bacterial superantigens (127).

In human SLE, evidence for preferential involvement of T-cell subpopulations expressing particular $V_\beta$ gene products is limited to a study finding some enrichment of oligoclonal T cells bearing select $V_\beta$ TCRs in lupus kidneys (128). The enlarged lymph nodes from some SLE patients who present with the histology of necrotizing lymphadenitis may be a promising tissue source for identifying a potential link between retroviral gene products and SLE.

### Sjögren's Syndrome

The enlarged salivary glands from patients with Sjögren's syndrome have been an accessible organ for studies of a potential role for bacterial or viral gene products and autoimmunity. The rate of EBV infection is increased among patients with Sjögren's syndrome, and increased levels of $V_\beta 13$ T cells have been detected in their salivary glands

(129). However, no clear role for a particular superantigen has been demonstrated.

## CONCLUSIONS

Superantigens are the protein products of some bacteria and viruses, particularly retroviruses, that have the capacity to directly bind to MHC class II molecules and to the protein products of certain TCR β chain gene families. The consequences of superantigens for the host immune system are profound, including T-cell activation, cytokine production, anergy or deletion of large T-cell subpopulations, and activation and maturation of B cells and other immune and inflammatory cells. Superantigens have been implicated as etiologic agents in TSS, and strong support exists for a pathogenic role for superantigens in rheumatic fever and psoriasis. Although not definitive, data from human patients and experimental models of IDDM, rheumatoid arthritis, and multiple sclerosis lend some support to a model in which superantigens trigger an initial T-cell activation and expansion, resulting in recruitment and persistent activation of autoreactive T cells at the site of disease. Although current data do not indicate a role for superantigen in SLE, the products of endogenous retroviruses may be logical candidates as pathologic agents in that prototype systemic autoimmune disease. Superantigens are a fascinating manifestation of the intricate interdependence of all organisms and a reminder that the remnants of retroviral genomes, as they are carried by microbes and mammals, play an active role in biology.

## REFERENCES

1. Peavy DL, Adler WH, Smith RT. The mitogenic effects of endotoxin and staphylococcal enterotoxin B on mouse spleen cells and human peripheral lymphocytes. *J Immunol* 1970;105:1453–1458.
2. Nauciel C. Mitogenic activity of purified streptococcal erythrogenic toxin on lymphocytes. *Ann Immunol* 1973;124:383–390.
3. Langford MP, Stanton GJ, Johnson HM. Biological effects of staphylococcal enterotoxin A on human peripheral lymphocytes. *Infect Immun* 1978;22:62–68.
4. Festenstein H. Immunogenetic and biological aspects of *in vitro* lymphocyte allo-transformation (MLR) in the mouse. *Transplant Rev* 1973;15:62–88.
5. Festenstein H, Kimura S. The Mls system: past and present. *J Immunogenet* 1988;15:183–196.
6. White J, Herman A, Pullen AM, et al. The V$_\beta$-specific superantigen staphylococcal enterotoxin B: Stimulation of mature T cells and clonal deletion in neonatal mice. *Cell* 1989;56:27–35.
7. Kappler J, Kotzin B, Herron L, et al. V$_\beta$-specific stimulation of human T cells by staphylococcal toxins. *Science* 1990;244:811–813.
8. Marrack P, Kappler J. The staphylococcal enterotoxins and their relatives. *Science* 1990;248:705–711.
9. Kappler JW, Staerz UD, White J, et al. Self-tolerance eliminates T cells specific for Mls-modified products of the major histocompatibility complex. *Nature* 1988;332:35–40.
10. Janeway CA, Chalupny J, Conrad PJ, et al. An external stimulus that mimics Mls locus responses. *J Immunogenet* 1988;15:161–168.
11. Abe R, Vacchio MS, Fox B, et al. Preferential expression of the T-cell receptor V$_\beta$3 gene by Mlsc reactive T cells. *Nature* 1988;335:827–830.
12. Janeway CA Jr, Yagi J, Conrad PJ, et al. T-cell responses to Mls and to bacterial proteins that mimic its behavior. *Immunol Rev* 1989;107:61–88.
13. MacDonald HR, Schneider R, Lees RL, et al. T-cell receptor V$_\beta$ use predicts reactivity and tolerance to Mlsa-encoded antigens. *Nature* 1991;349:524–526.
14. Acha-Orbea H, Shakhov AN, Scarpellino L, et al. Clonal deletion of V$_\beta$14 positive T cells in mammary tumor virus transgenic mice. *Nature* 1991;350:207–211.
15. Choi Y, Kappler JW, Marrack P. A superantigen encoded in the open reading frame of the 3' long terminal repeat of mouse mammary tumor virus. *Nature* 1991;350:203–207.
16. Dyson PJ, Knight AM, Fairchild S, et al. Genes encoding ligands for deletion of V$_\beta$11 T cells cosegregate with mammary tumor virus genomes. *Nature* 1991;349:531–532.
17. Frankel WN, Rudy C, Coffin JM, et al. Linkage of Mls genes to endogenous mammary tumor viruses of inbred mice. *Nature* 1991;349:526–528.
18. Woodland DL, Happ MP, Gollub KJ, et al. An endogenous retrovirus mediating deletion of αβT cells? *Nature* 1991;349:529–530.
19. Woodland DL, Lund FE, Happ MP, et al. Endogenous superantigen expression is controlled by mouse mammary tumor proviral loci. *J Exp Med* 1991;174:1255–1258.
20. Beutner U, Frankel WN, Cote MS, et al. Mls-1 is encoded by the long terminal repeat open reading frame of the mouse mammary tumor virus Mtv-7. *Proc Natl Acad Sci USA* 1992;89:5432–5436.
21. Pullen AM, Choi Y, Kushnir E, et al. The open reading frames in the 3' long terminal repeats of several mouse mammary tumor virus integrants encode V$_\beta$3-specific superantigens. *J Exp Med* 1992;175:41–47.
22. Acha-Orbea H, Held W, Waanders GA, et al. Exogenous and endogenous mouse mammary tumor virus superantigens. *Immunol Rev* 1993;131:5–25.
23. Fleischer B, Schrezenmeier H. T-cell stimulation by staphylococcal enterotoxins: clonally variable response and requirements for major histocompatibility complex class II molecules on accessory or target cells. *J Exp Med* 1988;167:1697–1707.
24. Fischer H, Dohlstein M, Lindvall M, et al. Binding of staphylococcal enterotoxin A to HLA-DR on B cell lines. *J Immunol* 1989;142:3151–3157.
25. Fraser JD. High-affinity binding of staphylococcal enterotoxins A and B to HLA-DR. *Nature* 1989;339:221–223.
26. Mollick JA, Cook RG, Rich RR. Class II MHC molecules are specific receptors for staphylococcus enterotoxin A. *Science* 1989;244:817–820.
27. Scholl PR, Diez A, Geha RS. Staphylococcal enterotoxin B and toxic shock syndrome toxin-1 bind to distinct sites on HLA-DR and HLA-DQ molecules. *J Immunol* 1989;143:2583–2588.
28. Choi YW, Herman A, DiGiusto D, et al. Residues of the variable region of the T-cell-receptor β-chain that interact with *S. aureus* toxin superantigens. *Nature* 1990;246:471–473.
29. Dellabona P, Peccoud J, Kappler J, et al. Superantigens interact with MHC class II molecules outside of the antigen groove. *Cell* 1990;62:1115–1121.
30. Kappler JW, Herman A, Clements J, et al. Mutations defining functional regions of the superantigen staphylococcal enterotoxin B. *J Exp Med* 1992;175:387–396.
31. Swaminathan S, Furey W, Pletcher J, et al. Crystal structure of staphylococcal enterotoxin-B, a superantigen. *Nature* 1992;359:801–806.
32. Kim J, Urban RG, Strominger JL, et al. Crystallographic structure of toxin shock syndrome toxin-1 complexed with a human class II major histocompatibility molecule, HLA-DR1. *Science* 1994;266:1870–1874.
33. Jardetsky TS, Brown JH, Gorga JC, et al. Three-dimensional structure of a human class II major histocompatibility molecule complexed with superantigen. *Nature* 1994;368:711–718.
34. Conrad B, Weldmann E, Trucco G, et al. Evidence for superantigen involvement in insulin-dependent diabetes mellitus aetiology. *Nature* 1994;371:351–355.
35. Herman A, Croteau G, Sekaly R-P, et al. HLA-DR alleles differ in their ability to present staphylococcal enterotoxins to T cells. *J Exp Med* 1990;172:709–717.
36. Hodtsev AS, Choi Y, Spanopoulou E, Posnett DN. *Mycoplasma* superantigen is a CDR3-dependent ligand for the T cell antigen receptor. *J Exp Med* 1998;187:319–327.
37. Abe J, Forrester J, Nakahara T, et al. Selective stimulation of human T cells with streptococcal erythrogenic toxins A and B. *J Immunol* 1991;146:3747–3750.

38. Tomai M, Kotb M, Majumdar G, et al. Superantigenicity of streptococcal M protein. *J Exp Med* 1990;172:359–362.

39. Tomai MA, Aelion JA, Dockter ME, et al. T cell receptor V gene usage by human T cells stimulated with the superantigen streptococcal M protein. *J Exp Med* 1991;174:285–288.

40. Watanabe-Ohnishi R, Aelion J, Le Gros HL, et al. Characterization of unique human TCR V beta specificities for a family of streptococcal superantigens represented by rheumatogenic serotypes of M protein. *J Immunol* 1994;152:2066–2073.

41. Fleisher B, Schmidt KH, Gerlach D, et al. Separation of mitogenic activity from streptococcal M protein. *Infect Immun* 1992;60:1767–1770.

42. Stuart PM, Woodward JG. *Yersinia enterocolitica* produces superantigen activity. *J Immunol* 1992;148:225–233.

43. Abe J, Takeda T, Watanabe Y, et al. Evidence for superantigen production by Yersinia pseudotuberculosis. *J Immunol* 1993;151:4183–4188.

44. Cole BC, Daynes RA, Ward JR. Stimulation of mouse lymphocytes by a mitogen derived from *Mycoplasma arthritidis*. I. Transformation is associated with an H-2 linked gene that maps to the I-E/I-C subregion. *J Immunol* 1981;127:1931–1939.

45. Tumang JR, Posnett DN, Cole BC, et al. Helper T cell dependent human B cell differentiation mediated by a *Mycoplasma* superantigen bridge. *J Exp Med* 1990;171:2153–2158.

46. Friedman SM, Crow MK, Tumang JR, et al. Characterization of human T cells reactive with the *Mycoplasma arthritidis*–derived superantigen (MAM): generation of a monoclonal antibody against V$_\beta$17, the T cell receptor product expressed by a large fraction of MAM-reactive human T cells. *J Exp Med* 1991;174:891–900.

47. Crow MK, Chu Z, Ravina B, et al. Human B cell differentiation induced by microbial superantigens: unselected peripheral blood lymphocytes secrete polyclonal immunoglobulin in response to Mycoplasma arthritidis mitogen. *Autoimmunity* 1992;14:23–32.

48. Tumang JR, Zhou J-L, Gietl D, et al. T helper cell–dependent, microbial superantigen-mediated B cell activation *in vivo*. *Autoimmunity* 1997;24:247–255.

49. Cole BC, Griffiths MM. Triggering and exacerbation of autoimmune arthritis by the *Mycoplasma arthritidis* superantigen MAM. *Arthritis Rheum* 1993;36:994–1002.

50. Knudtson KL, Sawitzke AD, Cole BC. The superantigen *Mycoplasma arthritidis* mitogen (MAM): physical properties and immunobiology. In: Leung DYM, Huber BT, Schlievert PM, eds. *Superantigens: molecular biology, immunology, and relevance to human disease*. New York: Marcel Dekker, 1997:339–367.

51. Hugin AW, Vacchio MS, Morse HC III. A virus-encoded "superantigen" in a retrovirus-induced immunodeficiency syndrome in mice. *Science* 1991;252:424-427.

52. Weissenberger J, Altmann A, Meuer S, et al. Evidence for superantigen activity of the Bel-3 protein of human foamy virus. *J Med Virol* 1994;44:59–66.

53. Torres RA, Johnson HM. Identification of an HIV-1 Nef peptide that binds to HLA class II antigens. *Biochem Biophys Res Commun* 1994;200:1059–1065.

54. Akolkar PN, Chirmule N, Gulwani-Akolkar B, et al. V beta-specific activation of T cells by the HIV glycoprotein gp160. *Scand J Immunol* 1995;41:487–498.

55. Ross SR. Immunobiology of MMTV superantigens. In: Leung DYM, Huber BT, Schlievert PM, eds. *Superantigens: molecular biology, immunology, and relevance to human disease*. New York: Marcel Dekker, 1997:15–35.

56. Golovkina TV, Chervonsky A, Dudley JP, et al. Transgenic mouse mammary tumor virus superantigen expression prevents viral infection. *Cell* 1992;69:637–645.

57. Held W, Shakhov AN, Izui S, et al. Superantigen-reactive CD4$^+$ T cells are required to stimulate B cell after infection with mouse mammary tumor virus. *J Exp Med* 1993;177:359–366.

58. Held W, Waanders GA, Shakhov AN, et al. Superantigen-induced immune stimulation amplifies mouse mammary tumor virus and allows virus transmission. *Cell* 1993;74:529–540.

59. Pucillo C, Cepeda R, Hodes RJ. Expression of a MHC class II transgene determines superantigenicity and susceptibility to mouse mammary tumor virus infection. *J Exp Med* 1993;178:1441–1445.

60. Chervonsky AV, Xu J, Barlow AK, et al. Direct physical interaction involving CD40 ligand on T cells and CD40 on B cells is required to propagate MMTV. *Immunity* 1995;3:139–146.

61. Nusse R. The int genes in mammary tumorigenesis and in normal development. *Trends Genet* 1988;4:291–295.

62. Sassaman DM, Dombroski BA, Moran JV, et al. Many human L1 elements are capable of retrotransposition. *Nat Genet* 1997;16:37–43.

63. Liebold DM, Swergold GD, Singer MF, et al. Translation of LINE-1 DNA elements *in vitro* and in human cells. *Proc Natl Acad Sci USA* 1990;87:6990–6994.

64. Indraccolo S, Gunzburg WH, Leib-Mosch C, Erfle V, Salmons B, Identification of three human sequences with viral superantigen-specific primers. *Mamm Genome* 1995;6:339–344.

65. Imberti L, Sottini A, Bettinardi A, et al. Selective depletion in HIV infection of T cells that bear specific T cell receptor V$_\beta$ sequences. *Science* 1992;254:860–862.

66. Laurence J, Hodtsev AS, Posnett DN. Superantigen implicated in dependence of HIV-1 replication in T cells on TCR V$_\beta$ expression. *Nature* 1992;358:255–259.

67. Lafon M. Superantigen in rabies virus and its involvement in paralysis. In: Leung DYM, Huber BT, Schlievert PM, eds. *Superantigens: molecular biology, immunology, and relevance to human disease*. New York: Marcel Dekker, 1997:85–102.

68. Lafon M, Lafage M, Martinez-Arends A, et al. Evidence for a viral superantigen in humans. *Nature* 1992;358:507–510.

69. Lafon M, Scott-Algara D, March PN, et al. Neonatal deletion and selective expansion of mouse T cells by exposure to rabies virus nucleocapsid superantigen. *J Exp Med* 1994;180:1207–1215.

70. Dobrescu D, Ursea B, Pope M, et al. Enhanced HIV-1 replication in V$_\beta$12 T cells due to human cytomegalovirus in monocytes: evidence for a putative herpesvirus superantigen. *Cell* 1995;82:753–763.

71. Sutkowski N, Palkama T, Ciurli C, et al. An Epstein-Barr virus–associated superantigen. *J Exp Med* 1996;184:971–980.

72. Denkers EY, Caspar P, Sher A. *Toxoplasma gondii* possesses a superantigen activity that selectively expands murine T cell receptor V beta 5-bearing CD8$^+$ lymphocytes. *J Exp Med* 1994;180:985–994.

73. Johnson LP, Tomai MA, Schlievert PM. Molecular analysis of bacteriophage involvement in group A streptococcal pyrogenic exotoxin A production. *J Bacteriol* 1986;166:623–627.

74. Betley MJ, Mekalanos JJ. Staphylococcal enterotoxin A is encoded by phage. *Science* 1985;229:185–187.

75. Fast DJ, Schlievert PM, Nelson RD. Toxic shock syndrome-associated staphylococcal and streptococcal pyrogenic toxins are potent inducers of tumor necrosis factor production. *Infect Immun* 1989;57:291–294.

76. Tumang JR, Cherniak EP, Gietl DM, et al. T helper cell–dependent, microbial superantigen-induced murine B cell activation: polyclonal and antigen-specific antibody responses. *J Immunol* 1991;147:432–438.

77. Schattner E, Elkon KB, Yoo D-H, et al. CD40 ligation induces Apo-1/Fas expression on human B lymphocytes and facilitates apoptosis through the Apo-1/Fas pathway. *J Exp Med* 1995;182:1557–1565.

78. Friedman SM, Posnett DN, Tumang JR, et al. A potential role for microbial superantigens in the pathogenesis of systemic autoimmune disease. *Arthritis Rheum* 1991;34:468–480.

79. Mourad W, Al-Daccak R, Chatila T, et al. Staphylococcal superantigens as inducers of signal transduction in MHC class II–positive cells. *Semin Immunol* 1993;5:47–55.

80. Mehindate K, Thibodeau J, Dohlsten M, et al. Cross-linking of major histocompatibility complex class II molecules by staphylococcal enterotoxin A superantigen is a requirement for inflammatory cytokine gene expression. *J Exp Med* 1995;182:1573–1577.

81. Luther SA, Gulbranson-Judge A, Acha-Orbea H, et al. Viral superantigen drives extrafollicular and follicular B cell differentiation leading to virus-specific antibody production. *J Exp Med* 1997;185:551–562.

82. Leung DYM, Meissner HC, Fulton DR, et al. Toxic shock syndrome toxin-secreting *Staphylococcus aureus* in Kawasaki syndrome. *Lancet* 1993;342:1385–1388.

83. Deresiewicz RL. Staphylococcal toxic shock syndrome. In: Leung DYM, Huber BT, Schlievert PM, eds. *Superantigens: molecular biology, immunology, and relevance to human disease*. New York: Marcel Dekker, 1997:435–479.

84. Musser JM. Streptococcal superantigen, mitogenic factor and pyrogenic exotoxin B expressed by *Streptococcus pyogenes*: structure and function. In: Leung DYM, Huber BT, Schlievert PM, eds. *Superantigens: molecular biology, immunology, and relevance to human disease*. New York: Marcel Dekker, 1997:281–310.

85. Kawasaki T. Acute febrile mucocutaneous syndrome with lymphoid involvement with specific desquamation of the fingers and toes in children. *Jpn J Allergy* 1967;16:178–222.

86. Rowley AH, Shulman ST. Kawasaki syndrome. *Pediatr Clin North Am* 1999;46:313–327.

87. Yoshioka T, Matsutani T, Iwagami S, et al. Polyclonal expansion of TCRBV2- and TCRBV6-bearing T cells in patients with Kawasaki disease. *Immunology* 1999;96:465–472.

88. Abe J, Kotzin BL, Jujo K, et al. Selective expansion of T cells expressing T-cell receptor variable regions $V_\beta2$ and $V_\beta8$ in Kawasaki disease. *Proc Natl Acad Sci USA* 1992;89:4066–4070.

89. Smith TJ, Terada N, Robinson CC, et al. Acute infectious mononucleosis stimulates the selective expression/expansion of $V_\beta6.1$-3 and $V_\beta7$ T cells. *Blood* 1993;81:1521–1526.

90. Hofer MF, Lester MR, Schlievert PM, et al. Upregulation of IgE synthesis by staphylococcal toxic shock syndrome toxin-1 in peripheral blood mononuclear cells from patients with atopic dermatitis. *Clin Exp Allergy* 1995;25:1218–1227.

91. Heise M, Chow K, Kanagawa O. Interaction between T cells and murine acquired immunodeficiency virus superantigen: effect of second signal on T cell reactivity to the MAIDS virus superantigen. *Int Immunol* 1993;5:583–590.

92. Resnick SD. Toxic shock syndrome: recent developments in pathogenesis. *J Pediatr* 1990;116:321–328.

93. Stevens DL, Tanner MH, Winship J, et al. Reappearance of scarlet fever toxin A among streptococci in the Rocky Mountain West: severe group A streptococcal infections associated with a toxic shock-like syndrome. *N Engl J Med* 1989;321:1–7.

94. Stevens DL. The flesh-eating bacterium: what's next? *J Infect Dis* 1999;179[Suppl 2]:S366–S374.

95. Holm SE, Norrby A, Bergholm AM, et al. Aspects of pathogenesis of serious group A streptococcal infections in Sweden, 1988–1989. *J Infect Dis* 1992;166:31–37.

96. Becker K, Roth R, Peters G. Rapid and specific detection of toxigenic *Staphylococcus aureus:* use of two multiplex PCR enzyme immunoassays for amplification and hybridization of staphylococcal enterotoxin genes, exfoliative toxin genes, and toxic shock syndrome toxin 1 gene. *J Clin Microbiol* 1998;36:2548–2553.

97. Chieu CH, Lin TY. Successful treatment of severe streptococcal toxic shock syndrome with a combination of intravenous immunoglobulin, dexamethasone, and antibiotics. *Infection* 1997;25:47–48.

98. Krakauer T, Stiles BG. Pentoxifylline inhibits superantigen-induced toxic shock and cytokine release. *Clin Diagn Lab Immunol* 1999; 6:594–598.

99. De Vriese AS, Colardyn FA, Philippe JJ, et al. Cytokine removal during continuous hemofiltration in septic patients. *J Am Soc Nephrol* 1999;10:846–853.

100. Suzuki H, Guinter TI, Koyasu S, et al. Positive selection of CD4+ T cells by TCR-specific antibodies requires low valency TCR cross-linking: implications for repertoire selection in the thymus. *Eur J Immunol* 1998;28:3252–3258.

101. Sommer N, Harcourt GC, Willcox N, et al. Acetylcholine receptor-reactive T lymphocytes from healthy subjects and myasthenia gravis patients. *Neurology* 1991;41:1270–1276.

102. Matzinger P. Tolerance, danger, and the extended family. *Annu Rev Immunol* 1994;12:991–1045.

103. Banchereau J, Bazan F, Blanchard D. The CD40 antigen and its ligand. *Annu Rev Immunol* 1994;12:881–922.

104. Hillson JL, Karr NS, Opplinger IR, et al. The structural basis of germline-encoded $V_H3$ immunoglobulin binding to staphylococcal protein A. *J Exp Med* 1993;178:331–336.

105. Levinson AI, Kozlowski LM. B-cell superantigens and their biologic implications. In: Leung DYM, Huber BT, Schlievert PM, eds. *Superantigens: molecular biology, immunology, and relevance to human disease.* New York: Marcel Dekker, 1997:405–433.

106. Jackow CM, Cather JC, Hearne V, et al. Association of erythrodermic cutaneous T-cell lymphoma, superantigen-positive *Staphylococcus aureus,* and oligoclonal T-cell receptor V beta gene expansion. *Blood* 1997;89:32–40.

107. Schwab JH, Brown RR, Anderle SK, et al. Superantigen can reactivate bacterial wall-induced arthritis. *J Immunol* 1993;150:4141–4149.

108. Brocke S, Gaur A, Piercy C, et al. Induction of relapsing paralysis in experimental allergic encephalomyelitis by bacterial superantigen. *Nature* 1993;365:642–644.

109. Soos JM, Schiffenbauer J, Johnson HM. Treatment of PL/J mice with the superantigen, staphylococcal enterotoxin B, prevents development of experimental allergic encephalomyelitis. *J Neuroimmunol* 1993;44:39–43.

110. Schiffenbauer J, Johnson HM, Butfiloski E, et al. Staphylococcal enterotoxins can re-activate experimental allergic encephalomyelitis. *Proc Natl Acad Sci USA* 1993;90:8543–8546.

111. Kawamura T, Nagata M, Utsugi T, et al. Prevention of autoimmune type I diabetes by CD4+ suppressor T cells in superantigen-treated non-obese diabetic mice. *J Immunol* 1993;151:4362–4370.

112. Kim C, Siminovitch KA, Ochi A. Reduction of lupus nephritis in MRL/lpr mice by a bacterial superantigen treatment. *J Exp Med* 1991;174:1431–1437.

113. Kotb M. Streptococcal M protein: role in post-streptococcal autoimmunity. In: Leung DYM, Huber BT, Schlievert PM, eds. *Superantigens: molecular biology, immunology, and relevance to human disease.* New York: Marcel Dekker, 1997:311–338.

114. Paliard X, West SG, Lafferty JA, et al. Evidence for the effects of a superantigen in rheumatoid arthritis. *Science* 1991;253:325–329.

115. Howell MD, Diveley JP, Lundeen KA, et al. Limited T-cell receptor beta-chain heterogeneity among interleukin 2 receptor-positive synovial T cells suggests a role for superantigen in rheumatoid arthritis. *Proc Natl Acad Sci USA* 1991;88:10921–10925.

116. Zagon G, Tumang JR, Li Y, et al. Increased frequency of $V_\beta17$-positive T cells in patients with rheumatoid arthritis. *Arthritis Rheum* 1994;10:1431–1440.

117. Li Y, Sun G-R, Tumang JR, et al. CDR3 sequence motifs shared by oligoclonal rheumatoid arthritis synovial T cells: evidence for an antigen-driven response. *J Clin Invest* 1994;94:2525–2531.

118. Bowness P, Moss PA, Rowland-Jones S, et al. Conservation of T cell receptor usage by HLA-B27–restricted influenza-specific cytotoxic T lymphocytes suggests a general pattern for antigen-specific major histocompatibility complex class I–restricted responses. *Eur J Immunol* 1993;23:1417–1421.

119. Conrad B, Weissmahr RN, Boni J, et al. Human endogenous retroviral superantigen as candidate autoimmune gene in type I diabetes. *Cell* 1997;90:303–313.

120. Galley KA, Danska JS. Peri-islet infiltrates of young non-obese diabetic mice display restricted TCR β-chain diversity. *J Immunol* 1995;154:2969–2982.

121. Lower R, Tonjes RR, Boller K, et al. Development of insulin-dependent diabetes mellitus does not depend on specific expression of the endogenous retrovirus HERV-K. *Cell* 1998;95:11–14.

122. Oksenberg J, Panzara MA, Begovich AB, et al. Selection for TCR $V_\beta$-$D_\beta$-$J_\beta$ gene rearrangements with specificity for a myelin protein peptide in the brain lesions of multiple sclerosis. *Nature* 1993;362:68–70.

123. Baker BS, Bokth S, Powles A, et al. Group A streptococcal antigen-specific T lymphocytes in guttate psoriatic lesions. *Br J Dermatol* 1993;128:493–499.

124. Leung DYM, Travers JB, Giorno R, et al. Evidence for a streptococcal superantigen-driven process in acute guttate psoriasis. *J Clin Invest* 1995;96:2106–2112.

125. Valdimarsson H, Sigmundsdottir H, Jonsdotti I. Is psoriasis induced by streptococcal superantigens and maintained by M-protein–specific T cells that cross-react with keratin? *Clin Exp Immunol* 1997;107:21–24.

126. Perez-Lorenzo R, Zambrano-Zaragoza JF, Saul A, et al. Autoantibodies to autologous skin in guttate and plaque forms of psoriasis and cross-reaction of skin antigens with streptococcal antigens. *Int J Dermatol* 1998;37:524–531.

127. Van Rappard-van der Veen FM, Rolink AG, Gleichmann E. Diseases caused by reactions of T lymphocytes towards incompatible structures of the major histocompatibility complex. VI. Autoantibodies characteristic of systemic lupus erythematosus induced by abnormal T-B cell cooperation across I-E. *J Exp Med* 1982;155:1555–1560.

128. Datta SK, Kaliyaperumal A, Desai-Mehta A. T cells of lupus and molecular targets for immunotherapy. *J Clin Immunol* 1997;17:11–20.

129. Massengill SF, Goodenow MM, Sleasman JW. SLE nephritis is associated with an oligoclonal expansion of intrarenal T cells. *Am J Kidney Dis* 1998;31:418–426.

130. Sumida T, Yonaha F, Maeda T, et al. T cell receptor repertoire of infiltrating T cells in lips of Sjögren's syndrome patients. *J Clin Invest* 1992;89:681–685.

*Textbook of the Autoimmune Diseases,*
Edited by R. G. Lahita, N. Chiorazzi, and W. H. Reeves,
Lippincott Williams & Wilkins, Philadelphia © 2000.

# CHAPTER 4

# Genetics

## Peter K. Gregersen

Our overall understanding of the genetic basis of human autoimmune disorders is undergoing rapid change. This trend is likely to accelerate during the next few years, in part because of the completion of the Human Genome Project (1) and because of increased knowledge about biologic systems at a molecular level. The genetics of most autoimmune disorders is complex, and the ultimate contribution of genetics depends on integrating genetic data with the underlying pathophysiology of autoimmunity. There will be no isolation of "the gene" for autoimmunity; for many forms of autoimmune disease, multiple genes probably confer risk for disease by virtue of the genetic polymorphisms that may be relatively common in the population.

During the past two decades, the major focus of genetic research in autoimmunity has been on the major histocompatibility complex (MHC). This work has been reviewed extensively (2–7) and therefore is not reiterated in great detail in this chapter. Despite the large amount of work done in this area, there remains debate concerning exactly which genes within the MHC are responsible for the disease associations with this region. Most of this discussion concerning human leukocyte antigens (HLA) therefore focuses on how the MHC association data can be extended to further define the genetic elements that are responsible for disease susceptibility. The unresolved issues around HLA are likely to presage the problems that will be encountered in the evaluation of non–HLA-linked genes in disease susceptibility.

## GENETICALLY COMPLEX DISORDERS AND THE CONCEPT OF DISEASE SUSCEPTIBILITY

A hallmark of genetically complex disorders is the fact that there is not a simple one to one correspondence between inheritance of particular genes and the expression of a disease phenotype, in part because multiple genes probably are involved and therefore no single one of them (i.e., particular HLA alleles) has high predictive power for disease. Even in the presence of disease alleles, disease penetrance is far below 100%. This fact is starkly illustrated by the fact that monozygous (MZ) twins (carrying identical alleles at all loci) have disease concordance rates that are in the 15% to 30% range for most autoimmune diseases (8–14). It is likely that different combinations of genes give rise to similar autoimmune disease phenotypes in different individuals or population groups. The involvement of a heterogeneous group of genes that have relatively low penetrance makes the problem complicated and leads to the concept of disease susceptibility.

In its most basic sense, genetic susceptibility to disease implies that the probability of developing the disease, over a lifetime, is greater in the presence of a disease allele (A), than in its absence: $P(D|A) > P(D|$ not $A)$. For most disease alleles involved in autoimmunity, the ratio of these two probabilities is quite low, generally less than 10. Because at least some disease alleles are probably common, this implies that there are large numbers of people with the disease who do not carry a given disease allele and large numbers of people who carry disease-associated alleles but never develop detectable disease. It also means that observations must be made on large numbers of individuals to observe a significant difference in these probabilities. This can be done most directly by performing cohort or case-control studies, although other approaches can also lead to the same information.

## NONGENETIC FACTORS

It is common to consider genes and environment as the major factors involved in disease susceptibility. For most human autoimmune diseases, few specific environmental exposures have been convincingly identified, and with some exceptions (15), those that have been implicated generally confer only modestly increased risk (16–18). This leaves open the possibility that other factors are involved in the final development of disease in a given individual. For example, it seems

P. K. Gregersen: Departments of Medicine and Pathology, New York University School of Medicine, New York, New York 10016; Division of Biology and Human Genetics, North Shore University Hospital, Manhasset, New York 11030.

unlikely that the low rate of concordance among MZ twins is entirely caused by differences in their environments, especially because most twins share their environments to a large degree. An alternative source of variation among MZ twins relates to chance events (19). Some of these stochastic events may occur early in development. For example, recombination events within the T-cell and B-cell receptor loci generate diversity within the immune system. Likewise, the use of genes on the X chromosome may vary dramatically among girls inheriting the same sets of chromosomes, even within MZ twin pairs (20). This kind of stochastic variation in gene usage among female MZ twins can lead to phenotypic differences, including discordance in expression of X-linked diseases, such as Duchenne's muscular dystrophy (21).

Monoallelic expression of genes may occur on autosomes and involve a wide variety of gene families, including cytokine genes (22,23) and genes involved in growth control (24). In many cases, the choice of which allele is expressed depends on the parental origin of the allele, a phenomenon is called *genomic imprinting* (25). In other instances, the choice of allelic expression appears to be stochastic (22,23). Even in parentally imprinted genes, there appears to be some variation in the strength of the imprint, which may have a stochastic component (26). The extent of variation of these events within and between individuals has not been established. However, it seems likely that such probabilistic events have some influence on disease expression and may partly explain the low MZ twin concordance rate for autoimmunity.

## ASSESSING THE STRENGTH OF THE GENETIC COMPONENT IN AUTOIMMUNITY

In the absence of knowledge about specific genes, the evidence for a genetic contribution to a complex phenotype such as autoimmunity depends almost entirely on epidemiologic data. These data involve comparison of disease prevalence in groups of individuals with different degrees of genetic relatedness. The most common types of groups used for such studies are genetically identical individuals (MZ twins), individuals who share approximately 50% of their genes in common (DZ twins and siblings), and unrelated individuals in the population whose overall degree of genetic similarity (at polymorphic loci) is relatively low, with about 0.1% difference over the entire genome (1). A 0.1% difference among unrelated subjects implies approximately 3 million base pair differences over the entire genome, assuming only single nucleotide polymorphisms.

The use of such family and background population prevalence data to calculate risk ratios has become a popular means of estimating the size of the genetic component in complex diseases (27). This method uses prevalence rates to calculate the relative risk of disease between two comparison populations, most often siblings of affecteds compared with the general population. This leads to a value called $\lambda_s$, or relative risk to sibs, calculated as follows:

$$\lambda_s = \frac{\text{Disease prevalence in siblings of affecteds}}{\text{Disease prevalence in general population}}$$

Obtaining a reliable value of $\lambda_s$ depends on having accurate estimates of disease prevalence in the two comparison groups. This is not a trivial matter. In the case of rheumatoid arthritis, for example, the estimation of population prevalence is fraught with potential sources of error. A firm diagnosis of rheumatoid arthritis is difficult to make in large surveys, with errors in both directions possible. Underestimation may occur because of the lack of reporting of a disease that is no longer active. Overestimation may result from inadequate distinction between rheumatoid arthritis and other forms of polyarthritis. Most such surveys are not sufficiently large or detailed to enable accurate stratification on the basis of age, sex, or disease severity. The severity issue may be especially important, because genetic background may be involved in this aspect of the rheumatoid arthritis phenotype. Similar problems may occur in estimates of population prevalence of systemic lupus erythematosus (SLE), in which mild disease may be overlooked, or variability in phenotypic expression may confound the issue. The accurate detection and assessment of disease phenotype are also involved in the determination of sibling affection rates.

Despite these difficulties, a range of values for $\lambda_s$ have been established for many of the common autoimmune disorders. Representative examples are shown in Table 4.1. With the exception of ankylosing spondylitis, most autoimmune disorders appear to have a $\lambda_s$ in the range of 10 to 20. Also shown in Table 4.1 are estimates for $\lambda_{MZ}$. Analogous to the calculation for $\lambda_s$, $\lambda_{MZ}$ is calculated by the following:

$$\lambda_{MZ} = \frac{\text{Disease prevalence cotwins of affecteds}}{\text{Disease prevalence in general population}}$$

The value $\lambda_{MZ}$ can be interpreted as an estimate of the maximal genetic risk for the disease. This assumes that all the increased risk to an MZ cotwin of an affected individual results from the fact that they share the same genetic polymorphisms. This is clearly not the case, because at least some environmental sharing probably contributes to the risk. However, it is notable that the estimated value for $\lambda_{MZ}$ is quite high for many autoimmune disorders, and this emphasizes the fact that MZ twin concordance rates must be interpreted in light of the background population prevalence of the disease. A relatively low MZ twin concordance rate does not necessarily imply a low genetic component to the disorder.

**TABLE 4.1.** *Estimates of $\lambda_s$ and $\lambda_{MZ}$ for some common autoimmune disorders*

| Disease | $\lambda_s$ | $\lambda_{MZ}$ |
|---|---|---|
| Systemic lupus | 20 | 250 |
| Rheumatoid arthritis | 3–10 | 20–60 |
| Multiple sclerosis | 20 | 250 |
| Type I diabetes | 15 | 60 |
| Ankylosing spondylitis | 54 | 500 |

Data from references 28 through 32.

## ASSESSING AUTOIMMUNE DISEASE GENES

### Testing for Disease Genes by Association

Until recently, the most common method of testing for the association of an autoimmune disease with a particular gene, such as an HLA allele, has been the case-control study. Such studies establish an estimate for the degree of risk an allele carries for developing disease—the estimated relative risk (RR). To understand why this is an estimate, it is helpful to first consider another study design, the cohort study. Cohort studies are the ideal way to establish whether a particular factor, in this case a particular genetic polymorphism, is associated with risk for a particular outcome (e.g., disease). In cohort studies, a group of subjects are identified who carry or do not carry the gene of interest. These subjects are then followed over time to determine if the frequency of disease is different between the two groups. The results are tabulated in a contingency table (Table 4.2). By examining this table, it can be seen that the fraction of individuals with the gene who develop disease can be calculated as a/(a + b). Likewise, the fraction of individuals who do not carry the gene but nevertheless develop disease, is given by c/(c + d). The ratio of these two quantities is the RR of developing disease if the gene is present. However, when the outcome (disease) is relatively rare in the population, this ratio [a/(a + b)] ÷ [c/(c + d)] can be estimated as a simple ratio of the cross-product, (a × d) ÷ (b × c).

In practice, cohort studies for relatively rare diseases such as autoimmunity are impractical. The alternative case-control design is used in which patients with the disease are identified and the frequency of the gene is measured and compared with population controls who do not have the disease. The results are again recorded in a contingency table (Table 4.3). In this case, the ratio of the cross-product, (a × d) ÷ (b × c), is called the odds ratio (OR). However, just as in cohort studies, when the disease is rare in the population, this value can be interpreted as the estimated RR, and this is often used for reporting results from case-control studies.

Large numbers of case-control studies have been carried out over the last two decades to investigate the association between HLA alleles and autoimmunity (2–7). In general, the estimated relative risks for HLA class II associations with autoimmune diseases are in the range of 10 or less. The major exception is the very high estimated relative risks for ankylosing spondylitis with B27, which are in the range of 50 or more (33). In the case of systemic lupus, the HLA associations are most closely related to the type of autoantibody rather than with the disease itself (7).

Although the fact of HLA association with autoimmune diseases is not in dispute, the significance of these observations remains unclear. It is therefore useful to consider the

**TABLE 4.2.** *Contingency table for cohort study*

| Group | Disease | No disease |
|---|---|---|
| Exposed | a | b |
| Not exposed | c | d |

**TABLE 4.3.** *Contingency table for case-control study*

| Group | Exposed | Not exposed |
|---|---|---|
| Disease | a | b |
| No disease | c | d |

possible reasons for observing a population association between a gene and a phenotype:

1. A false-positive association is caused by statistical error or inadequate matching between controls and affected individuals (i.e., population stratification).
2. The allele under examination is directly involved in disease pathogenesis.
3. A gene in linkage disequilibrium with the test allele is responsible for the association.

The first possibility is unlikely to explain the mass of data supporting the association between autoimmunity and HLA-linked genes. However, this problem does continue to confound individual studies. It becomes increasingly important as larger genetic studies are used to narrow genetic associations to particular genes within the MHC or to particular subgroups of patients. The pattern of association between HLA and disease can vary among different ethnic groups, and therefore careful matching of controls for this parameter is required. The use of historical, unrelated controls is not an acceptable practice. The use of family-based controls is becoming a popular means of avoiding the problems inherent in using unrelated control populations.

The second possibility is often the conclusion put forward in many studies reporting HLA associations (2–7). The underlying assumption is that the higher the estimated RR and the larger the number of cases explained by the association, the greater is the likelihood that the polymorphism under examination actually explains the association. This approach is best exemplified by the many studies showing an association between the "shared epitope" and rheumatoid arthritis (2,3,34). Similar arguments have been made concerning specific DQ polymorphisms and autoantibody production in lupus and Sjögren's syndrome (7). Overall, the case is probably most compelling for B27 having a direct role in the pathogenesis of ankylosing spondylitis (35). Purely genetic arguments alone can never prove the case for direct involvement of a particular polymorphism in susceptibility to a multifactorial disease. However, further genetic analysis can provide evidence against this hypothesis. Examples of this are discussed in the next section, Family-Based Association Studies.

Despite the fact that many workers assume that their test allele is directly relevant to disease pathogenesis, the success of genetic association studies critically depends on linkage disequilibrium, and this is likely to explain at least a proportion of the positive HLA associations with autoimmune disease reported. *Linkage disequilibrium* is the term used to describe the fact that, when genes are close together on the same chromosome, allelic variants of these genes tend to occur together in the population more frequently than expected by chance. For example, the HLA-A1 allele is present in approximately 17% of the Danish population, and the HLA-B8 allele is found in 12.7% of Danish individuals. If the distributions of these alleles are independent, one expects approximately 2.1% ($0.17 \times 0.128 = 0.021$) of individuals to carry both of these alleles. The observed frequency is 6.9%, far higher than predicted. This results from the fact that the A and B loci are close to one another on chromosome 6 (about 1,000,000 base pairs apart), and these alleles are frequently found together on the same haplotype in this population (often in the context of an extended haplotype, A1-B8-DR3).

Although linkage disequilibrium is detected by means of a statistically significant variation from expected associations between alleles in a population, it reflects the underlying physical linkage between genes in a region of the genome. Within the HLA region, linkage disequilibrium is common, and it has been easy to detect because of the highly polymorphic nature of the HLA genes; linkage disequilibrium within HLA can extend to a distance of 1 centimorgan (cM), or approximately 1,000,000 base pairs or more. However, the extent of linkage disequilibrium varies among different populations and may vary for different regions of the genome (36). There are few data on the extent of linkage disequilibrium outside of HLA and other disease-associated genetic regions (36,37).

The practical consequence of linkage disequilibrium is that allelic associations with disease may reflect the association of an entire genetic region with the disease; any gene or set of genes within that region may be responsible for the observed association. It is therefore impossible to definitively state that the allele being used to demonstrate association is directly involved in the phenotype. If the average extent of linkage disequilibrium is only 0.5 cM, it still implies the existence of 20 to 50 genes in the region that could explain the association.

**Family-Based Association Studies**

Because patterns of linkage disequilibrium and disease association may vary among different populations and ethnic groups, the issue of controls is extremely important when performing association studies. Great effort is required to recruit matched, unrelated controls for these studies. Family-based controls are an elegant solution to this problem.

In 1987, Falk and Rubinstein proposed the haplotype RR method of generating controls for risk calculations (38). Figure 4.1 shows a nuclear family, with an affected individual carrying alleles 1 and 3 at a candidate locus, X. Both parents are heterozygous at this locus, with 1,2 and 3,4 carried by the father and mother, respectively. The parental haplotypes carrying the 2 and 4 alleles are not inherited by the affected child. These two noninherited haplotypes therefore can be used to construct a genotype for a control "individual." Although the generation of this control genotype requires typing two people instead of one, it has a major advantage: the test alleles (those transmitted to the child) are derived from exactly the same population (the parents) as the control

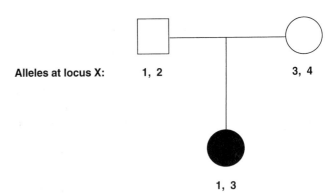

**FIG. 4.1.** The diagram of a simple nuclear family shows segregation of alleles at a marker locus X to an affected child. For family-based association studies, the noninherited parental alleles, 2 and 4, can be used as controls.

alleles. There can be no question of population stratification here, because in effect the same individuals are used as a source for the two groups of alleles (those found in affecteds and those found in controls). These data can be used to construct a contingency table, just like the one shown in Table 4.3.

A variant of this approach is called *transmission disequilibrium testing* (TDT) (39,40). Consider the family shown in Figure 4.1. For a heterozygous parent (such as 1,2 in the father), there is a probability of 0.5 that any given allele, such as allele 1, will be transmitted to a child. If this allele has no bearing on disease risk, the probability of transmission (T) to an affected child is equal to the probability of nontransmission (NT). This is stated simply as $P(T|D) = P(NT|D)$, where D indicates the presence of disease in the child. However, if the allele being examined is associated with disease risk, then $P(T|D) > P(NT|D)$. By examining large numbers of heterozygous parents with affected offspring, transmission disequilibrium testing can establish differences in disease association between test alleles and control alleles, both derived from the same individuals (the parents). Like the haplotype RR method, the problem of population stratification is avoided.

The work of Mulcahy is an example of the potential for TDT to contribute insight into the HLA associations in autoimmunity. This study investigated the involvement in rheumatoid arthritis of tumor necrosis factor (TNF) genes, which are located telomeric to HLA-DR in the MHC complex. Using this method, Mulcahy (41) provided evidence that TNF alleles associated with the A1-B8-DR3 haplotype (TNFc1) are associated with rheumatoid arthritis, independent of the shared epitope. TNFc1 is also found on an extended MHC haplotype that bears A2, B44, and DRB1*0401 and was preferentially transmitted to probands in this study, suggesting that DR4 may not be the only susceptibility gene on this haplotype. A reanalysis of these data by the MASC (Marker Association Segregation Chi-square) method also supports the view that a simple association with the shared epitope does not explain the MHC data in rheumatoid arthritis (42). Although these data need to be replicated independently, the results cannot be easily dismissed as resulting from an error due to population stratification, because the TDT uses parental controls.

A role for TNF expression polymorphisms in autoimmune disease pathogenesis was first raised in the context of lupus (43). Since then, multiple case-control studies for and against this hypothesis have been published (44–48). In some cases, the TNF allelic associations in lupus appear to simply reflect linkage disequilibrium with MHC class II alleles or no association is observed; in others, it appears that a TNF polymorphism confers risk for SLE, independent of the MHC or the closely linked complement alleles. All of these studies are subject to concern about population stratification confounding the results. It is in the context of this uncertainty that the TDT may play an important role in the future for evaluating candidate genes within and outside of the MHC.

## Testing by Linkage Methods: Allele Sharing in Affected Sibling Pairs

Although association methods have been the predominant approach to looking for genetic susceptibility genes in human autoimmunity, linkage-based methods have largely dominated the field of genetics in general, particularly for single-gene disorders. Classic linkage analysis (49) in multiplex families is most appropriate for simple mendelian genetic disorders in which the mode of inheritance is known (e.g., dominant, recessive); a detailed discussion of this method is beyond the scope of this chapter. Familial Mediterranean fever (a recessive, single-gene disorder) is among the few rheumatic diseases that have been successfully defined using linkage analysis (50,51). Classic linkage analysis has also been used to confirm HLA involvement in ankylosing spondylitis (52). However, another linkage-based method, affected sibling pair (ASP) analysis, has been much more widely employed to search for genes involved in genetically complex disorders, for which the mode of inheritance and number of genes involved are uncertain.

ASP analysis depends on linkage between a marker locus and a disease locus within families. Consider the families shown in Figure 4.2, in which there are two siblings, each affected with a disease or phenotype. In these cases, the affected siblings *within each family* are highly likely (although not certain) to be carriers of the same disease alleles. This assumption is based on the fact that the $\lambda_s$ calculation is high enough to indicate a substantial genetic component to the disease and that the genes involved are not so heterogeneous and so common in the population that affected sib pairs within a family are likely to have the disease on the basis of inheriting different susceptibility genes.

In the family shown in Figure 4.2A, both siblings have inherited identical alleles at a marker locus, X. In this case, there is only a 25% probability of this happening by chance. For example, given the fact that the first born sibling (sib 1) is 1,3, sibling 2 could have inherited one of four genotypes (1,3; 2,3; 1,4; or 2,4) with equal probability. By a similar reasoning, there is a 50% probability that these two siblings

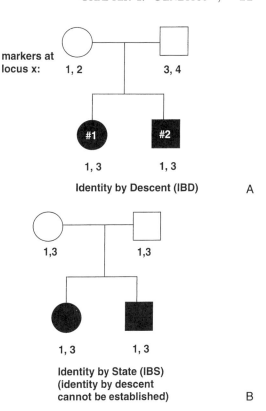

**FIG. 4.2.** Examples of families in which both sibling pairs are affected. **A:** The markers at locus X are completely informative in this family, and affected siblings are known to be identical by descent at this locus. The first-born (sib 1) and second-born (sib 2) children are indicated to assist discussion in the text. **B:** In this family, in which affected siblings are identical by state, it is uncertain whether there is sharing of any particular parental haplotype at locus X, because alleles 1 and 3 in each sibling could have come from different parents.

share only one allele and a 25% chance that they have nothing in common at this locus. If, however, the marker locus X is located very near to a disease gene, such affected siblings could be expected to share alleles more frequently than predicted by these mendelian segregation ratios. By examining large numbers of ASPs, it is possible to develop statistical evidence that this is the case for a given test marker locus, using a straightforward $\chi^2$ analysis, with the null hypothesis being that there is no increased sharing of alleles at the marker locus. This is the essence of ASP analysis (53,54).

In practice, this approach is complicated by a number of considerations. First, markers must be highly polymorphic to enable following their segregation in families. This problem has been solved through the use of microsatellite markers that contain highly variable tandem repeats of di-, tri-, or tetra-nucleotides (55). Nevertheless, not all marker loci are fully informative with respect to the segregation of parental chromosomes within a particular family. This is the case for the family in Figure 4.2B, in which the affected siblings have the same marker alleles, but it is not clear that each of these alleles came from the same chromosomes or even from the same parents. In this case, the siblings are said to be "identical by state" (IBS). This contrasts with family in Figure 4.2A, in which the siblings are identical by state and "identical by descent" (IBD). Families such as that shown in Figure 4.2B are uninformative with respect to marker X. For other marker loci, this family would still be useful for ASP analysis. When parents are unavailable for typing, statistical methods can be used to estimate the likelihood that identity by state actually reflects identity by descent (56). This calculation is heavily influenced by the frequency of the various alleles at the marker locus in the population.

How close to the disease gene does the marker have to be to be useful for ASP analysis? This depends on the likelihood that recombination between the marker locus and the disease locus occurs in the parents during meiosis. Recombination frequency between two loci is measured by the quantity $\theta$, also called the *recombination fraction*. When $\theta = 0.1$, it means that recombination between the two loci can be detected in 10% of meioses. In practice, if markers are placed at a distance of $\theta = 0.1$ or less from the disease locus, they are generally useful for detecting linkage. Although $\theta$ values are not solely dependent on physical distance, a $\theta$ value of 0.1 corresponds to roughly 10 million base pairs. The entire genome consists of $3.2 \times 10^9$ base pairs, and by using 300 to 400 markers, it is possible to be reasonably certain that one of them will be close enough to a disease locus to enable the detection of linkage. This has provided the rationale for many groups to proceed with a genome wide screen of ASPs for a variety of autoimmune disorders, including type I diabetes (57,58), multiple sclerosis (59–61), human SLE (62–65), and rheumatoid arthritis (66).

## Results of Genome Screens
## for Autoimmune Disease Genes

The linkage results from genome wide screens of ASPs have yielded complicated results, with often conflicting data from different groups. In part, this reflects the fact that these diseases are highly complex genetically, with many different loci making a contribution to susceptibility. Different populations may contain different sets of disease susceptibility alleles. Nevertheless, useful data are beginning to emerge.

A compilation of the major genetic screening studies using humans and mice indicates there may be substantial overlap in susceptibility loci for a variety of autoimmune disorders (67). A large number of these susceptibility loci overlap in a nonrandom fashion into 18 distinct clusters of genes. This fits with the observation that multiple autoimmune diseases may cluster within families (68). It also adds support for the proposition that rodent models of autoimmune diseases may be useful for predicting candidate genes in the analogous human disorders.

Perhaps the most tantalizing development has been the mapping of a susceptibility locus for human lupus to chromosome 1 (62–65). Early reports suggested this as a candidate region (69), and studies of murine lupus have also implicated a syntenic region (70). This latter observation led to a

focus on this region (1q31-1q42) by Tsao et al., and they observed striking linkage to 1q41-q42 using a relatively small number of ASPs (52) derived from 43 families (62). These workers went on to provide evidence that this linkage may result from a gene near or identical to poly(ADP-ribose) polymerase (PARP). Polymorphisms within this gene are strongly associated with lupus, as shown by transmission disequilibrium testing in sibling pairs and singleton families (71). This gene was specifically selected for testing as a candidate because it is involved in DNA repair and may play a role in regulating apoptosis (72). If these data are confirmed and extended to a precise mechanism for PARP in lupus pathogenesis, this success would provide an elegant example of how an interplay between modern genetic mapping, studies of basic pathophysiology, and animal disease models can lead to real progress in understanding human autoimmunity.

Nevertheless, it is wise to be cautious in coming to a conclusion that the PARP gene itself is involved in lupus susceptibility. A strong association between a disease and an allele does not necessarily imply involvement of that allele in disease pathogenesis. Association mapping depends on linkage disequilibrium between the test allele and the disease genes, and this may extend as far as 1 million base pairs, even in a diverse and relatively outbred (panmictic) population. The average 1 million base pair segment may contain as many as 30 to 100 genes. It is possible that the PARP associations with lupus merely reflect the involvement of another gene nearby. Consideration of the mapping studies in murine lupus emphasizes the complexity of disease gene mapping, because it now appears likely that there are possibly three different lupus susceptibility genes in the syntenic region of mouse chromosome 1 (68,71; Laurence Morel, personal communication, 1999). It is also clear from these murine lupus studies that individual genes are more tightly linked to specific phenotypes (e.g., high IgG, nephritis) than to lupus itself (70,73). Several linkage studies suggest similar genetic heterogeneity in humans (63–65).

The work on type I diabetes (IDDM) may be another example of successful mapping of disease susceptibility genes. IDDM has received the most sustained attention of all the autoimmune disorders and is a paradigm for large-scale screening for genetic susceptibility loci. A large number of genetic regions have been tentatively implicated in this disease. One study of 356 families (57) concluded that, in addition to the MHC, at least two other chromosomal regions contain genes that have a substantial influence on diabetes susceptibility: chromosome 10p13-q11 (IDDM10) and 16q22-q24. Many other regions have lower levels of statistical support in linkage analysis; for some of these, data on association indicate that the weak evidence for linkage nevertheless reflects the presence of a susceptibility locus. For example, the regions around the insulin gene (chromosome 11p15) and the CTLA-4 gene (chromosome 2q33) fall into this category (74–77). However, another larger study of 679 ASPs failed to provide support for many of these regions and raised the possibility that a new region on chromosome 1q may contribute to IDDM susceptibility (58). It is likely that at least some of these regions will ultimately yield specific information about the genetic polymorphisms involved in disease pathogenesis. The fact that this has not yet occurred reflects underlying genetic complexity of the problem and indicates that, outside of HLA, individual genes apparently make a very modest contribution to overall genetic risk for IDDM.

Genetic mapping studies of rheumatoid arthritis have lagged behind many of the other autoimmune disorders, in part because of a perception that the genetic risk for the disease may be lower than for other autoimmune diseases. Estimates for $\lambda_s$ as low as 2 or 3 have been reported (78), with up to 50% of the risk ascribed to MHC genes, implying a need for very large numbers of sibling pairs to detect linkage (79). These estimates are probably overly pessimistic (29). The only large ASP study reported has yielded modest evidence for a susceptibility locus on chromosome 3, which overlaps with the IDDM9 locus implicated in diabetes and contains candidate genes of potential interest, CD80 and CD86 (66). By stratifying families according to MHC type, the same group has developed evidence for a second region on chromosome 1, which contains an interesting candidate gene, TNF receptor 2 (80). These results need to be replicated and confirmed using association methods.

Another interesting issue raised by the study of rheumatoid arthritis is the question of how genetic background may influence disease severity. A number of studies have indicated that shared epitope–positive DR alleles may provide particular risk for severe disease (81,82). Rodent models of rheumatoid arthritis strongly suggest that separate genes may control disease severity and chronicity (83). This presents significant challenges for doing human genetic studies, because it implies that patient populations should be carefully stratified for disease severity when doing genetic analysis. Efforts to gather large numbers of well characterized sibling pairs with rheumatoid arthritis are underway in the United States and Europe (66,84,85).

### Considering Gene Interactions in Genetic Analysis

Because of the statistical complexities, the functional approach to genetic screening in most studies has been to evaluate each locus sequentially for evidence of linkage, as if each locus acted in isolation to confer risk (29). This is not the case, as is evident from studies of mouse models and human disease. For example, in murine lupus, independently segregating loci can act to inhibit or enhance the effects of other loci on disease susceptibility (70). Genetic susceptibility must be considered along with genetically protective alleles, which may exist elsewhere in the genome and interact in complex ways. This phenomenon is called *epistasis* and may present significant difficulties when trying to map complex traits (86). Along these lines, it has been argued that stratifying the population for MHC type may be required to detect the effects of certain susceptibility loci in autoimmune dis-

ease. One of the more intriguing examples is the effect of stratifying for IDDM patients who carry DR3/X. Strikingly, this genetic subgroup of patients has a much higher sex ratio (>1 to 2.1), and it is only in this group that significant linkage to Xp13-p11 can be detected (87). This suggests a role for a recessive X-linked susceptibility allele whose penetrance depends on DR3.

## CONCLUSIONS

Despite the rapid progress in genetic mapping technology, we are still in the very early stages of applying genetic principles to the dissection of genetically complex disorders such as autoimmunity. Future trends are likely to include the analysis of extremely large populations (thousands) of individuals (79), the development of very-high-throughput techniques using thousands of genetic markers (88), and the development of novel laboratory (89,90) and statistical approaches to detecting susceptibility genes that by themselves confer low but measurable risk. Although the study of genetics alone cannot solve the problem of autoimmunity, it is likely to spark the development of new hypotheses that can be tested and integrated into an overall scheme of disease mechanisms. To yield its potential, genetics should play an interactive role with other cellular and molecular approaches to understanding autoimmune pathogenesis.

## REFERENCES

1. Collins FS, Patrinos A, Jordan E, et al. New goals for the U.S. Human Genome Project: 1998–2003. *Science* 1998;282:682–689.
2. Nepom GT. Major histocompatibility complex-directed susceptibility to rheumatoid arthritis. *Adv Immunol* 1998;68:315–332.
3. Winchester R. The molecular basis of susceptibility to rheumatoid arthritis. *Adv Immunol* 1994;56:389–466.
4. Martin R. Genetics of multiple sclerosis—how could disease-associated HLA types contribute to pathogenesis? *J Neural Transm Suppl* 1997; 49:177–194.
5. Zamani M, Cassiman JJ. Reevaluation of the importance of polymorphic HLA class II alleles and amino acids in the susceptibility of individuals of different populations to type I diabetes. *Am J Med Genet* 1998;76:183–194.
6. She JX. Susceptibility to type I diabetes: HLA-DQ and DR revisited. *Immunol Today* 1996;17:323–329.
7. Reveille JD. The molecular genetics of systemic lupus erythematosus and Sjögren's syndrome. *Curr Opin Rheumatol* 1992;4:644–656.
8. Block SR, Winfield JB, Lockshin MD, et al. Studies of twins with systemic lupus erythematosus. *Am J Med* 1975;59:533–552.
9. Deapen D, Escalante A, Weinrib L, et al. A revised estimate of twin concordance in systemic lupus erythematosus. *Arthritis Rheum* 1992;35: 311–318.
10. Olmos P, Hern RA, Heaton DA, et al. The significance of the concordance rate for type I (insulin-dependent) diabetes in identical twins. *Diabetologia* 1988;31:747–750.
11. Ebers GC, Bulman DE, Sadovnick AD, et al. A population-based study of multiple sclerosis in twins. *N Engl J Med* 1986;315:1638–1642.
12. Aho K, Koskenvuo M, Tuominen J, et al. Occurrence of rheumatoid arthritis in a nationwide series of twins. *J Rheumatol* 1986;13:899–902.
13. Silman AJ, MacGregor AJ, Thomson W, et al. Twin concordance rates for rheumatoid arthritis: results from a nationwide study. *Br J Rheumatol* 1993;32:903–907.
14. Jarvinen P, Aho K. Twin studies in rheumatic diseases. *Semin Arthritis Rheum* 1994;24:19–28.
15. Conrad K, Mehlhorn J, Luthke K, et al. Systemic lupus erythematosus after heavy exposure to quartz dust in uranium mines: clinical and serological characteristics. *Lupus* 1996;5:62–69.

16. Symmons DP, Bankhead CR, Harrison BJ, et al. Blood transfusion, smoking, and obesity as risk factors for the development of rheumatoid arthritis: results from a primary care–based incident case-control study in Norfolk, England. *Arthritis Rheum* 1997;40:1955–1961.

17. Cooper GS, Dooley MA, Treadwell EL, et al. Hormonal, environmental, and infectious risk factors for developing systemic lupus erythematosus. *Arthritis Rheum* 1998;41:1714–1724.

18. Akerblom HK, Knip M. Putative environmental factors in type 1 diabetes. *Diabetes Metab Rev* 1998;14:31–67.

19. Gregersen PK. Discordance for autoimmunity in monozygotic twins. Are "identical" twins really identical? *Arthritis Rheum* 1993;36:1185–1192.

20. Monteiro J, Derom C, Vlietinck R, et al. Commitment to X inactivation precedes the twinning event in monochorionic MZ twins. *Am J Hum Genet* 1998;63:339–346.

21. Richards CS, Watkins SC, Hoffman EP, et al. Skewed X inactivation in a female MZ twin results in Duchenne muscular dystrophy. *Am J Hum Genet* 1990;46:672–681.

22. Hollander GA, Zuklys S, Morel C, et al. Monoallelic expression of the interleukin-2 locus. *Science* 1998;279:2118–2121.

23. Riviere I, Sunshine MJ, Littman DR. Regulation of IL-4 expression by activation of individual alleles. *Immunity* 1998;9:217–228.

24. Morison IM, Reeve AE. A catalogue of imprinted genes and parent-of-origin effects in humans and animals. *Hum Mol Genet* 1998;7:1599–1609.

25. Hall JG. Genomic imprinting: nature and clinical relevance. *Annu Rev Med* 1997;48:35–44.

26. Ohlsson R, Tycko B, Sapienza C. Monoallelic expression: "there can only be one." *Trends Genet* 1998;14:435–438.

27. Risch N. Linkage strategies for genetically complex traits. I. Multilocus models. *Am J Hum Genet* 1990;46:222–228.

28. Vyse TJ, Todd JA. Genetic analysis of autoimmune disease. *Cell* 1996;85:311–318.

29. Seldin MF, Amos CI, Ward R, et al. The genetics revolution and the assault on rheumatoid arthritis. *Arthritis Rheum* 1999;42:1071–1079.

30. Risch N. Assessing the role of HLA linked and unlinked determinants of disease. *Am J Hum Genet* 1987;40:1–14.

31. Hochberg MC. The application of genetic epidemiology to systemic lupus erythematosus. *J Rheumatol* 1987;14:867–869.

32. Brown MA, Kennedy LG, MacGregor AJ, et al. Susceptibility to ankylosing spondylitis in twins: the role of genes, HLA, and the environment. *Arthritis Rheum* 1997;40:1823–1828.

33. Van der Linden SM, Khan MA. The risk of ankylosing spondylitis in HLA-B27 positive individuals: a reappraisal. *J Rheumatol* 1984;11:727–728.

34. Gregersen PK, Silver J, Winchester RJ. The shared epitope hypothesis: an approach to understanding the molecular genetics of rheumatoid arthritis susceptibility. *Arthritis Rheum* 1987;30:1205–1213.

35. Arnett FC, Chakraborty R. Ankylosing spondylitis: the dissection of a complex genetic disease. *Arthritis Rheum* 1997;40:1746–1748.

36. Freimer NB, Service SK, Slatkin M. Expanding on population studies. *Nat Genet* 1997;17:371–373.

37. Laan M, Paabo S. Demographic history and linkage disequilibrium in human populations. *Nat Genet* 1997;17:435–438.

38. Falk CR, Rubinstein P. Haplotype relative risks: an easy reliable way to construct a proper control sample for risk calculations. *Ann Hum Genet* 1987;51:227–233.

39. Spielman RS, McGinnis RE, Ewens WJ. Transmission test for linkage disequilibrium: the insulin gene region and insulin-dependent diabetes mellitus (IDDM). *Am J Hum Genet* 1993;52:506–516.

40. Schaid DJ. Transmission disequilibrium, family controls, and great expectations. *Am J Hum Genet* 1998;63:935–941.

41. Mulcahy B, Waldron-Lynch F, McDermott MF, et al. Genetic variability in the tumor necrosis factor–lymphotoxin region influences susceptibility to rheumatoid arthritis. *Am J Hum Genet* 1996;59:676–683.

42. Genin E, Babron MC, McDermott MF, et al. Modelling the major histocompatibility complex susceptibility to RA using the MASC method. *Genet Epidemiol* 1998;15:419–430.

43. Jacob CO, Lewis GD, McDevitt HO. MHC class II–associated variation in the production of tumor necrosis factor in mice and humans: relevance to the pathogenesis of autoimmune diseases. *Immunol Res* 1991;10:156–168.

44. Wilson AG, Duff GW. Genetics of tumour necrosis factor in systemic lupus erythematosus. *Lupus* 1996;5:87–88.

45. Hajeer AH, Worthington J, Davies EJ, et al. TNF microsatellite a2, b3, and d2 alleles are associated with systemic lupus erythematosus. *Tissue Antigens* 1997;49[3 Pt 1]:222–227.

46. Chen CJ, Yen JH, Tsai WC, et al. The TNF2 allele does not contribute towards susceptibility to systemic lupus erythematosus. *Immunol Lett* 1997;55:1–3.

47. Sturfelt G, Hellmer G, Truedsson L. TNF microsatellites in systemic lupus erythematosus—a high frequency of the TNFabc 2-3-1 haplotype in multicase SLE families. *Lupus* 1996;5:618–622.

48. Rudwaleit M, Tikly M, Khamashta M, et al. Interethnic differences in the association of tumor necrosis factor promoter polymorphisms with systemic lupus erythematosus. *J Rheumatol* 1996;23:1725–1728.

49. Ott J. *Analysis of human genetic linkage.* Baltimore: Johns Hopkins University Press, 1992.

50. Pras E, Aksentijevich I, Gruberg L, et al. Mapping of a gene causing familial Mediterranean fever to the short arm of chromosome 16. *N Engl J Med* 1992;326:1509–1513.

51. The International FMF Consortium. Ancient missense mutations in a new member of the RoRet gene family are likely to cause familial Mediterranean fever. *Cell* 1997;90:797–807.

52. Rubin LA, Amos CI, Wade JA, et al. Investigation the genetic basis for ankylosing spondylitis: Linkage studies with the major histocompatibility complex region. *Arthritis Rheum* 1994;37:1212–1220.

53. Risch N. Linkage strategies for genetically complex traits. II. The power of affected relative pairs. *Am J Hum Genet* 1990;16:229–241.

54. Amos CI. Robust tests for linkage. In: *Current protocols in genetics. Supplement 8.* New York: John Wiley and Sons, 1995:1.8.1–1.8.32.

55. Todd JA. La carte des microsatellites est arrivee! *Hum Mol Genet* 1992;1:663–666.

56. Amos CI, Dawson DV, Elston RC. The probabilistic determination of identity-by-descent sharing for pairs of relatives from pedigrees. *Am J Hum Genet* 1990;47:842–853.

57. Mein CA, Esposito L, Dunn MG, et al. A search for type 1 diabetes susceptibility genes in families from the United Kingdom. *Nat Genet* 1998;19:297–300.

58. Concannon P, Gogolin-Ewens KJ, Hinds DA, et al. A second-generation screen of the human genome for susceptibility to insulin-dependent diabetes mellitus. *Nat Genet* 1998;19:292–296.

59. Ebers GC, Kukay K, Bulman DE, et al. A full genome search in multiple sclerosis. *Nat Genet* 1996;13:472–476.

60. Kuokkanen S, Gschwend M, Rioux JD, et al. Genomewide scan of multiple sclerosis in Finnish multiplex families. *Am J Hum Genet* 1997;61:1379–1387.

61. Chataway J, Feakes R, Coraddu F, et al. The genetics of multiple sclerosis: principles, background and updated results of the United Kingdom systematic genome screen. *Brain* 1998;121[1 Pt 10]:1869–1887.

62. Tsao BP, Cantor RM, Kalunian KC, et al. Evidence for linkage of a candidate chromosome 1 region to human systemic lupus erythematosus. *J Clin Invest* 1997;99:725–731.

63. Moser KL, Neas BR, Salmon JE, et al. Genome scan of human systemic lupus erythematosus: evidence for linkage on chromosome 1q in African-American pedigrees. *Proc Natl Acad Sci USA* 1998;95:14869–14874.

64. Gaffney PM, Kearns GM, Shark KB, et al. A genome-wide search for susceptibility genes in human systemic lupus erythematosus sib-pair families. *Proc Natl Acad Sci USA* 1998;95:14875–14879.

65. Shai R, Quismorio FP Jr, et al. Genome-wide screen for systemic lupus erythematosus susceptibility genes in multiplex families. *Hum Mol Genet* 1999;8:639–644.

66. Cornelis F, Faure S, Martinez M, et al. New susceptibility locus for rheumatoid arthritis suggested by a genome-wide linkage study. *Proc Natl Acad Sci USA* 1998;95:10746–10750.

67. Becker KG, Simon RM, Bailey-Wilson JE, et al. Clustering of nonmajor histocompatibility complex susceptibility candidate loci in human autoimmune diseases. *Proc Natl Acad Sci USA* 1998;95:9979–9984.

68. Bias WB, Reveille JD, Beaty TH, et al. Evidence that autoimmunity in man is a Mendelian dominant trait. *Am J Hum Genet* 1986;39:584–602.

69. Harley JB, Sheldon P, Neas B, et al. Systemic lupus erythematosus: considerations for a genetic approach. *J Invest Dermatol* 1994;103 [Suppl 5]:144S–149S.

70. Wakeland EK, Morel L, Mohan C, et al. Genetic dissection of lupus nephritis in murine models of SLE. *Clin Immunol* 1997;17:272–281.

71. Tsao BP, Cantor RM, Grossman JM, et al. ADPRT alleles from the chromosome 1q41-q42 linked region are associated with SLE. *Arthritis Rheum* 1998;41:S80(abst).

72. Kumari SR, Mendoza-Alvarez H, Alvarez-Gonzalez R. Functional interactions of p53 with poly(ADP-ribose) polymerase (PARP) during

apoptosis following DNA damage: covalent poly(ADP-ribosyl)ation of p53 by exogenous PARP and noncovalent binding of p53 to the M(r) 85,000 proteolytic fragment. *Cancer Res* 1998;58:5075–5078.

73. Vyse TJ, Kotzin BL. Genetic susceptibility to systemic lupus erythematosus. *Annu Rev Immunol* 1998;16:261–292.

74. Bell GI, Horita S, Karam JH. A polymorphic locus near the human insulin gene is associated with insulin-dependent diabetes mellitus. *Diabetes* 1984;33:176–183.

75. Bennett ST, Lucassen AM, Gough SC, et al. Susceptibility to human type 1 diabetes at IDDM2 is determined by tandem repeat variation at the insulin gene minisatellite locus. *Nat Genet* 1995;9:284–292.

76. Marron MP, Raffel LJ, Garchon HJ, et al. Insulin-dependent diabetes mellitus (IDDM) is associated with CTLA4 polymorphisms in multiple ethnic groups. *Hum Mol Genet* 1997;6:1275–1282.

77. Van der Auwera BJ, Vandewalle CL, Schuit FC, et al. CTLA-4 gene polymorphism confers susceptibility to insulin-dependent diabetes mellitus (IDDM) independently from age and from other genetic or immune disease markers: the Belgian Diabetes Registry. *Clin Exp Immunol* 1997;110:98–103.

78. Rigby AS, Voelm L, Silman AJ. Epistatic modeling in rheumatoid arthritis: an application of the Risch theory. *Genet Epidemiol* 1993;10:311–320.

79. Risch N, Merikangas K. The future of genetic studies of complex human diseases. *Science* 1996;273:1516–1517.

80. Cornelis F for the European Consortium on RA Families. New susceptibility locus on chromosome 1 for rheumatoid arthritis. *Arthritis Rheum* 1998;41:S242.

81. Weyand CM, Hicok KC, Conn DL, et al. The influence of HLA-DRB1 genes on disease severity in rheumatoid arthritis. *Ann Intern Med* 1992;117:801–806.

82. Criswell LA, Mu H, Such CL, King MC. Inheritance of the shared epitope and long-term outcomes of rheumatoid arthritis among community-based Caucasian females. *Genet Epidemiol* 1998;15:61–72.

83. Kawahito Y, Cannon GW, Gulko PS, et al. Localization of quantitative trait loci regulating adjuvant-induced arthritis in rats: evidence for genetic factors common to multiple autoimmune diseases. *J Immunol* 1998;161:4411–4419.

84. Hay EM, Ollier WE, Silman AJ. The Arthritis and Rheumatism Council's national family material repository. *Br J Rheumatol* 1993;32:443–444.

85. Gregersen PK. The North American Rheumatoid Arthritis Consortium—bringing genetic analysis to bear on disease susceptibility, severity, and outcome. *Arthritis Care Res* 1998;11:1–2.

86. Frankel WN, Schork NJ. Who's afraid of epistasis? *Nat Genet* 1996;14:371–373.

87. Cucca F, Goy JV, Kawaguchi Y, et al. A male-female bias in type 1 diabetes and linkage to chromosome Xp in MHC HLA-DR3–positive patients. *Nat Genet* 1998;19:301–302.

88. Service RF. DNA chips survey an entire genome. *Science* 1998;281:1122.

89. Barcellos LF, Klitz W, Field LL, et al. Association mapping of disease loci, by use of a pooled DNA genomic screen. *Am J Hum Genet* 1997;61:734–747.

90. Cheung VG, Gregg JP, Gogolin-Ewens KJ, et al. Linkage-disequilibrium mapping without genotyping. *Nat Genet* 1998;18:225–230.

*Textbook of the Autoimmune Diseases,*
Edited by R. G. Lahita, N. Chiorazzi, and W. H. Reeves,
Lippincott Williams & Wilkins, Philadelphia © 2000.

# CHAPTER 5

# Inflammation

Steven B. Abramson

Inflammation has been defined as the local reaction of tissue to injury. This may result in a complicated sequence of events that produces vasodilation, leakiness of the microvasculature with exudation of fluid and protein, and local infiltration of inflammatory cells. Inflammatory processes are critical to host defense against invading microorganisms and to wound healing in which the cellular constituents clear debris from injured sites and promote tissue repair. The phagocytic cells in particular are essential for the removal of foreign or dead particulate matter at sites of tissue injury. Inflammatory mediators released by phagocytes, such as degradative enzymes and the free radicals superoxide anion and nitric oxide, contribute to the capacity of these cells to degrade macromolecules within exudative effusions. However, the inflammatory response is a calculated risk for the host. When persistent, unregulated, and triggered in response to aberrant stimuli, it can lead to destruction of host tissue. Such is the case in many rheumatic syndromes, from crystal-induced arthropathies to autoimmune diseases, in which the normal host machinery is subverted, giving rise to local or widespread organ injury.

In addition to the infiltration and activation of leukocytes, inflammatory processes are characterized by the participation of soluble intercellular signaling molecules, including immunoglobulins, complement components, coagulation factors, cytokines, and chemokines. This chapter reviews some key elements that characterize the inflammatory response, several of which may serve as future targets for biologic or pharmacologic therapy of rheumatic diseases.

## ACUTE INFLAMMATION: THE RELEASE OF MEDIATORS FROM PHAGOCYTIC CELLS

### Chemotaxis and Phagocytosis

Neutrophils and monocyte/macrophages, are the body's "professional phagocytes." Activation of these cell may be

S. B. Abramson: Departments of Medicine and Pathology, New York University School of Medicine, New York, New York 10021; Department of Rheumatology, Hospital for Joint Diseases, New York, New York 10003.

triggered by the engagement of particles, such as invading microorganisms, or in response to soluble stimuli that engage specific cell-surface receptors. Soluble stimuli include bacterial chemoattractants, activated complement components (e.g., C5a), lipid mediators (e.g., leukotriene $B_4$), and chemokines (e.g., interleukin-8 [IL-8]). These mediators provoke directed migration (*chemotaxis*) and direct leukocytes out of the circulation and along a chemical gradient to the inflammatory site. Typically, such chemoattractants engage specific cell-surface receptors characterized by seven transmembrane spanning regions that are coupled to a GTP-binding protein signaling pathway (1).

After directed migration along a chemoattractant gradient, phagocytosis is initiated by the attachment or binding of target particles to the neutrophil surface. Attachment is followed by enclosure of the particle within a plasma membrane pouch. On closure, this pouch becomes a vacuole in the cytoplasm, called a phagosome. In most instances, soon after particle ingestion, primary or secondary lysosomes fuse with the phagosome, which are then called phagolysosomes. Fusion of the respective membranes permits entry of lysosomal contents into the phagosome and the shielded enzymatic degradation of ingested material, an important aspect of the scavenging function of neutrophils and macrophages. Phagocytosis can deliver a microbial prey to a sequestered compartment in which the noxious action of host cytotoxins (e.g., degradative enzymes) can be confined.

### Opsonization

Macrophages and neutrophils "recognize" certain serum-derived molecules when these molecules coat particles to be phagocytized. These molecules, antibodies or complement components (originally called opsonins from the Greek word for "to prepare food for") bind to bacteria, cells, or other surfaces and increase the efficiency of phagocytosis. The phagocytes recognize antibody- and complement-coated particles because they have surface receptors for immunoglobulin and for the C3 fragments C3b and iC3b. Using this strategy, phagocytes can consume a wide variety of different particles, because the stimulus to phagocytosis depends not on the characteristics of the organism but instead on recognition of the two major opsonins by specific cell-surface receptors.

Phagocytic cells express receptors for the complement fragment C3b (designated CR3) and its inactivated cleavage product iC3b (designated CD11b/CD18). CR1 and CD11b/CD18 play important roles in the clearance of particles, such as opsonized bacteria, to which C3b or iC3b are bound. This clearance mechanism is also essential for the removal of immune complexes that covalently bind C3b and iC3b (2). CD11b/CD18 is also the major neutrophil adhesion molecule responsible for neutrophil adherence to vascular endothelium and to other neutrophils. Intercellular adhesion molecule-1 (ICAM-1), expressed on resting and activated endothelial cells, is a ligand for the CD11b/CD18 and other CD18 integrins. Interaction between CD18 and ICAM-1, together with the ligation of selectin molecules with their carbohydrate counterreceptors, modulates the adhesion of neutrophils to vascular endothelium and their egress to the extravascular space (3). In diseases such as systemic lupus erythematosus (SLE), characterized by circulating immune complexes and complement activation, there is upregulation of endothelial cell adhesion molecules, indicating activation (4).

Neutrophils, monocytes/macrophages, platelets, B lymphocytes, and natural killer cells all express receptors for immune complexes. There are three types of receptors for multimeric IgG that bind these complexes through their Fc fragments: FcRI, FcII, and FcIII. FcγR polymorphisms affect phagocytic function and may therefore contribute to disease susceptibility factors in the development of autoimmunity (5,6).

## Degranulation

Phagocytic proteases are sequestered within lysosomal granules and generally do not pose a threat to the host. However, the extracellular release of granule contents may promote inflammation and damage at tissue sites. Degranulation may be provoked by soluble stimuli (e.g., C5a, IL-8, immune complexes). Degranulation is augmented when neutrophils encounter stimuli deposited on a surface; lysosomal release unfolds by a process of reverse endocytosis, which has been called "frustrated phagocytosis." This exuberant release of lysosomal enzymes from neutrophils may be relevant to the pathogenesis of tissue injury in diseases characterized by the deposition of immune complexes on cell surfaces or on extracellular surfaces such as vascular basement membranes or articular cartilage as in rheumatoid arthritis (7).

## Toxic Oxygen Radicals

When phagocytic leukocytes are activated, oxygen can be transformed into superoxide anion by a multiprotein complex assembled at the plasma membrane, designated the NADPH oxidase. This complex, which includes membrane-bound cytochrome $b_{558}$, two cytoplasmic proteins (GP67, GP47), and the low-molecular-weight GTP-binding protein, transfers an extra electron to molecular oxygen, generating a highly reactive and toxic free radical. Superoxide anion is a significant mediator of inflammation that causes tissue injury and irreversible modification of macromolecules (8).

Some of the toxic oxygen metabolites produced by neutrophils are generated by the myeloperoxidase–hydrogen peroxide–halide system. Myeloperoxidase is a highly cationic enzyme present in the azurophilic granules that catalyzes the reaction of hydrogen peroxide with a halide such as chloride to form hypohalous acids (e.g., hypochlorous acid). These products are capable of killing a variety of microorganisms and are cytotoxic to host cells (9).

## Macrophages as Secretory Cells in Inflammation

Although neutrophils and macrophage/monocytes are capable of chemotaxis, phagocytosis, and the release of toxic mediators, the macrophage/monocyte role in inflammation is more complex (8,10). These cells express the three major classes of Fc receptors and $\beta_1$, $\beta_2$, and $\beta_3$, integrins that facilitate phagocytosis of opsonized particles, intercellular adhesion, and adhesion to extracellular matrix proteins. Monocytes are recruited into tissues from the circulation in response to chemotactic factors (e.g., C5a, IL-8, transforming growth factor-β [TGF-β], fragments of collagen and fibronectin) produced at inflammatory sites. Recruitment requires the expression of adhesion molecules on activated vascular endothelium (e.g., intercellular adhesion molecule-1 [ICAM-1], vascular cell adhesion molecule-1 [VCAM-1]) that are recognized by counterligands of the circulating monocyte (e.g., lymphocyte function antigen-1 [LFA], very late activation (VLA) antigen-4 [VLA-4]). When monocytes emigrate into tissues they can be transformed into activated macrophages after exposure to cytokines such as interferon-γ, IL-1, and tumor necrosis factor (TNF). Macrophage activation results in an increase in cell size, increased synthesis of proteolytic enzymes, and the secretion of a variety of inflammatory products.

Macrophages secrete up to 100 substances, ranging from free radicals such as superoxide anion to large macromolecules such as fibronectin (8). Some products are secreted in response to inflammatory stimuli, and others are constitutively released. When stimulated by exposure to immune complexes, endotoxin, IL-1, or C3b-coated particles, macrophages and monocytes exhibit a procoagulant activity. The procoagulant products include tissue factor (identified as a receptor for factor VII), factor X activator, prothrombin activator, and vitamin K–dependent clotting factors II, VII, IX, and X. Monocytes in rheumatic disease patients display increased procoagulant activity that may contribute to fibrin deposition at sites of inflammation and has been implicated in the formation of crescent formation in glomerulonephritis.

### Cytokines

Macrophages secrete a variety of polypeptide hormones that regulate immune function, inflammation, and wound healing and repair. Macrophages, for example, produce three cytokines—IL-1α, IL-1β, and TNF-α—that have overlapping functions and are capable of inducing each others' release by macrophages themselves (8). Macrophages also produce the cytokine neutrophil-activating peptide-1/IL-8, which is a potent neutrophil chemoattractant. The production of IL-8, induced by IL-1α, IL-1β, and TNF-α, has been described in a variety of tissues, including alveolar macrophages, renal mesangial cells, and psoriatic skin lesions. IL-8 is a member of a family of macrophage inflammatory proteins (MIPs) or chemokines. In addition to IL-8, the superfamily of chemokines include macrophage (or monocyte) chemotactic protein-1 (MCP-1), MCP-2, MCP-3, RANTES ("regulated on activation, normally T-cell expressed and secreted"), MIP-1α, and MIP-1β, which act on monocytes but not neutrophils and have additional activities affecting basophil and eosinophil granulocytes and T lymphocytes (11).

### Products of Arachidonate

In addition to the capacity to secrete diverse biologically active proteins, monocytes and macrophages are significant sources of lipid mediators of inflammation that are derived from arachidonic acid. Arachidonic acid is metabolized through two distinct enzymatic pathways, the cyclooxygenase pathway and the lipoxygenase pathway, generating prostaglandins and leukotrienes, respectively.

Prostaglandin G/H synthase, or cyclooxygenase, is the initial enzyme in the prostaglandin pathway and is the target enzyme for inactivation by nonsteroidal antiinflammatory drugs (12). There are two isoforms of this enzyme that, although products of two distinct genes, are highly homologous. The gene for COX-1 is constituitively expressed in most cells. Expression of the gene for COX-2 is induced by a variety of cytokines and growth factors and is inhibited by dexamethasone. COX-2 has also been identified at noninflammatory sites, including the renal medulla, osteoblasts, ovary, and the central nervous system. Arachidonic acid is also metabolized by the lipoxygenase pathway of enzyme activation that generates such mediators of acute inflammation as leukotriene $B_4$; the sulfidopeptide leukotrienes $LTC_4$, $D_4$, and $E_4$; and the lipoxins $LXA_4$ and $LXB_4$ (13).

### Nitric Oxide

Macrophages are also among the cellular sources of reactive nitrogen intermediates such as nitric oxide. Nitric oxide, although originally identified as a product of endothelial cells that accounts for "endothelium-derived relaxation factor" activity, is a highly reactive molecule with diverse biologic functions. The exposure of macrophages to cytokines (e.g.,

IL-1β, interferon-γ) markedly increases nitric oxide production. Activities of nitric oxide that may be important in the inflammatory response include vasodilation and its capacity to react with superoxide anion to form toxic peroxynitrite compounds. The inhibition of nitric oxide synthesis can reduce the severity of disease in streptococcal cell wall induced arthritis in Lewis rats (14). The production of nitric oxide by synovial macrophages and articular chondrocytes has been demonstrated in human rheumatoid arthritis and osteoarthritis (15–17).

### Platelets as Inflammatory Cells

Platelets, which are derived from marrow megakaryocytes, are involved in hemostasis, wound healing, and cellular responses to injury. The platelet may also act as an inflammatory cell; for example, platelets chemotax to a variety of stimuli, including platelet-activating factor (PAF) and collagen fragments; endocytose immune complexes through Fc receptors; release inflammatory mediators on activation and aggregation; are activated by phlogistic agents (e.g., complement activation products), play a role in animal models of inflammatory disease; and have been identified in localization and activation at tissue injury sites in human inflammatory diseases. There is evidence for platelet activation in immunologically mediated diseases such as asthma, cold urticaria, scleroderma, and SLE (18).

## ACTIVATION OF THE COMPLEMENT SYSTEM

Inflammatory disease of blood vessels and tissues in rheumatic diseases often involves complement activation in the presence or absence of immune complex deposition. Complement cleavage products, particularly C3a, C5a, and C5b-9, are key mediators in the promotion of local tissue injury. The complement system is composed of at least 20 plasma proteins that participate in a variety of host defense and immunologic reactions. Each complement component is cleaved by means of a limited proteolytic reaction that proceeds by means of the classical or alternative pathway.

The alternative pathway is more primitive and may be activated by contact with a variety of substances, including polysaccharides (e.g., endotoxin) found in the cell walls of microorganisms. Activation of the classical pathway by immune complexes requires binding of the first complement component, C1, to sites on the Fc portions of immunoglobulins, particularly of the IgG1, IgG3, and IgM isotypes.

### Activation of C3

Activation of the third component of complement is central to the classical and alternative pathways. C3 is cleaved by convertases to two active products, C3a and C3b. C3a, released into the fluid phase, provokes the release of histamine from mast cells and basophils, causes smooth muscle contraction, and induces platelet aggregation. C3b has two functions; C3b is part of the C5 convertase, which continues the complement cascade, and C3b is also the major opsonin of the complement system. It binds to immune complexes and to a variety of activators such as microbial organisms. The binding of C3b to these particles facilitates the attachment of the particle to the C3b receptor on cells, complement receptor 1 (CR1), which is present on erythrocytes, neutrophils, monocytes, B lymphocytes, and glomerular podocytes. CR1 on phagocytes potentiates phagocytosis. CR1 on erythrocytes, which accounts for approximately 90% of CR1 in blood, facilitates the clearance of immune complexes from the circulation by transporting erythrocyte-bound complexes to the liver and spleen for removal. A new biologic role for C3a and C3a desArg has been described in the regulation of TNF-$\alpha$ and IL-1$\beta$ synthesis in nonadherent peripheral blood mononuclear cells (PBMCs) (19). C3a and C3a desArg suppressed endotoxin-induced synthesis of TNF-$\alpha$ and IL-1$\beta$. In contrast, in adherent PBMCs, C3a and C3a desArg enhanced endotoxin-induced production of these cytokines. C3a and C3a desArg may enhance cytokine synthesis by adherent monocytes at local inflammatory sites, while inhibiting the systemic synthesis of proinflammatory cytokines by circulating cells.

### Activation of C5

In addition to its role as an opsonin, C3b also forms part of the C5 convertase, which leads to the generation of C5a and C5b. C5a, like C3a, is an anaphylatoxin, capable of activating basophils and mast cells. C5a is also among the most potent biologic chemoattractants for neutrophils (discussed later). C5b, which attaches to the surface of cells and microorganisms, is the first component in the assembly of the membrane attack complex (MAC), or C5b-9.

### Membrane Attack Complex

The MAC, or the terminal complement assembly of C5b-9, has long been known to lyse bacteria. However, assembly of MAC on homologous leukocytes is not a cytotoxic event. After insertion of MAC into a leukocyte membrane, the cell sheds a small membrane-bound vesicle containing the MAC complex. What is less appreciated is that insertion of MAC into the cell membrane triggers cell activation before it is shed (20,21). MAC acts as an ionophore, provoking increases in cytosolic calcium and consequently triggering cell functions (22). These include generation of toxic oxygen products and activation of the cyclooxygenase (e.g., platelets, monocyte/macrophages, synoviocytes) and the lipoxygenase pathway of arachidonate metabolism. The deposition of MAC increases the surface expression of P-selectin on the endothelial cell surface, promoting adhesion to circulating neutrophils (23). *In vivo* evidence that vascular endothelium represents a site of C5b-9 deposition has been demonstrated in immune vasculitis (24–26) and infarcted myocardium (27). Mechanisms by which C5b-9 activates vascular endothelium

and promotes upregulation of surface adhesion molecules is discussed in the following section.

## COMPLEMENT, LEUKOCYTES, AND ACTIVATED ENDOTHELIUM

Autoimmune vasculitis commonly is caused by the local deposition of immune complexes in blood vessel walls, which results in complement activation and the generation of anaphylatoxins (e.g., C4a, C3a, C5a) and chemotaxins (C5a) (28,29). The resulting infiltration of vessel walls by polymorphonuclear leukocytes leads histologically to leukocytoclastic vasculitis and the release of lysosomal enzymes and oxygen radicals to tissue injury (30–32). One study suggests that the inflammatory response to immune complexes also requires cell-bound Fc receptors with subsequent amplification by cellular mediators and complement (33).

Some patients with SLE have small vessel disease and inflammatory vasculopathy in the absence of local immune complex deposition, particularly patients with central nervous system involvement (34–36). Several lines of investigation suggest another mechanism for this complement-mediated vascular injury in SLE, one not dependent on immune complex deposition (37–42). Immune reactants, including complement component and cytokines such as IL-1$\beta$ and TNF-$\alpha$, stimulate upregulation on the endothelial cell surface of ICAM-1 and E-selectin, which are the counter-receptors for the neutrophil adhesion molecule CD11b/CD18 and sialyl Lewis$^X$, respectively (43). In SLE, during periods of disease flare, circulating neutrophils are activated to increase their adhesiveness to vascular endothelium, as indicated by upregulation of the surface $\beta_2$ integrin CD11b/CD18 (44,45). The surface expression of three distinct endothelial cell adhesion molecules (E-selectin, VCAM-1, and ICAM-1) is also upregulated in patients with SLE (36). Endothelial cell activation was most marked in patients with disease exacerbations characterized by significant elevations of plasma C3a desArg, and the activation reversed with improvement in disease activity (36). In these studies, endothelial cell adhesion molecule upregulation was observed in otherwise histologically normal skin and was notable for the absence of local immune complex deposition (36). These data suggest that excessive complement activation in association with primed endothelial cells can induce neutrophil–endothelial cell adhesion and predispose to leukocyte-induced inflammatory vasculopathy during SLE disease flares.

### REFERENCES

1. Snyderman R, Uhing RJ. Chemoattractant stimulus-response coupling. In: Goldtsein IM, Snyderman R, eds. *Inflammation: basic principles and clinical correlates.* New York: Raven Press, 1992:421–439.
2. Schifferli JA, Ng YC, Peters DK. The role of complement and its receptor in the elimination of immune complexes. *N Engl J Med* 1986;315:488–495.
3. Lawrence MB, Springer TA. Leukocytes role on a selection of physiologic flow rates: distinction from and prerequisite for adhesion through integrins. *Cell* 1991;65:859–873.

4. Belmont HM, Abramson SB, Lie JT. Pathology and pathogenesis of vascular injury in systemic lupus erythematosus: interactions of inflammatory cells and activated endothelium. *Arthritis Rheum* 1996;39:9–22.

5. Salmon JE, Edberg JC, Brogle NL, Kimberly RP. Allelic polymorphisms of human Fc receptor IIA and Fcγ receptor IIIB: Independent mechanisms for differences in human phagocyte function. *J Clin Invest* 1992;89:1274–1281.

6. Van de Winkel J, Capel P. Human IgG Fc receptor heterogeneity: molecular aspects, clinical implications. *Immunol Today* 1993;14:215–221.

7. Pillinger MH, Abramson SB. The neutrophil in rheumatoid arthritis. *Rheum Dis Clin North Am* 1995;21:691–714.

8. Nathan CF. Secretory products of macrophages. *J Clin Invest* 1987;79: 319–326.

9. Johnson RJ, Lovett D, Lehrer RI, et al. Role of oxidants and proteases in glomerular injury. *Kidney Int* 1994;45:352–359.

10. Nikolic-Paterson DJ, Lan HY, Hill PA, Atkins RC. Macrophages in renal injury. *Kidney Int* 1994;45:S79–S82.

11. Schall TJ, Bacon KB. Chemokines, leukocyte trafficking and inflammation. *Curr Opin Immunol* 1994;6:865–873.

12. Baird NR, Morrison AR. Amplification of the arachidonic acid cascade: implications for pharmacologic intervention. *Am J Kidney Dis* 1993;21: 557–564.

13. Hamberg M, Samuelsson B. Prostaglandin endoperoxides: novel transformations of arachidonic acid in human platelets. *Proc Natl Acad Sci USA* 1974;71:3400–3404.

14. McCartney-Francis N, Allen JB, Mizel DE, et al. Suppression of arthritis by an inhibitor of nitric oxide synthase. *J Exp Med* 1993;178: 749–754.

15. Amin AR, Di Cesare PE, Vyas P, et al. The expression and regulation of nitric oxide synthase in human osteoarthritis-affected chondrocytes: evidence for up-regulated neuronal nitric oxide synthase. *J Exp Med* 1995;182:2097–2102.

16. Sakurai H, Kohsaka H, Liu M-F, et al. Nitric oxide production and inducible nitric oxide synthase expression in inflammatory arthritides. *J Clin Invest* 1996;96:2357–2363.

17. Clancy RM, Abramson SB. Nitric oxide: a novel mediator of inflammation. *Soc Exp Biol Med* 1995;210:93–101.

18. Ginsberg MH. Role of platelets in inflammation and rheumatic disease. *Adv Inflamm Res* 1986;2:53–71.

19. Takabayashi T, Vannier E, Clark BD, et al. A new biologic role for C3a and C3a desArg: regulation of TNF-alpha and IL-1 beta synthesis. *J Immunol* 1996;156:3455–3460.

20. Stein JM, Luzio JP. Membrane sorting during vesicle shedding from neutrophils during sublytic complement attack. *Biochem Soc Trans* 1989;16:1082–1083.

21. Morgan BP, Dankert JR, Esser AF. Recovery of human neutrophils from complement attack: removal of the membrane attack complex by endocytosis and exocytosis. *J Immunol* 1987;138:246–253.

22. Morgan BP. Complement membrane attack on nucleated cells: resistance, recovery and non-lethal effects. *Biochem J* 1989;264:1–14.

23. Hattori R, Hamilton KK, McEver RP, et al. Complement proteins C5b-9 induce secretion of high molecular weight multimers of endothelial von Willebrand factor and translocation of granule membrane. *J Biol Chem* 1989;264:9053–9060.

24. Biesecker G, Katz S, Koffler D. Renal localization of the membrane attack complex in systemic lupus erythematosus nephritis. *J Exp Med* 1981;154:1779–1794.

25. Biesecker G, Lavin L, Zisking M, et al. Cutaneous localization of the membrane attack complex in discoid and systemic lupus erythematosus. *N Engl J Med* 1982;306:264–270.

26. Kissel JT, Mendell JR, Rammohan KW. Microvascular deposition of complement membrane attack complex in dermatomyositis. *N Engl J Med* 1986;314:329–334.

27. Schafer H, Mathey D, Hugo F, et al. Deposition of the terminal C5b-9 complement complex in infarcted areas of human myocardium. *J Immunol* 1986;137:1945–1949.

28. Ishizaka K. Gamma globulin and molecular mechanisms in hypersensitivity reations. In: Kallos P, Waksman BH, eds. *Progress in allergy,* vol VII. New York: Karger, 1963;32–106.

29. Frank MM, Ellman L, Green I, et al. Site of deposition of C3 in arthus reactions of C4-deficient guinea pigs. *J Immunol* 1973;110:1447–1451.

30. Koeffler P, Schur P, Kunkel H. Immunological studies concerning the nephritis of systemic lupus erythematosus. *J Exp Med* 1967;126: 607–624.

31. Fauci TY, Haynes BF, Katz P. The spectrum of vasculitis. *Ann Intern Med* 1978;89:660–676.

32. Arthus M. Injections repetees de serum de cheval chez la lapin. *Soc Biol* 1903.

33. Sylvestre DL, Ravetch JV. Fc receptors initiate the Arthus reaction: redefining the inflammatory cascade. *Science* 1994;265:1095–1098.

34. Belmont HM, Hopkins P, Edelson HS, et al. Complement Activation during systemic lupus erythematosus: C3a and C5a anaphylatoxins circulate during exacerbations of disease. *Arthritis Rheum* 1986;29: 1085–1089.

35. Hopkins P, Belmont M, Buyon J, et al. Increased plasma anaphylotoxins in systemic lupus erythematosus predict flares of the disease and may elicit the adult cerebral distress syndrome. *Arthritis Rheum* 1988;31: 632–641.

36. Belmont HM, Buyon J, Giorno R, Abramson SB. Upregulation of endothelial cell adhesion molecules characterizes disease activity in systemic lupus erythematosus: the Shwartzman phenomenon revisited. *Arthritis Rheum* 1994;37:376–383.

37. Jacob HS, Craddock PR, Hammerschmidt DE, Moldow CF. Complement-induced granulocyte aggregation: an unsuspected mechanism of disease. *N Engl J Med* 1980;302:789–794.

38. Hammerschmidt DE, Weaver LJ, Hudson LD, et al. Association of complement activation and elevated plasma C5a with adult respiratory distress syndrome. *Lancet* 1980;1:947–949.

39. Hakim R, Breillatt J, Lazarus M, et al. Complement activation and hypersensitivity reactions to hemodialysis membranes. *N Engl J Med* 1984;311:878–882.

40. Craddock P, Fehr J, Dalmasso A, et al. Hemodialysis leukopenia. *J Clin Invest* 1977;59:879–888.

41. Chenoweth DE, Cooper SW, Hugli TE, et al. Complement activation during cardiopulmonary bypass. *N Engl J Med* 1981;304:497–505.

42. Perez HD, Horn JK, Ong R, Goldstein I. Complement (C5)–derived chemotactic activity in serum from patients with pancreatitis. *J Lab Clin Med* 1983;101:123–129.

43. Pober JS, Gimbrone M, Lapierre D, et al. Overlapping patterns of activation of human endothelial cells by interleukin-1, tumor necrosis factor and immune interferon. *J Immunol* 1986;137:1893–1896.

44. Buyon JP, Shadick N, Berkman R, et al. Surface expression of gp165/95, the complement receptor CR3, as a marker of disease activity in systemic lupus erythematosus. *Clin Immunol Immunopathol* 1988;46:141–149.

45. Philips MR, Abramson SB, Weissmann G. Neutrophil adhesion and autoimmune vascular injury. *Clin Aspects Autoimmun* 1989;3:6–15.

*Textbook of the Autoimmune Diseases,*
Edited by R. G. Lahita, N. Chiorazzi, and W. H. Reeves,
Lippincott Williams & Wilkins, Philadelphia © 2000.

# CHAPTER 6

# Cell Adhesion

Anna Huttenlocher

Chronic inflammatory disorders such as rheumatoid arthritis, diabetes, and multiple sclerosis are characterized by the presence of leukocytes and other inflammatory cells within the affected tissues. At sites of inflammation, leukocyte recruitment and function requires adhesive interactions between cells and between cells and the extracellular matrix (ECM). These interactions are mediated by cell-surface adhesion receptors, including integrins, selectins, and members of the immunoglobulin superfamily. Cell-surface adhesion receptors play a critical role during inflammation by mediating leukocyte extravasation and recruitment and by participating in the adhesive and signaling pathways required for effective leukocyte activation and cytotoxic cell functions. During the past decade, considerable progress in defining the roles of cell-surface adhesion receptors during inflammation has enabled development of therapeutic agents designed to block the recruitment and activity of leukocytes during inflammation, with potential application to a wide variety of inflammatory disorders. However, more needs to be learned about adhesion receptor function in normal and pathologic conditions to allow development of effective and specific cell adhesion–targeted therapies for autoimmune disorders. This chapter reviews the advances that have been made in understanding cell adhesion receptor function, with an emphasis on autoimmune disorders.

Given the complexity of cell adhesive interactions, it is not surprising that they are mediated by a diverse set of cellular receptors. Specific cell adhesion involves interaction between cell-surface adhesion receptors (many are glycoproteins) and their ligands. Three major families of cell-surface adhesion receptors participate in inflammatory processes: integrins, immunoglobulin-like proteins (i.e., immunoglobulin superfamily), and selectins (Fig. 6.1). Other cell-surface receptors that may potentially participate during inflammation are briefly discussed, including members of the cadherin, proteoglycan, a disintegrin and metalloprotease (ADAM) fami-

lies. These receptor families together are capable of mediating many different types of attachments, including stable, firm adhesions and transient, weak attachments. These attachments may be between cells of similar type (i.e., homophilic), between different types (i.e., heterophilic), or between cells and the ECM (Table 6.1). Members of the selectin family, for example, mediate transient heterophilic cell-cell adhesion and participate in the rolling and tethering of leukocytes along the endothelial surface. Members of the cadherin family promote stable homophilic cell-cell adhesion in highly structured tissues such as skin and muscle. Integrins are capable of participating in stable and transient adhesions in diverse processes, including leukocyte extravasation and activation.

In addition to their well-established role as adhesive molecules, cell-surface adhesion receptors function as receptors for cellular signaling, similar to growth factor and cytokine receptors (1). Adhesion receptors transmit signals from the extracellular environment, which are integrated with other cellular signals to coordinate many aspects of cell behavior, including the decision to proliferate, undergo apoptosis, migrate, or differentiate (2–7). By functioning as adhesive and signaling receptors, cell adhesion receptors play a central role in regulating leukocyte functions in normal and pathologic conditions. Examples of how cell-surface adhesion receptors may participate during inflammation include leukocyte recruitment to inflammatory sites, leukocyte proliferation and activation, leukocyte survival, antigen presentation, phagocytosis, cytotoxic T-cell functions, and regulation of gene expression (e.g., matrix metalloproteinases).

Cell adhesion receptor function is understandably highly regulated and dynamic. Cytokines, chemokines, and growth factors play a central role in regulating the function of cell-surface adhesion receptors. Mechanisms of regulation include changes in cell-surface expression, receptor affinity, receptor avidity (i.e., clustering), or changes in the association of the cytoplasmic domains of adhesion receptors with specific regulatory and signaling molecules. The process of inside-out signaling plays an important role in regulating the function of some cell adhesion receptors, including integrins

A. Huttenlocher: Departments of Pediatrics and Pharmacology, University of Wisconsin, Madison, Wisconsin 53706; Department of Pediatrics, University of Wisconsin, Madison, Wisconsin 53792.

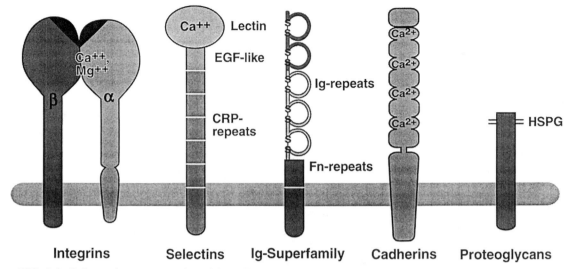

**FIG. 6.1.** Schematic representation of the different families of cell-surface adhesion receptors. (Adapted from Horwitz AF, Hunter T. Cell adhesion: integrating circuitry. *Trends Cell Biol* 1996;6:460–461.)

(8). Inside-out signaling involves an alteration in cell adhesion receptor function on the outside of the cell (i.e., receptor affinity or avidity) by changes from within the cell. Modulation of integrin affinity or avidity provides a rapid mechanism to regulate cell adhesion and is a particularly important mechanism for turning leukocyte adhesion on and off during processes such as leukocyte extravasation. Explanation of the mechanisms that regulate cell adhesion receptor function can contribute to our understanding of the pathogenesis of autoimmune diseases and the development of new treatment approaches.

## INTEGRINS

The integrins are a family of cell adhesion receptors involved in adhesive interactions between cells and between cells and the ECM. Integrins are $\alpha\beta$ transmembrane glycoproteins that

**TABLE 6.1.** *Receptor-mediated attachments*

| Adhesion receptor | Ligand | Type |
|---|---|---|
| Integrins | Matrix components | Stable and transient |
| | IgSF | Calcium dependent |
| | Cadherin | |
| Cadherin | Cadherin | Stable |
| | Integrin | Calcium dependent |
| IgSF | Integrin | Transient |
| | IgSF | Calcium independent |
| Selectins | Mucins | Transient |
| | Sialyl lewis$^x$ | Calcium dependent |
| Proteoglycans | ECM components | Stable and transient |
| | Cell surface receptors | Calcium independent |
| | Growth factors | |

IgSF, immunoglobulin superfamily; ECM, extracellular matrix.

bind to the ECM and to members of the immunoglobulin superfamily. Integrins are in many ways the most diverse and versatile of the cell-surface adhesion receptor families, with different members displaying various ligand specificities and functions. Integrins function as structural receptors, linking the ECM to the actin cytoskeleton, and as signal transduction receptors capable of regulating specific cellular processes (1). Integrins participate in normal and pathologic inflammatory responses by performing an adhesive function (e.g., leukocyte–endothelial cell adhesion) and by participating in signal transduction pathways that modulate T-cell activation and gene expression. The importance of integrins to normal cellular functions is demonstrated by studies using transgenic mice in which disruption of integrin expression (e.g., $\alpha_5$, $\beta_1$) is not compatible with normal embryonic development (1). Inherited deficiency of the $\beta_2$ integrin in leukocyte adhesion deficiency (LAD) points to the importance of $\beta_2$ integrin expression for normal immune function (9,10). Patients with LAD present with severe, recurrent bacterial infections because of failure of their leukocytes to adhere to the endothelium and extravasate into areas of inflammation. This section presents the advances made in characterizing the structure and function of integrins and their implications for the pathogenesis of autoimmune diseases.

### Integrin Structure

Integrins are transmembrane glycoproteins that contain two noncovalently linked subunits, an $\alpha$ and $\beta$ chain (1). The $\alpha$ chains are approximately 120 to 180 kd, and $\beta$ chains are 90 to 110 kd. Integrins bind to multiple ligands, including ECM proteins, proteins on the surface of cells, and activated complement components. The integrin family contains approximately 16 $\alpha$ and 8 $\beta$ chains, and the subunits combine to form receptors (more than 20 total) with different ligand specificities and functions (Table 6.2). Integrins are separated into dif-

**TABLE 6.2.** *Integrin family and ligands*

| Integrin heterodimer | Ligand |
|---|---|
| $\alpha_1\beta_1$ | COL I, COL IV, LM |
| $\alpha_2\beta_1$ | COL I (DGEA), COL IV, LM |
| $\alpha_3\beta_1$ | COL I, FN, LM-1, LM-5 |
| $\alpha_4\beta_1$ | CS-1 FN (EILDV), VCAM-1 |
| $\alpha_5\beta_1$ | FN (RGD) |
| $\alpha_6\beta_1$ | LM |
| $\alpha_7\beta_1$ | LM, FN |
| $\alpha_8\beta_1$ | TN |
| $\alpha_9\beta_1$ | ? |
| $\alpha_v\beta_1$ | FN (RGD), VN (RGD) |
| $\alpha_L\beta_2$ | ICAM-1, ICAM-2, ICAM-3 |
| $\alpha_M\beta_2$ | ICAM-1, factor X, FBG, C3bi |
| $\alpha_X\beta_2$ | FBG (GPRP), C3bi |
| $\alpha_d\beta_2$ | ICAM-3 |
| $\alpha_{IIb}\beta_3$ | FBG (RGD, KQAGDV), FN, TSP, vWF |
| $\alpha_v\beta_3$ | VN (RGD), FN (RGD), FBG, TSP, vWF |
| $\alpha_6\beta_4$ | LM |
| $\alpha_v\beta_5$ | FN, VN |
| $\alpha_v\beta_6$ | FN |
| $\alpha_4\beta_7$ | CS-1 FN (EILDV), VCAM-1 |
| $\alpha_E\beta_7$ | Cadherin |
| $\alpha_v\beta_8$ | TN |

COL, collagen; CS-1, domain of fibronectin; ECM, extracellular matrix; FBG, fibrinogen; FN, fibronectin; ICAM, intercellular adhesion molecule; LFA, lymphocyte function antigen; LM, laminin; MAdCAM-1, mucosal addressin cell adhesion molecule-1; TN, ; TSP, thrombospondin; VCAM, vascular cell adhesion molecule; VLA, very late activation antigen; VN, vitronectin.

ferent subfamilies, with the $\beta$ chain determining the specific subfamily. Some of the $\alpha$ chains form specific associations with a given $\beta$ chain ($\alpha_{IIb}$), and other $\alpha$ subunits interact with multiple $\beta$ chains ($\alpha_v$, $\alpha_6$, $\alpha_3$, $\alpha_4$). The ligand-binding functions of different integrins are also highly variable. Some integrins, such as $\alpha_5\beta_1$ integrin, bind only one ligand (FN-RGD in this case), but others, such as $\alpha_v\beta_3$ integrin or $\beta_2$ integrin, are promiscuous and able to recognize many different ligands. This versatility in the integrin family allows for remarkable specificity and diversity in its functions.

Integrins contain a large extracellular amino-terminal domain, a transmembrane domain, and a short cytoplasmic carboxyl-terminal domain (Fig. 6.1). The association of the $\alpha$ and $\beta$ subunits is required for ligand-binding function and for the expression of the subunits on the cell surface. The extracellular domain of the $\alpha$ subunit contains seven homologous 60–amino acid domains, three or four of which contain EF-hand–like calcium-binding motifs that participate in ligand binding. Certain integrins, including $\alpha_M$, $\alpha_L$, $\alpha_1$, and $\alpha_2$ integrin subunits, have an inserted 20–amino acid "intervening domain" referred to as an I domain (11). The I domains of $\alpha_L$ and $\alpha_M$ bind to divalent cations and may serve as ligand binding sites in these integrins (12). The I domains of $\alpha$L and $\alpha_M$ were crystallized in the presence of divalent cation and were found to contain six $\beta$ strands surrounded by seven $\alpha$ helices (13). At the surface of the I domain, there is a metal

coordination site that is involved in metal-dependent ligand binding, referred to as the MIDAS motif (i.e., metal ion-dependent adhesion site). The $\alpha$ subunit cytoplasmic domain is short (20 to 50 amino acids) and contains a membrane-proximal conserved sequence, GFFKR (14). The extracellular domain of the $\beta$ subunit also contains an amino-terminal A-like domain with a MIDAS motif (13). This region is likely to be involved in ligand binding and in stabilizing the noncovalent association between the $\alpha$ and $\beta$ chains. Studies suggest that the extracellular domain of the $\beta$ subunit is primarily responsible for ligand recognition of RGD/LDV motifs, although the $\alpha$ extracellular domain participates in the recognition of other ligands (15). The C-terminal region of the extracellular domain contains a cysteine-rich region with intrachain disulfide bonding. The $\beta$ subunit, like the $\alpha$ subunit, spans the membrane once and usually contains a short cytoplasmic domain (40 to 60 amino acids) (14).

**Leukocyte Integrins**

Many different members of the integrin family are expressed on the surface of leukocytes (16) (Table 6.3). The $\beta_2$ integrins are only found on leukocytes and are commonly referred to by their cluster of differentiation (CD) nomenclature, CD11a,b,c,d/CD18 (17,18). These integrins are also referred to as lymphocyte function-associated antigen-1 (LFA-1, also called CD11a/CD18 or $\alpha_L\beta_2$) (19,20); Mac-1 (CD11b/CD18 or $\alpha_{M9}\beta_2$) (21,22), and GP150/95 (CD11c/CD18) (23). The ligands for the $\beta_2$ integrin receptors are primarily coreceptors on the surface of other cells, including members of the immunoglobulin family, cell adhesion molecules (ICAMs) and vascular cell adhesion molecules (VCAMs). ECM proteins may also be recognized by the $\beta_2$ integrins, particularly by the very promiscuous $\alpha_M\beta_2$. The $\alpha_M\beta_2$ integrin recognizes cell-surface ligands (e.g., ICAMs) and many extracellular proteins, including fibrinogen, clotting factors, and complement components (18). The $\beta_2$ integrins participate in a wide variety of leukocyte functions, including cell migration and extravasation, phagocytosis, targeted cell killing, and T-cell activation.

Other subfamilies that are expressed on the surface of leukocytes include $\beta_1$, $\beta_3$, and $\beta_7$ integrins (Table 6.3). The $\beta_1$ integrins are expressed on the surface of many leukocytes, and their expression patterns are developmentally regulated. Although several of the $\beta_1$ integrins ($\alpha_4\beta_1$, $\alpha_5\beta_1$, and $\alpha_6\beta_1$) are expressed on the surface of resting and activated lymphocytes, other $\beta_1$ integrins ($\alpha_1\beta_1$, $\alpha_2\beta_1$, and $\alpha_3\beta_1$4) appear to be specifically expressed on the surface of activated lymphocytes (24). One of the $\beta_1$ integrins, $\alpha_4\beta_1$ integrin, plays a role in leukocyte extravasation and provides a costimulatory signal for T-cell activation by binding to fibronectin or the immunoglobulin superfamily member VCAM-1. By binding VCAM-1, $\alpha_4\beta_1$ integrin mediates leukocyte rolling and the subsequent integrin-mediated firm adhesion to the endothelial surface during leukocyte extravasation (25,26). The $\alpha_v\beta_3$

**TABLE 6.3.** *Leukocyte integrins*

| Integrin | Ligand | Distribution | Functions |
|---|---|---|---|
| $\alpha_1\beta_1$ (VLA-1) | LN, COL | Activated T/B cells | Cell-ECM adhesion |
| $\alpha_2\beta_1$ (VLA-2) | LN, COL | Activated T cells, B cells | Cell-ECM adhesion |
| $\alpha_3\beta_1$ (VLA-3) | LN, COL, FN | Activated T cells, thymocytes | Cell-ECM adhesion |
| $\alpha_4\beta_1$ (VLA-4) | VCAM-1 | Lymphocytes, monocytes | Cell-ECM adhesion |
|  | FN (CS-1) | Eosinophils | T-cell homing |
| $\alpha_5\beta_1$ (VLA-5) | FN (RGD) | Lymphocytes, monocytes, thymocytes, neutrophils | Cell-ECM adhesion |
| $\alpha_6\beta_1$ (VLA-6) | LN | Leukocytes, thymocytes | Cell-ECM adhesion |
| $\alpha_L\beta_2$ (LFA-1) | ICAM-1, 2, 3 | Leukocytes, thymocytes | Leukocyte-ECM adhesion; T cell–APC adhesion |
| $\alpha_M\beta_2$ (Mac-1) | ICAM-1 | Myeloid cells | Cell-ECM adhesion |
|  | iC3b, FBG, factor X | Activated B cells | Leukocyte-ECM adhesion, phagocytosis |
| $\alpha_X\beta_2$ (p150,95) | FBG, iC3b | Myeloid cells, activated B cells, dendritic cells | Cell-ECM adhesion |
|  |  |  | Leukocyte-ECM adhesion, phagocytosis |
| $\alpha_d\beta_2$ | ICAM-3 | Myeloid cells, lymphocytes | Leukocyte adhesion |
| $\alpha_v\beta_3$ | VN, FBG, FN, vWF | Monocytes, neutrophils | Cell-ECM adhesion |
| $\alpha_4\beta_7$ | FN | Lymphocytes | Lymphocyte homing to mucosa |
|  | VCAM-1 |  |  |
|  | MAdCAM-1 |  |  |
| $\alpha_E\beta_7$ | E-cadherin | Lymphocytes | Leukocyte adhesion |

APC, antigen-precenting cell; COL, collagen; CS-1, domain of fibronectin; ECM, extracellular matrix; FBG, fibrinogen; FN, fibronectin; ICAM, intercellular adhesion molecule; LFA, lymphocyte function antigen; LN, ; MAdCAM-1, mucosal addressin cell adhesion molecule-1; VCAM, vascular cell adhesion molecule; VLA, very late activation antigen; VN, vitronectin; vWF, von Willebrand factor.

integrins, which are expressed on the surface of many cells, including monocytes and neutrophils, participate in many different cell functions, including bone remodeling (i.e., osteoclast function) (27), angiogenesis (28), and neutrophil migration (29). Other integrins commonly expressed on the surface of leukocytes include the $\beta_7$ integrins. The $\alpha_4\beta_7$ integrin binds to VCAM-1 and the CS-1 domain of fibronectin and participates in leukocyte homing to Peyer's patches (30), whereas the $\alpha_E\beta_7$ integrin binds to E-cadherin and mediates adhesion of lymphocytes (primarily CD8+ T cells) to epithelial cells in the intestine (31).

## Integrin Regulation

Leukocyte adhesion is highly regulated, with most leukocytes circulating in the vasculature in a nonadherent state and becoming adherent only under specific conditions. Activation of integrin-mediated adhesion plays a central role in promoting leukocyte adhesion during inflammation. Integrin function may be regulated by changes in cell-surface expression, integrin affinity, integrin clustering, or by alterations in integrin signaling.

Changes in integrin expression on the cell surface provides a mechanism to regulate integrin-mediated adhesion (32). Receptor expression levels may be regulated by an increase in gene expression (over hours) or more rapidly by the recruitment of adhesion receptors from cytoplasmic stores to the cell surface (Table 6.4). For example, stimulation of lymphocytes with proinflammatory mediators increases the

**TABLE 6.4.** *Mechanisms that regulate the function of cell adhesion molecules*

| Mechanism | Family | Examples |
|---|---|---|
| Receptor expression |  |  |
| New synthesis | Integrin | $\alpha_5\beta_1$ |
|  |  | $\alpha_4\beta_1$ |
|  | Selectin | E-selectin |
|  | IgSF | ICAMs |
|  |  | VCAM |
| Recruitment (stores) | Selectin | P-selectin |
|  | Integrin | $\alpha_{IIb}\beta_3$ |
|  |  | $\alpha_M\beta_2$ |
| Receptor avidity | Integrin | $\alpha_L\beta_2$ |
|  | Proteoglycan | CD44 |
| Receptor affinity | Integrin | $\alpha_{IIb}\beta_3$ |
|  |  | $\alpha_M\beta_2$ |
|  |  | $\alpha_L\beta_2$ |
| Alternative splicing | Integrin | $\beta_1$ |
|  |  | $\beta_3$ |
|  |  | $\alpha_6$ |
|  | Proteoglycan | CD44 |
|  | IgSF | ICAM-1 |
| Glycocylation | Proteoglycan | CD44 |
|  | Integrin | $\alpha_5\beta_1$ |
|  | IgSF | ICAM-1 |
| Proteolysis | Selectin | L-selectin |
|  |  | P-selectin |

ICAM, intracellular adhesion molecule; IgSF, immunoglobulin superfamily; VCAM, vascular cell adhesion molecule.

Some data from Ginsberg M, Diaz-Gonzalez F. Cell adhesion molecules and endothelial cells in arthritis. In: Koopman WJ, ed., Arthritis and allied conditions: a textbook of rheumatology, 1997:479–491.

expression of $\beta_2$ integrin gradually at a transcriptional level. Alternatively, rapid increases in surface expression of the $\beta_2$ integrin can occur after activation of neutrophils by recruitment from cytoplasmic stores. The concentration of cell-surface integrin regulates basic processes such as cell migration, for which optimal cell function (migration in this case) is promoted at intermediate integrin expression levels (7,33).

Modulation of integrin affinity or clustering provides a rapid mechanism to turn leukocyte adhesion on or off. In response to inflammatory mediators, leukocyte integrins may undergo a conformational change that promotes enhanced ligand binding (i.e., a high-affinity conformation). The first evidence for activation-induced conformational changes in the integrin extracellular domain came from studies showing that specific antibodies recognize leukocyte integrins only after activation and induction of adhesion. By enhancing ligand binding function the high-affinity conformation promotes the firm leukocyte–endothelial adhesion that occurs during leukocyte extravasation. In contrast to leukocyte integrins, integrins on the surface of other cells, fibroblasts for example, are capable of promoting cell adhesion without receptor activation. Leukocyte adhesion may also be rapidly regulated by changes in integrin clustering on the cell surface (i.e., changes in receptor avidity) (34). Certain adhesion-promoting factors, including phorbol esters, stimulate adhesion in leukocytes by an increase in receptor avidity but not affinity (35). It is likely that a combination of changes in receptor affinity and avidity contribute to the increase in leukocyte adhesion that occurs after leukocyte activation.

Activation of leukocyte adhesion is regulated by a process known as inside-out signaling. Inside-out signaling involves the modulation of integrin-mediated ligand binding function on the outside of the cell by changes from within the cell (8,36). There is evidence that inside-out signaling plays an important role in regulating integrin-mediated adhesion during leukocyte extravasation and activation. For example, the the T-cell receptor (TCR)–CD3 complex on leukocytes mediate a weak but specific adhesion to the corresponding major histocompatibility complex (MHC)–antigen complex on target cells; this interaction activates leukocyte $\alpha_L\beta_2$ integrins that then promote firm adhesion to ICAM, allowing stabilization of T-cell–target cell binding (37,38). The integrin ligand binding function is regulated by many different cytoplasmic and cell-surface proteins, including $\beta_3$ endonexin (39), a surface protein CD98 (40), cytohesin-1 (41), and members of the RAS family of small GTP-binding proteins (42,43). Mutational analysis of the cytoplasmic domains of the $\alpha_{IIb}\beta_3$ integrin (8,44) and the $\alpha_L\beta_2$ integrin (45,46) have also demonstrated that the extracellular integrin ligand binding affinity is in large part under the control of the integrin cytoplasmic domain.

Integrin function is also regulated by the specific associations of the integrin cytoplasmic domain with cytoskeletal and signaling molecules (47). A model for the types of interactions that occur between the integrins and the actin cytoskeleton is the focal adhesion. Despite the fact that rapidly moving cells, such as leukocytes, do not form organized focal adhesions, it is thought that focal adhesions represent the general kinds of interactions that occur between integrins and the cytoskeleton. The focal adhesion functions as a structural center linking the ECM to the actin cytoskeleton and as a signaling center that recruits specific cytoplasmic signaling molecules. The $\beta$ integrin cytoplasmic domain is required for the localization of integrins to focal adhesions, and disruption of this interaction perturbs integrin-mediated adhesion (14,38,48). Direct binding between the $\beta_1$ integrin cytoplasmic domain has been demonstrated for several focal adhesion proteins, including talin (49), $\alpha$-actinin (50), and focal adhesion kinase (FAK) (51).

In addition to participating in inside-out signaling, integrins modulate cell behavior by ligand-induced signaling (i.e., outside-in signaling) (2–6). Integrin receptors, like growth factor or cytokine receptors, participate in signal transduction cascades that affect diverse cell functions, including gene expression, cell proliferation, migration, apoptosis, and differentiation. Studies demonstrate that recognition and signaling through different integrins may have very different effects on cell behavior and gene expression. An example with direct implications for rheumatic diseases is the differential effects of the $\alpha_4\beta_1$ and $\alpha_5\beta_1$ integrin signaling on the expression of matrix metalloproteinases in synovial fibroblasts. Binding of the $\alpha_5\beta_1$ integrin in fibroblasts to the RGD sequence of fibronectin promotes the expression of matrix metalloproteinases (MMPs) while signaling through the $\alpha_4\beta_1$ integrin through the CS-1 domain of fibronectin suppresses the expression of MMPs (52). Binding of lymphocytes to VCAM-1 may also trigger MMP production in T cells (53).

The cytoplasmic domain of the integrin receptor, like the T-cell receptor, does not have intrinsic enzymatic activity. However, by associating with cytoplasmic proteins, including many signaling molecules, integrin receptor engagement may affect common signal transduction pathways, including the activation of mitogen-activated protein kinase (MAPK) (54), protein tyrosine phosphorylation (55), pH changes (56), calcium fluxes (57,58), and alterations in inositol lipid pathways (5). There has been significant progress in defining integrin-mediated signaling pathways. The focal adhesion, which serves as a model for the integrin signaling complex, contains cytoskeletal proteins such as vinculin, talin, $\alpha$-actinin, and paxillin and signaling molecules such as FAK, protein kinase C (PKC), and members of the SRC family of protein kinases. On ligand binding, additional signaling molecules, including growth factor receptor–bound protein-2 (GRB-20), phosphoinositide 3-kinase, CRK, and the guanine nucleotide exchange factor SOS, become associated with the focal adhesion proteins. Downstream molecules activated by the formation of this complex include the RAS, RAF, and MAPK pathways, reminiscent of growth factor and T-cell receptor signaling pathways (Fig. 6.2). The $\alpha_L\beta_2$ integrin/ligand interactions are capable of stimulating T-cell activation at a level comparable to the CD28/B7 interaction (59).

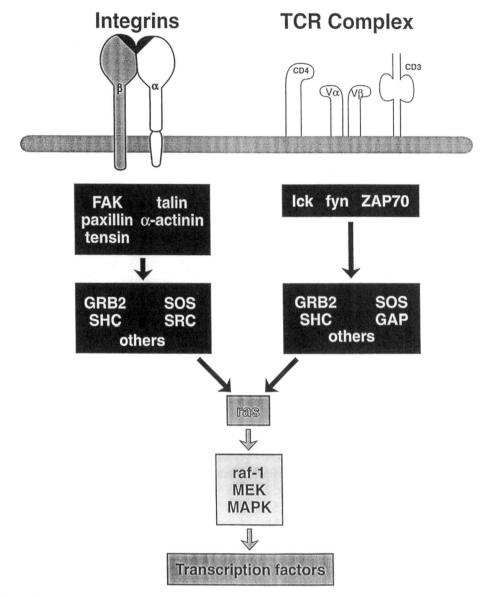

**FIG. 6.2.** Schematic representation of some of the signaling events involved in T-cell receptor (TCR) and integrin pathways. Similar molecules are involved in downstream signaling from integrins and the TCR, allowing synergy between these signaling pathways.

## IMMUNOGLOBULIN SUPERFAMILY

The immunoglobulin superfamily mediates calcium-independent heterophilic cell-cell adhesion (60) (Table 6.5). Members of this large and diverse family include T-cell receptors; cell-surface proteins such as CD2, CD4, and CD8; immunoglobulins; and class I and class II MHC receptors. Some of the members of the immunoglobulin superfamily participate in leukocyte adhesive functions, including intercellular adhesion molecule-1 (ICAM-1) (61), ICAM-2, ICAM-3, vascular cell adhesion molecule-1 (VCAM-1), CD31, and mucosal addressin cell adhesion molecule-1 (MAdCAM-1) (Table 6.5). These receptors generally mediate heterophilic cell-cell adhesion by binding to integrins on the surface of leukocytes. In contrast, the cell-surface receptor

CD31 mediates homophilic calcium-independent adhesion (leukocyte CD31–endothelial cell CD31) and heterophilic calcium-dependent adhesion by binding to $\alpha_v\beta_3$ integrin and cell-surface proteoglycans (62). Members of the immunoglobulin superfamily play an important role in leukocyte extravasation and homing and in the activation of leukocytes.

### Immunoglobulin Superfamily Structure

Members of the immunoglobulin superfamily are characterized by the presence of one or more immunoglobulin homology regions. The immunoglobulin domains have 60 to 100 amino acids arranged in two β sheets that are connected by a conserved disulfide bridge (Fig. 6.1). The ICAMs are type I membrane glycoproteins that contain a heavily *N*-glycocy-

**TABLE 6.5.** *Immunoglobulin superfamily*

| Receptor | Ligand | Distribution |
|---|---|---|
| ICAM-1 (CD54) | $\alpha_M\beta_2$ $\alpha_L\beta_2$ $\alpha_X\beta_2$ | Resting and activated leukocytes, resting and activated endothelial cells, other cells |
| ICAM-2 (CD102) | $\alpha_M\beta_2$ $\alpha_L\beta_2$ | Resting and activated leukocytes, resting and activated endothelial cells |
| ICAM-3 (CD50) | $\alpha_L\beta_2$ $\alpha_d\beta_2$ | Resting and activated leukocytes |
| ICAM-4 | $\alpha_M\beta_2$ $\alpha_L\beta_2$ | Red blood cells |
| VCAM | $\alpha_4\beta_1$ $\alpha_4\beta_7$ | Activated endothelial cells |
| MAdCAM-1 | $\alpha_4\beta_7$ L-selectin | Endothelial cells |
| PECAM-1 (CD31) | $\alpha_v\beta_3$ | Endothelial cells |

ICAM, intercellular adhesion molecule; MAdCAM-1, mucosal addressin cell adhesion molecule-1; PECAM, platelet/endothelial cell adhesion molecule; VCAM, vascular cell adhesion molecule.

lated extracellular domain, span the membrane once, and contain a short cytoplasmic domain. The different members of the family have variable numbers of immunoglobulin domains. For example, ICAM-1 and ICAM-3 contain five immunoglobulin domains, whereas ICAM-2 and ICAM-4 contain only two. The integrin ligand binding sites usually are in the amino-terminal domains. The crystal structure of ICAM-2 reveals a specific integrin-recognition surface that appears to be involved in recognizing I-domain–containing integrins such as LFA-1 (63).

### Immunoglobulin Superfamily Function

Members of the immunoglobulin superfamily, including the ICAMs and VCAM-1, serve as cellular ligands for the $\beta_1$ and $\beta_2$ integrins. By binding integrins, members of the immunoglobulin superfamily play an important role in leukocyte extravasation in normal immune surveillance and during acute and chronic inflammation (64,65). The importance of ICAM-1 to normal immune function is demonstrated by ICAM-1 knockout mice, which exhibit prominent defects in inflammatory responses, including defects in neutrophil emigration in response to inflammatory stimuli (66). Later studies demonstrated that crosses between ICAM-deficient mice and Fas (lpr) mice have improved survival and reduced renal injury, suggesting that ICAM-1 plays an important role in the pathogenesis of chronic inflammation (67). The ICAMs and VCAM usually are expressed on the surface of endothelial cells, although they may be expressed on the surface of other cell types. For example, ICAM-1 is also expressed on the surface of leukocytes, epithelial cells, and fibroblasts, and ICAM-2 is expressed on the surface of leuko-

cytes and platelets (65). ICAM-3 usually is not expressed on the surface of endothelial cells but is usually found on resting leukocytes, where it has been proposed to play a role in initiating leukocyte proliferation (68). These differences in expression reflect the distinct functions mediated by the different members of the immunoglobulin superfamily. For example, ICAM-2 appears to mediate primarily the adhesion and extravasation of leukocytes across unstimulated endothelium, and VCAM-1, which is expressed specifically on the surface of activated endothelial cells, mediates leukocyte extravasation across activated endothelium by binding to the $\alpha_4\beta_1$ integrin on leukocytes (69). CD31 is also important to leukocyte adhesion and migration across the endothelial surface by mediating homophilic binding to CD31 and heterophilic binding to the $\alpha_v\beta_3$ integrin (70). There is evidence that binding of endothelial cell CD31 to $\alpha_v\beta_3$ integrin on the surface of leukocytes promotes leukocyte migration by inhibiting firm $\beta_2$ integrin–mediated leukocyte–endothelial cell adhesion (71). In addition to playing an important role during leukocyte extravasation, ICAM–LFA-1 interactions also provide a costimulatory signal for the activation of T cells (72).

### Immunoglobulin Superfamily Regulation and Signaling

Immunoglobulin superfamily function is primarily regulated at the level of cell-surface expression. Distinct patterns of regulation are demonstrated by different members of the family (65). Some members of the family are constitutively expressed and are not inducible (e.g., ICAM-2), and others are expressed only after exposure to proinflammatory mediators (e.g., VCAM-1). ICAM-1, in contrast, is constitutively expressed on the endothelium at low levels and is further induced after exposure to proinflammatory mediators. The expression of ICAM-1 and VCAM-1 is regulated by cytokines, including interleukin-1 (IL-1), tumor necrosis factor (TNF), and interferon-$\gamma$ (IFN-$\gamma$). The function of the immunoglobulin superfamily members probably is regulated by other mechanisms, although they have not been clearly defined. It is known that there is a direct association between the cytoplasmic domains of ICAM-1 and ICAM-2 with actin-binding proteins such as $\alpha$-actinin, although the functional significance of these associations is unknown (73,74). Study results suggest that, in addition to performing an adhesive function, members of the immunoglobulin superfamily participate in cell signaling and affect T-cell activation. For example, like other cell-surface receptors, signaling through ICAM-1 activates the RAF/MAPK pathway (75).

### SELECTINS

The selectins mediate calcium-dependent heterophilic cell-cell adhesion (76). The three members of the family—L-selectin, P-selectin, and E-selectin—participate in leukocyte–endothelial cell and leukocyte-platelet interactions by binding to carbohydrate moieties on cell-surface glycopro-

**TABLE 6.6.** *Selectin family*

| Receptor | Ligand | Distribution |
|---|---|---|
| P-selectin | Sialyl Lewis$^x$ | Platelets |
| | PSGL-1 | Activated endothelial cells |
| E-selectin | Sialyl Lewis$^x$ | Activated endothelial cells |
| | ESL-1 | |
| L-selectin | Sialyl Lewis$^x$ | Neutrophils |
| | GlyCAM-1 | Lymphocytes |
| | CD34 | Monocytes |
| | MAdCAM-1 | Eosinophils |

ESL-1, E-selectin ligand-1; GlyCAM-1, glycan-bearing cell adhesion molecule-1; MAdCAM-1, mucosal addressin cell adhesion molecule-1; PSGL-1, P-selectin glycoprotein ligand-1.

teins (Table 6.6). Each of the selectins bind to specific cell-surface carbohydrates and bind to the tetrasaccharide sialyl Lewis$^x$ (77). The importance of selectin-ligand interactions to normal immune function is demonstrated by a primary immunodeficiency syndrome, leukocyte adhesion deficiency type II (78). Patients with LAD type II have a defect in fucose metabolism and do not express the functional sialyl Lewis$^x$ determinant. As a result of this deficiency, patient's leukocytes fail to accumulate normally in areas of inflammation, and patients present with recurrent infections.

## Selectin Structure

The extracellular domain of selectins contains an amino-terminal lectin domain, followed by an epidermal growth factor (EGF)–like domain and a variable number of complement regulatory repeats (Fig. 6.1) (79). The receptors span the membrane once and have a short cytoplasmic domain. The C-type lectin domain contains the ligand binding site and requires the presence of calcium for its carbohydrate-binding function. Although the EGF-like domain is not directly involved in ligand binding, it appears to be required for optimal ligand binding by the lectin domain. The cytoplasmic domain, like other cell adhesion molecules, is short and does not contain intrinsic enzymatic activity.

## Selectin Function

The three members of the selectin family have distinct tissue distributions and functions, although they all participate in leukocyte–endothelial adhesion and leukocyte extravasation (80,81). In general, the adhesion mediated by selectins is transient and of low affinity. The weak attachments supported by selectins promote tethering of leukocytes to the endothelial surface and under conditions of flowing blood support leukocyte rolling, an early step in the inflammatory process. The rapid, transient attachments promoted by selectins appear to be required for the subsequent stable attachments mediated by integrins. The importance of selectins to normal immune function is supported by studies of selectin knock out mice that show major defects in their inflammatory responses (82).

Each member of the selectin family has distinct tissue distributions and functions. All members of the family recognize the carbohydrate moiety sialyl Lewis$^x$ and bind with higher affinity to specific ligands (76). For example, L-selectin specifically recognizes sulfated glycosaminoglycans on cell-surface proteoglycans, including glycan-bearing cell adhesion molecule-1 (GlyCAM-1) on the surface of high endothelial venules (HEVs) in lymph nodes (83), MAdCAM-1 on the endothelium in the gastrointestinal system (84,85), and CD34 (86), a proteoglycan on the surface of endothelial cells and bone marrow cells. P-selectin specifically recognizes P-selectin glycoprotein ligand-1 (PSGL-1), a transmembrane glycoprotein with a large, mucin-like ectodomain that is expressed on the surface of neutrophils and specific lymphocyte subsets (87). E-selectin binds to E-selectin ligand-1 (ESL-1), a transmembrane protein that is identical to fibroblast growth factor (FGF) receptors (88). In myeloid cells, the ESL-1 is sialylated and fucosylated and therefore serves as an E-selectin ligand only on these cells.

L-selectin, initially described as a "lymphocyte homing receptor," is expressed constitutively on the surface of leukocytes, particularly naive T cells, where it participates in the homing to the HEVs in lymphoid organs (79,89). The selectin ligand GlyCAM-1, a proteoglycan with sulfated glycosaminoglycans, is specifically expressed on the HEVs of lymph nodes, where it supports the homing of naive L-selectin expressing leukocytes. Lymph nodes of mice deficient in L-selectin have reduced numbers of leukocytes. In contrast to naive T cells, activated and memory T cells express lower levels of L-selectin on their surfaces and therefore do not tend to preferentially home to these areas. However, L-selectin is present on the surface of neutrophils, where it participates in the migration of leukocytes into areas of inflammation by mediating leukocyte rolling along the blood vessel wall (90). P-selectin and E-selectin are expressed on the surface of activated endothelium. By binding to carbohydrate moieties on leukocyte glycoproteins, E-selectin and P-selectin mediate the transient rolling and tethering of leukocytes along the endothelial surface in areas of inflammation. This initial transient selectin-mediated adhesion permits the subsequent stable adhesion promoted by integrin-ICAM interactions.

## Selectin Regulation and Signaling

Like members of the immunoglobulin superfamily, selectins are regulated primarily by changes in cell-surface expression. In contrast to P-selectin and E-selectin, L-selectin is expressed constitutively and usually is not induced by the expression of proinflammatory mediators. Exposure to inflammatory mediators or binding to its counter receptor promotes shedding of the cell-surface L-selectin by a proteolytic mechanism (91). Selectin shedding may serve as a mechanism to limit the inflammatory response by competing with cell-surface receptor for ligand binding. There is evidence that serum levels of soluble L-selectin correlate with disease activity in certain inflammatory disorders (92). In contrast to L-selectin, the expression of E-selectin and P-selectin is not constitutive but is induced by the presence of inflammatory mediators, including TNF and IL-1. Increased expression of E-selectin occurs after a few hours of exposure to cytokines, suggesting transcriptional regulation (93). In contrast, P-selectin expression increases rapidly by direct recruitment from cytoplasmic stores (e.g., Weibel-Palade bodies in endothelial cells). P selectin, like L-selectin, may be shed from the cell surface during inflammation (79).

Association of the selectin cytoplasmic domain with regulatory proteins also plays a role in modulating selectin-mediated adhesive function. Studies have shown that the selectin cytoplasmic domain is required for leukocyte adhesion to the endothelium (94). Ligand binding through E-selectin promotes the association of its cytoplasmic domain with the actin cytoskeleton. The selectin cytoplasmic domain associates with actin-binding proteins found in integrin-receptor complexes, including FAK, paxillin, vinculin, and $\alpha$-actinin but not talin (95). The cytoplasmic domain of selectins may also activate specific signal transduction pathways, including the MAPK pathway (96). The role of selectin-mediated adhesion in cellular signaling has not been clearly defined, although selectin-mediated adhesion has been shown to modulate the activity of $\beta_2$ integrins (97–100).

## OTHER FAMILIES OF CELL ADHESION RECEPTORS

Several other families of cell-surface adhesion receptors may also participate in the inflammatory response, including the proteoglycans, cadherins, and the ADAM family. Proteoglycans are a diverse family of proteins that contain a core protein to which one or more glycosaminoglycan (GAG) chains are attached (101) (Fig. 6.1). CD44 is an integral membrane proteoglycan that participates in the inflammatory response by mediating cell-cell and cell-matrix interactions during cell adhesion and migration (102). Perturbing CD44 function may interfere with interactions between T cells and B cells, neutrophil phagocytosis, leukocyte migration, and the development of an inflammatory response. CD44, like other proteoglycans, binds to growth factors and chemokines. CD44 binds to the chemokine macrophage inflammatory protein-1$\beta$ (MIP-1$\beta$), which promotes the activation of $\alpha_4\beta_1$ integrin during leukocyte extravasation.

Cadherins are calcium-dependent cell-surface glycoproteins that generally mediate stable homophilic cell-cell adhesion (103) and play an important role in maintaining tissue structure and integrity. Cadherins are essential for establishing intercellular adhesion required for normal embryonic development (104). Disruption of cadherin-mediated cell-cell adhesion therefore results in distortion of tissue structure during development and is associated with an increase in carcinoma cell invasion and metastasis (105,106). The importance of cadherin-mediated cell-cell adhesion in maintaining vascular integrity is supported by the observation that its disruption promotes leukocyte extravasation (107). Disruption of cadherin-mediated adhesion in the gut by means of expressing a dominant negative cadherin promotes the development of inflammatory bowel disease in mice (108). Cadherins also participate in leukocyte adhesion by binding to $\alpha_E\beta_7$ integrin on the surface of leukocytes (31).

The ADAM family is a cell-surface adhesion receptor family that participates in cell-cell and cell-matrix interactions (109,110). This family of receptors contains a disintegrin-like domain and an MMP-like domain. Members of the ADAM family probably function as cell adhesion receptors by binding to integrins and other ligands and as cell-surface MMPs. The ADAM family members may mediate cell-cell adhesion by binding to $\alpha_v\beta_3$ integrins by their disintegrin domain (111). The MMP domain of the ADAM family member TACE is a TNF-$\alpha$–converting enzyme (112). TACE specifically cleaves surface TNF-$\alpha$ into its active, soluble form. Further studies must be performed to characterize how the adhesive and MMP activities of ADAM family members may participate in the pathogenesis of inflammation.

## LEUKOCYTE–ENDOTHELIAL CELL ADHESION

The recruitment of leukocytes during inflammation is a complex process that involves the coordinated actions of adhesion receptors and cytokines in an "adhesion cascade." Remarkable specificity in recruitment is provided by the involvement of specific adhesion receptors and inflammatory mediators during leukocyte homing and extravasation. The recruitment of leukocytes during inflammation may be separated into stages with the involvement of distinct classes of cell adhesion receptors (113) (Fig. 6.3 and Table 6.7). These stages include selectin-mediated leukocyte rolling or tethering along the endothelial surface; leukocyte integrin activation; integrin-mediated firm leukocyte adhesion; and leukocyte transmigration across the endothelium into the surrounding tissue.

Adhesion receptor function is dynamically regulated during leukocyte extravasation. Soluble factors, such as cytokines, play an important role in regulating adhesion receptor expression and activation (71). For example, IL-1 and TNF from macrophages and IFN-$\gamma$ from T cells induce the expression of endothelial adhesion receptors, including ICAM-1, VCAM, P-selectin, and E-selectin. Other inflammatory mediators released from activated endothelium include small chemotactic peptides or chemokines (Table 6.8). Chemokines, including $\alpha$-chemokines (with a cysteine–amino acid [X]–cysteine, or CXC, structure), attract neutrophils, and $\beta$-chemokines (with a CC structure) attract mononuclear cells, eosinophils, and basophils. Chemokines also promote leukocyte adhesion and transmigration by activating leukocyte integrins (114).

Specificity in leukocyte recruitment is provided by the presence of specific inflammatory mediators and by the types of adhesion receptors that are expressed on the leukocyte and endothelial surfaces (89). For example, naive T cells that con-

## Stage I: Rolling
### Selectins

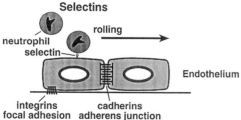

## Stage II: Firm Adhesion   Diapedesis
### Integrins/Ig SF        Integrins/CD31

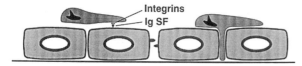

## Stage III: Migration
### Integrins/CD44

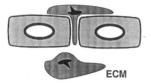

**FIG. 6.3.** Adhesive events that occur during leukocyte transmigration. The initial stage involves selectin-mediated cell rolling under conditions of flowing blood. Subsequently, firm adhesion between the endothelium and leukocyte is mediated by integrins on leukocytes and members of the immunoglobulin superfamily on the endothelium. The leukocytes then invade through the endothelium (i.e., diapedesis), a process mediated by integrins and the immunoglobulin superfamily member CD31. The final stage involves the migration of leukocytes through the surrounding extracellular matrix, which is mediated by multiple receptors, including CD44 and integrins.

**TABLE 6.7.** *Participation of cell-surface receptors during leukocyte extravasation*

| |
|---|
| Rolling |
| $\quad$ E-, P- and L-selectin and ligands |
| $\quad$ $\alpha_4\beta_1$ integrin : VCAM |
| $\quad$ CD44 : HA |
| $\quad$ $\alpha_4\beta_7$ : MAdCAM |
| Integrin activation |
| $\quad$ CD31 : CD31 |
| $\quad$ Chemokines and receptors |
| $\quad$ Selectins |
| Firm integrin-mediated adhesion |
| $\quad$ $\alpha_L\beta_2$ : ICAM-1 |
| $\quad$ $\alpha_M\beta_2$ : ICAM |
| $\quad$ $\alpha_4\beta_1$ : VCAM-1 |
| $\quad$ $\alpha_4\beta_7$ : MAdCAM-1 |
| Leukocyte transmigration |
| $\quad$ $\alpha_L\beta_2$ : ICAM-1 |
| $\quad$ $\alpha_M\beta_2$ : ICAM |
| $\quad$ $\alpha_v\beta_3$ : CD31 |
| $\quad$ $\alpha_4\beta_1$ : VCAM-1 |

ICAM, intercellular adhesion molecule; MAdCAM-1, mucosal addressin cell adhesion molecule-1; VCAM, vascular cell adhesion molecule.

tinually recirculate through the lymphoid system express high levels of L-selectin on their surface and therefore specifically target to the HEVs in lymphoid tissue. In contrast, memory T cells or other leukocytes, which express lower levels of L-selectin on their surface, tend to target to areas on the endothelium that are activated and express high levels of E-selectin and P-selectin.

Selectins mediate the initial transient attachment between leukocytes and the endothelial surface. Specifically, they promote tethering along the endothelial surface, and in flowing blood, these weak attachments promote leukocyte rolling. The $\alpha_4\beta_1$ integrins may also participate in these weak, transient attachments. Selectin-mediated adhesion and the presence of chemokines on the endothelial surface (bound to proteoglycans such as CD44) promote the activation of leukocyte integrins. The activation of leukocyte $\alpha_4\beta_1$ and $\beta_2$ integrins

**TABLE 6.8.** *Chemokines*

| Chemokines | Source | Target |
|---|---|---|
| CXC structure | | |
| $\quad$ IL-8 | Endothelial cells, monocytes, neutrophils, monocytes, T cells, synovial cells | Neutrophils, T cells |
| CC structure | | |
| $\quad$ RANTES | T cells | T cells, monocytes, eosinophils |
| $\quad$ MIP-1$\alpha$ | Monocytes, T/B cells, macrophages | T cells |
| $\quad$ MCP-1 | Monocytes, endothelial cells, fibroblasts | Monocytes, basophils |

CC, cysteine–cysteine; CXC, cysteine–amino acid–cysteine; IL-8, interleukin-8; MCP, macrophage (or monocyte) chemotactic protein; MIP, macrophage inflammatory protein; RANTES, regulated on activation, normally T-cell expressed and secreted chemokine.

Portions adapted from Imhof B, Dunon D. Basic mechanism of leukocyte migration. *Horm Metab Res* 1997;29:614–621.

promotes the binding to endothelial VCAM and ICAM, respectively. The integrin-mediated adhesion is strong and promotes the arrest of leukocytes on the endothelial surface. The final stage of leukocyte extravasation involves the rapid transmigration of leukocytes across the endothelium. Leukocyte diapedesis is promoted by $\beta_2$ integrin–ICAM, $\alpha_4\beta_1$-VCAM, and $\alpha_v\beta_3$ integrin-CD31 interactions. There is evidence that the $\alpha_v\beta_3$-CD31 interactions weaken the firm adhesions mediated by the $\beta_1$ and $\beta_2$ integrins, allowing movement of cells across the endothelium (62).

The endothelial surface plays an active role in orchestrating the inflammatory response. In response to cytokines, endothelial cells rapidly present P-selectin on their surfaces from cytoplasmic stores and within hours express other adhesion molecules, including E-selectin, VCAM-1, and ICAM. In response to TNF and IL-1, endothelial cells produce other inflammatory mediators, including chemokines, leukotriene LTB$_4$, and platelet-activating factor, which further amplify the inflammatory response. Endothelial cells may also play an important role by localizing inflammatory mediators to specific areas by the direct binding of chemokines to proteoglycans on their surface. Less is known about whether disruption of the endothelial barrier is required for leukocyte extravasation. Some studies suggest that neutrophil transendothelial migration occurs at tricellular corners (an area that normally has decreased cadherin expression) and does not involve disruption of cadherin-mediated adhesion (115). However, other studies have shown that disruption of cadherin-mediated endothelial cell adhesions promotes leukocyte extravasation (107). Mechanisms to limit the inflammatory response are also provided by the endothelium. These include the proteolytic shedding of surface adhesion molecules, including the selectins and VCAM.

## ADHESION MOLECULES: CLINICAL AND THERAPEUTIC IMPLICATIONS

Chronic inflammatory disorders, such as rheumatoid arthritis, diabetes, and multiple sclerosis, are characterized by the presence of leukocytes and other inflammatory cells within the affected tissues. The recruitment, retention, and persistent activity of these inflammatory cells is a cell-adhesion–dependent process. However, unlike leukocyte adhesion deficiency, in which an inherited defect in $\beta_2$ integrin expression directly contributes to disease pathogenesis, there are no clear examples in which inherited defects in adhesion receptors directly contribute to the pathogenesis of autoimmune disorders. However, the affected tissues in patients with many chronic inflammatory disorders, including lupus and rheumatoid arthritis, show increased expression of many adhesion receptors, including selectins, integrins, and immunoglobulin superfamily members. For example, increased $\beta_2$ integrin expression on the surface of leukocytes has been identified in patients with rheumatoid arthritis or lupus (24,92). The levels of $\beta_2$ integrin expression have been found to correlate directly with disease activity in patients with lupus (116). It

is likely that the changes in cell adhesion receptor expression that occur in many systemic inflammatory disorders are the result of altered expression or activity of cytokines or other inflammatory mediators rather than a primary defect in adhesion receptor expression or function.

It is intriguing to speculate about the possible role that abnormal adhesion receptor expression or function may play in the pathogenesis of autoimmune diseases. There is direct evidence that small changes in integrin expression levels or integrin affinity can result in striking changes in the ability of cells to migrate *in vitro* (117,118), suggesting that altered integrin expression or function may contribute directly to abnormal leukocyte adhesion or migration *in vivo* and therefore to the development of chronic inflammation. Supporting this possibility is the finding that ectopic expression of the $\beta_1$ integrin in the skin of transgenic mice promotes a disorder resembling psoriasis with epidermal hyperproliferation and inflammation (119). Patients with Down's syndrome express increased $\beta_2$ integrin on the surface of their leukocytes, which promotes increased leukocyte adhesion. It is an intriguing possibility that the increase in leukocyte adhesion may contribute to the susceptibility of these patients to autoimmune disorders such as rheumatoid arthritis (120,121). Evidence for ICAM-1 polymorphisms in multiple sclerosis suggests that specific cell adhesion receptor polymorphisms may contribute to the genetic background and susceptibility of patients with autoimmune disorders (122).

In the pathogenesis of chronic inflammatory disorders, adhesion receptors may play a role in endothelial cell–leukocyte adhesion, migration of leukocytes, regulation of MMP gene expression (which contributes to tissue damage), leukocyte activation, regulation of cell survival, and angiogenesis. The patterns of adhesion receptor expression have been studied extensively for a number of inflammatory disorders, including rheumatoid arthritis (24). Studies of rheumatoid arthritis patients have demonstrated increases in many different adhesion receptors on the surface of synovial endothelium, leukocytes, and macrophages, including $\beta_2$ integrins, ICAMs, selectins, and VCAM-1 (123). It is unknown whether these expression patterns are specific to rheumatoid arthritis or instead reflect the general state of active inflammation in affected patients. If specific patterns of adhesion receptor expression are found in different inflammatory disorders, this observation may be informative in terms of understanding the contribution of adhesion receptors to specific types of inflammatory disorders and may contribute to the development of specific adhesion receptor–targeted therapies for different inflammatory disorders.

Progress in cell adhesion receptor research has had important implications for the development of new diagnostic and therapeutic approaches for autoimmune disorders. Diagnostic applications include the use of soluble adhesion receptors as markers of disease activity (reviewed elsewhere [24,124]). These studies have suggested that specific soluble adhesion molecules are upregulated in different disorders. In rheumatoid arthritis, selectin levels are elevated in the synovial fluid and serum, although expression in the synovial fluid appears to correlate most closely with disease activity. Serum levels of ICAM-3 appear to correlate closely with disease activity in patients with rheumatoid arthritis. In patients with systemic lupus erythematosus, soluble ICAM and selectins were not useful markers of disease activity, but serum VCAM levels correlated with disease activity, particularly in patients with active nephritis. In patients with Wegener's granulomatosis, the serum levels of ICAM-1 correlated with disease activity and renal involvement.

Although less well studied, another potential application of adhesion receptor research is in the development of new imaging approaches. In animal models of arthritis, indium-tagged E-selectin monoclonal antibodies have been used to successfully image inflamed joints, suggesting that similar approaches may be used to identify organ involvement in patients with autoimmune disorders (125).

In addition to serving as a useful diagnostic tool, tailored disruption of adhesion receptors has the potential for being an important therapeutic target. Research investigating the use of adhesion-targeted therapies for a number of medical conditions are being actively investigated by pharmaceutical companies (Table 6.9). In support of adhesion-targeted therapies for rheumatic diseases is the observation that many of current medications affect adhesion receptor expression or function (92) (Table 6.8). For example, nonsteroidal antiinflammatory drugs disrupt $\beta_2$ integrin–mediated adhesion in neutrophils (126). Corticosteroids diminish ICAM-1 and E-selectin expression on activated endothelium and downregulate lymphocyte $\beta_2$ integrins (92). Methotrexate decreases integrin-mediated adhesion and decreases selectin expression and function (Table 6.10). The anti-TNF-$\alpha$ therapies affect synovial expression of VCAM-1 and E-selectin and downregulate the serum levels of soluble E-selectin and VCAM-1 (127).

Studies using animal models suggest that directly targeting adhesion receptors may also be a useful therapeutic approach. For example, blocking $\beta_2$ integrin or ICAM-1 function reduces inflammation and tissue injury in several animal models of inflammation, including antigen-induced arthritis, diabetes mellitus, and glomerulonephritis (24,92,128). Blocking $\alpha_4\beta_1$ integrins also has a significant antiinflammatory effect and, in combination with $\beta_2$-blocking antibodies, may completely inhibit the accumulation of leukocytes in areas of inflammation in animal models (129). Blocking the function of selectins or their ligands has also been useful in controlling inflammation in some animal models, but this approach may be most effective as combination therapy (130,131). These and other studies suggest that combination therapy targeting several different cell-surface adhesion receptors may be most useful (24). However, blocking cell-surface adhesion receptors such as the $\beta_2$ integrin may not be an effective long-term therapeutic approach because of the possible induction of profound immunosuppression similar to that observed in LAD patients.

A challenge for drug development is to devise treatments that target the specific cell adhesion molecules implicated in a particular disease process to avoid significant side effects. Specific patterns of cell adhesion molecule expression have been demonstrated for different disease processes, and early animal study results suggest some therapeutic benefit from specifically targeting the receptors implicated in a particular disease. Targeting specific members of the selectin family has disrupted disease progression in one type of disease but not another. For example, disrupting P-selectin but not E-selectin decreases lung injury in complement-induced disease, whereas the opposite is true for IgG immune complex–mediated lung injury (132). These observations may lead to the development of specific adhesion receptor targeting approaches, depending on the receptors implicated and the organ systems involved. Some clinical trials are in progress, and others are being planned to investigate the effects of blocking cell adhesion molecules on the progression of different autoimmune disorders (Table 6.9). For example, phase I/II trials of anti-ICAM monoclonal antibodies for patients with rheumatoid arthritis have been performed, and results suggest that there may be some therapeutic benefit for these patients (24). Some of these studies suggest that patients with early rheumatoid arthritis may have greater therapeutic benefit with the anti-ICAM antibodies than patients with long-standing disease (133).

**TABLE 6.9.** *Therapeutic approaches targeting cell adhesion molecules*

| Adhesion molecule | Cell type | Process or disorder being targeted |
|---|---|---|
| $\alpha_{IIb}\beta_3$ integrin[a] | Platelets | Prevention of restenoses after angioplasty, unstable angina |
| $\alpha_v\beta_3$ integrin[b] | Endothelial cells | Angiogenesis (tumor biology, diabetic retinopathy) |
| $\alpha_4\beta_1$ integrin | Leukocytes | Chronic inflammatory diseases (asthma[b], arthritis, insulin-dependent diabetes, multiple sclerosis) |
| $\beta_2$ integrins | Leukocytes | Acute and chronic inflammation (arthritis) |
| Selectins | Leukocytes, endothelial cells | Acute and chronic inflammation (arthritis) |
| ICAMs | Endothelial cells | Acute and chronic inflammation (rheumatoid arthritis[b]) |

ICAM, intercellular adhesion molecule.
[a] In clinical use.
[b] In clinical trials.

**TABLE 6.10.** *Effects of antiinflammatory medications on adhesion molecule expression and function*

| Drugs | Adhesion molecule effects |
|---|---|
| NSAIDs | Decrease in $\beta_2$ integrin-mediated adhesion, decrease in selectin function/expression |
| Corticosteroids | Decrease stimulated expression of E-selectin and ICAM-1 on endothelium |
| Sulfasalazine | Decrease in L-selectin function, decrease in $\beta_2$ integrin-mediated adhesion |
| Methotrexate | Decrease in L-selectin function, decrease in $\beta_2$ integrin-mediated adhesion |
| Colchicine | Decrease in E-selectin expression/function, decrease in L-selectin expression |
| Gold | Decrease in stimulated expression of E-selectin and VCAM-1/decrease E-selectin expression on synovial vascular endothelium |

Portions adapted from Cronstein BN, Weissmann G. The adhesion molecules of inflammation. Arthritis Rheum 1993; 36:147–157.

## CONCLUSIONS

Considerable progress has been made in characterizing the structure, function, and regulation of adhesion receptors. Adhesion molecules regulate many basic cellular processes, including cell migration, proliferation, and survival, which are central to the pathogenesis of autoimmune diseases. This investigative progress has implications for the development of new diagnostic and therapeutic approaches for a wide variety of inflammatory disorders. The challenge for future investigations is to identify specific adhesion therapies that block the inciting event but have limited long-term side effects. Although therapies blocking $\beta_2$-ICAM interactions show some evidence of therapeutic benefit, there is also the risk of long-term immunosuppression using these types of therapies. An attractive approach may be to develop combination therapies that target different components of the adhesion cascade, such as specific cytokines or adhesion molecules, to improve efficacy and potentially limit toxicity. The coming years promise to be informative in terms of understanding how adhesion molecules participate in the pathogenesis of chronic inflammation and in determining whether adhesion-targeted strategies can be therapeutically beneficial for patients with autoimmune diseases.

## REFERENCES

1. Hynes RO. Integrins: versatility, modulation and signaling in cell adhesion. *Cell* 1992;69:11–25.
2. Clark EA, Brugge JS. Integrins and signal transduction pathways: the road taken. *Science* 1995;268:233–239.
3. Damsky CH, Werb Z. Signal transduction by integrin receptors for extracellular matrix: cooperative processing of extracellular information. *Curr Opin Cell Biol* 1992;4:772–781.
4. Howe A, Aplin AE, Alahari SK, Juliano RL. Integrin signaling and cell growth control [In process citation]. *Curr Opin Cell Biol* 1998;10:220–231.
5. Yamada KM, Miyamoto S. Integrin transmembrane signaling and cytoskeletal control. *Curr Opin Cell Biol* 1995;7:681–689.
6. Schwartz MA, Schaller MD, Ginsberg MH. Integrins: emerging paradigms of signal transduction. *Annu Rev Cell Dev Biol* 1995;11:549–599.
7. Huttenlocher A, Sandborg RS, Horwitz AF. Adhesion in cell migration. *Curr Opin Cell Biol* 1995;7:697–706.
8. Ginsberg MH, Du X, Plow EF. Inside-out integrin signaling. *Curr Opin Cell Biol* 1992;4:766–771.
9. Fischer A, Lisowska-Grospierre B, Anderson DC, Springer TA. Leukocyte adhesion deficiency: molecular basis and functional consequences. *Immunodefic Rev* 1988;1:39–54.
10. Arnaout MA. Leukocyte adhesion molecules deficiency: its structural basis, pathophysiology and implications for modulating the inflammatory response. *Immunol Rev* 1990;114:145–180.
11. Michishita M, Videm V, Arnaout M. A novel divalent cation-binding site in the A domain of $\beta_2$ integrin CR3 (CD11b/CD18) is essential for ligand binding. *Cell* 1993;72:857–867.
12. Diamond MS, Garcia-Aguilar J, Bickford JK, Corbi AL, Springer TA. The I domain is a major recognition site on the leukocyte integrin Mac-1 (CD11b/CD18) for four distinct adhesion ligands. *J Cell Biol* 1993;120:1031–1043.
13. Lee JO, Rieu P, Arnaout MA, Liddington R. Crystal structure of the A-domain from the a-subunit of $\beta_2$ integrin complement receptor type 3 (CR3, CD11b/CD18). *Cell* 1995;80:631–638.
14. Sastry SK, Horwitz AF. Integrin cytoplasmic domains: mediators of cytoskeletal linkages and extra- and intracellular initiated transmembrane signaling. *Curr Opin Cell Biol* 1993;5:819–831.
15. Mould AP, Askari JA, Aota SI, et al. Defining the topology of integrin alpha$_5$beta$_1$-fibronectin interactions using inhibitory anti-alpha$_5$ and anti-beta$_1$ monoclonal antibodies: evidence that the synergy sequence of fibronectin is recognized by the amino-terminal repeats of the alpha5 subunit. *J Biol Chem* 1997;272:17283–17292.
16. Hemler M. VLA proteins in the integrin family: structures, functions and their role on leukocytes. *Annu Rev Immunol* 1991;8:365–400.
17. Gahmberg CG. Leukocyte adhesion: CD11/CD18 integrins and intercellular adhesion molecules. *Curr Opin Cell Biol* 1997;9:643–650.
18. Corbi AL. *Leukocyte integrins: structure, expression and function.* Austin, Texas: RG Landes, 1996.
19. Larson RS, Corbi AL, Berman L, Springer T. Primary structure of the leukocyte function-associated molecule-1 alpha subunit: an integrin with an embedded domain defining a protein superfamily. *J Cell Biol* 1989;108:703–712.
20. Springer TA, Teplow DB, Dreyer WJ. Sequence homology of the LFA-1 and Mac-1 leukocyte adhesion glycoproteins and unexpected relation to leukocyte interferon. *Nature* 1985;314:540–542.
21. Springer T, Galfre G, Secker DS, Milstein C. Mac-1: a macrophage differentiation antigen identified by monoclonal antibody. *Eur J Immunol* 1979;9:301–306.
22. Springer TA, Sastre L, Anderson DC. The LFA-1, Mac-1 leucocyte adhesion glycoprotein family and its deficiency in a heritable human disease. *Biochem Soc Trans* 1985;13:3–6.
23. Stacker SA, Springer TA. Leukocyte integrin P150,95 (CD11c/CD18) functions as an adhesion molecule binding to a counter-receptor on stimulated endothelium. *J Immunol* 1991;146:648–655.
24. Mojcik CF, Shevach EM. Adhesion molecules: a rheumatologic perspective. *Arthritis Rheum* 1997;40:991–1004.
25. Chan PY, Aruffo A. VLA-4 integrin mediates lymphocyte migration on the inducible endothelial cell ligand VCAM-1 and the extracellular matrix ligand fibronectin. *J Biol Chem* 1993;268:24655–24564.
26. Alon R, Kassner PD, Carr MW et al. The integrin VLA-4 supports tethering and rolling in flow on VCAM-1. *J Cell Biol* 1995;128:1243–1253.
27. Lakkakorpi PT, Horton MA, Helfrich MH et al. Vitronectin receptor has a role in bone resorption but does not mediate tight sealing zone attachment of osteoclasts to the bone surface. *J Cell Biol* 1991;115:1179–1186.
28. Brooks PC, Clark RA, Cheresh DA. Requirement of vascular integrin alpha v beta 3 for angiogenesis. *Science* 1994;264:569–571.
29. Lawson MA, Maxfield FR. Ca(2+)- and calcineurin-dependent recycling of an integrin to the front of migrating neutrophils. *Nature* 1995;377:75–79.
30. Hu MC, Crowe DT, Weissman IL, Holtzmann B. Cloning and expression of mouse integrin beta p(beta 7): a functional role in Peyer's

patch-specific lymphocyte homing. *Proc Natl Acad Sci USA* 1992;89:8254–8258.

31. Cepek KL, Shaw SK, Parker CM et al. Adhesion between epithelial cells and T lymphocytes mediated by E-cadherin and the alpha E beta 7 integrin. *Nature* 1994;372:190–193.

32. Shimizu Y, Van Seventer GA, Horgan KJ, Shaw S. Regulated expression and binding of three VLA (beta 1) integrin receptors on T cells. *Nature* 1990;345:250–253.

33. Palecek S, Loftus JC, Ginsberg MH, et al. Integrin-ligand binding properties govern cell migration speed through cell-substratum adhesiveness. *Nature* 1997;385:537–540.

34. van Kooyk Y, Weder P, Heije K, Figdor CG. Extracellular Ca$^{2+}$ modulates leukocyte function-associated antigen-1 cell surface distribution on T lymphocytes and consequently affects cell adhesion. *J Cell Biol* 1994;124:1061–1070.

35. Stewart MP, McDowall A, Hogg N. LFA-1–mediated adhesion is regulated by cytoskeletal restraint and by a Ca$^{2+}$-dependent protease, calpain. *J Cell Biol* 1998;140:699–707.

36. Kolanus W, Zeitlmann L. Regulation of integrin function by inside-out signaling mechanisms. *Curr Top Microbiol Immunol* 1998;231:33–49.

37. Dustin ML, Springer TA. T-cell receptor cross-linking transiently stimulates adhesiveness through LFA-1. *Nature* 1989;341:619–624.

38. Diamond MS, Staunton DE, Marlin SD, Springer TA. Binding of the integrin Mac-1 (CD11b/CD18) to the third immunoglobulin-like domain of ICAM-1 (CD54) and its regulation by glycosylation. *Cell* 1991;65:961–971.

39. Kashiwagi H, Schwartz MA, Eigenthaler M, et al. Affinity modulation of platelet integrin alpha$_{IIb}$beta$_3$ by beta$_3$-endonexin, a selective binding partner of the beta3 integrin cytoplasmic tail. *J Cell Biol* 1997;137:1433–1443.

40. Fenczik CA, Sethi T, Ramos JW, et al. Complementation of dominant suppression implicates CD98 in integrin activation [see comments]. *Nature* 1997;390:81–85.

41. Kolanus W, Nagel W, Schiller B, et al. Alpha L beta 2 integrin/LFA-1 binding to ICAM-1 induced by cytohesin-1, a cytoplasmic regulatory molecule. *Cell* 1996;86:233–242.

42. Hughes PE, Renshaw PE, Pfaff M, et al. Suppression of integrin activation: a novel function of a Ras/Raf–initiated MAP kinase pathway. *Cell* 1997;88:521–530.

43. Zhang Z, Vouri K, Wang H, et al. Integrin activation by R-RAS. *Cell* 1996;85:61–69.

44. O'Toole TE, Katagiri Y, Faull RJ, et al. Integrin cytoplasmic domains mediate inside-out signal transduction. *J Cell Biol* 1994;124:1047–1059.

45. Hibbs ML, Jakes S, Stacker SA, et al. The cytoplasmic domain of the integrin lymphocyte function-associated antigen 1 beta subunit: sites required for binding to intercellular adhesion molecule 1 and the phorbol ester-stimulated phosphorylation site. *J Exp Med* 1991;174:1227–1238.

46. Lu CF, Springer TA. The alpha subunit cytoplasmic domain regulates the assembly and adhesiveness of integrin lymphocyte function-associated antigen-1. *J Immunol* 1997;159:268–278.

47. Yamada KM, Geiger B. Molecular interactions in cell adhesion complexes. *Curr Opin Cell Biol* 1997;9:76–85.

48. Hayashi Y, Haimovich B, Reszka A, et al. Expression and function of chicken integrin beta 1 subunit and its cytoplasmic domain mutants in mouse NIH 3T3 cells. *J Cell Biol* 1990;110:175–184.

49. Horwitz A, Duggan K, Buck C, et al. Interaction of plasma membrane fibronectin receptor with talin—a transmembrane linkage. *Nature* 1986;320:531–533.

50. Otey CA, Pavalko FM, Burridge K. An interaction between alpha-actinin and the beta 1 integrin subunit *in vitro*. *J Cell Biol* 1990;111:721–729.

51. Schaller M, Parsons T. Focal adhesion kinase and associated proteins. *Curr Opin Cell Biol* 1994;6:705–710.

52. Huhtala P, Humphries MJ, McCarthy JB, et al. Cooperative signaling by alpha 5 beta 1 and alpha 4 beta 1 integrins regulates metalloproteinase gene expression in fibroblasts adhering to fibronectin. *J Cell Biol* 1995;129:867–879.

53. Romanic AM, Madri JA. The induction of 72-kD gelatinase in T cells upon adhesion to endothelial cells is VCAM-1 dependent. *J Cell Biol* 1994;125:1165–1178.

54. Chen Q, Kinch MS, Lin TH, et al. Integrin-mediated cell adhesion activates mitogen-activated protein kinases. *J Biol Chem* 1994;269:26602–26605.

55. Guan JL, Shalloway D. Regulation of focal adhesion-associated protein tyrosine kinase by both cellular adhesion and oncogenic transformation. *Nature* 1992;358:690–692.

56. Schwartz MA, Lechene C, Ingber DE. Insoluble fibronectin activates the Na/H antiporter by clustering and immobilizing integrin alpha 5 beta 1, independent of cell shape. *Proc Natl Acad Sci USA* 1991;88:7849–7853.

57. Jaconi ME, et al. Multiple elevations of cytosolic-free Ca$^{2+}$ in human neutrophils: initiation by adherence receptors of the integrin family. *J Cell Biol* 1991;112:1249–1257.

58. Sjaastad MD, Nelson WJ. Integrin-mediated calcium signaling and regulation of cell adhesion by intracellular calcium. *Bioessays* 1997;19:47–55.

59. Dubey C, Croft M, Swain SL. Costimulatory requirements of naive CD4$^+$ T cells. ICAM-1 or B7-1 can costimulate naive CD4 T cell activation but both are required for optimum response. *J Immunol* 1995;155:45–57.

60. Williams AF, Barclay AN. The immunoglobulin superfamily—domains for cell surface recognition. *Annu Rev Immunol* 1988;6:381–405.

61. Staunton DE, Marlin SD, Stratowa C, et al. Primary structure of ICAM-1 demonstrates interaction between members of the immunoglobulin and integrin supergene families. *Cell* 1988;52:925–933.

62. Piali L, Hammel P, Uherek C, et al. CD31/PECAM-1 is a ligand for alpha v beta 3 integrin involved in adhesion of leukocytes to endothelium. *J Cell Biol* 1995;130:451–460.

63. Casasnovas JM, Springer TA, Lin JH, et al. Crystal structure of ICAM-2 reveals a distinctive integrin recognition surface. *Nature* 1997;387:312–315.

64. Gahmberg CG, Tolvanen M, Kotovuori P. Leukocyte adhesion—structure and function of human leukocyte beta$_2$-integrins and their cellular ligands. *Eur J Biochem* 1997;245:215–232.

65. Buck CA. Immunoglobulin superfamily: structure, function and relationship to other receptor molecules. *Semin Cell Biol* 1992;3:179–188.

66. Sligh J, Ballantyne CM, Rich SS, et al. Inflammatory and immune responses are impaired in mice deficient in intercellular adhesion molecule 1. *Proc Natl Acad Sci USA* 1993;90:8529–8533.

67. Bullard D, King PD, Hicks MJ, et al. Intercellular adhesion molecule-1 deficiency protects MRL/MpJ-Fas(lpr) mice from early lethality. *J Immunol* 1997;159:2058–2067.

68. Hogg N, Landis RC. Adhesion molecules in cell interactions. *Curr Opin Immunol* 1993;5:383–390.

69. Elices MJ, Osborn L, Takada Y, et al. VCAM-1 on activated endothelium interacts with the leukocyte integrin VLA-4 at a site distinct from the VLA-4/fibronectin binding site. *Cell* 1990;60:577–584.

70. Bogen S, Pak J, Garifallou M, et al. Monoclonal antibody to murine PECAM-1 (CD31) blocks acute inflammation *in vivo*. *J Exp Med* 1994;179:1059–1064.

71. Imhof B, Dunon D. Basic mechanism of leukocyte migration. *Horm Metab Res* 1997;29:614–621.

72. Van Seventer GA, Shimizu K, Horgan KJ, Shaw S. The LFA-1 ligand ICAM-1 provides an important costimulatory signal for T cell receptor–mediated activation of resting T cells. *J Immunol* 1990;144:4579–4586.

73. Carpen O, Pallai P, Staunton DE, Springer TA. Association of intercellular adhesion molecule-1 (ICAM-1) with actin-containing cytoskeleton and alpha-actinin. *J Cell Biol* 1992;118:1223–12234.

74. Heiska L, Kantor C, Parr T, et al. Binding of the cytoplasmic domain of intercellular adhesion molecule-2 (ICAM-2) to alpha-actinin. *J Biol Chem* 1996;271:26214–26219.

75. Holland J, Owens T. Signaling through intercellular adhesion molecule 1 (ICAM-1) in a B cell lymphoma line: the activation of Lyn tyrosine kinase and the mitogen-activated protein kinase pathway. *J Biol Chem* 1997;272:9108–9112.

76. Rosen SD, Bertozzi CR. Two selectins converge on sulphate: leukocyte adhesion. *Curr Biol* 1996;6:261–264.

77. Rosen S, Bertozzi C. The selectins and their ligands. *Curr Opin Cell Biol* 1994;6:663–673.

78. Etzioni A, Harlan JM, Pollack S, et al. Leukocyte adhesion deficiency (LAD) II: a new adhesion defect due to absence of sialyl Lewis X, the ligand for selectins. *Immunodeficiency* 1993;4:307–308.

79. Lasky LA. Selectins: interpreters of cell-specific carbohydrate information during inflammation. *Science* 1992;258:964–949.

80. McEver RP, Moore KL, Cummings RD. Leukocyte trafficking mediated by selectin-carbohydrate interactions. *J Biol Chem* 1995;270:11025–11028.

81. Lasky LA. Selectin-carbohydrate interactions and the initiation of the inflammatory response. *Annu Rev Biochem* 1995;64:113–139.

82. Mayadas T, Johnson RC, Rayburn H, et al. Leukocyte rolling and extravasation are severely compromised in P-selectin–deficient mice. *Cell* 1993;74:541–554.

83. Lasky LA, Singer MS, Dowbenko D, et al. An endothelial ligand for L-selectin is a novel mucin-like molecule. *Cell* 1992;69:927–938.

84. Berg EL, McEvoy LM, Berlin C, et al. L-selectin–mediated lymphocyte rolling on MAdCAM-1 [see comments]. *Nature* 1993;366:695–698.

85. Briskin MJ, McEvoy LM, Butcher EC. MAdCAM-1 has homology to immunoglobulin and mucin-like adhesion receptors and to IgA1. *Nature* 1993;363:461–464.

86. Baumheter S, Singer MS, Henzel W, et al. Binding of L-selectin to the vascular sialomucin CD34. *Science* 1993;262:436–438.

87. Sako D, Chang XJ, Barone KM, et al. Expression cloning of a functional glycoprotein ligand for P-selectin. *Cell* 1993;75:1179–1186.

88. Steegmaier M, Levinovitz A, Isenmann S, et al. The E-selectin-ligand ESL-1 is a variant of a receptor for fibroblast growth factor. *Nature* 1995;373:615–620.

89. Gallatin WM, Weissman IL, Butcher EC. A cell-surface molecule involved in organ-specific homing of lymphocytes. *Nature* 1983;304:30–34.

90. Watson SR, Fennie C, Lasky LA. Neutrophil influx into an inflammatory site inhibited by a soluble homing receptor-IgG chimaera. *Nature* 1991;349:164–167.

91. Kishimoto TK, Jutila MA, Berg EL, Butcher EC. Neutrophil Mac-1 and MEL-14 adhesion proteins inversely regulated by chemotactic factors. *Science* 1989;245:1238–1241.

92. Cronstein BN, Weissmann G. The adhesion molecules of inflammation. *Arthritis Rheum* 1993;36:147–157.

93. Springer TA. Traffic signals for lymphocyte recirculation and leukocyte emigration: the multistep paradigm. *Cell* 1994;76:301–314.

94. Kansas GS, Ley K, Munro JM, Tedder TF. Regulation of leukocyte rolling and adhesion to high endothelial venules through the cytoplasmic domain of L-selectin. *J Exp Med* 1993;177:833–838.

95. Yoshida M, Westlin WF, Wang N, et al. Leukocyte adhesion to vascular endothelium induces E-selectin linkage to the actin cytoskeleton. *J Cell Biol* 1996;133:445–455.

96. Hidari KI, Weyrich AS, Zimmerman GA, McEver RP. Engagement of P-selectin glycoprotein ligand-1 enhances tyrosine phosphorylation and activates mitogen-activated protein kinases in human neutrophils. *J Biol Chem* 1997;272:28750–28756.

97. Giblin PA, Hwang ST, Katsumoto TR, Rosen SD. Ligation of L-selectin on T lymphocytes activates beta$_1$ integrins and promotes adhesion to fibronectin. *J Immunol* 1997;159:3498–3507.

98. Simon SI, Burns AR, Taylor AD, et al. L-selectin (CD62L) cross-linking signals neutrophil adhesive functions via the Mac-1 (CD11b/CD18) beta 2-integrin. *J Immunol* 1995;155:1502–1514.

99. Sikorski MA, Staunton DE, Mier JW. L-selectin crosslinking induces integrin-dependent adhesion: evidence for a signaling pathway involving PTK but not PKC. *Cell Adhes Commun* 1996;4:355–367.

100. Gopalan PK, Smith CW, Lu H, et al. Neutrophil CD18-dependent arrest on intercellular adhesion molecule 1 (ICAM-1) in shear flow can be activated through L-selectin. *J Immunol* 1997;158:367–375.

101. Kjellen L, Lindahl U. Proteoglycans: structures and interactions [published erratum appears in *Annu Rev Biochem* 1992;61:after viii]. *Annu Rev Biochem* 1991;60:443–475.

102. Kincade PW, Zheng Z, Katoh S, Hanson L. The importance of cellular environment to function of the CD44 matrix receptor. *Curr Opin Cell Biol* 1997;9:635–642.

103. Takeichi M. Cadherins: a molecular family important in selective cell-cell adhesion. *Annu Rev Biochem* 1990;59:237–252.

104. Larue L, Ohsugi M, Hirchenhaim J, Kemler R. E-cadherin null mutant embryos fail to form a trophectoderm epithelium. *Proc Natl Acad Sci USA* 1994;91:8263–8267.

105. Huber O, Bierkamp C, Kemler R. Cadherins and catenins in development. *Curr Opin Cell Biol* 1996;8:685–691.

106. Perl AK, Wilgenbus P, Dahl U, et al. A causal role for E-cadherin in the transition from adenoma to carcinoma. *Nature* 1998;392:190–193.

107. Gotsch U, Borges E, Bosse R, et al. VE-cadherin antibody accelerates neutrophil recruitment *in vivo*. *J Cell Sci* 1997;110:583–538.

108. Hermiston ML, Gordon JI. Inflammatory bowel disease and adenomas in mice expressing a dominant negative N-cadherin. *Science* 1995;270:1203–1207.

109. Wolfsberg TG, Primakoff P, Myles DG, White JM. ADAM, a novel family of membrane proteins containing a disintegrin and metalloprotease domain: multipotential functions in cell-cell and cell-matrix interactions. *J Cell Biol* 1995;131:275–278.

110. Wolfsberg TG, Straight PD, Gerena RL, et al. ADAM, a widely distributed and developmentally regulated gene family encoding membrane proteins with a disintegrin and metalloprotease domain. *Dev Biol* 1995;169:378–383.

111. Zhang XP, Kamata T, Yokoyama K, et al. Specific interaction of the recombinant disintegrin-like domain of MDC-15 (metargidin, ADAM-15) with integrin alpha$_v$beta$_3$. *J Biol Chem* 1998;273:7345–7350.

112. Black RA, Rauch CT, Kozlosky CJ, et al. A metalloproteinase disintegrin that releases tumour necrosis factor-alpha from cells. *Nature* 1997;385:729–733.

113. Springer TA. Traffic signals on endothelium for lymphocyte recirculation and leukocyte emigration. *Annu Rev Physiol* 1995;57:827–872.

114. Lloyd A, Oppenheimer JJ, Kelvin DJ, Taub DD. Chemokines regulate T cell adherence to recombinant adhesion molecules and extracellular matrix proteins. *J Immunol* 1996;156:932–938.

115. Burns AR, Walker DC, Brown ES, et al. Neutrophil transendothelial migration is independent of tight junctions and occurs preferentially at tricellular corners. *J Immunol* 1997;159:2893–2903.

116. Buyon JP, Shadick N, Berkman R, et al. Surface expression of Gp 165/95, the complement receptor CR3, as a marker of disease activity in systemic Lupus erythematosus. *Clin Immunol Immunopathol* 1988;46:141–149.

117. Huttenlocher A, Ginsberg MH, Horwitz AF. Modulation of cell migration by integrin-mediated cytoskeletal linkages and ligand-binding affinity. *J Cell Biol* 1996;134:1551–1562.

118. Kuijpers TW, Mul EP, Blom M, et al. Freezing adhesion molecules in a state of high-avidity binding blocks eosinophil migration. *J Exp Med* 1993;178:279–284.

119. Carroll JM, Romero MR, Watt FM. Suprabasal integrin expression in the epidermis of transgenic mice results in developmental defects and a phenotype resembling psoriasis. *Cell* 1995;83:957–968.

120. Taylor GM, Williams A, D'Souza SW. Increased expression of lymphocyte functional antigen in Down syndrome [Letter] [published erratum appears in *Lancet* 1986;2:822]. *Lancet* 1986;2:740.

121. Taylor GM, Haigh H, Williams A, et al. Down's syndrome lymphoid cell lines exhibit increased adhesion due to the over-expression of lymphocyte function-associated antigen (LFA-1). *Immunology* 1988;64:451–456.

122. Mycko M, Kwinkowski M, Tronczynska E, et al. Multiple sclerosis: the increased frequency of the ICAM-1 exon 6 gene point mutation genetic type K469. *Ann Neurol* 1998;44:70–75.

123. Koch AE, Burrows JC, Haines GK, et al. Immunolocalization of endothelial and leukocyte adhesion molecules in human rheumatoid and osteoarthritic synovial tissues. *Lab Invest* 1991;64:313–320.

124. Sfikakis P, Tsokos G. Clinical use of the measurement of soluble cell adhesion molecules in patients with autoimmune rheumatic diseases. *Clin Diagn Lab Immunol* 1997;4:241–246.

125. Jamar F, Chapman PT, Harrison AA, et al. Inflammatory arthritis: imaging of endothelial cell activation with an Indium-111–labeled F(ab′)2 fragment of anti-E-selectin monoclonal antibody. *Radiology* 1995;194:843–850.

126. Abramson SB, Weissmann G. The mechanisms of action of nonsteroidal antiinflammatory drugs. *Arthritis Rheum* 1989;32:1–9.

127. Paleolog E, Hunt M, Elliott MJ, et al. Deactivation of vascular endothelium by monoclonal anti-tumor necrosis factor alpha antibody in rheumatoid arthritis. *Arthritis Rheum* 1996;39:1082–1091.

128. Albelda SM, Smith CW, Ward PA. Adhesion molecules and inflammatory injury. *FASEB J* 1994;8:504–512.

129. Issekutz AC, Issekutz TB. Monocyte migration to arthritis in the rat utilizes both CD11/CD18 and very late activation antigen 4 integrin mechanisms. *J Exp Med* 1995;181:1197–1203.

130. Ley K, Gaehtgens P, Fennie C, et al. Lectin-like cell adhesion molecule 1 mediates leukocyte rolling in mesenteric venules *in vivo*. *Blood* 1991;77:2553–2555.
131. Mulligan MS, Paulson JC, De Frees S, et al. Protective effects of oligosaccharides in P-selectin–dependent lung injury. *Nature* 1993; 364:149–151.
132. Mulligan MS, Watson SR, Fennie C, Ward PA. Protective effects of selectin chimeras in neutrophil-mediated lung injury. *J Immunol* 1993;151:6410–6417.
133. Kavanaugh AF, Davis LS, Jain RI, et al. A phase I/II open label study of the safety and efficacy of an anti-ICAM-1 (intercellular adhesion molecule-1; CD54) monoclonal antibody in early rheumatoid arthritis. *J Rheumatol* 1996;23:1338–1344.
134. Ginsberg M, Diaz-Gonzalez F. Cell adhesion molecules and endothelial cells in arthritis. In: Koopman WJ, ed. *Arthritis and allied conditions: a textbook of rheumatology*. Baltimore: Williams & Wilkins, 1997:479–491.
135. Horwitz AF, Hunter T. Cell adhesion: integrating circuitry. *Trends Cell Biol* 1996;6:460–461.

*Textbook of the Autoimmune Diseases,*
Edited by R. G. Lahita, N. Chiorazzi, and W. H. Reeves,
Lippincott Williams & Wilkins, Philadelphia © 2000.

# CHAPTER 7

# Immune Tolerance

## David E. Anderson and David A. Hafler

The immune system exists to protect the body from infection by a plethora of microorganisms, including bacteria, viruses, and parasites. This goal is accomplished by a variety of interdependent methods. The skin is an often overlooked but extremely effective barrier to infection and is one of several innate mechanisms of immunity. Natural killer cells, which appear to primarily recognize changes in the levels of major histocompatibility complex (MHC) class I molecules expressed on cells within the body, represent another form of innate immunity. Although they can protect the body against tumor cells or virally infected cells, which often have altered levels of MHC class I expression, they have no "memory" of a prior viral infection or particular type of tumor.

This contrasts with T cells and B cells, which comprise the specific immune response. A given T cell or B cell and its clonal progeny are all specific for a given foreign microbial antigen and can "remember" a prior encounter with that antigen and effectively remove it much more quickly on secondary exposure to the antigen. This phenomenon is the basis for vaccination. After vaccination with exposure to antigens from a particular virus or bacterium with adjuvant, there is activation and expansion of T cells and B cells with specific receptors for those particular antigens. When the same individual is exposed to the infectious virus or bacteria years later, the T cells and B cells that were previously activated and expanded are mobilized quickly and usually eliminate the infectious agent before it can do any harm to the body.

B cells and T cells respond to foreign antigens in fundamentally different ways. A B cell responds to a foreign antigen using a membrane-bound immunoglobulin molecule as its receptor. This membrane-bound immunoglobulin receptor directly recognizes conformationally dependent stretches (i.e., epitopes) of a portion of foreign bacterial or viral pro-

tein. Unlike B cells, T cells critically depend on antigen-presenting cells (APCs) such as macrophages, dendritic cells, and B cells for their activation. Helper T cells recognize short linear fragments of processed foreign antigens (i.e., peptides) presented on the surface of APCs by MHC class II molecules.

Although it is relatively easy to conceive of a protein fragment from a bacterium or virus as being foreign, it is not as readily apparent to the immune system. There is no inherent biochemical or structural difference between a protein fragment derived from a damaged cell within the body and a fragment of membrane from a virus. However, the immune system must manage to reliably and consistently be in an activated state only in response to the viral protein fragment and not the fragment from its own tissues. This explains the necessity for *immune tolerance*, which is the ability of the immune system to be tolerant of antigens from its own tissues but respond to antigens from environmental sources, including bacteria, viruses, and parasites.

When an individual's immune system begins to attack her or his own tissues, we assume that immune tolerance has broken down and autoimmunity has developed. Although there are many different autoimmune diseases, they do not all necessarily stem from similar defects in the maintenance of immune tolerance. Self antigens can induce tolerance by a variety of different mechanisms, and it is incumbent on us to determine which mechanisms are defective in particular autoimmune diseases.

## T-CELL TOLERANCE IMPOSED BY THYMIC SELECTION

T cells must be able to recognize self MHC molecules presenting foreign antigens, but during T-cell selection within the thymus, MHC molecules presenting predominantly self antigens are present to achieve this result. Two critical factors allow this goal to be achieved. First, T-cell reactivity to foreign antigens is accomplished by recognition of MHC molecules presenting cross-reactive self antigens, a process called *positive selection* that gives rise to thymocytes that are

D. E. Anderson: Department of Medical Microbiology and Immunology, University of California, Davis School of Medicine, Davis, California 95616.

D. A. Hafler: Department of Neurology (Neuroscience), Harvard Medical School, Boston, Massachusetts 02115; and Laboratory of Molecular Immunology, Center for Neurologic Disease, Brigham and Women's Hospital, Boston, Massachusetts 02115.

inherently autoreactive. Second, *negative selection* mediated by the same MHC complexes presenting self antigens eliminates all highly autoreactive thymocytes before they emigrate to the periphery as mature T cells. This process of negative selection is arguably the most important mechanism of ensuring immune tolerance. The following sections describe the evidence for positive and negative T-cell selection and then focus on these two critical aspects of T-cell selection, which are responsible for inducing central T-cell tolerance.

### Evidence for Positive and Negative Selection

The discovery of what has been called *MHC restriction* was made by several groups throughout the 1970s and led to the award of two Nobel prizes. In the early 1970s, Shreffler and Benaceraf determined there was a requirement for a common MHC molecule for effective T-cell and B-cell interactions in adoptive transfer models of immunity in which B cells or T cells from one inbred strain of mice were transferred into another strain of irradiated recipient mice. In 1973, Shevach demonstrated that proliferative responses to antigen required MHC-matched APCs used to present antigen to the responding T cells. Using an *in vitro* cytotoxic assay for CD8-positive (CD8$^+$) T cells, Doherty and Zinkernagel similarly demonstrated MHC restriction in the generation of antiviral cytotoxic T lymphocyte (CTL) responses. Technologic advances enabling the deletion of a particular gene (i.e., gene knockout mice) or the constitutive expression of a gene of interest (i.e., transgenic mice) allowed the role of the thymus in inducing central tolerance and imparting MHC restriction to be characterized more fully.

### Anatomy and Location of T-Cell Selection

T-cell specificity for self MHC molecules has been examined using a variety of approaches, including the use of MHC class I– and MHC class II–deficient mice and T-cell receptor (TCR) transgenic mice in which the fate of the T-cell repertoire with a single specificity can easily be evaluated. Bone marrow chimeric mice, in which bone marrow with a given MHC background from one mouse is used to reconstitute the immune system of a second strain of mice with a different, defined MHC specificity, have also been used extensively to elucidate the mechanisms of T-cell positive and negative selection.

Numerous investigations have collectively demonstrated that MHC restriction is determined by the MHC of the host thymus and is the result of positive selection. Taking advantage of MHC class II knockout mice and bone marrow chimeric mice expressing peptide–MHC class II complexes on thymic stromal cells or on bone-marrow–derived hematopoietic cells, Glimcher et al. (1) found that positive selection occurred only when peptide/MHC class II complexes were expressed by thymic stromal cells. In an elegant follow-up study, this group used their peptide/MHC class II knockout mice and selectively reintroduced MHC class II complexes

only on the thymic cortical epithelium (the medullary epithelium and bone marrow-derived cells were MHC II negative) (2). CD4$^+$ cells were positively selected but no clonal deletion occurred.

*In vitro* experiments demonstrated that cells from these mice proliferated vigorously to self APCs (were autoreactive), consistent with a lack of negative selection. Subsequent *in vivo* experiments demonstrated that adoptive transfer of these autoreactive T cells into irradiated syngeneic mice induced graft-versus-host disease (GVHD), and when transferred into nonirradiated syngeneic mice, induced hypergammaglobulinemia and autoantibody production (3). These results convincingly demonstrate that positive selection in the absence of negative selection leads to generation of a polyclonal, pathogenic, autoreactive T-cell repertoire.

Although Glimcher et al. found that bone marrow-derived dendritic cells were not involved in positive selection, they did play a role in negative selection. Several groups have confirmed that the thymic medullary epithelium mediates negative selection (4,5). These data further indicate that positive and negative selection occur in anatomically distinct sites.

### Cross-Reactive Basis of Selection

Allen et al. were the first to describe altered peptide ligands (APLs), which are peptides containing single amino acid substitutions that do not have appreciable effects on the binding of the peptides to the MHC molecule but that induce different signals in mature T cells through the TCR (6). They demonstrated the role of APLs in the selection of thymocytes (7,8), and one type of these APLs, antagonists, has been used by Hogquist et al. *in vitro* to encourage positive selection of thymocytes. The theories regarding the selection and imposed self-tolerance of peripheral mature T cells have implied that positive selection is based on extensive T-cell cross-reactivity. For example, a thymocyte with low to moderate affinity for self peptide *A* may be positively selected and leave the thymus without being negatively selected because its TCR does not have too high an affinity for peptide *A* presented by MHC to warrant negative selection. In the periphery, this same mature T cell does not have any measurable reactivity to peptide *A* presented by MHC but is activated by foreign peptide *B* presented by the same MHC molecule. This thymocyte/T cell responds with different degrees of reactivity to two different peptides. It may be that, for any given mature T cell, the self peptide used to select the cell as a thymocyte has great similarity to the foreign peptide to which the mature T cell responds; the selecting peptide may be an antagonist peptide of the mature T cell, differing from the agonist peptide used to activate the mature T cell by only one or two amino acid changes.

In some cases, however, the peptides used to select thymocytes may bear little or no homology to the agonist foreign peptides used to activate the T cells within the periphery (9). Using a novel technique, Kapler and Marrack's group created transgenic mice expressing a single peptide–MHC class II complex and found that a fairly diverse T-cell repertoire was generated in these mice (about 20% the normal number of T cells) (10). This group subsequently demonstrated that T cells that were selected on a single peptide–MHC class II complex reacted with a diverse set of peptides bound by the same selecting MHC molecule, emphasizing the considerable degeneracy in peptide recognition during positive selection and peripheral T-cell activation (10). Nevertheless, although there is degeneracy in peptide recognition that can induce positive selection, one peptide cannot select the entire TCR repertoire (11,12).

## Models of Positive and Negative Selection

Several models have been proposed to explain the mechanism by which a self-restricted, self-tolerant T-cell repertoire is generated. One model suggested that perhaps the stage of thymocyte development at which point a given thymocyte interacted with a peptide–MHC complex dictated whether it was positively or negatively selected. Another model suggested that certain peptides might have an inherent ability to positively select while others served to negatively select thymocytes. Over time, however, these models have been disproved and are not discussed further in this chapter.

The two primary models used to explain T-cell selection are slight conceptual variations of the same general mechanism. The differential avidity model of selection has been championed by the work of Ashton-Rickardt and Tonegawa. It postulates that the developmental fate of an immature thymocyte depends on the avidity of interactions between thymocyte TCRs and peptide–MHC molecules on thymic stromal cells (13,14). This theory postulates that activating (or agonist) peptides induce positive selection of thymocytes when at low concentrations (low avidity), and at higher doses, the same peptide encourages negative selection (high avidity). In the efficacy model of thymocyte selection advocated by Hogquist and Bevan, the quality of the signal a peptide–MHC complex induces in a thymocyte, in addition to the number of peptide–MHC complexes present, determines the outcome of the selection process for a given thymocyte. This group has used variants of peptides for which a given thymocyte is specific, called antagonists, which induce signals that inhibit rather than activate mature T cells expressing the same TCR found within the periphery. When these antagonist peptides were used in in vitro assays of thymocyte selection, this group found that while agonist peptides induced negative selection at all concentrations, including very low concentrations at which the Ashton-Rickardt group saw positive selection of thymocytes, the antagonist peptides were found to positively select thymocytes when present at concentrations above a certain threshold (15,16). A schematic incorporating the salient features of these two models is presented in Figure 7.1.

Several other groups have provided data to support the notion that the avidity of interaction between a thymocyte and selecting peptide–MHC complexes dictates the outcome of the selection process. Sebzda et al. (17) used the same TCR transgenic mice as Tonegawa's group but used $\beta_2$-microglobulin knockout mice instead of TAP knockout mice to eliminate contaminating endogenous peptide presentation by MHC molecules. Using only a peptide agonist (i.e., a defined viral peptide recognized by the TCR), they found that low concentrations mediated positive selection, whereas high concentrations led to negative selection. Cook et al. (18) showed that, rather than modulating the amount of peptide used to select a thymocyte with a TCR specific for the peptide–MHC complex, they could modulate the level of the MHC molecules and achieve a similar effect. TCR transgenic mice were bred to express different levels of MHC molecules on the thymic stroma; at low levels of selecting peptide–MHC complexes, the thymocytes were positively selected, whereas mice bred to express high levels of the selecting peptide–MHC molecules were found to negatively select most thymocytes.

In another study, surface plasmon resonance was used to directly measure the kinetics of TCR interactions with peptides known to positively and negatively select thymocytes (19). The results suggested that the affinity of the peptide for the TCR correlated with the outcome of selection, such that positive selection occurred over a 1-log range of peptide starting threefold below the affinity required for negative selection. However, the affinity of the TCR for peptide–MHC complex was not an absolute predictor of the outcome of selection, and the investigators suggested that clustering of coreceptors might play a role in the selection process by influencing the overall avidity of a T cell for an APC. The presence or absence of various coreceptors and adhesion molecules might just as easily affect the quality of the signals directed through the TCR.

Two additional models have been postulated to explain T-cell selection and the induction of central T-cell tolerance. A "gemisch" of peptides may be responsible for positive selection of thymocytes. The selection of any one TCR may not depend one self peptide; rather, the summation of each peptide–MHC complex of very low affinity may add up to high ligand density and positive selection. In this way, none of the cooperating, selecting ligands would be individually detected as agonists or antagonists (9). Alternately, Matzinger suggested that, although thymocytes require negative selection to prevent widespread autoimmunity mediated by recent thymic emigrants, thymocytes may not go through any positive selection process. Instead, peripheral tissue damage from physical trauma or insult or by microbial infection may induce some kind of danger signal to the immune system encouraging the activation of T cells (20). Little direct evidence has supported these alternate models of T-cell selection.

## Role of Apoptosis in Negative Selection

The term apoptosis describes a common series of morphologic changes that accompanied the death of cells from a wide variety of tissues. Apoptosis is different from cell necrosis in many important ways. It requires new gene expression

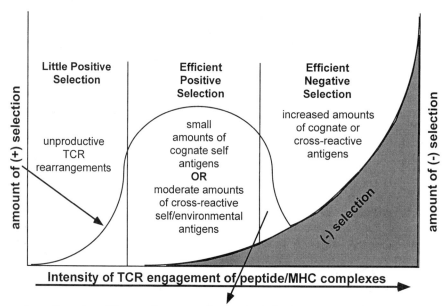

A small number of thymocytes are positively selected yet escape negative selection (central tolerance). Factors which allow for escape from negative selection include a lack or insufficient amount of autoantigen in the thymus or inefficient binding and presentation of autoantigen by the MHC molecules.

**FIG. 7.1.** The same peptide–major histocompatibility complex (MHC) molecule complexes can lead to positive or negative selection of T cells, depending on the number of complexes present during the T-cell selection process. T cells that do not react with peptide–MHC complexes or that encounter few complexes form low-avidity interactions and undergo apoptosis. T cells with an intermediate avidity of interaction with antigen-presenting cells (APCs) presenting greater numbers of peptide–MHC complexes are positively selected. T cells that react with self-peptide–MHC complexes with high avidity because of very-high-affinity T-cell receptors (TCRs) or large numbers of self/MHC complexes are negatively selected and deleted by an apoptotic process. This system generates a T-cell population that recognizes the self-MHC molecules in the periphery but deletes the T cells that strongly react with self-MHC molecules presenting self-peptides. The T cells in the periphery are capable of recognizing self-MHC molecules presenting a wide spectrum of foreign (nonself) peptides.

and is triggered by the appearance or loss of an external signal that leads to the activation of an internal cell death program. In contrast, cell necrosis does not appear to require the expression of new mRNAs or proteins and is believed to be initiated by cellular damage that disrupts osmotic balance. Perhaps most importantly, as a cell undergoes apoptosis it may break up into apoptotic bodies, but these are sealed and maintain their osmotic gradients; there is no spilling of intracellular contents and no provocation of inflammation (21).

During T-cell selection, apoptosis eliminates precursor cells with nonrearranged or aberrantly rearranged nonfunctional receptors (i.e., thymocytes that are not positively selected) and is responsible for the deletion of autoreactive T cells in the thymus by means of negative selection. Using three-color immunofluorescence and fluorescence-activated cell sorting (FACS) analysis on frozen human thymic tissue and freshly isolated human thymocytes, Le et al. (22) documented the role of apoptosis in central tolerance. They found that most apoptotic thymocytes were localized to the cortical-medullary junction, where anatomically negative selection is known to occur.

## Central Tolerance and Autoimmunity

Based on the fundamental investigations into how central tolerance functions to prevent the development of autoreactive T cells, many ideas have emerged to explain autoimmune diseases. Wraith et al. theorized that low affinity interactions between autoantigens and MHC molecules may undermine the efficacy of their presentation in the thymus, enabling autoreactive T cells to escape self-tolerance. To test this theory, his group used TCR transgenic mice specific for the central nervous system (CNS) autoantigen myelin basic protein (MBP) p1-11 and APLs based on this MBP epitope that had greater binding affinity for MHC class II molecules. Consistent with their theory, they found that the *in vivo* administration of the APLs resulted in deletion of T cells while administration of native peptide had no effect (23). Other groups have suggested similar explanations for the tendency of certain strains of mice to be more susceptible to certain autoimmune diseases, such as diabetes in nonobese diabetic (NOD) mice (24,25). Autoreactive cells can be found in the peripheral blood of normal individuals and patients with autoimmune diseases such as multiple sclerosis (26). The presence of autoreactive cells in the periphery alone is an insufficient explanation for the development of autoimmunity. The pool of autoreactive cells is much larger in patients with autoimmune diseases, they are in a different functional state (27–29), they have different effector profiles, or they have different thresholds of activation.

## PERIPHERAL MECHANISMS OF T-CELL TOLERANCE

### T-Cell Anergy

Efficient T-cell activation depends on two signals: an antigen-specific signal delivered through the TCR and a second costimulatory signal that induces secretion of T-cell growth factors such as interleukin-2 (IL-2). The best characterized costimulatory pathway is the B7 pathway (30,31). Two related B7 costimulatory molecules, B7.1 and B7.2, are expressed on APCs, although with different kinetics and expression patterns. B7.2 is found on most APCs at low but constitutive levels, whereas B7.1 usually is absent until an APC becomes activated, at which time it upregulates the expression of both molecules. These molecules direct signals into T cells through two receptors, CD28 and cytotoxic T-lymphocyte–associated molecule-4 (CTLA-4). Signals directed through CD28 enhance T-cell activation, and signals delivered through CTLA-4 attenuate T-cell activation (32,33).

The consequence of T-cell activation with peptide–MHC class II complexes in the absence of B7 costimulation was first reported by Jenkins and Schwartz (34). When ECDI-treated splenocytes (which effectively fixes the cell surface and inactivates many surface molecules) were used in vitro as APCs, they failed to stimulate proliferation by antigen-specific normal T-cell clones and instead induced a state of long-term unresponsiveness called anergy. This T-cell unresponsiveness was also induced in vivo by the intravenous administration of antigen-coupled splenocytes prepared by ECDI treatment. The results were not caused by extensive MHC class II complex alteration, because anti-MHC class II monoclonal antibodies prevented this anergy induction, suggesting that antigen presentation was taking place and needed for the anergy induction. The investigators proposed that the ECDI treatment impaired an additional APC signal necessary to induce IL-2 production and T-cell proliferation. However, the anergic state did not seem to involve inhibition of the IL-2 receptor pathway, because T-cell clones unable to respond to antigen–MHC restimulation responded normally to exogenous IL-2.

Extensive research has been conducted by a multitude of groups trying to induce anergy to prevent rejection in various models of transplantation and ameliorate a wide range of autoimmune diseases. Miller et al. used a system similar to the one used by Jenkins and Schwartz to demonstrate that chemical cross-linking of APCs pulsed with a variety of autoantigens and viral antigens known to induce various forms of experimental autoimmune encephalomyelitis (EAE),

a rodent model of multiple sclerosis, can induce tolerance and ameliorate or delay EAE (35–37). Working with human T-cell clones, Boussiotis et al. (38) found that stimulation of T-cell clones with fibroblasts expressing only MHC class II molecules (i.e., no B7.1 or B7.2 molecules present) resulted in anergy induction. If unmanipulated APCs were incubated with CTLA-4 immunoglobulin (CTLA4Ig) and mixed with T cells, an anergic state was similarly induced. In this case, the CTLA4Ig, a chimeric molecule with the binding domain of the high-affinity B7 receptor CTLA-4 fused to the constant portion of an immunoglobulin heavy chain, present in the cultures binds to the B7 molecules present on APCs and prevents delivery of a costimulatory signal to the responding T cells in the culture.

The immunosuppressive effects of in vivo CTLA4Ig administration have been well documented (39–41). It can induce T-cell tolerance, inhibit primary and secondary T-cell responses, and inhibit antibody production. It has been used in several models of autoimmune disease, and it was used in the treatment of mice with an experimental form of lupus and found to block autoantibody production and prolong life, even when treatment was delayed until the most advanced stage of clinical illness (42). Arima et al. (43) examined the effects of CTLA4Ig administration on the induction of EAE in Lewis rats. CTLA4Ig administration eight times before or immediately after immunization with spinal cord homogenate was able to prevent the development of EAE, and this was reversed by the administration of rIL-2 (suggesting that the cells were rendered anergic). However, administration of CTLA4Ig twice after immunization with spinal cord homogenate slightly enhanced the severity of disease, suggesting that blocking the CD28 pathway is most useful before T cells have been activated or clonally expanded.

CTLA4Ig administration has shown considerable promise in transplantation. Bluestone et al. (44) demonstrated that CTLA4Ig administration to mice receiving human pancreatic islets induced long-term, donor-specific tolerance (i.e., graft acceptance greater than 45 days, compared with 5 days for controls). Although CTLA4Ig treatment alone has shown promise in transplantation for the treatment of autoimmune diseases, a combination of CTLA4Ig and blocking monoclonal antibodies directed against CD40 or CD40L have shown considerably greater in vivo effects. This effect presumably is related to the fact that CD40 engagement on APCs induces upregulation of the B7 costimulatory molecules. One group demonstrated convincingly that, although administration of CTLA4Ig or anti-CD40 monoclonal antibodies could inhibit alloreactive mixed lymphocyte reactions in vitro and prevent skin graft rejection in vivo to some extent alone, they were extremely potent when combined (45). Another group similarly compared the administration of antihuman CD40L monoclonal antibody and CTLA4Ig alone or together in their ability to prevent renal allograft rejection in rhesus macaques. The allografts were mismatched for MHC class I and MHC class II antigens. Administration of anti-CD40L monoclonal antibody and CTLA4Ig was more effective than either agent alone, and there was no generalized immunosuppression in that *in vitro* mixed lymphocyte reactions were normal. Two monkeys receiving the optimal regimen were healthy for more than 150 days (46).

Sarvetnick's group has shown that anti-CD40L monoclonal antibodies given at 3 weeks of age to NOD mice, which develop spontaneous diabetes at about 10 weeks of age, prevented insulitis and diabetes. When measured *in vitro*, the monoclonal antibody treatment reduced antigen-specific T-cell proliferation and interferon-γ (IFN-γ) production (47).

### Activation-Induced Peripheral Cell Death

Lenardo et al. first characterized what has been called activation-induced cell death (AICD) (48). They noticed that suppressed T-cell proliferation *in vitro* at high antigen doses correlated with high IL-2 production and apoptosis. To explore this observation further, T cells were stimulated with antigen, placed in various concentrations of IL-2 for 2 days, and subsequently restimulated with antigen. They found that apoptosis occurred to degrees correlating with the amount of IL-2 present before antigen restimulation. Using TCR transgenic mice specific for an encephalitogenic MBP peptide, this group found that repeated immunizations of soluble MBP or MBP peptide could delete up to 80% of the MBP-specific T cells. The investigators argued that T cells "sensed" the intensity of an immune response by the level of cell cycling after initial antigen stimulation and that further antigen stimulation attenuated the immune response by decreasing the number of responding cells and downmodulating the amount of IL-2 production.

Using IL-2 receptor α-chain (CD25) knockout mice crossed with TCR transgenic mice, Van Parijs et al. (49) found that, as expected, these cells proliferated and survived less well than wild-type T cells and did not differentiate into effector cells. Stimulation in the presence of IL-15 compensated for this defect to some extent, probably because it signals through a common IL-2 receptor γ chain. Most importantly, these mice did not undergo AICD; IL-15 could not compensate for IL-2 and did not therefore increase the degree of AICD in the CD25 knockout TCR transgenic mice. These results confirmed *in vivo* that IL-2 responsiveness is necessary for AICD.

Many *in vitro* and *in vivo* models of AICD have found that signaling through CD28 on T cells can provide protection against apoptosis (50–53). This protection has been found to correlate with an increase in the intracellular expression of the antiapoptotic molecule Bcl-xl (member of the murine B-cell leukemia–lymphoma [Bcl] gene product family). Because it is clear that IL-2 is required to initiate and sustain an immune response and to help terminate a T-cell immune response through AICD, the role of costimulation in AICD could change depending on to what extent activation versus apoptosis was being favored by the IL-2 induced by the costimulatory signal. CD28 costimulation probably has roles in initiating a primary response, in maintaining T-cell viability

during a primary response, and in terminating excess antigen-specific T cells at the conclusion of an immune response.

One mechanism by which IL-2 may encourage AICD of T cells is through the upregulation of Fas ligand (FasL). In IL-2 receptor γ-chain knockout mice, there is a defect in peripheral CD4+ T-cell deletion (54). There is also a lack of FasL expression on activation, presumably explaining the lack of peripheral apoptosis. The data suggest there is a requirement for the common γ chain to convey the IL-2 signal into the cell for upregulation of FasL and subsequent AICD. Several reports demonstrated that the interaction between Fas and FasL on single T-cell clones or hybridomas could induce apoptosis after TCR triggering and T-cell activation (55–57). Abbas and Marshak-Rothstein demonstrated that mice with functional defects in the expression of Fas or FasL failed to undergo AICD and succumbed to massive lymphoproliferation and autoimmune disease (58). The kinetics of FasL expression are consistent with the notion that it plays a critical role in AICD, because it is almost exclusively expressed by activated T cells (59).

Immune privileged sites, such as the eyes or testes, may be protected by FasL expression on tissues within these sites (60,61). In an elegant study, Griffith et al. (62) used normal and gld mice (FasL-deficient mice) and showed that viral infection resulted in T-cell inflammation in the eyes of gld mice but not in those of normal mice because of apoptosis in the normal mice. Fas+ but not Fas− tumor cells were killed when placed in the anterior chamber of normal mice, further emphasizing that FasL expression may contribute to immune privilege.

Marrack et al. studied the mechanism of superantigen-mediated AICD *in vivo*. In mice injected with superantigen, T cells activated by the superantigen proliferate extensively and then rapidly die. The investigators found that lipopolysaccharide (LPS) administration was capable of preventing superantigen-driven T-cell death and that TNF-α mediated part of the effect (63). Another group elucidated the mechanism by which LPS protected CD4+ T cells from superantigen-mediated AICD. A small number of T cells were transferred into a syngeneic host, and the fate of the cells was tracked after immunization of the mice with the antigen for which the cells were specific. Co-injection of LPS significantly enhanced the clonal expansion of the transferred cells, their migration in germinal centers, and the help they provided for antibody production. Most importantly, the proinflammatory cytokines IL-1 and TNF-α could substitute for LPS, suggesting that the adjuvant effects of LPS are mediated in large part by proinflammatory cytokines (64).

### T-Cell Suppression by Cytokines

CD4+ helper T cells can be broadly categorized into one of several subsets according to the cytokines produced by the T cells after activation (65,66). Helper T cells type 1 (T$_H$1) secrete proinflammatory cytokines such as IFN-γ, TNF-α, and lymphotoxin (LT), which enhance APC activation and the clearance of many intracellular pathogens, whereas $T_H2$ cells secrete cytokines such as IL-4, IL-5, and IL-13. These cytokines aid in antibody class switching and elimination of many bloodborne infectious agents (65). The cytokines produced by each helper T-cell subset can themselves negatively regulate the differentiation of the other subset. IFN-γ produced by $T_H1$ cells inhibits the differentiation of naive T cells into $T_H2$ cells, and IL-4 secreted by $T_H2$ cells can inhibit the differentiation of $T_H1$ cells. The cytokines IL-10 and TGF-β, secreted by regulatory T cells type 1 ($T_R1$) and $T_H3$ cells, respectively, are potent suppressors of T-cell activation. IL-10 is potent at inhibiting LPS-induced macrophage cytokine production (67,68), and a combination of IL-4 and IL-10 can inhibit a delayed-type hypersensitivity reaction *in vivo* (69). *In vivo* administration of recombinant human interleukin-10 (rhIL-10) to humans has further demonstrated the ability of IL-10 to inhibit proinflammatory cytokine production (70). TGF-β can inhibit T-cell proliferation by a variety of mechanisms (71). The strategy of encouraging the development of $T_H2$, $T_R1$, or $T_H3$ T cells in an effort to inhibit pathogenic $T_H1$ cells has been called *immune deviation.*

Oral tolerance is being tested as a way to suppress the immune response in patients with autoimmune diseases such as multiple sclerosis, rheumatoid arthritis, and diabetes. Weiner and Hafler have conducted numerous studies demonstrating that the primary effect of oral tolerance is the expansion of antigen-specific T cells that secrete TGF-β (72,73). In one study, Weiner et al. examined brain tissue for cytokine expression in lesions from Lewis rats at the peak of EAE (74). $T_H1$ cytokines were present during peak disease but were diminished when rats were fed MBP. TGF-β also was present. In a phase II clinical study of the effects of oral administration of bovine MBP to patients with the relapsing-remitting form of multiple sclerosis, T-cell lines generated from patients fed oral MBP were found to secrete significantly more TGF-β in response to MBP than T-cell lines from patients not fed oral MBP (75).

Although inducing TGF-β secretion from autoreactive T cells by the oral administration of autoantigens is one form of inducing immune suppression, many studies have demonstrated that shifting autoreactive T cells toward a $T_H2$ phenotype shows promise in the prevention of $T_H1$-mediated autoimmune diseases (76). In one study, neuroantigen-specific T cells were differentiated *in vitro* into $T_H1$ or $T_H2$ phenotypes and then adoptively transferred into syngeneic mice and assessed for their ability to induce EAE (77). The data indicated that $T_H1$ but not $T_H2$ cells consistently induced disease and that $T_H2$ cells administered together with $T_H1$ cells could not prevent disease. However, another study demonstrated that the adoptive transfer of $T_H2$ MBP-specific T cells into syngeneic mice could reduce the incidence and eliminate EAE relapse (78). Another elegant study confirmed these results (79). EAE-susceptible SJL mice were immunized with the protein keyhole limpet hemocyanin (KLH) in incomplete Freund's adjuvant (IFA) to induce $T_H2$ cells reactive to KLH. EAE was then induced in the same mice using whole guinea pig myelin in complete Freund's adjuvant (CFA), which is known to induce proinflammatory cytokines and potent disease. The investigators found, when they included KLH with the whole myelin–CFA immunogen in mice that had been preimmunized with the KLH in IFA, that the disease was prevented or its severity greatly reduced. These results indicated that the cytokine microenvironment at the time autoreactive T cells are primed or activated could influence their pathogenicity. Moreover, $T_H2$ cytokines appeared to protect against disease, and this influence was effective even when cells were primed systemically rather than within the CNS. Consistent with this finding, Racke et al. (80) demonstrated that *in vivo* administration of IL-4 to mice ameliorated EAE clinical disease, induced $T_H2$ MBP-reactive T cells, diminished demyelination, and reduced inflammatory cytokines.

Two reports suggested future directions for modulating $T_H1$-mediated autoimmune diseases by cytokine-mediated suppression. Shaw et al. (81) described an attempt to ameliorate EAE induced in an adoptive transfer system by transducing a MBP-specific T-cell hybridoma with IL-4 and adoptively transferring it to mice. The investigators demonstrated a beneficial effect for local delivery of IL-4 in the CNS during the induction of disease. A similar study used a proteolipid protein (PLP)–specific T-cell clone transfected with IL-10 (82). The clone could significantly inhibit EAE disease induction or severity and to some extent ameliorate disease after onset.

### T-Cell Ignorance and Immune Privileged Sites

Several sites within the body have been designated by some investigators as immune privileged sites because of the relative difficulty of B-cell and T-cell migration into the sites. The CNS has been touted in the past as a prime example, particularly because of the tight endothelial junctions that help form the blood–brain barrier. However, experimental data have shown that T-cell migration into such sites occurs routinely and can do so with little pathogenic consequence (83).

There are probably several reasons that autoreactive T cells within an organ expressing the autoantigen may not necessitate an autoimmune response. Expression of FasL by the target tissue may induce apoptosis in autoreactive T cells. Alternately, the T cells may be rendered anergic. Goodnow et al. suggests that multiple mechanisms of tolerance exist and that self-reactive T cells do not necessarily cause tissue destruction when they encounter self antigen within an organ, a phenomena called clonal ignorance (84). In this study, the protein, Hen Egg Lysozyme (HEL), was expressed on the thyroid epithelium, pancreatic islet cells, or systemically in the presence of TCR transgenic T cells specific for HEL. The researchers found that the mechanisms used to induce tolerance depended on the location and concentration of antigen. When the self antigen was expressed in the thyroid or pancreas, T cells were less tolerant, and thyroiditis or insulitis

**TABLE 7.1.** *Mechanisms of T-cell tolerance*

| Type of tolerance | Mechanism | Relevant molecules or ligands |
|---|---|---|
| Central | Deletion by apoptosis | MHC molecules presenting (self) autoantigens |
| Peripheral | Anergy | B7.1/2:CD28 and CD40:CD40L pathways |
| | Activation-induced cell death (AICD) | IL-2, FasL |
| | Immune deviation/T-cell suppression | Antiinflammatory cytokines (IL-4, IL-10, TGF-β) |
| | Immune privilege | FasL |

occurred, although there was no destruction of self tissue; there was almost total deletion of T cells when HEL was expressed systemically. Other groups have seen similar influences of the site and concentration of antigen exposure to autoreactive T cells on the tolerance induced.

Hammerling's group (85) generated transgenic mice that expressed a foreign nonself MHC class I molecule on hepatocytes. Low levels of the MHC class I molecule were detected on mouse hepatocytes, but high levels could be induced by LPS treatment. The group found that, rather than simply ignoring the foreign tissue-specific antigen, T cells downregulated their expression of antigen-specific TCRs and were tolerant. When MHC class I expression was increased by LPS treatment, a portion of the previously tolerant cells appeared to be deleted. They concluded that the dose of antigen influences the degree of tolerance induced and that tolerant T cells are not necessarily refractory to further contact with the tolerogen and even greater tolerance induction or deletion. Tolerance, they hypothesize, may be the result of multiple interactions with antigen. Similarly, in another system, TCR transgenic T cells specific for male antigen were injected into thymectomized mice with various ratios of male and female bone marrow cells (86). The investigators found that, when antigen persisted, anergy was induced with high concentrations of antigen but that exhaustion occurred at lower antigen concentrations.

Most autoreactive T cells are deleted within the thymus by MHC complexes presenting a myriad of self antigens. This form of T-cell tolerance is called *central tolerance*. However, some presumably lower-affinity autoreactive T cells escape central tolerance and exist within the periphery of healthy, normal individuals without causing pathology because of the many peripheral mechanisms of tolerance. The many mechanisms of T-cell tolerance are summarized in Table 7.1.

## B-CELL TOLERANCE

Activation of B cells and antibody isotype class switching critically depend on T-cell help delivered by surface costimulatory molecules, such as CD40L expressed by activated T cells, or in the form of cytokines secreted by $T_H2$ cells, such as IL-4 and IL-5. Because of this dependence on T cells for complete maturation and activation, T-cell tolerance indirectly implies B-cell tolerance. However, several mechanisms ensure autoreactive B cells are not given the chance to receive aberrant T-cell help. These mechanisms are presented in Table 7.2 and discussed in the following sections.

### B-Cell Affinity Maturation

Within the paracortex of lymph nodes (or an analogous structure in the spleen), resting T cells can be found along with specialized APCs (i.e., follicular dendritic cells) that are presumably responsible for the initial stimulation of the T cells (87). Once stimulated, these T cells move to the paracortex–primary follicular junctions that are dominated by naive B cells that express mostly surface IgM or IgD receptors. In response to cytokines secreted by antigen-stimulated T cells nearby, a few antigen-specific B-cell clones divide to form germinal centers, made up mainly of these B-cell blasts and a few activated CD4+ T cells. Activated T cells with similar antigen specificity can then encourage the survival and expansion of B cells. Within these germinal centers, follicular dendritic cells capture and present intact antigen to B cells. Several days after an immune response has begun, antigen–antibody complexes may also bind to follicular dendritic cells. At this point, somatic mutations occur, ultimately leading to the generation of higher-affinity germinal center B cells. This process, called *affinity maturation*, is based on competition among the different B-cell clones with similar specificities. Those that after somatic mutations have a higher affinity for the antigen with which they interact compete for the antigen more effectively and continue their antigen-dependent clonal expansion. This is analogous to the process of positive selection of T cells; only cells that can productively engage antigen are given the chance to mature into competent lymphocytes of the periphery.

### Clonal Versus Receptor Selection

In an elegant series of papers, Nemazee's group has demonstrated that two mechanisms of immune tolerance are used within the bone marrow when immature B cells encounter self antigen and that the mechanism employed depends on the maturation state of the B cell. The first mechanism used to impart B-cell tolerance is referred to as *receptor editing*. If an immature self-reactive B-cell encounters self antigen in the bone marrow, the process promotes rearrangement of the second immunoglobulin receptor light chain in the hope of altering the B-cell receptor (BCR) specificity. In one study, two thirds of autoreactive immature B cells were found to undergo receptor editing without any significant apoptosis (88). Another study found that, later in B-cell development after receptor editing has occurred, immature B-cell engagement with self antigen leads to apoptosis within the bone marrow (89). Constitutive transgenic expression of the anti-

**TABLE 7.2.** *Mechanisms of B-cell tolerance*

| Type of tolerance | Mechanism | Relevant molecules or ligands |
|---|---|---|
| Central | Receptor editing | Early B-cell engagement of self antigen |
| | Clonal deletion | Late B-cell engagement of self antigen |
| Peripheral | Lack of T-cell help | CD40:CD40L pathway and cytokines (IL-4, IL-5) |
| | Deletion | Membrane-bound self antigen |
| | Anergy | Soluble self antigen |

apoptotic molecule BCL-2 could not prevent central tolerance imparted by self antigen expression within the bone marrow, but it did enhance the receptor editing process (90).

## B-Cell Clonal Deletion Versus Anergy

The bone marrow is the primary lymphoid organ responsible for development of B cells, and the secondary lymphoid organs, such as the spleen and lymph nodes, are specialized for generation of immune responses by B cells on antigen recognition. The lymph nodes drain most intercellular spaces by afferent lymphatic flow, and Peyer's patches, the appendix, and mesenteric nodes drain the intestines. Foreign antigens that enter the blood are cleared by the spleen.

The clever use of transgenic mice by Nemazee and Goodnow elucidated several mechanisms by which B-cell tolerance is induced. Nemazee and Burki (91) generated transgenic mice expressing anti-MHC membrane-bound immunoglobulin receptors that produced high levels of anti-MHC class I antibodies detectable in their sera. However, when they crossed them to mice expressing the same MHC class I autoantigen, the B cells were deleted. This mechanism of tolerance involving the deletion of autoreactive B-cell clones differed from another form of B-cell tolerance first described by Nossal and Pike (92). These investigators described the presence of B cells with autoantigen-specific immunoglobulin receptors that were functionally incapable of responding to antigen; this form of tolerance was referred to as *anergy*. Goodnow et al. confirmed both of these results using a similar system but with an elegant twist. They generated several different lines of transgenic mice. They generated transgenic mice that expressed a protein, HEL, in a membrane or soluble form and produced B-cell transgenic mice in which all the membrane immunoglobulin receptors were specific for the HEL antigen. When the BCR transgenic mice were crossed to the two different types of HEL transgenic mice, the autoreactive immature B cells were eliminated in the bone marrow on recognition of membrane-bound antigens, confirming the results of Nemazee et al. However, in mice in which the autoantigen was secreted into the serum, the B cells were not

deleted; they instead were anergized (93,94). When anergized, the B cells were found to downregulate the expression of their surface immunoglobulin receptors, and they had a greatly shortened lifespan of just 3 to 4 days. The work of these groups demonstrated that the induction of B-cell tolerance depends on the form in which antigen is recognized by an autoreactive B cell.

Using these same double-transgenic systems, the research groups discovered an additional mechanism of ensuring B-cell tolerance. When anergic B cells were transferred into mice with a diverse repertoire of B-cell receptors (e.g., non–immunoglobulin receptor transgenic mice) but that expressed soluble HEL protein systemically (which ensured the induction of anergy in HEL-specific B cells), Cyster et al. (95) found that the anergic B cells had an altered pattern of migration from the bone marrow. After leaving the bone marrow and being rendered anergic by engagement of soluble HEL in the periphery, the anergic B cell eventually migrated into the spleen. Within the spleen, however, these cells moved only to the outer part of the T-cell area, the periarteriolar lymphocyte sheath (PALS). Because they were anergic, they could not receive antigenic or costimulatory signals from the few T cells present in this area, signals that would encourage the B cells to proceed into the follicles, where extensive T-cell help and B-cell somatic hypermutation occurs.

## IMMUNE TOLERANCE AND AUTOIMMUNE DISEASES

There are many mechanisms by which the immune system seeks to ensure immune tolerance. Central tolerance of T cells and B cells involves primarily a deletional mechanism mediated by apoptosis. However, autoimmune T cells and B cells do exist in the periphery of normal individuals and experimental animals, but no autoimmune disease arises. Peripheral mechanisms of tolerance also play a significant role in preventing the development of autoimmunity. One of the biggest challenges to immunologists studying autoimmune diseases is to determine which mechanisms of ensuring tolerance have failed so that the appropriate treatment can be used for the disease.

For example, suppose that a failure to delete autoreactive T cells within the thymus proves to be responsible for a given autoimmune disease. If so, therapies are available and actively being refined that can delete autoreactive T cells within the thymus. Bone marrow chimerism, in which an allogeneic source of bone marrow from a healthy donor is transplanted into a diseased individual, has been shown to induce very efficient deletion of autoreactive cells (96). Bone marrow transplantation is being explored for the treatment of several autoimmune diseases, including multiple sclerosis and rheumatoid arthritis (97–99). If, however, there are defects in peripheral tolerance mechanisms, treatments using CTLA4Ig and anti-CD40L monoclonal antibodies may be capable of inducing anergic states in autoreactive T cells.

Alternately, oral tolerance may be used to suppress the autoreactive response or shift it toward a more benign type of response. Tremendous amounts of knowledge have been gained regarding the many ways in which the immune response can ensure a self-tolerant state, but little is known about which mechanisms are subverted in various auto-immune diseases.

## REFERENCES

1. Markowitz J, Auchincloss HJ, Gursby M, et al. Class II–positive hematopoietic cells cannot mediate positive selection of CD4+ T lymphocytes in class II–deficient mice. *Proc Natl Acad Sci USA* 1993; 90:2779–2783.
2. Laufer T, DeKoning J, Markowitz J, et al. Unopposed positive selection and autoreactivity in mice expressing class II MHC only on thymic cortex. *Nature* 1996;383:81–85.
3. Laufer TM, Fan L, Glimcher LH. Self-reactive T cells selected on thymic cortical epithelium are polyclonal and are pathogenic *in vivo*. *J Immunol* 1999;162:5078–5084.
4. Surh C, Sprent J. T-cell apoptosis detected in situ during positive and negative selection in the thymus. *Nature* 1994;372:100–103.
5. Oukka M, Colucci-Guyon E, Tran P, et al. CD4 T cell tolerance to nuclear proteins induced by medullary thymic epithelium. *Immunity* 1996;4:545–553.
6. Evavold BD, Allen PM. Separation of IL-4 production from Th cell proliferation by an altered T cell receptor ligand. *Science* 1991;252: 1308–1310.
7. Allen P. Peptides in positive and negative selection: a delicate balance. *Cell* 1994;76:593–596.
8. Vidal K, Hsu B, Williams C, et al. Endogenous altered peptide ligands can affect peripheral T cell responses. *J Exp Med* 1996;183:1311–1312.
9. Bevan M. In thymic selection, peptide diversity gives and takes away. *Immunity* 1997;7:175–178.
10. Ignatowicz L, Kappler J, Marrack P. The repertoire of T cells shaped by a single MHC/peptide ligand. *Cell* 1996;84:521–529.
11. Grubin C, Kovats S, deRoos P, et al. Deficient positive selection of CD4 T cells in mice displaying altered repertoires of MHC class II–bound self-peptides. *Immunity* 1997;7:197–208.
12. Surh C, Lee D, Fung-Leung W, et al. Thymic selection by a single MHC/peptide ligand produces a semidiverse repertoire of CD4+ T cells. *Immunity* 1997;7:209–219.
13. Ashton-Rickardt PG, Bandeira A, Delaney JR, et al. Evidence for a differential avidity model of T cell selection in the thymus. *Cell* 1994; 76:651–663.
14. Girao C, Hu Q, Sun J, et al. Limits to the differential avidity model of T cell selection in the thymus. *J Immunol* 1997;159:4205–4211.
15. Hogquist KA, Jameson SC, Health WR, et al. T cell receptor antagonist peptides induce positive selection. *Cell* 1994;76:17–27.
16. Hogquist K, Jameson S, Bevan M. Strong agonist ligands for the T cell receptor do not mediate positive selection of functional CD8+ T cells. *Immunity* 1995;3:79–86.
17. Sebzda E, Wallace V, Mayer J, et al. Positive and negative thymocyte selection induced by different concentrations of a single peptide. *Science* 1994;263:1615–1618.
18. Cook J, Wormstall E, Hornell T, et al. Quantitation of the cell surface level of Ld resulting in positive versus negative selection of the 2C transgenic T cell receptor *in vivo*. *Immunity* 1997;7:233–241.
19. Alam S, Travers P, Wung J, et al. T-cell-receptor affinity and thymocyte positive selection. *Nature* 1996;381:616–620.
20. Langman R, Cohn M. Terra firma: a retreat from danger. *J Immunol* 1996;157:4273–4276.
21. Cohen J. Apoptosis. *Immunol Today* 1993;14:126–130.
22. Le P, Maecher H, Cook J. *In situ* detection and characterization of apoptotic thymocytes in human thymus: expression of bcl-2 *in vivo* does not prevent apoptosis. *J Immunol* 1995;154:4371–4378.
23. Liu G, Farichild P, Smith R, et al. Low avidity recognition of self-antigen by T cells permits escape from central tolerance. *Immunity* 1995;3: 407–415.
24. Kanagawa O, Martin S, Vaupel B, et al. Autoreactivity of T cells from nonobese diabetic mice: an I-Ag7-dependent reaction. *Proc Natl Acad Sci USA* 1998;95:1721–1724.
25. Ridgway WM, Fasso M, Fathman CG. A new look at MHC and auto-immune disease. *Science* 1999;284:749–751.
26. Ota K, Matsui M, Milford E, et al. T-cell recognition of an immunodominant myelin basic protein epitope in multiple sclerosis. *Nature* 1990;346:183–187.
27. Scholz C, Patton K, Anderson D, et al. Expansion of autoreactive T cells in multiple sclerosis is independent of exogenous B7 costimulation. *J Immunol* 1998;160:1532–1538.
28. Zhang J, Markovic S, Raus J, et al. Increased frequency of IL-2 responsive T cells specific for myelin basic protein and proteolipid protein in peripheral blood and cerebrospinal fluid of patients with multiple sclerosis. *J Exp Med* 1994;179:973–984.
29. Lovett-Racke A, Trotter J, Lauber J, et al. Decreased dependence of myelin basic protein-reactive T cells on CD28-mediated costimulation in multiple sclerosis patients. *J Clin Invest* 1998;101:725–730.
30. Lenschow D, Bluestone JA. CD28/B7 system of T cell costimulation. *Annu Rev Immunol* 1996;14:233–258.
31. Tivol E, Schweitzer AN, Sharpe AH. Costimulation and autoimmunity. *Curr Opin Immunol* 1996;8:822–830.
32. Linsley P. Distinct roles for CD28 and cytotoxic T lymphocyte–associated molecule-4 receptors during T-cell activation? *J Exp Med* 1995;182: 289–292.
33. Thompson CB, Allison JP. The emerging role of CTLA-4 as an immune attenuator. *Immunity* 1997;7:445–450.
34. Jenkins MK, Pardoll DM, Mizuguchi J, et al. T-cell unresponsiveness *in vivo* and *in vitro*: fine specificity of induction and molecular characterization of the unresponsive state. *Immunol Rev* 1987;95:113–135.
35. Karpus W, Pope J, Peterson J, et al. Inhibition of Theiler's virus-mediated demyelination by peripheral immune tolerance induction. *J Immunol* 1995;155:947–957.
36. Kennedy K, Smith W, Miller S, et al. Induction of antigen-specific tolerance for the treatment of ongoing, relapsing autoimmune encephalomyelitis: a comparison between oral and peripheral tolerance. *J Immunol* 1997;159:1036–1044.
37. Vandenbark A, Celnik B, Vainiene M, et al. Myelin antigen-coupled splenocytes suppress experimental autoimmune encephalomyelitis in Lewis rats through a partially reversible anergy mechanism. *J Immunol* 1995;155:5861–5867.
38. Boussiotis V, Barber D, Nakaria T, et al. Prevention of T cell anergy by signaling through the gamma c chain of the IL-2 receptor. *Science* 1994;266:1039–1042.
39. Linsley PS, Wallace PM, Johnson J, et al. Immunosuppression *in vivo* by a soluble form of the CTLA-4 T cell activation molecule. *Science* 1992;257:792–795.
40. Milich D, Chen M, Hughes J, et al. The secreted hepatitis B precore antigen can modulate the immune response to the nucleocapsid: a mechanism for persistence. *J Immunol* 1998;160:2013–2021.
41. Wallace P, Rodgers J, Leytze G, et al. Induction and reversal of long-lived specific unresponsiveness to a T-dependent antigen following CTLA4Ig treatment. *J Immunol* 1995;154:5885–5895.
42. Finck B, Linsley P, Wofsy D. Treatment of murine lupus with CTLA4Ig. *Science* 1994;261:1225–1227.
43. Arima T, Rehman A, Hickey W, et al. Inhibition by CTLA4Ig of experimental allergic encephalomyelitis. *J Immunol* 1996;156:4916–4924.
44. Lenschow DJ, Zeng Y, Thistlethwaite Jr, et al. Long-term survival of xenogeneic pancreatic islet grafts induced by CTLA4lg. *Science* 1992;257:789–792.
45. Larsen C, Elwood E, Alexander D, et al. Long-term acceptance of skin and cardiac allografts after blocking CD40 and CD28 pathways. *Nature* 1996;381:434–438.
46. Kirk A, Harlan D, Armstrong N, et al. CTLA-Ig and anti-CD40 ligand prevent renal allograft rejection in primates. *Proc Natl Acad Sci USA* 1997;94:8789–8794.
47. Balasa B, Krahl T, Patstone G, et al. CD40 ligand-CD40 interactions are necessary for the initiation of insulitis and diabetes in nonobese diabetic mice. *J Immunol* 1997;159:4620–4627.
48. Critchfield J, Racke M, Zuniga-Pflucker J, et al. T cell deletion in high antigen dose therapy of autoimmune encephalomyelitis. *Science* 1994; 263:1139–1143.

49. Van Parijs L, Biuckians A, Ibragimov A, et al. Functional responses and apoptosis of CD25 (IL-2R alpha)-deficient T cells expressing a transgenic antigen receptor. *J Immunol* 1997;158:3738–3745.

50. Noel P, Biose L, Thompson C. CD28 costimulation prevents cell death during primary T cell activation. *J Immunol* 1996;157:636–642.

51. Boise L, Minn A, Noel P, et al. 1995; CD28 costimulation can promote T cell survival by enhancing the expression of Bcl-XL. *Immunity* 1995;3:87–98.

52. Mueller D, Seiffert S, Fang W, et al. Differential regulation of bcl-2 and bcl-x by CD3, CD28, and the IL-2 receptor in cloned CD4$^+$ helper T cells: a model for the long-term survival of memory cells. *J Immunol* 1996;156:1764–1771.

53. Radvanyi L, Shi Y, Vaziri H, et al. CD28 costimulation inhibits TCR-induced apoptosis during a primary T cell response. *J Immunol* 1996;156:1788–1798.

54. Nakajima H, Leonard W. Impaired peripheral deletion of activated T cells in mice lacking the common cytokine receptor gamma-chain: defective Fas ligand expression in gamma-chain–deficient mice. *J Immunol* 1997;159:4737–4744.

55. Brunner T, Mogil R, LaFace D, et al. Cell-autonomous Fas (CD95)/Fas-ligand interaction mediates activation-induced apoptosis in T-cell hybridomas. *Nature* 1995;373:441–444.

56. Dhein J, Walczak H, Baumler C, et al. Autocrine T-cell suicide mediated by APO-1/(Fas/CD95). *Nature* 1995;373:438–441.

57. Ju S, Panka D, Cui H, et al. Fas (CD95)/FasL interactions required for programmed cell death after T-cell activation. *Nature* 1995;373:444–448.

58. Ettinger R, Wang J, Bossu P, et al. Functional distinctions between MRL-lpr and MRL-gld lymphocytes: normal cells reverse the gld but not lpr immunoregulatory defect. *J Immunol* 1994;152:1557–1568.

59. Nagata S, Golstein P. The Fas death factor. *Science* 1995;267:1449–1456.

60. Streilein J. Unraveling immune privilege. *Science* 1996;270:1158–1159.

61. Streilein J, Ksander B, Taylor A. Immune deviation in relation to ocular immune privilege. *J Immunol* 1997;158:3557–3560.

62. Griffith T, Brunner T, Fletcher S, et al. Fas ligand-induced apoptosis as a mechanism of immune privilege. *Science* 1996;270:1189–1192.

63. Vella A, McCormack J, Linsley P, et al. Lipopolysaccharide interferes with the induction of peripheral T cell death. *Immunity* 1995;2:261–270.

64. Pape K, Khoruts A, Mondino A, et al. Inflammatory cytokines enhance the *in vivo* clonal expansion and differentiation of antigen-activated CD4$^+$ T cells. *J Immunol* 1997;159:591–598.

65. Abbas A, Murphy K, Sher A. Functional diversity of helper T lymphocytes. *Nature* 1996;383:787–793.

66. O'Garra A. Cytokines induce the development of functionally heterogeneous T helper cell subsets. *Immunity* 1998;8:275–283.

67. Fiorentino D, Zlotnik A, Mosmann T, et al. IL-10 inhibits cytokine production by activated macrophages. *J Immunol* 1991;147:3815–3822.

68. Wang P, Wu P, Siegel M, et al. IL-10 inhibits transcription of cytokine genes in human peripheral blood mononuclear cells. *J Immunol* 1994;153:811–816.

69. Powrie F, Menon S, Coffman R. Interleukin-4 and interleukin-10 synergize to inhibit cell-mediated immunity *in vivo*. *Eur J Immunol* 1993;23:3043–3049.

70. Pajkrt D, Camoglio L, Tiel-van Buul M, et al. Attenuation of proinflammatory response by recombinant human IL-10 in human endotoxemia: effect of timing of recombinant human IL-10 administration. *J Immunol* 1997;158:3971–3977.

71. Bright J, Kerr L, Sriram S. TGF-beta inhibits IL-2–induced tyrosine phosphorylation and activation of Jak-1 and Stat-5 in T lymphocytes. *J Immunol* 1997;159:175–183.

72. Chen Y, Inobe J, Weiner H. Induction of oral tolerance to myelin basic protein in CD8-depleted mice: both CD4$^+$ and CD8$^+$ cells mediated active suppression. *J Immunol* 1995;155:910–916.

73. Weiner H. Oral tolerance: immune mechanisms and treatment of autoimmune diseases. *Immunol Today* 1997;18:335–343.

74. Khoury SJ, Hancock WW, Weiner HL. Oral tolerance to myelin basic protein and natural recovery from experimental autoimmune encephalomyelitis are associated with down-regulation of inflammatory cytokines and differential upregulation of TGF-β, IL-4 and PGE expression in the brain. *J Exp Med* 1992;176:1355–1364.

75. Fukaura H, Kent S, Pietrusewicz M, et al. Induction of circulating myelin basic protein and proteolipid protein-specific transforming growth factor-β1-secreting Th3 T cells by oral administration of myelin in multiple sclerosis. *J Clin Invest* 1996;98:70–77.

76. Nicholson L, Kuchroo V. Manipulation of the Th1/Th2 balance in autoimmune disease. *Curr Opin Immunol* 1996;8:837–842.

77. Khoruts A, Miller S, Jenkins M. Neuroantigen-specific Th2 cells are inefficient suppressors of experimental autoimmune encephalomyelitis induced by effector Th1 cells. *J Immunol* 1995;155:5011–5017.

78. Cua D, Hinton D, Stohlman S. Self-antigen-induced Th2 responses in experimental allergic encephalomyelitis (EAE)-resistant mice: Th2-mediated suppression of autoimmune disease. *J Immunol* 1995;155:4052–4059.

79. Falcone M, Bloom B. A T helper cell 2 (Th2) immune response against non-self antigens modifies the cytokine profile of autoimmune T cells and protects against experimental allergic encephalomyelitis. *J Exp Med* 1997;185:901–907.

80. Racke M, Bonomo A, Scott D, et al. Cytokine-induced immune deviation as a therapy for inflammatory autoimmune disease. *J Exp Med* 1994;180:1961–1966.

81. Shaw M, Lorans J, Dhawan A, et al. Local delivery of interleukin-4 by retrovirus-transduced T lymphocytes ameliorates experimental autoimmune encephalomyelitis. *J Exp Med* 1997;185:1711–1714.

82. Mathisen P, Yu M, Johnson J, et al. Treatment of experimental autoimmune encephalomyelitis with genetically modified memory T cells. *J Exp Med* 1997;186:159–164.

83. Williams K, Hickey W. Traffic of hematogenous cells through the central nervous system. *Curr Top Microbiol Immunol* 1995;202:221–245.

84. Akkaraju S, Ho W, Leong D, et al. A range of CD4 T cell tolerance: partial inactivation to organ-specific antigen allows nondestructive thyroiditis or insulitis. *Immunity* 1997;7:255–271.

85. Ferber I, Schonrich G, Schenkel J, et al. Levels of peripheral T cell tolerance induced by different doses of tolerogen. *Science* 1994;263:674–676.

86. Rocha B, Grandien A, Freitas A. Anergy and exhaustion are independent mechanisms of peripheral T cell tolerance. *J Exp Med* 1995;181:993–1003.

87. Weissman I. Developmental switches in the immune system. *Cell* 1994;76:207–218.

88. Melamed D, Nemazee D. Self-antigen does not accelerate immature B cell apoptosis but stimulates receptor editing as a consequence of developmental arrest. *Proc Natl Acad Sci USA* 1997;94:9267–9272.

89. Melamed D, Benschop R, Cambier J, et al. Developmental regulation of B lymphocyte immune tolerance compartmentalized clonal selection from receptor selection. *Cell* 1998;92:173–182.

90. Lang J, Arnold B, Hammerling G, et al. Enforced Bcl-2 expression inhibits antigen-mediated clonal elimination of peripheral B cells in an antigen dose-dependent manner and promotes receptor editing in autoreactive, immature B cells. *J Exp Med* 1997;186:1513–1522.

91. Nemazee D, Burki K. Clonal deletion of B lymphocytes in a transgenic mouse bearing anti-MHC class I antibody genes. *Nature* 1989;337:562–566.

92. Nossal G, Pike B. Clonal anergy: persistence in tolerant mice of antigen-binding B lymphocytes incapable of responding to antigen or mitogen. *Proc Natl Acad Sci USA* 1980;77:1602–1606.

93. Goodnow CC. Transgenic mice and analysis of B-cell tolerance. *Annu Rev Immunol* 1992;10:489–518.

94. Fulcher D, Basten A. Reduced life span of anergic self-reactive B cells in a double-transgenic model. *J Exp Med* 1994;179:125–134.

95. Cyster J, Hartley S, Goodnow C. Competition for follicular niches excludes self-reactive cells from the recirculating B-cell repertoire. *Nature* 1994;371:389–395.

96. Nikolic B, Sykes M. Bone marrow chimerism and transplantation tolerance. *Curr Opin Immunol* 1997;9:634–640.

97. Burt R, Burns W, Miller S. Bone marrow transplantation for multiple sclerosis: returning to Pandora's box. *Immunol Today* 1997;18:559–561.

98. Fassas A, Anagnostopoulos A, Kazis A, et al. Peripheral blood stem cell transplantation in the treatment of progressive multiple sclerosis: first results of a pilot study. *Bone Marrow Transplant* 1997;20:631–638.

99. Krance R, Brenner M. BMT beats autoimmune disease. *Nat Med* 1998;4:153–155.

*Textbook of the Autoimmune Diseases,*
Edited by R. G. Lahita, N. Chiorazzi, and W. H. Reeves,
Lippincott Williams & Wilkins, Philadelphia © 2000.

# CHAPTER 8

# Autoantibodies

Westley H. Reeves, Hanno B. Richards, and Minoru Satoh

The classic studies of hemolytic antibodies by Paul Ehrlich early in the 20th century laid the foundation for our current concepts of autoimmunity. Soon after 1900, he coined the term *autoimmunity* to signify an immune response against self and introduced the concept of *horror autotoxicus.* By this term, he suggested that there are powerful mechanisms protecting the organism against autoimmunity. Although these mechanisms were originally thought to prevent autoimmunization entirely, it became clear over the intervening one-half century that autoimmunity is a relatively common occurrence. Autoimmunity may be mediated primarily by T cells, as in the case of experimental autoimmune encephalomyelitis (1), or by B cells (autoantibodies), as in systemic lupus erythematosus (SLE) (2).

This chapter focuses on the production of autoantibodies and their role in disease pathogenesis. Although autoantibodies are the products of B cells, their production in many cases also requires autoreactive T cells. Not all autoantibodies cause autoimmune disease. In some instances, a pathogenic role is clear, but in others, autoantibodies may serve as a marker of an autoimmune process without having a direct role in disease pathogenesis.

## CLASSIFICATION OF AUTOANTIBODIES

Autoantibodies to a variety of normal cellular and extracellular constituents have been described (Table 8.1). It is useful to classify them according to whether they are directed against components of all cells or components unique to particular organs or tissues. Organ-specific autoantibodies are commonly associated with limited autoimmune disorders, such as autoimmune thyroiditis, diabetes mellitus, or paraneoplastic syndromes. In contrast, autoantibodies against the nuclear or cytoplasmic antigens found in all cells

are typical of systemic autoimmune conditions, such as SLE, polymyositis/dermatomyositis (PM/DM), or systemic sclerosis (SSc).

## DETECTION OF AUTOANTIBODIES

Highly specific and sensitive assays are available for detecting many types of autoantibodies. Widely used techniques include immunofluorescence, enzyme-linked immunosorbent assays (ELISAs), double immunodiffusion, agglutination assays, immunoblotting, and immunoprecipitation. A brief discussion of these assays follows, emphasizing advantages and pitfalls.

### Immunofluorescence

The fluorescent antinuclear antibody (FANA) assay is a classic example of the detection of autoantibodies by immunofluorescence techniques. Antinuclear antibodies are a hallmark of systemic autoimmune diseases such as SLE and SSc (3). The FANA test detects autoantibodies in a test serum against a variety of nuclear antigens, including proteins, nucleic acids, and nucleic acid–protein complexes. As illustrated in Figure 8.1 Top, human Hep-2 cells (laryngeal carcinoma cell line) adherent to a microscope slide are fixed and permeabilized, and they are then incubated with the patient's serum. The slide is washed to remove unbound antibodies and incubated with fluorescent antiimmunoglobulin antibodies. The slide is then viewed using a fluorescence microscope, and nuclear staining is scored by intensity and pattern at various serum dilutions. The staining pattern depends on the location of the target antigen, such as diffuse (homogeneous), speckled, nucleolar, and centromere (Fig. 8.1 Bottom). This technique also is useful for detecting autoantibodies against cytoplasmic antigens, such as mitochondria, ribosomes, or tRNA synthetases. The advantages of the FANA assay are its sensitivity and simplicity, making it an ideal screening assay for SLE and other systemic autoimmune diseases. However, the specificity is relatively low, as discussed later.

W. H. Reeves, H. B. Richards, M. Satoh: Department of Medicine, University of Florida, Gainesville, Florida 32610.

**TABLE 8.1.** *Classification of diseases associated with autoantibodies*

*Diseases with organ-specific autoantibodies*
Endocrine disease
    Insulin-dependent diabetes mellitus: glutamic acid decarboxylase, insulin
    Autoimmune thyroiditis
        Graves' disease: thyroid-stimulating hormone
        Hashimoto's thyroiditis: thyroid microsomal antibodies
Liver disease
    Autoimmune hepatitis (lupoid hepatitis): anti-smooth muscle antibodies
Gastrointestinal tract disease
    Pernicious anemia: anti-parietal cell antibodies
Blood disease
    Autoimmune hemolytic anemia: warm autoantibodies, cold agglutinins
    Autoimmune thrombocytopenia: anti-platelet antibodies
    Autoimmune neutropenia: anti-neutrophil antibodies
    Autoimmune coagulopathies: clotting factors (e.g., factor VIII), $\beta_2$-glycoprotein I
Skin disease
    Vitiligo (anti-melanocyte antibodies)
    Bullous pemphigoid: anti-hemidesmosome antigens (BPAG1, BPAG2)
    Pemphigus vulgaris: desmoglein 1
Central nervous system disease
    Myasthenia gravis: acetylcholine receptor
    Paraneoplastic cerebellar syndromes (Stiff man syndrome): glutamic acid decarboxylase
Renal disease
    Goodpasture's syndrome: glomerular basement membrane
    Tubulointerstitial nephritis: proton translocating ATPase
Vascular disease
    Vasculitis: myeloperoxidase, proteinase III

*Diseases with non–organ-specific autoantibodies*
Systemic lupus erythematosus: nuclear and ribosomal antigens
Systemic sclerosis: nucleolar antigens
Polymyositis/dermatomyositis: tRNA synthetases and other cytoplasmic antigens
Primary biliary cirrhosis: mitochondria, nuclear envelope
Sjögren's syndrome: cytoplasmic and nuclear antigens
Rheumatoid arthritis: IgG (Fc), nuclear antigens

## Enzyme-Linked Immunosorbent Assay

ELISAs, like the FANA assay, are relatively simple, rapid, sensitive tests for autoantibodies that are useful for screening purposes (4). In a typical ELISA, plastic wells of a microtiter plate are coated with a purified antigen. Diluted test serum is added, followed by enzyme- or radioactively labeled anti-immunoglobulin antibodies. Binding of the second antibody is detected by adding a substrate for the enzyme, forming a colored product. The product is quantitated by determining absorbance in a spectrophotometer. In view of their high sensitivity, ELISAs must be standardized carefully to avoid measuring nonspecific binding.

A major drawback of ELISAs is that results depend on the purity of the antigen used to coat the wells. Variations on the standard ELISA technique have been employed, such as the double-sandwich or antigen-capture assay (4), in which antigen is affinity purified onto the wells using a monoclonal antibody. This approach allows the antigen to be highly purified but has the disadvantage that sera containing anti-immunoglobulin antibodies, such as rheumatoid factors, may bind to the monoclonal antibody itself, leading to false-positive results.

## Double Immunodiffusion

Double immunodiffusion in agarose gels (Ouchterlony) is a early immunochemical test that still is used widely (5). The test is performed by placing antigen and antibody into wells punched out from an agarose gel. Each reactant diffuses radially through the agarose gel, with concentration decreasing as a geometric function of distance from the well. An insoluble precipitin line, consisting of immune complexes, forms where the antigen and antibody meet in approximately equal concentrations. The precipitin line can be viewed directly in the gel. If two serum samples contain the same specificity, their precipitin lines fuse, forming a curved "line of identity." Double immunodiffusion is employed extensively for autoantibody screening in SLE and other systemic autoimmune diseases. Anti-Sm, nRNP, Ro (SS-A), La (SS-B), topoisomerase I, ribosomal P, and other serum autoantibodies can be detected in this manner (3). The advantage of this test is its simplicity and specificity. The main disadvantages are that it is relatively labor intensive and of lower sensitivity than alternatives, such as ELISA.

## Agglutination Immunoassays

Agglutination assays are based on the ability of an antibody to agglutinate large particles, such as red blood cells or latex beads, coated with the corresponding antigen (6). Pentavalent IgM antibodies agglutinate particles several hundred times more efficiently than IgG antibodies because they can bind to more than one site on a single particle and have the potential to cross-link sites on a larger number of different particles. A latex bead agglutination test is used for detecting antiimmunoglobulin antibodies (rheumatoid factors) (7). The direct and indirect antiglobulin (Coombs') tests (8) are hemagglutination assays used in the diagnosis of autoimmune hemolytic anemia. The advantages of agglutination techniques include ease of use, rapidity, and high sensitivity. The technique is limited by the requirement for purified antigens and the ability to link them to inert particles, such as latex beads.

## Immunoblotting

The immunoblot (Western blot) technique is in some respects analogous to ELISA. Instead of coating the antigen on plastic, the proteins in a crude or purified antigen preparation are separated according to molecular weight by sodium dodecyl

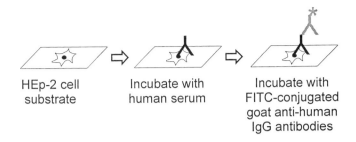

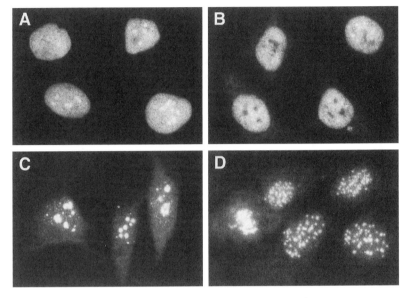

FIG. 8.1. Fluorescent antinuclear antibody assay. **Top:** In this diagram of the assay, Hep-2 cells (human laryngeal carcinoma cell line) are grown on a coverslip, washed, and fixed. The cells are then incubated with human test serum, followed by fluorescently tagged goat anti-human immunoglobulin antibodies. **Bottom:** Slides are viewed with fluorescence microscopy, and the distribution and intensity of fluorescent staining at different dilutions are scored. Illustrated are the typical patterns: diffuse (**A**), speckled (sparing the nucleolar regions) (**B**), nucleolar (**C**), and centromere (**D**). In panel **D**, the staining of centromeres lined up along the metaphase plate of a mitotic cell, which distinguishes anticentromere staining from other speckled patterns.

sulfate (SDS)–polyacrylamide gel electrophoresis and transferred electrophoretically to a suitable membrane, such as nitrocellulose (9). The membrane is then incubated with diluted test serum, followed by an enzyme-labeled second antibody. A substrate that forms an insoluble product is used so that the colored reaction product is deposited on the membrane. Radioactive or chemiluminescent detection systems also may be employed. This technique permits reactivity of the test serum with individual proteins in a complex mixture to be assayed. The technique is very sensitive but more demanding technically than other assays. A major drawback is that Western blot assays do not define relationships among the various components of a particle, because the test is performed after dissociating the antigen. Many antigenic determinants are conformational, and may be destroyed by the harsh detergents used in SDS-polyacrylamide gel electrophoresis.

### Immunoprecipitation

Although gel diffusion and ELISA allow detection of autoantibodies to native antigenic determinants, the composition of the antigenic particles and fine specificities of the autoantibodies cannot readily be determined. Western blot, although useful for defining fine specificities, is of limited value for detecting antibodies against conformational epi-

topes. For this reason, immunoprecipitation of radiolabeled cell extracts has become an important research tool for examining autoantibody specificities.

Radiolabeled antigens are allowed to form immune complexes with autoantibodies, which are purified onto protein A–Sepharose beads. After dissociating the immune complexes from the beads, the radiolabeled proteins are separated by SDS-polyacrylamide gel electrophoresis and detected by autoradiography (3). A similar approach can be used to analyze the nucleic acid components of small ribonucleoprotein particles (10).

### IMPORTANCE OF AUTOANTIBODIES IN DISEASE PATHOGENESIS

A distinction must be made between autoimmunity and autoimmune disease. Although autoantibody production is a frequent manifestation of autoimmune reactions, it does not always lead to autoimmune disease. Autoantibodies cause disease by mechanisms analogous to those involved in allergic reactions. Four types of hypersensitivity reactions were classified by Gell and Coombs (11). Two of them, type II (antibody-mediated cytotoxic hypersensitivity) and type III (immune complex–mediated hypersensitivity) are relevant to the induction of disease by autoantibodies. Prototypes of each mechanism are considered in the following sections.

## Type II Hypersensitivity

Autoantibody-mediated cytotoxicity is an important mechanism in the pathogenesis of a number of autoimmune conditions. Autoantibodies against cell-surface antigens may initiate cell destruction by complement-mediated lysis, phagocytosis, or antibody-dependent cell-mediated cytotoxicity (ADCC). Examples are the autoimmune hemolytic anemias and autoimmune thrombocytopenia. Alternatively, autoantibodies may bind to surface receptors and activate or inhibit their function. Anti-TSH receptor autoantibodies in Graves' disease are representative of agonistic autoantibodies, whereas antiacetylcholine receptor autoantibodies in myasthenia gravis illustrate antagonistic autoantibodies.

### Autoimmune Hemolytic Anemia: Type IIA Hypersensitivity

Autoimmune hemolytic anemias (AIHA) are a diverse group of clinical syndromes mediated by different types of autoantibodies against red blood cells. The mechanism of hemolysis depends on the type of autoantibodies produced (Table 8.2). Autoimmune hemolysis has been classified into two groups on the basis of thermal reactivity of the autoantibodies (12–14). Warm autoantibodies react optimally at temperatures of 35 to 40°C, whereas cold agglutinins and other cold-reactive autoantibodies begin to react at 28 to 32°C and exhibit maximal reactivity at 4°C. Warm autoantibodies are typically polyclonal IgG, although they rarely may be IgM or IgA. Most are IgG1 subclass antibodies reactive with Rh antigens that are detectable using the direct antiglobulin (Coombs') test (12,13). Erythrophagocytosis mediated by Fc receptors located on hepatic Kupffer cells and splenic marginal zone macrophages is the major mechanism of red blood cell destruction in most patients with warm autoantibodies (15,16).

Fc receptors for IgG are multimeric cell-surface receptors that mediate phagocytosis, ADCC, activation of tyrosine kinases, release of inflammatory mediators, and transcription of cytokine genes (17). Three types of stimulatory Fc receptors appear to be involved in the pathogenesis of AIHA: the high-affinity FcγRI receptor, which binds monomeric IgG, and the FcγRIIA and FcγRIII receptors, which because of their low affinity can bind only multivalent immune complexes (15,17) (Table 8.3). Inhibitory Fc receptors, such as FcγRIIB, also have been reported (18).

Fc receptors that trigger phagocyte activation, endocytosis, and phagocytosis have one or more intracytoplasmic immunoreceptor tyrosine-based activation motifs (ITAMs) (18). FcγRI (CD64) and FcγRIIIA (CD16) are multichain receptors consisting of an IgG binding α subunit plus a γ subunit bearing an ITAM (18,19). In contrast, FcγRIIA is a single chain IgG receptor bearing an intrachain ITAM within the cytoplasmic domain.

Activated macrophages from γ-chain–deficient mice are defective in expression of FcγRI and FcγRIII, lack phagocytic activity, and have defective ADCC (19). The γ-chain–deficient mice are resistant to the development of experimental immune hemolytic anemia induced by IgG rabbit antimouse red blood cell antibodies (15). Complement fixation and uptake of red blood cells by phagocyte complement receptors may play only a secondary role, because experimental immune hemolytic anemia develops normally in C3-deficient mice (16).

In striking contrast to warm autoantibody-mediated AIHA, AIHA induced by cold agglutinins is complement mediated (13,14). FcγR-mediated erythrophagocytosis is not involved, because these autoantibodies are IgMs, which cannot be taken up by reticuloendothelial cell Fc receptors. Idiopathic cold agglutinin disease generally is associated with an IgM paraprotein recognizing a red blood cell antigen, most often the I antigen (Table 8.2). Unlike IgG, which must be cross-linked, pentavalent IgM fixes complement efficiently without cross-linking. On binding to the surface of red blood cells at low temperature, IgM cold agglutinins activate C1, C4, C2, and C3b. On warming, the antibody can dissociate, but C3b remains fixed irreversibly. This can lead to recruitment of the terminal components of the complement cascade (C5-C9) and intravascular hemolysis, C3b receptor-mediated hepatic reticuloendothelial cell phagocytosis, or conversion of the red blood cell C3b to C3d by the C3b inactivator complex associated with phagocyte C3b receptors. Red blood cells bearing surface C3d molecules are not phagocytosed and have a normal life span.

### Graves' Disease: Type IIB Hypersensitivity

Autoantibodies against cell-surface receptors may bind to functional or nonfunctional sites. There may be a general predilection for autoantibodies to recognize active or func-

**TABLE 8.2.** *Autoimmune hemolytic anemia*

| Classification | Autoantibody | Usual antigen | Mechanism of hemolysis |
|---|---|---|---|
| Warm autoantibodies | Polyclonal IgG | Usually Rh antigen | FcγR I, II, or III mediated uptake of IgG-coated RBC in spleen |
| Cold agglutinin AIHA: "idiopathic" | Cold reacting monoclonal IgM | I antigen | CR1 (C3b receptor), CR3, CR4, liver reticuloendothelial cells |
| Cold agglutinin AIHA: infection | Cold reacting polyclonal IgM | i or I antigen | CR1 (C3b receptor), CR3, CR4, liver reticuloendothelial cells |
| Paroxysmal cold hemoglobinuria | Cold reacting polyclonal IgG | P antigen | Complement-mediated intravascular hemolysis |

**TABLE 8.3.** *Fcγ receptors with immunoreceptor tyrosine-based activation motifs*

| | FcγRI (CD64) | FcγRIIA (CD32) | FcγRIIIA (CD16) |
|---|---|---|---|
| α chain | 72 kd | 40 kd | 50–80 kd |
| Structure | $\alpha_\beta\gamma_2$ | Single chain | $\alpha_\gamma2$, $\alpha_{\gamma\zeta}$ |
| ITAM | γ chain | Intrachain | γ chain |
| Endocytosis | + | + | + |
| Phagocytosis | + | + | + |
| ADCC | + | ? | + |
| NF-κB induction | + | + | ? |
| Subclass specificity | IgG1 = 3 > 4 ≫ 2, 4 | IgG1 = 3 ≫ 2, 4 | IgG1 = 3 ≫ 2, 4 |
| Affinity for IgG | $10^8 M^{-1}$ | $2 \times 10^6 M^{-1}$ | $5 \times 10^5 M^{-1}$ |
| Cell types | Mφ, M, PMN | Mφ, M, PMN, P | Mφ, M, NK, T |

Mφ, macrophages; M, monocytes; PMN, polymorphonuclear leukocytes; P, platelets; NK, natural killer cells; T, T-lymphocyte subset; ITAM, immunoreceptor tyrosine-based activation motif; ADCC, antibody-dependent cell-mediated cytotoxity.
Data from references 17, 18, and 237.

tional sites of autoantigens (20). Such antibodies may inhibit function or stimulate it. Graves' disease, a common organ-specific autoimmune thyroid disease characterized by autoantibody-mediated hyperthyroidism, is the prototype of autoimmune disease induced by stimulatory (agonistic) autoantibodies (21). The production of thyroid-stimulating autoantibodies in Graves' disease has been recognized since 1956 (22). Autoantibodies to the thyroid-stimulating hormone receptor (TSHR) cause hyperthyroidism in these patients. The direct pathogenic role of anti-TSHR autoantibodies is demonstrated by the passive transplacental transfer of IgG thyroid-stimulating autoantibodies to the fetus, resulting in transient neonatal Graves' disease (23).

Stimulatory autoantibodies in Graves' disease inhibit the binding of [$^{125}$I]-labeled TSH to its receptor by binding to a conformational epitope of the extracellular domain of the TSHR (24,25). Until recently, detection of anti-TSHR antibodies depended on the TSH binding inhibition assay because of the difficulty in expressing an appropriately glycosylated TSHR protein that retains immunoreactivity. This difficulty was overcome by expressing the recombinant C-terminally truncated extracellular domain as a secreted glycoprotein in Chinese hamster ovary cells (26). A soluble protein consisting of amino acids 1 through 261 of the TSHR reverses the inhibition of [$^{125}$I]-labeled TSH binding to its receptor caused by Graves' disease autoantibodies and effectively neutralizes autoantibody activity. This protein does not bind to TSH, reflecting the fact that the TSH binding domain of the TSHR is discontinuous, involving multiple segments throughout the extracellular domain. Autoantibodies appear to interact with TSHR somewhat differently than the natural ligand. Nevertheless, they stimulate signaling through the TSH receptor, enhancing the production of thyroid hormone. Although agonistic autoantibodies are more common, antagonistic autoantibodies also have been reported (22,27). The latter are associated with hypothyroidism and exemplify a second form of type II hypersensitivity mediated by blocking autoantibodies.

### Myasthenia Gravis: Type IIB Hypersensitivity

Myasthenia gravis is an example of a disease caused by antagonistic autoantibodies (28). The disease in humans is caused by spontaneous development of autoantibodies that block the acetylcholine receptor (AChR), causing muscular weakness and fatigue. Immunization of experimental animals with AChR from the electric organs of *Torpedo* species causes a similar syndrome. Like Graves' disease, transplacental passage of IgG autoantibodies results in transient neonatal myasthenia gravis (29). Moreover, the disease can be transferred passively by injecting mice with the immunoglobulin fraction of myasthenic serum (30).

The neuromuscular syndrome typical of myasthenia gravis is caused by autoantibodies against AChR, which are found at postsynaptic membranes of neuromuscular junctions (28). The AChR binds acetylcholine released from a nerve ending and transiently opens a calcium channel. The signal is terminated by the action of acetylcholine esterase in the basal lamina between the nerve ending and the postsynaptic membrane. AChRs are large, multisubunit structures composed of two α subunits, plus one β, one γ, and one δ subunit. These subunits form a central pore that serves as the calcium channel. The acetylcholine binding site is formed by the two α subunits.

Despite extensive sequence homology between the subunits of the AChR, most autoantibodies are specific for a major antigenic region located on the α subunit (31). This region is located on the extracellular domain but is distinct from the acetylcholine binding site. Along with nearby regions located on the β and γ subunits, it is the main target of autoantibodies raised by immunizing animals with *Torpedo* AChR and those occurring spontaneously in myasthenia gravis patients (31). Fortunately, autoantibodies to the acetylcholine binding site are absent, because such antibodies rapidly cause death in experimental animals (28). Although slight effects have been reported (28), direct inhibition of receptor function is not the major effect of anti-AChR autoantibodies. Instead, they cause disease primarily by downmodulating the receptor and by complement-mediated lysis of the cells bearing AChR. Intermolecular cross-linking of AChR by antibodies is thought to be critical for antigenic modulation.

## Type III Hypersensitivity

The second major mechanism by which autoantibodies cause disease is through the formation of immune complexes (i.e., type III hypersensitivity). Immune complexes are formed when an antibody binds noncovalently to its cognate antigen. Antigen–antibody complexes have different properties from those of the antigen or the immunoglobulin component alone (32,33). The two main consequences of immune complex formation are complement fixation and binding to Fc or complement receptors on phagocytic cells. Clearance is facilitated by the binding of immune complexes to C3b receptors (CR1) on the surface of red blood cells, which retain the complexes in the circulation until their removal by phagocytic cells in the spleen or liver.

Immune complex formation is a normal consequence of humoral immunity that removes foreign antigens from the circulation. Efficient removal of immune complexes by Fc or complement receptor–mediated uptake in phagocytic cells usually prevents their deposition elsewhere. Immune complexes may activate the classical or alternative complement pathway. Monomeric IgG binds C1q weakly, but the strength of complement activation is proportional to the number of IgG molecules associated with the complex. Likewise, the uptake of immune complexes by Fcγ receptors is enhanced by increasing the number of IgG molecules associated with the complex.

Besides mediating uptake of immune complexes by complement receptors, complement plays a major role in maintaining immune complexes in a soluble form, preventing their deposition in tissues (34). C3b is bound to the solubilized immune complexes, facilitating their clearance by the erythrocyte complement receptor CR1. The properties of complement receptors mediating uptake of immune complexes are summarized in Table 8.4. This efficient immune complex transport and removal by Fc and complement receptors can be overwhelmed, leading to tissue deposition and immune complex disease. This may result from overproduction of immune complexes, blockade of the phagocytic function of the reticuloendothelial system, or depletion of complement, leading to inefficient solubilization of immune complexes. Serum sickness and SLE are prototypes of human disease thought to be caused in this manner.

### Systemic Lupus Erythematosus: Type III Hypersensitivity

Early studies of serum sickness led to the description of immune complex disease (35). The major clinical features of serum sickness, including fever, glomerulonephritis, vasculitis, urticaria, and arthritis, appear 7 to 21 days after primary immunization or 2 to 4 days after secondary immunization with a foreign protein. They are caused by a humoral immune response to the heterologous protein, resulting in high levels of circulating immune complexes and hypocomplementemia (36). The immune complexes deposit in tissues, causing inflammatory lesions closely resembling those seen in SLE.

The Arthus reaction is another example of immune complex–mediated disease that may be relevant to the pathogenesis of SLE (33). The classic Arthus reaction is induced by repeated cutaneous injections of horse serum into rabbits. In later studies, specific antibody is injected intradermally, and the cognate antigen is administered intravenously, resulting in the local formation of immune complexes (i.e., reverse passive Arthus reaction) (37). Immune complex deposition is manifested by edema, hemorrhage, and neutrophil infiltration. Fc receptors appear to play a primary role, although the response is amplified by complement activation (37). The reverse passive Arthus reaction is attenuated in Fc receptor γ-chain–deficient mice but is relatively intact in cobra venom factor–treated (complement depleted) mice or C3-, C4-, or C5-deficient mice (16). The histopathologic changes in the kidneys and blood vessels of SLE patients closely resemble those in chronic serum sickness and the Arthus reaction, respectively.

Like acute serum sickness, active lupus nephritis frequently is associated with hypocomplementemia (38,39). Immunoglobulin and complement deposits are seen in the blood vessels, skin, and renal glomeruli of lupus patients (40) (Fig. 8.2), leading to proliferative glomerulonephritis and effacement of the normal glomerular architecture (Fig. 8.3). Preformed immune complexes may be deposited, or immune complexes may develop in situ as a consequence of the interaction of cationic antigens with heparan sulfate glycos-

**TABLE 8.4.** *Complement receptors*

| Characteristic | CR1 | CR2 | CR3 | CR4 | C1qRP |
|---|---|---|---|---|---|
| Alternate name | CD35 | CD21 | CD11b/CD18 | CD11c/CD18 | — |
| Specificity | C3b, C4b | C3d, C3dg, iC3b | iC3b | iC3b | C1q |
| Subunits | Single chain, 4 allotypes (160–260 kd) | Single chain (140 kd) | CD11b (165 kd); CD18 (95 kd) | CD11c (150 kd); CD18 (95 kd) | Single chain (126 kd) |
| Cell types | RBC, Mφ, B, FDC, PMN | B, FDC | Mφ, FDC, PMN | Mφ, PMN | B, Mφ, P, En |
| Function | Transport of immune complexes | B-cell activation, EBV receptor | Phagocytosis | Phagocytosis | Phagocytosis |

RBC, red blood cells; Mφ, macrophages; B, B lymphocytes; FDC, follicular dendritic cells; PMN, polymorphonuclear leukocytes; P, platelets; En, endothelial cells; EBV, Epstein–Barr virus.

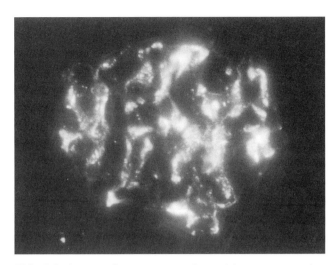

**FIG. 8.2.** Immunofluorescence of renal immune complex deposition in lupus. Direct immunofluorescence staining shows extensive mesangiocapillary IgG deposits in a renal glomerulus from a mouse with pristane-induced lupus. Frozen tissue was stained with fluorescein isothiocyanate (FITC)–conjugated goat antimouse IgG antibodies.

aminoglycan in the glomerular basement membrane (32, 41,42). Alternatively, autoantibodies cross-reactive with basement membrane antigens may cause *in situ* immune complex formation (41). The association of lupus-like disease with deficiencies of the early complement components,

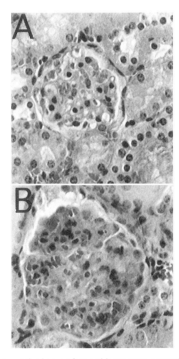

**FIG. 8.3.** Histopathology of renal immune complex disease in lupus. Sections cut from paraformaldehyde-fixed renal tissue were stained with hematoxylin and eosin. **A:** Glomerulus from a normal BALB/c mouse. **B:** Glomerulus from a mouse of the same strain with pristane-induced lupus. Notice the increased glomerular size, increased cellularity and mesangial matrix, and obliteration of the normal capillary loop architecture.

especially C2 and C4 (43,44), is consistent with the role of the classical and alternative complement pathways in solubilizing immune complexes (34). Complement deficiencies may promote enhanced tissue deposition of immune complexes (i.e., classical pathway) or diminish the efficiency of solubilizing glomerular immune deposits after they are formed (i.e., alternative pathway) (34).

The similar appearance of immune complex deposits in the glomeruli of SLE patients, MRL/*lpr* and (NZB/NZW)F1 mice with spontaneous lupus-like disease, and mice with pristane-induced lupus (45) also argues that immune complexes play a central role in the pathogenesis of SLE. This idea is supported further by the absence of nephritis in immunoglobulin-deficient lupus mice (46) and the induction of renal lesions by certain monoclonal anti-DNA antibodies (47–49). The role of complement in murine lupus nephritis is less clear. C5-deficient NZB background mice develop immune complex-mediated glomerulonephritis, suggesting that terminal complement activation may not play a critical role (50). The (NZB/W)F1 mice treated with a monoclonal antibody against C5 that prevents generation of C5a and the membrane attack complex (C5b-9) have milder proteinuria, less mesangial matrix deposition, and longer survival compared with control mice treated with an irrelevant monoclonal antibody, despite similar anti-DNA antibody production and glomerular IgG and C3 deposition (51). Fc receptors also are likely to play a role in the pathogenesis of lupus nephritis. Abnormal Fc receptor function was reported in SLE some time ago (52), although it is unclear whether this is a primary or secondary defect. Certain Fc receptor polymorphisms are associated with more severe lupus nephritis (53).

## AUTOANTIBODIES AS MARKERS OF A DISEASE PROCESS

It is not surprising that pathogenic autoantibodies are useful as disease-specific markers, but it is less obvious why other autoantibodies with no apparent role in disease pathogenesis also are pathognomonic for particular autoimmune disease subsets. For example, some antinuclear antibodies are highly specific markers for subsets of systemic autoimmune disease, despite having no apparent role in disease pathogenesis. These have been used extensively in the immunodiagnosis of systemic autoimmunity.

The FANA assay was one of the earliest diagnostic tests for systemic autoimmunity. It is extremely sensitive but of relatively low diagnostic specificity (54). Of 276 FANA-positive individuals studied by Shiel and Jason, 18.8% had SLE; 10.9% drug-induced lupus; 21.7% other collagen vascular diseases, such as scleroderma or polymyositis, 10.1% autoimmune thyroiditis; 5.8% other organ-specific autoimmune diseases; 8.3% infections; 2.9% neoplasms; and 24.3% other conditions or "idiopathic" autoantibodies (55). Some otherwise normal individuals produce low-titer antinuclear antibodies (56,57). The prevalence of a positive FANA result is 3% to 5% in randomly selected, healthy Caucasians (57). The production of antinuclear antibodies is strongly age dependent, increasing to 10% to 37% in healthy individuals older than 65 years (56) (Fig. 8.4). Although antinuclear antibodies are not unusual in healthy individuals, the titers are generally much lower (≤1 : 40) than in patients with systemic autoimmune diseases. Conversely, a patient with a negative FANA result has less than a 3% chance of having SLE. Although of limited utility in confirming the diagnosis of systemic autoimmune disease, the FANA is valuable for excluding the diagnosis of lupus.

Since the development of the FANA test, more specific autoantibody tests have been developed. Autoantibodies specific for SLE, SSc, PM/DM, primary biliary cirrhosis (PBC), and other systemic autoimmune disorders have been identified. In some cases, detection of these autoantibodies is essentially diagnostic. The reason for the disease specificity of this subset is unclear; in many cases, the autoantibodies are not pathogenic. Some of the clinically useful autoantibody markers for SLE, SSc, PM/DM, and PBC are discussed as examples of marker autoantibodies.

### Systemic Lupus Erythematosus

Antinuclear antibody production is the immunologic hallmark of SLE. The diversity of FANA patterns produced by sera from patients with SLE (Fig. 8.1 Bottom) led to efforts to classify the autoantibodies responsible for different patterns of reactivity (3). Anti-double-stranded DNA (anti-dsDNA) antibodies are found in about 70% of SLE patients' sera at some point during their disease and are 95% specific for that diagnosis (54,58). Consistent with the immune complex-mediated pathogenesis of lupus discussed earlier, anti-dsDNA antibodies and complement frequently exhibit a reciprocal pattern, with high levels of anti-dsDNA antibodies and hypocomplementemia during exacerbations and the reverse pattern during remissions. However, this pattern is not seen in all patients. Although somewhat controversial, it is widely accepted that certain anti-dsDNA autoantibodies contribute directly to disease pathogenesis by forming immune complexes that deposit in the glomeruli (59), reacting with planted antigens in the glomerular basement membrane (60), or cross-reacting with glomerular antigens (41,49). Injection of some mouse monoclonal anti-DNA antibodies induces renal disease, consistent with the possibility that they are involved in the pathogenesis of nephritis (47,48).

Anti-Sm antibodies are produced by approximately 25% of lupus patients and, like anti-dsDNA, are virtually pathognomonic for SLE (61–63). There is little or no evidence that they cause disease. Antibodies to the ribosomal P0, P1, and P2 antigens also are highly specific but less sensitive markers of the disease (64,65) (Table 8.5). They are associated with neuropsychiatric manifestations (66), but it is uncertain whether they cause central nervous system disease (67).

Anti-dsDNA, Sm, and ribosomal P are highly unusual in drug-induced lupus, whereas anti-ssDNA and antihistone antibodies are associated with drug-induced lupus, SLE, and other systemic autoimmune diseases and therefore are not "marker" autoantibodies. Anti-dsDNA, Sm, and ribosomal P also are associated with lupus-like disease in mice. It is unclear why these antibodies are specific for lupus. Autoantibodies may contribute directly to the disease process (41,47,48) or may reflect autoimmune mechanisms unique to the pathogenesis of SLE.

### Systemic Sclerosis

SSc is an autoimmune disorder characterized by progressive fibrosis of the skin and internal organs, including the kidneys, lungs, and intestinal tract. It is associated with widespread vascular lesions and a characteristic subset of autoantibodies. A nucleolar pattern on FANA (Fig. 8.1 Bottom) testing sug-

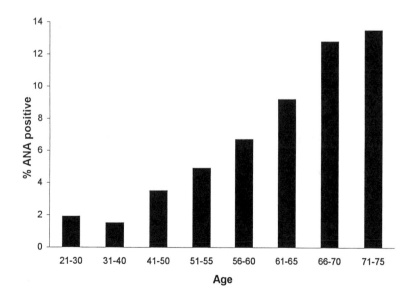

**FIG. 8.4.** The prevalence of antinuclear antibodies increases with age. The percent of antinuclear antibody (ANA)–positive sera is shown as a function of age in years. Notice the gradual increase from about 2% to nearly 14% as age increases from between 21 and 30 years to between 71 and 75 years. (Data from Hooper B, Whittingham S, Mathews JD, et al. Autoimmunity in a rural community. *Clin Exp Immunol* 1972;12:79.)

**TABLE 8.5.** *Autoantibody markers for systemic autoimmune disease subsets*

| Autoantibody | Disease specificity | Prevalence[a] | Clinical associations |
|---|---|---|---|
| α-dsDNA | SLE | 70% | Nephritis, active disease |
| α-Sm | SLE | 25% | High specific for SLE |
| α-ribosomal P | SLE | 15% | Neuropsychiatric involvement |
| α-topoisomerase I | SSc | 15% | Proximal (severe) scleroderma |
| α-RNA polymerase I, II, III | SSc | 20% | Severe disease; anti-RNAP I/III more specific than II |
| α-fibrillarin | SSc | 5% | Highly specific for SSc |
| α-Th | SSc | 5% | Highly specific for SSc |
| α-Jo-1 (tRNA[his] synthetase) | PM/SM | 20% | Antisynthetase syndrome |
| α-PL-7 (tRNA[thr] synthetase) | PM/DM | 3% | Antisynthetase syndrome |
| α-PL-12 (tRNA[ala] synthetase) | PM/DM | 3% | Antisynthetase syndrome |
| α-SRP | PM/DM | 4% | Severe myositis |

dsDNA, double-stranded DNA; PM/DM, polymyositis/dermatomyositis; SLE, systemic lupus erythematosus; SSc, systemic sclerosis.

[a] Approximate prevalence of autoantibody in associated disease subset.

gests the diagnosis of SSc (3,68,69). Several nucleolar antigens have been identified as targets of autoantibodies, including fibrillarin (U3 small nucleolar ribonucleoprotein) (70), the To/Th (7-2 small ribonucleoprotein) antigen (71), the transcription factor NOR-90 (hUBF) (72), and RNA polymerases I and III (73,74) (Table 8.5). The nucleoplasmic and nucleolar enzyme topoisomerase I (Scl-70) also is an important diagnostic marker (69).

Antitopoisomerase I and anti-RNA polymerase autoantibodies are associated with severe disease and therefore are useful prognostically (75,76). Antitopoisomerase I antibodies are highly specific for the diagnosis of scleroderma. Their prevalence in SSc is 15% to 30%, and they are found at higher frequency in patients with proximal than with limited skin involvement. The detection of anti-RNA polymerase II antibodies along with antitopoisomerase I antibodies is associated with even more severe disease and a poor prognosis (75). However, unlike anti-RNA polymerase I/III antibodies, which are found only in SSc, anti-RNA polymerase II antibodies are also associated with SLE (77). Autoantibodies to RNA polymerases I, II, or III are detected in 28% of Japanese and 16% of African-American scleroderma patients but only 8% of Caucasians, mainly because of a low frequency of anti-RNA polymerase II antibodies in this group. Antifibrillarin antibodies are found in 5% to 8% of SSc patients (68–70). Although specific for SSc, it is unclear whether these antibodies are associated with a particular subset of the disease.

Anticentromere antibodies (Fig. 8.1 Bottom) are a useful marker for a mild variant of SSc called CREST syndrome (*c*alcinosis, *R*aynaud's phenomenon, *e*sophageal hypomotility, *s*clerodactyly, *t*elangiectasias) (78). These autoantibodies recognize primarily CENP-B, a major centromere protein (79). Although common in the CREST subset, anticentromere antibodies are not as specific as other SSc markers (80,81). These antibodies occasionally are found in individuals with Raynaud's phenomenon without overt collagen vascular disease, some of whom subsequently develop CREST syndrome (82).

**Polymyositis and Dermatomyositis**

Polymyositis is an inflammatory muscle disorder of autoimmune origin that is characterized by proximal muscle weakness (sometimes with muscle pain), elevated muscle enzyme levels (e.g., creatine kinase, aldolase), and typical abnormalities on electromyography. The same abnormalities are found in dermatomyositis, along with skin involvement, typically with Gottron's papules (i.e., violaceous papules on the dorsal aspect of the interphalangeal joints), telangiectasias, and a heliotrope rash over the upper eyelids. Autoantibodies to certain cytoplasmic antigens, many of which are tRNA synthetases, are diagnostic markers for PM/DM (Table 8.5). Anti-tRNA synthetase antibodies are rare in the absence of myositis (<1%). The most common myositis-associated autoantibody is anti-histidyl-tRNA synthetase (anti-Jo-1), which is detected in 20% of adult myositis patients (83). Other synthetases also are recognized by autoantibodies in PM/DM, including threonyl (anti-PL-7), alanyl (anti-PL-12), isoleucyl (anti-OJ), and glycyl (anti-EJ) tRNA synthetases (83). All of the antisynthetase autoantibodies are associated with myositis, interstitial lung disease, Raynaud's phenomenon, mechanic's hands (i.e., roughened skin over the fingertips), arthritis, and fever, a constellation designated *antisynthetase autoantibody syndrome* (83,84). Autoantibodies to the signal recognition particle also are disease specific but are not associated with antisynthetase autoantibody syndrome. They may be a marker for severe myositis (83). Viral infections may play a role in triggering the autoantibodies characteristic of PM/DM, possibly because of the formation of immunogenic complexes of aminoacyl tRNA synthetases with tRNA-like structures on picornaviral genomes (83). However, there is little direct evidence to support this intriguing possibility.

**Primary Biliary Cirrhosis**

PBC is an autoimmune liver disease characterized by damage to the bile duct epithelium and the production of antimitochondrial autoantibodies (85). It affects primarily middle-aged women, resulting in cholestasis, severe pruritus, and jaundice terminating in cirrhosis. The major autoantigens in this disease are components of the inner mitochondrial multienzymatic complex M2, especially the dihydrolipoamide acetyltransferase component (E2) of pyruvate dehydrogenase (86–88). Occasionally, patients have autoantibodies to non-M2 mitochondrial antigens, such as M4 or M9. Antimitochondrial antibodies produce a characteristic particulate cytoplasmic staining pattern that is readily distinguishable from the more diffuse staining exhibited by myositis autoantibodies.

Autoantibodies to E2 can be detected by Western blotting in 96% of sera from patients with PBC (85). Although these antibodies occasionally are produced by patients with infections or drug-induced hepatitis (86) or even by asymptomatic individuals, a high percentage of them eventually develop PBC (89,90). Despite the strong linkage of anti-E2 autoantibodies with PBC, when this specificity is generated by immunizing mice, rats, guinea pigs, rabbits, or monkeys with recombinant E2, these animals fail to develop liver disease (91).

The reason that particular autoantibodies such as anti-E2, Sm, topoisomerase I, or aminoacyl tRNA synthetases are uniquely associated with certain disease subsets is unknown. These autoantibodies may mediate disease directly in an obscure manner. Many recognize multiple epitopes on their target autoantigens, raising the possibility that a subset could cross-react with another antigen, leading to disease. Alternatively, autoantibody specificity could reflect a unique feature of the pathogenic process, without the autoantibodies themselves causing disease. In either case, understanding the origins of autoantibodies is an important step in defining the pathogenesis of autoimmune diseases such as SLE, SSc, PM/DM, and PBC.

## ORIGINS OF AUTOANTIBODIES

In-depth understanding of the origins of autoantibodies remains elusive despite intensive study. The B-cell subsets responsible for autoantibody production are heterogeneous, as is the requirement for T cells, antigen drive, and somatic hypermutation. Current knowledge about the origins of autoantibodies is summarized in the next section.

### B-Cell Subsets Responsible for Autoantibody Production

Two major B-cell subsets have been defined. Conventional (B2) B cells are responsible for most high-affinity IgG antibodies and are derived in the bone marrow, but they undergo antigen-induced differentiation in the germinal centers of peripheral lymphoid organs (e.g., lymph nodes, spleen). The B1 subset is thought to be a distinct lineage enriched in the peritoneal cavity that is self-renewing and characterized by a unique phenotype (CD23$^-$, IgM$^{hi}$, IgD$^{lo}$, often but not always CD5$^+$). B1 cells produce mainly low-affinity, often polyreactive IgM antibodies (92–94) and are responsible for most

of the serum IgM. Total IgM levels are reduced in CD19-deficient mice, consistent with the fact that formation of B1 cells critically depends on CD19 expression (95). Disruption of CR2 (CD21) also reduces B1 cell numbers but has little effect on serum IgM levels (96). CD19 and CR2 are components of the B-cell coreceptor complex, which acts synergistically with surface immunoglobulin to promote B-cell activation (Fig. 8.5).

Autoantibodies are produced by both B-cell subsets, but their characteristics differ. For example, anti-DNA antibodies and rheumatoid factors produced by the B2 subset tend to be high-affinity IgG autoantibodies exhibiting little cross-reactivity with other antigens, whereas autoantibodies produced by the CD5$^+$ B-cell subset tend to be low-affinity, polyreactive IgMs (97,98). The CD5$^+$ B-cell subset is expanded in human rheumatoid arthritis and Sjögren's syndrome in association with rheumatoid factor production (99,101). CD5$^+$ B-cell tumor cells frequently secrete autoantibodies (102). This subset also is expanded in some autoim-

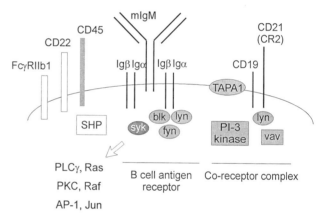

FIG. 8.5. B-cell activation. Some of the molecules mediating B-cell activation are illustrated. The B-cell antigen receptor illustrated consists of surface IgM (sIgM) in association with two additional molecules involved in signaling: Igα (CD79α) and Igβ (CD79β). These proteins both have immunoreceptor tyrosine–based activation motifs (ITAMs) that become tyrosine phosphorylated upon antigen binding. The receptor tyrosine kinases blk, lyn, and fyn associate with the B-cell antigen receptor and, upon receptor aggregation, phosphorylate two tyrosines in the ITAM of region of Igβ. This leads to recognition and activation of the Syk tyrosine kinase, which initiates intracellular signaling via multiple substrates and pathways, including the Ras/ERK/Raf pathway, calcium pathways, protein kinase C (PKC), and additional mitogen-activated protein kinases. These pathways ultimately lead to the activation of DNA-binding factors (e.g., AP-1 and Jun) that activate the transcription of specific genes. The B-cell coreceptor complex, consisting of CD21 (CR2), CD19, and TAPA 1 enhances the efficiency of these reactions, in part through interactions with vav and phosphatidylinositol 3-kinase (PI-3 kinase). Signaling mediated by the B-cell receptor and coreceptor is held in check by the tyrosine phosphatase SHP-1, which becomes activated as a consequence of triggering either FcγRIIb or CD22. CD22 is a negative regulator of antigen receptor signaling; tyrosine-containing motifs within its cytoplasmic domain may participate in recruiting lyn, syk, PI-3 kinase and phospholipase C γ (PLCγ). CD45 is a positive regulator of antigen receptor signaling and mediates tyrosine-specific dephosphorylation of lyn or related Src-family kinases.

mune mice, including NZB and moth-eaten mice (92). NZB mice develop AIHA, anti-ssDNA autoantibodies, and a mild lupus-like syndrome. Moth-eaten mice have a defect in the SH2 domain containing tyrosine phosphatase SHP-1, which plays a major role in regulating B-cell receptor signaling (Fig. 8.5); have nearly 100% CD5+ B cells; and develop immune complex disease and autoantibodies (103,104). However, expansion of the B1 subset is not a universal finding in autoimmune disease, because MRL/*lpr* mice have low or normal frequencies of these cells (92).

## Molecular Analysis of Autoantibody Generation

Immunoglobulins with specificity for self antigens can be created during V/D/J recombination, in which case their variable regions are in a germline configuration (105), or they can arise as a consequence of antigen-stimulated somatic mutation and affinity maturation of the variable regions of immunoglobulins that do not initially exhibit autoreactivity (106,107). The relative importance of each mechanism in generating pathogenic autoantibodies has been the object of intensive study and considerable debate. After autoreactive B cells are generated, they are censored by a variety of mechanisms, as reviewed elsewhere (108). In general, high-affinity autoantibodies arising through V/D/J recombination are censored in the bone marrow, whereas those arising through somatic mutation, which takes place mainly in germinal centers of secondary lymphoid organs, are censored in the periphery. Autoreactive B cells are inactivated by clonal deletion (i.e., apoptosis) or rendered anergic by the lack of critical costimulatory signals (108). B cells expressing high-affinity receptors for self antigens are more efficiently censored than those expressing low-affinity receptors, which may escape censoring altogether.

### Natural Autoantibodies

Natural autoantibodies are IgM immunoglobulins encoded by germline genes that display polyreactivity and low affinity for antigen (109,110). They frequently are derived from the B1 subset (92), may be selected by self antigens, and can be produced without a requirement for T-cell help (111). Because of their low affinity for self antigen or differential susceptibility of the B1 and B2 subsets to censoring (112), the B cells producing natural autoantibodies are not deleted or anergized and can secrete polyreactive autoantibodies. The physiologic and pathophysiologic relevance of these autoantibodies is controversial (109,110), but there is growing evidence that natural autoantibodies or antibodies, produced by the organism in the absence of antigenic stimulation, may play a critical role in primary immune responses.

It has been suggested that the formation of immune complexes of antigens with polyreactive natural antibodies activates C3, generating iC3b/C3dg and promoting the binding of the complexes to CR2 on the B-cell surface (113). The uptake of these complexes induces expression of the potent costimulatory molecule B7 (CD80). C3-deficient mice,

guinea pigs, dogs, or humans are deficient in generating primary antibody responses (114), further supporting the idea that the binding of immune complexes to CR2 play a role in antibody production.

CR2 is part of a complex of proteins, consisting of CD19, CD21, and TAPA-1 (CD81) (Fig. 8.5), that amplifies B-cell responses to certain T-cell–dependent antigens (115). The binding of C3 to CR2 on mature B cells is associated with phosphorylation of tyrosine residues in the cytoplasmic domain of CD19, priming the cells for activation through cross-linking of surface immunoglobulin (95,116,117). Coligation of CD19 and the B-cell antigen receptor is a link between innate immunity and T-cell–dependent antibody responses. CD19-deficient mice have a profound defect in B-cell responses to T-cell–dependent protein antigens, lack germinal centers, and exhibit an absence of antibody affinity maturation (95). In addition to defective conventional antibody responses, CD19 −/− mice have greatly reduced B1 cells, possibly reflecting inefficient selection by self antigens (95). B1 cells and natural autoantibodies may play an important role in normal antigen-directed B-cell development. Amplification of T-cell–dependent antibody responses is held in check by CD22 and FcγRIIB by means of interactions with the tyrosine phosphatase SHP-1 (Fig. 8.5) (115). FcγRIIB may play a key regulatory role by allowing antibody production to be downmodulated by a product of the immune response: IgG-containing immune complexes. Consistent with that idea, disruption of FcγRIIB causes defective regulation of IgM, IgG, and IgA levels (118).

Although it seems likely that B1 cells and natural antibodies are involved in physiologic responses of B cells to T-cell–dependent antigens, their role in the pathogenesis of autoimmune disease is less clear. Some nonpolyreactive autoantibodies with a germline configuration are derived preferentially from the B1 subset, such as those recognizing murine red blood cells treated with the proteolytic enzyme bromelain (92). These autoantibodies are encoded primarily by two V region gene combinations ($V_H11$ and $V_H12$) preferentially expressed by B1 cells and are not represented in the immunoglobulin repertoire induced by immunization with conventional foreign antigens (112). The frequent association of autoimmune disease with expansion of the B1 cell subset, as in NZB, moth-eaten (SHP-1 deficient), and Lyn-deficient mice, may reflect an exaggeration of the physiologic role of natural autoantibodies in enhancing primary antibody responses by conventional B cells. Although moth-eaten and Lyn-deficient mice develop a syndrome with some features of lupus, many of the characteristic autoantibodies are not seen in these strains, possibly because many of the latter are derived from the conventional (B2) subset.

### Conventional Autoantibodies

The generation of autoantibodies by somatic mutation of nonautoreactive immunoglobulin variable (V) regions, presumably within germinal centers, has been well documented (106). Unlike low-affinity, polyreactive anti-ssDNA autoantibodies produced by the B1 subset, which frequently bear germline Ig variable region sequences and may be only weakly dependent on T-cell help, conventional autoantibodies bear numerous somatic mutations and do not develop in the absence of T cells. Conventional autoantibodies appear to be of major importance in the development of immune damage mediated by type II and type III hypersensitivity-like reactions (112,119). Moreover, conventional B cells are the primary source of the autoantibodies in *lpr* mice (120).

The strongest evidence that autoantibodies are generated through a process of antigen-driven B-cell activation is the high degree of somatic mutations in anti-DNA, anti-Sm, and rheumatoid factor autoantibody V regions (119,121,122). The high frequency of replacement versus silent mutations found in anti-DNA and anti-Sm clones and their nonrandom distribution argues that these autoantibodies are selected on the basis of receptor specificity. In contrast to antibodies against bromelain-treated red blood cells, which are in the germline configuration, autoantibodies to untreated mouse erythrocytes are encoded by a wide variety of somatically mutated immunoglobulin variable regions, consistent with T-cell help and antigen drive (123). With the caveat that somatic hypermutation and germinal center formation occasionally occur in the course of T-cell–independent responses (124), the analysis of autoantibody V regions strongly points to T-cell involvement.

## Role of T Cells and Antigen

The role of T cells in autoantibody production in lupus has been studied intensively. Indirect evidence for T-cell–dependent autoantibody production is provided by the predominance of IgG2a antinuclear antibodies in MRL mice (125). The importance of T cells also is indicated by the lower levels of autoantibodies in MRL/*lpr* or NZB/W mice treated with anti-CD4 antibodies or CTLA4Ig (126,127) and by the necessity for cognate T-cell and B-cell interactions in autoantibody production (128).

### T-Cell Subsets Participating in Autoantibody Production

Early evidence for the influence of T cells on autoantibody production came from studies in athymic (nude) mice, which lack T-cell–dependent antibody responses (129). Nude mice are resistant to the induction of T-cell–dependent experimental autoimmune diseases such as autoimmune thyroiditis, orchitis, glomerulonephritis, and encephalomyelitis (130). Moreover, (NZB/W)F1 nude mice do not develop anti-DNA autoantibodies or renal disease typical of SLE, despite exhibiting B-cell hyperresponsiveness (131), and are unresponsive to immunization with bacterial DNA (132). In pristane-induced lupus, anti-Sm antibodies cannot be induced in nude mice (133). Treatment of MRL/*lpr* or (NZB/W)F1 mice with anti-CD4 antibodies abrogates the production of anti-DNA antibodies (126,134), and these antibodies fail to

develop in CD4-deficient, lupus-prone mice (135). Similarly, autoantibody production is reduced in mice deficient in $\alpha\beta$ T cells (136) or class II major histocompatibility complex (MHC) molecules (137). Although most autoantibodies in murine lupus depend on the $\alpha\beta$ T-cell subset, some are produced by mice having only $\gamma\delta$ T cells (136,138).

Autoreactive T cells have been identified in human SLE (139–142), and in lupus mice, both $\alpha\beta$ and $\gamma\delta$ T-cell receptor–bearing cells responsive to histones have been implicated in anti-DNA antibody production and acceleration of the renal disease (143). Considerable evidence shows that T cells are involved in autoantibody production and that cognate T-cell and B-cell interactions play a crucial role. The latter are mediated, in part, by CD28-B7 and CD40-CD40 ligand interactions.

### CD28/B7 Costimulatory Pathway

Ligation of the T-cell antigen receptor is insufficient by itself to activate naive T cells to proliferate or differentiate. A costimulatory signal delivered by antigen presenting cells also is required (144,145). In the absence of this second signal, T-cell receptor occupancy by antigen causes unresponsiveness (i.e., anergy) or cell death. The best characterized costimulatory molecules are B7.1 and B7.2, which are expressed on the surface of macrophages, dendritic cells, activated B cells, and other antigen presenting cells (146,147). The CD28 molecule is the only receptor for B7.1 and B7.2 on naive T cells, but after activation, the higher affinity CTLA-4 receptor also is expressed (147,148). The primary role of CTLA-4 may be to downregulate antigen-specific T-cell responses, although it can have T-cell stimulatory or inhibitory effects in different situations (148).

CTLA-4 deficient or CD28 deficient mice have impaired IgG responses to T-cell–dependent antigens (147). Humoral immune responses to exogenous antigens also are profoundly inhibited by a fusion protein consisting of the extracellular domain of CTLA-4 bound to the immunoglobulin C$\gamma$1 chain (CTLA4Ig) (149), and treatment of (NZB/W)F1 mice with CTLA4Ig before the onset of autoimmunity dramatically reduces anti-dsDNA autoantibody production and prolongs survival (127). Moreover, B7.2-CD28/CTLA-4 interactions are critical for germinal center formation and somatic hypermutation (150). Evidence strongly indicates that the CD28/B7 costimulatory system plays an important role in autoantibody production.

### CD40L/CD40 System

CD40 is a surface receptor expressed constitutively on B cells and certain other cell types belonging to the tumor necrosis factor receptor (TNFR) family. It binds to a ligand (CD40L, CD154) expressed on activated CD4$^+$ T cells that is a T-cell surface protein related to tumor necrosis factor (TNF) (151,152). CD40L expression is induced on helper T cells activated by antigen and is restricted to T cells in the outer periarteriolar lymphoid sheath (PALS) regions of the spleen (152) and is essential for the formation of germinal centers in response to thymus-dependent antigens. Germinal centers, the primary site of isotype switching and somatic mutation, are absent in CD40L- or CD40-deficient mice (153,154) and in patients with hyper-IgM syndrome, a severe immunodeficiency resulting from CD40L mutations (155). Patients with hyper-IgM syndrome and CD40L-deficient mice fail to produce high-affinity IgG, IgA, or IgE antibodies and have defective memory B-cell generation in response to thymus-dependent antigens (156,157). CD40–CD40L interactions are believed to play a critical role in promoting B-cell development into memory cells instead of plasma cells (157).

In view of the importance of isotype switching, somatic mutation, and affinity maturation in autoantibody production, it is not surprising that CD40L deficiency abrogates the production of anti-dsDNA autoantibodies and rheumatoid factor in the lupus-like syndrome of MRL mice (158). Glomerulonephritis also is milder in CD40L-deficient MRL/lpr mice and is ameliorated in (SWR × NZB)F1 mice treated with anti-CD40L antibodies (158,159). When anti-CD40L treatment is combined with CTLA4Ig treatment, long-lasting inhibition of autoantibody production and glomerulonephritis can be achieved in (NZB/W)F1 mice (160), which may be of potential therapeutic significance.

### Role of Cytokines

Cytokines are small, soluble proteins secreted by cells that alter the function of the producing cells themselves or other cells. Cytokines produced by helper T cells have been implicated in the pathogenesis of many autoimmune diseases (161,162). For instance, cytokines produced by the type 2 helper T-cell ($T_H2$) subset (i.e., interleukin (IL)-4, IL-5, and IL-10) may enhance autoantibody production in lupus (161–165). The $T_H1$ cytokines IL-2 and IFN-$\gamma$ may promote nephritis, nitric oxide production, and autoantibody production in MRL mice (166,167). Different subsets of cytokines may be involved in different aspects of autoimmunity under different conditions.

The importance of cytokines in the pathogenesis of autoimmunity has become increasingly clear. IL-4 overproduction in IL-4 transgenic mice promotes the production of antinuclear and antismooth muscle autoantibodies, autoimmune hemolytic anemia, and the development of nephritis (168). IL-4 also influences autoantibody production in mercuric chloride–treated mice, although its main effect may be to skew the predominant isotype toward IgG1 (169). In (NZB/W)F1 mice, treatment with anti-IL-10 antibodies reduces the production of IgG anti-dsDNA antibodies and delays the onset of renal disease (163). The latter effect is abrogated by anti-TNF-$\alpha$ antibodies, suggesting that neutralization of IL-10 delays the onset of autoimmunity by upregulating TNF-$\alpha$ production.

$T_H1$ cytokines also appear to play a role in autoantibody production and immune complex disease in murine lupus.

Treatment of (NZB/W)F1 mice with anti-IFN-$\gamma$ antibodies or soluble IFN-$\gamma$ receptors inhibits the development of glomerulonephritis and delays the onset of anti-dsDNA antibody production, while having little effect on autoantibody levels (170,171). IgG2a and IgG3 anti-dsDNA antibody levels, but not IgG1, are reduced in MRL/lpr IFN-$\gamma$ knockout mice, suggesting that, although IFN-$\gamma$ is not essential for anti-dsDNA autoantibody production, it influences the predominant isotype of the anti-DNA response (172,173). Renal disease appears to be milder in MRL/lpr mice deficient in $T_H1$ (IFN-$\gamma$ or $T_H2$ (IL-4) cytokines (173).

The proinflammatory cytokine IL-6 also may play a role in autoantibody production. IL-6 is a pleiotropic cytokine thought to be of pivotal importance to immune regulation through its action on B and T cells (174,175). It acts primarily on the late phase of B-cell differentiation. IL-6 production by macrophages has been implicated in the pathogenesis of anti-DNA antibodies and nephritis in (NZB/W)F1 mice (176,177). In pristane-induced lupus, anti-dsDNA antibody production is abrogated in IL-6–deficient mice (178). Moreover, patients with IL-6–secreting tumors, such as atrial myxomas, produce autoantibodies (175,179). It may be significant that elderly individuals produce increased amounts of IL-6 (180) and have a higher frequency of antinuclear antibodies (Fig. 8.4).

### EFFECTS OF GENETIC BACKGROUND AND ENVIRONMENTAL TRIGGERS

Genetic background and environmental stimuli are involved in autoantibody production. The relative importance of each is variable, with genetic background playing a more important role in some instances and the environment in others.

### Genetic Background

There is considerable evidence that autoimmunity and autoantibody production is in part genetically determined (181,182). Although the precise genetic defects are not known, they may affect some of the same immunologic systems discussed previously. For instance, genetic defects in SHP-1 or Lyn promote autoantibody production by the B1 subset (183), and humans and mice with certain cytokine defects are predisposed to autoimmunity (168,175). One of the best characterized genetic defects influencing autoantibody formation is the lpr mutation in mice (184). This mutation affects Fas, a key protein in the lymphocyte apoptosis pathway that may be important in removing autoreactive lymphocytes in the periphery (108). The lpr mutation acts primarily as an accelerating factor that promotes the development of autoimmunity (i.e., autoantibodies and kidney disease) on an MRL background. Gene mapping techniques have identified loci in the (NZB/W)F1 model that promote the production of antichromatin antibodies (185).

In the near future, this approach may lead to identification of genes involved in the induction of autoantibody production or in regulating the levels of these antibodies. Other than MHC-linked genes, the genes responsible for autoantibody production in humans and mice are not characterized (186).

### Environmental Triggers

The induction of autoantibody production by a wide variety of environmental stimuli, including chemicals, viruses, and sunlight, has been reported. For example, although human lupus is believed to be primarily a genetic disorder, the induction of autoantibodies and features of lupus by drugs is relatively common. Most frequently, the offending drug is procainamide, quinidine, hydralazine, methyldopa, or isoniazid, but many others have been implicated (187). The lupus syndrome induced by drugs such as procainamide differs in key respects from the idiopathic SLE syndrome (188). For instance, glomerulonephritis is rare, and the marker autoantibodies anti-dsDNA and anti-Sm usually are absent.

Autoantibody production can be induced in experimental animals by heavy metals. For instance, autoantibodies associated with scleroderma are induced in SJL and other H-2$^s$ mice by mercuric chloride (189). MHC-linked genes and cytokines promote the production of antifibrillarin autoantibodies in mercuric chloride–treated mice. The Hg(II) ion is highly reactive with sulfhydryl groups and more weakly with hydroxyl, carbonyl, and phosphoryl groups (190). The binding of Hg(II) to protein side chains may form metal-protein complexes that are so stable they alter the unfolding of proteins inside endosomes, leading to the enhanced presentation of cryptic epitopes (189). Experimental evidence that mercury induces a conformational change in the fibrillarin molecule, probably by interacting with cysteines, has been obtained (190). However, there is little evidence that mercury or other heavy metals contribute to the antifibrillarin response in human scleroderma. Nevertheless, the induction of antifibrillarin antibodies by mercury in mice provides a valuable model for understanding autoantibody specificity.

Autoantibody production also has been reported after cosmetic surgery in patients injected with paraffin or silicone (191). Although silicone breast implants have been suggested to promote the development of connective tissue diseases, controlled epidemiologic studies failed to confirm this association (192). However, the possibility of an association with autoantibody production in humans has not been excluded.

Further evidence that autoantibodies can be induced by "inert" foreign substances is provided by the lupus-like syndrome caused by pristane, an isoprenoid alkane derived from mineral oil. Intraperitoneal injection of pristane in nonautoimmune prone mice, such as BALB/c, induces the production of anti-Sm, dsDNA, ribosomal P, and other autoantibodies, and it produces an immune complex–mediated glomerulonephritis closely resembling lupus nephritis (45,193). Although the types of autoantibodies induced differ somewhat between strains, the widespread susceptibility among mouse strains suggests that the lupus-like syndrome developing in these mice is largely independent of genetic background. Pristane is taken up by macrophages in the peritoneal cavity, resulting in IL-6 production (194,195). In susceptible strains, this leads to plasmacytoma development (196). IL-6 plays a critical role in the induction of anti-dsDNA antibodies by pristane (178), as in (NZB/W)F1 mice (176,177).

## PROPOSED MECHANISMS OF AUTOANTIBODY PRODUCTION

The underlying causes of autoantibody production in human autoimmune disease are incompletely defined. However, it has become increasingly clear that multiple pathways may lead to autoantibody formation, some of which are described in the following sections.

### Polyclonal Activation

One of the proposed mechanisms of autoantibody production is polyclonal B-cell activation. This idea stems from from observations that microbial substances, such as lipopolysaccharide or peptidoglycan, can stimulate resting peripheral B cells to secrete polyclonal immunoglobulins, some of them recognizing self antigens (197,198). For reasons that are incompletely understood, autoantibodies with rheumatoid factor or anti-ssDNA activity are produced frequently in this manner, possibly with implications for SLE (199). Moreover, lipopolysaccharide exacerbates autoimmune disease (i.e., nephritis) in lupus-prone mice (200). Most autoantibodies generated in response to polyclonal B-cell activators, such as lipopolysaccharide, are probably natural autoantibodies. Although polyclonal activation frequently precedes the onset of lupus, there is overwhelming evidence that many autoantibodies are not generated in this manner (122,201–203). However, polyclonal B-cell activation may be a prerequisite for generating more specific autoantibodies (204,205).

### Molecular Mimicry

Immunologic cross-reactivity of one antigen with another, called *molecular mimicry* (206), is way of generating autoantibodies. Molecular mimicry may contribute to autoimmunity in two ways. An immune response to a foreign antigen cross-reactive with self may cause autoimmunity directly (206). Alternatively, the same epitope may be shared by more than one self antigen, and an immune response to one of them may lead to autoimmunity against another.

Viral infections frequently precipitate autoantibody production or autoimmune disease (207). Immunologic cross-reactivity of a viral antigen with self can lead to the production of autoantibodies. For example, immunologic cross-reactivity has been shown between herpes simplex virus and intermediate filaments (208) and between a retroviral p30$^{gag}$ protein and the U1 small nuclear ribonucleoprotein (snRNP) 70K protein (209). Immunization of mice with murine leukemia virus (MuLV) p30$^{gag}$ protein induces autoantibodies recognizing the cross-reactive portion of the U1-70K protein, suggesting that retroviral infection may play a role in the pathogenesis of autoantibodies to the U1 snRNP.

Examples of molecular mimicry between self proteins also have been described. For instance, the Sm antigens B′, B, and D share two regions of sequence homology, designated Sm motifs 1 and 2 (210). As a consequence, cross-reactive antibodies are prominent in the immune response to U1 snRNPs (211). For example, the monoclonal antibody Y12 recognizes an epitope shared by the Sm-B and B′ proteins, a conformational epitope of Sm-D, and a conformation-dependent epitope formed by the complex of Sm-E, -F, and -G (212,213).

Autoantibodies that recognize a common posttranslational modification shared by more than one protein also have been reported. For example, monoclonal antibodies against phosphoamino acids, such as phosphotyrosine, have been produced by immunization and recognize a wide variety of phosphoproteins (214). Specific recognition of the phosphorylated form of RNA polymerase has been reported in human systemic autoimmunity and may explain the strong linkage between autoantibodies to the phosphorylated form of RNA polymerase II and autoantibodies to the phosphoprotein topoisomerase I in scleroderma patients (75).

## Altered Self Hypothesis

Immunization with a foreign protein can induce autoimmunity to the homologous self protein. For example, immunization with foreign thyroglobulin has been used to induce thyroiditis and autoantibodies to thyroglobulin (215), and immunization with bovine collagen can induce autoimmunity to type II collagen, with anticollagen antibodies and an IL-6–dependent rheumatoid arthritis–like syndrome (216,217). Heymann nephritis (218,219) and experimental myasthenia gravis (28) are induced in an analogous manner.

The binding of a foreign antigen to a self protein also can induce autoimmunity. The interaction of the p53 tumor suppressor protein with simian virus 40 (SV40) large T antigen is an example. SV40 large T antigen (SVT) transforms cells by binding to and inactivating p53. Rodents with SV40-induced tumors develop autoantibodies against p53 (220,221). Similarly, although mice are tolerant to murine p53, when immunized with p53/SVT complexes, they produce high levels of autoantibodies to p53 (222), possibly because T cells specific for SVT provide help to B cells specific for self p53 (intermolecular-intrastructural help [223]). Alternatively, the binding of SVT to self p53 may alter its processing by antigen presenting cells, leading to the presentation of cryptic self peptides to which tolerance is incomplete (224). The observation that, after priming with p53/SVT complex, autoantibody production can be boosted with murine p53 alone supports the latter possibility.

The "cryptic epitope" hypothesis could have far-reaching implications for autoimmunity because there are so many ways of generating altered self. These include the binding of a metal ion or drug to a self protein (189), abnormal degradation of self proteins (225), and alteration of a protein's structure by somatic mutation (226). The latter may explain autoantibody production in certain neoplastic diseases. For example, autoantibodies to p53 are produced by 9% to 15% of breast cancer patients, generally in association with mutations that enhance the stability of p53 by promoting the formation of p53–heat shock protein-70 (HSP70) complexes (227–229).

## Idiotype–Antiidiotype Mechanism

An antiidiotypic antibody is defined as an antibody recognizing determinants found on the variable region of another antibody (230). In view of the diversity of the immunoglobulin repertoire, certain idiotypes may mimic foreign or self antigens (231). Mimicry of the internal image of a foreign or self antigen by an antibody could generate antiidiotypic antibodies recognizing the original antigen. Autoantibodies can be produced in this way experimentally (232), a strategy that has been used in vaccine development (233). Antialanyl tRNA synthetase and anti-tRNA$^{ala}$ antibodies in polymyositis are an example of autoantibody production by this route (234,235). A subset of autoantibodies recognize the active site of alanyl tRNA synthetase and can inhibit its activity (234). Antibodies to tRNA$^{ala}$ are associated with antialanyl tRNA synthetase antibodies, and the two specificities appear to have an idiotype–antiidiotype relationship.

## Role of Apoptotic Cells in Autoantibody Production

Several autoantigens recognized by autoantibodies produced in SLE or SSc are present in apoptotic blebs and are degraded by interleukin-1β converting enzyme–like proteases. Cleavage by these enzymes may define a class of autoantigens (236). However, because apoptosis is a normal part of embryonic development, the fragments of autoantigens produced during "normal" apoptosis could induce tolerance. Nevertheless, abnormal apoptosis events could generate cryptic self peptides. Reports that a number of scleroderma-specific autoantigens, including topoisomerase I, the large subunit of RNA polymerase II, and human upstream binding factor (hUBF or NOR-90) are uniquely fragmented by reactive oxygen species in a metal (iron or copper)–dependent manner raise the possibility that metal-catalyzed oxidation reactions may target a subset of antigens for autoimmunity (225).

## CONCLUSIONS

Autoantibodies may be produced in the presence or absence of autoimmune disease. They are important clinically as markers of specific disease processes and sometimes are involved in disease pathogenesis. They can induce disease directly by binding to their target antigens and initiating immune injury or indirectly through immune complex formation. Autoantibodies are produced by B1 and B2 (conventional) B cells. However, many of the specific autoantibodies associated with autoimmune diseases appear to be antigen selected and require T-cell help, characteristics most commonly associated with conventional B-cell responses. B1 cells, however, may play a key role in the early phase of autoantibody production, analogous to their role in primary antibody responses to exogenous antigens. Autoantibody formation may be triggered by polyclonal B-cell activation, molecular mimicry, altered self, or other mechanisms. Which of these mechanisms predominates in the development of autoantibodies in various human diseases remains to be determined.

## ACKNOWLEDGMENTS

*We gratefully acknowledge the assistance of Dr. J. Charles Jennette (renal histopathology) and Ms. Melody Shaw (indirect immunofluorescence) in preparing the figures. Work was supported by research grants AR40391 and AR44731 from the Public Health Service and a Biomedical Science Grant from the Arthritis Foundation; Dr. Richards is an Arthritis Foundation Postdoctoral Fellow.*

## REFERENCES

1. Liblau RS, Singer SM, McDevitt HO. Th1 and Th2 CD4$^+$ T cells in pathogenesis of organ-specific autoimmune diseases. *Immunol Today* 1995;16:34–38.
2. Kotzin BL. Systemic lupus erythematosus. *Cell* 1996;85:303–306.
3. Tan EM. Autoantibodies to nuclear antigens (ANA): their biology and medicine. *Adv Immunol* 1982;33:167–240.
4. Carpenter AB. Enzyme-linked immunoassays. In: Rose NR, Conway de Macario E, Folds JD, et al., eds. *Manual of clinical laboratory immunology.* Washington, DC: American Society for Microbiology Press, 1997:20–29.
5. Johnson AM. Immunoprecipitation in gels. In: Rose NR, Friedman H, Fahey JL., eds. *Manual of clinical laboratory immunology.* Washington, DC: American Society for Microbiology Press, 1986:14–24.
6. Kasahara Y. Agglutination immunoassays. In: Rose NR, Conway de Macario E, Folds JD, et al., eds. *Manual of clinical laboratory immunology.* Washington, DC: American Society for Microbiology Press, 1997:7–12.
7. Wener MH, Mannik M. Rheumatoid factors. In: Rose NR, Conway de Macario E, et al., eds. *Manual of clinical laboratory immunology.* Washington, DC: American Society for Microbiology Press, 1997: 942–948–948.
8. Petz LD. Autoimmune hemolytic anemias. In: Rose NR, Conway de Macario E, Folds JD, et al., eds. *Manual of clinical laboratory immunology.* Washington, DC: American Society for Microbiology Press, 1997:1018–1025.
9. Towbin H, Staehelin T, Gordon J. Electrophoretic transfer of proteins from polyacrylamide gels to nitrocellulose sheets: procedure and some applications. *Proc Natl Acad Sci USA* 1979;76:4350–4354.
10. Lerner MR, Steitz JA. Antibodies to small nuclear RNAs complexed with proteins are produced by patients with systemic lupus erythematosus. *Proc Natl Acad Sci USA* 1979;76:5495–5499.
11. Coombs RR. Immunopathology. *Br Med J* 1968;1:597–602.
12. Engelfriet CP, Overbeeke MA, von dBE. Autoimmune hemolytic anemia. *Semin Hematol* 1992;29:3–12.
13. Winkelstein A, Kiss JE. Immunohematologic disorders. *JAMA* 1997;278: 1982–1992.
14. Nydegger UE, Kazatchkine MD, Miescher PA. Immunopathologic and clinical features of hemolytic anemia due to cold agglutinins. *Semin Hematol* 1991;28:66–77.
15. Clynes R, Ravetch JV. Cytotoxic antibodies trigger inflammation through Fc receptors. *Immunity* 1995;3:21–26.
16. Sylvestre D, Clynes R, Ma M, et al. Immunoglobulin G–mediated inflammatory responses develop normally in complement-deficient mice. *J Exp Med* 1996;184:2385–2392.
17. Ravetch JV. Fc receptors: rubor redux. *Cell* 1994;78:553–560.
18. Daeron M. Fc receptor biology. *Annu Rev Immunol* 1997;15:203–234.
19. Takai T, Li M, Sylvestre D, Clynes R, Ravetch JV. FcR gamma chain deletion results in pleiotropic effector cell defects. *Cell* 1994;76: 519–529.
20. Chan EK, Tan EM. Human autoantibody-reactive epitopes of SS-B/La are highly conserved in comparison with epitopes recognized by murine monoclonal antibodies. *J Exp Med* 1987;166:1627–1640.
21. Baker JR. Autoimmune endocrine disease. *JAMA* 1997;278:1931–1937.
22. Rees Smith B, McLachlan SM, Furmaniak J. Autoantibodies to the thyrotropin receptor. *Endocr Rev* 1988;9:106–121.
23. Volpe R. Thyrotropin receptor autoantibodies. In: Peter JB, Shoenfeld Y, eds. *Autoantibodies.* Amsterdam: Elsevier, 1996:822–829.
24. Manley SW, Bourke JR, Hawker RW. The thyrotrophin receptor in guinea-pig thyroid homogenate: interaction with the long-acting thyroid stimulator. *J Endocrinol* 1974;61:437–445.
25. Smith BR, Hall R. Thyroid-stimulating immunoglobulins in Graves' disease. *Lancet* 1974;2:427–430.
26. Chazenbalk GD, Jaume JC, McLachlan SM, et al. Engineering the human thyrotropin receptor ectodomain from a non-secreted form to a secreted, highly immunoreactive glycoprotein that neutralizes autoantibodies in Graves' patients' sera. *J Biol Chem* 1997;272: 18959–18965.
27. Matsuura N, Yamada Y, Nohara Y, et al. Familial neonatal transient hypothyroidism due to maternal TSH-binding inhibitor immunoglobulins. *N Engl J Med* 1980;303:738–741.
28. Lindstrom J. Immunobiology of myasthenia gravis, experimental autoimmune myasthenia gravis, and Lambert-Eaton syndrome. *Annu Rev Immunol* 1985;3:109–131.
29. Keesey J, Lindstrom J, Cokely H, Herrmann C. Anti-acetylcholine receptor antibody in neonatal myasthenia gravis. *N Engl J Med* 1977; 296:55.
30. Toyka KV, Drachman DB, Pestronk A, et al. Myasthenia gravis: passive transfer from man to mouse. *Science* 1975;190:397–399.
31. Tzartos SJ, Lindstrom JM. Monoclonal antibodies used to probe acetylcholine receptor structure: localization of the main immunogenic region and detection of similarities between subunits. *Proc Natl Acad Sci USA* 1980;77:755–759.
32. Mannik M. Immune complexes. In: Lahita RG, ed. *Systemic lupus erythematosus.* New York: Churchill Livingstone, 1992:327–341.
33. Belmont HM, Abramson SB, Lie JT. Pathology and pathogenesis of vascular injury in systemic lupus erythematosus. *Arthritis Rheum* 1996;39:9–22.
34. Schifferli JA, Woo P, Peters DK. Complement-mediated inhibition of immune precipitation. I. Role of the classical and alternative pathways. *Clin Exp Immunol* 1982;47:555–562.
35. Dixon FJ, Feldman JD, Vazquez JJ. Experimental glomerulonephritis: the pathogenesis of a laboratory model resembling the spectrum of human glomerulonephritis. *J Exp Med* 1961;113:899–919.
36. Roujeau JC, Stern RS. Severe adverse cutaneous reactions to drugs. *N Engl J Med* 1994;331:1272–1285.
37. Sylvestre DL, Ravetch JV. Fc receptors initiate the Arthus reaction: redefining the inflammatory cascade. *Science* 1994;265:1095–1098.
38. Vaughan JH, Bayles TB, Favour CB. The response of serum gamma globulin level and complement titer to adrenocorticotrophic hormone (ACTH) therapy in lupus erythematosus disseminatus. *J Lab Clin Med* 1961;37:698–702.
39. Lloyd W, Schur PH. Immune complexes, complement, and anti-DNA in exacerbations of systemic lupus erythematosus (SLE). *Medicine (Baltimore)* 1981;60:208–217.
40. Koffler D, Schur PH, Kunkel HG. Immunological studies concerning the nephritis of systemic lupus erythematosus. *J Exp Med* 1967; 126:607–624.
41. Lefkowith JB, Gilkeson GS. Nephritogenic autoantibodies in lupus: current concepts and continuing controversies. *Arthritis Rheum* 1996;39:894–903.
42. Kramers C, Hylkema MN, van Bruggen MCJ, et al. Anti-nucleosome antibodies complexed to nucleosomal antigens show anti-DNA reactivity and bind to rat glomerular basement membrane *in vivo. J Clin Invest* 1994;94:568–577.

43. Agnello V. Complement deficiency states. *Medicine (Baltimore)* 1978;57:1–23.
44. Walport MJ, Davies KA, Morley BJ, et al. Complement deficiency and autoimmunity. *Ann N Y Acad Sci* 1997;815:267–281.
45. Satoh M, Kumar A, Kanwar YS, et al. Antinuclear antibody production and immune complex glomerulonephritis in BALB/c mice treated with pristane. *Proc Natl Acad Sci USA* 1995;92:10934–10938.
46. Shlomchik MJ, Madaio MP, Ni D, et al. The role of B cells in lpr/lpr-induced autoimmunity. *J Exp Med* 1994;180:1295–1306.
47. Vlahakos DV, Foster MH, Adams S, et al. Anti-DNA antibodies form immune deposits at distinct glomerular and vascular sites. *Kidney Int* 1992;41:1690–1700.
48. Ohnishi K, Ebling FM, Mitchell B, et al. Comparison of pathogenic and non-pathogenic murine antibodies to DNA: antigen binding and structural characteristics. *Int Immunol* 1994;6:817–830.
49. Raz E, Brezis M, Rosenmann E, et al. Anti-DNA antibodies bind directly to renal antigens and induce kidney dysfunction in the isolated perfused rat kidney. *J Immunol* 1989;142:3076–3082.
50. Lanier BG, McDuffie FC, Holley KE. Role of C5 in the nephritis of NZB/W mice. *J Immunol* 1971;106:740–746.
51. Wang Y, Hu Q, Madri JA, et al. Amelioration of lupus-like autoimmune disease in NZB/W F1 mice after treatment with a blocking monoclonal antibody specific for complement component C5. *Proc Natl Acad Sci USA* 1996;93:8563–8568.
52. Frank MM, Hamburger MI, Lawley TJ, et al. Defective reticuloendothelial system Fc-receptor function in systemic lupus erythematosus. *N Engl J Med* 1979;300:518–523.
53. Salmon JE, Millard S, Schachter LA, et al. Fc gamma RIIA alleles are heritable risk factors for lupus nephritis in African Americans. *J Clin Invest* 1996;97:1348–1354.
54. Edworthy SM, Zatarain E, McShane DJ, et al. Analysis of the 1982 ARA lupus criteria data set by recursive partitioning methodology: new insights into the relative merit of individual criteria. *J Rheumatol* 1988;15:1493–1498.
55. Shiel WC, Jason M. The diagnostic associations of patients with antinuclear antibodies referred to a community rheumatologist. *J Rheumatol* 1989;16:782–785.
56. Hooper B, Whittingham S, Mathews JD, et al. Autoimmunity in a rural community. *Clin Exp Immunol* 1972;12:79–87.
57. Hawkins BR, O'Connor KJ, Dawkins RL, et al. Autoantibodies in an Australian population. I. Prevalence and persistence. *J Clin Lab Immunol* 1979;2:211–215.
58. Weinstein A, Bordwell B, Stone B, et al. Antibodies to native DNA and serum complement (C3) levels: application to diagnosis and classification of systemic lupus erythematosus. *Am J Med* 1983;74:206–216.
59. Koffler D, Agnello V, Carr RI, et al. Anti-DNA antibodies and the renal lesions of patients with systemic lupus erythematosus. *Transplant Proc* 1969;1:933–938.
60. Rumore PM, Steinman CR. Endogenous circulating DNA in systemic lupus erythematosus: occurrence as multimeric complexes bound to histone. *J Clin Invest* 1990;86:69–74.
61. Tan EM, Kunkel HG. Characteristics of a soluble nuclear antigen precipitating with sera of patients with systemic lupus erythematosus. *J Immunol* 1966;96:464–471.
62. Hardin JA, Mimori T. Autoantibodies to ribonucleoproteins. *Clin Rheum Dis* 1985;11:485–505.
63. Craft J. Antibodies to snRNPs in systemic lupus erythematosus. *Rheum Dis Clin North Am* 1992;18:311–335.
64. Miyachi K, Tan EM. Antibodies reacting with ribosomal ribonucleoprotein in connective tissue diseases. *Arthritis Rheum* 1979;22:87–93.
65. Elkon KB, Bonfa E, Brot N. Antiribosomal antibodies in systemic lupus erythematosus. *Rheum Dis Clin North Am* 1992;18:377–390.
66. Bonfa E, Golombek SJ, Kaufman LD, et al. Association between lupus psychosis and anti-ribosomal P protein antibodies. *N Engl J Med* 1987;317:265–271.
67. Teh LS, Isenberg DA. Antiribosomal P protein antibodies in systemic lupus erythematosus. *Arthritis Rheum* 1994;37:307–315.
68. Reimer G, Steen VD, Penning CA, et al. Correlates between autoantibodies to nucleolar antigens and clinical features in patients with systemic sclerosis (scleroderma). *Arthritis Rheum* 1988;31:525–532.
69. Kuwana M, Kaburaki J, Okano Y, et al. Clinical and prognostic associations based on serum antinuclear antibodies in Japanese patients with systemic sclerosis. *Arthritis Rheum* 1994;37:75–83.
70. Okano Y, Steen VD, Medsger TAJ. Autoantibody to U3 nucleolar ribonucleoprotein (fibrillarin) in patients with systemic sclerosis. *Arthritis Rheum* 1992;35:95–100.
71. Okano Y, Medsger TA. Autoantibody to Th ribonucleoprotein (nucleolar 7-2 RNA protein particle) in patients with systemic sclerosis. *Arthritis Rheum* 1990;33:1822–1828.
72. Rodriguez-Sanchez J, Gelpi C, Juarez C, et al. A new autoantibody in scleroderma that recognizes a 90-kDa component of the nucleolus organizing region of chromatin. *J Immunol* 1987;139:2579–2584.
73. Hirakata M, Okano Y, Pati U, et al. Identification of autoantibodies to RNA polymerase II: occurrence in systemic sclerosis and association with autoantibodies to RNA polymerase I and III. *J Clin Invest* 1993;91:2665–2672.
74. Okano Y, Steen VD, Medsger TA. Autoantibody reactive with RNA polymerase III in systemic sclerosis. *Ann Intern Med* 1993;119:1005–1013.
75. Satoh M, Kuwana M, Ogasawara T, et al. Association of autoantibodies to topoisomerase I and the phosphorylated (IIO) form of RNA polymerase II in Japanese scleroderma patients. *J Immunol* 1994;153:5838–5848.
76. Rothfield NF. Autoantibodies in scleroderma. *Rheum Dis Clin North Am* 1992;18:483–498.
77. Satoh M, Ajmani AK, Ogasawara T, et al. Autoantibodies to RNA polymerase II are common in systemic lupus erythematosus and overlap syndrome. Specific recognition of the phosphorylated (IIO) form by a subset of human sera. *J Clin Invest* 1994;94:1981–1989.
78. Fritzler MJ, Kinsella TD, Garbutt E. The CREST syndrome: a distinct serologic entity with anticentromere antibodies. *Am J Med* 1980;69:520–526.
79. Earnshaw WC, Machlin PS, Bordwell BJ, et al. Analysis of anticentromere autoantibodies using cloned autoantigen CENP-B. *Proc Natl Acad Sci USA* 1987;84:4979–4983.
80. Goldman JA. Anicentromere antibody in patients without CREST and scleroderma: association with active digital vasculitis, rheumatic and connective tissue disease. *Ann Rheum Dis* 1989;48:771–775.
81. Wade JP, Sack B, Schur PH. Anticentromere antibodies—clinical correlates. *J Rheumatol* 1988;15:1759–1763.
82. Weiner ES, Hildebrandt S, Senecal JL, et al. Prognostic significance of anticentromere antibodies and anti-topoisomerase I antibodies in Raynaud's disease. *Arthritis Rheum* 1991;34:68–77.
83. Targoff IN. Autoantibodies in polymyositis. *Rheum Dis Clin North Am* 1992;18:455–482.
84. Love LA, Leff RL, Fraser DD, et al. A new approach to the classification of idiopathic inflammatory myopathy: myositis-specific autoantibodies define a useful homogeneous patient group. *Medicine (Baltimore)* 1991;70:360–374.
85. O'Donohue J, Williams R. Primary biliary cirrhosis. *Q J Med* 1996;89:5–13.
86. Berg PA, Klein R. Antimitochondrial antibodies in primary biliary cirrhosis. *J Hepatol* 1986;2:123–131.
87. Klein R, Pointner H, Zilly W, et al. Antimitochondrial antibody profiles in primary biliary cirrhosis distinguish at early stages between a benign and a progressive course: a prospective study on 200 patients followed for 10 years. *Liver* 1997;17:119–128.
88. Van de Water J, Gershwin ME, Leung P, et al. The autoepitope of the 74-kD mitochondrial autoantigen of primary biliary cirrhosis corresponds to the functional site of dihydrolipoamide acetyltransferase. *J Exp Med* 1988;167:1791–1799.
89. Metcalf JV, Mitchison HC, Palmer JM, et al. Natural history of early primary biliary cirrhosis. *Lancet* 1996;348:1399–1402.
90. Mitchison HC, Lucey MR, Kelly PJ, et al. Symptom development and prognosis in primary biliary cirrhosis: a study in two centers. *Gastroenterology* 1990;99:778–784.
91. Krams SM, Surh CD, Coppel RL, et al. Immunization of experimental animals with dihydrolipoamide acetyltransferase, as a purified recombinant polypeptide, generates mitochondrial antibodies but not primary biliary cirrhosis. *Hepatology* 1989;9:411–416.
92. Hardy RR, Hayakawa K. CD5 B cells, a fetal B-cell lineage. *Adv Immunol* 1994;55:297–337.
93. Herzenberg LA, Stall AM, Lalor PA, et al. The LY-1 B cell lineage. *Immunol Rev* 1986;93:81–102.
94. Shirai T, Hirose S, Okada T, et al. CD5+ B cells in autoimmune disease and lymphoid malignancy. *Clin Immunol Immunopathol* 1991;59:173–186.
95. Rickert RC, Rajewsky K, Roes J. Impairment of T-cell–dependent B-cell responses in B-1 cell development in CD19-deficient mice. *Nature* 1995;376:352–355.

96. Ahearn JM, Fischer MB, Croix D, et al. Disruption of the Cr2 locus results in a reduction in B-1a cells and an impaired B cell response to T-dependent antigen. *Immunity* 1996;4:251–262.

97. Casali P, Notkins AL. CD5+ B lymphocytes, polyreactive antibodies and the human B-cell repertoire. *Immunol Today* 1989;10:364–368.

98. Casali P, Burastero SE, Balow JE, et al. High-affinity antibodies to ssDNA are produced by CD-5 cells in systemic lupus erythematosus patients. *J Immunol* 1989;143:3476–3483.

99. Hardy RR, Hayakawa K, Shimizu M, et al. Rheumatoid factor secretion from human Leu-1+ B cells. *Science* 1987;236:81–83.

100. Plater-Zyberk C, Maini RN, Lam K, et al. A rheumatoid arthritis B cell subset expresses a phenotype similar to that in chronic lymphocytic leukemia. *Arthritis Rheum* 1985;28:971–976.

101. Dauphinee M, Tovar Z, Talal N. B cells expressing CD5 are increased in Sjögren's syndrome. *Arthritis Rheum* 1988;31:642–647.

102. Sthoeger ZM, Wakai M, Tse DB, et al. Production of autoantibodies by CD5-expressing B lymphocytes from patients with chronic lymphocytic leukemia. *J Exp Med* 1989;169:255–268.

103. Pani G, Siminovitch KA, Paige CJ. The motheaten mutation rescues B-cell signaling and development in CD45-deficient mice. *J Exp Med* 1997;186:581–588.

104. Sidman CL, Shultz LD, Hardy RR, et al. Production of immunoglobulin isotypes by Ly-1+ B cells in viable motheaten and normal mice. *Science* 1986;232:1423–1425.

105. Sanz I, Dang H, Takei M, et al. $V_H$ sequence of a human anti-Sm autoantibody: evidence that autoantibodies can be unmutated copies of germline genes. *J Immunol* 1989;142:883–887.

106. Diamond B, Scharff MD. Somatic mutation of the T15 heavy chain gives rise to antibody with autoantibody specificity. *Proc Natl Acad Sci USA* 1984;81:5841–5844.

107. Davidson A, Shefner R, Livneh A, et al. The role of somatic mutation of immunoglobulin genes in autoimmunity. *Annu Rev Immunol* 1987;5:85–108.

108. Goodnow CC, Cyster JG, Hartley SB, et al. Self-tolerance checkpoints in B lymphocyte development. *Adv Immunol* 1995;59:279–368.

109. Avrameas S, Ternynck T. Natural autoantibodies: the other side of the immune system. *Res Immunol* 1995;146:235–248.

110. Coutinho A, Kazatchkine MD, Avrameas S. Natural autoantibodies. *Curr Opin Immunol* 1995;7:812–818.

111. Lymberi P, Blancher A, Clavas P, et al. Natural autoantibodies in nude and normal outbred (Swiss) and inbred (BALB/c) mice. *J Autoimmun* 1989;2:283–295.

112. Izui S. Autoimmune hemolytic anemia. *Curr Opin Immunol* 1994;6:926–930.

113. Thornton BP, Vetvicka V, Ross GD. Natural antibody and complement-mediated antigen processing and presentation by B lymphocytes. *J Immunol* 1994;152:1727–1737.

114. Bottinger EC, Bitter-Suermann D. Complement and the regulation of humoral immune responses. *Immunol Today* 1987;8:261–264.

115. Doody GM, Dempsey PW, Fearon DT. Activation of B lymphocytes: integrating signals from CD19, CD22 and Fc gamma RIIb1. *Curr Opin Immunol* 1996;8:378–382.

116. Cambier JC, Pleiman CM, Clark MR. Signal transduction by the B cell antigen receptor and its coreceptors. *Annu Rev Immunol* 1994;12:457–486.

117. Tedder TF, Zhou LJ, Engel P. The CD19/CD21 signal transduction complex of B lymphocytes. *Immunol Today* 1994;15:437–442.

118. Takai T, Ono M, Hikida M, et al. Augmented humoral and anaphylactic responses in Fc gamma RII–deficient mice. *Nature* 1996;379:346–349.

119. Shlomchik M, Mascelli M, Shan H, et al. Anti-DNA antibodies from autoimmune mice arise by clonal expansion and somatic mutation. *J Exp Med* 1990;171:265–298.

120. Reap EA, Sobel ES, Cohen PL, et al. Conventional B cells, not B-1 cells, are responsible for producing autoantibodies in lpr mice. *J Exp Med* 1993;177:69–78.

121. Bloom DD, Davignon JL, Retter MW, et al. V region gene analysis of anti-Sm hybridomas from MRL/Mp-lpr/lpr mice. *J Immunol* 1993;150:1591–1610.

122. Shlomchik MJ, Marshak-Rothstein A, Wolfowicz CB, et al. The role of clonal selection and somatic mutation in autoimmunity. *Nature* 1987;328:805–811.

123. Reininger L, Shibata T, Ozaki S, et al. Variable region sequences of pathogenic anti-mouse red blood cell autoantibodies from autoimmune NZB mice. *Eur J Immunol* 1990;20:771–777.

124. Wang D, Wells SM, Stall AM, et al. Reaction of germinal centers in the T-cell–independent response to the bacterial polysaccharide alpha(1→6)dextran. *Proc Natl Acad Sci USA* 1994;91:2502–2506.

125. Eisenberg RA, Craven SY, Cohen PL. Isotype progression and clonality of anti-Sm autoantibodies in MRL/Mp-lpr/lpr mice. *J Immunol* 1987;139:728–733.

126. Wofsy D, Seaman WE. Successful treatment of autoimmunity in NZB/NZW F1 mice with monoclonal antibody to L3T4. *J Exp Med* 1985;161:378–391.

127. Finck BK, Linsley PS, Wofsy D. Treatment of murine lupus with CTLA4Ig. *Science* 1994;265:1225–1227.

128. Sobel ES, Kakkanaiah VN, Kakkanaiah M, et al. T-B collaboration for autoantibody production in lpr mice is cognate and MHC-restricted. *J Immunol* 1994;152:6011–6016.

129. Holub M. *Immunology of nude mice.* Boca Raton: CRC Press, 1989:1–160.

130. Bernard CCA. The nude mouse in autoimmunity. In: Fogh J, Giovanella BC, eds. *The nude mouse in experimental and clinical research.* New York: Academic Press, 1982:323–344.

131. Mihara M, Ohsugi Y, Saito K, et al. Immunologic abnormality in NZB/NZW F1 mice. Thymus-independent occurrence of B cell abnormality and requirement for T cells in the development of autoimmune disease, as evidenced by an analysis of the athymic nude individuals. *J Immunol* 1988;141:85–90.

132. Gilkeson GS, Pritchard AJ, Pisetsky DS. Cellular requirements for anti-DNA production induced in mice by immunization with bacterial DNA. *Eur J Immunol* 1990;20:1789–1794.

133. Richards HB, Satoh M, Jennette JC, et al. Disparate T cell requirements of two subsets of lupus-specific autoantibodies in nude mice. *Clin Exp Immunol* 1999;115:547–553.

134. Santoro TJ, Portanova JP, Kotzin BL. The contribution of L3T4+ T cells to lymphoproliferation and autoantibody production in MRL-lpr/lpr mice. *J Exp Med* 1988;167:1713–1718.

135. Koh DR, Ho A, Rahemtulla A, et al. Murine lupus in MRL/lpr mice lacking CD4 or CD8 T cells. *Eur J Immunol* 1995;25:2558–2562.

136. Peng SL, Madaio MP, Hughes DPM, et al. Murine lupus in the absence of αβ T cells. *J Immunol* 1996;156:4041–4049.

137. Jevnikar AM, Grusby MJ, Glimcher LH. Prevention of nephritis in major histocompatibility complex class II-deficient MRL-lpr mice. *J Exp Med* 1994;179:1137–1143.

138. Peng SL, Madaio MP, Hayday AC, Craft J. Propagation and regulation of systemic autoimmunity by gamma/delta T cells. *J Immunol* 1996;157:5689–5698.

139. Hoffman RW, Takeda Y, Sharp GC, et al. Human T cell clones reactive against U-small nuclear ribonucleoprotein autoantigens from connective tissue disease patients and healthy individuals. *J Immunol* 1993;151:6460–6469.

140. Okubo M, Yamamoto K, Kato T, et al. Detection and epitope analysis of autoantigen-reactive T cells to the U1–small nuclear ribonucleoprotein A protein in autoimmune disease patients. *J Immunol* 1993;151:1108–1115.

141. Crow MK, DelGuidice-Asch G, Zehetbauer JB, et al. Autoantigen-specific T-cell proliferation induced by the ribosomal P2 protein in patients with systemic lupus erythematosus. *J Clin Invest* 1994;94:345–352.

142. Rajagopalan S, Zordan T, Tsokos GC, et al. Pathogenic anti-DNA autoantibody-inducing T helper cell lines from patients with active lupus nephritis: isolation of CD4-8- T helper cell lines that express the gamma delta T-cell antigen receptor. *Proc Natl Acad Sci USA* 1990;87:7020–7024.

143. Mohan C, Adams S, Stanik V, et al. Nucleosome: a major immunogen for pathogenic autoantibody-inducing T cells of lupus. *J Exp Med* 1993;177:1367–1381.

144. Harding FA, McArthur JG, Gross JA, et al. CD28-mediated signalling co-stimulates murine T cells and prevents induction of anergy in T-cell clones. *Nature* 1992;356:607–609.

145. Thompson CB. Distinct roles for the costimulatory ligands B7-1 and B7-2 in T helper cell differentiation. *Cell* 1995;81:979–982.

146. Linsley PS, Brady W, Grosmaire L, et al. Binding of the B cell activation antigen B7 to CD28 costimulates T cell proliferation and interleukin 2 mRNA accumulation. *J Exp Med* 1991;173:721–730.

147. Lenschow DJ, Walunas TL, Bluestone JA. CD28/B7 system of T cell costimulation. *Annu Rev Immunol* 1996;14:233–258.

148. Bluestone JA. Is CTLA-4 a master switch for peripheral T cell tolerance? *J Immunol* 1997;158:1989–1993.

149. Linsley PS, Wallace PM, Johnson J, et al. Immunosuppression *in vivo* by a soluble form of the CTLA-4 T cell activation molecule. *Science* 1992;257:792–795.

150. Han S, Hathcock K, Zheng B, et al. Cellular interaction in germinal centers: roles of CD40 ligand and B7-2 in established germinal centers. *J Immunol* 1995;155:556–567.

151. Banchereau J, Bazan F, Blanchard D, et al. The CD40 antigen and its ligand. *Annu Rev Immunol* 1994;12:881–922.

152. Laman JD, Claassen E, Noelle RJ. Functions of CD40 and its ligand, gp39 (CD40L). *Crit Rev Immunol* 1996;16:59–108.

153. Xu J, Foy TM, Laman JD, et al. Mice deficient for the CD40 ligand. *Immunity* 1994;1:423–431.

154. Kawabe T, Naka T, Yoshida K, et al. The immune responses in CD40-deficient mice: impaired immunoglobulin class switching and germinal center formation. *Immunity* 1994;1:167–178.

155. Aruffo A, Farrington M, Hollenbaugh D, et al. The CD40 ligand, gp39, is defective in activated T cells from patients with X-linked hyper-IgM syndrome. *Cell* 1993;72:291–300.

156. Foy TM, Laman JD, Ledbetter JA, et al. GP39-CD40 interactions are essential for germinal center formation and the development of B cell memory. *J Exp Med* 1994;180:157–163.

157. Liu YJ, Banchereau J. Regulation of B-cell commitment to plasma cells or to memory B cells. *Semin Immunol* 1997;9:235–240.

158. Ma J, Xu J, Madaio MP, et al. Autoimmune lpr/lpr mice deficient in CD40 ligand: spontaneous Ig class switching with dichotomy of autoantibody responses. *J Immunol* 1996;157:417–426.

159. Mohan C, Shi Y, Laman JD, et al. Interaction between CD40 and its ligand gp39 in the development of murine lupus nephritis. *J Immunol* 1995;154:1470–1480.

160. Daikh DI, Finck BK, Linsley PS, et al. Long-term inhibition of murine lupus by brief simultaneous blockade of the B7/CD28 and CD40/gp39 costimulation pathways. *J Immunol* 1997;159:3104–3108.

161. Romagnani S. Lymphokine production by human T cells in disease states. *Annu Rev Immunol* 1994;12:227–257.

162. Hagiwara E, Klinman DM. Abnormalities in cytokine production and responsiveness in autoimmune disease. In: Snapper CM, ed. *Cytokine regulation of humoral immunity: basic and clinical aspects.* Chichester, UK: John Wiley & Sons, 1996:409–430.

163. Ishida H, Muchamuel T, Sakaguchi S, et al. Continuous administration of anti-interleukin 10 antibodies delays onset of autoimmunity in NZB/W F1 mice. *J Exp Med* 1994;179:305–310.

164. Herron LR, Coffman RL, Bond MW, et al. Increased autoantibody production by NZB/NZW B cells in response to IL-5. *J Immunol* 1988;141:842–848.

165. Goldman M, Druet P, Gleichmann E. T$_H$2 cells in systemic autoimmunity: insights from allogeneic diseases and chemically induced autoimmunity. *Immunol Today* 1991;12:223–227.

166. Takahashi S, Fossati L, Iwamoto M, et al. Imbalance towards Th1 predominance is associated with acceleration of lupus-like autoimmune syndrome in MRL mice. *J Clin Invest* 1996;97:1597–1604.

167. Huang FP, Feng GJ, Lindop G, et al. The role of interleukin 12 and nitric oxide in the development of spontaneous autoimmune disease in MRL/MP-lpr/lpr mice. *J Exp Med* 1996;183:1447–1459.

168. Erb KJ, Ruger B, von Brevern M, et al. Constitutive expression of interleukin (IL)-4 *in vivo* causes autoimmune-type disorders in mice. *J Exp Med* 1997;185:329–339.

169. Ochel M, Vohr HW, Pfeiffer C, et al. IL-4 is required for the IgE and IgG1 increase and IgG1 autoantibody formation in mice treated with mercuric chloride. *J Immunol* 1991;146:3006–3011.

170. Jacob CO, van der Meide PH, McDevitt HO. *In vivo* treatment of (NZB × NZW)F1 lupus-like nephritis with monoclonal antibody to gamma interferon. *J Exp Med* 1987;166:798–803.

171. Ozmen L, Roman D, Fountoulakis M, et al. Experimental therapy of systemic lupus erythematosus: the treatment of NZB/W mice with mouse soluble interferon-gamma receptor inhibits the onset of glomerulonephritis. *Eur J Immunol* 1995;25:6–12.

172. Haas C, Le Hir M. IFN-gamma is essential for the development of autoimmune glomerulonephritis in MRL/lpr mice. *J Immunol* 1997;158:5484–5491.

173. Peng SL, Moslehi J, Craft J. Roles of interferon-gamma and interleukin-4 in murine lupus. *J Clin Invest* 1997;99:1936–1946.

174. Akira S, Taga T, Kishimoto T. Interleukin-6 in biology and medicine. *Adv Immunol* 1993;54:1–78.

175. Hirano T, Taga T, Yasukawa K, et al. Human B-cell differentiation factor defined by an anti-peptide antibody and its possible role in autoantibody production. *Proc Natl Acad Sci USA* 1987;84:228–231.

176. Alarcon-Riquelme ME, Moller G, Fernandez C. Macrophage depletion decreases IgG anti-DNA in cultures from (NZB × NZW)F1 spleen cells by eliminating the main source of IL-6. *Clin Exp Immunol* 1993;91:220–225.

177. Finck BK, Chan B, Wofsy D. Interleukin-6 promotes murine lupus in NZB/NZW F1 mice. *J Clin Invest* 1994;94:585–591.

178. Richards HB, Satoh M, Shaw M, et al. IL-6 dependence of anti-DNA antibody production: evidence for two pathways of autoantibody formation in pristane-induced lupus. *J Exp Med* 1998;188:985-990.

179. Jourdan M, Bataille R, Seguin J, et al. Constitutive production of interleukin-6 and immunologic features in cardiac myxomas. *Arthritis Rheum* 1990;33:398–402.

180. Fagiolo U, Cossarizza A, Scala E, et al. Increased cytokine production in mononuclear cells of healthy elderly people. *Eur J Immunol* 1993;23:2375–2378.

181. Bias WB, Reveille JD, Beaty TH, et al. Evidence that autoimmunity in man is a mendelian dominant trait. *Am J Hum Genet* 1991;39:584–602.

182. Theofilopoulos AN. The basis of autoimmunity. Part II. Genetic predisposition. *Immunol Today* 1995;16:150–159.

183. Hibbs ML, Tarlinton DM, Armes J, et al. Multiple defects in the immune system of lyn-deficient mice, culminating in autoimmune disease. *Cell* 1995;83:301–311.

184. Cohen PL, Eisenberg RA. Lpr and gld: single gene models of systemic autoimmunity and lymphoproliferative disease. *Annu Rev Immunol* 1991;9:243–269.

185. Wu J, Longmate JA, Adamus G, et al. Interval mapping of quantitative trait loci controlling humoral immunity to exogenous antigens: evidence that non-MHC immune response genes may also influence susceptibility to autoimmunity. *J Immunol* 1996;157:2498–2505.

186. Arnett FC. The genetic basis of lupus erythematosus. In: Wallace DJ, Hahn BH, eds. *DuBois' lupus erythematosus.* Philadelphia: Lea & Febiger, 1993:13–36.

187. Hess E. Drug-related lupus. *N Engl J Med* 1988;318:1460–1462.

188. Blomgren SE, Condemi JJ, Vaughan JH. Proacainamide-induced lupus erythematosus. *Am J Med* 1972;52:338–3348.

189. Griem P, Gleichmann E. Metal ion induced autoimmunity. *Curr Opin Immunol* 1995;7:831–838.

190. Pollard KM, Lee DK, Casiano CA, et al. The autoimmunity-inducing xenobiotic mercury interacts with the autoantigen fibrillarin and modifies its molecular and antigenic properties. *J Immunol* 1997;158:3521–3528.

191. Kumagai Y, Shiokawa Y, Medsger TAJ, et al. Clinical spectrum of connective tissue disease after cosmetic surgery: observations on eighteen patients and a review of the Japanese literature. *Arthritis Rheum* 1984;27:1–12.

192. Hochberg MC, Perlmutter DL, Medsger TA, et al. Lack of association between augmentation mammoplasty and systemic sclerosis (scleroderma). *Arthritis Rheum* 1996;39:1125–1131.

193. Satoh M, Reeves WH. Induction of lupus-associated autoantibodies in BALB/c mice by intraperitoneal injection of pristane. *J Exp Med* 1994;180:2341–2346.

194. Nordan RP, Potter M. A macrophage-derived factor required by plasmacytomas for survival and proliferation *in vitro*. *Science* 1986;233: 566–569.

195. Shacter E, Arzadon GK, Williams J. Elevation of interleukin-6 in response to a chronic inflammatory stimulus in mice: inhibition by indomethacin. *Blood* 1992;80:194–202.

196. Anderson PN, Potter M. Induction of plasma cell tumours in BALB/c mice with 2,6,10,14-tetramethylpentadecane (pristane). *Nature* 1969; 222:994–995.

197. Dziarski R. Preferential induction of autoantibody secretion in polyclonal activation by peptidoglycan and lipopolysaccharide: *in vitro* studies. *J Immunol* 1982;128:1018–1025.

198. Dziarski R. Preferential induction of autoantibody secretion in polyclonal activation by peptidoglycan and lipopolysaccharide. II. *In vivo* studies. *J Immunol* 1982;128:1026–1030.

199. Klinman DM, Steinberg AD. Systemic autoimmune disease arises from polyclonal B cell activation. *J Exp Med* 1987;165:1755–1760.

200. Hang L, Slack JH, Amundson C, et al. Induction of murine autoimmune disease by chronic polyclonal B cell activation. *J Exp Med* 1983;157:874–883.

201. Van Rappard-Van der Veen FM, Kiesel U, Poels L, et al. Further evidence against random polyclonal antibody formation in mice with lupus-like graft-vs-host disease. *J Immunol* 1984;132:1814–1820.

202. Chou CH, Ali SA, Roubey R, et al. Onset and regulation of lamin B autoantibody production is independent of the level of polyclonal activation. *Autoimmunity* 1991;8:297–305.

203. Reininger L, Shibata T, Schurmans S, et al. Spontaneous production of anti-mouse red blood cell autoantibodies is independent of the polyclonal activation in NZB mice. *Eur J Immunol* 1990;20:2405–2410.

204. Klinman D. Polyclonal B cell activation in lupus-prone mice precedes and predicts the development of autoimmune disease. *J Clin Invest* 1990;86:1249–1254.

205. Klinman DM, Eisenberg RA, Steinberg AD. Development of the autoimmune B cell repertoire in MRL-lpr/lpr mice. *J Immunol* 1990;144:506–511.

206. Oldstone MBA. Molecular mimicry and autoimmune disease. *Cell* 1987;50:819–820.

207. Gianani R, Sarvetnick N. Viruses, cytokines, antigens, and autoimmunity. *Proc Natl Acad Sci USA* 1996;93:2257–2259.

208. Fujinami RS, Oldstone MBA, Wroblewska Z, et al. Molecular mimicry in virus infection: crossreaction of measles virus phosphoprotein or of herpes simplex virus protein with human intermediate filaments. *Proc Natl Acad Sci USA* 1983;80:2346–2350.

209. Query CC, Keene JD. A human autoimmune protein associated with U1 RNA contains a region of homology that is cross-reactive with retroviral p30$^{gag}$ antigen. *Cell* 1987;51:211–220.

210. Hermann H, Fabrizio P, Raker VA, et al. snRNP Sm proteins share two evolutionarily conserved sequence motifs which are involved in Sm protein-protein interactions. *EMBO J* 1995;14:2076–2088.

211. Habets WJ, Sillekens PTG, Hoet MH, et al. Small nuclear RNA-associated proteins are immunologically related as revealed by mapping of autoimmune reactive B-cell epitopes. *Proc Natl Acad Sci USA* 1989;86:4674–4678.

212. Hirakata M, Craft J, Hardin JA. Autoantigenic epitopes of the B and D polypeptides of the U1 snRNP: analysis of domains recognized by the Y12 monoclonal anti-Sm antibody and by patient sera. *J Immunol* 1993;150:3592–3601.

213. Brahms H, Raker VA, van Venrooij WJ, et al. A major, novel systemic lupus erythematosus autoantibody class recognizes the E, F, and G Sm snRNP proteins as an E-F-G complex but not in their denatured states. *Arthritis Rheum* 1997;40:672–682.

214. Wang JYJ. Antibodies for phosphotyrosine: analytical and preparative tool for tyrosyl-phosphorylated proteins. *Anal Biochem* 1988;172:1–7.

215. Vladutiu AA, Rose NR. Cellular basis of the genetic control of immune responsiveness to murine thyroglobulin in mice. *Cell Immunol* 1975;17:106–113.

216. Klareskog L. What can we learn about rheumatoid arthritis from animal models? *Springer Semin Immunopathol* 1989;11:315–333.

217. Alonzi T, Fattori E, Lazzaro D, et al. Interleukin 6 is required for the development of collagen-induced arthritis. *J Exp Med* 1998;187:461–468.

218. Farquhar MG, Saito A, Kerjaschki D, et al. The Heymann nephritis antigenic complex: megalin (gp330) and RAP. *J Am Soc Nephrol* 1995;6:35–47.

219. Kerjaschki D, Neale TJ. Molecular mechanisms of glomerular injury in rat experimental membranous nephropathy (Heymann nephritis). *J Am Soc Nephrol* 1996;7:2518–2526.

220. Lane DP, Crawford LV. T antigen bound to a host protein in SV40-transformed cells. *Nature* 1979;278:261–263.

221. Linzer DIH, Levine AJ. Characterization of a 54 k dalton cellular SV40 tumor antigen present in SV40-transformed cells and uninfected embryonal carcinoma cells. *Cell* 1979;17:43–52.

222. Dong X, Hamilton KJ, Satoh M, et al. Initiation of autoimmunity to the p53 tumor suppressor protein by complexes of p53 and SV40 large T antigen. *J Exp Med* 1994;179:1243–1252.

223. Craft J, Fatenejad S. Self antigens and epitope spreading in systemic autoimmunity. *Arthritis Rheum* 1997;40:1374–1382.

224. Cibotti R, Kanellopoulos JM, Cabaniols JP, et al. Tolerance to a self protein involves its immunodominant but does not involve its subdominant determinants. *Proc Natl Acad Sci USA* 1992;89:416–420.

225. Casciola-Rosen L, Wigley F, Rosen A. Scleroderma autoantigens are uniquely fragmented by metal-catalyzed oxidation reactions: implications for pathogenesis. *J Exp Med* 1997;185:71–79.

226. Soussi T. The humoral response to the tumor-suppressor gene-product p53 in human cancer: implications for diagnosis and therapy. *Immunol Today* 1996;17:354–356.

227. Crawford LV, Pim DC, Bulbrook RD. Detection of antibodies against the cellular protein p53 in sera from patients with breast cancer. *Int J Cancer* 1982;30:403–408.

228. Davidoff AM, Iglehart JD, Marks JR. Immune response to p53 is dependent upon p53/HSP70 complexes in breast cancers. *Proc Natl Acad Sci USA* 1992;89:3439–3442.

229. Schlichtholz B, Legros Y, Gillet D, et al. The immune response to p53 in breast cancer patients is directed against immunodominant epitopes unrelated to the mutational hot spot. *Cancer Res* 1992;52:6380–6384.

230. Kunkel HG, Posnett DN, Pernis B. Anti-immunoglobulins and their idiotypes: are they part of the immune network? *Ann N Y Acad Sci* 1984;324–329.

231. Plotz PH. Autoantibodies are anti-idiotype antibodies to antiviral antibodies. *Lancet* 1983;2:824–826.

232. Cleveland WL, Wassermann NH, Sarangarajan R, et al. Monoclonal antibodies to the acetylcholine receptor by a normally functioning auto-anti-idiotypic mechanism. *Nature* 1983;305:56–57.

233. Moller G. Anti-idiotype antibodies as immunogens. *Immunol Rev* 1987;90:5–155.

234. Mathews MB, Bernstein RM. Myositis autoantibody inhibits histidyl-tRNA synthetase: a model for autoimmunity. *Nature* 1983;304:177–179.

235. Bunn CC, Bernstein RM, Mathews MB. Autoantibodies against alanyl-tRNA synthetase and tRNA (ala) coexist and are associated with myositis. *J Exp Med* 1986;163:1281–1291.

236. Casciola-Rosen LA, Anhalt GJ, Rosen A. DNA-dependent protein kinase is one of a subset of autoantigens specifically cleaved early during apoptosis. *J Exp Med* 1995;182:1625–1634.

237. Ravetch JV, Kinet JP. Fc receptors. *Annu Rev Immunol* 1991;9:457–492.

*Textbook of the Autoimmune Diseases,*
Edited by R. G. Lahita, N. Chiorazzi, and W. H. Reeves,
Lippincott Williams & Wilkins, Philadelphia © 2000.

# CHAPTER 9

# Cytokines in Autoimmunity

Jorge Alcocer-Varela and Xavier Valencia

Autoimmunity is regarded as the inability of the immune system to distinguish between self and nonself. The immune system has the capacity to maintain a state of equilibrium, although it responds to a diverse array of foreign antigens and despite its permanent exposure to self antigens. During the past decade, much progress has been made in the understanding of processes that lead from a normal autoimmune state, in which no clinical manifestations exist, to an autoimmune disease. It has been hypothesized that, after an infection, immune response spreads to tissue-specific autoantigens in genetically predisposed subjects, eventually determining progression to disease. Molecular mimicry between microbial or viral and self antigens may in some instances initiate autoimmunity. Local release of inflammatory cytokines after infection probably plays a pivotal role in determining loss of tolerance to self autoantigens and the pathogenic activation of autoreactive cells (1–3).

T-cell tolerance to self antigens cannot solely be accounted for intrathymic clonal deletion or induction of anergy in peripheral T cells. In several experimental systems, expression of the pathogenic capacity of potentially self-reactive T cells was actively prevented by other T cells with an immunoregulatory role (4,5).

Primary exposure of naive CD4$^+$ T cell to antigen results in differentiation to a defined helper subset. The preferential development of a particular helper T-cell subset correlates directly with susceptibility or resistance to certain disease states. Various factors influence the differentiation of particular T$_H$ response, including antigen type, antigen dose, the type of antigen-presenting cell (APC), and the presence of cytokines. The primary helper T-cell types are T$_H$1 and T$_H$2, which are characterized by distinct patterns of cytokine secretion.

This chapter considers cytokine participation in the pathogenesis of autoimmune diseases by analyzing evidence for their participation in these diseases. Each disease shows some similar and some distinct features, some of which are shared with other autoimmune diseases (5–8). Figure 9.1 shows some of the immunoregulatory networks that may be pertinent to the understanding of autoimmune disease.

## T$_H$1 AND T$_H$2 T-CELL SUBSETS

Among the factors known to play an important role in determining the T$_H$1-T$_H$2 balance are antigen and costimulation. Low and high antigen concentrations tend to induce T$_H$2 responses preferentially, whereas intermediate doses induce T$_H$1 responses. The mechanism responsible for these effects is poorly understood. It is possible that certain concentrations of antigen induce a state of tolerance that preferentially shuts off T$_H$1 responses (9–11).

During the presentation of antigens, the type of APC also has a profound effect on the resultant immune response. Langerhans cells and dendritic cells induce T$_H$1 proliferation, whereas B cells tend to induce a T$_H$2 response (12). A major factor in this dichotomy in APC function is the elaboration of particular cytokines on antigen encounter (13).

T$_H$1 cells secrete interleukin-2 (IL-2), tumor necrosis factor-α (TNF-α), and interferon-γ (IFN-γ) and are involved in cell-mediated inflammatory responses. T$_H$2 cells secrete IL-4, IL-5, IL-6, IL-8, IL-10, and IL-13 and favor humoral responses and allergy (14). An important feature of these helper T-cell subsets is the ability of one subset to regulate the activities of the other. The balance between these cells can play a major role in the type of disease manifestation observed. The establishment of this balance depends on many factors, including the antigen structure, the APCs, and the cytokine environment. This feature is critical for understanding the adverse effects induced by cytokines. There is much evidence that the cytokine products of each helper T-cell subset inhibit the differentiation and effector functions of the other. For example, IFN-γ has been shown to prevent T$_H$2

J. Alcocer-Varela: Departments of Immunology and Rheumatology, Instituto Nacional Nutricion, Mexico, DF 14000, Mexico.

X. Valencia: Division of Rheumatology and Immunology, Harvard Medical School, Brigham and Women's Hospital, Boston, Massachusetts 02115.

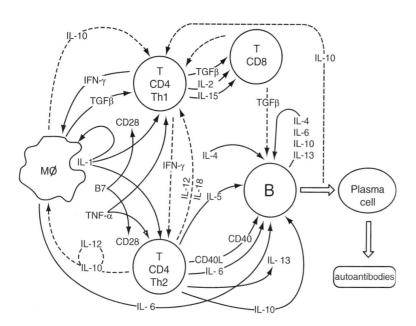

**FIG. 9.1.** Immunoregulatory pathways in humans. Interplays of various activation *(solid lines)* and inhibition systems *(dashed lines)* are shown. Many cytokines have stimulating or inhibitory activities that are influenced by the microenvironment of a cell. Several cytokines are inhibited by soluble receptors; some cytokines inhibit other cytokines.

cell proliferation, whereas IL-10 inhibits the synthesis of $T_H1$ cytokines (14,15). Emergence of a $T_H2$-type response typically results in the inhibition of $T_H1$ differentiation and the downregulation of $T_H1$-mediated immune responses.

## CURRENT CONCEPTS OF CYTOKINES

*Cytokine* is a generic name for a diverse group of soluble proteins and peptides, which act as regulators at low concentrations (nanomolar to picomolar) and which, under normal or pathologic conditions, modulate the functional activities of individual cells and tissues. These molecules also mediate interactions between cells directly and regulate processes taking place in the extracellular environment. The biologic activities of cytokines can be measured by a variety of bioassays employing factor-dependent cell lines or antibodies (enzyme-linked immunoabsorbent assay [ELISA]); using modern techniques of molecular biology, it is possible to measure message amplification phenotyping and to detect the presence of cytokine-specific mRNAs (16).

Many genes encoding cytokines can give rise to a variety of forms of cytokines by means of alternative splicing, yielding molecules with slightly different but biologically significant bioactivities. The expression patterns of different forms of cytokines or of members of a cytokine family are overlapping only partially, suggesting a specific role for each factor.

Almost all cytokines are pleiotropic effectors showing multiple biologic activities. Several cytokines have overlapping activities, and a single cell frequently interacts with multiple cytokines with similar responses. A consequence of this functional overlap is that one factor frequently may functionally replace another altogether or at least partially compensate for the lack of another mediator. Because most cytokines have ubiquitous biologic activities, their physiologic significance as normal regulators or in pathologic situations is often difficult to assess (17,18). Table 9.1 lists the cytokines and their main functions.

Cytokines show stimulating or inhibitory activities and may synergize or antagonize the actions of other factors. A single cytokine may also under certain circumstances elicit reactions that are the reverse of those under other circumstances. The type, the duration, and the extent of cellular activities induced by a particular cytokine can be influenced considerably by the microenvironment of a cell, depending, for example, on the cell cycle phase, the type of APCs, cytokine concentrations, the combination of other cytokines present at the same time, and even on the temporal sequence of several cytokines acting on the same cell. Cytokine signals can travel quickly to remote areas of a multicellular organism. They can reach numerous target cells and can be degraded quickly. It can be assumed that cytokines play an important role in all sorts of cell to cell communication processes, although many of the mechanisms of their actions are still unknown. They also play a central role in neuroimmunologic, neuroendocrinologic, and neuroregulatory processes. Cytokines are important regulators of mitosis, differentiation, migration, cell survival, and cell death. Several infectious agents exploit the cytokine repertoire of organisms to evade immune responses of the host (19,20).

Viruses appear to affect the activities of cytokines by inhibiting the synthesis and release of cytokines from infected cells, by interfering with the interaction between cytokines and their receptors, by inhibiting signal transmission pathways of cytokines, and by synthesizing virus-encoded cytokines that antagonize the effects of host cytokines mediating antiviral processes. The biologic activities of cytokines are mediated by specific membrane receptors, which can be expressed on virtually all cell types. Some receptors are expressed constitutively, but their expression is also subject to several regulatory mechanisms (20).

TABLE 9.1. *Cytokines and their main functions*

| Cytokine | Producer cells | Main actions |
|---|---|---|
| IL-1 $\alpha/\beta$ | Monocytes/macrophages<br>Endothelial cells<br>Fibroblasts<br>Neurons<br>Glial cells<br>Keratinocytes<br>Epithelial cells | Induces prostaglandin synthesis by endothelial cells<br>Induces collagenase synthesis in sinovim and cartilage<br>T-cell activation, IL-2 production, and RIL-2 expression<br>Induces GM-CSF and IL-4 production by activated T cells<br>Stimulates B-cell proliferation and differentiation<br>Synergistic action with other cytokines activating NK cells |
| IL-2 | T cells | T-cell proliferation and differentiation<br>Stimulates cytolytic activity of NK cells<br>Stimulates B-cell proliferation and Ig synthesis<br>Associated with its receptor, it is involved in signals transduction<br>Activates NK and LAK cells<br>Induces cell-mediated immune responses<br>Stimulates neutrophil and macrophage functions |
| IL-3 | T cells<br>Thymic epithelial cells<br>Keratinocytes<br>Neurons<br>Mast cells | Stimulates growth and differentiation of myelomonocytic lineage<br>Stimulates erythroid progenitors |
| IL-4 | T cells<br>Macrophages<br>Mast cells<br>Basofils<br>B cells<br>Bone marrow stroma | Induces naive T-cell differentiation to $T_H2$ cells<br>B-cell growth and differentiation<br>Promotes isotype switch (IgG4 and IgE)<br>Stimulates endothelial cells and fibroblasts |
| IL-5 | T cells<br>Mast cells | Eosinophil growth and differentiation<br>Chemotactic for eosinophils |
| IL-6 | T cells<br>Monocytes/macrophages<br>Fibroblasts<br>Hepatocytes<br>Endothelial cells<br>Neurons | Activates hematopoietic progenitor cells<br>Induces megakaryocyte development<br>Induces growth and differentiation of T and B cells, hepatocytes and keratinocytes<br>Stimulates acute-phase protein production by hepatocytes |
| IL-7 | Bone marrow stroma<br>Fetal liver cells | Growth of pre-B and pro-B cells<br>T-cell proliferation<br>NK and LAK cell enhancing activity |
| IL-8 | Monocytes<br>T cells<br>Fibroblasts<br>Endothelial cells<br>Keratinocytes<br>Hepatocytes<br>Chondrocytes<br>Neutrofils<br>Epithelial cells | Chemotactic for neutrophils, T cells, and basophils<br>Induces release of lisosomal enzymes<br>Induces neutrophil adhesion to endothelial cells |
| IL-9 | T cells | Mast cell enhancing activity<br>Stimulates hematopoiesis<br>Enhances T-cell survival *in vitro* |
| IL-10 | T cells<br>B cells<br>Monocytes/macrophage<br>Keratinocytes<br>Dendritic cells | Inhibits antigen presentation by macrophages<br>Inhibits macrophage proinflammatory cytokine production<br>Induces B-cell activation, Ig synthesis<br>Increases antibody responses |
| IL-11 | Fibroblasts<br>Stroma fibroblasts | Synergistic activity with IL-3 and IL-4 in megakaryocyte development<br>Stimulates acute-phase protein production |
| IL-12 | B cells<br>T cells<br>Macrophages | Stimulates T-cell differentiation to $T_H1$ cells<br>Stimulates NK-cell growth and activation |
| IL-13 | T cells | B-cell growth and differentiation<br>Inhibits monocyte inflammatory cytokine production<br>IgG4 and IgE switch |
| IL-14 | T cells | Induces growth of activated B cells<br>Inhibits Ig production by activated B cells |

**TABLE 9.1.** *Continued*

| Cytokine | Producer cells | Main actions |
|---|---|---|
| IL-15 | T cells | Induces B-cell growth and differentiation |
| | Bone marrow stroma | Induces T-cell proliferation |
| IL-16 | T cells | CD4⁺ T growth factor |
| | | Chemotactic factor for T CD4⁺ cells |
| IL-17 | T cells | Induces IL-6 and IL-8 production by fibroblasts |
| | | Increases adhesion molecule expression by fibroblasts |
| IL-18 | Phagocytic cells | Augments IFN-γ production by T cells, NK cytotoxicity, and T-cell proliferation |
| IFN-α/β | T cells | Antiviral activity |
| | B cells | Stimulates macrophage functions |
| | Monocytes/macrophages | Regulates MHC class I and II expression |
| | Fibroblasts | |
| IFN-γ | T cells | Macrophage activation |
| | NK cells | Increases MHC expression |
| G-CSF | T cells | Stimulates neutrophil activation and differentiation |
| | Macrophages | Stimulates differentiation of granulocyte-macrophage colony |
| | Neutrophils | |
| | Endothelial cells | |
| | Fibroblasts | |
| GM-CSF | Macrophages | Stimulates stem cell development |
| | T cells | Stimulates differentiation of myelomonocytic lineage |
| | Endothelial cells | |
| | Mast cells | |
| | Neutrophils | |
| | Eosinophils | |
| | Fibroblasts | |
| TGF-β | Chondrocytes | Stimulates extracellular matrix proteins |
| | Osteoblasts | Tissue repair |
| | Osteoclasts | Activates osteoblasts and inhibits osteoclasts |
| | Platelets | Inhibits NK functions |
| | Fibroblasts | Inhibits T- and B-cell proliferation |
| | Macrophages | Synergistic action with IL-4 in IgA secretion |
| | NK cells | |
| | Hepatocytes | |
| TNF-α | Neutrophils | Regulates the gene expression of growth factors, cytokines, transcription factors, receptors, and acute-phase proteins |
| | Activated lymphocytes | |
| | NK cells | Helps resistance to infections and neoplasm growth |
| | LAK cells | Local inflammation |
| | Astrocytes | Endothelial activation |
| | Endothelial cells | |
| | Smooth muscle cells | |
| TNF-β | Lymphocytes | Functions similar to TNF-α |

CM-CSF, granulocyte–macrophage colony–stimulating factor; G-CSF, granulocyte colony–stimulating factor; IL, interleukin; IFN, interferon; LAK, lymphokine-activated killer; MHC, major histocompatibility complex; NK, natural killer; TGF, transforming growth factor; T$_H$, help T cell; TNF, tumor necrosis factor.

Cytokine receptors share a number of characteristics. Many of them are multisubunit structures that bind ligands and act as signal transducers because of their intrinsic tyrosine kinase activity. Several receptors often share common signal-transducing receptor components in the same family, which in part explains the functional redundancy of cytokines. This redundancy and the ubiquitous cellular distribution of certain cytokine receptors have hampered attempts to define critical responsive cell populations and the physiologically important cell-specific functions of cytokines *in vivo* (21).

## T$_H$1 AND T$_H$2 CYTOKINES

Since 1986, when Mosmann et al. reported the existence of two different CD4⁺ T cells based on the cytokines they pro-

duce, the T$_H$1/T$_H$2 model has evolved to encompass several newly discovered cytokines and major new functions (22–24). T$_H$1 cytokines and T$_H$2 cytokines refer to the patterns of cytokines secreted by two subpopulations of murine CD4⁺ T cells that determine the outcome of an antigenic response toward humoral or cell-mediated immunity.

Cells other than T cells expressing CD4 are capable of producing T$_H$1 and T$_H$2 cytokines. These cells include CD8⁺ T cells, monocytes, natural killer (NK) cells, B cells, eosinophils, mast cells, basophils, dendritic cells and other cells. T$_H$1 cytokines include IL-2, IFNγ, IL-12, IL-18, and TNF-β. T$_H$2 cytokines include IL-4, IL-5, IL-6, IL-10, and IL-13 (25,26).

The most potent cytokine inducer of T$_H$2 cells is IL-4. Several types of immune cells can produce IL-4 in the initial immune response, including NK1.1$^+$CD4$^+$ T cells, γδ T cells, CD8$^+$ T cells, and mast cells (27,28).

IL-10 inhibits the induction of T$_H$1 immunity and enables the elaboration of a T$_H$2 response. Because IL-10 can be produced by certain APCs (15,29), it has been hypothesized that, under the influence of transforming growth factor-β (TGF-β), the preferential production of IL-10 by APCs leads to the development of T$_H$2 immunity in autoimmune diseases. It has been hypothesized that the autoregulatory effects of IL-10 on APC function might be a critical factor in the ability of an APC to present antigen in a suppressive manner (29).

In direct contrast to IL-4 or IL-10, IL-12 strongly induces the development of T$_H$1 cells (30). Activation of monocytes/macrophages usually results in elaboration of the proinflammatory cytokine IL-12 (30). One effect of IL-12 is direct stimulation of T$_H$1 differentiation. Another effect is the stimulation of IFN-γ production by T and NK cells. IFN-γ is a potent inducer of T$_H$1 immunity by the additional stimulation of IL-12 secretion and the inhibition of IL-4 (24,25,31).

T$_H$1-cell development depends on IL-12 produced by APCs. The interaction of the CD40 ligand on T cells with CD40 on dendritic cells results in very high production of IL-12 (32,33), favoring the development of a T$_H$1 response. Because of the potent proinflammatory and immunoregulatory functions of IL-12, the immune system has developed feedback mechanisms for antagonizing its action. IL-10 negatively regulates IL-12 p40 transcription. In B-cell lines, the nuclear factor NF-κB appears to play a crucial role in the regulation of IL-12 p40 production. Molecular analysis of the promoter region of the human gene for p40 has also identified a member of the ETS family of transcription factors as a major regulatory factor (32).

Another exogenous factor also influencing the development of undifferentiated CD4$^+$ T cells toward the T$_H$1 or T$_H$2 phenotype is TGF-β (34). Murine T$_H$2 cells, but not T$_H$1 cells, also express P600, the human counterpart of which has been identified as IL-13 (35). A novel cytokine inducing the synthesis of IFN-γ in T$_H$1 cells has been identified as IL-18 (36).

T$_H$1 and T$_H$2 cells not only produce a different set of cytokines but also appear to express different activation markers preferentially. CD30, a member of the TNF receptor superfamily, is mainly expressed by T$_H$2-like and cytotoxic T cells, whereas the product of lymphocyte activation gene-3 (LAG-3), a member of the immunoglobulin superfamily, preferentially associates with T$_H$1-type cells (37). It has been identified a stable cell-surface marker (STL2) expressed on T$_H$2 but not T$_H$1 (38).

The different patterns of cytokine secretion correspond with different functions as immune effectors. T$_H$1 cells promote cell-mediated effector responses. T$_H$2 cells are mainly helper cells that influence B-cell development and augment humoral responses such as the secretion of antibodies, predominantly of Ig E, by B cells. Both types of helper T cells influence each other by the cytokines they secrete; IFN-γ, for example, can downregulate T$_H$2 clones, and T$_H$2 cytokines, such as IL-10, can suppress T$_H$1 functions. IFN-γ can inhibit

the proliferation of murine T$_H$2 cells but not that of T$_H$1 clones. It appears that these functional subsets are mutually antagonistic such that the decision about which subset predominates within an infection may also determine its outcome.

T$_H$1-type and T$_H$2-type responses in humans may play an important role in certain diseases. T$_H$1-type responses are involved in the pathogenesis of organ-specific autoimmune disorders and acute allograft rejection and in some chronic inflammatory disorders of the gastrointestinal tract, such as gastric antritis and Crohn's disease. In contrast, allergic reactions involving IgE and mast cells result from the development and activation of allergen-specific T$_H$2 cells. Different types of helper T-cell populations resembling those observed in mice are found also in humans. However, the differences in cytokine expression seem to be quantitative rather than qualitative.

## CYTOKINES IN SYSTEMIC LUPUS ERYTHEMATOSUS

### Immune Dysregulation

Systemic lupus erythematosus (SLE) is the prototype of human autoimmune disease, characterized by multisystem involvement and autoantibodies to nuclear, cytoplasmic, and cell-surface autoantigens. The mechanism responsible for the breakdown of self-tolerance is unknown. This disease has a multifactorial pathogenesis, with genetic and environmental precipitating factors. The immune dysregulation that characterizes the disease is complex but has two main characteristics. One is B-lymphocyte hyperactivity and immunoglobulin repertoire changes, causing increased spontaneous production of immunoglobulins and autoantibody production (39). The mechanism by which B lymphocytes remain inappropriately activated for years during SLE or other autoimmune diseases are still poorly understood and may involve several agents acting in concert: genetic background, environmental factors such as drugs, hormonal influences, viral infections, and abnormal production of cytokines (40–42). The other is an impaired cell-mediated immunity. This includes decreased T-cell proliferative responses in autologous mixed lymphocyte reactions or after stimulation with mitogens, defective costimulatory signals, and several defects in the production of cytokines. The impaired cell-mediated immunity results from T-lymphocyte and APC dysfunctions (43–45).

### Cytokine Regulation

Since 1982, when we reported a defect in the production of and response to IL-2 by mononuclear cells from SLE patients, the production of cytokines in this disease has become the object of numerous studies (46–48). Cytokines have been suggested to play an important role in the immune dysregulation observed in SLE patients and murine lupus-prone strains. Some of the T-cell abnormalities found in SLE patients can be attributed to decreased activity of IL-2.

Whether caused by an intrinsic T-cell alteration or not, a defect in IL-2 regulation occurs in patients with SLE and contributes to the complex disturbances of the immune system of SLE patients.

Although the origin of this abnormality is unknown, several mechanisms have been proposed to explain it: a primary defect of CD4 cells; a suppressive effect of the activity of IL-2 by CD8 cells by means of specific antibodies against IL-2 or by other cytokines; exhaustion of T cells because of their activation *in vivo*; and deficiency of other cytokines that participate in T cells activation. It was later shown that this was not an intrinsic defect, because it recovered after the cells were rested (49). It was also shown that SLE monocytes had defective production of (47,49) and response to IL-1 (49).

Multiple cytokine-mediated alterations have been demonstrated in SLE patients. Abnormal (increased or decreased) production of IL-1, TNF-α, IL-2, IL-3, IL-4, IL-5, IL-6, IL-10, TGF-β, and IFN-γ have been reported (50). Moreover, some of these cytokines (IL-1, TNF-α, IL-6, and IFN-γ) have been found in renal tissue of these patients, suggesting a local pathogenic effect (51).

Although peripheral blood mononuclear cells from SLE patients produce decreased amounts of IL-6 on stimulation, B lymphocytes from SLE patients spontaneously produce IL-6 and constitutively express IL-6 receptors (52). *In vitro* inhibition of this autocrine loop by anti-IL-6 receptor antibodies decreases the spontaneous production of autoantibodies. Anti-TNF-α antibodies also decrease production of immunoglobulins by cultured peripheral blood mononuclear cells of SLE patients, but circulating TNF-α is not detected in such patients. A correlation has been demonstrated for the serum levels of TNF-α receptors, IL-1 receptor antagonist (IL-1ra), and clinical disease activity. Overexpression of TNF-α mRNA in bone marrow cells also has been observed in these patients (53).

The elevated levels of TNF-α and IL-10 observed in SLE patients reflects the hyperactivation of cells that are responsible for the overproduction of autoantibodies. Once induced, these cytokines act as proinflammatory effectors through their biologic properties, including stimulation of a cascade of other soluble factors that amplify the initial stimulus and lead to the progression of the disease. Abnormal IFN-α production has been found in SLE patients (54). This cytokine has pleiotropic effects on the immune system, and its defective production can induce autoimmune manifestations. It has a role in upregulation of major histocompatibility complex (MHC) class II molecules and in this way contributes to the pathogenesis of autoimmunity.

The B-cell hyperactivity found in SLE and in other autoimmune diseases may be related to a generic increase in $T_H2$ cytokines, an increase caused by IL-4, IL-6, and IL-10. However, the IL-6 production in SLE may result from the hyperactivity of cells other than T cells, and increased IL-10 production results from monocytes and B cells rather than T lymphocytes (55). The autocrine and paracrine effects of IL-10 may be crucial to the B-cell hyperactivity and particularly to autoantibody production. IL-10 is a potent stimulator of B lymphocytes, and it stimulates the production of anti-DNA autoantibodies by peripheral blood mononuclear cells from SLE patients (56). It is also a potent inhibitor of APC and T-lymphocyte functions. Increased production of IL-10 could explain the two main characteristics of the immune dysregulation of SLE. Consistent with this concept, several reports demonstrated increased production of IL-10 in SLE patients (57,58).

Immune dysregulation partially mimicking that of SLE has been described in healthy relatives of SLE patients. Some of these relatives display autoreactive B-lymphocyte hyperactivity, although the autoantibodies produced are of low affinity and are not pathogenic. A larger proportion of the relatives display impaired cell-mediated immunity, decreased IL-2 production, and polyclonal B lymphocyte hyperactivity (59). Relatives of SLE patients have a dysregulation of IL-10 production similar to that of patients. This finding strongly suggests that IL-10 gene dysregulation may belong to the background predisposing to the disease rather than representing a simple marker of immune activation (60).

IL-12 is another cytokine that appears to play a role in polyclonal B-cell activation observed in SLE. Its presence in mononuclear cell cultures is able to downregulate the spontaneous immunoglobulin production; this inhibiting activity does not seem to be mediated through IFN-γ secretion (61).

The decreased production of lymphocyte-derived TGF-β in SLE cannot be normalized by the addition of IL-2 and TNF-α or by antagonism of IL-10. Abnormal production of each of these cytokines in SLE could be important in the perpetuation of B-cell hyperactivity (62).

## CYTOKINES IN RHEUMATOID ARTHRITIS

### Pathogenesis of Rheumatoid Arthritis

Although much work has been done, the pathogenesis of rheumatoid arthritis (RA) remains obscure. There are well-recognized susceptibility factors that involve hormonal factors that could account for the disease predominance in women and the genetic contribution to the disease that is clearly contained within the class II MHC locus, especially in the DR1 and DR4 disease-susceptible haplotypes. These haplotypes are found in more than 80% of RA patients of Caucasian origin and constitute one of the strongest pieces of evidence to support the theory that T lymphocytes are important at some point in the pathogenesis of RA by shaping the T-cell receptor (TCR) repertoire or in the presentation of an inducing microbial or autoantigenic peptide. Although many infectious agents have been implicated in the cause of RA over the years, including viruses, mycoplasmal organisms, and mycobacteria, none has been proved to be causative.

RA is considered to be a heterogeneous and systemic disease; it extends throughout the synovial joint and in some cases well beyond the joint. One characteristic finding in RA synovitis is the increase in cellularity, which is most evident in the synovial membrane that becomes infiltrated by cells thought to be recruited from the blood. Characteristically, the lining layer (intima) increases from one to two cells thick to a layer six to eight cells thick composed mostly of activated type A synoviocytes (i.e., macrophage type) along with type B synoviocytes (i.e., fibroblast type). In rheumatoid synovitis, there is also formation of lymphoid aggregates resembling germinal centers in the deeper portions of the synovium around blood vessels containing activated endothelial cells that form high endothelial venules, the site where most activated T cells extravasate (62,63). The most abundant cells in the synovial membrane during the early stages of the disease are macrophages and T lymphocytes, but plasma cells, dendritic cells, and activated fibroblasts are also found. This histologic picture changes according to the chronicity of the disease; in later stages, the type B synoviocytes and macrophages predominate, with fewer number of T cells (64). Many of these cells are activated and express abundantly class II human leukocyte antigen (HLA) and adhesion molecules of relevance in antigen presentation (65–67).

The histologic hallmark of RA, the pannus, is the major site of irreversible tissue damage and originates at the junction of the synovium lining the joint capsule with the cartilage and bone. This tissue is rich in transformed type B synoviocytes and macrophages. The cells of the pannus invade over the underlying cartilage and into the subchondral bone, causing the erosion of these tissues that is characteristic of the disease (68). Cartilage destruction results from the activity of matrix metalloproteinases (MMPs), which are proteolytic enzymes produced and secreted by macrophage-type synoviocytes and type B synoviocytes in response to proinflammatory cytokines such as IL-1 and TNF-α. Collagenase (MMP-1) and stromelysin-1 (MMP-3), whose production is increased, have been found to be important in the destructive process in RA (69). The activity of MMP is regulated to some extent by tissue inhibitors of metalloproteinases (TIMPs); these bind irreversibly the enzyme to form a 1 : 1 complex with the MMP. These TIMPs are produced predominantly by type B synoviocytes and to a lesser extent by the macrophage-type synoviocytes. Two immunoregulatory cytokines, TGF-β and IL-10, that are produced in RA synovium inhibited the production of proinflammatory cytokines that induce MMPs and induced the production of their natural inhibitors, TIMPs (70,71).

## Cytokine Expression in Rheumatoid Arthritis

Much of the initial data reporting the levels of cytokines were obtained from studies performed in the synovial fluid of RA patients. Many studies investigated a limited number of cytokines from each joint (72,73), and as such, the production of IL-1 was first documented in this compartment (74). The relevance of cytokines initially found in the synovial fluid to the pathogenesis of the disease is unclear. The synovial fluid is composed of a complex mixture of molecules, including a large concentration of hyaluronan, other proteo-

glycans, serum proteins, and degradative enzymes, many of which inhibit or degrade cytokine function. The information gained from these studies therefore is unlikely to be of relevance to the pathogenesis of RA.

Cytokine expression in synovium probably is of greater relevance to the origin of RA, because most investigators agree that this is the principal site of immune and inflammatory activity. Cytokines interact, and it has been suggested that they should be considered as a network (75). The importance of simultaneously detecting multiple cytokines is illustrated by T-lymphocyte cytokines, for which patterns of cytokine production have profound implications to the outcome of immune responses. Although *in vivo* evidence shows that few T cells secrete the very restricted cytokine patterns originally described as $T_H1$ and $T_H2$ subsets (76,77), it is clear that cell-mediated immune responses are dominated by $T_H1$ cytokines such as IFN-γ and humoral responses by $T_H2$ cytokines such as IL-4 (78). This subject is covered in more detail elsewhere in this chapter.

The initial data on cytokine expression in the synovial membrane in RA were generated by Northern or Southern hybridization, which provided abundant information on the different cytokines expressed in RA synovium. However, these techniques have been replaced by more sensitive methods such as reverse transcriptase–polymerase chain reaction (RT-PCR). The RT-PCR provides a useful method for detecting the expression of a large number of cytokine mRNA species from sites of human disease that provide limited sample size. This technique is useful for detecting mRNA expressed at low levels, such as T-lymphocyte mRNA. Most of the RA tissue used in these studies has come from operative joint replacement, a procedure that usually is done during the late stages of disease. The tissue samples therefore can be expected to have a different cellular profile from that of early-stage disease.

### Proinflammatory Cytokines

IL-1 and TNF-α protein were readily detected in synovial fluid (79–81). In the synovial tissue at the mRNA levels, these cytokines can be detected by blotting and by *in situ* hybridization (82). Immunostaining with monoclonal antibodies specific for these cytokines demonstrated expression predominantly in macrophage-type synoviocytes (83). Later, they were also detected in short-term culture of synovial cells, and IL-1 and TNF-α were detected in a bioassay of synovial membrane cultures; they were present in quantities able to signal a biologic response effectively (84). Laboratory and clinical evidence suggest that TNF-α has a particularly relevant role in the pathogenesis of RA (85,86). TNF-α induces the release of MMP from neutrophils, synovial fibroblasts, and chondrocytes (87–89); induces the expression of endothelial adhesion molecules involved in the migration of leukocytes to extravascular sites of inflammation (90); and stimulates the release of other proinflammatory cytokines, specifically IL-1 secretion (84,91).

TNF-α concentrations are increased in the synovial fluid of patients with active RA (79,83), and increased plasma levels of this cytokine are associated with joint pain (92). Later, as other proinflammatory cytokines and growth factor complementary DNA (cDNA) were cloned, it became important to study the presence and relevance of TNF-α in RA, and the mRNA and protein were detected initially in RA synovial fluid. Among these cytokines were IL-6 (93–95), interferon-α (IFN-α) (81), granulocyte-macrophage colony-stimulating (GM-CSF) (96), macrophage colony-stimulating factor (M-CSF) (97), and leukemia inhibitory factor (LIF) (98–100). Most studies used osteoarthritis tissue or fluid as controls, and usually the same array of cytokines were produced, although at a lower level.

IL-6 derived from synovial fibroblasts during active disease has been established as the cytokine that induces the hepatic synthesis of acute-phase proteins in RA (101). Interleukin-12, a monocyte derived proinflammatory cytokine is a potentially relevant cytokine in RA, because it has a role in skewing the immune response toward $T_H1$ (102). It is likely that IL-12 could be involved early in the RA process, when $CD4^+$ $T_H1$ lymphocytes predominate in the inflammatory infiltrate. In later stages of the disease, IL-12 appeared to be important in maintaining the $T_H1$ preponderance in the immune response and in controlling cytokine production; this was confirmed in studies of RA patients (103,104).

The cells that form most of the hyperplastic pannus are the type B or fibroblast-type synoviocytes, and the cytokines identified as major contributors in this hyperplasia include platelet-derived growth factor (PDGF) (105,106), fibroblast growth factor (FGF) (105,107), and TGF-β (106,108–110). Which of these predominantly drives the hyperplastic response is debatable, but the data point to a additive effects of PDGF and FGF. Later data concerning the role of the newly cloned IL-15, which has an IL-2 activity, demonstrate its participation in RA. Studies showed that IL-15–activated T cells stimulated the secretion of TNF-α by macrophages through a cell-contact–dependent mechanism, and this effect was seen in peripheral blood T cells and in synovial T cells from RA patients (111). These findings are interesting because IL-2 has the opposite effects in this study, despite sharing the γ chain of their receptors.

In another study, IL-15 was found to be a chemoattractant for T cells in RA, and its expression was demonstrated by immunostaining in the lining layer of the synovial membrane. These investigators (112) also found that synovial fluid T lymphocytes proliferate in response to IL-15, demonstrating that continued responsiveness to IL-15 is a feature of T cells after entry into the synovial compartment. The investigators concluded that IL-15 can recruit and activate T lymphocytes in the synovial membrane, thereby contributing to RA pathogenesis (112). These findings need to be confirmed before considering IL-15 as the predominant cytokine in directing the immune response in RA.

### Chemokines

The prominent features of the rheumatoid synovial microenvironment, such as the selective accumulation of memory T cells bearing the activation markers $VLA4^+$ and $CD45R0^+$ and activated macrophages in the membrane and of polymorphonuclear cells in the fluid, suggest an important role for leukocyte chemoattractant molecules such as chemokines. The superfamily of chemokines consists of an array of cytokines unparalleled in biology: the current roster approaches 50 related proteins. These proteins range in size from 68 to 120 amino acids (in the natural form) and can be conveniently divided into at least three structural branches: C, CC, and CCC, according to variations in a shared cysteine motif (113). The largest branch, that of the CC or β chemokines, has nearly 20 members in humans. The smallest branch, the C class, has but one. The CXC is a chemokine branch can be further subdivided by structure and function. Further dissection of this still growing family of cytokines is beyond the scope of this chapter, but the topic is reviewed elsewhere (114).

Chemokines are released by the cells present in abundant numbers in RA, including endothelial cells, synovial fibroblasts, macrophages, and lymphocytes. Members of all three chemokine superfamilies have been implicated in the pathogenesis of RA. The first chemokine to be described in RA was IL-8 (115), and it initially was correlated with the increased angiogenesis common in early stages of the disease. Using immunohistochemical analysis, several groups reported the expression of epithelial cell–derived neutrophil-activating peptide-78 (ENA-78) (116), macrophage inflammatory protein-1α (MIP-1α) (117), monocyte chemotactic protein-1 (MCP-1) (118), and regulated on activation, normally T cell expressed and secreted (RANTES) (119), predominantly associated with synovial tissue macrophages and, to a lesser extent, with the activated endothelium (i.e., high endothelial venules) and type B synoviocytes.

### Chemokine Receptors

Chemokine receptors are members of the large family of serpentine receptors with seven transmembrane domains that couple to *Bordetella pertussis* toxin-sensitive heterotrimeric G proteins for signal transduction (120,121). The two subfamilies of receptors, CXCR and CCR, interact with CXC or CC chemokines, and cross-selectivity has not been observed. Because the predominant leukocyte infiltration in RA is composed of T cells and macrophages, β chemokines are likely to be important in the accumulation of these cells in the RA synovium. Most T cells infiltrating the synovial membrane in RA are activated or memory T lymphocytes and particularly important for the migration of activated or memory T cells are the CXCR3 ligands IP-10 (IFN-γ–inducible 10-kd protein) and MIG (monocyte/macrophage-activating, IFN-γ–inducible protein) and the CCR5 ligands RANTES, MIP-

1α, and MIP-1β. It was demonstrated by inmunostaining of T cells in RA synovial fluid that virtually all such T cells expressed CXCR3 and about 80% expressed CCR5, representing a high enrichment over levels of CXCR3+ and CCR5+ T cells in peripheral blood, which were 35% and 15%, respectively (122). The investigators concluded that these results demonstrate that the chemokine receptors CXCR3 and CCR5 are markers for T cells associated with certain inflammatory reactions, particularly T_H1-type reactions, as is seen in RA (52; B. Moser, personal communication, 1999).

Identifying the nature of this lymphocyte subset migration is important for understanding the cellular and molecular mechanisms of inflammation and for designing strategies for selective immunosuppression. These are encouraging results for identification of a particular subset of potentially pathogenic T cell in RA, although we still need to determine whether the actions of IP-10 or MIG, resulting in the recruitment of CXCR3+ lymphocytes, are the reason for the distinctive phenotype of migrating cells or whether another chemokine such as a CCR5 ligand is responsible. An alternative explanation for the high expression of CXCR3 or CCR5 on inflammatory cells is upregulation by inflammatory cytokines after extravasation, an environment existing in RA.

### Antiinflammatory Cytokines

Among this group of cytokines, the ones with proved relevance to RA are TGF-β, IL-4, IL-10, and IL-13. Several groups have reported TGF-β to be abundant in its precursor, inactive form and in the active form in rheumatoid synovium (123–125). However, there is controversy about the role of TGF-β in RA, because studies using animal models of joint inflammation have shown a proinflammatory effect instead of an antiinflammatory one (126). In another study, the administration of anti-TGF-β into the joints of rats with arthritis decreased the inflammation (127). This cytokine is likely to be important in the reparative and fibrotic process in the joints because it inhibits the production of MMPs such as collagenase (123), induces TIMP (128), and stimulates the production of type I and type XI collagen. Locally secreted TGF-β may promote reparative processes in arthritic synovial connective tissue and tissue repair by inhibiting cartilage and bone destruction. The disruption in the balance between these activities would result in different outcomes of the initial stimulus for TGF-β secretion. In chronic lesions, the overproduction of TGF-β could participate in the ongoing damage by recruiting inflammatory macrophages and activating synovial fibroblasts with the potential for tissue destruction.

Initial studies of the expression of IL-4 demonstrated that this T-cell–derived antiinflammatory cytokine is absent in the RA synovium (129). This indicated that the T_H2 pattern of cytokines is not abundant in RA and that the T_H1 type predominates in this disease (130). However, with the advent of more sensitive techniques such as PCR, some investigators were able to detect IL-4 mRNA (131–133). The net effect of this low level of IL-4 production in the RA joint is unknown, although some researchers have proposed this virtual lack of IL-4 in RA as a potential therapeutic target for these patients (134).

IL-10 is regarded as a T_H0 cytokine, because it has profound antiinflammatory and immunoregulatory effects, and it is secreted in a subset of human T cells that differentiate under the influence of IL-12 into an IFN-γ/IL-10 subset (135). It has been extensively documented in RA peripheral blood (55) and synovial joints by RT-PCR of biopsy specimens and identified in synovial cell culture of RA patients (136,137). Among its antiinflammatory effects relevant to RA are inhibition of IL-1β secretion (although IL-4 is more potent in this effect), induction of soluble TNF-α receptors (TNFRs) production, and downregulation of the membrane-bound TNF-α receptor (138), producing a net effect of less biologic activity for TNF-α. Among the proinflammatory activities is stimulation of B-cell activity, which may be important in driving the production of rheumatoid factor (139), and possible prevention of apoptosis of B and T lymphocytes (72,140). Because IL-10 is abundant in the RA joint, it may have a role in sustaining the survival of T cells there.

IL-13, a product of activated T cells, has multiple biologic actions, primarily on B cells and monocytes. It inhibits the production of proinflammatory cytokines, chemokines, and hematopoietic growth factors by activated human monocytes. In studies of RA patients, it has been found to be consistently produced in synovial fluid lymphocytes, and IL-13 levels were significantly higher than those of IL-4 (140). The investigators also demonstrated *in vitro* the inhibitory effect of IL-13 in the secretion of IL-1β and TNF-α by synovial fluid macrophages from RA subjects. These findings suggest that IL-13 may have a therapeutic potential in the treatment of patients with RA, although they should be confirmed first.

### Cytokine Regulation in Rheumatoid Arthritis

Since the start of studies of cytokine expression in RA, a different pattern of cytokine regulation emerged from that found for *in vitro* activated cells. An important distinction was the consistent pattern of cytokine production, with virtually all samples analyzed producing essentially the same pattern; the level of IL-1α was relatively high, in contrast to *in vitro* stimulated macrophages, in which IL-1β predominates over IL-1α) (142). The presence of cytokines in all rheumatoid synovial membrane samples suggested that, unlike what is reported in normal cells stimulated *in vitro*, in which cytokine expression is transient, cytokine expression in rheumatoid synovium probably was prolonged or continuous. The signal that drives this cytokine pattern in RA was later found to be TNF-α (84).

TNF-α was shown to be the major regulator of IL-1 in RA synovium and of other relevant proinflammatory cytokines such as GM-CSF, which is responsible for maintaining the increased MHC class expression on RA synoviocytes (96). TNF-α emerged as the key cytokine regulator of the proinflammatory cytokine cascade. What regulates TNF-α production in RA joints is remains unsolved, although some data from treatment studies suggest that the process may be T-cell mediated, because depletion of T cells in the joint leads to decreased TNF-α production. However, the specific T-cell–derived signals to the monocytic cells, the principal source of TNF-α, remains unknown. The important role of TNF-α in the pathogenesis of RA was subsequently confirmed in therapeutic clinical trials in which the biologic effects of this cytokine were affected. The first strategy was to use neutralizing monoclonal antibodies, anti-TNF-α. With the intent of diminishing the risk of immunogenicity, the trials used a biologic treatment consisting of a chimeric monoclonal antibody (75% human immunoglobulin). This monoclonal antibody (cA2) was effective in improving all indices of disease activity used to monitor the study subjects. The indices included relevant validated outcome measures such as the number of swollen and tender joints and laboratory evidence of inflammatory activity such as the erythrocyte sedimentation rate (ESR) and C-reactive protein (CRP) (143) levels. The cA2 effects lasted a median of 12 weeks in this study. The magnitude of the clinical response with this agent was convincingly reproduced in a randomized, double-blind, placebo-controlled trial (144). During follow-up of these patients, important adverse effects were found; infectious episodes were increased compared with the placebo-treated group, although the investigators reported the infections were not life threatening. An unexpected development of IgM-class anti-dsDNA antibodies was documented in 6% the cA2 treatment group without clinical SLE, and in all cases the antibody levels resolved over several months. The origin and potential pathogenicity of these antibodies remain unsolved.

To exert a more selective blockade of the TNF-α cascade in another study, RA patients were treated with a recombinant TNFR p75-Fc fusion molecule (145). This approach was based on the knowledge that there are two distinct cell-surface TNF-α receptors, designated p55 and p75 (146,147). Soluble, truncated versions of the membrane TNFRs, consisting of only the extracellular, ligand-binding domain, are present in body fluids and are thought to be involved in regulating TNF activity (148,149). These soluble TNFRs have been detected in synovial tissue and at the junction between cartilage and pannus (150,151), and their levels are increased in the serum and synovial fluid of RA patients (152–155). The results of the randomized, double-blind trial with TNFR p75-Fc fusion protein (145) in RA patients demonstrated its efficacy. Treatment with TNFR-Fc for 3 months reduced disease activity as assessed by a number of clinical end points, biochemical markers of disease, and quality of life reports in this trial. The investigators postulated that the mechanism of action of this biologic agent probably involves its ability to inhibit competitively TNF-α binding to cell-surface TNFR. An important advantage was that patients so treated did not

develop antibodies that neutralized the therapeutic agent, possibly because the chimeric protein contained only human amino acid sequences. The researchers observed only minor adverse effects, such as injection-site reactions and mild upper respiratory symptoms such as cough, rhinitis, and pharyngitis. Overall, the safety-efficacy profile of TNFR-Fc seems promising. Further long-term studies are needed to establish its role in the contemporary treatment strategies for RA.

IL-1 activity is modulated by IL-1 receptor antagonist (IL-1ra), the only cytokine receptor antagonist known (156). IL-1ra has a high affinity for type I and II membrane IL-1 receptor, but because of the ability of IL-1 to activate cells at very low receptor occupancy rates, a high molar excess (about 100 : 1) of IL-1ra is required to antagonize the biologic activity of IL-1. Expression of IL-1ra is upregulated at mRNA and protein levels in RA (157) and is localized to CD68+ macrophages within the synovium. The ratio of IL-1ra to IL-1 in RA is 1.2 : 3.6 (158), well below the 100-fold excess required to neutralize IL-1 bioactivity, which produces the net effect of increased bioactive IL-1 in RA patients.

## CYTOKINES IN INSULIN-DEPENDENT DIABETES MELLITUS

Insulin-dependent diabetes mellitus (IDDM) is an organ-specific autoimmune disorder in humans and results from the inflammatory destruction of insulin-secreting pancreatic β cells. The clinical onset of diabetes is preceded by periinsulitis and insulitis. Insulitis is characterized by infiltration of the pancreatic islets of Langerhans by T cells, B cells, and macrophages (159,160). Genetic and environmental factors (e.g., viral infections) play a role in the development of this highly prevalent autoimmune disease. The various stages leading to the destruction of insulin-secreting cells probably take place over months or years in humans, because immunologic markers of antiislet autoimmunity (i.e., autoantibodies directed against islet antigens like antiglutamate decarboxylase [GAD] or antiinsulin) can be detected well before clinical onset of the disease. This long preclinical phase suggests the possibility of effective development of prophylactic treatment to delay or halt progression toward insulin deficiency. However, to provide intervention at the adequate moment through appropriate therapeutic measures requires an understanding of the immunologic mechanisms controlling the various stages of the autoimmune process and their chronology. We emphasize the data relevant to human IDDM, but animal models are mentioned when deemed necessary.

Evidence suggesting a role of functionally polarized T cells, differing by their cytokine secretion patterns, in regulating immune responses directed against a variety of antigens has provided the framework for a new hypothesis concerning the development of autoimmunity in IDDM. The possibility that an imbalance between the helper T lymphocytes ($T_H1$ and $T_H2$) favors the activation of immune effectors against insulin-secreting cells remains controversial.

Most studies using experimental models favor the role of $T_H1$ lymphocytes in the development of autoimmunity to pancreatic β cells (161–163). Whether such a T-cell imbalance is directly responsible for triggering the autoimmune process is uncertain, but an attractive approach to interrupting the harmful autoimmune process and providing protection against the disease is to artificially favor the activation of $T_H2$ over $T_H1$ regulatory T cells.

## $T_H1$ and $T_H2$ Lymphocyte Subtypes

Effector functions in the immune system are carried out by lymphocytes, which produce antibodies, and T lymphocytes, which secrete a variety of cytokines and focus cytolytic activity on target cells in response to recognition of processed antigens. The various helper T-cell subsets were initially identified in cloned murine T cells (161) and subsequently characterized in humans (162). The current concept of helper T-cell subsets in humans is that $T_H1$ cells promote inflammatory cellular immune responses and are biased toward secretion of IFN-γ, IL-2, and possibly TNF-β. $T_H2$ cells are biased toward secretion of IL-4, IL-5, IL-6, IL-10, and IL-13; induce humoral immunity; and inhibit $T_H1$ responses.

Studies of human autoimmune diseases such as Crohn's disease, multiple sclerosis, Graves' ophthalmopathy, and Hashimoto's thyroiditis have demonstrated a $T_H1$ cytokine profile. Conversely, skin T cells in systemic sclerosis are $T_H2$ (164). The role of $T_H1$ and $T_H2$ cells in T-cell regulation raises a number of issues in autoimmunity, especially in IDDM, a model of spontaneous autoimmune disease in animals (nonobese diabetic [NOD] mouse and biobreeding [BB] rat) and humans. Is there an initial imbalance during the early phase of autoimmunity or a progressive switch from a $T_H2$ to a $T_H1$ response that may offer a clue to disease development? Kinetics of the autoimmune process in human IDDM and the chronology of events leading to diabetes are considerably less well known in view of the lack of histologic access to the pancreas. Autoantibodies directed against pancreatic antigens (e.g., antiglutamate decarboxylase, antiinsulin), although highly predictive of diabetes outcome, are detected months to years before clinical onset of diabetes (165,166), but it has not been possible to correlate the presence of autoantibodies with the process that leads to the selective destruction of pancreatic β cells. Some subjects who carry antibodies never develop diabetes, and others lose autoantibodies with time and correct anomalies of carbohydrate metabolism (167).

## Characterization of Helper T Lymphocytes Involved in Insulin-Dependent Diabetes Mellitus

Several lines of evidence suggest that the progression of the autoimmune process in the NOD mouse and the BB rat follows a $T_H1$ response profile. Most data indicate IFN-γ predominates over IL-4 gene expression and secretion within the lymphocytic infiltrate invading the pancreatic islets *in situ* or islets grafted under the kidney capsule in NOD mice

(168–170), although not all investigators concur with these findings (171). A predominant $T_H1$ response in the IDDM process is further supported by the prevention of cyclophosphamide-induced diabetes in the NOD mouse by the injection of anti-IFN-γ antibodies (172) The transgenic expression of IFN-γ on β cells under the control of the rat insulin promoter has been shown to trigger the development of insulitis and diabetes in cases of conventional murine genetic backgrounds and the activation of islet-specific cytotoxic T cells (173,174). In a transgenic model in which a viral protein was expressed by β cells and diabetes was induced by systemic infection with the corresponding virus, the presence of IFN-γ was essential to disease development (175). However, inactivation of the IFN-γ gene in the NOD mouse delayed but did not prevent the onset of diabetes (176), indicating that compensating mechanisms can take over the $T_H1$ cytokine defect.

In humans, the systematic study of the pancreatic infiltrate is not readily accessible, but studies have shown the expression of IFN-γ in pancreatic tissue from patients with IDDM who died of ketoacidosis, and no $T_H2$ cytokines were detected (177). These difficulties in obtaining lymphocytes directly from human islet infiltrate and procuring human islet cells as a source of antigen have been major limitations in physiologic studies of islet-specific T lymphocytes. Studies performed after nonspecific activation of peripheral T cells by mitogens have uniformly reported a reduction in the ability of lymphocytes to produce IL-4 or a reduction in the IL-4/IFN-γ ratio compared with controls (178,179). Other studies performed after stimulation of peripheral T cells from recent-onset IDDM patients by human islet cells (140) or extracts of insulinoma membrane (180) have failed to detect IFN-γ secretion despite significant T-cell proliferation. However, these latter results were not replicated in a later study in which the levels of macrophage-derived cytokines such as IL-1, TNF-α, and IL-12 were measured in supernatants of stimulated peripheral blood lymphocytes in high-risk relatives of IDDM patients who had antiislet cell antibodies (i.e., anti-GAD and antiinsulin). The investigators found a correlation between the levels of antiislet antibodies and the levels of IL-12 produced by these subject T cells, supporting the view of $T_H1$ predominance in the early stages of the disease process (181).

In a study of a series of at-risk nonprogressors (defined by genetic susceptibility and the presence of antiislet antibodies) and IDDM patients (including five identical twin or triplet sets discordant for the disease), the diabetic siblings had a statistically significant lower frequency of $CD4^-CD8^-$ $Va24JaQ^+$ T cells compared with their nondiabetic siblings (182). These T-cell subsets are the initial source of IL-4. The investigators demonstrated that the few $CD4^-CD8^-$ $Va24JaQ^+$ T cells found in diabetic patients were biased toward a $T_H1$ cytokine pattern, secreting high levels of IFN-γ but negligible levels of IL-4, in sharp contrast to the high levels of IL-4 secreted by these T cells in nonprogressor siblings. This is the first study to clearly demonstrate that human IDDM is associated with an extreme $T_H1$ phenotype for

Va24JaQ$^+$ T cells and a decrease in their circulating frequency and indicates they may be functionally related to the resistance or progression of this autoimmune disease in humans.

### Cytokines Secreted in Response to Islet Autoantigens

The autoantigens responsible for triggering the autoimmune reaction directed against insulin-secreting cells have not been definitely identified. Numerous antigens are involved in the course of the diabetic autoimmune process. Purified or recombinant GAD and insulin have been used to study the anti-β-cell T cell *in vitro*. In humans, islet cell antibodies are useful markers of autoimmunity to β cells. However, overwhelming evidence from animal models suggests that the autoimmune reaction is mediated by T lymphocytes and that the production of antibodies is a secondary phenomenon. Proliferation of mononuclear cells (including T lymphocytes) in the presence of GAD has been detected in the blood of recent-onset diabetic patients or subjects at risk for developing the disease (183). In at-risk individuals, an inverse relationship exists between the level of anti-GAD antibodies and detection of a proliferative T-cell response (184), implying the possible existence of a $T_H1/T_H2$ balance. However, cytokines produced by CD4$^+$ T lymphocytes on GAD recognition have not been studied. Conversely, GAD-specific cytotoxic T cells have been characterized in recent-onset diabetic patients as producing IFN-γ (185). Cytokine secretion accompanying T-lymphocyte responses to other pancreatic autoantigens has not been reported, possibly because of the low sensitivity of techniques used to measure cytokine production (e.g., ELISA) and the low precursor frequency of autoantigen-specific lymphocytes in the blood (186).

### Immunotherapy and $T_H1/T_H2$ Balance in Insulin-Dependent Diabetes Mellitus

Studies performed in mouse models such as NOD support the idea of disease prevention or modulation by manipulating $T_H2$ responses through injecting IL-4 or interfering with $T_H1$ responses by administering anti-IFN-γ (172,187). Conflicting results have been obtained in mice by enhancing the expression of IL-10, which inhibits the production of $T_H1$ cytokines and proliferation of $T_H1$ lymphocytes induced by macrophages. However, transgenic expression of IL-10 in β cells accelerated development of insulitis and diabetes in the NOD model (188). In humans, immunotherapy with cytokines has not been attempted for IDDM. However, cytokines may prove nonspecific for modulating islet cell–specific T cells and favor deleterious immune reactions (e.g., viral reactivation, parasitic infiltration, allergic phenomena) (189). Although this has not been the case in the nonprogressors studied by Hafler who had extremely high levels of IL-4 in their blood and no evidence of immunosuppression or atopy, further follow-up is necessary to exclude this possibility.

Evidence supports the concept of IDDM being a $T_H1$-driven disease. It is still necessary to define the initial trigger of this biased response against the pancreatic β cells. Ongoing trials enlisting humans using orally administered insulin to prevent diabetes are based on the concept of antigen-driven bystander suppression. Regulatory cells elicited in the gut by orally administered antigens are thought to migrate to the pancreas, creating a tolerogenic environment and downregulating the local inflammatory process. This protective mechanism seems to depend essentially on TGF-β. This cytokine produced by $T_H1$ or $T_H2$ cells has regulatory potential in $T_H1$- and $T_H2$-mediated autoimmune diseases (190).

## CONCLUSIONS

Chronicity and destructive potential are characteristic features of the inflammatory response in the tissues of patients with rheumatic diseases. The past decade in research has been dominated by a shift from premolecular to molecular techniques. A major effort has been made to determine which cytokines and inflammatory mediators are produced at the site of disease. Tissue-residing and -infiltrating cells secrete proinflammatory cytokines *in situ,* which probably have a critical role in amplifying and maintaining inflammation (Fig. 9.1). The migration of inflammatory cells into the tissue is an important component of the disease; adhesion molecules facilitate tissue infiltration, and they affect cell activation and cell-cell and cell-matrix interactions.

The paradigm that RA is an antigen-driven and T-cell–mediated disease has prompted attempts to use T-cell–depleting reagents as therapeutic agents. Although T cells can be eliminated in peripheral blood, the overall therapeutic benefits have been minimal and accompanied by major side effects. The lack of therapeutic efficacy is combined with the persistence and selective proliferation of T cells in the joint, reemphasizing the role of tissue-infiltrating T cells in the disease. Studies of the composition of the T-cell infiltrate have demonstrated heterogeneity, indicating that the frequency of disease-relevant T cells is probably low. Pathologic T-cell function may be much more systemic than previously suspected. The relevance of modulation of the cytokine network in RA stimulated reevaluation of the mechanisms of action of established antirheumatic drugs, and methotrexate was found to increase the expression of IL-4 and IL-10 at the gene level in RA treated patients (159).

One of the remaining challenging questions being addressed is the possibility that better therapeutic results may be obtained in controlling RA by combination therapy. More than one cytokine could be targeted simultaneously, or a proinflammatory cytokine blockade could be combined with anti-T-cell therapy. A potentially useful approach could be the combination of the existing biologics with disease-modifying drugs of proven efficacy, such as methotrexate and Azulfidine or cyclosporine.

The many specific activities of individual cytokines have been the basis for current concepts of therapeutic intervention, particularly the treatment of hematopoietic malfunctions and tumor therapy. Applications involve the support of chemotherapy and radiation therapy, bone marrow transplantation, and general immunostimulation. Although some cytokines are in clinical use, physicians must be aware that knowledge about them is limited and that the *in vivo* modulation of the activity of any one factor may not have the desired effect. Nevertheless, our new and growing understanding of the biologic mechanisms governing cytokine actions is an important contribution to medical knowledge. The biochemistry and molecular biology of cytokine actions explain some well-known and some obscure clinical aspects of diseases. Knowledge that cytokines create regulatory hierarchies and provide independent or interrelated regulatory mechanisms that can confer distinct and interactive developmental functions lays a solid, albeit rather complicated, foundation for current and future clinical experiences.

## REFERENCES

1. Wicker L, Wekerle H. Autoimmunity. *Curr Opin Immunol* 1995;7: 783–785.
2. Ohashi PS, Sarvetnick N. A bias from tolerance to immunity [Editorial]. *Curr Opin Immunol* 1997;9:815–817.
3. Hafler DA, Flavell R. How to know thy self. *Curr Opin Immunol* 1996;8:805–807.
4. Nicholson LB, Kuchroo V. Manipulation of the Th1/Th2 balance in autoimmune disease. *Curr Opin Immunol* 1996;8:837–842.
5. O'Garra A, Steinman L, Gijbels K. CD4+ T-cell subsets in autoimmunity. *Curr Opin Immunol* 1997;9:872–883.
6. Seder RA, Paul WE. Acquisition of lymphokine-producing phenotype by CD4+ T cells. *Annu Rev Immunol* 1994;12:635–673.
7. Romagnani S. Lymphokine production by human T cells in disease states. *Annu Rev Immunol* 1994;12:227–257.
8. Pfeiffer C, Stein J, Southwood S, et al. Altered peptide ligands can control CD4 T lymphocyte differentiation *in vivo*. *J Exp Med* 1995;181: 1569–1574.
9. Paul WE, Seder SA. Lymphocyte responses and cytokines. *Cell* 1994;76:241–245.
10. Chang T, Shea CM, Urioste S, et al. Heterogeneity of helper/inducer T. lymphocytes. III. Responses of IL-2 and IL-4 production (Th1 and Th2) clones to antigens presented by different accessory cells. *J Immunol* 1990;145:2803–2808.
11. Chambers CA, Allison JP. Co-stimulation in T cell responses. *Curr Opin Immunol* 1997;9:396–404.
12. Gajewski TF, Pinnas M, Wong T, et al. Murine Th1 and Th2 clones proliferate optimally in response to distinct antigen-presenting cell populations. *J Immunol* 1991;146:1750–1758.
13. Carter LL, Dutton RW. Type 1 and type 2: a fundamental dichotomy for all T-cell subsets *Curr Opin Immunol* 1996;8:336–342.
14. Charlton B, Lafferty KJ. The Th1/Th2 balance in autoimmunity. *Curr Opin Immunol* 1995;7:793–798.
15. Howard M, O'Garra A. Biological properties of interleukin-10. *Immunol Today* 1992,13:198–200.
16. Cherwinski HM, Schumacher JH, Brown KD, et al. Two types of mouse helper T-cell clone III—further differences in lymphokine synthesis between Th1 and Th2 clones revealed by RNA hybridization: functionally monospecific bioassays and monoclonal antibodies. *J Exp Med* 1987 166:1229–1244.
17. Mosmann TR, Coffman RL. T_H1 and T_H2 cells:different patterns of lymphokine secretion lead to different functional properties. *Annu Rev Immunol* 1989;7:145–173.
18. Mosmann TR, Coffman RL. Heterogeneity of cytokine secretion patterns and functions of helper T cells. *Adv Immunol* 1989;46:111–147.
19. Wilder RL. Neuroendocrine-immune system interactions and autoimmunity. *Annu Rev Immunol* 1995;13:307–338.
20. Von Herrath MG, Oldstone MBA. Virus-induced autoimmune disease. *Curr Opin Immunol* 1996;8:878–885.
21. Miyajima A, Kitamura T, Harada N, et al. Cytokine receptors and signal Transduction. *Annu Rev Immunol* 1992;10:295–331.
22. Mosmann TR, Cherwinski H, Bond MW, et al. Two types of murine helper T cell clone. I. Definition according to profiles of lymphokine activities and secreted proteins. *J Immunol* 1986;136:2348–2357.
23. Miossec P. Cytokine-induced autoimmune disorders. *Drug Saf* 1997;17:93–104.
24. Muraille E, Leo O. Revisiting the Th1/Th2 paradigm. *Scand J Immunol* 1998;47:1–9.
25. Romagnani S. The Th1/Th2 paradigm. *Immunol Today* 1997;18: 263–266.
26. Brennan FM, Feldmann M. Cytokines in autoimmunity. *Curr Opin Rheumatol* 1996;8:872–877.
27. Secrist H, DeKruyff RH, Umetsu DT. Interleukin 4 production by CD4+ T cells from allergic individuals is modulated by antigen concentration and antigen-presenting cell type. *J Exp Med* 1995;181: 1081–1089.
28. Palmer EM, van Seventer GA. Human T helper cell Differentiation is regulated by the combined action of cytokines and accessory cell dependent costimulatory signals. *J Immunol* 1997;158:2654–2662.
29. Cohen SB, Parry SL, Feldmann M, et al. Autocrine and paracrine regulation of human T cell IL-10 production. *J Immunol* 1997;158: 5596–5602.
30. Trinchieri F. Interleukin-12 and its role in the generation of Th1 cells. *Immunol Today* 1993;14:335–338.
31. Meyaard L, Hovenkamp E, Otto SA, et al. IL-12 induced IL-10 production by human T cells as a negative feedback for IL-12 induced immune responses. *J Immunol* 1996;156:2776–2782.
32. Adorini L, Sinigaglia F. Pathogenesis and immunotherapy of autoimmune diseases. *Immunol Today* 1997;18:209–211.
33. Van Kooten C, Banchereau J. Functions of CD40 on B cells, dendritic cells and other cells. *Curr Opin Immunol* 1997;9:330–337.
34. Massague J. The transforming growth factor-β family. *Annu Rev Cell Biol* 1990;6:597–641.
35. Zurawski G, De Vries JE. Interleukin 13, an interleukin 4–like cytokine that acts on monocytes and B cells, but not on T cells. *Immunol Today* 1994;15:19–26.
36. Tomura M, Marui S, Mu J, et al. Differential capacities of CD4+, CD8+ and CD4− CD8− T cell subsets to express IL-18 receptor and produce IFNγ in response to IL-18. *J Immunol* 1998,160:3759–3765.
37. Del Prete G, De Carli M. D'Elios MM, et al. CD30-mediated signaling promotes the development of human T helper 2–like T cells. *J Exp Med* 1995;182:1655–1661.
38. Xu D, Chan WL, Leung BP, et al. Selective expression of a stable cell surface molecule on type 2 but not type 1 helper T cells. *J Exp Med* 1998;187:787–794.
39. Steinberg AD. Insights into the basis of systemic lupus. *J Autoimmun* 1995;8:771–785.
40. Nepom GT, Erlich H. MHC class II molecules and autoimmunity. *Annu Rev Immunol* 1991;9:493–525.
41. Ansar-Ahmed S, Penhale WJ, Talal N. Sex hormones, immune responses, and autoimmune disease. Mechanisms of sex hormone action. *Am J Pathol* 1985;12:531–551.
42. Kreig AM, Steinberg AD. Retroviruses and autoimmunity. *J Autoimmun* 1990;3:137–166.
43. Handwerger BS. T-cell and B-cell function in lupus. *Curr Opin Rheumatol* 1991;3:757–779.
44. Ulfgren AK, Lindblad S, Klareskog L, et al. Detection of cytokine producing cells in the synovial membrane from patients with rheumatoid arthritis. *Ann Rheum Dis* 1995;54:654–661.
45. Via CS, Tsokos GC, Bermas B, et al. T cell-antigen–presenting cell interactions in human systemic lupus erythematosus: evidence for heterogeneous expression of multiple defects. *J Immunol* 1993;151:3 914–3922.
46. Alcocer-Varela J, Alarcon-Segovia D. Decreased production of and response to interleukin-2 by cultured lymphocytes from patients with systemic lupus erythematosus. *J Clin Invest* 1982;69:1388–1392.
47. Linker-Israeli M. Cytokine abnormalities in human lupus. *Clin Immunol Immunopathol* 1992;63:10–12.
48. Llorente L, Richaud-Patin Y, Fior R, et al. Spontaneous production of interleukin-10 by B lymphocytes and monocytes in systemic lupus erythematosus. *Eur Cytokine Netw* 1993;4:421–430.
49. Crispin JC, Alcocer-Varela J. Interleukin-2 and systemic lupus erythematosus—fifteen years later. *Lupus* 1998;7:214–222.

50. Segal R, Bermas BL, Dayan M, et al. Kinetics of cytokine production in experimental systemic lupus erythematosus. *J Immunol* 1997; 158:3009–3016.

51. Handwerger BS, da Silva RL, Via CV. The role of cytokines in the immunopathogenesis of lupus. *Springer Semin Immunopathol* 1994; 16:153–170.

52. Nagafushi H, Suzuki Y, Mizuchima Y, et al. Constitutive expression of IL-6 receptors and their role in the excessive B cell function in patients with systemic lupus erythematosus. *J Immunol* 1993;151: 6525–6534.

53. Alvarado C, Alcocer-Varela, J, Richaud-Patin, Y, et al. Differential oncogene and TNF-α mRNA expression in bone marrow cells from systemic lupus erythematosus patients. *Scand J Immunol* 1998;48: 551–556.

54. Tsokos GC, Boumpas DT, Smith PL, et al. Deficient γ-interferon production in patients with systemic lupus erythematosus. *Arthritis Rheum* 1986;29:1210–1215.

55. Llorente L, Zou W, Levy Y, et al. *In vivo* production of interleukin-10 by non-T cells in rheumatoid arthritis, Sjögren's syndrome and systemic lupus erythematosus: a potential mechanism of B lymphocyte hyperactivity and autoimmunity. *Arthritis Rheum* 1994;11:1647–1655.

56. Llorente L, Zou W, Levy Y, et al. Role of interleukin 10 in the B lymphocyte hyperactivity and autoantibody production of human systemic lupus erythematosus. *J Exp Med* 1995;181:839–844.

57. Mongan AE, Ramdahim S, Warrington RJ. Interleukin-10 response abnormalities in systemic lupus erythematosus. *Scand J Immunol* 1997;46:406–412.

58. Mehrian R, Quismorio FP, Strassmann G, et al. Synergistic effect between IL-10 and bcl-2 genotypes in determining susceptibility to systemic lupus erythematosus. *Arthritis Rheum* 1998;41:596–602.

59. Sakane T, Murakawa Y, Suzuki N, et al. Familial occurrence of impaired interleukin-2 activity and increased peripheral blood B cells actively secreting immunoglobulins in systemic lupus erythematosus. *Am J Med* 1989;86:385–390.

60. Llorente L, Richaud-Patin Y, Couderc J, et al. Dysregulation of interleukin-10 production in relatives of patients with systemic lupus erythematosus. *Arthritis Rheum* 1997;40:1429–1435.

61. Houssiau FA, Mascart-Lemone F, Goldman M, et al. Interleukin 12 inhibits *in vitro* immunoglobulin production by SLE peripheral blood mononuclear cells. *Clin Exp Rheumatol* 1996;14 (suppl 5–16):S44.

62. Ohtsuka K, Dixon Gray J, Stimmler MM, et al. Decreased production of TGF-β by lymphocytes from patients with systemic lupus erythematosus. *J Immunol* 1998;160:2539–2545.

63. Harris ED Jr. Rheumatoid arthritis: pathophysiology and implications for therapy. *N Engl J Med* 1990;322:1277–1289.

64. Cush JJ, Lipsky PE. Phenotypic analysis of synovial tissue and peripheral blood lymphocytes isolated from patients with rheumatoid arthritis. *Arthritis Rheum* 1988;31:1230–1238.

65. Johnson BA, Haines GK, Harlow LA, et al. Adhesion molecule expression in human synovial tissue. *Arthritis Rheum* 1993;36:137–146.

66. Morales-Ducret J, Wayner E, Elices MJ, et al. α4/β1 Integrin (VLA4) ligands in arthritis. I. Vascular cell adhesion molecule 1 expression in synovium and on fibroblast-like synoviocytes. *J Immunol* 1992;149: 1424–1431.

67. Thomas R, Davis LS, Lipsky PE. Rheumatoid synovium is enriched in mature antigen-presenting dendritic cells. *J Immunol* 1994;152: 2613–2623.

68. Allard SA, Muirden KD, Camplejohn KL, et al. Chondrocyte-derived cells and matrix at the rheumatoid cartilage-pannus junction identified with monoclonal antibodies. *Rheumatol Int* 1987;7:153–159.

69. Menard HA, El-Amine M. The calpastatin system in rheumatoid arthritis. *Immunol Today* 1996;17:545–547.

70. Vincenti MP, Clark IM, Brinckerhoff CE. Using inhibitors of metalloproteinases to treat arthritis. *Arthritis Rheum* 1994;37:1115–1126.

71. Ladner UM. Molecular and cellular interactions in rheumatoid synovium. *Curr Opin Rheumatol* 1996;8:210–220.

72. Brennan FM, Field M, Chu CQ, et al. Cytokine expression in rheumatoid arthritis. *Br J Rheumatol* 1991;30[Suppl 1]:76–80.

73. Miossec P, Naviliat M, DaeAngeac AD, et al. Low levels of interleukin-4 and high levels of transforming growth factor β in rheumatoid joints. *Arthritis Rheum* 1990;33:1180–1187.

74. Fontana A, Hentgartner H, Fehr K, et al. Interleukin-1 activity in the synovial fluid of patients with rheumatoid arthritis. *Rheumatol Int* 1982;2:49–56.

75. Balkwill FR, Burke F. The cytokine network. *Immunol Today* 1989;10:299–304.

76. Mosmann TR. Cytokines: is there a biological meaning? *Curr Opin Immunol* 1991;3:311–314.

77. Yamamura M, Uyemura K, Deans RJ, et al. Defining protective responses to pathogens: cytokines profiles in leprosy patients. *Science* 1991;254:277–279.

78. Kelso A. Th1 and Th2 subsets: paradigm lost? *Immunol Today* 1995;16:374–379.

79. Saxne T, Palladino MA Jr, Heinegard D, et al. Detection of tumor necrosis factor α but not tumor necrosis factor β in rheumatoid arthritis synovial fluid and serum. *Arthritis Rheum* 1988;31:1041–1045.

80. Hopkins SJ, Humphreys M, Jayson MI. Cytokines in synovial fluid I. The presence of biologically active and immunoreactive IL-1. *Clin Exp Immunol* 1988;72:422–427.

81. Hopkins SJ, Meager A. Cytokines in synovial fluid II. The presence of tumor necrosis factor and interferon. *Clin Exp Immunol* 1988;73: 88–92.

82. Wood NC, Dickens E, Symons JA, et al. *In situ* hybridization of interleukin-1 in CD14 positive cells in rheumatoid arthritis. *Clin Immunol Immunopathol* 1992;62:295–300.

83. Chu CR, Field M, Feldmann M, et al. Localization of tumor necrosis factor α in synovial tissues and at the cartilage-pannus junction in patients with rheumatoid arthritis. *Arthritis Rheum* 1991;34: 1125–1132.

84. Brennan FM, Chantry D, Jackson A, et al. Inhibitory effect of TNFα antibodies on synovial cell interleukin-1 production in rheumatoid arthritis. *Lancet* 1989;2:244–247.

85. Arend WP, Dayer JM. Inhibition of the production and effects of interleukin-1 and tumor necrosis factor α in rheumatoid arthritis. *Arthritis Rheum* 1995;38:151–160.

86. Brennan FM, Feldmann M. Cytokines in autoimmunity. *Curr Opin Immunol* 1992;4:754–759.

87. Shingu M, Nagai Y, Isayama T, et al. The effects of cytokines on metalloproteinase inhibitors (TIMP) and collagenase production by human chondrocytes and TIMP production by synovial cells and endothelial cells. *Clin Exp Immunol* 1993;94:145–160.

88. MacNaul KL, Chartrain N, Lark M, et al. Differential effects of IL-1 and TNFα on the expression of stromelysin, collagenase and their natural inhibitor, TIMP, in rheumatoid human synovial fibroblasts. *Matrix Suppl* 1992;1:198–199.

89. Ahmadzadeh N, Shingu M, Nobunaga M. The effect of recombinant tumor necrosis factor α on superoxide and metalloproteinase production by synovial cells and chondrocytes. *Clin Exp Rheumatol* 1990;8:387–391.

90. Moser RB, Schleiffenbaum B, Groscurth P, et al. Interleukin-1 and tumor necrosis factor stimulate human vascular endothelial cells to promote transendothelial neutrophil passage. *J Clin Invest* 1989;83: 444–455.

91. Nawroth PP, Bank I, Handley D, et al. Tumor necrosis factor/cachecton interacts with endothelial cell receptors to induce the release of interleukin-1. *J Exp Med* 1986;163–1363.

92. Beckham JC, Caldwell DS, Peterson BL, et al. Disease severity in rheumatoid arthritis: relationships of plasma tumor necrosis factor-α, soluble interleukin-2 receptor, soluble CD4/CD8 ratio, neopterin, and fibrin D-dimer to traditional severity and functional measures. *J Clin Immunol* 1992;12:353–361.

93. Hirano T, Matsuda T, Turner M, et al. Excessive production of interleukin 6/B-cell stimulatory factor-2 in rheumatoid arthritis. *Eur J Immunol* 1988;18:1797–1801.

94. Field M, Chu C, Feldmann M, et al. Interleukin-6 localization in the synovial membrane in rheumatoid arthritis. *Rheumatol Int* 1991;11: 45–50.

95. Helle M, Boeije L, deGroot E, et al. Detection of IL-6 in biological fluids: synovial fluids and sera. *J Immunol Methods* 1991;138:47–56.

96. Alvaro-Garcia JM, Zvaifler NJ, Brown CB, et al. Cytokines in chronic inflammatory arthritis, VI. Analysis of the synovial cells involved in granulocyte-macrophage colony-stimulating factor production and gene expression in rheumatoid arthritis and its regulation by IL-1 and TNFα. *J Immunol* 1991;146:3365–3371.

97. Firestein GS, Xu WD, Townsend K, et al. Cytokines in chronic inflammatory arthritis I. Failure to detect T cell lymphokines (interleukin 2 and interleukin 3) and presence of macrophage colony-stimulating factor (CSF-1) and a novel mast cell growth factor in rheumatoid synovitis. *J Exp Med* 1988;168:1573–1586.

98. Lotz M, Moats T, Villeger PM. Leukemia inhibitory factor is expressed in cartilage and synovium and can contribute to the pathogenesis of arthritis. *J Clin Invest* 1992;90:888–896.

99. Dechanet J, Taupin JL, Rissoan MC, et al. Interleukin-4 but not interleukin-10 inhibits the production of leukemia inhibitory factor by rheumatoid synovium and synoviocytes. *Eur J Immunol* 1994;24: 3222–3228.

100. Waring PM, Carroll GJ, Kandiah DA, et al. Increased levels of leukemia inhibitory factor in synovial fluid from patients with rheumatoid arthritis and other inflammatory arthritides. *Arthritis Rheum* 1993;36:911–915.

101. Okamoto H, Masahiro Y, Morita Y, et al. The synovial expression and serum levels of interleukin-6, interleukin-11, leukemia inhibitory factor, and oncostatin M in rheumatoid arthritis. *Arthritis Rheum* 1997;40: 1096–1105.

102. Manetti R, Parronchi P, Giudizi MG, et al. Natural killer cell stimulatory factor (NKSF/IL-12) induces Th1-type specific immune responses and inhibits the development of IL-4 producing Th cells. *J Exp Med* 1993:177:1199–1204.

103. Bucht A, Larsson P, Weisbrot L, et al. Expression of interferon-γ (IFN-γ), IL-10, IL-12 and transforming growth factor β (TGF-β) mRNA in synovial fluid cells from patients in the early and late phases of rheumatoid arthritis (RA). *Clin Exp Immunol* 1996;103:357–367.

104. Kotake S, Schumacher HR Jr, Yarboro CH, et al. *In vivo* gene expression of type 1 and type 2 cytokines in synovial tissues from patients in early stages of rheumatoid, reactive, and undifferentiated arthritis. *Proc Assoc Am Physicians* 1997;109:286–301.

105. Remmers EF, Sano, H, Lafyatis R, et al. Production of platelet derived growth factor B chain (PDGF-B/c-sis) mRNA and immunoreactive PDGF b-like polypeptide by rheumatoid synovium: coexpression with heparin binding acidic fibroblast growth factor-1. *J Rheumatol* 1991; 18:7–13.

106. Goddard DH, Grossman SL, Moore ME. Autocrine regulation of rheumatoid arthritis synovial cell growth *in vitro*. *Cytokine* 1990;2: 149–155.

107. Sano H, Forough R, Maier JA, et al. Detection of high levels of heparin binding growth factor-1 (acidic fibroblast growth factor) in inflammatory arthritis joints. *J Cell Biol* 1990;110:1417–1426.

108. Bucala R, Ritchin C, Winchester R, Cerami A. Constitutive production of inflammatory and mitogenic cytokines by rheumatoid synovial fibroblasts. *J Exp Med* 1991;173:569–574.

109. Thornton SC, Por SB, Penny R, et al. Identification of the major fibroblast growth factors released spontaneously in inflammatory arthritis as platelet derived growth factor and tumor necrosis factor-α. *Clin Exp Immunol* 1991;86:79–86.

110. Goddard DH, Grossman SL, Williams WV, et al. Regulation of synovial cell growth: coexpression of transforming growth factor β and basic fibroblast growth factor by cultured synovial cells. *Arthritis Rheum* 1992;35:1296–1303.

111. McInnes IB, Leug BP, Sturrock RD, et al. Interleukin-15 mediates T-cell dependent regulation of tumor necrosis factor-α production in rheumatoid arthritis. *Nat Med* 1997;3:189–195.

112. McInnes IB, al-Mughales J, Field M, et al. The role of interleukin-15 in T-cell migration and activation in rheumatoid arthritis. *Nat Med* 1996;2:175–182.

113. Schall TJ, Bacon KB. Chemokines, leukocyte trafficking, and inflammation. *Curr Opin Immunol* 1994;6:865–873.

114. Moser B, Loetscher M, Piali L, et al. Lymphocyte responses to chemokines. *Int Rev Immunol* 1998;16:323–344.

115. Seitz M, Dewald B, Gerber N, et al. Enhanced production of neutrophil activating peptide-1/interleukin-8 in rheumatoid arthritis. *J Clin Invest* 1991;87:463–469.

116. Koch AE, Kunkel SL, Harlow LA, et al. Epithelial neutrophil activating peptide-78: a novel chemotactic cytokine for neutrophils in arthritis. *J Clin Invest* 1994;94:1012–1018.

117. Koch AE, Kunkel SL, Harlow LA, et al. Macrophage inflammatory protein-1α. *J Clin Invest* 1994;93:921–928.

118. Koch AE, Kunkel SL, Harlow LA, et al. Enhanced production of monocyte chemoattractant protein-1 in rheumatoid arthritis. *J Clin Invest* 1992;90:772–779.

119. Rathanaswami P, Hachicha M, Sadick M, et al. Expression of the cytokine RANTES in human rheumatoid synovial fibroblasts. Differential regulation of RANTES and interleukin-8 genes by inflammatory cytokines. *J Biol Chem* 1993;268:5834–5839.

120. Murphy PM. The molecular biology of leukocyte chemoattractant receptors. *Annu Rev Immunol* 1994;12:593–633.

121. Raport CJ, Scweickart VL, Chantry D, et al. New members of the chemokine receptor gene family. *J Leukoc Biol* 1996;59:18–23.

122. Qin S, Rottman JB, Myers P, et al. The chemokine receptors CXCR3 and CCR5 mark subsets of T cells associated with certain inflammatory reactions. *J Clin Invest* 1998;101:746–754.

123. Lafyatis R, Thomson NL, Remmers ER, et al. Transforming growth factor-β production by synovial tissues from rheumatoid arthritis patients and streptococcal cell wall arthritis rats. Studies on secretion by synovial fibroblast-like cells and immunohistological localization. *J Immunol* 1989;143:1142–1148.

124. Lotz MKJ, Carson DA. Transforming growth factor-β and cellular immune responses in synovial fluids. *J Immunol* 1990;144:4189–4194.

125. Chu CQ, Field M, Abney E, et al. Transforming growth factor-β1 in rheumatoid synovial membrane and cartilage/pannus junction. *Clin Exp Immunol* 1991;86:380–386.

126. Fava RA, Olsen NJ, Postlehwaite AE, et al. Transforming growth factor-β1 (TGFβ1) induced neutrophil recruitment to synovial tissues: implications for TGF-β driven synovial inflammation and hyperplasia. *J Exp Med* 1991;173:1121–1132.

127. Wahl SM, Hunt DA, Wakefield IM, et al. Transforming growth factor-β (TGF-β) induces monocyte chemotaxis and growth factor production. *Proc Natl Acad Sci USA* 1987;84:5788–5792.

128. Wright JK, Cawston TE, Hazelman BL. Transforming growth factor-β stimulates the production of tissue inhibitor of metalloproteinases (TIMP) by human synovial and skin fibroblasts. *Biochim Biophys Acta* 1991;1094:207–210.

129. Cohen SBA, Katsikis PD, Chu CQ, et al. High IL-10 production by the activated T cell population within the rheumatoid synovial membrane. *Arthritis Rheum* 1995;38:946–952.

130. Mitenburg AJ, van Laar JM, de Kuiper R, et al. T cells cloned from human rheumatoid synovial membrane functionally represent the Th1 subset. *Scand J Immunol* 1992;35:603–610.

131. Quayle AJ, Chromarat P, Miossec P, et al. Rheumatoid inflammatory T-cell clones express Th1 but also Th2 and mixed (Th0 like) cytokine patterns. *Scand J Immunol* 1993;38:75–82.

132. Simon AK, Seipelt E, Sieper J. Divergent T-cell cytokine patterns in inflammatory arthritis. *Proc Natl Acad Sci USA* 1994;91:8562–8565.

133. Sew Hoy MD, Williams JL, Kirkham BW. Symmetrical synovial fluid cell cytokine messenger RNA expression in rheumatoid arthritis: analysis by reverse transcription/polymerase chain reaction. *Br J Rheumatol* 1997;36:170–173.

134. Miossec P, Briolay J, Dechanet J, et al. The inhibition of the production of proinflammatory cytokines and immunoglobulins by interleukin-4 in an *ex vivo* model of rheumatoid synovitis. *Arthritis Rheum* 1992;35:874–883.

135. Pohl-Koppe A, Balashov KE, Steere AC, et al. Identification of a T cell subset capable of both IFN-γ and IL-10 secretion in patients with chronic *Borrelia burgdorferi* infection. *J Immunol* 1998;160:1804–1810.

136. Katsikis P, Chu CQ, Brennan FM, et al. Immunoregulatory role of interleukin 10 (IL-10) in rheumatoid arthritis. *J Exp Med* 1994;179: 1517–1527.

137. Cush JJ, Splawski JB, Thomas R, et al. Elevated interleukin-10 levels in patients with rheumatoid arthritis. *Arthritis Rheum* 1995;38:96–104.

138. Joyce DA, Gibbons D, Green P, et al. Two inhibitors of proinflammatory cytokine release, IL-10 and IL-4, have contrasting effects on release of soluble p75 TNF receptor by cultured monocytes. *Eur J Immunol* 1994;24:2699–2705.

139. Rousset F, Garcia E, Deference T, et al. IL-10 is a potent growth and differentiation factor for activated human B lymphocytes, *Proc Natl Acad Sci USA* 1992;89:1890–1893.

140. Harrison LC, De Aizpurua H, Luodovaris T, et al. Reactivity to human islets and fetal pig proislets by peripheral blood mononuclear cells from subjects with preclinical and clinical insulin-dependent diabetes. *Diabetes* 1991;40:1128–1133.

141. Isomaki P, Luukkainen R, Toivanen P, et al. The presence of interleukin-13 in rheumatoid synovium and its antiinflammatory effects on synovial fluid macrophages from patients with rheumatoid arthritis. *Arthritis Rheum* 1996;39:1693–1702.

142. Dinarello CA. The interleukin-1 family: 10 years of discovery. *FASEB J* 1994;8:1314–1325.

143. Elliot MJ, Maini RN, Feldmann M, et al. Treatment of rheumatoid arthritis with chimeric monoclonal antibodies to TNFα. *Arthritis Rheum* 1993;36:1681–1690.

144. Elliot MJ, Maini RN, Feldmann M, et al. Randomized double blind comparison of a chimaeric monoclonal antibody to tumor necrosis factor α (cA2) versus placebo in rheumatoid arthritis. *Lancet* 1994;344:1105–1110.

145. Moreland LW, Baugartner CW, Schiff MH, et al. Treatment of rheumatoid arthritis with a recombinant human tumor necrosis factor receptor (p75)-Fc fusion protein. *N Engl J Med* 1997;337:141–147.

146. Smith CA, Davis T, Anderson D, et al. A receptor for tumor necrosis factor defines an unusual family of cellular and viral proteins. *Science* 1990;248:1019–1023.

147. Loetscher H, Pan YC, Lahm HW, et al. Molecular cloning and expression of the human 55-kd tumor necrosis factor receptor. *Cell* 1990;61:351–359.

148. Engelman H, Aderka D, Rubinstein M, et al. A tumor necrosis factor-binding protein purified to homogeneity from human urine protects cells from tumor necrosis factor toxicity. *J Biol Chem* 1989;264:11974–11980.

149. Olsson I, Lantz M, Nilsson E, et al. Isolation and characterization of a tumor necrosis factor binding protein from urine. *Eur J Haematol* 1989;42:270–275.

150. Deleuran BW, Chu CQ, Field M, et al. Localization of tumor necrosis factor receptors in the synovial tissue and cartilage-pannus junction in patients with rheumatoid arthritis: implications for local actions of tumor necrosis factor-α. *Arthritis Rheum* 1992;35:1170–1178.

151. Westacott CI, Atkins RM, Dieppe PA, et al. Tumor necrosis factor-α expression on chondrocytes isolated from human articular cartilage. *J Rheumatol* 1994;21:1710–1715.

152. Roux-Lombard P, Punzi L, Hasler F, et al. Soluble tumor necrosis factor receptors in human inflammatory synovial fluids. *Arthritis Rheum* 1993;36:485–498.

153. Barrera P, Boerbooms AM, Janssen EM, et al. Circulating soluble tumor necrosis factor receptors, interleukin-2 receptors, tumor necrosis factor-α, and interleukin-6 levels in rheumatoid arthritis: longitudinal evaluation during methotrexate and azathioprine therapy. *Arthritis Rheum* 1993;36:1070–1079.

154. Chikanza IC, Roux-Lombard P, Dayer JM, et al. Tumor necrosis factor soluble receptors behave as acute phase reactants following surgery in patients with rheumatoid arthritis, chronic osteomyelitis and osteoarthritis. *Clin Exp Immunol* 1993;92:19–22.

155. Cope AP, Aderka D, Doherty M, et al. Increased levels of soluble tumor necrosis factor receptors in the sera and synovial fluid of patients with rheumatic diseases. *Arthritis Rheum* 1992;35:1160–1169.

156. Arend WP, Dayer JM. Cytokines and cytokine inhibitors or antagonists in rheumatoid arthritis. *Arthritis Rheum* 1990;33:305–315.

157. Firestein GS, Berger AE, Tracey DE, et al. IL-1 receptor antagonist protein production and gene expression in rheumatoid arthritis and osteoarthritis synovium. *J Immunol* 1992;149:1054–1062.

158. Firestein GS, Boyle DL, Yu C, et al. Synovial interleukin-1 receptor antagonist and interleukin-1 balance in rheumatoid arthritis. *Arthritis Rheum* 1994;37:644–652.

159. Constantin A, Loubet-Lescoulie P, Lambert N, et al. Antiinflammatory and immunoregulatory action of methotrexate in the treatment of rheumatoid arthritis. *Arthritis Rheum* 1998;41:48–57.

160. Kikutani H, Makino S. The murine autoimmune diabetes model: NOD and related strains. *Adv Immunol* 1992;51:285–322.

161. Mosmann TR, Schumacher JH, Street NF, et al. Diversity of cytokine synthesis and function of mouse CD4⁺ T cells. *Immunol Rev* 1991;123:209–229.

162. Romagnani S. Biology of human Th1 and Th2 cells. *J Clin Immunol* 1995;15:121–129.

163. Kallmann BA, Huther M, Tubes M, et al. Systematic bias of cytokine production toward cell-mediated immune regulation in IDDM and toward humoral immunity in Graves' disease. *Diabetes* 1997;46:237–243.

164. Romagnani S. Th1 and Th2 in human diseases. *Clin Immunol Immunopathol* 1996;80:225–235.

165. Roll U, Christie MR, Fuchtenbusch M, et al. Perinatal autoimmunity in offspring of diabetic parents. *Diabetes* 1996;45:967–973.

166. Verge CF, Gianani R, Kawasaki E, et al. Prediction of type I diabetes in first-degree relatives using a combination of insulin, GAD, and ICA51bdc/IA-2 autoantibodies. *Diabetes* 1996;45:926–933.

167. Leslie EDG, Pyke DA. Escaping insulin-dependent diabetes. *Br Med J* 1991;302:1103–1104.

168. Shehadeh NN, Larosa F, Lafferty KJ. Altered cytokine activity in adjuvant inhibition of autoimmune diabetes. *J Autoimmunity* 1993;6:291–300.

169. Ravinovitch A, Suarez-Pinzon WL, Sorensen O, et al. IFNγ gene expression in pancreatic islet-infiltrating mononuclear cells correlates with autoimmune diabetes in nonobese diabetic mice. *J Immunol* 1995;15:4487–4482.

170. Suarez-Pinzon W, Rajotte RV, Mosmann TR, et al. Both CD4⁺ and CD8⁺ T cells in syngeneic islet grafts in NOD mice produce interferon-γ during β-cell destruction. *Diabetes* 1996;45:1350–1357.

171. Anderson JT, Cornelius JG, Jarpe AJ, et al. Insulin-dependent diabetes in the NOD mouse model. II. β-Cell destruction in autoimmune diabetes is a Th2 not a Th1 mediated event. *Autoimmunity* 1993;15:113–122.

172. Debray-Sachs M, Carnaud C, Boitard C, et al. Prevention of diabetes in NOD mice treated with antibody to murine IFNγ. *J Autoimmun* 1991;4:237–248.

173. Sarvetnick N, Liggitt D, Pitts SL, et al. Insulin-dependent diabetes mellitus induced in transgenic mice by ectopic expression of class II MHC and interferon-γ. *Cell* 1988;52:773–782.

174. Sarvetnick N, Shizuru J, Liggitt D, et al. Loss of pancreatic islet tolerance induced by β-cell expression of interferon-γ. *Nature* 1990;346:844–847.

175. Von Herrath MG, Oldstone MB. Interferon-γ is essential for destruction of β cells and development of insulin-dependent diabetes mellitus. *J Exp Med* 1997;185:531–539.

176. Hultgren B, Huang X, Dybdal N, et al. Genetic absence of γ-interferon delays but does not prevent diabetes in NOD mice. *Diabetes* 1996;45:812–817.

177. Huang X, Yuan J, Goddard A, et al. Interferon expression in the pancreas of patients with type I diabetes. *Diabetes* 1995;44:658–664.

178. Berman MA, Sandborg CI, Wang Z, et al. Decreased IL-4 production in new onset type I insulin-dependent diabetes mellitus. *J Immunol* 1996;157:4690–4696.

179. Katz JD, Benoist C, Mathis D. T helper cell subsets in insulin-dependent diabetes. *Science* 1995;268:1185–1188.

180. Roep BO, Kallan AA, Duinkerken G, et al. T-cell reactivity to β-cell destruction in IDDM. *Diabetes* 1995;44:278–283.

181. Szelachowska M, Kretowski A, Kinalska I. Increased *in vitro* interleukin-12 production by peripheral blood in high-risk IDDM first degree relatives. *Horm Metab Res* 1997;29:168–171.

182. Wilson BS, Kent SC, Patton KT, et al. Extreme Th1 bias of invariant Va24JaQ T cells in type 1 diabetes. *Nature* 1998;391:177–181.

183. Atkinson MA, Kaufman DL, Campbell L, et al. Response of peripheral-blood mononuclear cells to glutamate decarboxylase in insulin-dependent diabetes. *Lancet* 1992;339:458–459.

184. Harrison LC, Honeyman MC, De Aizpurua HJ, et al. Inverse relation between humoral and cellular immunity to glutamic acid decarboxylase in subjects at risk of insulin-dependent diabetes. *Lancet* 1993;341:1365–1369.

185. Panina-Bordignon P, Lang R, Van Endert PM, et al. Cytotoxic T cells specific for glutamic acid decarboxylase in autoimmune diabetes. *J Exp Med* 1995;181:1923–1927.

186. Roep BO. T-cell responses to autoantigens in IDDM. *Diabetes* 1996;45:1147–1156.

187. Rapoport MJ, Jaramillo A, Zipris D, et al. Interleukin-4 reverses T cell proliferative unresponsiveness and prevents the onset of diabetes in nonobese diabetic mice. *J Exp Med* 1993;178:87–99.

188. Wogensen L, Lee MS, Sarvetnick N. Production of interleukin-10 by islets cells accelerates immune-mediated destruction of β cells in nonobese diabetic mice. *J Exp Med* 1994;179:1379–1384.

189. Tepper RI, Levinson DA, Stanger BZ, et al. IL-4 induces allergic-like inflammatory disease and alters T cell development in transgenic mice. *Cell* 1990;62:457–467.

190. Bridoux F, Badou A, Saoudi A, et al. Transforming growth factor β (TGF-β)–dependent inhibition of helper cell 2 (Th2)–induced autoimmunity by self-major histocompatibility complex (MHC) class II-specific, regulatory CD4⁺ T cell lines. *J Exp Med* 1997;185:1769–1775.

Textbook of the Autoimmune Diseases,
Edited by R. G. Lahita, N. Chiorazzi, and W. H. Reeves,
Lippincott Williams & Wilkins, Philadelphia © 2000.

# CHAPTER 10

# The Complement System and Autoimmunity

V. Bala Subramanian, M. Kathryn Liszewski, and John P. Atkinson

The complement system is an ancient system of interacting proteins that forms an essential part of the host's immune and inflammatory responses to infection and tissue injury. More than 30 proteins involved in this system have been identified. Many of these proteins participate directly in the cascade of activation; others, some cell bound and some secreted, have regulatory functions that impose strict temporal and spatial control of complement activation; and a third group serves as receptors for complement activation protein fragments.

This chapter first provides a brief overview of the workings of the complement system. The second section highlights the autoimmune syndromes observed with specific complement deficiencies. In the third section, we speculate on how complement deficiency predisposes to systemic lupus erythematosus (SLE) and other autoimmune diseases. In the last section, we describe some inhibitors of complement activation on the horizon for potential use in therapy of human diseases.

The complement cascade may be activated by any of three known pathways (Fig. 10.1 and Table 10.1) described subsequently. The aim is to generate multimolecular enzymes that have the capacity to cleave and thereby activate C3 and C5. Deposition of active cleavage products of C3 (C3b) promotes adherence and phagocytosis of targets (phenomenon of opsonization). Further, activation of C5 leads to the formation of the membrane attack complex (MAC; C5b–9) that perturbs cell membranes, including sufficient injury to produce cell lysis.

V. B. Subramanian: Department of Medicine, Division of Rheumatology, Washington University School of Medicine, St. Louis, Missouri 63110; Barnes–Jewish Hospital, One Barnes–Jewish Hospital Plaza, St. Louis, Missouri 63110.

M. K. Liszewski: Department of Medicine, Division of Rheumatology, Washington University School of Medicine, St. Louis, Missouri 63110.

J. P. Atkinson: Department of Internal Medicine, Division of Rheumatology, Washington University School of Medicine, St. Louis, Missouri 63110-1093; Department of Internal Medicine, Barnes–Jewish Hospital, St. Louis, Missouri 63110-1093.

The *classical pathway* is primarily activated by antigen–antibody (Ag–Ab, or immune) complexes. It can also be activated by C-reactive proteins in complex with bacterial capsular polysaccharides and some viruses and gram-negative bacteria by means of a direct interaction with C1q. The classical pathway is an effector of humoral immunity and is concerned with the processing and safe disposal of the resulting complexes. This pathway is triggered by the binding of C1q in definitive stoichiometry to Ag-Ab complexes that contain immunoglobulin G (IgG$_1$, IgG$_2$, IgG$_3$) or M. This binding leads to a conformational change in C1q that results in sequential activation of C1r and C1s. C1s then cleaves C4 and C2. The larger cleavage products, C4b and C2a, together form the classical pathway C3 convertase (C4b2a). The convertase is anchored to the target by C4b, whereas C2a carries the catalytic (serine protease) domain. The activated C3 (C3b) generated by this bimolecular enzyme complex opsonizes and solubilizes Ag-Ab complexes and is also capable of binding to C4b2a to form a C5 convertase (C4b2aC3b).

The *alternative pathway* is phylogenetically older and represents an antibody-independent system of host defense. It amplifies on foreign surfaces such as the cell membranes of microorganisms, but the nature of biochemical determinants on surfaces that inhibit or promote alternative pathway engagement are not well understood. To be able to act quickly, independent of the Ab, this pathway maintains a constant state of readiness (tickover) and a capacity for positive feedback (amplification loop). The state of readiness is maintained by a continuous low-grade spontaneous hydrolysis of the C3 thioester bond, which leads to its binding directly to nonspecific accepter molecules in plasma, such as water to form C3(H$_2$O), or to cell surfaces, such as microorganisms (1). This can, within 1 second of finding the target, complex with factor B [C3(H$_2$O)B]. Factor B so bound is susceptible to cleavage by factor D to form an alternative pathway C3 convertase [C3(H$_2$O)Bb]. Properdin stabilizes this enzyme complex (half-life of seconds to minutes). This complex activates C3 to C3b to generate more C3 convertases (C3bBb). This amplification loop facilitates the deposition of

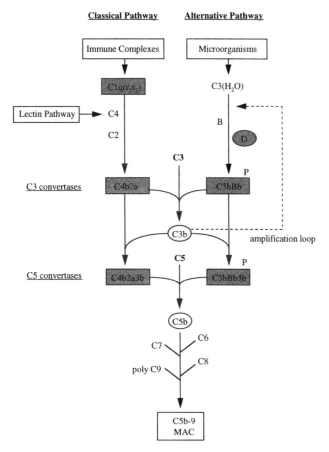

**Classical Pathway**   **Alternative Pathway**

**FIG. 10.1.** Overview of the complement cascade. This diagram emphasizes the parallel nature of the activation scheme for the two major pathways leading to a common membrane attack complex (MAC). The serine proteases are indicated by the shaded boxes. Both pathways independently activate C3 and then C5. C3b is the major opsonic fragment, whereas C5b is the entrance to the MAC. The classical pathway is most commonly activated by the binding of immune complexes to the C1 complex, whereas the alternative pathway is triggered when activated C3 deposits on a target, such as a microorganism. Activated C3, the initiator of the alternative pathway, can be formed in two ways: by the classical pathway or by the spontaneous tickover of C3. The latter occurs because within C3 is an unstable thioester bond. This turnover results in a fluid-phase convertase (as shown), or the activated "C3" may bind directly to a target. The amplification loop is then employed to augment C3b deposition. Amplification is permitted on a dangerous target but is inhibited on self. In the lectin pathway, mannan-binding lectin, by means of its associated proteases, cleaves C4 and C2 in a fashion analogous to its cleavage by C1. Properdin becomes associated with and thereby stabilizes the alternative pathway C3 and C5 convertases. B, factor B; D, factor D; P, Properdin.

large numbers of C3b on the target for opsonization or subsequent lysis. In addition, the attachment of a second C3b to the C3bBb complex produces a C5 convertase and thereby an entry to the MAC.

The *lectin pathway* (2), described recently, differs from the classical pathway only in the initiation step. Here, mannan-binding lectin (MBL) (or other collectins, such as bovine conglutinin, surfactant protein-A, and so forth) binds to mannose or glucosamine-rich surfaces and activates complement (3). MBL, like C1q, has a globular head that has C-type lectin domains capable of binding sugar-rich surfaces of microbes. Although MBL with a suitable target can activate C1r and C1s, it appears to activate C4 and C2 by means of one or more distinct proteases known as MBL-associated serine proteases (MASPs). These proteases, MASP-1 (4,5) and MASP-2 (6), are structurally and functionally homologous to C1r and C1s.

The *terminal part of complement activation* is common to all three pathways. The active C3b generated by the convertases binds in turn to the respective convertases to form C5 convertases. When C5 is cleaved to C5b, the MAC is assembled through sequential nonproteolytic reactions. C5b acts as receptor for C6, which it has to bind to before the "C6 receptor site" decays within 2 minutes. C5b6 can bind C7 while still bound to the target, or it can be released into circulation to find C7 and insert into other cell membranes (reactive lysis[1]) (7). The binding of C7 leads to conformational changes in the complex, which irreversibly converts a hydrophilic C5b6 complex to an amphipathic C5b67 complex capable of inserting into cell membranes. This stable complex can bind C8 and C9 on the cell surface. Binding of C8 creates small pores on the membrane and low-grade lysis (8), but for rapid lysis, multimeric C9 binding is essential. Binding of one molecule of C9 exposes a binding site for a second C9 molecule, which, in turn, can bind more C9. Thus, C5b–9 complex forms a tubular pore in the cell membrane surrounded by 10 to 16 C9 molecules (9) and leads to osmotic cell lysis.

The complement pathway, with its proinflammatory and destructive capabilities, requires tight regulation so that foreign surfaces are "attacked" and so that host tissue is "protected." Table 10.2 summarizes the regulatory proteins and their functions. Their importance in modulating complement activation is highlighted by their abuse by microorganisms to gain entry [measles (10–12), Epstein–Barr virus (13), echovirus (14), and others (15)], to evade complement-mediated lysis by acquiring host regulators [human immunodeficiency virus (HIV) (16,17), β-hemolytic streptococci (18), *Schistosoma* species (19)], or by synthesis of self proteins that mimic the host's regulatory proteins, such as virulence factors [vaccinia (20), herpes simplex virus (21)]. Their efficiency in preventing complement activation in plasma and on self tissue is being exploited for therapeutic use in xenotransplantation (22,23) and in the treatment of inflammatory diseases (24,25).

Classical pathway initiation is controlled by C1 inhibitor (1-Inh), which is a member of a group of *ser*ine protease *in*hibitors (SERPINs). It binds to C1r and C1s in 1:1:2 ratio (C1r:C1s:C1-Inh) that dissociates from the Ab-C1q complex (26). C1-Inh does not influence appropriate activation of C1 by IgM or IgG on an antigenic surface. With its constant surveillance, it prevents fluid-phase activation of C1 and excessive complement activation on a target. The alternative pathway, because of its continuous tickover, is mainly regulated

_____

[1] C5b67, a stable amphipathic complex, when released into circulation, can insert into any cell membrane and sequentially bind C8 and C9 to bring about cell lysis. This type of cell lysis, remote from early activation events, is termed *reactive lysis*.

**TABLE 10.1.** *Components of the cascade*

| Component | Chromosomal location | Molecular weight (kd) | Serum concentration (μg/mL) |
|---|---|---|---|
| Classical pathway | | | |
| C1 | | | |
|   C1q | 1p34 | 410 (6 × A, B, C)[a] | 75 |
|   C1r | 12p13 | 85 | 50 |
|   C1s | 12p13 | 85 | 50 |
| C4 | 6p21 | 210 | 200–500 |
| C2 | 6p21 | 110 | 20 |
| | | | |
| Lectin pathway[b] | | | |
| MBL | 10q11 | 32 | 150 (wide range) |
| MASP-1 | 3q27 | 83 | 6μg/mL |
| MASP-2 | 1p36 | 80 | ? |
| | | | |
| Alternative pathway | | | |
| Factor B | 6p21 | 93 | 200 |
| Factor D | ? | 25 | 1–2 |
| Properdin | Xp11 | 220 | 25 |
| | | | |
| C3 | 19/p13 | 195 | 550–1200 |
| | | | |
| Terminal pathway | | | |
| C5 | 9q33 | 190 | 70 |
| C6 | 5p12 | 128 | 60 |
| C7 | 5p12 | 121 | 60 |
| C8 | | | |
|   α, β | 1p32 | 64, 64 | 60 |
|   γ | 9q34 | 22 | 9 |
| C9 | 5p13 | 79 | 60 |

[a] C1q is composed of six arms, and each arm consists of three intertwined equal peptide chains, termed A, B, and C.

[b] MASP, MBL-associated serine protease; MBL, mannan-binding lectin.

at the level of the C3 convertase feedback loop. The classical and alternative pathway C3 convertases efficiently convert C3 to C3b. C4-binding protein (C4BP), factor H, factor I, decay-accelerating factor (DAF; CD55), membrane cofactor protein (MCP; CD46), and complement receptor type one (CR1; CD35) function to check this activation in plasma and on host tissue (reviewed in 27). C4BP binds C4b, and factor H binds C3b in fluid phase. They act as cofactors for the cleavage of C3b and C4b into inactive products by the serine protease factor I as well as dissociate their ligands from their respective convertases. On self tissue, DAF disassociates C3 and C5 convertases of both pathways, whereas MCP acts as a cofactor in cleavage of C3b and C4b by factor I. CR1 has both cofactor and decay-accelerating activities.

S protein (vitronectin) and clusterin (SP-40,40) regulate the MAC in the fluid phase. These proteins bind to the metastable site of C5b–7, thus preventing its insertion into the cell membranes, even if these complexes fix C8 and C9. Additionally, S protein can bind C8 and C9 and prevent C9 polymerization, which is crucial for lytic pore formation. On the other hand, CD59 is responsible for protecting host cells from deposited MAC. CD59, which has binding sites for C8 and C9, incorporates into forming MACs and prevents deposition of the first C9 and its subsequent polymerization.

Homologous restriction factor, another glycoprotein that, like DAF and CD59, is bound to cell membranes by a GPI-anchor, has also been shown to have weak MAC inhibitory (1/100 of CD59) activity by different groups. It is possible, however, that some of these results may have been caused by contamination with polymeric forms of CD59. All membrane-bound complement regulators, except CR1, show wide tissue distribution.

The small cleavage products released from the activation of C3, C4, and C5 (C3a, C4a, and C5a, respectively) are anaphylatoxins. Their effect is regulated by plasma carboxypeptidases (reviewed in 28).

Table 10.3 summarizes the complement receptors. Four types of receptor molecules have been identified for the major cleavage fragments of C3. Complement receptor type one (CR1; CD35) is the receptor for C3b and C4b (13,27,29). It is expressed on erythrocytes, most leukocytes, dendritic cells, some astrocytes, and glomerular podocytes. It is the immune-adherence receptor and helps to bind and transport C3b and C4b opsonized immune complexes and particles to the tissue phagocytes. By virtue of its cofactor activity for cleavage of C3b, it generates ligands for other complement receptors (Fig. 10.2). Complement receptor type two (CR2; CD21) binds C3d, C3dg, and iC3b (13,30–32). It is expressed on

**TABLE 10.2.** *Complement regulatory proteins*

| | Chromosomal location | Molecular weight (kd) | Serum concentration (µg/mL) or tissue distribution | Function |
|---|---|---|---|---|
| **Initiation step** | | | | |
| C1 inhibitor | 11q11 | 105 | 120–200 | Inactivates C1r and C1s; a SERPIN |
| | | | | |
| **Amplification step** | | | | |
| Factor I | 4q25 | 88 | 35 | Cleaves C3b and C4b; requires a cofactor |
| Membrane cofactor protein | 1q 3.2 | 45–70 | Most cells except erythrocytes | Cofactor for factor I–mediated cleavage of C4b and C3b |
| Decay-accelerating factor | 1q 3.2 | 70 | Most cells | Destabilizes C3 and C5 convertases |
| C4-binding protein | 1q 3.2 | 560 | 250 | Cofactor for factor I cleavage of C4b; destabilizes CP C3 and C5 convertases |
| Factor H | 1q 3.2 | 150 | 500 | Cofactor for factor I cleavage of C3b; destabilizes AP C3 and C5 convertases and CP C5 convertase |
| Complement receptor 1 | 1q 3.2 | 190–280 | Erythrocytes, mononuclear phagocytes, most B lymphocytes and 15% of T lymphocytes, follicular-dendritic cells, glomerular podocytes, astrocytes | Receptor for C3b and C4b; cofactor activity for C3b and C4b and decay acceleration for C3 and C5 convertases of both pathways |
| Properdin | Xp11 | 112–224 | 25 | Stabilizes AP convertases |
| **Membrane attack** | | | | |
| S protein | 17q | 75–80 | 250–450 | Blocks fluid-phase MAC |
| Clusterin | 8p21 | 80 | 35–105 | Blocks fluid-phase MAC |
| CD59 | 11p13 | 18 | All cells | Blocks MAC on host cells |
| **Other** | | | | |
| Anaphylatoxin inactivator | ? | 305 | 35 | Inactivates C3a, C4a, C5a (partially) |

AP, alternative pathway; CP, classical pathway; MAC, membrane attack complex; SERPIN, serine protease inhibitor.

premature and mature B lymphocytes, thymocytes, follicular–dendritic cells, and nasopharyngeal epithelial cells. It plays an important role in signaling B cells to proliferate and produce antibody (33). It is also the B lymphocyte receptor for Epstein–Barr virus (34,35). CD23 (36) and interferon-α (37) may also be ligands of CR2. Complement receptors CR3 (CD11b; CD18) and CR4 (CD11c; CD18) belong to the integrin family and share a common β chain. iC3b is a ligand for both receptors, although there is evidence that they also bind to noncomplement ligands (38–44). By binding of iC3b-coated target, they, in cooperation with CR1, enhance phagocytosis.

A wide range of cellular proteins appear to bind C1q, but which of them constitutes a true receptor is debatable. Three putative receptors for C1q have been described. One binds the globular head of C1q (gC1q-R) (45) and is expressed on

most tissues. gC1q-R shows no sequence homology to any known protein. The second binds to the collagenous portion of C1q (cC1qR) and is known to be the same as calreticulin, a calcium-binding intracellular protein found in the endoplasmic reticulum of all cells (46). Engagement of these two receptors with aggregated C1q is reported to trigger a variety of biologic effects, including enhanced ingestion in phagocytes as well as oxygen burst in neutrophils, eosinophils, and endothelial and vascular smooth muscle cells (47). The third, C1qRp, most fulfills the criteria for a membrane receptor and is known to enhance phagocytosis on interaction with C1q (48).

The cellular responses of the anaphylatoxins C3a, C4a, and C5a are also receptor mediated. C3a and C5a receptors (28), recently cloned, are members of the rhodopsin supergene family and are much more widely expressed than was suggested by initial studies at the protein level.

**TABLE 10.3.** *Complement receptors*

| Receptor | Molecular weight (kd) | Chromosomal location | Distribution | Function |
|---|---|---|---|---|
| C1qRp | 126 | ? | Mononuclear phagocytes | Enhances phagocytosis mediated via C1q, MBL, SP-A |
| CR1 | 220 (190, 250, 280) | 1q32 | Erythrocytes, mononuclear phagocytes, dendritic cells, most B lymphocytes and 15% of T lymphocytes, glomerular podocytes, astrocytes | Receptor for C3b and C4b; cofactor for factor I; accelerates dissociation of AP and CP C3 and C5 convertases; processing of IC; phagocytosis; antigen localization |
| CR2 | 140 (150) | 1q32 | B lymphocytes, dendritic cells, nasopharyngeal epithelial cells | Receptor for C3d; immune regulation; lowers threshold for B-cell activation; EBV receptor |
| CR3 | α 165 β 95 | 16p11 21q22 | Mononuclear phagocytes, NK cells | Receptor for iC3b; phagocytosis of iC3b-coated particles; cell adhesion; member of leukocyte integrin family |
| CR4 | α 150 β 95 | 16p11 21q22 | Myeloid cells, dendritic cells, NK cells, activated B lymphocytes, cytotoxic T lymphocytes, platelets | Receptor for iC3b; functions in cell adhesion; integrin |
| C3aR | 95 | 12p13 | Mast cells, granulocytes, T lymphocytes, monocytes | Depending on cell type: chemotaxis, chemokinesis, cell adhesion, aggregation, release of lysosomal contents; mast cell activation; immune regulation |
| C5aR | 43 | 19q13 | Neutrophils, eosinophils, monocytes, macrophages, lung vascular smooth muscle cells, endothelial cells, bronchoalveolar epithelial cells, astrocytes, parenchymal liver cells | Depending on cell type: chemotaxis, cell adhesion; degranulation or release of granular enzymes and histamine; influence on humoral and cellular immune response |

AP, alternative pathway; CP, classical pathway; EBV, Epstein–Barr virus; IC, immune complexes; MBL, mannan-binding lectin; NK, natural killer; SP-A, surfactant protein A.

## BIOLOGIC FUNCTIONS OF THE COMPLEMENT SYSTEM

### Opsonization and Lysis

The brisk deposition of large numbers of C3b by either pathway (opsonization) marks targets such as bacteria, viruses, and effete red blood cells for ingestion by circulating or tissue phagocytes. Receptors for C3 fragments, specifically CR1 and CR3, participate in and enhance ingestion by mononuclear phagocytes. Alternatively, further activation of C5 and deposition of MAC result in cell lysis. Insertion of large numbers of MAC on nucleated cells often results in cell death but, at sublytic concentration, MAC can lead to cell activation (49). In endothelial cells, it leads to production of procoagulant and proinflammatory mediators, expression of cell adherence molecules and platelet-activating factor on neutrophils and monocytes, and generation of reactive oxygen species, prostaglandins, and cytokines.

### Immune Complex Clearance

Under normal physiologic conditions, the processing and disposal of immune complexes is an efficient mechanism wherein complement is a crucial player. The relative rarity of immune complex diseases in infectious illnesses attests to the workings of this process. Waxman et al. (50) showed that, in baboons, systemic complement depletion results in rapid deposition of immune complexes in kidney and lungs (instead of in the liver and spleen, as in complement-sufficient animals), whereby they can potentially set up an inflammatory response. The efficient deposition of large numbers of C3b on immune complexes containing IgG or IgM (IgA-containing immune complexes fix C1q poorly, although aggregated IgA can fix C3 by means of the alternative pathway) prevents abnormal tissue deposition of immune complexes. First, deposition of C3b solubilizes large aggregates by breaking the Fc-Fc interactions; second, C3b-bound

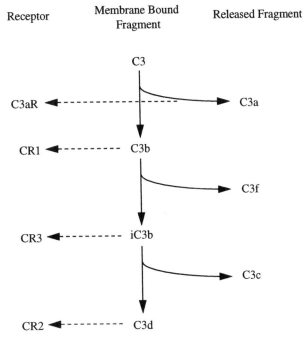

Receptor  Membrane Bound  Released Fragment
Fragment

**FIG. 10.2.** Proteolytic cleavage of C3. The chart depicts the cleavage fragments and their receptors. C3a is an approximately 10,000-dalton fragment released from the amino terminus of the α chain by the C3 convertases. It is an anaphylatoxin. The much larger C3b fragment becomes covalently bound to a target, where it is a ligand for CR1, and it may also form part of a C5 convertase. C3f is a 3,000-dalton fragment released by serine protease factor I. This reaction requires a cofactor. Factor H, CR1, and membrane cofactor protein (MCP) can all serve in this role. This reaction leads to the formation of iC3b—the major ligand for the integrin-related CR3. Only CR1 can efficiently serve as a cofactor for the next cleavage of iC3b to C3c and C3d. C3d remains attached covalently to the target (an immunologic scar) and is a ligand for CR2.

immune complexes bind to C3b receptors (CR1) on circulating blood cells, a process referred to by Nelson as *immune adherence* (51,52). Hebert's group, using a primate model, demonstrated that erythrocyte CR1 was pivotal in binding and transporting immune complexes to the liver and spleen, where they transferred the complexes to the mononuclear cells for phagocytosis, whereas erythrocytes themselves returned to circulation—a process referred to as *primate erythrocyte immune complex clearance mechanism* (53,54).

### Release of Proinflammatory Peptides

Activation of complement by noxious agents, such as microorganisms, biomaterials, or immune complexes, results in release of small complement peptides, C3a, C4a and C5a, which are key participants in the inflammatory response of the host (28,55–57). These small complement peptides are similar in structure and mediate a similar set of activities but with different potencies (C5a>>C3a>>C4a). As anaphylatoxins, they lead to mast cell degranulation, increase vascular permeability, and affect smooth muscle contraction (58–60). Their anaphylatoxic effects are short lived and localized as a result of inactivation by cleavage of the termi-

nal arginine by plasma carboxyl peptidases (to form the *desArg* form). C5a desArg, however, retains its chemotactic activity, and like C5a, its chemotactic activity is enhanced by vitamin D–binding protein (61). C3a and C4a lack chemotactic activity. C5a and C5a desArg also augment cell adherence, production of reactive oxygen species, degranulation, and release of intracellular enzymes from granulocytes, similar to sublytic amounts of C5b–9 deposition. Some of the minor C3 cleavage fragments are also thought to release leukocytes from bone marrow and to cause leukocytosis. Another kinin-like byproduct of C2 cleavage is thought to be responsible for the angioedema seen in C1 inhibitor deficiency.

### Immune Regulation

Although viewed mainly as a component of the innate immune system and as an effector of adaptive immunity, there is mounting evidence that the complement system plays an important role in the afferent arm of adaptive immunity (62,63). The recognition of pathogens by the innate immune system results in complement activation and covalent attachment of C3. The importance of complement in antibody production was first demonstrated by Pepys (64). More than a decade ago, Melchers et al. (65) showed that C3d-CR2 (CD21) interaction regulates antibody production by B cells. Ligation of CR2 (CD21) lowers the threshold for B-cell activation (33,66). C3d coupling to antigen is sufficient to accomplish this activation, and the number of C3d molecules attached proportionately reduces the amount of antigen required for a secondary response (67). The recent development and characterization of mice deficient in C3, C4, and CR1 and CR2 (discussed later) has provided further understanding of how the complement system bridges innate and acquired immunity.

### GENETICS OF COMPLEMENT COMPONENTS AND REGULATORY PROTEINS

Most of the complement proteins, their receptors, and their regulators have been cloned, and their genes have been localized to at least 14 different chromosomes (Tables 10.1 to 10.3). The clustering of the genes for the components of C3-cleaving enzymes (C4, C2, factor B—HLA class III) and of the C3- and C4-binding and regulatory proteins (CR1, CR2, factor H, C4bp, MCP, and DAF—the so-called regulators of complement activation [RCA] gene cluster) on chromosome 6p and 1q regions, respectively, is notable.

### HLA Class III

The genes for C2 and factor B, the two genes for C4, and the 21-hydroxylase pseudogene are clustered within $1 \times 10^6$ base pairs (bp) of DNA on the short arm of chromosome 6, flanked by HLA class II region on the centromeric side and class I region on the telomeric side (Fig. 10.3) (68). As with HLA class I and class II genes, these complement genes express a high degree of polymorphism (complotypes) and, because of their close linkage, are usually inherited as a group. Factor B

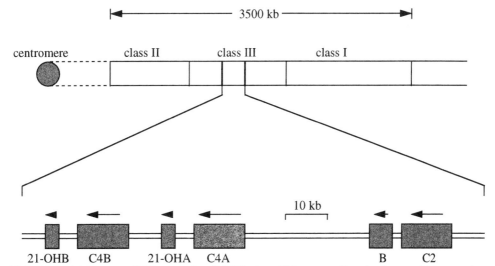

**FIG. 10.3.** Major histocompatibility complex (MHC) class III locus on the short arm of human chromosome 6. Arrows indicate the direction of transcription. 21-OH, 21-hydroxylase (A and B).

and C2 genes are tightly linked, separated from each other by only 421 bp, and they demonstrate an overall similarity in structure. Their genes, however, differ considerably in size (factor B is 6 kb, whereas C2 is 18 kb), mostly as a result of variation in intronic regions.

For C2, three allelic forms have been identified: C2C (the most common, with a gene frequency of more than 95%), C2A, and C2B. Additional polymorphisms have been identified by restriction fragment length polymorphisms (RFLP) (69). Complotypes missing the gene for C2 have been identified at a frequency of about 2%, with homozygous deficiency occurring at a gene frequency of 0.01% in the white population. For factor B, four allelic forms have been identified: S, F, F1, and S1, with gene frequencies of 0.71, 0.27, 0.01, and 0.01, respectively. Several other rare polymorphisms (69) have been demonstrated by RFLP. Complotypes lacking factor B have not yet been identified.

The two C4 genes in the class III region code for the functionally active C4A and C4B isotypes. These two proteins, each comprising 1725 amino acids, are more than 99% identical (70–73). Four amino acid differences in positions 1101 to 1106, near the thioester bond, are responsible for the electrophoretic (fast versus slow), serologic (C4A carrying Rodgers' blood group antigen and C4B carrying Chido's) and hemolytic (C4B is several-fold more active than C4A in whole complement assay) variation. Besides their isotypic differences, C4A and C4B each demonstrate additional polymorphisms that give rise to more than 40 C4A and C4B alleles. The alleles sequenced thus far appear to be the result of single amino acid differences in the region of the molecule containing the thioester (the C4d fragment).

Particular sets of class I and II genes appear to be closely linked to the class III genes that have become entrapped in the linkage group. Deletions and duplications of C4 and 21-hydroxylase genes are common (72–78). Thus, on some complotypes, there may be one C4A gene and two C4B genes.

These deletions and duplications, in addition to the high frequency of null alleles at either locus, could be accounted for by unequal crossover. C4A and C4B null alleles can also result from intact but noncoding genes, presumably a result of point mutations, frame shifts, or C4A-to-C4B gene conversions (78). Although a variety of extended haplotypes have been identified, C4A null on the background of B8-DR3 is the most common in whites. The serum level of C4 is the result of expression of two C4A and two C4B alleles. Complete C4 deficiency (C4D) (a null homozygote) possesses null alleles in all four loci and therefore expresses no C4 protein. More common are null alleles at either the C4A or C4B locus, with reduced C4 levels, usually in the lower end of the normal range. On activation, C4A is more efficient in binding amino groups and consequently more efficient in metabolizing certain types of immune complexes than is C4B (79,80). C4B binds hydroxyl groups better and demonstrates enhanced hemolytic activity in assays because sheep erythrocytes are a hydroxyl-rich substrate. The two isotypes also differ in their ability to serve as ligands for the C3b and C4b receptors (81,82).

**The Regulators of Complement Activation Gene Cluster**

The RCA gene cluster comprises a group of proteins (CR1, CR2, MCP, DAF, factor H and C4BP) clustered on the long arm of chromosome 1 (Fig. 10.4). These proteins share structural and functional features (83). Structurally, they all contain repeating motifs of about 60 amino acids, called *complement control proteins* (CCPs) or *short consensus repeats*. These repeats have a framework of 10 to 18 highly conserved residues, including 4 cysteines, the pairings of which promote a double-loop structure of the module and are responsible for the 20% to 40% homology between repeats. These repeats can generally be mapped to boundaries defined by intron–exon junctions, although there are exceptions.

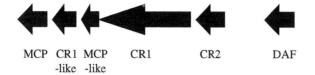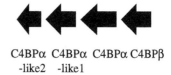

MCP  CR1  MCP      CR1          CR2          DAF            C4BPα C4BPα C4BPα C4BPβ
     -like -like                                           -like2  -like1

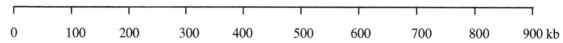

0      100    200    300    400    500    600    700    800    900 kb

**FIG. 10.4.** The regulators of complement activation (RCA) gene cluster on the long arm of human chromosome 1. Factor H (not shown) lies 5 to 10 cM from this complex. Note that the direction of transcription is the same for all proteins. The term *like* refers to a partial duplication of the original gene; for so-designated proteins, a mRNA species has yet to be demonstrated, but there are no stop codons in the exons, which suggests that these partial duplicates are unlikely to be pseudogenes. C4BP, C4-binding protein (α and β chain); CR1, complement receptor type 1; CR2, complement receptor type 2; DAF, decay-accelerating factor; MCP, membrane cofactor protein.

Functionally, the proteins encoded by the genes in the RCA cluster all bind C3b and C4b or their cleavage fragments. Proteins such as factor B and C2, encoded by genes outside the RCA cluster, also have CCP motifs and bind C3b and C4b. Other proteins containing CCPs, such as coagulation factor XIII, the selectins, and interleukin-2 receptor, are not known to bind complement fragments.

## COMPLEMENT DEFICIENCY AND AUTOIMMUNE DISEASES

One of the paradoxes of autoimmune diseases is that, although the complement system contributes much to inflammation and organ damage, both inherited and acquired deficiencies of complement proteins predispose to autoimmune conditions. Studies suggest that the predisposition to SLE becomes higher as the deficiency involves progressively earlier components of the complement activation pathway. Thus, C1q deficiency appears to confer highest susceptibility (84), which clinically also tends to be more severe and early in onset. Although C1r, C1s, and C4 deficiencies also show high prevalence of disease, C2 deficiency is associated with development of disease in only about one-third of patients (85); it is unclear whether this is related to the ability of classical pathway to bypass C2 (86,87). By contrast, few patients with C3 deficiency have autoimmune problems, which generally present as mild, lupus-like disease.

Relative to complement deficiency and autoimmune disease, concerns about ascertainment bias have been addressed by population studies by the Swiss (88) and the Japanese (89). These studies demonstrated that, although the prevalence differed in the two racial groups, early complement component deficiencies were not found in their normal blood donors. The possible mechanisms for the predisposition to autoimmune diseases in complement deficiency states are discussed later in this chapter.

### C1q Deficiency

Berkel et al. first described the case of a 10-year-old Turkish boy in whom recurrent skin lesions, infections, and glomerulonephritis were related to complete C1q deficiency (90). Since then, more than 30 cases of C1q deficiency presenting with SLE or SLE-like conditions have been reported (84,91,92). The molecular basis of this defect has been identified in only a few of these patients. In each of these instances, the defect is due to a point mutation in any of the three genes encoding C1q. These mutations lead to a premature stop codon resulting in deficiency of protein or to a single amino acid substitution (glycine to arginine) causing expression of normal levels of a dysfunctional protein (summarized in 88).

As in the case of the Turkish boy, C1q deficiency clinically presents at a young age (median, 7 years) and affects more boys than girls (84,91). Patients have SLE or SLE-like disease, proliferative glomerulonephritis with immunoglobulin deposits with or without C3 deposition, and chronic infections. Other patients have been identified with poikiloderma congenita, vasculitis, or discoid lupus. Only one subject identified with C1q deficiency, a sibling of three patients with C1q deficiency, has remained healthy so far. Many patients with C1q deficiency have detectable antinuclear antibody (ANA), and most of these patients show antibodies against extractable nuclear antigens. Anti-DNA antibodies are seen less often. Rheumatoid factor and circulating immune complexes may also be positive in these patients.

### C1r and C1s Deficiencies

C1r and C1s deficiencies generally occur together, probably because of the close proximity of their genes on chromosome 12. Some patients have complete deficiency of both components, whereas others have complete absence of one component and decreased levels of the other (93–95). Clinical features, as in C1q deficiency, are either of SLE or SLE-like disease. Most reported cases have no detectable ANA or rheumatoid factor.

## C4 Deficiency

Inherited deficiency of C4 may result from the involvement of C4A or C4B or both (C4A*Q0, C4B*Q0). Complete C4 deficiency is a rare occurrence, with only a dozen or so kindred (with about 40 patients) reported in the literature (96–103). It is caused by a homozygous defect in both C4A and C4B genes and results in undetectable levels of C4 in serum. More than 90% of affected patients demonstrate clinical evidence of SLE.

Homozygous deficiency of either C4A or C4B (reviewed in 104) is more common and is seen in about 1% to 3% of the general population. Although total C4 levels may be in the low-normal range, these patients possess no detectable levels of the respective isoform. The association of homozygous C4A deficiency with SLE, reported by many groups, is interesting. In contrast to the general population, 15% of patients with SLE show C4A deficiency (105), but the significance of this association has been confounded by a strong linkage disequilibrium between C4A null alleles and HLA-DR3 and HLA-B8 in patients with SLE (75,76,106,107). C4A null allele has been found in SLE on the background of other extended haplotypes and appears to be an independent risk factor for SLE. In particular, extended haplotypes distinct from DR3-B8 are seen in the Chinese and Japanese populations with C4A null state (108–110). The clinical expression of SLE, in homozygous C4A deficiency, is no different from SLE in other patients, although some studies have noted less neurologic and renal involvement and more photosensitivity.

The association of SLE with a C4B null state is less obvious and may be related to racial factors. Although C4A null alleles are more prevalent in SLE in white, African-American, and Japanese populations, C4B null alleles are associated with SLE in white French populations (111) and in Australian aborigines (112). The Chinese demonstrate association of SLE with both C4A and C4B null alleles. More obvious is the increased prevalence of homozygous C4B deficiency in children with bacteremia (113) and meningitis (114). The physiologic basis of the clinical expression in C4A and C4B null states may be related to the efficiency of C4A in forming amide links (important in immune complex processing) and of C4B in forming hydroxyl bonds (important in interaction with bacterial surface polysaccharides).

Partial or heterozygous deficiency of C4A or C4B is more common in the general population. In patients with SLE, however, the frequency of C4A, and not C4B, deficiency is increased. A variety of other diseases, such as chronic active hepatitis, insulin-dependent diabetes mellitus (115), subacute sclerosing panencephalitis (116), and HIV-related syndromes (117), have been found in association with partial C4A deficiency. IgA nephropathy, Henoch–Schönlein purpura (118),

juvenile dermatomyositis, and scleroderma (119,120) have been reported to be associated with heterozygous C4A or C4B deficiency. C4 deficiency is also associated with higher anti-Ro and anticardiolipin antibodies in African Americans (121).

## C2 Deficiency

Genetic deficiency of C2 is the most common of known complete complement deficiencies of the activation pathways. Heterozygous deficiency is seen in 1% and homozygous deficiency in 0.01% of the general population (122). Type I deficiency is caused by a 28 bp genomic deletion in exon 6. The ensuing frame shift and premature stop codon result in undetectable serum levels of C2 (123). This is generally inherited in an autosomal dominant manner on the background of A25, B18, C2Q0, BFS, C4A4, C4B2, DR2 extended haplotype (124,125). Recently, another type I deficiency that is inherited with a different extended haplotype has been described in which the 28-bp deletion on one allele is associated with a 2-bp deletion on exon 2 of the other allele (126). In C2 deficiency type II, point mutations result in a dysfunctional protein that may be detected in peripheral blood at normal or subnormal levels (127). Lack of this classical pathway component leads to suboptimal opsonic and bactericidal activity, but only a subset of these patients have increased frequency of bacterial infections with encapsulated organisms.

In contrast to C1q and C4 deficiency, only one-third of the C2-deficient population presents with SLE (85). These patients demonstrate many characteristic features of SLE, although progressive nephritis and central nervous system involvement appear less commonly. Photosensitive cutaneous rash at a young age is a typical finding. ANA and anti-DNA antibodies are less common in C2 deficiency–related SLE, but the incidence of anti-Ro is higher. Another one-third of patients express manifestations of other rheumatic diseases, such as discoid lupus, dermatomyositis, glomerulonephritis, or vasculitis.

Although some patients with heterozygous C2 deficiency have been diagnosed with SLE and juvenile rheumatoid arthritis, the association appears to be weak.

## C3 Deficiency

C3 has two well-known polymorphic alleles, C3F and C3S, based on fast and slow mobility on electrophoretic gels, as well as several rare variants. Rare hypomorphic variants C3*f and C3*s are associated with significantly reduced levels of C3 in blood and have been described in healthy subjects as well as in patients with glomerulonephritis (128), cutaneous vasculitis (129), and recurrent hemolytic uremic syndrome (130). More commonly, inherited C3 deficiency is caused either by a point mutation in the donor splice site of intron 18 of the C3 gene (described in the first patient—a Caucasoid boy) (131) or by an 800-bp genomic deletion spanning exons 22 and 23 (as noted in Afrikaaner patients) (132). More than 15 families with C3 deficiency have been described

(133–135), including a recent report of a family with compound heterozygous C3 deficiency (136). Clinically, patients may present with the following:

- Systemic infections resulting from encapsulated bacteria (pneumococci, meningococci, hemophilus), such as meningitis, septicemia, upper and lower respiratory tract infections, and osteomyelitis. Predisposition to these infections is related to the opsonic, chemotactic, and bactericidal defects in the absence of C3.
- Generalized inflammatory rash that follows infections, the pathophysiology of which is unclear. Biopsy of the skin shows neutrophilic infiltrate without any immune complexes.
- SLE or immune complex–type disease, particularly membranoproliferative glomerulonephritis, although some patients have vasculitis. The lupus-like illness may be associated with ANA, anti-dsDNA, and the presence of circulating immune complexes (133).

The relatively milder form of rheumatologic problems in C3 compared with C1q, C4 or C2 deficiency underlines the physiologic importance of the early components in "defense" against immune complex diseases.

### C5 to C9 Deficiencies

The terminal complement component deficiencies result in absence of serum hemolytic and bactericidal activity. This predisposes these patients to recurrent infections, particularly neisserial. Few cases of SLE have been reported in association with these deficiencies (137–142), and these patients have no distinguishing features in their SLE. The relative rarity of rheumatic illnesses in association with terminal component deficiency suggests that there is not a causal relationship. The molecular nature of many of these deficiencies is beginning to be defined.

### Acquired Complement Deficiencies

Although deficiency of early components of the complement pathway predisposes to SLE, patients with SLE unrelated to complement deficiency show depressed levels of these early components. Consumption of the components secondary to activation by immune complexes outstrips their synthesis. Many studies have correlated clinical activity of lupus with low complement (C1q, C4, C2, C3) levels and $CH_{50}$. Serial measurement of these parameters also demonstrate that increases in their levels coincide with clinical improvement of lupus, but the utility of these measurements must be established for each patient.

Deficiency of regulatory proteins (e.g., C1 inhibitor) resulting in complement depletion and disease is discussed later in this chapter.

Two other distinct forms of acquired complement deficiency are of interest. They are related to the presence of autoantibodies, one to C1q and the other to the alternative pathway C3 convertase. Antibodies to C1q are not uncommon in patients with SLE and are also frequently found in patients with hypocomplementemic urticarial vasculitic syndrome (HUVS). These IgG antibodies (143–145) are targeted against a neoepitope in the C1q collagenous region that is exposed after C1 activation. They are associated strongly with classical pathway activation and consumption of the early complement components and present clinically as SLE or more characteristically as HUVS with urticarial vasculitis, arthritis, bronchitis, and glomerulonephritis. In some patients, anti-C1q antibodies present with membranoproliferative glomerulonephritis in the absence of features of SLE or HUVS. Whether anti-C1q antibodies are pathogenic is not clear; however, when these antibodies are purified from patients' sera and injected in mice, they form immune complexes in the glomeruli, in the presence of human C1q (146). The mechanism for the development of these autoantibodies in selected patients remains unknown.

Proteins that bind and stabilize the C3 convertase C3bBb were first discovered in patients with lipodystrophy and low C3 levels (and normal C2 and C4 levels) who presented with membranoproliferative glomerulonephritis (147). These proteins are autoantibodies targeted against a neoepitope on the convertase; they prevent decay (147,148) of the enzyme complex and have been termed *C3 nephritic factors*. Stabilization of the convertase results in increased C3 cleavage, low C3 levels, and inflammation. If classical pathway convertase is stabilized (C4 nephritic factor), the presentation is like that of SLE (149–151).

Finally, there is some evidence pointing to the possibility that drugs such as hydralazine and isoniazid induce SLE by binding to and inhibiting C4 activity (152).

### Mannan-Binding Lectin Deficiency

Variant alleles that result in absent or low levels of MBL are relatively common and predispose to recurrent infections, although an association with SLE has also been reported (48,153).

## DEFICIENCY OF REGULATORY PROTEINS

The function of the regulatory proteins is to prevent excessive and abnormal activation of complement, such as in the fluid phase, and to protect host tissue during appropriate complement activation by microorganisms and immune complexes. Deficiency of these proteins results in excessive complement activation and inflammatory damage to the host tissue.

### Angioedema (C1 Inhibitor Deficiency)

C1 inhibitor deficiency is associated with the syndrome of angioneurotic edema, which consists of recurrent bouts of swelling of subcutaneous tissue, of the mucosa of intestinal walls and, most seriously, of the airway. The deficiency can be inherited or acquired. Most patients (85%) with autosomally dominant inherited deficiency show very low or absent serum levels of C1 inhibitor (type I deficiency), whereas others (15%) show normal or increased levels of a functionally inactive protein (type II deficiency).

C1 inhibitor gene, which is 17 kb long and located on chromosome 11 (154–156), has limited homology to the related proteins of the SERPIN superfamily and exhibits some unusual features which are of relevance in the cause of deficiency (reviewed in 157). First, its introns and the flanking regions are relatively abundant in Alu sequences, which are common sites of recombination that result in deletions and duplications. Twenty percent of known molecular defects in C1 inhibitor deficiency are due to such deletions or duplications. Second, the sequence through a region of exon 8 forms a partial palindrome, and another short region of exon 5 consists of triplet repeats. Both these regions are susceptible to mutations, deletions, and duplications, which account for a number of reported C1 inhibitor deficiencies. Third, most C1 inhibitor deficiencies result from single base changes that have been found throughout the coding sequence of the gene (most of them within exon 8). These molecular defects result in premature stop codons and protein deficiency or, in some cases, generation of a dysfunctional protein.

Two forms of acquired C1 inhibitor deficiency have been recognized. Type I acquired angioedema is seen in association with lymphoproliferative disorders and a few other malignancies. There is a suggestion that C1 inhibitor depletion may be due to highly efficient complement activation by antibodies directed against the idiotypes of circulating immunoglobulins in these lymphoproliferative disorders (158). Type II acquired angioedema is due to circulating autoantibodies against C1 inhibitor, which make the protein prone to proteolytic cleavage (159–161).

The clinical syndrome of angioedema is similar with both hereditary and acquired defects (162,163). As mentioned, patients have recurrent episodes of acute localized edema of skin and mucus membranes with predilection to affect face, extremities, gastrointestinal tract, and larynx. Skin edema is nonpitting and may be associated with a nonpruritic erythema marginatum–like rash. Intestinal edema presents as acute, severe, abdominal cramping and is usually associated with nausea and vomiting and sometimes diarrhea.

Attacks may be precipitated by stress, trauma, or illness but most often occur without any identifiable event. Attacks in women tend to increase in frequency during menstruation and diminish during the third trimester of pregnancy. Symptoms usually resolve within 72 hours. Laryngeal edema is life-threatening.

Although there is evidence that a fragment of C2 may be responsible for the edema, analysis of C1 inhibitor mutants with reduced C1r and C1s inhibitory activity in a family with no angioedema suggests that bradykinin may be the primary mediator of angioedema. By virtue of its role in regulation of the contact system, C1 inhibitor may be important in protection from endotoxic shock associated with gram-negative sepsis (164–166). Androgenic compounds, such as danazol

and stanozolol, lead to increased C1 inhibitor synthesis by the normal gene (the reason for much less than 50% of serum levels in these heterozygous individuals is an enigma). It takes 7 to 10 days of treatment to obtain protective serum levels of the C1 inhibitor. Severe acute attacks are treated by infusion of C1 inhibitor, which is also useful as prophylaxis before dental or other surgical procedures.

A number of patients with hereditary angioedema have been reported to have lupus. This predisposition is likely related to unregulated C1 activity and consumption of C4 and C2. Many of these patients have very low or undetectable C4 and C2 levels chronically and are serologically and clinically similar to C4- and C2-deficient patients.

## Paroxysmal Nocturnal Hemoglobinuria: CD55 (Decay-Accelerating Factor) and CD59 Deficiencies

Paroxysmal nocturnal hemoglobinuria (PNH) is a rare acquired clonal hematologic disorder of stem cells characterized by episodic intravascular hemolysis and hemoglobinuria (not necessarily nocturnal). It is often exacerbated by infections and is associated with a varying degree of hematopoietic failure and venous thrombosis. The disease was first recognized more than 100 years ago (167). Since then, patients were found to have erythrocytes unusually susceptible to complement-mediated lysis. Experiments in recent decades demonstrated that increased lysis is related to lack of normal decay of C3bBb deposited on red blood cells (168) and the deposition of much smaller amounts of C3 for a given degree of lysis compared with normal red blood cells (169). The former defect was shown to be caused by the absence of DAF (CD55) (170,171) and the latter by a lack of regulation of polymeric C9 assembly (CD59 deficiency) (172) on these cells. Many other proteins, such as leukocyte alkaline phosphatase and erythrocyte acetylcholinesterase, are also deficient on these cells. All these proteins are attached to the cell membrane by glycosylphosphatidylinositol (GPI) anchor.

The molecular basis for PNH has been linked to the more than 100 defects identified in the *Pig-A* gene, which is located on the short arm of the X chromosome (reviewed in 173). Most of the known defects are caused by insertion or deletion of one, two, or a few nucleotides that results in a premature stop codon and an inactive gene product. In the absence of this gene product that has homology to glycosyl transferases, cells are unable to add *N*-acetyl glucosamine to phosphatidylinositol, and no GPI anchor is made. About 20% of known defects are missense mutations, resulting in an abnormal protein that is capable of producing small amounts of a GPI anchor.

In PNH, intravascular hemolysis is explained by the absence of the membrane regulators of complement (CD59 deficiency is more significant than CD55 deficiency), and venous thrombosis may be caused by abnormal platelet activation and the lack of monocyte urokinase receptor. The hematopoietic defect, however, is not easily explained. The current hypothesis suggests the presence of a second defect relative to marrow cell suppression. If the suppressive influence was sufficient, both normal and PNH clones would be suppressed. As the influence decreases, such as in disease states or during therapy, the PNH clone would have a growth and survival advantage and replace the normal marrow (174,175).

Treatment of PNH is primarily empirical—steroids, by their modifying effect on complement activation, can help some patients (176,177). The hematopoietic defect can be relieved to an extent by treatment with antithymocyte globulin and cyclosporine. The only definitive treatment is with bone marrow transplantation. In the future, PNH may be a candidate for cure by gene therapy.

## Complement Receptor Type I Deficiency

CR1 has received much scrutiny in relation to SLE because of its role in immune complex clearance. Wilson et al. (178) correlated low and high erythrocyte CR1 copy numbers with a *cis*-acting Hind III restriction fragment length polymorphism (RFLP) of 6.9 kb and 7.4 kb, respectively. Earlier studies established a correlation between expression of low copy of CR1 per erythrocyte and SLE. Although several studies suggested that reduced numbers of CR1 on erythrocytes were inherited in SLE (reviewed in 179), subsequent studies showing loss of CR1 from transfused erythrocytes (180) and no increased frequency of 6.9 kb RFLP fragment in SLE patients (181) conclusively demonstrated that inherited deficiency of CR1 is not a susceptibility factor for SLE and that reduced erythrocyte CR1 copy numbers are acquired in SLE. Other studies have shown similar fluctuations in CR1 copy numbers in hemolytic anemias, acquired immunodeficiency syndrome, PNH, rheumatoid arthritis, and Sjögren's syndrome (reviewed in 179).

CR1 exhibits a size polymorphism in which four codominantly inherited alleles give rise to several phenotypes. Although the smallest allele has decreased functional capacity (182) and has correlated with SLE is several families (183), larger surveys have not found an association between this allele and SLE (184).

## Factor H Deficiency

Factor H is encoded by a single gene located in the RCA gene cluster. Three different factor H–related mRNAs, found in relatively equal abundance in the liver (185), are responsible for the full length (155 kd) and the truncated (49 and 39 to 43 kd) forms of the protein present in serum.

Factor H deficiency has been described in about 10 families. The inheritance follows an autosomal recessive pattern. The most common clinical manifestations are membranoproliferative glomerulonephritis, hemolytic uremic syndrome, and recurrent meningococcal infections (186–191). Most of the reported cases have shown depressed $CH_{50}$ or total hemolytic complement activity, $AP_{50}$ (total alternative pathway activity), C3, factor B, and C5 levels from unregu-

lated complement activation, with factor H levels between 10% and 50% of normal serum concentration. Homozygous deficiency with less than 1% detectable functional factor H is known as well in a patient with near-normal levels of a dysfunctional protein. Several homozygous deficient siblings of patients remain healthy. This may be explained by the presence of truncated forms of the protein or the small amounts of 155-kd factor H in circulation. More careful analysis of the truncated proteins in these kindred will clarify the issue. The molecular basis for factor H deficiency has been reported in only one patient, in whom the protein secretion was blocked by point mutations in the framework cysteine residues of two CCPs (192). Plasma exchange and infusion of fresh-frozen plasma to replenish the deficient factor may be helpful. In a variety of Yorkshire pigs with factor H deficiency, exogenous factor H therapy is effective in the treatment of the lethal glomerulonephritis (193).

## C4BP Deficiency

Only a single family with C4BP deficiency has been reported (194). The propositus, a 33-year-old woman who had 15% levels of C4BP, presented with angioedema and Behçet's disease. Her healthy father and a sister have 25% of normal levels of the protein. The molecular basis for this deficiency is unknown. The relationship of this deficiency to the clinical presentation is also difficult to establish from this single case.

## Properdin Deficiency

Properdin deficiency is a rare X-linked recessive disorder that is manifested by susceptibility to meningococcal disease with a high mortality rate. Most of the cases reported are due to point mutations resulting in no detectable (type 1) (195) or low (type 2) (196) levels of circulating protein. One Dutch family with normal levels of a mutated, dysfunctional protein has also been described (197).

## Factor I Deficiency

Like those with properdin deficiency, the most common clinical problem in patients with factor I deficiency is also a susceptibility to recurrent neisserial infections. Although the molecular basis for this deficiency is unknown, RFLPs that allow for carrier detection have been identified (198).

## LESSONS FROM ANIMAL MODELS

Guinea pigs deficient in C4, C2, and C3 are grossly disease free. It may be relevant that, unlike humans and mice, no spontaneous development of SLE has been reported in the guinea pig. Dogs with C3 deficiency develop immune complex renal disease, and pigs lacking factor H die from membranoproliferative glomerulonephritis (as seen in humans). Study of these animals has been instructive; however, the development of mice with targeted deficiencies of complement components will likely most enhance our understanding of complement biology. Mice with C1q (199), C3 (200), C4 (200), factor B (201), and CR1 and CR2 (CD21 and CD35) (202,203) gene knockouts have been developed. C1q-deficient mice show SLE-like disease with a range of ANAs and promise to be a good model system to study the relation between complement deficiency and autoimmune disease. Although none of the other knockout mice show any distinct disease phenotype, studies using mice lacking C3, C4, and CR1 and CR2 have already proved useful in defining the role of the complement system as a link between innate and adaptive immunity (63).

## HOW DOES COMPLEMENT DEFICIENCY CAUSE AUTOIMMUNE DISEASE?

### Infection and Systemic Lupus Erythematosus

Although complement deficiency may be the single best known genetic predisposition to autoimmune conditions such as SLE, the linkage between complement deficiency and infection is most direct. The natural question is whether susceptibility to infection is or is not related to the development of SLE in these patients. Arguments can be made for both.

On encountering foreign organisms, the complement cascade is activated by natural antibodies, MBL (204), C-reactive proteins (205), or other surface determinants. The inability to coat microbes with C3b or form lytic complexes, in a complement-deficient person, may lead to persistent and possibly invasive infections. The ensuing tissue damage, along with an altered humoral immune response (discussed later), could predispose to antibody production against self tissue. If recurrent or chronic, this would lead to autoimmune syndromes. In addition, there are solid examples of molecular mimicry whereby an antibody generated against the infective agent cross-reacts with self tissue, causing inflammatory damage. Arguments against this idea arise from the fact that no such agent has been demonstrated to induce SLE and that it does not explain why C1q and complete C4 deficiency more constantly cause SLE than C3 or C2 deficiency. Because the clinical and the autoantibody profile observed in most SLE patients with and without complement deficiency is similar, the speculation about the need for a "hit" by an environmental agent such as a retroviral infection in a host with subtle or obvious immunodeficiency, in the causation of SLE, remains attractive (206).

### Defective Immune Complex Processing

C3b and C4b deposition, which disrupts the lattices and maintains immune complex solubility, if impaired because of complement deficiency, would be expected to result in immune complex deposition in abnormal sites (such as the kidney)—a hallmark of SLE. Also contributing would be the inability of erythrocyte CR1 to bind, process, and transport these complexes to the tissue phagocytes, which catabolize these complexes and present antigenic peptides to T cells.

Inflammation caused by the immune complexes would release autoantigens and further drive the autoimmune response (207–210).

Evidence for this hypothesis comes from studies showing abnormal clearance of immune complexes in patients with inherited and acquired complement deficiencies (50,211–214). Notable are the abnormalities in uptake of immune complexes by the liver phagocytes and the absence of uptake by the spleen (214). The latter could potentially lead to defects in adaptive immunity, discussed later.

### Abnormal Humoral Immune Response

It has been known for more than a decade that humoral immunity is impaired in people with early complement component deficiency, particularly at a low antigenic dose. In C3-deficient patients, Ochs et al. (215) noted that a similar antibody response was evoked by primary and secondary immunizations and that there was failure in class switching from IgM to IgG. To some extent, increasing the antigenic dose could overcome these defects.

These defects could be explained by poor antigen trapping by follicular–dendritic cells or could be a threshold problem. Recent experiments demonstrate that, in the absence of C3 fragments on antigens, there is poor antigen localization by follicular cells (33), which, like B cells, possess CR1, CR2, and CR3; that C3d decreases the antigenic threshold for B-cell response in a dose-dependent fashion (67); and that C3d-CD21 interaction is essential for a normal humoral immune response (202,203,216,217). It is, however, paradoxical to hypothesize that poor antibody response could predispose to SLE, which is characterized by plethora of autoantibodies! Although the mechanism is unclear, the problem may lie in faulty negative selection of autoreactive B cells from primary follicles. Gene knockout animal models will help define any role for complement in this regard.

### Presentation of Novel Antigens

One hypothesis assumes a primary role for the complement system in housekeeping and suggests that, in complement-deficient states, the inability to dispose of damaged tissue safely after inflammation (such as that resulting from infections, ischemia, or ultraviolet ray exposure) (207,218), or to process apoptotic tissue (such as apoptotic blebs created in keratinocytes after ultraviolet ray exposure) (219), results in presentation of novel nuclear antigens. This could set up a vicious cycle of autoantibody production, immune complex formation, and further tissue damage. These issues are being addressed in mice with targeted deficiency of C1q.

## COMPLEMENT INHIBITORS AS THERAPEUTIC AGENTS

The central role that complement plays in inducing tissue injury in SLE and other autoimmune diseases has led to a major effort to identify therapeutic tools to modulate complement activation. Replacement of complement components in the rare patient with complete deficiency who is relatively refractory to standard therapy has achieved success in C2 deficiency (220) and a more predictable success in episodic angioedema with use of C1 inhibitor (221–224). In animal models, cobra venom factor has reproducibly provided a means to inactivate the complement system. Its use in humans is limited by its high immunogenicity. Several novel agents with complement inhibitory activity have been developed. Three recombinant proteins that have been studied extensively in animals are promising. They are soluble CR1 (sCR1), an MCP-DAF hybrid (complement activation blocker type 2 [CAB-2]), and a humanized monoclonal antibody to C5 (5G1.1). Two are in human trials (sCR1 and 5G1.1).

Soluble CR1 (24,225) is a recombinant form of CR1 that lacks the transmembrane and the cytoplasmic tail. By virtue of its cofactor activity for C3b and C4b cleavage and its decay-accelerating activity toward C3 and C5 convertases, it is a potent complement inhibitor. In animal models of inflammation, it is effective in reducing tissue injury in immune complex, ischemia-reperfusion, and autoantibody mediated syndromes. In phase I and II human clinical trials it has been effective in inhibiting complement. Effort is underway to determine active sites on CR1 and to construct a smaller and more active form of this protein (226–229).

CAB-2 (230) is a recombinantly produced soluble hybrid protein composed of the CCP repeats of MCP (CD46) and DAF (CD55). It exploits the combined abilities of these two proteins in blocking complement activation at the level of the convertases. This protein has proved effective in many of the same animal model systems as sCR1.

Antibody to C5 (231) is a single-chain humanized monoclonal reagent that appears to be nonantigenic. It binds C5 and blocks its cleavage, so that no C5a or C5b is produced. This antibody has been highly effective in various disease models of animals, including NZB and NZW mouse model of SLE, in which it prevents renal disease and death. In phase I clinical trials, it has been shown to inhibit C5a and MAC formation in patients undergoing cardiopulmonary bypass or hemodialysis.

## CONCLUSION

The complement system plays a crucial role in the host's innate and adaptive immune defense. In autoimmune states and when unregulated, it is also the cause of inflammatory damage to self tissue. In recent years, great progress has been made in the understanding of genetics and biochemistry of the complement proteins. Their biologic role in immune response and autoimmunity is under intense study in mice and in humans. Inherited deficiency of early complement components is still the best known single genetic correlate with autoimmune disease such as SLE. The technique of gene targeting will enable further understanding of the function of these proteins and may lead to an answer to the question of how a single protein deficiency of C1q, C4, or C2 causes SLE. The introduction of complement inhibitors in therapeutics may provide new ways to tackle autoimmune and inflammatory diseases.

## REFERENCES

1. Lachmann PJ, Nichol PAE. Reaction mechanism of the alternative pathway of complement fixation. *Lancet* 1973;1:465–467.
2. Matsushita M. The lectin pathway of the complement system. *Microbiol Immunol* 1996;40:887–893.
3. Lu J, Thiel S, Wiedemann H, et al. Binding of the pentamer/hexamer forms of mannan-binding protein to zymosan activates the proenzyme C1r₂C1s₂ complex, of the classical pathway of complement, without development of C1q. *J Immunol* 1990;144:2287–2294.
4. Terai I, Kobayashi K, Matsushita M, et al. Human serum mannose-binding lectin (MBL)-associated serine protease-1 (MASP-1): determination of levels in body fluids and identification of two forms in serum. *Clin Exp Immunol* 1997;110:317–323.
5. Endo Y, Sato T, Matsushita M, et al. Exon structure of the gene encoding the human mannose-binding protein-associated serine protease light chain: comparison with complement C1r and C1s genes. *Int Immunol* 1996;8:1355–1358.
6. Thiel S, Vorup-Jensen T, Stover CM, et al. A second serine protease associated with mannan-binding lectin that activates complement. *Nature* 1997;386:506–510.
7. Lachmann PJ, Thompsen RA. Reactive lysis: the complement mediated lysis of unsensitized cells. The characterization of activated reactor as C5b and the participation of C8 and C9. *J Exp Med* 1970;131:643–657.
8. Podack ER. Assembly and function of the terminal components In: Ross GD, ed. *Immunobiology of the complement system.* Orlando, FL: Academic Press, 1986:115–137.
9. Tschopp J. Ultrastructure of the membrane attack complex of complement: heterogeneity of the complex caused by different degrees of C9 polymerisation. *J Biol Chem* 1984;259:7857–7863.
10. Naniche D, Varior-Krishnan G, Cervoni F, et al. Human membrane cofactor protein (CD46) acts as a cellular receptor for measles virus. *J Virol* 1993;67:6025–6032.
11. Dorig RE, Marcil A, Chopra A, et al. The human CD46 molecule is a receptor for measles virus (Edmonston strain). *Cell* 1993;75:295–305.
12. Manchester M, Valsamakis A, Kaufman R, et al. Measles virus and C3 binding sites are distinct on membrane cofactor protein (MCP; CD46). *Proc Natl Acad Sci U S A* 1995;92:2303–2307.
13. Ahearn JM, Fearon DT. Structure and function of the complement receptors, CR1 (CD35) and CR2 (CD21). *Adv Immunol* 1989;46:183–219.
14. Bergelson JM, Chan M, Solomon KR, et al. Decay-accelerating factor (CD55), a glycosylphosphatidylinositol-anchored complement regulatory protein, is a receptor for several echoviruses. *Proc Natl Acad Sci U S A* 1994;91:6245–6248.
15. Bergelson JM, Mohanty JG, Crowell RL, et al. Coxsackievirus B3 adapted to growth in RD cells binds to decay-accelerating factor (CD55). *J Virol* 1995;69:1903–1906.
16. Montefiori DC, Cornell RJ, Zhou JY, et al. Complement control proteins, CD46, CD55, and CD59, as common surface constituents of human and simian immunodeficiency viruses and possible targets for vaccine protection. *Virology* 1994;205:82–92.
17. Saifuddin M, Parker CJ, Peeples ME, et al. Role of virion-associated glycosylphos-phatidylinositol-linked proteins CD55 and CD59 in complement resistance of cell line-derived and primary isolates of HIV-1. *J Exp Med* 1995;182:501–509.
18. Hortsmann RP, Sievertsen HJ, Knobloch J, et al. Antiphagocytic activity of streptococcal M protein: selective binding of complement control factor H. *Proc Natl Acad Sci U S A* 1988;85:1657–1641.
19. Horta MF, Ramalho Pinto FJ. Role of human decay-accelerating factor in the evasion of *Schistosoma mansoni* from the complement-mediated killing *in vitro. J Exp Med* 1991;174:1399–1406.
20. Kotwal GJ, Moss B. Vaccinia virus encodes a secretory polypeptide structurally related to complement control proteins. *Nature* 1988;335:176–178.

21. Fries LF, Friedman HM, Cohen GH, et al. Glycoprotein C of herpes simplex virus 1 is an inhibitor of the complement cascade. *J Immunol* 1986;137:1636–1641.

22. McCurry KR, Kooyman DL, Alvarado CG, et al. Human complement regulatory proteins protect swine-to-primate cardiac xenografts from humoral injury. *Nature Med* 1995;1:423–427.

23. Rooney IA, Liszewski MK, Atkinson JP. Using membrane-bound complement regulatory proteins to inhibit rejection. *Xenobiotica* 1993;1:29–35.

24. Moore FD Jr. Therapeutic regulation of the complement system in acute injury states. *Adv Immunol* 1994;56:267–299.

25. Kalli KR, Hsu P, Fearon DT. Therapeutic uses of recombinant complement protein inhibitors. *Springer Semin Immunopathol* 1994;15:417–431.

26. Perkins JJ, Smith KF, Amatayakul S, et al. Two-domain structure of the native and reactive center cleaved forms of C1 inhibitor of human complement by neutron scattering. *J Mol Biol* 1990;214:751–763.

27. Liszewski MK, Farries T, Lublin D, et al. Control of the complement system. *Adv Immunol* 1996;61:201–283.

28. Ember JA, Jagels MA, Hugli TE. The human complement system in health and disease In: Volanakis JE, Frank MM, eds. *Characterization of complement anaphylatoxins and their biological responses.* New York: Marcel Dekker, 1998:241–284.

29. Ross GD. Complement receptor type 1. *Curr Top Microbiol Immunol* 1992;178:31–44.

30. Ross GD, Polley MJ, Rabellino EM, et al. Two different complement receptors on human lymphocytes: one specific for C3b and one specific for C3b inactivator-cleaved C3b. *J Exp Med* 1973;138:798–811.

31. Eden A, Miller GW, Nussenzweig V. Human lymphocytes bear membrane receptors for C3b and C3d. *J Clin Invest* 1973;52:3239–3242.

32. Weis JJ, Tedder TF, Fearon DT. Identification of a 145,000 $M_r$ membrane protein as the C3d receptor (CR2) of human B lymphocytes. *Proc Natl Acad Sci U S A* 1984;81:881–885.

33. Fearon DT, Carter RH. The CD19/CR2/TAPA-1 complex of B lymphocytes: linking natural to acquired immunity. *Annu Rev Immunol* 1995;13:127–149.

34. Frade R, Barel M, Ehlin-Henriksson B, et al. gp140, The C3d receptor of human B lymphocytes, is also the Epstein–Barr virus receptor. *Proc Natl Acad Sci U S A* 1985;82:1490–1493.

35. Fingeroth JD, Weiss JJ, Tedder TF, et al. Epstein–Barr virus receptor of human B lymphocytes is the C3d receptor CR2. *Proc Natl Acad Sci U S A* 1984;81:4510–4514.

36. Aubry J-P, Pochon S, Graber P, et al. CD21 is a ligand for CD23 and regulates IgE production. *Nature* 1992;358:505–507.

37. Delcayre AX, Salas F, Mathur S, et al. Epstein Barr virus/complement C3d receptor is an interferon a receptor. *EMBO J* 1991;10:919–926.

38. Wright SD, Weitz JL, Huang AJ, et al. Complement receptor type three (CD11b/CD18) of human polymorphonuclear leukocytes recognizes fibrinogen. *Proc Natl Acad Sci U S A* 1988;85:7734–7738.

39. Wright SD, Jong MTC. Adhesion-promoting receptors on human macrophages recognize *Escherichia coli* by binding to lipopolysaccharide. *J Exp Med* 1986;164:1876–1888.

40. Ross GD, Cain JA, Lachmann PJ. Membrane complement receptor type three (CR3) has lectin-like properties analogous to bovine conglutinin and functions as a receptor for zymosan and rabbit erythrocytes as well as a receptor for iC3b. *J Immunol* 1985;134:3307–3315.

41. Galon J, Gauchat J-F, Mazieres N, et al. Soluble Fcγ receptor type III (FcγRIII,CD16) triggers cell activation through interaction with complement receptors. *J Immunol* 1996;157:1184–1192.

42. Smith CW, Marlin SD, Rothlein R, et al. Cooperative interactions of LFA-1 and Mac-1 with intercellular adhesion molecule-1 in facilitating adherence and transendothelial migration of human neutrophils *in vitro. J Clin Invest* 1989;83:2008–2017.

43. Relman D, Tuomanen E, Falkow S, et al. Recognition of a bacterial adhesion by an integrin: macrophage CR3 ($a_MB_2$,CD11b/CD18) binds filamentous hemagglutinin of Bordetella pertussis. *Cell* 1990;61:1375–1382.

44. Russell DG, Wright SD. Complement receptor type 3 (CR3) binds to an Arg-Gly-Asp-containing region of the major surface glycoprotein, gp63, of *Leishmania promastigotes. J Exp Med* 1988;168:279–292.

45. Ghebrehiwet B, Lim B-L, Peerschke EIB, et al. Isolation, cDNA cloning, and overexpression of a 33 kDa cell surface glycoprotein that binds to the globular "heads" of C1q. *J Exp Med* 1994;179:1809–1821.

46. Malhotra R, Thiel S, Reid KBM, et al. Human leucocyte C1q receptor binds to other soluble proteins with collagen domains. *J Exp Med* 1990;173:955–959.

47. Tenner A. C1q interaction with cell surface receptors. *Behring Inst Mitt* 1989;84:220–229.

48. Nepomuceno RR, Henschen-Edman HA, Burgess WH, et al. cDNA cloning and primary structure analysis of C1qR(P), the human C1q/MBL/SPA receptor that mediates enhanced phagocytosis *in vitro. Immunity* 1997;6:119–129.

49. Hattori R, Hamilton KK, McEver RP, et al. Complement proteins C5b-9 induce secretion of high molecular weight multimers of endothelial von Willebrand factor and translocation of granule membrane protein GMP-140 to the cell surface. *J Biol Chem* 1989;264:9053–9060.

50. Waxman FJ, Hebert LA, Comacoff JB, et al. Complement depletion accelerates the clearance of immune complexes from the circulation of primates. *J Clin Invest* 1984;74:1329–1340.

51. Nelson RA. The immune adherence phenomenon. *Science* 1953;118:733–737.

52. Nelson DS. Immune adherence. *Adv Immunol* 1963;3:131.

53. Cornacoff JB, Hebert LA, Smead WL, et al. Primate erythrocyte-immune complex-clearing mechanism. *J Clin Invest* 1983;71:236–247.

54. Hebert LA, Cosio FG. The erythrocyte-immune complex-glomerulonephritis connection in man. *Kidney Int* 1987;31:870-877.

55. Gerard NP, Gerard C. The chemotactic receptor for human C5a anaphylatoxin. *Nature* 1991;349:614–617.

56. Boulay F, Mery L, Tardif M, et al. Expression cloning of a receptor for C5a anaphylatoxin on differentiated HL-60 cells. *Biochem* 1991;30:2993–2999.

57. Crass T, Raffetseder U, Martin U, et al. Expression cloning of the human C3a anaphylatoxin receptor (C3aR) from differentiated U-937 cells. *Eur J Immunol* 1996;26:1944–1950.

58. Lepow IH, Willms-Kretschmer RA, Patrick RA, et al. Gross and ultra-structural observations of lesions produced by intradermal injection of human C3a in man. *Am J Pathol* 1970;61:13–20.

59. Wuepper KD, Bikosch VA, Muller-Eberhard HJ, et al. Cutaneous responses to human C3 anaphylatoxin in man. *Clin Exp Immunol* 1972;11:13–20.

60. Vallota EH, Muller-Eberhard HJ. Isolation and characterization of a new and highly active form of C5a anaphylatoxin from epsilon-aminocaproic acid-containing porcine serum. *J Exp Med* 1973;137:1109–1123.

61. Kew RR, Fisher JA, Webster RO. Co-chemotactic effect of Gc-globulin (vitamin D binding protein) for C5a. *J Immunol* 1995;155:5369–5374.

62. Fearon DT, Locksley RM. The instructive role of innate immunity in the acquired immune response. *Science* 1996;272:50–54.

63. Carroll MC, Prodeus AP. Linkages of innate and adaptive immunity. *Curr Opin Immunol* 1998;10:36–40.

64. Pepys MB. Role of complement in induction of antibody production *in vivo:* effect of cobra venom factor and other C3-reactive agents on thymus dependent and thymus independent antibody responses. *J Exp Med* 1974;140:126–145.

65. Melchers F, Erdei A, Schulz T, et al. Growth control of activated, synchronized murine B cells by the C3d fragment of human complement. *Nature* 1985;317:264–267.

66. Carter RH, Fearon DT. CD19: lowering the threshold for antigen receptor stimulation of B lymphocytes. *Science* 1992;256:105–107.

67. Dempsey PW, Allison ME, Akkaraju S, et al. C3d of complement as a molecular adjuvant: bridging innate and acquired immunity. *Science* 1996;271:348–350.

68. Carroll MC, Campbell RD, Bentley DR, et al. A molecular map of the human major histocompatibility complex class III region linking complement genes C4, C2 and factor B. *Nature* 1984;307:237–241.

69. Campbell RD. Molecular genetics of C2 and factor B. *Br Med Bull* 1987;43:37–49.

70. Campbell RD, Law SKA, Reid KBM. Structure, organization and regulation of the complement genes. *Annu Rev Immunol* 1988;6:161–195.

71. Arnett FC, Moulds JM. HLA class III molecules and autoimmune rheumatic diseases. *Clin Exp Rheumatol* 1991;9:289–296.

72. Belt KT, Carroll MC, Porter RR. The structural basis of the multiple forms of human complement component C4. *Cell* 1984;36:907–914.

73. Yu CY, Belt KT, Giles CM. Structural basis of the polymorphism of human complement component C4A and C4B: gene size, reactivity and antigenicity. *EMBO J* 1986;5:2873–2881.

74. Belt KT, Yu CY, Carroll MC, Porter RR. Polymorphism of human complement component C4. *Immunogenetics* 1985;21:173–180.

75. Carroll MC, Palsdittir A, Belt KT. Deletion of complement C4 and steroid 21-hydroxylase genes in the HLA class III region. *EMBO J* 1985;4:2547–2552.

76. Schneider PM, Carroll MC, Alper CA. Polymorphism of the human complement C4 and steroid 21-hydroxylase genes: restriction fragment length polymorphisms revealing structural deletions, homoduplications, and size variants. *J Clin Invest* 1986;78:650–657.

77. Tokunaga K, Saueracker G, Kay PH. Extensive deletions and insertions in different MHC supratypes detected by pulsed field gel electrophoresis. *J Exp Med* 1988;168:933–940.

78. Partanen J, Campbell RD. Restriction fragment analysis of non-deleted complement C4 null genes suggests point mutations in C4A null alleles but gene conversions in C4B null alleles. *Immunogenetics* 1989;30:520–523.

79. Law SK, Dodds AW, Porter RR. A comparison of the properties of two classes, C4A and C4B, of the human complement component C4. *EMBO J* 1984;3:1819–1823.

80. Isenman DE, Young JR. The molecular basis for the difference in immune hemolysis activity of the Chido and Rodgers isotypes of human complement component C4. *J Immunol* 1984;132:3019–3027.

81. Reilly BD. Quantitative analysis of C4Ab and C4Bb binding to the C3b/C4b receptor (CR1, CD35). *Clin Exp Immunol* 1997;110: 310–316.

82. Gatenby PA, Barbosa JE, Lachmann PJ. Differences between C4A and C4B in the handling of immune complexes: the enhancement of CR1 binding is more important than the inhibition of immunoprecipitation. *Clin Exp Immunol* 1990;79:158–163.

83. Hourcade D, Holers VM, Atkinson JP. The regulators of complement activation (RCA) gene cluster. *Adv Immunol* 1989;45:381–416.

84. Bowness P, Davies KA, Norsworthy PJ, et al. Hereditary C1q deficiency and lupus. *Q J Med* 1994;87:455–464.

85. Ruddy S. Component deficiencies: the second component. *Prog Allergy* 1986;39:250–266.

86. Farries TC, Knutzen Steuer KL, Atkinson JP. The mechanism of activation of the alternative pathway of complement by cell-bound C4b. *Mol Immunol* 1990;27:1155–1161.

87. Farries TC, Steuer-Knutzen KL, Atkinson JP. Evolutionary implications of a new bypass activation pathway of the complement system. *Immunol Today* 1990;11:78–80.

88. Hassig A, Borel JF, Ammann P. Essentielle hypocomplementemia. *Pathol Microbiol* 1964;27:542–547.

89. Inai S, Akagaki Y, Moriyama T. Inherited deficiencies of the late-acting complement components other than C9 found among healthy blood donors. *Int Arch Allergy Appl Immunol* 1989;90:274–279.

90. Berkel AJ, Sanal O, Thesen R, et al. A case of selective C1q deficiency. *Turk J Pediatr* 1977;19:101–108.

91. Topaloglu A, Bakkaloglu A, Slingsby JH, et al. Molecular basis of hereditary C1q deficiency associated with SLE and IgA nephropathy in a Turkish family. *Kidney Int* 1996;50:635–642.

92. Slingsby JH, Norsworthy P, Pearce G, et al. Homozygous hereditary C1q deficiency and systemic lupus erythematosus: a new family and the molecular basis of C1q deficiency in three families. *Arthritis Rheum* 1996;39:663–670.

93. Moncada B, Day B, Good RA, et al. Lupus-erythematosus-like syndrome with a familial defect of complement. *N Engl J Med* 1972;286:689–693.

94. Rich KC Jr, Hurley J, Gewurz H. Inborn C1r deficiency with a mild lupus-like syndrome. *Clin Immunol Immunopathol* 1979;13:77–84.

95. Lee SL, Wallace SL, Barone R, et al. Familial deficiency of two subunits of the first component of complement. *Arthritis Rheum* 1978;21:958–967.

96. Schaller JG, Gilliland BG, Ochs HD, et al. Severe systemic lupus erythematosus with nephritis in a boy with deficiency of the fourth component of complement. *Arthritis Rheum* 1977;20:1519–1525.

97. Tappeiner G, Scholz S, Linert J. Hereditary deficiency of the fourth component of complement (C4): study of a family. *Colloque INSERM* 1978;800:399–404.

98. Ballow M, McLean RH, Einarson M. Hereditary C4 deficiency: genetic studies and linkage to HLA. *Transplant Proc* 1979;11: 1710–1712.

99. Tappeiner G, Hintner H, Schloz S, et al. Systemic lupus erythematosus in hereditary deficiency of the fourth component of complement. *J Am Acad Dermatol* 1982;7:66–79.

100. Tappeiner G. Disease states in genetic complement deficiencies. *Int J Dermatol* 1982;21:175–191.

101. Urowitz MB, Gladman DD, Minta JO. Systemic lupus erythematosus in a patient with C4 deficiency. *J Rheumatol* 1981;8:741–746.

102. Kjellman M, Laurell A-B, Low B. Homozygous deficiency of C4 in a child with a lupus erythematosus syndrome. *Clin Genet* 1982;22: 331–339.

103. Mascart-Lemone F, Hauptmann G, Goetz J, et al. Genetic deficiency of the fourth component of complement presenting with recurrent infections and a SLE-like disease: genetical and immunological studies. *Am J Med* 1983;75:295–304.

104. Atkinson JP. Systemic lupus erythematosus In: Lahita RG, ed. Genetic susceptibility and class III complement genes. New York: Churchill Livingstone, 1992:87–102.

105. Fielder AH, Walport MJ, Batchelor JR, et al. Family study of the major histocompatibility complex in patients with systemic lupus erythematosus: importance of null alleles of C4A and 4B in determining disease susceptibility. *Br Med J* 1983;286:425–428.

106. Kemp ME, Atkinson JP, Skanes VM, et al. Deletion of C4A genes in patients with systemic lupus erythematosus. *Arthritis Rheum* 1987; 30:1015–1022.

107. Goldstein R, Arnett FC, McLean RH, et al. Molecular heterogeneity of complement component C4-null and 21-hydroxylase genes in systemic lupus erythematosus. *Arthritis Rheum* 1988;31:736–744.

108. Yukiyama Y, Tokunaga K, Takeuchi F. Genetic polymorphism of complement in patients with systemic lupus erythematosus II. The fourth (C4) and the seventh (7) components of complement. *Jpn J Rheumatol* 1988;1:271–276.

109. Zhao X-Z, Zhang JJ, Tian YW. Allotypic differences and frequencies of C4 null alleles (C4Q0) detected in patients with systemic lupus erythematosus (SLE). *Chin Sci Bull* 1989;34:237–240.

110. Dunckley H, Gatenby PA, Hawkins BR, et al. Deficiency of C4A is a genetic determinant of systemic lupus erythematosus in three ethnic groups. *J Immunogenet* 1987;14:209–218.

111. Gougerot A, Stoppa-Lyonnet D, Poirier JC, et al. HLA markers and complotypes: risk factors in systemic lupus erythematosus. *Ann Dermatol Venereol* 1987;114:329–334.

112. Christiansen FT, Zhang WJ, Griffiths M, et al. MHC encoded complement deficiency, ancestral haplotypes and SLE: C4 deficiency explains some but not all of the influence of the MHC. *J Rheumatol* 1991;18:1350–1358.

113. Bishof NA, Welch TR, Beischel LS. C4B deficiency: a risk factor for bacteremia with encapsulated organisms. *J Infect Dis* 1990;162: 248–250.

114. Rowe PC, McLean RH, Wood RA, et al. Association of homozygous C4b deficiency with bacterial meningitis. *J Infect Dis* 1989;160: 448–451.

115. Raum D, Awdeh Z, Alper CA. BF types and the mode of inheritance of insulin-dependent diabetes mellitus (IDDM). *Immunogenetics* 1981;12:59–74.

116. Rittner C, Meier EMM, Stradmann B, et al. Partial C4 deficiency in subacute sclerosing panencephalitis. *Immunogenetics* 1984;20:407–412.

117. Steel CM, Beatson D, Cuthbert RJG, et al. HLA haplotype A1 B8 DR3 as a risk factor for HIV-related disease. *Lancet* 1988;1:1185–1188.

118. McLean RH, Wyatt RJ, Julian BA. Complement phenotypes in glomerulonephritis: increased frequency of homozygous null C4 phenotypes in IgA nephropathy and Henoch–Schonlein purpura. *Kidney Int* 1984;26:855–860.

119. Moldenhauer E, Schmidt R, Heinrichs M. Scleroderma: possible significance of silent alleles at the C4B locus. *Arthritis Rheum* 1984; 27:711–712.

120. Briggs DC, Welsh K, Pereira RS. A strong association between null alleles at the C4A locus in the major histocompatibility complex and systemic sclerosis. *Arthritis Rheum* 1986;29:1274–1277.

121. Hauptmann G, Toppeiner G, Schifferli JA. Inherited deficiency of the fourth component of complement. *Immunodeficiency Reviews* 1988;1: 3–22.

122. Sullivan KE, Petri MA, Schmeckpeper BJ, et al. Prevalence of a mutation causing C2 deficiency in systemic lupus erythematosus. *J Rheumatol* 1994;21:1128–1133.

123. Johnson CA, Densen P, Hurford R, et al. Type I human complement C2 deficiency: a 28 base pair gene deletion causes skipping of exon 6 during RNA splicing. *J Biol Chem* 1992;267:9347–9353.

124. Awdeh ZL, Raum DD, Glass D, et al. Complement-human histocompatibility antigen haplotypes in C2 deficiency. *J Clin Invest* 1981; 67:581–583.

125. Hauptmann G, Tongio MM, Goetz J. Association of the C2-deficiency gene (C2*Q0) with the C4A*4, C4B*2 genes. *J Immunogenet* 1982; 9:127–132.

126. Wang X, Circolo A, Lokki ML, et al. Molecular heterogeneity in deficiency of complement protein C2 type 1. *Immunology* 1998;93:184–191.

127. Johnson CA, Densen P, Wetsel RA, et al. Molecular heterogeneity of C2 deficiency. *N Engl J Med* 1992;326:871–874.

128. McLean RH, Weinstein A, Damjanov I, et al. Hypomorphic variant of C3, arthritis, and chronic glomerulonephritis. *J Pediatr* 1978;93:937–943.

129. McLean RH, Weinstein A, Chapitis J, et al. Familial partial deficiency of the third component of complement (C3) and the hypocomplementemic cutaneous vasculitis syndrome. *Am J Med* 1980;68:549–558.

130. Wyatt RJ, Jones D, Stapleton FB, et al. Recurrent hemolytic-uremic syndrome with the hypomorphic fast allele of the third component of complement. *J Pediatr* 1985;107:564–566.

131. Botto M, Fong FY, So AK, et al. Molecular basis of hereditary C3 deficiency. *J Clin Invest* 1990;86:1158–1163.

132. Botto M, Fong FY, So AK. Homozygous hereditary C3 deficiency due to a partial gene deletion. *Proc Natl Acad Sci U S A* 1992;89: 4957–4961.

133. Botto M, Walport MJ. Hereditary deficiency of C3 in animals and humans. *Int Rev Immunol* 1993;10:37–50.

134. Nilsson UR, Nilsson B, Storm KE, et al. Hereditary dysfunction of the third component of complement associated with a systemic lupus erythematosus-like syndrome and meningococcal meningitis. *Arthritis Rheum* 1992;35:580–586.

135. Peleg D, Harit-Bustan H, Katz Y, et al. Inherited C3 deficiency and meningococcal disease in a teenager. *Pediatr Infect Dis J* 1992;11: 401–404.

136. Katz Y, Wetsel RA, Schlesinger M, et al. Compound heterozygous complement C3 deficiency. *Immunology* 1995;94:5–7.

137. Tedesco F, Silvani CM, Agelli M. A lupus-like syndrome in a patient with deficiency of the sixth component of complement. *Arthritis Rheum* 1981;24:1438–1440.

138. Trapp RG, Mooney H, Husain I. Hereditary complement (C6) deficiency with discoid lupus/Sjögren's syndrome. *Arthritis Rheum* 1980; 23:757.

139. Mooney E. Complement factor 6 deficiency associated with lupus. *J Am Acad Dermatol* 1984;11:896–897.

140. Zeitz HJ, Miller GW, Lint TF. Deficiency of C7 with systemic lupus erythematosus. *Arthritis Rheum* 1981;24:87–93.

141. Jasin HE. Absence of the eighth component of complement in association with systemic lupus erythematosus-like disease. *J Clin Invest* 1977;60:709–715.

142. Pickering RJ, Rynes RI, LoCascio N. Identification of the subunit of the eighth component of complement (C8) in a patient with systemic lupus erythematosus and absent C8 activity: patient and family studies. *Clin Immunol Immunopathol* 1982;23:323–334.

143. Wener MH, Uwatoko S, Mannik M. Antibodies to the collagen-like region of C1q in sera of patients with autoimmune rheumatic diseases. *Arthritis Rheum* 1989;32:544–551.

144. Uwatoko S, Aotsuka S, Okawa M, et al. Characterization of C1q-binding IgG complexes in systemic lupus erythematosus. *Clin Immunol Immunopathol* 1984;30:104–116.

145. Siegert C, Daha M, Westedt ML, et al. IgG autoantibodies against C1q are correlated with nephritis, hypocomplementemia, and dsDNA antibodies in systemic lupus erythematosus. *J Rheumatol* 1991;18: 230–234.

146. Uwatoko S, Gauthier VJ, Mannik M. Autoantibodies to the collagen-like region of C1q deposit in glomeruli via C1q immune deposits. *Clin Immunol Immunopathol* 1991;61:268–273.

147. Walport MJ, Davies KA, Botto M, et al. C3 nephritic factor and SLE: report of four cases and review of the literature. *Q J Med* 1994;87: 609–615.

148. Wisnieski JJ, Nathanson MH, Anderson JE, et al. Metabolism of C4 and linkage analysis in a kindred with hereditary incomplete C4 deficiency. *Arthritis Rheum* 1987;30:919–926.

149. Halbwachs L, Leveille M, Lesavre PH, et al. Nephritic factor of the classical pathway of complement: immunoglobulin G autoantibody directed against the classical pathway C3 convertase enzyme. *J Clin Invest* 1980;65:1249–1256.

150. Fujita T, Sumita T, Yoshida S, et al. C4 nephritic factor in a patient with chronic glomerulonephritis. *J Clin Lab Immunol* 1987;22:65–70.

151. Gigli I, Sorvillo J, Mecarelli-Halbwachs L, et al. Mechanism of action of the C4 nephritic factor: deregulation of the classical pathway C3 convertase. *J Exp Med* 1981;154:1–12.

152. Sim E, Gill EW, Sim RB. Drugs that induce systemic lupus erythematosus inhibit complement component. *Lancet* 1984;1:422–424.

153. Davies EJ, Snowden N, Hillarby MC. Mannose-binding protein gene polymorphism in systemic lupus erythematosus. *Arthritis Rheum* 1995;38:110–114.

154. Carter PE, Dunbar B, Fothergill JE. Genomic and cDNA cloning of the human C1 inhibitor: intron-exon junctions and comparison with other serpins. *Eur J Biochem* 1988;173:163–169.

155. Carter P, Duponchel C, Tosi M, et al. Complete nucleotide sequence of the gene for human C1 inhibitor with an unusually high density of Alu elements. *Eur J Biochem* 1991;197:301–308.

156. Theriault A, Whaley K, McPhaden A, et al. Regional assignment of the human C1-inhibitor gene to 11q11-q13.1. *Hum Genet* 1989;84:477–479.

157. Davis AE III. The human complement system in health and disease In: Volanakis JE, Frank MM, eds. *C1 inhibitor gene and hereditary angioedema*. New York: Marcel Dekker, 1998:455–480.

158. Geha RS, Quinti I, Austen KF, et al. Acquired C1-inhibitor deficiency associated with antiidiotypic antibody to monoclonal immunoglobulins. *N Engl J Med* 1985;312:534–540.

159. Jackson J, Sim RB, Whelan A, et al. An IgG autoantibody which inactivates C1-inhibitor. *Nature* 1986;323:722–724.

160. Alzenz J, Bork K, Loos M. Autoantibody-mediated acquired deficiency of C1 inhibitor. *N Engl J Med* 1987;316:1360–1366.

161. Malbran A, Hammer C, Frank MM, et al. Acquired angioedema: observations on the mechanism of action of auto-antibodies directed against C1 esterase inhibitor. *J Allergy Clin Immunol* 1988;81: 1199–1204.

162. Donaldson VN, Rosen FS. Hereditary angioneurotic edema: a clinical survey. *Pediatrics* 1966;37:1017–1027.

163. Frank MM, Gelfand F, Atkinson JP. Hereditary angioedema: clinical syndrome and its management. *Ann Intern Med* 1976;84:580–593.

164. Nuijens JH, Eerenberg-Belmer AJM, Huijbregts CCM, et al. Proteolytic inactivation of plasma C1 inhibitor in sepsis. *J Clin Invest* 1989;84:443–450.

165. Hack CE, Ogilvie AC, Eisele B, et al. Initial studies on the administration of C1-esterase inhibitor to patients with septic shock or with a vascular leak syndrome induced by interleukin-2 therapy. *Prog Clin Biol Res* 1994;388:335–357.

166. Aasen AO, Smith-Erichsen N, Amundsen E. Plasma kallikrein-kinin system in septicemia. *Arch Surg* 1983;118:343–346.

167. Gull WW. A case of intermittent haematinuria, with remarks. *Guys Hosp Rep* 1866;12:381.

168. Parker CJ, Baker PJ, Rosse WF. Increased enzymatic activity of the alternative pathway convertase when bound to the erythrocytes of paroxysmal nocturnal hemoglobinuria. *J Clin Invest* 1982;69:337–346.

169. Rosse WF, Logue GL, Adams J, et al. Mechanisms of immune lysis of the red cells in hereditary erythroblastic multinuclearity with a positive acidified serum test and paroxysmal nocturnal hemoglobinuria. *J Clin Invest* 1974;53:31–43.

170. Nicholson-Weller A, March JP, Rosenfeld SI, et al. Affected erythrocytes of patients with paroxysmal nocturnal hemoglobinuria are deficient in the complement regulatory protein, decay accelerating factor. *Proc Natl Acad Sci U S A* 1983;80:5066–5070.

171. Pangburn MK, Schreiber RD, Muller-Eberhard HJ. Deficiency of an erythrocyte membrane protein with complement regulatory activity in paroxysmal nocturnal hemoglobinuria. *Proc Natl Acad Sci U S A* 1983;80:5430–5434.

172. Holguin MH, Frederick LR, Bernshaw NJ, et al. Isolation and characterization of a membrane protein from normal human erythrocytes that inhibits reactive lysis of the erythrocytes of paroxysmal nocturnal hemoglobinuria. *J Clin Invest* 1989;84:7–17.

173. Rosse WF. The human complement system in health and disease In: Volanakis JE, Frank MM, eds. *Paroxysmal nocturnal hemoglobinuria and complement*. New York: Marcel Dekker, 1998:481–497.

174. Frickhofen N, Liu JM, Young NS. Etiologic mechanisms of hematopoietic failure. *Am J Pediatr Hematol Oncol* 1990;12:385–395.

175. Baranski BG, Young NS. Autoimmune aspects of aplastic anemia. *In Vivo* 1988;2:91–94.

176. Firkin F, Goldberg H, Firkin BG. Glucocorticoid management of paroxysmal nocturnal hemoglobinuria. *Aust Ann Med* 1968;17:127–134.

177. Rosse WF. Treatment of paroxysmal nocturnal hemoglobinuria. *Blood* 1982;60:20–23.

178. Wilson JG, Murphy EE, Wong WW. Identification of a restriction fragment length polymorphism by a CR1 cDNA that correlates with the number of CR1 on erythrocytes. *J Exp Med* 1986;164:50–59.

179. Walport MJ, Lachmann PJ. Erythrocyte complement receptor type 1, immune complexes, and the rheumatic diseases. *Arthritis Rheum* 1988;31:153–158.

180. Walport M, Ng YC, Lachmann PJ. Erythrocytes transfused into patients with SLE and hemolytic anemia lose complement receptor type 1 from their cell surface. *Clin Exp Immunol* 1987;69:501–507.

181. Moldenhauer F, David J, Fielder AHL. Inherited deficiency of erythrocyte complement receptor type 1 does not cause susceptibility to systemic lupus erythematosus. *Arthritis Rheum* 1987;30:961–966.

182. Wong WW, Farrell SA. Proposed structure of the F' allotype of human CR1: loss of a C3b binding site may be associated with altered function. *J Immunol* 1990;146:656–662.

183. Van Dyne S, Holers VM, Lublin DM, et al. The polymorphism of the C3b/C4b receptor in the normal population and in patients with systemic lupus erythematosus. *Clin Exp Immunol* 1987;68:570–579.

184. Moulds JM, Reveille JD, Arnett FC. Structural polymorphisms of complement receptor 1 (CR1) in systemic lupus erythematosus (SLE) patients and normal controls of three ethnic groups. *Clin Exp Immunol* 1996;105:302–305.

185. Schwaeble W, Schwalger H, Broolmans RA, et al. Human complement factor H: tissue specificity in the expression of three different mRNA species. *Eur J Biochem* 1991;198:399–404.

186. Levy M, Halbwachs-Mecarelli L, Gubler MC, et al. H deficiency in two brothers with atypical dense intramembranous disease. *Kidney Int* 1986;30:949–956.

187. Thompson RA, Winterborn MH. Hypocomplementaemia due to a genetic deficiency of B1H globulin. *Clin Exp Immunol* 1981;46:110–119.

188. Wyatt RJ, Julian BA, Weinstein A, et al. Partial H deficiency and glomerulonephritis in two families. *J Clin Immunol* 1982;2:110–117.

189. Lopez-Larrea C, Dieguez MA, Enguix A, et al. A familial deficiency of complement factor H. *Biochem Soc Trans* 1987;15:648–649.

190. Nielsen HE, Koch C, Magnusson P, et al. Complement deficiencies in selected groups of patients with meningococcal disease. *Scand J Infect Dis* 1989;21:389–396.

191. Nielsen HE, Kristensen KC, Koch C, et al. Hereditary complete deficiency of complement factor H associated with recurrent meningococcal disease. *Scand J Immunol* 1989;30:711–718.

192. Ault BH, Schmidt BZ, Fowler NL, et al. Human factor H deficiency. *J Biol Chem* 1997;272:25168–25175.

193. Hogasen K, Jansen JH. Porcine membranoproliferative glomerulonephritis (MPGN) type II is reversed by factor H substitution therapy. *J Am Soc Nephrol* 1997;8:474–475.

194. Trapp RG, Fletcher M, Forristall J, et al. C4 binding protein deficiency in a patient with atypical Behçet's disease. *J Rheumatol* 1987;14:135–138.

195. Westberg J, Nordin Fredrikson G, Truedsson L, et al. Sequence-based analysis of properdin deficiency: identification of point mutations in two phenotypic forms of an X-linked immunodeficiency. *Genomics* 1995;29:1–8.

196. Nielsen HE, Koch C. Congenital properdin deficiency and meningococcal infection. *Clin Immunol Immunopathol* 1987;44:134–139.

197. Nordin Fredrikson G, Westberg J, Kuijper EJ, et al. Molecular characterization of properdin deficiency type III. *J Immunol* 1996;157:3666–3671.

198. Kolble K, Buckle V, Lefranc G. Physical mapping of complement factor I gene in normal and deficient genomes. *Complement Inflamm* 1989;6:355.

199. Botto M, Nash J, Taylor P, et al. Immune complex processing in a murine model of C1q deficiency (abst). *Mol Immunol* 1996;33 (Suppl 1):71.

200. Wessels MR, Butko P, Ma M, et al. Studies of group B streptococcal infection in mice deficient in complement component C3 or C4 demonstrate an essential role for complement in both innate and acquired immunity. *Proc Natl Acad Sci U S A* 1995;92:11490–11494.

201. Matsumoto M, Fukuda W, Circolo A, et al. Abrogation of the alternative complement pathway by targeted deletion of murine factor B. *Proc Natl Acad Sci U S A* 1997;94:8720–8725.

202. Molina H, Holers VM, Li B, et al. Markedly impaired humoral immune response in mice deficient in complement receptors 1 and 2. *Proc Natl Acad Sci U S A* 1996;93:3357–3361.

203. Ahearn JM, Fischer MB, Croix D, et al. Disruption of the CR2 locus results in a reduction in B-1a cells and in an impaired B cell response to T-dependent antigen. *Immunity* 1996;4:251–262.

204. Epstein J, Eichbaum Q, Sheriff S, et al. The collectins in innate immunity. *Curr Opin Immunol* 1996;8:29–35.

205. Szalai AJ, Agrawal A, Greenhough TJ, et al. C-reactive protein: structural biology, gene expression, and host defense function. *Immunol Res* 1997;16:127–136.

206. Atkinson JP. Some thoughts on autoimmunity. *Arthritis Rheum* 1995;38:301–305.

207. Walport MJ, Davies KA, Morley BJ, et al. Complement deficiency and autoimmunity. *Ann N Y Acad Sci* 1997;815:267–281.

208. Atkinson JP, Schneider PM. Systemic lupus erythematosus In: Lahita RG, ed. *Genetic susceptibility and class III complement genes.* New York: Churchill Livingstone, 1999:91–104.

209. Schifferli JA, Peters DK. Complement, the immune-complex lattice and the pathophysiology of complement-deficiency syndromes. *Lancet* 1983;2:957–959.

210. Atkinson JP. Systemic vasculitis. In: LeRoy EC, ed. *Immune complexes and the role of complement.* New York: Marcel Dekker, 1992:525–546.

211. Lobatto S, Daha MR, Breedveld FC, et al. Abnormal clearance of soluble aggregates of human immunoglobulin G in patients with systemic lupus erythematosus. *Clin Exp Immunol* 1988;72:55–59.

212. Davies KA, Peters AM, Beynon HL, et al. Immune complex processing in patients with systemic lupus erythematosus: *in vivo* imaging and clearance studies. *J Clin Invest* 1992;90:2075–2083.

213. Halma C, Daha MR, Camps JAJ, et al. Deficiency of complement component C3 is associated with accelerated removal of soluble [123]I-labelled aggregates of IgG from the circulation. *Clin Exp Immunol* 1992;90:394–400.

214. Davies KA, Erlendsson K, Beynon HLC, et al. Splenic uptake of immune complexes in man is complement-dependent. *J Immunol* 1993;151:3866–3873.

215. Ochs HD, Wedgwood RJ, Heller SR, et al. Complement, membrane glycoproteins, and complement receptors: their role in regulation of the immune response. *Clin Immunol Immunopathol* 1986;40:94–104.

216. Fischer M, Ma M, Goerg S, et al. Regulation of the B cell response to T-dependent antigens by classical pathway complement. *J Immunol* 1996;157:549–556.

217. Croix D, Ahearn J, Rosengard A, et al. Antibody response to a T-dependent antigen requires B cell expression of complement receptors. *J Exp Med* 1996;183:1857–1864.

218. Lachmann PJ, Walport MJ. Autoimmunity and autoimmune disease In: Evered D, Whelan J, eds. *Deficiency of the effector mechanisms of the immune response and autoimmunity.* New York: Wiley & Sons, 1987:129–136.

219. Korb LC, Ahearn JM. C1q binds directly and specifically to surface blebs of apoptotic human keratinocytes. *J Immunol* 1997;158:4525–4528.

220. Steinsson K, Erlendsson K, Valdimarsson H. Successful plasma infusion treatment of a patient with C2 deficiency and systemic lupus erythematosus: clinical experience over 45 months. *Arthritis Rheum* 1989;32:906–918.

221. Bergamaschini L, Cicardi M, Tucci A, et al. C1 inhibitor concentrate in the therapy of hereditary angioedema. *Allergy* 1983;38:81–84.

222. Gadek JE, Hosea SW, Gelfand JA, et al. Replacement therapy in hereditary angioedema: successful treatment of acute episodes of angioedema with partly purified C1 inhibitor. *N Engl J Med* 1980;302:542–546.

223. Sim TC, Grant JA. Hereditary angioedema: its diagnostic and management perspectives. *Am J Med* 1990;88:656–664.

224. Waytes AT, Rosen FS, Frank MM. Treatment of hereditary angio-edema with a vapor-heated C1 inhibitor concentrate. *N Engl J Med* 1996;334:1630–1634.
225. Moore FD Jr, Klickstein LB. The use of complement C3 receptors In: Austen KF, Burakoff SJ, Rosen FS, et al, eds. *The use of recombinant, soluble forms of the membrane complement C3 receptors, CR1 and CR2, as inhibitors of serum complement activation and function.* Cambridge, MA: Blackwell Scientific, 1996:311–323.
226. Krych M, Hourcade D, Atkinson JP. Sites within the complement C3b/C4b receptor important for the specificity of ligand binding. *Proc Natl Acad Sci U S A* 1991;88:4353–4357.
227. Krych M, Clemenza L, Howdeshell D, et al. Analysis of the functional domains of complement receptor type 1 (C3b/C4b receptor; CD35) by substitution mutagenesis. *J Biol Chem* 1994;269:13273–13278.
228. Subramanian VB, Clemenza L, Krych M, et al. Substitution of two amino acids confers C3b binding to the C4b binding site of CR1 (CD35): analysis based on ligand binding by chimpanzee erythrocyte complement receptor. *J Immunol* 1996;157:1242–1247.
229. Krych M, Hauhart R, Atkinson JP. Structure-function analysis of the active sites of complement receptor type 1. *J Biol Chem* 1998;273: 8623–8629.
230. Higgins PJ, Ko J-L, Lobell R, et al. A soluble chimeric complement inhibitory protein that possesses both decay-accelerating and factor I cofactor activities. *J Immunol* 1997;158:2872–2881.
231. Thomas TC, Rollins SA, Rother RP, et al. Inhibition of complement activity by humanized anti-C5 antibody and single-chain Fv. *Mol Immunol* 1996;33:1389–1401.

*Textbook of the Autoimmune Diseases,*
Edited by R. G. Lahita, N. Chiorazzi, and W. H. Reeves,
Lippincott Williams & Wilkins, Philadelphia © 2000.

# CHAPTER 11

# Immune Complexes and Autoimmunity

Kevin A. Davies

## IMMUNE COMPLEXES: WHAT ARE THEY AND WHEN DO THEY FORM *IN VIVO?*

### Normal Physiology

Immune complexes (IC) comprise any combination of antibody and antigen. The composition of ICs is highly variable. In addition to antigen and antibody, there may be complement proteins associated with IC, covalently bound in the cases of C3 and C4, or noncovalently bound in the case of C1q. The biologic and physicochemical properties of an IC vary according to the antibody isotype and according to the antigen, which may be soluble or particulate, such as bacteria or cells.

IC formation is a physiologic consequence of an adaptive humoral immune response. Binding of antibody to antigen is designed to promote removal of foreign antigens, the stimulation of an appropriate adaptive immune response, and the development of specific immunologic memory by the focusing of complexes to "professional" antigen-presenting cells within the immune system.

### Pathophysiology

ICs are also an important cause of pathologic tissue damage. This occurs in two situations. The first of these is when antigen persists as a consequence of ineffective clearance by the formation of ICs. This may occur in various circumstances, for example, when the antigen is an autoantigen that cannot be removed from the body or, in the case of persistent infection, when the immune response does not effectively control the infection and there is persistent production of antigens from the infectious agent. The second circumstance in which ICs cause tissue injury is when the physiologic clearance mechanisms are overwhelmed by formation of a large amount of ICs, for example, in serum sickness. Failure to

eliminate potentially harmful ICs may result in their persistence, either in the circulation or in the tissues, with potentially phlogistic effects. Alternatively, failure of effective antigen presentation in ICs to professional antigen-presenting cells (e.g., in the spleen) may result in an abnormal immune response, a consequence of which may be the failure of antigen clearance or the development of persistent autoimmunity. These mechanisms are discussed in detail later.

## CLEARANCE AND PROCESSING OF IMMUNE COMPLEXES

Both Fc receptors and complement play crucial roles in the processing of ICs. Incorporation of complement proteins into ICs modifies the lattice structure (see later). Covalently incorporated cleavage products of components C3 and C4 can then influence the fate of ICs by serving as ligands, first for receptors on cells that transport ICs through the body and, second, for receptors on cells within the reticuloendothelial system that take up and process the complexes. Cellular uptake of ICs results in the catabolism of foreign antigen and presentation to T and B lymphocytes, leading to a specific immune response to that antigen. ICs may be classified into those that contain soluble antigens, such as proteins, and those that contain particulate antigens, such as cells and bacteria. The clearance mechanisms are not the same for soluble and particulate ICs, and the different processes involved are reviewed later.

### Clearance of Soluble Immune Complexes

#### *Role of Complement in the Modification of Immune Complex Structure*

The incorporation of proteins of the complement system into ICs is a key element in the way in which complement mediates IC processing and was first recognized during the 1940s with the finding that immune precipitates contain more nitrogen when formed in normal, compared with heat-treated, serum (1). It was subsequently demonstrated that the pres-

K. A. Davies: Rheumatology Section, Division of Medicine, Imperial College School of Medicine, Hammersmith Hospital, London, U.K. W12 0NN.

ence of complement reduces the rate of immune precipitation, a phenomenon rediscovered 20 years later by investigators developing radioimmunoassays, who observed that complement interferes with the precipitation reaction (2,3). It was later discovered that complement not only inhibits the formation of immune precipitates but also can solubilize immune precipitates that have already formed (4).

Inhibition of immune precipitation is primarily mediated through activation of the classical pathway of complement (5,6). Solubilization of immune precipitates, on the other hand, is mediated by the alternative pathway (4). The capacity of complement to inhibit immune precipitation has been studied in several *in vitro* model systems. For example, it was demonstrated that complexes formed between bovine serum albumin (BSA) and rabbit anti-BSA at 37°C are kept soluble more easily when formed in antibody excess. During the first minutes of the reaction, ICs are kept soluble by classical pathway components alone, but in the later stages, the alternative pathway is essential (6).

Binding of C3 fragments is necessary for maintaining IC solubility. C3 and C4 binding is covalent and, in the case of ovalbumin and rabbit antiovalbumin ICs studied *in vitro,* has been shown to involve amide bonds between C3b and the immunoglobulin G (IgG) heavy chain (7).

How do complement proteins facilitate the modification of IC solubility? Two possible explanations have been adduced. The first is that the incorporation of complement proteins into the lattice reduces the valency of antibody for antigen by occupying sites of interaction between antibody and antigen (reviewed in 8). The second possibility is that complement incorporation interferes with noncovalent Fc–Fc interactions, which promote the rapid aggregation of ICs (9).

A number of properties of the antibody component of an IC determines the efficiency of inhibition of immune precipitation. For example, only antibody isotypes that activate the classical pathway induce complement-mediated inhibition of immune precipitation. Thus, inhibition of immune precipitation occurs with IgG and IgM complexes but not with IgA complexes (10). The ability of an IC to activate the classical pathway of complement does not parallel precisely its ability to incorporate C3b into the lattice. This is of some clinical relevance because, for example, complexes of monoclonal IgM rheumatoid factor and IgG, found in patients with mixed essential cryoglobulinemia (see Cryoglobulinemia and Hepatitis Infection), deplete complement rapidly but do not effectively incorporate C3 into the complex (11).

The formation of immune precipitates can activate the alternative pathway of complement. Solubilization of immune precipitates is associated with covalent binding of C3b to antigen and antibody molecules. A fraction of antibody may be released from the complex during solubilization, although the mechanism whereby bound C3b interferes with primary antigen–antibody bonds is unclear. This solubilization reaction is relatively inefficient, requiring a considerable amount of complement activation (about one molecule of C3b needs to bind per antibody molecule to induce solubilization) (12).

Because less than 10% of activated C3 binds to an immune aggregate, large quantities of complement are consumed during solubilization, which may result in deposition of the membrane attack complex and release of potentially proinflammatory complement split products and anaphylatoxins into the tissues. The degree of complement activation required for solubilization can be generated only by alternative pathway amplification; insoluble immune aggregates appear to form "protected" surfaces to which factor H has little access, thereby providing sites where amplification of complement activation is favored (13). All the proteins of the alternative pathway, including properdin, are required. Activation of the classical pathway alone is neither necessary nor sufficient to solubilize immune precipitates, although partial solubilization by classical pathway activation has been demonstrated *in vitro* using immune precipitates (14,15).

To summarize, there are two important differences between the processes of inhibition of IC precipitation and solubilization of precipitates. First, the capacity of the complement system to inhibit immune precipitation is 10 times greater than its capacity for solubilization, probably reflecting the ease of prevention of Fc–Fc interactions and lattice enlargement, compared with disruption of a lattice that is already formed. Second, the reactions differ in their inflammatory potential because inhibition of immune precipitation generates smaller amounts of the anaphylatoxins C3a and C5a than does solubilization (16).

### Complement Receptor Type 1 and Immune Complex Transport

ICs that enter the circulation, or are formed within it, may have to travel some distance around the body before reaching one of the organs of the fixed mononuclear phagocytic system. There is evidence that most ICs travel through the circulation bound to receptors on the surface of circulating cells (erythrocytes in primates) rather than free in plasma. When ICs arrive in the organs of the fixed mononuclear phagocytic system, they are transferred from the carrier cell to fixed macrophages.

This binding of IC to receptors on carrier cells was first described for complement-coated microorganisms more than 80 years ago. Pneumococci were injected intravenously into immune rabbits, and the clustering of bacteria around platelets in blood taken by cardiac puncture was observed (17). Rieckenberg (18) found that the serum of rats that had recovered from infection with *Trypanosoma brucei* caused platelets to adhere to *T. brucei in vitro*. It was subsequently found in humans and other primates that red blood cells, rather than platelets, are the main cell in blood to which opsonized trypanosomes would bind in this "immune adherence" reaction (19).

The role of complement in mediating these binding reactions was initially suggested by Russian scientists in the 1920s, who observed that heat-inactivated serum would not mediate binding (20). It was then shown specifically that erythrocyte adherence reactions could be abolished by heat treatment of sera or by dilute ammonia (which facilitates inactivation of C4 (21–23). The observation that treatment of serum with cobra venom factor prevented adherence reactions showed an essential role for C3 (23). Many of these early observations were published mainly in minor European and British journals and were overlooked between the late 1930s and early 1950s. No mention is made of any of the work on complement-dependent adherence reactions described previously in two major reviews on the complement system published at this time (24,25).

It was Nelson, in 1953, who rediscovered adherence reactions between human erythrocytes and specifically opsonized treponemes and pneumococci (26). He confirmed the complement-dependent nature of these reactions and first coined the term *immune adherence*. The modern era of studies on this phenomenon followed the isolation by Fearon (27) of the molecule responsible for the adherence reactions of human erythrocytes, the C3b/iC3b receptor (complement receptor type 1 [CR1]; CD35). This receptor bound large ICs and was shown to play a role in the transport of soluble ICs *in vivo* in primates (28).

CR1 is a receptor for C3b and iC3b and has a number of different biologic activities, including the uptake by phagocytic cells of C3b and iC3b-coated ICs and particles; the activation of B cells by antigen in the form of complement-coated ICs; action as a cofactor for factor I–mediated cleavage of C3b to iC3b and then C3dg; and function as the key transport molecule for ICs, both soluble and particulate. It is the last of these functions that is of crucial importance in understanding the role of IC processing in autoimmunity, and our discussion focuses on this area.

The sites of CR1 expression vary substantially among different species. In humans and other primates, most CR1 in the circulation is located in a clustered form on erythrocytes. The number of CR1 molecules per red blood cell is very low, varying between 50 and about 1,000 receptors per cell in humans (29,30). This compares with 5,000 to 50,000 receptors per neutrophil (numbers vary depending on the state of cellular activation) (31). Red blood cells, however, play an important role in the binding and transport of C3b and iC3b-coated ICs and particles through the circulation, for two reasons. The first is the vast majority of red blood cells, compared with other cell types (about 1,000 erythrocytes for every neutrophil). The second is the spatial organization of CR1 on the cell surface, which on red blood cells is clustered (32). This facilitates high-avidity interactions with ligand, as compared with neutrophils and lymphocytes, on which the receptor is expressed as cell-surface monomers. In other species, a hybrid molecule sharing the activities expressed by human CR1 and CR2 is expressed on leukocytes and platelets (33).

In light of the key role that CR1 plays in the binding and transport of ICs, there has been a great deal of interest in polymorphisms of the molecule in autoimmune disease. There are two types of genetic polymorphism of CR1, each

of which may show functional variation in respect to the transport of ICs. The first is a structural polymorphism. Four alleles of CR1 have been characterized, with molecular weights of about 210 kd (F′ [or C] allotype), about 250 kd (F [or A] allotype), about 290 kd (S [or B] allotype), and about 330 kd. This variation of about 40 kd between allelic variants results from the variable internal repetition of the long homologous repeats forming the structural core of the receptor. The 210 kd (F′ [or C]) allotype has reduced binding affinity for C3b dimers, corresponding to absence of one long homologous repeat containing a C3b-binding site (34). This uncommon variant appears to have an increased prevalence among patients with systemic lupus erythematosus (SLE) (35), although it is very uncommon even in this population. The potential contributory role of abnormalities in CR1 function in the pathophysiology of autoimmune disease is discussed in detail under Defects in Complement Receptor Type 1.

CR1 also exhibits a numerical polymorphism of expression on red blood cells in the normal population, with numbers varying between 50 and 500 CR1 molecules per erythrocyte. This numerical variation of CR1 expression on erythrocytes was first identified after the discovery of normal subjects whose erythrocytes failed to show immune adherence and was subsequently shown to be an inherited trait (36). Studies have confirmed the numerical polymorphism by direct enumeration of the receptor using radioligand-binding assays (37).

### How Do Immune Complexes Interact With Other Circulating Cells?

Neutrophils have both complement and Fc receptors, and on resting polymorphonuclear neutrophil (PMN) testing, the number of CR1 molecules per cell is about 10-fold higher than that per erythrocyte (33), raising the possibility that PMNs may have a role in IC binding and transport. The kinetics of the interaction between neutrophil CR1 and IC binding is different from the kinetics of erythrocyte CR1 and IC binding (38). Nonopsonized ICs react very slowly with PMNs, and precoating the complexes with C3b accelerates the reaction only marginally.

Only CR1 appears to be involved in this efficient binding because it is inhibited by a monoclonal anti-CR1 antibody. Despite the the greater numbers of CR1 molecules per cell, neutrophils do not bind C3b-coated ICs better than erythrocytes, a discrepancy largely explained by electron microscopic studies showing that CR1 molecules are not clustered on PMNs. Activation of neutrophils with C5a, interleukin-8 (IL-8), and *N*-formyl-met-leu-phe (FMLP) does not modify this distribution, despite stimulating a 5- to 10-fold increase in the total number of CR1 molecules expressed on the PMN surface (39). These observations suggest that in primates, at least, CR1-dependent binding of ICs to circulating leukocytes is not of major importance in IC processing. In fact, one of the primary roles of erythrocyte CR1 may be in preventing potentially harmful interactions among ICs, leukocytes, and vascular endothelium by maintaining the complexes within the central stream of the vessel, a hypothesis supported by *in vitro* observations that erythrocyte CR1 can protect cultured human umbilical vascular endothelial cells from IC- and PMN-mediated injury (40).

### Soluble Immune Complex Processing: In Vivo *Studies*

The main site of clearance of ICs is the fixed mononuclear phagocytic system. In most species, including primates, rodents, and lagomorphs, the liver and spleen are the primary sites in the circulation in which tissue macrophages are located (41). Pulmonary intravascular macrophages are also found in pigs, cows, sheep, goats, and cats, and these have been shown to be important in the clearance of both particles (42) and soluble ICs (43).

Important findings that have emerged from the study of the mechanisms of IC processing include the identification of the sites of processing of ICs; the finding that the nature of the antigen in the complex may influence clearance kinetics; observations that IC uptake by the mononuclear phagocytic system is saturable; and characterization of receptors on circulating cells that act as transport receptors for ICs in the circulation. For example, in rodents and lagomorphs, soluble ICs, injected intravenously, are predominantly removed in the liver and spleen (44–47), as in humans, but the complexes are not transported in the circulation bound to erythrocytes, which in these species do not bear CR1. Platelets in these species carry C3b receptors, and in one study, rapid *in vivo* binding of ICs to platelets was observed after intravenous injection (44).

Evidence for the importance of the antigen component as well as antibody in determining the mode and kinetics of clearance of ICs has derived from studies of the clearance in mice of ICs containing as antigen either orosomucoid or ceruloplasmin or their desialylated derivatives (48). The asialo-orosomucoid–containing complexes are cleared 20-fold more rapidly than those containing the sialylated molecule, and blocking studies showed that the rapid clearance phase is mediated by a hepatocyte carbohydrate receptor. The importance of receptors (e.g., the recently described family of "scavenger" receptors), other than those designed to bind complement proteins or immunoglobulin, in the clearance of IC in humans remains to be elucidated.

IC clearance mechanisms have been shown to be saturable in rabbits injected with escalating doses of soluble ICs. After saturation of hepatic uptake, spillover of ICs into other organs was observed (46). The extent to which this mechanism may operates in human disease remains unclear.

The first *in vivo* demonstration of the physiologic importance of erythrocyte complement receptor type 1 in IC clearance was in a series of studies performed in baboons (49–51). Radiolabeled ICs comprising BSA or anti-BSA were initially employed and were shown to localize mainly in the liver (52). In decomplemented animals, the ICs did not bind to red blood cells and were cleared more rapidly, depositing in other

organs, including the kidney. IgA-containing complexes, which fixed complement poorly, failed to bind to baboon erythrocyte CR1, were cleared rapidly, and localized in other organs (51).

A number of model ICs have been employed to explore the *in vivo* processing of exogenously administered soluble ICs in humans. The three main models that have been employed are heat-aggregated IgG, tetanus toxoid (TT) or anti-TT, and hepatitis B surface antigen (HBsAg) or anti-HBsAg ICs. Radiolabeled heat-aggregated IgG injected intravenously into healthy subjects was shown by scintigraphy to be cleared mainly in the liver and spleen (53).

The roles of complement and CR1 in soluble IC clearance mechanisms in humans were first studied *in vivo* using [125]I-labeled tetanus–toxoid or antitetanus–toxoid complexes (54). ICs bound to erythrocyte CR1 receptors in a complement-dependent manner, and CR1 number correlated with the level of uptake. In subjects with low CR1 numbers and hypocomplementemia, there was a rapid initial disappearance of ICs. A second phase of clearance was nearly monoexponential, and the observed elimination rate correlated inversely with CR1 numbers and the binding of ICs to red blood cells. Important differences were seen between control subjects and patients with SLE, and these are discussed in more detail later.

Extensive *in vivo* studies of soluble IC clearance have also been performed using a different model, the [123]I-labeled HBsAg and anti-HBsAg ICs. The fate of these complexes was monitored by blood sampling and external scanning to define the sites and kinetics of processing in healthy subjects, in patients with SLE, and in a single patient with homozygous C2 deficiency (55,56). In healthy subjects, complexes were cleared in the liver and spleen. Most of the injected complexes bound rapidly to red blood cells. In all subjects, there was a close correlation between *in vivo* binding to red blood cells and CR1 number. Results of studies using this model in SLE patients are discussed further under Processing of Immune Complexes in Patients With Abnormal CR1 and Complement Function.

A major criticism of the studies of IC processing described previously is that they all involve the exogenous administration of large ICs prepared *in vitro,* in the absence of complement, and may not therefore be representative of potentially pathogenic ICs that may form *in vivo*. Similar results have, however, been obtained from studies performed with ICs that form *in vivo*, both in an animal model and in humans. For example, the successive infusion of human anti–double-stranded DNA (anti-dsDNA) antibodies and dsDNA into monkeys and rabbits led to rapid formation of ICs that bound to red blood cell CR1 (57). The formation and fate of IC formed *in vivo* in patients receiving radioimmunotherapy has also been studied (58). The successive administration of a radiolabeled mouse antitumor antibody and a human anti-mouse antibody was shown to result in the formation of ICs comprising the two antibody species. Rapid clearance of complexes was observed with significant binding of the complexed material to red blood cell CR1. Systemic complement activation and a 30% fall in erythrocyte CR1 numbers were observed. Clearance took place primarily in the liver.

## Clearance of Particulate Complexes

### Clearance of an Autoantigen: Red Blood Cells

Autoimmune hemolysis and pathologic platelet destruction within the fixed macrophage system are important clinical features of SLE and are discussed in detail elsewhere in the volume. The site of clearance of particulate ICs depends on the class of antibody bound to the antigen. Studies of autoimmune hemolytic anemia, which constitutes an important clinical example of a persistent IC disease involving a particulate autoantigen, erythrocytes, demonstrate this well. Cold agglutinin disease is mediated by IgM anti-I antibodies, which stimulate efficient classical pathway activation and fixation of C4 and C3 to erythrocytes.

The role of anti-I and complement in mediating cell lysis was first studied in a rabbit model (59). IgM cold agglutinin was injected into C3-depleted and C6-deficient rabbits. The latter developed thrombocytopenia, neutropenia, and a decrease in hemoglobin and packed cell volume, with only minimal hemoglobinemia, but a rapid decrease in plasma C3 levels. Circulating red blood cells could be readily agglutinated with anti-C3 antibodies, and *in vivo* immune adherence of platelets to red blood cells occurred. In the C3-depleted animals, injection of the anti-I IgM produced no significant hematologic changes.

It has also been possible to model the fate of erythrocytes in cold agglutinin disease in nonhuman primates using radiolabeled cells coated with an IgM cold agglutinin (60). The main site of red blood cell uptake is the liver, and transient retention of cells in this organ is thought to be mediated by reversible binding to complement receptors. In patients with cold agglutinin disease, circulating red blood cells are characterized by morphologic change to a microspherocytic form, associated with the presence of several thousand C3dg molecules bound per cell.

In IgG-mediated warm hemolytic anemia, on the other hand, uptake of erythrocytes occurs predominantly in the spleen by Fc-dependent pathways. $^{51}$Cr-labeled incompatible red blood cells, transfused into recipients with noncomplement fixing antibodies, were removed from the circulation monoexponentially, with a half-time of 18 to 20 minutes (61). Splenic uptake exhibited similar kinetics. No uptake was detectable elsewhere, notably in the liver. Because the spleen removes cells exclusively and receives only a relatively small fraction of the cardiac output, it was reasoned that the splenic extraction efficiency is very high. It was subsequently shown that the site of sensitized red blood cell destruction is dependent on the degree of antibody coating, with more heavily coated cells being destroyed predominantly by the liver (62).

Radiolabeled erythrocytes, coated with antibody (IgG), have been extensively studied as a probe of mononuclear phagocytic function in various diseases (63). In humans and other species, these cells are cleared primarily in the spleen. The mechanisms by which this probe exhibits primarily splenic clearance, whereas soluble ICs (see earlier) and cells coated with IgM and C3 localize predominantly in the liver, are poorly understood. Tissue macrophages in the liver and spleen bear both Fc and complement receptors (CR1, CR3, and CR4) (64), whereas follicular dendritic cells within the spleen and lymph nodes also bear the C3dg receptor, CR2. The Fc receptors on monocytes and macrophages primarily involved in interactions with ICs or immunoglobulin aggregates are the relatively low-affinity receptors, FcγRII and FcγRIII (65,66).

Evidence from *in vitro* experiments performed using magnetic anti-IgG probes indicates that the potential "availability" of IgG on red blood cells to interact with fixed cellular receptors may be different depending on whether the immunoglobulin is distributed at multiple sites on the red blood cell surface, adjacent to the cell membrane, or presented in ICs bound to clustered CR1, away from the erythrocyte cell membrane (67). In the latter case, it has been postulated that IgG may be "safely" stripped from the cells as a consequence of interaction with fixed macrophages, with little associated damage to the red blood cell. In the instance of the antibody-coated erythrocytes used to study the function of the fixed macrophage system in the type of *in vivo* study discussed previously, multiple, more intimate contacts with receptors on fixed macrophages may result in cellular destruction, especially in the spleen (reviewed in 68).

It is also possible that the anatomy of the splenic circulation favors the uptake of particulate rather than soluble ICs. The hematocrit in the spleen is relatively high compared with that in major arteries and veins (69). The converse applies in the sinusoids of the liver, which have a low hematocrit in comparison with major blood vessels. This reflects observations that hepatic sinusoidal macrophages are efficient at clearing soluble ICs from plasma and that splenic macrophages play an important role in handling IgG-coated erythrocytes. After splenectomy, the peripheral blood contains abnormal red blood cells bearing denatured hemoglobin, known as *Heinz bodies,* and nuclear remnants, known as *Howell–Jolly bodies,* clearly illustrating the physiologic role of the spleen in the processing of abnormal red blood cells (70).

### Bacterial and Endotoxin Clearance

Mortality and morbidity resulting from infection are major problems in patients with SLE. Many factors have been implicated, including the use of corticosteroids and immunosuppressive drugs. SLE patients with hypocomplementemia and low red blood cell CR1 numbers may also be susceptible both to gram-positive and gram-negative infections because of defective clearance of bacteria and endotoxin. Bacterial clearance *in vivo* has not been studied experimentally in humans but has been evaluated in a variety of animal models.

A number of important interspecies differences have been observed, and care is required in extrapolating observations in animal models to the human situation.

Variations in the site of clearance may have a major influence on the pathophysiologic consequences of bacteremia. For example, pigs are extremely susceptible to the development of adult respiratory distress syndrome (ARDS) (71). Equivalent doses (on a weight basis) of *Pseudomonas aeruginosa* administered in parallel to pigs and dogs were well-tolerated by the latter but were associated with acute pulmonary failure in pigs, in which there was selective lung uptake of the organisms. Complement depletion, but not neutrophil depletion, abrogated the development of ARDS. These findings suggest that the susceptibility of pigs to ARDS may be specifically related to the pulmonary vascular location of the mononuclear phagocytic system and to the local release of inflammatory mediators.

The role of natural antibody and complement in the clearance of endotoxin from the circulation remains unclear. Recently reported experiments in mice rendered C3 or C4 deficient by gene targeting have demonstrated defective lipopolysaccharide (LPS) clearance in the complement-deficient animals and enhanced mortality (72). RAG-/- mice, which are unable to produce immunoglobulin, also exhibit defective LPS processing (73). Attempts in humans to enhance LPS clearance and to reduce mortality in septic shock by the administration of exogenous IgM antilipid A antibodies have proved largely unsuccessful (reviewed in 74), even though the reagents used have been shown *in vitro* to complex with LPS, fix complement, and mediate binding to erythrocyte CR1 (75,76).

## ROLE OF THE COMPLEMENT SYSTEM IN IMMUNE COMPLEX–MEDIATED AUTOIMMUNE DISEASE

The complement system plays both beneficial and deleterious roles in autoimmune disease. There is a large amount of evidence showing that complement causes inflammatory injury to tissues in patients and experimental animals, in which ICs form in the circulation or locally in tissues. It is also clear, however, that either inherited or acquired deficiencies of classical pathway complement proteins in humans are associated with increased susceptibility to the development of IC disease typical of SLE.

### Complement Deficiency and Systemic Lupus Erythematosus

#### Clinical Observations

Inherited homozygous deficiency of C1q, C1r, C1s, C4, or C2 has been strongly associated with the development of SLE. There is a hierarchy of severity and susceptibility to SLE according to the position of the missing protein in the pathway of classical pathway complement activation. More than 90% of patients with homozygous C1q deficiency develop SLE, typically at an early age (77). Disease is characterized by severe rashes, with a significant proportion of patients developing glomerulonephritis or cerebral SLE. A wide range of autoantibodies to extractable nuclear antigens, including anti-Ro, anti-Sm, and anti-RNP, are found in these patients, although anti-dsDNA antibodies are much less common.

About one third of patients with C2 deficiency develop SLE (78), and the autoantibody profile tends to be restricted to the presence of anti-Ro antibodies. The severity of disease is similar to that seen in SLE patients without homozygous complement deficiency. C3 deficiency, on the other hand, is usually not associated with the development of full-blown SLE and typically presents with recurrent pyogenic infections (79). Up to one third of C3-deficient patients develop a prominent rash in association with pyogenic infections, which in one case was associated with a dense neutrophilic cutaneous infiltrate (80).

SLE-associated autoantibodies are only exceptionally identified in patients with C3 deficiency, although about one fourth of C3-deficient patients develop mesangiocapillary glomerulonephritis. Deficiency of two of the alternative pathway control proteins, factor I and factor H, is associated with severe secondary C3 deficiency caused by failure of regulation of the alternative pathway and amplification loop of C3 cleavage (81). These patients show a similar phenotype to C3 deficiency and typically suffer from recurrent pyogenic infections with only occasional development of glomerulonephritis without significant autoantibody formation.

Many studies have shown associations between specific gene products of the major histocompatibility complex (MHC) (reviewed elsewhere in the volume) and the development of SLE and other autoimmune diseases. It is frequently extremely difficult to determine which associations between MHC gene products and specific diseases are primary and which are due to other linked genes in the MHC because of the phenomenon of linkage disequilibrium. All four complement genes located in the Class III region of the MHC (C4A, C4B, C2, and factor B) exhibit extensive genetic polymorphism, which in the case of C4A and C4B includes frequent "null" alleles that do not encode the production of a protein product. The observation that homozygous complement deficiency was associated with SLE raised the possibility that null alleles of C4 might show an association with the disease. This was found to be the case (82,83), and the results of early studies have been confirmed in a number of different ethnic populations (84), strengthening the likelihood that the C4 null allele is the relevant gene. However, the association between C4A null alleles and SLE is not confirmed by all studies and remains controversial (85).

An increased prevalence of alleles of mannose-binding lectin (MBL) has been associated with reduced serum levels of the protein among two populations of patients with SLE (86). The significance of these results is not certain, and the role of MBL in the pathophysiology of IC-mediated autoimmune disease remains to be defined.

There has been an increased prevalence of antinuclear antibodies and of the development of SLE and a range of other autoimmune disorders (including glomerulonephritis, Sjögren's syndrome, inflammatory bowel disease, and thyroiditis) (87,88) in patients with hereditary angioedema resulting from heterozygous C1 inhibitor deficiency. These patients show prolonged reduction in C4 and C2 levels because of partially unregulated activity of C1r and C1s, and disordered regulation of both cell-mediated and humoral immunity has been described in these patients (89). Similarly, patients with prolonged acquired C3 deficiency resulting from the presence of the autoantibody C3 nephritic factor may develop SLE many years after presentation with partial lipodystrophy or mesangiocapillary glomerulonephritis with dense deposits (90).

These associations of acquired complement deficiency and IC-mediated autoimmune disease strongly support the hypothesis that complement has a key role in the pathophysiology of these conditions. However, the possibility remains that the associations of complement deficiency with SLE are a result of the ascertainment artifact, as a consequence of the fact that complement levels are mainly measured in patients with diseases associated with complement activation. This would mean that any examples of complement deficiency detected would inevitably be associated with those conditions. Extensive surveys have shown that inherited homozygous complement deficiency is extremely rare in healthy populations (91,92).

Further evidence for the role of complement and ICs in autoimmunity comes from a number of animal models of complement deficiency that have been described. For example, dogs from a colony with C3 deficiency develop a similar pattern of glomerulonephritis to that seen in C3-deficient humans (93). Pigs have been discovered in Norway that develop a severe, mesangiocapillary glomerulonephritis of early onset; these animals have been shown to have hereditary factor H deficiency (94). Mice with targeted deletions of C4 (95), C3 (72), C1q (79), factor B (96), and the Cr2 locus (97) have been developed. Our own data show that C1q-deficient mice develop antinuclear antibodies, and a significant proportion of these animals die with crescentic glomerulonephritis (98).

### Possible Mechanisms

A number of physiologic activities of the complement system may explain the clinical associations of hypocomplementemia and autoimmune disease discussed previously. One of the most important of these is the role of complement in the processing of ICs. Defective IC processing and clearance may result in the inefficient clearance of ICs by the fixed mononuclear phagocytic system with deposition of ICs in many tissues, causing inflammation, the release of autoantigens, and stimulation of an autoimmune response. Direct evidence for the abnormal processing of ICs in hypocomplementemic patients is discussed in detail later.

Two other roles of the complement system may also be relevant in the pathophysiology of SLE. Complement has an important role in antigen processing and presentation in germinal centers and in host defense against infection. Detailed discussion of these areas is beyond the scope of the present review, which relates primarily to the role of ICs in autoimmunity. However, it is worth considering the possibility that the classical pathway of complement normally provides defense against an infectious agent that induces SLE. Complement proteins are known to play an important role in host defense against pyogenic infections. It seems unlikely, however, that this is a major factor in the induction of SLE because other abnormalities of host defense associated with recurrent pyogenic disease are not associated with development of the disease. There is evidence for a role of complement in host defense against C-type retroviruses (99,100), and it remains an unproven possibility that SLE is an autoimmune response that follows infection by an unidentified virus of this type.

### Do Primary or Secondary Defects Exist in Immune Complex Clearance and Processing Mechanisms?

#### Defects in Complement Receptor Type 1

We have already discussed the role of CR1 in the clearance of soluble and particulate ICs. The number of receptors per red blood cell varies widely among healthy subjects, and the level of expression is under genetic control at the CR1 locus (30,36). The molecular mechanism of this has not been established, but a restriction fragment length polymorphism within the CR1 gene is correlated with high or low expression of CR1 on red blood cells (101,102). Patients with SLE express reduced numbers of receptors per cell compared with healthy subjects (37). This raises the possibility that low expression of CR1 might constitute a disease susceptibility gene for the development of SLE. A number of studies, however, showed that low expression of CR1 in SLE and in certain other conditions associated with complement activation on erythrocytes or in the fluid phase is due to acquired mechanisms (37).

#### Fc Receptor Function

It has long been questionable that defects in mononuclear phagocytic function predispose to the development of SLE by impairment of IC clearance. This hypothesis originally stemmed from experimental studies of the clearance of colloidal carbon particles in animals (41), which showed that uptake by the mononuclear phagocytic system was saturable. ICs injected into rabbits also showed saturable uptake in the liver, followed by spillover into other organs (46). Despite these experimental data in animals, however, there is no firm evidence that demonstrates that saturation of soluble IC clearance mechanisms occurs in human disease.

A number of different methods have been used to study whether there is indeed impaired processing of ICs in SLE by the mononuclear phagocytic system. Studies of the clearance of IgG-coated erythrocytes by the spleen showed delayed uptake in SLE, and correlations were found between clearance rate, disease activity, and levels of circulating ICs in patients with SLE (103,104). As discussed previously, however, IgG-coated erythrocytes may not be an appropriate surrogate measure for Fc- and complement-dependent clearance mechanisms of soluble ICs. The clearance of soluble ICs in a C2-deficient patient with SLE was totally corrected by complement repletion, largely excluding a primary defect in mononuclear phagocytic function as the explanation for defective IC clearance in that patient (56).

Mononuclear phagocytic cell function in SLE may also be addressed by studying genetic variation in Fc and complement receptors. Support for the idea that Fc receptor function is abnormal in SLE has come from recent studies of a functionally important polymorphism of the Fc receptor, FCγRIIa. An allotypic variant of FcγRIIa, FcγRIIa-HR (FcγRIIa-R131), has been shown *in vitro* to reduce the capacity of phagocytic cells to bind and internalize IgG-containing ICs and IgG-opsonized erythrocytes (105). This receptor mainly binds $IgG_2$. A number of groups have addressed the question of whether there is an overrepresentation of this allotypic variant in patients with SLE, either by genotype analysis or by determination of receptor phenotype on peripheral blood leukocytes by fluorescence-activated cell sorter analysis using specific monoclonal antibodies. An excess of FcγRIIa-R131 homozygotes was found in African-American patients with SLE nephritis (106) and in Dutch patients with SLE (107). We were unable to confirm this finding, however, in groups of white, Afro-Caribbean, or Chinese patients with SLE (108). Further studies are needed to test whether this polymorphic variant of FcγRIIa is a disease susceptibility gene for SLE or, more specifically, for SLE nephritis.

### Processing of Immune Complexes in Patients With Abnormal CR1 and Complement Function

The *in vivo* clearance of soluble ICs in human disease has been studied using all of the three models described earlier, that is, IgG aggregates (AIgG), tetanus toxoid complexes, and anti-HBsAg–HBsAg complexes. Important differences in the clearance of radiolabeled aggregated γ-globulin were seen between healthy subjects and patients with SLE (109). The mean half-time for initial clearance of AIgG was shorter in patients than in control subjects, and binding of AIgG to erythrocytes was significantly lower in patients than in control subjects. Liver and spleen uptake ratios were also significantly higher in patients than in control subjects, attributable to reduced splenic uptake of AIgG. Accelerated clearance of AIgG was also observed in two C3-deficient patients studied using the same model complexes (110).

Similar observations were made in patients with SLE and hypocomplementemia in studies that employed [125]I-labeled tetanus toxoid–antitetanus toxoid complexes as probes of the pathways of IC processing (54). The most striking finding was the enhanced rapid initial clearance of complexes in patients with SLE and low complement levels, most marked in a patient with C1q deficiency.

The explanation for these results, notably for the rapid initial clearance of ICs in hypocomplementemic patients, came from our own studies using [123]I-labeled HBsAg–anti-HBsAg ICs. As in healthy subjects, the liver and spleen were the main sites of complex uptake. The initial clearance of ICs from blood was more rapid, however, in patients with SLE than in control subjects because of more rapid uptake in the liver. In SLE patients, however, there was significant release of complexes from the liver after 30 to 40 minutes, which was not seen in control subjects. Binding of ICs to erythrocytes was greatly reduced in these patients as a consequence of hypocomplementemia and reduced CR1 numbers. As discussed previously, in a C2-deficient patient studied before and after therapy with fresh-frozen plasma, there was no uptake of ICs in the spleen before therapy but both the kinetics and sites of complex clearance reverted to normal after normalization of classical pathway complement activity (56).

To summarize, the main findings of these studies of *in vivo* IC processing in SLE patients are as follows:

- More rapid initial clearance of complexes from the circulation takes place in patients than in control subjects, followed by release of ICs back into the circulation.
- The splenic uptake of ICs is reduced in patients.

It is possible that the impaired uptake of complexes in the spleen in SLE may be related to the mode of delivery of ICs to the fixed mononuclear phagocytic system. Reduced binding to red blood cell CR1 was observed in all three models in SLE patients, with a resultant increase in the numbers of complexes delivered to the fixed macrophage system in the fluid phase. As discussed previously, the anatomy of the spleen favors the uptake of particles (68). The hematocrit in the splenic vasculature is relatively high compared with that in the major blood vessels, and splenic macrophages play a key role in the processing of IgG-coated erythrocytes (discussed under Clearance of Particulate Complexes). It might therefore be expected that ICs bound to red blood cell CR1 would be selectively processed in the spleen, whereas complexes presented in the fluid phase would localize to the liver.

The explanation for the observed release of ICs back into the circulation from the liver is unclear. One possibility is that only complexes that are able to interact efficiently with both complement receptors and Fc receptors on fixed macrophages, with subsequent internalization and processing, are retained efficiently within the liver and spleen. ICs bearing relatively little C3b, which are delivered in the fluid phase, may bind rapidly to the relatively low-affinity Fcγ receptors (II and III), but ligation of these receptors alone may be insufficient to trigger efficient internalization of the complexes.

## Role of Immune Complexes and Complement in Causing Inflammation

### Background

ICs induce tissue injury primarily by activation of the complement system. Three main mechanisms are involved:

1. Complement proteins attached covalently (C3 and C4) or noncovalently (C1q) to ICs may ligate receptors on leukocytes and lymphocytes, triggering these cells to express effector activities.
2. Formation of the membrane attack complex may cause direct cellular damage or, at sublytic levels, may stimulate local cell activation.
3. Complement activation may cause anaphylatoxin generation.

The architecture of the affected tissues is an important factor in determining the nature of IC-mediated inflammatory tissue injury. A good example of this is in glomerular renal inflammation, in which the glomerular basement membrane is a barrier to the exit of leukocytes from glomerular capillaries. Tissue injury in membranous glomerulonephritis, in which ICs form in the subepithelium, is induced by the complement membrane attack complex in the absence of inflammatory leukocytes (111). On the other hand, when ICs form or are deposited in the subendothelium, as in SLE or Goodpasture's disease, tissue injury is induced by a combination of leukocytes and complement (112).

The study of animals with gene-targeted deletions of complement receptors and Fc receptors has greatly facilitated further exploration of the triggering mechanisms of inflammation by ICs. One model system that has been widely used to study the mechanisms of inflammation induced by ICs is the reverse passive Arthus reaction. In this model, antibody is injected into the skin or introduced into the lungs of an animal that has been injected intravenously with antigen. In skin, the reverse passive Arthus reaction is dependent on both Fc- and complement-mediated pathways (113–115). Complement depletion alone does not significantly reduce the inflammatory response. Deficiency of FcγRIII diminishes the response to a variable degree, which correlates inversely with the level of hemolytic complement expressed in individual animals (114). Complete abolition of the response is seen only in FcγRIII animals after depletion of complement with cobra venom factor. These observations are similar to those made some years ago in C5-deficient and cobra venom factor–treated mice, which showed that, at low concentrations of antibody, complement-dependent inflammatory pathways dominated, whereas at high concentrations, complement-independent pathways played a more crucial role (115).

The results of studies of the reverse passive Arthus reaction in the lung are similar to those in the skin. In this model, however, complement depletion or deficiency of C5 appear to block the inflammatory response more effectively than in the skin (116). A role for the anaphylatoxin, C5a, or the membrane attack complex may be inferred from the observation that C5 deficiency has some protective effect against the Arthus reaction in the lung (114), as in the skin.

Several lines of evidence support an important role for mast cells in triggering tissue injury in response to ICs in the Arthus reaction. Studies performed in a strain of mice lacking mast cells as a result of deficiency of stem cell factor, c-kit, showed a markedly reduced reverse passive Arthus reaction (117). Reconstitution studies have been performed in these animals with mast cells derived from animals deficient or sufficient in the Fc receptor γ chain (118). The Arthus response was only effectively restored to normal in mice reconstituted with mast cells bearing FcγRIII, showing that ICs in this model trigger mast cells to release their mediators and cause inflammation by ligation of this Fc receptor.

Intrapulmonary IC formation has also been studied in mice with gene-targeted deletions of either the NK-1r substance P receptor or the C5a receptor (119). The induction of the inflammatory response after intrapulmonary IC formation was abrogated in NK-1r-/- mice and was also absent in C5aR-/- mice. These observations suggest an additional role for the tachykinin, substance P, in IC-mediated inflammation. Substance P, found in C-type nerve fibers, is also found in macrophages and mast cells, as is the NK-1 receptor.

### In Situ *Immune Complex Formation and the Deposition of Complexes From the Circulation*

The relative importance of *in situ* IC formation and of the deposition of IC from the circulation in causing inflammation has long been the subject of debate. In solution, when antigen meets antibody at equivalence or in antibody excess, rapid precipitation occurs. This reaction requires intact IgG molecules, as distinct from F(ab′)₂ fragments, suggesting that Fc–Fc interactions are important in promoting precipitation (120). Large complexes also promote the aggregation of small complexes on their surface (9). Such interactions bring the reacting molecules into close proximity; this is followed by formation of an "infinite lattice" of alternating antigen–antibody bonds, resulting in the precipitation of an insoluble IC. Such a lattice can also build up on an antigen or antibody located within tissues, either as an intrinsic component, or "planted" from the circulation. *In situ* formation of ICs in this way has been demonstrated in experimental glomerulonephritis, in which planted antigen (or antibody), exposed successively to further antibody and antigen, leads to the development of large, microscopically visible deposits (121).

Continuous overproduction of antibody, often antigen driven, is a major factor in the pathophysiology of autoimmune diseases, such as SLE, and in infections, such as bacterial endocarditis, in which ICs are thought to play an important role. In these diseases, ICs are formed in large antibody excess and are likely to be large, complement-activating aggregates. Immobilization of these ICs in tissues, either from *in situ* formation or deposition from the bloodstream, causes inflammation and organ injury. The complement system has a role in limiting such injury by inhibiting the formation of large ICs, as discussed previously, and by promoting their safe disposal by the mononuclear phagocytic system.

### Role of Autoantibodies to Complement Components in Amplifying Immune Complex–mediated Tissue Damage

A number of autoantibodies to complement components may have a role in amplifying the phlogistic effects of ICs. The two best characterized examples are C3 nephritic factor (C3 NeF) and antibodies to the collagenous part of the C1q molecule [anti-C1q(CLR)].

C3 NeF is an IgG autoantibody directed against neoantigenic determinants on the alternative pathway C3 convertase, C3bBb. C3 NeF stabilizes the enzyme, causing dysregulated complement activation, leading to a severe secondary deficiency of C3 (122). C3 NeF is associated clinically with partial lipodystrophy and type II membranoproliferative glomerulonephritis, in which electron-dense deposits occur in the glomerulus. These deposits do not generally contain immunoglobulin, although C3 is usually demonstrable. The mechanism of the association of C3 NeF with glomerulonephritis is not understood. One hypothesis is that C3 NeF causes secondary C3 deficiency, which in turn is responsible for the development of nephritis, a hypothesis supported by observations that homozygous C3 deficiency is associated in some humans and in dogs with development of mesangiocapillary glomerulonephritis, although not with the typical electron-dense deposits that define type II mesangiocapillary glomerulonephritis. The mechanism of the association of C3 deficiency with glomerulonephritis also remains uncertain. Attempts to induce renal injury in experimental animals rendered hypocomplementemic by nonimmune mechanisms have been generally unsuccessful (123,124), and nephritis in the context of NeF may coexist with normal complement levels (122).

Another possible explanation for the association of C3 Nef with glomerulonephritis is that C3 NeF can activate complement locally in the kidney. This explanation could also account for the association of factor H and I deficiencies with glomerulonephritis, in which C3, locally synthesized in the kidney may undergo unregulated activation and cause local tissue injury. In support of this hypothesis are *in vitro* experiments showing that heat-killed kidney cells may activate complement and bind an NeF-stabilized C3 convertase (125). There is also a report of a patient with mesangiocapillary glomerulonephritis, hypocomplementemia, and systemic candidiasis. The glomerular deposits in this patient contained both C3 and *Candida albicans,* a known alternative pathway activator (126).

There is increasing interest in antibodies to C1q in autoimmune disease. The pathogenic role of these anti-C1q IgG autoantibodies to neoepitopes on the collagenous part of the C1q molecule is also poorly understood. The antibodies exhibit a number of specific clinical associations, notably with SLE and hypocomplementemic urticarial vasculitis syndrome (127,128), and are strongly associated with classical pathway complement activation, causing very low levels of C3, C4, and C1q. It is possible that they may augment activation of the complement system by ICs in tissues. This idea is supported by recent observations that anti-C1q antibodies, purified from two patients with SLE, deposited in mouse glomeruli in the presence of human C1q (129). A range of other autoantibodies to complement neoantigens has also been described. For example, IgG autoantibodies that stabilize the classical pathway convertase, C4b2a, have been reported in a patient with poststreptococcal glomerulonephritis and in some patients with SLE (130,131).

## IMMUNE COMPLEXES IN SPECIFIC DISEASES

### Glomerulonephritis

Immune deposits in the inflamed glomerulus are typically found in one of three locations: the mesangium, the subendothelium, or the subepithelium. Mesangial and subendothelial deposits are associated with proliferative lesions, whereas subepithelial deposits are characteristic of membranous glomerulonephritis. Glomerular pathology, particularly that associated with SLE, is often complex, and mixed lesions frequently occur (132). Subepithelial immune deposits are generally thought to develop as a result of *in situ* IC formation (133). It is much less clear whether mesangial and subendothelial deposits form *in situ,* from deposited circulating ICs, or from a mixture of both (see *In Situ* Immune Complex Formation and the Deposition of Complexes From the Circulation).

### Subepithelial Immune Complexes

Subepithelial IC formation has been extensively studied in the rat. Heymann's nephritis is a model of membranous nephropathy in this species, in which subepithelial granular IC deposits result from the binding of free antibody to an antigen expressed on the surface of glomerular epithelial cells (134). Complement-dependent (C5–9) tissue injury results (135). This pattern of glomerular injury can result from IC formation with either fixed or planted glomerular antigens. The original Heymann's nephritis involves a fixed glomerular antigen, a glycoprotein (GP330) localized along the epithelial cell membrane and coated pits (136). Binding of divalent antibody is thought to cause antigenic modulation and redistribution of the IC on the surface of the cell, with resultant capping and shedding of the aggregates into the nearby slit pore areas and lamina rara externa (137). An analogous mechanism is likely to operate in idiopathic membranous nephritis in humans, although the relevant autoantigen has not been characterized.

Many different autoantibodies occur in patients with SLE and glomerulonephritis. The precise role of these autoantibodies in this context, however, remains unclear. In animal models, polyspecific anti-DNA antibodies have been shown to bind directly to cell membrane antigens (138) and to localize under certain conditions in glomeruli (139). It is, however, difficult experimentally to induce the formation of subepithelial deposits containing exogenous antigens by the infusion of ICs (140). Highly cationic, preformed IC can produce this picture, possibly as a result of the attraction of cationic antigens or antibodies to oppositely charged glomerular structures. The subepithelial localization of immune deposits may result from filtration forces, whereas granularity may result from condensation of IC-containing polyvalent antigens into larger deposits, which may be detectable by electron microscopy (141).

In SLE, one of the main candidate antigens for involvement in IC formation is dsDNA, an anionic antigen, and the localization of injected DNA to glomeruli has been demonstrated experimentally (142). The cationic nature of anti-DNA antibodies may also be of importance, and cationic anti-DNA antibodies have been successfully eluted from mice with SLE nephritis (143,144).

### Subendothelial and Mesangial Complex Formation

Circulating macromolecules have potential access to both these sites, and trapping of circulating IC may have an important role to play in immune deposit. This hypothesis is supported by studies showing the localization of injected IC to mesangium. It has proved difficult, however, to induce glomerular injury after the injection of preformed ICs (145). When initial antigen localization to the mesangium is succeeded by further accretion of antibody, immune deposit formation results, with induction of a focal proliferative nephritis (146). Direct antibody-induced mesangial cell damage has also been demonstrated experimentally (147).

Experimentally, glomerulonephritis associated with subendothelial deposits is similarly difficult to induce by the injection of preformed ICs. It is possible, however, to produce subendothelial deposit formation experimentally by induction of antigen expression on the endothelial cell surface, followed by subsequent infusion of an appropriate antibody (148), but such deposits are then rapidly shed into the circulation.

### Infectious Disease

A number of well-documented associations between IC disease and infection have been described. Two examples of considerable clinical importance are cryoglobulinemia associated with viral hepatitis and subacute bacterial endocarditis. Classical pathway complement consumption is characteristic of both conditions.

### Cryoglobulinemia and Hepatitis Infection

A cryoglobulin comprises an antibody or an IC, the physicochemical properties of which cause it to precipitate from serum at temperatures below 37°C. Cryoglobulinemia may occur in a range of autoimmune disorders, including SLE, rheumatoid arthritis, and Sjögren's syndrome, and is also associated with infections and lymphoproliferative disorders. Cryoglobulins may be classified into three types (149): type 1—monoclonal paraproteins of IgG or IgM isotype, which typically occur in patients with myeloma, chronic lymphocytic leukemia, or Waldenström's macroglobulinemia; type 2—comprising a monoclonal rheumatoid factor, which is typically seen in mixed essential cryoglobulinemia, but also in association with autoimmune or lymphoproliferative disorders; and type 3—"mixed cryoglobulinemia," comprising polyclonal IgG or IgM and complement.

Mixed cryoglobulinemia can occur in association with infections such as Epstein–Barr virus, cytomegalovirus kalaazar, and infective endocarditis. Hepatitis B and hepatitis C virus (HCV) infections are commonly associated with type 2 cryoglobulinemia, particularly in the southern part of Europe (150–153). Of 63 French patients with mixed cryoglobulinemia, anti-HCV antibodies were detected in the serum of 33, whereas 30 patients tested negative (152). Cryoglobulin levels were higher in the anti-HCV–positive group, hemolytic complement activity was lower, and symptoms, particularly those affecting the skin, were more severe. HCV RNA sequences were detected in the majority of sera, and cryoprecipitates were derived from the anti-HCV–positive group, but HBV DNA was not detectable in any of the cryoprecipitates studied. In an analysis of 113 consecutive anti-HCV–positive patients studied in Cambridge, UK, 21 had detectable cryoglobulins, of which 19 of 21 were type 3 and 2 of 21 type 2 (154). HCV RNA was also detected in the majority of cryoprecipitates. Cryoglobulins were detected in 24 of 65 Japanese patients with hepatitis C (155).

### Infective Endocarditis

The best example of IC disease occurring in the context of a chronic bacterial infection is infective endocarditis resulting from chronic bacterial colonization of cardiac valvular structures, most commonly by streptococci (156–158). Chronic bacteremia of any cause may be associated with IC formation. For example, circulating ICs were detected in the serum of 40% patients with bacteremia due to infection of an intravascular catheter or access device and in the serum of 70% patients with *Staphylococcus aureus* bacteremia related to chronic deep tissue infection (159), in whom chronic hypocomplementemia may also be a feature. The hypocomplementemia observed in infective endocarditis is caused partly by classical pathway activation by ICs and probably also by activation of complement by the bacteria. Vegetations on mitral and aortic valves removed at surgery from patients with *Streptococcus viridans* endocarditis have been shown to contain immunoglobulin, C3, and bacterial antigens. Both endocardial and subendocardial deposition of C5b–9 have also been demonstrated (160). Antisarcolemmal antibodies that cross-react with bacterial antigens have been demonstrated in infective endocarditis, and there is evidence that these cross-reactive antibodies have complement-dependent cytolytic potential *in vitro* (161). As is the case in many infections, however, direct attempts to demonstrate bacterial antigens or antimicrobial antibodies in circulating ICs have generally proved unsuccessful (162).

The persistence of circulating ICs in infective endocarditis may be associated with tissue injury, typically vasculitis affecting the skin, arthritis, or glomerulonephritis (163), and it has been demonstrated *in vitro* that the serum of patients with endocarditis and high levels of ICs exhibits defective complement-mediated inhibition of immune precipitation (164). Rheumatoid factors are frequently detected in endocarditis. Various groups have demonstrated a fall in both IC and rheumatoid factor levels and a rise in the ability of serum to inhibit immune precipitation after successful treatment of infective endocarditis (158,164).

## Immune Complexes and Extrarenal Tissue Injury in Systemic Lupus Erythematosus

Direct injury to blood vessels is thought to be important in the mediation of tissue injury in a variety of different organs, and many conditions are described as "vasculitic" in nature. Complement activation by ICs has an important role in the mediation of cellular injury to blood vessels, particularly in SLE (165). The precise role of IC in the induction of vascular injury, however, is still unclear. Deposition of IC within vessel walls results in complement activation and the release of chemotactic factors, particularly C5 fragments, as discussed previously. Intravascular aggregation of neutrophils may occur, and the subsequent inflammatory response produces endothelial damage, an increase in vascular permeability, and ultimately tissue necrosis.

Neutrophil–endothelium interactions and their role in the induction of inflammation have been reviewed by Mason and Haskard (166). Localization of neutrophils to the pulmonary vasculature is well described in a variety of situations in association with complement activation and IC formation and may result in leukostatic occlusion in the pulmonary arterioles (167). It has also been suggested that one of the potential benefits of IC carriage in the circulation by erythrocyte CR1 (see earlier) is that as a consequence of red blood cell binding, ICs remain in the central jet stream in small vessels, away from the vascular endothelium, where they may be trapped, with potentially harmful consequences (40).

ICs have been implicated in a variety of cardiac diseases. In SLE pericarditis, complement activation, anti-DNA and antinuclear antibodies, and ICs have all been detected in pericardial fluid (168–171). Complement components and immunoglobulins have also been demonstrated in cardiac valvular lesions in SLE (172). There is experimental evidence in animals that IC deposition may induce endothelial damage in coronary vessels, with a subsequent predisposition to atheroma formation (173), and a similar mechanism has been postulated in humans (174).

In the lung, there is conflicting evidence relating to the importance of ICs in the mediation of both acute pneumonitis and chronic interstitial lung disease. Immune deposits, including DNA–anti-DNA complexes, have been described in lung tissue from patients with both conditions (175–178). Other observers, however, have failed to demonstrate ICs in the lungs of SLE patients with pulmonary hemorrhage (179–181).

In the skin, ICs in SLE and related conditions are typically observed at the dermoepidermal junction. An experimental model has been described in which mice were immunized with DNA pretreated with ultraviolet radiation and subsequently exposed to ultraviolet light. Specific antibodies to the altered DNA were produced, and anti-DNA– and DNA-containing immune deposits occurred in the skin (182). As in the kidney, the site of IC localization may be strongly influenced by charge. The dermoepidermal junction possesses a fixed negative charge. Joselow et al. (183) demonstrated that the injection of preformed IC, made in antigen excess with cationic antibodies, induced immune deposit formation at this site after 1 to 4 hours. Immunization of mice with cationized rabbit IgG produced similar results. In humans, Landry and Sams (184) demonstrated antibodies to structural components of the dermoepidermal junction as well as antinuclear antibodies in skin eluates obtained from SLE patients.

In the central nervous system (CNS), a variety of disease processes have been attributed to IC formation or deposition. In patients with SLE, infarction and hemorrhage are often attributed to IC-mediated vasculitis (185). In such patients, however, hypercoagulability resulting from the presence of anticardiolipin antibodies may also have a role in precipitating thrombotic events (186), discussed in detail in Chapter 34. Both antibodies and ICs (including DNA–anti-DNA complexes) have been demonstrated in the choroid plexus of patients with CNS SLE, but similar observations have been made in patients with asymptomatic disease, suggesting that nonspecific IC trapping at this site may occur (187–189). Depression of C4 levels (190–191) and increased levels of fluid-phase C5b–9 have also been described in the cerebrospinal fluid (CSF) of SLE patients with CNS disease (192). Seibold et al. (193) reported the presence of IC in the CSF of 33 of 34 patients with definite cerebral SLE, compared with 1 of 12 patients without CNS disease, and in 4 of 90 multiple sclerosis patients. Other investigators have described anti-DNA–DNA complexes in the CSF (194). The relevance of these findings to the immunopathogenesis of cerebral SLE remains unclear.

## REFERENCES

1. Heidelberger M. Quantitative chemical studies on complement or alexin. I. A method. *J Exp Med* 1941;73:691–694.

2. Morgan CR, Sorenson RL, Lazarow A. Further studies of an inhibitor of the two antibody immunoassay system. *Diabetes* 1964;13:579–584.

3. Utiger RD, Daughaday WH. Studies on human growth hormone. I. A radioimmunoassay for human growth hormone. *J Clin Invest* 1962; 41:254–261.

4. Miller GW, Nussenzweig V. A new complement function: solubilization of antigen-antibody aggregates. *Proc Natl Acad Sci U S A* 1975; 72:418–422.

5. Schifferli JA, Morris SM, Dash A, Peters DK. Complement-mediated solubilization in patients with systemic lupus erythematosus, nephritis or vasculitis. *Clin Exp Immunol* 1981;46:557–564.

6. Schifferli JA, Bartolotti SR, Peters DK. Inhibition of immune precipitation by complement. *Clin Exp Immunol* 1980;42:387–394.

7. Hong K, Takata Y, Sayama K, et al. Inhibition of immune precipitation by complement. *J Immunol* 1984;133:1464–1470.

8. Lachmann PJ, Walport MJ. Deficiency of the effector mechanisms of the immune response and autoimmunity. In: Whelan J, ed. *Autoimmunity and autoimmune disease*. Ciba Foundation Symposium #129. Chichester, UK: Whiley Ltd, 1987:149–171.

9. Moller NP, Steengaard J. Fc mediated immune precipitation. I. A new role of the Fc portion of IgG. *Immunology* 1983;38:631–640.

10. Johnson A, Harkin S, Steward MW, et al. The effects of immunoglobulin isotype and antibody affinity on complement-mediated inhibition of immune precipitation and solubilization. *Mol Immunol* 1987;24: 1211–1217.

11. Ng YC, Peters DK, Walport MJ. Monoclonal rheumatoid factor-IgG immune complexes: poor fixation of opsonic C4 and C3 despite efficient complement activation. *Arthritis Rheum* 1987;31:99–107.

12. Takahashi M, Tack BF, Nussenzweig V. Requirements for the solubilization of immune aggregates by complement: assembly of a factor B-dependent C3-convertase on the immune complexes. *J Exp Med* 1977; 145:86–100.

13. Fries LF, Gaither TA, Hammer CH, et al. C3b covalently bound to IgG demonstrates a reduced rate of inactivation by factors H and I. *J Exp Med* 1984;160:1640–1655.

14. Spath PJ, Pascual M, Meyer Hanni L, et al. Solubilization of immune precipitates by complement in the absence of properdin or factor D. *FEBS Lett* 1988;234:131–134.

15. Volanakis JE. Complement-induced solubilization of C-reactive protein-pneumococcal C-polysaccharide precipitates: evidence for covalent binding of complement proteins to C-reactive protein and to pneumococcal C-polysaccharide. *J Immunol* 1982;128:2745–2750.

16. Schifferli JA, Steiger G, Paccaud JP. Complement mediated inhibition of immune precipitation and solubilization generate different concentrations of complement anaphylatoxins (C4a, C3a, C5a). *Clin Exp Immunol* 1986;64:407–414.

17. Bull CG. The agglutination of bacteria in vivo. *J Exp Med* 1915; 22:484–491.

18. Rieckenberg H. Eine neue immuninitasreaktion bei experimenteller trypanosomen-infection: die blutpattchen-probe. *Immunitatsforsch* 1917;26:53–64.

19. Duke HL, Wallace JM. "Red-cell adhesion" in trypanosomiasis of man and animals. *Parasitology* 1930;22:414–456.

20. Kritschewsky IL, Tscherikower RS. Uber anti-korper, die microorganismen mit blutpattchen beladen (thrombozytobarinen). *Z Immunitatsforsch* 1925;42:131–149.

21. Gordon J, Whitehead HR, Wormall A. The action of ammonia on complement: the fourth component. *Biochem J* 1926;20:1028–1035.

22. Wallace JM, Wormall A. Red cell adhesion in trypanosomiasis of man and other animals. II Some experiments on the mechanism of the reaction. *Parasitology* 1931;23:346–359.

23. Brown HC, Broom JC. Studies in trypanosomiasis. II. Observations on the red cell adhesion test. *Trans R Soc Trop Med Hyg* 1938;32: 209–222.

24. Osborne TWB. *Complement or alexin*. London: Oxford University Press, 1937.

25. Ecker EE, Pillemer L. Complement. *Ann N Y Acad Sci* 1942;43:63–83.

26. Nelson RA Jr. The immune adherence phenomenon: an immunologically specific reaction between micro-organisms and erythrocytes leading to enhanced phagocytosis. *Science* 1953;118:733–737.

27. Fearon DT. Identification of the membrane glycoprotein that is the C3b receptor of the human erythrocyte, polymorphonuclear leukocyte, B lymphocyte, and monocyte. *J Exp Med* 1980;152:20–30.

28. Hebert LA, Cosio FG. The erythrocyte-immune complex-glomerulonephritis connection in man. *Kidney Int* 1987;31:877–885.

29. Walport MJ, Ross GD, Mackworth-Young C, et al. Family studies of erythrocyte complement receptor type 1 levels: reduced levels in patients with SLE are acquired, not inherited. *Clin Exp Immunol* 1985;59:547–554.

30. Wilson JG, Wong WW, Schur PH, et al. Mode of inheritance of decreased C3b receptors on erythrocytes of patients with systemic lupus erythematosus. *N Engl J Med* 1982;307:981–986.

31. Fearon DT, Collins LA. Increased expression of C3b receptors on polymorphonuclear leukocytes induced by chemotactic factors and by purification procedures. *J Immunol* 1983;130:370–375.

32. Paccaud J-P, Carpentier J-L, Schifferli JA. Direct evidence for the clustered nature of complement receptors type 1 on the erythrocyte membrane. *J Immunol* 1988;141:3889–3894.

33. Fearon DT. Cellular receptors for fragments of the third component of complement. *Immunol Today* 1984;5:105–110.

34. Wong WW. Structural and functional correlation of the human complement receptor type 1. *J Invest Dermatol* 1990;94:64S–67S.

35. Van Dyne S, Holers VM, Lublin DM, et al. The polymorphism of the C3b/C4b receptor in the normal population and in patients with systemic lupus erythematosus. *Clin Exp Immunol* 1987;68:570–579.

36. Klopstock A, Schartz J, Bleiberg Y, et al. Hereditary nature of the behaviour of erythrocytes in immune adherence-haemagglutination phenomenon. *Vox Sang* 1965;10:177–187.

37. Walport MJ, Lachmann PJ. Erythrocyte complement receptor type 1, immune complexes and the rheumatic diseases. *Arthritis Rheum* 1987;31:153–158.

38. Paccaud JP, Carpentier JL, Schifferli JA. Difference in the clustering of complement receptor type 1 (CR1) on polymorphonuclear leukocytes and erythrocytes: effect on immune adherence. *Eur J Immunol* 1990;20:283–289.

39. Paccaud JP, Schifferli JA, Baggiolini M. NAP-1/IL-8 induces up-regulation of CR1 receptors in human neutrophil leukocytes. *Biochem Biophys Res Commun* 1990;166:187–192.

40. Beynon HLC, Davies KA, Haskard DO, et al. Erythrocyte complement receptor type 1 and interactions between immune complexes, neutrophils and endothelium. *J Immunol* 1994;153:3160–3167.

41. Biozzi G, Benacerraf B, Halpern BN. Quantitative study of the granulopectic activity of the reticuloendothelial system II. *Br J Exp Pathol* 1953;34:441–457.

42. Niehaus GD, Shumacker PR, Saba TM. Reticuloendothelial clearance of blood-borne particulates: relevance to experimental lung microembolization and vascular injury. *Ann Surg* 1980;191:479–487.

43. Davies KA, Chapman PT, Norsworthy PJ, et al. Clearance pathways of immune complexes in the pig: insight into the adaptive nature of antigen clearance in humans. *J Immunol* 1995;155:5760–5768.

44. Taylor RP, Kujala G, Wilson K, et al. In vivo and in vitro studies of the binding of antibody/dsDNA immune complexes to rabbit and guinea pig platelets. *J Immunol* 1985;134:2550–2558.

45. Edberg JC, Kujala GA, Taylor RP. Rapid immune adherence reactivity of nascent, soluble antibody/DNA immune complexes in the circulation. *J Immunol* 1987;139:1240–1244.

46. Haakenstad AO, Mannik M. Saturation of the reticuloendothelial system with soluble immune complexes. *J Immunol* 1974;112:1939–1948.

47. Finbloom DS, Plotz PH. Studies of reticuloendothelial function in the mouse with model immune complexes. II. Serum clearance, tissue uptake and reticuloendothelial saturation in NZB/W mice. *J Immunol* 1979;123:1600–1603.

48. Finbloom DS, Magilavy DB, Harford JB, et al. Influence of antigen on immune complex behavior in mice. *J Clin Invest* 1981;68:214–224.

49. Cornacoff JB, Hebert LA, Smead WL, et al. Primate erythrocyte-immune complex-clearing mechanism. *J Clin Invest* 1983;71:236–247.

50. Waxman FJ, Hebert LA, Cornacoff JB, et al. Complement depletion accelerates the clearance of immune complexes from the circulation of primates. *J Clin Invest* 1984;74:1329–1340.

51. Waxman FJ, Hebert LA, Cosio FG, et al. Differential binding of immunoglobulin A and immunoglobulin G1 immune complexes to primate erythrocytes in vivo: immunoglobulin A immune complexes bind less well to erythrocytes and are preferentially deposited in glomeruli. *J Clin Invest* 1986;77:82–89.

52. Cornacoff JB, Hebert LA, Birmingham DJ, et al. Factors influencing the binding of large immune complexes primate erythrocyte CR1 receptor. *Clin Immunol Immunopathol* 1984;30:255–264.

53. Lobatto S, Daha MR, Voetman AA, et al. Clearance of soluble aggregates of immunoglobulin G in healthy volunteers and chimpanzees. *Clin Exp Immunol* 1987;68:133.

54. Schifferli JA, Ng YC, Estreicher J, et al. The clearance of tetanus toxoid/anti-tetanus toxoid immune complexes from the circulation of humans. Complement- and erythrocyte complement receptor 1-dependent mechanisms. *J Immunol* 1988;140:899–904.

55. Davies KA, Peters AM, Beynon HLC, et al. Immune complex processing in patients with systemic lupus erythematosus: in vivo imaging and clearance studies. *J Clin Invest* 1992;90:2075–2083.

56. Davies KA, Erlendsson K, Beynon HLC, et al. Splenic uptake of immune complexes in man is complement-dependent. *J Immunol* 1993;151:3866–3873.

57. Edberg JC, Kujala GA, Taylor RP. Rapid immune adherence reactivity of nascent, soluble antibody/DNA immune complexes in the circulation. *J Immunol* 1987;139:1240.

58. Davies KA, Hird V, Stewart S, et al. A study of in vivo immune complex formation and clearance in man. *J Immunol* 1990;144:4613–4620.

59. Brown DL, Lachmann PJ, Dacie JV. The in vivo behavior of complement-coated red cells: studies in C6-deficient, C3-depleted, and normal rabbits. *Clin Exp Immunol* 1970;7:401–422.

60. Atkinson JP, Frank MM. Studies on the in vivo effects of antibody: interaction of IgM antibody and complement in the immune clearance and destruction of erythrocytes in man. *J Clin Invest* 1974;54:339–348.

61. Hughes-Jones NC, Mollison PL, Mollison PN. Removal of incompatible red cells by the spleen. *Br J Haematol* 1957;3:125–133.

62. Mollison PL, Crome P, Hughes-Jones NC, et al. Rate of removal from the circulation of red cells sensitised with different amounts of antibody. *Br J Haematol* 1965;11:461–470.

63. Frank MM, Lawley TJ, Hamburger MI, et al. Immunoglobulin G Fc receptor-mediated clearance in autoimmune diseases. *Ann Intern Med* 1983;98:206–218.

64. Smedsrod B, Pertoft H, Eggertsen G, et al. Functional and morphological characterization of cultures of Kupffer cells and liver endothelial cells prepared by means of density separation in Percoll, and selective substrate adherence. *Cell Tissue Res* 1985;241:639–649.

65. Ross GD, Newman SL. Regulation of macrophage functions by complement, complement receptors, and IgG-Fc receptors. In: Bellanti JA, Herscowitz HB, eds. *The reticuloendothelial system: a comprehensive treatise,* Vol 6. New York: Plenum, 1984:173–200.

66. Unkeless JC, Fleit H, Mellman IS. Structural aspects and heterogeneity of immunoglobulin Fc receptors. *Adv Immunol* 1981;31:247–270.

67. Reist CJ, Wright JD, Labuguen RH, et al. Human IgG in immune complexes bound to human erythrocyte CR1 is recognized differently than human IgG bound to an erythrocyte surface antigen. *J Immunol Methods* 1993;163:199–208.

68. Peters AM. Splenic blood flow and blood cell kinetics. *Clin Haematol* 1983;12:421–447.

69. Weiss L. The spleen. In: Weiss L, ed. *Cell and tissue biology,* 2nd ed. Baltimore: Urban and Schwarzenberg, 1988:517.

70. Robertson DA, Bullen AW, Hall R, et al. Blood film appearances in the hyposplenism of coeliac disease. *Br J Clin Pract* 1983;37:19–22.

71. Crocker SH, Eddy DO, Obenauf RN, et al. Bacteremia: host specific lung clearance and pulmonary failure. *J Trauma* 1981;21:215–220.

72. Wessels MR, Butko P, Ma M, et al. Studies of group B streptococcal infection in mice deficient in complement component C3 or C4 demonstrate an essential role for complement in both innate and acquired immunity. *Proc Natl Acad Sci U S A* 1995;92:11490–11494.

73. Reid R, Prodeus AP, Khan W, et al. Natural antibody and complement are critical for endotoxin clearance from the circulation. *Mol Immunol* 1996;33:78(abst).

74. Lynn WA, Cohen J. Adjunctive therapy for septic shock: a review of experimental approaches. *Clin Infect Dis* 1995;20:143–158.

75. Seelen MA, Athanassiou P, Lynn WA, et al. The anti-lipid A monoclonal antibody E5 binds to rough gram-negative bacteria, fixes C3, and facilitates binding of bacterial immune complexes to both erythrocytes and monocytes. *Immunology* 1995;84:653–661.

76. Tonoli M, Davies KA, Norsworthy PJ, et al. The anti-lipid antibody HA-1A binds to rough gram-negative bacteria, fixes complement and facilitates binding to erythrocyte CR1(CD35). *Clin Exp Immunol* 1993;92:232–238.

77. Bowness P, Davies KA, Norsworthy PJ, et al. Hereditary C1q deficiency and systemic lupus erythematosus. *Q J Med* 1994;87:455–464.

78. Ruddy S. Component deficiencies. 3. The second component. *Prog Allergy* 1986;39:250–267.

79. Botto M, Fong KY, So AK, et al. Homozygous hereditary C3 deficiency due to a partial gene deletion. *Proc Natl Acad Sci U S A* 1992;89:4957–4961.

80. Botto M, Walport MJ. Hereditary deficiency of C3 in animals and humans. *Int Rev Immunol* 1993;10:37–50.

81. Vyse TJ, Spath PJ, Davies KA, et al. Hereditary complement factor I deficiency. *Q J Med* 1994;87:385–401.

82. Fielder AH, Walport MJ, Batchelor JR, et al. Family study of the major histocompatibility complex in patients with systemic lupus erythematosus: importance of null alleles of C4A and C4B in determining disease susceptibility. *Br Med J Clin Res* 1983;286:425–428.

83. Christiansen FT, Dawkins RL, Uko G, et al. Complement allotyping in SLE: association with C4A null. *Aust N Z J Med* 1983;13:483–488.

84. Howard PF, Hochberg MC, Bias WB, et al. Relationship between C4 null genes, HLA-D region antigens, and genetic susceptibility to systemic lupus erythematosus in Caucasian and black americans. *Am J Med* 1986;81:187–193.

85. Hartung K, Baur MP, Coldewey R, et al. Major histocompatibility complex haplotypes and complement C4 alleles in systemic lupus erythematosus: results of a multicenter study. *J Clin Invest* 1992;90:1346–1351.

86. Davies EJ, Snowden N, Hillarby MC, et al. Mannose-binding protein gene polymorphism in systemic lupus erythematosus. *Arthritis Rheum* 1995;38:110–114.

87. Donaldson VH, Hess EV, McAdams AJ. Lupus-erythematosus-like disease in three unrelated women with hereditary angioneurotic edema [Letter]. *Ann Intern Med* 1977;86:312–313.

88. Brickman CM, Tsokos GC, Balow JE, et al. Immunoregulatory disorders associated with hereditary angioedema. I. Clinical manifestations of autoimmune disease. *J Allergy Clin Immunol* 1986;77:749–757.

89. Brickman CM, Tsokos GC, Chused TM, et al. Immunoregulatory disorders associated with hereditary angioedema. II. Serologic and cellular abnormalities. *J Allergy Clin Immunol* 1986;77:758–767.

90. Walport MJ, Davies KA, Botto M, et al. C3 nephritic factor and SLE. *Q J Med* 1994;87:609–615.

91. Inai S, Akagaki Y, Moriyama T, et al. Inherited deficiencies of the late-acting complement components other than C9 found among healthy blood donors. *Int Arch Allergy Appl Immunol* 1989;90:274–279.

92. Hassig A, Borel JF, Ammann P, et al. Essentielle hypokomplementamie. *Pathol Microbiol* 1964;27:542.

93. Cork CL, Morris JM, Olson JL, et al. Membranoproliferative glomerulonephritis in dogs with a genetically determined deficiency of the third component of complement. *Clin Immunol Immunopathol* 1991;60:455–470.

94. Hogasen K, Jansen JH, Mollnes TE, et al. Hereditary porcine membranoproliferative glomerulonephritis type II is caused by factor H deficiency. *J Clin Invest* 1995;95:1054–1061.

95. Fischer MB, Ma M, Goerg S, et al. Regulation of the B cell response to T-dependent antigens by classical pathway complement. *J Immunol* 1996;157:549–556.

96. Matsumoto M, Fukada W, Goellner J, et al. Generation and characterization of mice deficient for factor B. *Mol Immunol* 1996;33:63–60.

97. Ahearn JM, Fischer MB, Croix D, et al. Disruption of the Cr2 locus results in a reduction in B-1a cells and in an impaired B cell response to T-dependent antigens. *Immunity* 1996;4:251–262.

98. Botto M, Dell'Agnola C, Bygrave AE, et al. Homozygous C1q deficiency causes glomerulonephritis associated with multiple apoptotic bodies. *Nat Genet* 1998;19:56–59.

99. Takeuchi Y, Cosset FL, Lachmann PJ, et al. Type C retrovirus inactivation by human complement is determined by both the viral genome and the producer cell. *J Virol* 1994;68:8001–8007.

100. Rother RP, Fodor WL, Springhorn JP, et al. A novel mechanism of retrovirus inactivation in human serum mediated by anti-alpha-galactosyl natural antibody. *J Exp Med* 1995;182:1345–1355.

101. Cornillet P, Philbert F, Kazatchkine MD, et al. Genomic determination of the CR1 (CD35) density polymorphism on erythrocytes using polymerase chain reaction amplification and HindIII restriction enzyme digestion. *J Immunol Methods* 1991;136:193–197.

102. Moldenhauer F, David J, Fielder AHL, et al. Inherited deficiency of erythrocyte complement receptor type 1 does not cause susceptibility to systemic lupus erythematosus. *Arthritis Rheum* 1987;30:961–966.

103. Frank MM, Hamburger MI, Lawley TJ, et al. Defective reticuloendothelial system Fc-receptor function in systemic lupus erythematosus. *N Engl J Med* 1979;300:518–523.

104. Hamburger MI, Lawley TJ, Kimberly RP, et al. A serial study of splenic reticuloendothelial system Fc-receptor function in systemic lupus erythematosus. *Arthritis Rheum* 1982;25:48.

105. Salmon JE, Brogle NL, Edberg JC, et al. Allelic polymorphisms of human Fcγ receptor IIA and Fcγ receptor IIIB: independent mechanisms for differences in human phagocyte function. *J Clin Invest* 1992;89:1274–1281.

106. Salmon JE, Millard S, Schachter LA, et al. Fcγ RIIA alleles are heritable risk factors for lupus nephritis in African Americans. *J Clin Invest* 1996;97:1348–1354.

107. Duits AJ, Bootsma H, Derksen RHWM, et al. Skewed distribution of IgG Fcγ receptor IIa is associated with renal disease in systemic lupus erythematosus patients. *Arthritis Rheum* 1995;39:1832–1836.

108. Botto M, Theodoridis E, Thompson EM, et al. Fcγ RIIa polymorphism in systemic lupus erythematosus (SLE): no association with disease. *Clin Exp Immunol* 1996;104:264–268.

109. Halma C, Breedveld FC, Daha MR, et al. Elimination of soluble ¹²³I-labeled aggregates of IgG in patients with systemic lupus erythematosus: effect of serum IgG and numbers of erythrocyte complement receptor type 1. *Arthritis Rheum* 1991;34:442–452.

110. Halma C, Daha MR, Camps JA, et al. Deficiency of complement component C3 is associated with accelerated removal of soluble ¹²³I-labelled aggregates of IgG from the circulation. *Clin Exp Immunol* 1992;90:394–400.

111. Cochrane CJ. Mediation of immunologic glomerular injury. *Transplant Proc* 1969;1:949–956.

112. Henson PM, Cochrane CG. The effects of complement depletion on experimental tissue injury. *Ann N Y Acad Sci* 1975;256:426–440.

113. Sylvestre DL, Ravetch JV. Fc receptors initiate the Arthus reaction: redefining the inflammatory cascade. *Science* 1994;265:1095–1098.

114. Hazenbos WLW, Gessner JE, Hofhuis FMA, et al. Impaired IgG dependent anaphylaxis and Arthus reaction in Fc gamma RIII (CD16) deficient mice. *Immunity* 1996;5:181–188.

115. Ben-Efraim S, Cinader B. The role of complement in the passive cutaneous reaction of mice. *J Exp Med* 1964;120:925–942.

116. Larsen GL, Mitchell BC, Henson PM. The pulmonary response of C5 sufficient and deficient mice to immune complexes. *Am Rev Respir Dis* 1981;123:434–439.

117. Zhang Y, Ramos BF, Jakschik BA. Augmentation of reverse Arthus reaction by mast cells in mice. *J Clin Invest* 1991;88:841–846.

118. Sylvestre DL, Ravetch JV. A dominant role for mast cell Fc receptors in the Arthus reaction. *Immunity* 1996;5:387–390.

119. Bozic CR, Lu B, Hopken UE, et al. Neurogenic amplification of immune complex inflammation. *Science* 1996;273:1722–1725.

120. Rodwell JD, Tang LH, Schumaker VN. Antigen valence and Fc-localised secondary forces in antibody precipitation. *Mol Immunol* 1980;17:1591–1597.

121. Wilson CB, Dixon FJ. Renal response to immunological injury. In: Brenner BM, Rector FC, eds. *The kidney*, 4th ed. Philadelphia: WB Saunders, 1986:800–890.

122. Ng YC. C3 nephritic factor and membranoproliferative glomerulonephritis. In: Pusey CD, ed. Immunology of renal diseases. Dordrecht/Boston/London: Kluwer Academic Publishers, 1991:215–227.

123. Verroust PJ, Wilson CB, Dixon FJ. Lack of nephritogenicity of systemic activation of the alternative complement pathway. *Kidney Int* 1974;6:157–169.

124. Simpson IJ, Moran J, Evans DJ, et al. Prolonged complement activation in mice. *Kidney Int* 1978;13:467–471.

125. Baker PJ, Adler S, Yang Y, et al. Complement activation by heat-killed human kidney cells: formation, activity and stabilization of cell-bound C3 convertases. *J Immunol* 1984;133:877–881.

126. Chesney RW, Oregan S, Guyda HJ, et al. Candida endocrinopathy syndrome with membranoproliferative glomerulonephritis: demonstration of glomerular candida antigen. *Clin Nephrol* 1976;5:232–238.

127. Wisnieski JJ, Baer AN, Christensen J, et al. Hypocomplementemic urticarial vasculitis syndrome: clinical and serologic findings in 18 patients. *Medicine (Baltimore)* 1995;74:24–41.

128. Wisnieski JJ, Jones SM. Comparison of autoantibodies to the collagen-like region of C1q in hypocomplementaemic urticarial vasculitis syndrome and systemic lupus erythematosus. *J Immunol* 1992;148:1396–1403.

129. Uwatoko S, Gauthier VJ, Mannik M. Autoantibodies to the collagen-like region of C1q deposit in glomeruli via C1q immune deposits. *Clin Immunol Immunopathol* 1991;61:268–273.

130. Halbwachs L, Leveille M, Lesavre P, et al. Nephritic factor of the classical pathway of complement: immunoglobulin autoantibody directed against the classical pathway C3 convertase enzyme. *J Clin Invest* 1980;65:1249–1256.

131. Daha MR, Hazavoet HM, van Es LA, et al. Stabilization of the classical pathway convertase C42 by a factor (F-42) isolated from sera of patients with SLE. *Immunology* 1980;40:417–424.

132. Appel GB, Silva FG, Pirani CL. Renal involvement in systemic lupus erythematosus (SLE): a study of 56 patients emphasising histologic classification. *Medicine* 1978;57:371–410.

133. Mannik M. Mechanisms of tissue deposition of immune complexes. *J Rheumatol* 1987;14:35–42.

134. Van Damme BJC, Fleuren GJ, Bakker WW, et al. Experimental glomerulonephritis in the rat induced by antibodies to tubular antigens. IV. Fixed glomerular antigens in the pathogenesis of heterologous immune complex glomerulonephritis. *Lab Invest* 1978;38:502–510.

135. Salant DJ, Belok S, Madaio MP, et al. A new role for complement in experimental membranous nephropathy in rats. *J Clin Invest* 1980;66:1339–1350.

136. Kerjaschki D, Farquar MG. Immunocytochemical localisation of the Heymann nephritis antigen (GP330) in glomerular epithelial cells of normal Lewis rats. *J Exp Med* 1983;157:667–685.

137. Camussi G, Brentjens JR, Noble B. Antibody-induced redistribution of Heymann's antigen on the surface of cultured glomerular visceral epithelial cells: possible role in the pathogenesis of Heymann glomerular nephritis. *J Immunol* 1985;135:2409–2416.

138. Shoenfeld Y, Rauch J, Massicotte H, et al. Polyspecificity of monoclonal lupus autoantibodies produced by human-human hybridomas. *N Engl J Med* 1983;308:414–420.

139. Madaio MP, Carlson J, Cataldo J, et al. Murine monoclonal anti-DNA antibodies bind directly to glomerular antigens and form immune deposits. *J Immunol* 1987;138:2883–2889.

140. Couser WG, Salant DJ. In-situ immune complex formation and glomerular injury. *Kidney Int* 1980;17:1–13.

141. Agodoa LYC, Gauthier VJ, Mannik M. Precipitating antigen-antibody systems are required for the formation of sub-epithelial electron dense immune deposits in rat glomeruli. *J Exp Med* 1983;158:1259–1271.

142. Izui S, Lambert PH, Miescher PA. In vitro demonstration of a particular affinity of glomerular basement membrane and collagen for DNA: a possible basis for a local formation of DNA-anti-DNA complexes in systemic lupus erythematosus. *J Exp Med* 1976;144:428–443.

143. Ebling F, Hahn BH. Restricted subpopulations of DNA antibodies in kidneys of mice with systemic lupus: comparison of antibodies in serum and renal eluates. *Arthritis Rheum* 1980;23:392–403.

144. Dang H, Harbeck RJ. Comparison of anti-DNA antibodies from serum and kidney eluates of NZB X NZW F1 mice. *J Clin Lab Immunol* 1982;9:139–145.

145. Couser WG, Salant DJ. Immunopathogenesis of glomerular capillary wall injury in nephrotic states. *Contemp Iss Nephrol* 1982;9:47–83.

146. Mauer SM, Sutherland DER, Howard RJ. The glomerular mesangium. III. Acute immune mesangial injury: a new model of glomerulonephritis. *J Exp Med* 1973;137:553–570.

147. Yamamoto T, Wilson CB. Antibody-induced mesangial damage: the model, functional alterations and effects of complement. *Kidney Int* 1986;29:296(abst).

148. Matsuo S, Caldwell P, Brentjens J, et al. Nephrotoxic serum glomerulonephritis induced in the rabbit by anti-endothelial cell antibodies. *Kidney Int* 1985;27:217(abst).

149. Brouet JC. Cryoglobulinaemias. *Presse Med* 1983;12:2991–2996.

150. Pawlotsky JM, Dhumeaux D, Bagot M. Hepatitis C virus in dermatology: a review. *Arch Dermatol* 1995;131:1185–1193.

151. Dupin N, Chosidow O, Lunel F, et al. Essential mixed cryoglobulinemia: a comparative study of dermatologic manifestations in patients infected or noninfected with hepatitis C virus. *Arch Dermatol* 1995;131:1124–1127.

152. Cacoub P, Fabiani FL, Musset L, et al. Mixed cryoglobulinemia and hepatitis C virus. *Am J Med* 1994;96:124–132.

153. Galli M, Monti G, Invernizzi F, et al. Hepatitis B virus-related markers in secondary and in essential mixed cryoglobulinemias: a multicentric study of 596 cases. The Italian Group for the Study of Cryoglobulinemias (GISC). *Ann Ital Med Int* 1992;7:209–214.

154. Wong VS, Egner W, Elsey T, et al. Incidence, character and clinical relevance of mixed cryoglobulinaemia in patients with chronic hepatitis C virus infection. *Clin Exp Immunol* 1996;104:25–31.

155. Tanaka K, Aiyama T, Imai J, et al. Serum cryoglobulin and chronic hepatitis C virus disease among Japanese patients. *Am J Gastroenterol* 1995;90:1847–1852.

156. Maisch B. Autoreactive mechanisms in infective endocarditis. *Springer Semin Immunopathol* 1989;11:439–456.

157. Petersdorf RG. Immune complexes in infective endocarditis [Editorial]. *N Engl J Med* 1976;295:1534–1535.

158. McKenzie PE, Hawke D, Woodroffe AJ, et al. Serum and tissue immune complexes in infective endocarditis. *J Clin Lab Immunol* 1980;4:125–132.

159. Landoy Z, West TE, Vladutiu AO, et al. Evaluation of a Cordia-IC enzyme-linked immunosorbent assay kit for the detection of circulating immune complexes. *J Clin Microbiol* 1985;22:279–282.

160. Williams RC Jr, Kilpatrick K. Immunofluorescence studies of cardiac valves in infective endocarditis. *Arch Intern Med* 1985;145:297–300.

161. Maisch B, Mayer E, Schubert U, et al. Immune reactions in infective endocarditis. II. Relevance of circulating immune complexes, serum inhibition factors, lymphocytotoxic reactions, and antibody-dependent cellular cytotoxicity against cardiac target cells. *Am Heart J* 1983; 106:338–344.

162. Burton Kee J, Morgan Capner P, Mowbray JF. Nature of circulating immune complexes in infective endocarditis. *J Clin Pathol* 1980;33: 653–659.

163. Weetman AP, Matthews N, O'Hara SP, et al. Meningococcal endocarditis with profound acquired hypocomplementaemia. *J Infect* 1985;10:51–56.

164. Kerr MA, Wilton E, Naama JK, et al. Circulating immune complexes associated with decreased complement-mediated inhibition of immune precipitation in sera from patients with bacterial endocarditis. *Clin Exp Immunol* 1986;63:359–366.

165. Abramson S, Belmont HM, Hopkins P, et al. Complement activation and vascular injury in systemic lupus erythematosus. *J Rheumatol* 1987;14(Suppl 13):43–46.

166. Mason JC, Haskard DO. The clinical importance of leukocyte and endothelial cell adhesion molecules in inflammation. *Vasc Med Rev* 1994;5:249–275.

167. Lewis SL, Van Epps DE, Chenoweth DE. C5a receptor modulation on neutrophils and monocytes from chronic hemodialysis and peritoneal dialysis patients. *Clin Nephrol* 1986;26:37–44.

168. Hunder CG, Mullen BJ, McDuffie FC. Complement in pericardial fluid of lupus erythematosus: studies of two patients. *Ann Intern Med* 1974;80:453–458.

169. Dubois EL. *Lupus erythematosus: a review of the current status of discoid and systemic lupus erythematosus and their variants.* Los Angeles: University of Southern California Press, 1974.

170. Goldenberg DL, Leff G, Grayzel AI. Pericardial tamponade in systemic lupus erythematosus: with absent hemolytic complement activity in pericardial fluid. *N Y State J Med* 1975;75:910–912.

171. Michet CJ, Hunder CG: Pericarditis. In: Ansell BM, Simkin PA, eds. *The heart and rheumatic disease.* Cornwall: Butterworths International Medical Reviews—Rheumatology, 1984:1–26.

172. Shapiro RF, Gamble CN, Wisner KB. Immunopathogenesis of Libman Sacks endocarditis: assessment by light and immunofluorescent microscopy in two patients. *Ann Rheum Dis* 1977;36:508–515.

173. Hardin NH, Minnick CR, Murphy GE. Experimental induction of atheroarteriosclerosis by the synergy of allergic injury to arteries and lipid-rich diet. *Am J Pathol* 1973;73:301–326.

174. Bennet RM: Myocardial involvement. In: Ansell BM, Simkin PA, eds. *The heart and rheumatic diseases.* Cornwall: Butterworths International Medical Reviews—Rheumatology 2, 1984:27–64.

175. Inoue T, Kanayana Y, Ohe A. Immunopathologic studies of pneumonitis in systemic lupus erythematosus. *Ann Intern Med* 1979; 91:30–34.

176. Pertschuk LP, Moccia LF, Rosen Y. Acute pulmonary complications in systemic lupus erythematosus: immunofluorescence and light microscopic study. *Am J Clin Pathol* 1977;68:553–557.

177. Churg A, Franklin W, Chan KL. Pulmonary haemorrhage and immune-complex deposition in the lung: complications in a patient with systemic lupus erythematosus. *Arch Pathol Lab Med* 1980; 104:388–391.

178. Eisenberg H, Dubois EL, Sherwin RP. Diffuse interstitial lung disease in systemic lupus erythematosus. *Ann Intern Med* 1973;79:37–45.

179. Castadena S, Herrero-Beaumont G, Abuad JM: Pulmonary hemorrhage in lupus erythematosus without evidence of an immunologic cause. *Arch Intern Med* 1985;145:2128–2129.

180. Desnoyers MR, Bernstein S, Cooper AG. Pulmonary hemorrhage in lupus erythematosus without evidence of an immunologic cause. *Arch Intern Med* 1984;144:1398–1400.

181. Marino CT, Pertschuk LP. Pulmonary hemorrhage in systemic lupus erythematosus. *Arch Intern Med* 1981;141:201–203.

182. Natali PG, Tan EM. Experimental skin lesions in mice resembling systemic lupus erythematosus. *Arthritis Rheum* 1973;16:579–589.

183. Joselow SA, Gown A, Mannik M: Cutaneous deposition of immune complexes in chronic serum sickness of mice induced with cationised or unaltered antigen. *J Invest Dermatol* 1985;85:559–563.

184. Landry M, Sams WM. Systemic lupus erythematosus: studies of the antibodies bound to skin. *J Clin Invest* 1973;52:1871–1880.

185. McCune WJ, Golbus J. Neuropsychiatric lupus. *Rheum Dis Clin North Am* 1988;14:149–167.

186. Harris EN, Boey ML, Mackworth-Young CG. Anticardiolipin antibodies: detection by radioimmunoassay and association with thrombosis in systemic lupus erythematosus. *Lancet* 1983;8361:1211–1214.

187. Boyer RS, Sun NCJ, Verity A. Immunoperoxidase staining of the choroid plexus in systemic lupus erythematosus. *J Rheumatol* 1980;7:645–650.

188. Lambert P, Garret R, Lampert A. Ferritin immune complexes in the choroid plexus. *Acta Neuropathol* 1977;38:83.

189. Lampert PW, Oldstone MBA. Host immunoglobulin G and complement deposits in the choroid plexus during spontaneous immune complex disease. *Science* 1973;180:408.

190. Hadler NM, Gerwin RD, Frank MM, et al. The fourth component of complement in the cerebrospinal fluid in systemic lupus erythematosus. *Arthritis Rheum* 1973;16:507–521.

191. Petz LD, Sharp GC, Cooper NR. Serum and cerebrospinal fluid complement and serum autoantibodies in systemic lupus erythematosus. *Medicine* 1971;50:259.

192. Sanders ME, Alexander EL, Koski CL. Detection of activated terminal complement (C5b-9) in cerebrospinal fluid from patients with central nervous system involvement of primary Sjögren's syndrome or systemic lupus erythematosus. *J Immunol* 1987;138:2095–2099.

193. Seibold JR, Buckingham RB, Medsger TA. Cerebrospinal fluid immune complexes in systemic lupus erythematosus involving the central nervous system. *Semin Arthritis Rheum* 1982;12:68–76.

194. Keefe EB, Bardana EJ, Harbeck RJ. Lupus meningitis: antibody to deoxyribonucleic acid (DNA) and DNA anti-DNA complexes in cerebrospinal fluid. *Ann Intern Med* 1974;80:58–60.

*Textbook of the Autoimmune Diseases,*
Edited by R. G. Lahita, N. Chiorazzi, and W. H. Reeves,
Lippincott Williams & Wilkins, Philadelphia © 2000.

# CHAPTER 12

# Molecular Mimicry

Lori J. Albert, Yi-Xue Zhao, and Robert D. Inman

---

Autoimmune disease occurs when a specific immune response is mounted against self. Autoimmune diseases are characterized by the presence of self-reactive T cells and antibodies against self antigens, reflecting a loss of tolerance to self that results in organ injury and disease. There are important unresolved issues in understanding the origins of autoimmunity: how tolerance is broken, how autoreactive T and B cells arise, and what determines target organ specificity. Most elusive of all is the nature of the inciting event. In recent years, a multifactorial view of autoimmunity has become appreciated by investigators in this field. Many of these diseases have a clear association with certain major histocompatibility complex (MHC) haplotypes as well as other genetic factors. A persistent theme in understanding autoimmunity, however, has been the effort to find a link between autoimmune diseases and infection as the inciting event. Since it was first recognized that acute rheumatic fever (ARF) was initiated by a streptococcal infection three decades ago, there have been many theoretical and experimental arguments supporting infection as the triggering event in autoimmune disease.

A current working model for the pathogenesis of autoimmune disease has evolved, in part, from the idea that an infectious organism can be responsible for the disease. The susceptible person acquires an infection, and immunogenic peptides derived from the pathogen are bound by the host MHC and presented to T cells. However, if the epitopes that the infectious agent expresses are immunologically similar to host determinants, but still possess enough minor antigenic differences to induce an immune response, tolerance to self may be broken, and the pathogen-specific response generated

will cross-react with self antigens (Fig. 12.1). This theory has been called *molecular mimicry.*

The term molecular mimicry was originally used in 1964 by Damian (1), who suggested that some protein antigens from parasites and host share sufficient structural homology that immunoreactive T and B cells would not be elicited. The mimicry concept was also used by Snell in 1968 to explain persistent viral infection (2). He proposed that viruses encode antigens similar enough to host MHC that the host effectively regards an infecting virus as "self" and will not mount an immune response, thus allowing the virus to persist. It is interesting to observe that both tolerance and aberrant autoimmunity have been proposed as the logical consequence of molecular mimicry.

In this chapter, we examine the evidence for molecular mimicry as a valid paradigm for the development of autoimmune disease. The first section of this chapter provides an overview of the basic elements of the molecular mimicry hypothesis: tolerance induction in the host and the survival of autoreactive T and B lymphocytes, mechanisms by which microbial mimics of host epitopes might break tolerance, and a conceptual framework for evaluating the evidence for molecular mimicry in disease pathogenesis. The next section addresses molecular mimicry as a mechanism to explain the appearance of autoimmune phenomena that follow an infection with an identified organism. This discussion provides clinical experience relevant to the argument that mimicry by infectious organisms plays a role in the development of autoimmune disease. Evidence for mimicry is taken from examples of bacterial, viral, and parasitic infections that result in autoimmune sequelae. In the final section, the hypothesis that autoimmune diseases are initiated by infectious organisms through a mechanism involving molecular mimicry is examined in the context of specific autoimmune diseases. The evidence for putative pathogens and the experimental and clinical support for the proposed mimicry are examined for diabetes mellitus, rheumatoid arthritis (RA), multiple sclerosis (MS), and the spondyloarthropathies (SpA).

L. J. Albert: Department of Medicine, University of Toronto, Toronto, Ontario M5G 2C4, Canada; Department of Medicine, Division of Rheumatology, University Health Network, Toronto Western Hospital, Toronto, Ontario M5T 2S8, Canada.

Y.-X. Zhao: POC.KIT Corporation, Toronto, Ontario M9W 5T4, Canada.

R. D. Inman: Departments of Medicine and Immunology, University of Toronto, Toronto, Ontario M5G 2C4, Canada; Arthritis Center of Excellence, Toronto Western Hospital, Toronto, Ontario M5T 2S8, Canada.

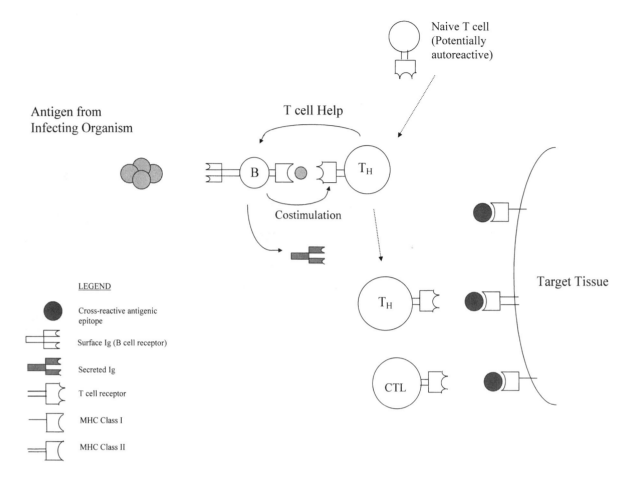

**FIG. 12.1.** The molecular mimicry hypothesis. Foreign, microbial agents (bacteria, virus, nematode) gain access to the host by way of mucous membranes, gut, or circulation. An immune response is initiated against these pathogens after processing and presentation of multiple epitopes by antigen-presenting cells, including B cells. If these epitopes bear similarities to host epitopes (*shaded circles in diagram*), the immune response is directed against the host as well. This is mediated through "ignorant" autoreactive T and B cells, which become activated on exposure to the mimicking antigenic epitopes. B cells present these mimicking epitopes in the context of class II major histocompatibility complex. The complex is recognized by T helper (*T_H*) cells, which become activated in the presence of appropriate costimulatory signals. Tissue damage is mediated by the local elaboration of cytokines and recruitment of other inflammatory cells. Cross-reactive antibody production by B cells requires reciprocal help from $T_H$ cells. Cytotoxic T lymphocytes (*CTL*) recognize mimicked antigens in the context of class I MHC on the surface of target tissues and directly induce tissue damage. Previously unrecognized, or "cryptic," epitopes may be released after tissue damage, leading to amplification of this response.

## OVERVIEW

### Specificity and Degeneracy in Immune Recognition

Antigen-presenting cells (APC) constantly sample their environment and do not distinguish between self and foreign antigens. In fact, a significant proportion of peptides eluted from MHC molecules are self peptides (3). The responsibility of discriminating self from nonself falls to the T cells (4). The fundamental basis for productive T-cell responses, T-cell tolerance, or T-cell death is the recognition by the T-cell antigen receptor (TCR) of an antigenic peptide, 8 to 15 amino acids in length, bound to an MHC molecule on the surface of the APC (reviewed in 5; 6,7). This trimolecular recognition event must have the flexibility to allow recognition of the universe of foreign antigens, while retaining enough specificity to avoid immunity against self.

The crystallographic characterization of the MHC–peptide complex has revealed that antigenic peptides bind in a cleft between two α-helices on the membrane-distal surface of both MHC class I and II molecules (8,9). Analysis of peptides eluted from MHC molecules has revealed that hundreds of different peptides can be bound by a single MHC molecule (10). The main requirement for binding is the presence of identical or similar amino acid residues at several specific positions along the peptide sequence (11,12). The side chains of these residues insert into "pockets" in the MHC molecule that are lined by amino acids that vary between the different MHC alleles, thus supporting the notion of an allele-specific "motif" (13,14). These "anchor" residues, however, need not occur in exactly the same location in all the peptides binding to a particular MHC because peptides are permitted to kink to allow the correct residues to be inserted into the pockets in the groove (15). Thus, this flexibility in binding characteristics creates a "promiscuous" MHC–peptide array of relationships.

There is also flexibility in the T-cell recognition of these peptide antigens (reviewed in 4). There is evidence that a range of nonhomologous peptides are able to stimulate a single TCR. The response of the T cell can vary between activation or anergy, depending on the ligand. The ligands thus recognized can be functionally classified as agonists, partial agonists, and antagonists. This has important implications for both tolerance induction and potential cross-reactive immune responses.

Antibody responses are thought to be capable of recognizing the universe of peptides derived from all proteins. This necessitates an extensive antibody repertoire, which is generated by somatic recombination of immunoglobulin variable-region genes. Diversity is further enhanced by a process of somatic hypermutation in B cells (reviewed in 5; 16). There is thus generated an extensive range of recognition of antigens. To some extent, antibody specificity involves T-cell specificity, by the requirement of helper T cells for most productive B-cell responses to antigen (reviewed in 17). However, the broad diversity in the repertoire of antigen receptors for both B cells and T cells, while conferring defense mechanisms against exogenous antigens, also sets the stage for autoreactivity. This risk is minimized through negative selection and the induction of tolerance.

## Tolerance Induction

T-cell tolerance induction occurs mainly through selection in the thymus. Immature pre–T cells arising from the bone marrow mature in the thymus by the sequential rearrangement of constant and variable gene segments that encode the TCR, such that each cell expresses a unique, rearranged TCR-$\alpha\beta$ heterodimer. Evidence to date suggests that the affinity of the newly expressed TCR for a peptide–MHC complex expressed on the surrounding APCs determines the ultimate fate of the thymocyte (18). Those thymocytes expressing a TCR with low avidity for a self peptide–MHC complex are positively selected and are ultimately allowed to differentiate into a mature single-positive T cell, either CD4$^+$ or CD8$^+$. Thymocytes expressing TCR that have no avidity for self peptide–MHC complexes do not survive and die locally by apoptosis. This process of positive selection ensures that the T-cell repertoire is composed of cells that recognize peptides in the context of host MHC. The population of positively selected thymocytes includes some cells that have a relatively strong avidity for self peptide–MHC complexes. This strong signal drives these cells to clonal deletion, likely through an apoptotic fate similar to that of those thymocytes with no recognition signal. Thus, potentially autoreactive cells are negatively selected and deleted from the repertoire (18).

B-lymphocyte tolerance to self antigens occurs centrally, in the bone marrow, primarily through clonal deletion of immature cells that express high-affinity immunoglobulin M (IgM) receptors for autoantigens (19). Unlike T cells, however, there is a 1- to 2-day delay after antigen recognition, during which secondary gene rearrangements can replace self-reactive light chains with other specificities, which is called *receptor editing.*

Although more than 95% of developing T cells die during thymic maturation, some autoreactive T cells escape into the peripheral T-cell pool (20,21). Similarly, self-reactive B-cell clones can escape the bone marrow (19). This is the result of selection processes that must strike a balance between comprehensive recognition of the universe of pathogen-derived epitopes and elimination of T-cell and B-cell receptors that react with self antigens. However, peripheral mechanisms of tolerization are operative for both T and B cells. Autoreactive T cells may escape the thymus because certain tissue antigens may not be represented in the thymus during selection or because the TCR has low avidity for the antigen. To deal with these survivors, at least two mechanisms of tolerance are available (reviewed in 22). The first is clonal elimination, which is determined by the amount of antigen and the frequency of antigen-specific T cells; the second is induction of anergy, which occurs when an antigen is presented in the absence of adequate costimulatory signals. Autoreactive B cells can also be eliminated or anergized in peripheral lymphoid tissue by several mechanisms that depend on the avidity of antigen binding to B-cell receptors and whether antigen is soluble or immobilized on follicular dendritic cells (19).

Some T cells, however, are not deleted in the thymus nor tolerized extrathymically because the self antigens that they recognize are normally not presented at threshold levels for recognition or are not immediately accessible to circulating T cells. These T cells are considered to be "ignorant" of their cognate antigens, and the antigens for which they are specific are considered "cryptic" epitopes (23; reviewed in 19). This point is illustrated by the lymphocytic choriomeningitis virus–rat insulin promotor (LCMV-RIP) transgenic mouse model (20,24). In this model, expression of the glycoprotein or nucleoprotein of LCMV is directed to pancreatic $\beta$ cells of host mice by use of the RIP in the transgene construct. Viral proteins thus become self proteins. If mature mice are infected with LCMV, this leads to the development of an antiviral CD8$^+$ cytotoxic T-cell response and the development of diabetes. Thus, potentially autoreactive T cells ignore their cognate antigen expressed in the pancreatic $\beta$ cells until primed through systemic infection with LCMV.

B cells, like T cells, are not tolerized to cryptic epitopes. Another source of autoreactive B cells are those anergic B cells released from bone marrow. These lymphocytes are thought to have an antigen receptor that has been "retuned," making them more difficult to reactivate than naive B cells, particularly by T-cell–independent routes (19). Data suggest, however, that anergic B cells retain the ability to be reactivated by strong cross-linking of antigen receptors (25).

## Infection and Breaking of Tolerance

The development of autoimmunity implies that ignorant or anergic populations of autoreactive lymphocytes have become activated. This could be the result of cryptic epitopes being revealed or the priming of autoreactive cells by other stimuli. Can infection lead to the activation of autoreactive lymphocytes? There are some examples of human disease in which a prior infection with a specific pathogen leads to important nonseptic sequelae. As discussed later, in rheumatic fever and reactive arthritis, immune-mediated chronic inflammation is initiated by a bacterial infection. There are also some supportive experimental models. Mice transgenic for a TCR specific for myelin basic protein (an autoantigen implicated in MS) develop the inflammatory, demyelinating condition of experimental allergic encephalomyelitis (EAE) spontaneously under normal housing conditions. They remain healthy, however, if housed in pathogen-free conditions (26). A similar situation was observed for the HLA-B27 transgenic rat model that shows decreased frequency of spontaneous arthropathy and other features of Reiter's syndrome under pathogen-free housing conditions (27). These models indicate that exposure to microbial pathogens somehow figures importantly in the development of autoimmunity. There is also evidence that systemic infection may be sufficient to activate preexisting self-reactive T cells (28).

How might infection provide the stimulus for the breaking of tolerance? Although molecular mimicry is the primary focus of this review, there are several other potential mechanisms (5). Infection may result in tissue damage and thus expose T cells to previously cryptic antigens. A second possibility is that local inflammation may stimulate the expression of MHC molecules and costimulatory molecules on tissue cells, thus allowing T-cell activation and an immune response to proceed. A third possibility is that infectious agents may bind to self proteins and thus act as a carrier to allow B cells that express an autoreactive receptor to receive inappropriate T-cell help. A fourth mechanism invokes bacterial superantigens, which could directly stimulate polyclonal T-cell activation and overcome clonal anergy or ignorance, allowing autoreactive T cells to emerge. It has also been suggested that exposure to bacterial antigens may drive the development of a pathogenic $T_H1$ response (29). These various pathways do not implicate molecular mimicry per se, but they should be recognized as other ways in which infection could potentially disrupt immunologic homeostasis in the periphery and lead to autoimmunity.

## Infection and Molecular Mimicry

The key to the molecular mimicry hypothesis is that the immune system sees homology between determinants in infecting pathogens and host tissues. Thus, a first order of evidence to support infection producing autoimmune disease must be the demonstration of homology. Because of the promiscuous nature of immune recognition discussed previously, knowledge of sequence homology alone is not sufficient to predict T-cell reactivity. Furthermore, Roudier et al. (30) have made some pertinent calculations regarding the likelihood of finding perfect matches for random peptides in protein databases. They calculated that on the basis of chance alone, one can expect to find any five–amino acid motif on up to 10 proteins in the computer sequence databases. The shorter the homologous sequence, the greater the likelihood of perfect matches occurring by chance alone. Thus, to support a pathogenic role for these homologous sequences, there must be some evidence of functional cross-reactivity.

There is abundant evidence for shared epitopes based on cross-reactivity of antibodies between microbial antigens and host epitopes (31,32; *vide infra*). As discussed later, such evidence has been generated by many investigators using both polyclonal and monoclonal antibodies, in the cases of both autoimmune sequelae of infection and autoimmune disease, implicating a putative pathogen. This type of approach is usually based on a presupposition of clinical evidence for a connection between a particular pathogen and a disease process. This often arises from temporal or geographic clustering of cases of infection and autoimmunity.

Identifying mimicry of T-cell epitopes may prove to be more enlightening for understanding the induction of autoimmune diseases than for examining cross-reacting antibodies alone. Studies on autoimmune ovarian disease in mice have highlighted the importance of T-cell help in driving the autoantibody response (reviewed in 33). Furthermore, immune destruction mediated directly by activated autoreactive T cells is crucial to the pathogenesis of many autoimmune diseases. This is interesting in view of the facts that relatively fewer autoreactive T cells escape the thymus than do B cells from the bone marrow (19), that T-cell diversity is not influenced by postselective receptor mutation, and that T cells recognize only peptide epitopes, whereas B cells recognize a much broader spectrum of antigens.

The approach to finding foreign epitopes homologous to self TCR epitopes has involved characterizing the immunodominant self epitope for a specific autoimmune disease, defining the relevant protein sequence, and using protein databases to identify candidate pathogens. For example, T-cell clones from some subjects with MS were shown to react to the peptide of myelin basic protein, MBP(85-99). This analysis provided the basic information on the residues crucial for MHC class II binding and for TCR recognition. Wucherpfennig and Strominger (34) used this information to develop a set of criteria for a protein sequence database screen, based on the knowledge of degeneracy of amino acid side chains. Viral and bacterial peptides thus selected from the database were then synthesized and tested for their ability to activate the MBP(85-99)-specific T-cell clones. Using this technique, it was demonstrated that specific microbial peptides can indeed act as mimics of the MBP(85-99) peptide. Importantly, this study reinforces the contribution of flexibility in the trimolecular recognition complex to the development of cross-reactivity. The activating peptides would not necessarily have been predicted based on homologous linear sequence alignments between the MBP peptide and viral antigens. As discussed later, the flexibility and degeneracy of TCR recognition was further confirmed by a recent study (35) that demonstrated that from a library of randomly generated peptides, cross-reactive stimulatory peptides for an antigen-specific human T-cell clone could be found; peptides of both human and microbial origin were identified, and some were even more potent ligands than the autoantigen used to establish the T-cell clone.

The evidence that peptides with a degree of sequence homology can effectively activate autoreactive T-cell clones from patients supports the basic premise of the molecular mimicry hypothesis. However, there are still unknown factors. Are the predicted cross-reacting epitopes generated from natural proteins during antigen processing, and can they elicit responses *in vivo?* Presumably, antagonist peptides are also generated naturally. What determines the balance of T-cell activation and apoptosis? If the balance favors antagonist epitopes, this might explain the relatively rare occurrence of autoimmune disease. T-cell activation is now known to be a multifaceted process that requires at least two signals. The signal partner for antigen recognition is costimulation. What roles do costimulation and other modulating factors, such as local cytokines, play in activation of autoreactive T cells? Experimental studies in this field generally make use of T-cell clones, which are generated by repeated stimulation with the specific antigen and T-cell growth factors *in vitro.* Of necessity, these analyses examine the response of cells that are at the effector stage, and may not reflect the response of naive cells *in vivo* (18,36). It is also important to consider the influence of "epitope spreading" (37) on the specificity of T cells derived from patients. The T-cell response is initially focused on a limited number of immunodominant epitopes, but with the generation of the immune response over time, there is spreading to previously cryptic epitopes recognized by T cells. Because in the clinical setting, we are limited to studying established disease, the importance of the selected cross-reactive epitopes in the early events of disease induction remains unresolved, and perhaps unresolvable.

The demonstration of homologous and cross-reactive epitopes constitutes only circumstantial evidence for the molecular mimicry hypothesis. Functional cross-reactivity should be demonstrated to produce disease. In certain rats, arthritis can be induced by injection of complete Freund's adjuvant containing killed *Mycobacterium tuberculosis* in oil, and the arthritis produced can be transmitted by a T-cell clone whose target antigen is mycobacterial 65-kD heat shock protein (HSP65) (38,39). This mycobacterum-specific T-cell clone was found to cross-react with the link protein of proteoglycan found in joints. Models of experimental uveitis (reviewed in 40) and ovarian autoimmune disease (reviewed in 33) are also described in which immunization with microbial peptides produced the experimental disease. Injection of a hepatitis B virus (HBV) protein sharing homology with MBP into rabbits induced antibody and cell-mediated cross-reactivity with MBP, and also produced an inflammatory central nervous system (CNS) disease (41). Perhaps the most compelling evidence to date is the study by Zhao et al. (42) on the autoimmune disease of the eye triggered by herpes simplex virus type 1 (HSV-1). As discussed later, this disease is clearly mediated by T cells that cross-react with a viral epitope and an endogenous host protein.

**Criteria for Molecular Mimicry**

In summary, to validate the molecular mimicry hypothesis as a mechanism of induction of autoimmune disease, several criteria must be met. First, there must be some evidence to implicate a particular pathogen or a particular pathogenic epitope. This may come from epidemiologic associations for the former. For the latter, it may come about indirectly, based either on information about MHC-binding motifs or on retrospective reasoning from defined antigen specificities of T-cell clones derived from patients. Second, there must be demonstration of sequence homology or predicted conformational identity between self determinants and pathogen epitopes. This is actually inherent in the process of identifying the pathogen if the starting point is the antigen recognition pattern of the TCR from patient-derived T-cell clones. Third, it should be shown that the pathogenic epitope can induce cross-reactive antibodies or T-cell responses as well as pathology in some experimental model. The fourth criterion, and perhaps the most stringent, is that the cross-reacting self determinants have to be relevant to what is known about the biology of the clinical disease process (e.g., they should be expressed in target organs). Finally, it should be demonstrated that primary reactivity against these determinants produces clinical disease. At present, these criteria are not fulfilled for any of the autoimmune diseases. Nevertheless, this provides a useful framework for critically evaluating the evidence available on the specific diseases.

In a critical analysis of this issue, it should be added that there are certain difficulties inherent in looking to infection as the cause of chronic autoimmune disease. As discussed in the next section, there are clear examples of autoimmunity arising secondary to well-defined infectious diseases. There are intrinsic hurdles, however, in confidently attributing chronic autoimmune disease to an inciting infection. The infectious process may be resolved long before the autoimmune disease declares itself, thus making it difficult to identify reliable associations between particular pathogens and particular diseases. Alternatively, the infection may itself be occult and beyond the limits of our current technology to detect. Thus, it is difficult to exclude the possibility that a particular autoimmune disease is the result of an immune response against persistent viable or even nonviable organisms and that mimicry is merely an epiphenomenon. Mimicry might also arise as a secondary phenomenon as a result of alteration of host determinants through tissue injury and the creation of neoepitopes. Finally, in the case of retroviruses, not only can integration into the genome alter host determinants and fundamentally change the definition of self but also retroviruses provide the potential for unique mechanisms to interfere with host immunity, through altered expression or regulation of immunoregulatory genes (43).

## AUTOIMMUNITY AS A SEQUELA OF INFECTION

### Acute Rheumatic Fever

ARF is a well-characterized febrile syndrome affecting heart, joints, skin, and CNS that occurs after infection with a group A β-hemolytic streptococcus. It was recognized early that the organism could not be cultured from these affected target organs and that the course of the disease was not altered by antibiotic therapy. With the advent of immunofluorescence as a new technique for clinical immunology in the 1960s, ARF was one of the first diseases to be studied systematically, and it became the paradigm of an autoimmune disease triggered by an infection. It was soon recognized that sera of patients with ARF contained autoantibodies to heart tissue (44) and that the heart cross-reactive antibodies were directed against an antigen in the membrane of the organism (45). Heart cross-reactive antibodies were also observed in patients undergoing cardiac surgery, but only in the ARF patients was the reactivity against the myocardium absorbed out with streptococcal organisms.

Similar heart cross-reactive antibodies appeared in the sera of experimental animals inoculated with group A streptococci. The cross-reacting determinants of the organism were purified and characterized by the use of heart-reactive antibodies that were affinity purified against sarcolemmal sheaths of cardiac myofibers (46). The antigen isolated in this manner appeared to be composed of four polypeptides that were 22 to 32 kd. Dale and Beachy (47,48) undertook an extensive series of studies as part of a search for a streptococcal vaccine free of cross-reactivity with host tissues and thus free of rheumatogenic potential. It is ironic that this quest for agents *free* of molecular mimicry gave birth to three decades of research studying agents *expressing* molecular mimicry.

The major virulence factor for group A streptococci is the M protein, an α-helical coiled coil fibrillar molecule found on the streptococcal surface that enables the organism to resist phagocytic attack, most likely through its ability to restrict the deposition of C3b on the bacterial surface. Type 5 streptococcal M protein was shown to express three epitopes that cross-react with the sarcolemmal membrane of human myocardium (47). Rabbit antibodies against the pepsin-extracted and purified M protein showed reactivity with heart tissue by indirect immunofluorescence. By Western blot analysis, these antisera reacted with the heavy chains of myosin but not with actin or tropomyosin (48). The latter reaction was of interest because it had previously been shown that the streptococcal M protein exhibits a 7–amino acid periodicity that is structurally similar to the tropomyosin molecule (49). Rabbit antibodies against the type 5 M protein

opsonized type 5 streptococci, indicating that the M protein epitopes were expressed on the surface of the organism. It was also observed that sera from patients with ARF had higher titers of antibodies to myosin than that of healthy subjects or of patients with poststreptococcal glomerulonephritis (50). This group of investigators subsequently used synthetic peptides to produce opsonic, protective antibodies that lacked heart cross-reactivity (51).

An alternative approach in studying ARF was to use monoclonal antibodies directed against the group A streptococci (52). Western blot analysis of such monoclonal antibodies showed reactivity with the heavy chain of skeletal myosin (53). Whole, heat-killed group A streptococci absorbed out antimyosin and anti–M protein reactivity in parallel. The monoclonal antibody bound to both skeletal muscle and ventricular myosin. The exact nature of the cross-reacting streptococcal antigen was not defined, and on Western blots, the monoclonal antibody detected several membrane-associated components of group A streptococci.

Cross-reactions with myosin were mapped initially to a region within the N-terminal half of the M5 protein molecule (54,55). One IgM monoclonal antibody reacting with myosin and this region of the M protein was shown to lead to lysis of rat heart cells in tissue culture (56). This is one of few direct attempts to address the biologic significance of these cross-reacting antibodies. To address cross-reactivity with the surface-exposed C-repeat region, rabbits were immunized with overlapping peptides of the region of the M6 protein (57). The antipeptide antisera reacted in an enzyme-linked immunosorbent assay (ELISA) with denatured forms of several mammalian coiled coil proteins, including myosin and cardiac tropomyosin, but these cross-reactive antibody titers were weak, and reactivity with the native proteins could not be demonstrated.

A novel approach to identifying the streptococcal genes encoding myosin cross-reactive antigens used ARF serum to screen a genomic library of M-protein–negative *Streptococcus pyogenes* (58). This identified a 67-kd protein that reacted with myosin-specific, affinity-purified antibodies from ARF patients, but also reacted with sera from patients with uncomplicated streptococcal infections. Sequencing revealed regions of homology with the β chains of both murine and human MHC class II haplotypes. Moreover, mouse anti-IA sera reacted with the recombinant protein. This suggested that a streptococcal protein distinct from M protein had structural and antigenic similarities to MHC class II antigens as well as myosin. It is noteworthy, however, that there is no simple HLA susceptibility association with ARF.

Studies have also addressed the basis for ARF sera binding to the sarcolemmal sheath of cardiac myofibers, a localization suggested by the original immunofluorescence studies of heart-reactive antibodies. Purified sarcolemmal sheaths were extracted and yielded a 39-kd polypeptide that was reactive with ARF sera but not with sera from other streptococcus-infected patients. Sequencing of this protein indicated that it was human cardiac tropomyosin (59).

To identify more precisely the peptides accounting for M protein–myosin cross-reactivity, Cunningham et al. (56) analyzed antipeptide responses in mice. MRL/++ mice immunized with the NT4 peptide of the M protein developed a significant myocarditis (60). Treatment with either anti-CD4 or anti-Ia$^k$ monoclonal antibody inhibited the cardiac inflammation. Because it was known that NT4 cross-reacts with cardiac myosin, the effect of the streptococcal peptide on coxsackievirus-induced myocarditis was studied. Inducing tolerance to the NT4 peptide significantly reduced the viral myocarditis, implicating a degree of molecular mimicry among NT4, coxsackievirus B3, and myosin. This suggested that rheumatic heart disease and viral myocarditis might use similar immune response pathways.

To identify T-cell epitopes relevant to this cross-reactivity, BALB/c mice were immunized with human cardiac myosin, and the dominant myosin cross-reactive T-cell epitopes of M5 protein were identified with a panel of 23 overlapping peptides. Of the six peptides identified by T-cell proliferation, three revealed a sequence highly homologous with a site conserved in cardiac myosin. Immunization of BALB/c mice with these peptides demonstrated inflammatory infiltrates in the myocardium and allowed identification of myosin cross-reactive B-cell epitopes. The M5 peptides elicited higher antibody response to cardiac myosin than the skeletal myosin.

These studies support the notion that M proteins may break tolerance to unique and pathogenic epitopes of human cardiac myosin and that this sequence of events may be important in the pathogenesis of rheumatic carditis (61). These experimental studies have brought the concept of molecular mimicry closer to functional relevance, but the comparable analysis of identifying human T-cell epitopes that are cross-reactive, or indeed the isolation of pathogenic T-cell populations in patients, still awaits further study. It should also be noted that ARF in adult patients primarily takes the form of poststreptococcal polyarthritis, with only rare cardiac manifestations. Whether molecular mimicry may account for the noncardiac features of ARF is unresolved, and the autoantigens in joints, skin, and CNS remain unknown. Nevertheless, ARF still stands as the classic example of a nonseptic chronic inflammatory disease triggered by a bacterial infection.

## Viral Myocarditis

It has been recognized since the 1980s that the experimental myocarditis induced by coxsackievirus B3 (CVB3) is commonly accompanied by autoimmune features (62,63). Autoantibodies to cardiac isoforms of myosin develop after CVB3 infection and correlate with the animal's susceptibility to viral myocarditis. The range of antibodies to different cardiac antigens seen in the mice parallels that seen in patients with human myocarditis (64). There are strain-specific alterations in the local immune pathways in this model, with DBA/2 mice developing predominantly a T$_H$2-dependent humoral response, compared with BALB/c mice, which develop a preferential T$_H$1-dependent, CD8$^+$CTL response (65).

Molecular mimicry between proteins of the virus and the mammalian heart has been invoked as an important contributor to the immunopathology of this model. To address the role of cross-reacting antibodies, neutralizing monoclonal antibodies were generated against CVB3 (66). Several such antibodies were found to induce myocarditis subsequent to intraperitoneal inoculation of mice. Immunocytochemical assays demonstrated significant binding of monoclonal antibodies to the surface of normal cultured murine cardiac fibroblasts. The best predictors for myocarditic potential of a given monoclonal antibody were the capacity for stimulation of fibroblasts to produce a chemoattractant for macrophages and the capacity for recognition of epitopes on murine or human cardiac myosins. Thus, the pathogenic potential of these cross-reactive monoclonal antibodies is clearly established in this experimental model. As mentioned previously, monoclonal antibodies directed against the streptococcal M5 protein were shown to both neutralize CVB3 and cross-react with cardiac proteins, suggesting that myocarditis triggered by two very different pathogens may be mediated by similar immunologic mechanisms (67).

Evidence exists for molecular mimicry at the T-cell level as well in myocarditis. It has been shown that CD4$^+$ T cells recovered from CVB3-infected mice react with the NT4 peptide of the streptococcal M5 protein (68). The unresolved question is whether these cross-reactive T cells are primarily directed to myosin antigens released locally as a result of myocyte necrosis, or whether at the T-cell level, there exists mimicry among CVB3, myosin, and streptococci as well. Analysis of T-cell hybridomas from CVB3-infected mice identified clones that reacted not only to the virus but also to myosin and NT4 (69). Some clones, however, reacted only to CVB3 and myosin, suggesting some mimicking epitopes that are distinctive for the virus and the heart alone.

Several aspects of this model are noteworthy when considering the biologic significance of molecular mimicry. Tissue tropism in coxsackievirus infections is likely determined by host factors, in particular organ-specific viral receptors (70). Cardiotropic CVB3 employs receptors that are heart specific, whereas hepatotropic (hepatitis-inducing) or β-tropic (diabetes-inducing) CVB3 variants use surface molecules specific for hepatocytes or β cells, respectively. Second, myocyte CVB3 can cause myocyte necrosis directly, without invoking host immune response as effector mechanisms (71,72). In virulent strains of CVB3, the immune response may be more protective than pathogenic. Local cell death by necrosis (as opposed to apoptosis) creates a microenvironment replete with proinflammatory cytokines, which can further amplify local tissue injury. Third, tolerance to self can alternatively be subverted by immunization with myosin and complete Freund's adjuvant (73). This experimental myocarditis closely resembles viral myocarditis in its clinical and pathologic features and has generated a series of studies to identify the crucial cytokines involved (74) and the specific myocarditogenic peptides of myosin (75).

For purposes of this discussion, this model serves to illustrate that if tolerance to self myosin is overcome, an immune-mediated myocarditis can ensue. If in the course of virus-induced myocyte necrosis there is a release of cardiac myosin, a similar scenario could follow without invoking molecular mimicry in a mechanistic way. The endogenous alarm signal generated by cell necrosis may be the parallel of the exogenous signal provided by the use of adjuvant. The myocarditis occurring after immunization with the strepto-coccal NT4 peptide requires complete Freund's adjuvant, and in general, the more injurious the adjuvant, the more robust the immune response.

Finally, an observation from a clinical trial in myocarditis addresses the question of the pathogenic role of molecular mimicry. This trial compared conventional treatment of myocarditis with immunosuppressive regimens (steroids, and either azathioprine or cyclosporine) (76). There was no difference in outcome between the treatment groups. Furthermore, those patients with markers of immune activation, either humoral or cellular, had a better outcome, regardless of their treatment group. The conclusion may be drawn from this observation that the immune response in these patients, far from playing a deleterious role, is actually contributing to host defense and healing. This clinical observation stands as a challenge, albeit indirect, to the clinical significance of the autoimmune phenomena seen in myocarditis.

## Chagas' Disease

*Trypanosoma cruzi* infects up to 18 million people in Latin America, and mortality is primarily a consequence of heart failure during the chronic phase of the infection. Chagas' disease is thought to be the single most common cause of heart failure in the world. Although the precise etiology of Chagas' disease is not understood, initiation of an autoimmune attack on the heart and nervous tissue has been supported by several lines of investigation. Early studies described the generation of certain monoclonal antibodies that cross-react with mammalian neurons and myocardium and with *T. cruzi* parasites as evidence supporting molecular mimicry in the cellular events underlying this disorder. It is recognized that there is a scarcity of parasites in the chronic inflammatory lesions in the heart despite a slow increase in the severity of the cardiac disease over time. Characterization of putative autoantigens that share epitopes with parasite molecules has further strengthened the autoimmune theory (77–79).

An observation proposed as strong support for autoimmunity in Chagas' disease documented that mice with chronic *T. cruzi* infection vigorously rejected normal syngeneic heart transplants (80). This was cited as evidence that *T. cruzi* induces antiheart T-cell responses capable of destroying normal heart tissue and that such responses could account for tissue destruction in the native heart. A report revisiting this experiment, however, calls this conclusion into

question (81). In this study, neonatal hearts transplanted into mice chronically infected with *T. cruzi* did not exhibit signs of autoimmune rejection or indeed any significant inflammatory response. Transplanted hearts established in mice before systemic infection with *T. cruzi* do become parasitized, and the ensuing inflammatory response is identical to that observed in native hearts of *T. cruzi*–infected mice in terms of cell types, cytokines, and adhesion molecules. The features of this response are very different from those observed in allogeneic heart rejection. These data appear to demonstrate that, in this model, parasitization of heart tissue is both necessary and sufficient for the induction of tissue damage in Chagas' disease and that this may constitute evidence against the autoimmune etiology of the disease.

By comparison with this experimental model, analysis of sera from patients with Chagas' disease has identified antibodies that cross-react with the carboxy-terminal part of the ribosomal PO protein of *T. cruzi* and the second extracellular loop of the human $\beta_1$-adrenergic receptor. Using competitive ELISA and Western blot analysis, cross-reactivity of peptides appear to validate molecular mimicry between these antigens (82). In support of the pathogenic significance of this phenomenon, these cross-reacting antibodies have been shown to exert chronotropic effects on neonatal rat cardiomyocytes *in vitro* (83). The presumption is that such autoantibodies functionally interfering with G-protein–coupled receptors of the heart could explain the electrophysiologic disturbances of heart function, which in many cases are the cause of sudden death in chagasic patients.

The immunodominant peptide of the *T. cruzi* ribosomal P proteins (R13) shares sequence homology not only with the extracellular loop of the $\beta_1$-adrenergic receptor but also with human ribosomal P proteins, which are in turn the target of anti-P autoantibodies in systemic lupus erythematosus (84). The profile of reactivity for these different autoantibodies differs significantly, however, with chagasic anti-P autoantibodies, demonstrating much greater affinity for the trypanosomal P protein than the human P protein, whereas lupus anti-P antibodies were the reverse. Although chagasic anti-P antibodies showed chronotropic activity on cardiomyocytes *in vitro,* their lupus counterparts had no such functional effects. It was concluded that the adrenergic-stimulating activity of anti-P antibodies may play a direct role in the induction of functional myocardial impairments observed in Chagas' disease. Although implicating a pathophysiologic role for these autoantibodies, these analyses remain confined to an *in vitro* system and have yet to be validated *in vivo* or in the clinical setting.

## Herpes Keratitis

One of the challenges in the studies of molecular mimicry has been to establish the pathogenic significance of cross-reacting determinants of host and pathogen. Herpes stromal keratitis (HSK) is a disease triggered by herpes simplex virus type 1 (HSV-1) infection. This infection initiates a T-cell–dependent destruction of corneal tissue and is a leading cause of human blindness (85,86).

Using a murine model of HSK, a study examined whether pathogenic T-cell clones might also recognize HSV epitopes. It had been demonstrated in earlier studies by this group of investigators that murine resistance to HSK lay in sequence homology between a gene encoding an IgG$_2$ antibody and that encoding a protein expressed in corneal cells. Resistant strains of mice were thus tolerant of the corneal autoantigen and were resistant to HSK. The more recent report identified this homologous sequence also to be present in the herpes protein UL6 (42). This suggested an experimental approach to test the functional significance of this mimicry. It was demonstrated that T cells from mice infected with HSV containing native UL6 caused disease, whereas T cells from mice infected with UL6-negative HSV did not. In addition, more than 75% of animals infected with the native virus developed autoimmune keratitis, whereas less than 20% with the mutant (UL6-negative) virus infection did so.

This study raises the possibility that virus-induced autoimmunity may reflect a balance of two opposing mimicry mechanisms. Genetic polymorphism affecting the sequence or local expression of a protein can generate endogenous host proteins that can tolerize to autoantigens. This can result in *decreased* susceptibility to virus-induced autoimmune disease. If the infecting virus expresses a molecular mimic (as in UL6-positive HSV), however, this can result in *increased* virus-induced autoimmunity by activation and recruitment of autoreactive T cells. Whether human T cells mediate keratitis by a similar mechanism has not been determined, and the host factors that confer immunogenetic susceptibility to this disease in humans remain unknown. Furthermore, the nature of the corneal autoantigen has not been identified.

## MOLECULAR MIMICRY IN THE AUTOIMMUNE DISEASES

### Diabetes Mellitus

Insulin-dependent diabetes mellitus (IDDM) is a chronic disorder that results from destruction of the insulin-producing β cells of the pancreatic islets. The incidence of disease shows regional variability and ranges from 1 to 2 per 100,000 population per year in Japan to a more than 40 per 100,000 population per year in parts of Finland (87). IDDM is believed to be an autoimmune disease in its origin. The initial phase of disease is clinically silent, and evidence suggests that T lymphocytes and other inflammatory cells invade the islets during this period, eventually destroying them (87–89). A lymphocytic infiltrate is observed in the pancreas of the recently diagnosed diabetic patient, and islet-reactive autoantibodies are detected months or years before the onset of clinical disease. The pathogenic process then becomes clinically overt, manifested by the inability to maintain glucose homeostasis, with resulting hyperglycemia, polyuria, and ketoacidosis.

Several genes map the risk for diabetes, but the concordance in identical twins is less than 50% (90), suggesting that environmental factors may trigger the disease. Ninety-five percent of IDDM patients express HLA-DR3, HLA-DR4, or both (87,91,92). In whites, genes such as *HLA-DQB*0302* are also a high risk genotype. Interestingly, the nonobese diabetic (NOD) mouse, an animal model of IDDM, has a highly analogous genetic predisposition to develop spontaneous autoimmune diabetes (93), with the most important contributor being the unique I-A$^{g7}$, which is structurally similar to the human susceptibility alleles (91,94).

The NOD mouse represents a good model of the overall progression of human IDDM as well as the polygenic and environmental factors that influence it (95). Insulitis in the inbred NOD strain appears spontaneously at about 3 to 4 weeks of age and is well established by 10 weeks of age. Progression to overt diabetes occurs in 80% of female mice between 10 and 30 weeks of age. The insulitis is mediated predominantly by CD4$^+$ T cells, which are polyclonal (96). This insulitis is necessary but not sufficient for diabetes development, as evidenced by the fact that male NOD mice do not develop overt diabetes despite having insulitis. Diabetes in the NOD mouse, as in humans, is characterized by the presence of autoreactive T and B cells, directed against a range of islet autoantigens, including glutamic acid decarboxylase (GAD) (97,98), insulin (99; reviewed in 88) and islet cell antigen p69 (ICA69) (100).

Molecular mimicry is an attractive possible mechanism for the induction of insulitis in NOD mice at 3 weeks of age. The onset of insulitis coincides with weaning. At this time, new food proteins and microbial antigens are introduced into the gut and challenge the immune system. Thus, many potentially cross-reactive bacteria would be available to trigger autoimmunity. This model, however, does not explain the discrepancy between the nearly universal development of histopathologic insulitis and the development of frank disease in only a proportion of female mice (88). Furthermore, it has been shown that when animals are housed under specific pathogen-free conditions, there is 100% incidence of diabetes (101,102). This strongly suggests that the development of disease is endogenous and not related to externally derived pathogens. Mice made transgenic for the TCR from a diabetogenic T-cell clone derived from an NOD mouse develop rampant insulitis and eventually diabetes (103). Characterization of the disease in these mouse highlights two checkpoints in disease development: first, the interval before development of insulitis; second, the time to development of aggressive β-cell destruction. It is unknown whether mimicry plays any part in the progression through these stages.

Viral mimicry as a mechanism for the induction of diabetes has been studied using the LCMV-RIP transgenic mouse (20,24). Pancreatic β cells in these mice are induced to express the nucleoprotein or glycoprotein of LCMV by the use of the RIP in the transgene construct. The viral gene product thus becomes a self antigen. In these mice, there is no spontaneous diabetes. After infection of adult animals with LCMV, however, more than 95% of these transgenic mice develop an antiviral (i.e., anti-self) CD8⁺ cytotoxic T-lymphocyte response that leads to IDDM (20,24). The development of diabetes is accelerated in double transgenic mice having TCR specific for LCMV, likely because of the the larger number of responding T cells (20).

This model serves to demonstrate that autoreactive T cells against islet autoantigens can indeed exist in ignorance, and that viral infection can specifically break ignorance of self antigen and initiate the autoimmune disease. In this case, however, the β-cell–specific antigen is created by the transgene construct and is the same antigen used to induce disease (i.e., LCMV nucleoprotein or glycoprotein). The "perfect" mimicry inherent in this system restricts its generalizability to the question of molecular mimicry at large.

A hypothesis for the human disease, extrapolated from this model, proposes that a virus with tropism for β cells in the islets of Langerhans chronically infects those cells after an infection *in utero* or in early life. An immune response induced by a subsequent infection by the same virus, or one with immunologically cross-reactive determinants, would then lead to a chronic immune response directed at the β cells (24).

The initiation of an inflammatory response directed against β cells as a result of viral mimicry of self antigens is clearly a complex process. As suggested by the studies in these transgenic animals, autoreactive cells against islet autoantigens must exist, but their ignorance is maintained in the uninfected animals because glycoprotein- or nucleoprotein-specific cytotoxic T lymphocytes (CTLs) do not receive appropriate activation signals from the islets in the pancreas.

Other studies using the transgenic animals point to the importance of cytokines and costimulatory molecules in breaking peripheral ignorance to self antigens in this model (reviewed in 104). For example, mice coexpressing the costimulatory molecule B7-1 with LCMV glycoprotein in the islets develop spontaneous diabetes with no other manipulation (104).

Mimicry related to viral infection in human IDDM has drawn support from some clinical studies. A small number of IDDM cases are thought to occur years after *in utero* viral infection such as congenital rubella syndrome (105). Other associations between viral infections and IDDM have been established through epidemiologic studies examining immunity to members of the enterovirus family, particularly to coxsackievirus B (106). Although data on coxsackievirus antibodies are controversial (106,107), some studies reported an increased prevalence of anti–coxsackievirus B IgM antibodies in newly diagnosed IDDM patients compared with control subjects, consistent with a recent coxsackievirus B infection at the time of diagnosis. Of note, the anti–coxsackievirus B IgM antibodies were more common among IDDM patients with the susceptibility allele HLA-DR3 (108). There has also been a single report describing the isolation of a strain of coxsackievirus B from the pancreas of a child, newly diagnosed with IDDM, that could transfer the disease to IDDM prone mice (109). However, a recent coxsackievirus B infection would not explain the onset of immunologic evidence for β-cell reactivity long before the onset of clinical disease. Nevertheless, evidence for mimicry related to coxsackievirus B has been actively pursued. This has been supported by the finding of sequence homology between human GAD65 and a coxsackievirus B protein (110).

GAD65 is an enzyme that is selectively concentrated in neurons secreting the neurotransmitter γ-aminobutyric acid (GABA) and in pancreatic β cells (111). GAD65 is a major target of autoimmunity in IDDM. Autoantibodies directed against GAD65 are present in 70% to 80% of newly diagnosed IDDM patients and are associated with increased risk for IDDM (112). GAD autoimmunity is also present in NOD mice, and reactivity against GAD is one of the earliest detectable immune alterations in these mice (97). When the primary sequence of human GAD65 became available, a search of protein databases revealed that the region of the protein corresponding to amino acids 250 to 273 shares sequence homology with the region corresponding to amino acids 28 to 50 of CoxP2-C, an enzyme involved in the replication of coxsackievirus B (110). Within these regions, there is a six–amino acid stretch (PEVKEK) that is identical between the two proteins.

Cross-reactivity between CoxP2-C and GAD65 was examined in mice by surveying a panel of 10 murine MHC class II alleles for presentation of synthetic peptides derived from the similarity sequence of human GAD65 and CoxP2-C (GAD ssp and Cox ssp) (113). Both GAD ssp and Cox ssp were dominant determinants, inducing T-cell proliferation, but only in the context of the diabetes-associated NOD MHC class II allele. The T-cell response was also cross-reactive between Cox and GAD ssp. The GAD65 and CoxP2-C ssp were shown to be generated as dominant determinants *in vivo* after immunization with full-length GAD65 and CoxP2-C, with behavior similar to the synthetic peptides. Taken together, these data provide support for molecular mimicry as the basis for the cross-reactivity that was observed. The restriction of T-cell cross-reactivity to a specific MHC susceptibility allele is consistent with the MHC association in human disease. The structural similarity between NOD and human MHC class II susceptibility alleles for IDDM suggests that cross-reactive T-cell recognition of GAD65 and CoxP2-C could play a role in the pathogenesis of human IDDM.

The corresponding T-cell–reactive epitopes of GAD65 in humans have been further delineated (114). The response of peripheral blood mononuclear cells (PBMC) to a panel of overlapping synthetic peptides was measured in PBMC isolated from control subjects, newly diagnosed IDDM patients, and subjects at risk for IDDM. The latter were defined as first-degree relatives of an IDDM patient who were positive for islet cell autoantibodies or insulin autoantibodies. PBMC responsiveness to GAD peptides was observed in all three groups, but there was an elevated frequency of immune responsiveness to peptides containing the GAD65 and CoxP2-C ssp, which was seen in at-risk and newly diagnosed IDDM subjects but not in control subjects. HLA typing of responding subjects suggested that reactivity to GAD showed some association with HLA-DR3 and HLA-DR4, but the numbers were too small to make a confident association. PBMC from three subjects who reacted against one of the two GAD65 peptides also proliferated in response to coxsackievirus peptides, whereas PBMC from control subjects did not. These data appear to be consistent with the study in mice discussed previously; however, the findings have yet to be confirmed in a larger population.

As discussed by Solimena and De Camilli (108), linking diabetes to coxsackievirus through a mechanism involving mimicry with GAD65 may be premature. As noted previously, the findings of cross-reactivity in humans must be extended to larger numbers of subjects studied. Although the findings in the NOD mouse are more compelling, actual coxsackievirus infection has not been associated with the development of diabetes in this model. Furthermore, a search of databases identified 17 viruses with some homology to various fragments of GAD65 (115). It is therefore difficult to conclude, based on the evidence to date, that cross-reactivity between GAD peptides and coxsackievirus specifically is important in the pathogenesis of IDDM.

Indeed, two recent studies do not favor GAD65 and CoxP2-C cross-reactivity. Richter et al. (116) used human monoclonal antibodies known to be specific for a set of diabetes-associated GAD65 epitopes to look for cross-reactivity in a panel of viruses implicated in the development of IDDM. This group was not able to detect antibody cross-reactivity between GAD65 and B4-2C proteins, nor with 60-kD HSP (HSP60) or antigens from several viruses. Endl et al. (89) analyzed a panel of human GAD65-specific T-cell lines generated from recent-onset IDDM patients for the response to a set of overlapping peptides derived from the human GAD65 sequence. There were several naturally processed GAD65 epitopes that were recognized by the T-cell lines, however, and the immunodominant epitope defined for several cell lines did not contain the GAD and CoxP2-C ssp, although it did span a region of homology. Thus, the evidence that cross-reactivity between CoxP2-C and GAD is important to the development of diabetes remains controversial.

Molecular mimicry of dietary cow milk proteins has also been suggested as a trigger for IDDM. Although this hypothesis is controversial and the foreign antigen invoked is not an infectious pathogen, the evidence is still important to consider in weighing the potential contribution of mimicry to induction of diabetes. Bovine serum albumin (BSA) was first suggested as a candidate trigger for IDDM on the basis of epidemiologic evidence (reviewed in 117). Additionally, patients and rodent models were shown to have elevated anti-BSA antibodies that precipitate the protein p69 from β-cell lysates. The p69, or ICA69, is a a neuroendocrine protein of unknown function that appears to be a target autoantigen in IDDM (reviewed in 100). The 17-amino-acid BSA peptide

(ABBOS) peptide (position 152 to 169) has been proposed as the reactive, disease-associated epitope in BSA (118).

Karjalainen et al. (118) demonstrated elevated serum concentrations of IgG anti-BSA antibodies (but not antibodies to other milk proteins) in patients with diabetes compared with control subjects. Most of these antibodies were specific for the ABBOS peptide. Subsequently, it was shown that proliferative T-cell responses to BSA and the ABBOS peptide were present in most patients with recent-onset IDDM (119). Miyazaki et al. (117) expanded further on these data by testing various cow milk proteins and found that T cells from children with recent-onset diabetes showed specific sensitization only to BSA, and within the BSA molecule to the ABBOS peptide. They also extended these T-cell responses to show reactivity to recombinant p69 and identified a common sequence motif that is shared by p69 and ABBOS. It was demonstrated that the sequence of the relevant p69 region carrying this motif is conserved in diabetic patients. Thus, it was hypothesized that the ABBOS peptide is immunogenic only in hosts with IDDM-associated class II (DR and DQ) haplotypes that are able to bind and present this antigen. The immature gut of infants exposed to dietary cow milk absorbs large protein fragments, which would include the ABBOS peptide, and immunity to this peptide would be generated in these susceptible patients. Mimicry between ABBOS and p69 would potentially result in self-reactive immunity under conditions of immune recognition of p69. Viral infection creates such conditions because p69 is upregulated on the surface of β cells in the presence of interferon-γ, which is released systemically during infection. Thus, unrelated infectious events would induce the expression of p69 on the surface of β cells, transiently exposing some of these cells to immune attack. The long course preceding clinical diabetes might be explained by the temporary nature of such episodes of p69 expression on β cells.

This hypothesis has been considered controversial. Data from Atkinson et al. (120) showed no increased responsiveness of PBMC to BSA or ABBOS peptides, challenging the original observation. Cavallo and colleagues (121) later suggested that bovine casein was the target antigen in BSA based on sequence identity between casein and the β-cell glucose transporter GLUT-2 and on a higher frequency of lymphocyte proliferation in response to bovine casein in diabetics compared with control subjects or patients with autoimmune thyroid disease. Furthermore, stimulation of PBMC from patients with IDDM has been reported to be induced by insulin, several islet cell antigens, and GAD (reviewed in 120). This widespread reactivity calls into question the relevance of anti-BSA and anti-ABBOS immunity to the pathogenesis of IDDM. Finally, there is no evidence in NOD mice, nor in the Bio Breeding rat, another model of spontaneous diabetes, that immune response to BSA plays a role in diabetes induction (122). Thus, the role of BSA as a pathogenic molecular mimic in IDDM remains unresolved.

## Rheumatoid Arthritis

RA is a relatively common autoimmune disease with a prevalence of about 1% in white populations. It is characterized by a chronic inflammation of the synovial joints with infiltration by T cells, macrophages, and plasma cells, all of which show signs of activation (123,124). The target autoantigen in RA is still unknown; however, antibodies to self antigens, such as IgG (125), type II collagen (126–128), and heat shock proteins (HSPs) (39,129), have been described. The development of autoantibodies against the Fc portion of IgG, known as *rheumatoid factors,* is one of the immunologic hallmarks of the disease.

Susceptibility to RA is specifically associated with the MHC class II alleles DRB1*0401, DRB1*0404, and DRB1*0101 (130). The DRβ chains encoded by these genes possess a "shared epitope" formed by a short stretch of amino acids (at positions 67 to 74) of the third hypervariable region (HV3) that is highly conserved among RA-associated alleles (131,132). This can take the form of QKRAA (glutamine, lysine, arginine, alanine, alanine) or QRRAA. Because DRB1*0402, a closely related molecule not associated with RA, differs from the RA-linked DRB1*0401 and DRB1*0404 molecules only in the 67 to 74 region (at positions 67, 70, and 71), this part of the molecule is likely to have a crucial role in disease susceptibility. This epitope appears to impart a specific pattern of peptide binding (133). The shared epitope, however, is neither necessary nor sufficient for the development of RA. Within the RA patient population, the presence of the shared epitope has been associated with rheumatoid factor seropositivity and more aggressive disease (132,134). Thus, this epitope may be important in the immune response to different antigenic triggers and may modulate the course of the disease rather than influence primary susceptibility to the disease. Understanding the potential role of this motif in pathogenesis has been an important research theme in RA.

A number of potential microbial triggers of RA have been proposed on the basis of antibody cross-reactivity and sequence homology. The 100-kd glycoprotein of Epstein–Barr virus (EBV) has sequence similarity with the shared epitope of DRB1. Patients with serologic evidence of a previous infection with EBV have been shown to have antibodies to the QKRAA motif (135,136). Patients with RA have also been shown to have heightened immunoreactivity to EBV compared with control subjects (137,138). Mimicry between EBV nuclear antigen-1 (EBNA-1) and type I collagen has also been implicated in the pathogenesis of RA (139). There have also been reports of elevated antibody levels against *Proteus mirabilis* in RA patients with active disease (140). Furthermore, sequences in *P. mirabilis* hemolysin have been identified that have homology with sequences in type II collagen that are known to bind to the RA-associated DR motifs (133) but not to the nonassociated DRB1*0402. Evidence for functional cross-reactivity, however, has been limited for these pathogens.

There is a considerable body of evidence for HSPs as putative triggering agents in RA. The family of HSPs (reviewed in 141) comprises a set of proteins that are produced when a cell is confronted with a sudden increase in temperature. HSPs can be induced by other stresses (metabolic, toxic, or physical), and many are expressed constitutively and have multiple functions. HSPs may act as scavengers for denatured or abnormal proteins and can act as chaperones in protein folding. They are highly conserved evolutionarily with respect to structure and function. Furthermore, they appear to be major antigens of many pathogens (141). HSPs are therefore excellent candidates for immunologic mimicry.

In one model, arthritis was induced in rats by injection of complete Freund's adjuvant containing killed *Mycobacterium tuberculosis* in oil. This adjuvant arthritis (AA) can be transmitted by a T-cell clone that has as its target antigen amino acids 180 to 188 of the HSP65 (39,142), which is the mycobacteria member of the widely distributed HSP60 family. HSP65 has a low degree of homology with its human counterpart in this region, but there is homology with a region of the link protein of rat proteoglycan, a constituent of cartilage. Subsequent studies, however, showed that the homologous peptide from link protein does not stimulate the arthritogenic T-cell clone (143). T cells isolated from rats with streptococcal cell wall (SCW)–induced arthritis also recognize antigens from *M. tuberculosis* and can transfer arthritis to naive animals (144). Although HSP65 did not originally appear to be involved in the antigenic cross-reactivity, a subsequent study showed that pretreatment of rats with HSP65 completely prevented the development of SCW arthritis (145). Furthermore, prior immunization with one of the T-cell clones identified in AA can also generate resistance to the induction of AA and SCW arthritis. Thus, these studies suggest a role for HSP65 in the regulation of these experimental models of arthritis, and this has led to investigation of the role of HSP65 in RA.

Elevated antibodies against HSP65 have been demonstrated in some studies of patients with RA (reviewed in 146). Antibody reactivity has not been consistently found, however, and no correlation between antibody levels and age, gender, disease duration, or HLA-DR haplotypes has been demonstrated. T cells from rheumatoid synovial fluid (SF) have been shown to have elevated proliferative responses to an acetone-precipitable fraction of *M. tuberculosis* as well as to recombinant mycobacterial HSP65 (reviewed in 147). These responses are more marked in SF than in peripheral blood and have been found both early and late in disease. This reactivity was found not to be confined to mycobacterial antigens, however, and for HSP65, it was more pronounced in patients with reactive arthritis than in those with RA (148). Furthermore, elevated proliferative responses to mycobacteria can be found in mononuclear cells from nonautoimmune inflammatory sites (147), and responses to HSP65 are more frequent than for SF-derived T cells. This suggests that HSP65 may not be a major antigen recognized by SF T cells. However, the fine specificity of SF T cells in RA is only beginning to be established. In one study, two T-cell clones derived from rheumatoid synovium were demonstrated to have two epitopes for recognition that were mapped to one of the homology regions shared by mycobacterial and human HSP (149).

Nevertheless, the more relevant question in terms of RA pathogenesis is whether there is reactivity against HSP60, the human homolog of HSP65. HSP60 shares sequence homology with a wide range of autoantigens (150). Thus, a response generated against HSP60 through mimicry by mycobacterial HSP65 could cross-react with tissue antigens and might contribute to RA pathogenesis. Rheumatoid synovial tissue itself has also been demonstrated to express HSP60 (151,152) and could thus be the target of this immune response. Although both SF-derived T-cell and PBMC from patients with juvenile chronic arthritis show substantial proliferative responses to recombinant HSP60, however, those from RA patients do not (153,154). Thus, on the basis of the available data, it is difficult to establish with confidence a case for pathogenic molecular mimicry with HSP65.

Other efforts to define mimicry between host and microbial HSP in RA have examined cross-reactivity with the HV3 shared epitope of DRB1. The 40-kd HSP or dnaJ class of HSPs from *Escherichia coli* and several other bacteria contains the QKRAA sequence of the shared epitope (155,156). Albani et al. (157) addressed the potential for mimicry between dnaJ proteins and the shared epitope by examining cellular and humoral immune responses to the QKRAA-containing region of *E. coli* dnaJ in adults with early RA, control subjects, and patients with other autoimmune diseases. PBMC from patients with early RA or juvenile RA but not from control subjects proliferated in response to recombinant intact dnaJ. Only the PBMC from RA patients, as well as their corresponding synovial mononuclear cells, responded specifically to a synthetic peptide, dnaJp1, containing the QKRAA epitope at the amino terminus. Of the RA patients that were HLA typed, all expressed alleles containing the shared epitope. T cells from control subjects who were also DRB1*0401 positive did not respond to the dnaJ-derived peptide homologous to the 0401 binding site. Despite this, peptide binding was shown to be equivalent for class II molecules extracted from a responding DRB1*0401 RA patient and from nonresponding DRB1*0401-positive or DRB1*0701-positive control subjects. Interestingly, it was noted that peptides of self origin did not bind as well as exogenously derived dnaJ peptides.

In a subsequent study, T-cell responses against self peptides were not detected (158). Thus, the presence of the RA-associated sequence motif on HLA-DR is not sufficient to induce a cellular immune response to the dnaJ epitope expressed by the peptide because DRB1*0401-positive control subjects did not respond. It was proposed that differences between patients and controls in cellular reactivity to dnaJ peptides are thus due to divergent T-cell repertoires rather than to specific differences in peptide binding to HLA class II molecules. Both RA patients and control subjects had comparable levels of antibodies (IgG) to recombinant *E. coli* dnaJ, indicating prior exposure in all populations. However, a dnaJ peptide inhibited antibody binding to dnaJ to a greater degree in RA patients, implying that RA patients focus the antibody responses to different epitopes on dnaJ than do control subjects.

On the basis of the evidence for cellular cross-reactivity of PBMC from RA patients with HSP from *E. coli*, a multistep hypothesis for molecular mimicry in induction and perpetuation of RA has been proposed (158). In the first step, HLA-derived peptides encompassing the shared epitope sequence randomly select T cells that bind the self-derived peptide at low avidity. This is supported by the demonstration of tolerance to self peptides from the third hypervariable region of HLA-DRB1*0401 in RA patients and control subjects (159). These positively selected T cells can, at some later time, be activated after encountering and binding with higher avidity to peptides of microbial origin expressing the shared epitope. Intermittent exposure of the systemic immune system to bacterial antigens at mucosal surfaces might lead to the activation of previously quiescent QKRAA-specific T cells.

Alternative support for cross-reactivity of epitopes comes from *in vitro* binding studies (160). Extracts of bacterial proteins were screened for binding to affinity columns prepared with peptides from the third hypervariable (HV3) region of HLA-DRB1*0401. It was demonstrated that dnaK, the 70-kd HSP from *E. coli*, binds peptides from the HV3 region. This was not a surprising finding because any QKRAA-containing peptide is capable of binding dnaK (dnaJ, which carries QKRAA, is a natural ligand of dnaK). When HLA-DR molecules were immunoprecipitated from HLA-DRB1*0401 homozygous cell lines, they coprecipitated with a 70-kd protein that was shown to be the constitutive human HSP, HSP73. Similar findings were demonstrated for DRB1*1001, which contains the RRRAA motif, but not for lymphoblastoid lines homozygous for non–RA-associated alleles. It was also shown that HSP73 targets HLA-DRB1*0401 to lysosomes, suggesting that this interaction may influence the behavior of the class II alleles in processing and presentation of self peptide. Favoring this is the localization of genes encoding HSP70 to the human MHC class III region between the loci for complement and tumor necrosis factor (161), the demonstration that heat shock enhances antigen processing (reviewed in 162), and the demonstration of at least one hsp70 family member that is localized in cytoplasmic vesicles and appears to play a role in antigen presentation (163). DRB1*0401 may also present peptides from HSP73 itself, which could trigger responses to self HSP70 or proteins with homologous sequences in other tissues. For example, a dominant epitope on human type II collagen has been identified as having linear sequence homology to HSP70 (164).

These studies of molecular mimicry in RA have not yet reached a definitive conclusion. Using current techniques of molecular biology, which combine the HLA susceptibility to the disease, the crucial role of the T cell in disease pathogenesis, and probable candidate autoantigens, however, studies have continued to provide intriguing clues about the inciting events in RA.

## Multiple Sclerosis

MS is a demyelinating disease of the CNS with a variable clinical course. A relapsing–remitting course is common, but one third of MS patients have a chronic progressive course leading to paralysis, visual loss, and bowel and bladder dysfunction. The prevalent hypothesis for most investigators has been that the disease has an infectious trigger and that it is sustained by an ongoing autoimmune response, but neither the microbial triggers nor the autoantigens have been definitively characterized. Elevated antibody levels against a number of viruses have been described: HBV, HSV-1, measles virus, EBV, and human herpes virus type 6 (165,166). Viruses have been recovered from the cerebrospinal fluid (CSF) in several studies (167,168). The strongest candidate autoantigens have been MBP and proteolipid (PLP). MBP has been extensively studied because of its role in postinfectious encephalomyelitis and its ability to induce EAE, an animal model of MS. EAE is a demyelinating disease of the CNS mediated by MBP-reactive $CD4^+$ T cells, which recognize distinct MBP peptides in the context of predominantly class II I-A antigens. PLP can also induce EAE, and EAE can be transferred by PLP-specific T cells. Several studies have demonstrated a higher frequency of MBP-reactive and PLP-reactive T cells in PBMC of MS patients compared with control subjects, and there is an accumulation of such cells in the CSF of these patients (169,170).

Infection may lead to local damage of the CNS, which in turn may expose a previously sequestered autoantigen to the immune system, initiating a secondary immune attack an the altered CNS tissues. Molecular mimicry, however, has been proposed by a number of investigators to explain the link between infection and autoimmunity in the pathogenesis of MS. MBP demonstrates sequence homologies with several viruses, including HBV polymerase, the nucleoprotein and hemagglutinin of influenza virus, the core protein of polyomavirus, the polyprotein of poliomyelitis virus, and the EC-LF2 protein of EBV, among others (41). PLP demonstrates homologies with decapeptides from measles virus and rubella virus (171). Autoantibodies to MBP and PLP have been demonstrated in the serum and CSF of MS patients, but there have been few studies evaluating molecular mimicry between B-cell epitopes of pathogen and host proteins. One group found high-affinity antibodies to transaldolase in serum and CSF of MS patients and subsequently demonstrated cross-reactivity of these antibodies with the gag protein of the immunodeficiency virus type 1 by Western blot analysis (172). Despite this serologic support for a degree of mimicry, it is noteworthy that the immunopathology of MS points more toward a cell-mediated process than toward CNS-specific immunoglobulin deposition or immune complex–mediated local complement activation.

On the assumption that autoreactive T cells are playing the central role in MS pathogenesis, there has been interest in examining whether cross-reacting viral peptides could account for clonal expansion of MBP-reactive T cells. Structural characterization of the immunodominant MBP(85-99) peptide identified residues crucial to MHC binding and T-cell–receptor recognition (173). Based on these structural preconditions, a database search was undertaken in which the degeneracy of amino acid side chains required for T-cell activation were considered (34). A panel of 129 peptides that matched the molecular mimicry motif was tested on seven MBP-specific T-cell clones derived from two MS patients. Seven viral peptides (from EBV, influenza type A virus, human papillomavirus, reovirus, adenovirus, and HSV) and one bacterial peptide (from *Pseudomonas aeruginosa*) efficiently activated three of these clones. It was noted that the cross-reactivity would not have been predicted on the basis of linear sequence homology, sounding a note of caution for investigations into molecular mimicry solely on the basis of amino acid sequence.

While identifying a population of truly cross-reactive T cells from MS patients, the study served to illustrate that some T-cell receptors actually recognize, not a single peptide, but rather a limited repertoire of structurally related peptides derived from different antigens. That a diverse range of viral peptides are capable of stimulating MBP-specific T-cell clones suggests that a broad range of pathogens could potentially serve as the entry point for the generation of the local autoimmune response in MS. This might account for the difficulty in linking a single pathogen to the pathogenesis of MS (174).

The pathogenic potential of the T-cell cross-reactivity demonstrated so clearly in this study remains to be defined. Only two MS patients and only seven T-cell clones from these patients were studies. Thus, the frequency of the cross-reacting T cells in a given patient and their prevalence in the MS population at large remain unknown. Moreover, the search for cross-reacting peptides was intentionally restricted to pathogens with some clinical support for association with MS. In fact, there were more than 600 sequences of viral and bacterial origin that met the binding motif criteria, and there must be large numbers of peptides of nonmicrobial origin that would meet the criteria and that might have proved stimulatory for the MBP-reactive T-cell clones.

The degenerate antigen recognition of autoreactive T cells specific for MBP was confirmed in a study that used a random combinatorial peptide library to identify cross-reacting ligands (35). Screening of protein databases with the library information revealed not only MBP as a potential ligand for the T cells but also several peptides derived from both self and foreign antigens. Some of these synthetic peptides demonstrated greater stimulatory capability *in vitro* than did MBP. These observations introduce a level of complexity into the search for cross-reactive T-cell epitopes because neither sequence homology nor T-cell proliferation to candidate peptides may be considered truly monospecific.

One study that approached this issue in terms of frequency of cross-reactivity demonstrated that 29% of T-cell lines from MS patients (n = 10) but only 1.3% of T-cell lines from healthy donors (n = 2) showed cross-reactivity with MBP and human coronavirus strain 229E antigens (175). There was also evidence for reciprocal reactivity in T cells derived from the patients. The clinical impetus to study coronaviruses derived from antibody studies in MS patients demonstrating coronavirus gene expression on the brain tissue of some MS patients (176). Control viral antigens were not included in this study, however, and the presupposition was again made that MBP is the crucial, if not the dominant, auto-antigen in MS.

A comparison of T-cell epitopes with B-cell epitopes of MBP was reported (177). MBP autoantibodies were affinity purified from CNS lesions of 11 or 12 postmortem cases studied. Residues in the immunodominant region for auto-antibody binding were located in a 10–amino acid segment that also contained the MHC and TCR contact residues of the T-cell epitope. Based on the antibody-binding motif, micro-bial peptides were identified that bound the purified auto-antibodies. These peptides derived from a wide range of viruses and bacteria. A peptide from human papillomavirus that was previously found to activate an MBP-specific cell clone, for example, was bound by autoantibodies from all MS patients studied. Autoantibody binding of microbial peptides required sequence identity at four or five contiguous residues in the epitope center. Microbial peptides previously found to activate T-cell clones did not have a comparable homology to MBP because sequence identity was not required at MHC contacts. The observation that autoantibodies demonstrate fine specificity similar to autoreactive T cells provides some support for the approach of screening for cross-reactive pathogens using serologic evidence from patients. Such an approach may still shed light on a process that is ultimately T-cell mediated. This suggests that screening potential pathogens in MS may reasonably and more easily be done using autoantibodies than using T-cell clones.

The pathogenic potential for host and microbial cross-reactivities is enhanced by the demonstration of animal mod-els that recapitulate the immunopathology of the disease. Sequence homology between MBP and HBV polymerase (HBVP) was evaluated for pathogenic potential in such an *in vivo* situation (41). An eight–amino acid peptide from HBVP sharing sequence homology with MBP was used to immunize rabbits. The resulting CNS lesions of the rabbits displayed a histologic picture reminiscent of EAE. Serum antibodies from the immunized animals reacted with both MBP and HBVP, and PBMC from the animals showed a proliferative response to both MBP and HBVP. Animals immunized with viral peptides lacking sequence homology with the encephal-itogenic site of MBP did not develop CNS lesions. It is not evident, however, whether this phenomenon would be observed in mice, in which the mechanisms underlying EAE are defined much more precisely than is the case for rabbits. In the larger context of clinical immunology, it is noteworthy that CNS disease is not considered a manifestation of human HBV infection.

Transgenic animal studies have offered indirect clues to a microbial role in the development of EAE. Transgenic mice were constructed expressing genes encoding a rearranged T-cell receptor specific for MBP (26). T-cell tolerance was not induced in the periphery, and functional autoreactive T cells were found in the spleen and lymph nodes of these mice. EAE developed in these animals after administration of per-tussis toxin alone. Of interest, spontaneous EAE developed in transgenic mice housed in a nonsterile facility but not in those maintained in a sterile, specific pathogen-free facility. Thus, in animals with genetic predisposition to the autoim-mune disease, microbial agents appear to play a triggering role for disease activation. Although this is compatible with a molecular mimicry mechanism, it could also be that the infectious agent provokes changes in cytokine levels, levels of MBP expressed *in situ,* expression of homing receptors, or adhesion molecules expressed on autoreactive T cells, which in concert lead to the immunopathology in the CNS.

A different transgenic mouse model was developed pur-portedly to address the hypothesis that infection with a virus sharing antigenic epitopes with CNS antigens by molecular mimicry can elicit a virus-specific immune response that also recognizes self epitopes (178). Transgenic mice were devel-oped that expressed the nucleoprotein or glycoprotein of LCMV in oligodendrocytes through the use of the MBP pro-moter and the PLP gene. Intraperitoneal infection of these mice with LCMV led to infection of peripheral tissues but not CNS, and the virus was cleared in 14 days. After clearance of the virus, a chronic inflammation of the CNS resulted, with upregulation of MHC class I and II molecules locally. A sec-ond LCMV infection led to enhanced pathology in the CNS, with loss of myelin and clinical motor dysfunction. Infection with unrelated viruses (vaccinia virus, Pichinde virus) that cross-reacted with LCMV-specific memory T cells led to a comparable enhancement of the CNS disease. Thus, in this model, a peripheral infection with a virus sharing epitopes with a protein expressed on oligodendrocytes led to CNS immunopathology reminiscent of that seen in MS.

The cross-activation of memory T cells specific for a CNS autoantigen by subsequent viral infections may relate to the observation that MS can flare after infection with a variety of different viruses (179). As discussed previously for the LCMV-RIP transgenic model for diabetes mellitus (20,24), however, the infection with LCMV does not speak directly to the molecular mimicry hypothesis because in this instance, the identical factor (LCMV) serves at once as exogenous stimulus and endogenous autoantigen. Finally, evidence is lacking to show that viral infections of wild-type mice can reproduce the demyelination that is characteristic of EAE and MS. The cellular corollary of this, that T cells originally acti-vated by a naturally processed viral pathogen can recognize a CNS protein, is similarly lacking.

## Spondyloarthropathies

The SpAs include a group of different, but closely related, diseases: ankylosing spondylitis (AS), reactive arthritis,

Reiter's syndrome, psoriatic arthritis, and enteropathic arthritis. All of these subsets are characterized by a high frequency of spinal inflammation, oligoarthritis, inflammatory bowel, and eye and skin lesions. SpAs, in particular reactive arthritis, have been linked on clinical grounds to a variety of gram-negative enteric bacteria, including *Campylobacter jejuni*, *Yersinia enterocolitica*, *Shigella flexneri*, *Salmonella typhimurium*, and *Chlamydia trachomatis*. This has been supported by the finding of bacterial antigenic components and nuclear material in the target tissues (reviewed in 180). It has been well established that there exists a strong association between HLA-B27 and SpA (181), but the link between HLA-B27 and microbial infections in the pathogenesis of SpA remains unknown. Molecular mimicry between microbial antigens and HLA-B27 has been proposed to explain this connection.

Early evidence for molecular mimicry was based on the observation that antisera from rabbits immunized with HLA-B27+ human lymphocytes reacted against *Klebsiella aerogenes* (182). Subsequent studies showed that levels of anti–*Klebsiella pneumoniae* antibodies were higher in patients with AS than in control subjects (183). Subsequently, the development of monoclonal antibody provided support for antigenic similarity between HLA-B27 and antigens from several other arthritogenic bacteria. A monoclonal antibody, Ye-1, raised by immunizing animals with *Y. enterocolitica*, reacted with HLA-B27–positive cell lines (184). Another monoclonal antibody, Ye-2, reacted with a synthetic peptide derived from a subtype of HLA-B27 (185). Interestingly, Ye-2 recognized a synthetic peptide derived from bovine carbonic anhydrase, which has little amino acid homology to the HLA-B27 peptide, reinforcing the importance of conformational rather than linear epitopes for antibody binding. Reciprocal cross-reactivity was also demonstrated using monoclonal antibodies against HLA-B27 (B27M1 and B27M2), which recognize proteins from several bacteria, including *Y. enterocolitica*, *K. pneumoniae*, *S. flexneri*, *S. typhimurium*, and *E. coli* (186–188). Thus, these studies demonstrated serologic cross-reactivity between HLA-B27 and microbial antigens, implicating shared B-cell epitopes.

Further evidence for homology between HLA-B27 and enteric bacteria associated with SpA has been obtained by search of protein databases. A six–amino acid sequence (QTDRED) was found to be homologous between the HLA-B2705 gene product and *K. pneumoniae* nitrogen reductase (189). Sera from some HLA-B27 patients with Reiter's syndrome and AS bound the regions of both HLA-B2705 and nitrogenase, which contains the shared sequence (189,190). Rat antisera to several HLA-B2705 peptides and *K. pneumoniae* nitrogenase peptides were shown to bind synovial tissue of patients with both AS and reactive arthritis (191). Notably, the region of the HLA-B2705 antigen encompassing the homologous QTDRED sequence was strongly expressed on both synovial membrane lining cells and vascular endothelium of vessels in inflamed synovium of patients. A computer database search revealed homology between HLA-B2705 and another enzyme of *K. pneumoniae*, pulluanase (192). IgA and IgG antibody levels were elevated against synthetic peptides containing homology sequences shared by HLA-B27 and pulluanase. Increased antibody levels to pulluanase were also observed in AS patients.

Several other bacteria associated with SpA have also been identified as sharing amino acid sequence homology with HLA-B27. A plasmid, pHS-2, derived from arthritogenic strains of *S. flexneri*, encodes a sequence containing a stretch of amino acid homology with HLA-B27, although the expressed gene product has not been demonstrated (193). Affinity-purified anti-B2705 peptide antibodies strongly reacted against the peptide derived from pHS-2 (194). A leucine residue common to both HLA-B2705 and pHS-2 peptides was crucial for the cross-reactivity. Some evidence for sequence homology was also demonstrated for *Y. enterocolitica*. A *Yersinia* adhesin, Yad A, shares four amino acids (QTDR) with the first hypervariable region of HLA-B27 (195). Outer membrane proteins (Omph) of *Yersinia* and *Salmonella* were also found to share amino acid homology with HLA-B27 (196). Notably, these amino acid sequences are located in the same regions on the HLA-B27 molecule as a hexapeptide identical to *K. pneumoniae* nitrogenase and a pentapeptide shared with an *S. flexneri* protein (197). Clinical support was provided by the finding that some patients with reactive arthritis and AS had antibodies reactive against a panel of synthetic peptides bearing the homology sequence between HLA-B27 and Yad A or Omph. However, shorter stretches of amino acid sequence homology are more likely to occur on the basis of chance alone, as discussed previously.

The relatively common occurrence of sequence homology with HLA-B27 among enteric bacteria might relate to the pathogenic role of HLA-B27. The hypervariable regions of the HLA-B molecules were compared with the known sequenced protein for identical consecutive amino acid stretches (198). Unique among the HLA-B alleles, HLA-B27 shared an unexpected number of hexapeptides and pentapeptides with gram-negative bacterial proteins. Moreover, the enteric proteins appeared to satisfy the structural requirements for peptide binding to HLA-B27 in those regions of the sequence shared with HLA-B27. The mechanism by which these homologous sequences might mediate disease was then examined (199).

A model was proposed in which peptides that both mimic and bind HLA-B27 may constitute the molecular mechanism for SpA. The amino acid sequence of endogenous peptides found in the binding cleft of the HLA-B27 molecule had previously been used to define an HLA-B27 binding motif (200–202). The motif includes an invariant arginine in position 2 of a nonapeptide. HLA-B27 itself contains a nonapeptide sequence within the third hypervariable region that conforms to the binding motif. An assembly assay was used to study synthetic nonapeptides derived from sequences of enteric bacterial proteins homologous with the hypervariable regions of HLA-B27 and conforming to the HLA-B27–binding motif. The sequence of HLA-B2705 demonstrates a nonapeptide (LRRYLENGK), predicted to bind in the binding cleft of HLA-B27. Some nonapeptides from enteric organisms that share sequence homology with this nonapeptide of HLA-B27 also bound to HLA-B27. Thus, the bacteria that possess peptides that both mimic and bind HLA-B27 could alter the immune response in SpA. Similarly, peptides bound to or derived from histocompatibility alleles may operate in the HLA-B27–associated SpA. It could be hypothesized that the inflammatory response against self tissue results from the breakdown in tolerance of the host to self HLA-B27 and the endogenous peptides bound therein. Exposure of the host to enteric peptides homologous with HLA-B27 could evoke this response.

Despite the considerable amount of work devoted to exploring the potential for molecular mimicry in the pathogenesis of SpA, there has been no compelling evidence that such mimicry is of pathogenic significance in these diseases. For example, the possession of cross-reactive epitopes by bacteria does not correlate with an association between particular bacteria and arthritis (203). No antibody specific to the cross-reactive epitope has been demonstrated to have a direct role in inducing the manifestations of SpA. Moreover, a number of bacteria (e.g., *E. coli*) that share amino acid sequence with HLA-B27 do not appear to be arthritogenic based on clinical evidence. Thus, serologic cross-reactivity between a wide variety of bacterial proteins and HLA-B27 might be a relatively common phenomenon of limited pathologic significance. In addition, it has not been possible to demonstrate T-cell reactivity against peptides representing HLA-B27 antibody epitopes from patients with SpA (204). Thus, despite the fact that elevated levels of antibody reacting with the HLA-B27 peptide could be demonstrated, no evidence for T-cell–mediated immune reactivity could be found in the same patients. This challenges the molecular mimicry model in SpA because a T-cell–mediated immune response to the triggering microorganisms likely plays a crucial role in the pathogenesis of SpA (205).

Animal models have also been examined with respect to molecular mimicry between HLA-B27 and microbial proteins in the pathogenesis of SpA. Lewis rats transgenic for B2705 plus human $\beta_2$-microglobulin spontaneously develop an SpA-like disease, yet only a low proportion (15%) of these rats produced antibody to the HLA-B2705 peptide representing the potential cross-reacting epitope in the pHS-2 plasmid (206). The levels and distribution of the anti–HLA-B2705 or anti–pHS-2 peptide antibodies did not correlate directly with the presence of the experimental disease in the rat (206). In another approach, mice transgenic for HLA-B2705 and human $\beta_2$-microglobulin were immunized with a peptide, QTDRED, shared between HLA-B27 and *K. pneumoniae* nitrogenase (207). This peptide represents the epitope for serologic cross-reactivity, as discussed previously (190). Immunization with the cross-reactive peptide (the putative autoantigen) did not induce arthritis in the animals. In fact, the transgenic mice demonstrated tolerance to the epitope at both the T-cell and B-cell levels, in contrast to the nontransgenic litter mates, in which elevated humoral and cellular responses to the peptide were observed. This experimental model lends some support to the notion of mimicking peptides inducing tolerance rather than autoimmunity.

Molecular mimicry is clearly unresolved as an inciting mechanism in SpA. Although there has been a strong clinical correlation, as well as evidence for sequence homology and serologic cross-reactivity, there has been no clear demonstration of functional cross-reactivity. There are other theoretical issues with the hypothesis in this disease. First, class I HLA molecules, such as HLA-B27, are constitutively expressed on all nucleated cells in the body; thus, a direct mimicry mechanism between HLA-B27 and putative inciting organisms does not explain inflammation in the selected target tissues (e.g., spine, uveal tract of the eye, skin). Second, the SpAs are notable among the rheumatic diseases for the paucity of autoimmune phenomena demonstrable. Specific autoreactive T cells and autoantibodies against self antigens of target tissues have been difficult to demonstrate. Thus, autoimmunity itself and molecular mimicry as a mechanism have yet to be rigorously established in SpA.

## FUTURE DIRECTIONS

Molecular mimicry has persisted as an attractive hypothesis to explain the pathogenesis of autoimmune disease. Theoretically, the model integrates what is known about the development and breakdown of immunologic tolerance with the longheld clinical suspicion that microbial pathogens are culprits in the initiation of autoimmune disease. But using a grid to define criteria for molecular mimicry, does the evidence presented here validate the molecular mimicry hypothesis as a mechanism of induction of autoimmune disease? There is some supportive evidence, but for no one autoimmune disease have all the criteria been met.

The impetus to consider molecular mimicry in any one disease is based on a clinical suspicion that a pathogen is associated with the disease. Thus, the first criterion is automatically fulfilled for the diseases discussed. It is interesting, however, that investigators frequently invoke multiple different pathogens, and these are often common viruses or bacteria, complicating any confirmation of discreet, temporally related infectious events. The complexity is increased further by factors that have not been systematically considered in these studies. The interaction of innate and acquired immunity, the role of CTL, and the balance of $T_H1$ and $T_H2$ and their associated cytokines and costimulatory molecules need to be better understood to determine the host response to "arthritogenic" organisms. These studies must also take into account the fact that most people do not develop autoimmune disease after an infection. If infection does indeed trigger autoimmunity by means of molecular mimicry pathways, there may be multiple default pathways, as yet uncharacterized, that serve a protective role in most people and truncate an incipient autoimmune response.

The demonstration of sequence homology between candidate organisms and self determinants has probably been the most popular line of research in the molecular mimicry field. The significance of sequence homology, however, diminishes in proportion to the length of the homology sequence, and it has become clear that recognition of conformational identity, rather than simple sequence homology, is more relevant to T-cell activation. This has been addressed in studies determining the antigen specificity of patient-derived T-cell clones and testing synthetic, conformationally homologous peptides for T-cell activation before identifying the native protein in database screens. Although elegant, this approach is an unwieldy method for any large-scale screening of potential cross-reactive epitopes. Furthermore, as discussed for MS, T-cell responses to candidate peptides identified in this way may not even be monospecific, and identifying the single culprit may not be possible by this means.

Cross-reactive autoantibodies and T cells have been demonstrated in many of the autoimmune diseases. These are of unknown significance, however, when the various host determinants in disease pathogenesis are incompletely understood. For example, cross-reactivity generated against MHC-derived peptides does not explain the development of disease restricted to the joints or the β cells of the pancreas. Furthermore, there is limited evidence that these cross-reactive responses can be generated by naturally processed pathogens in the course of an infection and that these responses can produce target tissue injury.

Evidence for molecular mimicry will remain circumstantial until a comprehensive model system is developed in which a pathogen reproducibly activates T and B cells specific for homologous self determinants and until these activated cells can be shown to produce target tissue injury. An alternate approach to this problem may be to redirect the research focus toward gaining a better understanding of the normal host response to infection, with the development of autoimmunity viewed as a failure of the normal protective mechanisms. The role of molecular mimicry in such complex immune responses remains to be defined.

# REFERENCES

1. Damian RT. Molecular mimicry: antigen sharing by parasite and host and its consequences. *Am Nat* 1964;98:129–149.
2. Oldstone BA. Molecular mimicry and autoimmune disease. *Cell* 1987;50:819–820.
3. Chicz RM, Urban RG, Lane WS, et al. Predominant naturally processed peptides bound to HLA-DR1 are derived from MHC-related molecules and are heterogeneous in size. *Nature* 1992;358:764–768.
4. Kersh GJ, Allen PM. Essential flexibility in the T-cell recognition of antigen. *Nature* 1996;380:495–498.
5. Janeway CA Jr, Travers P, eds. *Immunobiology: the immune system in health and disease,* 2nd ed. New York: Current Biology/Garland Publishing, 1996.
6. Davis MM, Bjorkman PJ. T-cell antigen receptor genes and T-cell recognition. *Nature* 1988;334:395–402.
7. Guillet JG, Lai MZ, Briner TJ, et al. Interaction of peptide antigens and class II major histocompatibility antigens. *Nature* 1986;324:260–262.
8. Brown JH, Jardetzky TS, Gorga JC, et al. The three-dimensional structure of the human class II major histocompatibility antigen HLA-DR1. *Nature* 1993;364:33–39.
9. Garboczi DN, Ghosh P, Utz U, et al. Structure of the complex between human T-cell receptor, viral peptide and HLA-A2. *Nature* 1996;384:134–141.
10. Chicz RM, Urban RG, Gorga JC, et al. Specificity and promiscuity among naturally processed peptides bound to HLA-DR alleles. *J Exp Med* 1993;178:27–47.
11. Babbitt B, Allen PM, Matsueda G, et al. Binding of immunogenic peptides to Ia histocompatibility molecules. *Nature* 1985;317:359–361.
12. Buus S, Sette A, Colon SM, et al. The relation between major histocompatibility complex (MHC) restriction and the capacity of Ia to bind immunogenic peptides. *Science* 1987;235:1353–1358.
13. Falk K, Rotzsche O, Stevanovic S, et al. Allele-specific motifs revealed by sequencing of self peptides eluted from MHC molecules. *Nature* 1991;351:290–296.
14. Hunt DF, Henderson RA, Shabanowitz J, et al. Characterization of peptides bound to the class I MHC molecule HLA-A2.1 by mass spectrometry. *Science* 1992;255:1261–1263.
15. Guo H-C, Jardetzky TS, Lane WS, et al. Different length peptides bind to HLA-Aw68 similarly at their ends but bulge out in the middle. *Nature* 1992;360:364–366.
16. Kim S, Davis M, Sinn E, et al. Antibody diversity: somatic hypermutation of rearranged Vh genes. *Cell* 1981;27:573–581.
17. Parker DC. T cell-dependent B-cell activation. *Annu Rev Immunol* 1993;11:331–340.
18. Ohashi PS. T cell selection and autoimmunity: flexibility and tuning. *Curr Opin Immunol* 1996;8:808–814.
19. Goodnow CC. Balancing immunity and tolerance: deleting and tuning lymphocyte repertoires. *Proc Natl Acad Sci U S A* 1996;93:2264–2271.
20. Ohashi PS, Oehen S, Buerki K, et al. Ablation of "tolerance" and induction of diabetes by virus infection in viral antigen transgenic mice. *Cell* 1991;65:305–317.
21. Kawai K, Ohashi PS. Immunological function of a defined T-cell population tolerized to low-affinity self antigens. *Nature* 1995;374:68–69.
22. Kruisbeek AM, Amsen D. Mechanisms underlying T-cell tolerance. *Curr Opin Immunol* 1996;8:233–244.
23. Sercarz EE, Lehmann PV, Ametani A, et al. Dominance and crypticity of T cell antigenic determinants. *Annu Rev Immunol* 1993;11:729–766.
24. Oldstone MBA, Nerenberg M, Southern P, et al. Virus infection triggers insulin-dependent diabetes mellitus in a transgenic model: role of anti-self (virus) immune response. *Cell* 1991;65:319–331.
25. Bachmann MF, Rohrer UH, Kundig TM, et al. The influence of antigen organization on B cell responsiveness. *Science* 1993;262:1448–1451.
26. Goverman J, Woods A, Larson L, et al. Transgenic mice that express a myelin basic protein-specific T cell receptor develop spontaneous autoimmunity. *Cell* 1993;72:551–560.
27. Taurog JD, Richardson JA, Croft JT, et al. The germ free state prevents development of gut and joint inflammatory disease in HLA-B27 transgenic rats. *J Exp Med* 1994;180:2359–2364.
28. Rocken M, Urban JF, Shevach EM. Infection breaks T-cell tolerance. *Nature* 1992;359:79–82.
29. Segal BM, Klinman DM, Shevach EM. Microbial products induce autoimmune disease by an IL-12 dependent pathway. *J Immunol* 1997;158:5087–5090.
30. Roudier C, Auger I, Roudier J. Molecular mimicry reflected through database screening: serendipity or survival strategy? *Immunol Today* 1996;17:357–358.
31. Srinivasappa J, Saegusa J, Prabhadar BS, et al. Molecular mimicry: frequency of reactivity of monoclonal antiviral antibodies with normal tissues. *J Virol* 1986;57:397–401.
32. Bahmanyar S, Srinivasappa J, Casali P, et al. Antigenic mimicry between measles virus and human T lymphocytes. *J Infect Dis* 1987;156:526–527.
33. Tung KSK, Lou YH, Garza KM, et al. Autoimmune ovarian disease: mechanism of disease induction and prevention. *Curr Opin Immunol* 1997;9:839–845.
34. Wucherpfennig KW, Strominger JL. Molecular mimicry in T cell-mediated autoimmunity: viral peptides activate human T cell clones specific for myelin basic protein. *Cell* 1995;80:695–705.
35. Hemmer B, Fleckenstein BT, Vergelli M, et al. Identification of high potency microbial and self ligands for a human autoreactive class II restricted T cell clone. *J Exp Med* 1997;185:1651–1659.
36. Hausmann S, Wucherpfennig KW. Activation of autoreactive T cells by peptides from human pathogens. *Curr Opin Immunol* 1997;9:831–838.

37. Lehmann PV, Forsthuber T, Miller A, et al. Spreading of T-cell autoimmunity to cryptic determinants of an autoantigen. *Nature* 1992;358:155–157.

38. Holoshitz J, Naparstek Y, Ben-Nun A, et al. Line of T lymphocytes induce or vaccinate against autoimmune arthritis. *Science* 1983;219:56–58.

39. Van Eden W, Thole JER, van der Zee R, et al. Cloning of the mycobacterial epitope recognized by T lymphocytes in adjuvant arthritis. *Nature* 1988;331:171–173.

40. Singh VK, Nagaraju K. Experimental autoimmune uveitis: molecular mimicry and oral tolerance. *Immunol Res* 1996;15:323–346.

41. Fujinami RS, Oldstone MBA. Amino acid homology between the encephalitogenic site of myelin basic protein and virus: mechanism for autoimmunity. *Science* 1985;230:1043–1045.

42. Zhao Z-S, Granucci F, Yeh L, et al. Molecular mimicry by herpes simplex virus-type 1: autoimmune disease after viral infection. *Science* 1998;279:1344–1347.

43. Wu J, Zhou T, He J, et al. Autoimmune disease in mice due to integration of an endogenous retrovirus in an apoptosis gene. *J Exp Med* 1993;178:461–468.

44. Kaplan MH, Dallenbach FD. Immunologic studies of heart tissue. II. Occurrence of bound gamma globulin in auricular appendages from rheumatic hearts. Relationship to certain histopathologic features of rheumatic heart disease. *J Exp Med* 1961;113:1–12.

45. Zabriskie JB, Freimer EH. An immunological relationship between the group A streptococcus and mammalian muscle. *J Exp Med* 1966;124:661–678.

46. van de Rijn I, Zabriskie JB, McCarty M: Group A streptococcal antigens cross-reactive with myocardium: purification of heart-reactive antibody and isolation and characterization of the streptococcal antigen. *J Exp Med* 1977;146:579–599.

47. Dale JB, Beachy EH. Multiple, heart-cross-reactive epitopes of streptococcal M protein. *J Exp Med* 1985;161:113–122.

48. Dale JB, Beachy EH. Epitopes of streptococcal M protein shared with cardiac myosin. *J Exp Med* 1985;162:583–591.

49. Manjula BN, Fischetti VA. Tropomyosin-like seven residue periodicity in three immunologically distinct streptococcal M proteins and its implications for the antiphagocytic property of the molecule. *J Exp Med* 1980;151:695–708.

50. Dale JB, Beachy EH. Localization of protective epitopes of the amino terminus of type 5 streptococcal M protein. *J Exp Med* 1986;163:1191–1202.

51. Beachy EH, Gras-Masse H, Tarter A, et al. Opsonic antibodies evoked by hybrid peptide copies of types 5 and 24 streptococcal M proteins synthesized in tandem. *J Exp Med* 1986;163:1451–1458.

52. Cunningham MW, Krisher K, Graves DC. Murine monoclonal antibodies reactive with human heart and group A streptococcal membrane antigens. *Infect Immun* 1984;46:34–41.

53. Krisher K, Cunningham MW. Myosin: a link between streptococci and heart. *Science* 1985;277:413–415.

54. Dale JB, Beachy EH. Sequence of myosin-cross-reactive epitopes of streptococcal M protein. *J Exp Med* 1986;164:1785–1790.

55. Beachy EH, Bronze MS, Dale JB, et al. Protective and autoimmune epitopes of streptococcal M proteins. *Vaccine* 1988;6:192–196.

56. Cunningham MW, Antone SM, Gulizia JM, et al. Cytotoxic and viral neutralizing antibodies cross react with streptococcal M protein, enteroviruses and human cardiac myosin. *Immunology* 1992;89:1320–1324.

57. Vashishtha A, Frischetti V. Surface-exposed conserved region of the streptococcal M protein induces antibodies cross-reactive with denatured forms of myosin. *J Immunol* 1993;150:4693–4701.

58. Kil KS, Cunningham MW, Barnett LA. Cloning and sequence analysis of a gene encoding a 67-kilodalton myosin-cross-reactive antigen of streptococcus pyogenes reveals its similarity with class II major histocompatibility antigens. *Infect Immun* 1994;62:2440–2449.

59. Khanna AK, Nomura Y, Fischetti VA, et al. Antibodies in the sera of acute rheumatic fever patients bind to human cardiac tropomyosin. *J Autoimmunol* 1997;10:99–106.

60. Huber SA, Cunningham MW. Streptococcal M protein peptide with similarity to myosin induces CD4+ T cell-dependent myocarditis in MRL/++ mice and induces partial tolerance against coxsackieviral myocarditis. *J Immunol* 1996;156:3528–3534.

61. Cunningham MW, Antone SM, Smart M, et al. Molecular analysis of human cardiac myosin-cross-reactive B- and T-cell epitopes of the group A streptococcal M5 protein. *Infect Immunol* 1997;65:3913–3923.

62. Wolfgram LJ, Beisel KW, Herskowitz Z, et al. Variations in the susceptibility to coxsackievirus B3-induced myocarditis among different strains of mice. *J Immunol* 1986;136:1846–1852.

63. Neu N, Beisel KW, Traystmann MD, et al. Autoantibodies specific for the cardiac myosin isoform are found in mice susceptible to coxsackievirus B3 induced myocarditis. *J Immunol* 1987;138:2488–2492.

64. Neumann DA, Rose NR, Ansari AA, et al. Induction of multiple heart autoantibodies in mice with coxsackievirus B3- and cardiac myosin-induced autoimmune myocarditis. *J Immunol* 1994;152:343–350.

65. Huber S, Polgar J, Schultheiss P, et al. Augmentation of pathogenesis of coxsackievirus B3 infections by exogenous administration of interleukin-1 and interleukin-2. *J Virol* 1994;68:195–206.

66. Gauntt CJ, Arizpe HM, Higdon AL, et al. Molecular mimicry, anti-coxsackievirus B3 neutralizing monoclonal antibodies, and myocarditis. *J Immunol* 1995;154:2983–2995.

67. Cunningham MW, Antone SM, Gulizia JM, et al. Cytotoxic and viral neutralizing antibodies cross-react with streptococcal M protein, enteroviruses, and human cardiac myosin. *Proc Natl Acad Sci U S A* 1992;89:1320–1324.

68. Huber SA, Moraska A, Cunningham M. Alterations in major histocompatibility complex association of myocarditis induced by coxsackie B3 mutants selected with monoclonal antibodies to group A streptococci. *Proc Natl Acad Sci U S A* 1994;91:5543–5547.

69. Huber SA. Autoimmunity in myocarditis: relevance of animal models. *Clin Immunol Immunopathol* 1997;83:93–102.

70. Huber S, Haisch C, Lodge PA. Functional diversity in vascular endothelial cells: role in coxsackievirus tropism. *J Virol* 1990;64:4516–4520.

71. Herzum M, Ruppert V, Kuytz B, et al. Coxsackievirus B3 infection leads to cell death of cardiac myocytes. *J Mol Cell Cardiol* 1994;26:907–913.

72. McManus BM, Chow LH, Wilson JE, et al. Direct myocardial injury by enterovirus: a central role in the evolution of murine myocarditis. *Clin Immunol Immunopathol* 1993;68:159–169.

73. Neu N, Rose NR, Beisel BW, et al. Cardiac myosin induces myocarditis in genetically predisposed mice. *J Immunol* 1987;139:3630–3636.

74. Smith SC, Allen PM. Neutralization of endogenous tumor necrosis factor ameliorates the severity of myosin-induced myocarditis. *Circ Res* 1992;70:856–863.

75. Wegmann KW, Zhao W, Griffin AC, et al. Identification of myocarditogenic peptides derived from cardiac myosin capable of inducing experimental allergic myocarditis in the Lewis rat: the utility of a class II binding motif in selecting self-reactive peptides. *J Immunol* 1994;153:892–900.

76. Mason JW, O'Connell JB, Herskowitz A, et al. A clinical trial of immunosuppressive therapy for myocarditis. *N Engl J Med* 1995;333:269–275.

77. Van Voorhis WC, Eisen H. A surface antigen of Trypanosoma cruzi that mimics mammalian nervous tissue. *J Exp Med* 1989;169:641–652.

78. Cunha-Neto E, Duranti M, Gruber A. Autoimmunity in Chagas disease cardiopathy: biologic relevance of a cardiac myosin-specific epitope crossreactive to an immunodominant Trypanosoma cruzi antigen. *Proc Natl Acad Sci U S A* 1995;92:3541–3545.

79. Van Voorhis WC, Schlekewy L, Trong HL: Molecular mimicry by Trypanosoma cruzi: the Fl-160 epitope that mimics mammalian nerve can be mapped to a 12-amino acid peptide. *Proc Natl Acad Sci U S A* 1991;88:5993–5997.

80. Ribeiro dos Santos R, Rossi MA, Laus JL, et al. Anti-CD4 abrogates rejection and reestablishes long term tolerance to syngeneic newborn hearts grafted in mice chronically infected with Trypanosoma cruzi. *J Exp Med* 1992;175:29–39.

81. Tarleton RL, Zhang L, Downs MO. "Autoimmune rejection" of neonatal heart transplants in experimental Chagas disease is a parasite-specific response to infected host tissue. *Proc Natl Acad Sci U S A* 1997;94:3932–3937.

82. Ferrari I, Levin MJ, Wallukat G, et al. Molecular mimicry between the immunodominant ribosomal protein PO of Trypanosoma cruzi and a functional epitope on the human b1-adrenergic receptor. *J Exp Med* 1995;182:59–65.

83. Elies R, Ferrair I, Wallukat G, et al. Structural and functional analysis of the B cell epitopes recognized by anti-receptor autoantibodies in patients with Chagas disease. *J Immunol* 1996;157:4203–4211.

84. Kaplan D, Ferrari I, Bergami PL, et al. Antibodies to the ribosomal P proteins of Trypanosoma cruzi in Chagas disease possess functional autoreactivity with heart tissue and differ from anti-P autoantibodies in lupus. *Proc Natl Acad Sci U S A* 1997;94:10301.

85. Rouse BT: Virus-induced immunopathology. *Adv Virus Res* 1996; 47:353.

86. Streilein JW, Dana MR, Ksander BR. Immunity causing blindness: five different paths to herpes stromal keratitis. *Immunol Today* 1997;18:443–449.

87. Atkinson MA, Maclaren NK. The pathogenesis of insulin-dependent diabetes mellitus. *N Engl J Med* 1994;331:1428–1436.

88. Gazda LS, Charlton B, Lafferty KJ. Diabetes results from a late change in the autoimmune response of NOD mice. *J Autoimmunol* 1997;10: 261–270.

89. Endl J, Otto H, Jung G, et al. Identification of naturally processed T cell epitopes from glutamic acid decarboxylase presented in the context of HLA-DR alleles by T lymphocytes of recent onset IDDM patients. *J Clin Invest* 1997;99:2405–2415.

90. Barnett AH, Eff C, Leslie RDG, et al. Diabetes in identical twins: a study of 200 pairs. *Diabetologia* 1981;20:87–93.

91. Todd JA, Bell JI, McDevitt HO. HLA-DQ beta gene contributes to susceptibility and resistance to insulin-dependent diabetes mellitus. *Nature* 1987;329:599–604.

92. Sheehy MJ, Scharf SJ, Rowe JR, et al. A diabetes-susceptible HLA haplotype is best defined by a combination of HLA-DR and HLA-DQ alleles. *J Clin Invest* 1989;83:830–835.

93. Wicker LS, Todd JA, Peterson LB. Genetic control of autoimmune diabetes in the NOD mouse. *Annu Rev Immunol* 1995;13:179–200.

94. Lundberg AS, McDevitt HO. Evolution of major histocompatibility complex class II allelic diversity: direct descent in mice and humans. *Proc Natl Acad Sci U S A* 1992;89:6545–6549.

95. Makino S, Kunimoto K, Muraoka Y, et al. Breeding of a non-obese, diabetic strain of mice. *Exp Anim* 1980;29:1–6.

96. Nakano N, Kikutani, H, Nishimoto H, et al. T cell receptor V gene usage of islet B cell-reactive T cells is not restricted in non-obese diabetic mice. *J Exp Med* 1991;173:1091–1097.

97. Kaufman DL, Clare-Salzler M, Tian J, et al. Spontaneous loss of T-cell tolerance to glutamic-acid decarboxylase in murine insulin-dependent diabetes. *Nature* 1993;366:69–72.

98. Tisch R, Yang XD, Singer SM, et al. Immune response to glutamic acid decarboxylase correlates with insulitis in non-obese diabetic mice. *Nature* 1993;366:72–75.

99. Pontesilli O, Carotenuto P, Gazda LS, et al. Circulating lymphocyte populations and autoantibodies in non-obese diabetic (NOD) mice: a longitudinal study. *Clin Exp Immunol* 1987;70:84–93.

100. Karges W, Hammond-McKibben D, Gaedigk R, et al. Loss of self-tolerance to ICA69 in nonobese diabetic mice. *Diabetes* 1997;46: 1548–1556.

101. Oldstone MBA. Viruses as therapeutic agents. I. Treatment of non-obese insulin-dependent mice with virus prevents insulin-dependent diabetes mellitus while maintaining general immune competence. *J Exp Med* 1990;171:2077–2089.

102. Wilberz S, Partke JH, Dagnaes-Hansen F, et al. Persistent MHV (mouse hepatitis virus) infection reduces the incidence of diabetes mellitus in non-obese diabetic mice. *Diabetologia* 1991;34:2–5.

103. Katz JD, Wang B, Haskins K, et al. Following a diabetogenic T cell from genesis through pathogenesis. *Cell* 1993;74:1089–1100.

104. von Herrath MG, Guerder S, Lewicki H, et al. Coexpression of B7-1 and viral ("self") transgenes in pancreatic b cells can break peripheral ignorance and lead to spontaneous autoimmune diabetes. *Immunity* 1995;3:727–738.

105. Menser, MA, Forrest JM, Bransby RD: Rubella infection and diabetes mellitus. *Lancet* 1978;1:57–60.

106. Szopa TM, Titchener PA, Portwood ND, et al. Diabetes mellitus due to viruses-some recent developments. *Diabetologia* 1993;36:687–695.

107. Barrett-Connor E. Is insulin-dependent diabetes mellitus caused by coxsackievirus B infection? A review of the epidemiologic evidence. *Rev Infect Dis* 1985;7:207–215.

108. Solimena M, De Camilli P. Coxsackieviruses and diabetes. *Nature Med* 1995;1:25–27.

109. Yoon JW, Austin M, Onodera T, et al. Isolation of a virus from the pancreas of a child with diabetic ketoacidosis. *N Engl J Med* 1979; 300:1173–1179.

110. Kaufman DL, Erlander MG, Clare-Salzler M, et al. Autoimmunity to two forms of glutamate decarboxylase in insulin-dependent diabetes mellitus. *J Clin Invest* 1992;89:283–292.

111. Solimena M, Folli F, Aparisi R, et al. Autoantibodies to GABA-ergic neurons and pancreatic beta cells in stiff man syndrome. *N Engl J Med* 1990;322:1555–1560.

112. Harrison LC, Honeyman MC, DeAizpurua HJ, et al. Inverse relation between humoral and cellular immunity to glutamic acid decarboxylase in subjects at risk of insulin-dependent diabetes. *Lancet* 1993;341: 1365–1369.

113. Tian J, Lehmann PV, Kaufman DL. T cell cross-reactivity between coxsackievirus and glutamate decarboxylase is associated with a murine diabetes susceptibility allele. *J Exp Med* 1994;180:1979–1984.

114. Atkinson MA, Bowman MA, Campbell L, et al. Cellular immunity to a determinant common to glutamate decarboxylase and coxsackie virus in insulin-dependent diabetes. *J Clin Invest* 1994;94:2125–2129.

115. Jones DB, Armstrong NW. Coxsackie virus and diabetes revisited. *Nature Med* 1995;1:284.

116. Richter W, Mertens T, Schoel B, et al. Sequence homology of the diabetes-associated autoantigen glutamate decarboxylase with coxsackie B4-2C protein and heat shock protein 60 mediates no molecular mimicry of autoantibodies. *J Exp Med* 1994;180:721–726.

117. Miyazaki I, Cheung RK, Gaedigk R, et al. T cell activation and anergy to islet cell antigen in type I diabetes. *J Immunol* 1995;154:1461–1469.

118. Karjalainen J, Martin JM, Knip M, et al. A bovine albumin peptide as a possible trigger of insulin-dependent diabetes mellitus. *N Engl J Med* 1992;327:302–307.

119. Cheung R, Karjalainen J, Singal DP, et al. T cells from children with IDDM are sensitized to bovine serum albumin. *Scand J Immunol* 1994;40:623–628.

120. Atkinson MA, Bowman MA, Kao K-J, et al. Lack of immune responsiveness to bovine serum albumin in insulin-dependent diabetes. *N Engl J Med* 1993;329:1853–1857.

121. Cavallo MG, Fava D, Monetini L, et al. Cell-mediated immune response to b casein in recent onset insulin-dependent diabetes: implications for disease pathogenesis. *Lancet* 1996;348:926–928.

122. Malkani S, Nompleggi D, Hansen JW, et al. Dietary cow's milk protein does not alter the frequency of diabetes in the BB rat. *Diabetes* 1997;46:1133–1140.

123. Feldmann M, Brennan FM, Maini RN. Rheumatoid arthritis. *Cell* 1996;85:307–310.

124. Feldmann M, Brennan FM, Maini RN. Role of cytokines in rheumatoid arthritis. *Annu Rev Immunol* 1996;14:397–440.

125. Vaughan JH. Pathogenetic concepts and origins of rheumatoid factor in rheumatoid arthritis. *Arthritis Rheum* 1993;36:1–6.

126. Andriopoulos NA, Mestecky J, Miller EJ, et al. Antibodies to native and denatured collagens in sera of patients with rheumatoid arthritis. *Arthritis Rheum* 1976;19:613–617.

127. Clague RB, Shaw MJ, Holt PJ. Incidence of serum antibodies to native type I and type II collagens in patients with inflammatory arthritis. *Ann Rheum Dis* 1980;39:201–206.

128. Tarkowski A, Klareskog L, Carlsten H, et al. Secretion of antibodies to type I and type II collagen by synovial tissue cells in patients with rheumatoid arthritis. *Arthritis Rheum* 1989;32:1087–1092.

129. Winfield JB. Stress proteins, arthritis and autoimmunity. *Arthritis Rheum* 1989;32:1497–1504.

130. Nepom GT, Byers P, Seyfried C, et al. HLA genes associated with rheumatoid arthritis. *Arthritis Rheum* 1989;32:15–21.

131. Gregersen PK, Silver J, Winchester RJ. The shared epitope hypothesis: an approach to understanding the molecular genetics of susceptibility to rheumatoid arthritis. *Arthritis Rheum* 1987;30:1205–1213.

132. Nepom GT, Nepom BS. Prediction of susceptibility to rheumatoid arthritis by human leukocyte antigen genotyping. *Rheum Dis Clin North Am* 1992;18:785–792.

133. Hammer J, Gallazzi F, Bono E, et al. Peptide binding specificity of HLA-DR4 molecules: correlation with rheumatoid arthritis association. *J Exp Med* 1995;181:1847–1855.

134. Weyand CM, Hicok KC, Conn DL, et al. The influence of HLA-DRB1 genes on disease severity in rheumatoid arthritis. *Ann Intern Med* 1992;117:801–806.

135. Roudier J, Rhodes G, Petersen J, et al. The Epstein-Barr virus glycoprotein gp110, a molecular link between HLA DR4, HLA DR1 and rheumatoid arthritis. *Scand J Immunol* 1988;27:367–371.

136. Roudier J, Petersen J, Rhodes GH, et al. Susceptibility to rheumatoid arthritis maps to a T-cell epitope shared by the HLA-Dw4 DR beta-1 chain and the Epstein-Barr virus glycoprotein gp110. *Proc Natl Acad Sci U S A* 1989;86:5104–5108.

137. Yaq QY, Rickinson AB, Gaston JSH, et al. Disturbance of the Epstein-Barr virus-host balance in rheumatoid arthritis patients: a quantitative study. *Clin Exp Immunol* 1986;64:302–310.

138. Depper JM, Zvaifler NJ, Epstein-Barr virus: its relationship to the pathogenesis of rheumatoid arthritis. *Arthritis Rheum* 1981;24: 755–761.

139. Birkenfeld P, Haratz N, Klein G, et al. Cross-reactivity between the EBNA-1 p107 peptide, collagen and keratin: implications of the pathogenesis of rheumatoid arthritis. *Clin Immunol Immunopathol* 1990;54: 14–25.

140. Wilson C, Tiwana H, Ebringer A. HLA-DR4 restriction, molecular mimicry and rheumatoid arthritis. *Immunol Today* 1997;18:96–97.

141. Kaufmann SHE. Heat shock proteins and the immune response. *Immunol Today* 1990;11:129–146.

142. Cohen IR, Holoshitz J, Van Eden W, et al. T-lymphocyte clones illuminate pathogenesis and effect therapy of experimental arthritis. *Arthritis Rheum* 1985;28:841–845.

143. van der Zee R, van Eden W, Meloen RH, et al. Epitope mapping and characterization of a T cell epitope by the simultaneous synthesis of multiple peptides. *Eur J Immunol* 1989;19:43–47.

144. DeJoy SQ, Ferguson KM, Sapp TM, et al. Streptococcal cell wall arthritis: passive transfer of disease with a T cell line and crossreactivity of streptococcal cell wall antigens with *Mycobacterium tuberculosis*. *J Exp Med* 1989;170:369–382.

145. van den Broek MF, Hogervorst EJM, van Bruggen MCJ, et al. Protection against streptococcal cell wall-induced arthritis by pretreatment with the 65-kD mycobacterial heat shock protein. *J Exp Med* 1989;170:449–466.

146. Tishler M, Shoenfeld Y. Anti-heat shock protein antibodies in rheumatic and autoimmune diseases. *Semin Arthritis Rheum* 1996;26: 558–563.

147. Res PC, Telgt D, van Laar JM, et al. High antigen reactivity in mononuclear cells from sites of chronic inflammation. *Lancet* 1990; 336:1406–1408.

148. Gaston JSH, Life PF, Bailey LC, et al. In vitro responses to a 65 kilodalton mycobacterial protein by synovial T cells from inflammatory arthritis patients. *J Immunol* 1989;143:2494–2500.

149. Quayle AJ, Wilson KB, Li SG, et al. Peptide recognition, T cell receptor usage and HLA restriction elements of human heat-shock protein (hsp) 60 and mycobacterial 65-kDa hsp-reactive T cell clones from rheumatoid synovial fluid. *Eur J Immunol* 1992;22:1315–1322.

150. Jones DB, Coulson AF, Duff GW. Sequence homologies between hsp60 and autoantigens. *Immunol Today* 1993;14:115–118.

151. Karlsson-Parra A, Soederstroem K, Ferm M, et al. Presence of human 65 kD heat shock protein (hsp) in inflamed joints and subcutaneous nodules of RA patients. *Scand J Immunol* 1990;31:283–288.

152. de Graeff-Meeder ER, Voorhorst M, van Eden W, et al. Antibodies to the mycobacterial 65-kD heat shock protein are reactive with synovial tissue of adjuvant arthritic rats and patients with rheumatoid arthritis and osteoarthritis. *Am J Pathol* 1990;137:1013–1017.

153. de Graeff-Meeder ER, van der Zee R, Rijkers GT, et al. Recognition of human 60 kD heat shock protein by mononuclear cells from patients with juvenile chronic arthritis. *Lancet* 1991;337:1368–1372.

154. Gaston JS, Life PF, van der Zee R, et al. Epitope specificity and MHC restriction of rheumatoid arthritis synovial T cell clones which recognize a mycobacterial 65 kDa heat shock protein. *Int Immunol* 1991;3:965–972.

155. Van Asseldork M, Simons M, Visser H, et al. Cloning nucleotide sequence and regulatory analysis of the Lactococcus lactis dnaJ gene. *J Bacteriol* 1993;175:1637–1644.

156. Bardwell JCA, Tilly K, Craig E, et al. The nucleotide sequence of the Escherichia coli K12 dnaJ+ gene: a gene that encodes a heat shock protein. *J Biol Chem* 1986;261:1782–1785.

157. Albani S, Keystone EC, Nelson JL, et al. Positive selection in autoimmunity: abnormal immune responses to a bacterial dnaJ antigenic determinant in patients with early rheumatoid arthritis. *Nature Med* 1995;1:448–452.

158. Albani S, Carson DA. A multistep molecular mimicry hypothesis for the pathogenesis of rheumatoid arthritis. *Immunol Today* 1996;17: 466–470.

159. Salvat S, Auger I, Rochelle L, et al. Tolerance to a self-peptide from the third hypervariable region of HLA-DRB1*0401 in rheumatoid arthritis patients and normal subjects. *J Immunol* 1994;152:5321–5329.

160. Auger I, Escola JM, Gorvel JP, et al. HLA-DR4 and HLA-DR10 motifs that carry susceptibility to rheumatoid arthritis bind 70-kD heat shock proteins. *Nature Med* 1996;2:306–310.

161. Campbell RD, Trowsdale J. Map of the human MHC. *Immunol Today* 1993;14:349–352.

162. Williams DB, Watts TH. Molecular chaperones in antigen presentation. *Curr Opin Immunol* 1995;7:77–84.

163. Domanico S, Denagel D, Dahlseid J, et al. Cloning of the gene encoding peptide-binding protein 74 shows that it is a new member of the heat shock protein 70 family. *Mol Cell Biol* 1993;13:3598–3610.

164. Krco C, Pawelski J, Hardeers J, et al. Characterization of the antigenic structure of human type II collagen. *J Immunol* 1996;156:2761–2768.

165. Dhib-Jalubt S, Lewis K, Bradburn E, et al. Measles virus polypeptide-specific antibody profile in multiple sclerosis. *Neurology* 1990;40: 430–435.

166. Soldan SS, Perti R, Salem N, et al. Association of human herpes virus 6 (HHV-6) with multiple sclerosis: increased IgM response to HHV-6 early antigen and detection of serum HHV-6 DNA. *Nature Med* 1997;3:1394–1397.

167. Burks JS, DeVald BL, Jankovsky LD, et al. Two coronaviruses isolated from central nervous system tissue of two multiple sclerosis patients. *Science* 1980;209:933–934.

168. Perron H, Garson JA, Bedin F, et al. Molecular identification of a novel retrovirus repeatedly isolated from patients with multiple sclerosis. The Collaborative Research Group on Multiple Sclerosis. *Proc Natl Acad Sci U S A* 1997;94:7583–7584.

169. Olsson T, Wei Zhi W, Hojeberg B, et al. Autoreactive T lymphocytes in multiple sclerosis determined by antigen-induced secretion of interferon-gamma. *J Clin Invest* 1990;86:981–985.

170. Sun JB, Olsson T, Wang WZ, et al. Autoreactive T and B cells responding to myelin proteolipid protein in multiple sclerosis and controls. *Eur J Immunol* 1991;21:1461–1468.

171. Atkins GJ, Daly EA, Sheahan BJ, et al. Multiple sclerosis and molecular mimicry. *Neuropathol Appl Neurobiol* 1990;16:179–180.

172. Banki K, Colombo E, Sia F, et al. Oligodendrocyte-specific expression and autoantigenicity of transaldolase in multiple sclerosis. *J Exp Med* 1994;180:1649–1663.

173. Wucherpfennig KW, Sette A, Southwood S, et al. Structural requirements for binding of an immunodominant myelin basic protein peptide to DR2 isotypes and for its recognition by human T cell clones. *J Exp Med* 1994;179:279–290.

174. Allen I, Brankin B. Pathogenesis of multiple sclerosis: the immune diathesis and the role of viruses. *J Neuropathol Exp Neurol* 1993;52: 95–105.

175. Talbot PJ, Paquette JS, Ciurli C, et al. Myelin basic protein and human coronavirus 229E cross-reactive T cells in multiple sclerosis. *Ann Neurol* 1996;39:233–240.

176. Stewart JN, Mounir S, Talbot PJ. Human coronavirus gene expression in the brains of multiple sclerosis patients. *Virology* 1992;191: 502–505.

177. Wucherpfennig KW, Catz I, Hausmann S, et al. Recognition of the immunodominant myelin basic protein peptide by autoantibodies and HLA-DR2-restricted T cell clones from multiple sclerosis patients: identity of key contact residues in the B-cell and T-cell epitopes. *J Clin Invest* 1997;100:1114–1122.

178. Evans CF, Horwitz MS, Hobbs MV, et al. Viral infection of transgenic mice expressing a viral protein in oligodendrocytes leads to chronic central nervous system autoimmune disease. *J Exp Med* 1996;184: 2371–2384.

179. Anderson O, Lygner PE, Bergstrom T, et al. Viral infections trigger multiple sclerosis relapses: a prospective seroepidemiological study. *J Neurol* 1993;240:417–422.

180. Behar SM, Porcelli SA. Mechanisms of autoimmune disease induction: the role of the immune response to microbial pathogens. *Arthritis Rheum* 1995;38:458–476.

181. Lopez de Castro JA. The pathogenetic role of HLA-B27 in chronic arthritis. *Curr Opin Immunol* 1998;10:59–66.

182. Ebringer A, Cowling P, Ngwa-Suh N, et al. Cross-reactivity between Klebsiella aerogenes species and B27 lymphocyte antigens as an aetiological factor in ankylosing spondylitis. In: Dausset J, Svejaard A, eds. *HLA and disease*, Vol 58. Paris: INSERM, 1976:27.

183. Avakian H, Welsh J, Ebringer A, et al. Ankylosing spondylitis, HLA-B27 and Klebsiella. II. Cross-reactivity studies with human tissue typing sera. *Br J Exp Pathol* 1980;61:92–96.
184. Kono DH, Ogasawara M, Effros RB, et al. Ye-1, a monoclonal antibody that cross-reacts with HLA-B27 lymphoblastoid cell lines and an arthritis causing bacteria. *Clin Exp Immunol* 1985;61:503–508.
185. Yong Z, Zhang JJ, Schaack T, et al. A monoclonal anti-HLA-B27 antibody which is reactive with a linear sequence of the HLA-B27 protein is useful for the study of molecular mimicry. *Clin Exp Rheumatol* 1989;7:513–519.
186. Grumet FC, Fendly BM, Engleman EG. Monoclonal anti-HLA-B27 antibody (B27M1): production and lack of detectable typing difference between patients with ankylosing spondylitis, Reiter's syndrome, and normal controls. *Lancet* 1981;2:174.
187. Grumet FC, Fendly BM, Fish L, et al. Monoclonal antibody (B27M2) subdividing HLA-B27. *Hum Immunol* 1982;5:61–72.
188. Raybourne RB, Bunning VK, Williams KM. Reaction of anti-HLA-B monoclonal antibodies with envelope proteins of Shigella species: evidence for molecular mimicry in the spondyloarthropathies. *J Immunol* 1988;140:3489–3495.
189. Schwimmbeck PL, Yu DT, Oldstone MB. Autoantibodies to HLA B27 in the sera of HLA B27 patients with ankylosing spondylitis and Reiter's syndrome: molecular mimicry with Klebsiella pneumoniae as potential mechanism of autoimmune disease. *J Exp Med* 1987;166:173–181.
190. Ewing C, Ebringer R, Tribbick G, et al. Antibody activity in ankylosing spondylitis sera to two sites on HLA B27.1 at the MHC groove region (within sequence 65-85), and to a Klebsiella pneumoniae nitrogenase reductase peptide (within sequence 181-199). *J Exp Med* 1990;171:1635–1647.
191. Husby G, Tsuchiya N, Schwimmbeck PL, et al. Cross-reactive epitope with Klebsiella pneumoniae nitrogenase in articular tissue of HLA-B27+ patients with ankylosing spondylitis. *Arthritis Rheum* 1989;32:437–445.
192. Fielder M, Pirt SJ, Tarpey I, et al. Molecular mimicry and ankylosing spondylitis: possible role of a novel sequence in pullulanase of Klebsiella pneumoniae. *FEBS Lett* 1995;369:243–248.
193. Stieglitz H, Fosmirer S, Lipsky P. Identification of a 2-Md plasmid from Shigella flexneri associated with reactive arthritis. *Arthritis Rheum* 1989;32:937–946.
194. Tsuchiya N, Husby G, Williams RC Jr, et al. Autoantibodies to the HLA-B27 sequence cross-react with the hypothetical peptide from

the arthritis-associated Shigella plasmid. *J Clin Invest* 1990;86:1193–1203.
195. Skurnik M, Wolf-Watz H. Analysis of the yopA gene encoding the Yop1 virulence determinants of Yersinia spp. *Mol Microbiol* 1989;3:517–529.
196. Koski P, Rhen M, Kantele J, et al. Isolation, cloning, and primary structure of a cationic 16-kDa outer membrane protein of Salmonella typhimurium. *J Biol Chem* 1989;264:18973–18980.
197. Lahesmaa R, Skurnik M, Toivanen P. Molecular mimicry: any role in the pathogenesis of spondyloarthropathies? *Immunol Res* 1993;12:193–208.
198. Scofield RH, Warren WL, Koelsch G, et al. A hypothesis for the HLA-B27 immune dysregulation in spondyloarthropathy: contributions from enteric organisms, B27 structure, peptides bound by B27, and convergent evolution. *Proc Natl Acad Sci U S A* 1993;90:9330–9334.
199. Scofield RH, Kurien B, Gross T, et al. HLA-B27 binding of peptide from its own sequence and similar peptides from bacteria: implications for spondyloarthropathies. *Lancet* 1995;345:1542–1544.
200. Madden DR, Gorga JC, Strominger JL, et al. The structure of HLA-B27 reveals nonamer self-peptides bound in an extended conformation. *Nature* 1991;353:321–325.
201. Jardetzky TS, Lane WS, Robinson RA, et al. Identification of self peptides bound to purified HLA-B27. *Nature* 1991;353:326–329.
202. Ohno S. How cytotoxic T cells manage to discriminate nonself from self at the nonapeptide level. *Proc Natl Acad Sci U S A* 1992;89:4643–4647.
203. van Bohemen CG, Nabbe AJ, Grumet FC, et al. Lack of correlation between HLA-B27 like antigenic epitopes on Shigella flexneri and the occurrence of reactive arthritis. *Clin Exp Immunol* 1986;65:679–682.
204. Tsuchiya N, Husby G, Williams RC Jr. Studies of hormonal and cell-mediated immunity to peptides shared by HLA-B27.1 and Klebsiella pneumoniae nitrogenase in ankylosing spondylitis. *Clin Exp Immunol* 1989;76:354–360.
205. Sieper J, Braun J. Pathogenesis of spondyloarthropathies: persistent bacterial antigen, autoimmunity, or both? *Arthritis Rheum* 1995;38:1547–1554.
206. Tsuchiya N, Williams RC Jr. Molecular mimicry: hypothesis or reality? *West J Med* 1992;157:133–138.
207. Singh B, Dillion T, Lauzon J, et al. Tolerance to the HLA-B27 and Klebsiella pneumoniae crossreactive epitope in mice transgenic for HLA-B2705 and human beta 2-microglobulin. *J Rheumatol* 1994;21:670–674.

*Textbook of the Autoimmune Diseases,*
Edited by R. G. Lahita, N. Chiorazzi, and W. H. Reeves,
Lippincott Williams & Wilkins, Philadelphia © 2000.

# CHAPTER 13

# Costimulation in Autoimmunity

Amy J. Miga and Randolph J. Noelle

The initiation of the acquired immune responses is triggered by the recognition of antigen, whereas the amplification and control of this response is regulated through the activities of costimulatory molecules. Costimulatory molecules can synergistically upregulate or downregulate humoral and cell-mediated immune responses. The role of these molecules and the cells that express them are discussed in this chapter. In addition, recent studies demonstrating that costimulatory molecules are ideal targets for immune intervention in autoimmune disease are presented.

## CELL POPULATIONS

### Antigen-Presenting Cells

T cells are alerted to the presence of foreign (e.g., bacterial) or self or altered peptides (as in the case of tumor cells) when antigen is displayed on the surface of antigen-presenting cells (APCs). The T-cell receptor (TCR) for antigen recognizes short peptide fragments complexed with major histocompatibility complex (MHC) class I and class II molecules presented on the surface of APCs. The functions of the APC are to sample the extracellular environment as well as proteins produced within the APC, to degrade these proteins proteolytically to peptides, and to couple the derived peptides to MHC class I and II molecules for presentation on the cell surface. CD8[+] T cells (cytotoxic T cells) recognize peptides coupled to MHC I molecules, whereas CD4[+] T cells (helper T cells) recognize peptides complexed with MHC class II molecules. CD8[+] T lymphocytes mediate cellular responses to antigen, culminating in the destruction of virally infected cells or tumor cells. Essentially all nucleated cells express MHC class I and are therefore capable of being recognized and killed by cytotoxic T cells. Upon activation of CD4[+] helper T cells by peptide–MHC class II molecules, the T cells express surface proteins and produce cytokines that

can mediate the development of humoral and inflammatory immune responses.

There is a spectrum of APCs that function in triggering humoral and cell-mediated immunity. These include dendritic cells (DCs), Langerhans cells LCs), macrophages, and B cells.

### Dendritic Cells

DCs are potent stimulators of primary immune responses. As their name implies, DCs have long, dendritic processes that serve to increase the surface area where antigen is expressed. Although LCs are DCs found in the skin, interstitial DCs are found in organs such as the heart, lungs, liver, kidneys, and gastrointestinal tract (1). Within these tissues, DCs capture antigen; they then migrate to regional lymphoid organs where they present antigen to lymphocytes. It has been recognized that DCs mature during the course of the immune response. Initially, the resident interstitial DCs are active in sampling the environment and presenting antigen to the T-cell compartment. If antigen is recognized by the T cell, however, the DCs are triggered to halt sampling, and they mature to become more effective at triggering T-cell activation. The maturation of DCs involves the upregulation of a number of costimulatory molecules and the elaboration of cytokines that facilitate T-cell activation.

### Macrophages

Macrophages arise from monocytes and are professional APCs located throughout the body. These cells are highly phagocytic, using membrane extensions that engulf material to be phagocytosed. Macrophages bear Fc receptors that bind to the constant fragment (Fc fragment) of certain classes of antibody, offering another means by which these cells can participate in antigen uptake. During this process, the antibody simultaneously engages antigen and the Fc receptor. The binding of the antibody to the TCR enables the

A. J. Miga and R. J. Noelle: Department of Microbiology, Dartmouth Medical School, Lebanon, New Hampshire 03756.

macrophage to engulf more efficiently the antigen for which the antibody is specific. The Fc receptor also allows macrophages to participate in antibody-dependent cell-mediated cytotoxicity, as the bound antibody maintains the antigen in close proximity to the macrophage, rendering it more susceptible to lytic components released by the cell.

Macrophages are influenced by the expression of chemotactic factors that promote migration of these APCs to sites of inflammation. Like other APCs, they process antigen to be presented in the context of MHC molecules. Although absent in DCs, macrophages contain high levels of myeloperoxidase, cathepsin B, and dipeptidyl peptidase, enzymes that are involved in the degradation of peptides for subsequent loading onto MHC molecules (2). As with DCs, macrophage activation enhances their antigen-presenting capabilities by increasing MHC class II and adhesion molecule expression. They promote the immune response by elaborating hydrolytic enzymes, complement proteins, and proinflammatory cytokines (1).

### B Cells

B cells arise and mature within the bone marrow and can respond to antigen in a T-cell–independent or T-cell–dependent manner. The surface expression of immunoglobulin (Ig) constitutes the antigen receptor of the B cell and enables it to bind directly to antigen (e.g., toxins and bacterial or viral particles; Fig. 13.1). The B-cell membrane Ig (mIg) receptor engages antigen for which it is specific, and this is followed by activation, proliferation, and differentiation of the B cell. Its progeny give rise to memory B cells and Ig-secreting plasma cells. Although the role of B cells in mediating antibody production has long been known, their function as APCs was recognized more recently. In general, resting B

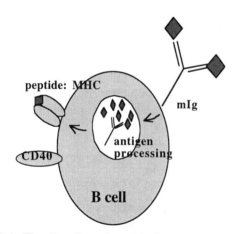

**FIG. 13.1.** The B cell: antigen binding and presentation. Membrane immunoglobulin binds directly to the antigen for which the B cell is specific. The antigen–antibody complex is internalized, followed by degradation of antigen into peptides. Peptides are loaded onto major histocompatibility complex molecules within the cell and exported for presentation on the cell surface.

cells are poor APCs because of their low level of costimulatory molecule expression. In contrast, once activated by cytokines and other factors, B cells can mature and become extremely proficient APCs. Unlike all other APCs, by virtue of the expression of mIg, B cells can capture antigen specifically, when antigen is at extremely low concentrations, triggering immune responses. B cells also express Fc receptors.

### T Cells

T lymphocytes arise from hematopoietic stem cells in the bone marrow and migrate to the thymus, where they mature and acquire their TCR. The TCR enables the T cell to recognize cells expressing altered self or foreign peptides on their surface, as in the case of tumor cells and infected cells, respectively. Surface expression of CD4 or CD8 glycoproteins facilitates the recognition of antigenic peptides and distinguishes T-helper ($T_H$) cells from cytotoxic T cells.

#### T-Helper Cells

$T_H$ cells display CD4 on their surface and engage peptides presented in the context of MHC class II. When triggered by the antigen–MHC complex, the TCR initiates a cascade of events that results in the elaboration of cytokines that influence the activity of other cells of the immune system, including their TCR and MHC expression, cytokine release, and proliferation. Distinct subsets of $T_H$ cells exist, and cytokines released by $T_H$ cells depend on their classification.

$T_H0$ cells are a subset of naive, uncommitted $T_H$ (CD4$^+$) cells (3). Antigen presentation by APCs induces $T_H0$ cell activation, and on activation, the $T_H0$ cells differentiate. $T_H0$ cells may preferentially differentiate into either $T_H1$ or $T_H2$ cells, depending on the cytokine environment, strength of the antigenic signal, and types of costimulatory molecules present. The distinguishing feature of $T_H1$ and $T_H2$ cells is the spectrum of cytokines that they produce. $T_H1$ cells are involved in cell-mediated inflammatory responses and enhance microbicidal activity in macrophages. They are generated in the presence of interleukin-12 (IL-12) and are typified by the release of interferon-γ (IFN-γ), IL-2, and tumor necrosis factor-β (TNF-β). IFN-γ promotes APC IL-12 release, thereby providing positive feedback for further $T_H1$-cell generation. IL-4 is required for the differentiation of $T_H2$ cells, which are characterized by the release of IL-4, IL-5, IL-6, and IL-10. An immune response dominated by either $T_H1$ or $T_H2$ cells promotes cell-mediated or humoral immunity, respectively. Cytokines released by $T_H1$ cells inhibit the generation of $T_H2$ cells, and vice versa.

#### T-Cytotoxic Cells

When activated, T-cytotoxic cells (Tc cells) differentiate into effector cells called *cytotoxic T lymphocytes* (CTLs), which are capable of killing virally infected or altered cells.

These cells are also involved in the rejection of foreign transplant tissue.

Surface expression of the CD8 glycoprotein enables the Tc cells to engage peptide presented in the context of MHC class I. Differentiation of and proliferation into CTLs is influenced by $T_H1$-derived cytokines, such as IFN-$\gamma$ and IL-2. The mechanism by which CTLs kill their targets involves the exocytosis of perforin-containing granules. As their name implies, the contents of these granules act to perforate the target cell membrane, thereby killing the cell.

### Naive Versus Memory T Cells

Initial exposure to antigen evokes a primary immune response, or priming, in which immune cells are activated, and an immune response ensues. Priming causes an increase in the precursor frequency of the antigen-specific lymphocyte populations. In addition to an increase in precursor frequency, the requirements for restimulation of memory lymphocytes is more lax than that of naive T cells. Furthermore, memory cells are differentiated to mediate effector function. All of these attributes taken together explain why memory cells are far more rapid and efficient at mounting immune responses.

### B Cells

#### B Cells, Plasma Cells, and Naive Versus Memory Cells

B cells that respond to antigen can differentiate into memory B cells or plasma cells. A primary immune response results in the secretion of IgM, whereas a memory response is characterized by the release of high-affinity Ig from a variety of Ig classes (e.g., IgG, IgA, and IgE). Although memory B cells respond to antigen with their surface Ig receptor as naive B cells do, they have a longer life span and can persist for months or even years.

Plasma cells lack the Ig receptor characteristic of naive and memory B cells. They are found within the bone marrow, spleen, and lymph nodes and secrete large amounts of soluble Ig during their short life span (only a few days or weeks). It is plasma cells that give rise to high levels of protective Ig.

#### T-Independent Versus T-Dependent Response

In a polymeric state, antigen can trigger the activation of B cells in the absence of T-cell involvement (T-independent response). Bacterial products, such as lipopolysaccharide, capsular proteins, and flagellin, can mediate a T-independent B-cell response (a response that does not require T cell help), which is typified by the release of soluble IgM and lack of memory B cells. For the elaboration of a variety of Ig isotypes and the generation of memory, B cells must respond in a T-dependent fashion. This involves cognate interactions between B and T cells (Fig. 13.2).

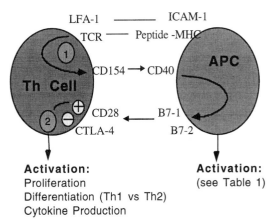

**FIG. 13.2.** Th cell–antigen-presenting cell (APC) interaction. Adhesion molecules (lymphocyte function antigen-1 [LFA-1] and intercellular adhesion molecule-1 [ICAM-1]) facilitate the interactions between T cells and APCs. T-cell receptor engagement of peptide major histocompatibility complex upregulates CD154 expression on the surface of the $T_H$ cell. CD154 triggers APC activation and expression of B7-1 and B7-2 costimulatory molecules. These reciprocally activate the $T_H$ cell, causing their proliferation, differentiation, and cytokine production.

## CELLULAR INTERACTIONS AND ANTIGEN PRESENTATION

### Antigen Presentation

Cognate interactions between T-cell APCs are crucial for the development of an effective immune response. B cells, monocytes, macrophages, and DCs are major populations of cells within the immune system. These are so-called *professional* APCs and serve to present antigen to T cells for subsequent T-cell activation. Fig. 13.2 illustrates the current model of $T_H$ cell–APC association (4,5). Foreign antigen is processed into peptides by the APC and presented on the cell surface bound to MHC class II self antigens. If a nearby $T_H$ cell is specific for the bound peptide, the TCR may engage it in the context of MHC class II. The literature often refers to TCR signaling by means of peptide MHC class II as *signal 1.* This interaction is stabilized by the adhesion molecules' lymphocyte function antigen-1 and intercellular adhesion molecule-1.

In addition to TCR-mediated signals, the APC must deliver a *costimulatory* signal to induce T-cell activation. B7-1 (CD80) and B7-2 (CD86) are members of the Ig superfamily and are potent monomeric costimulatory molecules. They interact with the T-cell costimulatory receptor CD28, a homodimer that is also an Ig family member. CD28 is expressed on resting and activated T cells, and its stimulation is referred to as *signal 2.*

CD154 and CD40 are two cell-surface proteins also involved in cognate T-cell–APC interactions. CD154 (gp39; CD40 ligand; CD40L) is a type II integral membrane protein expressed primarily on activated CD4$^+$ $T_H$ cells. Professional APCs express CD40 constitutively on their surface. Upon

T$_H$-cell activation, CD154 is transiently expressed and engages its receptor CD40. The 50-kd glycoprotein CD40 is a member of the tumor necrosis factor receptor family of molecules and is known to be a crucial player in the generation of humoral immune responses. Because CD40 signaling has been shown to promote costimulatory molecule expression, there has also been a keen interest in its participation in T-cell–mediated immunity.

### Initiation of Humoral Immunity: Activation of B Cells and the Role of CD40 in Antibody Production and Germinal Center Formation

Engagement of antigen by the mIg constitutes the first signal required for B-cell activation. When B cells have captured antigen through their mIg receptor, they process and present antigen for recognition by antigen-specific T cells (Fig. 13.1). As a result of TCR recognition of antigen, TCR stimulation induces expression of the cell-surface protein CD154, which then binds to its CD40 receptor on the B cell. Signaling through CD40 provides the B cell with a second signal, which drives T-cell–dependent B-cell proliferation and is crucial for germinal center formation. Germinal centers are the site of memory B-cell generation; hence, the CD40 pathway is crucial to the generation of primary and secondary antibody responses to T-cell–dependent antigens (Table 13.1) (6). As the B cells are triggered to respond, there is an increase in the expression of B7-1 and B7-2, which reciprocally triggers enhanced T$_H$-cell responses. Enhanced T-cell triggering results in cytokine production by the cognate T cells that can foster B-cell growth and differentiation as well as support T-cell expansion in an autocrine fashion.

Because triggering of CD40 by CD154 is crucial to mounting an effective humoral response, it is not surprising that mutations in the gene encoding CD154 cause a devastating immunodeficiency in humans. Defects in the CD154 molecule render humans with X-linked hyper-IgM (X-HIM) syn-

drome unable to signal through CD40 (7). Those with this immunodeficiency are unable to undergo Ig class switching and therefore lack serum IgA, IgG, and IgE. Therefore, although they produce normal or elevated levels of IgM antibody, these patients are deficient in other Ig isotypes, each of which mediates distinct effector functions. These patients must undergo γ-globulin therapy throughout their lifetime. Despite these efforts, however, X-HIM patients are prone to severe bacterial infections and have a shortened life expectancy.

### Initiation of Cell-Mediated Immunity: Activation of T Cells and Professional Antigen-Presenting Cells and Participation of CD154, CD40, B7-1, B7-2, IL-12, CD28

Just as the triggering of B cells by CD40 initiates humoral immunity, triggering of CD40 on other APCs can trigger the initiation of cell-mediated immunity. CD40 stimulation results in the upregulation of B7-1 and B7-2 costimulatory molecules on macrophages and DCs (Table 13.1). B7-1 and B7-2 engage the T$_H$-cell coreceptor CD28, thereby delivering a second signal (signal 2), which culminates in T-cell activation, proliferation, and cytokine production. Other inflammatory mediators (like TNF-α and lipopolysaccharide) can also induce maturational development of APCs. Therefore, the production of inflammatory mediators early during the innate immune response can facilitate the maturation of APCs that can enhance the acquired immune response.

In addition to B7-1 and B7-2 upregulation, APCs that are triggered to mature produce cytokines and chemokines (cytokines that chemoattract lymphocytes) that regulate T-cell differentiation. Compelling evidence implicates CD40 triggering as inducing IL-12, IL-8, and macrophage inflammatory protein (MIP)-1α production by monocytes, macrophages, and DCs. Furthermore, it has been shown that upregulated expression of costimulatory molecules and cytokine production can elicit a synergistic effect on T-cell activation.

### Downregulation of the Immune Response and the Role of CTLA-4

CTLA-4 is a glycoprotein that is homologous to the costimulatory receptor CD28, although it differs in its kinetics of expression and its affinity for costimulatory molecules. CD28 is found on most resting T cells and acts as a positive costimulator, whereas CTLA-4 is a downregulator of T-cell function. CTLA-4 is expressed only on activated T cells, binds ligands B7-1 and B7-2 with 10- to 20-fold higher affinity than its homolog, and acts to downregulate T-cell activity. During a normal immune response, T cells become activated, proliferate, and upregulate CTLA-4. Because CTLA-4 has a higher affinity for B7 molecules than does CD28, it can successfully compete for ligand binding. Mice that have been engineered to lack this receptor suffer from severe T-cell dysregulation. Shortly after birth, massive lymphoproliferation and tissue destruction occur. There is severe lymphocytic

**TABLE 13.1.** *Implications of antigen-presenting cell activation*

| Cell population | Activities upon activation |
|---|---|
| B cell | B-cell proliferation |
| | B7-1 and B7-2 costimulatory molecule expression |
| | Immunoglobulin isotype switching |
| | Memory B-cell and plasma cell generation |
| Differentiated cell (DC) | Enhanced peptide-MHC expression |
| | Decreased antigen uptake |
| | B7-1 and B7-2 costimulatory molecule expression |
| | IL-12 release |
| Macrophage | Enhanced peptide-MHC expression |
| | B7-1 and B7-2 costimulatory molecule expression |
| | IL-12 release |
| | Elaboration of inflammatory mediators |

IL-12, interleukin-12; MHC, major histocompatibility complex.

infiltration of the heart, pancreas, spleen, and other tissues, and the mice die by 3 to 4 weeks of age (8,9). This suggests that the CTLA-4 signal downregulates T-cell activation and proliferation and is therefore crucial in maintaining immunologic homeostasis.

## COSTIMULATORY MOLECULES IN AUTOIMMUNE DISEASE

### CD40

#### Multiple Sclerosis and Experimental Autoimmune Encephalomyelitis

Myelin is a membranous sheath that covers the axons of some neurons and insulates them during the transmission of nerve impulses. Produced by oligodendroglial cells, the myelin sheath is composed of proteins and lipids and can be severely affected by an attack by the immune system. Multiple sclerosis (MS) is a an autoimmune disease that destroys myelin within the central nervous system (CNS) and affects about 250,000 people in the United States (10). Although the cause of this disease remains elusive, autoreactive T cells participate in an immune response that results in inflammatory lesions along the myelin sheath and subsequent myelin destruction. Nerve transmission is impaired by demyelination and, as a result, patients with this disease may suffer from weakness, fatigue, limb paralysis, vision abnormalities, or other complications. The clinical course of MS may follow a relapsing–remitting profile, whereby neurologic deficits eventually resolve, or a relapsing–progressive or chronic–progressive course, in which there is steady progression of disease with or without relapse, respectively.

Experimental autoimmune encephalomyelitis (EAE) is an experimentally induced animal model of MS that shares clinical and histologic similarities with its human correlate. It is induced by immunizing rodents with myelin components. During EAE induction, the antigen is delivered emulsified in an adjuvant, such as complete Freund's adjuvant (CFA), which contains oil and killed mycobacterium. Such emulsion may slow the release of antigen over time, and the mycobacterial components are thought to enhance the inflammatory response. Macrophages are known to participate in the development of this inflammatory disease and, along with T cells, make up the majority of infiltrating cells in CNS tissue of both MS patients and EAE animals.

$T_H1$ cells are thought to be responsible for disease manifestations in both MS and EAE (11,12). Cytokine studies revealed that expression of $T_H1$-derived cytokines (IFN-$\gamma$ and TNF-$\beta$) correlates with disease and that IL-10 ($T_H2$ derived) is associated with recovery (13,14). These particular cytokines are considered crucial because IFN-$\gamma$–secreting $CD4^+$ $T_H1$ cells stimulate macrophage activation (15), thereby inducing a response mediated by oxygen radicals and nitric oxide. Although these effects are beneficial in eliminating bacteria during an infection, macrophage-derived toxic mediators (such as oxygen radicals) induce local tissue damage, causing extensive tissue destruction to joints (as in arthritis) or to myelin (as in MS and EAE).

As described previously, triggering of CD40 is known to activate T cells reciprocally by the upregulation of costimulatory molecules and their association with CD28. CD40 also promotes IL-12 release by APCs; this is significant because the IL-12 receptor is thought to synergize with CD28 in T-cell proliferation and cytokine production. These findings led Gerritse et al (16) to examine a potential role for CD154–CD40 interactions in both MS and EAE. In the immunohistochemical analysis of CNS brain lesions of MS patients, these investigators showed that $CD4^+$ and $CD154^+$ (activated) $T_H$ cells colocalized with CD40-bearing macrophages and B cells in areas of CNS perivascular infiltration. Such infiltrates, likely $T_H1$-type inflammatory cells, were not observed in patients with noninflammatory neurologic disease, thereby suggesting a potential role for this receptor–ligand pair in inflammatory disease.

Further studies by Gerritse et al (16) were done in a murine model of EAE. These investigators immunized mice with myelin components (active immunization), which involved subcutaneous injection of myelin peptide [proteolipid protein (PLP)] in CFA. The response that ensues results in the activation of myelin-reactive T cells, culminating in inflammatory lesions, myelin destruction, and impaired nerve transmission. Disease was assessed by the development of clinical signs of disease: limp tail, hind limb weakness, hind limb paralysis, full paralysis, and even death.

These animal studies investigated the *in vivo* relevance of the CD154–CD40 interaction in the initiation of EAE. Control mice received intraperitoneal injections of hamster Ig (HIg) on alternate days, whereas the experimental group was treated with a monoclonal antibody (mAb) that binds CD154 (anti-CD154). This mAb (MR-1) blocks the CD154–CD40 association, thereby preventing the CD40 signaling cascade and its downstream effects (17–19). The investigators found that disrupting the interaction between CD154 and CD40 with an anti-CD154 mAb abrogates development of actively induced murine EAE (16). It is likely that in the absence of a CD40 signal, APCs have a diminished capacity to express costimulatory molecules and IL-12, a cytokine important in the generation of $CD4^+$ $T_H1$ cells. $T_H$ cells thereby receive insufficient stimulation, and their priming is prevented, rendering them deficient in their ability to express cytokines and adhesion molecules required for CNS infiltration.

Gerritse et al (16) also examined the potential for anti-CD154 treatment when signs of clinical disease have been established. They showed that treatment with anti-CD154 after disease onset blocked disease progression. Thus, despite the presence of activated $T_H$ cells and CNS infiltration, blocking the CD40 signal still had beneficial effects. This suggests a role for CD154 beyond $T_H$-cell priming and that anti-CD154 can mediate inhibitory effects at one or many levels of disease. CD154 and CD40 could prove to be valuable targets for therapeutic intervention in MS patients. By thoroughly evaluating the role of CD154 and CD40 in disease induction and effector phases, researchers may help define the therapeutic potential of anti-CD154 in this and other immune-mediated diseases.

### Systemic Lupus Erythematosus

Systemic autoimmune diseases are characterized by autoreactivity against a wide range of target antigens and, as a result, may cause damage to a variety of organs and tissues. Systemic lupus erythematosus (SLE) is a systemic autoimmune disease characterized by the production of pathogenic autoantibodies and immune complexes. B cells of SLE patients generate autoantibodies in a CD4[+] T-cell–dependent manner, and their antigen specificity can be directed against a wide spectrum of components in the body, from red blood cells, neurons, and platelets to RNA, nuclear polypeptides, and DNA (1). SLE usually appears in women between 20 and 40 years of age, and its principal clinical manifestations include kidney dysfunction and a butterfly-shaped rash on the face (20). Other complications include weakness, pleurisy, pericarditis, and joint pain. Autoimmune hemolytic anemia can also occur as a result of anti–red blood cell autoantibodies that direct complement-mediated lysis. Similarly, deposition of immune complexes along blood vessel walls can result in activation of complement, which subsequently damages blood vessel walls, resulting in tissue damage and glomerulonephritis.

Scientists employ a murine model in studying the generation and treatment of human SLE. The F1 generation of New Zealand black mouse strain crossed to New Zealand white (NZB/WF1) spontaneously develops SLE and provides an animal model for this disease. As with humans, mice with SLE generate antibodies to red blood cells, nuclear proteins, and DNA and develop glomerulonephritis from immune complex deposition in the kidney. The autoantibody production in these lupus-prone mice cause them to develop spontaneous autoimmune hemolytic anemia and nephritis. These mice also have a shortened life span.

Because the pivotal role for CD154–CD40 interactions in B-cell proliferation, antibody production, and isotype switching had been well-established, Early et al (21) examined the therapeutic potential of an anti-CD154 mAb in SLE treatment. They found that initiation of anti-CD154 treatment at 4 months of age inhibited anti-DNA autoantibody production and renal disease and significantly prolonged survival of NZB/WF1 mice. Antibody treatment was associated with inhibition of renal damage and deposition of immune complexes. As with MS and EAE, anti-CD154 may be a powerful means of manipulating the immune system and inhibiting autoimmune disease. Data from T-cell studies led Koshy et al (22) to suggest a dysregulation in CD154 expression in SLE patients. They found that expression of CD154 on activated T cells from SLE patients was prolonged compared with CD154 levels from rheumatic disease control T cells cultured in the same manner. In addition, others have shown that B cells from SLE patients express CD154, suggesting

that B cell–B cell interactions may be responsible for dysregulated Ig production.

### Collagen-Induced Arthritis

Rheumatoid arthritis (RA) is among the most common autoimmune diseases, affecting both adults and children (20). This inflammatory disorder is characterized by joint stiffness and pain, malaise, and tissue damage and is associated with morbidity and accelerated mortality (23). There is infiltration of leukocytes into the synovial lining of joints, antibody production by B cells, deposition of anticollagen antibodies in articular cartilage, and complement-mediated destruction of the joint. The severe synovial inflammation can result in tissue damage and deformity. Although new and more efficacious treatments are being sought, current therapeutic approaches include nonsteroidal inflammatory agents, low-dose corticosteroids, and immunosuppressive drugs. Because of the clinical and histopathologic similarities to RA, collagen-induced arthritis (CIA) is a popular animal model used for the study of this inflammatory disease and investigation into potential therapeutic targets.

In 1977, Trentham et al. (24) reported that chronic inflammatory arthritis could be induced in rats by intradermal injection with native type II collagen emulsified in either CFA or incomplete Freund's adjuvant (IFA). Induced by autoantigen, arthritis develops 10 to 16 days after immunization in several strains of rats and mice and persists for 4 to 8 weeks (25). It results in the progressive formation of fibrous and bony ankylosis. Macrophages and activated CD4[+] T cells accumulate in the human RA synovium, and immunohistochemical analyses have shown that T-lymphocyte infiltration is significant in early CIA synovial lesions as well. The CIA synovium is infiltrated by macrophages, anticollagen antibodies are generated, and delayed-type hypersensitivity to collagen occurs (26). These features, in addition to chronic synovitis, make this an appropriate animal model for human RA.

T lymphocytes are required for generation of this disease. Further support for the interference of CD154–CD40 interactions in the treatment of autoimmune disease was presented by Durie et al. (27) in their studies of CIA. Although 75% to 80% of control animals developed CIA, no mice that received anti-CD154 exhibited signs of clinical disease. The extensive joint inflammation found in the control mice was not seen in the anti-CD154 treated group. Disruption of CD40 signaling with this mAb also inhibited the generation of anticollagen type II IgG antibodies, infiltration of inflammatory cells into the subsynovial tissue, and erosion of cartilage and bone.

### TNBS-Induced Colitis

Crohn's disease is one form of intestinal inflammation referred to as a *human inflammatory bowel disease* (IBD) and includes regional enteritis, Crohn's ileitis, and granulomatous colitis. Although the cause of this disease remains unknown, genetic and environmental factors may contribute

(28). Associated with severe abdominal pain, diarrhea, nutritional deficiencies, and weight loss, IBD is characterized by infiltration of macrophages and lymphocytes to the intestine and increased production of inflammatory mediators and IgG antibodies. Activated and memory T-cell populations in the lamina propria are increased, and patients with IBD have been shown to generate antibodies against epithelial cell antigens. These antibodies likely contribute to epithelial cell destruction. The severe tissue damage that occurs with this inflammatory response can lead to abdominal abscess formation, ulceration, and fistulas. Patients with Crohn's disease may also experience severe bleeding. Bowel obstruction, mucosal destruction, and other factors can contribute to the diarrhea. Although treatments are aimed at controlling inflammation (i.e., with antiinflammatory agents, steroids, or immunosuppressive drugs), many patients need to undergo surgery.

Rectal administration of mice with the haptenizing reagent 2,4,6-trinitrobenzene sulfonic acid (TNBS) induces a chronic colitis. This $T_H1$-mediated disease is known as *TNBS-induced colitis* and is used to study potential treatments in human IBD. Anti-CD154 treatment during disease induction prevented clinical and histologic evidence of disease and blocked IFN-γ production by lamina propria CD4+ T cells (29). The administration of recombinant IL-12 reversed the disease-inhibiting effect of anti-CD154, suggesting that the relevance of CD40 in this animal model may be due to its role in IL-12 release.

### Graft-Versus-Host Disease

Tissue typing and careful matching of donor and recipient MHC are crucial steps in the process of bone-marrow transplantation. Despite best efforts to match donors with recipients, however, T cells from the grafted donor bone marrow can sometimes recognize recipient peptide–MHC complexes (alloantigens) as "foreign" and attack the host as a result. The donor lymphocytes traffic to various organs, where they become activated and proliferate in response to host allogeneic MHC antigens. Tissue damage occurs as natural killer cells, CTLs, and macrophages are activated and inflammatory cytokines are released. This phenomenon is known as *graft-versus-host disease* (GVHD) and affects most transplant recipients. GVHD can be fatal, and those patients who survive may suffer from jaundice, diarrhea, or spleen enlargement.

To investigate the immunologic events associated with GVHD, this *in vivo* reaction is studied in mice by transferring immunocompetent lymphocytes into an immunocompromised recipient. Like their human counterpart, mice suffering from GVHD often exhibit splenomegaly as a result of T-cell proliferation and weight loss.

Acute and chronic forms of GVHD occur in humans and in mice. Acute GVHD occurs within about 60 days after transplantation when CTL activity causes skin, liver, and gut damage. Chronic GVHD is characterized by a later onset, whereby donor, alloreactive $T_H$ cells interact with host B cells and induce polyclonal B-cell activation and excessive autoantibody production. Therefore, whereas acute GVHD is associated with CTL activity, chronic GVHD is associated with polyclonal B-cell activation, increased Ig production, and the generation of autoreactive antibodies.

By manipulating the immune system with anti-CD154 administration, Durie et al. (30) have shown that blockade of the CD40 signal prevents acute and chronic GVHD. The ability of anti-CD154 to prevent the onset of chronic GVHD was assessed by the reduction of splenomegaly, hyperimmunoglobulin production, and anti-DNA autoantibodies. Anti-CD154 also blocked the generation of anti-host CTL responses and splenomegaly associated with acute GVHD.

### Insulin-Dependent Diabetes Mellitus

Throughout the pancreas, the β cells are organized into clusters known as the *islets of Langerhans*. Here, they produce insulin, a peptide hormone involved in glucose metabolism. Insulin-dependent diabetes mellitus (IDDM) is an organ-specific autoimmune disease in which T cells and autoantibodies target the pancreatic β cells. T cells and macrophages infiltrate the islets of Langerhans (insulitis), and the ensuing immune response destroys the β cells, causing decreased insulin production and elevated glucose levels.

An animal model for this disease is provided by the nonobese diabetic (NOD) mouse strain, which spontaneously develops a disease similar to its human counterpart. These mice often become diabetic by 7 months of age. Treatment before disease onset has been shown to be effective in completely preventing disease development; however, treatment with αCD154 early after the development of diabetes did not halt disease progression (31).

## B7-1 and B7-2

### Multiple Sclerosis and Experimental Autoimmune Encephalomyelitis

The participation of costimulatory molecules is not limited to the normal immune response. Overwhelming data illustrate that B7-1 and B7-2 are crucial to the generation and maintenance of a number of immune-mediated diseases.

Evidence that supports a role for B7-1 in inflammatory diseases of the CNS includes the well-documented upregulation of B7-1 in MS patients (32,33). Windhagen et al (34) examined cytokine and costimulatory molecule expression in both control and MS specimens. Their immunocytochemical and semiquantitative polymerase chain reaction (PCR) analyses revealed that B7-1 was upregulated early in the initiation of MS when compared with control specimens.

An alternative way to examine the role of costimulatory molecules in autoimmune diseases involves the use of blocking antibodies. Studies with antibodies that block B7-1 reveal that such treatment significantly inhibits clinical disease and

CNS pathology in EAE mice (35,36). Although costimulation appears to be involved in the initiation and maintenance of this autoimmune disease, it is unclear whether B7-1 and B7-2 participate in the same manner. Data that address this issue have been difficult to reconcile.

### Systemic Lupus Erythematosus

Nakajima et al. (37) were able to prolong survival of their lupus-prone NZB/W F1 mice by treating them early with a combination of anti–B7-1 and anti–B7-2 antibodies. Such treatment completely prevented autoantibody production and nephritis and corresponded with a decrease in anti-DNA antibodies as well as a decrease in IL-2, IFN-γ, IL-4, and IL-6 messenger RNA. Blocking B7-1 and B7-2 affords significant protection against this disease even when treatment is delayed until advanced illness (38).

### Collagen-Induced Arthritis

Knoerzer et al. (39) investigated the involvement of costimulatory molecules in their rat model of CIA. T-cell costimulation through B7-1 or B7-2 can be prevented by a soluble form of CTLA-4. By fusing the extracellular region of CTLA-4 with an IgG fusion partner, a soluble CTLA4Ig competes with CD28 for ligand binding and therefore blocks CD28-mediated costimulation. CTLA4Ig treatment before collagen immunization prevented clinical and histologic manifestations of disease. Such treatment inhibited anti-collagen antibody titers and prevented the erosion of articular cartilage and bone.

Webb et al. (40) also found that blocking B7-1 and B7-2 costimulation with CTLA4Ig prevented CIA in immunized mice. Such treatment inhibited the generation of anticollagen IgG1 and IgG2a antibodies and inhibited lymphocyte expansion within the draining lymph nodes. When given after disease onset, treatment with either CTLA4Ig or a combination of anti–B7-1 and anti–B7-2 mAb was effective in disease amelioration, suggesting a role for T cells in disease initiation as well as progression. These studies also support a role for CD28 in $T_H1$ responses because blocking costimulation inhibited $T_H1$ responses *in vitro*.

### Insulin-Dependent Diabetes Mellitus

Herold et al. (41,42) have shown that CD28-/- mice are resistant to the development of streptozotocin-induced diabetes mellitus. Diabetic mice exhibit upregulation of B7-2 on islet cells, and treatment with anti–B7-2 prevented insulitis and hyperglycemia. Although anti–B7-2 protected against disease, anti–B7-1 exacerbated it, suggesting that expression of these costimulatory molecules may influence the phenotype of the disease-causing T cells. Their data suggests that B7-1 and B7-2 may play a differential role in the development of disease.

### Experimental Autoimmune Myasthenia Gravis

Although some antibody-mediated autoimmune diseases are characterized by the deposition of antigen–antibody complexes, others are characterized by an alteration in receptor function. Myasthenia gravis is one such autoimmune disease and is caused by the production of antibodies directed against acetylcholine receptors (AChRs) on the motor end plates of muscles. The binding of these antibodies to the AChR impairs the binding of acetylcholine to its target. This causes muscle weakness, and muscle activation is further impaired as a result of complement-mediated degradation of the receptor. As with SLE, the generation of pathogenic anti-AChR antibodies is T-cell dependent.

Immunization of rodents with AChR induces experimental autoimmune myasthenia gravis. Reminiscent of the human disease, rodents generate anti-AChR antibodies and experience muscular weakness. The participation of costimulatory molecules in this disease has been illustrated by McIntosh et al. (43). CTLA4Ig treatment mediated a significant decrease in lymphoproliferation and antibody production. IL-2 and IFN-γ production was also suppressed.

### Graft-Versus-Host Disease

It has been hypothesized that the transplanted donor T cells require costimulatory molecule expression to mediate disease. Data from Blazar et al. (44) have supported this notion and have illustrated a role for costimulatory molecules in their murine model of GVHD. These investigators found that B7-1 expression was upregulated on donor CD4$^+$ thoracic duct lymphocytes after transplantation. B7-1 expression on donor T cells is required for GVHD-induced death, and administration of anti–B7-1 and anti–B7-2 antibodies inhibits CD4$^+$ and CD8$^+$ T-cell expansion and protects the animals from GVHD-induced death.

Studies by Via et al. (45) demonstrated that costimulation is crucial to the generation of CTLs. Blocking costimulatory molecules with CTLA4Ig inhibits donor T-cell activation and differentiation into effector cells that mediate disease. In both acute and chronic GVHD, cytokine production was suppressed, as was the expression of memory markers on donor T cells.

## Others

### Interleukin-12: Multiple Sclerosis and Experimental Autoimmune Encephalomyelitis

A disease-promoting role for IL-12 has been suggested because its expression precedes the onset of clinical disease and peak levels of IFN-γ (11,12). Immunocytochemical and semiquantitative PCR studies have indicated that IL-12 is upregulated early in the initiation of MS (34). The EAE mouse model has been used to elucidate further a role for this cytokine in MS.

PLP-stimulated lymph node cells were used to transfer EAE adoptively into syngeneic recipients (46). Treatment with anti–IL-12 inhibited disease induced by the adoptive transfer. Mice given IL-12–treated lymph node cells exhibited an increased expression of inducible nitric oxide synthase (iNOS), which is involved in nitric oxide generation. Leonard et al. (46) suggested that IL-12 may mediate iNOS expression and thereby contribute to CNS inflammation.

## CONCLUSION

Studies have underscored the importance of costimulatory molecules in the regulation of immune responses. Ligand-receptor pairs like CD154 and CD40 and B7-1 or B7-2 and CD28 play a crucial role in amplifying antigen-specific immune responses.

The initiation and progression of antibody-mediated immune responses requires antigen-specific (signal 1) and antigen-nonspecific (signal 2) signals. For B cells, the binding of antigen to the mIg receptor represents signal 1. To trigger efficient B-cell expansion and differentiation, engagement of CD40 (signal 2) is necessary. T-cell help for B cells is mediated through the CD154–CD40 interaction. Thus, CD40 signaling of B cells promotes B-cell expansion, Ig isotype switching and production, and memory B-cell formation. It has been implicated in antibody-mediated diseases, including SLE, CIA, and myasthenia gravis.

As with antibody-mediated immunity, cell-mediated immunity is also controlled by antigen-specific and antigen-nonspecific signals. The recognition of the MHC–peptide complex on the surface of APC by the TCR is signal 1, and engagement of CD28 represents signal 2. The successful triggering of signals 1 and 2 elicit T-cell clonal expansion, the production of cytokines, and the acquisition of T-cell effector functions.

The studies discussed in this chapter offer compelling evidence for the participation of costimulatory molecules in the generation and maintenance of normal immune responses and autoimmune-mediated diseases. Because of the central role of these costimulatory molecules in the progression of autoimmunity, they are important targets for therapeutic intervention in a wide range of diseases. Clinical trials using agents that can block the function of these molecules have been initiated, and in the coming years we will learn whether human autoimmune diseases can be managed by regulating the function of costimulatory molecules.

## REFERENCES

1. Kuby J. *Immunology,* 2nd ed. New York: W.H. Freeman, 1994.
2. Hart DNJ. Dendritic cells: unique leukocyte populations which control the primary immune responses. *Blood* 1997;90:3245–3287.
3. Swain SL. Regulation of the development of helper T cell subsets. *Immunol Res* 1991;10:177–182.
4. Foy TM, Aruffo A, Bajorath J, et al. Immune regulation by CD40 and its ligand GP39. *Annu Rev Immunol* 1996;14:591–617.
5. Thompson CB. Distinct roles for the costimulatory ligands B7-1 and B7-2 in T helper cell differentiation? *Cell* 1995;81:979–982.
6. Foy TM, Durie FH, Noelle RJ. The expansive role of CD40 and its ligand, gp39, in immunity. *Semin Immunol* 1994;6:259–266.
7. Allen RC, Armitage RJ, Conley ME, et al. CD40 ligand gene defects responsible for X-linked hyper-IgM syndrome [see Comments]. *Science* 1993;259:990–993.
8. Tivol EA, Borriello F, Schweitzer AN, et al. Loss of CTLA-4 leads to massive lymphoproliferation and fatal multiorgan tissue destruction, revealing a critical negative regulatory role of CTLA-4. *Immunity* 1995;3:541–547.
9. Waterhouse P, Penninger JM, Timms E, et al. Lymphoproliferative disorders with early lethality in mice deficient in CTLA-4 [see Comments]. *Science* 1995;270:985–988.
10. Steinmann L. Multiple sclerosis: a coordinated immunological attack against myelin in the central nervous system. *Cell* 1996;85:299–302.
11. Olsson T. Critical influences of the cytokine orchestration on the outcome of myelin antigen-specific T-cell autoimmunity in experimental autoimmune encephalomyelitis and multiple sclerosis. *Immunol Rev* 1995;144:245–268.
12. Olsson T. Cytokine-producing cells in experimental autoimmune encephalomyelitis and multiple sclerosis. *Neurology* 1995;45:S11–S15.
13. Issazadeh S, Ljungdahl A, Hojeberg B, et al. Cytokine production in the central nervous system of Lewis rats with experimental autoimmune encephalomyelitis: dynamics of mRNA expression for interleukin-10, interleukin-12, cytolysin, tumor necrosis factor alpha and tumor necrosis factor beta. *J Neuroimmunol* 1995;61:205–212.
14. Kennedy MK, Torrance DS, Picha KS, et al. Analysis of cytokine mRNA expression in the central nervous system of mice with experimental autoimmune encephalomyelitis reveals that IL-10 mRNA expression correlates with recovery. *J Immunol* 1992;149:2496–2505.
15. Janeway CA, Travers P. *Immunobiology: the immune system in health and disease,* 2nd ed. New York: Garland Publishing, 1994.
16. Gerritse K, Laman JD, Noelle RJ, et al. CD40-CD40 ligand interactions in experimental allergic encephalomyelitis and multiple sclerosis. *Proc Natl Acad Sci U S A* 1996;93:2499–2504.
17. Noelle RJ, Ledbetter JA, Aruffo A. CD40 and its ligand, an essential ligand-receptor pair for thymus-dependent B-cell activation. *Immunol Today* 1992;13:431–433.
18. Noelle RJ, Roy M, Shepherd DM, et al. A 39-kDa protein on activated helper T cells binds CD40 and transduces the signal for cognate activation of B cells. *Proc Natl Acad Sci U S A* 1992;89:6550–6554.
19. Noelle R, Snow EC. T helper cells. *Curr Opin Immunol* 1992;4: 333–337.
20. Paul WE. *Fundamental immunology,* 3rd ed. New York: Raven Press, 1993.
21. Early GS, Zhao W, Burns CM. Anti-CD40 ligand antibody treatment prevents the development of lupus-like nephritis in a subset of New Zealand black × New Zealand white mice: response correlates with the absence of an anti-antibody response. *J Immunol* 1996;157:3159–3164.
22. Koshy M, Berger D, Crow MK. Increased expression of CD40 ligand on systemic lupus erythematosus lymphocytes. *J Clin Invest* 1996;98: 826–837.
23. Kavanaugh AF, Lipsky PE. Rheumatoid arthritis. In: Rich RR, ed. *Clinical immunology: principles and practice.* St. Louis: CV Mosby, 1996:1093–1116.
24. Trentham DE, Townes AS, Kang AH. Autoimmunity to type II collagen an experimental model of arthritis. *J Exp Med* 1977;146:857–868.
25. Trentham DE, Dynesius-Trentham RA. Attenuation of an adjuvant arthritis by type II collagen. *J Immunol* 1983;130:2689–2692.
26. Brahn E. Animal models of rheumatoid arthritis: clues to etiology and treatment. *Clin Orthop* 1991;265:42–53.
27. Durie FH, Fava RA, Foy TM, et al. Prevention of collagen-induced arthritis with an antibody to gp39, the ligand for CD40. *Science* 1993;261:1328–1330.
28. Strober W, Neurath MF. Immunologic diseases of the gastrointestinal tract. In: Rich RR, eds. *Clinical immunology: principles and practice.* St. Louis: CV Mosby, 1996:1401–1428.
29. Kelsall BL, Stuber E, Neurath M, et al. Interleukin-12 production by dendritic cells: the role of CD40-CD40L interactions in Th1 T-cell responses. *Ann N Y Acad Sci* 1996;795:116–126.
30. Durie FH, Aruffo A, Ledbetter J, et al. Antibody to the ligand of CD40, gp39, blocks the occurrence of the acute and chronic forms of graft-vs-host disease. *J Clin Invest* 1994;94:1333–1338.

31. Balasa B, Krahl T, Patstone G, et al. CD40 ligand-CD40 interactions are necessary for the initiation of insulitis and diabetes in nonobese diabetic mice. *J Immunol* 1997;159:4620–4627.

32. Hafler DA, Weiner HL. Antigen-specific immunosuppression: oral tolerance for the treatment of autoimmune disease. *Chem Immunol* 1995;60:126–149.

33. Williams KC, Ulvestad E, Hickey WF. Immunology of multiple sclerosis. *Clin Neurosci* 1994;2:229–245.

34. Windhagen A, Newcombe J, Dangond F, et al. Expression of costimulatory molecules B7-1 (CD80), B7-2 (CD86), and interleukin 12 cytokine in multiple sclerosis lesions. *J Exp Med* 1995;182:1985–1996.

35. Perrin PJ, Scott D, Davis TA, et al. Opposing effects of CTLA4-Ig and anti-CD80 (B7-1) plus anti-CD86 (B7-2) on experimental allergic encephalomyelitis. *J Neuroimmunol* 1996;65:31–39.

36. Miller SD, Vanderlugt CL, Lenschow DJ, et al. Blockade of CD28/B7-1 interaction prevents epitope spreading and clinical relapses of murine EAE. *Immunity* 1995;3:739–745.

37. Nakajima A, Azuma M, Kodera S, et al. Preferential dependence of autoantibody production in murine lupus on CD86 costimulatory molecule. *Eur J Immunol* 1995;25:3060–3069.

38. Finck BK, Linsley PS, Wofsy D. Treatment of murine lupus with CTLA4Ig. *Science* 1994;265:1225–1227.

39. Knoerzer DB, Karr RW, Schwartz BD, et al. Collagen-induced arthritis in the BB rat: prevention of disease by treatment with CTLA-4-Ig. *J Clin Invest* 1995;96:987–993.

40. Webb LM, Walmsley MJ, Feldmann M. Prevention and amelioration of collagen-induced arthritis by blockade of the CD28 co-stimulatory pathway: requirement for both B7-1 and B7-2. *Eur J Immunol* 1996;26:2320–2328.

41. Herold KG, Lenschow DJ, Bluestone JA. CD28/B7 regulation of autoimmune diabetes. *Immunol Res* 1997;16:71–84.

42. Herold KC, Vezys V, Koons A, et al. CD28/B7 costimulation regulates autoimmune diabetes induced with multiple low doses of streptozotocin. *J Immunol* 1997;158:984–991.

43. McIntosh KR, Linsley PS, Drachman DB. Immunosuppression and induction of anergy by CTLA4Ig in vitro: effects on cellular and antibody responses of lymphocytes from rats with experimental autoimmune myasthenia gravis. *Cell Immunol* 1995;166:103–112.

44. Blazar BR, Sharpe AH, Taylor PA, et al. Infusion of anti-B7.1 (CD80) and anti-B7.2 (CD86) monoclonal antibodies inhibits murine graft-versus-host disease lethality in part via direct effects on CD4+ and CD8+ T cells. *J Immunol* 1996;157:3250–3259.

45. Via CS, Rus V, Nguyen P, et al. Differential effects of CTLA4Ig on murine graft-versus-host disease (GVHD) development: CTLA4Ig prevents both acute and chronic CVHD development but reverses only chronic GVHD. *J Immunol* 1996;157:4258–4267.

46. Leonard JP, Waldburger KE, Goldman SJ. Prevention of experimental autoimmune encephalomyelitis by antibodies against interleukin 12. *J Exp Med* 1995;181:381–386.

# SECTION II

## Autoimmune Disease and Organ Systems

*Textbook of the Autoimmune Diseases,*
Edited by R. G. Lahita, N. Chiorazzi, and W. H. Reeves,
Lippincott Williams & Wilkins, Philadelphia © 2000.

# CHAPTER 14

# Hematologic Disorders Associated With Autoimmunity

Richard D. Huhn and Harish P. G. Dave

## HEMATOPOIETIC (MARROW) FAILURE SYNDROMES

Theoretically, all subclasses of blood cells are derived from hematopoietic stem cells through stochastic or determinative proliferation followed by differentiation of their progeny (Fig. 14.1). Proliferation and differentiation are directed by the actions of cytokines and the anchorage of progenitor cells to marrow or reticuloendothelial cells mediated by various adhesion molecules. Hematopoietic cytokines may be stimulatory or inhibitory. The traditional colony-stimulating factors support the growth of colonies of blood cells *in vitro* (1). In contrast, many of the proinflammatory cytokines (e.g., tumor necrosis factor [TNF], transforming growth factor-β, interferon-α and interferon-γ) suppress hematopoiesis.

Marrow failure disorders are caused by damage or suppression of hematopoietic stem and progenitor cells. The most common cause of marrow failure is exposure to cytotoxic drugs (i.e., cancer chemotherapy) that cause apoptotic death of proliferative hematopoietic progenitor cells. Accidental (e.g., industrial) exposure to marrow toxins or radiation accounts for infrequent cases of hematopoietic failure. Otherwise, autoimmune mechanisms appear to be involved in the pathogenesis of most disorders of acquired and congenital hematopoietic failure.

### Approach to the Patient

Patients with marrow failure syndromes have one or more of several characteristic insidious constitutional symptoms and signs related to anemia, thrombocytopenia, or leukopenia. The history and examination should focus on cardiopul-

monary insufficiency, hemostatic problems, and infections. Environmental and occupational histories of toxin exposure may be useful in some situations. Bone marrow aspiration and biopsy should be performed for examination of tissue and cellular morphologies, iron staining, and cytogenetic studies in all new cases. Magnetic resonance imaging of marrow loci (e.g., vertebral column, pelvic bones) may occasionally be helpful in the differential evaluation of marrow failure by distinguishing adipose marrow replacement in acquired aplastic anemia from the hematopoietic hypercellularity characteristic of myelodysplastic syndromes (MDS) (2–6).

### Acquired Aplastic Anemia

Acquired aplastic anemia is an uncommon disease. Epidemiologic studies variably report incidence rates of 1.5 to 7 cases per 1 million population per year (7–13). Idiopathic aplastic anemia can present at any age from early childhood to old age; the age of onset appears to be bimodal, with peaks in the third decade and in elderly years (7). A history of an antecedent viral infection can often be elicited, but with the exception of acute viral hepatitis, such history has little utility in the differential diagnosis of marrow failure (14–20). A clear association between acute viral hepatitis and some cases of acquired aplastic anemia has been well described, but a specific etiologic agent has not been identified (17,19). In Southeast Asia, it is thought that fecal contamination of rice paddies may account for an increased regional incidence of acquired aplastic anemia related to viral pathogens (21,22). Although many prescription drugs have commonly been blamed for marrow failure in anecdotal reports and small case studies, very few drugs have been definitively associated with aplastic anemia (Table 14.1). As an example, chloramphenicol has historically been cited as a causal agent (23); however, despite an abundance of case reports, associations between chloramphenicol and aplastic anemia are variable in

R. D. Huhn: Coriell Institute for Medical Research, Camden, New Jersey 08103.

H. P. G. Dave: Division of Hematology–Oncology, George Washington University, Washington, DC 20037; Hematology Section, Laboratory of Molecular Hematology, Veterans Affairs Medical Center, Washington, DC 20422.

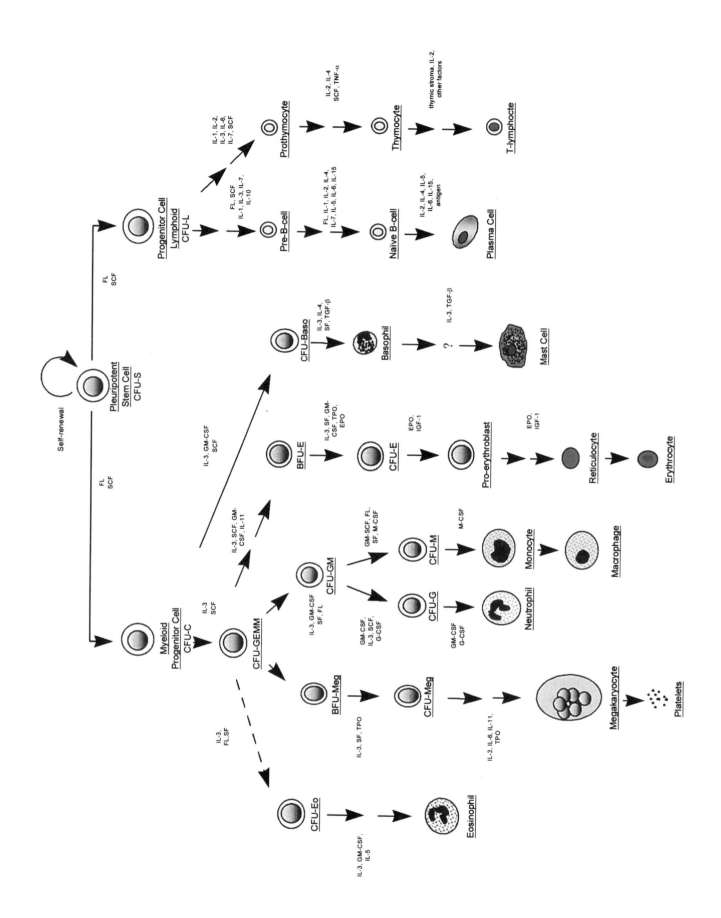

epidemiologic analyses (24). Likewise, a variety of anti-infective, antiinflammatory, and anticonvulsant drugs have been weakly associated with aplastic anemia, and it has been hypothesized that genetic background is in some way responsible for different susceptibilities to drug-induced or metabolite-induced marrow injury (25,26).

The initiating insult in the pathogenesis of idiopathic aplastic anemia remains obscure. Considerable evidence supports the involvement of autoimmune cytotoxic attack on marrow stem cells and progenitor cells. Site-directed lymphocyte infiltration of hematopoietic areas of marrow has been observed (27). Bone marrow cells from patients with severe aplastic anemia cultured in semisolid media supplemented with various combinations of hematopoietins yield severely reduced proportions of colony-forming cells. Removal of autologous T lymphocytes by rosetting or fluorescent cell sorting before culture inoculation reversibly restores the proportion of clonogenic cells toward normal (28–30). In aplastic anemia, expression of the proinflammatory cytokines interferon-γ and TNF-α by marrow mononuclear cells is increased (31–34). Inclusion of antiinterferon-γ or anti–TNF-α antibody in culture media ameliorates the suppression of hematopoiesis (33,35–38). CD34$^+$ (progenitor) cells from marrow of aplastic patients show increased expression of the fas protein, which may result from effects of proinflammatory cytokines and can activate signals for apoptosis (39–41). Thus, theoretically, one or more environmental insults, such as viral infection or toxin exposure, could render hematopoietic cells immunogenic, resulting in autoimmune targeting of hematopoietic cells, apoptotic death of stem or progenitor cells, and suppression of blood cell production.

### Clinical Presentation

Mild asymptomatic cases of aplastic anemia may occasionally be detected by an abnormal hemogram performed on routine general examination. More often, patients present with insidious symptoms and signs reflecting single or combined blood cytopenias. Moderate to severe anemia results in symptoms related to insufficient tissue oxygenation, such as fatigue, malaise, asthenia, poor mentation, headache, tinnitus, and cardiopulmonary insufficiency (exercise intolerance, palpitations, postural dizziness, angina, congestive heart failure). Severe granulocytopenia (i.e., neutrophil count less than 500/mm$^3$) results in impaired front-line host defenses, often leading to bacterial or fungal infections involving skin, oropharyngeal, and gut organisms, which are often invasive

and frequently life-threatening. Clinically significant lymphocytopenia occurs less frequently. Viral infections and so-called opportunistic infections are not prominent in the typical presentations of marrow failure disorders. Thrombocytopenia, if severe (i.e., platelet count less than 10,000/mm$^3$ to 20,000/mm$^3$) leads to microvascular hemorrhagic phenomena, such as petechiae, spontaneous bruising, epistaxis, and gingival bleeding. With prolonged severe thrombocytopenia, serious and life-threatening bleeding, such as gastrointestinal, urinary, and central nervous system hemorrhage, may occur.

Physical examination may reveal pallor, tachycardia, and tachypnea in the anemic patient. Severe anemia may lead to high-output cardiac congestion with signs of jugular venous distention, pulmonary rales, tachycardia with cardiac gallop, hepatomegaly with hepatojugular reflux, and dependent edema. Leukopenic patients may have fever and local or regional lymphadenopathy in conjunction with recurrent pharyngitis or skin infections, such as cellulitis or furunculosis. Occasionally, pneumonia is the presenting syndrome. Severely thrombocytopenic patients may have petechiae, ecchymoses, bloody gingival margins (especially common in patients with poor dental hygiene), stools testing positive for occult blood, frank melena, or hematuria. Gastrointestinal and central nervous system hemorrhages are unusual until severe thrombocytopenia has persisted for many months.

### Diagnostic Approach

The complete blood count and differential reveal a subnormal count of one or more blood cell lineages. The red blood cell (RBC) mean corpuscular volume (MCV) is often moderately elevated, and the RBC distribution width is usually increased. Examination of the peripheral smear is important because, in idiopathic aplastic anemia, blood cells usually have normal morphologies. Fragmented or spherical RBC forms are not characteristic features. Abnormalities of granulocytes, such as dysmorphic nuclei, cytoplasmic hypogranularity, and Auer rods, are more suggestive of vitamin and nutrient deficiencies, MDS, or acute leukemia. Platelet size may be reduced, but platelet function and cytoplasmic appearance are usually normal. Viral serologic studies may be useful for epidemiologic investigation but do not guide the treatment of individual patients. Serum levels of iron, vitamin B$_{12}$, and folate may detect an occasional case of vitamin and nutrient deficiency. Such deficiency is not likely to be etiologically

**FIG 14.1.** Simplified schema of the proliferation, lineage differentiation, and functional maturation of hematolymphoid cells under the influence of combinations of paracrine and humoral cytokines. Where more than one factor is designated, their individual or combined actions may be known to influence cells of the respective maturation stages. In addition to the designated cytokines, adhesion molecules expressed on stromal cells of the marrow and reticuloendothelial organs and blood vessel endothelial cells influence homing and maturation. (Adapted from Bagby GC Jr, Heinrich MC. Growth factors, cytokines, and the control of hematopoeisis. In: Hoffman R, Benz EJ Jr, Shattil SJ, et al., eds. *Hematology: basic principles and practice*, 3rd ed. New York: Churchill Livingstone, 2000:154–202.)

**TABLE 14.1.** *Classification of drugs and chemicals associated with aplastic anemia*

Agents that regularly produce marrow depression as major toxicity in commonly employed doses or normal exposures

Cytotoxic drugs used in cancer chemotherapy

   Alkylating agents (busulfan, melphalan, cyclophosphamide)
   Antimetabolites (antifolic compounds, nucleotide analogs)
   Antimitotics (vincristine, vinblastine, colchicine)
   Some antibiotics (daunorubicin, doxorubicin)
Benzene (and less often, benzene-containing chemicals: kerosene, carbon tetrachloride, Stoddard's solvent, chlorophenols)

Agents probably associated with aplastic anemia but with a relatively low probability relative to their use

   Chloramphenicol
   Insecticides
   Antiprotozoals: quinacrine and chloroquine
   Nonsteroidal antiinflammatory drugs, including phenylbutazone (see text), indomethacin, ibuprofen, sulindac, diclofenac, naproxen, piroxicam, fenoprofen, fenbufen, aspirin (?)
   Anticonvulsants, (hydantoins, carbamazepine, phenacemide, ethosuximide)
   Gold and arsenic (and other heavy metals, like bismuth, mercury)
   Sulfonamides as a class
   Some antibiotics
   Antithyroid (methimazole, methylthiouracil, propylthiouracil)
   Antidiabetes drugs (tolbutamide, carbutamide, chlorpropamide), carbonic anhydrase inhibitors (acetazolamide and methazolamide), mesalazine
   D-penicillamine
   2-Chlorodeoxyadenosine
   Estrogens (in pregnancy and in high doses in animals)

Agents more rarely associated with aplastic anemia

   Antibiotics (streptomycin, tetracycline, methicillin, ampicillin, mebendazole and albendazole, sulfonamides (see above), flucytosine, mefloquine, dapsone)
   Antihistamines (cimetidine, ranitidine, chlorpheniramine)
   Sedatives and tranquilizers (chlorpromazine, prochlorperazine, piperacetazine, chlordiazepoxide, meprobamate, methyprylon, remoxipride)
   Antiarrhythmics (tocainide, amiodarone)
   Allopurinol (may potentiate marrow suppression by cytotoxic drugs)
   Ticlopidine
   Methyldopa
   Quinidine
   Lithium
   Guanidine
   Canthaxanin
   Potassium perchlorate
   Thiocyanate
   Carbimazole
   Cyanamide
   Desferrioxamine
   Amphetamines

Young NS, Maciejewski JP. Aplastic anemia. In: Hoffman R, Benz EJ Jr, Shattil SJ, et al. *Hematology: basic principles and practice,* 3rd ed. New York: Churchill Livingstone, 2000:297–331.

relevant to the development of marrow failure but should be corrected because therapy may be impeded until the deficiency is corrected.

Bone marrow aspiration and biopsy should be performed for examination of histology and cell morphologies, iron staining, and cytogenetic studies in all new cases of marrow failure. In aplastic anemia, in contrast to most cases of MDS, the marrow cellularity is significantly reduced.[1] In severe aplastic anemia, the marrow space is composed mostly of large adipose cells with small islands of blood cell activity (Fig. 14.2). In the hematopoietic islands, lymphocytes and plasma cells may predominate as a result of dropout of normal myeloid elements and should not be misinterpreted as lymphoma or plasma cell infiltration. The aspirate smear shows marked myeloid and erythroid hypocellularity usually without dysplastic features.[2] Megakaryocytes are severely underrepresented on the aspirate smear. Initial evaluation should include the diepoxybutane test for chromosomal fragility of marrow leukocytes, which is positive in the congenital marrow failure disease of Fanconi anemia (see later). Cytogenetic abnormalities distinguish between idiopathic aplastic anemia and MDS (see later). Marrow examinations should be repeated as needed to evaluate changes in clinical status and responses to therapy.

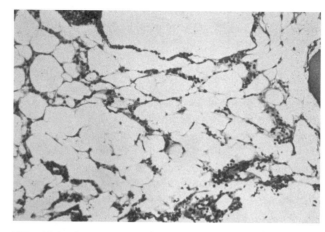

**FIG. 14.2.** Severe aplastic anemia. Bone marrow biopsy showing empty intertrabecular space with minimal residual cellular elements composed mostly of small lymphocytes. Rare small foci of residual hematopoeitic activity may be present. (Courtesy of the American Society of Hematology slide bank, 3rd ed.)

---

[1] Normal marrow cellularity varies inversely with age. Marrow cellularity in a young adult should be greater than about 60%, but the marrow of a healthy elderly person may be as low as 30% to 50%. More importantly, the cellularity may differ considerably between biopsy samples because of significant regional variability. Therefore, it may be important to examine several biopsy sections in questionable cases.
[2] Myelodysplasia with hypocellular marrow may occasionally masquerade as aplastic anemia or evolve from prolonged cases of aplastic anemia. Hypocellular MDS is discussed later in the context of the myelodysplastic syndromes.

*Treatment*

Mild cytopenias are best left untreated. In all cases, peripheral blood examinations should be performed periodically to observe for deterioration. Although aplastic anemia is seldom spontaneously reversible, it may smolder for quite some time in some patients, never to become clinically significant. More often, however, aplastic anemia presents with pronounced symptoms related to hematopoietic suppression, as described previously, and must be addressed expeditiously.

The most successful definitive treatments for acquired severe aplastic anemia are allogeneic bone marrow transplantation and intensive immunosuppression. Allogeneic transplantation can permanently replace diseased marrow and restore nearly normal hematopoietic function, with a long-term survival rate of about 70% (42–47). Although allotransplantation is becoming safer and more efficient with the development of methods to obtain and transplant progenitor or stem cells from donors' peripheral blood, the procedure is nonetheless arduous and entails a significant risk of acute and chronic graft-versus-host disease. Therefore, allogeneic transplantation for idiopathic aplastic anemia is recommended only for young patients who have not been heavily transfused and who have HLA-identical sibling donors. Intensive immunosuppression with antithymocyte globulin (ATG) or antilymphocyte globulin (ALG) with or without cyclosporine is equally successful for induction of remission but has a high rate of relapse (45,48–50). Fortunately, relapses can often be reversed by reinstitution of maintenance immunosuppression or by repeating the full regimen of ATG with cyclosporine (45). Reports suggesting that there may be a high rate of clonal hematopoietic abnormalities (e.g., MDS, acute myeloid leukemia) after treatment of aplastic anemia with ATG and cyclosporine supported by hematopoietic growth factors are highly controversial (51).

On the basis of observations that remissions of aplastic anemia may be obtained despite engraftment failure with bone marrow transplantation, studies of high-dose cyclophosphamide alone for treatment of severe aplastic anemia have been initiated (52–54). Patients so treated undergo long periods of severe neutropenia; nevertheless, the regimen is relatively well tolerated. The response rate approximates 70%. Trials comparing high-dose cyclophosphamide versus ATG plus cyclosporine are being conducted.

Corticosteroids should not be used because they do not improve hematopoiesis and yet superimpose additional nonspecific impairments of host defenses and metabolic side effects. Androgenic compounds, such as nandrolone decanoate, oxymetholone, and danazol, may improve blood cell production modestly and transiently (55–59). Although not curative, the androgenic steroids may enable short delays in the institution of specific therapy (i.e., allogeneic transplantation or immunosuppression). The hematopoietic growth factors, granulocyte colony-stimulating factor (G-CSF) and erythropoietin, stimulate granulocyte and erythrocyte production, respectively, but do not provide durable restoration

of marrow function (60,61). Hematopoietic factors should be used only in marrow failure disorders either when more definitive treatment (e.g., immunosuppression) has failed or when measures to improve severe cytopenias temporarily are urgently required.

Interleukin-10 (IL-10) is an immunomodulatory cytokine that suppresses the production of proinflammatory cytokines by activated T lymphocytes (62,63). IL-10 enhances colony formation by marrow cells of some patients with aplastic anemia (64). It is being investigated in clinical trials as an anti-inflammatory agent and awaits testing in patients with refractory marrow failure.

**Myelodysplastic Syndromes**

The MDS comprise several types of refractory hypoproliferative anemia with hypercellular bone marrow that may be accompanied by a variety of abnormal morphologic features (dysplasia) of the marrow hematopoietic cells (65–68). The French-American-British classification scheme subdivides MDS into five morphologic categories that correlate roughly with prognosis, as listed in Table 14.2. An International Prognostic Scoring system, incorporating evaluations of marrow blast cells, karyotypic abnormalities, and cytopenias, has improved the precision of prognosis (69). The most common dysplastic cell morphologies include dyserythropoiesis with binucleate and fragmented erythroblast nuclei; abnormal megakaryocytes with hypolobulated nuclei and abnormalities of cytoplasmic demarcation; and granulocyte dysplasia with nuclear hyposegmentation, pseudo–Pelger–Huët abnormality, and hypogranular cytoplasm (Fig. 14.3). The subclass of refractory anemia with ringed sideroblasts (RARS) is named for the abnormal prominence of erythroid cells with circumnuclear iron-containing siderotic granules in the marrow. The subclasses, refractory anemia with excess blasts

**TABLE 14.2.** *Median survival and time to 25% of patients evolving to acute myeloid leukemia as predicted by French-American-British (FAB) morphologic classification in myelodysplastic syndromes*

| FAB classification | Median survival (yr) | 25% Disease evolution (yr) |
|---|---|---|
| RARS | 6.9 | 10.1 |
| RA | 4.2 | 4.7 |
| RAEB | 1.5 | 1.4 |
| RAEB-t | 0.6 | 0.2 |
| CMML | 2.3 | 2.9 |

CMML, chronic myelomonocytic leukemia; RA, refractory anemia; RAEB, refractory anemia with excess blasts; RAEB-t, RAEB in transformation; RARS, refractory anemia with ringed sideroblasts.

Adapted from Greenberg P, Cox C, LeBeau MM, et al. International scoring system for evaluating prognosis in myelodysplastic syndromes [See Comments.] [ Published erratum appears in *Blood* 1998;91:1100.] *Blood* 1997;89:2079–2088, with permission.

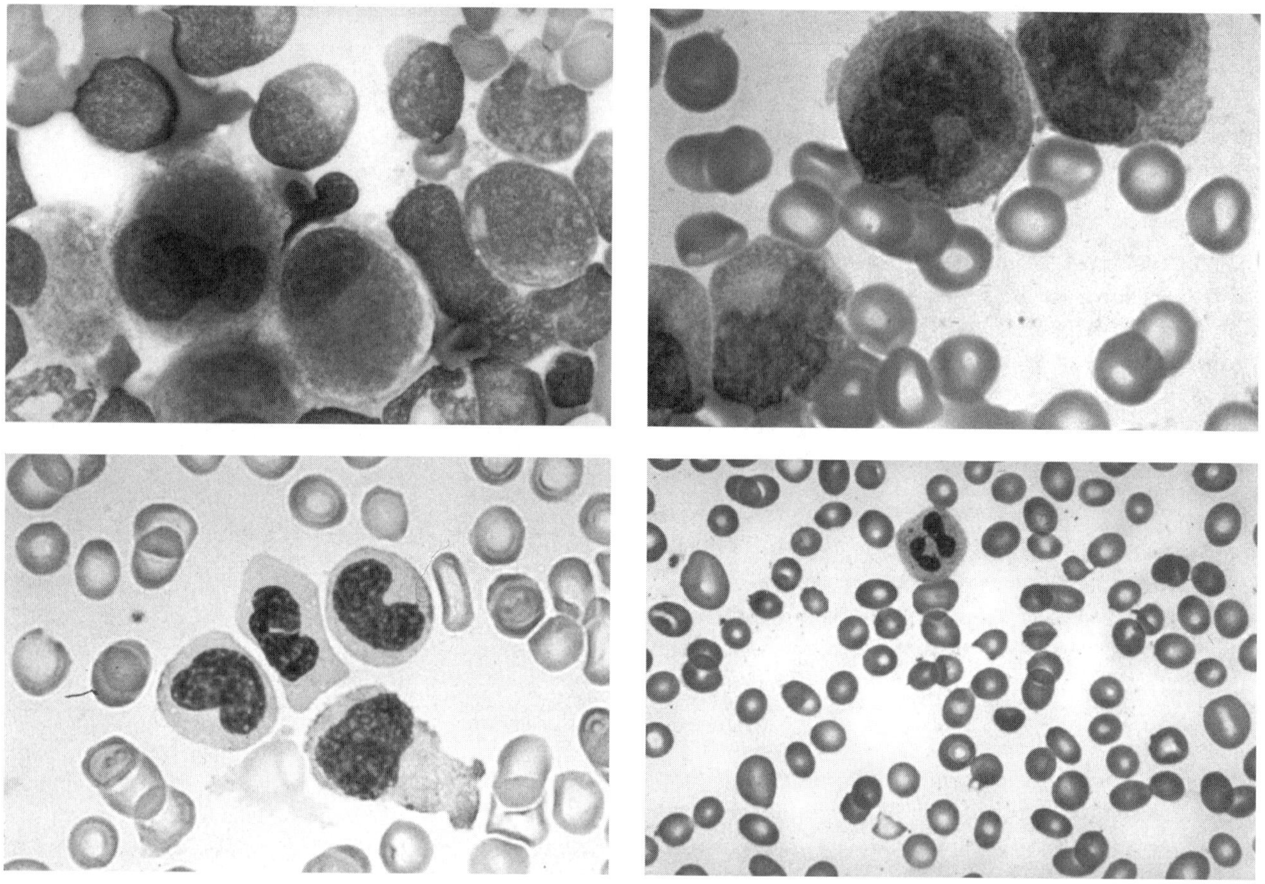

**FIG. 14.3.** Examples of myelodysplasia. **A:** Bone marrow aspirate: hypolobulated micromegakaryocytes and blast cells. **B:** Bone marrow aspirate: dysplastic promyelocytes with marked abnormalities of nuclear morphology. **C:** Bone marrow aspirate: dysplastic hypogranular neutrophils (one Pelger–Huët abnormality) and metamyelocyte. **D:** Peripheral blood smear: anisocytosis and poikilocytosis of erythrocytes with a hypogranular dysplastic neutrophil. (Courtesy of the American Society of Hematology slide bank, 3rd ed.).

(RAEB) and RAEB in transformation (RAEB-t), are defined by high percentages of marrow myeloblasts (5% to 20% and 20% to 30%, respectively) and are often accompanied by bizarre morphologic derangements (68). There are several nonrandom cytogenetic abnormalities frequently identified in primary MDS that may signify either good (e.g., 5q-, 20q-, Y-) or poor (e.g., chromosome 7 abnormalities, trisomy 8, complex cytogenetic abnormalities) prognoses (69,70). Cytogenetic abnormalities may be cryptic or complex and often signify molecular disorders of oncogenes or tumor suppressor genes (71–76). There is a high risk for certain types of MDS, such as RAEB and RAEB-t, to progress to acute leukemia—hence the now obsolete synonym "preleukemia." The morphologic and biologic distinctions between MDS and acute myeloid leukemia are often nebulous or arbitrary. Secondary leukemia is notoriously resistant to chemotherapy but may be amenable to allogeneic transplantation (77–82).

Several observations have been made that suggest that autoimmunity may be involved in the pathogenesis of cytopenias in some cases of MDS. First, autoimmune phenomena (including classically defined connective tissue disorders)

commonly accompany MDS (83–95). Second, marrow failure and phenotypic abnormalities of hematopoietic cells occur frequently in patients with autoimmune diseases (96–101). Third, immunosuppressive treatments have been reported to induce remissions in some cases of MDS (102–106). Hypocellular marrow, which is found in about one tenth to one fourth of MDS cases, may be an overt manifestation of autoimmune cytotoxicity directed against marrow progenitor cells (107–109). Theoretically, autoimmune attack against cells of dysplastic hematopoietic clone could result in damage to bystander cells (110,111). Alternatively, primary autoimmune attack on hematopoietic cells could induce cellular dysplasia through abstruse biochemical or molecular genetic mechanisms reminiscent of incomplete or aborted apoptosis (112–116). Mechanisms of autoimmunity in MDS have not been well characterized, but examination of the marrow of patients with aplastic anemia or pure red cell aplasia (PRCA) often shows dysplastic features during the early stages of disease recovery (117–122). Thus, hypoplastic MDS could represent a transitional stage in the evolution of some cases of aplastic anemia.

*Clinical Presentation*

The initial complaints of patients with MDS are usually symptoms related to anemia. Some patients have primary infectious or hemostatic complaints. Leukemic transformation with marrow hypercellularity may occasionally be accompanied by skeletal pain or fever with sweating. Physical examination reflects the consequences of the patients' specific cytopenias (refer to aplastic anemia, discussed earlier). The differential diagnosis of blood cytopenias with normal or hypercellular marrow includes hypersplenism related to hepatic disease, chronic infectious diseases, or hematolymphoid proliferative diseases, which should be excluded. Isolated thrombocytopenia is more likely to be a result of autoimmune destruction than marrow disease; a therapeutic trial of steroids before marrow examination may be prudent in such cases (123).

*Treatment*

The cornerstone of clinical care for patients with myelodysplasia is transfusion support for cytopenias. Nutrient and vitamin deficiencies should be corrected if identified. Refractory anemia is rarely responsive to pyridoxine (124–135). Hematopoietic growth factors are sometimes effective for palliative (albeit transient) elevations of blood cell counts in some patients who develop infection or high transfusion burden but are not curative and often lose effectiveness with continued use (136–144). Trials of various combinations of so-called maturational agents (chemotherapeutic and biomodulating agents, including low-dose cytosine arabinoside, thioguanine, low-dose etoposide, vincristine, retinoic acids, dihydroxycholecalciferol, $\beta$-hydroxybutyrate, interferon-$\alpha$, and IL-2) have been generally disappointing because of low response rates or short response durations (145–174). Furthermore, toxicities of some of the maturational agents include transient or prolonged worsening of cytopenias with increased risk for infection or increased transfusion requirements and intolerable constitutional side effects. Intensive chemotherapy and autologous hematopoietic cell transplantation may achieve high rates of hematologic responses in some patients, but relapses are common (80,175–180).

On the basis of empiric evidence for the pathogenic role of autoimmunity in MDS, immunosuppressive treatment with cyclosporine, ATG, or both has been studied in exploratory trials. In one trial, substantial hematologic responses to cyclosporine, including improvement of anemia and transfusion independence, were obtained in 82% of 17 patients with refractory anemia regardless of the cellularity of the bone marrow (102). In another report, responses to ATG were observed in nine of 14 patients (64%) with refractory anemia and in two of six patients (33%) with RAEB (106). Unfortunately, responses to ATG were not long-lived: the median response duration was 10 months (range, 3 to 38 months). Trials combining ATG and cyclosporine are ongoing.

The only established opportunity for cure of MDS is allogeneic bone marrow transplantation (with initial remission-induction chemotherapy, if required, for secondary acute leukemia) (80,181,182). Unfortunately, most patients with MDS are middle aged or elderly and thus are poor candidates for allotransplantation because of the arduous nature of conditioning regimens using intensive chemoradiotherapy, which result in higher morbidity and mortality rates. Considerable research into the biology of hematopoietic cell transplantation has demonstrated that engraftment of HLA-compatible hematopoietic cells may be possible using immunosuppressive, but nonablative, host conditioning (183). Trials have begun at several transplantation centers to study the engraftment and therapeutic efficacy of such "lite" allotransplantations for patients whose age or organ system impairments would be contraindications to the usual allotransplantation procedures (184–187). Employing purine analog-based immunosuppressive conditioning regimens, the procedures theoretically exploit graft-versus-leukemia effects to suppress or eliminate the abnormal cell clones. Early trial results have demonstrated extensive engraftment without apparent increases in the frequency or severity of graft-versus-host disease. Results of larger trials will show whether such procedures are truly efficacious. If successful, this will make allogeneic bone marrow transplantation and hence, cure, possible in older patients with MDS.

**Paroxysmal Nocturnal Hemoglobinuria**

Paroxysmal nocturnal hemoglobinuria (PNH) is a clonal disorder of hematopoietic cells in which patients are subject to episodic hemolysis and peculiar vascular thromboses (188–191). PNH cells are characterized by deficiency of expression of several membrane proteins anchored by glycophosphatidylinositol (GPI), including the complement defense proteins, decay-accelerating factor (CD55), membrane inhibitor of reactive lysis (CD59), and C8-binding protein (192–196). Erythrocytes in PNH are abnormally sensitive to complement-mediated cytolysis in acidic environments.

Deficiency of GPI-anchored proteins results from an acquired defect in the gene (*pig-a*) that is responsible for an early step in the biosynthesis of the anchor molecule (197–199). Transfection of the *pig-a* gene or transfer of GPI-anchored proteins into PNH cells corrects the biosynthetic defect (198,200). However, *pig-a* gene mutations are not sufficient for the development of PNH because clonal populations of cells with the PNH genotype may be found in healthy subjects as well (201).

PNH is etiologically associated with acquired aplastic anemia (110,117,190,202–206). In most patients with PNH, the marrow is demonstrably deficient in clonogenic cells, although some patients have a hypercellular marrow (207–209). Up to 80% of patients with long-standing PNH develop significant single-lineage or multilineage cytopenias, and a significant minority develop marrow aplasia (210).

Conversely, 10% or more of patients with acquired aplastic anemia who are successfully treated with intensive immunosuppression develop hematopoietic cell clones deficient in synthesis of GPI-anchored proteins (211). The GPI-deficient clones are not handicapped with respect to proliferation *in vitro* (191,209,212,213). Therefore, it has been postulated that an autoimmune attack on the marrow allows the PNH clone a proliferative advantage in the setting of suppression of normal hematopoiesis (214). Alternatively, marrow failure could theoretically develop as a result of exhaustion of the reserve of hematopoietic progenitors in the process of compensation for ineffective erythropoiesis (110).

### Clinical Presentation

Patients with PNH infrequently present with the primary complaint of episodic red urine. More often, anemia is discovered through laboratory evaluation of constitutional symptoms or thromboembolic events. Thrombosis tends to occur in peculiar sites, such as the hepatic veins (e.g., Budd–Chiari syndrome) or cerebral veins (e.g., sagittal sinus syndrome) (215–222). Other characteristic but less common sites of thrombosis are abdominal veins and dermal veins. Some patients may present with aplastic anemia (see earlier).

### Diagnostic Approach

Intravascular (and presumably intramedullary) hemolysis is the pathophysiologic hallmark of PNH. In some cases, hemolysis can be severe enough to produce hemoglobinemia and hemoglobinuria. Hemoglobinuria may be distinguished from hematuria by the absence of RBCs on urinary microscopic examination. Myoglobin (i.e., rhabdomyolysis) does not discolor the plasma. Aside from normocytic anemia, the hemogram is usually not abnormal. The peripheral blood smear has no characteristic features in PNH. The definitive diagnostic tests are Ham's acid hemolysis test, in which acidified plasma causes RBC lysis *in vitro* (expressed as a percentage of RBCs), and the flow cytometric assessment of GPI-anchored proteins (i.e., CD59, CD55, or both) on granulocytes or platelets (223–231).

### Treatment

Initial treatment with high-dose corticosteroids often ameliorates or prevents hemolytic episodes by suppressing complement activation (232–234). Chronic hemolysis leads to increased iron losses and folate requirement. Iron stores should be assessed (serum ferritin or marrow examination), and the replacement of iron and folate should be instituted if needed. Transfusions of packed RBCs may be required to treat or prevent fatigue and cardiopulmonary symptoms. Washing of donor RBCs, once thought to help prevent the occasional concomitant hemolysis of endogenous circulating erythrocytes, is now believed to be unnecessary (235). Acute throm-

bosis in critical vessels should be treated emergently with thrombolytic agents followed by heparin and maintenance therapy with warfarin (236–238).

On the basis of its apparent clinical relationship to acquired aplastic anemia, PNH has been treated with intensive immunosuppression (239–241). In general, treatment with ATG, cyclosporine, or both induces significant remissions in a substantial fraction of patients but does not eradicate the PNH (GPI-deficient) clone. Allogeneic hematopoietic cell transplantation, on the other hand, reverses the aplasia and eradicates the PNH clone, with resolution of episodic thromboses (218,242,243). Of course, allogeneic transplantation carries risks of substantial procedure-related morbidity, such as neutropenic infection and graft-versus-host disease, and, until recently, has been available only to the small proportion of young patients with related HLA-matched siblings. Autologous transplantation may be limited by the preferential mobilization of PNH stem cells by hematopoietic cytokines (244). Advances in transplantation of stem cells from mismatched or unrelated donors and umbilical cord blood cells and the use of nonmyeloablative conditioning regimens may lead to wider availability for patients with nonmalignant diseases, such as PNH (186,245–247). In the future, correction of the defective or missing *pig-a* gene in hematopoietic cells may be feasible (248,249).

## Acquired Pure Red Cell Aplasia

PRCA is a disorder of severely suppressed production or arrest of maturation of erythroid precursors leading to profound anemia unaccompanied by neutropenia or thrombocytopenia (250). PRCA is strongly associated with some viral infections, especially the B19 parvovirus, which infects the erythroid progenitor cell (251). The virus can be propagated in cultures of human bone marrow, blood, and fetal liver. Humoral immunity normally terminates the infection in immunocompetent patients and is lifelong. Pooled commercial immunoglobulin (which typically contains high titers of antiparvovirus antibody) can be used to treat persistent infection.

A noninfectious form of PRCA has been identified that appears to have an immunologic etiology. T lymphocytes or antibodies that suppress both autologous and normal erythropoiesis *in vitro* can often be demonstrated in primary acquired PRCA (252–261). Secondary PRCA may be associated with thymoma, hematologic neoplasms (especially lymphoma and chronic lymphocytic leukemia) and nonhematologic neoplasms, idiosyncratic reactions to drugs, infections, and pregnancy (262–269). PRCA may complicate autoimmune diseases, including systemic lupus erythematosus (SLE) and rheumatoid arthritis, and has been frequently reported in association with large granular lymphocyte (LGL) lymphoproliferative disorders (270–274). Chronic immunodeficiency may underlie a susceptibility to parvovirus infection leading to PRCA (275). Some cases of PRCA are associated with autoimmune hemolytic anemias, which should raise suspicion of a lymphoproliferative disorder (261,262, 276–280). Profound anemia can result from PRCA superimposed on hemolytic anemias (especially sickle cell anemia), in which erythropoiesis may be too handicapped to compensate for RBC destruction. Acquired PRCA is to be distinguished from congenital anemias (e.g., Fanconi anemia) in that residual erythropoiesis can be detected by marrow examination in those diseases.

*Clinical Presentation*

Anemic patients are weak and fatigued. The more rapid and severe the anemia, the more intense the symptoms. Such patients may have significant cardiopulmonary compromise manifested as mental confusion, dyspnea on exertion, chest pain, and signs of cardiac congestion, such as tachycardia with gallop, cardiomegaly, and dependent edema. In addition, symptoms may include those attributable to an underlying disorder, such as opportunistic infection, lymphoma, or autoimmune disease.

*Diagnostic Approach*

Anemia may be severe, often with blood hemoglobin levels below 7 g/dL. Erythrocytes of the peripheral blood usually are normochromic and normocytic. The reticulocyte count is severely reduced (less than 20,000/mm$^3$). Mild cytopenias of other lineages may coexist but are not usually prominent. Evidence of acute or reactivated infection with parvovirus B19 should be sought with serologic tests for anti-B19 immunoglobulin M (IgM) and IgG and by polymerase chain reaction amplification for B19 DNA. A bone marrow examination is especially important to distinguish viral and primary autoimmune PRCA from MDS with erythroid hypoplasia. In PRCA, the overall marrow cellularity is usually normal. Granulocytes and megakaryocytes and their precursors usually are normal in number and morphology. In contrast, the marrow of MDS shows dysplastic morphologic features of one or more cell lineages. In parvovirus-induced PRCA, erythroid precursors are rare, and the pronormoblasts are markedly enlarged and vacuolated (giant pronormoblasts) (281). A dramatic scarcity of erythroblasts and arrest of erythroid maturation are apparent in PRCA (Fig. 14.4). The iron stain shows normal to increased marrow iron stores. Computed tomography of the chest and abdomen should be performed to seek evidence of thymoma, lymphoma, or other malignancy.

*Treatment*

The anemia should be treated with transfusions as necessary to correct constitutional and cardiopulmonary symptoms. Vitamin and nutrient deficiencies should be treated if identified. Underlying malignancies, infectious diseases, and autoimmune disorders should be identified and treated specifically. Suspected drugs should be discontinued. Thereafter

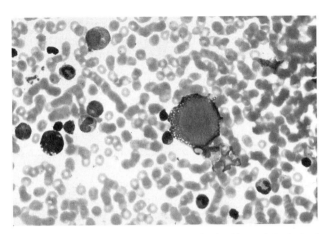

**FIG. 14.4.** Acquired pure red cell aplasia. Vacuolated giant pronormoblast characteristic of infection with parvovirus B19. (Courtesy of the American Society of Hematology slide bank, 3rd ed.).

(about 1 month), an absence of improvement in reticulocyte count or transfusion requirements strongly suggests PRCA of a primary autoimmune etiology for which immunosuppressive therapy should be considered. Although the response rate is limited and relapses may be frequent, initial treatment should be attempted with corticosteroids (to avoid the potential toxicities of more potent immunosuppressive agents) (282–287). Higher response rates may be obtained with cytotoxic agents, such as azathioprine or cyclophosphamide, administered by oral low-dose regimens (288,289). ATG is an alternative immunosuppressive agent that may be highly effective but entails acute toxicities (283,290–292). Cyclosporine has been reported to be effective in high proportions of small numbers of patients with both primary and leukemia-associated PRCA (265,283,293,294). Danazol, plasmapheresis, lymphocytopheresis, and intravenous immune globulin (IVIG) have been infrequently reported as effective treatments for PRCA but may reasonably be tried in refractory cases (287,295). No reports have yet been made of high-dose alkylator therapy or hematopoietic cell transplantation for acquired PRCA.

**Congenital Marrow Failure Syndromes**

Acquired aplastic anemia may be mimicked by certain uncommon congenital hematopoietic disorders presenting with the sudden or progressive failure of one or more lineages of blood cells. Fanconi's anemia is characterized by multilineage hematopoietic failure associated with anatomic anomalies (e.g., abnormalities or absence of bones of the arms and digits), chromosomal fragility, and a high risk of secondary malignancies (especially leukemias) (296–298). The diagnosis of Fanconi's anemia is supported by a positive test for chromosomal breakage in blood cells cultured in the presence of diepoxybutane or mitomycin C (299–303). Hematopoietic insufficiency in Fanconi's anemia may be improved by androgenic steroids, but cure may only be effected by allogeneic bone marrow transplantation (304,305).

Diamond–Blackfan anemia (DBA) is a congenital marrow failure disorder in which an intrinsic defect of erythropoietic progenitor cells leads to a progressive normocytic or macrocytic anemia (306–308). DBA is also associated with anatomic abnormalities (307). The intrinsic survival and proliferative defect of erythroid progenitors in DBA may be partially overcome by IL-3 *in vitro* (309–312). Clinical trials have shown that some patients may be responsive to this agent (310,311). Hematopoietic cell transplantation can be curative (313,314). Although DBA is often responsive to corticosteroids both *in vitro* and *in vivo,* there is no clear evidence for an immunologic etiology of either Fanconi's anemia or DBA. Other congenital hematopoietic failure disorders are exceptionally rare, for which the reader is referred to the cited authoritative texts.

## Chronic Neutropenia

### Large Granular Lymphoproliferative Disorders

Clonal expansion of LGLs of T-cell and natural killer (NK) cell phenotype, also known as LGL leukemia, may be associated with one or more autoimmune disorders (272,315–321). An inciting infection with an unknown viral pathogen is thought to play a role in the pathogenesis of LGL disorders because leukemic LGL cells constitutively express the cytotoxic proteins, perforin and Fas ligand, characteristic of activated cytotoxic T lymphocytes (315,322–324). Furthermore, about half of Western patients with T-lymphocyte LGLs have positive serologic tests for the specific epitope of the envelope protein of human T-cell leukemia virus type I, designated BA21 (325,326). No mutations of Fas or Fas ligand have been recognized in LGL leukemia cells (in contrast to the *lpr* mice, which have concomitant lymphoproliferative and autoimmune diseases) (324,327). Dysregulated apoptosis, however, may play a role in the expansion of LGL cells because they are resistant to Fas-mediated cell killing (322).

### Clinical Presentation

Both T-LGL and NK-LGL may be associated with hematopoietic suppression (274,320). T-LGL is more common among middle-aged and older patients (median age of onset, 55 years), constituting the majority of cases of T-cell chronic lymphocytic leukemia (315,328,329). T-LGL has a chronic course with insidious development of symptoms related to neutropenia. Recurrent neutropenic fevers or bacterial infections with organisms from the skin or gut (e.g., cellulitis, pharyngitis, perirectal abscess) are the most common presentations. A significant minority of patients may have mild to moderate anemia with corresponding fatigue and cardiopulmonary insufficiency. A small subset of patients may also have mild to moderate splenomegaly with or without hepatomegaly. Autoimmune disorders are frequently associated with T-LGL. Serologic abnormalities may include the rheumatoid factor, antinuclear antibodies, immune complexes, hypergammaglobulinemia, increased $\beta_2$-microglobulin, antineutrophil antibodies, and antiplatelet antibodies (321,330,331). T-LGL commonly accompanies rheumatoid arthritis, and a large proportion of patients with Felty's syndrome have evidence of clonal LGL expansion (332–338). Thus, the complex of erosive arthritis, hepatosplenomegaly, and neutropenia overlaps with (or may be equivalent to) Felty's syndrome.

LGL leukemia of NK cells is usually an acute systemic illness of younger adults, presenting with constitutional symptoms, extensive lymphadenopathy, and hepatosplenomegaly (339,340). NK-LGL is frequently refractory to chemotherapy and often has a rapidly fatal course.

### Diagnostic Approach

A modest absolute lymphocytosis (4000 to 10,000/μL with atypical lymphocytes often more than 500/μL) is frequently, but not uniformly, recognized on the complete blood count. The peripheral blood film must be examined to confirm the phenotypic classification of LGL. LGLs are recognized as irregular cells about 12 μm in diameter with pale blue cytoplasm and azurophilic granules, often reported as "atypical lymphocytes." The bone marrow examination may show either nodular or diffuse infiltration by LGLs, which can be identified by immunohistochemical staining. Flow cytometric immunophenotyping can distinguish between T-LGL cells ($CD3^+$, $CD8^+$, $CD16^+$, and $CD57^+$) and NK-LGL cells ($CD3^-$, $CD4^-$, $CD8^-$, $CD16^+$, and $CD56^+$) (317).

### Treatment

Treatment of T-LGL lymphoproliferative disorder is necessary only for patients who have symptomatic cytopenias. There is no standard treatment; however, several lympholytic approaches have been effective, including low-dose oral methotrexate, cyclosporine, and oral cyclophosphamide (320,341–346). Filgrastim (G-CSF) may help in prevention and treatment of infections by raising the granulocyte count (347).

### Cyclic Neutropenia

A disorder of periodic reduction of circulating neutrophils associated with increased risk of invasive bacterial infections is recognized as cyclic neutropenia (348–350). The disorder is most often recognized in children and is usually inherited in an autosomal dominant pattern (351,352). The inherited form is associated with cyclic impairment of myelopoiesis, with periodicity of about 21 days (353). Treatment with G-CSF is effective and significantly reduces the risk of infection by shortening the neutropenic cycles and elevating both the zenith and nadir neutrophil counts (353–355).

An acquired form of cyclic neutropenia in adults has been recognized in association with large granular lymphoproliferative syndrome (356–358). The cycling period may vary from about 14 to 21 days. This disorder has been described in the setting of various autoimmune, chronic inflammatory, and immunodeficiency disorders, such as Crohn's disease, ankylosing spondylitis, and common variable immunodeficiency syndrome (359–367). Expression of G-CSF receptors on neutrophils is quantitatively normal in cyclic neutropenia (368). Both cellular and humoral factors have been reported to regulate the cycling (369–372). It is tempting to speculate that this disorder is related to the LGL disorder characteristic of Felty's syndrome associated with an unmasking of the theoretically physiologic cycling of hematopoietic cell clones (373,374). Acquired cyclic neutropenia may be a premalignant manifestation of acute lymphoblastic leukemia or acute NK cell leukemia (375,376). Consistent with the hypothetical autoimmune lymphoproliferative etiology of acquired cyclic neutropenia, patients have been effectively treated with corticosteroids or cyclosporine (344,345,363,377,378). G-CSF is effective in raising the neutrophil count but has been reported to exacerbate symptoms of the underlying autoimmune disease (347,354,379–385).

## Amegakaryocytic Thrombocytopenia

Amegakaryocytic thrombocytopenia (AT) is an unusual syndrome of marrow failure involving isolated loss of megakaryocytes with peripheral thrombocytopenia (386,387). There is considerable pathologic and clinical overlap with other syndromes of acquired marrow failure disorders. AT may be considered analogous to acquired PRCA in that a single hematopoietic cell lineage is suppressed. Several cases of acquired AT progressing to aplasia have been reported (388–390). AT may be an initial presentation of non-Hodgkin's lymphoma (391). In contrast to PRCA, there is no convincing evidence for an infectious etiology of AT. Nutrient deficiencies, specifically of vitamin B$_{12}$, may be associated with relative megakaryocytic hypoplasia (392). Prolonged heavy alcohol consumption may cause a transient reduction of megakaryocytes (393,394).

In accordance with the current understanding of megakaryocyte physiology, serum thrombopoietin (TPO) levels are inversely related to megakaryocyte mass, and in contrast to autoimmune thrombocytopenia (AITP), TPO levels are elevated in AT (395–397). Acquired AT is often associated with evidence of autoimmunity (398–404). Several cases have been described in the setting of SLE (400,401). In some cases, either T-lymphocyte cell-mediated or humoral suppression of megakaryocytic colonies in semisolid cultures has been demonstrated (399,405–407).

### Clinical Presentation

As with other thrombocytopenic disorders, the predominant complaints reflect the insidious onset of hemostatic defects (easy bruising, spontaneous ecchymoses, gingival or nasal bleeding, petechiae). Bleeding does not occur until the platelet count falls below 20,000/mm$^3$ or less (sudden drops

in platelet count may be accompanied by bleeding at higher levels of thrombocytopenia). Concomitant symptoms of autoimmune disease may also be noted. A family history of hemostatic problems or marrow failure syndromes should suggest alternative etiologies. There are no specific findings on physical examination. Splenomegaly is not a diagnostic finding.

### Diagnostic Studies

The complete blood count and peripheral blood smear show severely reduced platelet counts with small to normal-sized platelets. In contrast, platelets in AITP are normal to large in size (408–410). The erythrocyte MCV may be elevated, but there are otherwise no characteristic abnormalities of other cell lines in the peripheral blood. Antinuclear antibody tests and other tests associated with concomitant autoimmune syndromes may be positive. The bone marrow examination shows severe reduction of megakaryocytes without other quantitative or morphologic (i.e., dysplastic) abnormalities (411). As for the initial evaluation of other marrow failure diseases, tests of acid hemolysis (Ham's test) and chromosomal fragility (diepoxybutane test) and cytogenetic studies should be performed to screen for alternative marrow failure etiologies.

### Treatment

Platelet transfusions should be used as required for bleeding or to maintain safe platelet counts. As predicted by its presumed autoimmune etiology, AT has most often been successfully treated by immunosuppressive therapy. Corticosteroids may be tried initially on an empiric basis (401,412). In the absence of a rapid response or when the situation is urgent because of bleeding, more potent immunosuppressive agents should be used. Both cyclosporine and ATG have effect (392,413–416). In addition, there have been reports of responses to vinca alkaloids and alkylating agents (403,417). Danazol may also produce responses (418,419). No reports have been made of allogeneic or autologous hematopoietic cell transplantation for AT.

## AUTOANTIBODY-MEDIATED CYTOLYTIC SYNDROMES

### Autoimmune Thrombocytopenia

#### Idiopathic Thrombocytopenic Purpura in Adults

AITP is a disorder of low blood platelet counts in which platelet destruction is caused by antiplatelet autoantibodies (420,421). Autoimmunity to platelets in AITP may involve both humoral and cellular immune mechanisms (422). In children, acute immune thrombocytopenia may follow viral infections and is usually self-limited (423). In contrast, AITP in adults is usually idiopathic (although it may be associated with autoimmune or lymphoproliferative diseases, e.g., SLE, non-Hodgkin's lymphoma) and is frequently chronic and refractory to treatment (420,423–426). AITP is characterized by shortened platelet survival, as determined by kinetic analysis of [111]In-labeled platelets *in vivo* (423,427). External scintigraphic imaging shows that platelets are sequestered (and presumably cleared) by the spleen and other sites of the reticuloendothelial system (423,428). Autoimmune platelet destruction is probably mediated by antibodies directed against platelet surface glycoproteins (427,429–431). Antibodies directed against glycoproteins IIb/IIIa and Ib/IX are detected on autologous platelets of 75% to 83% of patients; circulating autoantibodies against the same glycoprotein are identified in large proportions of cases (429–431). Rarely, antiplatelet glycoprotein antibodies may result in acquired platelet functional defects (e.g., acquired "thrombasthenia") (432–437). Antibody concentrations on patients' platelets decrease in response to effective treatment (429).

### Clinical Presentation

Thrombocytopenia is frequently asymptomatic until the platelet count falls below 30,000 to 50,000/μL. Patients may then complain of easy bruisability and large ecchymoses. Microvascular hemostatic defects manifested by spontaneous petechiae and gingival bleeding are seen as the platelet count drops further (typically below 20,000/μL) or when the platelet count drops rapidly. Some patients, especially those with thrombocytopenia of long standing, may not manifest symptoms despite platelet counts below 10,000/μL. In particular, serious hemostatic problems (e.g., gastrointestinal or central nervous system hemorrhage) are unusual until the platelet count has been severely reduced for a long time. Episodic waning of the platelet count may accompany or follow viral infections; even when there is no associated infectious syndrome, the periodic worsening may be accompanied by mild to moderate constitutional symptoms suggesting reactivation of an inflammatory process.

### Diagnostic Approach

Practice guidelines for the diagnosis and management of AITP were published by the American Society of Hematology (123). Isolated thrombocytopenia in an adult without quantitative or morphologic abnormalities of other cell lineages or evidence of underlying autoimmune or neoplastic disease is only rarely attributable to hematopoietic disorders (e.g., MDS). The peripheral blood smear should be examined carefully for evidence of intravascular hemolysis (schistocytes suggestive of disseminated intravascular coagulation [DIC], hemolytic uremic syndrome [HUS], or thrombotic thrombocytopenic purpura [TTP]). The smear must also be inspected for platelet clumping, a technical artifact that may give misleading false low counts on the automated cytometer. Examination of the bone marrow on initial presentation is not recommended in the absence of additional suspicious signs or symptoms; however, many practitioners would argue that the risk of missing a serious hematopoietic disorder or in-

volvement of the marrow with a neoplastic disease is high enough and serious enough to indicate marrow examination. In otherwise uncomplicated AITP, the marrow cellularity is usually normal or modestly increased. The most striking feature is the abundance of megakaryocytes. The following specific abnormalities argue against primary AITP: morphologic abnormalities of any cell lineages (i.e., myelodysplasia, megaloblastic anemia); increased blast cells or maturation arrest; infiltration by lymphocytes, plasma cells, or carcinoma cells; marrow fibrosis; and depletion of megakaryocytes. Similarly, the clinical finding of splenomegaly should lead to reconsideration of the diagnosis of AITP.

### Treatment

Corticosteroids are the standard initial treatment for AITP. A starting dose of prednisone should be in the range of 1 mg/kg/day (438,439). The dosage should be rapidly tapered by about one fourth as soon as a response is obtained. Thereafter, dosage tapering should be slow; a 2-week basis is frequently recommended. Exact methods of steroid dosage taper are often considered "an art" and may be individualized on the basis of therapeutic response. The objective is to reduce the dosage as soon as possible to a level below which the metabolic side effects of corticosteroids are prominent. Inability to wean the patient off corticosteroids indicates the need for alternative treatment. High-dose pulsed intravenous corticosteroids have been more effective in some reports, but it is not clear how to predict which patients will respond (440–447). Infusion of IVIG (e.g., 2 g/kg over 2 to 5 days) is frequently effective but is costly and may have to be repeated chronically (448–451). Alternatively, anti-D immune globulin (e.g., WinRho) is often effective but also requires repeated courses (452–454).

Splenectomy is recommended for steroid-refractory patients and for those with frequent relapses (455–457). Response to IVIG has been reported to predict effectiveness of splenectomy (458). A significant number of patients fail to respond or relapse after splenectomy. Failure of splenectomy should prompt a search for an accessory spleen by radionuclide scanning. After splenectomy, an initial appearance of erythrocyte Howell–Jolly bodies on the peripheral blood smear followed by their disappearance may indicate "regrowth" of an accessory spleen. About two thirds of patients have satisfactory responses to IVIG, splenectomy, or both; nearly one third of patients fail to respond to these standard therapies (458).

Chronic severe thrombocytopenia (platelet count less than 5000 to 20,000/mm³) is associated with a high risk of hemorrhage, especially mucosal bleeding, genitourinary bleeding, prolonged bleeding from cutaneous or internal injuries, and spontaneous ecchymoses (459). Chronic severe AITP that is refractory to treatment with steroids, IVIG, and splenectomy has a mortality rate of 4% to 16%, largely attributable to bleeding (420,424,460,461).

Many second-line treatments with various effectiveness have been reported. Patients with chronic autoimmune diseases that are refractory to conventional treatments may be successfully treated with various regimens of immunosuppressive cytotoxic agents (457,462–466). Danazol (an androgenic agent), cyclophosphamide, and azathioprine are among the most widely used of these agents. Responses have also been reported with anthracyclines, vinca alkaloids, dapsone, colchicine, cyclosporine, and interferon-α (465,467–475). Plasmapheresis with protein A column absorption is infrequently effective and is usually complicated by systemic inflammatory symptoms (476,477).

Unfortunately, low-dose oral cytotoxic regimens often fail to produce significant durable remissions for many patients. Prolonged treatment with low- to moderate-dose alkylating agents, such as cyclophosphamide, is also associated with increased risk of secondary myelodysplasia and leukemia, presumably as a result of chronic repeated mutational damage to stem cells (478). Higher doses of intravenous cyclophosphamide (pulse therapy) or combination chemotherapy can effectively induce durable remissions in some patients with otherwise refractory autoimmune disorders, including refractory AITP (463,479–482). The presumptive mechanism of effect of pulse cyclophosphamide is transient elimination of autoreactive T-lymphocyte clones; other mechanisms, such as alterations of lymphocyte subpopulations, may also contribute to the effect (483,484). Late relapses have been common after discontinuation of pulse cyclophosphamide treatments (485,486). Several trials have employed or proposed to employ yet higher doses of cyclophosphamide (i.e., "transplant doses") to treat autoimmune diseases in the anticipation of improved rates of durable remissions (54,487–489). Lim et al. (490) reported the successful treatment of two patients with refractory AITP using high-dose cyclophosphamide with autologous peripheral blood stem cell (PBSC) support. Both patients had previously failed to respond to corticosteroids, IVIG, and splenectomy. Their myelosuppression–immunosuppression regimen consisted of cyclophosphamide, 50 mg/kg/day with mesna for uroprotection. Complications were minimal; neutropenia resolved on days 11 and 13, respectively, and neither patient developed culture-proven infections. Although both patients required platelet transfusions in the peritransplantation period, complete remissions of AITP (platelet counts of more than 150,000/mm³) were achieved within 5 weeks of treatment. As of the publication date, complete remissions were maintained for more than 11 and 7 months, respectively. A systematic phase I and II trial of high-dose cyclophosphamide with autologous CD34-enriched (T-lymphocyte depleted) peripheral blood stem cell support for chronic severe AITP is being undertaken at the U.S. National Institutes of Health.

### Posttransfusion Purpura

In rare cases, acquired immune thrombocytopenia may develop about 1 week after transfusion of a blood product containing platelet material (i.e., packed RBCs, whole blood, plasma) (491–495). Typically, the patient is a multiparous woman; men and nulliparous women are at only minimal risk for posttransfusion purpura (PTP). Women whose prior pregnancies were complicated by neonatal alloimmune thrombocytopenia are not at significantly increased risk for PTP. PTP can masquerade as refractory thrombocytopenia after hematopoietic cell transplantation (496).

In PTP, the recipient develops isoantibodies against foreign epitopes on the donor platelets, which secondarily result in destruction of the recipients' own platelets. The mechanism of isoantibody formation is poorly understood. The sera of most PTP patients contains antibodies against the human platelet antigen-1a (HPA-1a); target antigens, including HPA-1b, glycoprotein IIb/IIIa, and others, have been identified uncommonly (495,497,498). Theoretically, platelet alloantigens accumulated during product storage, or antigen–antibody complexes resulting from alloreaction could bind to autologous bystander platelets, resulting in their targeting and lysis (498).

Thrombocytopenia mimicking idiopathic thrombocytopenia may be severe (frequently less than 10,000/mm³) and result in hemostatic complications, including hemorrhage. Significant thrombocytopenia (and bleeding) may last 2 to 6 weeks (492). Infusion of IVIG is usually effective within about 3 days (497,499–502). Corticosteroids may sometimes be effective (503). Random donor platelet transfusions often result in moderately severe allergic transfusion reactions and usually do not provide significant increments of platelet counts. Antigen-matched products may be supportive if the antigen is identified. For patients who require subsequent transfusions of blood products, it would appear prudent to limit reexposure to immunogenic antigens by using only antigen-matched blood products, if possible.

### Autoimmune Hemolytic Syndromes

#### Approach to the Patient

The patient with mild compensated hemolytic anemia may have minimal symptoms beyond mild fatigue, whereas the patient with severe hemolytic anemia presents with some degree of constitutional symptoms (often severe fatigue and malaise), cardiopulmonary insufficiency (e.g., dyspnea on exertion, cardiac congestive symptoms), and hyperbilirubinemia or frank jaundice. In acute hemolytic episodes with intravascular hemolysis, there may be back pain and dark urine. A history of prescription drugs, recent infectious illnesses, and systemic inflammatory (i.e., rheumatic) symptoms should be sought. The examination should concentrate on the heart and lungs, reticuloendothelial organs (liver, spleen, and lymph nodes), skin, and joints. Laboratory examination must include complete and differential blood counts. A microscopic examination of the peripheral blood smear is mandatory to detect evidence of RBC lysis (most commonly spherocytosis, but depending on the pathophysiology, poikilocytosis and occasionally schistocytosis may be seen) and erythropoietic compensation (polychromatophilia). Serum chemistries should be performed to identify hepatic dysfunction and renal failure.

### Warm-reacting Antibody-mediated Hemolysis

Antibodies directed against surface antigens of RBCs may arise spontaneously or in association with any of several autoimmune diseases. Reticuloendothelial destruction of antibody-bound erythrocytes then leads to varying degrees of anemia. Antibodies that react with erythrocytes at warm temperatures (in contradistinction to the cold-reacting antibodies, *vide infra*) are generally of the IgG class (504,505). Epitopes of RBC membrane proteins (e.g., band 3, glycophorin A) may be common targets, but individual patients' autoantigens are usually not identifiable (506–508). Hypothetically, mimicry of host self antigens by microbial epitopes could initiate autoimmunization (509–511). In chronic lymphoproliferative disorders, such antibodies may arise through antigen-independent polyclonal proliferation of IgG-producing B lymphocytes (330,512–519). Accordingly, there is a strong association of secondary autoimmune hemolytic anemia with various lymphoproliferative and immunodeficiency diseases, including chronic lymphocytic leukemia, Hodgkin's disease, multiple myeloma, Waldenström's macroglobulinemia, acquired immunodeficiency syndrome (AIDS), congenital immunodeficiency syndromes, and graft-versus-host disease (266,520–535). Treatment of lymphoproliferative disorders with nucleoside analog drugs has reportedly been associated with hemolytic anemia (536–542). Many drugs, of which α-methyldopa is the most notorious, have been implicated in the pathogenesis of autoimmune hemolytic anemia (543). With α-methyldopa, however, there is a much greater incidence of Coombs' test positivity than the rate of clinical hemolysis.

### Clinical Presentation

Autoimmune hemolytic anemia has an overall incidence of about 10 cases per 1 million population per year and is more common in women than in men (544). Although many etiologic associations have been reported, as discussed previously, most cases are sporadic. The severity of the clinical features reflects the severity of anemia and the intensity of hemolysis coupled with underlying disease manifestations. Active episodes are often heralded by malaise, myalgia, and other symptoms of systemic inflammation (545). There may be jaundice when hemolysis is brisk. Splenomegaly, occasionally large, may be a prominent finding in about one third of patients. In Evans' syndrome, hemolytic anemia may be accompanied by AITP, with attendant microvascular hemorrhage (see the previous section on AITP).

### Diagnostic Approach

In addition to anemia, examination of the peripheral blood film usually shows spherocytes with polychromasia reflect-

ing reticulocytosis. Some patients may have folate deficiency as a result of increased erythropoiesis and thus may not show reticulocytosis. Nucleated RBCs may seen on the smear if hemolysis is rapid. Hyperbilirubinemia and reduced haptoglobin levels signify brisk hemolysis. The direct antiglobulin test (DAT), or direct Coombs' test, detects erythrocyte-bound immunoglobulin or complement, and the indirect antiglobulin test detects antierythrocyte antibodies in serum. These tests must be carefully interpreted in the light of clinical information because false-positive and false-negative test results can confuse the differential diagnosis (546–551). Urine hemosiderin may be detectable. Infrequently, hemolytic anemia may be mediated by RBC antibody deposition that is undetectable by the DAT, especially if mediated by cold-reacting antibodies of wide thermal amplitude (552). A few patients with autoimmune hemolytic anemia may have a negative DAT because of the paucity of antibody molecules bound to the cell surface; such cases may be detected using a more sensitive reagent or the micro-Coombs' test.

### Treatment

Therapeutic transfusion should not be withheld from patients who have symptoms. The risk for acute intravascular hemolytic reactions is not to be underestimated but is more than counterbalanced by the adverse consequences of anemia, such as myocardial ischemia, high-output congestive heart failure, and cerebral hypoxia (553). Close collaboration between the clinician and the blood bank usually enables successful transfusion therapy through sophisticated methods of compatibility testing (554–556). Given the difficulties in cross-matching blood in the presence of a warm autoantibody, however, it would be reasonable and prudent to transfuse the severely anemic patient who has critical end-organ compromise with type-specific or "least-incompatible" packed RBCs.

Corticosteroid treatment may be effective, presumably through suppression of antierythrocyte antibody production and inhibition of reticuloendothelial destruction of antibody-coated erythrocytes (557). Corticosteroids have myriad adverse side effects and should be tapered and discontinued as soon as possible after induction of remission. Infusion of IVIG may be effective in a few patients with steroid-refractory disease (558–560). Successful treatment with danazol has also been reported. Patients with rapid hemolysis who are unresponsive or cannot be weaned from corticosteroids should be considered for splenectomy (561,562). Splenectomy increases the risk for infection by encapsulated bacteria (e.g., hemophilus, streptococcal pneumonia, meningococcal infection) for which preoperative immunizations should be administered. Immunosuppressive agents, such as cyclophosphamide, azathioprine, cyclosporine, and mycophenolate mofetil, may be effective for patients who do not respond to steroids and splenectomy, but these agents have not been systematically investigated (563–571). There have been a few reports of high-dose chemotherapy with stem cell support for autoimmune hemolytic anemia and Evans' syndrome, but the long-term treatment results are yet inconclusive (572,573).

### Cold Agglutinin Disease

Anti-RBC antibodies with higher affinity at colder temperatures, called *cold agglutinins,* may cause intermittent hemolysis after exposure of the patient to cold temperatures (574,575). The relationship between temperature and an antibody's affinity for RBCs is the so-called thermal amplitude (a conceptually poor but traditionally accepted descriptor). Such antibodies generally bind more avidly with decreasing temperature, with a peak affinity at about 4°C (576). Cold agglutinins may result from aberrant monoclonal antibody production or may occur in association with clonal lymphoproliferative diseases (primary cold agglutinin disease [CAD]). Cold agglutinins may also result from polyclonal immunoreactivity against cross-reactive or molecularly modified antigens during or after infection with various microbial agents, such as *Mycoplasma pneumoniae,* Epstein–Barr virus, or human immunodeficiency virus (HIV), which is referred to as *secondary CAD* (577–580). Sera of healthy people may occasionally be found to have low-titer cold agglutinins of low thermal amplitude and no clinical significance. Most cold agglutinins in primary CAD are directed against the erythrocyte I antigen; some may recognize the i antigen; rarely, the target may be other erythrocyte surface antigens (581–585).

Cold agglutinins bind to erythrocytes on cooling of the blood in the peripheral circulation and typically dissociate on reentry to the warmer central circulation. Most cold agglutinins are of the IgM class and fix complement efficiently before dissociation from target cells (575,586). Those of high thermal amplitude may persist at higher temperatures. Consequently, in CAD, most circulating erythrocytes do not have demonstrable surface-bound antibody but are opsonized by complement components (usually C3b or C4b). Hemolysis results from damage of complement-bound erythrocytes in the spleen, liver, or other tissues of the reticuloendothelial system (587,588). In contrast to warm-reacting antibody-mediated hemolysis, erythrocyte destruction in CAD is relatively slow. Nevertheless, the peripheral blood smear often shows considerable spherocytosis.

### Clinical Presentation

Idiopathic and malignancy-related CAD occur most often in middle-aged and older patients. Secondary CAD related to infection is more common in younger patients. Mild-to-moderate anemia is the usual presenting problem in CAD. Anemia is due to intermittent low-grade hemolysis, which is rarely brisk enough to produce episodic hemoglobinuria. Only rarely does a patient have hemolysis extensive enough to cause jaundice. Blood hemoglobin levels are not usually decreased below 7 g/dL; therefore, symptoms of cardiopulmonary insufficiency are not common in the absence of

concurrent medical disorders. Some patients develop acrocyanosis in the cold, and some of these patients may have to move to warmer climates to obtain relief. Symptoms and signs of a primary lymphoproliferative disorder or an infectious disease (e.g., a history of recent pneumonia in mycoplasma-associated secondary CAD) may predominate. Hepatosplenomegaly may be found in infectious mononucleosis, cytomegalovirus infection, subacute bacterial endocarditis, and other infectious diseases as well as in various lymphoproliferative diseases, but is neither a cause nor an effect of the hemolytic process of CAD.

### Diagnostic Approach

As noted, the complete blood count with differential shows mild to moderate anemia with normocytic RBC indices. In the absence of vitamin and nutrient deficiency or concurrent infection with parvovirus B19, there is a compensatory reticulocytosis, which may elevate the MCV and increase the RBC distribution width. Occasionally, an extremely high MCV (in the 180 fL range) may be reported by the passage of clumped RBCs in the cytometer. The peripheral smear may show significant agglutination (especially if the blood sample is not prewarmed). Rouleaux formation may be observed in cases of multiple myeloma, Waldenström's macroglobulinemia, and other lymphoproliferative disorders if not masked by RBC agglutination. There are no characteristic abnormalities of the WBC lineages specific to CAD, but circulating malignant lymphocytes may be found in chronic leukemias and various lymphomas. Serum chemistry may reveal increased bilirubin and lactate dehydrogenase (LDH), resulting from hemolysis. Serum protein electrophoresis may detect monoclonal IgM or IgG gammopathy in lymphoproliferative disorders. There is a high cold agglutinin titer. The DAT is positive for complement and may occasionally be positive for polyspecific antibody (589). The indirect antiglobulin test is negative. In the marrow, compensation for hemolysis may produce erythroid hyperplasia in addition to histologic abnormalities related to underlying lymphoproliferative disease or metastatic malignancy. Myeloid and megakaryocytic cells are not characteristically abnormal.

### Treatment

Secondary CAD related to mycoplasma or other infections usually does not become apparent until after the underlying clinical syndrome has defined itself. It is usually self-limited and mild and does not typically require specific therapy. Unlike warm antibody-mediated hemolytic anemia, primary CAD does not often respond to corticosteroids or splenectomy (590). Evidence for lymphoproliferative disease should be sought in all patients with noninfectious CAD. The patient should be maintained in a warm environment while there is ongoing hemolysis. Primary CAD may respond to immunosuppressive cytotoxic drugs, such as cyclophosphamide, chlorambucil, or fludarabine (591–596). Plasma exchange may be beneficial in some cases (597–600). Recurrence of the hemolytic disorder may herald relapse of the malignancy. Patients with significant anemia-related cardiopulmonary compromise may require transfusion. Cross-match testing must be performed carefully at 37°C to avoid misinterpretation. Infusion of blood products through a blood warmer may be required to avoid hemolysis (600).

### Paroxysmal Cold Hemoglobinuria

A self-limited syndrome of paroxysmal episodes of intravascular hemolysis after exposure to cold environments (paroxysmal cold hemoglobinuria) occurs rarely after some viral infections or in association with lymphoid malignancies or other autoimmune disorders (601–610). Postinfectious paroxysmal cold hemoglobinuria is mainly encountered in children (611–613). The syndrome is associated with constitutional symptoms, back pain, anemia, jaundice, and renal impairment. The hemolysis is caused by a cold-reacting antibody that fixes complement in the cold but completes the complement cascade upon warming after return to the central circulation (614,615). This antibody (Donath–Landsteiner antibody) was previously recognized more frequently in cases of tertiary syphilis. The DAT is usually negative in postinfectious paroxysmal cold hemoglobinuria. Because the syndrome is generally self-limited, supportive care with transfusions and avoidance of cold temperatures is usually the best therapeutic approach.

### Thrombotic Thrombocytopenic Purpura and Hemolytic Uremic Syndrome

Microangiopathic thrombocytopenia associated with fever, hemolytic anemia, neurologic abnormalities, and acute renal failure is the classic pentad of the TTP syndrome (616,617). HUS is a closely related disorder in which oliguric uremia is the most prominent feature associated with microangiopathic hemolysis and thrombocytopenia and can be thought of as microangiopathy localized to the kidneys (618). In both disorders, platelet thrombi cemented by von Willebrand's factor (vWF) occlude the microvasculature of various organs, resulting in both organ-specific clinical disorders and hemolysis with thrombocytopenia (619,620). In contrast to DIC, the thrombi of TTP and HUS are devoid of fibrin (621). The etiology of TTP is not understood. HUS is often associated with exposure to microbial toxins (e.g., shigella or *Escherichia coli* enterotoxin) or cancer chemotherapy (622–627). TTP and HUS are related closely in pathology and clinical presentation. Both syndromes may be incited by endothelial cell damage or disruption of the normal mechanisms that shield platelets from interaction with high-molecular weight multimers of vWF (628–635). Antibody directed against a vWF cleaving protease (which cleaves large multimers into smaller species) may be identified in acute nonrecurring TTP (631,636). In contrast, patients with familial TTP have reduced protease activity in the absence of a detectable in-hibitor. In acute HUS, cleaving protease activity is not reduced.

### Clinical Presentation

TTP and HUS may be superimposed on, or mimicked by, preexisting immune vascular disorders or infectious diseases (637). Most patients with TTP have features of anemia, thrombocytopenia, and neurologic disorders, with only 40% having the full pentad. Symptoms are often highly nonspecific and may include malaise and weakness in addition to one or more symptoms of the pentad. Neurologic manifestations are often protean and transient. HUS presents more typically with abdominal pain and is often associated with rapid development of anuria, hypotension, and renal failure.

### Diagnostic Studies

In addition to thrombocytopenia, the peripheral blood smear of TTP patients shows moderate to large numbers of schistocytes resulting from microvascular fragmentation. Serum LDH levels are elevated as a result of both intravascular hemolysis and tissue injury. Bone marrow examination does not contribute to the diagnosis of thrombotic microangiopathies but may be helpful in seeking evidence of marrow failure syndromes or disseminated malignancies. Skin biopsy of rash, when present, may help by showing intravascular thrombus formation. Infrequently, intravascular thrombosis may be detected in blood vessels in the bone marrow biopsy specimen. Plasma electrophoresis shows the presence of ultralarge species of vWF multimers.

### Treatment

Plasmapheresis is a highly effective therapy for TTP, although it is unclear whether the effect of plasma exchange is to remove a pathologic substance or to replace a defective plasma component (638–644). Corticosteroids and antiplatelet agents are often empirically administered to patients with TTP; the effectiveness of corticosteroids in HUS is undetermined (645–647). Other therapies for TTP, including immunosuppressive agents, staphylococcal protein A column plasma immunoadsorption, and splenectomy, should be considered for patients with refractory or recurrent TTP (648–654). The role of treatment modalities other than plasmapheresis has not been adequately tested.

## Autoimmune Neutropenia of Childhood

Autoimmune neutropenia of childhood (also known as *autoimmune neutropenia of infancy* and *chronic benign neutropenia of childhood*) is a syndrome of neutropenia and frequent minor infections resulting from autoimmune destruction of neutrophils caused by autoreactive antineutrophil antibodies (655–658). Autoimmune neutropenia occurs with an incidence of 1 in 100,000 population per year in young children. It is distinct from cyclic neutropenia and other intrinsic myelopoietic (progenitor cell) defects, alloimmune neonatal neutropenia, and secondary autoimmune neutropenia. Previously reported associations with parvovirus infections have been challenged (657,659). Antineutrophil antibodies are usually directed against the NA-1 or NA-2 antigens but are of unclear clinical and pathologic specificity (660,661). Antibody-coated neutrophils are destroyed by splenic sequestration in a manner analogous to the platelet destruction of AITP.

### Approach to the Patient

It is important to distinguish autoimmune neutropenia of infancy, which is relatively benign and short-lived (median duration, 20 months), from the congenital cytopenic syndromes, which are chronic, subject to serious infections, and have the propensity to transform into clonal disorders (658,662–668). Differential diagnostic considerations must include marrow failure (stem cell) and immunodeficiency disorders.

### Clinical Presentation

The peak incidence of autoimmune neutropenia of infants is between 8 to 11 months (658). Infection with skin, oropharyngeal, nasopharyngeal, and gut organisms frequently precedes the recognition of neutropenia. In particular, otitis, sinusitis, gingivitis, cellulitis, perirectal abscess, and vulvovaginal ulcers are the most common infections. Such infections are typically mild to moderate in severity.

### Diagnostic Approach

The differential diagnosis includes other causes of autoimmune neutropenia, such as Evans' syndrome and drug reactions; transient postinfectious neutropenia; immunodeficiency syndromes; and congenital or acquired aplastic anemia. In the autoimmune neutropenia of infancy, the lymphocyte, erythrocyte, and platelets counts are normal. Neutrophil morphology is normal. The bone marrow shows normal to increased cellularity with a loss of mature neutrophils (657,659). Antineutrophil antibodies may be detected by flow cytometry, immunofluorescence, or agglutination reactions (669,670).

### Treatment

Because the neutropenia is self-limited, prophylactic antibiotic treatment is not usually indicated. Infections are usually benign; treatment with appropriate antibiotics guided by physical examination and microbiologic tests is usually effective (657,658). Severe infections should be treated with combination broad-spectrum intravenous antibiotics. In problematic cases, intravenous immune globulin or corticosteroids may help slow neutrophil destruction (655,658). G-CSF may be used to increase neutrophil counts temporarily if required in the treatment of severe infections (657).

## IMMUNE-MEDIATED COAGULATION DISORDERS

### Antiphospholipid Antibody Syndromes

Antiphospholipid antibodies (APAs) must be considered in the differential diagnosis of recurrent or unusual venous or arterial thromboses (thrombophilia). The etiologies of thrombophilia compose a large and heterogenous group of pathophysiologic disorders. Primary "hypercoagulable" states are unusual; they include deficiencies or functional abnormalities of natural anticoagulants (e.g., antithrombin III, protein C, protein S, or plasminogen), elevated levels of plasminogen activator inhibitors, hyperhomocysteinemia, factor V Leiden (resistance to activated protein C), and the prothrombin G20210A mutation (671,671a). PNH is a rare cause of thrombosis at unusual sites, such as mesenteric and hepatic vessels (188). Common secondary causes of thrombosis include tissue injury (including surgery), inflammation, damage to blood vessel endothelium (e.g., atherosclerosis, hypoxia), autoimmune diseases (including the antiphospholipid syndromes), malignancy, pregnancy and estrogen and progesterone therapy, myeloproliferative disorders, and hyperlipidemia (672,673).

APAs are a heterogenous group of autoreactive antibodies directed against a variety of negatively charged phospholipids, including cardiolipin, phosphatidylserine, phosphatidylinositol, and phosphatidic acid complexed with coagulation factors or other plasma proteins (674). The first APA was the "reagin" associated with syphilis, described by Wasserman in 1906. Later, a plasma component was recognized in some patients with SLE that inhibited phospholipid-based coagulation assays (e.g., the activated partial thromboplastin time [aPTT]) (675). Such inhibitors are commonly labeled *lupus anticoagulants* (676). Lupus anticoagulant may be detectable in the plasma of more than 50% of SLE patients; however, APAs are often encountered in patients with other autoimmune, inflammatory, or infectious diseases (e.g., malignancy, HIV, syphilis) and chronic exposure to certain drugs, such as chlorpromazine, procainamide, and hydralazine (677,678). Some patients develop transient lupus anticoagulant after viral infection. Indeed, there may be a substantial prevalence of APAs among the general population (679,680). Although the classic lupus anticoagulant is an antibody directed against the complex of prothrombin with phospholipid and calcium ion, numerous antibodies directed against various peptide–phospholipid complexes (e.g., $\beta_2$-glycoprotein I and cardiolipin) have been identified (674,681). Therefore, the lupus anticoagulant, anticardiolipin antibody, and other such antibodies may be categorized together as APAs.

### Approach to the Patient

Patients with APAs may experience thrombotic or thromboembolic events in the absence of other predisposing factors (e.g., trauma, surgery, or malignancy). Recurrent fetal loss is a characteristic feature in women. History of prior episodes of thrombosis or family history of thromboembolic events supports primary thrombophilia rather than APA syndrome. Arthropathy, skin rash, lymphadenopathy, vasculitis, and renal disease point to possible secondary causes. A thorough evaluation of prescription and nonprescription drugs is important. Screening examinations for occult solid tumors or hematopoietic malignancy (e.g., stool guaiac test, chest radiographs, complete blood counts, prostate specific antigen) are appropriate in the absence of more probable causes.

### Clinical Presentation

Despite their inhibitory effect on coagulation *in vitro,* APAs are not generally associated with clinical hemorrhagic disorders. Rather, patients with APA are at increased risk for thrombosis and related complications, including both venous and arterial thromboses, recurrent fetal loss, and other obstetric complications, pulmonary infarction, livedo reticularis, myocardial infarction, transient ischemic attack, and stroke (682,683). APAs are found in a small proportion of patients with recurrent thrombosis independent of specific autoimmune diseases (684). Both the lupus anticoagulant and the anticardiolipin antibody may be implicated in recurrent thrombosis (685). Thrombocytopenia may be associated with lupus anticoagulant, presumably on the basis of concomitant autoreactive antiplatelet antibodies; conversely, APAs may be recognized in a significant proportion of patients with autoimmune (idiopathic) thrombocytopenia (686–689). The term *primary APA syndrome* encompasses thrombotic and obstetric complications associated with APAs but without connective tissue disease, whereas the *secondary APA syndrome* refers to patients with APA-related complications in the setting of autoimmune disease, such as SLE. A severe and unusual variant of the syndrome, characterized by disseminated microangiopathy with a mortality rate of about 60% as a result of multiorgan failure, is recognized as the catastrophic APA syndrome (690). DIC may accompany the catastrophic APA syndrome, but it is not clear whether DIC is the cause or the result of multiorgan system injury.

### Diagnostic Approach

The lupus anticoagulant is usually recognized by an abnormal prolongation of a phospholipid-dependent clotting assay, such as the aPTT (674). In the absence of anticoagulant drugs or factor deficiencies, the prothrombin time is ordinarily normal or only slightly prolonged. The presence of an inhibitor is then confirmed by an aPTT mixing study, in which the patient's plasma is diluted with an equal volume of normal plasma. Correction of the aPTT indicates a factor deficiency, whereas failure to correct substantially the prolonged aPTT is consistent with the presence of an inhibitor. The prolonged aPTT resulting from lupus anticoagulant may be distinguished from other inhibitors by correction with addition of phospholipid derived from platelet membranes (platelet neutralization procedure) or various other sources (691,692). In

patients with a normal aPTT, lupus anticoagulant can be detected by prolongation of clotting time in the diluted Russell's viper venom test, which is more sensitive for lupus anticoagulant than the aPTT (693–695). Although the lupus anticoagulant is a species of APA, the converse is not true; not all APAs function as anticoagulants. Anticardiolipin antibody is not identified by abnormal coagulation tests but rather by enzyme-linked immunosorbent assay (681). This assay has low specificity in that it may have a broad cross-reactivity *in vitro* with a variety of negatively charged phospholipids. Furthermore, the anticardiolipin titers may fluctuate significantly with time; negative tests should be repeated for patients with recurrent thrombotic events. Consultation with the laboratory hematopathologist or clinical hematologist is advised for selection of testing procedures to identify specific antibodies and interpretation of their clinical significance.

### Treatment

In the absence of a history of thrombosis, the lupus anticoagulant does not necessarily require treatment (696). APA thrombosis syndromes are sometimes classified on the basis of the sites of thrombosis (697) (Table 14.3). APA-associated thromboses are frequently recurrent if untreated (698,699). Treatment of the APA syndrome requires chronic anticoagulation. The addition of antiplatelet agents may not confer additional benefit when intensive anticoagulation is used (700). The most widely accepted treatment of patients with APA after documented thrombosis is intensive anticoagulation with warfarin. Although some authors have suggested a target INR of 3 or higher, it would be prudent to set a target INR of 2.5 until prospective clinical trials indicate otherwise (701,701a). The monitoring of aPTT in such patients receiving heparin is problematic because the APA may cause it to be spuriously prolonged. In that setting, chromogenic factor Xa levels or other assays that are insensitive to lupus anticoagulant are less likely to overestimate or underestimate the degree of anticoagulation (701). An alternative method of long-term anticoagulation in these patients is to use low-molecular-weight heparin (697), the dose of which is based on a body weight formula that obviates the need for clotting time monitoring. The benefit of preventing thrombosis appears to outweigh the risk for hemorrhage associated with chronic anticoagulation (700). Pregnant women with a history of APA-associated thrombosis or recurrent fetal loss should not receive warfarin (due to teratogenicity) but rather may be treated with aspirin and heparin or corticosteroids (702). It is unknown whether anticoagulation or antiplatelet prophylaxis will help prevent thrombosis in patients with asymptomatic serologic APA.

## Spontaneous Acquired Inhibitors of Coagulant Factors

### Approach to the Patient

The ordinary setting in which acquired coagulant factor inhibitors are encountered is in the hemophiliac patient who becomes alloimmunized by chronic factor replacement ther-

**TABLE 14.3.** *Classification and recommended therapy for anti-phospholipid antibody thrombosis syndromes*

| Type | Syndrome manifestations | Therapy |
|---|---|---|
| I | Peripheral venous syndromes<br>  Deep vein thrombosis with or without pulmonary embolus | IV or SC heparin followed by long-term SC heparin |
| II | Peripheral and central arterial syndromes<br>  Coronary artery thrombosis<br>  Peripheral artery thrombosis<br>  Aortic thrombosis<br>  Carotid artery thrombosis | IV or SC heparin followed by long-term SC heparin |
| III | Retinal and cerebrovascular syndrome<br>  Retinal artery thrombosis<br>  Retinal vein thrombosis<br>  Cerebrovascular thrombosis<br>  Transient cerebral ischemic attacks | *Retinal*<br>  Pentoxyphylline<br>*Cerebrovascular*<br>  Long-term low-dose warfarin plus low-dose ASA |
| IV | Mixed syndromes<br>  Mixtures of manifestations of types I, II, and III | Tailored to specific manifestations, according to above recommendations |
| V | Fetal wastage syndromes<br>  Placental vascular thrombosis<br>  Maternal thrombocytopenia | Low-dose ASA preconception, then low-dose ASA plus low-dose heparin postconception |
| VI | Anti-phospholipid antibody without apparent clinical manifestations | No clear indication |

ASA, acetylsalicylic acid; IV, intravenous; SC, subcutaneous.
Adapted from Bick RL. Antiphospholipid thrombosis syndromes: etiology, pathophysiology, diagnosis and management. *Int J Hematol* 1997;65:193–213.

apy. Some patients are encountered, however, with spontaneous hemorrhage or other hemostatic defects resulting from autoantibodies against coagulant factors (677,703). All patients with a history of spontaneous hemostatic disorders should undergo thorough hematologic assessment, including history of specific bleeding events and family history. A careful description of the type and timing of hemorrhage after hemostatic challenge (e.g., dental procedures, surgery, trauma, childbirth) may hold important clues. The physical examination should concentrate on the reticuloendothelial organs and lymph nodes because of the possible association with malignant lymphoproliferative syndromes. Laboratory testing should include a complete blood count with differential, routine coagulation tests (prothrombin time, aPTT, thrombin time), and ristocetin cofactor or ristocetin-induced platelet aggregation analysis (for vWF assessment).

*Clinical Presentation*

The possibility of a coagulant factor inhibitor should be considered in any patient with a spontaneous hemostatic disorder. Coagulopathy caused by a factor inhibitor has a clinical presentation similar to spontaneous or acquired factor deficiency. Late bleeding from surgical or traumatic sites, hemarthroses, and deep hematomas (including retroperitoneal bleeding) are suggestive of severe coagulation factor abnormalities. Spontaneous mucous membrane bleeding, petechiae, and easy bruising point to vascular or platelet disorders. Most spontaneous coagulation factor inhibitors have been described as IgG directed against factor VIII, resulting in a severe bleeding diathesis (704–708). However, inhibitors of factors V, VII, IX, X; fibrinogen; and vWF have also been described (709–728). Accelerated clearance of coagulant fac-

tors from plasma resulting from antibodies directed against nonenzymatic epitopes of coagulant factors may present as acquired factor deficiencies. Although most patients with spontaneous factor inhibitors have no identifiable underlying etiologic disease, occasional cases have been reported in association with various autoimmune and chronic inflammatory diseases and conditions, including rheumatoid arthritis, SLE, inflammatory bowel diseases, penicillin therapy, and other less frequent disorders (729–734). Factor V inhibitor may arise as a result of immunization by bovine thrombin used as surgical fibrin glue, often during cardiac surgery (735). Monoclonal gammopathies (e.g., paraproteins of monoclonal gammopathy of undetermined significance, multiple myeloma, chronic lymphocytic leukemia, and non-Hodgkin's lymphoma) rarely consist of antibodies that react with coagulant factors (725,726,736). The M proteins of multiple myeloma and Waldenström's macroglobulinemia may indirectly interfere with fibrin monomer conversion from fibrinogen or with fibrin polymerization; rarely, they may be true antibodies against fibrinogen or factor XIII (737,738).

*Diagnostic Approach*

If a coagulation test is prolonged, an inhibitor is demonstrated by the failure of mixing the patient's plasma with normal plasma to correct the test time (677). Specific factor assays can be performed to identify the target factor of the inhibitor. In contrast, the effective result of accelerated factor clearance caused by antibody–factor complex formation is a factor deficiency. Thus, mixing with normal plasma corrects the coagulation tests of patients with accelerated clearance as well as factor synthesis deficiencies (e.g., hepatocellular failure, vitamin K deficiency, or unsuspected exposure to anticoagulants, such as warfarin). Dysfibrinogenemia (related to hepatocellular disorders, chronic inflammatory diseases, and so forth) prolongs all coagulation test times, including the thrombin time (739).

### Treatment

Treatment of acute bleeding is the highest priority. Bleeding due to anticoagulant factors can have catastrophic consequences, including internal bleeding into the gastrointestinal tract or central nervous system. Hemostatic measures should include the usual compression, immobilization, and vasoocclusive methods as would be applied to any bleeding patient. Intramuscular injections should be avoided and venipunctures minimized. In the patient with factor VIII autoantibody who is bleeding acutely, porcine or high-purity human factor VIII may be infused at a dosage calculated to neutralize the autoantibody and replenish plasma factor VIII to about 30% activity (740). Repeated exposure to the porcine factor VIII can lead to development of antibodies against the porcine protein and effectively abrogate its efficacy. Unfortunately, if the autoantibody titer is very high, it may not be possible to surmount the factor neutralization with replacement therapy, and it becomes necessary to bypass the factor deficiency with factor IX complex concentrate (740,741). Use of that agent, especially if overdosed, may result in thrombosis or intravascular coagulation; thus, its use should be guided by an experienced clinical hematologist. Recombinant factor VIIa is available to treat patients with inhibitor to factor VIII and has fewer associated complications. Plasma exchange may be considered for patients with bleeding unresponsive to factor replacement (742–744).

In the long-term, therapy should be aimed at suppression of the autoantibody. An initial trial of IVIG may successfully reduce the factor neutralization; however, trials of more intensive immunosuppression regimens incorporating steroids, alkylating agents, antimetabolites, or vinca alkaloids are often necessary (741,745–750). Acquired factor V inhibitor has been treated with platelet transfusion (751).

## SECONDARY HEMATOLOGIC MANIFESTATIONS OF AUTOIMMUNE DISEASES

### Anemia of Chronic Disease

Anemia is the most common hematologic complication of chronic autoimmune and inflammatory conditions. Inflammatory diseases may be associated with several potential causes of anemia, such as blood loss caused by bleeding from inflamed foci (e.g., ulcerative colitis) or drugs (e.g., gastritis caused by nonsteroidal antiinflammatory drugs). The anemia of chronic disease (ACD; more appropriately termed the *anemia of chronic inflammation*) is a prominent cause of anemia in the setting of chronic illnesses, such as rheumatic diseases, cancer, and AIDS (752,753). The pathogenesis of ACD is multifactorial, characterized by hyporesponsiveness to

erythropoietin, impaired iron use, and a modest reduction of RBC survival (754–757). Proinflammatory cytokines, such as IL-1, TNF-$\alpha$, and interferon-$\gamma$, may be involved in the impairments of erythropoietin production and response as well as impaired iron use (758–762).

### Clinical Presentation

In the setting of a primary inflammatory disease, the hematocrit and hemoglobin may decline gradually and hence without concomitant constitutional complaints. The ACD generally does not present with any specific symptoms or signs unless it is very severe. In that instance, the patient may complain of fatigue, palpitations, dizziness, and exertional dyspnea. Most commonly, there is no complaint or one of mild fatigue only.

### Diagnostic Approach

In a patient with a chronic immune or inflammatory disorder, a mild to moderate normocytic or occasionally slightly microcytic anemia is likely to be caused by ACD. Assessment of iron-deficiency anemia, which often coexists with ACD, is the most important consideration. In ACD, both the serum iron and and transferrin levels are usually decreased, with a concomitant increase in iron saturation (763,764). In the absence of iron deficiency, the serum ferritin level may be modestly increased. Iron-deficiency anemia is associated with reduced serum iron levels and normal to increased serum transferrin levels, with a resulting reduction of serum iron saturation (764). The serum ferritin level is reduced in iron-deficiency anemia (765). Serum transferrin levels may sometimes help distinguish ACD from iron deficiency when used in conjunction with measurements of serum ferritin (766–768). Finding of iron deficiency should prompt a search for a site of bleeding. Deficiencies of serum vitamin $B_{12}$ and folate levels may coexist with ACD (769). The peripheral blood smear should be examined to eliminate suspicion of other causes of anemia, such as hemolysis (spherocytes), concurrent megaloblastic and iron-deficiency anemias (variable MCV with macrocytic RBCs, anisocytosis, and hyperlobulated neutrophils), and MDS (variety of dysplastic features). In the absence of reasonable suspicion of marrow disease, an aspirate or biopsy of the bone marrow is not indicated in the evaluation of ACD.

### Treatment

If the anemia is mild, specific treatment of ACD may not be required. Correction of the underlying inflammatory disease is the most important intervention. Vitamin and nutrient deficiencies should be corrected if identified. There is no role for the empiric use of iron supplementation if there is no evidence of concomitant iron-deficiency anemia. If transfusion is not urgently required, symptomatic anemia may be treated with recombinant human erythropoietin, beginning at a dosage of 100 to 150 U/kg given subcutaneously three times per week, with subsequent adjustment based on response (770–772). Erythropoietin is not effective if iron stores are deficient (773). Responses to erythropoietin may require several weeks (771).

**Pernicious Anemia**

Autoantibody-mediated destruction of gastric parietal cells, which is usually accompanied by histopathologically demonstrable lymphocytic and plasma cell infiltrates and the production of antibodies to intrinsic factor (IF), results in achlorhydria and loss of IF production (774–776). Pernicious anemia (PA) is the megaloblastic anemia resulting from cobalamin deficiency caused by the loss of gastric acid and defective IF secretion by atrophic gastric epithelium (777). Some reports suggest associations between gastritis resulting from *Helicobacter pylori* infection and the development of PA (777,778). Other complications of cobalamin deficiency include various peripheral and central neuropathic disorders (777). The body's extensive capacity for reutilization and storage of cobalamin explains the delayed onset of anemia and neuropathic disorders (779). There is a well-documented, albeit infrequent, association of PA with other autoimmune diseases, especially thyroiditis (780).

*Clinical Presentation*

Patients with cobalamin deficiency may present with complaints related to either or both anemia or neuropathies. The neuropathic syndromes of cobalamin deficiency are outside the scope of this chapter, and the reader is referred to authoritative textbooks of neurology for that information. Cobalamin deficiency results in a megaloblastic anemia (*vide infra*). Folate deficiency may also result in megaloblastic anemia, but in contrast to cobalamin deficiency, this is more likely to occur rapidly in malnourished patients. In MDS, hematopoietic cells may have megaloblastic features in the absence of cobalamin or folate deficiency (781). Most patients with PA are elderly; the peak age of diagnosis is 60 years of age or older (777). A significant number of cases, however, occur at both a younger age and in the nonwhite population. Although concurrent coronary artery disease is common in older patients, the slow decline of blood oxygen-carrying capacity in PA allows for cardiopulmonary compensation. Thus, symptoms may be minimal until the anemia becomes severe.

*Diagnostic Tests*

The complete blood count shows anemia, often severe. Megaloblastic anemias are characterized by macrocytic RBCs, which in the absence of concomitant iron deficiency, can result in extreme elevation of the MCV (sometimes to values more than 110 fL) (782). On the peripheral smear, hyperlobulated granulocytes (more than five lobes) may be identified and are pathognomonic of megaloblastic anemias.

Serum LDH may be elevated as a result of the hemolysis inherent in "ineffective erythropoiesis."

Testing for anti-IF antibodies has a strong positive predictive value in diagnosis of PA. The presence of anti-IF antibodies is diagnostic of PA. However, the sensitivity is in the order of 50% to 70%, and hence false negatives may occur (783–785).

In the evaluation of macrocytic anemias, serum cobalamin and RBC folate levels should be measured. Tissue cobalamin deficiency results in elevated levels of serum methylmalonic acid (MMA) and homocysteine (786–788). Hence, patients who have a low serum cobalamin level and elevated MMA but who have tested negative for anti-IF antibodies need to be further evaluated with a multistage Schilling's test to isolate the defective step in cobalamin absorption (789). In addition to atrophic gastritis with loss of IF, impaired cobalamin absorption may arise most commonly from cobalamin maldigestion. Less frequently, myriad other abnormalities (e.g., abnormal ileal receptors, defective transcobalamins, R-protein deficiency, tapeworm infestation, and so forth) may be responsible and require additional sophisticated testing (777).

A bone marrow examination is rarely necessary for evaluation of megaloblastic anemia, as in the case of significant hematologic disease with neurologic manifestations. The marrow morphology is cellular, with large erythroblasts having bizarre immature-appearing nuclei and dyssynchrony between nuclear and cytoplasmic maturation (megaloblasts). The cellular morphology may rarely be abnormal enough to be confused with acute erythroleukemia.

*Treatment*

Cobalamin deficiency is readily corrected by parenteral injection of vitamin $B_{12}$. A transient hypokalemia with cardiovascular complications resulting from rapid cellular proliferation on replacement of cobalamin has been described but is rarely experienced (790). RBC transfusion should be necessary only in cases of severe anemia with cardiopulmonary compromise or cerebral dysfunction and should be administered slowly to avoid congestive heart failure.

## HUMAN IMMUNODEFICIENCY VIRUS–RELATED AUTOIMMUNE SYNDROMES AND HEMATOLOGIC DISORDERS

Infection with HIV may result in any of several secondary hematologic disorders (791). Lymphopenia results directly from cytopathic effects of the virus (792–794). The most common and important secondary hematologic complications are related to direct suppression of hematopoiesis by infection of hematopoietic cells or supporting tissue; autoimmune marrow suppression or destruction of maturing blood cells; or inhibition of hematopoiesis by antiretroviral drugs (795–811). Azidothymidine and other nucleoside analogs often cause a macrocytic anemia (812). Antiinfective drugs, especially ganciclovir and trimethoprim–sulfamethoxazole (co-trimoxazole), are frequent causes of cytopenias (813–816). Marrow infiltration by HIV-related malignancies (e.g., lymphoma) and infection by opportunistic organisms (e.g., mycobacteria) can cause marrow suppression (808,817–825). The anemia of chronic inflammation, which is discussed separately, is also an important hematologic complication of HIV infection. Immunodeficiency may predispose to prolonged severe PRCA related to parvovirus B19 infection. In any individual patient, several mechanisms may be operating simultaneously.

HIV can infect essentially all of the significant component cells of the marrow stroma, including the macrophages, endothelial cells, and fibroblasts as well as megakaryocytes and multilineage progenitor cells (796,801,826–832). By direct and indirect mechanisms, including lymphocytic infiltration of marrow with CD8$^+$ (suppressor) cells, HIV infection of stromal cells can result in both the production of hematopoietic inhibitory substances (e.g., proinflammatory cytokines, such as TNF-α, IFN-γ, and transforming growth factor-β) and a decrease in production of stimulatory factors (e.g., granulocyte-macrophage colony-stimulating factor) (796, 833–835).

Peripheral destruction of mature blood cells by autoantibodies is one of the major causes of cytopenic complications in HIV infection. AITP may occur in 30% or more of HIV-infected patients (836,837). AITP is independent of hematopoietic suppression, although inhibition of megakaryocytopoiesis handicaps the marrow's ability to compensate for peripheral destruction. Immune hemolysis is unusual despite the high frequency of positive DATs in HIV-infected patients (535,838–840). Likewise, although antineutrophil antibodies can often be identified, neutropenia associated with HIV infection usually results from drug-induced or virus-induced myelopoietic suppression (841–843). APAs (particularly the lupus anticoagulant) occur with high frequency and are occasionally responsible for thrombotic events (844–847).

### Diagnostic Approach

In general, the various hematologic manifestations of HIV disease are similar in cause to their respective counterparts when not associated with HIV; therefore, the differential diagnostic considerations are similar to those in the respective syndromes discussed elsewhere in this chapter.

A careful inventory of the patient's medications may uncover a previously unsuspected pharmacologic cause for marrow suppression. On physical examination, palpable splenic enlargement, as may abe encountered in lymphoma or chronic infectious processes, may point toward hypersplenism as a cause of cytopenias. In addition, splenomegaly and lymphadenopathy should suggest the possibility of systemic lymphoma involving the marrow. Examination of the peripheral blood smear is important because it can hold clues to the etiology of cytopenias. For example, spherocyte RBC

forms suggest reticuloendothelial hemolysis (e.g., immune hemolysis), whereas schistocytes indicate microvascular RBC trauma (i.e., DIC or TTP). The neutrophils have dysplastic features, reflecting the frequent dysplastic bone marrow changes of HIV infection. On coagulation tests, the lupus anticoagulant may prolong the aPTT, which is not corrected by a one-to-one mix with normal plasma. Bone marrow abnormalities are not specific for HIV infection; an aspirate and biopsy should be performed if a secondary complication, such as lymphoma or opportunistic infection, is suspected. Hypercellularity with dysplastic morphology of one or more lineages is the most common marrow abnormality. Marrow involvement by fungal or mycobacterial organisms may be reflected by granulomas or fibrosis and warrants microbiologic investigation, such as special fungal and acid-fast bacillus stains and cultures. Lymphoid aggregates are common and nonspecific.

### Treatment

For the most part, recommended treatments for secondary hematologic complications of HIV are founded on experience with treatment of the respective syndromes unassociated with HIV, as discussed elsewhere in this chapter. Anemia of chronic inflammation is best managed by correction of underlying inflammatory or infectious diseases, if possible. Anemia and thrombocytopenia may remit if HIV replication is successfully suppressed by antiretroviral chemotherapy. PRCA resulting from parvovirus infection may respond to infusions of IVIG (848). If anemia is persistent, severe (i.e., hematocrit less than 25% to 30%) and symptomatic, a trial of erythropoietin may be warranted to lessen fatigue and reduce transfusion requirements (849,850). Patients with circulating erythropoietin levels of less than 500 mIU/mL are most likely to respond. Iron deficiency, which restrains the effect of erythropoietin on RBC production, should be corrected first. AITP may respond to a short course of therapy with corticosteroids. Responses of immune thrombocytopenia to infusions of IVIG or anti-D antibody may be impressive but are usually short-lived (851–853). Splenectomy is a less attractive option but may provide long-term responses of platelet counts and should be considered in patients with high CD4 counts (854). Cytotoxic drugs or other immunosuppressive agents may further inhibit host defenses. Granulocytopenia is usually a result of myelosuppressive drugs or progressive marrow suppression related to HIV infection rather than a treatable autoimmune process (855). Judicious treatment of patients with moderate to severe granulocytopenia with filgrastim may reduce neutropenic complications (849,856).

## HEMATOPOIETIC STEM CELL TRANSPLANTATION FOR AUTOIMMUNE DISEASES

The pathogenesis of autoimmunity involves the aberrant activation of T lymphocytes by self antigens, probably amplified by epitope spreading. Chronic autoimmune diseases refractory to first-line treatments can often be managed effectively with cytotoxic drugs. The effectiveness of cytotoxic drugs in autoimmune diseases is believed to be related to their lympholytic action. Theoretically, extensive depletion of lymphocytes could interrupt the cycle of autoimmunization and amplification. Unfortunately, intensive immunosuppression with cytotoxic drugs is accompanied by severe myelosuppression and the attendant risks related to blood cytopenias. Myelosuppression can be reliably overcome by support with hematopoietic progenitor or stem cells from the bone marrow or the PBSCs, which are capable of reconstituting marrow function. The clinical development of hematopoietic growth factors has enabled safe and convenient methods for mobilizing and harvesting PBSCs (857–859).

Immune reconstitution after transplantation may result in "reeducation" of T lymphocytes with tolerance to the previously immunogenic autoantigens (860–862). Depletion of T lymphocytes from the grafts (e.g., by immunomagnetic enrichment of myeloid stem cells) should reduce the probability of reinfusion of autoreactive immunocytes (863). Further, allotransplantation would be expected to install a new immune milieu partially or entirely (864,865). These theoretical principles have not been confirmed experimentally.

Many anecdotal accounts and cases have been reported of hematopoietic cell transplantation for patients with primary and secondary autoimmune diseases. Initial reports described resolution of coincidental autoimmune disorders in patients undergoing allogeneic and autologous transplantation for primary hematopoietic neoplasms (866–869). [In support of the theories of lymphocyte-mediation of autoimmunity, sporadic descriptions of inadvertent transmission of an autoimmune disorder from donor to recipient by allogeneic transplantation can also be found (870,871).] Systematic trials of allogeneic and autologous transplantation for refractory severe autoimmune diseases have been proposed, and a few are being executed (872).

The largest collective experience has been in patients with severe SLE, systemic sclerosis, rheumatoid arthritis, and multiple sclerosis (873,874). Euler et al. (875) described five patients with various autoimmune diagnoses who experienced early recurrence or persistence of their diseases after autologous transplantation with unmanipulated stem cell grafts. Subsequently, Burt et al. (876) reported an extensive series of autologous transplantations using CD34+ cell-enriched grafts in patients with various progressive autoimmune diseases. All patients obtained stabilization or improvement of their diseases. Among several reports of autologous hematopoietic stem cell transplantation for severe AITP with or without autoimmune hemolytic anemia, the responses have not been consistently correlated with lymphocyte depletion of the grafts (490,877,878). Overriding those considerations, however, has been the important observation that hematopoietic engraftment is efficient, and there have been minimal regimen-related toxicities in these patients. The demonstrated feasibility and safety of this approach to treatment of severe autoimmune disease should lead to larger trials and more extensive study of variations on the methods.

## REFERENCES

1. Bagby GC, Selleri C. Growth factors and the control of hematopoiesis. In: Hoffman R, Benz EJ Jr, Shattil SJ, et al., eds. *Hematology: basic principles and practice,* 2nd ed. New York: Churchill Livingstone, 1995;207–242.
2. Pathria MN, Issacs P. Magnetic resonance imaging of bone marrow. *Curr Opin Radiol* 1992;4:21–31.
3. Depaoli L, Davini O, Foggetti MD, et al. Evaluation of bone marrow cellularity by magnetic resonance imaging in patients with myelodysplastic syndrome. *Eur J Haematol* 1992;49:105–107.
4. Negendank W, Soulen RL. Magnetic resonance imaging in patients with bone marrow disorders. *Leuk Lymphoma* 1993;10:287–298.
5. Rozman M, Mercader JM, Aguilar JL, et al. Estimation of bone marrow cellularity by means of vertebral magnetic resonance. *Haematologica* 1997;82:166–170.
6. Takagi S, Tanaka O. The role of magnetic resonance imaging in the diagnosis and monitoring of myelodysplastic syndromes or leukemia. *Leuk Lymphoma* 1996;23:443–450.
7. Szklo M, Sensenbrenner L, Markowitz J, et al. Incidence of aplastic anemia in metropolitan Baltimore: a population-based study. *Blood* 1985;66:115–119.
8. Gordon-Smith EC, Issaragrisil S. Epidemiology of aplastic anaemia. *Baillieres Clin Haematol* 1992;5:475–491.
9. Yang C, Zhang X. Incidence survey of aplastic anemia in China. *Chin Med Sci J* 1991;6:203–207.
10. Mary JY, Baumelou E, Guiguet M. Epidemiology of aplastic anemia in France: a prospective multicentric study. The French Cooperative Group for Epidemiological Study of Aplastic Anemia. *Blood* 1990;75: 1646–1653.
11. Rawson NS, Harding SR, Malcolm E, et al. Hospitalizations for aplastic anemia and agranulocytosis in Saskatchewan: incidence and associations with antecedent prescription drug use. *J Clin Epidemiol* 1998;51:1343–1355.
12. Clausen N, Kreuger A, Salmi T, et al. Severe aplastic anaemia in the Nordic countries: a population based study of incidence, presentation, course, and outcome. *Arch Dis Child* 1996;74:319–322.
13. Kelly JP, Jurgelon JM, Issaragrisil S, et al. An epidemiological study of aplastic anaemia: relationship of drug exposures to clinical features and outcome. *Eur J Haematol Suppl* 1996;60:47–52.
14. Young NS. Pathogenesis and pathophysiology of aplastic anemia. In: Hoffman R, Benz EJ Jr, Shattil SJ, et al., eds. *Hematology: basic principles and practice,* 2nd ed. New York: Churchill Livingstone, 1995: 299–336.
15. Paquette RL, Kuramoto K, Tran L, et al. Hepatitis C virus infection in acquired aplastic anemia. *Am J Hematol* 1998;58:122–126.
16. Pardi DS, Romero Y, Mertz LE, et al. Hepatitis-associated aplastic anemia and acute parvovirus B19 infection: a report of two cases and a review of the literature. *Am J Gastroenterol* 1998;93:468–470.
17. Brown KE, Wong S, Young NS. Prevalence of GBV-C/HGV, a novel 'hepatitis' virus, in patients with aplastic anaemia. *Br J Haematol* 1997;97:492–496.
18. Rafel M, Cobo F, Cervantes F, et al. Transient pancytopenia after non-A non-B non-C acute hepatitis preceding acute lymphoblastic leukemia. *Haematologica* 1998;83:564–566.
19. Brown KE, Tisdale J, Barrett AJ, et al. Hepatitis-associated aplastic anemia [see Comments]. *N Engl J Med* 1997;336:1059–1064.
20. Kurtzman G, Young N. Viruses and bone marrow failure. *Baillieres Clin Haematol* 1989;2:51–67.
21. Issaragrisil S, Chansung K, Kaufman DW, et al. Aplastic anemia in rural Thailand: its association with grain farming and agricultural pesticide exposure. Aplastic Anemia Study Group. *Am J Public Health* 1997;87:1551–1554.
22. Issaragrisil S, Kaufman D, Thongput A, et al. Association of seropositivity for hepatitis viruses and aplastic anemia in Thailand [see Comments]. *Hepatology* 1997;25:1255–1257.
23. Risks of agranulocytosis and aplastic anemia: a first report of their relation to drug use with special reference to analgesics. The International Agranulocytosis and Aplastic Anemia Study. *JAMA* 1986;256: 1749–1757.

24. Kumana CR, Li KY, Chau PY. Worldwide variation in chloramphenicol utilization: should it cause concern? *J Clin Pharmacol* 1988;28: 1071–1075.

25. Yunis AA. Chloramphenicol-induced bone marrow suppression. *Semin Hematol* 1973;10:225–234.

26. Nagao T, Mauer AM. Concordance for drug-induced aplastic anemia in identical twins. *N Engl J Med* 1969;281:7–11.

27. Melenhorst JJ, van Krieken JH, Dreef E, et al. T cells selectively infiltrate bone marrow areas with residual haemopoiesis of patients with acquired aplastic anaemia. *Br J Haematol* 1997;99:517–519.

28. Nissen C, Cornu P, Gratwohl A, et al. Peripheral blood cells from patients wih aplastic anaemia in partial remission suppress growth of their own bone marrow precursors in culture. *Br J Haematol* 1980;45: 233–243.

29. Teramura M, Kobayashi S, Iwabe K, et al. Mechanism of action of antithymocyte globulin in the treatment of aplastic anaemia: in vitro evidence for the presence of immunosuppressive mechanism. *Br J Haematol* 1997;96:80–84.

30. Nakao S, Takamatsu H, Yachie A, et al. Establishment of a CD4+ T cell clone recognizing autologous hematopoietic progenitor cells from a patient with immune-mediated aplastic anemia. *Exp Hematol* 1995;23:433–438.

31. Liu H, Ding R, Jiang S, et al. Suppression of haematopoiesis by sera from patients with aplastic anemia. *Tokushima J Exp Med* 1996;43: 107–111.

32. Nistico A, Young NS. gamma-Interferon gene expression in the bone marrow of patients with aplastic anemia. *Ann Intern Med* 1994;120: 463–469.

33. Selleri C, Maciejewski JP, Sato T, et al. Interferon-gamma constitutively expressed in the stromal microenvironment of human marrow cultures mediates potent hematopoietic inhibition. *Blood* 1996;87: 4149–4157.

34. Tong J, Bacigalupo A, Piaggio G, et al. In vitro response of T cells from aplastic anemia patients to antilymphocyte globulin and phytohemagglutinin: colony-stimulating activity and lymphokine production. *Exp Hematol* 1991;19:312–316.

35. Hsu HC, Tsai WH, Chen LY, et al. Production of hematopoietic regulatory cytokines by peripheral blood mononuclear cells in patients with aplastic anemia. *Exp Hematol* 1996;24:31–36.

36. Hsu HC, Tsai WH, Chen LY, et al. Overproduction of inhibitory hematopoietic cytokines by lipopolysaccharide-activated peripheral blood mononuclear cells in patients with aplastic anemia. *Ann Hematol* 1995;71:281–286.

37. Schultz JC, Shahidi NT. Detection of tumor necrosis factor-alpha in bone marrow plasma and peripheral blood plasma from patients with aplastic anemia. *Am J Hematol* 1994;45:32–38.

38. Miura A, Endo K, Sugawara T, et al. T cell-mediated inhibition of erythropoiesis in aplastic anaemia: the possible role of IFN-gamma and TNF-alpha. *Br J Haematol* 1991;78:442–449.

39. Callera F, Garcia AB, Falcao RP. Fas-mediated apoptosis with normal expression of bcl-2 and p53 in lymphocytes from aplastic anaemia. *Br J Haematol* 1998;100:698–703.

40. Young NS. Immune pathophysiology of acquired aplastic anaemia. *Eur J Haematol Suppl* 1996;60:55–59.

41. Maciejewski JP, Selleri C, Sato T, et al. Increased expression of Fas antigen on bone marrow CD34+ cells of patients with aplastic anaemia. *Br J Haematol* 1995;91:245–252.

42. Margolis DA, Cammita BM. Hematopoietic stem cell transplantation for severe aplastic anemia. *Curr Opin Hematol* 1998;5:441–444.

43. Deeg HJ, Leisenring W, Storb R, et al. Long-term outcome after marrow transplantation for severe aplastic anemia. *Blood* 1998;91: 3637–3645.

44. Passweg JR, Socie G, Hinterberger W, et al. Bone marrow transplantation for severe aplastic anemia: has outcome improved? *Blood* 1997; 90:858–864.

45. Young NS, Barrett AJ. The treatment of severe acquired aplastic anemia. *Blood* 1995;85:3367–3377.

46. Cuthbert RJ, Shepherd JD, Nantel SH, et al. Allogeneic bone marrow transplantation for severe aplastic anemia: the Vancouver experience. *Clin Invest Med* 1995;18:122–130.

47. Paquette RL, Tebyani N, Frane M, et al. Long-term outcome of aplastic anemia in adults treated with antithymocyte globulin: comparison with bone marrow transplantation. *Blood* 1995;85:283–290.

48. Rosenfeld SJ, Kimball J, Vining D, et al. Intensive immunosuppression with antithymocyte globulin and cyclosporine as treatment for severe acquired aplastic anemia. *Blood* 1995;85:3058–3065.

49. Marsh J, Schrezenmeier H, Marin P, et al. Prospective randomized multicenter study comparing cyclosporin alone versus the combination of antithymocyte globulin and cyclosporin for treatment of patients with nonsevere aplastic anemia: a report from the European Blood and Marrow Transplant (EBMT) Severe Aplastic Anaemia Working Party. *Blood* 1999;93:2191–2195.

50. Marsh JC, Gordon-Smith EC. Treatment of aplastic anaemia with antilymphocyte globulin and cyclosporin. *Int J Hematol* 1995;62: 133–145.

51. Izumi T, Muroi K, Takatoku M, et al. Development of acute myeloblastic leukaemia in a case of aplastic anaemia treated with granulocyte colony-stimulating factor. *Br J Haematol* 1994;87:666–668.

52. Brodsky RA, Petri M, Smith BD, et al. Immunoablative high-dose cyclophosphamide without stem-cell rescue for refractory, severe autoimmune disease. *Ann Intern Med* 1998;129:1031–1035.

53. Brodsky RA. Biology and management of acquired severe aplastic anemia. *Curr Opin Oncol* 1998;10:95–99.

54. Brodsky R, Sensenbrenner LL, Jones RJ. Complete remission in severe aplastic anemia after high-dose cyclophosphamide without bone marrow transplantation. *Blood* 1996;87:491–494.

55. Selleri C, Catalano L, De Rosa G, et al. Danazol: in vitro effects on human hemopoiesis and in vivo activity in hypoplastic and myelodysplastic disorders. *Eur J Haematol* 1991;47:197–203.

56. Issaragrisil S, Visudhiphan S, Piankijagum A. Oxymetholone treatment in aplastic anemia. *J Med Assoc Thai* 1983;66:542–546.

57. Pizzuto J, Conte G, Sinco A, et al. Use of androgens in acquired aplastic anaemia: relation of response to aetiology and severity. *Acta Haematol* 1980;64:18–24.

58. Androgen therapy of aplastic anaemia: a prospective study of 352 cases. *Scand J Haematol* 1979;22:343–356.

59. Van Hengstum M, Steenbergen J, Haanen C. Clinical course in 28 unselected patients with aplastic anaemia treated with anabolic steroids. *Br J Haematol* 1979;41:323–333.

60. Welte K, Gabrilove J, Bronchud MH, et al. Filgrastim (r-metHuG-CSF): the first 10 years. *Blood* 1996;88:1907–1929.

61. Sonoda Y, Ohno Y, Fujii H, et al. Multilineage response in aplastic anemia patients following long-term administration of filgrastim (recombinant human granulocyte colony stimulating factor). *Stem Cells (Dayt)* 1993;11:543–554.

62. Moore KW, O'Garra A, de Waal Malefyt R, et al. Interleukin-10. *Annu Rev Immunol* 1993;11:165–190.

63. Huhn RD, Radwanski E, O'Connell SM, et al. Pharmacokinetics and immunomodulatory properties of intravenously administered recombinant human interleukin-10 in healthy volunteers. *Blood* 1996; 87:699–705.

64. Asano Y, Shibata S, Kobayashi S, et al. Effect of interleukin 10 on the hematopoietic progenitor cells from patients with aplastic anemia. *Stem Cells* 1999;17:147–151.

65. Heaney ML, Golde DW. Myelodysplasia. *N Engl J Med* 1999;340: 1649–1660.

66. Kouides PA, Bennett JM. Morphology and classification of myelodysplastic syndromes. *Hematol Oncol Clin North Am* 1992;6:485–499.

67. Varela BL, Chuang C, Woll JE, et al. Modifications in the classification of primary myelodysplastic syndromes: the addition of a scoring system. *Hematol Oncol* 1985;3:55–63.

68. Bennett JM, Catovsky D, Daniel MT, et al. Proposals for the classification of the myelodysplastic syndromes. *Br J Haematol* 1982;51: 189–199.

69. Greenberg P, Cox C, LeBeau MM, et al. International scoring system for evaluating prognosis in myelodysplastic syndromes [see Comments] [published erratum appears in *Blood* 1998;91:1100]. *Blood* 1997;89:2079–2088.

70. Toyama K, Ohyashiki K, Yoshida Y, et al. Clinical implications of chromosomal abnormalities in 401 patients with myelodysplastic syndromes: a multicentric study in Japan. *Leukemia* 1993;7:499–508.

71. Veldman T, Vignon C, Schrock E, et al. Hidden chromosome abnormalities in haematological malignancies detected by multicolour spectral karyotyping. *Nat Genet* 1997;15:406–410.

72. Hoglund M, Johansson B, Pedersen-Bjergaard J, et al. Molecular characterization of 12p abnormalities in hematologic malignancies: deletion of KIP1, rearrangement of TEL, and amplification of CCND2. *Blood* 1996;87:324–330.

73. Shimizu K, Ichikawa H, Tojo A, et al. An ets-related gene, ERG, is rearranged in human myeloid leukemia with t(16;21) chromosomal translocation. *Proc Natl Acad Sci U S A* 1993;90:10280–10284.
74. Srivastava A, Boswell HS, Heerema NA, et al. KRAS2 oncogene overexpression in myelodysplastic syndrome with translocation 5;12. *Cancer Genet Cytogenet* 1988;35:61–71.
75. Mise K, Abe S, Sato Y, et al. Localization of c-Ha-ras-1 oncogene in the t(7p-;11p+) abnormality of two cases with myeloid leukemia. *Cancer Genet Cytogenet* 1987;29:191–199.
76. Woloschak GE, Dewald GW, Bahn RS, et al. Amplification of RNA and DNA specific for erb B in unbalanced 1;7 chromosomal translocation associated with myelodysplastic syndrome. *J Cell Biochem* 1986;32:23–24.
77. Hamblin T. The treatment of acute myeloid leukaemia preceded by the myelodysplastic syndrome. *Leuk Res* 1992;16:101–108.
78. Bennett JM. Secondary acute myeloid leukemia [Editorial]. *Leuk Res* 1995;19:231–232.
79. Schiller G, Lee M, Paquette R, et al. Transplantation of autologous peripheral blood progenitor cells procured after high-dose cytarabine-based consolidation chemotherapy for adults with secondary acute myelogenous leukemia in first remission [In Process Citation]. *Leuk Lymphoma* 1999;33:475–485.
80. Anderson JE, Gooley TA, Schoch G, et al. Stem cell transplantation for secondary acute myeloid leukemia: evaluation of transplantation as initial therapy or following induction chemotherapy. *Blood* 1997;89: 2578–2585.
81. Gardin C, Chaibi P, de Revel T, et al. Intensive chemotherapy with idarubicin, cytosine arabinoside, and granulocyte colony-stimulating factor (G-CSF) in patients with secondary and therapy-related acute myelogenous leukemia. Club de Reflexion en Hematologie. *Leukemia* 1997;11:16–21.
82. de Witte T, Suciu S, Peetermans M, et al. Intensive chemotherapy for poor prognosis myelodysplasia (MDS) and secondary acute myeloid leukemia (sAML) following MDS of more than 6 months duration: a pilot study by the Leukemia Cooperative Group of the European Organisation for Research and Treatment in Cancer (EORTC-LCG). *Leukemia* 1995;9:1805–1811.
83. Enright H, Miller W. Autoimmune phenomena in patients with myelodysplastic syndromes. *Leuk Lymphoma* 1997;24:483–489.
84. Hamblin TJ. Immunological abnormalities in myelodysplastic syndromes. *Semin Hematol* 1996;33:150–162.
85. Enright H, Jacob HS, Vercellotti G, et al. Paraneoplastic autoimmune phenomena in patients with myelodysplastic syndromes: response to immunosuppressive therapy. *Br J Haematol* 1995;91:403–408.
86. Kuzmich PV, Ecker GA, Karsh J. Rheumatic manifestations in patients with myelodysplastic and myeloproliferative diseases [see Comments]. *J Rheumatol* 1994;21:1649–1654.
87. Jaeger U, Panzer S, Bartram C, et al. Autoimmune-thrombocytopenia and SLE in a patient with 5q-anomaly and deletion of the c-fms oncogene. *Am J Hematol* 1994;45:79–80.
88. Brooks PM. Rheumatic manifestations of neoplasia. *Curr Opin Rheumatol* 1992;4:90–93.
89. Pirayesh A, Verbunt RJ, Kluin PM, et al. Myelodysplastic syndrome with vasculitic manifestations. *J Intern Med* 1997;242:425–431.
90. Berthelot JM, Hamidou M, Dauty M, et al. Joint manifestations in myelodysplastic syndromes: a report of three cases presenting as polymyalgia rheumatica. *Rev Rhum Engl Ed* 1997;64:95–100.
91. Ohno E, Ohtsuka E, Watanabe K, et al. Behçet's disease associated with myelodysplastic syndromes: a case report and a review of the literature. *Cancer* 1997;79:262–268.
92. Hull DR, McMillan SA, Rea IM, et al. Antineutrophil cytoplasmic antibodies in myelodysplasia. *Ulster Med J* 1996;65:55–57.
93. Yano K, Eguchi K, Migita K, et al. Behçet's disease complicated with myelodysplastic syndrome: a report of two cases and review of the literature. *Clin Rheumatol* 1996;15:91–93.
94. Billstrom R, Johansson H, Johansson B, et al. Immune-mediated complications in patients with myelodysplastic syndromes: clinical and cytogenetic features. *Eur J Haematol* 1995;55:42–48.
95. Kohli M, Bennett RM. An association of polymyalgia rheumatica with myelodysplastic syndromes [see Comments]. *J Rheumatol* 1994;21: 1357–1359.
96. Ramakrishna R, Chaudhuri K, Sturgess A, et al. Haematological manifestations of primary Sjögren's syndrome: a clinicopathological study. *Q J Med* 1992;83:547–554.
97. Rosenthal NS, Farhi DC. Bone marrow findings in connective tissue disease. *Am J Clin Pathol* 1989;92:650–654.
98. Paolozzi FP, Goldberg J. Acute granulocytic leukemia following systemic lupus erythematosus. *Am J Med Sci* 1985;290:32–35.
99. Pereira RM, Velloso ER, Menezes Y, et al. Bone marrow findings in systemic lupus erythematosus patients with peripheral cytopenias. *Clin Rheumatol* 1998;17:219–222.
100. Yetgin S, Ozen S, Saatci U, et al. Myelodysplastic features in juvenile rheumatoid arthritis. *Am J Hematol* 1997;54:166–169.
101. Feng CS, Ng MH, Szeto RS, et al. Bone marrow findings in lupus patients with pancytopenia. *Pathology* 1991;23:5–7.
102. Jonasova A, Neuwirtova R, Cermak J, et al. Cyclosporin A therapy in hypoplastic MDS patients and certain refractory anaemias without hypoplastic bone marrow. *Br J Haematol* 1998;100:304–309.
103. Bucalossi A, Marotta G, Galieni P, et al. Successful treatment of a patient with refractory anemia by immunosuppressive therapy: another case of 'autoimmune myelodysplasia'? [Letter; see Comments]. *Acta Haematol* 1995;94:58.
104. Ferrara F, Copia C, Annunziata M, et al. Complete remission of refractory anemia following a single high dose of cyclophosphamide. *Ann Hematol* 1999;78:87–88.
105. Biesma DH, van den Tweel JG, Verdonck LF. Immunosuppressive therapy for hypoplastic myelodysplastic syndrome. *Cancer* 1997;79: 1548–1551.
106. Molldrem JJ, Caples M, Mavroudis D, et al. Antithymocyte globulin for patients with myelodysplastic syndrome. *Br J Haematol* 1997;99: 699–705.
107. Nand S, Godwin JE. Hypoplastic myelodysplastic syndrome. *Cancer* 1988;62:958–964.
108. Tuzuner N, Cox C, Rowe JM, et al. Hypocellular myelodysplastic syndromes (MDS): new proposals [see Comments]. *Br J Haematol* 1995; 91:612–617.
109. Fohlmeister I, Fischer R, Modder B, et al. Aplastic anaemia and the hypocellular myelodysplastic syndrome: histomorphological, diagnostic, and prognostic features. *J Clin Pathol* 1985;38:1218–1224.
110. Young NS. The problem of clonality in aplastic anemia: Dr Dameshek's riddle, restated. *Blood* 1992;79:1385–1392.
111. Burrows SR, Fernan A, Argaet V, et al. Bystander apoptosis induced by CD8+ cytotoxic T cell (CTL) clones: implications for CTL lytic mechanisms. *Int Immunol* 1993;5:1049–1058.
112. Heusel JW, Wesselschmidt RL, Shresta S, et al. Cytotoxic lymphocytes require granzyme B for the rapid induction of DNA fragmentation and apoptosis in allogeneic target cells. *Cell* 1994;76:977–987.
113. Ucker DS, Wilson JD, Hebshi LD. Target cell death triggered by cytotoxic T lymphocytes: a target cell mutant distinguishes passive pore formation and active cell suicide mechanisms. *Mol Cell Biol* 1994; 14:427–436.
114. Beresford PJ, Xia Z, Greenberg AH, et al. Granzyme A loading induces rapid cytolysis and a novel form of DNA damage independently of caspase activation. *Immunity* 1999;10:585–594.
115. Smyth MJ, Browne KA, Thia KY, et al. Hypothesis: cytotoxic lymphocyte granule serine proteases activate target cell endonucleases to trigger apoptosis. *Clin Exp Pharmacol Physiol* 1994;21:67–70.
116. Kawahara A, Enari M, Talanian RV, et al. Fas-induced DNA fragmentation and proteolysis of nuclear proteins. *Genes Cells* 1998;3: 297–306.
117. Narayanan MN, Geary CG, Freemont AJ, et al. Long-term follow-up of aplastic anaemia. *Br J Haematol* 1994;86:837–843.
118. Orazi A, Albitar M, Heerema NA, et al. Hypoplastic myelodysplastic syndromes can be distinguished from acquired aplastic anemia by CD34 and PCNA immunostaining of bone marrow biopsy specimens [see Comments]. *Am J Clin Pathol* 1997;107:268–274.
119. Negendank W, Weissman D, Bey TM, et al. Evidence for clonal disease by magnetic resonance imaging in patients with hypoplastic marrow disorders. *Blood* 1991;78:2872–2879.
120. de Planque MM, Kluin-Nelemans HC, van Krieken HJ, et al. Evolution of acquired severe aplastic anaemia to myelodysplasia and subsequent leukaemia in adults. *Br J Haematol* 1988;70:55–62.
121. Garcia-Suarez J, Pascual T, Munoz MA, et al. Myelodysplastic syndrome with erythroid hypoplasia/aplasia: a case report and review of the literature. *Am J Hematol* 1998;58:319–325.
122. Williamson PJ, Oscier DG, Bell AJ, et al. Red cell aplasia in myelodysplastic syndrome [see Comments]. *J Clin Pathol* 1991;44:431–432.

123. George JN, Woolf SH, Raskob GE, et al. Idiopathic thrombocytopenic purpura: a practice guideline developed by explicit methods for the American Society of Hematology [see Comments]. *Blood* 1996;88: 3–40.

124. May A, Fitzsimons E. Sideroblastic anaemia. *Baillieres Clin Haematol* 1994;7:851–879.

125. Brodsky RA, Hasegawa S, Fibach E, et al. Acquired sideroblastic anaemia following progesterone therapy. *Br J Haematol* 1994;87:859–862.

126. Rojer RA, Mulder NH, Nieweg HO. Response to pyridoxine hydrochloride in refractory anemia due to myelofibrosis. *Am J Med* 1978;65: 655–660.

127. Rosenberg SJ, Bennett JM. Pyridoxine-responsive anemia. *N Y State J Med* 1969;69:1430–1433.

128. Hoagland HC, Linman JW. Pyridoxine-responsive anemia: a preleukemic manifestation? *Minn Med* 1972;55:891–895.

129. Geschke W, Beutler E. Refractory sideroblastic and nonsideroblastic anemia: a review of 27 cases. *West J Med* 1977;127:85–92.

130. Harris JW. X-linked, pyridoxine-responsive sideroblastic anemia [Editorial; see Comments]. *N Engl J Med* 1994;330:709–711.

131. Murakami R, Takumi T, Gouji J, et al. Sideroblastic anemia showing unique response to pyridoxine. *Am J Pediatr Hematol Oncol* 1991;13: 345–350.

132. Kushner JP, Cartwright GE. Sideroblastic anemia. *Adv Intern Med* 1977;22:229-49:229–249.

133. Mason DY, Emerson PM. Primary acquired sideroblastic anaemia: response to treatment with pyridoxal-5-phosphate. *Br Med J* 1973;1: 389–390.

134. May A, Fitzsimons E. Sideroblastic anaemia. *Baillieres Clin Haematol* 1994;7:851–879.

135. Solomon LR, Hillman RS. Vitamin B6 metabolism in idiopathic sideroblastic anaemia and related disorders. *Br J Haematol* 1979;42: 239–253.

136. Ganser A, Hoelzer D. Treatment of myelodysplastic syndromes with hematopoietic growth factors. *Hematol Oncol Clin North Am* 1992;6: 633–653.

137. Gradishar WJ, Le Beau MM, O'Laughlin R, et al. Clinical and cytogenetic responses to granulocyte-macrophage colony-stimulating factor in therapy-related myelodysplasia. *Blood* 1992;80:2463–2470.

138. Estey EH, Kurzrock R, Talpaz M, et al. Effects of low doses of recombinant human granulocyte-macrophage colony stimulating factor (GM-CSF) in patients with myelodysplastic syndromes. *Br J Haematol* 1991;77:291–295.

139. Yoshida Y, Nakahata T, Shibata A, et al. Effects of long-term treatment with recombinant human granulocyte-macrophage colony-stimulating factor in patients with myelodysplastic syndrome. *Leuk Lymphoma* 1995;18:457–463.

140. Runde V, Aul C, Ebert A, et al. Sequential administration of recombinant human granulocyte-macrophage colony-stimulating factor and human erythropoietin for treatment of myelodysplastic syndromes. *Eur J Haematol* 1995;54:39–45.

141. Greenberg P, Negrin R, Nagler A, et al. Effects of prolonged treatment of myelodysplastic syndromes with recombinant human granulocyte colony-stimulating factor. *Int J Cell Cloning* 1990;8[Suppl 1]:293–300.

142. Nagler A, MacKichan ML, Negrin RS, et al. Effects of granulocyte colony-stimulating factor therapy on in vitro hemopoiesis in myelodysplastic syndromes. *Leukemia* 1995;9:30–39.

143. Willemze R, van der Lely N, Zwierzina H, et al. A randomized phase-I/II multicenter study of recombinant human granulocyte-macrophage colony-stimulating factor (GM-CSF) therapy for patients with myelodysplastic syndromes and a relatively low risk of acute leukemia. EORTC Leukemia Cooperative Group [published erratum appears in *Ann Hematol* 1992;64:312]. *Ann Hematol* 1992;64:173–180.

144. Yoshida Y, Hirashima K, Asano S, et al. A phase II trial of recombinant human granulocyte colony-stimulating factor in the myelodysplastic syndromes. *Br J Haematol* 1991;78:378–384.

145. Sastre JL, Ulibarrena C, Bustillo M, et al. Long-term disappearance of previous chromosomal abnormalities in myelodysplastic syndromes treated with low dose cytosine arabinoside and granulocyte/macrophage-colony stimulating factor [Letter]. *Haematologica* 1998;83:763–765.

146. Santini V, Ferrini PR. Differentiation therapy of myelodysplastic syndromes: fact or fiction? *Br J Haematol* 1998;102:1124–1138.

147. Cheson BD. Standard and low-dose chemotherapy for the treatment of myelodysplastic syndromes. *Leuk Res* 1998;22[Suppl 1]:S17–S21.

148. Nair R, Nair CN, Advani SH. All trans retinoic acid with low dose cytosine arabinoside in the treatment of myelodysplastic syndrome. *LeukLymphoma* 1998;29:187–192.

149. Ganser A, Karthaus M. Clinical use of hematopoietic growth factors in the myelodysplastic syndromes. *Leuk Lymphoma* 1997;26[Suppl 1]: 13–27.

150. Jack FR, Summerfield GP. Long term remission of acute myeloid leukaemia with trilineage myelodysplasia treated solely with low dose cytarabine. *Clin Lab Haematol* 1994;16:197–200.

151. Hellstrom-Lindberg E, Robert KH, Gahrton G, et al. Low-dose ara-C in myelodysplastic syndromes (MDS) and acute leukemia following MDS: proposal for a predictive model. *Leuk Lymphoma* 1994;12: 343–351.

152. Miller KB, Kim K, Morrison FS, et al. The evaluation of low-dose cytarabine in the treatment of myelodysplastic syndromes: a phase-III intergroup study [published erratum appears in *Ann Hematol* 1993;66:164]. *Ann Hematol* 1992;65:162–168.

153. Munshi NC, Tricot GJ. Single weekly cytosine arabinoside and oral 6-thioguanine in patients with myelodysplastic syndrome and acute myeloid leukemia. *Ann Hematol* 1997;74:111–115.

154. Spitzer TR, Lazarus HM, Crum ED, et al. Treatment of myelodysplastic syndromes with low-dose oral 6-thioguanine. *Med Pediatr Oncol* 1988;16:17–20.

155. Doll DC, Kasper LM, Taetle R, et al. Treatment with low-dose oral etoposide in patients with myelodysplastic syndromes. *Leuk Res* 1998;22:7–12.

156. Ogata K, Nomura T. Application of low-dose etoposide therapy for myelodysplastic syndromes. *Leuk Lymphoma* 1993;12:35–39.

157. Ogata K, Yamada T, Ito T, et al. Low-dose etoposide: a potential therapy for myelodysplastic syndromes. *Br J Haematol* 1992;82:354–357.

158. Hofmann WK, Ganser A, Seipelt G, et al. Treatment of patients with low-risk myelodysplastic syndromes using a combination of all-trans retinoic acid, interferon alpha, and granulocyte colony-stimulating factor. *Ann Hematol* 1999;78:125–130.

159. Ferrero D, Bruno B, Pregno P, et al. Combined differentiating therapy for myelodysplastic syndromes: a phase II study. *Leuk Res* 1996;20: 867–876.

160. Letendre L, Levitt R, Pierre RV, et al. Myelodysplastic syndrome treatment with danazol and cis-retinoic acid. *Am J Hematol* 1995;48: 233–236.

161. Ohno R. Differentiation therapy of myelodysplastic syndromes with retinoic acid. *Leuk Lymphoma* 1994;14:401–409.

162. Aul C, Runde V, Gattermann N. All-trans retinoic acid in patients with myelodysplastic syndromes: results of a pilot study. *Blood* 1993;82: 2967–2974.

163. Kurzrock R, Estey E, Talpaz M. All-trans retinoic acid: tolerance and biologic effects in myelodysplastic syndrome. *J Clin Oncol* 1993;11: 1489–1495.

164. Hellstrom E, Robert KH, Samuelsson J, et al. Treatment of myelodysplastic syndromes with retinoic acid and 1 alpha-hydroxy-vitamin D3 in combination with low-dose ara-C is not superior to ara-C alone: results from a randomized study. The Scandinavian Myelodysplasia Group (SMG). *Eur J Haematol* 1990;45:255–261.

165. Hast R, Axdorph S, Lauren L, et al. Absent clinical effects of retinoic acid and isoretinoin treatment in the myelodysplastic syndrome. *Hematol Oncol* 1989;7:297–301.

166. Mellibovsky L, Diez A, Perez-Vila E, et al. Vitamin D treatment in myelodysplastic syndromes. *Br J Haematol* 1998;100:516–520.

167. Motomura S, Fujisawa S, Tsunooka S, et al. Hematologic benefits of 1-hydroxyvitamin D3 in an elderly patient with chronic myelodysplastic syndrome [Letter]. *Am J Hematol* 1996;53:143–144.

168. Morosetti R, Koeffler HP. Differentiation therapy in myelodysplastic syndromes. *Semin Hematol* 1996;33:236–245.

169. Paquette RL, Koeffler HP. Differentiation therapy. *Hematol Oncol Clin North Am* 1992;6:687–706.

170. De Rosa L, Montuoro A, De Laurenzi A. Therapy of 'high risk' myelodysplastic syndromes with an association of low-dose Ara-C, retinoic acid and 1,25-dihydroxyvitamin D3. *Biomed Pharmacother* 1992;46:211–217.

171. Blazsek I, Musset M, Boule D, et al. Combined differentiation therapy in myelodysplastic syndrome with retinoid acid, 1 alpha,25 dihydroxy-vitamin D3, and prednisone. *Cancer Detect Prev* 1992;16:259–264.

172. Nand S, Stock W, Stiff P, et al. A phase II trial of interleukin-2 in myelodysplastic syndromes. *Br J Haematol* 1998;101:205–207.

173. Ogata K, Tamura H, Yokose N, et al. Effects of interleukin-12 on natural killer cell cytotoxicity and the production of interferon-gamma and tumour necrosis factor-alpha in patients with myelodysplastic syndromes. *Br J Haematol* 1995;90:15–21.

174. De Rosa G, Pezzullo L, Selleri C, et al. Low-dose interleukin-2 for treating postautologous transplant cytogenetic abnormality recurrency in a case of acute myeloid leukemia with hyperdiploidy [Letter]. *Blood* 1998;92:4484–4485.

175. de Witte T, Van Biezen A, Hermans J, et al. Autologous bone marrow transplantation for patients with myelodysplastic syndrome (MDS) or acute myeloid leukemia following MDS. Chronic and Acute Leukemia Working Parties of the European Group for Blood and Marrow Transplantation. *Blood* 1997;90:3853–3857.

176. Laporte JP, Isnard F, Lesage S, et al. Autologous bone marrow transplantation with marrow purged by mafosfamide in seven patients with myelodysplastic syndromes in transformation (AML-MDS): a pilot study. *Leukemia* 1993;7:2030–2033.

177. Ruutu T, Hanninen A, Jarventie G, et al. Intensive chemotherapy of poor prognosis myelodysplastic syndromes (MDS) and acute myeloid leukemia following MDS with idarubicin and cytarabine. *Leuk Res* 1997;21:133–138.

178. Hasle H, Arico M, Basso G, et al. Myelodysplastic syndrome, juvenile myelomonocytic leukemia, and acute myeloid leukemia associated with complete or partial monosomy 7. European Working Group on MDS in Childhood (EWOG-MDS). *Leukemia* 1999;13:376–385.

179. Gordon BG, Warkentin PI, Strandjord SE, et al. Allogeneic bone marrow transplantation for children with acute leukemia: long-term follow-up of patients prepared with high-dose cytosine arabinoside and fractionated total body irradiation. *Bone Marrow Transplant* 1997;20:5–10.

180. Fenaux P, Preudhomme C, Hebbar M. The role of intensive chemotherapy in myelodysplastic syndromes. *Leuk Lymphoma* 1992;8:43–49.

181. Demuynck H, Verhoef GE, Zachee P, et al. Treatment of patients with myelodysplastic syndromes with allogeneic bone marrow transplantation from genotypically HLA-identical sibling and alternative donors. *Bone Marrow Transplant* 1996;17:745–751.

182. Anderson JE, Appelbaum FR, Storb R. An update on allogeneic marrow transplantation for myelodysplastic syndrome. *Leuk Lymphoma* 1995;17:95–99.

183. Stewart FM, Zhong S, Wuu J, et al. Lymphohematopoietic engraftment in minimally myeloablated hosts. *Blood* 1998;91:3681–3687.

184. Khouri IF, Keating M, Korbling M, et al. Transplant-lite: induction of graft-versus-malignancy using fludarabine-based nonablative chemotherapy and allogeneic blood progenitor-cell transplantation as treatment for lymphoid malignancies. *J Clin Oncol* 1998;16:2817–2824.

185. Giralt S, Estey E, Albitar M, et al. Engraftment of allogeneic hematopoietic progenitor cells with purine analog-containing chemotherapy: harnessing graft-versus-leukemia without myeloablative therapy. *Blood* 1997;89:4531–4536.

186. Grigg A, Bardy P, Byron K, et al. Fludarabine-based non-myeloablative chemotherapy followed by infusion of HLA-identical stem cells for relapsed leukaemia and lymphoma [In Process Citation]. *Bone Marrow Transplant* 1999;23:107–110.

187. Slavin S, Nagler A, Naparstek E, et al. Nonmyeloablative stem cell transplantation and cell therapy as an alternative to conventional bone marrow transplantation with lethal cytoreduction for the treatment of malignant and nonmalignant hematologic diseases. *Blood* 1998;91:756–763.

188. Rosse WF. Paroxysmal nocturnal hemoglobinuria. In: Hoffman R, Benz EJ Jr, Shattil SJ, et al., eds. *Hematology: basic principles and practice,* 2nd ed. New York: Churchill Livingstone, 1995:370–381.

189. Dunn DE, Ware RE, Parker CJ, et al. Research directions in paroxysmal nocturnal hemoglobinuria. *Immunol Today* 1999;20[Suppl 4]:168–171.

190. Packman CH. Pathogenesis and management of paroxysmal nocturnal haemoglobinuria. *Blood Rev* 1998;12:1–11.

191. Luzzatto L, Bessler M. The dual pathogenesis of paroxysmal nocturnal hemoglobinuria. *Curr Opin Hematol* 1996;3:101–110.

192. Sun X, Funk CD, Deng C, et al. Role of decay-accelerating factor in regulating complement activation on the erythrocyte surface as revealed by gene targeting. *Proc Natl Acad Sci U S A* 1999;96:628–633.

193. Wilcox LA, Ezzell JL, Bernshaw NJ, et al. Molecular basis of the enhanced susceptibility of the erythrocytes of paroxysmal nocturnal hemoglobinuria to hemolysis in acidified serum. *Blood* 1991;78:820–829.

194. Rosse WF. The control of complement activation by the blood cells in paroxysmal nocturnal hemoglobinuria. *Blood* 1986;67:268–269.

195. Parker CJ, Wiedmer T, Sims PJ, et al. Characterization of the complement sensitivity of paroxysmal nocturnal hemoglobinuria erythrocytes. *J Clin Invest* 1985;75:2074–2084.

196. Hansch G, Hammer C, Jiji R, et al. Lysis of paroxysmal nocturnal hemoglobinuria erythrocytes by acid-activated serum. *Immunobiology* 1983;164:118–126.

197. Devetten MP, Liu JM, Ling V, et al. Paroxysmal nocturnal hemoglobinuria: new insights from murine Pig-a-deficient hematopoiesis. *Proc Assoc Am Physicians* 1997;109:99–110.

198. Dunn DE, Yu J, Nagarajan S, et al. A knock-out model of paroxysmal nocturnal hemoglobinuria: Pig-a(-) hematopoiesis is reconstituted following intercellular transfer of GPI-anchored proteins. *Proc Natl Acad Sci U S A* 1996;93:7938–7943.

199. Rotoli B, Boccuni P. The PIG-A gene somatic mutation responsible for paroxysmal nocturnal hemoglobinuria. *Haematologica* 1995;80:539–545.

200. Sloand EM, Maciejewski JP, Dunn D, et al. Correction of the PNH defect by GPI-anchored protein transfer. *Blood* 1998;92:4439–4445.

201. Araten DJ, Nafa K, Pakdeesuwan K, et al. Clonal populations of hematopoietic cells with paroxysmal nocturnal hemoglobinuria genotype and phenotype are present in normal individuals. *Proc Natl Acad Sci U S A* 1999;96:5209–5214.

202. Nagarajan S, Brodsky RA, Young NS, et al. Genetic defects underlying paroxysmal nocturnal hemoglobinuria that arises out of aplastic anemia. *Blood* 1995;86:4656–4661.

203. Griscelli-Bennaceur A, Gluckman E, Scrobohaci ML, et al. Aplastic anemia and paroxysmal nocturnal hemoglobinuria: search for a pathogenetic link. *Blood* 1995;85:1354–1363.

204. Schrezenmeier H, Hertenstein B, Wagner B, et al. A pathogenetic link between aplastic anemia and paroxysmal nocturnal hemoglobinuria is suggested by a high frequency of aplastic anemia patients with a deficiency of phosphatidylinositol glycan anchored proteins [published erratum appears in *Exp Hematol* 1995;23:181]. *Exp Hematol* 1995;23:81–87.

205. Tichelli A, Gratwohl A, Nissen C, et al. Late clonal complications in severe aplastic anemia. *Leuk Lymphoma* 1994;12:167–175

206. Nakao S, Yamaguchi M, Takamatsu H, et al. Expansion of a paroxysmal nocturnal hemoglobinuria (PNH) clone after cyclosporine therapy for aplastic anemia/PNH syndrome [Letter; see Comments]. *Blood* 1992;80:2943–2944.

207. Moore JG, Humphries RK, Frank MM, et al. Characterization of the hematopoietic defect in paroxysmal nocturnal hemoglobinuria. *Exp Hematol* 1986;14:222–229.

208. Backx B, Broeders L, Touw I, et al. Blast colony-forming cells in myelodysplastic syndrome: decreased potential to generate erythroid precursors. *Leukemia* 1993;7:75–79.

209. Maciejewski JP, Sloand EM, Sato T, et al. Impaired hematopoiesis in paroxysmal nocturnal hemoglobinuria/aplastic anemia is not associated with a selective proliferative defect in the glycosylphosphatidylinositol-anchored protein-deficient clone. *Blood* 1997;89:1173–1181.

210. Hillmen P, Lewis SM, Bessler M, et al. Natural history of paroxysmal nocturnal hemoglobinuria. *N Engl J Med* 1995;333:1253–1258.

211. Tichelli A, Gratwohl A, Wursch A, et al. Late haematological complications in severe aplastic anaemia. *Br J Haematol* 1988;69:413–418.

212. Ware RE, Nishimura J, Moody MA, et al. The PIG-A mutation and absence of glycosylphosphatidylinositol-linked proteins do not confer resistance to apoptosis in paroxysmal nocturnal hemoglobinuria. *Blood* 1998;92:2541–2550.

213. Brodsky RA, Vala MS, Barber JP, et al. Resistance to apoptosis caused by PIG-A gene mutations in paroxysmal nocturnal hemoglobinuria. *Proc Natl Acad Sci U S A* 1997;94:8756–8760.

214. Bessler M, Mason P, Hillmen P, et al. Somatic mutations and cellular selection in paroxysmal nocturnal haemoglobinuria. *Lancet* 1994;343:951–953.

215. Tomizuka H, Hatake K, Kitagawa S, et al. Portal vein thrombosis in paroxysmal nocturnal haemoglobinuria. *Acta Haematol* 1999;101:149–152.

216. Barker JE, Wandersee NJ. Thrombosis in heritable hemolytic disorders. *Curr Opin Hematol* 1999;6:71–75.

217. Ganguli SC, Ramzan NN, McKusick MA, et al. Budd-Chiari syndrome in patients with hematological disease: a therapeutic challenge. *Hepatology* 1998;27:1157–1161.

218. Graham ML, Rosse WF, Halperin EC, et al. Resolution of Budd-Chiari syndrome following bone marrow transplantation for paroxysmal nocturnal haemoglobinuria. *Br J Haematol* 1996;92:707–710.

219. Alfaro A. Cerebral venous thrombosis in paroxysmal nocturnal haemoglobinuria [Letter]. *J Neurol Neurosurg Psychiatry* 1992;55:412.

220. Arora A, Sharma MP, Buch P, et al. Paroxysmal nocturnal hemoglobinuria with hepatic vein thrombosis presenting as hepatic encephalopathy. *Indian J Gastroenterol* 1990;9:91–92.

221. Klein KL, Hartmann RC. Acute coronary artery thrombosis in paroxysmal nocturnal hemoglobinuria. *South Med J* 1989;82:1169–1171.

222. Valla D, Dhumeaux D, Babany G, et al. Hepatic vein thrombosis in paroxysmal nocturnal hemoglobinuria: a spectrum from asymptomatic occlusion of hepatic venules to fatal Budd-Chiari syndrome. *Gastroenterology* 1987;93:569–575.

223. Hartmann RC, Jenkins DE Jr, Arnold AB. Diagnostic specificity of sucrose hemolysis test for paroxysmal nocturnal hemoglobinuria. *Blood* 1970;35:462–475.

224. Rosse WF. Dr Ham's test revisited [Editorial]. *Blood* 1991;78:547–550.

225. Iwamoto N, Kawaguchi T, Takatsuki K, et al. Positivity of the sugar-water test in the screening for paroxysmal nocturnal hemoglobinuria [Letter]. *Blood* 1994;84:1349.

226. Sirchia G, Marubini E, Mercuriali F, et al. Study of two in vitro diagnostic tests for paroxysmal nocturnal haemoglobinuria. *Br J Haematol* 1973;24:751–759.

227. Jankovic S, Kraguljac N, Basara N, et al. Paroxysmal nocturnal hemoglobinuria: golden standards vs. modern technologies [Letter]. *Am J Hematol* 1995;50:66–67.

228. Schubert J, Alvarado M, Uciechowski P, et al. Diagnosis of paroxysmal nocturnal haemoglobinuria using immunophenotyping of peripheral blood cells. *Br J Haematol* 1991;79:487–492.

229. Vu T, Griscelli-Bennaceur A, Gluckman E, et al. Aplastic anaemia and paroxysmal nocturnal haemoglobinuria: a study of the GPI-anchored proteins on human platelets. *Br J Haematol* 1996;93:586–589.

230. Schubert J, Vogt HG, Zielinska-Skowronek M, et al. Development of the glycosylphosphatitylinositol-anchoring defect characteristic for paroxysmal nocturnal hemoglobinuria in patients with aplastic anemia. *Blood* 1994;83:2323–2328.

231. Bessler M, Fehr J. Fc III receptors (FcRIII) on granulocytes: a specific and sensitive diagnostic test for paroxysmal nocturnal hemoglobinuria (PNH). *Eur J Haematol* 1991;47:179–184.

232. Issaragrisil S, Piankijagum A, Tang-naitrisorana Y. Corticosteroids therapy in paroxysmal nocturnal hemoglobinuria. *Am J Hematol* 1987;25:77–83.

233. Rosse WF. Treatment of paroxysmal nocturnal hemoglobinuria. *Blood* 1982;60:20–23.

234. Dessypris EN, Clark DA, McKee LC Jr, et al. Increased sensitivity to complement or erythroid and myeloid progenitors in paroxysmal nocturnal hemoglobinuria. *N Engl J Med* 1983;309:690–693.

235. Brecher ME, Taswell HF. Paroxysmal nocturnal hemoglobinuria and the transfusion of washed red cells: a myth revisited. *Transfusion* 1989;29:681–685.

236. McMullin MF, Hillmen P, Jackson J, et al. Tissue plasminogen activator for hepatic vein thrombosis in paroxysmal nocturnal haemoglobinuria. *J Intern Med* 1994;235:85–89.

237. Kwan T, Hansard P. Recombinant tissue-plasminogen activator for acute Budd-Chiari syndrome secondary to paroxysmal nocturnal hemoglobinuria. *N Y State J Med* 1992;92:109–110.

238. Sholar PW, Bell WR. Thrombolytic therapy for inferior vena cava thrombosis in paroxysmal nocturnal hemoglobinuria. *Ann Intern Med* 1985;103:539–541.

239. Paquette RL, Yoshimura R, Veiseh C, et al. Clinical characteristics predict response to antithymocyte globulin in paroxysmal nocturnal haemoglobinuria. *Br J Haematol* 1997;96:92–97.

240. Doney K, Pepe M, Storb R, et al. Immunosuppressive therapy of aplastic anemia: results of a prospective, randomized trial of antithymocyte globulin (ATG), methylprednisolone, and oxymetholone to ATG, very high-dose methylprednisolone, and oxymetholone. *Blood* 1992;79:2566–2571.

241. Kusminsky GD, Barazzutti L, Korin JD, et al. Complete response to antilymphocyte globulin in a case of aplastic anemia-paroxysmal nocturnal hemoglobinuria syndrome [Letter]. *Am J Hematol* 1988;29:123.

242. Bemba M, Guardiola P, Garderet L, et al. Bone marrow transplantation for paroxysmal nocturnal haemoglobinuria. *Br J Haematol* 1999;105:366–368.

243. Saso R, Marsh J, Cevreska L, et al. Bone marrow transplants for paroxysmal nocturnal haemoglobinuria. *Br J Haematol* 1999;104:392–396.

244. Johnson RJ, Rawstron AC, Richards S, et al. Circulating primitive stem cells in paroxysmal nocturnal hemoglobinuria (PNH) are predominantly normal in phenotype but granulocyte colony-stimulating factor treatment mobilizes mainly PNH stem cells. *Blood* 1998;91:4504–4508.

245. Sykes M, Preffer F, McAfee S, et al. Mixed lymphohaemopoietic chimerism and graft-versus-lymphoma effects after non-myeloablative therapy and HLA-mismatched bone-marrow transplantation [see Comments]. *Lancet* 1999;353:1755–1759.

246. Aker M, Varadi G, Slavin S, et al. Fludarabine-based protocol for human umbilical cord blood transplantation in children with Fanconi anemia [see Comments]. *J Pediatr Hematol Oncol* 1999;21:237–239.

247. Denning-Kendall PA, Horsley H, Nicol A, et al. Clinical application of in vitro expansion of cord blood. *Bone Marrow Transplant* 1998;22[Suppl 1]:S63–65.

248. Nishimura J, Smith CA, Phillips KL, et al. Paroxysmal nocturnal hemoglobinuria: molecular pathogenesis and molecular therapeutic approaches. *Hematopathol Mol Hematol* 1998;11:119–146.

249. Takeda J, Miyata T, Kawagoe K, et al. Deficiency of the GPI anchor caused by a somatic mutation of the PIG-A gene in paroxysmal nocturnal hemoglobinuria. *Cell* 1993;73:703–711.

250. Erslev AJ, Soltan A. Pure red-cell aplasia: a review. *Blood Rev* 1996;10:20–28.

251. Brown KE, Young NS. Parvovirus B19 in human disease. *Annu Rev Med* 1997;48:59–67.

252. Charles RJ, Sabo KM, Kidd PG, et al. The pathophysiology of pure red cell aplasia: implications for therapy. *Blood* 1996;87:4831–4838.

253. Hanada T, Abe T, Nakamura H, et al. Pure red cell aplasia: relationship between inhibitory activity of T cells to CFU-E and erythropoiesis. *Br J Haematol* 1984;58:107–113.

254. Partanen S, Ruutu T, Vuopio P, et al. Acquired pure red-cell aplasia: a consequence of increased natural killer cell activity? *Leuk Res* 1984;8:117–122.

255. Abkowitz JL, Kadin ME, Powell JS, et al. Pure red cell aplasia: lymphocyte inhibition of erythropoiesis. *Br J Haematol* 1986;63:59–67.

256. Sivakumaran M. Th1/Th2 lymphocyte subsets in pure red cell aplasia [Letter]. *Br J Haematol* 1999;105:569–570.

257. Nezu M, Kawano E, Ishii H, et al. Pure red-cell aplasia requiring cytotoxic chemotherapy: presence of clonal T-lymphocytes without characteristics of chronic lymphocytic leukemia [Letter]. *Am J Hematol* 1996;53:145–147.

258. Sivakumaran M, Bhavnani M, Stewart A, et al. Is pure red cell aplasia (PRCA) a clonal disorder? *Clin Lab Haematol* 1993;15:1–5.

259. Morikawa K, Oseko F, Hara J, et al. Induction of non-MHC-restricted cytotoxicity in a patient with pure red cell aplasia: functional relevance to antigen-specific cytotoxic T cells. *Hematol Pathol* 1991;5:125–138.

260. Nagasawa M, Okawa H, Yata J. A B cell line from a patient with pure red cell aplasia produces an immunoglobulin that suppresses erythropoiesis. *Clin Immunol Immunopathol* 1991;61:18–28.

261. Mangan KF, Besa EC, Shadduck RK, et al. Demonstration of two distinct antibodies in autoimmune hemolytic anemia with reticulocytopenia and red cell aplasia. *Exp Hematol* 1984;12:788–793.

262. Nidorf D, Saleem A. Immunosuppressive mechanisms in pure red cell aplasia: a review. *Ann Clin Lab Sci* 1990;20:214–219.

263. Morgenthaler TI, Brown LR, Colby TV, et al. Thymoma. *Mayo Clin Proc* 1993;68:1110–1123.

264. Yoo D, Pierce LE, Lessin LS. Acquired pure red cell aplasia associated with chronic lymphocytic leukemia. *Cancer* 1983;51:844–850.

265. Gotic M, Basara N, Rolovic Z, et al. Successful treatment of refractory pure red cell aplasia secondary to chronic lymphocytic leukaemia with cyclosporine A: correlation between clinical and in vitro effects. *Nouv Rev Fr Hematol* 1994;36:307–309.

266. Diehl LF, Ketchum LH. Autoimmune disease and chronic lymphocytic leukemia: autoimmune hemolytic anemia, pure red cell aplasia, and autoimmune thrombocytopenia. *Semin Oncol* 1998;25:80–97.

267. Thompson DF, Gales MA. Drug-induced pure red cell aplasia. *Pharmacotherapy* 1996;16:1002–1008.
268. Pritsch O, Maloum K, Dighiero G. Basic biology of autoimmune phenomena in chronic lymphocytic leukemia. *Semin Oncol* 1998;25:34–41.
269. Chikkappa G, Pasquale D, Zarrabi MH, et al. Cyclosporine and prednisone therapy for pure red cell aplasia in patients with chronic lymphocytic leukemia [see Comments]. *Am J Hematol* 1992;41:5–12.
270. Linardaki GD, Boki KA, Fertakis A, et al. Pure red cell aplasia as presentation of systemic lupus erythematosus: antibodies to erythropoietin. *Scand J Rheumatol* 1999;28:189–191.
271. Kiely PD, McGuckin CP, Collins DA, et al. Erythrocyte aplasia and systemic lupus erythematosus. *Lupus* 1995;4:407–411.
272. Loughran TP Jr, Starkebaum G. Large granular lymphocyte leukemia: report of 38 cases and review of the literature. *Medicine (Baltimore)* 1987;66:397–405.
273. Lacy MQ, Kurtin PJ, Tefferi A. Pure red cell aplasia: association with large granular lymphocyte leukemia and the prognostic value of cytogenetic abnormalities [see Comments]. *Blood* 1996;87:3000–3006.
274. Garcia Vela JA, Perez V, Monteserin MC, et al. Pure red cell aplasia associated with large granular lymphocytic leukemia: a rare association in Western countries [Letter]. *Haematologica* 1998;83:664–665.
275. Ergas D, Resnitzky P, Berrebi A. Pure red blood cell aplasia associated with parvovirus B19 infection in large granular lymphocyte leukemia [Letter]. *Blood* 1996;87:3523–3524.
276. Tohda S, Nara N, Tanikawa S, et al. Pure red cell aplasia following autoimmune haemolytic anaemia: cell-mediated suppression of erythropoiesis as a possible pathogenesis of pure red cell aplasia. *Acta Haematol* 1992;87:98–102.
277. Estrov Z, Berrebi A, Kusminsky G, et al. Circulating mononuclear cells from pure red cell aplasia of chronic lymphocytic leukemia suppress in vitro erythropoiesis. *Acta Haematol* 1989;81:213–216.
278. Mangan KF, Chikkappa G, Farley PC. T gamma (T gamma) cells suppress growth of erythroid colony-forming units in vitro in the pure red cell aplasia of B-cell chronic lymphocytic leukemia. *J Clin Invest* 1982;70:1148–1156.
279. Akard LP, Brandt J, Lu L, et al. Chronic T cell lymphoproliferative disorder and pure red cell aplasia: further characterization of cell-mediated inhibition of erythropoiesis and clinical response to cytotoxic chemotherapy. *Am J Med* 1987;83:1069–1074.
280. Alter R, Joshi SS, Verdirame JD, et al. Pure red cell aplasia associated with B cell lymphoma: demonstration of bone marrow colony inhibition by serum immunoglobulin. *Leuk Res* 1990;14:279–286.
281. Koduri PR. Novel cytomorphology of the giant proerythroblasts of parvovirus B19 infection. *Am J Hematol* 1998;58:95–99.
282. Raghavachar A. Pure red cell aplasia: review of treatment and proposal for a treatment strategy. *Blut* 1990;61:47–51.
283. Kwong YL, Wong KF, Liang RH, et al. Pure red cell aplasia: clinical features and treatment results in 16 cases. *Ann Hematol* 1996;72:137–140.
284. Uchiyama M, Ichikawa Y, Komatsuda M, et al. Acquired chronic pure red cell aplasia successfully treated with intravenous pulse methylprednisolone therapy. *Intern Med* 1992;31:1277–1280.
285. Chowdhury KL, Jalali RK, Abrol A, et al. "Steroid responsive pure red cell aplasia." *Indian J Med Sci* 1990;44:333–336.
286. Ozsoylu S. High-dose intravenous methylprednisolone for pure red cell aplasia [Letter; see Comments]. *Am J Hematol* 1990;34:236–237.
287. Needleman SW. Durable remission of pure red cell aplasia after treatment with high-dose intravenous gammaglobulin and prednisone [see Comments]. *Am J Hematol* 1989;32:150–152.
288. Firkin FC, Maher D. Cytotoxic immunosuppressive drug treatment strategy in pure red cell aplasia. *Eur J Haematol* 1988;41:212–217.
289. Vilan J, Rhyner K, Ganzoni AM. Pure red cell aplasia: successful treatment with cyclophosphamide. *Blut* 1973;26:27–34.
290. Jacobs P, Wood L. Pure red cell aplasia: antilymphocyte globulin-mediated remission [Letter]. *S Afr Med J* 1993;83:538.
291. Jacobs P, Wood L. Pure red cell aplasia: stable complete remission following antilymphocyte globulin administration. *Eur J Haematol* 1988;40:371–374.
292. Abkowitz JL, Powell JS, Nakamura JM, et al. Pure red cell aplasia: response to therapy with anti-thymocyte globulin. *Am J Hematol* 1986;23:363–371.
293. Leonard EM, Raefsky E, Griffith P, et al. Cyclosporine therapy of aplastic anaemia, congenital and acquired red cell aplasia [see Comments]. *Br J Haematol* 1989;72:278–284.
294. Coutinho J, Lima M, dos Anjos Teixeira M, et al. Pure red cell aplasia associated to clonal CD8+ T-cell large granular lymphocytosis: dependence on cyclosporin A therapy. *Acta Haematol* 1998;100:207–210.
295. McGuire WA, Yang HH, Bruno E, et al. Treatment of antibody-mediated pure red-cell aplasia with high-dose intravenous gamma globulin. *N Engl J Med* 1987;317:1004–1008.
296. Alter BP. Arms and the man or hands and the child: congenital anomalies and hematologic syndromes. *J Pediatr Hematol Oncol* 1997;19:287–291.
297. D'Andrea AD, Grompe M. Molecular biology of Fanconi anemia: implications for diagnosis and therapy. *Blood* 1997;90:1725–1736.
298. Auerbach AD, Allen RG. Leukemia and preleukemia in Fanconi anemia patients: a review of the literature and report of the International Fanconi Anemia Registry. *Cancer Genet Cytogenet* 1991;51:1–12.
299. Auerbach AD. Fanconi anemia diagnosis and the diepoxybutane (DEB) test [Editorial]. *Exp Hematol* 1993;21:731–733.
300. Seyschab H, Friedl R, Sun Y, et al. Comparative evaluation of diepoxybutane sensitivity and cell cycle blockage in the diagnosis of Fanconi anemia. Blood 1995;85:2233–2237.
301. Cervenka J, Arthur D, Yasis C. Mitomycin C test for diagnostic differentiation of idiopathic aplastic anemia and Fanconi anemia. *Pediatrics* 1981;67:119–127.
302. Kuffel DG, Lindor NM, Litzow MR, et al. Mitomycin C chromosome stress test to identify hypersensitivity to bifunctional alkylating agents in patients with Fanconi anemia or aplastic anemia. *Mayo Clin Proc* 1997;72:579–580.
303. German J, Schonberg S, Caskie S, et al. A test for Fanconi's anemia. *Blood* 1987;69:1637–1641.
304. Gluckman E, Auerbach AD, Horowitz MM, et al. Bone marrow transplantation for Fanconi anemia. *Blood* 1995;86:2856–2862.
305. Flowers ME, Zanis J, Pasquini R, et al. Marrow transplantation for Fanconi anaemia: conditioning with reduced doses of cyclophosphamide without radiation [see Comments]. *Br J Haematol* 1996;92:699–706.
306. Willig TN, Ball SE, Tchernia G. Current concepts and issues in Diamond-Blackfan anemia. *Curr Opin Hematol* 1998;5:109–115.
307. Krijanovski OI, Sieff CA. Diamond-Blackfan anemia. *Hematol Oncol Clin North Am* 1997;11:1061–1077.
308. Halperin DS, Freedman MH. Diamond-blackfan anemia: etiology, pathophysiology, and treatment. *Am J Pediatr Hematol Oncol* 1989;11:380–394.
309. Freedman MH. Erythropoiesis in Diamond-Blackfan anemia and the role of interleukin 3 and steel factor. *Stem Cells (Dayt)* 1993;11[Suppl 2]:98–104.
310. Gillio AP, Faulkner LB, Alter BP, et al. Treatment of Diamond-Blackfan anemia with recombinant human interleukin-3 [see Comments]. *Blood* 1993;82:744–751.
311. Ball SE, Tchernia G, Wranne L, et al. Is there a role for interleukin-3 in Diamond-Blackfan anaemia? Results of a European multicentre study. *Br J Haematol* 1995;91:313–318.
312. Bastion Y, Bordigoni P, Debre M, et al. Sustained response after recombinant interleukin-3 in Diamond Blackfan anemia [Letter; see Comments]. *Blood* 1994;83:617–618.
313. Auerbach AD. Umbilical cord blood transplants for genetic disease: diagnostic and ethical issues in fetal studies. *Blood Cells* 1994;20:303–309.
314. Vettenranta K, Saarinen UM. Cord blood stem cell transplantation for Diamond-Blackfan anemia. *Bone Marrow Transplant* 1997;19:507–508.
315. Loughran TP. Large granular lymphocytic leukemia: an overview. *Hosp Pract (Off Ed)* 1998;33:133–138.
316. Loughran TP Jr, Kadin ME. Large granular lymphocyte leukemia. In: Beutler E, Shattil SJ, Coller BS, et al., eds. *Williams hematology,* 5th ed. New York: McGraw-Hill, 1995:1047–1049.
317. Loughran TP Jr. Clonal diseases of large granular lymphocytes. *Blood* 1993;82:1–14.
318. Starkebaum G, Loughran TP Jr, Gaur LK, et al. Immunogenetic similarities between patients with Felty's syndrome and those with clonal expansions of large granular lymphocytes in rheumatoid arthritis. *Arthritis Rheum* 1997;40:624–626.
319. Gentile TC, Loughran TP Jr. Resolution of autoimmune hemolytic anemia following splenectomy in CD3+ large granular lymphocyte leukemia. *Leuk Lymphoma* 1996;23:405–408.

320. Dhodapkar MV, Li CY, Lust JA, et al. Clinical spectrum of clonal proliferations of T-large granular lymphocytes: a T-cell clonopathy of undetermined significance? *Blood* 1994;84:1620–1627.

321. Gentile TC, Wener MH, Starkebaum G, et al. Humoral immune abnormalities in T-cell large granular lymphocyte leukemia. *Leuk Lymphoma* 1996;23:365–370.

322. Lamy T, Liu JH, Landowski TH, et al. Dysregulation of CD95/CD95 ligand-apoptotic pathway in CD3(+) large granular lymphocyte leukemia. *Blood* 1998;92:4771–4777.

323. Zambello R, Loughran TP Jr, Trentin L, et al. Serologic and molecular evidence for a possible pathogenetic role of viral infection in CD3-negative natural killer-type lymphoproliferative disease of granular lymphocytes. *Leukemia* 1995;9:1207–1211.

324. Perzova R, Loughran TP Jr. Constitutive expression of Fas ligand in large granular lymphocyte leukaemia. *Br J Haematol* 1997;97:123–126.

325. Loughran TP Jr, Hadlock KG, Yang Q, et al. Seroreactivity to an envelope protein of human T-cell leukemia/lymphoma virus in patients with CD3-(natural killer) lymphoproliferative disease of granular lymphocytes. *Blood* 1997;90:1977–1981.

326. Loughran TP Jr, Hadlock KG, Perzova R, et al. Epitope mapping of HTLV envelope seroreactivity in LGL leukaemia. *Br J Haematol* 1998;101:318–324.

327. Singer GG, Carrera AC, Marshak-Rothstein A, et al. Apoptosis, Fas and systemic autoimmunity: the MRL-lpr/lpr model. *Curr Opin Immunol* 1994;6:913–920.

328. Kingreen D, Siegert W. Chronic lymphatic leukemias of T and NK cell type. *Leukemia* 1997;11[Suppl 2]:S46–S49.

329. Kroft SH, Finn WG, Peterson LC. The pathology of the chronic lymphoid leukaemias. *Blood Rev* 1995;9:234–250.

330. Bassan R, Pronesti M, Buzzetti M, et al. Autoimmunity and B-cell dysfunction in chronic proliferative disorders of large granular lymphocytes/natural killer cells. *Cancer* 1989;63:90–95.

331. Sivakumaran M, Richards S. Immunological abnormalities of chronic large granular lymphocytosis. *Clin Lab Haematol* 1997;19:57–60.

332. Loughran TP Jr, Starkebaum G, Kidd P, et al. Clonal proliferation of large granular lymphocytes in rheumatoid arthritis. *Arthritis Rheum* 1988;31:31–36.

333. Kuipers JG, Jacobs R, Kemper A, et al. TCR1+ large granular lymphocyte proliferation in rheumatoid arthritis. *Rheumatol Int* 1994;14:163–168.

334. Bowman SJ, Sivakumaran M, Snowden N, et al. The large granular lymphocyte syndrome with rheumatoid arthritis: immunogenetic evidence for a broader definition of Felty's syndrome. *Arthritis Rheum* 1994;37:1326–1330.

335. Bowman SJ, Bhavnani M, Geddes GC, et al. Large granular lymphocyte expansions in patients with Felty's syndrome: analysis using anti-T cell receptor V beta-specific monoclonal antibodies. *Clin Exp Immunol* 1995;101:18–24.

336. Waase I, Kayser C, Carlson PJ, et al. Oligoclonal T cell proliferation in patients with rheumatoid arthritis and their unaffected siblings. *Arthritis Rheum* 1996;39:904–913.

337. Saway PA, Prasthofer EF, Barton JC. Prevalence of granular lymphocyte proliferation in patients with rheumatoid arthritis and neutropenia. *Am J Med* 1989;86:303–307.

338. Stanworth SJ, Green L, Pumphrey RS, et al. An unusual association of Felty syndrome and TCR gamma delta lymphocytosis. *J Clin Pathol* 1996;49:351–353.

339. Chan WC, Gu LB, Masih A, et al. Large granular lymphocyte proliferation with the natural killer-cell phenotype. *Am J Clin Pathol* 1992;97:353–358.

340. Gentile TC, Uner AH, Hutchison RE, et al. CD3+, CD56+ aggressive variant of large granular lymphocyte leukemia [see Comments]. *Blood* 1994;84:2315–2321.

341. Loughran TP Jr, Kidd PG, Starkebaum G. Treatment of large granular lymphocyte leukemia with oral low-dose methotrexate. *Blood* 1994;84:2164–2170.

342. Yamada O, Mizoguchi H, Oshimi K. Cyclophosphamide therapy for pure red cell aplasia associated with granular lymphocyte-proliferative disorders. *Br J Haematol* 1997;97:392–399.

343. Dhodapkar MV, Lust JA, Phyliky RL. T-cell large granular lymphocytic leukemia and pure red cell aplasia in a patient with type I autoimmune polyendocrinopathy: response to immunosuppressive therapy. *Mayo Clin Proc* 1994;69:1085–1088.

344. Sood R, Stewart CC, Aplan PD, et al. Neutropenia associated with T-cell large granular lymphocyte leukemia: long-term response to cyclosporine therapy despite persistence of abnormal cells. *Blood* 1998;91:3372–3378.

345. Bargetzi MJ, Wortelboer M, Pabst T, et al. Severe neutropenia in T-large granular lymphocyte leukemia corrected by intensive immunosuppression. *Ann Hematol* 1996;73:149–151.

346. Yamada O, Yun-Hua W, Motoji T, et al. Clonal T-cell proliferation causing pure red cell aplasia in chronic B-cell lymphocytic leukaemia: successful treatment with cyclosporine following in vitro abrogation of erythroid colony-suppressing activity. *Br J Haematol* 1998;101:335–337.

347. Weide R, Heymanns J, Koppler H, et al. Successful treatment of neutropenia in T-LGL leukemia (T gamma-lymphocytosis) with granulocyte colony-stimulating factor. *Ann Hematol* 1994;69:117–119.

348. Dale DC, Hammond WP 4th. Cyclic neutropenia: a clinical review. *Blood Rev* 1988;2:178–185.

349. Welte K, Dale D. Pathophysiology and treatment of severe chronic neutropenia. *Ann Hematol* 1996;72:158–165.

350. Dale DC. Immune and idiopathic neutropenia. *Curr Opin Hematol* 1998;5:33–36.

351. Palmer SE, Stephens K, Dale DC. Genetics, phenotype, and natural history of autosomal dominant cyclic hematopoiesis. *Am J Med Genet* 1996;66:413–422.

352. Souid AK. Congenital cyclic neutropenia. *Clin Pediatr (Phila)* 1995;34:151–155.

353. Schmitz S, Franke H, Wichmann HE, et al. The effect of continuous G-CSF application in human cyclic neutropenia: a model analysis. *Br J Haematol* 1995;90:41–47.

354. Dale DC. Hematopoietic growth factors for the treatment of severe chronic neutropenia. *Stem Cells (Dayt)* 1995;13:94–100.

355. Schmitz S, Franke H, Loeffler M, et al. Model analysis of the contrasting effects of GM-CSF and G-CSF treatment on peripheral blood neutrophils observed in three patients with childhood-onset cyclic neutropenia. *Br J Haematol* 1996;95:616–625.

356. Loughran TP Jr, Clark EA, Price TH, et al. Adult-onset cyclic neutropenia is associated with increased large granular lymphocytes. *Blood* 1986;68:1082–1087.

357. Loughran TP Jr, Hammond WP 4th. Adult-onset cyclic neutropenia is a benign neoplasm associated with clonal proliferation of large granular lymphocytes. *J Exp Med* 1986;164:2089–2094.

358. Bartlett NL, Longo DL. T-small lymphocyte disorders. *Semin Hematol* 1999;36:164–170.

359. Fata F, Myers P, Addeo J, et al. Cyclic neutropenia in Crohn's ileocolitis: efficacy of granulocyte colony-stimulating factor. *J Clin Gastroenterol* 1997;24:253–256.

360. Lamport RD, Katz S, Eskreis D. Crohn's disease associated with cyclic neutropenia. *Am J Gastroenterol* 1992;87:1638–1642.

361. Stevens C, Peppercorn MA, Grand RJ. Crohn's disease associated with autoimmune neutropenia. *J Clin Gastroenterol* 1991;13:328–330.

362. Couper R, Kapelushnik J, Griffiths AM. Neutrophil dysfunction in glycogen storage disease Ib: association with Crohn's-like colitis. *Gastroenterology* 1991;100:549–554.

363. Storek J, Glaspy JA, Grody WW, et al. Adult-onset cyclic neutropenia responsive to cyclosporine therapy in a patient with ankylosing spondylitis. *Am J Hematol* 1993;43:139–143.

364. Lassoued S, Roubinet F, Hamidou M, et al. Large granular lymphocytes and neutropenia in a patient with ankylosing spondylitis [Letter]. *Arthritis Rheum* 1989;32:355.

365. Parikh PM. Cyclic neutropenia in common variable immunodeficiency [Letter; see Comments]. *Indian Pediatr* 1994;31:1295–1297.

366. Agarwal BR, Currimbhoy Z. Resolution of cyclic neutropenia by intramuscular gamma globulin in a case of common variable immunodeficiency with predominantly antibody deficiency [see Comments]. *Indian Pediatr* 1994;31:320–322.

367. Tsuda M, Urakami T, Watanabe S, et al. Recombinant human granulocyte colony-stimulating factor therapy for cyclic neutropenia associated with common variable immunodeficiency. *Acta Paediatr Jpn* 1993;35:124–126.

368. Kyas U, Pietsch T, Welte K. Expression of receptors for granulocyte colony-stimulating factor on neutrophils from patients with severe congenital neutropenia and cyclic neutropenia. *Blood* 1992;79:1144–1147.

369. Cukrova V, Klamova H. Inhibitor of granulopoiesis in human cyclic neutropenia. *Folia Haematol Int Mag Klin Morphol Blutforsch* 1990; 117:647–652.

370. Smith JG, Seenan AK, Smith MA, et al. Cyclical neutropenia and T8 lymphocyte mediated stimulation of granulopoiesis. *Br J Haematol* 1985;60:481–489.

371. Ucci G, Danova M, Riccardi A, et al. Abnormalities of T cell subsets in a patient with cyclic neutropenia. *Acta Haematol* 1987;77:177–179.

372. Hara T, Ishii E, Ueda K, et al. Natural killer activity in human cyclic neutropenia [Letter]. *Br J Haematol* 1986;64:630–632.

373. Hearn T, Haurie C, Mackey MC. Cyclical neutropenia and the peripheral control of white blood cell production. *J Theor Biol* 1998;192: 167–181.

374. Haurie C, Dale DC, Mackey MC. Cyclical neutropenia and other periodic hematological disorders: a review of mechanisms and mathematical models. *Blood* 1998;92:2629–2640.

375. Lensink DB, Barton A, Appelbaum FR, et al. Cyclic neutropenia as a premalignant manifestation of acute lymphoblastic leukemia. *Am J Hematol* 1986;22:9–16.

376. Shepherd PC, Corbett GM, Allan NC. Neutropenia preceding acute lymphoblastic leukaemia [Letter]. *J Clin Pathol* 1988;41:703–704.

377. Platanias L, Raefsky E, Young N. Neutropenia associated with large granular lymphocytes responsive to corticosteroids in vitro and in vivo. *Eur J Haematol* 1987;38:89–94.

378. Garipidou V, Tsatalas C, Sinacos Z. Severe neutropenia in a patient with large granular lymphocytosis: prolonged successful control with cyclosporin A. *Haematologica* 1991;76:424–425.

379. Heussner P, Haase D, Kanz L, et al. G-CSF in the long-term treatment of cyclic neutropenia and chronic idiopathic neutropenia in adult patients. *Int J Hematol* 1995;62:225–234.

380. Walls J, Dessypris EN, Krantz SB. Case report: granulocyte colony-stimulating factor overcomes severe neutropenia of large granular lymphocytosis. *Am J Med Sci* 1992;304:363–365.

381. Fine KD, Byrd TD, Stone MJ. Successful treatment of chronic severe neutropenia with weekly recombinant granulocyte-colony stimulating factor. *Br J Haematol* 1997;97:175–178.

382. Hammond WP 4th, Price TH, Souza LM, et al. Treatment of cyclic neutropenia with granulocyte colony-stimulating factor. *N Engl J Med* 1989;320:1306–1311.

383. Cooper DL, Henderson-Bakas M, Berliner N. Lymphoproliferative disorder of granular lymphocytes associated with severe neutropenia: response to granulocyte colony-stimulating factor. *Cancer* 1993;72: 1607–1611.

384. Dale DC, Bonilla MA, Davis MW, et al. A randomized controlled phase III trial of recombinant human granulocyte colony-stimulating factor (filgrastim) for treatment of severe chronic neutropenia. *Blood* 1993;81:2496–2502.

385. Jakubowski A, Winton EF, Gencarelli A, et al. Treatment of chronic neutropenia associated with large granular lymphocytosis with cyclosporine A and filgrastim. *Am J Hematol* 1995;50:288–291.

386. Manoharan A, Williams NT, Sparrow R. Acquired amegakaryocytic thrombocytopenia: report of a case and review of literature. *Q J Med* 1989;70:243–252.

387. Hoffman R. Acquired pure amegakaryocytic thrombocytopenic purpura. *Semin Hematol* 1991;28:303–312.

388. King JA, Elkhalifa MY, Latour LF. Rapid progression of acquired amegakaryocytic thrombocytopenia to aplastic anemia. *South Med J* 1997;90:91–94.

389. Slater LM, Katz J, Walter B, et al. Aplastic anemia occurring as amegakaryocytic thrombocytopenia with and without an inhibitor of granulopoiesis. *Am J Hematol* 1985;18:251–254.

390. Geissler D, Thaler J, Konwalinka G, et al. Progressive preleukemia presenting amegakaryocytic thrombocytopenic purpura: association of the 5q- syndrome with a decreased megakaryocytic colony formation and a defective production of Meg-CSF. *Leuk Res* 1987;11:731–737.

391. Lugassy G. Non-Hodgkin's lymphoma presenting with amegakaryocytic thrombocytopenic purpura. *Ann Hematol* 1996;73:41–42.

392. Ghosh K, Sarode R, Varma N, et al. Amegakaryocytic thrombocytopenia of nutritional vitamin B12 deficiency. *Trop Geogr Med* 1988;40:158–160.

393. Levine RF, Spivak JL, Meagher RC, et al. Effect of ethanol on thrombopoiesis. *Br J Haematol* 1986;62:345–354.

394. Gewirtz AM, Hoffman R. Transitory hypomegakaryocytic thrombocytopenia: aetiological association with ethanol abuse and implications regarding regulation of human megakaryocytopoiesis. *Br J Haematol* 1986;62:333–344.

395. Nagasawa T, Hasegawa Y, Shimizu S, et al. Serum thrombopoietin level is mainly regulated by megakaryocyte mass rather than platelet mass in human subjects. *Br J Haematol* 1998;101:242–244.

396. Zent CS, Ratajczak J, Ratajczak MZ, et al. Relationship between megakaryocyte mass and serum thrombopoietin levels as revealed by a case of cyclic amegakaryocytic thrombocytopenic purpura. *Br J Haematol* 1999;105:452–458.

397. Mukai HY, Kojima H, Todokoro K, et al. Serum thrombopoietin (TPO) levels in patients with amegakaryocytic thrombocytopenia are much higher than those with immune thrombocytopenic purpura. *Thromb Haemost* 1996;76:675–678.

398. Koduri PR. Amegakaryocytic thrombocytopenia with a positive direct Coombs' test [see Comments]. *Am J Hematol* 1993;44:68–69.

399. Hoffman R, Briddell RA, van Besien K, et al. Acquired cyclic amegakaryocytic thrombocytopenia associated with an immunoglobulin blocking the action of granulocyte-macrophage colony-stimulating factor. *N Engl J Med* 1989;321:97–102.

400. Nagasawa T, Sakurai T, Kashiwagi H, et al. Cell-mediated amegakaryocytic thrombocytopenia associated with systemic lupus erythematosus. *Blood* 1986;67:479–483.

401. Sakurai T, Kono I, Kabashima T, et al. Amegakaryocytic thrombocytopenia associated with systemic lupus erythematosus successfully treated by a high-dose prednisolone therapy. *Jpn J Med* 1984;23: 135–138.

402. Griner PF, Hoyer LW. Amegakaryocytic thrombocytopenia in systemic lupus erythematosus. *Arch Intern Med* 1970;125:328–332.

403. Kouides PA, Rowe JM. Large granular lymphocyte leukemia presenting with both amegakaryocytic thrombocytopenic purpura and pure red cell aplasia: clinical course and response to immunosuppressive therapy. *Am J Hematol* 1995;49:232–236.

404. Rovira M, Feliu E, Florensa L, et al. Acquired amegakaryocytic thrombocytopenic purpura associated with immunoglobulin deficiency. *Acta Haematol* 1991;85:34–36.

405. Benedetti F, de Sabata D, Perona G. T suppressor activated lymphocytes (CD8+/DR+) inhibit megakaryocyte progenitor cell differentiation in a case of acquired amegakaryocytic thrombocytopenic purpura. *Stem Cells (Dayt)* 1994;12:205–213.

406. Gewirtz AM, Sacchetti MK, Bien R, et al. Cell-mediated suppression of megakaryocytopoiesis in acquired amegakaryocytic thrombocytopenic purpura. *Blood* 1986;68:619–626.

407. Katai M, Aizawa T, Ohara N, et al. Acquired amegakaryocytic thrombocytopenic purpura with humoral inhibitory factor for megakaryocyte colony formation. *Intern Med* 1994;33:147–149.

408. Corash L. The relationship between megakaryocyte ploidy and platelet volume. *Blood Cells* 1989;15:81–107.

409. Takubo T, Yamane T, Hino M, et al. Usefulness of determining reticulated and large platelets in idiopathic thrombocytopenic purpura. *Acta Haematol* 1998;99:109–110.

410. Illes I, Pfueller SL, Hussein S, et al. Platelets in idiopathic thrombocytopenic purpura are increased in size but are of normal density. *Br J Haematol* 1987;67:173–176.

411. Westerman DA, Grigg AP. The diagnosis of idiopathic thrombocytopenic purpura in adults: does bone marrow biopsy have a place? [see Comments]. *Med J Aust* 1999;170:216–217.

412. Canavan BF, Huhn RD, Kim HC, et al. Concurrent presentation of erythrocytic and megakaryocytic aplasia. *Am J Hematol* 1996;51:68–72.

413. Khelif A, Ffrench M, Follea G, et al. Amegakaryocytic thrombocytopenic purpura treated with antithymocyte globulin [Letter]. *Ann Intern Med* 1985;102:720.

414. Peng CT, Kao LY, Tsai CH. Successful treatment with cyclosporin A in a child with acquired pure amegakaryocytic thrombocytopenic purpura. *Acta Paediatr* 1994;83:1222–1224.

415. Trimble MS, Glynn MF, Brain MC. Amegakaryocytic thrombocytopenia of 4 years duration: successful treatment with antithymocyte globulin. *Am J Hematol* 1991;37:126–127.

416. Chan DK, O'Neill B. Successful trial of antithymocyte globulin therapy in amegakaryocytic thrombocytopenic purpura [Letter]. *Med J Aust* 1988;148:602–603.

417. el Saghir NS, Geltman RL. Treatment of acquired amegakaryocytic thrombocytopenic purpura with cyclophosphamide. *Am J Med* 1986; 81:139–142.

418. Kayser W, Euler HH, Schmitz N, et al. Danazol in acquired amegakaryocytic thrombocytopenic purpura: a case report. *Blut* 1985; 51:401–404.

419. Kashyap R, Choudhry VP, Pati HP. Danazol therapy in cyclic acquired amegakaryocytic thrombocytopenic purpura: a case report. *Am J Hematol* 1999;60:225–228.

420. George JN, El-Harake MA, Raskob GE. Chronic idiopathic thrombocytopenic purpura. *N Engl J Med* 1994;331:1207–1211.

421. Karpatkin S. Autoimmune (idiopathic) thrombocytopenic purpura. *Lancet* 1997;349:1531–1536.

422. Semple JW, Freedman J. Abnormal cellular immune mechanisms associated with autoimmune thrombocytopenia. *Transfus Med Rev* 1995;9:327–338.

423. George JN, El-Harake MA, Aster RH. Thrombocytopenia due to enhanced platelet destruction by immunologic mechanisms. In: Beutler E, Lichtman MA, Coller BS, et al., eds. *Williams hematology,* 5th ed. New York: McGraw-Hill, 1995:1314–1355.

424. George JN, El-Harake MA, Raskob GE. Chronic idiopathic thrombocytopenic purpura [see Comments]. *N Engl J Med* 1994;331: 1207–1211.

425. Baudard M, Pagnoux C, Audouin J, et al. Idiopathic thrombocytopenic purpura as the presenting feature of a primary bilateral adrenal non Hodgkin's lymphoma. *Leuk Lymphoma* 1997;26:609–613.

426. Stasi R, Stipa E, Masi M, et al. Prevalence and clinical significance of elevated antiphospholipid antibodies in patients with idiopathic thrombocytopenic purpura. *Blood* 1994;84:4203–4208.

427. George JN, Dale GL. Platelet kinetics. In: Beutler E, Lichtman MA, Coller BS, et al., eds. *Williams hematology,* 5th ed. New York: McGraw-Hill, 1995:1202–1205.

428. Stratton JR, Ballem PJ, Gernsheimer T, et al. Platelet destruction in autoimmune thrombocytopenic purpura: kinetics and clearance of Indium-111-labeled autologous platelets. *J Nucl Med* 1989;30:629–637.

429. Berchtold P, Wenger M. Autoantibodies against platelet glycoproteins in autoimmune thrombocytopenic purpura: their clinical signigicance and response to treatment. *Blood* 1993;81:1246–1250.

430. Kiefel V, Freitag E, Kroll H, et al. Platelet autoantibodies (IgG, IgM, IgA) against glycoproteins IIb/IIIa and Ib/IX in patients with thrombocytopenia. *Ann Hematol* 1996;72:280–285.

431. He R, Reid DM, Jones CE, et al. Spectrum of Ig classes, specificities, and titers of serum antiglycoproteins in chronic idiopathic thrombocytopenic purpura. *Blood* 1994;83:1024–1032.

432. Malik U, Dutcher JP, Oleksowicz L. Acquired Glanzmann's thrombasthenia associated with Hodgkin's lymphoma: a case report and review of the literature. *Cancer* 1998;82:1764–1768.

433. Fuse I, Higuchi W, Narita M, et al. Overproduction of antiplatelet antibody against glycoprotein IIb after splenectomy in a patient with Evans syndrome resulting in acquired thrombasthenia [see Comments]. *Acta Haematol* 1998;99:83–88.

434. Macchi L, Nurden P, Marit G, et al. Autoimmune thrombocytopenic purpura (AITP) and acquired thrombasthenia due to autoantibodies to GP IIb-IIIa in a patient with an unusual platelet membrane glycoprotein composition. *Am J Hematol* 1998;57:164–175.

435. Jallu V, Pico M, Chevaleyre J, et al. Characterization of an antibody to the integrin beta 3 subunit (GP IIIa) from a patient with neonatal thrombocytopenia and an inherited deficiency of GP IIb-IIIa complexes in platelets (Glanzmann's thrombasthenia). *Hum Antibodies Hybridomas* 1992;3:93–106.

436. Meyer M, Kirchmaier CM, Schirmer A, et al. Acquired disorder of platelet function associated with autoantibodies against membrane glycoprotein IIb-IIIa complex—1: glycoprotein analysis. *Thromb Haemost* 1991;65:491–496.

437. Niessner H, Clemetson KJ, Panzer S, et al. Acquired thrombasthenia due to GPIIb/IIIa-specific platelet autoantibodies. *Blood* 1986;68: 571–576.

438. Bellucci S, Charpak Y, Chastang C, et al. Low doses v conventional doses of corticoids in immune thrombocytopenic purpura (ITP): results of a randomized clinical trial in 160 children, 223 adults. *Blood* 1988;71:1165–1169.

439. Ozsoylu S. High-dose intravenous methylprednisolone for immune thrombocytopenic purpura [Letter]. *Blood* 1989;73:354–355.

440. Alpdogan O, Budak-Alpdogan T, Ratip S, et al. Efficacy of high-dose methylprednisolone as a first-line therapy in adult patients with idiopathic thrombocytopenic purpura. *Br J Haematol* 1998;103:1061–1063.

441. Caulier MT, Rose C, Roussel MT, et al. Pulsed high-dose dexamethasone in refractory chronic idiopathic thrombocytopenic purpura: a report on 10 cases. *Br J Haematol* 1995;91:477–479.

442. Godeau B, Zini JM, Schaeffer A, et al. High-dose methylprednisolone is an alternative treatment for adults with autoimmune thrombocytopenic purpura refractory to intravenous immunoglobulins and oral corticosteroids. *Am J Hematol* 1995;48:282–284.

443. Dubbeld P, van der Heul C, Hillen HF. Effect of high-dose dexamethasone in prednisone-resistant autoimmune thrombocytopenic purpura (ITP). *Neth J Med* 1991;39:6–10.

444. Andersen JC. Response of resistant idiopathic thrombocytopenic purpura to pulsed high-dose dexamethasone therapy [see Comments] [published erratum appears in *N Engl J Med* 1994;331:283]. *N Engl J Med* 1994;330:1560–1564.

445. Arruda VR, Annichino-Bizzacchi JM. High-dose dexamethasone therapy in chronic idiopathic thrombocytopenic purpura. *Ann Hematol* 1996;73:175–177.

446. Warner M, Wasi P, Couban S, et al. Failure of pulse high-dose dexamethasone in chronic idiopathic immune thrombocytopenia. *Am J Hematol* 1997;54:267–270.

447. Menichelli A, Del Principe D, Rezza E. Intravenous pulse methylprednisolone in chronic idiopathic thrombocytopenia. *Arch Dis Child* 1984;59:777–779.

448. Bussel JB, Pham LC, Aledort L, et al. Maintenance treatment of adults with chronic refractory immune thrombocytopenic purpura using repeated intravenous infusions of gammaglobulin [see Comments]. *Blood* 1988;72:121–127.

449. Bussel JB, Kimberly RP, Inman RD, et al. Intravenous gammaglobulin treatment of chronic idiopathic thrombocytopenic purpura. *Blood* 1983;62:480–486.

450. Emmerich B, Hiller E, Woitinas F, et al. Dose-response relationship in the treatment of idiopathic thrombocytopenic purpura with intravenous immunoglobulin. *Klin Wochenschr* 1987;65:369–372.

451. Seifried E, Pindur G, Stotter H, et al. Treatment of refractory chronic idiopathic thrombocytopenic purpura with high dose intravenous immunoglobulin. *Blut* 1984;48:369–376.

452. Bussel JB, Graziano JN, Kimberly RP, et al. Intravenous anti-D treatment of immune thrombocytopenic purpura: analysis of efficacy, toxicity, and mechanism of effect [see Comments]. *Blood* 1991;77: 1884–1893.

453. Gringeri A, Cattaneo M, Santagostino E, et al. Intramuscular anti-D immunoglobulins for home treatment of chronic immune thrombocytopenic purpura. *Br J Haematol* 1992;80:337–340.

454. Sagripanti A, Ferretti A, Giannessi D, et al. Anti-D treatment for chronic immune thrombocytopenic purpura: clinical and laboratory aspects. *Biomed Pharmacother* 1998;52:293–297.

455. Mazzucconi MG, Arista MC, Peraino M, et al. Long-term follow-up of autoimmune thrombocytopenic purpura (ATP) patients submitted to splenectomy. *Eur J Haematol* 1999;62:219–222.

456. Stasi R, Stipa E, Masi M, et al. Long-term observation of 208 adults with chronic idiopathic thrombocytopenic purpura. *Am J Med* 1995;98:436–442.

457. Dan K, Gomi S, Kuramoto A, et al. A multicenter prospective study on the treatment of chronic idiopathic thrombocytopenic purpura. *Int J Hematol* 1992;55:287–292.

458. Law C, Marcaccio M, Tam P, et al. High-dose intravenous immune globulin and the response to splenectomy in patients with idiopathic thrombocytopenic purpura [see Comments]. *N Engl J Med* 1997; 336:1494–1498.

459. Williams WJ. Classification and clinical manifestations of disorders of hemostasis. In: Beutler E, Lichtman MA, Coller BS, et al., eds. *Williams hematology,* 5th ed. New York: McGraw-Hill, 1995: 1276–1281.

460. Berchtold P, McMillan R. Therapy of chronic idiopathic thrombocytopenic purpura in adults. *Blood* 1989;74:2309–2317.

461. Cortelazzo S, Finazzi G, Buelli M, et al. High risk of severe bleeding in aged patients with chronic idiopathic thrombocytopenic purpura. *Blood* 1991;77:31–33.

462. Fauci AS, Young KR Jr. Immunoregulatory agents. In: Kelly WN, Harris ED Jr, Ruddy S, et al., eds. *Textbook of rheumatology,* 5th ed. Philadelphia: WB Saunders, 1997:805–827.

463. McMillan R. Therapy for adults with refractory chronic immune thrombocytopenic purpura. *Ann Intern Med* 1997;126:307–314.

464. Quiquandon I, Fenaux P, Caulier MT, et al. Re-evaluation of the role of azathioprine in the treatment of adult chronic idiopathic thrombocytopenic purpura: a report on 53 cases. *Br J Haematol* 1990;74: 223–228.

465. Schiavotto C, Castaman G, Rodeghiero F. Treatment of idiopathic thrombocytopenic purpura (ITP) in patients with refractoriness to or with contraindication for corticosteroids and/or splenectomy with immunosuppressive therapy and danazol. *Haematologica* 1993;78[6 Suppl 2]:29–34.

466. Reiner A, Gernsheimer T, Slichter SJ. Pulse cyclophosphamide therapy for refractory autoimmune thrombocytopenic purpura [see Comments]. *Blood* 1995;85:351–358.

467. Buelli M, Cortelazzo S, Viero P, et al. Danazol for the treatment of idiopathic thrombocytopenic purpura. *Acta Haematol* 1985;74:97–98.

468. McVerry BA, Auger M, Bellingham AJ. The use of danazol in the management of chronic immune thrombocytopenic purpura. *Br J Haematol* 1985;61:145–148.

469. Ahn YS, Mylvaganam R, Garcia RO, et al. Low-dose danazol therapy in idiopathic thrombocytopenic purpura. *Ann Intern Med* 1987;107: 177–181.

470. Cosgriff TM, Black ML, Stein W 3rd. Successful treatment of severe refractory idiopathic thrombocytopenic purpura with liposomal doxorubicin. *Am J Hematol* 1998;57:85–86.

471. Cervantes F, Montserrat E, Rozman C, et al. Low-dose vincristine in the treatment of corticosteroid-refractory idiopathic thrombocytopenic purpura (ITP) in non-splenectomized patients. *Postgrad Med J* 1980;56:711–714.

472. Hernandez F, Linares M, Colomina P, et al. Dapsone for refractory chronic idiopathic thrombocytopenic purpura. *Br J Haematol* 1995;90: 473–475.

473. Dubbeld P, Hillen HF, Schouten HC. Interferon treatment of refractory idiopathic thrombocytopenic purpura (ITP) [see Comments]. *Eur J Haematol* 1994;52:233–235.

474. Kumakura S, Ishikura H, Tsumura H, et al. A favourable effect of long-term alpha-interferon therapy in refractory idiopathic thrombocytopenic purpura. *Br J Haematol* 1993;85:805–807.

475. Proctor SJ. alpha Interferon therapy in the treatment of idiopathic thrombocytopenic purpura. *Eur J Cancer* 1991;[27 Suppl 4]:S63–S68.

476. Snyder HW Jr, Cochran SK, Balint JP Jr, et al. Experience with protein A-immunoadsorption in treatment-resistant adult immune thrombocytopenic purpura. *Blood* 1992;79:2237–2245.

477. Guthrie TH Jr, Oral A. Immune thrombocytopenia purpura: a pilot study of staphylococcal protein A immunomodulation in refractory patients. *Semin Hematol* 1989;26[2 Suppl 1]:3–9.

478. Baker GL, Kahl LE, Zee BC, et al. Malignancy following treatment of rheumatoid arthritis with cyclophosphamide: long-term case-control follow-up study. *Am J Med* 1987;83:1–9.

479. Reiner A, Gernsheimer T, Slichter SJ. Pulse cyclophosphamide therapy for refractory autoimmune thrombocytopenic purpura. *Blood* 1995;85:351–358.

480. Figueroa M, Gehlsen J, Hammond D, et al. Combination chemotherapy in refractory immune throbocytopenic purpura. *N Engl J Med* 1993;328:1226–1229.

481. Fox DA, McCune WJ. Immunosuppressive drug therapy of systemic lupus erythematosus. *Rheumatic Dis Clin North Am* 1994;20:265–299.

482. Figueroa M, Gehlsen J, Hammond D, et al. Combination chemotherapy in refractory immune thrombocytopenic purpura [see Comments]. *N Engl J Med* 1993;328:1226–1229.

483. Mackall CL, Fleisher TA, Brown MR, et al. Lymphocyte depletion during treatment with intensive chemotherapy or cancer. *Blood* 1994;84:2221–2228.

484. Mackall CL, Fleisher TA, Brown MR, et al. Age, thymopoiesis, and CD4+ T-lymphocyte regeneration after intensive chemotherapy. *N Engl J Med* 1995;332:143–149.

485. Valeri A, Radhakrishnan J, Estes D, et al. Intravenous pulse cyclophosphamide treatment of severe lupus nephritis: a prospective five-year study. *Clin Nephrol* 1994;42:71–78.

486. Pablos JL, Gutierrez-Millet V, Gomez-Reino JJ. Remission of lupus nephritis with cyclophosphamide and late relapses following therapy withdrawal. *Scand J Rheumatol* 1994;23:142–144.

487. Tyndall A, Black C, Finke J, et al. Treatment of systemic sclerosis with autologous heamopoietic stem cell transplantation. *Lancet* 1997;349:254.

488. Marmont AM, Van Bekkum CW. Stem cell transplantation for severe autoimmune diseases: new proposals but still unanswered questions. *Bone Marrow Transplant* 1997;16:497–498.

489. Snowden JA, Biggs JC, Brooks PM. Autologous blood stem cell transplantation for autoimmune diseases. *Lancet* 1996;348:1112–1113.

490. Lim SH, Kell J, Al-Sabah A, et al. Peripheral blood stem-cell transplantation for refractory autoimmune thrombocytopenic purpura. *Lancet* 1997;349:475.

491. Waters AH. Post-transfusion purpura. *Blood Rev* 1989;3:83–87.

492. Mueller-Eckhardt C. Post-transfusion purpura. *Br J Haematol* 1986; 64:419–424.

493. Porcelijn L, von dem Borne AE. Immune-mediated thrombocytopenias: basic and immunological aspects. *Baillieres Clin Haematol* 1998;11:331–341.

494. Vogelsang G, Kickler TS, Bell WR. Post-transfusion purpura: a report of five patients and a review of the pathogenesis and management. *Am J Hematol* 1986;21:259–267.

495. Mueller-Eckhardt C, Lechner K, Heinrich D, et al. Post-transfusion thrombocytopenic purpura: immunological and clinical studies in two cases and review of the literature. *Blut* 1980;40:249–257.

496. Evenson DA, Stroncek DF, Pulkrabek S, et al. Posttransfusion purpura following bone marrow transplantation. *Transfusion* 1995;35: 688–693.

497. Mueller-Eckhardt C, Kiefel V. High-dose IgG for post-transfusion purpura-revisited. *Blut* 1988;57:163–167.

498. Kickler TS, Ness PM, Herman JH, et al. Studies on the pathophysiology of posttransfusion purpura. *Blood* 1986;68:347–350.

499. Becker T, Panzer S, Maas D, et al. High-dose intravenous immunoglobulin for post-transfusion purpura. *Br J Haematol* 1985;61: 149–155.

500. Hamblin TJ, Naorose Abidi SM, Nee PA, et al. Successful treatment of post-transfusion purpura with high dose immunoglobulins after lack of response to plasma exchange. *Vox Sang* 1985;49:164–167.

501. Glud TK, Rosthoj S, Jensen MK, et al. High-dose intravenous immunoglobulin for post-transfusion purpura. *Scand J Haematol* 1983;31:495–500.

502. Mueller-Eckhardt C, Kuenzlen E, Thilo-Korner D, et al. High-dose intravenous immunoglobulin for post-transfusion purpura [Letter]. *N Engl J Med* 1983;308:287.

503. Weisberg LJ, Linker CA. Prednisone therapy of post-transfusion purpura. *Ann Intern Med* 1984;100:76–77.

504. Packman CH, Leddy JP. Acquired hemolytic anemia due to warm-reacting autoantibodies. In: Beutler E, Lichtman MA, Coller BS, et al., eds. *Williams hematology,* 5th ed. New York: McGraw-Hill, 1995: 677–685.

505. Namirska-Krzton H, Fabijanska-Mitek J, Seyfried H. Enzyme-linked antiglobulin test for the evaluation of the amount of IgG autoantibodies on red blood cells. *Clin Lab Haematol* 1995;17:221–224.

506. Victoria EJ, Pierce SW, Branks MJ, et al. IgG red blood cell autoantibodies in autoimmune hemolytic anemia bind to epitopes on red blood cell membrane band 3 glycoprotein. *J Lab Clin Med* 1990;115:74–88.

507. Leddy JP, Wilkinson SL, Kissel GE, et al. Erythrocyte membrane proteins reactive with IgG (warm-reacting) anti-red blood cell autoantibodies. II. Antibodies coprecipitating band 3 and glycophorin A. *Blood* 1994;84:650–656.

508. Leddy JP, Falany JL, Kissel GE, et al. Erythrocyte membrane proteins reactive with human (warm-reacting) anti-red cell autoantibodies. *J Clin Invest* 1993;91:1672–1680.

509. Kowal C, Weinstein A, Diamond B. Molecular mimicry between bacterial and self antigen in a patient with systemic lupus erythematosus. *Eur J Immunol* 1999;29:1901–1911.

510. Oldstone MB. Molecular mimicry and immune-mediated diseases. *FASEB J* 1998;12:1255–1265.

511. Davies JM. Molecular mimicry: can epitope mimicry induce autoimmune disease? *Immunol Cell Biol* 1997;75:113–126.

512. Kipps TJ, Carson DA. Autoantibodies in chronic lymphocytic leukemia and related systemic autoimmune diseases. *Blood* 1993;81: 2475–2487.

513. Youinou P, Le Corre R, Dueymes M. Autoimmune diseases and monoclonal gammopathies. *Clin Exp Rheumatol* 1996;[14 Suppl 14]: S55–S58.

514. Borche L, Lim A, Binet JL, et al. Evidence that chronic lymphocytic leukemia B lymphocytes are frequently committed to production of natural autoantibodies. *Blood* 1990;76:562–569.

515. Sthoeger ZM, Wakai M, Tse DB, et al. Production of autoantibodies by CD5-expressing B lymphocytes from patients with chronic lymphocytic leukemia. *J Exp Med* 1989;169:255–268.

516. Bataille R, Klein B, Durie BG. The relationship between autoimmune states and B cell proliferations [Editorial]. *J Rheumatol* 1989;16:1023–1024.

517. Leung PS, Gershwin ME. Immunoglobulin genes in autoimmunity. *Int Arch Allergy Immunol* 1993;101:113–118.

518. Mayer R, Stone K, Han A, et al. Malignant CD5 B cells: biased immunoglobulin variable gene usage and autoantibody production. *Int Rev Immunol* 1991;7:189–203.

519. Outschoorn I, Rowley MJ, Cook AD, et al. Subclasses of immunoglobulins and autoantibodies in autoimmune diseases. *Clin Immunol Immunopathol* 1993;66:59–66.

520. Efremov DG, Ivanovski M, Burrone OR. The pathologic significance of the immunoglobulins expressed by chronic lymphocytic leukemia B-cells in the development of autoimmune hemolytic anemia. *Leuk Lymphoma* 1998;28:285–293.

521. Centola M, Lin K, Sutton C, et al. Production of anti-erythrocyte antibodies by leukemic and nonleukemic B cells in chronic lymphocytic leukemia patients. *Leuk Lymphoma* 1996;20:465–469.

522. Costello RT, Xerri L, Bouabdallah R, et al. Leukopenia, thrombocytopenia, and acute autoimmune hemolytic anemia associated with an unusual (type 2/4) Hodgkin's disease: case report [Letter]. *Am J Hematol* 1996;52:333–334.

523. Shah SJ, Warrier RP, Ode DL, et al. Immune thrombocytopenia and hemolytic anemia associated with Hodgkin disease. *J Pediatr Hematol Oncol* 1996;18:227–229.

524. Majumdar G. Unremitting severe autoimmune haemolytic anaemia as a presenting feature of Hodgkin's disease with minimum tumour load. *Leuk Lymphoma* 1995;20:169–172.

525. Sierra RD. Coombs-positive hemolytic anemia in Hodgkin's disease: case presentation and review of the literature. *Mil Med* 1991;156:691–692.

526. Xiros N, Binder T, Anger B, et al. Idiopathic thrombocytopenic purpura and autoimmune hemolytic anemia in Hodgkin's disease. *Eur J Haematol* 1988;40:437–441.

527. Spitzer T, Crum E, Schacter L, et al. Sarcoidosis, Hodgkin's disease, and autoimmune hemolytic anemia. *Am J Med Sci* 1986;291:190–193.

528. Vaiopoulos G, Kyriakou D, Papadaki H, et al. Multiple myeloma associated with autoimmune hemolytic anemia. *Haematologica* 1994;79:262–264.

529. Crisp D, Pruzanski W. B-cell neoplasms with homogeneous cold-reacting antibodies (cold agglutinins). *Am J Med* 1982;72:915–922.

530. Tanaka T, Ueda N, Fujita M, et al. Macroglobulinemia Waldenström complicated by autoimmune hemolytic anemia, meningeal sign and femoral lysis. *Acta Pathol Jpn* 1979;29:777–789.

531. Rapoport AP, Rowe JM, McMican A. Life-threatening autoimmune hemolytic anemia in a patient with the acquired immune deficiency syndrome. *Transfusion* 1988;28:190–191.

532. Gonzalez CA. Successful treatment of autoimmune hemolytic anemia with intravenous immunoglobulin in a patient with AIDS. *Transplant Proc* 1998;30:4151–4152.

533. Puppo F, Torresin A, Lotti G, et al. Autoimmune hemolytic anemia and human immunodeficiency virus (HIV) infection [Letter; see Comments]. *Ann Intern Med* 1988;109:249–250.

534. Toy PT, Reid ME, Burns M. Positive direct antiglobulin test associated with hyperglobulinemia in acquired immunodeficiency syndrome (AIDS). *Am J Hematol* 1985;19:145–150.

535. Telen MJ, Roberts KB, Bartlett JA. HIV-associated autoimmune hemolytic anemia: report of a case and review of the literature [see Comments]. *J Acquir Immune Defic Syndr* 1990;3:933–937.

536. Sen K, Kalaycio M. Evan's syndrome precipitated by fludarabine therapy in a case of CLL [Letter]. *Am J Hematol* 1999;61:219.

537. Vick DJ, Byrd JC, Beal CL, et al. Mixed-type autoimmune hemolytic anemia following fludarabine treatment in a patient with chronic lymphocytic leukemia/small cell lymphoma. *Vox Sang* 1998;74:122–126.

538. Longo G, Gandini G, Ferrara L, et al. Fludarabine and autoimmune hemolytic anemia in chronic lymphocytic leukemia [Letter]. *Eur J Haematol* 1997;59:124–125.

539. Tsiara S, Christou L, Konstantinidou P, et al. Severe autoimmune hemolytic anemia following fludarabine therapy in a patient with chronic lymphocytic leukemia [Letter]. *Am J Hematol* 1997;54:342.

540. Robak T, Blasinska-Morawiec M, Krykowski E, et al. Autoimmune haemolytic anaemia in patients with chronic lymphocytic leukaemia treated with 2-chlorodeoxyadenosine (cladribine). *Eur J Haematol* 1997;58:109–113.

541. Myint H, Copplestone JA, Orchard J, et al. Fludarabine-related autoimmune haemolytic anaemia in patients with chronic lymphocytic leukaemia. *Br J Haematol* 1995;91:341–344.

542. Fleischman RA, Croy D. Acute onset of severe autoimmune hemolytic anemia after treatment with 2-chlorodeoxyadenosine for chronic lymphocytic leukemia [Letter]. *Am J Hematol* 1995;48:293.

543. Murphy WG, Kelton JG. Methyldopa-induced autoantibodies against red blood cells. *Blood Rev* 1988;2:36–42.

544. Schwartz RS, Silberstein LE, Berkman EM. Autoimmune hemolytic anemias. In: Hoffman R, Benz EJ Jr, Shattil SJ, et al., eds. *Hematology: basic principles and practice,* 2nd ed. New York: Churchill Livingstone, 1995:710–729.

545. Domen RE. An overview of immune hemolytic anemias. *Cleve Clin J Med* 1998;65:89–99.

546. Win N, Islam SI, Peterkin MA, et al. Positive direct antiglobulin test due to antiphospholipid antibodies in normal healthy blood donors. *Vox Sang* 1997;72:182–184.

547. Bordin JO, Souza-Pinto JC, Kerbauy J, Measurement of red blood cell antibodies in autoimmune hemolytic anemia. *Braz J Med Biol Res* 1991;24:895–899.

548. Wilson L, Wren MR, Issitt PD. Enzyme-linked antiglobulin test: variables affecting the test when measuring levels of red cell antigens. *Med Lab Sci* 1985;42:20–25.

549. Postoway N, Nance SJ, Garratty G. Variables affecting the enzyme-linked antiglobulin test when detecting and quantitating IgG red cell antibodies. *Med Lab Sci* 1985;42:11–19.

550. Chaplin H, Nasongkla M, Monroe MC. Quantitation of red blood cell-bound C3d in normal subjects and random hospitalized patients. *Br J Haematol* 1981;48:69–78.

551. Axelson JA, LoBuglio AF. Immune hemolytic anemia. *Med Clin North Am* 1980;64:597–606.

552. Curtis BR, Lamon J, Roelcke D, et al. Life-threatening, antiglobulin test-negative, acute autoimmune hemolytic anemia due to a non-complement-activating IgG1 kappa cold antibody with Pra specificity. *Transfusion* 1990;30:838–843.

553. Salama A, Berghofer H, Mueller-Eckhardt C. Red blood cell transfusion in warm-type autoimmune haemolytic anaemia [see Comments]. *Lancet* 1992;340(8834–8835):1515–1517.

554. Wright MS, Smith LA. Laboratory investigation of autoimmune hemolytic anemias. *Clin Lab Sci* 1999;12:119–122; quiz, 123–125.

555. Jefferies LC. Transfusion therapy in autoimmune hemolytic anemia. *Hematol Oncol Clin North Am* 1994;8:1087–1104.

556. Sokol RJ, Hewitt S, Booker DJ, et al. Patients with red cell autoantibodies: selection of blood for transfusion. *Clin Lab Haematol* 1988;10:257–264.

557. Meyer O, Stahl D, Beckhove P, et al. Pulsed high-dose dexamethasone in chronic autoimmune haemolytic anaemia of warm type. *Br J Haematol* 1997;98:860–862.

558. Flores G, Cunningham-Rundles C, Newland AC, et al. Efficacy of intravenous immunoglobulin in the treatment of autoimmune hemolytic anemia: results in 73 patients. *Am J Hematol* 1993;44:237–242.

559. Hilgartner MW, Bussel J. Use of intravenous gamma globulin for the treatment of autoimmune neutropenia of childhood and autoimmune hemolytic anemia. *Am J Med* 1987;83(4A):25–29.

560. Mitchell CA, Van der Weyden MB, Firkin BG. High dose intravenous gammaglobulin in Coombs positive hemolytic anemia. *Aust N Z J Med* 1987;17:290–294.

561. Akpek G, McAneny D, Weintraub L. Comparative response to splenectomy in Coombs-positive autoimmune hemolytic anemia with or without associated disease. *Am J Hematol* 1999;61:98–102.

562. Coon WW. Splenectomy in the treatment of hemolytic anemia. *Arch Surg* 1985;120:625–628.

563. Gombakis N, Trahana M, Athanassiou M, et al. Evans syndrome: successful management with multi-agent treatment including intermediate-dose intravenous cyclophosphamide [Letter]. *J Pediatr Hematol Oncol* 1999;21:248–249.

564. Majumdar G, Brown S, Slater NG, et al. Clinical spectrum of autoimmune haemolytic anaemia in patients with chronic lymphocytic leukaemia. *Leuk Lymphoma* 1993;9:149–151.

565. Panceri R, Fraschini D, Tornotti G, et al. Successful use of high-dose cyclophosphamide in a child with severe autoimmune hemolytic anemia. *Haematologica* 1992;77:76–78.

566. Zupanska B, Sylwestrowicz T, Pawelski S. The results of prolonged treatment of autoimmune haemolytic anaemia. *Haematologia (Budap)* 1981;14:425–433.

567. Silva VA, Seder RH, Weintraub LR. Synchronization of plasma exchange and cyclophosphamide in severe and refractory autoimmune hemolytic anemia. *J Clin Apheresis* 1994;9:120–123.

568. Goebel KM, Goebel FD, Gassel WD, et al. Immune response in patients with autoimmune thrombocytopenia and autoimmune haemolytic anaemia receiving azathioprine. *Klin Wochenschr* 1974;52:916–920.

569. Rackoff WR, Manno CS. Treatment of refractory Evans syndrome with alternate-day cyclosporine and prednisone. *Am J Pediatr Hematol Oncol* 1994;16:156–159.

570. Dundar S, Ozdemir O, Ozcebe O. Cyclosporin in steroid-resistant autoimmune haemolytic anaemia. *Acta Haematol* 1991;86:200–202.

571. Hershko C, Sonnenblick M, Ashkenazi J. Control of steroid-resistant autoimmune haemolytic anaemia by cyclosporine. *Br J Haematol* 1990;76:436–437.

572. Musso M, Porretto F, Crescimanno A, et al. Autologous peripheral blood stem and progenitor (CD34+) cell transplantation for systemic lupus erythematosus complicated by Evans syndrome. *Lupus* 1998;7: 492–494.

573. Martino R, Sureda A, Brunet S. Peripheral blood stem cell mobilization in refractory autoimmune Evans syndrome: a cautionary case report [Letter; see Comments]. *Bone Marrow Transplant* 1997;20:521.

574. Frank MM, Atkinson JP, Gadek J. Cold agglutinins and cold-agglutinin disease. *Annu Rev Med* 1977;28:291–298.

575. Rosse WF, Adams JP. The variability of hemolysis in the cold agglutinin syndrome. *Blood* 1980;56:409–416.

576. Feizi T. The monoclonal antibodies of cold agglutinin syndrome. *Med Biol* 1980;58:123–127.

577. Lind K, Benzon MW, Jensen JS, et al. A seroepidemiological study of Mycoplasma pneumoniae infections in Denmark over the 50-year period 1946-1995. *Eur J Epidemiol* 1997;13:581–586.

578. Konig AL, Kreft H, Hengge U, et al. Coexisting anti-I and anti-F1/Gd cold agglutinins in infections by Mycoplasma pneumoniae. *Vox Sang* 1988;55:176–180.

579. Horwitz CA, Moulds J, Henle W, et al. Cold agglutinins in infectious mononucleosis and heterophil-antibody-negative mononucleosis-like syndromes. *Blood* 1977;50:195–202.

580. Ciaffoni S, Luzzati R, Roata C, et al. Presence and significance of cold agglutinins in patients with HIV infection. *Haematologica* 1992;77: 233–236.

581. Jefferies LC, Carchidi CM, Silberstein LE. Naturally occurring anti-i/I cold agglutinins may be encoded by different VH3 genes as well as the VH4.21 gene segment. *J Clin Invest* 1993;92:2821–2833.

582. Silberstein LE, Jefferies LC, Goldman J, et al. Variable region gene analysis of pathologic human autoantibodies to the related i and I red blood cell antigens. *Blood* 1991;78:2372–2386.

583. Gottsche B, Salama A, Mueller-Eckhardt C. Autoimmune hemolytic anemia caused by a cold agglutinin with a new specificity (anti-Ju). *Transfusion* 1990;30:261–262.

584. Salama A, Pralle H, Mueller-Eckhardt C. A new red blood cell cold autoantibody (anti-Me) [published erratum appears in *Vox Sang* 1986;50:111]. *Vox Sang* 1985;49:277–284.

585. Roelcke D, Ebert W, Geisen HP. Anti-Pr3: serological and immunochemical identification of a new anti-Pr subspecificity. *Vox Sang* 1976; 30:122–133.

586. Kirschfink M, Fritze H, Roelcke D. Complement activation by cold agglutinins. *Vox Sang* 1992;63:220–226.

587. Zilow G, Kirschfink M, Roelcke D. Red cell destruction in cold agglutinin disease. *Infusionsther Transfusionsmed* 1994;21:410–415.

588. Kirschfink M, Knoblauch K, Roelcke D. Activation of complement by cold agglutinins. *Infusionsther Transfusionsmed* 1994;21:405–409.

589. Sokol RJ, Booker DJ, Stamps R. The pathology of autoimmune haemolytic anaemia. *J Clin Pathol* 1992;45:1047–1052.

590. Lahav M, Rosenberg I, Wysenbeek AJ. Steroid-responsive idiopathic cold agglutinin disease: a case report. *Acta Haematol* 1989;81: 166–168.

591. Jacobs A. Cold agglutinin hemolysis responding to fludarabine therapy [Letter]. *Am J Hematol* 1996;53:279–280.

592. Azuma E, Nishihara H, Hanada M, et al. Recurrent cold hemagglutinin disease following allogeneic bone marrow transplantation successfully treated with plasmapheresis, corticosteroid and cyclophosphamide. *Bone Marrow Transplant* 1996;18:243–246.

593. L'Abbate A, Maggiore Q, Caccamo A, et al. Suppression of post-apheresis autoantibody rebound in cryoglobulinemia and cold agglutinin hemolytic anemia. *Int J Artif Organs* 1983;[6 Suppl 1]:51–56.

594. Murphy S, LoBuglio AF. Drug therapy of autoimmune hemolytic anemia. *Semin Hematol* 1976;13:323–334.

595. Hippe E, Jensen KB, Olesen H, et al. Chlorambucil treatment of patients with cold agglutinin syndrome. *Blood* 1970;35:68–72.

596. Evans RS, Baxter E, Gilliland BC. Chronic hemolytic anemia due to cold agglutinins: a 20-year history of benign gammopathy with response to chlorambucil. *Blood* 1973;42:463–470.

597. Taft EG, Propp RP, Sullivan SA. Plasma exchange for cold agglutinin hemolytic anemia. *Transfusion* 1977;17:173–176.

598. Valbonesi M, Guzzini F, Zerbi D, et al. Successful plasma exchange for a patient with chronic demyelinating polyneuropathy and cold agglutinin disease due to anti-Pra. *J Clin Apheresis* 1986;3:109–110.

599. Pereira A, Mazzara R, Escoda L, et al. Anti-Sa cold agglutinin of IgA class requiring plasma-exchange therapy as early manifestation of multiple myeloma. *Ann Hematol* 1993;66:315–318.

600. Andrzejewski C Jr, Gault E, Briggs M, et al. Benefit of a 37 degree C extracorporeal circuit in plasma exchange therapy for selected cases with cold agglutinin disease. *J Clin Apheresis* 1988;4:13–17.

601. Heddle NM. Acute paroxysmal cold hemoglobinuria. *Transfus Med Rev* 1989;3:219–229.

602. Bird GW. Paroxysmal cold haemoglobinuria. *Br J Haematol* 1977;37: 167–171.

603. Boccardi V, D'Annibali S, Di Natale G, et al. Mycoplasma pneumoniae infection complicated by paroxysmal cold hemoglobinuria with anti-P specificity of biphasic hemolysin. *Blut* 1977;34:211–214.

604. Bell CA, Zwicker H, Rosenbaum DL. Paroxysmal cold hemoglobinuria (P.C.H.) following mycoplasma infection: anti-I specificity of the biphasic hemolysin. *Transfusion* 1973;13:138–141.

605. Sivakumaran M, Murphy PT, Booker DJ, et al. Paroxysmal cold haemoglobinuria caused by non-Hodgkin's lymphoma. *Br J Haematol* 1999;105:278–279.

606. Lau P, Sererat S, Moore V, et al. Paroxysmal cold hemoglobinuria in a patient with Klebsiella pneumonia. *Vox Sang* 1983;44:167–172.

607. Shirey RS, Park K, Ness PM, et al. An anti-i biphasic hemolysin in chronic paroxysmal cold hemoglobinuria. *Transfusion* 1986;26:62–64.

608. Sharara AI, Hillsley RE, Wax TD, et al. Paroxysmal cold hemoglobinuria associated with non-Hodgkin's lymphoma. *South Med J* 1994;87:397–399.

609. Lippman SM, Winn L, Grumet FC, et al. Evans' syndrome as a presenting manifestation of atypical paroxysmal cold hemoglobinuria. *Am J Med* 1987;82:1065–1072.

610. Andersen E, Skov F, Hippe E. A case of cold haemoglobinuria with later sarcoidosis: treatment with plasmapheresis and immunosuppressiva. *Scand J Haematol* 1980;24:47–50.

611. Vogel JM, Hellman M, Moloshok RE. Paroxysmal cold hemoglobinuria of nonsyphilitic etiology in two children. *J Pediatr* 1972;81: 974–977.

612. Wynn RF, Stevens RF, Bolton-Maggs PH, et al. Paroxysmal cold haemoglobinuria of childhood: a review of the management and unusual presenting features of six cases. *Clin Lab Haematol* 1998;20: 373–375.

613. Miyagawa Y, Yamada S, Komiyama A, et al. Measurement of Donath-Landsteiner antibody-producing cells in idiopathic nonsyphilitic paroxysmal cold hemoglobinuria (PCH) in children. *Blood* 1978;52: 97–101.

614. Ries CA, Garratty G, Petz LD, et al. Paroxysmal cold hemoglobinuria: report of a case with an exceptionally high thermal range Donath-Landsteiner antibody. *Blood* 1971;38:491–499.

615. Nordhagen R. Two cases of paroxysmal cold hemoglobinuria with a Donath-Landsteiner antibody reactive by the indirect antiglobulin test using anti-IgG [Letter; see Comments]. *Transfusion* 1991;31:190–191.

616. Moake JL. Thrombotic thrombocytopenic purpura and the hemolytic uremic syndrome. In: Hoffman R, Benz EJ Jr, Shattil SJ, et al., eds. *Hematology: basic principles and practice*, 2nd ed. New York: Churchill Livingstone, 1995:1879–1889.

617. Neild GH. Hemolytic uremic syndrome/thrombotic thrombocytopenic purpura: pathophysiology and treatment. *Kidney Int Suppl* 1998;64: S45–S49.

618. George JN, Gilcher RO, Smith JW, et al. Thrombotic thrombocytopenic purpura-hemolytic uremic syndrome: diagnosis and management. *J Clin Apheresis* 1998;13:120–125.

619. Moake JL. von Willebrand factor in the pathophysiology of thrombotic thrombocytopenic purpura. *Clin Lab Sci* 1998;11:362–364.

620. Galbusera M, Noris M, Rossi C, et al. Increased fragmentation of von Willebrand factor, due to abnormal cleavage of the subunit, parallels disease activity in recurrent hemolytic uremic syndrome and thrombotic thrombocytopenic purpura and discloses predisposition in families. The Italian Registry of Familial and Recurrent HUS/TTP. *Blood* 1999;94:610–620.

621. Asada Y, Sumiyoshi A, Hayashi T, et al. Immunohistochemistry of vascular lesion in thrombotic thrombocytopenic purpura, with special reference to factor VIII related antigen. *Thromb Res* 1985;38:469–479.

622. Besser RE, Griffin PM, Slutsker L. Escherichia coli O157:H7 gastroenteritis and the hemolytic uremic syndrome: an emerging infectious disease. *Annu Rev Med* 1999;50:355–367.

623. Palmisano J, Agraharkar M, Kaplan AA. Successful treatment of cis-platin-induced hemolytic uremic syndrome with therapeutic plasma exchange. *Am J Kidney Dis* 1998;32:314–317.

624. Gordon LI, Kwaan HC. Thrombotic microangiopathy manifesting as thrombotic thrombocytopenic purpura/hemolytic uremic syndrome in the cancer patient. *Semin Thromb Hemost* 1999;25:217–221.

625. Antunes I, Magina S, Granjo E, et al. Hemolytic-uremic syndrome induced by pentostatin in a patient with cutaneous T-cell lymphoma [Letter]. *Dermatology* 1999;198:179–180.

626. Fung MC, Storniolo AM, Nguyen B, et al. A review of hemolytic uremic syndrome in patients treated with gemcitabine therapy. *Cancer* 1999;85:2023–2032.

627. Flombaum CD, Mouradian JA, Casper ES, et al. Thrombotic microangiopathy as a complication of long-term therapy with gemcitabine. *Am J Kidney Dis* 1999;33:555–562.

628. Galbusera M, Benigni A, Paris S, et al. Unrecognized pattern of von Willebrand factor abnormalities in hemolytic uremic syndrome and thrombotic thrombocytopenic purpura. *J Am Soc Nephrol* 1999;10: 1234–1241.

629. Taylor CM, Williams JM, Lote CJ, et al. A laboratory model of toxin-induced hemolytic uremic syndrome. *Kidney Int* 1999;55:1367–1374.

630. Gordjani N, Sutor AH. Coagulation changes associated with the hemolytic uremic syndrome. *Semin Thromb Hemost* 1998;24:577–582.

631. Furlan M, Robles R, Galbusera M, et al. von Willebrand factor-cleaving protease in thrombotic thrombocytopenic purpura and the hemolytic-uremic syndrome [see Comments]. *N Engl J Med* 1998;339: 1578–1584.

632. Borghardt EJ, Kirchertz EJ, Marten I, et al. Protein A-immunoadsorption in chemotherapy associated hemolytic-uremic syndrome. *Transfus Sci* 1998;[19 Suppl]:5–7.

633. Tassinari D, Sartori S, Panzini I, et al. Hemolytic-uremic syndrome during therapy with estramustine phosphate for advanced prostatic cancer. *Oncology* 1999;56:112–113.

634. van der Heijden M, Ackland SP, Deveridge S. Haemolytic uraemic syndrome associated with bleomycin, epirubicin and cisplatin chemotherapy: a case report and review of the literature. *Acta Oncol* 1998;37:107–109.

635. Chow TW, Turner NA, Chintagumpala M, et al. Increased von Willebrand factor binding to platelets in single episode and recurrent types of thrombotic thrombocytopenic purpura. *Am J Hematol* 1998;57: 293–302.

636. Tsai HM, Lian EC. Antibodies to von Willebrand factor-cleaving protease in acute thrombotic thrombocytopenic purpura [see Comments]. *N Engl J Med* 1998;339:1585–1594.

637. Hess DC, Sethi K, Awad E. Thrombotic thrombocytopenic purpura in systemic lupus erythematosus and antiphospholipid antibodies: effective treatment with plasma exchange and immunosuppression [see Comments]. *J Rheumatol* 1992;19:1474–1478.

638. Moake JL. Thrombotic thrombocytopenic purpura today. *Hosp Pract (Off Ed)* 1999;34:53–59.

639. Furlan M, Robles R, Morselli B, et al. Recovery and half-life of von Willebrand factor-cleaving protease after plasma therapy in patients with thrombotic thrombocytopenic purpura. *Thromb Haemost* 1999; 81:8–13.

640. Knobl P, Rintelen C, Kornek G, et al. Plasma exchange for treatment of thrombotic thrombocytopenic purpura in critically ill patients. *Intensive Care Med* 1997;23:44–50.

641. Pereira A, Mazzara R, Monteagudo J, et al. Thrombotic thrombocytopenic purpura/hemolytic uremic syndrome: a multivariate analysis of factors predicting the response to plasma exchange. *Ann Hematol* 1995;70:319–323.

642. Ruggenenti P, Galbusera M, Cornejo RP, et al. Thrombotic thrombocytopenic purpura: evidence that infusion rather than removal of plasma induces remission of the disease. *Am J Kidney Dis* 1993;21: 314–318.

643. Onundarson PT, Rowe JM, Heal JM, et al. Response to plasma exchange and splenectomy in thrombotic thrombocytopenic purpura: a 10-year experience at a single institution. *Arch Intern Med* 1992; 152:791–796.

644. Rock GA, Shumak KH, Buskard NA, et al. Comparison of plasma exchange with plasma infusion in the treatment of thrombotic thrombocytopenic purpura. Canadian Apheresis Study Group [see Comments]. *N Engl J Med* 1991;325:393–397.

645. Bell WR, Braine HG, Ness PM, et al. Improved survival in thrombotic thrombocytopenic purpura-hemolytic uremic syndrome: clinical experience in 108 patients [see Comments]. *N Engl J Med* 1991;325: 398–403.

646. Bobbio-Pallavicini E, Gugliotta L, Centurioni R, et al. Antiplatelet agents in thrombotic thrombocytopenic purpura (TTP): results of a randomized multicenter trial by the Italian Cooperative Group for TTP. *Haematologica* 1997;82:429–435.

647. Sagripanti A, Carpi A, Rosaia B, et al. Iloprost in the treatment of thrombotic microangiopathy: report of thirteen cases. *Biomed Pharmacother* 1996;50:350–356.

648. Mazzel C, Pepkowitz S, Klapper E, et al. Treatment of thrombotic thrombocytopenic purpura: a role for early vincristine administration. *J Clin Apheresis* 1998;13:20–22.

649. Hand JP, Lawlor ER, Yong CK, et al. Successful use of cyclosporine A in the treatment of refractory thrombotic thrombocytopenic purpura. *Br J Haematol* 1998;100:597–599.

650. Bachman WR, Brennan JK. Refractory thrombotic thrombocytopenic purpura treated with cyclosporine [Letter]. *Am J Hematol* 1996;51: 93–94.

651. Gaddis TG, Guthrie TH Jr, Drew MJ, et al. Treatment of plasma refractory thrombotic thrombocytopenic purpura with protein A immunoabsorption. *Am J Hematol* 1997;55:55–58.

652. Drew MJ. Resolution of refractory, classic thrombotic thrombocytopenic purpura after staphylococcal protein A immunoadsorption. *Transfusion* 1994;34:536–538.

653. Pereira A, Monteagudo J, Bono A, et al. Effect of splenectomy on von Willebrand factor multimeric structure in thrombotic thrombocytopenic purpura refractory to plasma exchange. *Blood Coagul Fibrinolysis* 1993;4:783–786.

654. Castaman G, Rodeghiero F, Ruggeri M, et al. Long-lasting remission after high-dose intravenous immunoglobulins in a case of relapsing thrombotic thrombocytopenic purpura. *Haematologica* 1991;76: 511–512.

655. Bux J, Kissel K, Nowak K, et al. Autoimmune neutropenia: clinical and laboratory studies in 143 patients. *Ann Hematol* 1991;63:249–252.

656. Shastri KA, Logue GL. Autoimmune neutropenia [see Comments]. *Blood* 1993;81:1984–1995.

657. Bux J, Behrens G, Jaeger G, et al. Diagnosis and clinical course of autoimmune neutropenia in infancy: analysis of 240 cases. *Blood* 1998; 91:181–186.

658. Lalezari P, Khorshidi M, Petrosova M. Autoimmune neutropenia of infancy. *J Pediatr* 1986;109:764–769.

659. McClain K, Estrov Z, Chen H, et al. Chronic neutropenia of childhood: frequent association with parvovirus infection and correlations with bone marrow culture studies [see Comments]. *Br J Haematol* 1993; 85:57–62.

660. Madyastha PR, Glassman AB. Characterization of neutrophil agglutinins in primary autoimmune neutropenia of early childhood. *Ann Clin Lab Sci* 1988;18:367–373.

661. McCullough J, Clay ME, Priest JR, et al. A comparison of methods for detecting leukocyte antibodies in autoimmune neutropenia. *Transfusion* 1981;21:483–492.

662. Alter BP. Fanconi's anemia and malignancies. *Am J Hematol* 1996; 53:99–110.

663. dos Santos CC, Gavish H, Buchwald M. Fanconi anemia revisited: old ideas and new advances. *Stem Cells (Dayt)* 1994;12:142–153.
664. Strathdee CA, Buchwald M. Molecular and cellular biology of Fanconi anemia. *Am J Pediatr Hematol Oncol* 1992;14:177–185.
665. Alter BP. Bone marrow failure syndromes. *Clin Lab Med* 1999;19:113–133.
666. Touw IP. Granulocyte colony-stimulating factor receptor mutations in severe chronic neutropenia and acute myeloid leukaemia: biological and clinical significance. *Baillieres Clin Haematol* 1997;10:577–587.
667. Welte K, Boxer LA. Severe chronic neutropenia: pathophysiology and therapy. *Semin Hematol* 1997;34:267–278.
668. Touw IP, Dong F. Severe congenital neutropenia terminating in acute myeloid leukemia: disease progression associated with mutations in the granulocyte-colony stimulating factor receptor gene. *Leuk Res* 1996;20:629–631.
669. Bux J, Kober B, Kiefel V, et al. Analysis of granulocyte-reactive antibodies using an immunoassay based upon monoclonal-antibody-specific immobilization of granulocyte antigens. *Transfus Med* 1993;3:157–162.
670. Bux J, Sohn M, Hachmann R, et al. Quantitation of granulocyte antibodies in sera and determination of their binding sites. *Br J Haematol* 1992;82:20–25.
671. Bauer KA. Hypercoagulable states. In: Hoffman R, Benz EJ Jr, Shattil SJ, et al., eds. *Hematology: basic principles and practice*, 3rd ed. New York: Churchill Livingstone, 2000:2009–2039.
671a. Huisman MV, Rosendaal F. Thrombophilia. *Curr Opin Hematol* 1999;6:291–297.
672. Cogo A, Bernardi E, Prandoni P, et al. Acquired risk factors for deep-vein thrombosis in symptomatic outpatients. *Arch Intern Med* 1994;154:164–168.
673. Lensing AW, Prandoni P, Prins MH, et al. Deep-vein thrombosis [see Comments]. *Lancet* 1999;353:479–485.
674. Riley RS, Friedline J, Rogers JS 2nd. Antiphospholipid antibodies: standardization and testing. *Clin Lab Med* 1997;17:395–430.
675. Conley CL, Hartmann RC. A hemorrhagic disorder caused by circulating anticoagulant in patients with disseminated lupus erythematosus. *J Clin Invest* 1952;31:621–622.
676. Feinstein DI, Rapaport SI. Acquired inhibitors of blood coagulation. *Prog Hemost Thromb* 1972;1:75–95.
677. Feinstein DI. Inhibitors of blood coagulation. In: Hoffman R, Benz EJ Jr, Shattil SJ, et al, eds. *Hematology: basic principles and practice,* 3rd ed. New York: Churchill Livingstone, 2000:1963–1983.
678. Kunkel LA. Acquired circulating anticoagulants. *Hematol Oncol Clin North Am* 1992;6:1341–1357.
679. Fields RA, Toubbeh H, Searles RP, et al. The prevalence of anticardiolipin antibodies in a healthy elderly population and its association with antinuclear antibodies. *J Rheumatol* 1989;16:623–625.
680. Vila P, Hernandez MC, Lopez-Fernandez MF, et al. Prevalence, follow-up and clinical significance of the anticardiolipin antibodies in normal subjects. *Thromb Haemost* 1994;72:209–213.
681. Schultz DR. Antiphospholipid antibodies: basic immunology and assays. *Semin Arthritis Rheum* 1997;26:724–739.
682. Lockshin MD. Antiphospholipid antibody syndrome. *Rheum Dis Clin North Am* 1994;20:45–59.
683. Bick RL. Antiphospholipid thrombosis syndromes: etiology, pathophysiology, diagnosis and management. *Int J Hematol* 1997;65:193–213.
684. Ginsberg JS, Wells PS, Brill-Edwards P, et al. Antiphospholipid antibodies and venous thromboembolism. *Blood* 1995;86:3685–3691.
685. Kampe CE. Clinical syndromes associated with lupus anticoagulants. *Semin Thromb Hemost* 1994;20:16–26.
686. Nojima J, Suehisa E, Kuratsune H, et al. High prevalence of thrombocytopenia in SLE patients with a high level of anticardiolipin antibodies combined with lupus anticoagulant. *Am J Hematol* 1998;58:55–60.
687. Godeau B, Piette JC, Fromont P, et al. Specific antiplatelet glycoprotein autoantibodies are associated with the thrombocytopenia of primary antiphospholipid syndrome. *Br J Haematol* 1997;98:873–879.
688. Lipp E, von Felten A, Sax H, et al. Antibodies against platelet glycoproteins and antiphospholipid antibodies in autoimmune thrombocytopenia. *Eur J Haematol* 1998;60:283–288.
689. Hakim AJ, Machin SJ, Isenberg DA. Autoimmune thrombocytopenia in primary antiphospholipid syndrome and systemic lupus erythematosus: the response to splenectomy. *Semin Arthritis Rheum* 1998;28:20–25.
690. Asherson RA. The catastrophic antiphospholipid syndrome, 1998: a review of the clinical features, possible pathogenesis and treatment. *Lupus* 1998;[7 Suppl 2]:S55–S62.
691. Triplett DA. Many faces of lupus anticoagulants. *Lupus* 1998;[7 Suppl 2]:S18–S22.
692. Brandt JT, Barna LK, Triplett DA. Laboratory identification of lupus anticoagulants: results of the Second International Workshop for Identification of Lupus Anticoagulants. On behalf of the Subcommittee on Lupus Anticoagulants/Antiphospholipid Antibodies of the ISTH. *Thromb Haemost* 1995;74:1597–1603.
693. Pengo V, Biasiolo A, Rampazzo P, et al. dRVVT is more sensitive than KCT or TTI for detecting lupus anticoagulant activity of anti-beta2-glycoprotein I autoantibodies. *Thromb Haemost* 1999;81:256–258.
694. Triplett DA. Lupus anticoagulants: diagnostic dilemma and clinical challenge. *Clin Lab Sci* 1997;10:223–228.
695. Galli M, Finazzi G, Bevers EM, et al. Kaolin clotting time and dilute Russell's viper venom time distinguish between prothrombin-dependent and beta 2-glycoprotein I-dependent antiphospholipid antibodies. *Blood* 1995;86:617–623.
696. Lockshin MD. Which patients with antiphospholipid antibody should be treated and how? *Rheum Dis Clin North Am* 1993;19:235–247.
697. Bick RL, Baker WF. Antiphospholipid syndrome and thrombosis [In Process Citation]. *Semin Thromb Hemost* 1999;25:333–350.
698. Rosove MH, Brewer PM. Antiphospholipid thrombosis: clinical course after the first thrombotic event in 70 patients. *Ann Intern Med* 1992;117:303–308.
699. Krnic-Barrie S, O'Connor CR, Looney SW, et al. A retrospective review of 61 patients with antiphospholipid syndrome: analysis of factors influencing recurrent thrombosis. *Arch Intern Med* 1997;157:2101–2108.
700. Khamashta MA, Cuadrado MJ, Mujic F, et al. The management of thrombosis in the antiphospholipid-antibody syndrome [see Comments]. *N Engl J Med* 1995;332:993–997.
701. Moll S, Ortel TL. Monitoring warfarin therapy in patients with lupus anticoagulants. *Ann Intern Med* 1997;127:177–185.
701a. Greaves M. Antiphospholipid antibodies and thrombosis. *Lancet* 1999;353:1348–1353.
702. Khamashta MA. Management of thrombosis and pregnancy loss in the antiphospholipid syndrome. *Lupus* 1998;[7 Suppl 2]:S162–S165.
703. Hay CR. Acquired haemophilia. *Baillieres Clin Haematol* 1998;11:287–303.
704. Cohen AJ, Kessler CM. Acquired inhibitors. *Baillieres Clin Haematol* 1996;9:331–354.
705. Bouvry P, Recloux P. Acquired hemophilia. *Haematologica* 1994;79:550–556.
706. Geurs F, Baele G, Afschrift M. Acquired haemophilia in the elderly. *Acta Clin Belg* 1995;50:238–241.
707. Nilsson IM, Lamme S. On acquired hemophilia A: a survey of 11 cases. *Acta Med Scand* 1980;208:5–12.
708. Lottenberg R, Kentro TB, Kitchens CS. Acquired hemophilia: a natural history study of 16 patients with factor VIII inhibitors receiving little or no therapy. *Arch Intern Med* 1987;147:1077–1081.
709. Feinstein DI, Rapaport SI, McGehee WG, et al. Factor V anticoagulants: clinical, biochemical, and immunological observations. *J Clin Invest* 1970;49:1578–1588.
710. Knobl P, Lechner K. Acquired factor V inhibitors. *Baillieres Clin Haematol* 1998;11:305–318.
711. Brunod M, Chatot-Henry C, Mehdaoui H, et al. Acquired anti-factor VII (proconvertin) inhibitor: hemorrhage and thrombosis [Letter]. *Thromb Haemost* 1998;79:1065–1066.
712. Campbell E, Sanal S, Mattson J, et al. Factor VII inhibitor. *Am J Med* 1980;68:962–964.
713. Roberts HR, Cromartie R. Overview of inhibitors to factor VIII and IX. *Prog Clin Biol Res* 1984;150:1–18.
714. Collins HW, Gonzalez MF. Acquired factor IX inhibitor in a patient with adenocarcinoma of the colon. *Acta Haematol* 1984;71:49–52.
715. Berman BW, McIntosh S, Clyne LP, et al. Spontaneously acquired factor IX inhibitors in childhood. *Am J Pediatr Hematol Oncol* 1981;3:77–81.
716. Miller K, Neely JE, Krivit W, et al. Spontaneously acquired factor IX inhibitor in a nonhemophiliac child. *J Pediatr* 1978;93:232–234.
717. Matsunaga AT, Shafer FE. An acquired inhibitor to factor X in a pediatric patient with extensive burns. *J Pediatr Hematol Oncol* 1996;18:223–226.

718. Lankiewicz MW, Bell WR. A unique circulating inhibitor with specificity for coagulation factor X. *Am J Med* 1992;93:343–346.

719. Ness PM, Hymas PG, Gesme D, et al. An unusual factor-X inhibitor in leprosy. *Am J Hematol* 1980;8:397–402.

720. Rao LV, Zivelin A, Iturbe I, et al. Antibody-induced acute factor X deficiency: clinical manifestations and properties of the antibody. *Thromb Haemost* 1994;72:363–371.

721. Marciniak E, Greenwood MF. Acquired coagulation inhibitor delaying fibrinopeptide release. *Blood* 1979;53:81–92.

722. Hoots WK, Carrell NA, Wagner RH, et al. A naturally occurring antibody that inhibits fibrin polymerization. *N Engl J Med* 1981;304:857–861.

723. Goudemand J, Samor B, Caron C, et al. Acquired type II von Willebrand's disease: demonstration of a complexed inhibitor of the von Willebrand factor-platelet interaction and response to treatment. *Br J Haematol* 1988;68:227–233.

724. Bovill EG, Ershler WB, Golden EA, et al. A human myeloma-produced monoclonal protein directed against the active subpopulation of von Willebrand factor. *Am J Clin Pathol* 1986;85:115–123.

725. Mohri H, Tanabe J, Ohtsuka M, et al. Acquired von Willebrand disease associated with multiple myeloma: characterization of an inhibitor to von Willebrand factor. *Blood Coagul Fibrinolysis* 1995;6:561–566.

726. Mannucci PM, Lombardi R, Bader R, et al. Studies of the pathophysiology of acquired von Willebrand's disease in seven patients with lymphoproliferative disorders or benign monoclonal gammopathies. *Blood* 1984;64:614–621.

727. Soff GA, Green D. Autoantibody to von Willebrand factor in systemic lupus erythematosus. *J Lab Clin Med* 1993;121:424–430.

728. Stewart MW, Etches WS, Shaw AR, et al. vWf inhibitor detection by competitive ELISA. *J Immunol Methods* 1997;200:113–119.

729. Green D, Lechner K. A survey of 215 non-hemophilic patients with inhibitors to Factor VIII. *Thromb Haemost* 1981;45:200–203.

730. Hauser I, Schneider B, Lechner K. Post-partum factor VIII inhibitors: a review of the literature with special reference to the value of steroid and immunosuppressive treatment. *Thromb Haemost* 1995;73:1–5.

731. Solymoss S. Postpartum acquired factor VIII inhibitors: results of a survey. *Am J Hematol* 1998;59:1–4.

732. Seidler CW, Mills LE, Flowers ME, et al. Spontaneous factor VIII inhibitor occurring in association with chronic graft-versus-host disease. *Am J Hematol* 1994;45:240–243.

733. Preminger GM, Knupp CL, Hindsley JP Jr, et al. Spontaneously acquired anti-factor VIII antibodies: report of a patient with adenocarcinoma of the prostate. *J Urol* 1984;131:1182–1184.

734. Sugishita K, Nagase H, Takahashi T, et al. Acquired factor VIII inhibitor in a non-hemophilic patient with chronic hepatitis C viral infection. *Intern Med* 1999;38:283–286.

735. Banninger H, Hardegger T, Tobler A, et al. Fibrin glue in surgery: frequent development of inhibitors of bovine thrombin and human factor V. *Br J Haematol* 1993;85:528–532.

736. Mateo J, Martino R, Borrell M, et al. Acquired factor VIII inhibitor preceding chronic lymphocytic leukemia. *Ann Hematol* 1993;67:309–311.

737. O'Kane MJ, Wisdom GB, Desai ZR, et al. Inhibition of fibrin monomer polymerisation by myeloma immunoglobulin. *J Clin Pathol* 1994;47:266–268.

738. Gastineau DA, Gertz MA, Daniels TM, et al. Inhibitor of the thrombin time in systemic amyloidosis: a common coagulation abnormality. *Blood* 1991;77:2637–2640.

739. Galanakis DK. Fibrinogen anomalies and disease: a clinical update. *Hematol Oncol Clin North Am* 1992;6:1171–1187.

740. Sultan Y, Algiman M. Treatment of factor VIII inhibitors. *Blood Coagul Fibrinolysis* 1990;1:193–199.

741. Sohngen D, Specker C, Bach D, et al. Acquired factor VIII inhibitors in nonhemophilic patients. *Ann Hematol* 1997;74:89–93.

742. Slocombe GW, Newland AC, Colvin MP, et al. The role of intensive plasma exchange in the prevention and management of haemorrhage in patients with inhibitors to factor VIII. *Br J Haematol* 1981;47:577–585.

743. Pintado T, Taswell HF, Bowie EJ. Treatment of life-threatening hemorrhage due to acquired factor VIII inhibitor. *Blood* 1975;46:535–541.

744. Erskine JG, Burnett AK, Walker ID, et al. Plasma exchange in non-haemophiliac patients with inhibitors to factor VIIIC. *Br Med J (Clin Res Ed)* 1981;283:760.

745. Schwartz RS, Gabriel DA, Aledort LM, et al. A prospective study of treatment of acquired (autoimmune) factor VIII inhibitors with high-dose intravenous gammaglobulin. *Blood* 1995;86:797–804.

746. Herbst KD, Rapaport SI, Kenoyer DG, et al. Syndrome of an acquired inhibitor of factor VIII responsive to cyclophosphamide and prednisone. *Ann Intern Med* 1981;95:575–578.

747. Green D. Immunosuppression of factor VIII inhibitors in non-hemophilic patients. *Semin Hematol* 1993;30[2 Suppl 1]:28–31.

748. Hultin MB, Shapiro SS, Bowman HS, et al. Immunosuppressive therapy of Factor VIII inhibitors. *Blood* 1976;48:95–108.

749. Shaffer LG, Phillips MD. Successful treatment of acquired hemophilia with oral immunosuppressive therapy [see Comments] [published erratum appears in *Ann Intern Med* 1998;128:330]. *Ann Intern Med* 1997;127:206–209.

750. Green D, Schuette PT, Wallace WH. Factor VIII antibodies in rheumatoid arthritis: effect of cyclophosphamide. *Arch Intern Med* 1980;140:1232–1235.

751. Chediak J, Ashenhurst JB, Garlick I, et al. Successful management of bleeding in a patient with factor V inhibitor by platelet transfusions. *Blood* 1980;56:835–841.

752. Cash JM, Sears DA. The anemia of chronic disease: spectrum of associated diseases in a series of unselected hospitalized patients. *Am J Med* 1989;87:638–644.

753. Schilling RF. Anemia of chronic disease: a misnomer [Editorial; see Comments]. *Ann Intern Med* 1991;115:572–573.

754. Means RT Jr. Pathogenesis of the anemia of chronic disease: a cytokine-mediated anemia. *Stem Cells (Dayt)* 1995;13:32–37.

755. Krantz SB. Pathogenesis and treatment of the anemia of chronic disease. *Am J Med Sci* 1994;307:353–359.

756. Greendyke RM, Sharma K, Gifford FR. Serum levels of erythropoietin and selected other cytokines in patients with anemia of chronic disease. *Am J Clin Pathol* 1994;101:338–341.

757. Sears DA. Anemia of chronic disease. *Med Clin North Am* 1992;76:567–579.

758. Jongen-Lavrencic M, Peeters HR, Wognum A, et al. Elevated levels of inflammatory cytokines in bone marrow of patients with rheumatoid arthritis and anemia of chronic disease. *J Rheumatol* 1997;24:1504–1509.

759. Roodman GD. Mechanisms of erythroid suppression in the anemia of chronic disease. *Blood Cells* 1987;13:171–184.

760. Faquin WC, Schneider TJ, Goldberg MA. Effect of inflammatory cytokines on hypoxia-induced erythropoietin production. *Blood* 1992;79:1987–1994.

761. Means RT Jr, Dessypris EN, Krantz SB. Inhibition of human erythroid colony-forming units by interleukin-1 is mediated by gamma interferon. *J Cell Physiol* 1992;150:59–64.

762. Moldawer LL, Marano MA, Wei H, et al. Cachectin/tumor necrosis factor-alpha alters red blood cell kinetics and induces anemia in vivo. *FASEB J* 1989;3:1637–1643.

763. Mulherin D, Skelly M, Saunders A, et al. The diagnosis of iron deficiency in patients with rheumatoid arthritis and anemia: an algorithm using simple laboratory measures [see Comments]. *J Rheumatol* 1996;23:237–240.

764. Vreugdenhil G, Baltus CA, van Eijk HG, et al. Anaemia of chronic disease: diagnostic significance of erythrocyte and serological parameters in iron deficient rheumatoid arthritis patients. *Br J Rheumatol* 1990;29:105–110.

765. Balaban EP, Sheehan RG, Demian SE, et al. Evaluation of bone marrow iron stores in anemia associated with chronic disease: a comparative study of serum and red cell ferritin [see Comments]. *Am J Hematol* 1993;42:177–181.

766. Nielsen OJ, Andersen LS, Hansen NE, et al. Serum transferrin receptor levels in anaemic patients with rheumatoid arthritis. *Scand J Clin Lab Invest* 1994;54:75–82.

767. Ferguson BJ, Skikne BS, Simpson KM, et al. Serum transferrin receptor distinguishes the anemia of chronic disease from iron deficiency anemia. *J Lab Clin Med* 1992;119:385–390.

768. Mast AE, Blinder MA, Gronowski AM, et al. Clinical utility of the soluble transferrin receptor and comparison with serum ferritin in several populations. *Clin Chem* 1998;44:45–51.

769. Vreugdenhil G, Wognum AW, van Eijk HG, et al. Anaemia in rheumatoid arthritis: the role of iron, vitamin B12, and folic acid deficiency, and erythropoietin responsiveness. *Ann Rheum Dis* 1990;49:93–98.

770. Means RT Jr. Clinical application of recombinant erythropoietin in the anemia of chronic disease. *Hematol Oncol Clin North Am* 1994;8:933–944.

771. Pincus T, Olsen NJ, Russell IJ, et al. Multicenter study of recombinant human erythropoietin in correction of anemia in rheumatoid arthritis [see Comments]. *Am J Med* 1990;89:161–168.

772. Salvarani C, Lasagni D, Casali B, et al. Recombinant human erythropoietin therapy in patients with rheumatoid arthritis with the anemia of chronic disease. *J Rheumatol* 1991;18:1168–1171.

773. Nordstrom D, Lindroth Y, Marsal L, et al. Availability of iron and degree of inflammation modifies the response to recombinant human erythropoietin when treating anemia of chronic disease in patients with rheumatoid arthritis. *Rheumatol Int* 1997;17:67–73.

774. Betterle C, Mazzi PA, Pedini B, et al. Complement-fixing gastric parietal cell autoantibodies: a good marker for the identification of type A chronic atrophic gastritis. *Autoimmunity* 1988;1:267–274.

775. Kaye MD. Immunological aspects of gastritis and pernicious anaemia. *Baillieres Clin Gastroenterol* 1987;1:487–506.

776. Raptopoulou-Gigi M, Polyzonis M, Orphanou-Koumerkeridou H, et al. Immunohistological phenotyping of the stomach infiltrating lymphocytes in chronic gastritis. *Allergol Immunopathol (Madr)* 1990;18:87–89.

777. Toh BH, van Driel IR, Gleeson PA. Pernicious anemia [see Comments]. *N Engl J Med* 1997;337:1441–1448.

778. Negrini R, Savio A, Poiesi C, et al. Antigenic mimicry between Helicobacter pylori and gastric mucosa in the pathogenesis of body atrophic gastritis. *Gastroenterology* 1996;111:655–665.

779. Herbert H. Vitamin B-12. In: Ziegler EE, Filer LJ Jr, eds. *Present knowledge in nutrition,* 7th ed. Washington, DC: ILSI Press, 1999:191–205.

780. Centanni M, Marignani M, Gargano L, et al. Atrophic body gastritis in patients with autoimmune thyroid disease: an underdiagnosed association. *Arch Intern Med* 1999;159:1726–1730.

781. Greenberg PL. Myelodysplastic syndrome. In: Hoffman R, Benz EJ Jr, Shattil SJ, et al., eds. *Hematology: basic principles and practice,* 3rd ed. New York: Churchill Livingstone, 2000:1106–1129.

782. Antony AC. Megaloblastic anemias. In: Hoffman R, Benz EJ Jr, Shattil SJ, et al., eds. *Hematology: basic principles and practice,* 3rd ed. New York: Churchill Livingstone, 2000:446–485.

783. Rose MS, Chanarin I. Intrinsic-factor antibody and absorption of vitamin B12 in pernicious anaemia. *Br Med J* 1971;1:25–26.

784. Rose MS, Chanarin I. Studies on intrinsic factor antibodies. *Br J Haematol* 1968;15:325–326.

785. Conn DA. Intrinsic factor antibody detection and quantitation. *Med Lab Sci* 1986;43:48–52.

786. Carmel R, Rasmussen K, Jacobsen DW, et al. Comparison of the deoxyuridine suppression test with serum levels of methylmalonic acid and homocysteine in mild cobalamin deficiency. *Br J Haematol* 1996;93:311–318.

787. Allen RH, Stabler SP, Savage DG, et al. Diagnosis of cobalamin deficiency. I. Usefulness of serum methylmalonic acid and total homocysteine concentrations [see Comments]. *Am J Hematol* 1990;34:90–98.

788. Lindenbaum J, Savage DG, Stabler SP, et al. Diagnosis of cobalamin deficiency. II. Relative sensitivities of serum cobalamin, methylmalonic acid, and total homocysteine concentrations. *Am J Hematol* 1990;34:99–107.

789. Nickoloff E. Schilling test: physiologic basis for and use as a diagnostic test. *Crit Rev Clin Lab Sci* 1988;26:263–276.

790. Isaac G, Holland OB. Drug-induced hypokalaemia: a cause for concern. *Drugs Aging* 1992;2:35–41.

791. Coyle TE. Hematologic complications of human immunodeficiency virus infection and the acquired immunodeficiency syndrome. *Med Clin North Am* 1997;81:449–470.

792. Jaworowski A, Crowe SM. Does HIV cause depletion of CD4+ T cells in vivo by the induction of apoptosis? *Immunol Cell Biol* 1999;77:90–98.

793. Zunich KM, Lane HC. Immunologic abnormalities in HIV infection. *Hematol Oncol Clin North Am* 1991;5:215–228.

794. Holland HK, Spivak JL. The haematological manifestations of acquired immune deficiency syndrome. *Baillieres Clin Haematol* 1990;3:103–114.

795. Moses A, Nelson J, Bagby GC Jr. The influence of human immunodeficiency virus-1 on hematopoiesis. *Blood* 1998;91:1479–1495.

796. Moses AV, Williams S, Heneveld ML, et al. Human immunodeficiency virus infection of bone marrow endothelium reduces induction of stromal hematopoietic growth factors [see Comments]. *Blood* 1996;87:919–925.

797. Bain BJ. Pathogenesis and pathophysiology of anemia in HIV infection. *Curr Opin Hematol* 1999;6:89–93.

798. Stella CC, Ganser A, Hoelzer D. Defective in vitro growth of the hemopoietic progenitor cells in the acquired immunodeficiency syndrome. *J Clin Invest* 1987;80:286–293.

799. Steinberg HN, Crumpacker CS, Chatis PA. In vitro suppression of normal human bone marrow progenitor cells by human immunodeficiency virus. *J Virol* 1991;65:1765–1769.

800. Geissler RG, Ottmann OG, Kleiner K, et al. Decreased haematopoietic colony growth in long-term bone marrow cultures of HIV-positive patients. *Res Virol* 1993;144:69–73.

801. Chelucci C, Hassan HJ, Locardi C, et al. In vitro human immunodeficiency virus-1 infection of purified hematopoietic progenitors in single-cell culture. *Blood* 1995;85:1181–1187.

802. Neal TF, Holland HK, Baum CM, et al. CD34+ progenitor cells from asymptomatic patients are not a major reservoir for human immunodeficiency virus-1. *Blood* 1995;86:1749–1756.

803. von Laer D, Hufert FT, Fenner TE, et al. CD34+ hematopoietic progenitor cells are not a major reservoir of the human immunodeficiency virus. *Blood* 1990;76:1281–1286.

804. Kaczmarski RS, Davison F, Blair E, et al. Detection of HIV in haemopoietic progenitors. *Br J Haematol* 1992;82:764–769.

805. Sullivan PS, Hanson DL, Chu SY, et al. Epidemiology of anemia in human immunodeficiency virus (HIV)-infected persons: results from the multistate adult and adolescent spectrum of HIV disease surveillance project. *Blood* 1998;91:301–308.

806. Kreuzer KA, Rockstroh JK. Pathogenesis and pathophysiology of anemia in HIV infection. *Ann Hematol* 1997;75:179–187.

807. Stricker RB, Goldberg B. AIDS and pure red cell aplasia [Letter; see Comments]. *Am J Hematol* 1997;54:264.

808. Namiki TS, Boone DC, Meyer PR. A comparison of bone marrow findings in patients with acquired immunodeficiency syndrome (AIDS) and AIDS related conditions. *Hematol Oncol* 1987;5:99–106.

809. Goldsmith JC, Irvine W. Reversible agranulocytosis related to azidothymidine therapy. *Am J Hematol* 1989;30:263–264.

810. Gill PS, Rarick M, Brynes RK, et al. Azidothymidine associated with bone marrow failure in the acquired immunodeficiency syndrome (AIDS). *Ann Intern Med* 1987;107:502–505.

811. Ganser A, Greher J, Volkers B, et al. Inhibitory effect of azidothymidine, 2'-3'-dideoxyadenosine, and 2'-3'-dideoxycytidine on in vitro growth of hematopoietic progenitor cells from normal persons and from patients with AIDS. *Exp Hematol* 1989;17:321–325.

812. Richman DD, Fischl MA, Grieco MH, et al. The toxicity of azidothymidine (AZT) in the treatment of patients with AIDS and AIDS-related complex: a double-blind, placebo-controlled trial. *N Engl J Med* 1987;317:192–197.

813. Markham A, Faulds D. Ganciclovir: an update of its therapeutic use in cytomegalovirus infection. *Drugs* 1994;48:455–484.

814. Morbidity and toxic effects associated with ganciclovir or foscarnet therapy in a randomized cytomegalovirus retinitis trial. Studies of ocular complications of AIDS Research Group, in collaboration with the AIDS Clinical Trials Group. *Arch Intern Med* 1995;155:65–74.

815. Rieder MJ, King SM, Read S. Adverse reactions to trimethoprim-sulfamethoxazole among children with human immunodeficiency virus infection. *Pediatr Infect Dis J* 1997;16:1028–1031.

816. Hughes WT, LaFon SW, Scott JD, et al. Adverse events associated with trimethoprim-sulfamethoxazole and atovaquone during the treatment of AIDS-related Pneumocystis carinii pneumonia. *J Infect Dis* 1995;171:1295–1301.

817. Ziegler JL, Beckstead JA, Volberding PA, et al. Non-Hodgkin's lymphoma in 90 homosexual men; relation to generalized lymphadenopathy and the acquired immunodeficiency syndrome. *N Engl J Med* 1984;311:565–570.

818. Ioachim HL, Dorsett B, Cronin W, et al. Acquired immunodeficiency syndrome-associated lymphomas: clinical, pathologic, immunologic, and viral characteristics of 111 cases. *Hum Pathol* 1991;22:659–673.

819. Pich A, Navone R. Bone marrow involvement in Kaposi's disease: report of a case. *Panminerva Med* 1989;31:144–147.

820. Levin M, Hertzberg L. Kaposi's sarcoma of the bone marrow presenting with fever of unknown origin. *Med Pediatr Oncol* 1994;22: 410–413.

821. Conran RM, Granger E, Reddy VB. Kaposi's sarcoma of the bone marrow. *Arch Pathol Lab Med* 1986;110:1083–1085.

822. Farhi DC, Mason UG 3d, Horsburgh CR Jr. The bone marrow in disseminated Mycobacterium avium-intracellulare infection. *Am J Clin Pathol* 1985;83:463–468.

823. Nichols L, Florentine B, Lewis W, et al. Bone marrow examination for the diagnosis of mycobacterial and fungal infections in the acquired immunodeficiency syndrome. *Arch Pathol Lab Med* 1991;115: 1125–1132.

824. Riley UB, Crawford S, Barrett SP, et al. Detection of mycobacteria in bone marrow biopsy specimens taken to investigate pyrexia of unknown origin. *J Clin Pathol* 1995;48:706–709.

825. Wiley EL, Perry A, Nightingale SD, et al. Detection of Mycobacterium avium-intracellulare complex in bone marrow specimens of patients with acquired immunodeficiency syndrome. *Am J Clin Pathol* 1994; 101:446–451.

826. Bahner I, Kearns K, Coutinho S, et al. Infection of human marrow stroma by human immunodeficiency virus-1 (HIV-1) is both required and sufficient for HIV-1-induced hematopoietic suppression in vitro: demonstration by gene modification of primary human stroma. *Blood* 1997;90:1787–1798.

827. Canque B, Marandin A, Rosenzwajg M, et al. Susceptibility of human bone marrow stromal cells to human immunodeficiency virus (HIV). *Virology* 1995;208:779–783.

828. Zauli G, Re MC, Davis B, et al. Impaired in vitro growth of purified (CD34+) hematopoietic progenitors in human immunodeficiency virus-1 seropositive thrombocytopenic individuals. *Blood* 1992;79: 2680–2687.

829. Scadden DT, Zeira M, Woon A, et al. Human immunodeficiency virus infection of human bone marrow stromal fibroblasts. *Blood* 1990;76: 317–322.

830. Sakaguchi M, Sato T, Groopman JE. Human immunodeficiency virus infection of megakaryocytic cells. *Blood* 1991;77:481–485.

831. Kunzi MS, Groopman JE. Identification of a novel human immunodeficiency virus strain cytopathic to megakaryocytic cells. *Blood* 1993;81:3336–3342.

832. Chelucci C, Federico M, Guerriero R, et al. Productive human immunodeficiency virus-1 infection of purified megakaryocytic progenitors/precursors and maturing megakaryocytes. *Blood* 1998;91: 1225–1234.

833. Maury CP, Lahdevirta J. Correlation of serum cytokine levels with haematological abnormalities in human immunodeficiency virus infection. *J Intern Med* 1990;227:253–257.

834. Aukrust P, Liabakk NB, Muller F, et al. Serum levels of tumor necrosis factor-alpha (TNF alpha) and soluble TNF receptors in human immunodeficiency virus type 1 infection: correlations to clinical, immunologic, and virologic parameters [published erratum appears in *J Infect Dis* 1994;169:1186–1187]. *J Infect Dis* 1994;169:420–424.

835. Roux-Lombard P, Modoux C, Cruchaud A, et al. Purified blood monocytes from HIV 1-infected patients produce high levels of TNF alpha and IL-1. *Clin Immunol Immunopathol* 1989;50:374–384.

836. Ratner L. Human immunodeficiency virus-associated autoimmune thrombocytopenic purpura: a review [see Comments]. *Am J Med* 1989;86:194–198.

837. Bierling P, Bettaieb A, Oksenhendler E. Human immunodeficiency virus-related immune thrombocytopenia. *Semin Thromb Hemost* 1995;21:68–75.

838. Tongol JM, Gounder MP, Butala A, et al. HIV-related autoimmune hemolytic anemia: good response to zidovudine [Letter; see Comments]. *J Acquir Immune Defic Syndr* 1991;4:1163–1164.

839. De Angelis V, Biasinutto C, Pradella P, et al. Mixed-type auto-immune haemolytic anaemia in a patient with HIV infection. *Vox Sang* 1995;68:191–194.

840. De Angelis V, Biasinutto C, Pradella P, et al. Clinical significance of positive direct antiglobulin test in patients with HIV infection. *Infection* 1994;22:92–95.

841. Kaplan C, Morinet F, Cartron J. Virus-induced autoimmune thrombocytopenia and neutropenia. *Semin Hematol* 1992;29:34–44.

842. Ribera E, Ocana I, Almirante B, et al. Autoimmune neutropenia and thrombocytopenia associated with development of antibodies to human immunodeficiency virus. *J Infect* 1989;18:167–170.

843. Weinberg GA, Gigliotti F, Stroncek DF, et al. Lack of relation of granulocyte antibodies (antineutrophil antibodies) to neutropenia in children with human immunodeficiency virus infection. *Pediatr Infect Dis J* 1997;16:881–884.

844. Gris JC, Toulon P, Brun S, et al. The relationship between plasma microparticles, protein S and anticardiolipin antibodies in patients with human immunodeficiency virus infection. *Thromb Haemost* 1996; 76:38–45.

845. Rubbert A, Bock E, Schwab J, et al. Anticardiolipin antibodies in HIV infection: association with cerebral perfusion defects as detected by 99mTc-HMPAO SPECT. *Clin Exp Immunol* 1994;98:361–368.

846. Hassell KL, Kressin DC, Neumann A, et al. Correlation of antiphospholipid antibodies and protein S deficiency with thrombosis in HIV-infected men. *Blood Coagul Fibrinolysis* 1994;5:455–462.

847. Cohen AJ, Philips TM, Kessler CM. Circulating coagulation inhibitors in the acquired immunodeficiency syndrome. *Ann Intern Med* 1986;104:175–180.

848. Frickhofen N, Abkowitz JL, Safford M, et al. Persistent B19 parvovirus infection in patients infected with human immunodeficiency virus type 1 (HIV-1): a treatable cause of anemia in AIDS. *Ann Intern Med* 1990;113:926–933.

849. Hermans P. Haematopoietic growth factors as supportive therapy in HIV-infected patients. *AIDS* 1995;[9 Suppl 2]:S9–S14.

850. Glaspy JA, Chap L. The clinical application of recombinant erythropoietin in the HIV-infected patient. *Hematol Oncol Clin North Am* 1994;8:945–959.

851. Bussel JB, Haimi JS. Isolated thrombocytopenia in patients infected with HIV: treatment with intravenous gammaglobulin. *Am J Hematol* 1988;28:79–84.

852. Jahnke L, Applebaum S, Sherman LA, et al. An evaluation of intravenous immunoglobulin in the treatment of human immunodeficiency virus-associated thrombocytopenia. *Transfusion* 1994;34:759–764.

853. Smith N. Intravenous anti-D immunoglobulin in the management of immune thrombocytopenic purpura. *Curr Opin Hematol* 1996;3: 498–503.

854. Oksenhendler E, Bierling P, Chevret S, et al. Splenectomy is safe and effective in human immunodeficiency virus-related immune thrombocytopenia [see Comments]. *Blood* 1993;82:29–32.

855. Israel DS, Plaisance KI. Neutropenia in patients infected with human immunodeficiency virus. *Clin Pharm* 1991;10:268–279.

856. Scadden DT. Cytokine use in the management of HIV disease [see Comments]. *J Acquir Immune Defic Syndr Hum Retrovirol* 1997;[16 Suppl 1]:S23–S29.

857. Anderlini P, Donato M, Chan KW, et al. Allogeneic blood progenitor cell collection in normal donors after mobilization with filgrastim: the M.D. Anderson Cancer Center experience. *Transfusion* 1999;39: 555–560.

858. Shpall EJ. The utilization of cytokines in stem cell mobilization strategies. *Bone Marrow Transplant* 1999;[23 Suppl 2]:S13–S19.

859. Weaver CH, Birch R, Greco FA, et al. Mobilization and harvesting of peripheral blood stem cells: randomized evaluations of different doses of filgrastim. *Br J Haematol* 1998;100:338–347.

860. Guillaume T, Rubinstein DB, Symann M. Immune reconstitution and immunotherapy after autologous hematopoietic stem cell transplantation. *Blood* 1998;92:1471–1490.

861. Laurenti L, Sica S, Salutari P, et al. Assessment of hematological and immunological function during long-term follow-up after peripheral blood stem cell transplantation. *Haematologica* 1998;83:138–142.

862. Rosillo MC, Ortuno F, Moraleda JM, et al. Immune recovery after autologous or rhG-CSF primed PBSC transplantation. *Eur J Haematol* 1996;56:301–307.

863. Burt RK, Traynor AE, Cohen B, et al. T cell-depleted autologous hematopoietic stem cell transplantation for multiple sclerosis: report on the first three patients. *Bone Marrow Transplant* 1998;21:537–541.

864. Shenoy S, Mohanakumar T, Todd G, et al. Immune reconstitution following allogeneic peripheral blood stem cell transplants. *Bone Marrow Transplant* 1999;23:335–346.

865. Martinez C, Urbano-Ispizua A, Rozman C, et al. Immune reconstitution following allogeneic peripheral blood progenitor cell transplantation: comparison of recipients of positive CD34+ selected grafts with recipients of unmanipulated grafts. *Exp Hematol* 1999;27:561–568.

866. Tyndall A, Gratwohl A. Hemopoietic blood and marrow transplants in the treatment of severe autoimmune disease. *Curr Opin Hematol* 1997;4:390–394.

867. Marmont AM. Stem cell transplantation for severe autoimmune diseases: progress and problems. *Haematologica* 1998;83:733–743.

868. Cooley HM, Snowden JA, Grigg AP, et al. Outcome of rheumatoid arthritis and psoriasis following autologous stem cell transplantation for hematologic malignancy. *Arthritis Rheum* 1997;40:1712–1715.

869. Jondeau K, Job-Deslandre C, Bouscary D, et al. Remission of nonerosive polyarthritis associated with Sjögren's syndrome after autologous hematopoietic stem cell transplantation for lymphoma. *J Rheumatol* 1997;24:2466–2468.

870. Berisso GA, van Lint MT, Bacigalupo A, et al. Adoptive autoimmune hyperthyroidism following allogeneic stem cell transplantation from an HLA-identical sibling with Graves' disease. *Bone Marrow Transplant* 1999;23:1091–1092.

871. Karthaus M, Gabrysiak T, Brabant G, et al. Immune thyroiditis after transplantation of allogeneic CD34+ selected peripheral blood cells. *Bone Marrow Transplant* 1997;20:697–699.

872. Marmont AM, Van Bekkum DW. Stem cell transplantation for severe autoimmune diseases: new proposals but still unanswered questions. *Bone Marrow Transplant* 1995;16:497–498.

873. Tyndall A, Black C, Finke J, et al. Treatment of systemic sclerosis with autologous haemopoietic stem cell transplantation [Letter; see Comments]. *Lancet* 1997;349:254.

874. Snowden JA, Kearney P, Kearney A, et al. Long-term outcome of autoimmune disease following allogeneic bone marrow transplantation. *Arthritis Rheum* 1998;41:453–459.

875. Euler HH, Marmont AM, Bacigalupo A, et al. Early recurrence or persistence of autoimmune diseases after unmanipulated autologous stem cell transplantation [see Comments]. *Blood* 1996;88:3621–3625.

876. Burt RK, Traynor AE, Pope R, et al. Treatment of autoimmune disease by intense immunosuppressive conditioning and autologous hematopoietic stem cell transplantation. *Blood* 1998;92:3505–3514.

877. Skoda RC, Tichelli A, Tyndall A, et al. Autologous peripheral blood stem cell transplantation in a patient with chronic autoimmune thrombocytopenia. *Br J Haematol* 1997;99:56–57.

878. Marmont AM, van Lint MT, Occhini D, et al. Failure of autologous stem cell transplantation in refractory thrombocytopenic purpura. *Bone Marrow Transplant* 1998;22:827–828.

*Textbook of the Autoimmune Diseases,*
Edited by R. G. Lahita, N. Chiorazzi, and W. H. Reeves,
Lippincott Williams & Wilkins, Philadelphia © 2000.

# CHAPTER 15

# Autoimmunity of the Gastrointestinal Tract

Józefa Węsierska-Gądek, Walter Reinisch, and Edward Penner

## MORPHOLOGY AND TERMINOLOGY OF CHRONIC GASTRITIS

The importance of classification of chronic gastritis is the causal relation of some cases to pernicious anemia, peptic ulcer, and adenocarcinoma. By identifying combinations of morphologic features, topographic distribution of the abnormalities and the association with other variables, it is possible to define different subtypes (1). Chronic atrophic gastritis is recognized macroscopically by the loss of gastric mucosal folds and thinning of the gastric mucosa layer. Depending on the localization of the lesions, the disease can be classified into two types. Type A autoimmune gastritis is restricted to the fundus and body of the stomach, whereas type B gastritis involves the antrum and comprises also the fundus and the body. Type A gastritis is associated with pernicious anemia, autoantibodies to gastric parietal cells, and to intrinsic factor, achlorhydria, low serum pepsinogen levels, and elevated serum gastrin concentrations. The latter results from hyperplasia of gastrin-producing cells. Type B gastritis is generally associated with the *Helicobacter pylori* infection accompanied by low serum gastrin concentrations because of destruction of the gastrin-producing cells. One of the cardinal histologic features of all subtypes is inflammation, which is primarily chronic (i.e., composed of lymphocytes and plasma cells). However, inflammation may have a variable acute component of neutrophils.

## PERNICIOUS ANEMIA

Pernicious anemia, the most common cause of vitamin $B_{12}$ deficiency, is of diverse pathophysiologic origins (2). The

J. Węsierska-Gądek: Department of Cell Cycle Regulation, University of Vienna, Institute of Tumor Biology—Cancer Research, A-1090 Vienna, Austria.

Walter Reinisch: Department of Gastroenterology and Hepatology, Fourth Department of Internal Medicine, University of Vienna, A-1090 Vienna, Austria.

Edward Penner: Fourth Department of Internal Medicine, University of Vienna, A-1090 Vienna, Austria.

term *pernicious anemia* applies solely to the conditions associated with chronic atrophic gastritis. Pernicious anemia, originally described by Thomas Addison in 1849, was linked to the stomach by Austin Flint in 1860 (3). The discovery of a serum inhibitor of intrinsic factors, later identified as an autoantibody to intrinsic factor (4), and of autoantibodies to parietal cells (5) led to the deduction that immunologic disturbances underlay the gastritis that causes pernicious anemia. The risk of gastric carcinoids seems to be high in this patient group compared with a normal population, but the lesions are mostly relatively benign tumors (6).

### Pathologic Findings

Gastric biopsy specimens from patients with pernicious anemia show a mononuclear cellular infiltrate in the submucosa extending into the lamina propria between the gastric glands. The infiltrate includes plasma cells, T cells, and a population of non-T cells. The infiltrating plasma cells contain autoantibodies to the antigen of parietal cells and to intrinsic factor (7,8).

### Clinical Manifestations

The median age at diagnosis of pernicious anemia is 60 years because of the late onset and slow progression of the disease (9). There is a slight prevalence of women. The usual presentation is linked with symptoms of anemia. The vitamin $B_{12}$ deficiency results in several abnormalities of the digestive tract, such as smooth and red tongue caused by atrophic glossitis, diarrhea, and megaloblastosis of the epithelial cells. Vitamin $B_{12}$ deficiency may cause peripheral neuropathy and lesions in the posterior and lateral columns of the spinal cord and cerebrum. These lesions progress from demyelination to axonal degeneration and neuronal death. The most frequent manifestations of peripheral neuropathy include paresthesias and numbness. The manifestations of lesions in the spinal cord are, for example, loss of position sense and sensory ataxia spasticity. Cerebral symptoms range from mild personality defects and memory loss to psychosis.

**Immunologic Manifestations**

The most important feature of pernicious anemia is the presence of circulating autoantibodies directed against parietal cells in more than 90% patients. The autoantigen was found as a microsomal component in sections of human gastric mucosa by means of immunofluorescence and complement fixation techniques. It was further localized to the microvilli of the parietal cells. Later, the gastric H$^+$/K$^+$-adenosine triphosphatase (ATPase) acid pump was demonstrated to constitute the major autoantigen of the parietal cell (10–13). The ATPases are a highly conserved family of proteins responsible for the ATP-dependent transport of ions across the membranes of mammalian cells that includes Na$^+$/K$^+$-ATPase and Ca$^{2+}$-ATPase. These enzymes have a highly conserved 100-kd catalytic subunit ($\alpha$) that undergoes phosphorylation during reaction cycles and have a 60- to 90-kd glycoprotein subunit ($\beta$). The $\alpha$ and $\beta$ subunits are required for the ATPase activity. One major parietal cell autoantigen recognized by the human antibodies is the $\alpha$ subunit of the gastric H$^+$/K$^+$-ATPase. A second major parietal cell antigen targeted by the human autoantibodies is a 60- to 90-kd glycoprotein (14). The antibodies inhibited the enzymatic activity of H$^+$/K$^+$-ATPase, and their binding site was reported to be located on the cytoplasmic side of H$^+$/K$^+$-ATPase.

The $\alpha$ and $\beta$ subunits of human H$^+$/K$^+$-ATPase were cloned, and their nucleotide sequences have been determined. This made it possible to apply recombinant DNA techniques for generation of recombinant peptides and to characterize the epitopes on human H$^+$/K$^+$-ATPase. The major epitope is located in the NH$_2$-terminal part of the $\alpha$ subunit between residues 360 and 525 on the cytosolic side of the secretory membrane (15). Gastric H$^+$/K$^+$-ATPase appears to be the only parietal cell antigen recognized by circulating parietal cell autoantibodies. Immunoblotting and immunoprecipitation experiments revealed reactivity solely within the two subunits of this ATPase.

Identification of gastric H$^+$/K$^+$-ATPase as the autoantigen raises a question about the role of the ATPase in the immunopathogenesis of the gastric lesions. Development of an animal model of autoimmune gastritis, organ-specific autoimmune disease, represents a new experimental approach that could bring more insights into the pathogenesis of this disorder. Murine autoimmune gastritis can be generated in susceptible mice strains after neonatal thymectomy, treatment of newborn mice with cyclosporine, or immunization with gastric H$^+$/K$^+$-ATPase (16). However, transgenic expression of the $\beta$ subunit of the ATPase prevents experimental induced gastritis. These findings suggest that autoimmune gastritis occurs only when pathogenic T cells are transferred to immunocompromised mice and that the pathogenic T cells have been rendered tolerant after overexpression of $\beta$ subunit.

The antiparietal cell antibody commonly found in pernicious anemia often occurs in subjects with gastritis who do not have pernicious anemia. Antibody to intrinsic factor (IF) rarely occurs in atrophic gastritis that is not accompanied by vitamin B$_{12}$ malabsorption, and it has been suggested that such cases represent a predisease state (17,18). For that reason, it is considered to be more specific marker for pernicious anemia than antiparietal cell antibody. IF is a protein that is produced by gastric parietal cells and binds to and facilitates the absorption of vitamin B$_{12}$. Antibodies to IF are found in serum of about 55% of patients with pernicious anemia, many of whom have such antibodies in gastric secretion. The role of IF antibodies in the development of pernicious anemia is not clear. Although they prevent IF-mediated vitamin B$_{12}$ absorption and are almost exclusively confined to patients with pernicious anemia, nearly half such patients do not have IF antibodies in serum or gastric juice, and there are no apparent differences between those with and those without IF antibodies. Southern blot analysis of genomic DNA from patients with congenital pernicious anemia (lacking IF) revealed normal restriction fragment patterns, suggesting that a sizable gene deletion was not responsible for the IF deficiency (19).

**Mechanism of Vitamin B$_{12}$ Malabsorption**

Gastric parietal cells produce IF, a 60-kd glycoprotein that can bind dietary vitamin B$_{12}$. The complex of vitamin B$_{12}$ and IF is transferred to the distal ileum, where it is absorbed after binding to the specific receptors on the luminal membranes. IF deficiency leads to the malabsorption of vitamin B$_{12}$. At least two mechanisms are responsible for the absence of IF. The progressive destruction and loss of parietal cells impairs its secretion. Autoantibodies present in the gastric juice can block the vitamin B$_{12}$ binding site of the IF and prevent complex formation. Because the vitamin B$_{12}$ is required for DNA replication, the vitamin B$_{12}$ deficiency affects most frequently organs exhibiting rapid cell turnover such as the gastrointestinal tract and the bone marrow.

**Diagnostic Approach**

Examination of the peripheral blood reveals macrocytosis with hypersegmented polymorphonuclear leukocytes, leukopenia, anemia, thrombocytopenia, or pancytopenia. Determination of B$_{12}$ and folate concentrations in serum is the first important diagnostic test followed by a Schilling test. A low B$_{12}$ concentration and normal folate level are characteristic for pernicious anemia. An elevated concentration of fasting serum gastrin and low pepsinogen level are associated with pernicious anemia (20). If the diagnosis is not definite proof, examination of a bone marrow aspirate is necessary. Megaloblastic hemopoiesis documented by the presence of megaloblasts and large myeloid precursors is characteristic of the disease (21).

## Therapy

The standard therapy is regular monthly intramuscular injections of at least 100 μg of vitamin $B_{12}$ to restore its deficiency. For elderly patients with gastric atrophy, taking tablets containing 25 μg to 1 mg of vitamin $B_{12}$ daily has been recommended to prevent $B_{12}$ deficiency. This treatment remedies the anemia and may correct the neurologic complications.

## ACHLORHYDRIA

Achlorhydria or diffuse antral gastritis in its pure form is not primarily atrophic but is characterized by a mixed acute and chronic mucosal inflammation. It tends not to extend beyond the antrum and is strongly associated with the presence of *H. pylori*. The gram-negative gastric pathogen causes lifelong infections leading to gastritis and to gastric and duodenal ulceration and mucosa-associated lymphoid tissue (MALT) lymphoma (1,22–24).

### Pathophysiologic Characteristics of *Helicobacter pylori*–Infected Patients

Patients with *H. pylori*–induced antigastric antibodies differ in a number of histopathologic parameters from those without autoimmune manifestations. They develop antigastric autoantibodies of various specificity, have increased numbers of T cells infiltrating the corpus glandular epithelium, have increased numbers of polymorphonuclear leukocytes invading the corpus, have an elevated epithelial apoptosis rate in the corpus, and have increased occurrence and severity of corpus atrophy (25–29). Moreover, the patients have increased blood gastrin levels, accompanied by decreased acid secretion and a lowered pepsinogen I : II ratio.

### Autoantibodies to Gastric–Mucosal Antigens

Infection with *H. pylori* induces autoantibodies reactive with gastric parietal cell canaliculi. Parietal cells secrete gastric acid by a mechanism involving the proton pump (i.e., the gastric $H^+/K^+$-ATP-ase), which is localized in the apical secretory canaliculi (30). It has been shown that *H. pylori* lipopolysaccharide (LPS) expresses Lewis x and y blood group antigens, which are also present on gastric epithelial cells (31). It seemed plausible that an initial event for the epitope specificity of *H. pylori*–induced autoantibodies is molecular mimicry (32,33). It has been reported that animals immunized or infected with *H. pylori* develop antibodies directed against *H. pylori* LPS, parietal $H^+/K^+$-ATPase (32), and Lewis x/y antigens (34). However, infected patients develop antibodies reacting with *H. pylori* LPS and native gastric $H^+/K^+$-ATPase but not with Lewis x/y antigens. Binding to gastric $H^+/K^+$-ATPase or to canaliculi was not abolished by preadsorption with *H. pylori* cells. These data indicate that the infected patients develop autoantibodies driven by gastric $H^+/K^+$-ATPase, not because of molecular mimicry (34).

Moreover, several sera recognize a 45-kd glycoprotein, probably IF, implicating epitope spreading to other autoantigens.

### Putative Pathogenesis of *Helicobacter pylori*–Induced Autoimmunity

Infection with *H. pylori* results in gastric mucosal influx of $CD4^+T$ cells and in a type 1 helper T-cell ($T_H1$) response. In the gastric tissue, increased levels of interferon-γ (IFN-γ), tumor necrosis factor-α (TNF-α), interleukin-12 (IL-12), and corresponding mRNAs were detected (35,36). *H. pylori* infection may induce IL-12, which is responsible for selection of IFN-γ–producing $T_H1$ cells. IFN-γ results in aberrant expression of major histocompatibility complex (MHC) class II molecules on gastric epithelium instead of on professional antigen-presenting cells. Increased MHC class II molecules stimulate enhanced presentation of autoantigens such as gastric $H^+/K^+$-ATPase, leading to activation of the immune cascade. After increased autoantigen presentation, autoreactive T cells become activated, inducing autoantibodies and resulting in destruction of glands, such as by execution of FAS-FASL–mediated apoptosis.

Induction of autoimmunity after infection is not unique feature of *H. pylori* but a common characteristic of many pathogens. For example, *Campylobacter jejuni* induces Guillain-Barré syndrome.

### Diagnostic Approach

Type B gastritis (37–40) is characterized by a regenatory epithelium, depletion of mucus, lymphoid follicles, intestinal metaplasia, and focal atrophy. Rod-like microorganisms corresponding to *H. pylori* are observed on the surface.

### Therapy

Treatment of *H. pylori* infection consists of proton pump inhibitors (PPIs) and antibiotics, most notably clarithromycin and metronidazole. PPI therapy is widely used, but long-term treatment with these drugs in subjects who are *H. pylori* positive may increase their risk of developing gastric cancer.

## AUTOIMMUNE HEPATITIS

### Classification

Autoimmune hepatitis (AIH) (41,42) is an inflammatory liver disease characterized histologically by a dense mononuclear cell infiltrate in the portal tract and serologically by the presence of non–organ- and liver-specific autoantibodies and increased levels of immunoglobulin G (Fig. 15.1).

AIH is associated with circulating antibodies to cellular components. On the basis of different autoantibodies specificities, AIH is subdivided into three groups (43–47). Type I AIH is associated with antibodies to nuclear (ANA) and/or smooth muscle (SMA) autoantigens, whereas type II AIH is

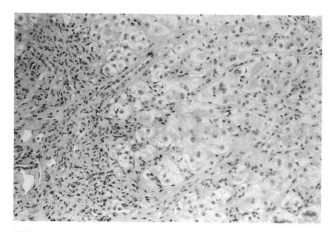

**FIG. 15.1.** Inflammatory reaction in autoimmune hepatitis (AIH).

characterized by antibodies to liver-kidney microsomal (LKM1) antigen. In addition, a substantial number of patients with AIH produce antibodies to a cytosolic soluble liver antigen (SLA) alone or in combination with ANA and/or SMA. Whether the latter patients represent a distinct AIH entity is controversial. However, this antibody had proved to be an extremely useful diagnostic marker and may help in identifying patients who are seronegative for other autoantibodies.

### Antinuclear Antibodies and Autoimmune Hepatitis

#### Heterogeneity of Antinuclear Antibodies

Patients with AIH spontaneously produce ANAs (45,48) that are directed against nucleic acids and various nuclear proteins of their own cells. Although the pathogenic role of such antibodies was not demonstrated, they represent specific disease markers and are useful biologic tools.

ANAs were initially recognized by the LE cell test and now can be easily detected by indirect immunofluorescence microscopy using tissue preparations as a substrate. Commercially available Hep-2 cells are most frequently used for routine screening for ANAs. The application of uniformly prepared cultured cell substrates or tissue sections from manufacturers offers the possibility to standardize the testing for ANAs. In the case of a positive reaction, the titer of ANAs after the sequential serum dilution can be determined, and the staining pattern can be clearly analyzed.

The frequency of ANAs in AIH is about 70% of cases at the time of presentation according to the earlier (42) and later studies (48). However, these data should be carefully considered regarding the results of a study of International Union of Immunological Societies (IUIS) Standardization Committee (49). According to this report, the ranges of frequencies of ANA positivity on Hep-2 cells for normal subjects strongly depends on serum dilution (49). The respective frequencies at serum dilution of 1 : 40, 1 : 80, 1 : 160, and 1 : 320 were 32%, 13%, 5%, and 3%, respectively, demonstrating the critical balance between sensitivity and specificity of the tests at different di-

lutions. The interpretation of the ANA frequency in AIH should be made in light of the previously described study findings to avoid overestimation.

The immunofluorescent patterns exhibited by ANA-positive human sera vary from homogenous, speckled, centromere, rimlike, and nuclear dots to nucleolar and may indicate the subcellular localization of target antigens (Fig. 15.2). In the case of a characteristic staining pattern such as rimlike or nucleolar, it can be expected that the autoantibodies are directed against constituents of the corresponding subnuclear structure as nuclear envelope or nucleoli. Homogenous or speckled nuclear staining is less informative, because these types of reactivity are common for several nuclear antigens. Moreover, most autoimmune sera are heterogeneous and contain different antibodies, resulting in overlapping staining patterns.

Indirect immunofluorescence is an easy and rapid assay for the detection of autoantibodies in the clinical routine, but it is not suitable for identification of responsive antigens. For this purpose, two other methods are employed: immunoblotting (often called Western blotting) and immunoprecipitation. Although both methods make use of electrophoresis and allow determination of the size and optionally charge of autoantigens, they are not equivalent but rather complementary. During immunoblotting assay, antigens immobilized on membrane are at least partially denatured, whereas immunoprecipitation tests are performed with native antigens. Other methods such as enzyme-linked immunosorbent assay (ELISA) or immunodots are also available. Although they are sensitive, they show greater variability than other assays (50). The quality of the antigen used as its purity or lack of proteolytic degradation cannot be directly verified. Because of these important limitations, both methods seem to be more suitable for quantitative estimations than for qualitative determinations.

The presence of circulating ANAs is one of the diagnostic criteria for AIH. ANAs are a heterogeneous group of antibodies (51,52) that are also detectable in other liver disorders. Four major groups of ANAs have been described in patients with AIH: anti-DNA, antihistones, antinucleoprotein particles, and antinonhistone proteins. For a better understanding of the properties and physiologic function of the autoantibodies, it is advisable to characterize their corresponding antigens.

### Anti-DNA Antibodies

Most cellular DNA occurs in the nucleus in form of complexes with various structural and regulatory proteins. Naked DNA is susceptible to degradation by endogenous nucleases or mechanical injury, and the formation of complexes with proteins protects DNA from them. Native DNA occurs mostly as a double-stranded helix and adopts different higher-order conformations, of which the B structure is the most common. Complex formation with nuclear proteins may alter the conformation of DNA. There are many DNA-binding proteins. Among these structural proteins are some such as the histones that bind nucleic acids independent of

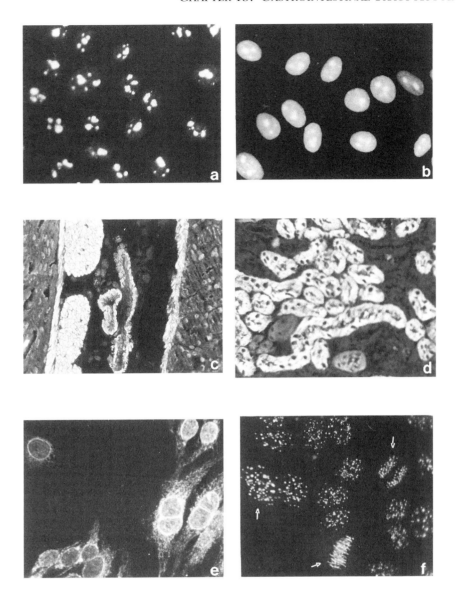

**FIG. 15.2.** Immunofluorescence patterns exhibited by autoimmune hepatitis sera. For detection of autoantibodies, HEp-2 cells **(A, E, F)**, HeLa cells **(B)**, or rodent tissue preparations were used. **A:** Nucleolar staining pattern. **B:** Homogenous plus nucleolar pattern. **C:** Pattern shown by antismooth muscle antibodies (SMAs). **D:** liver-kidney microsomal (LKM) antigen. **E:** Rimlike pattern. **F:** Centromere pattern, with cells in different stages of the cell cycle *(arrows)*.

sequence, and there are proteins that bind to specific sequences of DNA.

The classic B conformation is considered to be weakly immunogenic or nonimmunogenic. Immunogenic nucleic acid forms include single-stranded DNA and RNA, RNA-DNA hybrids (duplexes and triplexes) and Z-DNA. Modified DNA, such as methylated or carcinogen-substituted DNA, and DNA-protein complexes are thought to be potent immunogens (51,52).

There are two main types of anti-DNA antibodies (53–55). Antibodies targeting single-stranded DNA (ssDNA) recognize pyrimidine and purine bases in denatured DNA and are not reactive with double-stranded DNA (dsDNA). The lack

of reactivity with dsDNA is not surprising, because the bases are not accessible in native DNA. A second type of antibodies representing those reactive with dsDNA recognizes primarily the sugar-phosphate backbone and therefore is able to bind dsDNA or ssDNA.

Anti-DNA antibodies, found primarily in persons with systemic lupus erythematosus (SLE) (53–55) and implicated in the pathogenesis of the disease, were also observed in patients with AIH. Several studies have determined the frequency of anti-dsDNA antibodies in AIH (56,57).

Studies in the 1970s, based on liquid or solid phase immunoassays and commercial sources of antigen, ascertained a high frequency of positivity for anti-dsDNA in AIH patients, but positive results were also obtained for those with other liver disorders. Because the specificity of these assays depends strongly on the quality of the antigen used, it is impossible to exclude the possibility that even negligible contamination with ssDNA could lead to overestimation because of nonspecific reactivity. When more specific immunoassays for anti-dsDNA antibodies, such as Farr-type radioimmunoassays, membrane filtration, or *Crithidia luciliae* immunofluorescence, were used alone or in combination (58–60), the positivity rate was about 10% for AIH cases. In a later study (61), the frequency of anti-DNA antibodies in AIH determined by ELISA was about 50% (56 of 99 patients). Moreover, anti-DNA antibodies were detected in persons with chronic hepatitis B. The frequency and titers of anti-DNA antibodies of the IgG class in patients with AIH and chronic hepatitis B were similar. Mortality and response to therapy were not related to the presence or absence of these autoantibodies.

Anti-dsDNA antibodies occur seldom in AIH. Earlier assays and ELISA results tended to overestimate the frequency of positive results. Because the patients with or without antibodies could not be distinguished by clinical, histologic, and biochemical criteria, it has been suggested that the presence of anti-dsDNA antibodies in AIH is a nonspecific manifestation of inflammation.

### Antihistone Antibodies

Histones are abundant, highly conserved nuclear proteins (62). Because of the high content of arginine and lysine residues, they are positively charged and bind to DNA in chromatin in a sequence-independent mode. Histone proteins are involved in compacting DNA and formation of primary and higher-order chromatin structure. Five main classes of histones—H1, H2A, H2B, H3, and H4—occur in the nucleus in a highly organized nucleosomal structure (63). Each nucleosomal particle, representing the smallest chromatin unit, consists of about 200 base pairs of DNA wrapped twice around a histone core, which contains two of each of the H2A, H2B, H4, and H4 histones in an octameric configuration. The H1 histones are associated with linker DNA at sites where DNA enters and exits core particles and connects one nucleosome to the next. Moreover, because of its cooperative binding, histone H1 is involved in formation of higher-order chromatin structure.

The primary structure of molecules may vary within each of the five classes of histone proteins. H1 is most heterogeneous of the histones, encompassing multiple H1 subtypes. The expression of distinct H1 subtypes and their relative concentrations differs in tissue- and species-specific manner and varies during differentiation and throughout development (64,65). All H1 subtypes possess three structurally distinct domains. A central globular domain consisting of 75 amino acids is the most conserved and is flanked by randomly coiled amino- and carboxyl-terminal parts. The carboxyl-terminal segment, rich in lysine, alanine, and proline, is highly basic. The heterogeneity of H1 histone proteins may be of func-

tional importance in that the several H1 variants differentially regulate formation of the higher-order chromatin structure (65). The remaining histones occur also as subtypes. The variability of their primary structure has been determined. The major antigenic determinants in histones are known to occur in the variable regions of the amino and carboxyl termini (65–67). Because the regions are exposed on the surface of nucleosomes and are accessible to antibodies, the native chromatin structures may act as immunogens.

Autoantibodies to all classes of histone proteins are frequently found in autoimmune diseases and seem to be a characteristic feature of idiopathic and drug-induced SLE (66–69). With immunofluorescence, human sera positive for histones exhibit a homogenous nuclear staining pattern (Fig. 15.2B) correlating with the chromatin distribution. Antihistone antibodies in the free or DNA-complexed form have been detected in AIH patients' sera (70–72). The incidence of antihistone antibodies ranges from 25% to 35% (70–72). A detailed analysis using individual histones revealed the reactivity of AIH sera with all histones, but H2B was most prevalent. In one report, antihistone-positive cases were accompanied by active disease and associated with sicca syndrome (72). The available data indicate that antihistone antibodies are not a specific feature of AIH and are instead randomly generated in the course of inflammatory processes in the liver.

### Antibodies to Nonhistone Proteins

*Centromere Proteins.* Antibodies to centromere proteins exhibit (ACAs) an anticentromere staining pattern by immunofluorescence (73–75). The centromere plays a major role in segregation of eukaryotic chromosomes in mitosis by serving as the site for chromatid attachment and kinetochore assembly (76). A characteristic feature of the anticentromere antibodies (ACAs) is differential staining pattern of the interphase and mitotic cells that helps distinguish them from other autoantibodies.

The antibodies recognize at least three well-defined centromere proteins—CENP-A (17 kd), CENP-B (80 kd), and CENP-C (140 kd)—as shown by immunoblotting with human nuclear proteins or by ELISA and using purified recombinant proteins (75,77,78). These centromere antigens are DNA-binding proteins; a sequence-specific DNA activity has been found only for CENP-B (79). CENP-B, located in the central domain of the centromere, possess a DNA-binding domain in the $NH_2$ terminus and dimerization domain in the COOH terminus (80). CENP-C is a highly basic protein located in the inner kinetochore plate, playing an important role in the assembly of centromere (75,81). CENP-A protein shows a high degree of sequence identity with histone H3 and shares with it a similar organization (75,82–84).

ACAs occur frequently in scleroderma (70% to 80%) and are characteristic of the CREST syndrome (*c*alcinosis, *R*aynaud's phenomenon, *e*sophageal hypomotility, *s*clerdactyly, *t*elangiectasias). The frequency of ACA estimated by immunofluorescence, ELISA, or both assays was about 40% in cases of AIH. However, in our experience, the ACA determinations based solely on immunofluorescence (Fig. 15.2F) are not sufficiently substantiated by ELISA, and because of extreme variation, we were not able to reproduce the results (i.e., high percentage of anit–ACA-antibodies). This discrepancy can be explained by the overestimation if evaluation was based solely on immunofluorescence or ELISA. In our experience, the ACA determinations based solely on immunofluorescence pattern are not sufficiently substantiated and commercially available ELISA tests gave extremely varying results.

*Antilamin Antibodies.* Antibodies directed against nuclear lamins give a characteristic peripheral nuclear staining pattern by immunofluorescence, which is designated as rimlike (Fig. 15.2E). This type of reactivity indicates that antibodies recognize components of the nuclear envelope (85–87), but it does not detail the reactive antigens. The nuclear envelope, a supramolecular structure of interphase nucleus in eukaryotic cells, separates the nucleus from the cytoplasm (85–87). The most important function of the nuclear envelope is to give support for chromatin organized in the loops and to regulate exchange of macromolecules between the nucleus and cytoplasm.

The nuclear envelope consists of three morphologically and functionally distinct components: outer and inner nuclear membranes, the pore complexes, and the nuclear lamina. The outer nuclear membrane is connected with the rough endoplasmic reticulum. The outer and inner nuclear membranes are joined at multiple sites, where the nuclear pore complexes are anchored. At the nucleoplasmic side of the inner membrane, the nuclear lamina is attached.

The nuclear lamina, a proteinaceous meshwork, is composed of a relatively small number of proteins, which have been called lamins (85). Depending on the cell type and differentiation state, this structure contains one to six polypeptides that are immunologically related (85,88). In most terminally differentiated mammalian cells, three major lamins (A, B, and C) are commonly expressed in nearly equimolar concentrations. The nuclear lamins have similar sizes, ranging from 60 to 70 kd. Sequence analysis of complementary DNA encoding lamin A and C revealed that these two proteins have identical primary structures up to the amino acid in position 566, and they differ only in the carboxyl terminus (89,90). Six terminal amino acids are unique for lamin C, whereas lamin A is extended at the carboxyl terminus for an additional fragment of 98 residues. Although lamin B gives a tryptic peptide map distinct from that of lamins A and C, it is structurally homologous to the latter. The nuclear lamins share structural homology with intermediate filaments (90). The nuclear lamins form in the interphase nucleus a highly polymerized network anchored at the inner side of the nuclear membrane.

Dramatic structural reorganization of the lamina occurs during mitosis, when it is transiently and reversibly disassembled in the early prophase (85). The lamins become dispersed throughout the cytoplasm and lose their association with chromosomes concomitant with disintegration of the nuclear envelope. When the nuclear envelope reforms during telophase, the lamins progressively polymerize and reassemble. Disassembly and reformation of the nuclear lamina network is mediated by a sequential hyperphosphorylation and dephosphorylation cycles of some of the nuclear lamins (85,91).

Autoantibodies to nuclear lamins have occurred in sera of patients with various autoimmune diseases (92–96). Although the characteristic peripheral staining of the nucleus is indicative for the presence of antilamin autoantibodies, their identity can be conclusively proved by immunoblotting using nuclear pore complexes–lamina fraction or purified nuclear lamins as antigen source. Antilamin antibodies were first described in sporadic cases of a heterogeneous group of patients with linear scleroderma, SLE, and neutropenia (92,93). We have observed such antibodies primarily in AIH (94). In our study comprising 51 patients with AIH and 37 cases of primary biliary cirrhosis (PBC), antilamin antibodies were found in 23% of AIH patients but only in a few cases of PBC. This low incidence in PBC was reminiscent of the sporadic occurrence of antilamin antibodies in systemic rheumatic disease. The antilamin seropositivity was ascertained by immunoblotting after one- and two-dimensional separation of antigens. The use of stringent conditions during immunoblotting allowed detection of high-affinity antibodies and eliminated the risk of the overestimation of positivity. AIH sera reacted preferentially with lamins A and C. Antibodies directed against all three lamins or against lamin B occurred less frequently. Antilamin antibodies in AIH were restricted to the patients with active disease. The relatively high frequency of antilamin antibodies in AIH was confirmed by other groups (95,96).

The occurrence of antibodies directed against the minor constituent of nuclear lamina, lamin $B_2$, in sera of AIH patients has been described (97). The reactivity with four distinct domains of lamin $B_2$ was examined in detail and compared with that exhibited by sera of patients with autoimmune rheumatic disorders. Most of the tested AIH sera were reactive with at least two domains of lamin $B_2$, including the carboxyl-terminal region. None of them recognized a fragment encompassing the nuclear localization sequence that is less conserved and rather specific for lamin $B_2$. Sera of patients with autoimmune rheumatic diseases mostly recognized only one domain. Some differences in the specificity between distinct disorders could be observed. These findings suggest that recognition of particular lamin protein domains by antibodies in patients' sera differs with pathology.

### Microsomal Autoantigens in Autoimmune Hepatitis

In 1973, Rizetto et al. (98) described an autoantibody in sera from a small percentage of AIH patients that stained the proximal renal tubes and the cytoplasm of hepatocytes in rat kidney and liver sections and was detected by indirect immunofluorescence (Fig. 15.2D). The staining pattern differed from that of antimitochondrial antibodies (AMAs). Because the highest reactivity was observed with microsomal fraction, these autoantibodies were defined as liver-kidney microsomal (LKM) antibodies (98–101). The reactive antigen was characterized by immunoblotting using proteins of isolated human microsomes as antigen. Analysis of immunoblots performed with AIH sera that were LKM positive by immunofluorescence revealed a 50-kd protein as the major antigen (102,103). Further screening of human liver cDNA libraries combined with immunoprecipitation led to identification of human cytochrome P450 2D6 (CYP2D6) as the main 50-kd microsomal antigen (104,105), called LKM1. Incubation of native sera or affinity-purified LKM1 antibodies with isolated microsomes or recombinant cytochrome CYP2D6 protein resulted in the inhibition of enzymatic activity, thereby indicating that circulating LKM1 antibodies may impair enzyme function (106).

CYP2D6 is a member of a drug-metabolizing enzyme superfamily (107,108) that is responsible for the metabolism of different types of agents, including β-blocking agents, antidepressants, antiarrhythmics, and antihypertensive drugs such as debrisoquine. Human liver CYP2D6 is an enzyme form that metabolizes debrisoquine and several other drugs subjected to the same genetic polymorphism. About 10% of the Caucasian population fails to express CYP2D6 in the liver and consequently shows a deficiency for drug metabolism mediated by that enzyme. The lack of enzyme expression was caused by defective alleles (109).

The immunodominant B-cell epitope of CYP2D6 has been localized within a linear sequence of 8 amino acids in the CYP2D6 molecule (110). The sequence of this epitope is highly conserved for class 2D cytochrome P450s. LKM1 antibodies are restricted to the immunoglobulin subclasses IgG1 and IgG4. Anti-CYP2D6 antibodies were found in patients with idiopathic AIH.

Although the CYP2D6 is mainly localized in microsomes, there are some lines of evidence that this enzyme is at least partially anchored in the hepatocyte plasma membrane. First indications came from Lenzi et al. (111), who showed that a LKM-positive AIH serum stained by immunofluorescence methods the surface of isolated rabbit hepatocytes. A similar observation for human hepatocytes was made by Loeper et al. (112,113). Moreover, they isolated the plasma membrane fraction from human hepatocytes and examined it for the presence of CYPs. The specific content of CYP in plasma membrane was 9% of that in microsomes. The anchorage of a small portion of cellular CYPs in the human hepatocyte plasma membrane seems to be specific and not caused by microsomal contamination. The activities of two specific markers of the endoplasmatic reticulum—NADPH-cytochrome c reductase and glucose-6-phosphatase—in the plasma membrane fraction were less than 1% of their respective specific activities in microsomal fraction, excluding microsomal contamination. Several CYP forms (1A2, 2C, 2D6, 2E1, and 3A4) were detected among plasma membrane proteins by immunoblotting techniques. The CYP in the plasma membrane fraction was complete, consisting of its protein and its heme moiety.

From the immunofluorescence assay and immunoperoxidase labeling, it is clear that at least some CYP epitopes are exposed on the outer surface of plasma membrane. Anti-LKM human sera and anti-CYP2D6 rabbit polyclonal antibodies recognize plasma membrane CYP2D6 in situ. This finding may have important implications. Functional plasma membrane CYPs may form reactive metabolites that covalently bind to these and other proteins. CYP modified by the covalent binding of reactive metabolites represents a new antigen and may trigger the formation of anti-CYP antibodies. Because of the CYP2D6 epitope presentation on the outer surface of hepatocytes, specific autoantibodies may be generated that participate with cytotoxic T cells in the immunologic destruction of hepatocytes in some forms of AIH.

Although CYP2D6 is the most prevalent antigen recognized by anti-LKM1 sera, a minor group of patients react with microsomal antigens that differ from CYP2D6. Another anti-LKM autoantibody exhibiting a slightly different staining pattern in liver and kidney sections was found in hepatitis cases caused by the diuretic drug ticrynafen (tienilic acid) (114,115) and was designated LKM2. This type of drug-induced hepatitis is mainly restricted to some countries, such as France and the United States, in which ticrynafen has been prescribed. These anti-LKM2 autoantibodies are directed against a human liver CYP2C9, which selectively transforms tienilic acid into a reactive metabolite. After withdrawal of the drug, the liver disease decreased, and the titers of anti-LKM2 antibodies markedly declined.

LKM3 antibodies, originally reported to occur in about 10% of patients with chronic hepatitis D (116), were also found in some patients with AIH (117). Anti-LKM3 antibodies recognize an antigen of about 55-kd and pI 8.0, which is expressed at low concentration in neonatal liver and which is easily inducible by agents such as phenobarbital and dioxin. Screening of a human liver cDNA library led to identification of cDNA encoding the LKM3 antigen (117). The sequence of this cDNA was highly homologous with that of uridine diphosphate-glucoronosyltransferase (UGT) of family 1. Characterization of the autoepitope revealed that most anti-LKM3–positive sera react with the carboxyl-terminal part of the enzyme (118). The carboxyl-terminal domain of UGT is encoded by exons 2 through 5, which are common to all members of family 1 UGTs. Using recombinant UGT expressed in a baculovirus system, an enzyme immunoassay was developed. Determination of the autoantibodies' specificity revealed that anti-UGT antibodies in chronic hepatitis D differ from those of the genuine AIH in that the titers are lower and that they recognize different epitopes. Anti-UGT–positive AIH sera react exclusively with family 1 UGTs. A subset of AIH patients develop autoantibodies to both microsomal antigens: CYP2D6 and UGT.

Another type of antimicrosomal autoantibody, reacting with the endoplasmic reticulum of liver preparations but not with that of kidney sections and therefore called antiliver microsome (anti-LM) autoantibody, was detected in patients with dihydralazine-induced hepatitis (119). These antibodies are directed against human liver CYP1A2, an enzyme involved in the metabolic activation of dihydralazine. The anti-LKM antibodies associated with ethanol-induced hepatitis recognize the hydroxyethyl radical-CYP2E1 adducts (120).

### Soluble Liver Antigen

Many AIH patients have antibodies directed against cytosolic SLA (121). SLA was originally defined as a nonspecies, non–organ-specific antigen despite its highest concentration in liver and kidney (121). According to the published protocol (121,122), it was isolated from rat liver as a 150,000 g supernatant after extensive ultracentrifugation of a homogenate. SLA is a heterogeneous fraction consisting of at least a hundred extremely soluble proteins. Wächter et al. (123) reported that anti-SLA–positive AIH sera preferentially react with cytokeratins 8 and 18 and proposed that both cytokeratins are target antigens in SLA. Cytokeratins are expressed in a cell- and tissue-specific manner (124,125), and as members of an intermediate-filament family, they are poorly soluble. This property is routinely used for isolation of cytokeratins, which are readily pelleted after centrifugation for 20 minutes at 3500 g, even in the presence of nonionic detergents and high salt concentrations. Because the protocol used for isolation of SLA is based on extensive ultracentrifugation steps that allow the separation of organelles and cytoskeleton from soluble cytosol proteins, it seems unlikely that cytokeratins represent the target antigens. We characterized SLA and showed that the major antigen belongs to the superfamily of glutathione *S*-transferase (GST) (126), multifunctional enzymes with similar or overlapping specificities (127,128). By microsequencing of the reactive protein spots, at least three distinct GST subunits (Ya, $Yb_1$, and Yc) between 25 and 27-kd were identified as antigen targets. Further analysis with affinity purified GSTs revealed that 25 of 31 SLA-positive AIH cases reacted with the enzyme. When tested with isolated GSTs, the various titers of antibodies and different reactivities of individual sera toward distinct GST subtypes became apparent. The differential reactivity of the sera with subunits suggests that autoantibodies can distinguish epitopes characteristic for distinct variants and offers evidence for determinant spreading rather that epitope cross-reactivity.

GSTs constitute more than 5% of the total liver proteins (127) that can be extracted from the rat liver and are extremely soluble. GSTs are involved in hepatic detoxification of cytotoxic compounds and carcinogens, and they act as carrier proteins in biliary secretion (127,128). Aside from the catalytic role, the enzymes may be considered as binding proteins that prevent genotoxic agents from interacting with DNA. Mammalian GSTs are encoded by at least four gene families; cytosolic GSTs appear to be products of three families, whereas microsomal GST is genetically distinct (127). The importance of this enzyme family in the function of healthy liver makes them an interesting target for a liver disease–specific antigen. It cannot be excluded that these enzymes become exposed or released or that there is an alteration in synthesis in response to liver damage during initiation of disease (129).

### Diagnostic Approach

No disease manifestations are pathognomonic of AIH, and its diagnosis requires the confident exclusion of other conditions. AIH has been defined as an unresolved, predominantly periportal hepatitis that is usually accompanied by hypergammaglobulinemia and tissue autoantibodies and that is responsive to immunosuppressive therapy in most instances. Because these criteria do not enable a simple diagnosis of AIH, the International Hepatitis Group put forward a set of findings necessary for the diagnosis of AIH (46) (Table 15.1).

### Therapy

Not all patients with a diagnosis of AIH need therapy. Treatment benefits have been established for patients with severe disease, but treatment guidelines are lacking for individuals with minimal or no symptoms. Prednisolone with or without azathioprine is effective in the management of AIH. Combination therapy is generally preferred, because it is associated with fewer side effects than monotherapy with prednisolone. Basically, treatment starts with 30 mg of prednisolone plus 50 mg of azathioprine daily, and the dosage is then reduced according to the liver function tests. In the monotherapy regimen, prednisolone is started at 60 mg daily. With this regimen, remission is achieved in two thirds of patients after 2 years of therapy.

## PRIMARY BILIARY CIRRHOSIS

PBC is a chronic liver disease that occurs predominantly in women. It is characterized by obliteration of small intrahepatic bile ducts and portal inflammation leading to fibrosis and eventually to cirrhosis (130–133) (Fig. 15.3). Although the disease is far less prevalent than viral and alcoholic liver disorders, it represents one of the most common indications for liver transplantation worldwide.

The cause of PBC remains obscure. It may develop in a susceptible individual after exposure to an environmental trigger. Common presenting symptoms are pruritus, nonspecific complaints such as lethargy, and right upper quadrant pain; less frequently, patients have signs of hepatic failure, such as ascites, jaundice, variceal and bleeding. PBC evolves through four stages: an asymptomatic state in patients with normal liver function test results (PBC is suspected by demonstration of antimitochrondrial antibodies), asymptomatic patients with abnormal liver test results, symptomatic patients, and those with decompensated disease.

Since PBC was first regarded as an immune-mediated disease, research has focused on the role of autoantibodies in the pathogenesis of this enigmatic disease (134–136). Using complement fixation and then indirect immunofluorescence tests, it was recognized that almost all patients with PBC pro-

**TABLE 15.1.** *Diagnostic criteria for autoimmune hepatitis*

| Definite autoimmune hepatitis | Probable autoimmune hepatitis |
|---|---|
| Normal serum alpha$_1$-antitrypsin,[a] copper and ceruloplasmin[a] levels | Abnormal serum copper or ceruloplasmin levels but Wilson's disease excluded |
| Seronegativity of IgM anti-HAV, HBsAg,[a] IgM anti-HBc,[a] and anti-HCV[a] (RIBA nonreactive) | Anti-HCV may be present but not active true infection |
| Seronegativity for cytomegalovirus and Epstein–Barr virus | Same requirement |
| No parenteral blood exposure | Same requirement |
| Average ethanol ingestion <35 g daily for men and 25 g for women | <50 g daily for men and 40 g daily for women |
| No recent use of hepatotoxic drugs | Recent use but active disease after drug withdrawal |
| Any serum aminotransferase[a] abnormality (must exceed alkaline phosphatase[a] elevation) | Same requirement |
| Gamma globulin,[a] IgG, or total globulin level >1.5 times normal | Any elevation acceptable |
| SMA,[a] ANA,[a] or anti-LKM1[a] >1:80 in adults or 1:20 in children | Titers at least 1:40 in adults and 1:10 in children |
| Liver biopsy examination[a] showing moderate-to-severe piecemeal necrosis with or without lobular hepatitis or central–portal bridging necrosis | Seronegativity acceptable if other liver-related autoantibodies are present |
| No biliary lesions, granulomas, copper deposition, or other features suggesting different diagnosis | Same histologic requirements |

ANA, antinuclear antibodies; HBsAG, hepatitis B surface antigen; HCV, hepatitis C virus; LKM1, liver–kidney microsomal antigen; SMA, smooth muscle antigens.

[a] Denotes most cost-effective tests for diagnosis in adults.

duce autoantibodies that are not organ or species specific and that are directed against mitochondrial antigens (134–136). Later, these PBC-associated AMAs were shown to react with trypsin-sensitive antigens on the inner mitochondrial membrane (135); they were designated as M2 antigens. Moreover, sera of approximately 50% of PBC patients contain antibodies to nuclear structures. When viewed by means of indirect immunofluorescence microscopy, two distinct antibody staining patterns can be identified, those showing staining of the nuclear periphery (rimlike pattern) and another group exhibiting multiple nuclear dots.

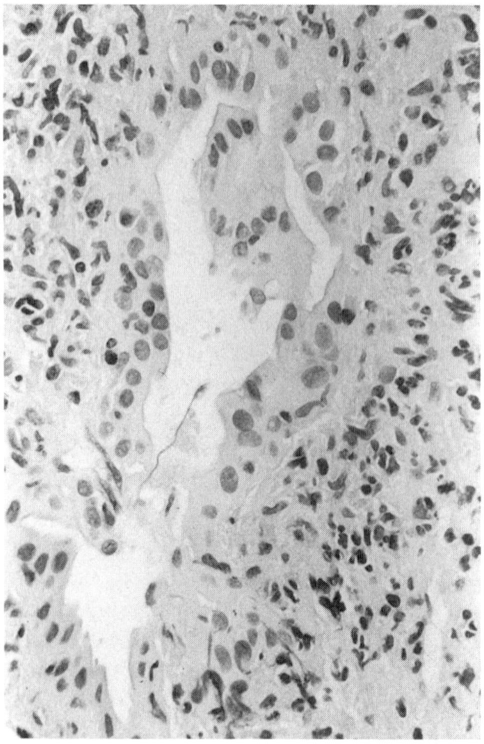

**Antimitochondrial Antibodies**

AMAs provide the major criterion in the diagnosis of PBC. They are routinely detected by indirect immunofluorescence tests and can be further characterized by immunoblotting and ELISA. Immunofluorescence is typically performed using Hep-2 cells or commercially available rodent tissue sections (Fig. 15.4). The indirect immunofluorescence test for AMA have serious drawbacks. While recognizing the positivity or negativity for AMA, it tells nothing about the antigen targets. In some cases, interpretation of staining patterns is difficult because of nonspecific findings or the presence of other antibodies, resulting in overlapping patterns. Other anticytoplasmatic antibodies that are frequently confused with AMA are antibodies to CYP2D6. To unequivocally identify the autoantibodies, an immunoblotting test using mitochondrial preparations is the method of choice. Immunoblotting experiments demonstrate that there is usually reactivity with one or more mitochondrial autoantigens; a 74-kd protein is most frequently recognized (137,138). Other antigens of different molecular masses (i.e., 56, 48, 41, and 36-kd) were less common.

In the late 1980s, the cloning and sequencing of a cDNA selected by screening a rat liver cDNA library with sera from PBC patients led to identification of the mitochondrial antigens (139–142). The targets of AMAs are members of a functionally related enzyme family, the 2-oxo-acid dehydrogenase complex (2-OADC), that includes the E2 subunits of the pyruvate dehydrogenase complex (PDC), the branched-chain 2-oxo-acid dehydrogenase complex (BCOADC) and

**FIG. 15.3.** Histologic appearance of a liver biopsy sample from a patient with primary biliary cirrhosis.

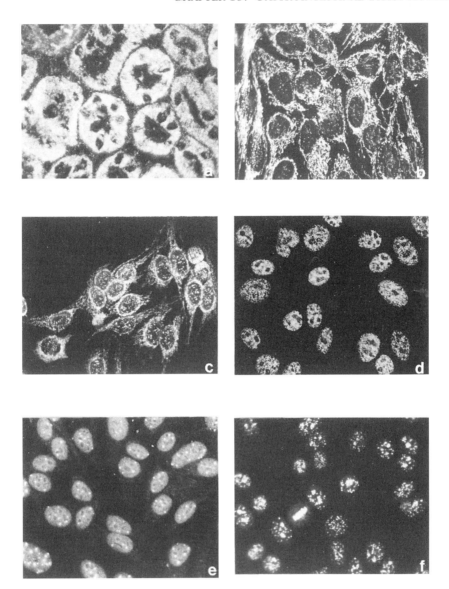

**FIG. 15.4.** Immunofluorescence patterns displayed by sera from patients with primary biliary cirrhosis (PBC). For detection of autoantibodies, rodent tissue preparations **(A)** or HEp-2 cells **(B–F)** were used. **A, B:** Antimitochondrial antibodies. **C:** Staining pattern shown by anti-gp210–specific serum. **D:** Speckled staining pattern. **E:** Nuclear dots stained by anti-Sp-100–positive PBC serum. **F:** Anticentromere staining.

the 2-oxoglutarate dehydrogenase complex (2-OGDC). Some sera also recognize the E1α subunit of the pyruvate dehydrogenase complex and protein X. Each of the enzyme complexes consists of three subunits E1, E2, and E3. These three 2-OADCs have key roles in intermediary metabolism, and their E2 components are highly conserved in evolution. The E2 components of different complexes exhibit a high degree of structural homology. PBC sera do not always react with all mitochondrial autoantigens; the pattern of reactivity tends to differ from patient to patient. The specificity of AMAs displayed by PBC sera is summarized in Table 15.2. It is

**TABLE 15.2.** *Specificity of antimitochondrial antibodies in primary biliary cirrhosis sera*

| Antigen | Molecular weight | Reactivity (%) |
|---|---|---|
| PDC-E2 | 74 | 92 |
| BCOADC-E2 | 56 | 54 |
| OGDC-E2 | 48 | 66 |
| Protein X | 52 | ? |
| PDC-E1α | 41 | 66 |
| PDC-E1β | 36 | 1–7 |

remarkable that the PBC sera predominantly recognize the E2 component of each enzyme complex, which is a lipoamide acetyltransferase for the PDC and BCOADC and a succinyl transferase for the OGDC, probably because of their homology. Three-dimensional structure of the E2 component of PDC offered insights into the mode of autoimmune recognition (143).

In addition to indirect immunofluorescence and immunoblotting, ELISA using recombinant mitochondrial antigens has been successfully employed in the serologic diagnosis of PBC (144,145). ELISA permits screening of a large number of specimens and has proved to be highly sensitive and specific. Moreover, the use of "designer molecules," different antigens exposed as single hybrid proteins, permits testing of multiple sera for antigen and epitope specificity in a highly efficient way (145).

There are, however, several caveats in AMA testing. Almost 10% of PBC patients are negative for AMAs; for them, the diagnosis still rests on the clinical features, biochemistry, and histologic findings. Neither positivity for AMA nor its titer relate to the severity of disease and cannot be applied in the follow-up of the clinical course.

## Antimitochondrial Antibodies and Disease

Despite characterization of the mitochondrial autoantigens, it remains difficult to reconcile their role within the disease process, a granulomatous destruction that is limited to the small intrahepatic bile ducts. Several hypotheses have been put forward to explain the possible participation of AMAs in the pathogenesis of PBC. One possibility includes the abnormal expression of mitochondrial proteins on bile duct epithelial cells, and another postulates an abnormal translocation of the 2-OADC enzymes. The most attractive hypothesis favors abnormal expression of pyruvate dehydrogenase or a cross-reactive molecule in the involved segments of the bile ducts.

## Antibodies Against Constituents of the Nuclear Pores

Nuclear pore complexes are integral components of a nuclear envelope, a proteinaceous structure separating the nucleus from the cytoplasm (146). The nuclear pores, morphologically and functionally distinct from other components of the nuclear envelope, consist of several proteins, with glycoproteins being the most frequent constituents (147,148). PBC sera exhibiting a rimlike staining pattern can recognize proteins of the nuclear envelope (149–151). About one third of PBC patients develop autoantibodies against glycoprotein 210 (gp210), an integral member of the nuclear pores (152,153). "Mature" gp210 is composed of three main domains (154–157). A large 1,783–amino acid amino-terminal domain is located in the perinuclear space between the outer and inner nuclear membrane. A short hydrophobic segment consisting of 20 amino acids spans the outer nuclear membrane, and the 58–amino acid carboxyl-terminal tail domain faces the cytoplasm. gp210 contains asparagine-linked high

mannose-type oligosaccharides (154,155). The carbohydrate residues are not randomly distributed within the gp210 molecule, but they are restricted to its amino-terminal part (156,157). Autoantibodies against gp210 recognize at least two different epitopes. About one third of anti-gp210–positive PBC sera react with a short 15–amino acid fragment within the carboxyl-terminal part of gp210 (158). Most gp210-seropositive PBC sera recognize an epitope located within the large glycosylated luminal amino-terminal domain (153,159). Carbohydrate residues are an essential part of the epitope. About 65% of anti-gp210–positive PBC sera lose their affinity for gp210 on its enzymatic deglycosylation (153,159).

The complete gp210 sequence has been determined for the rat (155) but not for humans. A comparison of a short, partial sequence of human gp210 revealed considerable differences from that of rats. The cDNA coding for rat gp210 was in the past cloned into the expression vector, allowing generation of the recombinant protein in *Escherichia coli*. Unfortunately, the bacterially expressed gp210 recombinant protein lacks posttranslational modifications and therefore is not suitable for application as an antigen for screening anti-gp210 antibodies. It remains unknown whether the sequence encompassing the epitopes exhibits homology between humans and rats.

Anti-gp210 antibodies seem to be highly specific for PBC, and their detection may be useful, especially in diagnosing individuals without AMAs. Antibodies against p62 protein, another component of nuclear pores, have been described in about 30% of PBC sera (160). The p62 protein belongs to a group of mammalian nuclear pore glycoproteins that are modified at approximately 10 to 20 sites with *O*-linked *N*-acetylglucosamine (161). These proteins are involved in nucleocytoplasmic transport. p62 represents the best characterized member of this family. The *N*-acetylglucosamine residues are attached to the serine/threonine stretch in the central part of protein. Deglycosylation of p62 did not affect its reactivity with PBC sera, indicating that recognized sugar moieties are not an integral part of the immunodeterminant. These antibodies, also detected by other groups, appear to represent a distinct entity and do not colocalize with anti-gp210 (160,162–164).

Anti-gp210– and anti-p62–positive PBC patients show features, in terms of clinical data, biochemistry, and morphology, similar to those of PBC patients who are solely positive for AMAs (165). Several studies have shown that these antibodies might be of special value in the diagnosis of PBC in patients who are seronegative for AMAs (165).

## Antibodies Showing Nuclear Dot Staining

ANAs featuring the nuclear dot pattern have been widely observed in PBC sera (166). This staining pattern is defined by multiple nuclear dots of variable size and with wide distribution over the cell nucleus, although sparing the nucleolar region. This pattern is characteristic, but it may be erroneously classified as that of ACAs, which occur in roughly 15% of PBC sera. However, the staining characteristics are quite different. First, centromere antigens are mostly of uniform size, and nuclear dots vary in size and number in the individual cell. Second, antibodies giving the nuclear dot pattern in distinction to ACAs give the same staining pattern of the interphase and the mitotic cells.

## Antibodies to Sp-100

Sp-100 was identified as a target antigen of antibodies, showing dotlike intranuclear localization by means of immunofluorescence microscopy (167). It is an acidic nuclear protein (pI 5.2), with an electrophoretic mobility corresponding to 100 kd. Isolation and cloning of the Sp-100 full-length cDNA revealed a sequence encoding a protein of 480 amino acids with a predicted molecular mass of 50-kd (168). The Sp-100 sequence demonstrates two regions with similarities to known proteins, one to the antigen binding site of the human MHC class 1 molecules and another to several transcriptional regulatory factors, including the human immunodeficiency virus (HIV) nef-1 protein. Determination of epitope mapping with different truncated Sp-100 recombinant proteins revealed at least three nonoverlapping major autoantigenic determinants that were recognized by most PBC sera. One domain, which contains the sequence similarity with the HIV nef-1 protein, was recognized by all anti-Sp-100–positive sera (169). The biologic function of Sp-100 protein is unknown. Infection of Hep-2 cells with influenza A virus or mitogenic stimulation of peripheral blood lymphocytes affected expression of the Sp-100 protein. Notable enhancement of the Sp-100–specific mRNA and of protein expression was observed during cultivation of human cells in the presence of three different types of interferons (IFNs), whereas no such effect occurred after treatment with TNF-α (170). These findings characterize Sp-100 protein as a new member of cytokine-modulated proteins.

Another protein giving the nuclear dot pattern, the promyelocytic leukemia (PML) antigen, colocalizes with Sp-100 and shows a disease specificity similar to that of Sp-100 antibodies (171). The PML autoantigen, discovered in the context of leukemic transformation, is expressed in the form of many COOH-terminally spliced variants and is enhanced by IFNs. Both proteins are covalently modified by PIC1/SUMO-1, a small ubiquitin-like protein (172). This modification may play a regulatory role in the structure and function of these autoantigens.

## Anticentromere Antibodies

The frequency of ACAs in PBC is 10% to 50%, depending on the tests used for their determination (74,173,174). In our experience, ACAs are observed in about 15% of PBC sera. Detailed information on the structure and function of autoantigens is given the "Antibodies to Nonhistone Proteins" section (page 234).

## Diagnostic Approach

The diagnosis of PBC is normally straightforward. It includes a cholestatic laboratory profile, diagnostic or compatible morphology, and a positive test for AMA and sometimes for gp210.

## Therapy

Almost all immunosuppressive drugs have been tried in controlled trials of medical therapy for PBC. Steroids led to the biochemical and morphologic improvements but also to considerable side effects. Other drugs such as azathioprine, cyclosporin, and methotrexate have shown marginal efficacy in routine therapy. However, several placebo-controlled trials have shown that ursodeoxycholic acid (UDCA), a hydrophilic bile acid, improves the symptoms, biochemistry, and histology. Use of this drug prolongs survival and retards liver transplantation. UDCA is the drug of choice for treating PBC, but liver transplantation has a definite place in the treatment of the end-stage PBC, with 5-year survival rates approaching 80%.

## INFLAMMATORY BOWEL DISEASE

Inflammatory bowel disease (IBD) is the second most common chronic inflammatory disorder, after rheumatoid arthritis, and comprises at least two entities: Crohn's disease (CD) and ulcerative colitis (UC). CD and UC are differentiated by differences in clinical presentation, course, diagnostic criteria, response to treatment options, and prognosis. The available data suggest that the diseases develop on different, heterogeneous polygenic backgrounds under the influence of acquired or environmental factors, which have not been clearly identified. However, because both diseases share a number of epidemiologic, pathophysiologic, macroscopic, and microscopic features and because no standard has been established for differentiating them, discrimination continues to be based on a combination of clinical and diagnostic observations (175,176).

CD is a chronic, relapsing disease that can affect the entire gastrointestinal tract and is characterized by a focal, asymmetric, transmural, and occasionally granulomatous inflammation. It has the potential for systemic and extraintestinal complications. CD is a lifetime affliction and recurs after resective surgery. In UC, the relapsing inflammatory process is confined to the mucosa and superficial submucosa of the colon and rectum, extending typically in a continuous manner proximally from the rectum. UC is a surgically curable disease.

Sulphasalazine or 5-aminosalicylic acid, glucocorticoids, and immunosuppressive drugs are standard therapies for IBD. Advances in understanding the pathogenetic mechanisms of CD and UC led to the introduction of antiinflammatory and immunosuppressive strategies that may challenge the application of current treatment regimens in the near future (177).

## Epidemiology

The incidence and prevalence rates of IBD vary substantially, depending on differences in racial and ethnic groups, and they are associated with the socioeconomic development, which points to the importance of genetic and environmental factors in the pathogenesis of CD and UC. The incidence of IBD is highest among whites, relatively low in blacks, and lowest among Asians (178). Jews have increased incidence and prevalence rates for IBD compared with other ethnic groups in the same locations. A North–South gradient has been observed, with higher rates found in Northern European countries. Overall, the prevalence of CD has increased in Western Europe and the United States and is estimated at 30 to 50 cases per 100,000 persons, with an incidence of 1 to 10 cases per 100,000 persons. The incidence rate of UC is 2 to 6 cases per 100,000 persons, with a prevalence that has remained relatively constant over the last five decades at 40 to 100 cases per 100,000 persons (179). The frequencies of UC and CD in men and women are essentially equivalent, with differences found among racial and ethnic groups. CD and UC can manifest at any age but is most common in teenagers and young adults, and a second smaller increase in incidence occurs in the fifth and sixth decades.

## Genetics

Family and epidemiologic studies strongly support the assumption that neither CD nor UC has a simple mendelian pattern of recessive inheritance, even with variable penetrance, but that both diseases are related polygenic disorders. The higher concordance rates of IBD, particularly CD, in identical compared with nonidentical twins; the 10-fold increased risk of IBD among relatives with CD and UC, particularly siblings, versus spouses; and differences in disease prevalence in different ethnic groups and migrants have provided strong evidence that genetic predisposition is important in the pathogenesis of IBD (180–182). Susceptibility to CD in families may involve a gene that is imprinted, because there is a higher risk of transmission from the mother than from the father (183). Concordance for disease type (i.e., inflammatory, stricturing, or fistulizing) and site has been observed in affected family members with CD (184,185). Evidence for the existence of genetic anticipation in CD has been provided by pointing out that the age at onset is lower and disease more extensive in siblings than in offspring of affected parent-child pairs (186,187). Later findings of clinical differences between familial and sporadic CD need to be further substantiated (188).

Molecular genetic studies have provided novel information regarding susceptibility genes involved in the pathogenesis of CD and UC. Genes encoding MHC antigens, cytokines, and adhesion molecules have been analyzed. Associations of haplotypes of the MHC as determinants of disease susceptibility and behavior in IBD have been extensively investigated, as in many other diseases with a suspected autoimmune origin or pathogenesis, and seem to be more important in UC than in CD. HLA class II associations with UC are complex, and separate alleles confer susceptibility or resistance. For Japanese and Jewish patients, several studies have shown an increased frequency with haplotype DR2, but for Caucasian populations, the results are more conflicting. The equivocal results with HLA-DR2 appear to be caused by positively and negatively associated subspecifities in this group. HLA-DRB1 may even predict extensive disease or extraintestinal manifestations in UC. The incidence of DRB1*15 allele was increased among UC patients having a positive family history (189).

Hugot et al. reported the first genome-wide screening for susceptibility genes in IBD (190). A locus on chromosome 16, designated IBD1, was identified that could account for at least 10% of susceptibility to CD. Putative candidate genes included in this region are the interleukin-4 receptor and CD11 integrin. A subsequent two-stage genome-wide search for susceptibility genes revealed striking evidence for linkage between IBD and regions on chromosomes 12, 7, and 3. Individual markers on chromosomes 2 and 6 were linked with susceptibility to UC, but not to CD. These data have provided the most rigorous evidence that CD and UC are related polygenic disorders, sharing some susceptibility genes (191). This idea is further strengthened by the finding that no single standard differentiates CD from UC. Strong positional candidates on chromosomes 7 are hepatocyte growth factor, epidermal growth factor receptor, and *MUC3*, a gene encoding the protein backbone of an intestinal secretory mucin. The region on chromosome 3 includes the $G\alpha_{i2}$ gene encoding a subunit of an inhibitory guanine nucleotide–binding protein. Knockout mice deficient for $G\alpha_{i2}$ develop a lethal diffuse colitis, complicated by adenocarcinoma of the colon (192).

Genetic heterogeneity and subgrouping of IBD patients has been advocated by analysis of genetic and subclinical markers. Perinuclear antineutrophil cytoplasmic antibodies (pANCAs) are the most established subclinical markers in IBD, with a high degree of specificity for UC and associated primary sclerosing cholangitis (PSC) compared with CD or other colitides (193). These antibodies are directed against granule proteins of neutrophils such as proteinase-3, myeloperoxidase, cathepsin G, elastase, lactoferrin, or bactericidal/permeability-increasing protein, and they probably reflect a genetic susceptibility because of the finding of increased levels in unaffected relatives of patients with UC (194–196). The pANCAs in the serum of patients with UC may reflect a genetically determined dysregulation of immunoglobulin production. Several findings argue against a pathogenic role of pANCA in UC, but demonstration that these antibodies also recognize a cytoplasmic antigen expressed in the neuroendocrine cells of the pancreas, retinal cells, and nonepithelial cells of the gastrointestinal tract, skin, and lung could point to an autoimmune-mediated colonic inflammation elicited by these autoantibodies (197,198).

Antibodies to the mannan portion of yeast, anti-*Saccharomyces cerevisiae* antibodies (ASCAs), occur in up to 70% of patients with CD and in 20% of their healthy first-degree relatives but only 5% of patients with UC (199). ASCA combined with ANCA may help differentiate UC from CD, and heterogeneity may help to stratify patients with CD (200). Goblet cell antibodies (GABs) have a prevalence of approximately 30% among patients with CD and UC. The high prevalence among first-degree relatives suggest that GABs may represent another marker characterizing susceptibility to IBD (201).

Genetic polymorphism in the gene coding for the antiinflammatory cytokine interleukin-1 receptor antagonist (IL-1RA) has been associated with UC by demonstrating an overexpression of its allele 2. This has been interpreted as a possible genetic predisposition for severity of the inflammatory course but the concept has been challenged by others (202–204). A mucosal imbalance of the proinflammatory cytokine IL-1 and IL-1RA has been demonstrated in IBD, supporting the pathogenic importance of this antagonizing system for the perpetuation of intestinal inflammation (205). Associations of polymorphisms of TNF microsatellites and intercellular adhesion molecule 1 gene with CD have been inconclusive (206–208).

Impairment of the epithelial barrier function leading to increased intestinal permeability against antigens and proinflammatory molecules has been found by many groups in patients with CD and described as an predictive factor for clinical relapse. However, the role of this epithelial dysfunction as an genetic marker of disease susceptibility remains to be established (209,210). Additional candidate genes for a genetic contribution to IBD are those encoding mucin apoproteins or mucin glycosylating proteins. Alterations in mucin glycoproteins have been found consistently in patients with UC and unaffected identical twins of patients with UC but not in patients with CD (211).

Models of unrestrained mucosal inflammation in gene-targeted mice provide a novel approach to investigate susceptibility genes for IBD. Chronic intestinal inflammation in mice results from deletions of the T-cell receptor, MHC class II molecules, IL-2, IL-10, or the G protein $G\alpha_{i2}$, leading to lymphoid abnormalities from abnormal T-cell development or regulation and from cytokine deficiency (212). From these models, the sensitive regulation of the gut-associated lymphoid tissue that requires a delicate balance between response and anergy can be delineated. The enhanced susceptibility of mice deficient in intestinal trefoil factor or transforming growth factor-β (TGF-β) to colonic injury demonstrates the importance of locally produced growth factors to mucosal homeostasis and healing (213,214). Chimeric mice expressing a dominant negative N-cadherin mutant transgene develop colitis, presumably resulting from altered epithelial cell-cell and cell-matrix interactions that cause an influx of foreign antigens across the damaged mucosa (215). None of the current models is the exact representation of human IBD, suggesting that the human disease may not result from a single genetic defect but reflect insults caused by the alterations of various genes (216).

## Environmental Risk Factors

Various environmental factors have been considered in the cause of IBD. Smoking is the most extensively studied environmental risk factor, reported to have opposing effects on the disease severity of CD and UC. Smoking has a protective effect on UC but is deleterious for CD, a discrepancy that may help to clarify the pathogenesis of IBD (217,218). The use of nonsteroidal antiinflammatory drugs (NSAIDs) has been associated with an increased risk of flare-ups of colitis and the need for admission to hospital due to IBD (219). Oral contraceptives, refined sugar, domestic hygiene, and perinatal and childhood infections have been associated with IBD, but further evaluation is required to confirm the consistency of and define the strength of these associations (220).

Several circumstances, such as the improvement of IBD by fecal diversion, bowel rest, or an elemental diet and the importance of the intestinal flora for the development of colitis in genetically altered mice, suggest a pathogenetic role of microbial agents or their products in IBD (221,222). Infectious agents under investigation include *Mycobacterium paratuberculosis*, *Listeria monocytogenes*, *Streptococcus* spp., and abnormal *E. coli*, but the evidence supporting these bacteria as etiologic factors is inconclusive. Epidemiologic and basic scientific data have led to the hypothesis that CD is a chronic, granulomatous vasculitis with resultant focal ischemia caused by a persistent, perinatal infection of the vascular endothelium with measles virus (223–225). However, the data have not been validated by other groups (226,227).

The consumption of fish has been suggested as a protective dietary factor in IBD. The antiinflammatory omega-3 fatty acids in fish oil may be particularly important, and initial clinical trials with these substances provide evidence of their effectiveness (228). Appendectomy protects against developing UC, apparently because of its important role in antigen presentation and immune activation within the gut-associated lymphoid tissue (229). Data from T-cell receptor (TCR)-α–deficient mice, a genetic model of UC, support the protective role of appendectomy (230).

## Pathogenesis and Immune Mechanisms of Inflammatory Bowel Disease

The cause of IBD is unknown, but preferred theories describe pathogenic or resident luminal bacteria that constantly stimulate the mucosal immune system, leading to a chronic inflammatory response on the basis of genetically determined host susceptibility factors (Fig. 15.5). As an initial step in the pathogenesis of IBD, the breakdown of the intestinal mucosal barrier by infections, toxins, or NSAIDs results in the exposure of lamina propria immune cells to luminal bacteria, bacterial products (including superantigens), cell wall components and toxins, dietary antigens, or possibly self-antigens,

| Initiating events → | Perpetuating events → | Impaired mucosal balance → | Mediators of tissue damage |
|---|---|---|---|
| Infections | Luminal bacteria | Genetic susceptibility | Cytokines: TNF-α, IFN-γ |
| Toxins | Bacterial products | CD4+ lymphocytes | Chemokines: IL-8, ENA-78 |
| NSAIDs | Dietary antigens | Imbalance IL-1/IL-1RA | Neutrophils, eosinophils |
| Multifocal gastrointestinal | Autoantigens | Imbalance Th1/Th2 | Macrophages |
| infarction? | Smoking (CD) | Imbalance pro-/anti- | Eicosanoids |
| | | inflammatory cytokines | Nitrogen and reactive oxygen |
| | | oral tolerance ↓ | metabolites |
| | | Epithelial permeability ↑ | Proteases |
| | | Mucin abnormality | Complement |

**FIG. 15.5.** Proposed model of pathogenesis of inflammatory bowel disease. (Adapted from Sartor RB. Pathogenesis and immune mechanisms of chronic inflammatory bowel disease. *Am J Gastroenterol* 1997;12:5S–11S.)

which perpetuate the inflammatory process. Macrophages and helper T-lymphocyte subsets become activated and release proinflammatory cytokines and chemokines that recruit other inflammatory cells, such as monocytes, lymphocytes, neutrophils, and eosinophils to the intestinal process. A self-perpetuating inflammatory cascade causes a disturbance between proinflammatory mediators and immunosuppressive mechanisms, leading to the net result of tissue injury and functional abnormalities. CD and UC appear to have its distinct constellation of genetic factors, immunologic characteristics, and pathologic findings (175).

Cell-mediated immune responses to gut antigens are actively prevented by subpopulations of regulatory T cells, mediating their inhibitory function by the cytokines IL-10 and TGF-β (231). Observations suggest that counterregulatory CD4+ T-cell subsets are essential for the development of IBD (232). The demonstration of activated CD4+ lymphocytes in patients with IBD, the symptomatic exacerbation of CD after high-dose IL-2 treatment, the ability of therapeutic agents that modulate lymphocyte activation and of allogenic bone marrow transplantation to ameliorate disease activity, and the apparent requirement for CD4+ T cells in murine models of IBD offer evidence for this hypothesis (233,234). The adoptive transfer of the subpopulation of CD45RB$^{hi}$ CD4+ T cells from normal mice to T-cell–lacking severe combined immunodeficiency (SCID) mice results in the development of a severe and chronic pancolitis in the recipient mice because of the differentiation of transferred cells to type 1 helper T (T$_H$1) cells, producing increased amounts of IFN-γ, IL-2, and TNF-α (235). CD4+ T$_H$1 lymphocytes also appear to be the effector cells responsible for the intestinal inflammation in other gene-targeted mice models of IBD and in chronic intestinal lesions of patients with CD, whereas a T$_H$2 profile of IL-4 and IL-10 production has been shown in early CD and UC (236–239). Lamina propria lymphocytes are expanded oligoclonally in patients with IBD, with the presence of interindividual TCR β-chain complementary determining region-3 patterns, implying an individually distinct selective pressure on the TCR in response to the antigen/MHC complex, which may be determined by the HLA haplotype (240,241). TCR-γδ T cells are also strikingly expanded in the lamina propria of patients with IBD and are a major source of IFN-γ (242). The increased integrin expression on lamina propria lymphocytes may confer the enhanced lymphocyte homing capabilities of these cells to the activated endothelial cells in IBD intestine (243,244).

Controversial reports have been published about the concomitance of active IBD in immunocompromised patients with acquired immunodeficiency syndrome (AIDS). The recurrence of CD after solid organ transplantation despite immunosuppressive therapy and in transplanted bowel in a patient with short-bowel syndrome argue against a major role of T cells in the pathogenesis of IBD (245–247).

In normal intestinal mucosa, most macrophages are resident and display a mature phenotype, whereas in IBD, a monocyte-like (CD14+,L1+) subset of newly recruited cells is present, primed for the production of TNF-α (248). Monocyte-derived macrophages demonstrate upregulation of the costimulatory molecules CD80 and CD86, which are crucial for enhanced antigen-presenting capacity and may be implicated in breaking the immunologic tolerance to luminal antigens in IBD (249). Nuclear factor kappa B (NF-κB), a transcription factor known to regulate the synthesis of inflammatory cytokines such as IL-1, TNF-α, and IL-8, is activated in the macrophages and epithelial cells of inflamed intestinal mucosa (250). Local administration of antisense oligonucleotides to the P65 subunit of NF-κB abrogated clinical and histologic signs of inflammation in mice with transmural granulomatous colitis, pointing to the potential therapeutic utility of this molecular approach in patients with IBD (251).

The presence of neutrophils in intestinal lamina propria because of chemotactic mediators such as IL-8, leukotriene

B$_4$, platelet-activating factor, and formyl-methionyl-leucyl-phenylalanine is a characteristic finding in IBD lesions (252–256). Through their release of reactive oxygen products and the ensuing oxidation of sulfhydryls, peroxidation of membrane lipids, and degradation of proteins, carbohydrates, hyaluronic acid, and mucin, neutrophils are important contributors to mucosal damage and pathogenesis of IBD (257,258). Proteins of neutrophil granules are found in increased quantities in the lesions and stools of IBD patients (259–261). Neutrophil-derived 5′-adenosine monophosphate is involved in the development of diarrhea by stimulating the chloride secretion of intestinal epithelial cells (262). Evidence exists for the pathogenetic role of eosinophils in IBD, including increased concentrations of eosinophil granule proteins measured in whole-gut lavage fluid (263).

Altered cytokine and chemokine production is a hallmark of IBD, and lymphocyte-dependent models of IBD and cytokine polymorphisms are related to disease severity or the need to surgery. In the normal mucosa, proinflammatory and antiinflammatory cytokines are balanced, whereas in IBD, the production of several proinflammatory cytokines is increased (212,264). The key aggressive regulatory cytokines appear to be IL-1, TNF-α, IL-12, and IFN-γ, whereas IL-4, IL-10, and TGF-β are immunosuppressive (265). IL-12 is expressed by CD intestinal lamina propria mononuclear cells, consistent with the hypothesis of an IL-12–driven expansion of CD4$^+$ T cells of the T$_H$1 phenotype in the pathogenesis of IBD (266,267). The T$_H$1 cytokine IFN-γ, which is produced in increased amounts in intestinal IBD lesions, acts directly by injuring epithelial tight junctions and indirectly by activating macrophages to produce inflammatory mediators such as reactive oxygen and nitrogen intermediates and cytokines such IL-1, IL-12, and TNF-α and by induction of MHC class II molecules and costimulatory molecules (268). The number of TNF-α–producing cells is also increased in IBD. In CD, TNF-α–positive cells can be detected throughout the mucosa, whereas in UC, only subepithelial macrophages produce TNF-α (269,270). Despite the increased local production of TNF-α, serum concentrations are low, even in active disease (271). A mucosal imbalance of IL-1 and IL-1RA has been described for CD. IL-1 and TNF-α stimulate the production of many proinflammatory mediators, including other cytokines, arachidonic acid metabolites, and proteases, and both are involved in activating T lymphocytes.

The importance of a balanced cytokine production for mucosal immunologic homeostasis is underlined by mouse models in which the immunosuppressive genes for IL-10 and TGF-β have been deleted, producing severe colitis (272,273). IL-10 downregulates the production of multiple proinflammatory cytokines by T lymphocytes and monocytes, and it antagonizes T-cell differentiation toward the T$_H$1 phenotype (274). Administration of IL-10 significantly inhibited development of colitis in SCID mice restored with CD45RB$^{hi}$ CD4$^+$ T cells and might be beneficial in patients with CD.

Increased amounts of phospholipase A$_2$–activating protein, the rate-limiting enzyme in the production of arachidonic acid and of arachidonic acid metabolites, have been detected in the inflamed intestinal mucosa of patients with IBD (275). Chemotactic leukotrienes, especially leukotriene B$_4$, may account for most neutrophil recruitment and activation in IBD, but a pivotal role of leukotriene B$_4$ in UC was challenged by disappointing trials with inhibitors of its synthesis and action (276). Prostaglandins are produced by the cyclooxygenase (COX) pathway and exhibit proinflammatory and antiinflammatory effects. COX-1 is a constitutive enzyme thought to produce cytoprotective prostaglandins, and COX-2 represents the inducible form of cyclooxygenase, leading to the production of proinflammatory prostaglandins. COX-2 mRNA increases with endoscopic disease activity, but COX-1 mRNA remains unchanged (277). Prostaglandin E$_2$ may contribute to diarrhea by promoting intestinal electrolyte and fluid secretion. The elevated expression of inducible nitric oxide synthase protein and production of nitric oxide in the mucosa of patients with active CD and UC may provide a protective effect, as shown for acetic acid–induced murine colitis (278,279). Nitrogen and reactive oxygen metabolites may also be mediators of secretory diarrhea in IBD (280).

Nerve-immune interactions may have a significant role in the process of inflammatory changes in IBD. Neuropeptides regulate many of the inflammatory responses and modulate the functional effects of cytokines and other mediators. Substance P has received considerable attention because of its stimulatory effects on various immunocompetent cells, and increased innervation with sustance P– containing nerve fibers has been demonstrated in UC (281). Decreased levels of the immune-inhibitory somatostatin have been described in active IBD (282). Immunoneutralization of nerve growth factor and neurotrophin-3 significantly worsened the chronic trinitrobenzene sulfonic acid (TNBS)–induced colitis in the rat, suggesting an important protective role for neurotrophins in chronic inflammation of the colon (283).

The inflammatory response in IBD involves immune cells, epithelial cells, mesenchymal cells, neurons, and vascular endothelial cells, which are targets of cytokines and other mediators and contribute to the clinical manifestations in IBD (284). In UC, sCD95L or CD95L$^+$ mononuclear cells mediate epithelial apoptosis, which may be involved in the breakdown of the epithelial barrier function, facilitating the invasion of pathogenic microorganisms (285). The protective function of epithelial integrity against chronic enterocolitis is supported by chimeric mice with a dominant negative N-cadherin that develop intestinal inflammation when the crypt architecture is disrupted. Intestinal epithelial cells express the nonpolymorphic antigen-presenting molecule CD1d, and upon exposure to IFN-γ, major histocompatibility complex class II molecules (286,287). Enterocytes may evolve to nonclassic antigen-presenting cells, a development that has been related to the abnormal T-lymphocyte activation patterns in IBD (288). Defective expression of GP180, a novel CD8 ligand on intestinal epithelial cells in IBD patients, appears to be critical to the failure of intestinal epithelial cells to activate tolerance-inducing CD8$^+$ suppressor T cells. Gut epithelial cells are able to secrete an array of cytokines in a stereotypic response to pathogens, contributing to the cytokine milieu of the lamina propria (289). Enterocytes produce, among others, IL-15, which is a cofactor for IL-12–induced IFN-γ production, and chemotactic epithelial neutrophil-activating peptide 78 (290,291). IL-1, TNF-α, and insulin-like growth factor regulate development of fibrosis by stimulating proliferation of intestinal smooth muscle cells and fibroblasts, contributing to stricture formation and obstruction in CD (292,293).

The assumption that UC and CD are autoimmune diseases has little immunologic documentation. In UC, antitropomyosin antibodies cross-reacting with epithelial cells in the colon, bile ducts, and eye have been described, but this reaction may be of a secondary, nonpathogenic nature (294).

## Histopathology

Features that are useful for evaluation of histologic abnormalities in colorectal biopsy specimens from chronic idiopathic IBD patients are mucosal architecture, lamina propria cellularity, neutrophil infiltration, and epithelial irregularity. In most cases, a combination of crypt architectural distortion, decreased crypt density, irregular mucosal surface, transmucosal or discontinuous increased lamina cellularity, and epithelial damages (including flattening, vacuolation, focal cell loss, erosion, and ulceration) is characteristic in chronic idiopathic IBD and much less notable in infective-type colitis or other causes of colorectal inflammation (295,296). Large numbers of neutrophils, especially crypt abscesses, suggest chronic idiopathic IBD. The presence of epithelioid granulomas, defined as a discrete collection of at least five epithelioid cells (activated histiocytes with homogeneous eosinophilic cytoplasm) with or without accompanying multinuclear giant cells, is one of the histopathologic hallmarks of CD, although it is not a sensitive feature, because it occurs in only 18% of biopsy specimens from patients with known CD (297).

The differential diagnosis between UC and CD by means of histopathology depends mainly on the more severe architectural abnormality (i.e., crypt distortion, decreased crypt density, or a frankly villous surface) and greater density and transmucosal distribution of lamina propria cellularity in active UC (Fig. 15.6). Mucin depletion because of a reduction in the number of goblet cells or depleted mucin within cells is specific only for severe UC. In CD, variable, milder, discontinuous architectural abnormalities and epithelioid granulomas are accurate features. Polymorph infiltration is found in UC and CD, although focal infiltration is more often seen in CD (Figs. 15.7 and 15.8).

The histopathologic features found in IBD are characteristic but nonspecific. The histologic appearances of the biopsy specimen alone are not sufficient to predict accurately the final diagnosis in up to 30% of cases of UC and up to 60% of cases of CD. The final diagnosis depends on a combination

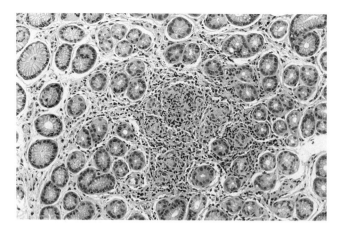

**FIG. 15.6.** Crohn's disease of the colon as revealed by a small epithelioid granuloma in the center of the micrograph. There is only a mild increase in the number of inflammatory cells. The crypts appear slightly distorted (hematoxylin and eosin stain; original magnification ×400). (Courtesy of G. Oberhuber)

of clinical, radiologic, and endoscopic findings and on examination of sequential biopsy specimens from multiple sites. A terminal ileal biopsy specimen may be useful if CD is suspected. The designation of indeterminate colitis is extended to cases for which it is not possible to make a distinction between UC and CD (298).

Microscopic colitis defines a clinicopathologic syndrome that manifests as chronic watery diarrhea in the presence of histologic inflammation but absence of definite endoscopic or radiologic abnormality. Lymphocytic and collagenous forms of colitis are included in this syndrome, but IBD, autoimmune disease, graft-versus-host disease, and drug-induced

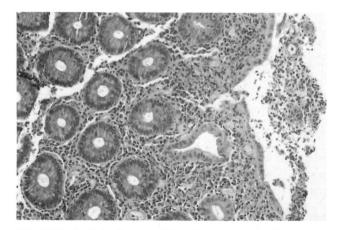

**FIG. 15.7.** Crohn's disease of the colon as revealed by an aphthous lesion. It is characterized by a subepithelial accumulation of inflammatory cells with accompanying epithelial degeneration, especially at the surface. Notice the cellular debris at the luminal side of the biopsy (hematoxylin and eosin stain; original magnification ×600). (Courtesy of G. Oberhuber)

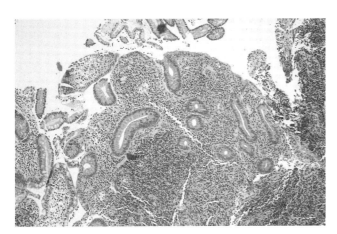

**FIG. 15.8.** Mucosal biopsy of the sigmoid colon shows the typical lesion of ulcerative colitis. It is characterized by architectural changes such as crypt distortion and elongation, and the number of goblet cells is decreased. The lamina propria is densely infiltrated by inflammatory cells, with a predominance of plasma cells. Notice the lymphoid aggregate at the basal side of the mucosa (hematoxylin and eosin stain; original magnification ×200). (Courtesy of G. Oberhuber)

inflammation also may present with microscopic colitis. In lymphocytic colitis, the number of intraepithelial lymphocytes is increased from less than 5 per 100 epithelial cells in normal mucosa to more than 20 per 100 (299). In collagenous colitis, the subepithelial collagen layer of normally 3 μm exceeds 10 μm, although it may be patchy and confined to the proximal colon (300,301). Whether lymphocytic and collagenous colitis represent single diseases or reflect the spectrum of a common pathogenesis and have a possible relationship with UC and CD is unclear. Empirical antiinflammatory therapy with 5-aminosalicylic acid may be useful (302).

## Clinical Course

### Crohn's Disease

Clinical presentation of patients with CD is heterogeneous because of the diversity of intestinal involvement and complications developing during the course of the disease and because of their functional and morphologic impairment after bowel resection. CD may affect any region of the gastrointestinal tract, with rare locations including the oral cavity, esophagus, stomach, and duodenum. In nearly 40% of patients, disease is confined to the small intestine, usually the terminal ileum; in 30%, the large bowel is affected, and in another 30%, the large bowel and small intestine are involved.

Phenotypic classification of CD has been accomplished according to anatomic location (i.e., duodenojejunoileitis, ileitis, ileocolitis, and colonic and perianal disease), disease extent, steroid responsiveness, number of surgical resections, extraintestinal manifestations, and pANCA status. Grouping according to an inflammatory, fibrostenotic, or fistulizing pattern of CD has been proposed, and these groups have different clinical outcomes (303). The Working Party for the World Congress of Gastroenterology in Vienna 1998 developed a simple classification of CD based on the objective variables of age at diagnosis, location, and behavior. Age at diagnosis represents to some extent a genetic component of CD, location delineates disease anatomy, and behavior describes the biology of the disease in terms of the occurrence of specific pathologic features (304) (Table 15.3).

The onset of CD often is insidious, and it can even occur without gastrointestinal manifestations, especially in children. Suspicion should be raised by a characteristic history of chronic or nocturnal diarrhea, abdominal pain, and weight loss. Depending on disease location, diarrhea is often small in volume and associated with rectal urgency and tenesmus in patients with colonic disease or of large volume in cases of small bowel CD. Diarrhea in CD represents the combination of effects such as mucosal inflammation, impaired motility, bile salt catharsis due to severe inflammation, surgical resection of terminal ileum, malabsorption, bacterial overgrowth, and partial obstruction. Decreased bile salt absorption and deconjugation due to bacterial overgrowth in the setting of stricture formation may lead to steatorrhea. Patients with ileocolonic CD often have abdominal pain in the right lower quadrant that is associated with abdominal distention, satiety, nausea, and vomiting because of partial intermittent, ileal obstruction. Patients with CD limited to the colon commonly present with hematochezia, perianal complications, and extraintestinal complications involving skin, eyes, or joints (305). Anorexia, abdominal pain, nausea, malabsorption, and intestinal cytokine production result in weight loss. Low-grade fever is often associated with ileocecal disease; high fevers may occur with severe disease and suppurative complications. Occasionally, there may be a fulminant onset or toxic megacolon that cannot be distinguished from severe UC, but free intestinal perforation is less common than in UC because of thickening of bowel wall (176).

On physical examination, evidence of an abdominal mass caused by thickened and adherent bowel loops, an indurated mesentery, enlarged lymph nodes or an abscess, and abdominal tenderness, especially in the right lower quadrant in ileocecal disease, should be sought. Anemia, leukocytosis, and thrombocytosis are common laboratory findings. Megaloblastic anemia may ensue because of vitamin $B_{12}$ and folic acid malabsorption. Hypocalcemia, hypomagnesemia, and hypoproteinemia indicate severe malabsorption.

Diffuse jejunoileitis is a variant of CD that can be complicated by multifocal stenoses, bacterial overgrowth, malabsorption, steatorrhea, and protein-losing enteropathy (306). Severe manifestations caused by gastric or duodenal ulceration and stricture-associated obstructions occur in only 1% to 5% of all patients with CD (307,308). However, focally enhanced gastritis has been found in 25% of patients with CD who had normal endoscopic findings (309). Rare esophageal CD is associated with dysphagia, odynophagia, chest pain, and dyspepsia.

**TABLE 15.3.** *Vienna classification of Crohn's disease*

| | |
|---|---|
| Age at diagnosis[a] | A1: <40 years |
| | A2: ≥40 years |
| Location[b] | L1: Terminal ileum[c] |
| | L2: Colon[d] |
| | L3: Ileocolon[e] |
| | L4: Upper GI[f] |
| Behavior | B1: Nonstricturing nonpenetrating[g] |
| | B2: Stricturing[h] |
| | B3: Penetrating[i] |

Further data to be collected:

Patient's name: _____ Date of birth: ____/____/____ Sex: female ☐ male ☐
Ethnicity: Caucasian ☐ black ☐ Asian ☐ other: _____ Jewish: yes ☐ no ☐ partly ☐
Family history of IBD: 1st degree relatives[j] ☐ other[k] ☐ none ☐
Extraintestinal manifestation: yes ☐ no ☐

[a] The age when diagnosis of Crohn's disease was first definitively established by radiology, endoscopy, pathology, or surgery.

[b] The maximum extent of disease involvement at any time before the first resection. Minimum involvement for a location is defined as any aphthous lesion or ulceration. Mucosal erythema and edema are insufficient. For classification at least both, a small bowel and a large bowel examination, are required. Use only one box.

[c] Disease limited to the terminal ileum (the lower third of the small bowel) with or without spillover into cecum.

[d] Any colonic location between cecum and rectum with no small bowel or upper gastrointestinal (GI) involvement.

[e] Disease of the terminal ileum with or without spillover into cecum and any location between ascending colon and rectum.

[f] Any disease location proximal to the terminal ileum (excluding the mouth), regardless of additional involvement of the terminal ileum or colon

[g] Inflammatory disease that never has been complicated at any time in the course of disease

[h] Stricturing disease is defined as the occurrence of constant luminal narrowing demonstrated by radiologic, endoscopic, or surgical-pathologic methods with prestenotic dilatation or obstructive signs/symptoms without presence of penetrating disease at any time in the course of disease.

[i] Penetrating disease is defined as the occurrence of intraabdominal or perianal fistulas, inflammatory masses, or abscesses at any time in the course of disease. Perianal ulcers are also included. Excluded are postoperative intraabdominal complications and perianal skintags.

[j] Parents, siblings or children.

[k] Second or third degree; no spouses.

Abscesses complicating preexisting CD occur in 21% of patients because of occlusion of blind tracts (i.e., sinuses). Abscesses mostly arise spontaneously, sometimes postoperatively between intestinal loops, between intestine and peritoneum, in the mesentery, or in intrahepatic or intrasplenic sites, eventually extending into the iliopsoas and the retroperitoneum.

In CD, inflammation may extend through the serosa, leading to adherence to adjacent intraabdominal and pelvic structures. Fistulas may develop as pathologic communications between the luminal gastrointestinal tract and other bowel segments, organs, or skin, particularly in the perianal region, and usually occur proximal to a stricture. Enteroenteric fistulas are often small and incidental findings but are occasionally large enough to cause diarrhea, malabsorption, and weight loss. Pneumaturia, recurrent urinary tract infections, and even fecaluria are features of enterovesical fistulas. Rectovaginal fistulas are characterized by foul vaginal discharge or even gas or stool passage through the vagina.

Muscular hyperplasia, fibrosis, adhesions, and inflammatory infiltration result in intestinal obstruction, particularly of the small intestine, in up to 30% of patients. Crampy mid-abdominal pain and diarrhea that worsens after meals and improves with fasting are associated symptoms. In approximately 25% of patients, especially those with Crohn's colitis, perianal CD is present as involvement of the anal canal, complicated by perianal fissures, abscesses, or fistulas protruding to scrotum, vulva, or groin.

CD has a naturally remitting and recurring course. The placebo response rate varies from 8% to 44% of patients with active CD and approximately 30% of patients who achieved remission relapse within 1 year (310). An aggressive perforating CD characterized by abscesses or fistula formation with a short duration of disease before surgery has been differentiated from nonperforating CD, which takes an indolent clinical course associated with obstruction and bleeding (311). Upper respiratory tract and enteric intercurrent infections, cigarette smoking, the use of NSAIDs, the failure to comply with the maintenance regimen, and mesalamine sensitivity are factors exacerbating CD (312). The issue of stressful life events or psychologic predispositions initiating or exacerbating IBD remains controversial. Seasonal variations in onset and exacerbations for UC, but not CD, have been found and suggest the influence of environmental allergens (313).

## Ulcerative Colitis

UC is a chronic disease characterized by mucosal inflammation limited to the colon. It involves the rectum and may extend proximally in a circumferential and uninterrupted pattern to involve parts or all of the large intestine. During the first attack, disease is limited to the rectum in approximately 30% of patients, extends to the hepatic flexure in about 40%, and involves the entire colon (extensive disease) in the remaining 30% (314). The classic feature of a continuous nature of colonic inflammation in UC has been blurred by the finding of skip areas, most often in the periappendiceal region in 75% of patients with left-sided UC (315). The hallmark clinical symptom of UC is bloody diarrhea with frequent bowel movements, often small in volume and associated with mucopus. In distal UC, blood is often present on the outside of the stool or may be passed without accompanying stool, whereas in cases of extensive disease, blood is typically mixed with the stool. Crampy lower abdominal pain, rectal urgency, and tenesmus are common. Weight loss, fever, and signs of toxicity are features of severe illness. Extensive disease, increased disease severity, and older age are parameters negatively influencing the outcome of the first UC attack (316).

UC is a spontaneously remitting disease with a placebo remission rate of approximately 10% and a placebo benefit rate of approximately 30% (317). However, in less than 8% of patients, no recurrence occurs after an initial acute attack during the next 10 years (318). The likelihood of relapse is not affected by colonic involvement or severity of the first attack, but an inverse correlation has been shown between age and recurrence (319). Intercurrent infection is a precipitating risk factor and seasonality to relapses from August to January has been observed (320,321).

Free perforation, massive hemorrhage, and toxic dilation are major complications of severe UC. Colonic perforation, most often in the sigmoid colon, occurs more often during the first attack of UC, because of the initial lack of muscularis hypertrophy and fibrosis, which develop over time and result in benign colonic strictures. Malignant strictures have to be identified. Toxic megacolon is the most serious complication, typically occurring in pancolitis and resulting from the extension of the inflammatory process beyond the submucosa to the muscularis, leading to colonic atony and distention. Antimotility agents, barium enema examinations, colonoscopy, and hypokalemia are risk factors for the development of this clinical setting. Patients present with fever, dehydration, tachycardia, hypotension, rebound tenderness over the colon, and reduced or absent bowel sounds. The patient may have anemia, leukocytosis, hypoalbuminemia, electrolyte disturbances, and metabolic acidosis.

## Diagnostic Approach

No single standard has been established for the diagnosis of IBD, and the discrimination of UC and CD continues to be based on a combination of clinical, laboratory, endoscopic, histopathologic, and radiographic observations (322,323) (Table 15.4). The potential heterogeneity of the clinical presentations makes the diagnosis of CD, especially colonic disease, particularly difficult. In 10% to 20% of IBD cases, the definite allocation to UC or CD remains impossible by macroscopic and microscopic findings, and these are classified as indeterminate colitis (298,324). However, a precise diagnosis is required because the diseases differ in their natural course and complications, because of the opposing effect of cigarette smoking on disease severity (217,218), and the response to therapy. The high recurrence risk for CD within the ileal reservoir after ileal pouch–anal anastomosis underscores the necessity of a correct differential diagnosis (325).

Contrast radiography and endoscopy are often used in a complementary fashion as diagnostic tools. Upper or lower gastrointestinal tract endoscopy is used to assess disease location, extent, and severity, along with obtaining tissue for pathologic evaluation (326). Endoscopic biopsy can establish the diagnosis of IBD, occasionally distinguish between UC and CD, exclude acute self-limited colitis, or identify dysplasia or cancer as part of a surveillance examination (327). In 70% to 80% of colonoscopies, the intubation of the terminal ileum is successful, enabling the accurate endoscopic and histologic evaluation of this common site for CD. The accuracy of colonoscopy performed by experienced endoscopists in differentiating UC from CD is 85% to 90% (328,329). Contrast radiography is more effective in detecting colonic distensibility, strictures, and fistulas, but barium enema and colonoscopy are contraindicated in patients with moderate or severe UC because of the risk of toxic megacolon or colonic perforation. A combination of colonoscopy, if possible with ileoscopy of the terminal ileum, multiple colonic biopsies, and small bowel follow-through is appropriate to ascertain a diagnosis of CD or UC. The additional performance of gastroscopy with antral-corpeal biopsies can evaluate possible involvement of the upper gastrointestinal tract in CD and may help reduce uncertainties in deciding between CD and UC because of the frequent histologic finding of gastric minilesions in CD (309).

The earliest endoscopic finding of CD is the appearance of a red halo around a lymph follicle with microscopic, but not macroscopic, ulceration; it seems to precede visible aphthoid ulcers and suggests that these lesions originate from follicle-associated epithelium (330). Advanced endoscopic features of CD include aphthoid ulcerations, deep linear, serpiginous or fissure-like ulcers, strictures, fissures, and fistulas (Figs. 15.9 and 15.10). Linear ulceration with intervening areas of intact mucosa, often heaped because of inflammatory infiltration, produces a cobblestone appearance. CD involvement of the colon is usually segmental, and the rectum can be spared. Skip areas are often present between lesions, but occasionally Crohn's colitis may be diffuse, with rectal involvement. Benign strictures are usually concentric and smooth, whereas malignant strictures are more likely to be rigid, nodular, or eccentric. Generally, the endoscopic appearance of CD does not correlate with clinical disease activity and should not be

**TABLE 15.4.** *Differentiation of Crohn's disease and ulcerative colitis by anatomic, clinical, endoscopic, and histopathologic features*

| Characteristic | Crohn's disease | Ulcerative colitis |
|---|---|---|
| Disease location | | |
|   Upper gastrointestinal tract | Occurs | Absent |
|   Ileal involvement | 70%, narrowed | 15%, dilated, "backwash ileitis" |
|   Rectal involvement | Occurs | 95–100% |
|   Perianal disease | Common | Absent |
|   Postoperative recurrence | Common | Absent |
| Clinical presentation | | |
|   Influence of smoking on course of disease | Negative | Positive |
|   Weight loss | Common | Occurs |
|   Fever | Occurs | In severe cases |
|   Abdominal pain | Common | Occurs |
|   Tenesmus | Occurs | Common |
|   Hematochezia | Occurs | Common |
|   Right lower quadrant abdominal mass | Common | Absent |
| Complications | | |
|   Colonic distention | Rare | In severe cases |
|   Stricture | Common | Rare |
|   Abscess | Common | Rare |
|   Fistulas | Common | Rare |
|   Primary sclerosing cholangitis | Rare | Occurs |
|   Pyoderma gangrenosum | Rare | Occurs |
|   Erythema nodosum | Occurs | Rare |
|   Right hydronephrosis | Occurs | Absent |
| Endoscopic features | | |
|   Mucosal involvement | Discontinuous | Continuous |
|   Mucosal granularity, friability | Occurs | Common |
|   Cobblestoning | Common | Absent |
|   Ulcers | In normal mucosa | In abnormal mucosa |
|   Correlation between clinical and endoscopic activity | Absent | Reasonable |
| Histopathologic features | | |
|   Epitheloid granuloma | Occurs | Absent |
|   Crypt distortion, decreased crypt density | Occurs | Common |
|   Lamina propria cellularity | Focal | Dense |
|   Mucin depletion | Occurs | Common |

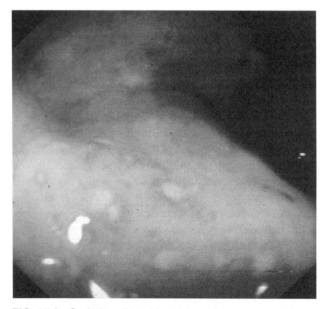

**FIG. 15.9.** Crohn's colitis with aphthous lesions among areas of macroscopically intact mucosa. (Courtesy of Schöfl)

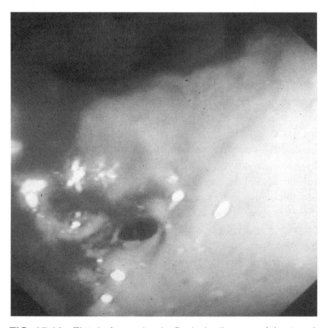

**FIG. 15.10.** Fistula formation in Crohn's disease of the terminal ileum. (Courtesy of Schöfl)

used to assess symptoms or response to therapy (331). However, colonoscopic evaluation of a surgical anastomosis can be used to predict the likelihood of clinical recurrence (332). Endoscopic findings described in gastroduodenal CD have included patchy or streaky mucosal reddening, edema, single or multiple nodularities, cobblestoning, erosions, and ulcers (333).

A complete examination of the small intestine is possible by two radiologic methods. For the small bowel follow-through assessment, patients drink a barium suspension, whereas for enteroclysis, a small bowel enema and air contrast are applied by a tube passed orally into the third portion of the duodenum or proximal jejunum. Data have shown that small bowel follow-through assessment is safer than enteroclysis for diagnosing the presence and extent of CD, is preferred by patients, and does not miss gastroduodenal disease (334), whereas previous studies described excellent sensitivity and specificity for enteroclysis (335). Linear ulcers located along the mesenteric border of the small intestine, displayed as a long, thin, linear barium collection opposite to an relatively uninvolved small bowel, are an important sign of CD (336). Detailed views of strictures, long segments of luminal narrowing, fistulas, sinus tracts, inflammatory masses, ulcerations, and a cobblestone appearance are important features of small bowel radiography (Figs. 15.11 and 15.12). Analogous lesions can be demonstrated in the colon by double-contrast radiography using a barium enema. For the evaluation of a stenosed bowel segment, contrast examination of the colon is particularly important. However, radiologic features of CD are not specific and may be observed in cases of bacterial infections such as *Yersinia* ileitis or tuberculosis (337).

In UC, endoscopy is the most accurate method of determining the extent of colonic disease. The lesions involve the distal rectum and proceed proximally in a continuous and circumferential pattern. Endoscopic findings in UC include a

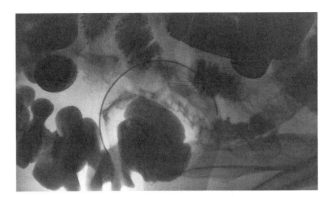

FIG. 15.12. Enteroclysis of ileal Crohn's disease with a cobblestone appearance. (Courtesy of E. Schober)

loss of the typical vascular pattern because of edema, erythema, granularity, and friability (Fig. 15.13). In severe UC, ulceration with a mucopurulent exudate and spontaneous bleeding may be apparent. Regenerative or residual inflammatory mucosa may be prominent as pseudopolyps (326). Endoscopic and histologic rectal sparing is unusual for UC and more often is associated with CD, unless topical steroids have been used in treatment. In cases of UC, clinical activity, endoscopic activity, and histology show a reasonable correlation, and the persistence of active inflammatory lesions determined by histologic examination in the setting of endoscopic remission predicts early relapse (338).

Plain radiographs in supine and upright positions should be performed for every patient with severe UC to detect colonic dilatation. A diameter of 5.5 cm or greater in the segment of

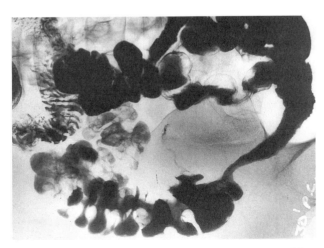

FIG. 15.11. Small bowel follow-through assessment of ileocolonic Crohn's disease with narrowing of the terminal ileum and fistula formation of the cecum. (Courtesy of E. Schober)

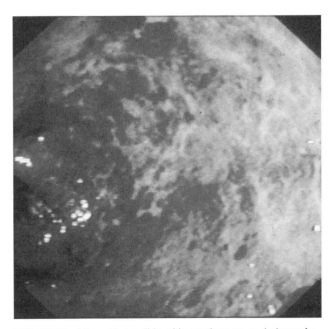

FIG. 15.13. Ulcerative colitis with continuous and circumferential loss of the typical vascular pattern because of granularity and friability. (Courtesy of Schöfl)

the colon, which is highest in the abdominal cavity in the corresponding position, most commonly in the transverse colon, is an important sign in the diagnosis of toxic megacolon. Barium enema results in early UC may be normal or show limited distensibility, with a slightly irregular or granular mucosa. In more severe disease, coarse granularity, nodularity, pseudopolyps, and ulcerations are discernible. Severe proctitis results in enlargement of the presacral space. Backwash ileitis can be observed in 15% to 20% of patients with pancolitis. In long-standing UC, the colon is shortened and has a tubular appearance because of loss of haustral markings. Suspicion of colon cancer should be raised in the cases of masses, flattened or rigid areas, and strictures.

Transabdominal bowel sonography (TABS) is a safe and useful diagnostic method to obtain information about transmural changes of the small and large bowel, excluding the rectosigmoid, in patients with IBD (339). TABS is an accurate method for the detection of intestinal complications in CD, such as strictures, intraabdominal fistulas, or abscesses (340). Computed tomography or magnetic resonance imaging are also appropriate to discriminate intraabdominal masses and abscesses (341). Enteroclysis spiral computed tomography (CT) is an accurate method for the detection of mucosal and extramucosal abnormalities in patients with CD (342). Radiolabeled leukocyte scans can assist assessment of localization, extent, and degree of active inflammation in IBD (343).

An increased prevalence of pANCAs has been described for the sera of patients with UC (344). However, the significant proportion of pANCA-negative UC patients and the identification of a small subgroup of CD patients with pANCA positivity as a specific clinical phenotype with features of UC limits the clinical utility of this serologic marker for differentiation of the diseases (345). The combination of ASCAs with ANCAs may become a useful diagnostic tool for differentiating UC from CD.

## Disease Activity

Assessment of disease activity is essential for planning management of IBD, for evaluating treatment, and for determining prognosis (346). Clinical and endoscopic activity indices are available for UC and CD, but they are largely used in clinical and drug studies.

As initially proposed by Truelove and Witts, a three-degree evaluation of clinical severity in UC is usually performed (347) (Table 15.5). During a first attack, UC is mild in more than 50% of patients (most often in patients with distal disease), moderate in approximately 25%, and severe in approximately 20%. Other clinical indices such as the severe clinical activity index proposed by Rachmilewitz and more quantitative activity scores (including endoscopy) are available (348,349). Overall, frequency and the amount of blood in stools, abdominal pain, incontinence, and signs of toxicity are important symptoms to describe the clinical activity in UC. Combination with the description of possible extrain-

**TABLE 15.5.** *Evaluation of inflammatory bowel disease severity*

Crohn's disease
*Mild to moderate Crohn's disease* applies to ambulatory patients able to tolerate oral alimentation without manifestations of dehydration, toxicity (high fevers, rigors), abdominal tenderness, painful mass, or obstruction.
*Moderate to severe Crohn's disease* applies to patients who have failed to treatment for mild to moderate disease or those with prominent symptoms of fever, significant weight loss (more than 10%), abdominal pain and tenderness (without rebound), intermittent nausea or vomiting (without obstructive findings), or significant anemia.
*Severe or fulminant Crohn's disease* refers to patients with persisting symptoms despite the introduction of steroids on an outpatient basis or individuals presenting with high fever, persistent vomiting, evidence of intestinal obstruction, rebound tenderness, cachexia, or evidence of an abscess.
*Remission* refers to patients who are asymptomatic or without inflammatory sequelae and includes patients who have responded to acute medical intervention or undergone surgical resections without gross residual disease. Patients requiring systemic steroids are usually not considered to be in remission.

Ulcerative colitis
*Mild disease* applies to patients who have four stools daily or less, without or only with small amounts of blood, no systemic signs of toxicity, and a normal erythrocyte sedimentation rate.
*Moderate disease* applies to patients who have more than four stools daily but have minimal signs of toxicity.
*Severe disease* is defined as six or more bloody stools daily and evidence of toxicity as demonstrated by fever, tachycardia, anemia, or an elevated erythrocyte sedimentation rate to 30 mm/hour or more.

*a* The criteria for Crohn's disease (CD) are formulated according to the working definitions of the American College of Gastroenterology for the development of guidelines in the management of CD. The three-degree evaluation of ulcerative colitis is adapted from the criteria of Truelove and Witts (347).

testinal manifestations, abdominal tenderness, and endoscopic findings permits a good evaluation of disease severity.

Defining disease activity in CD is complicated by the heterogeneous patterns of disease location and complications and by the lack of a standard indicator of clinical disease. The discrepancy between histologic investigation, endoscopic appearance, and symptoms or clinical indices is often profound (331,350,351). Disease severity may be established on clinical parameters differentiating localized inflammatory, obstructive, or fistulizing processes; systemic and extraintestinal manifestations; and the global impact of the disease on the individual's quality of life as outlined in the working definitions of the American College of Gastroenterology for the development of guidelines in the management of CD (352) (Table 15.5).

Different indices have been developed to rate disease activity in CD, but the most commonly used measurement is the CD activity index (CDAI) (353). The CDAI was developed to objectively assess response to therapy by incorporating variables that have been identified by multiple regression analysis to best predict disease activity. The included items are the number of liquid or very soft stools, abdominal pain, general well-being, extraintestinal manifestations, abdominal mass, use of antidiarrheal drugs, hematocrit, and body weight. The total score is obtained by summing the products of the grade of each variable and its weighting factor, and the total ranges from 0 to 600. Scores below 150 indicate remission, and scores above 450 signify severe illness. The considerable impact of subjective elements on the CDAI and its impairment by complications such as stenosis or functional disorders after bowel resection, the need for registration of symptoms for 7 days, and the inclusion of the hematocrit (known to be a poor measure of disease activity) has lead to the criticism that the CDAI is a measure of illness rather than of inflammatory activity.

An index including, apart from stool consistency, only objective variables and biochemical values was developed by Van Hees et al. (354). Disease-specific instruments to measure quality of life factors in IBD have been designed (355). The 32-item IBD questionnaire (IBDQ) measures four quality of life dimensions: bowel, systemic, social, and emotional factors. The only validated endoscopic CD activity index is the CD endoscopic index of severity (CDEIS), assessing the percentage of CD-affected mucosal surface in five segments of the intestine: rectum, sigmoid and left colon, transverse colon, right colon, and ileum. However, no relation between clinical activity and endoscopic severity exits (356). An endoscopic score to evaluate the severity of postoperative recurrence of CD was introduced by Rutgeerts et al. (332).

Acute-phase reactants (e.g., orosomucoid, C-reactive protein), erythrocyte sedimentation rate, platelet count, and serum albumin have been used as nonspecific parameters to monitor inflammatory activity in IBD (357,358). Based on the increasing notions of the pathophysiologic mechanisms engaged in IBD, other markers of inflammation have been tested to assess disease activity such as cytokines (e.g., IL-6, IL-8) and soluble cytokine receptors (e.g., IL-2R) (264). Fecal excretion of lactoferrin and increased gut permeability have also been considered for evaluation of disease activity in patients with IBD (359,360).

## Recurrence of Crohn's Disease After Resection

After curative resection with ileocolonic anastomosis, CD recurs within months in the neoterminal ileum, beginning as aphthous lesions (361,332). One year after surgery, endoscopic and radiologic recurrence rates of 27% to 75% have been described (362). Patients with severe endoscopic or radiologic findings become symptomatic within 1 to 3 years. Recurrence is triggered by the fecal stream and luminal bacteria (363). Adverse risk factors for early recurrence are aggressive disease, high preoperative inflammatory disease activity, multiple bowel resections, and smoking (364,365).

## Extraintestinal Manifestations

Extraintestinal manifestations affect 25% to 30% of patients with IBD, with joint involvement occurring most frequently, followed by skin lesions, PSC, and ocular manifestations (366,367). The pathogenesis of the extraintestinal disorders is largely unknown, but some, such as erythema nodosum and peripheral arthritis, appear directly related to the severity of and medical response to the colonic inflammation, whereas others, such as PSC, ankylosing spondylitis, sacroiliitis and sometimes pyoderma gangrenosum, may progress independently of the colitis activity. The disorders may manifest before, at the same time, or after the onset of colonic symptoms, as well as after colectomy (368).

Peripheral arthritis, occurring in 25% of cases, is the most common extraintestinal manifestation of IBD and is characterized by asymmetric pain or painful swelling involving the knees, hips, ankles, elbows, and wrists without bony destruction or evidence of other rheumatic diseases. Enteropathic peripheral arthropathy without axial involvement can be subdivided into a pauciarticular, large joint arthropathy that is most commonly associated with relapsing IBD and a bilateral, symmetric polyarthopathy that is associated with persistent symptoms (369). The migration of activated, intestinal lymphoblasts to synovial tissue by means of the vascular adhesion protein-1 of endothelial cells may be a mechanism of reactive arthritis in IBD (370). Effective anticolitic therapy usually results in improvement of peripheral arthritis. NSAIDs may relief arthritic pain but carry the risk of triggering a relapse of IBD.

Ankylosing spondylitis with or without sacroiliitis, mostly associated with positivity for HLA-B27, affects 2% to 6% of patients with UC. Patients present with low back pain, morning stiffness, and a stooped posture. The treatment comprises physical rehabilitation, sulfasalazine, and NSAIDs (371).

Pyoderma gangrenosum, more frequently associated with UC, and erythema nodosum, more often occurring in CD, are the most striking skin manifestations of IBD and are seen in 15% of patients. Erythema nodosum is characterized by raised, tender nodules, usually occurring over the anterior surface of the tibia. Pyoderma gangrenosum manifests as an expanding, often large, and deep ulcer with a necrotic base on the leg. Whereas erythema nodosum improves with effective therapy of colitis, no predictably successive therapy exists for pyoderma gangrenosum. Various medications, including local, oral, or intravenous corticosteroids, sulphasalazine, azathioprine, cyclosporine, or dapsone, have been tested empirically.

Ocular manifestations occur in about 5% of patients with IBD. In UC, the serious condition of anterior uveitis, presenting as eye pain, photophobia, blurred vision, and conjunctival injection, is prominent in 0.5% to 3% of patients. It requires an urgent diagnosis by slit-lamp examination and therapy with topical corticosteroids. Scleritis and episcleritis presenting as scleral injection and burning are milder ocular complications that are more frequently seen in CD.

PSC is the major hepatic disease in IBD, occurring in 3% to 5% of patients with UC and in a smaller percentage of the patients with CD. Approximately 75% of patients with PSC have associated IBD. The manifestations of the disease may vary from asymptomatic intrahepatic limitations to progressive intrahepatic and extrahepatic periductal fibrosis accompanied by cholestasis, secondary bacterial cholangitis, cholangiocarcinoma, and liver cirrhosis with hepatic insufficiency and portal hypertension (372). The clinical course of PSC does not parallel activity of the colitis, and the disease may progress or occur after colectomy. Controversy exists regarding PSC as a risk factor for the development of right-sided colorectal dysplasia or cancer in patients with UC (373,374). The presence of PSC has important implications for surgical treatment of colitis, because proctocolectomy with ileostomy may lead to peristomeal varices, and ileal pouch–anal anastomosis is associated with a higher frequency of pouchitis. Orthotopic liver transplantation is the only life-sustaining and potentially curative therapy for PSC. Ursodeoxycholic acid has improved biochemical liver function test results but failed to prolong survival without liver transplantation in cases of advanced disease. The effect of ursodeoxycholic acid on the course of early PSC cannot be excluded (375). Up to 30% of patients with IBD have asymptomatic elevations of the liver functions without PSC (376). Other hepatic complications of IBD include fatty liver because of weight loss and malnutrition.

Thromboembolic complications occur in 1% to 39% of patients with IBD and are associated with a high mortality rate (319,377). Activation of blood coagulation, with increased serum levels of factors V and VIII and fibrinogen, as well as decreased levels of protein C, protein S, antithrombin III, and factor XIII, has been recognized, but no consistent abnormalities have been observed in all patients. Platelet dysfunction and thrombocytosis may be related to the risk of thromboembolism (378). A thrombotic pathogenesis of IBD with mesenteric microvascular occlusion has been suggested. The epidemiologic finding that inherited disorders of coagulation appear to protect against IBD is consistent with this hypothesis (379). Factor XIII substitutions and heparin are beneficial in patients with active UC, but this approach is not routinely practiced.

Clinically significant renal or urologic complications occur in 10% to 15% of patients with IBD and may be related to complications of the intestinal disease process (e.g., macalculous hydronephrosis, fistula formation, abscess), metabolic or inflammatory consequences of the disease (e.g., urolithiasis, amyloidosis), medication side effects (e.g., renal tubular damage from 5-ASA), or interpreted as extraintestinal manifestation of IBD (e.g., renal tubular and glomerular nephropathies) (380–382). Pancreatitis, pancreatic dysfunction, and focal white matter lesions in the brain have been associated with IBD (383,384). Rare pulmonary complications, especially in patients with UC, include pulmonary infiltrates with eosinophilia, bronchiolitis obliterans, pulmonary nodules, and serositis. However, pulmonary function abnormalities have been observed in 55% of patients with UC but are not related to a family history of pulmonary disease or to current or previous smoking status (385).

Osteopenia, osteoporosis, and osteomalacia are frequent metabolic bone diseases in IBD, occurring in more than 50% of cases. Dual-energy x-ray absorptiometry has provided a practical tool for diagnosis. Several mechanisms may be involved in IBD-associated bone disease. Vitamin D and calcium deficiency due to malabsorption and reduced intake may activate bone turnover. Treatment with corticosteroids may exert catabolic effects on the bone, and patients with a total lifetime steroid dosage of more than 5 to 10 g of prednisone or equivalent doses should be considered at increased risk for osteoporosis. During acute phases of IBD, immobilization may predispose the patient to high-turnover bone disease. The generation of cytokines such as IL-1 and IL-6 in the inflamed intestinal mucosa may directly induce bone degradation (386).

CD may be complicated by metabolic disorders related to small bowel malabsorption such as nephrolithiasis (from hyperoxaluria after intestinal resection), cholelithiasis, or anemia (from iron deficiency). Anemia in more than 80% of patients with IBD is caused by iron deficiency due to chronic intestinal blood loss and folate or vitamin $B_{12}$ malabsorption. Inadequate erythropoietin production based on the intestinal overproduction of antagonizing proinflammatory cytokines may also contribute to this symptom (387). In some cases, hemolysis or myelosuppression occurs. Anemia occurs in about one third of patients with CD and, in its severe form, as defined as a hemoglobin concentration of 10.5 g/dL, in approximately 15% of cases.

**Differential Diagnosis**

IBD must be differentiated from other specific or idiopathic IBDs that may mimic or sometimes complicate the clinical course. Stools should be examined for the presence of enteric pathogens, ova and parasites, and *Clostridium difficile* toxin. A serologic exclusion of amebic infection must be performed (176) (Table 15.6).

Especially in patients at risk for AIDS, intestinal tuberculosis should be differentiated from CD. Tuberculosis may involve the entire gastrointestinal tract, but the ileocecal region is the most common site of infection that may lead to the development of inflammatory mass, fistulization, bowel narrowing, and lymph node enlargement. Fistula and intestinal stenosis may also result from chronic fungal infections such as actinomycosis or blastomycosis. *Yersinia* ileitis may resemble Crohn's ileitis, and various bacterial pathogens such as *Salmonella, Shigella, Campylobacter jejuni,* or *E. coli* O157:H7 can cause an UC-like illness. Lymphogranuloma, infection with *Chlamydia,* herpesvirus, and cytomegalovirus and syphilis or gonorrhea may lead to proctitis in homosexual men. In HIV-infected patients, opportunistic infections such as *Mycobacterium avium* complex, *Cryptosporidium, Microsporidium,* and *Isospora* may cause diarrhea and abdominal pain.

**TABLE 15.6.** *Differential diagnosis of inflammatory bowel disease*

*Salmonella, Shigella*
*E. coli* 0157:H7
*Campylobacter jejuni, Yersinia enterocolitica*
Tuberculosis
Amebiasis, giardiasis, *Plesiomonas, Aeromonas*
Gonorrhea, syphilis, lymphogranuloma venereum
*Chlamydia*
Herpes simplex, cytomegalovirus
*Cryptosporidium, Microsporidium,* or *Isospora*
*Clostridium difficile*
Actinomycosis, blastomycosis
Diverticulitis
Radiation enteritis
Ischemic bowel disease
Diversion colitis
Solitary rectal ulcer syndrome
Cathartic colon
Irritable bowel syndrome
Drug-induced colitis
Collagenous and lymphocytic colitis
Carcinoma, lymphoma
Carcinoid syndrome
Eosinophilic enteritis
Vasculitis
Behçet's syndrome

Diverticulitis may be confused clinically and radiographically with CD, but endoscopy is helpful, because in CD, the abnormality of mucosa is more evident. Radiation enteritis may appear many years after therapy is completed and can be complicated by stricturing or fistulization. Apart from mucosal granularity, friability, and ulcerations, telangiectases are often observed in late radiation colitis. The spectrum of ischemic bowel disease may encompass early edematous lesions to gangrenous bowel. Hypercoaguable states in the setting of neoplastic or hematologic disorders, severe cardiac or peripheral vascular disease, and vasculitides can predispose to ischemic colitis, which typically centers on the splenic flexure and often spares the rich vascularly supplied rectum. Diversion colitis may develop in a segment of the colon that has been surgically bypassed and results from depriving the intestinal epithelium of the metabolic fuel (e.g., glutamine, short-chain fatty acids) derived from the intestinal lumen. As a consequence, the mucosal barrier is compromised and penetrated by luminal proinflammatory mediators.

Solitary rectal ulcer syndrome, cathartic colon, irritable bowel syndrome, collagenous and lymphocytic colitis, and colitis induced by drugs such as NSAIDs, gold, estrogen, and allopurinol occasionally mimic IBD.

### Fertility and Pregnancy in Inflammatory Bowel Disease

Women with IBD are often at their peak of reproductive life and therefore likely to undergo pregnancy. Fertility of women with IBD appears to be normal, but a significant proportion of patients avoid sexual activity and pregnancy because of dyspareunia and emotional or cosmetic reasons. The incidence of spontaneous abortions, stillbirths, prematurity, and congenital abnormalities is comparable to that for a normal population of patients with inactive disease, but in the case of active disease, increased frequencies have been described (388). Physicians' efforts should be directed at inducing remission before women become pregnant. Male infertility due to sulfasalazine-induced, reversible oligospermia, decreased motility, and abnormal sperm forms may contribute to decreased numbers of pregnancies in IBD couples.

Pregnancy does not increase the risk of relapse for a patient with IBD when the disease is quiescent at the time of conception. However, for patients with active IBD at the time of conception, approximately one third will improve, one third will worsen, and one third will remain the same. New-onset IBD during pregnancy is no more severe than that in nonpregnant women and occurs most often during the first trimester or in the postpartum period. Sigmoidoscopy and biopsy are not contraindicated to diagnose and evaluate the course of IBD during pregnancy. Colonoscopy and radiologic examinations should be avoided, especially in the first trimester. Steroids and sulphasalazine should be used in pregnancy in the same way as they are in nonpregnant women. The new salicylates and azathioprine are most probably safe during pregnancy. Cyclosporine may be chosen as an alternative to surgery in treating steroid-refractory UC (389).

### Inflammatory Bowel Disease in Children

About 2% of all patients with IBD present before the age of 10 years, but 30% develop symptoms between the ages of 10 and 19 years. The classic gastrointestinal symptoms of bloody diarrhea, abdominal pain, and weight loss, as well as distribution of bowel involvement and response to therapy, are similar in children and adults. However, growth failure is a unique feature in pediatric IBD, particularly those with CD. Absolute height deficits are reported in 10% to 40% of these patients, and height velocities may be reduced in 88%. Growth retardation can be the first symptom of IBD and is often already present before other symptoms become apparent. The inflammatory process, accompanied by an increased caloric requirement, malabsorption, and malnutrition, plays a more important role in the occurrence of growth faltering than steroid treatment (390). Growth failure is an important marker of disease activity and the success of therapy (391). Enteral nutrition with an elemental or semi-elemental liquid diet is used as an alternative to corticosteroids in treating pediatric IBD, and energy and protein intake can be increased to 150% of recommended daily allowances for height and age (392). Depression and delayed puberty are also signs of ongoing IBD in children and adolescents (393).

### Therapy

Treatments for IBD with sulfasalazine or 5-aminosalicylic acid (5-ASA), glucocorticosteroids, and immunosuppressants are based on antiinflammatory or immune-modulating mechanisms. Progress in the understanding of the pathogenetic mechanisms of IBD has produced promising therapy strategies. However, a curative conservative management is still lacking because of the obscurity of the cause of the diseases.

Before establishment of therapy, the differential diagnosis must consider CD and UC, the extent and location of disease, and disease activity, and complications must be identified. The therapeutic recommendations are formulated according to the guidelines for the management of CD and UC in adults developed under the auspices of the American College of Gastroenterology and its Practice Parameters Committee (352,394).

### Management of Crohn's Disease

CD is neither medically nor surgically curable. Therapeutic approaches aim to maintain clinical remission, optimize quality of life, and minimize short- and long-term toxicity. The medical guidelines presented are primarily organized according to disease severity with modifications, where applicable according to disease location and are divided into acute and maintenance phases (395) (Table 15.7).

#### Mild to Moderate Active Crohn's Disease

Sulfasalazine and 5-ASA represented major advances in the treatment of IBD. In sulfasalazine, the antiinflammatory 5-ASA is attached by an azobond to the antibiotic sulfapyridine, which is split and released by colonic bacteria. The demonstration that side effects of sulfasalazine are mostly attributed to the sulfonamide component and that 5-ASA is the active moiety of this compound led to the development of new oral 5-ASA formulations. In some of the new drugs, the

sulfapyridine has been replaced, and 5-ASA has been linked by a nitrogen bridge to another carrier, such as another 5-ASA in olsalazine or 4-amino-benzoyl-β-alanine in balsalazide. In oral delayed-release preparations of 5-ASA (mesalamine), 5-ASA is not linked to a carrier but is coated with a semipermeable ethyl cellulose membrane or with acrylic resin, which retards release of the active molecule, especially in the colon. The therapeutic activity of sulfasalazine and 5-ASA in IBD is attributed to several mechanisms, including inhibition of platelet-activating factor, of the 5-lipoxygenase products prostaglandin $E_2$ and thromboxane $B_2$, and of interleukin-1 and TNF-α release. A reactive oxygen metabolite scavenging function, a suppression of antibody secretion, and an inhibition of the impaired epithelial barrier function induced by IFN-γ have been described (257,396–398). Intolerance to the sulfapyridine moiety of sulfasalazine is not uncommon and may result in nausea, vomiting, dyspepsia, anorexia, and headache. More severe, but less common adverse reactions to aminosalicylates include allergic reactions, diarrhea, pancreatitis, hepatoxicity, eosinophilia, cytopenia, hemolytic or megaloblastic anemia, coagulation disorders, renal disorders (e.g., renal tubular dysfunction, interstitial nephritis), pericarditis, myocarditis, lung disorders, rheumatologic and neurologic disorders, and male hypofertility.

Sulfasalazine at daily divided doses of 3 to 6 g is more effective than placebo in the control of active ileocolonic or colonic CD, but it is not consistently effective in patients with disease limited to the small intestine alone. Treatment with different oral 5-ASA formulations at doses of 3.2 to 4.8 g daily in divided doses may be of similar or even superior efficacy compared with sulfasalazine (399,400). Response to initial therapy should be evaluated after several weeks. Active therapy should be continued to the point of symptomatic remission, and patients in remission should be entered into a maintenance program. Symptoms of gastroduodenal disease have been reported to respond to acid-reduction therapy with omeprazole (401). Jejunoileitis is often complicated by small bowel bacterial overgrowth that responds to antibiotics (402).

#### Moderate to Severe Active Crohn's Disease

After exclusion of infection or abscess, patients with persistent symptoms under treatment with oral sulfasalazine or 5-ASA and patients with moderate-severe clinical presentation should be treated with glucocorticosteroids (equivalent to 0.5 to 0.75 mg/kg of prednisone), which are the most effective therapy for active CD and are superior to sulfasalazine (403–405). Generally, doses are tapered by 5 to 10 mg/week until 20 mg and by 2.5 to 5 mg/week from 20 mg to discontinuation. Clinical remission induced by oral steroids is not paralleled by major improvement of endoscopic lesions, pointing to the uselessness of endoscopic monitoring of steroid therapy (406). Prednisone and prednisolone are effective in the induction of remission but have many short-term adverse effects. Nearly one half of the patients treated

**TABLE 15.7.** *Treatment of Crohn's disease*

| Severity | Treatment |
|---|---|
| Mild to moderate | Oral sulfasalazine or 5-ASA |
| Moderate to severe | Oral steroids or oral budesonide (elemental or nonelemental dietary therapy; azathioprine, 6-mercaptopurine) |
| Severe or fulminant | Oral or intravenous steroids; surgery |
| Steroid-dependent and steroid-refractory disease | Azathioprine and 6-mercaptopurine; anti-TNF-α antibody |
| Perianal disease | Oral metronidazole or ciprofloxacin; oral steroids (addition of azathioprine and 6-mercaptopurine); intravenous cyclosporine (?); surgery |
| Maintenance | Azathioprine and 6-mercaptopurine, oral 5-ASA (?); anti-TNF-α antibody (?) |

5-ASA, 5-aminosalicylic acid; TNF, tumor necrosis factor.

acutely with steroids become steroid dependent or steroid resistant after the acute course, causing adrenal suppression and long-term toxicity, including osteoporosis, aseptic necrosis, cataracts, or hypertension (407).

Oral application formulations of budesonide, a semisynthetic topical active glucocorticoid with low systemic activity because of its rapid hepatic inactivation, have been developed as substitutes for conventional glucocorticosteroids. In a dosage of 9 mg/day, the controlled ileal release form of budesonide (Entocort) is similarly effective to induce remission in active ileal and right ileocolonic CD compared with systemic glucocorticoids and superior to sustained release mesalamine but less toxic (408–410). In smaller studies, efficacy was also shown for an oral, pH-dependent–release budesonide (Budenofalk) in treating active CD (411).

Glucocorticoids exert extensive antiinflammatory and immunosuppressive actions by inhibiting the expression and action of most cytokines and other mediators by multiple mechanisms. The activated glucocorticoid-receptor complex can bind and inactivate proinflammatory transcription factors (e.g., AP-1, NF-κB), upregulate the expression of cytokine inhibitory proteins (e.g. I-κB), and reduce the half-life time of cytokine mRNAs (412,413).

The application of total elemental diets and liquid polymeric diets implemented by oral administration or by nasogastric (nasoenteric) tubes by reducing antigenic stimulation with luminal contents has been investigated in CD. Although placebo-controlled trials of total enteral nutrition in CD have not been conducted, this therapy does appear to have a therapeutic benefit (414). However, meta-analysis confirms that steroids are more effective than elemental or nonelemental dietary therapy (415,416). Nutritional therapy is indicated in children with growth retardation.

Patients with more extensive disease and without indications for surgery should be treated concurrently with azathioprine or 6-mercaptopurine, which can enhance the short-term response to steroids (417).

### Severe or Fulminant Crohn's Disease

Patients with severe or fulminant disease should be hospitalized. Intraabdominal abscesses should be evaluated by ultrasound or CT and need percutaneous or surgical drainage. Surgical consultation is also warranted for patients with obstruction. In patients with inflammatory disease who failed to respond to oral steroids, parenteral corticosteroids equivalent to 40 to 60 mg of prednisone are administered in divided doses or as a continuous infusion. After induction of remission, parental steroid therapy can be gradually transferred to an oral regimen. Nutritional support by elemental feeding or parenteral hyperalimentation is indicated for patients unable to tolerate an oral diet for more than 5 to 7 days. Patients with evidence of obstruction because of inflammatory narrowing, fibrotic stricture, or an adhesive process should be treated with bowel rest (418). Differentiation of the obstructive cause is based on prior radiologic or endoscopic studies, the clinical course, and laboratory signs of inflammation. Adhesive obstructions typically respond to nasogastric suction. Fibrostenotic disease may respond initially to bowel rest and steroids, but obstructive symptoms often recur with steroid tapering.

Dehydrated patients are resuscitated with fluid and electrolytes. Blood transfusions are indicated in the setting of active hemorrhage or symptomatic anemia. Broad-spectrum antibiotic therapy is indicated in the presence of inflammatory mass.

### Perianal Disease

Nonsuppurative perianal complications of CD have a good response to metronidazole alone or in combination with ciprofloxacin (419,420). Perianal fistulas need continuous metronidazole treatment to minimize recurrent drainage, which is limited by the development of neurologic side effects (421,422). There is increasing evidence that immunosuppressive agents and intravenous cyclosporine are beneficial in treating perianal fistulas (423).

### Maintenance Therapy in Crohn's Disease

Corticosteroids should not be used as long-term agents to prevent relapse of CD because of their side effects. Trials with controlled ileal release budesonide also have been disappointing regarding a consistent maintenance benefit (424).

The immunomodulating purine analogues 6-mercaptopurine (6-MP) and its prodrug azathioprine (AZA) are the only medications that provide maintenance benefits after a latent period of 2 to 6 months, allowing reduction in steroid doses in patients with steroid dependence (425,426). Doses varied in the different trials, but AZA at 2.5 mg/kg and 6-MP at 1.5 mg/kg have been effective and generally well tolerated. Mucosal healing was demonstrated with AZA in patients with steroid-refractory Crohn's ileitis recurring after operation (427). The complete blood count must be monitored carefully early in the course of treatment and long term at a minimum of every 3 months because of the risk of initial or delayed leukopenia (429). It remains to be determined whether leukopenia is necessary to induce an optimal response (430). Pancreatitis occurs in 4% to 15% of patients; fever, rash, nausea, diarrhea, and opportunistic infections, especially in combination with steroids, have also been observed. The risk of malignancy is not increased relative to the general population (431). Teratogenesis has not been observed in humans. A concomitant therapy with allopurinol should be avoided because of competitive inhibition of metabolic pathways. The benefit of continuing therapy with 6-MP and AZA over 4 to 5 years has yet to be defined (432). In addition to the steroid-sparing effect of AZA, this drug has healed fistulas in two thirds of patients. Promising results with 6-MP have been presented concerning the prevention of clinical, endoscopic, and radiographic postoperative relapse (433).

Results from a trial of intramuscular injection of the folate analogue methotrexate (25 mg/week) demonstrated efficacy in discontinuing or tapering prednisone in 39% of active steroid-dependent patients, but further controlled studies are needed to clarify its effects for long-term remission (434,435). Potential side effects include mild nausea, rash, leukopenia, thrombocytopenia, allergic pneumonitis, and hepatic fibrosis. The drug should not be used during pregnancy (436).

Cyclosporine, an immunosuppressant undecapeptide derived from a soil fungus, is used in organ transplantation for its selective depression of helper T-cell function and inhibition of IL-2 release. Oral cyclosporine is not indicated for therapy of active CD (437,438). However, closure of a fistula may become an indication for continuous intravenous cyclosporine (439).

Oral tacrolismus appears to be effective as a rapidly bridging therapy to long-term treatment with AZA or 6-MP, but much more study is needed to determine the role of tacrolismus in IBD (440).

The efficacy of mesalamine for the maintenance of remission in patients with CD has been investigated in several controlled trials, but the benefit is controversial. Doses above 3 g/day may be considered to reduce the likelihood of recurrence after surgical resection, but the overall benefit is only borderline. The issue of mesalamine in the maintenance treatment of CD in a postmedical setting is less clear. By subgroup analysis, it appears that women, patients with ileal disease, and patients with prolonged disease duration have some benefit from mesalamine, but its effect seems to diminish as time passes. Long-term steroid-sparing activity of mesalamine has not been documented (441–446). Mesalamine is safe for the management of IBD during pregnancy. The exposure to mesalamine during pregnancy increased preterm deliveries and decreased birth weight but did not result in major or minor malformations (447,448).

### Management of Ulcerative Colitis

The goals of treatment in UC are induction and maintenance of clinical and mucosal remission (449). The endoscopically delineation of the proximal margin of inflammation determines the therapeutic management in UC. A distal inflammation, limited to below the splenic flexure, is within the reach of topical therapy, whereas extensive disease extending proximal to the splenic flexure requires systemic medication (Table 15.8).

### Mild to Moderate Distal Ulcerative Colitis

Topical mesalamine and oral therapy with aminosalicylates are equally effective in achieving and maintaining remission in mild to moderate distal colitis (450–453). A topical approach should always be the first choice in treating proctitis or distal colitis. Advantages of topical therapy include a quicker response time and a less frequent dosing schedule. Topical vehicles applied as suppositories reach about 10 cm proximally, foam reaches 15 to 20 cm, and enemas reach up to the splenic flexure. 5-ASA suppositories (500 mg twice daily) are effective in the treatment and maintenance of proctitis. In patients with left-sided colitis 5-ASA enemas (2 to 4 g daily) are the first choice in inducing and maintaining remission (454). Conventional topical corticosteroids (100-mg hydrocortisone enema, 10% cortisone foam) and rectal budesonide (2-mg budsonide enema) are clearly superior to placebo but less effective than rectal 5-ASA for inducing remission of symptoms, endoscopy, and histology and have not proven effective in maintaining remission (455). The addition of oral 5-ASA to topical therapy in patients with distal UC may be more effective than either therapy alone (456).

Refractory distal colitis is defined as active distal inflammation unresponsive within 4 to 6 weeks to topical treatment with 5-ASA or corticosteroids with oral salicylates or sulfasalazine (457). Dosage increases and a drug switch of 5-ASA to corticosteroids and *vice versa* are logical. Topical administration of cyclosporine, nicotine tartrate, lidocaine, or other anesthetics are possible but need confirmation. Oral or intravenous application of steroids may become necessary.

### Mild to Moderate Extensive Ulcerative Colitis

Patients with mild to moderate extensive colitis should begin therapy with oral sulfasalazine in daily doses titrated up to 4 to 6 g/day or an alternative aminosalicylate in doses up to 4.8 g/day (458). Approximately 80% of patients intolerant to sulfasalazine tolerate mesalamine and olsalazine (459). Data

**TABLE 15.8.** *Treatment of ulcerative colitis*

| Severity | Distal disease | Extensive disease |
| --- | --- | --- |
| Mild | Topical 5-ASA or steroids | Oral sulfasalazine or 5-ASA |
| Moderate | Topical 5-ASA or steroids plus oral sulfasalazine or 5-ASA | Oral steroids (addition of azathioprine or 6-mercaptopurine) |
| Severe | Topical 5-ASA or steroids with increased dose and duration; topical 5-ASA and steroids; oral steroids | Intravenous steroids (plus intravenous cyclosporin) Surgery |
| Maintenance | Topical 5-ASA | Oral sulfasalazine or 5-ASA |

5-ASA, 5-aminosalicylic acid.

indicate that oral balsalazide is more effective and better tolerated than mesalamine in the treatment of active UC (460). Responses to oral sulfasalazine and oral aminosalicylates are dose related, with up to 80% of patients manifesting clinical remission or improvement within 4 weeks. There is insufficient evidence to confirm a benefit of 5-ASA preparations over sulfasalazine for active or maintenance therapy, but sulfasalazine is not as well tolerated as 5-ASA in active disease despite their relatively similar tolerances in maintenance therapy.

Patients refractory to oral aminosalicylates should be treated with oral prednisone (40 to 60 mg/day) until significant clinical improvement, with a subsequent dose taper of 5 to 10 mg/week until 20 mg and then of 2.5 to 5 mg/week to discontinuation (461). For patients who do not respond to or cannot be weaned from steroids, AZA (1.5 to 2.5 mg/kg/day) has demonstrated effectiveness in achieving and maintaining remission (462,463). Budesonide may also be beneficial for patients with steroid-dependent UC (464).

### Severe Ulcerative Colitis

Severe UC is a potentially life-threatening condition, with a mortality, including surgical mortality, that is less than 2% because of the improvements of clinical management. Patients who continue to present with severe symptoms despite optimally dosed oral therapy with steroids and aminosalicylates, as well as topical medications, and patients with evidence of toxicity should be hospitalized and treated with intravenous steroids equivalent to 300 mg of hydrocortisone or 48 mg of methylprednisolone for 7 to 10 days. Patients without prior steroid medication alternatively may profit by intravenous adrenocorticotropic hormone (465–468). Therapy with aminosalicylates should not be initiated during an episode of acute, severe colitis because of possible allergic reactions confusing the clinical picture. Vital signs should be taken repeatedly, and frequent abdominal examination and abdominal radiographs should be performed to detect signs of peritoneal irritation and the presence of small bowel gas and colonic dilation. Patients should receive adequate intravenous fluid and electrolyte replacements. In patients with toxic megacolon, oral nutrition should be stopped, and bowel decompression should be instituted with the passage of a long tube; the patient also should be rolled to a prone position for 15 minutes every 2 to 3 hours to allow redistribution of colonic air. Relief from colonic distention is usually experienced within 24 to 48 hours (469). Adjunctive parenteral nutrition may be useful, but total parenteral nutrition shows no benefit (470). Broad-spectrum antibiotics may be used empirically (471). Surgical consultation should be obtained at the time of admission, because a coordinated effort by gastroenterologists and surgeon can reduce mortality (472). Anticholinergic and narcotic medications have to be avoided in this setting for the fear of worsening colonic atony or dilation.

Up to 35% of patients fail to respond to intravenous steroids (473). Eight or more stools per 24 hours or four to five stools per 24 hours together with C-reactive protein levels above 45 mg/L predict in 85% of patients the need for colectomy after a 3 days therapy with intravenous glucocorticoids (474). Additional management with intravenous cyclosporine in a dose of 4 mg/kg/day has proved effective at reducing the immediate colectomy rate in 80% of patients, but the long-term benefit is much less certain, and one third of patients require surgery within the next 6 months and 60% of patients after 12 months (475–477). Response to intravenous cyclosporine should be seen within 7 days at cyclosporine levels between 300 and 500 ng/mL. Monotherapy with intravenous cyclosporine (4 mg/kg) has also been as effective as 50 mg of an intravenous prednisolone equivalent (478). Major side effects of intravenous cyclosporine were observed in up to 50% of patients, with induction of renal insufficiency being the most frequent (479). Seizures have been associated with low serum magnesium and cholesterol levels because of the cyclosporin hydrophobic vehicle. Administration of intravenous cyclosporine should be performed with careful monitoring of renal function, blood pressure, and magnesium and cholesterol levels. Opportunistic infections, such as *Pneumocystis carinii* pneumonia and cytomegalovirus, have been described (480). Two series demonstrate that 6-MP is beneficial to maintain the initial response to intravenous cyclosporine (481). The efficacy of microemulsion cyclosporine capsules (Neoral) for response maintenance of severe steroid refractory UC remains to be determined. Intravenous and oral tacrolismus may also be successful as an alternative to cyclosporine for patients with severe UC.

### Maintenance Therapy in Ulcerative Colitis

Oral sulfasalazine, olsalazine, mesalamine, or balsalazide are all effective as a maintenance regimen in extensive UC by reducing relapse rate fourfold (482–486). Unlike sulfasalazine, use of larger doses of 5-ASA is generally well tolerated. The optimal 5-ASA dose is probably 2 g/day. Although the maximum length of maintenance therapy has not been established, permanent treatment is recommended. In distal UC remission can be maintained by topical therapy with 5-ASA suppositories or enemas (487,488). In patients with remissions not adequately sustained by aminosalicylates, AZA or 6-MP may be useful, but the risk-benefit ratio of indefinite use of these drugs is unknown. In patients with UC encouraging results for methotrexate were reported in open trials and series, whereas a later controlled trial with oral dosing did not show any benefit when compared with placebo (489).

### Alternative Treatments for Inflammatory Bowel Disease

In the past few years, new therapeutic concepts for IBD have been formulated based on the increasing insights in the pathophysiology of these diseases aimed at targeting proinflammatory mediators or molecules, aggressive luminal agents, and genetically determined defects. The most significant issue is the introduction of immunomodulatory treatments using cytokines and anticytokines.

An important role for TNF-α as a pivotal proinflammatory mediator in CD has emerged, which resulted in the development of therapeutic strategies that target TNF-α. Several studies have addressed the potential effect of anti-TNF-α treatment in CD. Administration of the high-affinity human (75%) mouse (25%) chimeric antibody cA2 against TNF-α to patients with treatment-resistent active CD caused clinical response in 65% and remission in 33% of patients (490). The incidences of short-term side effects in the anti-TNF-α–treated group and the placebo group did not differ. Retreatment with cA2 was effective to maintain remission after an initial treatment with cA2 pointing to its benefit for maintenance therapy (491). The same molecule has also shown efficacy for closure of enterocutaneous fistulas (492). The long-term risk profile of cA2 needs to be further evaluated, but especially the potential development of lymphoma seems to be unlikely. The precise mechanism of action is unknown, whether mainly antiinflammatory by neutralizing TNF-α or immune modulatory by altering the function of leukocytes bearing surface TNF-α. The clinical effects of cA2 therapy correlated with downregulation of the production of the $T_H1$ cytokine IFN-γ by CD2 stimulated lamina propria mononuclear cells, whereas no effect was observed on cytokine production by stimulated peripheral blood mononuclear cells indicating that the primary defect in immune regulation in CD is confined to the mucosal compartments (493). TNF-α antibodies also bind to membrane expressed TNF-α, altering the function of the TNF-α–producing cell and inducing its killing by complement activation (494). Another genetically engineered human antibody to TNF-α, CDP571, has shown effectiveness as a single infusion in patients with active CD (495). Anti-TNF-α seems to be a promising therapeutic strategy in patients who do not respond to standard treatment. The therapeutic efficacy in UC has been controversially described and needs further evaluation (496,497).

IL-10 is a cytokine with antiinflammatory and immunosuppressive properties. Gene-targeted IL-10–deficient mice develop a chronic intestinal inflammatory disease reminiscent of CD. IL-10 administered as a daily bolus injection over 1 week is safe, well tolerated, and may be clinically efficacious in 50% of patients with active steroid-resistent CD (498). The safety of subcutaneous IL-10 treatment was confirmed, but remission was observed in only 29% of treated patients with active CD (499).

The safety and activity of human recombinant IL-11 was evaluated in patients with active CD, and the average percent change from baseline in CDAI score could be significantly reduced (500). An attempt to block leukocyte recruitment to the site of inflammation by ISIS 2302 (ICAM-1 antisense oligonucleotide) in the treatment of steroid-dependent patients with CD may be promising (501). Depleting anti-CD4 antibodies showed only moderate efficacy in CD (502).

The long-lasting local expression and efficacy of antiinflammatory cytokine genes within the intestinal mucosa has been demonstrated by the local transfer of an adenovirus–IL-4 vector in rats with TNBS colitis (503).

Heparin has emerged as a possible therapy for IBD, targeting a potential endothelial dysfunction in regulation of coagulation, inflammation, and vascular repair as an important pathogenetic mechanism in UC (504).

Transdermal nicotine and nicotine enemas induced clinical response in active UC but were paralleled by common side effects (218,505). To improve the safety of nicotine, rectal enema and delayed-release oral nicotine formulations have been developed. To prove the benefit of sucralfate enemas in UC further, larger clinical trials are needed (506).

Despite the concept that luminal bacteria may play a role in the pathogenesis of IBD, antibiotic treatment has been used empirically in IBD for many years. Controlled clinical trials have been generally scarce and studies often lacked adequate statistical power. Data from open studies suggest the efficacy of metronidazole in perianal CD (419,421). A remission-prolonging effect of metronidazole after resection has been suggested (507). Metronidazole has also shown efficacy in controlling active CD, most pronounced in patients with ileocolonic disease (508). Metronidazole may be an alternative in some patients with active CD not responding to sulphasalazine (509). Administration of metronidazole can be complicated by gastrointestinal intolerance and metallic taste, as well as in the long term by peripheral neuropathy, necessitating careful attention to symptoms or signs of paresthesias or neurologic abnormalities. The quinolone antibiotic ciprofloxacin could become an alternative to metronidazole and has been shown efficacy for mild to moderate attacks of CD (510,511). Infection or abscess requires appropriate antibiotic therapy or drainage (percutaneous or surgical).

### Adjunctive Therapy in Inflammatory Bowel Disease

Most patients with CD having anemia respond to intravenous iron alone. Erythropoietin has additional effects on hemoglobin concentrations (512). Vitamin D and calcium supplementation prevents bone loss in patients with CD and hormone replacement therapy is beneficial in perimenopausal and postmenopausal women with IBD. Biphosphonates may become alternatives for treatment of metabolic bone disease in IBD (513).

### Cancer Surveillance in Inflammatory Bowel Disease

Patients with UC are at increased risk of colorectal cancer in the range of 0.5% to 1% per year after 10 years of extensive disease, and the carcinoma is frequently preceded by dysplasia (514). Dysplasia is characterized by cellular atypia, such as nuclear stratification, loss of nuclear polarity, and nuclear or cellular pleomorphism. Molecular markers such as Ki-67, DPC-4, and DYS may become useful for refining the diagnosis of dysplasia or may eventually provide an alternative method for predicting colorectal cancer (515). The presence of low-grade dysplasia is a risk factor with a 20% chance that colon contains cancer, whereas the risk with high-grade dysplasia is up to 40%.

Colitis-associated cancers are more often multiple, broadly infiltrating, anaplastic, uniformly distributed throughout the colon, and they occur in much younger patients than colorectal cancer in the general population. Endoscopic surveillance has been evaluated to detect cancer at an earlier and potential curable stage. In the absence of randomized studies comparing different surveillance protocols, the American College of Gastroenterology recommends an annual surveillance colonoscopy with multiple biopsies at regular intervals of approximately 10 cm in patients with a disease duration of 8 to 10 years (394,516). Uninflamed areas, masses, strictures, and flat lesions should be also biopsied. Chemoprevention of UC-associated colorectal cancer has been suggested by a possible protective effect of folic acid (517).

The risk of colorectal cancer in colonic CD is approximately three times that of unaffected patients, especially in younger patients with long disease duration (518). Surveillance programs therefore may be as appropriate in Crohn's colitis as in UC (519). An increased risk of adenocarcinoma of the small intestine has been observed in CD, notably in patients with young age at diagnosis and patients with extensive small bowel disease (520). However, the overall mortality and lifetime risk due to intestinal cancer seems to be not increased in patients with CD (521).

### Surgical Indications and Treatment

Although CD recurs in 50% to 80% of patients within 10 years after resection, surgery often proves to be the swiftest, safest, and most effective route to physical and psychosocial rehabilitation (522,523). For more than two thirds of patients with CD, surgical intervention is indicated. Complications such as obstructing stenoses, suppurative complications, massive hemorrhage, or perforation and intractable disease require surgical intervention. Patients with unresponsive fulminant disease who fail to improve within 7 to 10 days of intensive inpatient management should also be considered surgical candidates. Open laparotomy is the standard procedure for resections in IBD. However, laparoscopic colorectal surgery can be advantageous for treatment of terminal ileal CD, but the definite role of this approach has not clearly emerged (524,525). Strictureplasty has proved an safe and effective treatment for patients with multiple, symptomatic small bowel strictures (526). Nearly 40% of patients with CD will require at least a temporary stoma during their lives, with anorectal disease being the primary indication. Revision surgery for stomal complications is more common after colostomy than ileostomy (527). In selected patients with perianal CD abscess, incision and drainage, fissurectomy, and fistulotomy with Seton drainage are successful, sphincter-sparing techniques. Resection and drainage of intraabdomi-

nal abscesses may be preferable to attempted percutaneous drainage and staged resection with anastomosis (528).

The cumulative colectomy rates for UC after 10 years differ between 10% to 30% and depend on the severity of the first attack, the extent of disease at diagnosis and younger age at onset (529,530). Exsanguinating hemorrhage, frank perforation, and documented or strongly suspected carcinoma (high-grade dysplasia or low-grade dysplasia in a mass lesion) are absolute indications for surgery in UC (531–534). Low-grade dysplasia in flat mucosa may also be indicative for surgery, because the 5-year predictive value of such lesions for cancer or high-grade dysplasia is approximately 50%. Patients with severe acute UC unresponsive to intravenous cyclosporine within 7 days require colectomy. Because of the classic dictum of inherent curability by excisional surgery, colectomy should be evaluated at any point for patients with significant deterioration in medical therapy and medically intractable symptoms to regain quality of life (535).

One-, two-, or three-step proctocolectomy with Brooke ileostomy is the standard operation for UC. The procedure is curative and carries the lowest risk of complications. The cosmetically more appealing ileal pouch anal anastomosis (IPAA) preserves the muscularis mucosa of the rectum despite colectomy and maintains bowel continuity. However, the technical failure rate reported approaches 5% to 6%. Acute and chronic pouchitis episodes are seen in up to 50% to 60% and 5% to 10% of patients, respectively (536). Possible etiologic factors for pouchitis include bacterial overgrowth, fecal stasis, mucosal ischemia, intestinal malabsorption, and immune-mediated inflammation (537). The presence of extraintestinal manifestations, PSC, and p-ANCA have been associated with an increased risk of pouchitis, whereas smoking appears to have a protective effect (538,539). Pouchitis is characterized mainly by watery, foul-smelling diarrhea, sometimes containing blood, accompanied by abdominal cramps, urgency, anal soiling, and incontinence. General malaise and low-grade fever may be present. Endoscopically, the mucosal changes can be diffuse or patchy with edematous, hyperemic, granular lesions and punctate ulcers.

The broad-spectrum antibiotics metronidazole or ciprofloxacin are the mainstay of treatment (540,541). Pouchitis intractable to antibiotics requires antiinflammatory or immunosuppressive therapy similar to UC. Even without development of pouchitis, metaplastic, colonic-like changes appear in the pouch mucosa by 6 months after the operation. In long-standing ileoanal pouch severe mucosal atrophy can develop with a risk of neoplastic transformation (542,543). Pouch mucosa should be controlled by endoscopic and histologic surveillance. Generally, IPAA should be avoided in patients with CD because of the risk of disease recurrence within the ileal reservoir and its accompanying debilitating symptoms. However, the controversial notion that IPAA is an acceptable procedure in established CD has been advocated (544–546).

## Prognosis

The mortality rate is increased for patients with CD and UC compared with the general population; the increased rate is mainly attributed to IBD-related complications. The principal causes of death in CD are sepsis, perforation, and pulmonary embolism (547,548). Patients with CD have an increased extraintestinal cancer risk of 10% over an unaffected population with the most common tumor type being squamous cell cancer of the skin (549). In UC deaths from colorectal cancer, asthma, and non–alcohol-related liver diseases contribute to an increased mortality rate (550). In studies from southern Europe general mortality was not increased in CD and significantly lower than expected in UC because of a reduced risk of cardiovascular and possibly smoking related deaths (551,552).

## REFERENCES

1. Whitehead R. The classification of chronic gastritis: current status. *J Clin Gastroenterol* 1995;21[Suppl 1]:131–134.
2. Toh B-H, Van Driel IR, Gleeson PA. Pernicious anemia. *N Engl J Med* 1997;337:1441–1448.
3. Castle WB. Development of knowledge concerning the gastric intrinsic factor and its relation to pernicious anemia. *N Engl J Med* 1953;249: 603–614.
4. Taylor KB. Inhibition of intrinsic factor by pernicious anaemia sera. *Lancet* 1959;2:106–108.
5. Taylor KB, Roitt IM, Doniach D, et al. Autoimmune phenomena in pernicious anemia sera: gastric antibodies. *Br Med J* 1962;2:1347–1352.
6. Kokkola A, Sjöblom SM, Haapiainen R, et al. The risk of gastric carcinoma and carcinoid tumours in patients with pernicious anaemia. *Scand J Gastroenterol* 1998;33:88–92.
7. Baur S, Fisher JM, Strickland RG, Taylor KB. Autoantibody-containing cells in the gastric mucosa in pernicious anaemia. *Lancet* 1968;2: 887–894.
8. Kaye MD, Whorwell PJ, Wright R. Gastric mucosal lymphocyte subpopulations in pernicious anemia and in normal stomach. *Clin Immunol Immunolpathol* 1983;28:431–440.
9. Carmel R. Reassessment of the relative prevalences of antibodies to gastric parietal cell and to intrinsic factor in patients with pernicious anaemia: influence of patient age and race. *Clin Exp Immunol* 1992; 89:74–77.
10. Karlsson FA, Burman P, Loof L, Mardh S. Major parietal cell antigen in autoimmune gastritis with pernicious anemia is the acid-producing H$^+$,K$^+$ adenosine triphosphatase of the stomach. *J Clin Invest* 1988;81: 475–479.
11. Burman P, Karlsson FA, Loof L, et al. H$^+$,K-ATPase antibodies in autoimmune gastritis: observation on the development of pernicious anemia. *Scand J Gastroenterol* 1991;26:207–214.
12. Gleeson PA, Toh BH. Molecular targets in pernicious anaemia. *Immunol Today* 1991;12:233–238.
13. Toh B-H, Gleeson PA, Simpson RJ, et al. The 60- to 90-kDa parietal cell autoantigen associated with autoimmune gastritis is a ( subunit of the gastric H$^+$/K$^+$-ATPase (proton pump). *Proc Natl Acad Sci USA* 1990;87:6418–6422.
14. Callaghan JM, Khan MA, Alderuccio F, et al. α and β subunits of the gastric H$^+$/K($^+$)-ATPase (proton pump). *Autoimmunity* 1993;16: 289–295.
15. Song YH, Ma JY, Mardh S, et al. Localization of a pernicious anaemia autoantibody epitope on the α-subunit of human H,K-adenosine triphosphatase. *Scand J Gastroenterol* 1994;29:122–127.
16. Alderuccio F, Toh B-H, Tan SS, et al. An autoimmune disease with multiple molecular targets abrogated by the transgenic expression of a single autoantigen in the thymus. *J Exp Med* 1993;178:419–426.
17. Strickland RG, Mackay IR. Natural history of atrophic gastritis. *Lancet* 1974;2:777–778.
18. Cummins D, Ardeman S. Intrinsic factor antibodies and pernicious anaemia. *Lancet* 1991;338:383–384.
19. Hewitt JE, Gordon MM, Taggart RT, et al. Human gastric intrinsic factor: characterization of cDNA and genomic clones and localization to human chromosome 11. *Genomics* 1991;10:432–440.
20. Stockbrugger R, Angervall L, Lundquist G. Serum gastrin and atrophic gastritis in achlorhydria patients with and without pernicious anemia. *Scand J Gastroenterol* 1976;11:713–719.
21. Chanarin I. How to diagnose (and not misdiagnose) pernicious anaemia. *Blood Rev* 1987;1:280–283.
22. Appelmelk BJ, Faller G, Claeys D, et al. Bugs on trial: the case of *Helicobacter pylori* and autoimmunity. *Immunol Today* 1998;19:296–299.
23. McColl KEL. What remaining questions regarding *Helicobacter pylori* and associated diseases should be addressed by future research? *Gastroenterology* 1997;113:158–162.
24. Tytgat GN. Practical management issues for the *Helicobacter pylori*–infected patient at risk of gastric cancer. *Aliment Pharmacol Ther* 1998;12[Suppl 1]:123–128.
25. Negrini R, Lisato L, Zanella I, et al. *Helicobacter pylori* infection induces antibodies cross-reacting with human gastric mucosa. *Gastroenterology* 1991;101:437–445.
26. Negrini R, Savio A, Poiesi C, et al. Antigenic mimicry between *Helicobacter pylori* and gastric mucosa in pathogenesis of body atrophic gastritis. *Gastroenterology* 1996;111:655–665.
27. Faller G, Steininger H, Eck M, et al. Antigastric autoantibodies in *Helicobacter pylori* gastritis: prevalence, *in situ* binding sites and clues for clinical relevance. *Virchows Arch* 1996;427:483–486.
28. Faller G, Steininger H, Kranzlein J, et al. Antigastric autoantibodies in *Helicobacter pylori* infection: implications of histological and clinical parameters of gastritis. *Gut* 1997;619–623.
29. Steininger H, Faller G, Dewald E, et al. Apoptosis in chronic gastritis and its correlation with antigastric autoantibodies. *Virchows Arch* 1998;433:13–18.
30. Pettitt JM, Toh BH, Callaghan JM, et al. Gastric parietal cell development: expression of the H$^+$/K$^+$-ATPase subunits coincides with the biogenesis of the secretory membranes. *Immunol Cell Biol* 1993;71: 191–200.
31. Appelmelk BJ, Negrini R, Moran AP, Kuipers EJ. Molecular mimicry between *Helicobacter pylori* and the host. *Trends Microbiol* 1997;5: 70–73.
32. Appelmelk BJ, Simoons-Smit I, Negrini R, et al. Potential role of molecular mimicry between *Helicobacter pylori* lipopolysaccharide and host Lewis blood group antigens in autoimmunity. *Infect Immun* 1996; 64:2031–2040.
33. Moran AP. The role of lipopolysaccharide in *Helicobacter pylori* pathogenesis. *Aliment Pharmacol Ther* 1996;10[Suppl 1]:39–50.
34. Claeys D, Faller G, Appelmelk BJ, et al. The gastric H$^+$,K$^+$-ATPase is a major autoantigen in chronic *Helicobacter pylori* gastritis with body mucosa atrophy. *Gastroenterology* 1998;115:340–347.
35. D'Elios MM, Manghetti M, Almerigogna F, et al. Different cytokine profile and antigen-specificity repertoire in *Helicobacter pylori*–specific T cell clones from the antrum of chronic gastritis patients with or without peptic ulcer. *Eur J Immunol* 1997;27:1751–1755.
36. Blanchard TG, Czinn SJ. Immunological determinants that may affect the *Helicobacter pylori* cancer risk. *Aliment Pharmacol Ther* 1998;12 [Suppl 1]:83–90.
37. El-Omar EM, Oien K, El-Nujumi, A et al. *Helicobacter pylori* infection and chronic gastric acid hyposecretion. *Gastroenterology* 1997;113:15–24.
38. Sauerbruch T, Schreiber MA, Schussler P, Permanetter W. Endoscopy in the diagnosis of gastritis: diagnostic value of endoscopic criteria in relation to histologic diagnosis. *Endoscopy* 1984;16:101–104.
39. Andrew A, Wyatt JI, Dixon MF. Observer variation in the assessment of chronic gastritis according to the Sydney system. *Histopathology* 1994;25:317–322.
40. Dixon MF, Genta RM, Yardley JH, Correa P. Classification and grading of gastritis. International Workshop on the Histopathology of Gastritis, Houston, 1994. *Am J Surg Pathol* 1996;20:1161–1181.
41. Mackay IR, Taft CO, Cowling DS. Lupoid hepatitis. *Lancet* 1956;2:1323–1326.
42. Mackay IR, Weiden S, Hasker J. Autoimmune hepatitis. *Ann N Y Acad Sci* 1965;124:767–780.
43. Desmet VJ, Gerber M, Hoofnagle JH, et al. Classification of chronic hepatitis: diagnosis, grading and staging. *Hepatology* 1994;19: 1513–1520.

44. Czaja AJ. The variant forms of autoimmune hepatitis. *Ann Intern Med* 1996;125:588–598.

45. Krawitt EL. Autoimmune hepatitis. *N Engl J Med* 1996;334:897–903.

46. Johnson PI, McFarlane IG. Meeting report: International Autoimmune Hepatitis Group. *Hepatology* 1993;18:998–1005.

47. Czaja AJ, Manns MP. The validity and importance of subtypes in auto-immune hepatitis: a point of view. *Am J Gastroenterol* 1995;90: 1206–1211.

48. Czaja AJ, Nishioka M, Morshed S, Hachiya T. Patterns of nuclear immunofluorescence and reactivities to recombinant nuclear antigens in autoimmune hepatitis. *Gastroenterology* 1994;107:200–207.

49. Tan EM, Feltkamp TEW, Smolen JS, et al. Range of antinuclear antibodies in "healthy" individuals. *Arthritis Rheum* 1997;40:1601–1611.

50. Emlen W, O'Neill L. Clinical significance of antinuclear antibodies: comparison of detection with immunofluorescence and enzyme-linked immunosorbent assay. *Arthritis Rheum* 1997;40:1612–1618.

51. Tan EM. Autoantibodies to nuclear antigens (ANA): their immunobiology and medicine. *Adv Immunol* 1982;33:167–240.

52. Tan EM, Chan EKL, Sullivan KF, et al. Antinuclear antibodies (ANAs): diagnostically specific immune markers and clues towards the understanding of systemic autoimmunity. *Clin Immunol Immunol-pathol* 1988;47:121–141.

53. Schwartz RS, Stollar BD. Origins of anti-DNA autoantibodies. *J Clin Invest* 1985;75:321–327.

54. Pisetsky DS, Grudier JP, Gilkeson GS. A role for immunogenic DNA in the pathogenesis of systemic lupus erythematosus. *Arthritis Rheum* 1990;33:153–159.

55. Stollar BD. The origin and pathogenic role of anti-DNA antibodies. *Curr Opin Immunol* 1990;2:607–612.

56. Jain S, Markham T, Thomas HC. Double-stranded DNA-binding capacity of serum in acute and chronic liver disease. *Clin Exp Immunol* 1976;26:35–41.

57. Peretz A, Mascart-Lemone F, Nuttin G, Famaey JP. Chronic active hepatitis with a high level of anti-ds-DNA detected by a solid phase radioimmunoassay. *Clin Rheumatol* 1982;1:208–211.

58. Smeenk R, van der Lelij G, Swaak T. Specificity in systemic lupus erythematosus of antibodies to double-stranded DNA measured with the polyethylene glycol precipitation assay. *Arthritis Rheum* 1982;25: 631–638.

59. Gurian LE, Rogoff TM, Ware AJ, et al. The immunologic diagnosis of chronic active "autoimmune" hepatitis: distinction from systemic lupus erythematosus. *Hepatology* 1985;5:397–402.

60. Leggett BA, Collins RV, Cooksley WGE, et al. Evaluation of the Crithidia assay to distinguish between chronic active hepatitis and systemic lupus erythematosus. *J Gastroenterol Hepatol* 1987;21: 202–211.

61. Wood JR, Czaja AJ, Beaver SJ, et al. Frequency and significance of antibody to double-stranded DNA in chronic active hepatitis. *Hepatology* 1986;6:976–980.

62. Isenberg I. Histones. *Annu Rev Biochem* 1979;48:159–191.

63. McGhee JD, Felsenfeld G. Nucleosome structure. *Annu Rev Biochem* 1980;49:1115–1156.

64. Cole RD. A minireview of microheterogenity in H1 histone and its possible significance. *Anal Biochem* 1984;136:24–30.

65. Lennox RW. Differences in evolutionary stability among H1 subtypes: implication for the roles of H1 subtypes in chromatin. *J Biol Chem* 1984;259:669–672.

66. Hardin JA, Thomas JO. Antibodies to histones in systemic lupus erythematosus: localization of prominent autoantigens on histones H1 and H2B. *Proc Natl Acad Sci USA* 1983;80:7410–7414.

67. Gohill J, Fritzler MJ. Antibodies in procainamide-induced and systemic lupus erythematosus bind the C-terminus of histone 1 (H1). *Mol Immunol* 1987;24:275–285.

68. Węsierska-Gądek J, Penner E, Lindner H, et al. Autoantibodies against different histone H1 subtypes in systemic lupus erythematosus. *Arthritis Rheum* 1990;33:1273–1278.

69. Vila JL, Juarez C, Illa I, et al. Autoantibodies against the H1° subtype of histone H1. *Clin Immunol Immunopathol* 1987;45:499–503.

70. Penner E. Nature of immune complexes in autoimmune chronic active hepatitis. *Gastroenterology* 1987;92:304–308.

71. Czaja AJ, Ming C, Shirai M, Nishioka M. Frequency and significance of antibodies to histones in autoimmune hepatitis. *J Hepatol* 1995;23: 32–38.

72. Konikoff F, Swissa M, Shoenfeld Y. Autoantibodies to histones and their subfractions in chronic liver diseases. *Clin Immunol Immunopathol* 1989;51:77–82.

73. Meyer O, Haim T, Ryckewaert A. Significance of anti-centromere antibodies: clinical value. *Rev Rhum Mal Osteoartic* 1983;50:262–266.

74. Guldner HH, Lakomek HJ, Bautz FA. Human anti-centromere sera recognise a 19.5 kD non-histone chromosomal protein from HeLa cells. *Clin Exp Immunol* 1984;58:13–20.

75. Earnshaw W, Bordwell B, Marino C, Rothfield N. Three human chromosomal autoantigens are recognized by sera from patients with anti-centromere antibodies. *J Clin Invest* 1986;77:426–430.

76. Kipling D, Warburton PE. Centromeres, CENP-B and Tigger too. *Trends Genet* 1997;13:141–145.

77. Earnshaw WC, Machlin PS, Bordwell BJ, et al. Analysis of anticentromere autoantibodies using cloned autoantigen CENP-B. *Proc Natl Acad Sci USA* 1987;84:4979–4983.

78. Earnshaw WC, Rothfield NF. Identification of a family of human centromere proteins using autoimmune sera from patients with scleroderma. *Chromosoma* 1985;91:313–321.

79. Muro Y, Masumoto H, Yoda K, et al. Centromere protein B assembles centromeric alpha-satellite DNA at the 17-bp sequence, CENP-B-box. *J Cell Biol* 1992;116, 585–596.

80. Iwahara J, Kigawa T, Kitagawa K, et al. A helix-turn-helix structure unit in human centromere protein B (CENP-B). *EMBO J* 1998;17: 827–837.

81. Sugimoto K, Yata H, Muto Y, Himeno M. Human centromere protein C (CENP-C) is a DNA-binding protein which possesses a novel DNA-binding motif. *J Biochem (Tokyo)* 1994;116:877–881.

82. Sullivan KF, Hechenberger M, Masri K. Human CENP-A contains a histone H3 related histone fold domain that is required for targeting to the centromere. *J Cell Biol* 1994;127:581–592.

83. Valdivia MM, Figueroa J, Iglesias C, Ortiz M. A novel centromere monospecific serum to a human autoepitope on the histone H3-like protein CENP-A. *FEBS Lett* 1998;422:5–9.

84. Palmer DK, O'Day K, Trong HL, et al. Purification of the centromere-specific protein CENP-A and demonstration that it is s distinctive histone. *Proc Natl Acad Sci USA* 1991;88:3734–3738.

85. Gerace L, Comeau C, Benson M. Organization and modulation of nuclear lamina structure. *J Cell Sci Suppl* 1984;1:137–160.

86. Newport JW, Forbes DJ. The nucleus: structure, function, and dynamics. *Annu Rev Biochem* 1987;56:535–565.

87. Gerace L, Burke B. Functional organization of the nuclear envelope. *Annu Rev Cell Biol* 1988;4:335–374.

88. Kaufmann SH. Additional members of the rat liver lamin polypeptide family. *J Biol Chem* 1989;264:13946–13955.

89. Fisher DZ, Chaudhary N, Blobel G. cDNA sequencing of nuclear lamins A and C reveals primary and secondary structural homology to intermediate filament proteins. *Proc Natl Acad Sci USA* 1986;83: 6450–6454.

90. McKeon FD, Kirschner MW, Caput D. Homologies in both primary and secondary structure between nuclear envelope and intermediate filament proteins. *Nature* 1986;319:463–468.

91. Heald R, McKeon F. Mutations of phosphorylation sites in lamin A that prevent nuclear lamina disassembly in mitosis. *Cell* 1990;61: 579–589.

92. McKeon FD, Tuffanelli DI, Fukuyama K, Kirschner MW. Autoimmune response directed against conserved determinants of nuclear envelope proteins in a patient with linear scleroderma. *Proc Natl Acad Sci USA* 1983;80:4374–4378.

93. Reeves WH, Chaudhary N, Salerno A, Blobel G. Lamin B autoantibodies in sera of certain patients with systemic lupus erythematosus. *J Exp Med* 1987;165:750–762.

94. Węsierska-Gądek J, Penner E, Hitchman E, Sauermann G. Antibodies to nuclear lamins in autoimmune liver disease. *Clin Immunol Immunopathol* 1988;49:107–115.

95. Lassoued K, Guilly M-N, Danon F, et al. Antinuclear autoantibodies specific for lamins. *Ann Intern Med* 1988;108:829–833.

96. Konstantinov K, Halberg P, Wiik A, et al. Clinical manifestation in patients with autoantibodies specific for nuclear lamin proteins. *Clin Immunol Immunopathol* 1992;62:112–118.

97. Brito J, Biamonti G, Caporali R, Montecucco C. Autoantibodies to human nuclear lamin B2 protein. *J Immunology* 1994;153:2268–2277.

98. Rizzetto M, Swana G, Doniach D. Microsomal antibodies in active chronic hepatitis and other disorders. *Clin Exp Immunol* 1973;15: 331–344.

99. Smith MGM, Williams R, Walker G, et al. Hepatic disorders associated with liver/kidney microsomal antibodies. *Br Med J* 1974;2:80–84.

100. Homberg JC, Abuaf N, Bernard O, et al. Chronic active hepatitis associated with antiliver/kidney microsome antibody type 1: a second type of "autoimmune" hepatitis. *Hepatology* 1987;7:1333–1339.

101. DeLemos-Chiarandini C, Alvarez F, Bernard O, et al. Anti-liver-kidney microsome antibody is a marker for the rat hepatocyte endoplasmic reticulum. *Hepatology* 1987;7:468–475.

102. Alvarez F, Bernard O, Homberg JC, et al. Anti-liver-kidney microsomes antibody recognizes a 50,000 molecular weight protein of the endoplasmic reticulum. *J Exp Med* 1985;161:1231–1236.

103. Kyriatsoulis A, Manns M, Gerken G, et al. Distinction between natural and pathological autoantibodies by immunoblotting and densitometric subtraction: liver-kidney microsomal antibody (LKM) positive sera identify multiple antigens in human liver tissue. *Clin Exp Immunol* 1987;79:53–60.

104. Manns M, Johnson EF, Griffin KJ, et al. The major target antigen of liver kidney microsomal autoantibodies in idiopathic autoimmune hepatitis is cytochrome P450db1. *J Clin Invest* 1989;83:1066–1072.

105. Zanger UM, Hauri HP, Loeper J, et al. Antibodies against human cytochrome P450db1 in autoimmune hepatitis type II. *Proc Natl Acad Sci USA* 1988;85:8256–8260.

106. Manns M, Zanger U, Gerken G,, et al. Patients with type II autoimmune hepatitis express functionally intact cytochrome P450db1 that is inhibited by LKM-1 autoantibodies *in vitro* but not *in vivo*. *Hepatology* 1990;12:127–132.

107. Battula N, Sagara J, Gelboin HV. Expression of P1-450 and P3-450 DNA coding sequences as enzymatically active cytochromes P-450 in mammalian cells. *Proc Natl Acad Sci USA* 1987;84:4073–4077.

108. Wang PP, Beaune P, Kaminsky LS, et al. Purification and characterization of six cytochrome P-450 isozymes from human liver microsomes. *Biochemistry* 1983;22:5375–5383.

109. Gonzales FJ, Skoda RC, Kimura S, et al. Characterization of the common genetic defect in humans deficient in debrisoquine metabolism. *Nature* 1988;331:442–446.

110. Manns MP, Griffin KJ, Sullivan KF, et al. LKM-1 autoantibodies recognize a short linear sequence in P450 IID6. *J Clin Invest* 1991;88:1370–1378.

111. Lenzi M, Bianchi FB, Cassani F, et al. Liver cell surface expression of the antigen reacting with liver kidney microsomal antibody LKM). *Clin Exp Immunol* 1984;55:36–40.

112. Loeper J, Descatoire V, Maurice M, et al. Presence of cytochrome P450 hepatocyte plasma membrane: recognition by several autoantibodies. *Hepatology* 1990;12:909(abst).

113. Loeper J, Descatoire V, Maurice M, et al. Cytochrome P450 in human hepatocyte plasma membrane: recognition by several autoantibodies. *Gastroenterology* 1993;104:203–216.

114. Homberg JC, Andre C, Abuaf N, et al. A new anti-liver-kidney microsome antibody (anti-LKM-2) in tienilic acid–induced hepatitis. *Clin Exp Immunol* 1984;55:561–570.

115. Beaune PH, Dansette PM, Mansuy D, et al. Human anti-endoplasmic reticulum autoantibodies appearing in a drug-induced hepatitis are directed against a human liver cytochrome P-450 that hydroxlates the drug. *Proc Natl Acad Sci USA* 1987;84:551–555.

116. Crivelli O, Lavarini C, Chiaberge E, et al. Microsomal autoantibodies in chronic infection with the HbsAg associated delta agent. *Clin Exp Immunol* 1983;54:232–238.

117. Philipp T, Durazzo M, Trautwein C, et al. Recognition of uridine diphosphate glucuronosyl transferase by LKM-3 antibodies in chronic hepatitis. *Lancet* 1994;344:578–581.

118. Manns MP. Cytoplasmic antigens. In: McFarlane IG, Williams R, eds. *Molecular basis of autoimmune hepatitis*. Heidelberg: Springer-Verlag, 1996:59–74.

119. Bourdi M, Larrey D, Nataf J, et al. Anti-liver endoplasmic reticulum antibodies are directed against human cytochrome P450 1A2. *J Clin Invest* 1991;85:1967–1973.

120. Clot P, Albano E, Eliasson E, et al. Cytochrome P450 2E1 hydroxyethyl radical adducts as the major antigen in autoantibody formation among alcoholics. *Gastroenterology* 1996;111:206–216.

121. Manns M, Gerken G, Kyriatsoulis A, et al. Characterisation of a new subgroup of autoimmune chronic active hepatitis by autoantibodies against a soluble liver antigen. *Lancet* 1987;1:292–294.

122. DeDuwe C, Pressman BC, Gianetto R, et al. Tissue fractionation studies: intracellular distribution patterns of enzymes in rat liver tissues. *Biochem J* 1955;60:604–610.

123. Wächter B, Kyriatsoulis A, Lohse AW, et al. Characterization of liver cytokeratin as a major target antigen of anti-SLA antibodies. *J Hepatol* 1990;11:232–239.

124. Franke WW, Schiller D, Moll R, et al. Diversity of cytokeratins: differentiation specific expression of cytokeratin polypeptides in epithelial cells and tissues. *J Mol Biol* 1981;153:933–959.

125. Moll R, Franke WW, Schiller DL, et al. The catalog of human cytokeratins: patterns of expression in normal epithelia, tumors and cultures cells. *Cell* 1982;31:11–24.

126. Węsierska-Gądek J, Grimm R, Hitchman E, Penner E. Members of glutathione *S*-transferase gene family are antigens in autoimmune hepatitis. *Gastroenterology* 1998;114:329–335.

127. Hayes JD, Pulford DJ. The glutathione *S*-transferase supergene family: regulation of GST* and the contribution of the isoenzymes to cancer chemoprotection and drug resistance. *Crit Rev Biochem Mol Biol* 1995;30:445–600.

128. Smith GJ, Ohl VS, Litwack G. Ligandin, the glutathione *S*-transferases, and chemically induced hepatocarcinogenesis: a review. *Cancer Res* 1977;37:8–14.

129. Hayes PC, Hussey AJ, Keating J, et al. Glutathione *S*-transferase levels in autoimmune chronic active hepatitis: a more sensitive index of hepatocellular damage than aspartate transaminase. *Clin Chem Acta* 1988;172:211–216.

130. Kaplan MM. Primary biliary cirrhosis. *N Engl J Med* 1987;316:521–528.

131. Gershwin ME, Mackay IR. Primary biliary cirrhosis: paradigm or paradox for autoimmunity. *Gastroenterology* 1991;100:882–833.

132. Coppel RL, Gershwin ME. Primary biliary cirrhosis: the molecule and the mimic. *Immunol Rev* 1995;144:17–49.

133. Mackay IR, Primary biliary cirrhosis showing a high titer of autoantibody. *N Engl J Med* 1958;258:185–187.

134. Walker JG, Doniach D, Roitt IM, Sherlock S. Serological tests in diagnosis of primary biliary cirrhosis. *Lancet* 1965;1:827–829.

135. Berg PA, Doniach D, Roitt IM. Mitochondrial antibodies in primary biliary cirrhosis. I. Localisation of the antigen to mitochondrial membranes. *J Exp Med* 1967;126:277–290.

136. Gershwin ME, Coppel RL, Mackay IR. Primary biliary cirrhosis and mitochondrial autoantigens—insights from molecular biology. *Hepatology* 1988;8:147–151.

137. Mendel-Hartvig I, Nelson BD, Loof L, Totterman TH. Primary biliary cirrhosis : further biochemical and immunological characterization of mitochondrial antigens. *Clin Exp Immunol* 1985;62:371–379.

138. Lindenborn-Fotinos J, Baum H, Berg PA. Mitochondrial autoantibodies in primary biliary cirrhosis: species and nonspecies specific determinants of the M2 antigen. *Hepatology* 1985;5:763–769.

139. Gershwin ME, Mackay IR, Sturges A, Coppel RL. Identification and specificity of a cDNA encoding the 70 kD mitochondrial antigen recognized in primary biliary cirrhosis. *J Immunol* 1987;138:3525–3531.

140. Coppel RL, McNeilage LJ, Surh CD, et al. Primary structure of the human M2 mitochondrial autoantigen of primary biliary cirrhosis: dihydrolipoamide acetyltransferase. *Proc Natl Acad Sci USA* 1988;85:7317–7321.

141. Yeaman SJ, Danner DJ, Fussey SPM, et al. Primary biliary cirrhosis: identification of two major M2 mitochondrial autoantigens. *Lancet* 1988;1:1067–1070.

142. Surh CD, Danner DJ, Ahmed A, et al. Reactivity of PBC sera with a human fetal liver cDNA clone of branched chain alpha-keto acid dehydrogenase (BCKD) dihydrolipoamide acyltransferase, the 52 kD mitochondrial autoantigen. *Hepatology* 1988;9:63–68.

143. Howard MJ, Fuller C, Broadhurst RW. Three-dimensional structure of the major autoantigen in primary biliary cirrhosis. *Gastroenterology* 1998;115:139–146.

144. Van de Water J, Cooper A, Surh CD, et al. Detection of autoantibodies to recombinant mitochondrial proteins in patients with primary biliary cirrhosis. *N Engl J Med* 1989;320:1377–1380.

145. Moteki S, Leung PS, Coppel RL. Use of a designer triple expression hybrid clone for three different lipoyl domain for the detection of antimitochondrial autoantibodies. *Hepatology* 1996;24:97–103.

146. Gerace L, Burke B.Functional organization of the nuclear envelope. *Annu Rev Cell Biol* 1988;4:335–374.

147. Hurt EC. The nuclear pore complex. *FEBS Lett* 1993;325:76–80.

148. Pante N, Aebi U. The nuclear pore complex. *J Cell Biol* 1993;122:977–984.

149. Penner E, Węsierska-Gądek J, Hitchman E, Sauermann G. Proteins of the nuclear envelope as antigens in lupoid hepatitis. *Hepatology* 1987;7:1115(abst).

150. Lassoued K, Danon F, Andre C, et al. Antibodies directed to a 200 kD polypeptide(s) of the nuclear envelope: a new serologic marker associated with primary biliary cirrhosis. *Hepatology* 1987;7:1115(abst).

151. Lassoued K, Guilly M-N, Andre C, et al. Autoantibodies to a 200 kD polypeptide of the nuclear envelope: a new serologic marker of primary biliary cirrhosis. *Clin Exp Immunol* 1988;74:283–288.

152. Courvalin J-C, Lassoued K, Bartnik E, et al. The 210 kD nuclear envelope polypeptide recognized by human autoantibodies in primary biliary cirrhosis is the major glycoprotein of the nuclear pore. *J Clin Invest* 1990;86:279–285.

153. Węsierska-Gądek J, Hohenauer H, Hitchman E, Penner E. Autoantibodies from patients with primary biliary cirrhosis preferentially react with the amino-terminal domain of nuclear pore complex glycoprotein gp210. *J Exp Med* 1995;182:1159–1162.

154. Gerace L, Ottaviano Y, Kondor-Koch C. Identification of a major polypeptide of the nuclear pore complex. *J Cell Biol* 1982;95:826–837.

155. Wozniak RW, Bartnik E, Blobel G. Primary structure analysis of an integral membrane glycoprotein of the nuclear pore. *J Cell Biol* 1989;108:2083–2092.

156. Greber UF, Senior A, Gerace L. A major glycoprotein of the nuclear pore complex is a membrane-spanning polypeptide with a large luminal domain and a small cytoplasmic tail. *EMBO J* 1990;9:1495–1502.

157. Wozniak RW, Blobel G. The single transmembrane segment of gp210 is sufficient for sorting to the pore membrane domain of the nuclear envelope. *J Cell Biol* 1992;119:1441–1449.

158. Nickowitz RE, Worman HJ. Autoantibodies from patients with primary biliary cirrhosis recognize a restricted region within the cytoplasmic tail of nuclear pore membrane glycoprotein gp210. *J Exp Med* 1993;178:2237–2242.

159. Węsierska-Gądek J, Hohenauer H, Hitchman E, Penner E. Anti-gp210 antibodies in sera of patients with primary biliary cirrhosis: identification of a 64 kD fragment of gp210 as a major epitope. *Hum Antibodies Hybridomas* 1996;7:167–174.

160. Węsierska-Gądek J, Hohenauer H, Hitchman E, Penner E. Autoantibodies against nucleoporin p62 constitute a novel marker of primary biliary cirrhosis. *Gastroenterology* 1996;110:840–847.

161. Davis LI, Blobel G. Nuclear pore complex contains a family of glycoproteins that includes p62: glycosylation through a previously unidentified cellular pathway. *Proc Natl Acad Sci USA* 1987;84:7552–7556.

162. Miyachi K, Shibata M, Onozuka Y, et al. Primary biliary cirrhosis sera recognize not only gp210 but also proteins of the p62 complex bearing *N*-acetylglucosamine residues from rat liver nuclear envelope. *Mol Biol Rep* 1996;23:227–234.

163. Itoh S, Ichida T. Yoshida T, et al. Autoantibodies against gp210 kDa glycoprotein of the nuclear pore complex as a prognostic marker in patients with primary biliary cirrhosis. *J Gastroenterol Hepatol* 1998;13:257–265.

164. Worman HJ, Courvalin J-C. Autoantibodies against nuclear envelope proteins in liver disease. *Hepatology* 1991;14:1269–1279.

165. Invernizzi P, Podda M, Battezzati PM, et al. Autoantibodies to nuclear pore complex proteins (anti-p62 and anti-gp210) in primary biliary cirrhosis: a marker of adverse disease? *Hepatology* 1998;28:546(abst).

166. Szostecki C, Guldner HH, Will H. Autoantibodies against "nuclear dots" in primary biliary cirrhosis. *Semin Liver Dis* 1997;17:71–78.

167. Szostecki C, Krippner H, Penner E, Bautz FA. Autoimmune sera recognize a 100 kD nuclear protein antigen (Sp-100). *Clin Exp Immunol* 1987;68:108–116.

168. Szostecki C, Guldner HH, Netter HJ, Will H. Isolation and characterization of cDNA encoding a human nuclear antigen predominantly recognized by autoantibodies from patients with primary biliary cirrhosis. *J Immunol* 1990;15:4338–4347.

169. Szostecki C, Will H, Netter HJ, Guldner HH. Autoantibodies to the nuclear Sp100 protein in primary biliary cirrhosis and associated diseases: epitope specificity and immunoglobulin class distribution. *Scand J Immunol* 1992;36:555–564.

170. Guldner HH, Szostecki C, Grotzinger T, Will H. IFN enhance expression of Sp100, an autoantigen in primary biliary cirrhosis. *J Immunol* 1992;149:4067–4073.

171. Zuchner D, Sternsdorf T, Szostecki C, et al. Prevalence, kinetics, and therapeutic modulation of autoantibodies against Sp100 and promyelocytic leukemia protein in a large cohort of patients with primary biliary cirrhosis. *Hepatology* 1997;26:1123–1130.

172. Sternsdorf T, Jensen K, Will H. Evidence for covalent modification of the nuclear dot-associated proteins PML and Sp100 by PIC1/SUMO-1. *J Cell Biol* 1997;139:1621–1634.

173. Parveen S, Morshed SA, Nishioka M. High prevalence of antibodies to recombinant CENP-B in primary biliary cirrhosis: nuclear immunofluorescence patterns and ELISA reactivities. *J Gastroenterol Hepatol* 1995;10:438–445.

174. Chou MJ, Lee SL, Chen TY, Tsay GJ. Specificity of antinuclear antibodies in primary biliary cirrhosis. *Ann Rheum Dis* 1995;148–151.

175. Sartor RB. Pathogenesis and immune mechanisms of chronic inflammatory bowel disease. *Am J Gastroenterol* 1997;12:5S–11S.

176. Rubin PH, Present DH Differential diagnosis of chronic ulcerative colitis and Crohn's disease of the colon: one, two or many diseases? In: Kirsner JB, Shorter RG, eds. *Inflammatory bowel disease.* 4th ed. Baltimore: Williams & Wilkins, 1995:355–379.

177. Rutgeerts P. Medical therapy of inflammatory bowel disease. *Digestion* 1998;59:453–469.

178. Yang H, Rotter JI. Genetics of inflammatory bowel disease. In: Targan SR, Shanahan F, eds. *Inflammatory bowel disease: from bench to bedside.* Baltimore: Williams & Wilkins, 1994:32–64.

179. Calkins BM. Inflammatory bowel disease. In: Everhart JE, ed. *Digestive diseases in the United States: epidemiology and impact.* Bethesda: National Institute of Health, 1994.

180. Tysk C, Lindberg E, Jarnerot G, Floderus-Myrhed B. Ulcerative colitis and Crohn's disease in an unselected population of monozygotic and dizygotic twins: a study of heritability and the influence of smoking. *Gut* 1988;29:990–996.

181. Satsangi J, Jewell DP. The genetics of inflammatory bowel disease. *Gut* 1997;40:572–574.

182. Dignass A, Goebell H. Genetics of inflammatory bowel disease. *Curr Opin Gastroenterol* 1995;11:292–297.

183. Akolkar PN, Gulwani-Akolkar B, Heresbach D, et al. Differences in risk of Crohn's disease in offspring of mothers and fathers with inflammatory bowel disease. *Am J Gastroenterol* 1997;92:2241–2244.

184. Bayless TM, Tokayer AZ, Polito JM II, et al. Crohn's disease: concordance for site and clinical type in affected family members—potential hereditary influences. *Gastroenterology* 1996;111:573–579.

185. Peeters M, Nevens H, Baert F, et al. Familial aggregation in Crohn's disease: increased age-adjusted risk and concordance in clinical characteristics. *Gastroenterology* 1996;111:597–603.

186. Polito JM II, Rees RC, Childs B, et al. Preliminary evidence of genetic anticipation in Crohn's disease. *Lancet* 1996;347:798–800.

187. Satsangi J, Grootscholten C, Holt H, Jewell DP. Clinical patterns of familial inflammatory bowel disease. *Gut* 1996;38:738–741.

188. Sachar D. Crohn's disease a family affair [Editorial]. *Gastroenterology* 1996;111:813–815.

189. Cho JH, Brant SR. Genetics and genetic markers in inflammatory bowel disease. *Curr Opin Gastroenterol* 1998;14:283–238.

190. Hugot J-P, Laurent-Puig P, Gower-Rousseau C, et al. Mapping of a susceptibility locus for Crohn's disease on chromosome 16. *Nature* 1996;379:821–823.

191. Satsangi J, Parkes M, Louis E, et al. Two-stage genome-wide search in inflammatory bowel disease: evidence for susceptibility loci on chromosomes 3, 7, and 12. *Nat Genet* 1996;14:199–202.

192. Rudolph U, Finegold MJ, Rich SS, et al. Ulcerative colitis and adenocarcinoma of the colon in Gα$_{i2}$-deficient mice. *Nat Genet* 1995;10:143–149.

193. Oudkerk Pool M, Roca M, Reumaux D, et al. The value of pANCA as a serological marker for ulcerative colitis in different European regions. *Eur J Gastroenterol Hepatol* 1994;6:399–403.

194. Seibold F, Slametschka D, Gregor M, Weber P. Neutrophil autoantibodies: a genetic marker in primary sclerosing cholangitis and ulcerative colitis. *Gastroenterology* 1994;107:532–536.

195. Shanahan F, Duerr RH, Rotter JI, et al. Antineutrophil autoantibodies in ulcerative colitis: familial aggregation and genetic heterogeneity. *Gastroenterology* 1992;103:456–461.

196. Shanahan F. Neutrophil autoantibodies in inflammatory bowel disease: are they important? *Gastroenterology* 1994;107:586–589.

197. Gionchetti P, Vecchi M, Rizzello F, et al. Lack of effect of antineutrophil cytoplasmic antibodies associated with ulcerative colitis on superoxide anion production from neutrophils. *Gut* 1997;40:102–104.

198. Gordon LK, Eggena MP, Targan SR, Braun J. Tissue expression of antigens recognized by the ulcerative colitis marker antibody pANCA. *Gastroenterology* 1997;112:A982 (abst).

199. Sendid B, Quinton JF, Charrier G, et al. Anti-*Saccharomyces cerevisiae* mannan antibodies in familial Crohn's disease. *Am J Gastroenterol* 1998;93:1306–1310.

200. Quinton JF, Sendid B, Reumaux S, et al. Anti-*Saccharomyces cerevisiae* mannan antibodies combined with anti-neutrophil cytoplasmic autoantibodies in inflammatory bowel disease: prevalence and diagnostic role. *Gut* 1998;42:788–791.

201. Folwaczny C, Noehl K, Tschöp K, et al. Goblet cell antibodies in patients with inflammatory bowel disease and their first-degree relatives. *Gastroenterology* 1997;113:101–106.

202. Mansfield JC, Holden H, Tarlow JK, et al. Novel genetic association between ulcerative colitis and the anti-inflammatory cytokine interleukin-1 receptor antagonist. *Gastroenterology* 1994;106:637–642.

203. Roussomoustakaki M, Satsangi J, Welsh K, et al. Genetic markers may predict disease behaviour in patients with ulcerative colitis. *Gastroenterology* 1997;112:1845–1853.

204. Hacker UT, Gomolka M, Keller E, et al. Lack of association between an interleukin-1 receptor antagonist gene polymorphism and ulcerative colitis. *Gut* 1997;40:623–627.

205. Casini-Raggi V, Kam L, Chong YJT, et al. Mucosal imbalance of IL-1 and IL-1 receptor antagonist in inflammatory bowel disease. *J Immunol* 1995;154:2434–2440.

206. Plevy SE, Targan SR, Yang H, et al. Tumor necrosis factor microsatellites define a Crohn's disease–associated haplotype on chromosome 6. *Gastroenterology* 1996;110:1053–1060.

207. Louis E, Satsangi J, Roussomoustakaki M, et al. Cytokine gene polymorphisms in inflammatory bowel disease. *Gut* 1996;39:705–710.

208. Yang H, Vora DK, Targan SR, et al. Intercellular adhesion molecule I gene associations with immunological subsets of inflammatory bowel disease. *Gastroenterology* 1995;109:440–448.

209. Munkholm P, Langholz E, Hollander D, et al. Intestinal permeability in patients with Crohn's disease and ulcerative colitis and their first degree relatives. *Gut* 1994;35:68–72.

210. Wyatt J, Vogelsang H, Hübl W, et al. Intestinal permeability and the prediction of relapse in Crohn's disease. *Lancet* 1993;341:1437–1439.

211. Podolsky DK, Isselbacher KJ. Glycoprotein composition of colonic mucosa: specific alterations in ulcerative colitis. *Gastroenterology* 1984;87:991–9999.

212. Elson CO, Sartor RB, Tennyson GS, Riddell RH. Experimental models of inflammatory bowel disease. *Gastroenterology* 1995;109:1344–1367.

213. Mashimo H, Wu DC, Podolsky DK, Fishman MC. Impaired defense of intestinal mucosa in mice lacking intestinal trefoil factor. *Science* 1996;274:262–265.

214. Kulkarni AB, Huh C-G, Becker D, et al. Transforming growth factor $\beta_1$ null mutation in mice causes excessive inflammatory response and early death. *Proc Natl Acad Sci USA* 1993;90:770–774.

215. Hermiston ML, Gordon JI. Inflammatory bowel disease and adenomas in mice expressing a dominant negative N-cadherin. *Science* 1995;270:1203–1207.

216. Morales VM, Snapper SB, Blumberg RS. Probing the gastrointestinal immune function using transgenic and knockout technology. *Curr Opin Gastroenterol* 1996;12:577–583.

217. Cosnes J, Carbonell F, Beugerie L, et al. Effects of cigarette smoking on the long-term course of Crohn's disease. *Gastroenterology* 1996;110:424–431.

218. Thomas GAO, Rhodes J, Mani V, et al. Transdermal nicotine as maintenance therapy for ulcerative colitis. *N Engl J Med* 1995;332:988–992.

219. Evans JMM, McMahon AD, Murray FE, et al. Non-steroidal anti-inflammatory drugs are associated with emergency admission to hospital for colitis due to inflammatory bowel disease. *Gut* 1997;40:619–622.

220. Koutroubakis I, Manousos ON, Meuwissen SGM, Pena AS. Environmental risk factors in inflammatory bowel disease. *Hepatogastroenterology* 1996;43:381–393.

221. Rutgeerts P, Geboes K, Peeters M, et al. Effect of faecal stream diversion on recurrence of Crohn's disease in the neoterminal ileum. *Lancet* 1991;338:771–774.

222. Sartor RB, Rath HC, Sellon RK. Microbial factors in chronic intestinal inflammation. *Curr Opin Gastroenterol* 1996;12:327–333.

223. Ekbom A, Wakefield AJ, Zack M, Adami HO. Perinatal measles infection and subsequent Crohn's disease. *Lancet* 1994;344:508–510.

224. Wakefield AJ, Sawyerr AM, Dhillon AP, et al. Pathogenesis of Crohn's disease: multifocal gastrointestinal infarction. *Lancet* 1989;2:1057–1062.

225. Wakefield AJ, Ekbom A, Dhillon AP, et al. Crohn's disease: pathogenesis and persistent measles infection. *Gastroenterology* 1995;108:911–916.

226. Patriarca PA, Beeler JA. Measles vaccination and inflammatory bowel disease. *Lancet* 1995;345:1062–1063.

227. Feeney M, Clegg A, Winwood P, et al. A case-control study of measles vaccination and inflammatory bowel disease. *Lancet* 1997;350:764–746.

228. Belluzzi A, Brignola C, Campieri M, et al. Effect of an enteric-coated fish-oil preparation on relapses in Crohn's disease. *N Engl J Med* 1996;334:1557–1560.

229. Rutgeerts P, D'Haens G, Hiele M, et al. Appendectomy protects against ulcerative colitis. *Gastroenterology* 1994;106:1251–1253.

230. Mizoguchi A, Mizoguchi E, Chiba C, Bhan AK. Role of appendix in the development of inflammatory bowel disease in TCR-alpha mutant mice. *J Exp Med* 1996;184:707–715.

231. Groux H, O'Garra A, Bigler M, et al. A CD4⁺ T-cell subset inhibits antigen-specific T-cell responses and prevents colitis. *Nature* 1997;389:737–742.

232. Powrie F. T cells in inflammatory bowel disease: protective and pathogenetic roles. *Immunity* 1995;3:1587–1595.

233. Sparano JA, Brandt LJ, Dutcher JP, et al. Symptomatic exacerbation of Crohn's disease after treatment with high-dose interleukin-2. *Ann Intern Med* 1993;118:617–618.

234. Lopez-Cubero SO, Sullivan KM, McDonald GB. Course of Crohn's disease after allogeneic marrow transplantation. *Gastroenterology* 1998;114:433–440.

235. Powrie F, Leach MW, Mauze S, et al. Inhibition of T$_H$1 responses prevents inflammatory bowel disease in SCID mice reconstituted with CD45RB$^{high}$CD4⁺ T cells. *Immunity* 1994;1:553–562.

236. Simpson SJ, Mizoguchi E, Allen D, et al. Evidence that CD4⁺, but not CD8⁺, T cells are responsible for the murine interleukin 2–deficient colitis. *Eur J Immunol* 1995;25:2618–2625.

237. Mullin GE, Lazenby AJ, Harris ML, et al. Increased interleukin-2 messenger RNA in the intestinal mucosal lesions of Crohn's disease but not ulcerative colitis. *Gastroenterology* 1992;102:1620–1607.

238. Desreumaux P, Brandt E, Gambiez L, et al. Distinct cytokine patterns in early and chronic ileal lesions of Crohn's disease. *Gastroenterology* 1997;113:118–126.

239. Hornquist CE, Lu X, Rogers-Fani PM, et al. G$\alpha_{i2}$ deficient mice with colitis exhibit a local increase in memory CD4⁺ T cells and proinflammatory Th1-type cytokines. *J Immunol* 1997;158:1068–1077.

240. Saubermann LJ, Probert CSJ, Turner J, et al. Intraindividual T-cell receptor (TCR) β-chain patterns are present among activated intestinal T-cells in patients with inflammatory bowel disease. *Gastroenterology* 1997;112:A1084(abst).

241. Chott A, Probert CS, Lamprecht A, et al. A common TCR β-chain frequently expressed by CD8⁺ intestinal lymphocytes in ulcerative colitis is rarely found in Crohn's disease and other inflammatory disorders. *Gastroenterology* 1997;112:A949(abst).

242. McVay LD, Li B, Biancaniello R, et al. Changes in human mucosal γδ T cell repertoire and function associated with the disease process in inflammatory bowel disease. *Mol Med* 1997;3:182–203.

243. Yacyshyn BR, Lazarovits A, Tsai V, Matejko K. Crohn's disease, ulcerative colitis, and normal intestinal lymphocytes express integrins in dissimilar patterns. *Gastroenterology* 1994;107:1364–1371.

244. Binion DG, West GA, Ina K, et al. Enhanced leucocyte binding by intestinal microvascular endothelial cells in inflammatory bowel disease. *Gastroenterology* 1997;112:1895–1907.

245. Pospai D, René E, Fiasse R, et al. Crohn's disease stable remission after human immunodeficiency virus infection. *Dig Dis Sci* 1998;43:412–419.

246. Befeler AS, Lissoos T, Schiano TD, et al. Clinical course and management of inflammatory bowel disease after liver transplantation. *Transplantation* 1998;65:393–396.

247. Sustento-Reodica N, Ruiz P, Rogers A, et al. Recurrent Crohn's disease in transplanted bowel. *Lancet* 1997;349:688–591.

248. Rugtveit J, Nilsen EM, Bakka A, et al. Cytokine profiles differ in newly recruited and resident subsets of mucosal macrophages from inflammatory bowel disease. *Gastroenterology* 1997;112:1493–1505.

249. Rugtveit J, Bakka A, Brandtzaeg P. Differential distribution of B7.1 (CD80) and B7.2 (CD86) costimulatory molecules on mucosal macrophage subsets in human inflammatory bowel disease (IBD). *Clin Exp Immunol* 1997;110:104–113.

250. Rogler G, Brand K, Vogl D, et al. Nuclear factor kappa B is activated in macrophages and epithelial cells of inflamed intestinal mucosa. *Gastroenterology* 1998;115:357–369.

251. Neurath M, Pettersson S, Meyer zum Buschenfelde KM, Strober W. Local administration of antisense phosphorothioate oligonucleotides to the p65 subunit of NF-kappa B abrogates established experimental colitis in mice. *Nature* Med 1996;2:998–1004.

252. Hallgren R, Colombel JF, Dahl R, et al. Neutrophil and eosinophil involvement of the small bowel in patients with celiac disease and Crohn's disease: studies on the secretion rate and immunohistochemical localization of granulocyte granule constituents. *Am J Med* 1989;86:56–64.

253. Mazzucchielli L, Hauser C, Zgraggen K, et al. Expression of interleukin-8 gene in inflammatory bowel disease is related to the histologic grade of active inflammation. *Am J Pathol* 1994;144:997–1007.

254. Anton PA, Targan SR, Shanahan F. Increased neutrophil receptors for and response to the proinflammatory bacterial peptide formylmethionyl-leucyl-phenylalanin in Crohn's disease. *Gastroenterology* 1989;97:20–28.

255. Lobos EA, Sharon P, Stenson WF. Chemotactic activity in inflammatory bowel disease: role of leukotriene B₄. *Dig Dis Sci* 1987;32:1380–1388.

256. Sobhani I, Hochlaf S, Denizott Y, et al. Raised concentrations of platelet activating factor in colonic mucosa of Crohn's disease patients. *Gut* 1992;33:1220–1225.

257. Ahnfelt-Ronne I, Neilson OH, Christensen A, et al. Clinical evidence supporting the radical scavenger mechanism of 5-aminosalicylic acid. *Gastroenterology* 1990;98:1162–1169.

258. Simmonds NJ, Allen RE, Stevens TRJ, et al. Chemoluminescence assay of mucosal reactive oxygen metabolites in inflammatory bowel disease. *Gastroenterology* 1992;103:186–196.

259. Monajemi H, Meenan J, Lamping R, et al. Inflammatory bowel disease is associated with increased mucosal levels of bactericidal/permeability-increasing protein. *Gastroenterology* 1996;110:733–739.

260. Roseth AG, Fagerhol MK, Aadland E, Schjonsby H. Assessment of the neutrophil dominating protein calprotectin in feces: a methodologic study. *Scand J Gastroenterol* 1992;27:793–798.

261. Andus T, Gross V, Caesar I, et al. PMN elastase in assessment of patients with inflammatory bowel diseases. *Dig Dis Sci* 1993;38:1638–1634.

262. Madara JL, Patapoff TW, Gillece-Castro B, et al. 5′-Adenosine monophosphate is the neutrophil derived paracrine factor that elicits chloride secretion from T84 intestinal epithelial monolayers. *J Clin Invest* 1993;91:2320–2325.

263. Gelbmann CM, Barrett KE. Role of inflammatory cell types in IBD. In: Schölmerich J, Kruis W, Goebell H, et al, eds. *Falk Symposium 67: Inflammatory bowel disease: pathophysiology as a basis of treatment.* Lancaster, UK: Kluwer, 1993:62–79.

264. Sartor RB. Cytokines in intestinal inflammation: pathophysiological and clinical considerations. *Gastroenterology* 1994;106:533–539.

265. Deventer SJH. Cytokines and cytokine-based therapies. *Curr Opin Gastroenterol* 1998;14:317–321.

266. Monteleone G, Biancone L, Marasco R, et al. Interleukin 12 is expressed and actively released by Crohn's disease intestinal lamina propria mononuclear cells. *Gastroenterology* 1997;112:1169–1178.

267. Parronchi P, Romagnani P, Annunziato F, et al. Type 1 T-helper cell predominance and interleukin-12 expression in the gut of patients with Crohn's disease. *Am J Pathol* 1997;150:823–832.

268. Madara JL, Stafford J. Interferon-γ directly affects barrier function of cultured intestinal epithelial monolayers. *J Clin Invest* 1989;83:724–727.

269. Reinecker H-C, Steffen M, Witthoeft T, et al. Enhanced secretion of tumour necrosis factor-alpha, IL-6, and IL-1β by isolated lamina propria mononuclear cells from patients with ulcerative colitis and Crohn's disease. *Clin Exp Immunol* 1993;94:174–181.

270. Murch SH, Braegger CP, Walker-Smith JA, MacDonald TT. Location of tumour necrosis factor alpha by immunohistochemistry in chronic inflammatory bowel disease. *Gut* 1994;35:7105–7109.

271. Van Deventer SJH. Tumour necrosis factor and Crohn's disease. *Gut* 1997;40:443–448.

272. Kuhn R, Lohler J, Rennick D, Rajewsky K, Muller W. Interleukin–10-deficient mice develop chronic enterocolitis. *Cell* 1993;75:263-74.

273. Shull MM, Ormsby I, Kier AB, et al. Targeted disruption of the mouse transforming growth factor-β1 gene results in multifocal inflammatory disease. *Nature* 1992;359:693–699.

274. Moore KW, O'Garra A, de Waal Malefyt R, et al. Interleukin-10. *Annu Rev Immunol* 1993;11:165–190.

275. Peterson JW, Dickey DW, Saini SS, et al. Phospholipase A₂ activating protein and idiopathic inflammatory bowel disease. *Gut* 1996;39:698–704.

276. Dotan I, Rachmilewitz D. Inflammatory mediators in inflammatory bowel disease. *Curr Opin Gastroenterol* 1998;14:295–299.

277. Singer II, Kawka DW, Schloemann S, et al. Cyclooxygenase 2 is induced in colonic epithelial cells in inflammatory bowel disease. *Gastroenterology* 1998;115:297–306.

278. Kimura H, Miura S, Shigematsu T, et al. Increased nitric oxide production and inducible nitric oxide synthase activity in colonic mucosa of patients with active ulcerative colitis and Crohn's disease. *Dig Dis Sci* 1997;42:1047–1054.

279. McCafferty DM, Mudget JS, Swain MG, Kubes P. Inducible nitric oxide synthase plays a critical role in resolving intestinal inflammation. *Gastroenterology* 1997;112:1022–1027.

280. Gaginella TS, Kachur JF, Tamai H, Keshavarazian A. Reactive oxygen and nitrogen metabolites as mediators of secretory diarrhea. *Gastroenterology* 1995;109:2019–2028.

281. Watanabe T, Kubota Y, Muto T. Substance P containing nerve fibers in rectal mucosa of ulcerative colitis. *Dis Colon Rectum* 1997;40:718–725.

282. Yamamoto H, Morise K, Kusugami K, et al. Abnormal neuropeptide concentration in rectal mucosa of patients with inflammatory bowel disease. *J Gastroenterol* 1996;31:525–532.

283. Reinshagen M. Role of neurotrophin-3 and nerve growth factor in chronic experimental colitis in the rat. *Gastroenterology* 1996; A1111 (abst).

284. Stenson WF. The tissue reaction in inflammatory bowel disease. In: Kirsner JB, Shorter RG, eds. *Inflammatory bowel disease.* 4th ed. Baltimore: Williams & Wilkins, 1995:177–189.

285. Strater J, Wellisch I, Riedl S, et al. CD95 (APO-1/Fas)-mediated apoptosis in colon epithelial cells: a possible role in ulcerative colitis. *Gastroenterology* 1997;113:160–167.

286. Balk SP, Burke S, Polischuk JE, et al. Beta 2-microglobuline-independent MHC class Ib molecule expressed by human intestinal epithelium. *Science* 1994;265:259–262.

287. Mayer L, Eisenhardt D, Salomon P, et al. Expression of class II molecules on intestinal epithelial cells in humans. *Gastroenterology* 1991;100:3–12.

288. Mayer L, Eisenhardt D. Lack of induction of suppressor T cells by intestinal epithelial cells from patients with inflammatory bowel disease. *J Clin Invest* 1990;86:1255–1262.

289. Jung HC, Eckmann L, Yang SK, et al. A distinct array of proinflammatory cytokines is expressed in human colon epithelial cells in response to bacterial invasion. *J Clin Invest* 1995;95:55–65.

290. Zgraggen K, Walz A, Mazzucchelli L, et al. The C-X-C chemokine ENA-78 is preferentially expressed in intestinal epithelium in inflammatory bowel disease. *Gastroenterology* 1997;113:808–816.

291. Reinecker HC, MacDermott RP, Mirau S, et al. Intestinal epithelial cells both express and respond to interleukin 15. *Gastroenterology* 1996;111:1706–1713.

292. Stallmach A, Schuppan D, Riese HH, et al. Increased collagen type III synthesis by fibroblasts isolated from strictures of patients with Crohn's disease. *Gastroenterology* 1992;102:1920–1929.

293. Graham MF, Willey A, Adams J, et al. Interleukin-1β down-regulates collagen and augments collagenase expression in human intestinal smooth muscle cells. *Gastroenterology* 1996;110:344–350.

294. Bhagat S, Das KM. A shared and unique peptide in the human colon, eye, and joint detected by a monoclonal antibody. *Gastroenterology* 1994;107:103–108.

295. Nostrant TT, Kumar NB, Appelmann HD. Histopathology differentiates acute self-limited colitis from ulcerative colitis. *Gastroenterology* 1987;92:318–328.

296. Jenkins D, Balsitis M, Gallivan S, et al. Guidelines for the initial biopsy diagnosis of suspected chronic idiopathic inflammatory bowel disease. The British Society of Gastroenterology Initiative. *J Clin Pathol* 1997;50:93–105.

297. Seldenrijk CA, Morson BC, Meuwissen SGM, et al. Histopathological evaluation of colonic mucosa biopsy specimens in chronic inflammatory bowel disease: diagnostic implications. *Gut* 1991;32:1514–1520.

298. Price AB. Overlap in the spectrum of non-specific inflammatory bowel disease—"colitis indeterminate." *J Clin Pathol* 1978;31:567–577.

299. Lazenby AJ, Yardley JH, Giardiello FM, et al. Lymphocytic ("microscopic") colitis: a comparative histopathological study with particular reference to collagenous colitis. *Hum Pathol* 1989;20:18–28.

300. Lazenby AJ, Yardley JH, Giardiello FM, Bayless TM. Pitfalls in the diagnosis of collagenous colitis: experience with 75 cases from a registry of collagenous colitis at the Johns Hopkins Hospital. *Hum Pathol* 1990;21:905–910.

301. Tanaka M, Mazzoleni G, Riddell RH. Distribution of collagenous colitis: utility of flexible sigmoidoscopy. *Gut* 1992;33:65–70.

302. Zins BJ, Sandborn WJ, Tremaine WJ. Collagenous and lymphocytic colitis: subject review and therapeutic alternatives. *Am J Gastroenterol* 1995;90:1394–1400.

303. Sachar DB, Andrews HA, Farmer RG, et al. Proposed classification subgroups in Crohn's disease. *Gastroenterol Int* 1992;5:141–154.

304. Gasché C, Schölmerich J, Brynskov J, et al. A simple classification of Crohn's disease. *Am J Gastroenterol* 2000 (in press).

305. Ogorek CP, Fisher RS. Differentiation between Crohn's disease and ulcerative colitis. *Med Clin North Am* 1994;78:1249–1258.

306. Tan WC, Allan RN. Diffuse jejunoileitis of Crohn's disease. *Gut* 1993;34:1374–1378.

307. Schumacher G, Sandstedt B, Kollberg B. A prospective study of first attacks of inflammatory bowel disease and infectious colitis: clinical findings and early diagnosis. *Scand J Gastroenterol* 1994;29:265–274.

308. Lossing A, Langer B, Jeejeebhoy KN. Gastroduodenal Crohn's disease: diagnosis and selection of treatment. *Can J Surg* 1983;26:358–360.

309. Oberhuber G, Püspök A, Österreicher C, et al. Focally enhanced gastritis: a frequent type of gastritis in patients with Crohn's disease. *Gastroenterology* 1997;112:698–706.

310. Meyer S, Janowitz HD. "Natural history" of Crohn's disease: an analytic review of the placebo lesson. *Gastroenterology* 1984;87:1189–1192.

311. Greenstein AJ, Lachmann P, Sachar DB, et al. Perforating and nonperforating indications for repeated operations in Crohn's disease: evidence for two clinical forms. *Gut* 1988;29:588–592.

312. Miner PB. Factors influencing the relapse of patients with inflammatory bowel disease. *Am J Gastroenterol* 1997;92:1S–4S.

313. Moum B, Aadland E, Vatn MH, Ekbom A. Seasonal variation of onset of ulcerative colitis. *Gut* 1996;38:376–378.

314. Singleton JW. Clinical features, course, and laboratory findings in ulcerative colitis. In: Kirsner JB, Shorter RG, eds. *Inflammatory bowel disease.* 4th ed. Baltimore: Williams & Wilkins, 1995:355–379.

315. D'Haens G, Geboes K, Peeters M, et al. Patchy cecal inflammation associated with distal ulcerative colitis: a prospective endoscopic study. *Am J Gastroenterol* 1997;92:1275–1279.

316. de Dombal FT, Watts JM, Watkinson G, Goligher JC. The early course and prognosis of ulcerative colitis. *Proc R Soc Med* 1965;58:711–713.

317. Ilnyckyj A, Shanahan F, Anton PA, et al. Quantification of the placebo response in ulcerative colitis. *Gastroenterology* 1997;112:1854–1858.

318. Broström O. Prognosis in ulcerative colitis. *Med Clin North Am* 1990;74:201–218.

319. Edwards FC, Truelove SC. The course and prognosis of ulcerative colitis. *Gut* 1964;5:1–15.

320. Hermens DJ, Miner PB Jr. Exacerbation of ulcerative colitis. *Gastroenterology* 1991;101:254–262.

321. Riley SA, Mani V, Goodman MJ. Why do patients with ulcerative colitis relapse? [Letter] *Gut* 1990;31:179.

322. Podolsky DK. Inflammatory bowel disease. *N Engl J Med* 1991;325:928–937, 1008–1016.

323. Reinisch W, Heider K-H, Oberhuber G, et al. Poor diagnostic value of colonic CD44v6 and its serum soluble form to differentiate Ulcerative colitis and Crohn's disease. *Gut* 1998;43:375–382.

324. Wells AD, McMillan I, Price AB, et al. Natural history of indeterminate colitis. *Br J Surg* 1991;78:179–181.

325. Hyman NH, Fazio VW, Tuckson WB, Lavery IC. Consequences of ileal pouch-anal anastomosis for Crohn's colitis. *Dis Colon Rectum* 1991;34:653–657.

326. Waye JD. Endoscopy of inflammatory bowel disease. In: Kirsner JB, Shorter RG, eds. *Inflammatory bowel disease.* 4th ed. Baltimore: Williams & Wilkins, 1995:555–582.

327. Riddell RH. Pathology of idiopathic inflammatory bowel disease. In: Kirsner JB, Shorter RG, eds. *Inflammatory bowel disease.* 4rd ed. Baltimore: Williams & Wilkins, 1995:517–552.

328. Quinn PG, Binion DG, Connors PJ. The role of endoscopy in inflammatory bowel disease. *Med Clin North Am* 1994;78:1331–1352.

329. Pera A, Bellando P, Caldera T, et al. Colonoscopy in inflammatory bowel disease: diagnostic accuracy and proposal of an endoscopic score. *Gastroenterology* 1987;92:181–185.

330. Fujimura Y, Kamoi R, Ida M. Pathogenesis of aphthoid ulcers in Crohn's disease: correlative findings by magnifying colonoscopy, electron microscopy and immunohistochemistry. *Gut* 1996;38:724–732.

331. Modigliani R, Mary Y-J, Simon JF, et al. (Group détude therapeutiques des affections inflammatoires digestives). Clinical, biological and endoscopic picture of attacks of Crohn's disease: evolution on prednisolone. *Gastroenterology* 1990;98:811–818.

332. Rutgeerts P, Geboes K, Vantrappen G, et al. Predictability of the postoperative course of Crohn's disease. *Gastroenterology* 1990;99:956–963.

333. Yardley JH, Hendrix TR. Gastroduodenal Crohn's disease: the focus is on focality [Editorial]. *Gastroenterology* 1997;112:1031–1043.

334. Bernstein CN, Boult IF, Greenberg HM, et al. A prospective randomized comparison between small bowel enteroclysis and small bowel follow-through in Crohn's disease. *Gastroenterology* 1997;13:390–398.

335. Maglinte DDT, Lappas JC, Kelvin FM, et al. Small bowel radiography: how, when and why? *Radiology* 1987;163:297–305.

336. Herlinger H, Rubesin SE, Furth EE. Mesenteric border linear ulcer in Crohn's disease: historical, radiologic, and pathologic perspectives. *Abdom Imaging* 1998;23:122–126.

337. Carlson HC, Maccarty LM. Radiology of inflammatory bowel disease. In: Kirsner JB, Shorter RG, eds. *Inflammatory bowel disease.* 4th ed. Baltimore: Williams & Wilkins, 1995:583–640.

338. Riley SA, Mani V, Goodman MJ, et al. Microscopic activity in ulcerative colitis: what does it mean? *Gut* 1991;32:174–178.

339. Hata J, Haruma K, Suenaga K, et al. Ultrasonographic assessment of inflammatory bowel disease. *Am J Gastroenterol* 1992;87:443–447.

340. Gasché C, Moser G, Turetschek K, et al. Transabdominal bowel sonography for the detection of intestinal complications in Crohn's disease. *Gut* 1999;44:112–117.

341. Gore RM, Balthazar EJ, Ghahremani GG, Miller FH. CT features of ulcerative colitis and Crohn's disease. *Am J Roentgenol* 1996;167:3–15.

342. Schober E, Turetschek K, Oberhuber G, et al. Enteroclysis spiral CT: diagnostic yield in the preoperative assessment of Crohn's disease. *Radiology* 1996;201:1358(abst).

343. Schölmerich J, Schmidt E, Schümichen C, et al. Scintigraphic assessment of bowel involvement and disease activity in Crohn's disease using technetium 99m–hexamethyl propylene amine oxine as leucocyte label. *Gastroenterology* 1988;95:1287–1293.

344. Shanahan F, Duerr RH, Rotter JI, et al. Neutrophil autoantibodies in ulcerative colitis: familial aggregation and genetic heterogeneity. *Gastroenterology* 1992;103:456–461.

345. Vasiliauskas EA, Plevy SE, Landers CJ, et al. Perinuclear antineutrophil cytoplasmic antibodies in patients with Crohn's disease define a clinical subgroup. *Gastroenterology* 1996;110:1810–1819.

346. Kjeldsen J, Schaffalitzky de Muckadell OB. Assessment of disease severity and activity in inflammatory bowel disease. *Scand J Gastroenterol* 1993;28:1–9.

347. Truelove SC, Witts LJ. Cortisone in ulcerative colitis: Final report on a therapeutic trial. *BMJ* 1955;2:1041–1048.

348. Rachmilewitz D. Coated mesalazine (5-aminosalicylic acid) versus sulphasalazine in the treatment of active ulcerative colitis: a randomized trial. *BMJ* 1989;298:82–86.

349. Powell-Tuck J, Bown RL, Lennard-Jones JE. A comparison of oral prednisolone given as single or multiple daily doses for active proctocolitis. *Scand J Gastroenterol* 1978;13:833–837.

350. Olaison G, Sjödahl R, Tagesson C. Glucocorticoid treatment in ileal Crohn's disease: relief of symptoms but not of endoscopically viewed inflammation. *Gut* 1990;31:325–328.

351. Goodman MJ, Skinner JM, Truelove SC. Abnormalities in the apparently normal bowel mucosa in Crohn's disease. *Lancet* 1976;1:275–278.

352. Hanauer SB, Meyers S. Management of Crohn's disease in adults. *Am J Gastroenterol* 1997;92:559–566.

353. Best WR, Becktel JM, Singleton JW, Kern F. Development of a Crohn's disease activity index—National Crohn's Disease Study. *Gastroenterology* 1976;70:439–444.

354. Van Hees PAM, Van Elteren PH, Van Lier HJJ, Van Tongeren JHM. An index of inflammatory activity in patients with Crohn's disease. *Gut* 1980;21:279–286.

355. Irvine EJ, Feagan B, Rochon J, et al. Quality of life: a valid and reliable measure of therapeutic efficacy in the treatment of inflammatory bowel disease. *Gastroenterology* 1994;106:287–296.

356. Mary JY, Modigliani R. Development and and validation of an endoscopic index of the severity for Crohn's disease: a prospective multicenter study. *Gut* 1989;30:983–99.

357. Lobo AJ, Sobala GM, Juby LD, et al. Evaluation of indices of disease activity in Crohn's disease by consensus analysis. *Eur J Gastroenterol Hepatol* 1991;3:663–666.

358. André C, Descos L, Landais P, Fermanian J. Assessment of appropriate laboratory measurements to supplement the Crohn's disease activity index. *Gut* 1981;22:571–574.

359. Sugi K, Saitoh O, Hirata I, Katsu K. Fecal lactoferrin as a marker for disease activity in inflammatory bowel disease: comparison with other neutrophil-derived proteins. *Am J Gastroenterol* 1996;91:927–934.

360. Pironi L, Miglioli M, Ruggeri E, et al. Relationship between intestinal permeability to [$^{51}$Cr]EDTA and inflammatory activity in asymptomatic patients with Crohn's disease. *Dig Dis Sci* 1990;35:582–588.

361. Rutgeerts P, Geboes K, Vantrappen G. Natural history of recurrent Crohn's disease at the ileocolonic anastomosis after curative surgery. *Gut* 1984;25:666–672.

362. McLeod RS, Wolff BG, Steinhart AH, et al. Risk and significance of endoscopic/radiologic evidence of recurrent Crohn's disease. *Gastroenterology* 1997;113:1823–1827.

363. D'Haens G, Geboes K, Peeters M, et al. Early lesions of recurrent Crohn's disease caused by infusion of intestinal contents in excluded ileum. *Gastroenterology* 1998;114:262–267.

364. Sachar DB, Wolfson DM, Greenstein AJ, et al. Risk factors for postoperative recurrence of Crohn's disease. *Gastroenterology* 1983;85:917–921.

365. Borley NR, Mortensen NJ, Jewell DP. Preventing postoperative recurrence of Crohn's disease. *Br J Surg* 1997;84:1493–1502.

366. Greenstein AJ, Janowitz HD, Sachar DB. The extraintestinal complications of Crohn's disease and ulcerative colitis: a study of 700 patients. *Medicine (Baltimore)* 1976;55:401–412.

367. Weiss A, Mayer L. Extraintestinal manifestations of inflammatory bowel disease. In: Allan RN, Rhodes JM, Hanauer SB, et al, eds. *Inflammatory bowel disease.* New York: Churchill Livingstone, 1997:623–632.

368. Lamers CBHW. Treatment of extraintestinal manifestations of ulcerative colitis. *Eur J Gastroenterol Hepatol* 1997;9:850–853.

369. Orchard TR, Wordsworth BP, Jewell DP. Peripheral arthropathies in inflammatory bowel disease: their articular distribution and natural history. *Gut* 1998;42:387–391.

370. Salmi M, Rajala P, Jalkane S. Homing of mucosal leucocytes to joints: distinct endothelial ligands in synovium mediate leucocyte-subtype adhesion. *J Clin Invest* 1997;99:2165–2172.

371. De Vos M, Mielants H, Cuvelier C, et al. Long-term evolution of gut inflammation in patients with spondylarthropathy. *Gastroenterology* 1996;110:1696–1703.

372. Wiesner RH. Current concepts in primary sclerosing cholangitis. *Mayo Clin Proc* 1994;69:969–982.

373. Marchesa P, Lashner BA, Lavery IC, et al. The risk of cancer and dysplasia among ulcerative colitis patients with primary sclerosing cholangitis. *Am J Gastroenterol* 1997;92:1285–1288.

374. Nuako KW, Ahlquist DA, Sandborn WJ, et al. Primary sclerosing cholangitis and colorectal carcinoma in patients with chronic ulcerative colitis: a case-control study. *Cancer* 1998;82:822–826.

375. Kaplan MM. Toward better treatment of primary sclerosing cholangitis [Editorial]. *N Engl J Med* 1997;336:719–721.

376. Heikius B, Niemelä S, Lehtola J, et al. Hepatobiliary and coexisting pancreatic duct abnormalities in patients with inflammatory bowel disease. *Scand J Gastroenterol* 1997;32:153–161.

377. Jackson LM, O'Gorman PJ, O'Connell, et al. Thrombosis in inflammatory bowel disease: clinical setting, procoagulant profile and factor V Leiden. *Q J Med* 1997;90:183–188.

378. Collins CE, Rampton DS. Platelet dysfunction: a new dimension in inflammatory bowel disease. *Gut* 1995;36:5–8.

379. Thompson NP, Wakefield AJ, Pounder RE. Inherited disorders of coagulation appear to protect against inflammatory bowel disease. *Gastroenterology* 1995;108:1011–1015.

380. El-Serag HB, Zwas F, Bonheim NA, et al. The renal and urologic complications of inflammatory bowel disease. *Inflamm Bowel Dis* 1997;3:217–224.

381. Kreisel W, Wolf LM, Grotz W, Grieshaber M. Renal tubular damage: an extraintestinal manifestation of chronic inflammatory bowel disease. *Eur J Gastroenterol Hepatol* 1996;8:461–468.

382. Lovat LB, Madhoo S, Pepys MB, Hawkins PN. Long-term survival in systemic amyloid A amyloidosis complicating Crohn's disease. *Gastroenterology* 1997;112:1362–1365.

383. Gschwantler M, Kogelbauer G, Klose W, et al. The pancreas as a site of granulomatous inflammation in Crohn's disease. *Gastroenterology* 1995;108:1246–1249.

384. Geissler A, Andus T, Roth M, et al. Focal white matter lesions in brain of patients with inflammatory bowel disease. *Lancet* 1995;345:897–898.

385. Godet PG, Cowie R, Woodman RC, Sutherland LR. Pulmonary function abnormalities in patients with ulcerative colitis. *Am J Gastroenterol* 1997;92:1154–1156.

386. Andreassen H, Rungby J, Dahlerup F, Mosekilde L. Inflammatory bowel disease and osteoporosis. *Scand J Gastroenterol* 1997;32:1247–1255.

387. Gasché C, Reinisch W, Lochs H, et al. Anemia in Crohn's disease. Importance of inadequate erythropoietin production and iron deficiency. *Dig Dis Sci* 1994;39:1930–1934.

388. Burakoff R. Fertility and pregnancy in inflammatory bowel disease. In: Kirsner JB, Shorter RG, eds. *Inflammatory bowel disease.* 4th ed. Baltimore: Williams & Wilkins, 1995:492–436.

389. Modigliani R. Drug therapy for ulcerative colitis during pregnancy. *Eur J Gastroenterol Hepatol* 1997;9:854–857.

390. Motil KJ, Grand R, Davis-Kraft L, et al. Growth failure in children with inflammatory bowel disease: a prospective study. *Gastroenterology* 1993;105:681–691.

391. Saha MT, Ruuska T, Laippala P, Lenko HL. Growth of prepubertal children with inflammatory bowel disease. *J Pediatr Gastroenterol Nutr* 1998;26:310–314.

392. Wilschanski M, Sherman P, Pencharz P, et al. Supplementary enteral nutrition maintains remission in paediatric Crohn's disease. *Gut* 1996;38:543–548.

393. Calenda KA, Grand RJ. Clinical manifestations of pediatric inflammatory bowel disease. In: Kirsner JB, Shorter RG, eds. *Inflammatory bowel disease.* 4th ed. Baltimore: Williams & Wilkins, 1995:695–714.

394. Kornbluth A, Sachar DB. Ulcerative colitis practice guidelines in adults. *Am J Gastroenterol* 1997;92:204–211.

395. Feagen BG, McDonald JW, Koval JJ. Therapeutics and Inflammatory bowel disease: a guide of the interpretations of randomized controlled trials. *Gastroenterology* 1996;110:275–283.

396. Williams JG, Hallett MB. Effect of sulphasalazine and its derivative metabolite, 5-aminosalicylic acid, on toxic oxygen metabolite production by neutrophils. *Gut* 1989;30:1581–1587.

397. Bissonnette EY, Enciso JA, Befus AD. Inhibitory effects of sulfasalazine and its metabolites on histamine release and TNF-α production by mast cells. *J Immunol* 1996;156:218–223.

398. Di Paolo MC, Merrett MN, Crotty B, Jewell DP. 5-Aminosalicylic acid inhibits the impaired epithelial barrier function induced by gamma interferon. *Gut* 1996;38:115–119.

399. Tremaine WJ, Schroeder KW, Harrison JM, Zinsmeister AR. A randomized, double-blind placebo-controlled trial of the oral mesalamine (5-ASA) preparation, Asacol, in the treatment of symptomatic Crohn's colitis and ileocolitis. *J Clin Gastroenterol* 1994;19:278–282.

400. Gross V, Roth M, Fischbach W, et al. Comparison between high dose 5-aminosalicylic acid (5-ASA) and 6-methylprednisolone in active Crohn's disease. *Gastroenterology* 1994;106:A694(abst).

401. Valori RM, Cockel R. Omeprazole for duodenal ulceration in Crohn's disease. *Br Med J* 1990;300:438–439.

402. Meyers S, Sachar DB. Medical therapy of Crohn's disease. In: Kirsner JB, Shorter RG, eds. *Inflammatory bowel disease.* 4th ed. Baltimore: Williams & Wilkins, 1995:695–714.

403. Malchow H, Ewe K, Brandes JW, et al. European Cooperative Crohn's Disease Study (ECCDS): results of drug treatment. *Gastroenterology* 1984;86:249–266.

404. Summers RW, Switz DM, Sessions JT Jr, et al. National Cooperative Crohn's Disease Study's results of drug treatment. *Gastroenterology* 1979;77:847–869.

405. Salomon P, Kornbluth A, Aisenberg J, Janowitz HD. How effective are current drugs for Crohn's disease? A meta-analysis. *J Clin Gastroenterol* 1992;14:211–215.

406. Landi B, Anh TN, Cortot A, et al. Endoscopic monitoring of Crohn's disease: a prospective, randomized clinical trial. *Gastroenterology* 1992;102:1647–1653.

407. Reinisch W, Gasché C, Wyatt J, et al. Steroid dependency in Crohn's disease [Letter]. *Lancet* 1995;345:859.

408. Rutgeerts P, Lofberg R, Malchow H, et al. A comparison of budesonide with prednisolone for active Crohn's disease. *N Engl J Med* 1994;331:842–845.

409. Greenberg GR, Feagan BG, Martin F, et al. Oral budesonide for active Crohn's disease. *N Engl J Med* 1994;331:836–841.

410. Thomsen OO, Cortot A, Jewell D, et al. A comparison of budesonide and mesalamine for active Crohn's disease. *N Engl J Med* 1998;339:370–374.

411. Gross V, Caesar I, Andus T, et al. Dose-finding study with oral budesonide in patients with active Crohn's ileocolitis. *Gastroenterology* 1997;112:A986(abst).

412. Brattsand R. Overview of newer glucosteroid preparations for inflammatory bowel disease. *Can J Gastroenterol* 1990;4:407–414.

413. Brattsand R, Linden M. Cytokine modulation by glucocorticoids: mechanisms and actions in cellular studies. *Aliment Pharmacol Ther* 1996;10[Suppl 2]:81–90.

414. Steinhart AH, Greenberg GR. Nutrition in inflammatory bowel disease. *Curr Opin Gastroenterol* 1997;13:140–145.

415. Griffiths AM, Ohlsson A, Sherman PM, Sutherland LR. Meta-analysis of enteral nutrition as a primary treatment of active Crohn's disease. *Gastroenterology* 1995;108:1056–1067.

416. Messori A, Trallori G, Dalbasio G, et al. Defined-formula diets versus steroids in the treatment of active Crohn's disease: a meta-analysis. *Gastroenterology* 1996;31:267–272.

417. Present DH, Korelitz BI, Wisch N, et al. Treatment of Crohn's disease with 6-mercaptopurine: a long-term randomized double blind study. *N Engl J Med* 1980;302:981–987.

418. Greenberg GR, Fleming CR, Jeejeebhoy KN, et al. Controlled trial of bowel rest and nutritional support in the management of Crohn's disease. *Gut* 1988;29:1309–1315.

419. Bernstein LH, Frank MS, Brandt LJ, Boley SJ. Healing of perianal Crohn's disease with metronidazole. *Gastroenterology* 1980;79:357–365.

420. Solomon MJ, McLeod RS, O'Connor BI. Combination ciprofloxacin and metronidazole in severe perianal Crohn's disease. *Can J Gastroenterol* 1993;7:571–573.

421. Brandt LJ, Bernstein LH, Boley SJ, Frank MS. Metronidazole for perineal Crohn's disease: a follow-up study. *Gastroenterology* 1982;83:38–37.

422. Duffy LF, Daum F, Fisher SE, et al. Peripheral neuropathy in Crohn's disease patients treated with metronidazole. *Gastroenterology* 1985;88:681–684.

423. Present DH, Lichtiger S. Efficacy of cyclosporine in treatment of fistulae of Crohn's disease. *Dig Dis Sci* 1994;39:374–380.

424. Greenberg GR, Feagan BG, Martin F, et al. Oral budesonide as maintenance treatment for Crohn's disease: a placebo-controlled, dose-ranging study. *Gastroenterology* 1996;110:45–51.

425. Korelitz BI, Adler DJ, Mendelsohn RA, et al. Long-term experience with 6-mercaptopurine in the treatment of Crohn's disease. *Am J Gastroenterol* 1993;8:1198–1205.

426. Pearson DC, May GR, Fick GH, Sutherland LR. Azathioprine and 6-mercaptopurine in Crohn's disease: a meta-analysis. *Ann Intern Med* 1995;122:132–142.

427. D'Haens G, Geboes K, Ponette E, et al. Healing of severe recurrent ileitis with azathioprine therapy in patients with Crohn's disease. *Gastroenterology* 1997;112;1475–1481.

428. Sandborn WJ, Van Os EC, Zins BJ, et al. An intravenous loading dose of azathioprine decreases the time to response in patients with Crohn's disease. *Gastroenterology* 1995;109:1808–1817.

429. Connell WR, Kamm MA, Ritchie JK, Lennard-Jones JE. Bone marrow toxicity caused by azathioprine in inflammatory bowel disease:27 years of experience. *Gut* 1993;34:1081–1085.

430. Colonna T, Korelitz BI. The role of leukopenia in the 6-mercaptopurine–induced remission of refractory Crohn's disease. *Am J Gastroenterol* 1994;89:362–366.

431. Connell WR, Kamm MA, Dickson M, et al. Long-term neoplasia risk after azathioprine treatment in inflammatory bowel disease. *Lancet* 1994;343:1249–1252.

432. Bouhnik Y, Lémann M, Mary J-Y, et al. Long-term follow-up of patients with Crohn's disease treated with azathioprine or 6-mercaptopurine. *Lancet* 1996;347:215–219.

433. Korelitz B, Hanauer S, Rutgeerts P, et al. Post-operative prophylaxis with 6-MP, 5-ASA, or placebo in Crohn's disease: a 2 year multicenter trial. *Gastroenterology* 1998;114:A1011.

434. Feagan B, Rocon J, Fedorak R, et al. Methotrexate for the treatment of Crohn's disease. *N Engl J Med* 1995;332:292–297.

435. Lémann M, Chamiot-Prieur C, Mesnard B, et al. Methotrexate for the treatment of refractory Crohn's disease. *Aliment Pharmacol Ther* 1996;10:309–314.

436. Connell WR. Safety of drug therapy for inflammatory bowel disease in pregnant and nursing women. *Inflamm Bowel Dis* 1996;2:33–47.

437. Stange EF, Modigliani R, Pena AS, et al. European trial of cyclosporine in chronic active Crohn's disease: a 12-month study. The European Study Group. *Gastroenterology* 1995;109:774–782.

438. Feagan BG, McDonald JWD, Rochon J, Kinnear D, et al. Low-dose cyclosporine for the treatment of Crohn's disease. *N Engl J Med* 1994;330:1846–1851.

439. Hanauer SB, Smith MB. Rapid closure of Crohn's disease fistulas with continuous intravenous cyclosporin A. *Am J Gastroenterol* 1993;88:646–649.

440. WJ Sandborn. Preliminary report on the use of oral tacrolismus (FK506) in the treatment of complicated proximal small bowel and fistulizing Crohn's disease. *Am J Gastroenterol* 1997;92:876–879.

441. Cammà C, Giunta M, Roselli M, Cottone M. Mesalamine in the maintenance treatment of Crohn's disease: a meta-analysis adjusted for confounding variables. *Gastroenterology* 1997;113:1465–1473.

442. De Franchis R, Omodei P, Ranzi T, et al. Controlled trial of oral 5-aminosalicylic acid for the prevention of early relapse in Crohn's disease. *Aliment Pharmacol Ther* 1997;11:845–852.

443. Sutherland LR, Martin F, Bailey JR, et al. A randomized, placebo-controlled, double-blind trial of mesalamine in the maintenance of remission of Crohn's disease. *Gastroenterology* 1997;112:1069–1077.

444. Modigliani R, Colombel F, Dupas L, et al. Mesalamine in Crohn's disease with steroid-induced remission: effect on steroid withdrawal and remission maintenance. *Gastroenterology* 1996;110:688–693.

445. Brignola C, Cottone M, Pera A, et al. Mesalamine in the prevention of endoscopic recurrence after intestinal resection for Crohn's disease. *Gastroenterology* 1995;108:345–349.

446. D'Haens G, Rutgeerts P. Maintenance and prophylactic therapy for Crohn's disease. *Curr Opin Gastroenterol* 1997;13:312–316.

447. Habal FM, Hui G, Greenberg GR. Oral 5-aminosalicylic acid for inflammatory bowel disease in pregnancy: safety and clinical course. *Gastroenterology* 1993;105:1057–1060.

448. Diav-Citrin O, Park YH, Veerasuntharam G, et al. The safety of mesalamine in human pregnancy: a prospective controlled cohort study. *Gastroenterology* 1998;114:23–28.

449. Kornbluth A, Sachar DB. Ulcerative colitis practice guidelines in adults. *Am J Gastroenterol* 1997;92:204–211.

450. Hanauer SB. Medical therapy of ulcerative colitis. *Lancet* 1993;1:412–417.

451. Sninsky CA, Cort DH, Shanahan F, et al. Oral mesalamine (Asacol) for mildly to moderately active ulcerative colitis: a multi-center study. *Ann Intern Med* 1991;115:350–355.

452. Schroeder KW, Tremaine WJ, Ilstrup DM. Coated oral 5-aminosalicylic therapy for mildly to moderately ulcerative colitis: a randomized trial. *N Engl J Med* 1987;317:1625–1629.

453. Meyers S, Sachar DB, Present DH, Janowitz HD. Olsalazine sodium in the treatment of ulcerative colitis among patients intolerant of sulfasalazine: a prospective, randomized, placebo-controlled, double-blind, dose-ranging clinical trial. *Gastroenterology* 1987;93:2255–2262.

454. Campieri M, Corbelli C, Gionchetti P, et al. Spread and distribution of 5-ASA colonic foam and 5-ASA enema in patients with ulcerative colitis. *Dig Dis Sci* 1992;37:1890–1897.

455. Marshall JK, Irvine EJ. Rectal corticosteroids versus alternative treatments in ulcerative colitis: a meta-analysis. *Gut* 1997;40:775–781.

456. d'Albasio G, Pacini F, Camarri E, et al. Combined therapy with 5-aminosalicylic acid tablets and enemas for maintaining remission in ulcerative colitis: a randomized double-blind study. *Am J Gastroenterol* 1997;92:1143–1147.

457. Jarnerot G, Lennard-Jones J, Bianchi-Porro G, et al. Medical treatment of refractory distal ulcerative colitis. *Gastroenterol Int* 1991;4:93–98.

458. Sutherland LR, Roth DE, Beck PL. Alternatives to sulfasalazine: a meta-analysis of 5-ASA in the treatment of ulcerative colitis. *Inflamm Bowel Dis* 1997;3:65–78.

459. Giaffer MH, O'Brian CJ, Holdsworth CD. Clinical tolerance to three 5-aminosalicylic acid releasing preparations in patients with inflammatory bowel disease intolerant or allergic to sulfasalazine *Aliment Pharmacol Ther* 1992;6:51–61.

460. Green JRB, Lobo AJ, Holdsworth CD, et al. Balsalazide is more effective and better tolerated than mesalamine in the treatment of acute ulcerative colitis. *Gastroenterology* 1998;114:15–22.

461. Kornbluth AA, Salomon P, Sacks HS, et al. Meta-analysis of the effectiveness of current drug therapy of ulcerative colitis. *J Clin Gastroenterol* 1993;16:215–218.

462. Kirk AP, Lennard-jones JE. Controlled trial of azathioprine in chronic ulcerative colitis. *Br Med J* 1982;284:1291–1292.

463. Hawthorne AB, Logan RFA, Hawkey CJ, et al. Randomized controlled trial of azathioprine withdrawal in ulcerative colitis. *Br Med J*, 1992; 305:20–22.

464. Lofberg R, Danielsson A, Suhr O, et al. Oral budesonide versus prednisolone in patients with active extensive and left-sided ulcerative colitis. *Gastroenterology* 1998;110:1713–1718.

465. Truelove SC, Willoughby CP, Lee G, Kettlewell MG. Further experience in the treatment of severe attacks of ulcerative colitis. *Lancet* 1978;2:1086–1088.

466. Jarnerot G, Rolny P, Saulbergh-Gertzen H. Intensive intravenous treatment of ulcerative colitis. *Gastroenterology* 1985:89:1005–1013.

467. Kaplan HP, Portnoy B, Binder HJ, et al. A controlled evaluation of intravenous adrenocorticotropic hormone and hydrocortisone in the treatment of acute colitis. *Gastroenterology* 1975;69:91–95.

468. Rosenberg W, Ireland A, Jewell D. High-dose methylprednisone in the treatment of active ulcerative colitis. *J Clin Gastroenterol* 1990;12: 40–41.

469. Present DH, Wolfson D, Gelernt IM, et al. Medical decompression of toxic megacolon by "rolling": a new technique of decompression with favorable long-term follow-up. *J Clin Gastroenterol* 1988;10: 485–490.

470. McIntyre DB, Powell-Tuck J, Wood SR. Controlled trial of bowel rest in the treatment of severe acute colitis. *Gut* 1986;27:481–485.

471. Marion JF, Present DH. The modern medical management of acute, severe ulcerative colitis. *Eur J Gastroenterol Hepatol* 1997;9:831–835.

472. Jewell DP, Caprilli R, Mortensen N, et al. Indication and timing of surgery for severe ulcerative colitis. *Gastroenterol Int* 1991;4:161–164.

473. Kornbluth AA, Marion JF, Salomon P, Janowitz HD. How effective is current medical therapy for severe ulcerative colitis and Crohn's colitis? An analytical review of selected trials. *J Clin Gastroenterol* 1995;20: 280–284.

474. Travis SP, Farrant JM, Ricketts C, et al. Predicting outcome in severe ulcerative colitis. *Gut* 1996;38:905–910.

475. Lichtiger S, Present DH, Kornbluth A, et al. Cyclosporine in severe ulcerative colitis refractory to steroid therapy. *N Engl J Med* 1994; 330:1841–1845.

476. Kornbluth A, Lichtiger S, Present DH, et al. Long term results of oral cyclosporine in patients with severe ulcerative colitis: a double-blind, randomized, multi-center trial. *Gastroenterology* 1994;106:A714(abst).

477. Baert F, Hanauer S. CyA in severe steroid-resistant UC: long-term results of therapy. *Gastroenterology* 1994;106:A648(abst).

478. D'Haens G, Lemmens L, Hiele M, et al. Intravenous cyclosporine A (CyA) monotherapy versus intravenous methylprednisolone (MP) monotherapy in severe ulcerative colitis: a randomized double blind controlled trial. *Gastroenterology* 1998;114:A963(abst).

479. Mahadevan U, Kornbluth AA, Goldstein E, et al. Is cyclosporine (CS) induced nephrotoxicity permanent or progressive in patients with inflammatory bowel disease. *Gastroenterology* 1997;112:A1030(abst).

480. Stein R, Cohen R, Hanauer S. Complications during cyclosporine therapy for inflammatory bowel disease. *Gastroenterology* 1997;112: A1098(abst).

481. Marion JF, Present DH. 6-MP maintains cyclosporine induced response in patients with severe ulcerative colitis. *Am J Gastroenterol* 1996;91:1975(abst).

482. Azad Khan AK, Howes DT, Piris J, Truelove SC. Optimum dose of sulphasalazine for maintenance treatment in ulcerative colitis. *Gut* 1980;21:232–240.

483. Riley SA, Mani V, Goodman MJ, et al. Comparison of delayed release 5-aminosalicylic acid (mesalazine) and sulphasalazine as maintenance treatment for patients with ulcerative colitis. *Gastroenterology* 1988; 94:1383–1389.

484. Rutgeerts P. Comparative efficacy of coated, oral 5-aminosalicylic acid (Claversal) and sulphasalazine for maintaining remission of ulcerative colitis. *Aliment Pharmacol Ther* 1989;3:183–191.

485. Green JRB, Swan CHJ, Rowlinson A, et al. Comparison doses of balsalazide in maintaining ulcerative colitis in remission over 12 months. *Aliment Pharmacol Ther* 1992;6:647–652.

486. Ireland A, Mason CH, Jewell DP. Controlled trial comparing olsalazine and sulphasalazine for the maintenance of ulcerative colitis. *Gut* 1988;29:835–837.

487. Trallori G, Messori A, Scuffi C, et al. 5-aminosalicylic acid enemas to maintain remission in left-sided colitis: a meta- and economic analysis. *J Clin Gastroenterol* 1995;20:257–259.

488. Marteau P, Crand J, Foucault M, Rambaud JC. Use of mesalazine slow release suppositories 1 g three times per week to maintain remission of ulcerative colitis: a randomized double blind placebo controlled multicentre trial study. *Gut* 1998;42:195–199.

489. Oren R, Arber N, Odes S, et al. Methotrexate in chronic active ulcerative colitis: a double-blind, randomized, Israeli multicenter trial. *Gastroenterology* 1996;110:1416–1421.

490. Targan SR, Hanauer SB, Van Deventer SJH, et al. A short-term study of chimeric monoclonal antibody cA2 to tumor necrosis factor α for Crohn's disease. *N Engl J Med* 1997;337:1029–1035.

491. Rutgeerts P, D'Haens G, van Deventer SJH, et al. Retreatment with anti-TNF-α chimeric antibody (cA2) effectively maintains cA2-induced remission in Crohn's disease. *Gastroenterology* 1997;112: A1078.

492. van Deventer SJH, van Hogezand R, Present D, et al. Controlled study of anti-TNF treatment for enterocutaneous fistulae complicating Crohn's disease. *Gut* 1997;41[Suppl 3]:A2(abst).

493. Plevy SE, Carramanzana NM, Deem RL, et al. Clinical improvement in Crohn's disease patients treated with anti-TNF alpha correlates with downregulated mucosal T helper 1 responses. *Gastroenterology* 1996; 110:A993(abst).

494. Scallon BJ, Moore MA, Trinh H, et al. Chimeric anti-TNF-alpha monoclonal antibody cA2 binds recombinant transmembrane TNF-alpha and activates immune effector functions. *Cytokine* 1995;7:251–259.

495. Stack WA, Mann SD, Roy AJ, et al. Randomised controlled trial of CDP571 antibody to tumour necrosis factor-α in Crohn's disease. *Lancet* 1997;349:521–524.

496. Evans RC, Clarke L, Heath P, et al. Treatment of ulcerative colitis with an engineered human anti-TNF-alpha antibody CDP571. *Aliment Pharmacol Ther* 1997;11:1031–1035.

497. Sands BE, Podolsky DK, Tremaine WJ, et al. Chimeric monoclonal anti-tumor necrosis factor antibody (cA2) in the treatment of severe steroid-refractory ulcerative colitis (UC). *Gastroenterology* 1996;110: A1008.

498. Van Deventer SJH, Elson CO, Fedorak RN. Multiple doses of intravenous interleukin 10 in steroid-refractory Crohn's disease. *Gastroenterology* 1997;113:383–389.

499. Fedorak RN, Gangl A, Elson CO, et al. Safety, tolerance, and activity of multiple doses of subcutaneous recombinant human interleukin-10 (rHuIL-10) in patients with mild to moderate active Crohn's disease. *Gut* 1997;41[Suppl 3]:A16(abst).

500. Bank S, Sninsky C, Robinson M, et al. Safety and activity evaluation of rhIL-11 in subjects with active Crohn's disease. *Gastroenterology* 1997;122:A927.

501. Yacyshyn B, Woloschuk B, Yacyshyn MB, et al. Efficacy and safety of ISIS 2302 (ICAM-1 antisense oligonucleotide) treatment of steroid-dependent Crohn's disease. *Gastroenterology* 1997;112:A1123.

502. Stronkhorst A, Radema S, Yong SL, et al. CD4 antibody treatment in patients with active Crohn's disease: a phase 1 dose finding study. *Gut* 1997;40:320–327.

503. Hogaboam CM, Vallance BA, Kumar A, et al. Therapeutic effects of interleukin 4 gene transfer in experimental inflammatory bowel disease. *J Clin Invest* 1997;100:2766–2776.

504. Gaffney PR, Doyle CT, Gaffney A, et al. Paradoxical response to heparin in 10 patients with ulcerative colitis. *Am J Gastroenterol* 1995;90: 220–223.

505. Sandborn WJ, Tremaine WJ, Leighton JA, et al. Nicotine tartrate liquid enemas for mildly to moderately active left-sided ulcerative colitis unresponsive to first-line therapy: a pilot study. *Aliment Pharmacol Ther* 1997;11:663–671.

506. Winter TA, Marks IN. Sucralfate enemas in ulcerative colitis [Letter]. *Aliment Pharmacol Ther* 1997;11:821–822.

507. Rutgeerts P, Hiele M, Geboes K, et al. Controlled trial of metronidazole treatment for prevention of Crohn's recurrence after ileal resection. *Gastroenterology* 1995;108:1617–1621.

508. Sutherland L, Singleton J, Sessions J, et al. Double blind, placebo controlled trial of metronidazole in Crohn's disease. *Gut* 1991;32:1071–1075.

509. Ursing B, Alm T, Barany F, et al. A comparative study of metronidazole and sulfasalazine for active Crohn's disease in Sweden. II. Result. *Gastroenterology* 1982;83:550–562.

510. Colombel JF, Lémann M, Cassagnou M, et al. A controlled trial comparing ciprofloxacin with mesalazine for the treatment of active Crohn's disease. *Gastroenterology* 1997;112:A951(abst).

511. Prantera C, Zannoni F, Scribano ML, et al. A randomized, controlled clinical trial of metronidazole plus ciprofloxacin. *Am J Gastroenterol* 1996;91:328–332.

512. Gasché C, Dejaco C, Waldhoer T, et al. Intravenous iron and erythropoietin for anemia associated with Crohn's disease—a randomized, controlled trial. *Ann Intern Med* 1997;126:782–787.

513. Vogelsang H, Ferenci P, Resch H, et al. Prevention of bone mineral loss in patients with Crohn's disease by long-term oral vitamin D supplementation. *Eur J Gastroenterol Hepatol* 1995;7:609–614.

514. Sugita A, Sachar DB, Bodian C, et al. Colorectal cancer in ulcerative colitis: influence of anatomical extent and age at onset on colitis-cancer interval. *Gut* 1991;32:167–169.

515. Wright CL, Riddell RH. The pathology and politics of dysplasia in ulcerative colitis. *Curr Opin Gastroenterol* 1998;14:11–14.

516. Vermulapalli R, Lance P. Cancer surveillance in ulcerative colitis: more of the same or progress? *Gastroenterology* 1994;107:1196–1199.

517. Lashner BA, Provencher KS, Seidner DL, et al. The effect of folic acid supplementation on the risk for cancer or dysplasia in ulcerative colitis. *Gastroenterology* 1997;112:29–32.

518. Ekbom A, Helmik C, Zack M, Adami HO. Increased risk of large bowel cancer in Crohn's disease with colonic involvement. *Lancet* 1990;336:357–359.

519. Rubio CA, Befrits R. Colorectal adenocarcinoma in Crohn's disease. *Dis Colon Rectum* 1997;40:1072–1078.

520. Lashner BA. Risk factors for small bowel cancer in Crohn's disease. *Dig Dis Sci* 1992;37:1179–1184.

521. Munkholm P, Langholz E, Davidsen M, Binder V. Intestinal cancer risk and mortality in patients with Crohn's disease. *Gastroenterology* 1993;105:1716–1723.

522. Meyers S, Walfish JS, Sachar DB, et al. Quality of life after surgery for Crohn's disease: a psychosocial survey. *Gastroenterology* 1980;78:1–6.

523. Ritchie JK. The results of surgery for large bowel Crohn's disease. *Ann R Coll Surg Engl* 1990;72:155–157.

524. Sardinha TC, Wexner SD. Laparoscopy for inflammatory bowel disease: pros and cons. *World J Surg* 1998;22:370–374.

525. Fazio VW, Strong SA. Surgical treatment of inflammatory bowel disease. *Curr Opin Gastroenterol* 1997;13:317–324.

526. Hurst RD, Michelassi F. Strictureplasty for Crohn's disease: techniques and long-term results. *World J Surg* 1998;22:359–363.

527. Post S, Herfarth C, Schumacher H, et al. Experience with ileostomy and colostomy in Crohn's disease. *Br J Surg* 1995;82:1629–1633.

528. Ayuk P, Williams N, Scott N, et al. Management of intra-abdominal abscesses in Crohn's disease. *Ann R Coll Surg Engl* 1996;78:5–10.

529. Sinclair TS, Brunt PW, Mowat NAG. Nonspecific proctocolitis in northeastern Scotland: a community study. *Gastroenterology* 1983;85:1–11.

530. Leijonmarck CE, Persson PG, Hellers G. Factors affecting the colectomy rate in ulcerative colitis: an epidemiologic study. *Gut* 1990;31:329–333.

531. Nugent FW, Haggit RC, Gilpin PA. Cancer surveillance in ulcerative colitis. *Gastroenterology* 1991;100:1241–1248.

532. Bernstein CN, Shanahan F, Weinstein WM. Are we telling patients the truth about surveillance colonoscopy in ulcerative colitis. *Lancet* 1994;343:71–74.

533. Connell WR, Lennard-Jones JE, Williams CB, et al. Factors affecting the outcome of endoscopic surveillance for cancer in ulcerative colitis. *Gastroenterology* 1994;107:934–944.

534. Woolrich AJ, DaSilva MD, Korelitz BE. Surveillance in the routine management of ulcerative colitis: the predictive value of low grade dysplasia. *Gastroenterology* 1992;103:431–438.

535. Kelly KA, Pemberton JH, Wolff BG, Dozois RR. Ileal pouch-anal anastomosis. *Curr Probl Surg* 1992;29:65–131.

536. Heppell J, Kelly K. Pouchitis. *Curr Opin Gastroenterol* 1998;14:322–326.

537. Sandborn WJ. Pouchitis following ileal pouch anal anastomosis: definition, pathogenesis, and treatment. *Gastroenterology* 1994;107:1856–1860.

538. Penna C, Dozois R, Tremaine W, et al. Pouchitis after ileal pouch-anal anastomosis for ulcerative colitis occurs with increased frequency in patients with associated primary sclerosing cholangitis. *Gut* 1996;38:234–239.

539. Merrett MN, Mortensen N, Kettlewell M, Jewell DO. Smoking may prevent pouchitis in patients with restorative proctocolectomy for ulcerative colitis. *Gut* 1996;38:362–364.

540. Hurst RD, Molinari M, Chung TP, et al. Prospective study of the incidence, timing and treatment of pouchitis in 104 consecutive patients after proctocolectomy. *Arch Surg* 1996;131:497–500.

541. Madden MV, McIntyre AS, Nicholls RJ. Double-blind trial of metronidazole versus placebo in chronic unremitting pouchitis. *Dig Dis Sci* 1994;39:1193–1196.

542. Ståhlberg D, Gullberg K, Liljeqvist L, et al. Pouchitis following pouch operation for ulcerative colitis: incidence, cumulative risk, and risk factors. *Dis Colon Rectum* 1996;39:1012–1018.

543. Gullberg K, Ståhlberg D, Liljeqvist L, et al. Neoplastic transformation of the pelvic pouch mucosa in patients with ulcerative colitis. *Gastroenterology* 1997;112:1487–1492.

544. Sagar PM, Dozois RR, Wolff BG: Long-term results of ileal pouch-anal anastomosis in patients with Crohn's disease. *Dis Colon Rectum* 1996;39:893–898.

545. Panis Y, Poupard B, Nemeth J, et al. Ileal pouch/anal anastomosis for Crohn's disease. *Lancet* 1996;347:854–857.

546. Phillips RKS. Ileal pouch-anal anastomosis for Crohn's disease. *Gut* 1998;43:303–308.

547. Ekbom A, Helmick CG, Zack M, et al. Survival and causes of death in patients with inflammatory bowel disease: a population-based study. *Gastroenterology* 1992;103:954–960.

548. Weterman IT, Beimond I, Pena AS. Mortality and causes of death in Crohn's disease: review of 50 years' experience in Leiden University Hospital. *Gut* 1990;31:1387–1390.

549. Ekbom A, Helmick C, Zack M, Adami HO. Extracolonic malignancies in inflammatory bowel disease. *Cancer* 1991;67:2015–2019.

550. Persson PG, Bernell O, Leijonmarck CE, et al. Survival and cause-specific mortality in inflammatory bowel disease: a population-based cohort study. *Gastroenterology* 1996;110:1339–1345.

551. Cottone M, Magliocco A, Rosselli M, et al. Mortality in patients with Crohn's disease. *Scand J Gastroenterol* 1996;31:372–375.

552. Palli D, Trallori G, Saieva C, et al. General and cancer specific mortality of a population based cohort of patients with inflammatory bowel disease: the Florence study. *Gut* 1998;42:175–179.

*Textbook of the Autoimmune Diseases,*
Edited by R. G. Lahita, N. Chiorazzi, and W. H. Reeves,
Lippincott Williams & Wilkins, Philadelphia © 2000.

# CHAPTER 16

# Autoimmunity and the Heart

Sanjeev Trehan and David O. Taylor

The immunologic cardiovascular diseases comprise a heterogenous group of conditions that may result in serious morbidity and mortality because of cardiac ischemia, progressive cardiac dysfunction from congestive heart failure, and life-threatening arrhythmias. The immunologic disorders are systemic in nature, with symptoms masked in ambiguous, scarce, and nonspecific physical findings that contribute to the diagnostic challenge for the clinician. The past quarter century of extensive research efforts in this arena has yielded information on few specific mediators and the origins of some of the conditions, but the pathophysiologic role of immunologic mechanisms in common cardiac conditions such as congestive heart failure and atherosclerosis remains a mystery.

Acute myocarditis and dilated cardiomyopathy may occur as isolated conditions or in association with other systemic immunologic inflammatory illness. Most patients with myocarditis or cardiomyopathy do not have any established etiopathologic basis, although infectious agents, including viruses, bacteria, and rickettsiae, have been incriminated as primary pathogens or as inducers of an immunologic inflammatory response. The following sections discuss the primary cardiac disorders with proved and possible immunologic bases, rheumatologic conditions with cardiac involvement, and the autoimmune phenomena associated with cardiac transplantation.

## MYOCARDITIS AND DILATED CARDIOMYOPATHY

The World Health Organization along with the International Society and Federation of Cardiology Task Force on Cardiomyopathies (1) classified cardiomyopathies whenever possible by etiologic or pathogenetic factors. This classification recognizes chronic viral, postinfectious autoimmune, and primary autoimmune forms of dilated cardiomyopathy. Although it is stated that myocarditis is diagnosed by established histologic, immunologic, and immunohistochemical criteria, with the exception of the Dallas criteria (2), the remaining immunologic and immunohistochemical criteria remained to be defined. Myocarditis, regardless of the etiopathologic factors, remains an inflammatory cardiomyopathy associated with cardiac dysfunction.

### Etiology and Epidemiology

A wide variety of infectious and noninfectious causes are associated with myocarditis (Tables 16.1 through 16.3). Several epidemiologic observations linking these agents with myocarditis have been substantiated by application of serologic, polymerase chain reaction (PCR), or *in situ* hybridization methods. The incidence of infectious myocarditis in the general population is largely unknown. In prospective studies of a defined population over several years, an incidence of 0.02% was found. These were unequivocal cases of clinical myocarditis confirmed by myocardial enzyme leak and characteristic electrocardiographic (ECG) changes (3). ECG abnormalities suggesting asymptomatic myocardial involvement in the absence of enzymatic release have been found in 1.2% of military transcripts during a course of other acute infectious diseases (4). During an epidemic of influenza A, the incidence rose to 7.7% (5). In a prospective trial of 2,310 consecutive patients admitted to a large infectious disease hospital in Sweden, 8% showed ECG abnormalities suggesting myocarditis (6). The exact incidence of myocarditis is difficult to estimate, but approximately 5% of the virus-infected population may experience symptoms that suggest cardiac involvement. Although the list of possible etiologic agents is large, the enteroviruses, specifically Coxsackie B virus, is the most commonly identified etiologic agent of inflammatory cardiomyopathy, and among healthy active adults, at least 50% have detectable serum antibodies indicating prior infection

S. Trehan: Department of Internal Medicine, University of Utah Health Sciences Center, Salt Lake City, Utah 84132; Division of Cardiology, University Hospital, Salt Lake City, Utah 94132.

D. O. Taylor: Department of Medicine, Division of Cardiology, University of Utah Health Sciences Center, Salt Lake City, Utah 84132.

**TABLE 16.1.** *Common causes of myocarditis*

Infections
    Adenovirus
    Coxsackievirus
    Cytomegalovirus
    Epstein–Barr virus
    Human immunodeficiency virus type 1
    *Borrelia* (Lyme's disease)
    Toxoplasmosis
Drugs
    Amphetamines
    Anthracyclines (especially Adriamycin)
    Catecholamines
    Cocaine
    Cyclophosphamide
    Interleukin-2
Hypersensitivity
    Hydrochlorothiazide
    Methyldopa
    Penicillins
    Sulfadiazine
    Sulfamethoxizole
Systemic diseases
    Crohn's disease
    Kawasaki's disease
    Sarcoidosis
    Systemic lupus erythematosus
    Ulcerative colitis
    Cardiac rejection
    Giant cell myocarditis
    Peripartum myocarditis

with the Coxsackie B virus (7,8). The World Health Organization surveyed viral infections related to cardiovascular disease globally, and in a 10-year period from 1975 through 1985, the Coxsackie B virus was associated with the highest incidence of cardiovascular disease (34.6 cases per 1,000 persons), followed by influenza B (17.4 per 1,000), influenza A (11.7 per 1,000), Coxsackie A (9.1 per 1,000), and cytomegalovirus (8.0 per 1,000) (9).

The predominance of enteroviruses among myocarditis-associated agents has been substantiated by several laboratory and clinical studies (10–12). Other agents such as adenoviruses, Epstein–Barr virus (EBV), *Mycoplasma*, and *Chlamydia* have also been associated with cardiovascular disease. Martin et al. (12) demonstrated specific viral genome sequences in the endomyocardial biopsies of 26 (68%) of 38 patients with acute myocarditis; they identified adenovirus in 15, enterovirus in 8, herpes simplex in 2, and cytomegalovirus (CMV) in 1 patient. The control patients did not demonstrate any viral genome sequences.

CMV is a recognized cause of acute infectious myocarditis, although it is rare in healthy individuals (13,14). Maisch et al., using *in situ* hybridization techniques, demonstrated CMV-specific nucleotide sequences in 15% of patients with acute pericarditis. In transplant recipients, CMV infection is fairly common and has been reported to affect the transplanted heart (15,16).

## Bacterial Myocarditis

Myocarditis is a well-recognized complication of *Corynebacterium diphtheriae* infection, although this is now rare in the Western world (17). Myocardial dysfunction is also associated with *Salmonella* septicemia, although it is rarely clinically severe. It is mostly related to the toxemia of the severe infection, which is also observed with meningococcal and nonrheumatic streptococcal infections.

Perhaps the best-recognized agent responsible for myocarditis is the β-hemolytic streptococci, which results in rheumatic fever that is still seen in the Western world with a low frequency of sporadic cases occurring in regional clusters. The incidence in the United States is less than 2 cases per 100,000 persons, but in the developing world, rheumatic heart disease continues to be the leading cause of cardiac hospitalization in the 5- to 25-year-old age group (18).

Myocarditis is a complication with *Borrelia burgdorferi* infection (Lyme's disease) and is reported in up to 8% of the cases often characterized by development of atrial ventricular block and rarely progressing to left ventricular dysfunction and cardiomegaly (19). *Mycoplasma pneumoniae* infection has been associated with myocarditis. Lewes et al. demonstrated asymptomatic myocardial involvement as documented by ECG changes in one third of the cases with acute mycoplasmal infection (20). *Chlamydia* infections have also been associated with myocarditis, especially among small children who often have fatal outcomes (21). *Chlamydia pneumoniae* infection has been detected in a few cases of mild myocarditis and has been associated with respiratory infection resulting in sudden death in a young athlete (22).

## Other Causative Agents

*Trypanosoma cruzi* (Chagas' disease) is a well-recognized cause of myocarditis and cardiomyopathy in South America. *Toxoplasma gondii* poses a significant problem among cardiac transplant recipients, because many of them lack antibodies to this agent and develop myocarditis (23). Toxoplasmosis also poses a major threat to patients with acquired immunodeficiency syndrome (AIDS), and myocarditis has frequently occurred in human immunodeficiency virus–infected populations with or without concomitant *Toxoplasma* infection. In two autopsy studies of AIDS patients, myocarditis was found in almost one half of the cases, and in another study, 54% of 102 prospectively studied patients with AIDS had echocardiographic evidence of myocardial dysfunction (24–26).

## Pathophysiology of Viral Myocarditis

### Animal Models

The most widely accepted models for study of human myocarditis are those of enteroviral myocarditis induced by Coxsackie virus B3 (CVB3) and the encephalomyocarditis virus

**TABLE 16.2.** *Uncommon infectious causes of myocarditis*

Viral
  Arbovirus (dengue fever, yellow fever)
  Arenavirus (Lassa fever)
  Coronavirus
  Echovirus
  Encephalomyocarditis virus
  Hepatitis B
  Herpesvirus
  Influenza virus
  Junin virus
  Mumps virus
  Poliomyelitis virus
  Rabies
  Respiratory syncytial virus
  Rubella virus
  Rubeola virus
  Vaccinia virus
  Varicella virus
  Variola virus
Bacterial
  Brucellosis
  *Campylobacter jejuni*
  *Chlamydia trachomatis*
  *Clostridium*
  Diphtheria
  *Francisella* (tularemia)
  Gonoccus
  Haemophilus
  *Legionella*
  *Listeria*
  Meningococcus
  Mycobacteria (*tuberculosis, avium-intercellulare, leprae*)
  *Mycoplasma*
  Pneumococcus
  Psittacosis
  *Salmonella*
  *Staphylococcus*
  *Streptococcus*
  *Tropheryma whippelii* (Whipple's disease)

Fungal
  *Aspergillus*
  Actinomycetes
  *Blastomyces*
  *Candida*
  *Coccidioides*
  *Cryptococcus*
  *Fusarium oxysporum*
  *Histoplasma*
  Mucormycosis
  *Nocardia*
  *Sporothrix*
Rickettsial
  *Rickettsia rickettsii* (Rocky Mountain spotted fever)
  *Coxiella burnetii* (Q fever)
  Scrub typhus
  Typhus
Spirochetal
  *Leptospira*
  Syphilis
Helminthic
  *Cysticercus*
  *Echinococcus*
  *Schistosoma*
  *Toxocara* (visceral larva migrans)
  *Trichinella*
Protozoal
  *Entamoeba*
  *Leishmania*

(EMC). Induction of chronic murine myocarditis by CVB3 requires murine strains of certain genetic background and virus with a cardiovirulence capacity (27,28). Infection of syngeneic weanling mice with CVB3 results in cardiac infection lasting about a week, beyond which the virus cannot be cultured, but there is evidence that the viral RNA persists for several months after the initial infection (29,30). Several mechanisms have been hypothesized to explain the induction of chronic inflammatory response in myocytes by the viral infection:

1. Persistent infection of the cell affects dysregulatory processes that stimulate inflammation and resultant myocyte destruction (31).
2. The virus-induced myocyte injury releases or exposes hitherto hidden or cryptic antigens to immune cells, leading to autoimmune effector molecule synthesis and a maintained inflammatory response (32,33).
3. The CVB3 virion or other viral proteins share epitopes with internal or plasma membrane proteins of normal cells

(i.e., molecular mimicry) and stimulate immune responses that participate in autoimmune reactions (34).

These mechanisms are not mutually exclusive, and all may be operative concurrently. The CVB3 and CVB4 share epitopes with human cardiac myocyte sarcolemmal proteins (35,36), human and mouse cardiac myosins (37,38), streptococcal M protein (37), adenine nucleotide translocator (ANT) protein (39), and other proteins on normal mouse myocytes and fibroblasts (40). A large number of target epitopes have been proposed, including β-adrenergic receptor (41), laminin (42), branched chain ketoacid dehydrogenase (43), and heat shock protein 60 (HSP60) (44), and although antibodies to these antigens are frequently associated with myocarditis, the clinical significance and causal relationship is undetermined. This antibody response may be an epiphenomenon existing as an adjunct to the principal pathologic process.

Cytotoxic lymphocytes (CTLs) from mice with CVB3-induced myocarditis can recognize and kill *in vitro* neonatal myocytes, fibroblasts, and endothelial cells infected with the

**TABLE 16.3.** *Uncommon noninfectious causes of myocarditis*

| | |
|---|---|
| Drug induced | Toxins |
|   Toxic myocarditis |   Arsenic |
|     Amphetamines |   Carbon monoxide |
|     Arsenic |   Copper |
|     Chloroquine |   Iron |
|     Emetine |   Lead |
|     5-Fluorouracil |   Mercury |
|     Interferon-α |   Phosphorus |
|     Lithium |   Scorpion stings |
|     Paracetamol |   Snake venom |
|     Thyroid hormone |   Spider bites |
|   Hypersensitivity myocarditis |   Wasp stings |
|     Acetazolamide | Systemic diseases |
|     Allopurinol |   Arteritis (giant cell, Takayasau) |
|     Amphotericin B |   Beta-thalassemia major |
|     Carbamazepine |   Churg-Strauss vasculitis |
|     Cephalothin |   Cryoglobulinemia |
|     Chlorthalidone |   Dermatomyositis |
|     Colchicine |   Diabetes mellitus |
|     Diclofenac |   Hashimoto's thyroiditis |
|     Diphenhydramine |   Mixed connective tissue disease |
|     Furosemide |   Myasthenia gravis |
|     Indomethacin |   Periarteritis nodosa |
|     Isoniazid |   Pernicious anemia |
|     Lidocaine |   Pheochromocytoma |
|     Methysergide |   Polymyositis |
|     Oxyphenbutazone |   Rheumatoid arthritis |
|     *Para*-aminosalicyclic acid |   Scerloderma |
|     Phenindione |   Sjögren's syndrome |
|     Phenylbutazone |   Thymoma |
|     Phenytoin |   Wegener's granulomatosis |
|     Procainamide | Other causes |
|     Pyribenzamine |   Eosinophilic myocarditis |
|     Ranitadine |   Genetic defects |
|     Reserpine |   Granulomatous myocarditis |
|     Spironolactone |   Head trauma |
|     Streptomycin |   Hypothermia |
|     Tetracycline |   Hyperpyrexia |
|     Trimethaprim |   Ionizing radiation |
| |   Mononuclear myocarditis |

same strain of the virus (45), suggesting recognition of a novel tissue antigen induced by the infection. There is also evidence for cross-reactive, concurrent recognition of unrelated cardiac epitopes, because the CTLs also lyse uninfected myocytes *in vitro* (46). One of the proposed mechanisms for cytolysis is the production of perforin, a pore-forming protein, by the lymphocytes. The perforins, when inserted into myocyte membrane, induce a lethal increase in the cell's permeability (47). Coxsackievirus-infected mice also develop additional immune sensitization to cardiac heavy-chain myosin, possibly because of the release of sequestered myosin antigens from the virus-damaged cells. Immunization of mice with the heavy-chain myosin and an adjuvant produces a histomorphologically similar picture to that of CVB3-induced myocarditis. The genetic susceptibility, kinetics, and cellular composition of the infiltrates in these two models are similar and suggest the role of endogenous antigens as epitopes for the inflammatory response (48).

### Role of Cellular Immunity

The pathways and cellular participants in the immunopathogenesis of viral myocarditis are characterized in Figure 16.1. The replicating viral particles can be readily identified in cardiac myocytes within a few hours of inoculation of CVB3 into mice (49,50). The viral particles reach a numerical peak in 3 to 4 days, and at 7 to 10 days, they usually are no longer detectable (51). The inflammatory infiltrate is detectable by day 5 and reaches a plateau by day 7 to 10. The early inflammatory infiltrate consists of lymphocytes, macrophages, neutrophils, and natural killer cells and their associated cytokines and humoral effectors (52–55). The natural killer cells are the first to appear and are detected in the activated state in 3 to 4 days. These cells are capable of lysing virus-infected cells *in vitro* (55). The T lymphocytes and macrophages follow the natural killer cells in the temporal sequence and become the predominant cells infiltrating the myocardium in 7 to 10 days.

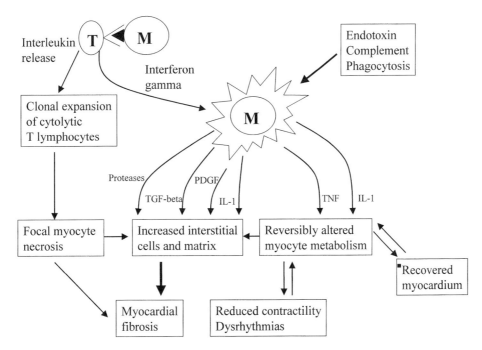

**FIG. 16.1.** Cellular pathways mediating reversible and irreversible immune injury to the heart. T lymphocyte (*T*), macrophages (*M*), transforming growth factor-beta (*TGF-beta*), platelet-derived growth factor (*PDGF*), interleukin-1 (*IL-1*), and tumor necrosis factor (*TNF*). (From Lange LG, Schreiner GF. Immune mechanisms of cardiac disease. *N Engl J Med* 1994;330:1129–1135, with permission.)

The severe combined immunodeficiency (SCID) mouse model has provided valuable insight into the early immune activity in response to the viral infection. SCID mice lack mature T and B lymphocyte function and develop extensive myocardial necrosis with pleomorphic infiltrates, rapid viral proliferation, and profound virus-associated myocytolysis when inoculated with CVB3 (56). Macrophage and natural killer cell activity is unaffected in the SCID mouse model and may participate in the myocytolytic activity, although direct viral myocytolysis predominates. Immunosuppressed mice also demonstrate similar characteristics, with higher viral loads, delayed clearance, and extensive myocyte necrosis, although direct viral myocytolysis is not common in immunocompetent mice (45,51,57–59). In the absence of a functional antiviral immune response, even noncardiovirulent strains have sufficient time to replicate and develop a cardiovirulent quasispecies that can cause fatal myocarditis (60). This may also explain the clinical observation that most severe and fatal cases of myocarditis develop in young children with immature and incompletely developed immune systems (61).

The virus-specific CTLs play a major role in the inflammatory response to the viral infection of the myocyte (51,59). The inflammatory response can be diminished significantly by T-lymphocyte depletion with antithymocyte globulin or thymectomy and irradiation (50,62). The CTL must recognize the foreign antigen associated with the syngeneic major histocompatibility complex (MHC) class I antigen that is found on immune derived cells. The CVB3-infected cells can readily express MHC class I antigens (63). The MHC class I

molecules provide peptide binding sites that evoke the effector responses on recognition of the foreign peptide by the antigen-specific receptors of the T lymphocyte (64). However, T-lymphocyte depletion and specific immunosuppression using cyclosporine has various effects depending on the murine model, virus, and time of therapy and is not uniformly beneficial (65–67). The virus cannot be cultured from cells after 7 to 10 days, but areas of inflammatory infiltrate and myocyte necrosis do demonstrate persistence of viral RNA, and the virus-specific CTLs may continue to see these as immunologic targets and hence perpetuate myocyte damage (68).

The infected myocyte can remain a target for the CTL even after the viral antigens are cleared because of expression of "neoantigens" induced by the virus or remain unsequestered because of the injury (69,70). Even nonviral antigens on infected myocytes can react with CTLs, such as those induced by actinomycin D (70), and new glycoproteins have been identified on the surface of CVB3-infected cells that can be recognized by the CTLs from other syngeneic infected mice (71). Observations suggest that costimulatory molecules B7.1, B7.2, and CD40 may be expressed on myocytes in patients with myocarditis and may make them into antigen-presenting cells (APCs) for CTLs and natural killer cells, thereby playing an important role in the direct myocardial damage caused by these lytic cells (72).

### Role of Humoral Immunity

Another mechanism for ongoing myocyte damage is the antibody-mediated autoimmune response. Because most proteins identified as cardiac autoantigens are intracellular, the mechanism by which these antibodies could harm normal intact myocytes becomes conceptually ambiguous. There are two proposed mechanisms. The first suggests that, after the antibody response is initiated, the circulating antibodies to intracellular antigens cross-react with the native membrane cardiac tissue proteins. After a small number of myocytes are damaged by the viral infection and release intracellular antigens, the resulting antibody response may affect normal myocytes, leading to global myocardial dysfunction. This hypothesis is supported by a number of cross-reacting antibodies, which have been previously described (35–44). The antibodies against the intracellular mitochondrial adenine nucleotide transferase protein cross-reacts with the myocyte sarcolemmal calcium ion channel protein, and binding of these channels can physiologically alter the metabolism and contractile function of the myocyte (73).

The alternate viewpoint suggests that CTLs and antibodies target uninfected myocytes by recognition of self antigens that were previously sequestered from immune surveillance. The processing and presentation of the self-immunogenic peptides complexed with the major histocompatibility complex are prerequisites in this hypothesis. Normal human cardiac myocytes do not express detectable levels of MHC class II antigens, and their constitutive expression of MHC class I molecules remains controversial (74). Myocardial inflammation such as that seen with viral myocarditis or transplant rejection can markedly increase the expression of MHC class I and II antigens by the myocytes (75–77). Increased MHC expression has also been demonstrated in endomyocardial biopsy specimens from patients with idiopathic dilated cardiomyopathy and myocarditis (78–80), and there may be a genetic predisposition to the immune regulatory dysfunction (81). There is also evidence for aberrant expression of intracellular antigens such as ANT and branched chain alpha-keto acid dehydrogenase (BCKD) on the surface of the myocytes (80).

The formation of antiidiotypic antibodies is an additional mechanism of immune regulation in which an antibody is formed to the idiotypic determinants (i.e., antigen recognition site) of the primary antibody. The antiidiotypic antibody may cross-react with unoccupied viral receptor sites on uninfected myocytes. This phenomenon has been demonstrated in the reovirus, polyomavirus, and the Coxsackie B virus models of myocarditis (82–84), and by the passive transfer of antiidiotypic B cells from a CVB3 myocarditic mouse to a syngeneic mouse and development of nonviral myocarditis (85).

### Role of Cytokines

The presence of a complex, cytokine-rich microenvironment is suggested by the heterogenous inflammatory cell populations in the hearts of infected mice. The cytokines perform a multitude of immunomodulatory functions, including regulation of antibody production, maintenance of self-tolerance (86,87), recruitment of ancillary cells in the inflammatory milieu (88,89), and maintenance of clonal expansion of CTLs (90,91). Certain cytokines regulate the collagenogenic and collagenolytic activity of fibroblasts (92). Although mounting evidence supports the negative inotropic effects or the blunting of catecholamine responses in myocytes exposed to various cytokines, no evidence suggests that the cytokines are directly responsible for myocytolysis (93). Barry (93), using an *in vitro* model, demonstrated that high concentrations of interleukin-1 (IL-1), tumor necrosis factor-$\alpha$ (TNF-$\alpha$), interferon-$\gamma$ (INF-$\gamma$), and IL-4 have no effect on myocyte survival over 24 hours, whereas the CTLs from a mixed lymphocyte reaction cause virtually 100% killing.

Gulick et al. demonstrated that cultured neonatal myocytes, when exposed to macrophage-derived IL-1 and TNF-$\alpha$, have reduced levels of cyclic AMP and have a reduced inotropic response to catecholamines (94). The mechanism for decreased responsiveness to catecholamines is believed to be modulated by increases in nitric oxide (NO) production, which is mediated by increased inducible NO synthase (iNOS) activity, and the blunting of the catecholamine response can be inhibited by the L-arginine analog $N^G$-monomethyl-L-arginine (L-NMMA) (95). The decreased contractile response of cardiac myocytes to $\beta$-adrenergic agonists after induction of iNOS also requires the presence of insulin and the coinduction of enzymes responsible for the production of tetrahydrobiopterin, a cofactor for NOS (96).

Other investigators have suggested that inflammatory cytokines may have direct negative inotropic effects independent of the responsiveness to the $\beta$-adrenergic agonists. High doses of IL-2 during chemotherapy have depressed myocardial function (97). Exposure of cardiac myocytes to endotoxin results in increased NO production and direct depression of contractility because of increased levels of cyclic GMP (98). TNF-$\alpha$ may produce negative inotropic effects by decreasing the $Ca^{2+}$ transiently, with no change in the L-type $Ca^{2+}$ current and independent of NO synthesis (99). The extent to which cytokines cause direct negative inotropic effects or attenuation of endogenous $\beta$-adrenergic agonist activity remains unclear, but there is no doubt of their ability to produce myocyte dysfunction and cardiac decompensation. Transgenic mice with overexpression of TNF-$\alpha$ develop biventricular dilatation and cardiac failure resulting in premature death. Pathologic specimens from these mice reveal globular, dilated hearts and transmural myocarditis with myocyte apoptosis (100).

Increased levels of intracellular adhesion molecule-1 (ICAM-1), IL-1$\alpha$, IL-1$\beta$, TNF-$\alpha$, and macrophage-stimulating factor have been demonstrated in patients with myocarditis and idiopathic dilated cardiomyopathy (101,102). In the CVB3 myocarditis model, the susceptibility of the animals can be increased by pretreatment with these cytokines (103). Transforming growth factor-$\beta$ (TGF-$\beta$) is identifiable by immunohistochemistry in the prenecrotic regions of infiltrates in the murine myocardium, and levels decrease when the macrophages and fibroblasts migrate to the necrotic foci. These growth factors may be responsible for recruitment of the immunologic effectors and may affect cardiac function directly (104). Intriguing features of cytokine activity are their effect on myocytes and their roles in secondary development of the myocyte hypertrophy and interstitial fibrosis characteristic of dilated cardiomyopathy (105). Among animals with different forms of viral myocarditis associated with similar degrees of initial myocyte necrosis, only those with persistent inflammation develop interstitial fibrosis, reflected by fibroblast proliferation and an increase in the amount of extracellular matrix. Myocardial fibrosis correlates well with the presence of T lymphocytes and macrophages, which in their activated state release fibrogenic cytokines such as fibroblast growth factor and TGF-β (106).

### Implications of Animal Models

Lymphocytic myocarditis animal models have conclusively demonstrated the association of viral infection and myocarditis, but the strength of this association in humans remains nebulous. The myocardial damage in murine models of viral myocarditis occurs in two distinct phases: an early phase of direct viral cytotoxicity in which virus-specific T-lymphocyte and antibody-mediated cytotoxicity predominate and a late or chronic phase in which the reactive CTLs, autoantibodies, cytokines, and microvascular damage mediate myocyte damage and dysfunction. The hypothetical mechanisms of virus-induced or precipitated autoimmune heart disease are presented in Figure 16.2.

Recognition that immune responses to specific viruses were important in the development of myocyte injury led to intensive research to design immunomodulatory and antiviral therapies. Pretreatment of mice with inactivated virus vaccine prevents the manifestations of EMC myocarditis (107). Administration of antiviral therapies reduces the virus load and attenuates the histologic findings of myocarditis (108, 109). The antiviral response can be augmented by IFN-α or the exogenous administration of IL-6 (110,111). Recombinant murine IFN-γ has improved the prognosis of acute murine myocarditis caused by ECM virus by suppressing viral replication (112).

The murine model has also been the subject of intensive study of clinically applied immunosuppressants such as corticosteroids (113), nonsteroidal antiinflammatory drugs (NSAIDs) (114,115), and cyclophosphamide (116), which have deleterious effects when given in the acute viremic phase. Cyclosporine, when administered in the early viremic phase, worsens myocardial injury, but in the late immune phase, it has a beneficial effect (117–119). Similar results have been reported with tacrolimus (FK 506) (120), and survival improves significantly when the immunosuppressants such as cyclosporine, azathioprine, and 15-deoxyspergualin are used in adjunct to immunomodulators such as IFN-α (121). Antibodies to TNF-α have improved survival and reduced myocardial injury (122). Cytokine inhibitors have had promising results in animal models, but results of human clinical trials have been inconsistent. Vesnarinone, a phosphodiesterase III inhibitor, has demonstrated beneficial hemodynamic effects. It inhibits the production of TNF-α and favorably modulates induction of iNOS (123). Amlodipine has increased survival of mice with viral myocarditis by inhibiting expression of iNOS and the production of NO in vivo and in vitro (124).

### Clinical Features and Diagnosis

#### Clinical Presentation

The manifestation of unexplained, progressive cardiac dysfunction or ventricular arrhythmias should alert the physician

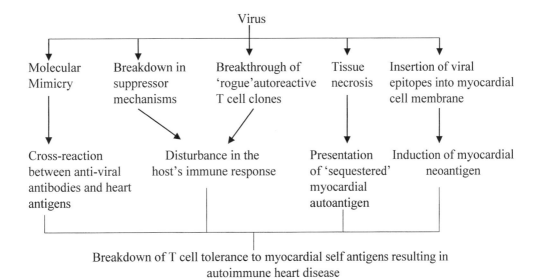

FIG. 16.2. Hypothetical mechanisms of virus induced or precipitated autoimmune heart disease. (From Caforio ALP. Postviral auto-immune heart disease—fact or fiction? *Eur Heart J* 1997;18:1051–1055, with permission.)

to the possibility of myocarditis, especially when routine cardiac diagnostic studies do not reveal a cause. The history of an antecedent viral infection or prodrome is frequently sought but seldom reported and rarely confirmed by convalescent serologies. The presence of mildly elevated levels of the MB isozyme fraction of creatine kinase (CK-MB) or troponin or of leukocytosis may further underscore the possibility of myocarditis.

Most patients with myocarditis probably remain asymptomatic and never seek medical attention. The high frequency of exposure to cardiotropic viruses and observation of a fairly high incidence of ECG abnormalities in apparently cardiac-healthy individuals supports this speculation (6). The incidence of myocarditis in an autopsy series after traumatic deaths in previously healthy individuals has been reported as 2.2% (125). In patients presenting with recent-onset heart failure and biopsy-proved myocarditis, 50% to 60% have had an antecedent flulike illness (126).

The most common presentation of myocarditis is an acute febrile syndrome associated with pericardial and systemic complaints. Symptoms of right and left ventricular failure and even of cardiogenic shock are frequently found in patients with biopsy-proved myocarditis, because it is these symptoms that lead to medical attention; however, the true incidence of heart failure in patients with myocarditis is probably much lower. One rather dramatic presentation of myocarditis is indistinguishable from an acute myocardial infarction, complete with chest pain, ECG features suggesting acute ischemic injury, enzymatic evidence of myocardial damage, and echocardiographic or ventriculographic evidence of global and regional wall motion abnormalities, but endomyocardial biopsy confirms myocarditis (127–129). Most patients presenting with this acute syndrome recover completely, although isolated instances of progressive myocyte loss and cardiac failure or sudden arrhythmic death have been reported (126). The segmental wall motion abnormalities result from virus-mediated injury, although local coronary arteritis or vasospasm have been suggested as possible culprits (130,131).

Children can present with syncope resulting from Stokes–Adams attacks from myopericarditis (132). Other atrial arrhythmias described with myocarditis include sinoatrial block, atrial standstill, atrioventricular block, intraatrial conduction abnormalities, atrial tachycardia, flutter, and fibrillation (133–138). Histologic evidence of myocarditis has been described in as many as two thirds of the patients with lone atrial fibrillation (139). Complete heart block has also been described in cases with viral infections such as EBV or mumps and with rickettsial infections (140–142).

Ventricular arrhythmias are frequently encountered with myocarditis, ranging from innocuous premature ventricular contractions to malignant and incessant ventricular tachycardia (143–145). Myocarditis has been incriminated as a cause of ventricular repolarization abnormalities in athletes with or without arrhythmias (145,146). Ventricular arrhythmias may also be precursors to sudden cardiac death of young athletes

with occult myocarditis (147). In autopsy series, myocarditis accounts for 17% to 25% of sudden deaths of young, healthy people (148–149). In a population-based retrospective study from Turin, Italy, an incidence of only 0.53% was reported for 17,162 autopsies performed over three decades (150), but the application of a standardized systematic histologic examination tends to give a higher incidence, usually in the range of 5%, for autopsies performed at a general hospital (151). Myocarditis is sometimes identified in cases of sudden infant death syndrome (152).

Myocarditis may be associated with myocardial thickening and fibrosis manifesting as diastolic dysfunction or restrictive cardiomyopathy and with asymmetric septal thickening resembling hypertrophic cardiomyopathy (153–155). Lieberman et al. (156) proposed a clinicopathologic description of myocarditis on the basis of the initial manifestations, endomyocardial biopsy results, and recovery (i.e., fulminant, acute, chronic active, or chronic persistent myocarditis).

### Physical Examination

The physical findings in cases of acute myocarditis depend on factors such as the extent of myocardial or pericardial involvement and the inciting agent (e.g., cardiotropic virus). Fever is common, and in the Myocarditis Treatment Trial (157), 18% of patients with myocarditis had fever. Sinus tachycardia frequently accompanies the febrile state but is often out of proportion to the fever and is more likely adrenergically mediated with the hemodynamic alterations from the failing heart. Significant ventricular dysfunction may also be associated with hypotension, gallops, murmurs of regurgitation, rales, jugular venous distention, hepatomegaly, ascites, pleural effusions, or peripheral edema, and with pericardial involvement, there may be friction rubs. The physical findings are not specific for myocarditis.

### Laboratory Findings

Patients with myocarditis frequently have serologic evidence of an inflammatory state, with elevation of nonspecific markers of inflammation such as the erythrocyte sedimentation rate, C-reactive protein, and elevated leukocyte counts. A fourfold increase in virus-specific IgG titers in the convalescent period is considered reliable evidence of recent infection and is found in 20% of patients with myocarditis (158,159). Other markers are elevated in myocarditis, including TNF-$\alpha$, ICAM-1, vascular cell adhesion molecule-1 (VCAM-1), interleukins, and soluble Fas (101,102,160,161), but they suffer from a lack of specificity for myocarditis.

Myocarditis, although associated with myocyte damage and necrosis, results in CK-MB elevation in only 12% of patients with biopsy-proved myocarditis (162). Lauer et al. (163) described CK-MB elevation in only one of five patients with histologic evidence of myocarditis, but the cardiac troponin T (cTnT) concentration was elevated in all five. The cTnT level was elevated in 28 patients, of whom 26 had immunohistologic evidence of myocarditis. The cTnT elevation is highly predictive for myocarditis (163).

### *Electrocardiography, Echocardiography, and Cardiac Scintigraphy*

Historically, acute myocarditis was diagnosed with the constellation of clinical symptoms, physical signs, and ECG abnormalities. Although no particular feature on the electrocardiogram is pathognomonic of acute myocarditis, sinus tachycardia, repolarization abnormalities, conduction abnormalities, and arrhythmias are common findings. Morgera et al. (164) reported ECG abnormalities in a series of 45 patients with biopsy-proved myocarditis: abnormal QRS duration in 45%; abnormal Q waves in 18%; left bundle branch block (LBBB) and right bundle branch block (RBBB) patterns in 18% and 13%, respectively; ST elevation in 16%; T-wave inversions in 16%; and advanced atrioventricular (AV) block in 16%. Among patients presenting earlier in the course of the disease with symptoms experienced for less than 1 month, 31% had advanced AV block, and 47% had ST elevation with T-wave inversions, which carries a poorer prognosis. Other predictors of poor outcome include LBBB, RBBB, and other conduction abnormalities that seem to suggest active, severe, and extensive myocarditis (165).

An echocardiogram is useful in assessing the extent of left ventricular systolic dysfunction, which may range from mild segmental hypokinesis to severe global hypokinesis or akinesis associated with severe congestive heart failure (166). The ventricular dimensions may remain normal or only mildly enlarged considering the extent of systolic dysfunction supporting the acuity of illness. There may be an increase in left ventricular sphericity, right ventricular elongation, an increase in wall thickness, and a left ventricular mass with the interstitial edema and compensatory hypertrophy (167,168). Restrictive filling patterns in the left ventricle identifying diastolic dysfunction have been reported consistently in cases of biopsy-proved myocarditis (168). Mural thrombi are common in diffusely hypokinetic ventricles (169). Pericardial effusions are reported for 10% of patients with myocarditis, but hemodynamic compromise with cardiac tamponade occurs infrequently (170).

Cardiac scintigraphy has been proposed as a convenient noninvasive test with high sensitivity to diagnose active myocarditis. Gallium-67 imaging, which identifies areas of increased inflammation, has been studied in clinical settings and found to have sensitivity and specificity rates of 83%, with a negative predictive value of 98% for the diagnosis of myocarditis (171). Indium-111 antimyosin monoclonal antibodies have been extensively studied to identify areas of myocyte damage in cases of acute myocarditis (172,173). It has extremely high sensitivity and often detects myocarditis, which on endomyocardial biopsy is not seen by routine histologic assessment but is detected by immunohistochemistry (174).

Contrast media–enhanced magnetic resonance imaging (MRI) of patients with myocarditis is an excellent tool for visualizing the location, activity, and extent of inflammation. Early in myocarditis (day 2), the enhancement of MRI signals is accentuated and focal, whereas later (day 84), this pattern seems to be attenuated and more diffuse (175).

### *Endomyocardial Biopsy and Cardiac Catheterization*

The use of endomyocardial biopsy for the diagnosis and management of myocarditis was first reported by Mason et al. (176). Subsequently, reports from several institutions documented myocarditis in patients presenting with unexplained heart failure or ventricular arrhythmias (Table 16.4), however there was considerable discordance in the diagnostic criteria used in these largely anecdotal reports. In preparation for a large, randomized, multicenter clinical trial of immunosuppressive therapy in myocarditis (157), standardized criteria were developed for diagnosis of myocarditis, better known as the *Dallas criteria*. This standard defines *active myocarditis* as "an inflammatory infiltrate of the myocardium with necrosis and/or degeneration of adjacent myocytes not typical of ischemic damage associated with coronary artery disease" (see Fig. 16.5A on page 286). Other causes of inflammation (e.g., connective tissue disorders, infection, drugs) should be excluded (2,206). The Dallas criteria also defined *borderline myocarditis* as an inflammatory infiltrate that is sparse and lacks myocyte injury, and on repeat biopsy, 67% of borderline myocarditis cases are found to histologically progress to active myocarditis (207).

One of the major limitations of endomyocardial biopsy is a sampling error. The inflammation in myocarditis tends to be patchy or focal. In an autopsy study of the right ventricular biopsy technique (10 samples taken from the apical septum), only 6 of 11 patients dying of myocarditis were correctly identified. Left ventricular biopsy missed the diagnosis in 8 of 11 (208). In another study using the standard four to six samples, the sensitivity of right ventricular endomyocardial biopsy was 50% (209). A negative biopsy finding does not exclude active myocarditis. In the Myocarditis Treatment Trial (MTT), only 10% of patients screened had histologic evidence of myocarditis; The European Study of Epidemiology and Treatment of Cardiac Inflammatory Disease (ESET-CID) demonstrated a 20% incidence of biopsy-proved myocarditis using the Dallas criteria and expanding with newer techniques of PCR and *in situ* hybridization (210).

The hemodynamic profiles of patients with acute myocarditis are representative of the extent of myocardial and pericardial involvement. Patients with significant ventricular dysfunction have elevated filling pressures with depressed cardiac outputs and stroke work indices. A restrictive hemodynamic profile can be seen and must be differentiated from that produced by postviral constrictive pericarditis. Pericardial effusion can occur, but cardiac tamponade is rare. Coronary arteriography is usually normal, although coronary vasculitis in animal models has been reported. The one major

**TABLE 16.4.** *Myocarditis determined by biopsy*

| Investigators | Year | No. biopsied | No. with myocarditis (%) | Reference |
|---|---|---|---|---|
| *In unexplained heart failure* | | | | |
| Mason et al. | 1980 | 400 | 7  (2) | 176 |
| Baandrup and Olsen | 1981 | 201 | 8  (4) | 177 |
| Fenoglio et al. | 1983 | 135 | 34 (25) | 178 |
| Rose et al. | 1984 | 76 | 0  (0) | 179 |
| Daly et al. | 1984 | 69 | 12 (17) | 180 |
| Parillo et al. | 1984 | 74 | 19 (26) | 181 |
| Regitz et al. | 1985 | 150 | 41 (27) | 182 |
| Cassling et al. | 1985 | 80 | 6  (7) | 183 |
| Salvi et al. | 1985 | 74 | 13 (18) | 184 |
| Dec et al. | 1985 | 27 | 18 (67) | 185 |
| Mortensen et al. | 1985 | 65 | 12 (18) | 186 |
| Hammond et al. | 1987 | 79 | 14 (18) | 187 |
| Meany et al. | 1987 | 123 | 40 (32) | 188 |
| Chow et al. | 1988 | 90 | 4  (4) | 189 |
| Hobbs et al. | 1989 | 148 | 31 (21) | 190 |
| Popma et al. | 1989 | 61 | 8 (13) | 191 |
| Maisch et al. | 1989 | 123 | 10  (8) | 192 |
| Vasiljevic et al. | 1990 | 85 | 10 (12) | 193 |
| Lieberman et al. | 1991 | 348 | 60 (17) | 194 |
| Herskowitz et al. | 1993 | 534 | 38 (26) | 195 |
| Kuhl et al. | 1996 | 170 | 9  (5) | 196 |
| Arbustini et al. | 1997 | 601 | 26  (4.3) | 197 |
| *In unexplained ventricular arrhythmias* | | | | |
| Strain et al. | 1983 | 18 | 3 (17) | 198 |
| Sugrue et al. | 1984 | 12 | 1  (8) | 199 |
| Take et al. | 1985 | 241 | 21  (9) | 200 |
| Hosenpud et al. | 1986 | 12 | 4 (33) | 201 |
| Yoshizato et al. | 1990 | 8 | 2 (25) | 202 |
| Sekiguchi et al. | 1992 | 43 | 9 (21) | 203 |
| Wiles et al. | 1992 | 33 | 3  (9) | 204 |
| Thongtang et al. | 1993 | 53 | 18 (36) | 205 |

exception is Kawasaki's disease, in which coronary artery aneurysms are frequently associated with myocarditis (211). Ventriculograms may demonstrate global or regional ventricular dysfunction, associated valvular regurgitation, and mural thrombi (212). Localized ventricular aneurysms with normal global systolic function have also been described (213).

**Natural History of Myocarditis**

The natural history of myocarditis is largely unknown, because most cases are subclinical and resolve without any significant residual cardiac dysfunction. Clinically apparent myocardial dysfunction, as seen with acute Coxsackie B viral infections, also resolves without residual dysfunction in most cases. An estimated 12% of patients with clinically suspected acute myocarditis eventually develop dilated cardiomyopathy (214). The murine myocarditis models frequently develop a pathologic process indistinguishable from the human form of idiopathic dilated cardiomyopathy.

The direct link between viral infection and myocarditis or dilated cardiomyopathy has not been conclusively proved. Definitive proof would be isolation of infectious virus from the heart tissue according to Koch's postulates, but this has

only been achieved in a few cases of acute fulminant myocarditis in neonates and infants (215,216). The indirect evidence for a viral cause of dilated cardiomyopathy relies on the animal models of virus-induced cardiomyopathy progressing to dilated cardiomyopathy, apparent progression of myocarditis in some patients to dilated cardiomyopathy, and increased enteroviral antibody titers in patients with dilated cardiomyopathy. The major limitations are that the relevance of disease in mice to humans is suspect, most cases of dilated cardiomyopathy do not have documented preceding myocarditis, and interpretation of epidemiologic serologic data is fraught with predicaments of uncertainty. Although Coxsackie B IgM antibodies are detected with greater frequency in patients with dilated cardiomyopathy than in normal control subjects, the frequency is similar to that for matched community controls and household contacts (217). Enteroviral genomic sequences are detected in the myocardium of 8% to 70% of patients with active myocarditis and 0% to 45% of patients with dilated cardiomyopathy, but in data derived from most published studies, the average detection frequencies are 25% for active myocarditis and 15% for dilated cardiomyopathy, which is not significantly different from the rate of 15% for healthy controls (218). In a meta-analysis of the association of enteroviruses with human heart disease, Baboonian concluded that, although the causative role of enteroviruses in acute myocarditis (particularly in children) was supported by an overall odds ratio of 4.4 (CI, 2.4–8.2), the association with dilated cardiomyopathy was only suggestive, with overall odds ratio of 3.8 (CI, 2.1–4.6) (219).

Although the link between myocarditis and dilated cardiomyopathy is unclear, certain prognostic factors are identifiable. The presence of an abnormal QRS complex on ECG correlates with severity of left ventricular damage and is an independent predictor of survival. Left atrial enlargement, atrial fibrillation, and LBBB also are associated with increased mortality (164). A higher baseline left ventricular ejection fraction (LVEF) is positively associated with survival, but intensity of conventional therapy at baseline is negatively associated with survival (157). Right ventricular dysfunction, as evidenced by abnormal right ventricular descent on an echocardiogram, was shown to be the most important predictor of death or of the need for cardiac transplantation in a group of 23 patients with biopsy-proved myocarditis who were followed long term (220). A net increase in LVEF (between initial and final ejection fractions) was associated with improved survival, whereas the baseline ejection fraction did not predict outcome. The presence and degree of left ventricular regional wall motion abnormalities did not affect the clinical course (220).

Light microscopic findings on biopsy have not been found to predict outcome in myocarditis. Less than 10% of biopsies repeated at 28 and 52 weeks continue to show evidence of ongoing or recurrent myocarditis, regardless of therapy. However, higher baseline serum antibodies to cardiac immune globulin G (IgG) by indirect immunofluorescence was associated with a better LVEF and a smaller left ventricular end diastolic dimension (157).

## Treatment of Myocarditis

### General Supportive Measures

General supportive measures for patients with myocarditis include a low-sodium diet, discontinuation of ethanol, and fluid restriction, especially in the presence of heart failure. Patients with myopericarditis may need analgesics for pain control. Recommendations for the limitation of physical activity are based on the murine model of CVB3 myocarditis, in which forced exercise during the acute phase of illness was associated with increased inflammatory and necrotic lesions and with increased mortality (221). The Task Force on Myopericardial Diseases recommends a convalescent period of approximately 6 months after the onset of clinical manifestations before a return to competitive sports (222).

### Conventional Therapy

The management of patients with presumed or confirmed myocarditis is primarily directed toward treatment of con-

gestive heart failure, arrhythmias, and symptoms from pericardial disease. Diuretics, vasodilators, and digoxin should be administered to patients with mild to moderate systolic dysfunction. Inotropic therapy and mechanical support with an intraaortic balloon pump or ventricular assist devices may be required for patients in refractory cardiogenic shock. Cardiac transplantation is reserved for patients who do not improve despite implementing these measures.

Although there are multiple studies on the use of angiotensin-converting enzyme inhibitors (ACEI) in heart failure (223), the utility of ACEI in myocarditis has been studied only in the murine model. Early treatment with captopril in a CVB3 myocarditis model resulted in less inflammatory infiltrate, myocardial necrosis, and calcification. Heart weight, heart to body weight ratio, and liver congestion diminished. Even with delayed therapy, a reduction in left ventricular mass and decreased liver congestion were evident (224). ACEI exert a potent vasodilator response, improve pump function, prevent ventricular remodelling, and may have antiarrhythmic properties; all patients with systolic dysfunction therefore should be placed on maximally tolerated doses of ACEI.

The use of β blockers in patients with mild to moderate heart failure due to dilated cardiomyopathy has been beneficial (225), but for their use in myocarditis, there are no trials in humans, and even among the nonmyocarditis heart failure population, the mortality benefit of β-blocker therapy has not been proved. Metoprolol-treated mice in an acute CVB3 murine myocarditis model have increased viral replication, myocyte necrosis, and 30-day mortality (226). Carteolol, a nonselective β blocker, has been studied in a chronic myocarditis model and found to have beneficial effects, with improved histologic scores and with reduced heart weight, heart volume, and liver congestion (227). It appears that β blockers should be avoided acutely, but in the chronic heart failure stage, the nonselective β blockers may be beneficial.

Antiarrhythmic therapy may be needed for control of ventricular and supraventricular dysrhythmias. Temporary and permanent pacemakers may be required in patients presenting with conduction system abnormalities. Because most patients with myocarditis have spontaneous resolutions, the antiarrhythmic therapy must be decided on individual basis and with a conservative approach. Patients who fail to improve despite histologic resolution of myocarditis may be candidates for aggressive electrophysiologic approaches and implantable defibrillators.

### Immunosuppressive Therapy

The data supporting an immunologic basis of myocarditis resulted in multiple treatment trials using immunosuppressants (Table 16.5). The conflicting results from these nonrandomized observations led to the development of the MTT (157). In a multicenter, prospective, randomized design, the MTT enrolled patients with heart failure of recent onset (<2 years), left ventricular dysfunction (LVEF <45%), and biopsy-proved

**TABLE 16.5.** *Selected nonrandomized trials of immunosuppressive treatment in myocarditis*

| Investigator | Year | Number treated | Treatment | Improved | Reference |
|---|---|---|---|---|---|
| Mason | 1980 | 8 | P + (A, P) | 4 (50%) | 176 |
| Fenoglio | 1983 | 18 | P, (A, P) | 7 (39%) | 178 |
| Daly | 1984 | 1 | P | 0 | 180 |
| Dec | 1985 | 9 | A + P | 4 (44%) | 185 |
| Mortensen | 1985 | 12 | A + P, CyA | 8 (67%) | 186 |
| Hobbs | 1989 | 34 | A + P, P, CyA | 25 (74%) | 190 |

A, azathioprine; P, prednisone; CyA, cyclosporine A.

myocarditis (per the Dallas criteria). The study screened 2,333 patients; 214 (10%) had endomyocardial biopsy evidence of myocarditis, and 111 patients had a qualifying LVEF value of less than 45%. Patients were randomized to three arms: prednisone plus cyclosporine, prednisone plus azathioprine, and no immunosuppressant treatment. All patients received conventional therapy for heart failure. The prednisone plus azathioprine group was subsequently eliminated because of limited numbers of patients. Patients were treated for 24 weeks, and the primary end point was LVEF at 28 weeks. Secondary analysis of other markers of left ventricular function, survival, and several immune parameters was performed.

At 28 and 52 weeks, no difference in LVEF was observed in treated patients compared with those not treated (Fig. 16.3). At 1 and 5 years, there was no difference in survival between groups or a need for cardiac transplantation (Fig. 16.4). On multivariate analysis, better baseline LVEF, less intensive conventional therapy, and shorter illness duration were independent predictors of improvement in LVEF during follow-up. Analysis of immunologic variables (e.g., cardiac IgG, circulating IgG, natural killer and macrophage activity, helper T cell level) suggested an association between better outcome and a more robust immune response. A higher level of cardiac IgG was associated with a higher LVEF and a smaller

left ventricular size. The mortality rate for the entire trial was 20% at 1 year and 56% at 4.3 years.

Gagliardi et al. (228) followed 20 children with biopsy-proved myocarditis who were treated with cyclosporine and prednisone. At one year, 10 of 20 patients still had histologic evidence of myocarditis. No patient died or required transplantation. However, there was no control group.

Certain subgroups may benefit from immunosuppressant therapy, including those with giant cell myocarditis (GCM), hypersensitivity myocarditis, or cardiac sarcoidosis. Using a multicenter database, Cooper (229) reviewed 63 patients with GCM. The rate of death or cardiac transplantation was 89%. Median survival was 5.5 months from symptom onset to death or transplantation. The median survival of patients treated with corticosteroids was 3.8 months, compared with 3.0 months for untreated patients. However, patients treated with corticosteroids and azathioprine had an average survival of 11.5 months. Cyclosporine in combination with cortico-

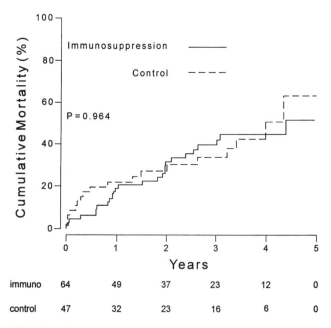

**FIG. 16.4.** Cumulative mortality in the Myocarditis Treatment Trial. The *solid line* represents patients treat by immunosuppression. The *dashed line* represents the control group. (Adapted from Mason JW, O'Connell JB, Herskowitz A, et al. A clinical trial of immunosuppressive therapy for myocarditis. *N Engl J Med* 1995;333:269–275, with permission.)

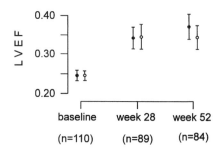

**FIG. 16.3.** Changes in left ventricular ejection fraction (*LVEF*) in the Myocarditis Treatment Trial. *Closed circles* represent patients treated by immunosuppression. *Open circles* represent the control group. (Adapted from Mason JW, O'Connell JB, Herskowitz A, et al. A clinical trial of immunosuppressive therapy for myocarditis. *N Engl J Med* 1995 333:269–275, with permission.)

steroids; corticosteroids plus azathioprine; or corticosteroids, azathioprine, and OKT3 survived an average of 12.6 months.

Other potential indications for a trial of immunosuppressant therapy include failure of myocarditis to resolve, progressive left ventricular dysfunction despite conventional therapy, continued active myocarditis demonstrated on biopsy, or fulminant myocarditis that does not improve within 24 to 72 hours of full hemodynamic support, including mechanical assistance. Myocarditis associated with a known immune mediated disease, such as systemic lupus erythematosus (SLE), may also benefit from immunosuppressive therapy.

Smaller studies have used different immunosuppressant regimens. Kühl et al. (230) treated 31 patients with biopsies classified as immunohistologically positive (i.e., more then two cells per high power field and expression of adhesion molecules), negative Dallas criteria, and left ventricular dysfunction. Patients were treated with conventional therapy for 3 months, followed by gradual tapering of methylprednisolone doses over 24 weeks (after biopsy and LVEF response). Therapy was associated with an improvement in ejection fraction in 64% and improved New York Heart Association functional class in 77%. Four patients (12%) had no change in their ejection fraction despite improvement in inflammatory infiltrates. However, study conclusions are limited by the absence of a control group.

Drucker et al. (231) retrospectively reviewed 46 children with congestive cardiomyopathy and Dallas criteria of borderline or definite myocarditis. Twenty-one patients were treated with intravenous IgG (2 g/kg over 24 hours) and were compared with 25 historical controls. Overall survival was not improved, although there was a trend toward improvement in 1-year survival in the treated group. In the IgG group, the left ventricular function was improved and persisted after adjustment for age, biopsy status, and use of ACEI and inotropes.

In a comparative study of IFN-α, thymomodulin, and conventional therapy for patients with biopsy-proved myocarditis or idiopathic dilated cardiomyopathy, an improvement in the treatment groups was reported for ejection fraction (at rest and during exercise), maximum exercise time, functional class, and ECG abnormalities (232). The use of intravenous immune globulin in 10 patients (NYHA III-IV) with symptoms of less than 6 months' duration resulted in an improvement in LVEF (Fig. 16.4) and functional improvement (NYHA I-II at 1 year of follow-up) in all nine patients who survived, regardless of biopsy results (233).

Perhaps alternative immunosuppressant regimens and different diagnostic criteria may be more successful in demonstrating the utility of immunosuppressants. The ESETCID (210) is a prospective, multicenter, placebo-controlled, double-blind study intended to address the natural course of myocarditis, myopericarditis, pericarditis, and postmyocarditic muscle disease; the underlying processes that lead to progression of disease; and the benefit of immunosuppressant therapy based on cause (i.e., autoimmune, enteroviral, or CMV induced). The primary end points are improvement in ejection fraction of more than 5% and improvement of more than 10% in exercise tolerance time with bicycle ergometry. The secondary end points are reduction in left ventricular end diastolic dimension volume index, resolution of inflammatory infiltrates, lifestyle improvement, elimination of myocardial viral DNA and RNA, reduction of arrhythmias, and evaluation of mortality and the need for cardiac transplantation. The treatment regimens include conventional therapy with diuretics, ACEI, digoxin, and antiarrhythmics or defibrillators; specific therapy for cytomegaloviral and enteroviral myocarditis; and prednisolone plus azathioprine for myocarditis without detectable virus.

### Cardiac Transplantation

In a small series (n = 12), the outcome of patients with active lymphocytic myocarditis confirmed by histologic examination of the explanted heart was significantly worse than controls undergoing transplantation for other diagnoses (234). This concern has not been validated in the analysis of outcome of 14,055 cardiac transplant recipients in the registry of the International Society for Heart and Lung Transplantation. One-year actuarial survival in all groups transplanted (i.e., idiopathic dilated cardiomyopathy, myocarditis, or peripartum cardiomyopathy versus other diagnoses) was 80% (236). Nonetheless, myocarditis may recur in the transplanted heart (235).

## VARIANTS OF MYOCARDITIS

### Giant Cell Myocarditis

GCM is a rare but frequently fatal disorder. It is defined histologically by extensive but patchy myocyte necrosis with areas of intense multicellular inflammatory infiltration that include histiocytes, lymphocytes, and the characteristic multinucleated giant cells (236–239) (Fig. 16.15B). Although multinucleated giant cells are present, they rarely form organized granulomas as seen with sarcoidosis; whether these two entities are distinct has been a subject of controversy (240,241). Litovsky et al. showed that GCM is characterized by myocytic destruction mediated by cytotoxic T cells, macrophagic giant cells, and eosinophils. In contrast, cardiac sarcoid is an interstitial granulomatous disease without myocytic necrosis (242).

Although the cause of GCM is unknown, it has been associated with a medley of autoimmune disorders and perhaps is immunologically mediated. Thymomas, SLE, rheumatoid arthritis, Wegener's granulomatosis, ulcerative colitis, chronic hepatitis, myasthenia gravis, myositis, pernicious anemia, Takayasu's arteritis, and lymphomas have been associated with GCM (243–251). The clinical presentation of GCM is similar to that of lymphocytic myocarditis, although arrhythmias and heart failure seem to predominate. Patients with GCM often present with conduction system abnormalities,

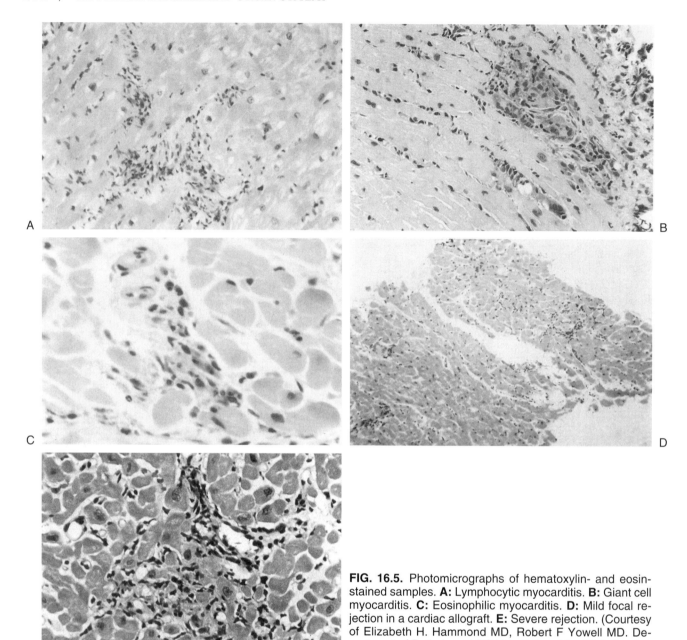

**FIG. 16.5.** Photomicrographs of hematoxylin- and eosin-stained samples. **A:** Lymphocytic myocarditis. **B:** Giant cell myocarditis. **C:** Eosinophilic myocarditis. **D:** Mild focal rejection in a cardiac allograft. **E:** Severe rejection. (Courtesy of Elizabeth H. Hammond MD, Robert F Yowell MD. Department of Pathology, LDS Hospital and the Utah Cardiac Transplant Program, Salt Lake City, UT.)

ventricular tachycardia, or even sudden death (243,252–254). Ventricular dysfunction with presentation as congestive heart failure is the other common manifestation (255,256). GCM has also manifested as asymmetric septal hypertrophy (257).

The natural history of GCM is obscure because of its rare occurrence, but isolated reports in the literature suggest that it carries a poor prognosis. Davidoff et al. (258) reported that 70% of GCM patients required cardiac transplantation or died during a 4-year follow-up period, compared with the 29% of lymphocytic myocarditis patients. Cooper et al. (259) described 63 patients with GCM collected in a worldwide registry. The registry patients had a 89% rate of death or need for transplantation, which was significantly worse than that

for the 111 patients with lymphocytic myocarditis seen in the MTT. The median survival was 5.5 months. The patients treated with immunosuppressive regimens, including cyclosporine, azathioprine, and prednisone, had an average cardiac survival of 12.3 months, compared with 3.0 months for the untreated patients. The rate of recurrent GCM in the transplanted patients was 25% (9 of 36).

The role of immunosuppressive therapy for GCM is unknown, but anecdotal and registry reports suggest possible benefit, and a trial of cyclosporine and prednisone with or without azathioprine must be attempted. Cardiac transplantation remains the last therapeutic resort for these patients, although there is risk of recurrent disease (259–261). This seems to be associated with abatement of immunosuppressive therapy after transplantation (262) and may represent atypical rejection in the allograft (263).

## Eosinophilic Myocarditis

The association of eosinophils with cardiac disease was first described by Loffler, who reported "endocarditis parietalis fibroplastica" associated with eosinophilia (264). Endocardial disease with eosinophilia is well recognized and extensively reviewed elsewhere (265,266), but the myocardial involvement is rare and frequently fatal, with the diagnosis often made postmortem. Endomyocardial biopsy is essential to the antemortem diagnosis of eosinophilic myocarditis (267) (Fig. 16.5C). Myocarditis may represent a fulminant necrotic form of the endocardial disease (268).

Eosinophils have the ability to secrete highly toxic cationic proteins into areas of inflammation, produce harmful oxygen radicals, and generate potent lipid mediators, leading myocyte necrosis as seen in proximity to degranulating eosinophils (269). Animal experiments have confirmed reduction in ventricular function in hypereosinophilic states and myocyte death when exposed to eosinophil-granule proteins (270). Eosinophilic myocardial infiltrates have been associated with profound eosinophilia caused by an allergic diathesis, parasitic infection, drug hypersensitivity, vasculitis, or Churg–Strauss syndromes (271–273), but eosinophilic myocarditis can occur in the absence of profound eosinophilia (274). Eosinophilic myocarditis may manifest as acute myocardial infarction, sudden death, cardiogenic shock, or nonspecific chest pain and dyspnea.

The natural history of eosinophilic myocarditis is usually swift and ominous, with rapid evolution to refractory heart failure or intractable arrhythmias leading to death. Biopsy-aided histologic confirmation is fundamental to antemortem diagnosis. Clinical improvement may occur with corticosteroid therapy (274).

## Cardiac Sarcoidosis

Sarcoidosis is a multiorgan, noncaseating granulomatous disorder of unknown origin. Histologically, it may involve the lung, lymph nodes, skin, liver, spleen, parotid glands, and the heart (275). Pulmonary manifestations are the predominant finding, with pulmonary hypertension and pulmonary fibrosis resulting in right heart failure (276). Asymptomatic cardiac involvement is common, with one fourth of the patients having sarcoid granulomas in the heart at autopsy (277). Characteristically, the noncaseating granulomas infiltrate the ventricular walls and become fibrotic. They may involve the conduction system. There may be transmural involvement with fibrous replacement of portions of the myocardium and aneurysm formation (278). The fibrous transition of granulomas may result in early diastolic dysfunction, but as the disease progresses and with extensive involvement, systolic impairment occurs.

The clinical presentation of cardiac sarcoidosis is variable and may depend on the amount of myocardium replaced with granulomas and the amount and location of scar tissue. Rhythm abnormalities and conduction disorders predominate (279). Patients with congestive heart failure may show clinical features of restrictive cardiomyopathy, dilated cardiomyopathy, or both (280). Papillary dysfunction with mitral regurgitation and pericardial involvement with effusive-constrictive disease have also been described (279). Myocardial scintigraphy with thallium 201 and gallium 67 is helpful in identifying patients with myocardial involvement (281). MRI has been proposed as a diagnostic modality (282,283). Histologic diagnosis with endomyocardial biopsy is corroborative, but a negative biopsy finding does not exclude the possibility because of sampling error. The finding of pulmonary involvement with bilateral hilar adenopathy and evidence of myocardial disease may suggest cardiac sarcoidosis in a young person.

Corticosteroids are indicated when myocardial involvement, conduction abnormalities, and ventricular arrhythmias are present (284). Patients with scintigraphic uptake of gallium 67 may be more responsive to corticosteroid therapy (285). Permanent pacemakers may be needed to treat the conduction abnormalities. Implantable defibrillators may be used in the prevention of sudden death (286). Heart failure is treated in the conventional manner, and heart transplantation is reserved for intractable heart failure (287). Heart and lung transplantations are performed infrequently for patients with pulmonary involvement, but there is a significant risk of recurrent disease (287).

## Peripartum Myocarditis and Cardiomyopathy

Virchow and Porak first reported the association of pregnancy with dilated cardiomyopathy in 1870 in an autopsy series (288). Peripartum myocarditis and cardiomyopathy (PMC) occurs in 1 of 3,000 to 15,000 pregnancies. The incidence is higher in Africa, and it increases with older age, multiparity, multiple gestations, and a history of PMC. PMC is a myocarditis of unknown cause, perhaps related to an infectious, autoimmune, or idiopathic process. The viral myocarditis hypothesis stems from the observations that pregnant mice are more susceptible to cardiotropic viruses; with increased viral replication (289) and with the increased hemodynamic burden of pregnancy, the myocardial lesions worsen (290). After delivery, the rapid degeneration of the uterus may result in fragmentation of tropocollagen by enzymatic degradation. This process releases actin, myosin, and their metabolites, and antibodies are formed that cross-react with the myocardium (288). Tocolytic therapy has been associated with cardiomyopathy (291).

The diagnosis of PMC must be made within 1 month before delivery of the fetus or 5 months later. The presentation is usually of decompensated ventricular systolic failure in the absence of any identifiable cardiac pathology. Therapy is tailored to the decompensated state with the use of diuretics, digoxin, and vasodilators (ACEI are contraindicated in pregnancy). Inotropic therapy may be needed for supporting those in cardiogenic shock, along with use of mechanical circulatory assist devices. Although there are anecdotal reports (292) of the benefit of immunosuppressive therapy, their routine use cannot be recommended; the only indication would be biopsy-proved fulminant myocarditis. Cardiac transplantation is a therapeutic option reserved for those with intractable heart failure, but transplantation should be delayed, because the short-term prognosis seems to be unfavorable because of increased allograft rejection, and the natural history of PMC suggests that one half the patients have spontaneous resolutions (293).

## RHEUMATIC CARDITIS: ACUTE RHEUMATIC FEVER

Acute rheumatic fever (ARF) is a multisystem, inflammatory disease that occurs 2 weeks to 6 months after a group A streptococcal pharyngitis. Societal improvements have resulted in a markedly diminished frequency and severity of ARF. The incidence of ARF in the United States is less than 2 cases per 100,000 persons, although there are isolated reports of local outbreaks. In the developing countries, ARF continues to be a major health threat, and rheumatic heart disease is the leading cause for cardiovascular related hospitalizations for the 5- to 25-year-old age group (18).

The pathophysiology of ARF remains mostly speculative, but it is believed that the streptococcal M protein cross-reacts with human cardiac myocytes, cartilages, chondrocytes, synovial cells, and subthalamic nuclei of the central nervous system. The virulence of the streptococcal infection depends on the serotype of the M protein, which determines its antigenic epitopes shared with the sarcolemmal proteins and cardiac myosin (294). The variations in virulence are responsible for the occasional local outbreaks in the developed countries with a low incidence of ARF.

Host factors are also responsible in the risk for rheumatic heart disease. There is a 50% attack recurrence rate for patients who have previously had rheumatic fever. There is a preponderance of human leukocyte antigen (HLA) DR1, DR3, DR4, DR7, DRW 53, and DQW 2 expression in most patients with rheumatic fever (295,296).

### Diagnosis and Clinical Presentation

The diagnosis of ARF is facilitated by application of Jones's criteria, first described in 1944 by T. Duckett Jones (297) and subsequently revised. The revised criteria are presented in Table 16.6. Rheumatic fever classically produces a pancarditis affecting the endocardium, myocardium, and pericardium. The incidence of carditis varies inversely with age, with 90% to 92% for children younger than 3 years, 50% for those between 3 and 6 years, 32% in adolescents between 14 and 17 years, and less than 15% in adults (18). The fulminant cases may resemble acute viral myocarditis with profound myo-

**TABLE 16.6.** *Guidelines for the diagnosis of initial attack of rheumatic fever (modified Jones criteria, 1992)*

Major manifestations
  Carditis
  Polyarthritis
  Chorea
  Erythema marginatum
  Subcutaneous nodules
Minor manifestations
  Clinical findings
    Arthralgia
    Fever
  Laboratory findings
    Elevated levels of acute phase reactants
      Erythrocyte sedimentation rate
      C-reactive protein
    Prolonged PR interval
Supporting evidence of antecedent group A streptococcal infection
  Positive throat culture or rapid streptococcal antigen
  Elevated or rising streptococcal antibody titer
If supported by evidence of recent group A streptococcal infection, the presence of two major or one major and two minor manifestations indicates a high probability of acute rheumatic fever.

From Special Writing Group of the Committee on Rheumatic Fever, Endocarditis, and Kawasaki Disease of the Council on Cardiovascular Disease in the Young of the American Heart Association. Guidelines for the diagnosis of rheumatic fever. Jones criteria, 1992 update. *JAMA* 1992;268:2069–2073.

cardial dysfunction. The most common finding is that of mitral regurgitation associated with mitral valvulitis. The murmur (Carey-Coombs) may be transient. Frequently, a pericardial friction rub is the only abnormality detected. Hemodynamically significant rheumatic valvular disease with mitral or aortic stenosis usually occurs with recurring attacks. No single laboratory test result is pathognomonic for the diagnosis of ARF, but evidence of preceding streptococcal infection may be obtained with throat swab culture (only in about 10%) or by detection of streptococcal antibodies, antistreptolysin O (ASO), or antideoxyribonuclease B (ADNase B). The other manifestations of ARF include migratory polyarthritis, erythema marginatum, subcutaneous nodules, and Sydenham's chorea. These has been extensively reviewed elsewhere (298).

Rheumatic carditis manifests within 3 weeks to 3 months of the preceding streptococcal infection, and most attacks last for less than 3 months, with 5% persisting beyond 6 months.

### Treatment

The patients with arthritis as a major component of ARF respond dramatically to treatment with aspirin. Even patients with mild carditis may be treated with aspirin alone (100 mg/kg/day in divided doses). Corticosteroids are reserved for the severe cases of rheumatic carditis. The evidence for long-term benefit of corticosteroid therapy is lacking, because the prevalence of apical systolic murmurs at 1 year or development of future valvular disease is not significantly different in the corticosteroid-treated patients and the aspirin-treated patients, but there is earlier resolution of murmurs and subcutaneous nodules in those treated with corticosteroids (299). Alternative NSAIDs have not been adequately assessed but may be beneficial in aspirin-intolerant patients.

The most effective treatment for ARF is primary prevention. Rheumatic fever does not occur if streptococcal pharyngitis is aggressively treated. Penicillin is extremely effective as a single injection of 1.2 MU of benzathine penicillin G or 125 to 250 mg of penicillin V given orally four times each day for 10 days. Erythromycin is the drug of choice in penicillin-allergic patients. Because recurrent streptococcal infections may reactivate carditis, secondary prophylaxis in patients with a history of rheumatic fever is recommended. Effective regimens include benzathine penicillin G (1.2 MU every 3 to 4 weeks) or penicillin V (250 mg orally twice daily), continued for 10 years or until age 25 for patients with prior history of carditis (300).

The M protein of the streptococcal cell wall has been identified and vaccination with this protein seems to be protective, without the inherent danger of causing cross-reactivity with the cardiac myocyte and resultant rheumatic complications. Large-scale clinical trials with this vaccine are pending (301,302).

## CARDIAC MANIFESTATIONS OF RHEUMATIC DISEASES

### Systemic Lupus Erythematosus

SLE is an autoimmune disease of unknown cause. It is mostly a disease of young women, with a peak incidence between ages 15 and 40, and it affects women five times more often than men. Its reported prevalence is 1 case per 2,000 individuals in the United States, and it has a strong familial component. The cardiovascular involvement in SLE has been extensively reviewed (303,304). The reported prevalence of cardiovascular involvement is 18% to 70% (305,306).

Pericarditis is the most common cardiovascular manifestation of SLE and is clinically apparent in 20% to 30% of lupus patients, with echocardiographic and autopsy evidence in a higher percentage (307–309). Histologically, the acute lesions display a fibrinous exudate, fibrinoid necrosis, and hematoxylin bodies, with obliteration of the pericardial space with fibrous adhesions as time progresses. Large effusions are rare, but small exudative effusions have been shown to contain antinuclear antibodies, lupus erythematosus cells, immune complexes, and a reduced level of complement (310). Pericarditis, which may be accompanied with pleuritis, occurs at any time during periods of active disease. Tamponade is a rare complication of SLE (311). Constrictive pericarditis has also been reported (312). Secondary bacterial pericarditis is not unusual, because these patients often are immunosuppressed with high-dose corticosteroids; *Staphylococcus aureus* is most frequently isolated, and these cases have a high mortality rate (313).

The treatment of SLE-related pericarditis depends on presenting symptoms and disease severity. Asymptomatic and hemodynamically insignificant pericardial effusions may be managed with watchful expectation and no therapy. Nonsteroidal antiinflammatory drugs are effective in managing the mildly symptomatic effusions, but for more severe cases, corticosteroid use may be warranted. Hemodynamically significant effusions are usually treated by pericardiocentesis, but recurrent cases may require a surgical window and aggressive medical therapy.

There are isolated reports of lupus-related cardiomyopathy. Studies comparing rest and exercise systolic and diastolic functions support the notion of lupus cardiomyopathy, but there are often confounding variables such as calciphylaxis-induced myopathy with chronic renal failure and secondary hyperparathyroidism, drug-related myopathy (colchicine), concomitant small vessel endarteritis, and a lack of myocardial lesions in SLE patients. Clinically evident congestive heart failure occurs infrequently. The diagnosis of lupus myocarditis can be made with endomyocardial biopsy, but treatment reports are largely anecdotal because of the infrequency of disease. Immunosuppression with corticosteroids or cyclophosphamide has produced favorable responses.

The classic valvular lesions of SLE were described by Libman and Sacks (314). Roldan et al. (315) reported that more than one half of patients with SLE demonstrate valvular abnormalities by echocardiography. The characteristic Libman–Sacks lesion is a small verrucous vegetation that is adherent to the endocardium, most frequently on the ventricular surface of the mitral leaflets at the valve rings and commissures. It may also involve the mural endocardium, chordae tendineae, and papillary muscles and can cover the valve surfaces. Histologically, the lesions display proliferating endothelial cells and myocytes with chronic inflammatory cells. Immunoglobulins and complement have been demonstrated on the endoluminal surface of vessels from verrucae (316). Verrucous endocarditis rarely produces clinical signs or symptoms. Innocuous murmurs from hyperdynamic flow states are common among SLE patients. Patients with Libman–Sacks endocarditis probably are at increased risk for bacterial endocarditis and thromboembolism (317). Nonrheumatic verrucous endocarditis may be treated with steroids if there is growth of lesions with other evidence of increased disease activity. The lesions usually heal with fibrosis and calcification. The increased use of steroids in the treatment of SLE may be responsible for the decrease in frequency of Libman–Sacks lesions. Echocardiographic evidence of valve thickening may be a reasonable indication for antibiotic prophylaxis for endocarditis, although firm evidence supporting their use is lacking.

The incidence of coronary artery disease in SLE patients has been increasing, with a concomitant rise in mortality from myocardial infarction and its sequelae. This increase may be related to arteritis or accelerated atherosclerosis resulting from corticosteroid therapy (318). Hypertension and hypercholesterolemia are common comorbidities and contribute to the increased coronary risk. The small vessel arteritis may lead to ischemic damage to the conduction system and resultant rhythm abnormalities. Transient supraventricular arrhythmias can be associated with pericardial inflammation and should be treated in the usual manner. Procainamide is probably best avoided, because it elicits a drug-induced lupus syndrome. The association between maternal lupus and congenital heart block in offspring is well recognized, especially when the maternal anti-Ro antibodies (SSA) are present (319). Fetal monitoring is advised for high-risk mothers if fetal bradycardia is detected.

### Rheumatoid Arthritis

Clinical heart disease occurs less frequently in patients with rheumatoid arthritis (RA), because they often are not active because of their skeletal disabilities. Cardiac manifestations are often recognized on random echocardiography or at autopsy.

Pericarditis is the most common cardiac manifestation of RA. Women are affected twice as often as men, and pericarditis typically occurs in patients with clinically active inflammatory disease with evidence of ongoing articular and extraarticular RA. The symptoms of pericarditis in RA patients are typical pain that may be partly pleuritic and positional, often accompanied with fever, orthopnea, paroxysmal nocturnal dyspnea, and edema. Pericardial friction rub may be evident on examination. Frank pulsus paradoxus and other signs suggestive of tamponade are rare. Echocardiography demonstrates effusion in 90% of RA patients with clinical pericarditis but also in 10% to 47% of asymptomatic patients (320,321). Aspirated pericardial fluid classically reveals an elevated leukocyte count and increased levels of protein, lactate dehydrogenase, and cholesterol but decreased levels of complement and glucose (322). Rheumatoid factor may also be detected. Resolution of pericarditis is slow and often takes several weeks to months. Pericarditis tends to portend poor long-term survival compared with that for patients without pericarditis, but the difference may only be representative of the extensive disease burden of these patients. Treatment options include NSAIDs, corticosteroids, gold salts, and methotrexate.

Valvular lesions in RA are rare and typically include cusp thickening and irregular fibrosis. Granulomatous involvement, when present, is usually found in the valve rings and cusps and occasionally in the aortic wall. The frequency of individual valve involvement is similar to that in cases of rheumatic fever: mitral (most common), aortic, tricuspid, and pulmonary (least common). The rarity of these lesions pathologically makes clinical disease even more uncommon. There is no evidence of increased mortality related to valvular disease in RA (323). Echocardiography has been used to identify valvular abnormalities in RA patients, but its clinical relevance is suspect. Most clinical reports describe aortic insufficiency, with mitral insufficiency occurring less often (324). Concomitant involvement of the pericardium and the conduction system has been reported, and the valvular disease is managed as valvular disease from other causes is.

The vasculitis seen with RA usually affects small dermal vessels and manifests as skin lesions. Coronary arteritis is rare and may occasionally result in myocardial infarction (325,326). Aortitis has also been associated with RA (327).

### Progressive Systemic Sclerosis

Progressive systemic sclerosis (PSS), also called scleroderma, is a disorder of unknown origin that affects multiple organ systems. It is characterized by a debilitating fibrosis of the cutaneous and visceral tissues. The most common feature of systemic sclerosis is its effect on the skin of the hands, face, and neck. However, for a given patient, survival is more closely linked to the visceral involvement of the disease, which may involve the lungs, gastrointestinal tract, kidneys, and the heart. The prevalence of systemic sclerosis has been estimated to be 0.1 to 13.4 per 100,000 in the general population (328). The use of serologic tests for autoantibodies (anticentromere and antitopoisomerase I) in addition to nailfold capillary microscopy to detect microvascular abnormalities may increase estimates of disease prevalence. Females are three times more likely to be affected than males.

The pericardium is commonly involved in patients with PSS, occurring in up to 70% of autopsy series (329,330). Clinically occurring pericarditis is recognized less frequently. Symptoms are typical of those experienced from pericarditis of other causes and include fever, chest pain, and dyspnea; they are accompanied by the findings of a friction rub and ECG changes (331). Tamponade and constrictive pericarditis are rare.

The overall mortality for PSS appears to be related to the progression of renal disease (332). Myocardial fibrosis is present in most of the patients at autopsy, although there is no evidence of systolic ventricular dysfunction. "Scleroderma heart" has been described as focally occurring fibrosis involving all four chambers but sparing the coronary arteries. The fibrosis is usually preceded by myocardial necrosis and localized inflammation with endothelial proliferation, intimal fibrosis, and medial hyperplasia in the small arterioles, implicating the microvasculature (333). Myocardial contraction band necrosis has been described in nearly one third of the patients, possibly because of ischemia from vasospasm (334). An advanced degree of fibrosis may result in restrictive physiology with abnormalities in diastolic function. Myocarditis has been described but is considered to be rare (335).

A miscellany of ECG abnormalities and arrhythmias have been reported in patients with PSS. Conduction defects such as bundle and fascicular blocks and first-, second-, and third-degree AV block are common. Disturbances of rhythm are frequent and include supraventricular and ventricular tachycardias and occasionally bradyarrhythmias. Myocardial fibrosis involving the sinoatrial node more often than the AV node and the His–Purkinje system have been described in autopsy studies (333). Pulmonary hypertension may develop in scleroderma and is more commonly associated with the limited disease variant (336).

Management of the specific cardiovascular complications of systemic sclerosis is similar to those caused by other disorders. D-penicillamine and other immunosuppressive therapy may be considered for refractory cardiac disease. ACEIs are attractive agents for control of hypertension and may have a beneficial effect on limiting fibrosis and improving myocardial perfusion abnormalities (337).

## Polymyositis and Dermatomyositis

Polymyositis and dermatomyositis (PM/DM) are in a spectrum of idiopathic inflammatory myopathies that often have cardiovascular involvement. The disease is characterized by progressive skeletal muscle weakness, elevated muscle enzymes, abnormal electromyogram findings, and inflammation or necrosis identified on muscle biopsy (338). Although PM/DM predominantly involves skeletal muscle, cardiac involvement, including conduction abnormalities, arrhythmias, mitral valve prolapse, congestive heart failure, and rarely pericarditis, have been reported.

Although early accounts of PM/DM rarely underscored the involvement of only the heart, cognizance about its cardiac manifestations has increased. Autopsy studies have found evidence of cardiac disease mostly confined to the myocardium. Myocarditis is present in approximately 25% (339,340). There is no correlation between the finding of myocarditis and development of congestive heart failure, because each can be seen in the absence of the other (341). Although myocarditis may play a role in the congestive heart failure of these patients, other factors such as diastolic dysfunction, hypertension, and ischemia may also be important. The use of corticosteroid therapy in the treatment of the primary disease may contribute to myocardial damage (342). The diagnosis of myocarditis in absence of biopsy often is confounded by CK-MB enzyme elevation, which may occur with regenerating skeletal muscle; however, the addition of specific cardiac markers such as troponin I has been helpful in differentiation of true myocardial injury.

The study of coronary arteries has demonstrated active vasculitis, intimal proliferation, medial sclerosis, and rarely arteritis obliterans (343), and myocardial infarction is rarely reported in PM/DM patients (339). The differentiation of primary disease from coexisting atherosclerosis and its possible acceleration by steroid use is always difficult. A high prevalence of mitral valve prolapse among PM/DM patients was found in an echocardiographic study of asymptomatic patients (344). Rarely, pericarditis has been reported in children with dermatomyositis and overlap syndromes.

The treatment of cardiac disorders with PM/DM should be focused on the primary disease. Immunosuppressive agents may be employed in addition to corticosteroids for cases of confirmed myocarditis.

## Seronegative Spondyloarthropathies

Seronegative spondyloarthropathies (SS) are a group of multisystem disorders that are associated with sacroiliac joint disease and a high incidence of the histocompatibility antigen HLA B27. This group of inflammatory spondyloarthropathies is accompanied by cardiac complications, specifically conduction blocks and lone aortic regurgitation. Mallory's 1936 description of aortic valvular regurgitation in two young men with a retrospectively clear diagnosis of SS was the first report of cardiac manifestations in this context (345). Three major pathologic changes seen in patients with SS are responsible for the development of aortic valvular insufficiency. Dilatation of the aortic root, fibrotic thickening and downward retraction of the bases of the cusps, and inward rolling of the edges of the cusps are pathognomonic features (346). The prevalence of aortic valve disease is 2% after 10 years of SS and 12% after 30 years of ankylosing spondylitis (347).

The treatment of severe aortic regurgitation is surgical, although there are concerns regarding proximal aortic dilatation, myocardial subaortic fibrosis, and concomitant restrictive lung disease. Rarely, there may be mitral insufficiency because of anterior leaflet dysfunction resulting from subaortic fibrosis of the anterior leaflet (348).

Conduction system disease in SS is manifested mainly as various degrees of heart block. The prevalence of heart block is approximately 8%, with a range of 1% to 15% (349). Heart block may be found in the presence of aortic disease or in isolation as the presenting feature of undiagnosed SS. Patients who are HLA B27 positive have a relative risk of 6.7 for needing a pacemaker, even in absence of clinically evident spondyloarthropathy (350). Electrophysiologic studies have found AV conduction abnormalities localized to the AV node and suprahisian region, in contrast to acquired heart block, which is most often infrahisian (351,352). The pathology of heart block appears to be the same fibrous infiltration that causes aortic root, valve, and ring disease. Myocarditis and pericarditis have been rarely reported in patients with ankylosing spondylitis and Reiter's syndrome (353).

## Systemic Vasculitis Syndromes

The inflammation of small and medium-sized arterioles is a hallmark of the systemic vasculitis syndromes, including polyarteritis nodosa, Wegener's granulomatosis, Kawasaki's disease, giant cell arteritis, Takayasu's arteritis, and Behçet's disease. The cardiovascular manifestations of these vasculitic syndromes range from coronary vasculitis resulting in angina, myocardial infarction, and resultant ischemic dysfunction to aortic and great vessel vasculitis, myocarditis, pericarditis, conduction abnormalities, and valvular dysfunction. Kawasaki's disease is a well recognized cause of aneurysmal coronary artery disease.

## CARDIAC TRANSPLANTATION AND POSTTRANSPLANTATION IMMUNE PHENOMENA

The past quarter century has seen the maturation of cardiac transplantation from a rare experiment to an accepted therapy for end-stage heart failure. The triumph of this enterprise has been primarily attributed to an improved understanding of the immunologic mechanisms associated with allograft rejection and our ability to modify these with the available armamentarium of immunosuppressive agents.

## Immunology of Rejection

### Acute Allograft Rejection

The primary immune response is allorecognition, a process by which the graft is recognized as foreign. The MHC is a genetic region that codes for specific products devoted to providing extracellular representation of foreign antigens. The MHC encoded class I and class II molecules provide peptide binding sites that evoke the effector responses on recognition of the foreign peptide by the antigen-specific receptors of the T lymphocyte (64).

Most T cells have T-cell receptors (TCR) with $\alpha$ and $\beta$ chains. The antigen, present in form of the peptide in the groove of MHC molecules, is identified by the TCR. CD4 and CD8 proteins on the reciprocal peripheral T lymphocytes react with class II and class I MHC molecules, respectively (354,355). It has been observed in animal experiments that rodents without any T cells do not reject transplanted organs, but when repopulated with CD4 cells alone, the same animals are able to reject allografts. The CD8 cells usually cannot do this. CD4 cells are necessary and sufficient to cause rejection, although they may recruit other cells (i.e., macrophages, cytotoxic T cells, natural killer cells, lymphokine-activated cells, B cells) into the process rather than causing the damage themselves (356,357).

Transplantation immunity can be induced by means of direct activation of T lymphocytes by the so-called passenger donor lymphocyte (PDL), a bone marrow–derived cell present within the allograft, or through an indirect pathway in which the peptides derived from allogeneic proteins are taken up and processed by specialized host APCs. The recognition of allogeneic "foreign" allopeptides is self–HLA restricted, which may restrict the ability of the activated effector cells to find target structures expressed on the allograft (358).

The importance of PDL for induction of immune responses has been highlighted in several reviews (359,360) and suggests that the activation of T cells does not only rely on the recognition of these cells as allogeneic but also on the immunostimulatory capacity of these cells. They must present donor MHC class II antigens with bound allopeptides to peripheral T cells (361) and provide reciprocal accessory bindings such as those between leukocyte function antigen, LFA-1 (CD11a/CD18), and intercellular adhesion molecule, ICAM-1 (CD54), and between CD28 and cytotoxic T-lymphocyte–associated molecule-4 (CTLA-4) with CD80 (B7) and B70/B7.2 (362,363). If the graft-derived PDLs lack immunostimulatory capacity, they have to be degraded and presented to the T cells as processed allogeneic peptides by the host immunostimulatory cells, the APCs (358). Murine experiments have shown that T-cell recognition of foreign peptides on cells that lack immunostimulatory capacity does not result in activation (364).

T-cell activation requires antigenic stimulation and a costimulatory signal. The TCR in association with the CD3 complex, consisting of four or five nonpolymorphic polypeptide chains, is involved in antigen-specific recognition and triggering of transmembrane signals leading to cellular activation and signal transduction (363). There appear to be two early signal transduction pathways that result in increased intracellular calcium. The calcium influx activates calcineurin, a calcium-sensitive phosphatase, that dephosphorylates the nuclear factor of activated T cells (NFAT-1). The transcription of IL-2 mRNA is under the regulatory control of NFAT-1, which activates the promoter region of the gene resulting in the production of IL-2 (363,365).

The TCR coupling to the tyrosine kinase pathway remains an enigma, but one of the substrates of tyrosine phosphorylation, a 70-kd tyrosine phosphoprotein (ZAP-70) associates with the CD3ζ subunit (366) and possibly has a role in augmentation of IL-2 production by means of the CD28 costimulation pathway, which stabilizes the AP-1 transactivating factor. The costimulation pathway is induced by surface proteins expressed on APCs (i.e., CD80 [B7.1/BB1]), which have reciprocal binding ligands on T cells in the form of CD28 and CTLA-4. This appears to be independent of an increase in cytosolic calcium or activation of protein kinase C (367–369). Functional anergy and consequent inadequacy of IL-2 may be induced by loss of the CD28 costimulatory signal (367).

After the process of allorecognition and subsequent signal transduction resulting in transcription of specific genes is complete, the next phase of the immune response to the allograft begins with clonal proliferation of cytotoxic lymphocytes, which occurs primarily because of the growth factor effects of IL-2. The synthesis of other cytokines such as IFN-γ, TNF-β, and B-cell growth factors (i.e., IL-4, IL-5, and IL-6) is also stimulated at a higher level by IL-2 (Fig. 16.6). The cytokines facilitate activation of macrophages and other inflammatory cells and the production of allospecific antigraft antibodies by B cells, which can recruit complement and cause damage to vascular endothelium (370,371). An additional function of cytokines is to increase the expression of class I and class II MHC antigens and expression of adhesion molecules such as ICAM-1, granule membrane protein-140 (GMP-140), and VCAM-1 in response to IFN-γ, TNF-β, and IL-1 (372,373). The capillary endothelia of rejecting cardiac allografts have increased expression of ICAM-1, VCAM-1, and MHC class II molecules (374). The combination of clonal expansion of allospecific cytotoxic T lymphocytes and the production of cytokines leads to the eventual cascade of rejection, culminating in graft death (Fig. 16.5D,E).

### Chronic Allograft Rejection

The immunology of chronic allograft rejection is less well understood because animal models are best suited only to

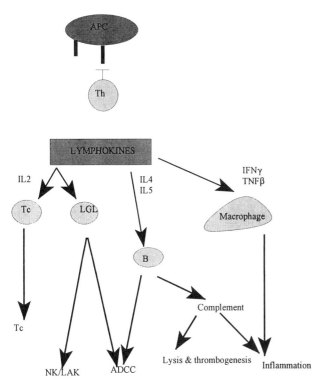

**FIG. 16.6.** The rejection cascade. The initial activation of helper T cells requires exposure to the major histocompatibility complex (MHC) class II–peptide complex on the antigen-presenting cell (*APC*), leading to production of a variety of lymphokines after the helper T cells are activated. The principal lymphokines involved in the rejection process are interleukin (*IL*)-2, interferon-γ (*IFN*-γ), tumor necrosis factor-β (*TNF*-β); IL-4, IL-5, and IL-6 are involved as B-cell growth factors. IL-2 is involved in the activation of cytotoxic T cells, natural killer (*NK*), and lymphokine-activated killer (*LAK*) cells, and it stimulates large granular lymphocytes (*LGLs*) to take up IgG antibodies on their surface receptors and participate in antibody-dependent cell-mediated cytotoxicity (*ADCC*). (Adapted from Rose ML, Yacoub M. *Immunology of heart and lung transplantation.* Kent: Edward Arnold Publications, 1993:4, with permission.)

study acute allograft rejection. In human transplantation, chronic allograft rejection and its associated graft dysfunction remain a major problem. Although the alloantigen-dependent mechanisms initiate the rejection processes, there are also alloantigen-independent factors such as graft ischemia and viral infections that contribute to chronic allograft dysfunction (375). There is probably a final common pathway for both processes, because alloantigen-independent factors also increase the risk for acute rejection, which is a known risk factor for chronic allograft dysfunction. It seems appropriate to attempt to block the T-cell responses in hope of inducing allograft tolerance and controlling the alloantigen-independent factors and therefore inhibiting development of chronic rejection. Blocking B7-CD28 interactions with CTLA-4 immunoglobulin seems to prolong graft survival and reduce graft atherosclerosis in animal models, as does treatment with mycophenolate mofetil (376,377). CMV can mediate allograft rejection through both alloantigen-independent

and alloantigen-dependent pathways. Experimental evidence suggests that aggressive treatment of CMV lessens the incidence of chronic rejection (378).

**Allograft Vasculopathy**

Cardiac allograft vasculopathy (CAV) remains a major cause of death in cardiac transplant recipients beyond the first year. It is a uniquely accelerated form of atherosclerosis that affects the vascular bed of the allograft but spares the native vessels throughout the body. The actuarial likelihood of angiographic CAV is 11%, 22%, and 45% at 1, 2, and 4 years, respectively (379). Intracoronary ultrasound is able to detect intimal thickening in 75% of transplant recipients at 1 year (380).

*Pathophysiology and Immunopathology*

The histopathologic pattern of CAV demonstrates a broad spectrum of abnormalities, ranging from the diffuse intimal proliferation to focal lipid-laden atherosclerotic plaques akin to those seen with native atherosclerosis. Early after transplantation, intimal proliferation with dense fibrous thickening predominates, but later, focal atherosclerotic plaques are often seen along with the intimal proliferative response. The obliterative arteriopathy seems to rapidly consume the smaller distal vessels and results in small, stellate infarctions (381). The cellular constituents of the intimal proliferative response are modified smooth muscle cells, macrophages, monocytes, and T lymphocytes (382).

The focal point of immunologic activity in the allograft remains the vascular endothelium, and the inciting event of CAV is subclinical endothelial injury. The evidence for increased expression of adhesion molecules was presented along with the MHC-dependent pathways. It appears that, besides the traditional immunologic mechanisms, there may be other factors, including MHC-independent ones that may play a role in development of CAV, because MHC-lacking mice or MHC-identical mice also develop CAV (383). Regardless of the initial mechanism, the final common pathway seems to be the clonal expansion of allospecific T lymphocytes and B lymphocytes, with a deluge of cytokine mediators (i.e., stimulatory such as IL-1, IL-2, IL-6, and TNF-α and growth factors such as platelet-derived growth factor, insulin-like growth factor-1, fibroblast growth factor, heparin-binding growth factors (HBGF), epidermal growth factor, granulocyte–macrophage colony-stimulating factor, and TGF-β) that promote the development of chronic graft vasculopathy (384).

Alloantigen-independent risk factors such as hyperlipidemia, glucose intolerance, insulin resistance, hypertension, CMV infections and ischemia or reperfusion injury at the time of graft harvest and implantation are likely cofactors in endothelial injury and subsequent graft vasculopathy.

*Diagnosis and Clinical Presentation*

The lack of innervation of the allograft results in painless ischemia and infarction. Most patients present with congestive heart failure or arrhythmias. Noninvasive screening methods, including thallium scintigraphy and stress echocardiography, are commonly used, but their sensitivity or specificity limits their reliable use. Coronary angiography remains the standard diagnostic modality for screening, and use of intracoronary ultrasound is gaining rapid ground as a choice diagnostic modality to assess the intimal proliferation.

### Treatment

There have been isolated but conflicting reports of the possible benefit of diltiazem and captopril in preventing CAV (385–387), but the most consistent evidence for a pharmacologic agent reducing the progression of CAV is for HMG-CoA reductase inhibitors (388,389). Immunosuppressive therapy with tacrolimus had shown promise in animal experiments, but in a large, randomized clinical trial, the preliminary data did not show any benefit in freedom from CAV in the tacrolimus-treated patients over those treated with cyclosporine. Mycophenolate mofetil and CTLA-4 immunoglobulin hold promise, but large-scale clinical trial data are awaited.

Meanwhile, with few preventive strategies, the only treatment for CAV remains revascularization or retransplantation. Angioplasty is associated with high restenosis rates (390), and long-term data on other newer devices are lacking.

## Posttransplantation Lymphoproliferative Disorder

Posttransplantation lymphoproliferative disorder (PTLD) occurs in fewer than 2% of transplant recipients. The presentation can be fulminant and fatal, refractory to any treatment, or relatively localized and benign, responding simply to reduction in immunosuppression. EBV, a lymphotropic virus that infects more than 90% of the population by adulthood, is thought to be the etiologic agent responsible for the development of lymphoproliferative lesions in immunosuppressed patients. The incidence of PTLD is low, approximately 1%, among patients who are seropositive for EBV before transplantation. The incidence of PTLD among patients who are seronegative for EBV before transplant and who receive an organ from an EBV-seropositive donor may be as high as 50% (391). There is a higher incidence of lung or gastrointestinal tract involvement but generally has a better prognosis than the other extranodal site PTLD (392). Treatment usually involves reduction of immunosuppression, administration of acyclovir, and chemotherapy for widespread disease.

## CONCLUSIONS

The wide variety of immunologic interactions with the heart includes primary cardiac afflictions such as lymphocytic myocarditis and its variants, rheumatic carditis, and other primarily immunologic disorders in which the heart becomes a target of the multisystem infirmities. Although the cardiovascular manifestations include ischemic, arrhythmic, and heart failure complications, the treatment must be individualized. The evidence for benefit of immunosuppressive therapy in most conditions is largely anecdotal and unproved in randomized clinical trials. Cardiac transplantation opens an entirely new arena of immunologic interactions, including acute and chronic allograft rejection and the long-term immunologic sequelae of progressive allograft vasculopathy and lymphoproliferative disorders.

## REFERENCES

1. Richardson P, McKenna WJ, Bristow M, et al. Report of the 1995 Word Organization/International Society and Federation of Cardiology Task Force on the Definition and Classification of Cardiomyopathies. *Circulation* 1996;93:841–842.
2. Aretz HT, Billingham ME, Edwards WD, et al. Myocarditis: histopathologic definition and classification. *Am J Cardiovasc Pathol* 1987;1:3–14.
3. Karjalainen J, Heikkila J, Nieminen M, et al. Etiology of mild acute infectious myocarditis: relation to clinical features. *Acta Med Scand* 1983;213:65–73.
4. Sahi T, Karjalainen J, Viitasalo MT, et al. Myocarditis in connection with viral infections in Finnish conscripts. *Ann Med Milit Fenn* 1982;57:198–203.
5. Karjalainen J, Nieminen M, Heikkila J. Influenza AI myocarditis in conscripts. *Acta Med Scand* 1980;207:27–30.
6. Bengtsson E. Electrocardiographic studies in patients with abnormalities in serial examinations with standard leads during acute infectious diseases. 1. Occurrence of abnormalities in STT complex of chest leads in resting electrocardiograms suggestive of localized myocardial lesions. *Acta Med Scand* 1957;159:395.
7. Walterson AP. Virological investigations in congestive cardiomyopathy. *Postgrad Med* 1978;54:505–507.
8. Kitaura Y. Virological study of idiopathic cardiomyopathy. *Jpn Circ J* 1981;45:279–294.
9. Grist NR, Reid D. Epidemiology of viral infections of the heart. In: Banatvala JE, ed. *Viral infections of the heart.* London: Hodder & Stoughton, 1993:23–31.
10. Vikerfors T, Stjerna A, Olcen P, et al. Acute myocarditis: serologic diagnosis, clinical findings and follow-up. *Acta Med Scand* 1988; 223:45–52.
11. Frisk G, Torfason EG, Diderholm H. Reverse radioimmune assays of IgM and IgG antibodies to coxsackie B viruses in patients with acute pericarditis. *J Med Virol* 1984;14:191–200.
12. Martin AB, Webber S, Fricker FJ, et al. Acute myocarditis: rapid diagnosis by PCR in children. *Circulation* 1994;19:330–339.
13. Wilson RSE, Morris TH, Russell RJ. Cytomegalovirus myocarditis. *Br Heart J* 1972;34:865–868.
14. Wink K, Schmitz H. Cytomegalovirus myocarditis. *Am Heart J* 1980; 100:667–672.
15. Wreghitt T, Cary N. Virus infections in heart transplant recipients and evidence for involvement of the heart. In: Banatvala JE, ed. *Viral infections of the heart.* London: Hodder & Stoughton, 1993:240–250.
16. Partanen J, Nieminen MS, Jrogerus L, et al. Cytomegalovirus myocarditis in transplanted heart verified by endomyocardial biopsy. *Clin Cardiol* 1991;14:846–849.
17. Havaldar PV. Diphtheria in the 80s: experience in a South Indian district hospital. *J Indian Medical Assoc* 1992;19:155–156.
18. Ledford DK. Immunologic aspects of vasculitis and cardiovascular disease. *JAMA* 1997;278:1962–1971.
19. McCallister HF, Klementowica PT, Andrew C, et al. Lyme carditis: an important cause of reversible heart block. *Ann Intern Med* 1989;110: 339–345.
20. Lewes D, Rainford DJ, Lane WF. Symptomless myocarditis and myalgia in viral and *Mycoplasma pneumoniae* infections. *Br Heart J* 1974; 36:924–932.
21. Odeh M, Oliven A. Chlamydial infections of the heart. *Eur J Microbiol Infect Dis* 1992;11:885–893.

22. Wesslen L, Pahlson C, Friman G, et al. Myocarditis caused by *Chlamydia pneumoniae* (TWAR) and sudden unexpected death in a Swedish elect orienteer. *Lancet* 1992;340:427–428.

23. Speirs GE, Hakim M, Calne RY, et al. Relative risk of donor transmitted *Toxoplasma gondii* infection in heart, liver and kidney transplant patients. *Clin Transplant* 1988;2:257–260.

24. Reilly JM, Cunnion RE, Anderson DW, et al. Frequency of myocarditis left ventricular dysfunction and ventricular tachycardia in acquired immune deficiency syndrome. *Am J Cardiol* 1988;62:789–793.

25. Anderson DW, Virmani R, Reilly JM, et al. Prevalent myocarditis at necropsy in acquired immune deficiency syndrome. *J Am Coll Cardiol* 1988;11:792–799.

26. Corallo S, Mutimelli MR, Moroni M, et al. Echocardiography detects myocardial damage in AIDS: prospective study in 102 patients. *Eur Heart J* 1988;9:887–892.

27. Gauntt C, Higdon A, Bowers D et al. What lessons can be learned from the animal model studies in viral heart diseases? *Scand J Infect Dis* 1993;88[Suppl]:49–65.

28. Herskowitz A, Wolfgram LJ, Rose NR, Beisel KW. Coxsackievirus B3 murine myocarditis: a pathologic spectrum of myocarditis in genetically defined inbred strains. *J Am Coll Cardiol* 1987;9:1311–1319.

29. Kyu B-S, Matsumori A, Sato Y, et al. Cardiac persistence of cardioviral RNA detected by polymerase chain reaction in a murine model of dilated cardiomyopathy. *Circulation* 1992;86:522–530.

30. Wee L, Liu P, Penn L, et al. Persistence of viral genome into late stages of murine myocarditis detected by polymerase chain reaction. *Circulation* 1992;86:1605–1614.

31. Kandolf R, Ameis D, Kirschner P, et al. In situ detection of enteroviral genomes in myocardial cells by nucleic acid hybridization: an approach to the diagnosis of viral heart disease. *Proc Natl Acad Sci USA* 1987;84:6272–6276.

32. Wolfgram LJ, Rose NR. Coxsackie virus infection as a trigger of cardiac autoimmunity. *Immunol Res* 1989;8:61–80.

33. Neumann DA, Rose NR, Ansari AA, et al. Induction of multiple heart autoantibodies in mice with coxsackie virus B3 and cardiac myosin induced autoimmune myocarditis. *J Immunol* 1994;152:343–350.

34. Oldstone MBA. Molecular mimicry and autoimmune disease. *Cell* 1987;50:819.

35. Beisel KW, Srinivasappa J, Prabhakar BS. Identification of a putative shared epitope between coxsackie virus B4 and alpha cardiac myosin heavy chain. *Clin Exp Immunol* 1991;86:49–55.

36. Maisch B, Bauer E, Cirst M, et al. Cytolytic crossreactive antibodies directed against cardiac membranes and viral proteins in coxsackie virus B3 and B4 myocarditis: characterization and pathogenetic relevance. *Circulation* 1993;87[Suppl IV]:IV-49–65.

37. Cunningham MW, Antone Sm, Gulizia JM, et al. Cytotoxic and viral neutralizing antibodies crossreact with streptococcal M protein, enteroviruses and human cardiac myosin. *Proc Natl Acad Sci USA* 1992;89:1320–1324.

38. Gauntt CJ, Higdon AL, Arizpe HM, et al. Epitopes shared between coxsackievirus B3 (CVB3) and normal heart tissue contribute to CVB3-induced murine myocarditis. *Clin Immunol Immunolpathol* 1993;68:129–134.

39. Schwimmbeck PL, Schwimmbeck NK, Schultheiss HP, et al. Mapping of antigenic determinants of adenine nucleotide translocator and coxsackie B3 virus with synthetic peptides: use for the diagnosis of viral heart disease. *Clin Immunol Immunolpathol* 1993;68:135–140.

40. Weller AH, Simpson K, Herzum M, et al. Coxsackie B3 induced myocarditis: virus receptor antibodies modulate myocarditis. *J Immunol* 1989;143:1843–1850.

41. Limas CJ, Goldenberg IF, Limas C. Autoantibodies against beta-adrenoreceptors in human dilated cardiomyopathy. *Circ Res* 1989;64:97–103.

42. Wolff PG, Kuhl U, Schultheiss HP. Laminin distribution and auto-antibodies to laminin in dilated cardiomyopathy and myocarditis. *Am Heart J* 1989;117:1303–1309.

43. Ansari AA, Herskowitz A, Danner DJ. Identification of mitochondrial proteins that serve as targets for autoimmunity. *Circulation* 1988;78[Suppl]:457(abst).

44. Latif N, Baker CS, Dunn MJ, et al. Frequency and specificity of anti-heart antibodies in patients with dilated cardiomyopathy detected using SDS-PAGE and Western blotting. *J Am Coll Cardiol* 1993;22:1378–1384.

45. Huber SA, Job LP, Woodruff JF. Lysis of infected myofibers by coxsackievirus B3 immune T lymphocytes. *Am J Pathol* 1980;98:681–694.

46. Huber SA, Lodge PA. Coxsackievirus B3 in Balb/c mice: evidence for autoimmunity to myocyte antigens. *Am J Pathol* 1984;116:21–29.

47. Seko Y, Shinkai Y, Kawasaki A, et al. Expression of perforins in infiltrating cells in murine hearts with acute myocarditis caused by coxsackievirus B3. *Circulation* 1991;84:788–795.

48. Neu N, Rose NR, Biesel KW, et al. Cardiac myosin induces myocarditis in genetically predisposed mice. *J Immunol* 1987;139:3630–3636.

49. Adesanya CO, Goldberg AH, Phear WPC, et al. Heart muscle performance after experimental viral myocarditis. *J Clin Invest* 1976;57:569–575.

50. Woodruff JF, Woodruff JJ. Involvement of T lymphocytes in the pathogenesis of Coxsackie virus B3 heart disease. *J Immunol* 1974;113:1726–1734.

51. Woodruff JF, Kilbourne ED. The influence of quantitated postweaning undernutrition on coxsackievirus B3 infection of adult mice. I. Viral persistence and increased severity of lesions. *J Infect Dis* 1970;121:137–163.

52. Godeny EK, Gauntt CJ. Interferon and natural killer cell activity in coxsackievirus B3 induced murine myocarditis. *Eur Heart J* 1987;8[Suppl J]:433–435.

53. In situ immune autoradiographic identification of cells in heart tissue of mice with coxsackievirus B3 induced myocarditis. *Am J Pathol* 1987;129:267–276.

54. Entman ML, Youker k, Shoji T, et al. Neutrophil induced oxidative injury of cardiac myocytes. *J Clin Invest* 1992;90;1335–1345.

55. Godeny EK, Gauntt CJ. Murine natural killer cells limit coxsackievirus B3 replication. *J Immunol* 1987:139:913–918.

56. Chow LH, Beisel KW, McManus BM. Enteroviral infection of mice with severe combined immunodeficiency: evidence for direct viral pathogenesis of myocardial injury. *Lab Invest* 1992;66:24–31.

57. Rager-Zisman B, Allison AC. Effects of immunosuppression on Coxsackie B3 virus in mice and passive protection by circulating antibody. *J Gen Virol* 1973;19:339–351.

58. Kilbourne ED, Wilson CB, Perrier D. The induction of gross myocardial lesions by Coxsackie (pleurodynia) virus and cortisone. *J Clin Invest* 1956;35:362–370.

59. Wong CY, Woodruff JJ, Woodruff JF. Generation of cytotoxic T lymphocytes during coxsackievirus B3 infection. II. Characterization of effector cells and demonstration of cytotoxicity against viral infected myofibers. *J Immunol* 1977;118:1165–1169.

60. Hufnagel G, Chapman N, Tracy S. A noncardiovirulent strain of coxsackievirus B3 causes myocarditis in mice with severe combined immunodeficiency syndrome. *Eur Heart J* 1995;16[Suppl O]:18–19.

61. Modlin J. Coxsackieviruses, echoviruses, and newer enteroviruses. In: Mandell G, Douglas R, Bennett J, eds. *Principles and practice of infectious diseases.* New York: Churchill Livingstone, 1990.

62. Lodge PA, Herzum M, Olszewski J, et al. Coxsackievirus B3 myocarditis: acute and chronic forms of the disease caused by different immunopathogenic mechanisms. *Am J Pathol* 1987;128:455–463.

63. Seko Y, Tsuchimochi H, Nakamura T, et al. Expression of major histocompatibility complex class I antigen in murine ventricular myocytes infected with coxsackievirus B3. *Circ Res* 1990;67:360–367.

64. Germain RN. MHC dependent antigen processing and peptide presentation: providing ligands for T lymphocyte activation. *Cell* 1994;76:287–289.

65. Monrad ES, Matsumori A, Murphy JC, et al. Cyclosporine therapy in experimental murine myocarditis with encephalomyocarditis virus. *Circulation* 1986;73:1058–1064.

66. O'Connell JB, Reap EA, Robinson JA. The effects of cyclosporine on acute murine Coxsackie B3 myocarditis. *Circulation* 1986;73:353–359.

67. Estrin M, Smith C, Huber S. Coxsackievirus B3 myocarditis. T-cell autoimmunity to heart antigens is resistant is resistant to cyclosporin-A treatment. *Am J Pathol* 1986;125:244–251.

68. Klingel K, Hohenadl C, Canu A, et al. Ongoing enterovirus induced myocarditis is associated with persistent heart muscle infection: quantitative analysis of virus replication, tissue damage, and inflammation. *Proc Natl Acad Sci USA* 1992;89:314–318.

69. Wilson Fm, Miranda QR, Chason JL, et al. Residual pathologic changes following murine Coxsackie A and B myocarditis. *Am J Pathol* 1969;55;253–265.

70. Huber SA, Heintz N, Tracy R. Coxsackievirus B3 induced myocarditis: virus and actinomycin D treatment of myocytes induces novel antigens recognized by cytolytic T lymphocytes. *J Immunol* 1988;141:3214–3219.

71. Lutton CW, Gauntt CJ. Coxsackievirus B3 infection alters the plasma membrane of neonatal skin fibroblasts. *J Virol* 1986;60:294–296.

72. Kawai S, Azuma M, Yagita H, et al. Expression of co-stimulatory molecules B7-1, B7-2, and CD40 in the heart of patients with acute myocarditis and dilated cardiomyopathy. *Circulation* 1998;97:637–639.

73. Morad M, Davies NW, Ulrich G, et al. Antibodies against ADP-ATP carrier enhance Ca$^{2+}$ current in isolated cardiac myocytes. *Am J Physiol* 1988;255:H960–H964.

74. Rose ML, Coles MI, Griffin RJ, et al. Expression of class I and class II major histocompatibility antigens in in normal and transplanted human heart. *Transplantation* 1986;41:776–780.

75. Herskowitz A, Ansari AA, Neumann DA, et al. Induction of major histocompatibility complex (MHC) antigens within the myocardium of patients with active myocarditis: a nonhistologic marker of myocarditis. *J Am Coll Cardiol* 1990;15:624–632.

76. Ansari AA, Tadros TS, Knopf WD, et al. Major histocompatibility complex class I and class II expression by myocytes in cardiac biopsies post-transplantation. *Transplantation* 1988;45:972–978.

77. Hammond EH, Menlove RL, Yowell RL, et al. Vascular HLA-DR expression correlates with pathologic changes suggestive of ischemia in idiopathic dilated cardiomyopathy. *Clin Immunol Immunopathol* 1993;68:197–203.

78. Hammond EH, Menlove RL, Anderson JL. Predictive value of immunofluorescence and electron microscopic evaluation of endomyocardial biopsies in the diagnosis and prognosis of myocarditis and idiopathic dilated cardiomyopathy. *Am Heart J* 1987;114:1055–1065.

79. Wang YC, Herskowitz A, Gu LB, et al. Influence of cytokines and immunosuppressive drugs on major histocompatibility complex class I/II expression by human cardiac myocytes in vitro. *Hum Immunol* 1991;31:1–11.

80. Ansari AA, Wang YC, Danner DJ, et al. Abnormal expression of histocompatibility and mitochondrial antigens by cardiac tissue from patients with myocarditis and dilated cardiomyopathy. *Am J Pathol* 1991;139:333–354.

81. Carlquist JF, Menlove Rl, Murray MB, et al. HLA class II (DR and DQ) antigen associations in idiopathic dilated cardiomyopathy. *Circulation* 1991;83:515–522.

82. Marriott SJ, Roeder DJ, Consigli RA. Anti-idiotypic antibodies to a polyomavirus monoclonal antibody recognize cell surface components of mouse kidney cells and prevent polyomavirus infection. *J Virol* 1987;61:2747–2753.

83. Erlanger BF, Cleveland WL, Wasserman NH, et al. Auto-anti-idiotype: a basis for auto-immunity and a strategy for antireceptor antibodies. *Immunol Rev* 1986;94:23–37.

84. Weremeichik H, Moraska A, Herzum M, et al. Naturally occurring anti-idiotypic antibodies: mechanisms of autoimmunity and immunoregulation? *Eur Heart J* 1991;12[Suppl D]:154–157.

85. Paque RE, Miller R. Anti-idiotype pulsed B cells in the induction and expression of autoimmune myocarditis. *Clin Immunol Immunopathol* 1993;68:111–117.

86. Neumann, Lane JR, Allen GS, et al. Viral myocarditis leading to cardiomyopathy: do cytokines contribute to pathogenesis? *Clin Immunol Immunopathol* 1993;68:181–190.

87. Kroemer G, Martinez AC. Cytokines and autoimmune disease. *Clin Immunol Immunopathol* 1991;61:275–295.

88. Entman ML, Youker K, Shappel SB, et al. Neutrophil adherence to isolated adult canine myocytes. *J Clin Invest* 1990;85:1497–1506.

89. Baggiolini M, Walz A, Kunkel SL. Neutrophil activating peptide-1/interleukin 8, a novel cytokine that activates neutrophils. *J Clin Invest* 1989;84:1045–1049.

90. Smith KA. Interleukin-2: inception, impact and implication. *Science* 1988;240:1169–1176.

91. Arai K, Lee F, Miyajima A, et al. Cytokines: coordinators of immune and inflammatory responses. *Annu Rev Biochem* 1990;59:783–836.

92. Postlewaite AE, Kang AH. Induction of fibroblast proliferation by human mononuclear leukocyte derived protein. *Arthritis Rheum* 1983;26:22–27.

93. Barry WH. Mechanisms of immune-mediated myocyte injury. *Circulation* 1994;89:2421–2432.

94. Gulick T, Pieper ST, Murphy MA, et al. Interleukin 1 and tumor necrosis factor inhibit cardiac myocyte beta adrenergic responsiveness. *Proc Natl Acad Sci USA* 1989;86:6753–6757.

95. Balligand JL, Ungureanu D, Kelly RA, et al. Abnormal contractile function due to induction of nitric oxide synthesis in rat cardiac myocytes follows exposure to activated macrophage conditioned medium. *J Clin Invest* 1993;91:2314–2319.

96. Smith TW, Balligand JL, Kaye DM, et al. The role of NO pathway in the control of cardiac function. *J Card Fail* 1996;2:S141–S148.

97. Beck AC, Ward JH, Hammond EH, et al. Cardiomyopathy associated with high-dose interleukin-2 therapy. *West J Med* 1991;155:293–296.

98. Brady AJ, Poole-Wilson PA, Harding SE, et al. Nitric oxide production within cardiac myocytes reduces their contractility in endotoxemia. *Am J Physiol* 1992;263(6 Pt 2):H1963–H1966.

99. Yokoyama T, Vaca L, Rossen RD, et al. Cellular basis for the negative inotropic effects of tumor necrosis factor-alpha in the adult mammalian heart. *J Clin Invest* 1993;92:2303–2312.

100. Bryant D, Becker L, Richardson J, et al. Cardiac failure in transgenic mice with myocardial expression of tumor necrosis factor-alpha. *Circulation* 1998;97:1375–1381.

101. Toyozaki T, Saito T, Takano H, et al. Increased serum levels of circulating intercellular adhesion molecule-1 in patients with myocarditis. *Cardiology* 1996;87:189–193.

102. Matsumori A, Yamada T, Suzuki H, et al. Increased circulating cytokines in patients with myocarditis and cardiomyopathy. *Br Heart J* 1994;72:561–566.

103. Huber SA, Polgar J, Schultheiss P, Schwimmbeck P. Augmentation of pathogenesis of coxsackievirus B3 infections in mice by exogenous administration of interleukin-1 and interleukin-2. *J Virol* 1994;68:195–206.

104. Ishido S, Sakaue M, Asaka K, Maeda S. Detection of transforming growth factor-β1 in Coxsackie B3 virus–induced murine myocarditis. *Acta Histochem Cytochem* 1995;28:137–142.

105. Herskowitz A, Neumann DA, Ansari AA. Concepts of autoimmunity applied to idiopathic dilated cardiomyopathy. *J Am Coll Cardiol* 1993;22:1385–1388.

106. Leslie KO, Schwarz J, Simpson K, et al. Progressive interstitial collagen deposition in coxsackievirus B3 myocarditis. *Am J Pathol* 1990;136:683–693.

107. Matsumori A, Crumpacker CS, Abelmann WH. Prevention of encephalomyocarditis virus myocarditis in mice by inactivated virus vaccine. In: Sekiguchi M, Olsen EGJ, Goodwin JF, eds. *Myocarditis and related disorders.* Tokyo: Springer-Verlag, 1995:228–229.

108. Matsumori A, Wang H, Abelmann WH, Crumpacker CS. Treatment of viral myocarditis with ribavirin in an animal preparation. *Circulation* 1985;71:834–839.

109. Kishimoto C, Crumpacker CS, Abelmann WH. Ribavirin treatment of murine coxsackievirus B3 myocarditis with analyses of lymphocyte subsets. *J Am Coll Cardiol* 1988;12:1334–1341.

110. Matsumori A, Crumpacker CS, Abelmann WH. Prevention of viral myocarditis with recombinant human leukocyte interferon alpha A/D in a murine model. *J Am Coll Cardiol* 1987;9:1320–1325.

111. Kanda T, McManus JEW, Nagai R, et al. Modification of viral myocarditis in mice by interleukin-6. *Circ Res* 1996;78:848–856.

112. Yamamoto N, Shibamori M, Ogura M, et al. Effects of intranasal administration of recombinant murine interferon-gamma on murine acute myocarditis caused by encephalomyocarditis virus. *Circulation* 1998;97:1017–1023.

113. Tomioka N, Kishimoto C, Matsumori A, Kawai C. Effects of prednisolone on acute viral myocarditis in mice. *J Am Coll Cardiol* 1986;7:868–872.

114. Costanzo-Nordin MR, Reap EA, O'Connell JB, et al. A nonsteroid antiinflammatory drug exacerbates Coxsackie B3 murine myocarditis. *J Am Coll Cardiol* 1985;6:1078–1082.

115. Rezkalla S, Khatib G, Khatib R. Coxsackievirus B3 murine myocarditis: Deleterious effects of nonsteroidal anti-inflammatory agents. *J Lab Clin Med* 1986;107:393–395.

116. Kishimoto C, Thorp KA, Abelmann WH. Immunosuppression with high doses of cyclophosphamide reduces the severity of myocarditis but increases the mortality in murine coxsackievirus B3 myocarditis. *Circulation* 1990;82:982–989.

117. O'Connell JB, Reap EA, Robinson JA. The effects of cyclosporine on acute murine Coxsackie B3 myocarditis. *Circulation* 1986;73:353–359.

118. Monrad ES, Matsumori A, Murphy JC, et al. Therapy with cyclosporine in experimental murine myocarditis with encephalomyocarditis virus. *Circulation* 1986;73:1058–1064.
119. Rezkalla S, Kloner RA, Khatib G, Khatib R. Effect of delayed cyclosporine therapy on left ventricular mass and myonecrosis during acute coxsackievirus murine myocarditis. *Am Heart J* 1990;120: 1377–1380.
120. McManus BM, Caruso HR, Stratta RJ, Wilson JE. Impact of FK 506 on myocarditis in the enteroviral murine model. *Transplant Proc* 1991;23:3365–3367.
121. Kanda T, Nagaoka H, Kaneko K, et al. Synergistic effects of tacrolimus and human interferon-α A/D in murine viral myocarditis. *J Pharmacol Exp Ther* 1995;274:487–493.
122. Yamada T, Matsumori A, Sasayama S. Therapeutic effect of anti-tumor necrosis factor-α antibody on the murine model of viral myocarditis induced by encephalomyocarditis virus. *Circulation* 1994;89: 846–851.
123. Matsui S, Matsumori A, Matoba Y, et al. Treatment of virus-induced myocardial injury with a novel immunomodulating agent, vesnarinone. *J Clin Invest* 1994;94:1212–1217.
124. Matsumori A. The use of cytokine inhibitors: a new therapeutic insight into heart failure. *Int J Cardiol* 1997;62[Suppl 1]:S3–S12.
125. Stevens PJ, Ground KE. Occurrence and significance of myocarditis in trauma. *Aerospace Med* 1970;41:776–780.
126. Herskowitz A, Campbell S, Deckers J, et al. Demographic features and prevalence of idiopathic myocarditis in patients undergoing endomyocardial biopsy. *Am J Cardiol* 1993;71:982–986.
127. Dec GW, Waldman H, Southern J, et al. Viral myocarditis mimicking acute myocardial infarction. *J Am Coll Cardiol* 1992;20:85–89.
128. Costanzo-Nordin MR, O'Connell JB, Subramanian R. Myocarditis confirmed by biopsy presenting as acute myocardial infarction. *Br Heart J* 1985;53:25–29.
129. Saffitz JE, Schwartz DJ, Southworth W, et al. Coxsackie viral myocarditis causing transmural right and left ventricular infarction without coronary narrowing. *Am J Cardiol* 1983;52:644–647.
130. Burch GE, Shewey LL. Viral coronary arteritis and myocardial infarction. *Am Heart J* 1976;92:11–14.
131. Ferguson DW, Farwell AP, Bradley WA, Rollings RC. Coronary artery vasospasm complicating acute myocarditis: a rare association. *West J Med* 1988;148:664–669.
132. Onoughi Z, Haba S, Kiyosawa N, et al. Stokes–Adams attacks due to acute nonspecific myocarditis in childhood. *Jpn Heart J* 1980;21: 307–315.
133. Frustaci A, Cameli S, Zeppilli P. Biopsy evidence of atrial myocarditis in an athlete developing transient sinoatrial disease. *Chest* 1995;108: 1460–1462.
134. Talwar KK, Radhakrishnan S, Chopra P. Myocarditis manifesting as persistent atrial standstill. *Int J Cardiol* 1988;20:283–286.
135. Straumanis JP, Wiles HB, Case CL. Resolution of atrial standstill in a child with myocarditis. *Pacing Clin Electrophysiol* 1993;16:2196–2201.
136. Nakazato Y, Nakata Y, Hisaoka T, et al. Clinical and electrophysiological characteristics of atrial standstill. *Pacing Clin Electrophysiol* 1995;18:1244–1254.
137. Liao PK, Seward JB, Hagler DJ, et al. Acute myocarditis associated with transient marked myocardial thickening and complete atrioventricular block. *Clin Cardiol* 1984;7:356–362.
138. Shah SS, Hellenbrand WE, Gallagher PG. Atrial flutter complicating neonatal Coxsackie B2 myocarditis. *Pediatr Cardiol* 1998;19: 185–186.
139. Frustaci A, Chimenti C, Bellocci F, et al. Histological substrate of atrial biopsies in patients with lone atrial fibrillation. *Circulation* 1997;96: 1180–1184.
140. Reitman MJ, Zirin HJ, DeAngelis CJ. Complete heart block in Epstein-Barr myocarditis. *Pediatrics* 1978;62:487–849.
141. Arita M, Ueno Y, Masuyama Y. Complete heart block in mumps myocarditis. *Br Heart J* 1981;46:342–344.
142. Salvi A, Grazia ED, Silvestri F, Camerini F. Acute rickettsial myocarditis and advanced atrioventricular block: diagnosis and treatment aided by endomyocardial biopsy. *Int J Cardiol* 1985;7:405–409.
143. Karjalainen J, Viitasalo M, Kala R, Heikkila J. 24-Hour electrocardiographic recordings in mild acute infectious myocarditis. *Ann Clin Res* 1984;16:34–39.
144. Tai Y-T, Law C-P, Fong P-C, et al. Incessant automatic ventricular tachycardia complicating acute Coxsackie B myocarditis. *Cardiology* 1992;30:339–344.
145. Zeppilli P, Santini C, Cameli S, et al. Brief report: healed myocarditis as a cause of ventricular repolarization abnormalities in athlete's heart. *Int J Sports Med* 1997;18:213–216.
146. Zeppilli P, Santini C, Palmieri V, et al. Role of myocarditis in athletes with minor arrhythmias and/or echocardiographic abnormalities. *Chest* 1994;106:373–380.
147. Maron BJ, Shirani J, Poliac LC, et al. Sudden death in young competitive athletes: clinical, demographic, and pathological profiles. *JAMA* 1996;276:199–204.
148. Phillips M, Robinowitz M, Higgins JR, et al. Sudden cardiac death in Air Force recruits: a 20-year review. *JAMA* 1986;256:2696–2699.
149. Gravanis MB, Sternby NH. Incidence of myocarditis: a 10-year autopsy study from Malmo, Sweden. *Arch Pathol Lab Med* 1991; 115:390–392.
150. Passarino G, Burlo P, Ciccone G, et al. Prevalence of myocarditis at autopsy in Turin, Italy. *Arch Pathol Lab Med* 1997;121:619–622.
151. Burlo P, Comino A, Di Gioia V, et al. [Adult myocarditis in a general hospital: observations on 605 autopsies]. *Pathologica* 1995;87: 646–649.
152. Shatz A, Hiss J, Arensburg B. Myocarditis misdiagnosed as sudden infant death syndrome (SIDS). *Med Sci Law* 1997;37:16–18.
153. Arvan S, Manalo E. Sudden increase in left ventricular mass secondary to acute myocarditis. *Am Heart J* 1988;116:200–202.
154. James KB, Lee K, Thomas JD, et al. Left ventricular diastolic dysfunction in lymphocytic myocarditis as assessed by Doppler echocardiography. *Am J Cardiol* 1994;73:282–285.
155. Kondo M, Takahashi M, Shimono Y, et al. Reversible asymmetric septal hypertrophy in acute myocarditis: serial findings of two-dimensional echocardiogram and thallium-201 scintigram. *Jpn Circ J* 1985; 49:589–593.
156. Lieberman EB, Herskowitz A, Rose NR, Baughman KL. A clinicopathologic description of myocarditis. *Clin Immunol Immunopathol* 1993;68:191–196.
157. Mason JW, O'Connell JB, Herskowitz A, et al. A clinical trial of immunosuppressive therapy for myocarditis. *N Engl J Med* 1995;333: 269–275.
158. Grist NR, Bell EJ. A six year study of Coxsackie B virus infections in heart disease. J Hyg (Lond) 1974;73:165–172.
159. Smith WG. Coxsackie B myopericarditis in adults. *Am Heart J* 1970;80:34–46.
160. Wojnicz, R, Kozielska K, Szczurek J, et al. HLA, ICAM-1 and VCAM-1 molecules in the endomyocardial biopsy specimens of patients with clinically suspected myocarditis. *Eur Heart J* 1997; 18 (abstract suppl):594.
161. Toyozaki T, Hiroe M, Saito T, et al. Levels of soluble Fas in patients with myocarditis, heart failure of unknown origin, and in healthy volunteers. *Am J Cardiol* 1998;81:798–800.
162. Myocarditis Treatment Trial (MTT) Investigators: Incidence and clinical characteristics of myocarditis. *Circulation* 1991;84[Suppl I]: II-2(abst).
163. Lauer B, Niederau C, Kuhl U, et al. Cardiac troponin T in patients with clinically suspected myocarditis. *J Am Coll Cardiol* 1997;30: 1354–1359.
164. Morgera T, DiLenarda A, Dreas L, et al. Electrocardiography of myocarditis revisited: Clinical and prognostic significance of electrocardiographic changes. *Am Heart J* 1992;124:455–467.
165. Take M, Sekiguchi M, Hiroe M, et al. Long-term follow-up of electrocardiographic findings in patients with acute myocarditis proven by endomyocardial biopsy. *Jpn Circ J* 1982;46:1227–1234.
166. Nieminen MS, Heikkla J, Karjalainen J. Echocardiography in acute infectious myocarditis: relation to clinical and echocardiographic findings. *Am J Cardiol* 1984;53:1331–1337.
167. Mendes LA, Picard MH, Dec GW, et al. Discordance of right and left ventricular remodeling in active myocarditis. *J Am Coll Cardiol* 1994;23:365A(abst).
168. James KB, Lee K, Thomas JD, et al. Left ventricular diastolic dysfunction in lymphocytic myocarditis as assessed by doppler echocardiography. *Am J Cardiol* 1994;73:282–285.
169. Kojima J, Miyazaki S, Fujiwara H, et al. Recurrent left ventricular mural thrombi in a patient with acute myocarditis. *Heart Vessels* 1988;4:120–122.
170. Pinamonti B, Alberti E, Cigalotto A, et al. Echocardiographic findings in myocarditis. *Am J Cardiol* 1988;62:285–291.

171. O'Connell JB, Henkin RE, Robinson JA, et al. Gallium-67 imaging in patients with dilated cardiomyopathy and biopsy proven myocarditis. *Circulation* 1984;70:58–62.

172. Yasuda T, Palacios IF, Dec GW, et al. Indium-111 monoclonal antimyosin antibody imaging in the diagnosis of acute myocarditis. *Circulation* 1987;76:306–311.

173. Khaw BA, Narula J. Non-invasive detection of myocyte necrosis in myocarditis and dilated cardiomyopathy with radiolabelled antimyosin. *Eur Heart J* 1995;16[Suppl O]:119–123.

174. Lauer B, Kuhl U, Souvatzoglu M, et al. Correlation of antimyosin-scintigraphy with histological and immunohistological findings in the endomyocardial biopsy in patients with clinically suspected myocarditis. *J Am Coll Cardiol* 1998;31:110A(abst).

175. Friedrich MG, Strohm O, Schulz-Menger J, et al. Contrast media-enhanced magnetic resonance imaging visualizes myocardial changes in the course of viral myocarditis. *Circulation* 1998;97:1802–1809.

176. Mason JW, Billingham ME, Ricci DR. Treatment of acute inflammatory myocarditis assisted by endomyocardial biopsy. *Am J Cardiol* 1980;45:1037–1044.

177. Baandrup U, Olsen EGJ. Critical analysis of endomyocardial biopsies from patients suspected of having cardiomyopathy. I: Morphological and morphometric aspects. *Br Heart J* 1981;45:475–486.

178. Fenoglio JJ, Ursell PC, Kellogg CF, et al. Diagnosis and classification of myocarditis by endomyocardial biopsy. *N Engl J Med* 1983;308: 12–18.

179. Rose AG, Fraser RC, Beck W. Absence of evidence of myocarditis in endomyocardial biopsy specimens from patients with dilated (congestive) cardiomyopathy. *S Afr Med J* 1984;66:871–874.

180. Daly K, Richardson PJ, Olsen EGJ, et al. Acute myocarditis. Role of histological and virological examination in the diagnosis and assessment of immunosuppressive treatment. *Br Heart J* 1984;51:30–35.

181. Parrillo JE, Aretz HT, Palacios I, et al. The results of transvenous endomyocardial biopsy can frequently be used to diagnose myocardial diseases in patients with idiopathic heart failure. *Circulation* 1984; 69:93–101.

182. Regitz V, Olsen EGJ, Rudolph W. Histologisch nachweisbare Myokarditis bei Patienten mit eingeschrankter linksventrikularer Funktion. *Herz* 1985;10:27–35.

183. Cassling RS, Linder J, Sears TD, et al. Quantitative evaluation of inflammation in biopsy specimens from idiopathically failing or irritable hearts: experience in 80 pediatric and adult patients. *Am Heart J* 1985;110:713–720.

184. Salvi A, Silvestri F, Gori D, et al. Endomyocardial biopsy: initial experience in 156 patients. *G Ital Cardiol* 1985;15:251–259.

185. Dec GW, Palacios IF, Fallon JT, et al. Active myocarditis in the spectrum of acute dilated cardiomyopathies: clinical features, histologic correlates, and clinical outcomes. *N Engl J Med* 1985;312:885–890.

186. Mortensen SA, Baandrup U, Buck J, et al. Immunosuppressive therapy of biopsy proven myocarditis: experiences with corticosteroids and cyclosporin. *Int J Immunother* 1985;1:35–45.

187. Hammond EH, Menlove RL, Anderson JL. Predictive value of immunofluorescence and electron microscopic evaluation of endomyocardial biopsies in the diagnosis and prognosis of myocarditis and idiopathic dilated cardiomyopathy. *Am Heart J* 1987;114:1055–1065.

188. Meany BT, Quigley PJ, Olsen EGJ, et al. Recent experience of endomyocardial biopsy in the diagnosis of myocarditis. *Eur Heart J* 1987;8:17–18.

189. Chow LC, Dittrich HC, Shabetai R. Endomyocardial biopsy in patients with unexplained congestive heart failure. *Ann Intern Med* 1988;109: 535–539.

190. Hobbs RE, Pelegrin D, Ratliff NB, et al. Lymphocytic myocarditis and dilated cardiomyopathy: treatment with immunosuppressive agents. *Cleve Clin J Med* 1989;56:628–635.

191. Popma JJ, Cigarroa RG, Buja LM, Hillis LD. Diagnostic and prognostic utility of right-sided catheterization and endomyocardial biopsy in idiopathic dilated cardiomyopathy. *Am J Cardiol* 1989;63:955–958.

192. Maisch B, Bauer E, Hufnagel G, et al. The use of endomyocardial biopsy in heart failure. *Eur Heart J* 1988;9:59–71.

193. Vasiljevic JD, Kanjuh V, Seferovic P, et al. The incidence of myocarditis in endomyocardial biopsy samples from patients with congestive heart failure. *Am Heart J* 1990;120:1370–1377.

194. Lieberman EB, Hutchins GM, Herskowitz A, et al. Clinicopathologic description of myocarditis. *J Am Coll Cardiol* 1991;18:1617–1626.

195. Herskowitz A, Campbell S, Deckers J, et al. Demographic features and prevalence of idiopathic myocarditis in patients undergoing endomyocardial biopsy. *Am J Cardiol* 1993;71:982–986.

196. Kuhl U, Noutsias M, Seeberg B, Schultheiss H-P. Immunohistological evidence for a chronic intramyocardial inflammatory process in dilated cardiomyopathy. *Heart* 1996;75:295–300.

197. Arbustini E, Gavazzi A, Dal Bello B, et al. Ten-year experience with endomyocardial biopsy in myocarditis presenting with congestive heart failure: frequency, pathologic characteristics, treatment and follow-up. *G Ital Cardiol* 1997;27:209–223.

198. Strain JE, Grose RM, Factor SM, et al. Results of endomyocardial biopsy in patients with spontaneous ventricular tachycardia but without apparent structural heart disease. *Circulation* 1983;68:1171–1181.

199. Sugrue DD, Holmes DR Jr, Gersh BJ, et al. Cardiac histologic findings in patients with life-threatening ventricular arrhythmias of unknown origin. *J Am Coll Cardiol* 1984;4:952–957.

200. Take M, Sekiguchi M, Hiroe M, et al. A clinicopathologic study on a cause of idiopathic cardiomyopathy and arrhythmia and conduction disturbance employing endomyocardial biopsy. *Heart Vessels Suppl* 1985;1:159–164.

201. Hosenpud JD, McAnulty JH, Niles NR. Unexpected myocardial disease in patients with life threatening arrhythmias. *Br Heart J* 1986;56: 55–61.

202. Yoshizato T, Edwards WD, Alboliras ET, et al. Safety and utility of endomyocardial biopsy in infants, children and adolescents: a review of 66 procedures in 53 patients. *J Am Coll Cardiol* 1990;15:436–442.

203. Sekiguchi M, Nishizawa M, Nunoda S, et al. Endomyocardial biopsy approach in cases with ventricular arrhythmias. *Postgrad Med J* 1992;68[Suppl 1]:S40–S43.

204. Wiles HB, Gillette PC, Harley RA, et al. Cardiomyopathy and myocarditis in children with ventricular ectopic rhythm. *J Am Coll Cardiol* 1992;20:359–362.

205. Thongtang V, Chiathiraphan S, Ratanarapee S, et al. Prevalence of myocarditis in idiopathic dysrhythmias: role of endomyocardial biopsy and efficacy of steroid therapy. *J Med Assoc Thai* 1993;76:368–373.

206. Aretz HT, Billingham ME, Edwards WD, et al. The utility of the Dallas Criteria for the histopathological diagnosis of myocarditis in endomyocardial biopsy specimens. *Circulation* 1993;88[Suppl I]: I-552(abst).

207. Dec GW, Fallon JT, Southern JF, Palacios I. "Borderline" myocarditis: an indication for repeat endomyocardial biopsy. *J Am Coll Cardiol* 1990;15:283–289.

208. Hauck AJ, Kearney DL, Edwards WD. Evaluation of postmortem endomyocardial biopsy specimens from 38 patients with lymphocytic myocarditis: implications for role of sampling error. *Mayo Clin Proc* 1989;64:1235–1245.

209. Chow LH, Radio SJ, Sears TE, et al. Insensitivity of right ventricular endomyocardial biopsy in the diagnosis of myocarditis. *J Am Coll Cardiol* 1989;14:915–920.

210. Hufnagel G, Maisch B. The European Study of Epidemiology and Treatment of Cardiac Inflammatory Disease (ESETCID)—first epidemiological results. *Eur Heart J* 1997;18(abstract suppl):594.

211. Kato H, Ichinose E, Kawasaki T. Myocardial infarction in Kawasaki disease: clinical analysis in 195 cases. *J Pediatr* 1986;108:923–927.

212. Hasumi M, Sekiguchi M, Morimoto S, et al. Ventriculographic findings in the convalescent stage in eleven cases with acute myocarditis. *Jpn Circ J* 1983;47:1310–1316.

213. Frustaci A, Maseri A. Localized left ventricular aneurysms with normal global function caused by myocarditis. *Am J Cardiol* 1992;70: 1221–1224.

214. O'Connell JB, Mason JW. Diagnosing and treating active myocarditis. *West J Med* 1989;150:431–435.

215. Woodruff JF. Viral myocarditis: a review. *Am J Pathol* 1980;101: 427–479.

216. Martin AB, Webber S, Fricker J, et al. Acute myocarditis. Rapid diagnosis by PCR in children. *Circulation* 1994;90:330–339.

217. Keeling PJ, Lukaszyk A, Poloniecki J, et al. A prospective case control study of antibodies to coxsackie B virus in idiopathic dilated cardiomyopathy. *J Am Coll Cardiol* 1994;23:593–598.

218. Martino TA, Liu P, Sole MJ. Enterovirus myocarditis and dilated cardiomyopathy: a review of clinical and experimental studies. In: Rotbart HA, ed. *Human enterovirus infections*. Washington, DC: American Society of Microbiology, 1995:291–350.

219. Baboonian C, Treasure T. Meta-analysis of the association of enteroviruses with human heart disease. *Heart* 1997;78:539–543.
220. Mendes LA, Dec GW, Picard MH, Palacios IF, Newell J, Davidoff R. Right ventricular dysfunction: an independent predictor of adverse outcome in patients with myocarditis. *Am Heart J* 1994;128:301–307.
221. Ilbäck N-G, Fohlman J, Friman G. Exercise in coxsackie B3 myocarditis: effects on heart lymphocyte subpopulations and the inflammatory reaction. *Am Heart J* 1989;117:1298–1302.
222. Maron BJ, Isner JM, McKenna WJ. Task Force 3: hypertrophic cardiomyopathy, myocarditis and other myopericardial diseases and mitral valve prolapse. *J Am Coll Cardiol* 1994;24:845–899.
223. Cohn JN. ACE inhibitors in non-ischemic heart failure: results from the MEGA trials. *Eur Heart J* 1995;16[Suppl O]:133–136.
224. Rezkalla S, Kloner RA, Khatib G, Khatib R. Beneficial effects of captopril in acute coxsackie virus B3 murine myocarditis. *Circulation* 1990;81:1039–1046.
225. Waagstein F. Adrenergic beta-blocking agents in congestive heart failure due to idiopathic dilated cardiomyopathy. *Eur Heart J* 1995;16[Suppl O]:128–132.
226. Rezkalla S, Kloner RA, Khatib G, Smith FE, Khatib R. Effect of metoprolol in coxsackie virus B3 murine myocarditis. *J Am Coll Cardiol* 1988;12:412–414.
227. Tominaga M, Matsumori A, Okada I, Yamada T, Kawai C. β-Blocker treatment of dilated cardiomyopathy: beneficial effects of carvedilol in mice. *Circulation* 1991;83:2021–2028.
228. Gagliardi MG, Bevilacqua M, Squitieri C, et al. Dilated Cardiomyopathy caused by acute myocarditis in pediatric patients: evolution of myocardial damage in a group of potential heart transplant candidates. *J Heart Lung Transplant* 1993;12:S224–S229.
229. Cooper LT, Berry GJ, Shabetai R for the Multicenter Giant Cell Myocarditis Study Group Investigators. Idiopathic giant-cell myocarditis—natural history and treatment. *N Engl J Med* 1997;336:1860–1866.
230. Kühl U, Schultheiss H-P. Treatment of chronic myocarditis with corticosteroids. *Eur Heart J* 1995;16:168–172.
231. Drucker NA, Colan SD, Lewis AB, et al. γ-Globulin treatment of acute myocarditis in the pediatric population. *Circulation* 1994;89:252–257.
232. Miric\fx M, Vasiljevic\fx J, Bojic\fx M, et al. Long-term follow up of patients with dilated heart muscle disease treated with human leucocytic interferon alpha or thymic hormones. *Heart* 1996;75:596–601.
233. Mc Namara DM, Rosenblum WD, Janosko KM, et al. Intravenous immune globulin in the therapy of myocarditis and acute cardiomyopathy. *Circulation* 1997;95:2476–2478.
234. O'Connell JB, Dec WG, Goldenberg IF, et al. Results of heart transplantation for active lymphocytic myocarditis. *J Heart Lung Transplant* 1990;9:351–356.
235. O'Connell JB, Breen TJ, Hosenpud JD. Heart transplantation in dilated heart muscle disease and myocarditis. *Eur Heart J* 1995;16[Suppl O]:137–139.
236. Davies MJ, Pomerance A, Teare RD. Idiopathic giant cell myocarditis—a distinctive clinicopathological entity. *Br Heart J* 1975;37:192–195.
237. Theaker JM, Gatter KC, Heryet A, et al. Giant cell myocarditis: evidence for the macrophage origin of the giant cells. *J Clin Pathol* 1985;38:160–164.
238. Fukuhara T, Morino M, Sakoda S, et al. Myocarditis with multinucleated giant cells detected in biopsy specimens. *Clin Cardiol* 1988;11:341–344.
239. Humbert P, Faivre R, Fellman D, et al. Giant cell myocarditis: an autoimmune disease? *Am Heart J* 1988;115:485–487.
240. Roberts WC, McAllister HA Jr, Ferrans VJ. Sarcoidosis of the heart. A clinicopathologic study of 35 necropsy patients (group 1) and review of 78 previously described necropsy patients (group 11). *Am J Med* 1977;63:86–108.
241. Johansen A. Isolated myocarditis versus myocardial sarcoidosis. *Acta Pathol Microbiol Scand* 1966;67:15–26.
242. Litovsky SH, Burke AP, Virmani R. Giant cell myocarditis: an entity distinct from sarcoidosis characterized by multiphasic myocyte destruction by cytotoxic T cells and histiocytic giant cells. *Mod Pathol* 1996;9:1126–1134.
243. de Jongste MJ, Oosterhuis HJ, Lie KI. Intractable ventricular tachycardia in a patient with giant cell myocarditis, thymoma and myasthenia gravis. *Int J Cardiol* 1986;13:374–378.
244. Kilgallen CM, Jackson E, Bankoff M, et al. A case of giant cell myocarditis and malignant thymoma: a postmortem diagnosis by needle biopsy. *Clin Cardiol* 1998;21:48–51.
245. Leib ML, Odel JG, Cooney MJ. Orbital polymyositis and giant cell myocarditis. *Ophthalmology* 1994;101:950–954.
246. Stevens AW, Grossman ME, Barr ML, et al. Orbital myositis, vitiligo, and giant cell myocarditis. *J Am Acad Dermatol* 1996;35(2 Pt 2):310–312.
247. Weidhase A, Grone HJ, Unterberg C, et al. Severe granulomatous giant cell myocarditis in Wegener's granulomatosis. *Klin Wochenschr* 1990;68:880–885.
248. McKeon J, Haagsma B, Bett JH, et al. Fatal giant cell myocarditis after colectomy for ulcerative colitis. *Am Heart J* 1986;111:1208–1209.
249. Ariza A, Lopez MD, Mate JL, et al. Giant cell myocarditis: monocytic immunophenotype of giant cells in a case associated with ulcerative colitis. *Hum Pathol* 1995;26:121–123.
250. Kloin JE. Pernicious anemia and giant cell myocarditis: new association. *Am J Med* 1985;78:355–360.
251. Hales SA, Theaker JM, Gatter KC. Giant cell myocarditis associated with lymphoma: an immunocytochemical study. *J Clin Pathol* 1987;40:1310–1313.
252. Singham KT, Azizah NW, Goh TH. Complete atrioventricular block due to giant cell myocarditis. *Postgrad Med J* 1980;56:194–196.
253. Lindvall K, Edhag O, Erhardt LR, et al. Complete heart block due to granulomatous giant cell myocarditis: report of 3 cases. *Eur J Cardiol* 1978;8:349–358.
254. Piette M, Timperman J. Sudden death in idiopathic giant cell myocarditis. *Med Sci Law* 1990;30:280–284.
255. Desjardins V, Pelletier G, Leung TK, et al. Successful treatment of severe heart failure caused by idiopathic giant cell myocarditis. *Can J Cardiol* 1992;8:788–792.
256. Nieminen MS, Salminen US, Taskinen E, et al. Treatment of serious heart failure by transplantation in giant cell myocarditis diagnosed by endomyocardial biopsy. *J Heart Lung Transplant* 1994;13:543–545.
257. Hori T, Fujiwara H, Tanaka M, et al. Idiopathic giant cell myocarditis accompanied by asymmetric septal hypertrophy. *Jpn Circ J* 1987;51:153–156.
258. Davidoff R, Palacios I, Southern J, et al. Giant cell versus lymphocytic myocarditis: a comparison of their clinical features and long-term outcomes. *Circulation* 1991;83:953–961.
259. Cooper LT Jr, Berry GJ, Shabetai R for the Multicenter Giant Cell Myocarditis Study Group Investigators. Idiopathic giant-cell myocarditis—natural history and treatment. *N Engl J Med* 1997;336:1860–1866.
260. Grant SC. Giant cell myocarditis in a transplanted heart. *Eur Heart J* 1993;14:1437.
261. Kong G, Madden B, Spyrou N, et al. Response of recurrent giant cell myocarditis in a transplanted heart to intensive immunosuppression. *Eur Heart J* 1991;12:554–557.
262. Gries W, Farkas D, Winters GL, et al. Giant cell myocarditis: first report of disease recurrence in the transplanted heart. *J Heart Lung Transplant* 1992;11(2 Pt 1):370–374.
263. Wolfsohn AL, Davies RA, Smith CO, et al. Giant cell myocarditis-like appearance after transplantation: an atypical manifestation of rejection? *J Heart Lung Transplant* 1994;13:731–733.
264. Loffler W. Endocarditis parietalis fibroplastica mit Bluteosinophilie, ein eigenartiges Krankheitsbild. *Schweiz Med Wochenschr* 1936;66:817–820.
265. Spry CJ, Take M, Tai PC. Eosinophilic disorders affecting the myocardium and endocardium: a review. *Heart Vessels Suppl* 1985;1:240–242.
266. Oakley CM, Olsen EGJ. Eosinophilia and heart disease (editorial). *Br Heart J* 1977;39:233–237.
267. Herzog CA, Snover DC, Staley NA. Acute necrotizing eosinophilic myocarditis. *Br Heart J* 1984;52:343–348.
268. Olsen EG, Spry CJ. Relation between eosinophilia and endomyocardial disease. *Prog Cardiovasc Dis* 1985;27:241–254.
269. Nakayama Y, Kohriyama T, Yamamoto S, et al. Electron-microscopic and immunohistochemical studies on endomyocardial biopsies from a patient with eosinophilic endomyocardial disease. *Heart Vessels Suppl* 1985;1:250–255.
270. Tai PC, Hayes DJ, Clark JB, et al. Toxic effects of human eosinophil products on isolated rat heart cells in vitro. *Biochem J* 1982;204:75–80.
271. Terasaki F, Hayashi T, Hirota Y, et al. Evolution to dilated cardiomyopathy from acute eosinophilic pancarditis in Churg–Strauss syndrome. *Heart Vessels* 1997;12:43–48.
272. Getz MA, Subramanian R, Logemann T, et al. Acute necrotizing eosinophilic myocarditis as a manifestation of severe hypersensitivity myocarditis: antemortem diagnosis and successful treatment. *Ann Intern Med* 1991;115:201–202.

273. Schuchter LM, Hendricks CB, Holland KH, et al. Eosinophilic myocarditis associated with high-dose interleukin-2 therapy. *Am J Med* 1990;88:439–440.

274. Galiuto L, Enriquez-Sarano M, Reeder GS, et al. Eosinophilic myocarditis manifesting as myocardial infarction: early diagnosis and successful treatment. *Mayo Clin Proc* 1997;72:603–610.

275. Newman LS, Rose CS, Maier LA. Sarcoidosis. *N Engl J Med* 1997;336:1224–1234.

276. Rizzato G, Pezzano A, Sala G, et al. Right heart impairment in sarcoidosis: hemodynamic and echocardiographic study. *Eur J Respir Dis* 1983;64:121–128.

277. Silverman KJ, Hutchins GM, Bulkley BH. Cardiac sarcoid: a clinicopathologic study of 84 unselected patients with systemic sarcoidosis. *Circulation* 1978;58:1204–1211.

278. Jain A, Starek PJ, Delany DL. Ventricular tachycardia and ventricular aneurysm due to unrecognized sarcoidosis. *Clin Cardiol* 1990;13:738–740.

279. Roberts WC, McAllister HA Jr, Ferrans VJ. Sarcoidosis of the heart: a clinicopathologic study of 35 necropsy patients (group I) and review of 78 previously described necropsy patients (group II). *Am J Med* 1977;63:86–108.

280. Sharma OP, Maheshwari A, Thaker K. Myocardial sarcoidosis. *Chest* 1993;103:253–258.

281. Hirose Y, Ishida Y, Hayashida K, et al. Myocardial involvement in patients with sarcoidosis: an analysis of 75 patients. *Clin Nucl Med* 1994;19:522–526.

282. Chandra M, Silverman ME, Oshinski J, et al. Diagnosis of cardiac sarcoidosis aided by MRI. *Chest* 1996;110:562–565.

283. Eliasch H, Juhlin-Dannfelt A, Sjogren I, et al. Magnetic resonance imaging as an aid to the diagnosis and treatment evaluation of suspected myocardial sarcoidosis in a fighter pilot. *Aviat Space Environ Med* 1995;66:1010–1013.

284. Shammas Rl, Movahed A. Sarcoidosis of the heart. *Clin Cardiol* 1993;16:462–472.

285. Okayama K, Kurata C, Tawarahara K, et al. Diagnostic and prognostic value of myocardial scintigraphy with thallium-201 and gallium-67 in cardiac sarcoidosis. *Chest* 1995;107:330–334.

286. Bajaj AK, Kopelman HA, Echt DS. Cardiac sarcoidosis with sudden death: treatment with the automatic implantable cardioverter defibrillator. *Am Heart J* 1988;116:557–560.

287. Padilla ML, Schilero GJ, Teirstein AS. Sarcoidosis and transplantation. *Sarcoidosis Vasc Diffuse Lung Dis* 1997;14:16–22.

288. Brown CS, Bertolet BD. Peripartum cardiomyopathy: a comprehensive review. *Am J Obstet Gynecol* 1998;178:409–414.

289. Farber PA, Glasgow LA. Factors modulating host resistance to virus infection. II: Enhanced susceptibility of mice to encephalomyocarditis virus infection during pregnancy. *Am J Pathol* 1968;53:463–478.

290. Takatsu T, Kitamura Y, Morita H, et al. Viral myocarditis and cardiomyopathy. In: Sekigushi M, Olsen EGJ, eds. *Cardiomyopathy.* Tokyo: University of Tokyo Press, 1978:34–35.

291. Lampert MB, Hibbard J, Weinest L, et al. Peripartum heart failure associated with prolonged tocolytic therapy. *Am J Obstet Gynecol* 1993;168:493–495.

292. Midei MG, Richardson PJ, Olsen EGJ, et al. Peripartum myocarditis and cardiomyopathy. *Circulation* 1990;81:922–928.

293. O'Connell JB, Costanzo-Nordin MR, Subramanian R, et al. Peripartum cardiomyopathy: clinical, hemodynamic, histologic and prognostic characteristics. *J Am Coll Cardiol* 1986;8:52–56.

294. Dale JB, Beachey EH. Sequence of myosin cross-reacting epitopes of streptococcal M protein. *J Exp Med* 1986;164:1785–1790.

295. Haffejee I. Rheumatic fever and rheumatic heart disease : the current state of its immunology, diagnostic criteria and prophylaxis. *Q J Med* 1992;84:641–658.

296. Carlquist JF, Ward RH, Meyer KJ, et al. Immune response factors in rheumatic heart disease: meta-analysis of HLA-DR associations and evaluation of additional class II alleles. *J Am Coll Cardiol* 1995;26:452–457.

297. Jones TD. Diagnosis of rheumatic fever. *JAMA* 1944;126:481–484.

298. da Silva NA, Pereira BA. Acute rheumatic fever: still a challenge. *Rheum Dis Clin North Am* 1997;23:545–568.

299. Rheumatic Fever Working Party (RFWP) of the MRC, Great Britain, and the Subcommittee of Principal Investigators of the American Council on Rheumatic Fever and Congenital Heart Disease, American Heart Association. The treatment of acute rheumatic fever in children: a cooperative clinical trial of ACTH, cortisone and aspirin. *Circulation* 1955;11:343–371.

300. Berrios X, del Campo E, Guzman B, et al. Discontinuing rheumatic fever prophylaxis in selected adolescents and young adults. A prospective study. *Ann Intern Med* 1993;118:401–406.

301. Dale JB, Chiang EY, Lederer JW. Recombinant tetravalent group A streptococcal M protein vaccine. *Immunology* 1993;151:2188–2194.

302. Dale JB, Simmons M, Chiang EC, et al. Recombinant, octavalent group A streptococcal M protein vaccine. *Vaccine* 1996;14:944–948.

303. Mandell BF. Cardiovascular involvement in systemic lupus erythematosus. *Semin Arthritis Rheum* 1987;17:126–141.

304. Ginzler EM. Clinical features and complications of systemic lupus erythematosus, and assessment of disease activity. *Curr Opin Rheumatol* 1990;2:703–707.

305. Jessar RA, Lamont-Havers W, Ragan C. Natural history of lupus erythematosus disseminatus. *Ann Intern Med* 1953;38:717–721.

306. Sturfelt G, Eskilsson J, Nived O, et al. Cardiovascular disease in systemic lupus erythematosus: a study of patients from a defined population. *Medicine (Baltimore)* 1992;71:216–223.

307. Badui E, Garcia-Rubi D, Robles E, et al. Cardiovascular manifestations in systemic lupus erythematosus: prospective study of 100 patients. *Angiology* 1985;36:431–441.

308. Cervera R, Font J, Paré C, et al. Cardiac disease in systemic lupus erythematosus: prospective study of 70 patients. *Ann Rheum Dis* 1992;51:156–159.

309. Michet CJ, Hunder GG. Pericarditis in systemic lupus erythematosus. In: Ansell BM, Simkin PA, eds. *The heart and rheumatic disease.* London: Butterworths, 1984:11–13.

310. Hunder GG, Mullen BJ, McDuffie FC, Complement in pericardial fluid of lupus erythematosus. *Ann Intern Med* 1974;80:453–458.

311. Lerer RJ. Cardiac tamponade as an initial finding in systemic lupus erythematosus. *Am J Dis Child* 1972;124:436–437.

312. Starkey RH, Hahn BH. Rapid development of constrictive pericarditis in a patient with systemic lupus erythematosus. *Chest* 1973;63:448–450.

313. Dorlon RE, Smith JM, Cook EH, et al. Staphylococcal pericardial effusion with tamponade in a patient with systemic lupus erythematosus. *J Rheumatol* 1982;9:813–814.

314. Libman E, Sacks B. A hitherto undescribed form of valvular and mural endocarditis. *Arch Intern Med* 1924;33:701–715.

315. Roldan CA, Shively BK, Crawford MH. An echocardiographic study of valvular heart disease associated with systemic lupus erythematosus. *N Engl J Med* 1997;335:1424.

316. Shapiro RF, Gamble CN, Wiesner KB, et al. Immunopathogenesis of Libman–Sacks endocarditis: assessment by light and immunofluorescent microscopy in two patients. *Ann Rheum Dis* 1977;36:508.

317. Doherty NE, Siegel RJ. Cardiovascular manifestations of systemic lupus erythematosus. *Am Heart J* 1985;110:1257–1265.

318. Haider YS, Roberts WC. Coronary arterial disease in systemic lupus erythematosus: quantification of degrees of narrowing in 22 necropsy patients (21 women) aged 16 to 37 years. *JAMA* 1980;70:775–781.

319. Singson BH, Akhter JE, Weinstein MM, et al. Congenital complete heart block and SSA antibodies: obstetrical implications. *Am J Obstet Gynecol* 1985;152:655–658.

320. Bacon PA, Gibson DG. Cardiac involvement in rheumatoid arthritis: an echocardiographic study. *Ann Rheum Dis* 1974;33:20–24.

321. Maione S, Valentini G, Giunta A, et al. Cardiac involvement in rheumatoid arthritis: an echocardiographic study. *Cardiology* 1993;83:234–239.

322. Franco AE and Levine HD. Rheumatoid pericarditis: report of 17 cases diagnosed clinically. *Ann Intern Med* 1972;77:837–844.

323. Reilly PA, Cosh JA, Maddison PJ, et al. Mortality and survival in rheumatoid arthritis: a 25-year prospective study of 100 patients. *Ann Rheum Dis* 1990;49:363–369.

324. Iveson JMI, Thadani U, Ionescu M, Wright V. Aortic valve incompetence and replacement in rheumatoid arthritis. *Ann Rheum Dis* 1975;34:312–320.

325. Swezey RL. Myocardial infarction due to rheumatoid arthritis. An antemortem diagnosis. *JAMA* 1967;199:855–857.

326. Voyles WF, Searles RP, Bankhurst AD. Myocardial infarction caused by rheumatoid vasculitis. *Arthritis Rheum* 1980;23:860–863.

327. Gravallese EM, Corson JM, Coblyn JS, et al. Rheumatoid aortitis: A rarely recognized but clinically significant entity. *Medicine (Baltimore)* 1989;68:95–106.

328. Masi AT, Rodnan GP, Medsger TA Jr, et al. Preliminary criteria for the classification of systemic sclerosis (scleroderma). *Arthritis Rheum* 1980;23:581–590.

329. D'Angelo WA, Fries JF, Masi AT, Shulman LE. Pathologic observations in systemic sclerosis (scleroderma): a study of fifty-eight autopsy cases and fifty-eight matched controls. *Am J Med* 1969;46:428–440.

330. McWhorter JE, LeRoy EC. Pericardial disease in scleroderma (systemic sclerosis). *Am J Med* 1974;57:566–575.

331. Botstein GR, LeRoy EC. Primary heart disease in systemic sclerosis (scleroderma): advances in clinical and pathologic features, pathogenesis, and new therapeutic approaches. *Am Heart J* 1981;102:913–919.

332. Bennett R, Bluestone R, Holt PJL, Bywaters EGL. Survival in scleroderma. *Ann Rheum Dis* 1971;30:581–588.

333. James TN. De subitaneis mortibus. VIII. Coronary arteries and conduction system in scleroderma heart disease. *Circulation* 1974;50: 844–856.

334. Bulkley BH, Ridolfi RL, Salyer WR. Myocardial lesions of progressive systemic sclerosis: a cause of cardiac dysfunction. *Circulation* 1976;53:483–490.

335. Kerr LD, Spiera H. Myocarditis as a complication in scleroderma patients with myositis. *Clin Cardiol* 1993;16:895–899.

336. Ueda N, Mimura K, Maeda H, et al. Mixed connective tissue disease with fatal pulmonary hypertension and a review of the literature. *Virchows Arch A* 1984;404:335–340.

337. Kahan A, Devaux JY, Amor B, et al. The effect of captopril on thallium 201 myocardial perfusion in systemic sclerosis. *Clin Pharmacol Ther* 1990;47:483–489.

338. Dalakas MC. Polymyositis, dermatomyositis, and inclusion-body myositis. *N Engl J Med* 1991;325:1487–1498.

339. Denbow CE, Lie JT, Tancredi RG, Bunch TW. Cardiac involvement in polymyositis: a clinicopathologic study of 20 autopsied patients. *Arthritis Rheum* 1979;22:1088–1092.

340. Oka M, Raasakka T. Cardiac involvement in polymyositis. *Scand J Rheum* 1978;7:203–208.

341. Haupt HM, Hutchins GM. The heart and cardiac conduction system in polymyositis-dematomyositis: a clinicopathologic study of 16 autopsied patients. *Am J Cardiol* 1982;50:998–1006.

342. Strongwater SL, Annesley T, Schnitzer TJ. Myocardial involvement in polymyositis. *J Rheumatol* 1983;10:459–463.

343. Askari AD. Cardiac abnormalities. *Clin Rheum Dis* 1984;10:131–149.

344. Gottdiener JS, Sherber HS, Hawley RJ, Engel WK. Cardiac manifestations in polymyositis. *Am J Card* 1978;41:1141–1149.

345. Mallory TB. Case records of the Massachusetts General Hospital. *N Engl J Med* 1936;214:690–698.

346. Bergfeldt L, Edhag O, Rajs J. HLA-B27–associated heart disease: clinicopathologic study of three cases. *Am J Med* 1984;77:961–967.

347. Graham DC, Smythe HA. The carditis and aortitis of ankylosing spondylitis. *Bull Rheum Dis* 1958;9:171–175.

348. Roberts WC, Hollingsworth JF, Bulkley BH, et al. Combined mitral and aortic regurgitation in ankylosing spondylitis: angiographic and anatomic features. *Am J Med* 1974;56:237–243.

349. Weed CL, Kulander BG, Mazzarella JA, Decker JL. Heart block in ankylosing spondylitis. *Arch Intern Med* 1966;117:800–817.

350. Bergfeldt L, Moller E. Complete heart block—another HLA-B27 associated disease manifestation. *Tissue Antigens* 1983;21:385–390.

351. Bergfeldt L, Vallin H, Edhag O. Complete heart block in HLA B27 associated disease: electrophysiological and clinical characteristics. *Br Heart J* 1984;51:184–188.

352. Nitter-Hauge S, Otterstad JE. Characteristics of atrioventricular conduction disturbances in ankylosing spondylitis (Mb. Bechterew). *Acta Med Scand* 1981;210:197–200.

353. Bergfeldt L. HLA B27 associated cardiac disease. *Ann Intern Med* 1997;127:621–629.

354. Hall BM. Transplantation overview: cells mediating allograft rejection. *Transplantation* 1991;51:1141–1151.

355. Parnes JR. Molecular biology and function of CD-4 and CD-8. *Adv Immunol* 1989;44:265–311.

356. Rose ML, Yacoub M. *Immunology of heart and lung transplantation.* Kent: Edward Arnold Publications, 1993:3–21.

357. Gracie JA, Sarawar SR, Bolton EM, et al. Renal allograft rejection in CD4⁺ T cell reconstituted athymic nude rats: the origin of CD4⁺ and CD8⁺ graft infiltrating cells. *Transplantation* 1990;50:996.

358. Moller E. Cell interactions and cytokines in transplantation immunity. *Transplant Proc* 1995;27:24–27.

359. Guttman RD, Lindquist RR, Ockner SA. Renal transplantation in the inbred rat. *Transplantation* 1969;8:472–484.

360. Austyn JM, Steinman RM. The passenger leukocyte—a fresh look. *Transplant Rev* 1988;2:139–176.

361. Sherman LA, Chattopadhyay S. The molecular basis of allorecognition. *Annu Rev Immunol* 1993;11:385–402.

362. Clark EA, Ledbetter JA. How B and T cells talk to each other. *Nature* 1994;367:425–428.

363. Krensky AM, Weiss A, Crabtree G, et al. T lymphocyte antigen interactions in transplant rejection. *N Engl J Med* 1990;322:510–517.

364. Ohashi PS, Oehen S, Burki K, et al. Ablation of tolerance and induction of diabetes by virus infection in viral antigen transgenic mice. *Cell* 1991;65:305–312.

365. Superdock KR, Helderman JH. Immunosuppressive drugs and their effects. *Semin Respir Infect* 1993;8:152–159.

366. Chan AC, Iwashima M, Turck CW, et al. ZAP-70: a 70 kd protein tyrosine kinase that associates with the TcR ζ chain. *Cell* 1992;71:649–662.

367. Schwartz RH. Costimulation of T lymphocytes: the role of CD28, CTLA-4, and B7/BB1 in interleukin 2 production and immunotherapy. *Cell* 1992;71:1065–1068.

368. Linsley PS, Brady W, Urnes M, et al: CTLA-4 is a second receptor for the B cell activation antigen B7. *J Exp Med* 1991;174:561–569.

369. Thompson CB, Lindsten T, Ledbetter JA, et al. CD28 activation pathway regulates the production of multiple T-cell derived lymphokines/cytokines. *Proc Natl Acad Sci USA* 1989;86:1333–1337.

370. Pober JS, Cotran RS. The role of endothelial cells in inflammation. *Transplantation* 1990;48:537–544.

371. Suthanthiran M, Strom TB. Renal transplantation. *N Engl J Med* 1994; 331:365–376.

372. Springer TA. Adhesion receptors of the immune system. *Nature* 1990;346:425–434.

373. May MJ, Ager A. ICAM-1 independent lymphocyte transmigration across high endothelium: differential upregulation by interferon γ, tumor necrosis factor α, and interleukin 1β. *Eur J Immunol* 1992;22: 219–226.

374. Lemstrom K, Koskinen P, Hayry P. Induction of adhesion molecules on the endothelia of rejecting cardiac allografts. *J Heart Lung Transplant* 1995;14:205–213.

375. Tilney NL, Paul LC. Antigen independent events leading to chronic graft dysfunction. In: Tilney NL, Strom TB, Paul LC, eds. *Transplantation biology: cellular and molecular aspects.* Philadelphia: Lippincott-Raven, 1996:629–637.

376. Russell ME, Hancock WW, Akalin E, et al. Chronic cardiac rejection in the LEW to F344 rat model. Blockade of CD28-B7 costimulation by CTLA4Ig modulates T cell and macrophage activation and attenuates arteriosclerosis. *J Clin Invest* 1996;97:833–838.

377. Morris RE, Wang J, Blum JR, et al. Immunosuppressive effects of the morpholinoethyl ester of mycophenolic acid (RS-61443) in rat and nonhuman primate recipients of heart allografts. *Transplant Proc* 1991;23:19–25.

378. Lemstrom K, Sihvola R, Bruggeman C, et al. Cytomegalovirus infection-enhanced cardiac allograft vasculopathy is abolished by DHPG prophylaxis in the rat. *Circulation* 1997;95:2614–2616.

379. Costanzo MR, Naftel DC, Pritzker MR, et al. Heart transplant coronary artery disease as detected by angiography: a multi-institutional study. *J Heart Lung Transplant* 1996;15:S39(abst).

380. Yeung AC, Davis SF, Hauptman PJ, et al. Incidence and progression of transplant coronary artery disease over one year: results of a multicenter trial with use of intravascular ultrasound. *J Heart Lung Transplant* 1995;14:S215–S220.

381. Johnson DE, Gao SZ, Schroeder JS, et al. The spectrum of coronary artery pathologic findings in human cardiac allografts. *J Heart Transplant* 1989;8:349–359.

382. Billingham ME. Pathology of graft vascular disease after heart lung transplantation and its relationship to obliterative bronchiolitis. *Transplant Proc* 1995;27:2013–2016.

383. Crisp SJ, Dunn MJ, Rose ML, et al. Antiendothelial antibodies in after heart transplantation: the accelerating factor in transplant associated coronary artery disease. *J Heart Lung Transplant* 1994;13:1381–1392.

384. Duquesnoy RJ, Demetris AJ. Immunopathology of cardiac transplant rejection. *Curr Opin Cardiol* 1995;10:193–206.

385. Schroeder JS, Gao SZ, Alderman EL, et al. A preliminary study of diltiazem in the prevention of coronary artery disease in heart-transplant recipients. *N Engl J Med* 1993;328:164–170.

386. Schroeder JS, Gao SZ. Calcium blockers and atherosclerosis: lessons from the Stanford Transplant Coronary Artery Disease/Diltiazem Trial. *Can J Cardiol* 1995;11:710–715.

387. Kobayashi J, Crawford SE, Backer CL, et al. Captopril reduces graft coronary artery disease in a rat heterotopic transplant model. *Circulation* 1993;88(5 Pt 2):II286–II290.

388. Southworth MR, Mauro VF. The use of HMG-CoA reductase inhibitors to prevent accelerated graft atherosclerosis in heart transplant patients. *Ann Pharmacother* 1997;31:489–491.

389. Ballantyne CM, Short BC, Bourge RC, et al. Lipid treatment and survival after heart transplantation. *J Am Coll Cardiol* 1998;

390. Halle AA, DiSciascio G, Massin EK, et al. Coronary angioplasty, atherectomy and bypass surgery in cardiac transplant recipients. *J Am Coll Cardiol* 1995;26:120–128.

391. Walker RC, Paya CV, Marshall WF, et al. Pretransplantation seronegative Epstein-Barr virus status is the primary risk factor for posttransplantation lymphoproliferative disorder in adult heart, lung, and other solid organ transplantations. *J Heart Lung Transplant* 1995;14:214–221.

392. Chen JM, Barr ML, Chadburn A, et al. Management of lymphoproliferative disorders after cardiac transplantation. *Ann Thorac Surg* 1993;56:527–538.

*Textbook of the Autoimmune Diseases,*
Edited by R. G. Lahita, N. Chiorazzi, and W. H. Reeves,
Lippincott Williams & Wilkins, Philadelphia © 2000.

# CHAPTER 17

# Immunologically Mediated Diseases of the Lung

Daniel E. Banks

The lung has a number of functions. It is at the interface of the external environment, and on the most elementary level, it behaves as a bellows, allowing the balanced exchange of oxygen and carbon dioxide. This role is critical, but another critical role is to protect the body from the adverse challenges of the outside environment. Because of its estimated surface area of approximately 100 m$^2$, it is particularly effective and particularly vulnerable.

This chapter focuses on events that affect the manner in which the lung reacts to agents in the ambient environment. These reactions are managed by the immune system, including a variety of immunocompetent cells and their products that typically reside in the reticuloendothelial system but interact with all organs. This chapter focuses on the role of these agents in the lung, including a summary of the important aspects of the immune system in the lung and description of the response to agents that may provoke and maintain airway hyperresponsiveness (primarily an airway response), to foreign agents that can induce interstitial pulmonary fibrosis (a parenchymal response), and to the unknown stimuli that induce primary pulmonary hypertension (a vascular response).

What appears to be one of the most intriguing aspects of the immunologic features of the lung is the recognition that there are only a few cells and a limited number of mediators (cytokines are perhaps the best described) available for the development of diseases. However, the manifestations of respiratory illnesses are most variable. The primary protective defenses of the lower respiratory tract are divided into three, with the macrophage participating in and often directing each aspect. These include resident defense mechanisms (i.e., alveolar macrophages, complement, surfactant, and a variety of other extracellular factors); the pulmonary inflammatory response (i.e., primarily macrophages and neutrophils); and specific immune responses involving macrophages, dendritic cells, and T and B lymphocytes.

D. E. Banks: Section of Pulmonary and Critical Care Medicine, West Virginia University School of Medicine, Morgantown, West Virginia 26506-9166; Department of Medicine, Ruby Memorial Hospital, Morgantown, West Virginia 16505.

## RESIDENT DEFENSE MECHANISMS

Alveolar macrophages are central in the lung's defense against foreign particles and pathogens in inspired air. They serve as the resident cellular defenders of the lung, and in combination with several other cells that communicate and amplify each other's role interact through humoral mediators, they are the first line of defense for the lung distal to the smaller bronchioles. They persist in the alveoli, interstitial spaces, intravascular spaces, and conducting airways and actively maintain the nonspecific defense of the lower respiratory tract by clearing organisms, particles, and debris that are recognized as present in the smaller airways and alveoli (1). Macrophages have multiple roles in the lung (Table 17.1) and are a major determinant of whether the lung can meet these challenges. These cells can interact with other cells through a number of secretory products (Table 17.2).

Perhaps the best estimates of the number of the different types of cells in the lung (including alveolar macrophages) are derived from work by Crapo et al. (2). Alveolar type I and type II epithelial cells (differentiation of these cells is primarily related to the ability of type II cells to produce surfactant) comprise approximately 8% and 7% of the cells in the lung, respectively. Capillary endothelial cells in the lung make up about one third of the total number of cells, and cells in the interstitial space account for approximately another third. The number of alveolar macrophages is greatly variable, ranging from 3% in nonsmokers to 19% in smokers, an increase that is apparently the result of airway inflammation (3).

Macrophages are a part of many organs and are members of the reticuloendothelial system. The alveolar macrophage is derived from bone marrow precursors. Promonocytes divide to produce monocytes (4), enter the blood stream, and inevitably enter the lung's interstitial space. When bone marrow monocytes are depleted by irradiation, alveolar macrophage numbers can be maintained by interstitial cell division and migration of these cells into the alveolus (5). In the healthy lung, this means of generating macrophages appears to be of little importance, but it probably plays an

**TABLE 17.1.** *Overview of macrophage roles*

- Phagocytize and possess the microbiologic potential of keeping the lung sterile
- Prevent allergy by ingesting and catabolizing foreign proteins
- Preserve and present antigens to lymphocytes and cooperate with other parts of the immune system
- Recognize and destroy neoplastic cells, preventing the development of cancer
- Ingest "elderly" type I and type II cells, red blood cells, and perhaps surfactant
- React with other cells in the pulmonary parenchyma (lymphocytes, neutrophils, and fibroblasts) and behave as secretory and regulatory cells that can initiate and prolong inflammatory responses and stimulate the production of matrix proteins

important role in clinically important chest infections. Chronic stimuli (e.g., cigarette smoke, inorganic dust exposure) dramatically increase the number of macrophages, stimulating movement of these cells from the intravascular spaces and the interstitium into the alveoli. These newly recruited macrophages and less mature macrophages appear more active than the resident macrophages (6). Overall, macrophages are a heterogeneous and functionally diverse population. They can be different sizes (they tend to increase in size as they age), and some appear more involved in phagocytosis while others are effective in mediator release, roles that appear to be identifiable by membrane surface receptors (7).

Macrophages protect the lung by phagocytosis, a process whereby the particle is "swallowed up" by the macrophage. This requires energy, and it begins with the opsonization or coating of the particles and follows with adherence of the particle to the macrophage cell membrane (usually a receptor mediated process) and then engulfment. The engulfed particles are invaginated within the cell and form discrete membrane lined "pouches" (i.e., phagosomes) that fuse with lysosomes and results in the release of enzymes (8).

The recognition and engulfment of invading organisms by the alveolar macrophages may be enhanced by many soluble products in the alveolar space. These include surfactant, a lipoprotein that has been primarily recognized to lower surface tension and opsonize particles but more recently shown to possess an immune-modulating action through its ability to stimulate phagocytosis and chemotaxis and to regulate cytokine release (9); fibronectin, a macrophage-derived growth factor that coats foreign particles and stimulates mesenchymal cell growth and adhesion to the extracellular matrix (10); immunoglobulins; and complement fragments. These soluble fragments (i.e., opsonins) allow attachment of microorganisms to the macrophage cell membrane and aid in engulfment (11). Fragments of complement, particularly C3b and C3bi, play an important role in this process.

To make phagocytosis most effective, the cell membrane of the macrophage has recognized receptors for the Fc part of IgG and for C3 components (12). The macrophage mannose

receptor (MMR) is found on resident macrophages but not on circulating monocytes. This marks a mature macrophage and binds mannosylated proteins, such as those that are a part of yeast or *Pneumocystis carinii* cell walls (13,14). Complement receptors and MMR appear to be important in binding *Mycobacterium tuberculosis* organisms to the macrophage, because there is apparently little interaction between the Fc receptor and this organism (15). With the isolation of a microorganism within a phagosome, there is a massive increase in oxygen consumption (i.e., respiratory burst), with the generation of superoxides, halogenated anions, and other toxic molecules. This phagocytic process is effective, and at least in the instance of *Staphylococcus aureus,* even in the absence of neutrophils, the organisms can be effectively cleared by macrophage function. However, other bacteria, notably *Klebsiella pneumoniae* and *Pseudomonas aeruginosa,* proliferate in the face of effective macrophage function when granulocytopenia occurs (16). The effectiveness of this phagocytic process can be modified, because macrophages stimulated by interferon-γ (IFN-γ), a product of activated T lymphocytes, limit *Legionella pneumophila* and *M. tuberculosis* growth within the cell (17), but this same agent appears to lessen the ability of mycobacteria to adhere to the macrophage (18). With stimulation, alveolar macrophages change shape, reflecting their functional change (Fig. 17.1). They can kill microorganisms extracellularly through the release of oxygen metabolites, reactive nitrogen intermediates, other substrates such as lysozyme and other proteolytic enzymes, arachidonic acid metabolites, and immunomodulatory cytokines (19).

## INFLAMMATORY RESPONSES

### Macrophages

Mediators that are important in effector cell function are listed in Tables 17.2 and 17.3. Macrophages are important amplifiers of the inflammatory response through their ability to release mediators that recruit other cells, and they largely mediate the cellular immune response. Macrophages have the potential to secrete more than 100 molecules; a partial list includes groups of molecules classified as cytokines, growth factors, enzymes and enzyme inhibitors, clotting factors, and complement (20) (Table 17.3). There is considerable overlap in the actions of many of these agents (21).

There are a number of chemotactic factors primarily secreted by alveolar macrophages that induce a nonspecific cellular influx into the lung. One of the key mediators of macrophage-mediated neutrophil influx is interleukin-8 (IL-8). In a process that is relevant to acute inflammation and to different types of noninfectious lung illnesses (22,23), IL-8 appears to be a major chemotactic agent for neutrophils and is a potent stimulant for the neutrophils to degranulate (24). In association with macrophages, fibroblasts express the gene for IL-8 release, a feature that is relevant in asbestosis and idiopathic pulmonary fibrosis (25). When histamine is released in

**TABLE 17.2.** *Selected clinically important cytokines released by lung effector cells*

*Interleukin-1* (IL-1) is produced by virtually all cells, including macrophages, neutrophils, B and T lymphocytes, and dendritic cells. Although there are at least 18 interleukins, the IL-1 family consists of dominant cytokines. IL-1 has an important role in the stimulation and activation of T and B cell proliferation, initiating lymphokine production and immunoglobulin synthesis, stimulating natural killer cells, activating neutrophils to produce cytokines, and inducing macrophages to manufacture tumor necrosis factor, IL-6, and granulocyte-macrophage colony-stimulating factor. IL-1 is an important factor in infection, responsible for fever, lethargy, and anorexia. It serves as a chemoattractant for other cells in the inflammatory process. Many of the IL-1 effects are attributable to its induction of arachidonic acid metabolism, with the resultant production of thromboxanes and prostaglandins (eicosanoid metabolites), agents that are potent mediators of inflammation.

*Tumor necrosis factor* (TNF) is primarily produced by macrophages but can also be manufactured by other cells. TNF was originally reported to be cytotoxic against tumor cells and to stimulate the antitumor responses of immune cells. Since then, a variety of roles have been recognized. It plays a role in stimulating the release of mediators that permit the movement of neutrophils into areas of inflammation. It stimulates other macrophages to release IL-6 (important in B-cell growth and differentiation) and IL-8 (a stimulant for neutrophil chemotaxis and neutrophil activation). Its metabolic action blocks lipoprotein lipase enzyme activity, resulting in cachexia in patients with cancer and sepsis. There are major overlaps in the functions of the two proinflammatory cytokines, IL-1 and TNF. Both are important in production of the endothelial adhesion molecules, ICAM-1 and E-selectin, needed for the early steps in neutrophil adhesion to the activated endothelium and eventual migration across the endothelium into the pulmonary parenchyma.

*Interleukin-4* (IL-4) *and interleukin-10* (IL-10) are released by lymphocytes. These cytokines have antiinflammatory activity, and when added to *in vitro* cell cultures, they suppress cytokine production by stimulated cytokines, lessen albumin leak into the parenchyma, and decrease neutrophil influx into the pulmonary parenchyma. Lessening macrophage stimulation is associated with downregulation of IL-1, IL-6, IL-8, TNF, and ICAM-1 expression. IL-4 is secreted by activated CD4Q+ T cells and by mast cells. It is mitogenic for B cells and promotes these activated B cells to produce IgE antibodies. This cytokine appears to be a critical mediator in allergic asthma because it also promotes the induction of type 2 helper-T cells, cells that control the activities of eosinophils and mast cells. In like manner, IL-10 has an inhibitory role in cytokine production by natural killer cells and macrophages. As well as being an inhibitor of proinflammatory cytokines, it behaves as a mitogen for mast cells, T cells, and B cells, and it promotes B-cell antibody production.

*Interleukin-6* (IL-6) is produced by a variety of cells, including macrophages, activated T and B lymphocytes, monocytes, endothelial cells, and fibroblasts. Expression of IL-6 is regulated by TNF, IL-1, platelet-derived growth factor, and agents that activate T and B cells. It plays a major role in B-cell division and differentiation, and it acts with the cytokines TNF and IL-1 to stimulate T cells. It has not been found to stimulate the release of other cytokines.

*Interleukin-8* (IL-8) is produced by activated macrophages, fibroblasts, neutrophils, and endothelial and epithelial cells. IL-8 plays a crucial role in attracting specific types of cells to sites of injury and inflammation and it appears to be most important in attracting neutrophils by stimulating the expression of leukocyte integrins, which promote the binding of neutrophils to endothelium. Similarly, these cytokines bind to the membranes of cells already in the lung matrix and attract cells to this environment. Expression of IL-8 is induced by proinflammatory cytokines such as IL-1, TNF, and interferon-γ.

*Transforming growth factor-β* (TGF-β) is produced by many cell types, including stimulated macrophages and T lymphocytes. TGF-β describes a family of peptides that may stimulate fibrosis and matrix development and inhibit B-cell immunoglobulin secretion. TGF has some properties that potentiate inflammation, attract neutrophils and monocytes, and stimulate adhesion protein production by monocytes. Although it was initially recognized as a primary growth factor for fibroblasts, it also possesses antifibrogenic activity and downregulates the immune response. It inhibits B- and T-cell proliferation and the corresponding cytokine and lymphokine production. It has an antiproliferative action on macrophages, endothelial cells, and lymphocytes.

*Colony-stimulating growth factors* are produced by a wide variety of cells. Granulocyte colony-stimulating factor (G-CSF) is produced by macrophages and fibroblasts. Granulocyte-macrophage colony-stimulating factor (GM-CSF) is produced by T lymphocytes, macrophages, fibroblasts, and endothelial cells. G-CSF stimulates production of neutrophils and monocytes/macrophages. GM-CSF stimulates production of monocytes/macrophages and is a factor in promoting the maturity of dendritic cells. Macrophages that develop in the presence of GM-CSF are more functionally active.

*Platelet-derived growth factor* (PGDF) is produced by macrophages. PGDF and fibronectin are competence factors ("encourage" cells to initiate the cell cycle) that initiate proliferation and stimulation of fibroblast activities.

the lung (as in late-phase asthma), IL-8 is released from vascular endothelial cells, and *in vitro* can exert a chemotactic effect for neutrophils, eosinophils, and basophils. This effect is magnified by the presence of tumor necrosis factor-α (TNF-α) and IL-1 (also produced by macrophages) (26,27). Similarly, human alveolar macrophage-derived chemotactic factor for neutrophils has been described (28).

It appears that alveolar macrophages are effective metabolizers of arachidonic acid compared with circulating monocytes, converting this substrate through the 5-lipoxygenase pathway to one of several leukotrienes. The most active is LTB$_4$, a metabolite that is chemotactic to neutrophils and activates neutrophil metabolism (29).

Alveolar macrophages recovered from patients with sarcoidosis possess 1α-hydroxylase activity and metabolize 1,25(OH)$_2$D$_3$ from 25-hydroxylase vitamin D$_3$. The presence of IFN-γ, produced by activated macrophages and lymphocytes, stimulates this reaction, which is blocked by corticosteroid therapy. Receptors for 1,23(OH)$_2$D$_3$ reside on T lymphocytes and inhibit the proliferation of T lymphocytes,

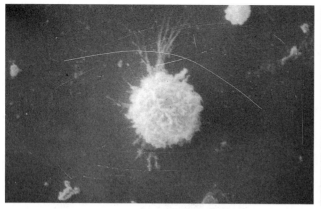
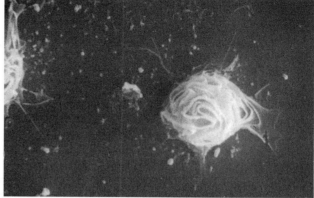

A

B

**FIG. 17.1.** The transmission electron micrographs of alveolar macrophages, collected by bronchoalveolar lavage, show a control **(A)** and stimulated cell **(B)**, with marked cell surface ruffling.

thereby limiting cytokine production. In the context of sarcoidosis, this may limit progression of the disease. Whether the alveolar macrophage can metabolize 25-hydroxylase vitamin $D_3$ in the healthy lung is not clear (30,31).

Alveolar macrophages produce a number of antiproteases and proteases that appear to be consequential in inflammation and the development of emphysema. These proteases can degrade extracellular matrix in the lung. Circulating monocytes contain the serine proteases, neutrophil elastase and cathepsin G, which are stored in macrophage granules and can be rapidly released. When these cells develop into alveolar macrophages, these proteinases change, and the synthesis of a number of matrix metalloproteinases begin. The activity of these cells is zinc dependent and can be blocked by tissue inhibitors of metalloproteinases (32,33).

### Polymorphonuclear Leukocytes

For the neutrophil to exert its inflammatory effect, it must reach the alveolus. This means that circulating neutrophils must adhere to and migrate across the vascular endothelial cells into the extracellular space and then migrate across airway epithelial cells into the alveolus. Cytokines play a crucial role in this process. *In vitro* studies have shown negligible transmigration across vascular endothelial cells in the absence of cytokines, but formyl-methionyl-leucyl-phenylalanine (FMLP), IL-8, and C5A are all effective chemoattractants (34), as are a number of other mediators, including leukotriene $B_4$, and TNF-$\alpha$. It appears that migration across the endothelial cells is mediated in a different manner from migration across epithelial cells. When IL-1$\beta$ was added to the media, neutrophil migration depended on IL-8 and platelet-activating factor, whereas migration across epithelial cells depended only on IL-8.

For a normal cellular response, there must be an accumulation of white blood cells in the affected area, the result of diapedesis of these neutrophils through the vessel walls into the inflamed area; normal underlying neutrophil function; and normal underlying tissue function (35,36). The key moment in migration of the neutrophil into the alveolus is its

attachment to the vascular endothelial cell. This particular process is mediated by a number of adhesion molecules (integrins, selectins, and intracellular adhesion molecules [ICAMs]) that play different roles in the neutrophil's initial "rolling along the endothelial cell" and allows for the two different cells to stick together, with the neutrophil becoming firmly adhered to the endothelial cell, and then stimulating the migration of the neutrophil through the cell junctions into the extracellular space (37). When the neutrophil arrives at the inflammatory focus, these cells participate in a respiratory burst. Through an energy-dependent mechanism, these cells release various amounts of oxygen metabolites, including $O_2^-, H_2O_2$, and $O\cdot$, and a variety of enzymes. The neutrophil also participates in arachidonic acid metabolism, releasing many of the products from the lipoxygenase pathway (notably $LTB_4$) (38).

When neutrophils are "activated," neutrophils change their shape and display pseudopodia, their metabolic rate is accelerated, superoxide radicals are formed, lysosomal release is begun, and membrane adhesion energy processes increase. Four mechanisms of neutrophil activation have been identified and have the potential to convert a "benign" circulating neutrophil into a cell that can initiate and perpetuate the inflammatory process. These include chemotactic agents such as lipopolysaccharides, cytokines (one of the important cytokines is platelet activating factor), endotoxins, complement, which directly stimulate receptors located on the neutrophil; endothelial cell contact; depletion of deactivators such as adenosine; and mechanical shear stress (39).

### Specific Immune Responses

When the lung is minced, enzyme digested, and cells purified, several distinct types of cells can be isolated in addition to those described previously. These include the interstitial macrophages and the dendritic cells (lymphocytes are described later).

Interstitial macrophages can also be recovered by serial lung lavage procedures, where the initial recovered cells are mature, fully active alveolar macrophages, and the later

**TABLE 17.3.** *Selected clinically important products released by macrophages*

*Enzymes*

*Lysosyme* is a nonmucin component of the airway lining. It catalyzes the cell wall constituents of most bacteria and is a part of the nonspecific immunity of the airway. It lyses most bacteria and is toxic to fungi. Although the antibacterial effect appears to be its most important feature, this enzyme also can diminish the tissue-damaging effects of inflammation by lessening the chemotaxis and production of free radicals by stimulated neutrophils.

*Beta-glucuronidase,* a lysosomal enzyme, is an acid hydrolase. This enzyme, in an acidic environment that is recognized as part of the inflammatory process, is able to degrade collagen, proteoglycans, and other ground substances such as chondroitin sulfate.

*Angiotensin-converting enzyme* is produced by activated macrophages. Levels are increased in patients with sarcoidosis and in smokers. It appears to play a role in the breakdown of bradykinin to an inactive peptide. Bradykinin potentiates vascular permeability, vasodilation, and activation of phospholipases that activate arachidonic acid metabolism.

Macrophage and neutrophil *elastases* may play important roles in the development of emphysema. The lung is protected from elastolytic damage by $\alpha_1$-antitrypsin and $\alpha_2$-macroglobulin. The airways are protected by the mucous layer. Elastase is primarily a neutrophil product, but macrophages can produce an elastase-like metalloproteinase and may ingest and later release neutrophil elastase. Oxidants (e.g., cigarette smoke) inactivate $\alpha_1$-antitrypsin, and antioxidants (e.g., superoxide dismutase, glutathione) protect the lung from injury.

*Collagenase and collagenase inhibitor* (which is active on the interstitial collagenases) are produced by macrophages. Metalloproteinases, including collagenases and gelatinases, denature collagen. Serine proteases include elastases and cathepsin, and they promote fibrinolysis during bouts of acute or chronic inflammation.

*Biologically active lipids*

*Cyclooxygenase and lipoxygenase metabolites* are metabolites of arachidonic acid. They can be derived from cell membrane phospholipids (specifically arachidonic acid), and when further broken down, they yield eicosanoids. These are recognized as prostaglandins (through the cyclooxygenase pathway) and leukotrienes (through the 5-lipoxygenase pathway). These eicosanoids are also secreted by macrophages through stimulation by IgE or IgG immune complexes. In general, products of the cyclooxygenase pathway inhibit macrophage production of interleukin-1 and tumor necrosis factor (and therefore may be described as antifibrogenic), whereas products of the 5-lipoxygenase pathway promote cytokine production and can be described as profibrogenic. Overall, the antifibrogenic effect includes functions such as inhibition of fibroblast proliferation, collagen synthesis, and cytokine production, and the profibrogenic actions can be described as promoting collagen synthesis and chemo-

taxis. Perhaps the most effective of the cyclooxygenase products is prostaglandin $D_2$ ($PGD_2$), which promotes local vasodilation and vascular permeability, as well as attracting neutrophils. Among the lipoxygenase products, there are four primary leukotrienes, leukotriene $B_4$ ($LTB_4$), $LTC_4$, $LTD_4$, and $LTE_4$. $LTB_4$ is an important cellular chemoattractant, and the others make up what was known as the "slow-reacting substance of the anaphylaxis," an agent that induced smooth muscle contraction, bronchoconstriction, and airway secretions.

*Platelet-activating factor* (PAF) is produced by alveolar macrophages, mast cells, neutrophils, eosinophils, and platelets. PAF is a complex, biologically active lipid stored in the cell. PAF has the potential to aggregate platelets with the release of platelet granules, and it can attract and activate neutrophils (at least partly through the release of $LTB_4$) and eosinophils so that they may release potent chemotaxins. It can cause activation and degranulation of neutrophils, activate complement, and stimulate the production and release of arachidonic acid metabolites, as well as perpetuate the inflammatory process within the lung. In these ways it plays a role in inducing bronchospasm and pulmonary edema.

*Proteins*

*Antiproteases* can protect lung tissue. Instillation of a collagenase inhibitor (tissue inhibitor of metalloproteinases [TIMP]) into the lung significantly decreases the amount of lung injury, the neutrophil response, and the overall inflammatory response. The lung is also protected from elastolytic damage by $\alpha_1$-antitrypsin and $\alpha_2$-macroglobulin, which bind most proteases and have been shown to bind and inhibit the proteolytic effects of elastase.

*Fibronectin,* a glycoprotein, is produced by alveolar macrophages. It is released into the extracellular matrix to promote fibroblast recruitment and growth.

*Complement components* are part of the immune defenses of the lower respiratory tract. Optimal phagocytosis by macrophages depends on opsonization and on the milieu in the alveolar lining fluids. These other elements in the alveolar lining fluid include complement components, most importantly C3b.

*Antioxidants*

*Antioxidants* transform free radical species (such as those derived from oxygen or lipid) into less reactive species, limiting their toxicity. There are a number of antioxidants in the alveolar lining fluid, including catalase, superoxide dismutase, and plasma proteins such as albumin, ceruloplasmin, and reduced glutathione. Of these, the most important molecule appears to be superoxide dismutase, which in the reduced state is an effective scavenger of toxic oxygen free radicals. This agent appears to be effective when it is extracellular (also present in the alveolar lining fluid is glutathione reductase and peroxidase, important elements of the redox cycle), and it protects when it is located within the cell.

recovered "interstitial macrophages" or cells separated by "mincing," are similar in terms of their antigenic markers, cytokine release, phagocytosis and surface receptors, but are much more able to replicate and present antigen to T lymphocytes (40,41).

Dendritic cells appear to have as their origin bone marrow monocytes. They have been recognized as "loosely adherent" cells (with a relatively pleomorphic morphology), which were initially recognized as occasional cells that might be isolated when the lung was minced, but more recently have been understood to be a part of a contiguous network of such cells throughout the airway epithelium and alveolar septal walls (42). These cells serve as "sensors" for foreign antigens that are not usually presented to the immune system until they interact with lymph node. These cells present the antigens that they have sequestered to T cells after further differentiation mediated by granulocyte–macrophage colony-stimulating factor (GM-CSF) (43). Dendritic cells appear to be the most active antigen presenting cells residing in the respiratory tract and they proliferate in response to dusts or bacterial exposures in the lung (acute and chronic stimuli), thereby improving surveillance for antigen exposure (44,45), and accelerating T-cell proliferation (46).

## Lymphocytes

Lymphocytes are circulating cells that are able to obtain and keep an "immunologic memory" for specific antigens. The presence of specific receptors on the surface of these lymphocytes separates them into T and B cells, and effect cell-mediated and humorally mediated immune function, respectively. T lymphocytes play an important role in delayed-type hypersensitivity, allograft reaction, tumor immunity, graft-versus-host reactions and cytotoxicity (their ability to kill other cells). B lymphocytes secrete specific antibodies in response to exposure to a specific antigen and are particularly effective in presenting the antigens that bind specifically to their surface immunoglobulins. A third type of cell, natural killer (NK) cells, provide nonspecific cytotoxic aid against virus and tumor-infected cells. On the basis of cell surface markers, mature T cells are considered to be helper/inducer cells ($CD4^+$) or cytotoxic/suppressor cells ($CD8^+$).

After activation, T lymphocytes secrete a number of lymphokines that attract, activate, and promote the growth and differentiation of other leukocytes. Based on animal studies, and confirmed by human *in vivo* studies, ($CD4^+$) or helper T cell ($T_H$) clones can be divided based of their membrane receptors and their cytokine profile (47,48). For example, $T_H1$ clones produce IL-2 and IFN-$\gamma$ but not IL-4 or IL-5, whereas $T_H2$ clones produce IL-4, IL-5, and granulocyte-macrophage colony-stimulating factor (GM-CSF) (Table 17.4).

## IMMUNOLOGICALLY MEDIATED CHEST ILLNESSES

The immune system of the lung plays a major role in all of the illnesses that affect the lung. Investigators are faced with a considerable challenge when attempting to show different diseases as models of illnesses where examples can be cited. We have chosen to address three models for the development of lung disease. The first is a review the development and presentations of asthma (the immunologic response of the airways), an increasingly complex process that is primarily driven by airway inflammation. The second is the interaction of the lung with the external environment in the development of interstitial lung disease (the immune responses associated

**TABLE 17.4.** *Lymphocyte functions*

*T lymphocytes:* Mature $CD4^+$ T cells secrete cytokines that stimulate the behavior of other lymphocytes. Functional subsets of $CD4^+$ cells ($T_h1$ and $T_h2$) participate in T-cell–mediated or B-cell–mediated immunity. Mature $CD8^+$ T cells can regulate processes through the expression of cytokines that suppress cell function and behave as cytotoxic cells.

*B lymphocytes:* Mature activated B cells differentiate into groups of plasma cells, which are members of a discrete clone of cells that produce immunoglobulins of a singular isotype (e.g., IgM, $IgG_{1-4}$, IgA, or IgE) specific for different antigens. B cells can be identified by the immunoglobulin receptors on the cell surface, whereas plasma cells are SIg negative.

*Natural killer cells:* These lymphocytes are distinct from T or B lymphocytes. They possess specific cell markers and are important in immune surveillance. They have several functions, including elaboration of proinflammatory cytokines (especially IFN-$\gamma$) and a cytotoxic effect whereby they are able to kill antibody-coated cells through an immunoglobulin-mediated action.

with alveolar injury). These dusts primarily cause injury through free radical generation, and through a sophisticated series of events under the proper host conditions, result in the formation of the silicotic nodule, the coal macule, or the abestos-induced fibrotic lung (identical to the histologic process that occurs in idiopathic pulmonary fibrosis). In these situations, it appears that the role of the immune system is to amplify the inflammatory response to optimize the lung's response. However, in this attempt to rid the lung of these "essentially nonmetabolizable" potentially fibrogenic external stimuli, the result becomes fibrosis and progressive lung scarring. The final model involves the rare disease *primary pulmonary hypertension*, a process whereby the pulmonary vasculature is modified and the vessels narrow and decrease in number as the result of a progressive obliterative vasculitis. Of important interest is the recognition that the natural history of this diseases can potentially be altered by infusion of specific prostaglandin.

## Asthma

Asthma is characterized by the presence of chronic airway inflammation that transiently increases during exacerbations (49–51). Documentation of the degree of airway inflammation has been perhaps best studied using inhalation challenge with the agent in question, followed by fiberoptic bronchoscopy where saline was infused into the alveolar space and aspirated (bronchoalveolar lavage [BAL]) bronchial biopsies were also performed (52). Specialized examination of induced sputum, although less well tested than evaluation of BAL cells and fluid or bronchial wall histology, may also be a useful noninvasive method to investigate inflammatory cells in the airways of asthmatic subjects (53,54).

The presence of airway inflammation is translated into the symptoms of dyspnea, cough, wheezing, chest tightness; clinical complaints that are typically worse at night or early morning. The severity of asthma correlates well with the degree of airways hyperresponsiveness. When asthma is mild and airways hyperresponsiveness is minimal, the patient typically experiences mild respiratory symptoms. In such individuals, symptoms wax and wane based on exposure to allergic factors. In those with more marked airway hyperresponsiveness, asthma can be a severe disabling illness associated with persistent, unrelenting respiratory complaints, to the point being of life-threatening. In such individuals, with such an excessive degree of airway hyperresponsiveness, irritants, perhaps more rather than allergens, are responsible for a worsening of the clinical status. A predominantly younger percentage of asthmatics have asthma associated with atopy, a genetic predisposition for the development of an IgE-mediated response to common allergens. Elevated total IgE correlates with symptomatic asthma in this group (55). Older individuals effected by this illness are often without an allergic diathesis.

Airway inflammation is a primary contributor to acute bronchoconstriction, airway edema, the development of mucus plugs, and airway wall remodeling. The sum of these changes translate into a measurable degree of airway hyperresponsiveness (which can be routinely measured in competent respiratory laboratories), airflow obstruction, respiratory symptoms and disease chronicity. In the airway, these measurable clinical features of asthma can be correlated with airway histologic changes and, in the most severe situation, the histologic changes are most prominent. There is a spectrum of histologic changes that vary with the severity of asthma. Denudation of the airway epithelium, connective tissue deposition beneath the basement membrane, edema, mast cell formation, and inflammatory cell infiltration, specifically with neutrophils, eosinophils, and lymphocytes, may present (56). In the most extreme situation, i.e., those who die from severe chronic asthma, autopsy reveals extensive airway changes. The previously described features are exaggerated and histologic examination shows hypertrophic smooth muscle, a thickened basement membrane, infiltration of the lamina propria by monocytes, eosinophils and mast cells, vasodilation and leakage of fluid into the alveolar spaces, and diffuse mucus plugging (containing mucus, serum proteins, cellular debris and inflammatory cells) of the bronchioles and large airways. The lung parenchyma shows focal areas of alveolar destruction adjacent to areas of intact alveolar walls and the bronchial smooth muscle is hyperplastic and disarrayed. It is likely that bronchial walls are thickened by persistent edema or an increased amount of subepithelial collagen and this, in addition to the decreased airway lumen diameter caused by a similar degree of smooth muscle shortening, provokes further clinical impairment (57,58). In this instance airway inflammation becomes a malignant process.

### Histologic Changes in the Airways of Asthmatics

Although there is no difference between the percentage of the basement membrane covered by epithelial cells or in the width of the intercellular spaces between columnar cells in healthy asthmatics and controls, the intercellular spaces between the basal cells are wider in asthmatics (59). Because the attachment of most columnar epithelial cells to the basement membrane is mediated through basal cells, the wider spaces between basal cells may adversely effect adhesion of columnar cells to the basement membrane, contributing to the influx of inflammatory cells into the epithelial and subepithelial layers and to the induction of epithelial fragility (60). Recent data have suggested that a marker of epithelial cell injury, cytokeratin 19 (a specific cytoskeletal structure of simple epithelia), is increased in airway inflammatory disease, and is thought to exist free in the airways as a result of metabolism by neutrophil elastase (61).

Overall, it appears that there has been an important underestimation of the role of the epithelial cells and their importance in protecting the asthmatic from potentially immune-altering injury. An intact epithelium is more than a passive barrier; it limits the inflammatory responses by degrading or inhibiting proinflammatory mediators and proteins and by actively producing consequential mediators such as IL-6, GM-CSF, and others under some conditions (62) (Fig. 17.2).

Although the width of the true basement membrane is similar in asthmatics and controls (63,64), a thickened reticular layer of the basement membrane has been described in young asthmatics with mild asthma, a feature that likely represents an early histologic change of asthma. This finding appears to be specific for asthma, because in chronic bronchitis, a disease that also causes airway inflammation with T lymphocyte activation, the thickness of the basement membrane does not differ from controls (65). In a human model of asthma resulting from a sensitizing workplace agent (e.g., toluene diisocyanate), cessation of exposure to such a sensitizer for approximately 6 months resulted in the lessening of the thickness of the reticular layer of the basement membrane, although the airway inflammatory cell infiltrate persisted (66). After a considerable time away from exposure (6 to 21 months), subepithelial fibrosis and the number of mast cells and fibroblasts declined, but the number of eosinophils and mononuclear cells and the degree of airway responsiveness to methacholine did not change (67). The association between the thickness of the reticular layer of the basement membrane

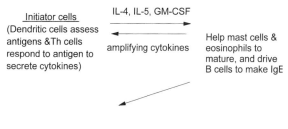

**FIG. 17.2.** Important mediators and their actions in allergic asthma.

and the number of mast cells and fibroblasts, suggests a role for these resident cells in the development of this subepithelial fibrosis. In the absence of removal from exposure to the sensitizing agent(s), basement membrane fibrosis may contribute to persistent abnormalities in lung function (68).

Several investigations have attempted to identify the differences (histologic and otherwise) between atopic and nonatopic asthma. Humbert et al. showed similar airway cellularity in atopic and nonatopic asthma and compared the molecular immunopathology of atopic and nonatopic asthma and showed increased of cells expressing mRNA encoding IL-4 and IL-5 and increased numbers of IL-4 and IL-5 immunoreactive cells within the bronchial mucosa (69) of both groups. These data differ from work by Walker et al., which showed a distinctly different pattern of T-cell activation and cytokine production in the BAL fluid of intrinsic nonatopic asthmatics compared with atopic asthmatics (70). BAL fluid analysis from the allergic asthmatic showed elevated levels of IL-4 and IL-5 (consistent with a $T_H2$ cell mediated process), while the intrinsic asthmatics had elevated BAL fluid levels of IL-2 and IL-5 but not IL-4. Although it appears that the differences and similarities in these two "varieties" of asthma have not been fully described, some data suggest that there are differences in mechanisms in intrinsic versus extrinsic asthma (71).

### Allergic Aspects of Asthma

The diagnosis of respiratory allergy usually depends on an adequate history and demonstration of IgE to the suspected allergen. Although the presence of an IgE antibody is not equivalent to clinical asthma (e.g., those with hay fever and without respiratory symptoms may have elevated IgE levels), those with allergic asthma typically have specific IgE antibodies to the offending allergens (72). There are a great number of potential allergens in the environment, with their prevalence differing by geographic location, but it appears that the most prevalent outdoor allergen may be ragweed while the most common indoor allergen is house dust mite (73,74). Exposure to these allergens in the sensitized individual induces airway inflammation and leads to overt asthma with a persistent increase in airway hyperresponsiveness. Several nonallergic exposures, such as exercise, cold air, and irritants such as smoke and perfumes, can provoke asthma in the allergic asthmatic and typically cause a time-limited episode of bronchospasm.

Lymphocytes previously were considered to play a role in IgE-mediated immunity mainly through the induction and regulation of IgE by B lymphocytes (75). However, T lymphocytes are now recognized to act as effector cells in atopic asthma by releasing cytokines that recruit and activate other inflammatory cells, causing inflammation independent from B-cell function and IgE production. In addition to their role as helper cells for the production of humoral antibodies by B cells, activated CD4+ lymphocytes may be considered to be inflammatory cells that interact in a major network involving all cells in the airway. Activated T cells may therefore initiate and propagate allergic inflammation in the airways and participate directly in the events responsible for asthma exacerbations (76–79). However, a number of cells produce IL-3, IL-4, IL-5, GM-CSF, and other relevant cytokines (80,81). T-lymphocyte activation and local accumulation of activated eosinophils in the bronchial wall occurs in asthma of diverse severity and cause, including atopic and nonatopic varieties (82–85). Different subsets of CD8+ T cells also can participate in B-cell suppression or act as cytotoxic cells for exogenous and endogenous antigens. These cells are MHC (HLA-DR) class I restricted but can respond to soluble exogenous antigens or haptens (86).

T lymphocytes modulate eosinophil adherence, chemotaxis, survival, and activation, and stimulate these cells to cause tissue damage. In the airways in atopic asthmatics, an increased number of activated CD25+ T lymphocytes (lymphocytes expressing the IL-2 receptor), activated eosinophils, and mast cells are observed. Activated lymphocytes and eosinophils in bronchial biopsies suggest that a T lymphocyte–eosinophil interaction is important, a hypothesis further supported by the findings of cells expressing IL-5 messenger RNA in bronchial biopsies of atopic asthmatics. IL-5 is a most important eosinophil regulating cytokine that promotes the development, activation, and survival of eosinophils. It is the predominant eosinophil-active lymphokine present in BAL fluids during allergen-induced late phase inflammation and its concentration in the airway mucosa of asthmatics correlates with markers of T lymphocyte and eosinophil activation (87,88). The role of IL-4 in allergic asthmatics has been further delineated. Inhalation of this cytokine provoked an increase in airway hyperresponsiveness and marked sputum eosinophilia (and a marked increase in neutrophils) (89). The recognition of the importance of these two cytokines in asthma may well lead to important clinical intervention.

The addition of eosinophils to the airway milieu heightens the degree of bronchial hyperresponsiveness. Eosinophils secrete a number of basic proteins (e.g. major basic protein, eosinophilic cationic protein, eosinophil peroxidase) that effectively increase vascular permeability, bronchoconstriction, and shedding of airway epithelial cells (90).

The role of the macrophage in asthma is less clearly understood. These cells express an enhanced ability to present antigen to T lymphocytes, and they produce superoxide anions, cytokines (e.g., GM-CSF, TNF-α, IL-6), and eicosanoid mediators (91). They also have low-affinity receptors for IgE on the alveolar macrophage cell surface (92). Analysis of BAL fluid in the asthmatic shows an increased number of macrophages compared with controls. An important mediator, IL-8, is produced by macrophages and stromal cells, such as epithelial and endothelial cells, as a result of cytokine networking between these cells and cytokine producing T cells. It behaves as a chemotactic cytokine for polymorphonuclear leukocytes. GM-CSF is also important in eosinophil development, activation, and in the amplification of eosinophilic inflammation.

Airway inflammation is associated with cell membrane breakdown. This results in generation of leukotrienes, lipid mediators that are derived from the arachidonic acid pathway. Of these, perhaps leukotriene $B_4$ ($LTB_4$) is most relevant to neutrophil function as instillation of $LTB_4$ results in a tremendous influx of neutrophils, enhances neutrophil–endothelial cell interactions, and stimulates neutrophil function, presumably accelerating the rate of inflammation (93). It may well be that the neutrophil is most important in acute severe asthma (status asthmaticus), as BAL from mechanically ventilated asthmatics showed a significantly elevated level of neutrophils, dramatically more compared with the BAL features in stable asthma (94).

### Nonallergic Features of Asthma

Several important nonimmune mechanisms play a role in the development of airway inflammation. There is an extensive distribution of autonomic motor and sensory nerve fibers in the airway walls that contain potent neurotransmitters that have the ability to alter airway smooth muscle tone, bronchial blood flow, microvascular permeability, and the secretion by glands and epithelium (95). In addition to what are recognized as classic neurotransmitters of the autonomic nervous system (i.e., acetylcholine released by the parasympathetic nerves and epinephrine released by the sympathetic nerves), the role of neuropeptides released from sensory and motor nerve fibers has been better described, but the role of neurogenic mediators in the pathogenesis of asthma is not clear (96). A traditional, but unproved hypothesis, has been that there was an imbalance between autonomic mechanisms of airway excitatory and inhibitory influences to the asthmatic condition (97). It appears that it is more complex than this, with neurotransmitters acting to affect airway inflammation and mediators of airway inflammation acting on the nerves of the lungs to alter neurotransmitter release.

The cholinergic nervous system is dominant in the human lung, and stimulation of these nerves (by irritants or cold) provokes bronchospasm and stimulate these nerves. This causes the release of acetylcholine and there has been great interest among investigators in determining whether cholinergic mechanisms are exaggerated in asthma. Asthmatics react excessively to cholinergic agonists, such as methacholine, but other agents, such as leukotrienes, also induce hyperresponsiveness, leading one to conclude that this might not be a specific response. Importantly, atropine (an anticholinergic drug) is an important inhaled therapeutic agent in obstructive lung disease, but less so in asthma compared with fixed states of airways obstruction. This leads one to postulate that the role of these neurogenic mediators are not a determining factor of the state of the airways in asthma (98).

Alternatively, with the clear evidence of improvement in symptoms and airway caliber after inhalation of sympathetic agents (epinephrine and its derivatives that act through β receptors on the smooth muscle cell membrane) there is a good reason to think that there are deficits in the adrenergic

system in the lung in asthma. It appears that epinephrine affects the cholinergic ganglia, suggesting influence of the cholinergic system by adrenergic input (99). However, the presence of asthma is not associated with increased or diminished circulating epinephrine levels, even during acute exacerbations (100). Similarly, β blockers can provoke an episode of bronchospasm in asthmatics, but not in those without asthma, leading investigators to consider that defects exist in the β receptor. *In vitro* data are available to show asthmatic human bronchial smooth muscle is less responsive to isoproterenol compared with nonasthmatic tissue (101).

The nonadrenergic, noncholinergic (NANC) nervous system in the lung regulates airway function through the release of proteins (mainly peptides but also nitric oxide and adenosine) that can alter airway diameter. This system is complex, including sensory and motor nerves, and compared with the cholinergic and sympathetic systems, relatively little is known about the structure and function of this system. Neuropeptides are synthesized in nerve cell bodies, transported by axoplasmic flow to the terminal ends of the nerves and are released when the appropriate stimulus occurs. NANC bronchodilator nerves produce vasoactive intestinal peptide (VIP), a peptide that is released from nerve terminals in smooth muscle. It appears to be closely associated with the cholinergic system and appears to block release and "antagonize" acetylcholine-mediated contraction of smooth muscle, thereby lessening the cholinergic effect (102). In an *in vitro* animal model where other potentially opposing proteins are absent, VIP serves as a potent bronchodilator (103). There is less VIP density in airway smooth muscle of asthmatics (104), but this might be explained by breakdown of this protein by enzymes released from inflammatory cells.

The sensory nerve fibers supply airway epithelium, airway smooth muscles and glands and blood vessels. These fibers contain several neuropeptides [calcitonin gene–related peptide (CGRP), substance P, and neurokinin A (NKA)]. CGRP is often found in conjunction with these other tachykinins. It is a potent vasodilator of bronchial vessels and appears to play a role in the airway hyperemia of asthma (105). VIP and SP are often localized in the same neuron, suggesting that release of these two peptides is engendered by the same stimulus (even though their action is considerably different) (106). Release of SP causes a bronchoconstrictor effect (although much less than the bronchoconstrictive action of NKA) mediated through an identified cellular receptor, and through another receptor, SP induces its most recognized effect, i.e., microvascular leakage from bronchial blood vessels and mucus secretion from submucosal glands and goblet cells in airways, features most important in asthma (107). Importantly, the airways of asthmatics contain more SP than that found in nonasthmatics (108). These two tachykinins are broken down by a neutral endopeptidase, an enzyme localized in the airway epithelium. At least in *in vitro* studies, when the airway epithelium is damaged, the effect of these peptides is magnified, a situation similar to that found in asthma (109). When such epithelium denudation occurs, the nerve fibers may also be more likely to be exposed to airway stimuli, with an increased susceptibility to irritant exposures, and thereby more prone to bronchoconstriction and edema.

### Neuronal Response Leading to Inflammation

There is evidence suggesting that the neuronal response does not greatly influence mild asthma, but probably is very consequential in chronic asthma. Insight into mechanisms has been stimulated by the recognition that capsaicin pretreatment depletes sensory neuropeptides. Pretreatment with capsaicin in an animal model of allergens prevented airway hyperresponsiveness (although it has little impact on antibody response, lipoxygenase product levels in tissue, or airway mucosal eosinophilia) (110), whereas there was no effect with such pretreatment in an acute model of allergen exposure (111). Not only has SP been recognized to be increased in BAL fluid of asthmatics at baseline and after antigen challenge (112), but in asthmatics who produced sputum after hypertonic saline inhalation, consistent with what may be anticipated considering what is known regarding the effects of SP (airways smooth muscle contraction with increased secretions and mucous plugging and airway wall edema).

### Combined Mechanisms in Asthma

An increasing number of cytokines have been recognized to participate in the immune process. It may be that the dominant controlling cell is the macrophage and much of its control of the immunologic processes are the result of its "suppression" of some of the important cells in the lung. Holt (113) has postulated that the handling of nonpathogenic antigens (such as pollens) includes a combination of dendritic cells and T cells. There is an important interaction between the dendritic cell and T cell, whereby initial antigen processing is the role of the dendritic cell and then presentation to the T cell. With the lung's constant exposure to antigens, the alveolar macrophage cannot possibly interact with all of these T lymphocytes and initiate an inflammatory response. Macrophages suppress an apparently important amount of activity of these stimulated lymphocytes through production of transforming growth factor-$\beta$ (TGF-$\beta$) and IL-1, and other mediators, which possess a downregulating effect on lymphocytes and an important antiinflammatory effect (114,115). Aubas investigated the ability of alveolar macrophages to modulate the lymphoproliferative response to T-cell mitogens in a population of peripheral blood mononuclear cells and showed that the ability of these to control T lymphocytes was less effective in asthmatics (116).

On another front of the immune response, when nonpathogenic antigens such as pollens are encountered, the antigen is presented by the dendritic cell to a certain type of helper T cell ($T_H$). Although the process is not well understood, it appears there the genetic predisposition of the host plays a most important role in the manner in which the antigen is handled. In nonatopics, the antigen is presented to $T_H1$ cells, which secrete IFN-$\gamma$ and suppress $T_H2$ lymphocytes. In atopics, the antigen is presented to $T_H2$ cells, which produce IL-4 and IL-5, cytokines which are B-cell growth factors. This predisposes to the production of IgE antibody. In an animal model, when lung macrophages are depleted, and an immune response delivered into the lung, there is a dramatic increase in systemic levels of IgE and a large influx of primarily CD4$^+$ cells into the airways (117). Overall, neuropeptides appear to play a relatively lesser response, particularly in those asthmatics with mild, occasional disease. Macrophages, dendritic cells, and lymphocytes possess receptors for neuropeptides and interact with these agents.

There remain a number of other inadequately explained aspects of our understanding of the pathogenesis of asthma. For example, why are $\beta$ receptors less responsive to stimulation in asthmatics? What is the importance of airway wall thickening, the result of cellular infiltration, collagen deposition and blood vessel engorgement, and resulting in fibrosis? How do two of the well-recognized features of inflammation, i.e., persistent mucous secretions in the airways and associated airway obstruction, affect the state of asthma and its prognosis?

## Environmental Factors in Interstitial Lung Disease

Although the immune system plays a critical role in the development of dust-induced interstitial lung disease, a variety of factors modify the host response to inhaled dusts. Silicosis, coal workers' pneumoconiosis, and the asbestos-related chest diseases result from long-term inhalational exposure to excessive amounts of inorganic dusts in the workplace. At least with silica and coal dust inhalation, the result is interstitial lung disease; with asbestos exposure, the results can be more complex, and although exposure may lead to interstitial lung disease, the worker may also develop pleural thickening, mesothelioma, lung cancer, and unexplained exudative pleural effusions with sufficient exposure. A detailed discussion of these illnesses is beyond the scope of this chapter (118).

Using silica as an example, the duration and amount of exposure and content of free crystalline silica in the dust are critical determinants of the development and progression of silicosis (119). Over time, the dust burden within the lung is the result of an equilibrium between dust deposition and dust clearance, the result of removal of particles and fibers in the expired air, mucociliary clearance of exogenous materials from the upper airways, and phagocytosis by alveolar macrophages with subsequent clearance by the mucociliary escalator or the pulmonary lymphatics. Particles less than 1 μm in diameter are most pathogenic and are retained in the lung (120). Fiber deposition in the lung is largely ruled by fiber diameter, with fiber length being less important, although there is considerable variability. Fibers up to 300 micrometers long can be found in the lung as long as their diameter is less than 5 μm. The typical fiber length of asbestos bodies is 20 to 50 μm, although many fibers less than 5 μm long can also be found (121).

Host factors that lead to the development of disease or alter the progression of illness are difficult to quantitate and are probably of less importance than dust characteristics. For example, although specific HLA haplotype associations with silicosis have been reported in a Japanese population (122) and HLA haplotype associations with coal workers' pneumoconiosis have been reported in a German population (123), it is difficult to be sure that HLA-based predispositions to fibrosis exist. Perhaps more importantly, when it comes to dust clearance from the lung, the adequacy of the lymphatic drainage in the lung is very important. Experimental exposure to a high concentration of quartz dust produced an alveolar proteinosis response in specific pathogen–free rats but resulted in only the typical granulomatous and fibrotic changes in ordinary stock rats (12). The different histologic response appears to be the degree of development of the lymphatic system, apparently much more developed in the specific pathogen–free rats. Even smoking may somehow alter the way that the lung handles dust as investigators have reported differences in the pulmonary response to hard rock mining exposures by smoking status (125).

Several potential mechanisms for fibrosis are attributed to dust inhalation:

1. Overwhelming of the clearance mechanisms with accumulations of an excessive amount of dust [this appears to be most relevant in association with coal dust exposure (a dust with considerably less fibrogenic potential than silica), which results in the formation of a lesion recognized as the coal macule located in the respiratory bronchiole]
2. Direct cytotoxicity of fibers and dusts—a common theme among these dusts is the presence of free radicals on the surface of the particle or fiber
3. Release of oxidants, enzymes, and cell membrane constituents from alveolar macrophages in association with cell death after particle and fiber exposure
4. Stimulation of cytokine release from alveolar macrophages with subsequent cytokine networking (126)—such cytokine secretion leads to recruitment of effector cells such as neutrophils and monocytes and to stimulation of fibroblast proliferation and collagen synthesis in the area of dust deposition.

### Silicosis

Interactions between alveolar macrophages and inhaled silica are dominant in the development of silicosis. Early work on the pathogenesis of silica-induced lung injury focused on cell damage and cell death occurring after ingestion of silica by alveolar macrophages (127,128). Lung injury was thought the result of ongoing cell digestion caused by the release of intracellular proteolytic enzymes after the disruption and death of the alveolar macrophage. This deadly process is "never ending," because intracellular silica released from the dying macrophage was phagocytized by other macrophages in an attempt to block the inflammatory process attributed to this particle. Current work supports elements of this hypothesis, as silica has recently been shown to induce apoptosis in alveolar macrophages (129).

Inhaled silica stimulates the alveolar macrophage. This cell initiates inflammation and fibrosis through a process of cytokine networking involving macrophages, lymphocytes, neutrophils, fibroblasts, epithelial cells and potentially other cells (130). Silica particles stimulate the alveolar macrophage to secrete cytokines apparently because of their ability to react with water to form hydroxyl radicals. This causes cell membrane lipid peroxidation (and the production of very active leukotrienes, the result of arachidonic acid metabolism) (131,132). The freshly crushed silica forms more hydroxl radicals, is more cytotoxic, produces more lipid peroxidation, and causes alveolar macrophages to produce more superoxide and hydrogen peroxide than does stored or "aged" silica. Signal transduction leading to cytokine production is likely to be mediated at least in part by calcium, as exposure to silica increases cytosolic free calcium in the alveolar macrophages (133,134).

Alveolar macrophages stimulated *in vitro* by silica or evaluated *ex vivo* after *in vivo* exposure to silica are recognized to secrete proinflammatory and profibrogenic mediators such as IL-1 (135,136), IL-6, TNF-α (137,138), TGF-β (a factor that induces the synthesis of extracellular matrix proteins and angiogenesis) (139), fibronectin (140), platelet-derived growth factor (PDGF, a macrophage growth factor that stimulates migration and growth of fibroblasts), and insulin-like growth factor-1 (IGF-1). The presence of these mediators in the tissue milieu are a part of an important network that can alter the activity of other cells. For example, not only macrophages, but pulmonary stromal cells such as endothelial and smooth muscle cells amplify local inflammation by secretion of chemokines such as IL-8 after stimulation by macrophage-derived IL-1 and TNF-α (141). Silica may also stimulate chemokine secretion by alveolar epithelial cells by direct action on these cells (142).

TNF appears to be particularly important in the pathogenesis of silicosis. Increased levels of lung TNF-α mRNA can be demonstrated by *in situ* hybridization in mice after intratracheal instillation of silica. Deposition of extracellular matrix protein (expressed as an increase in hydroxyproline) can be prevented in this model by pretreatment with anti-TNF-α antibodies or blockade of the TNF-α receptor (143). TNF-α–deficient mice show less inflammation and collagen accumulation in the lungs after instillation of silica when compared with healthy mice (144).

The profibrogenic cytokine TGF-β also is important in the pathogenesis of silicosis and can be localized by immunohistochemical staining in peribronchiolar fibrotic lesions, hyaline centers of nodules, progressive massive fibrosis (PMF) lesions, fibroblasts, and alveolar macrophages of human silicotic lungs (145).

## Coal Workers' Pneumoconiosis

Coal workers' pneumoconiosis (CWP) is the result of coal dust induced cell damage with activation of the fibrotic process. Coal dust is much less fibrogenic than silica. A mixture of 10 % silica and 90 % coal is far more cytotoxic to macrophages than pure coal dust (146). However, like silica, when coal dust is cleaved, surface free radicals are measurable. The free radicals generated by crushing anthracite coal (the hardest coal with the most carbon content) are more numerous than those generated from crushing bituminous coal, and in a manner consistent with epidemiologic data, exposure to anthracite coal is associated with a higher risk for development and progression of disease than is exposure to bituminous coal (147).

Long-term coal dust exposure increases the number of alveolar lining cells that can be recovered and a measurable elevation of the number of circulating blood monocytes with an increased rate of mitosis (148,149). This suggests that dust inhalation induces the recruitment of cells into the alveolus from the capillaries and lung interstitium. Recruited young macrophages appear to be more phagocytically active than older macrophages and clear particles more effectively. Although alveolar macrophages in animals are activated after chronic exposure to coal dust, there is relatively little lung damage. Protein and lysosomal enzyme levels in the acellular lavage fluid of these animals are not increased. However, when as little as 2 % silica is added, the fibrosis begins (150).

A number of investigators have applied BAL to evaluate mechanisms of CWP. Lapp showed no difference in BAL total or differential cell counts, IgA or IgG concentration, or spontaneous or stimulated PMA stimulated alveolar macrophage chemoluminescence in miners (without pneumoconiosis) compared with controls (151). In these two groups, there was no difference in the BAL total protein levels, and even though particle-stimulated chemoluminescence was decreased in miners, scanning electron microscopy showed a marked increase in alveolar macrophage cell surface ruffling, a feature consistent with macrophage activation. Transmission electron microscopy showed particles within these macrophages to be consistent with coal.

Others have also recognized the comparative inertness of the BAL fluid in miners with coal dust exposure. Investigators found no significant difference between nonsmoking miners with CWP and controls in the number of cells recovered, BAL cell differentials, and in the release of superoxide anion or hydrogen peroxide from alveolar macrophages. When compared with alveolar lining fluid findings in controls, BAL levels of fibronectin and alveolar-macrophage–derived growth factor (AMDGF), a factor important in mesenchymal cell proliferation) were elevated and no different from the values obtained in subjects with asbestosis and silicosis. Although fibrosis has not been a major part of the pathology of simple CWP, there is evidence of the presence of fibronectin in pneumoconiotic lesions (152).

In contrast, Wallaert demonstrated a significantly increased number of total cells in the BAL recovered from miners with simple and complicated CWP (153). Alveolar cells from miners with simple CWP and an advanced form of this illness, progressive massive fibrosis (PMF), spontaneously released significantly more superoxide, as contrasted to the comparison group. When these alveolar cells were stimulated with phorbol myristic acetate (PMA), only the cells recovered from the miners with PMF showed significantly increased amounts of superoxide release.

Coal-activated macrophages secrete a wide variety of mediators that attract and stimulate macrophages and neutrophils and then stimulate them to release reactive oxygen species, leukotrienes through breakdown of arachidonic acid in the cell membrane, and proteolytic enzymes (154). Excessive release of these reactive oxygen species overcomes the naturally protective antioxidant system and begins inflammation. Similarly, the previously described macrophage-derived inflammatory factors act as chemotactic agents for neutrophils, and increase neutrophil adherence and reactive enzyme release (platelet-derived growth factor and platelet activating factor). Secretion of many of these factors by activated macrophages may enhance fibroblast growth or stimulate the production of collagen. Because of the relatively lesser fibrogenic potential of coal dust, it appears that the lymphatic clearance system must first be overwhelmed before there is a sufficient stimulus for clinically important macrophage product release. The histologic features of silicosis and CWP are compared in Figure 17.3.

## Asbestos

Inflammation begins almost immediately after asbestos fiber exposure. Inhaled fibers are primarily deposited in the bifurcations of the conducting airways, with lesser amounts in the alveolar parenchyma (155). In an animal model, after just an hour of asbestos exposure, there is active uptake of fibers by type I epithelial cells, with high focal concentrations of cytokines, mitogenic factors, and toxic factors, all leading to cell proliferation. Within 48 hours, activated alveolar macrophages are recognized at the alveolar duct bifurcations and stimulation of fibroblasts begin. Depending on the dose and duration of exposure, this focal lesion may progress, forming a localized peribronchiolar fibrosing alveolitis that may inevitably progress to diffuse scarring.

Macrophage-derived cytokines regulate the development and progression of asbestos induced fibrosis. Fibronectin is a glycoprotein produced by the macrophage that has the potential to recruit fibroblasts and initiate fibroblast proliferation. Levels of this cytokine are significantly increased in the BAL fluid of asbestos-exposed worker (156). In asbestos workers without disease, but with asbestos-induced alveolitis, and in those with asbestosis, levels of fibronectin and procollagen 3 (a marker of collagen production) in BAL are significantly elevated. In contrast, excessive levels of these two macrophage-derived substances are not increased after exposure to inert dusts.

In addition to fibronectin, alveolar macrophages recovered from workers with asbestosis release exaggerated quantities

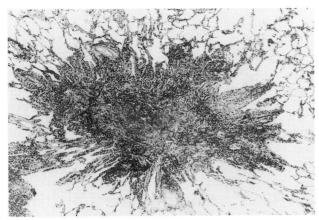
A

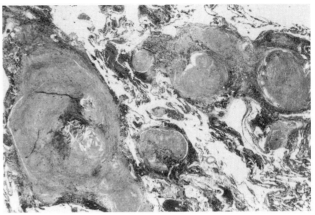
B

**FIG. 17.3. A:** The macular lesion of coal workers' pneumoconiosis (CWP). Near the center of this macule is a collection of coal dust–laden macrophages that completely fill alveolar spaces and extend into the connective tissue surrounding the respiratory bronchioles. A small amount of collagen is deposited, and focal emphysema is seen in the nearby areas. A bronchiole and an accompanying artery are seen in the right upper portion. Collections of coal dust–laden macrophages are evident in the perivascular areas. **B:** Chronic nodular silicosis. Among the mature silicotic nodules, the largest has a central area of necrosis. Each of the nodules in the figure shows a "sworled" pattern of fibrosis of laminated collagen. Around the periphery of the smaller nodules is a cellular infiltrate, the site of active inflammation where enlargement of the nodules occurs. Silica and silicates were seen in the fibrotic area by polarizing microscopy. The small nodules appear to coalesce. These illustrations reflect the different histologic features of silicosis and CWP. Although silicosis is overtly fibrotic, the coal macule appears to be primarily an accumulation of dust at the bifurcation of the respiratory bronchiole, with the gradual development of fibrosis in this setting. The inability to clear these particles, perhaps because of lymphatic blockage attributable to an excessive amount of dust related to the rate of clearance, results in this localized accumulation.

of growth factors, including PDGF, IGF-1, and fibroblast growth factor (FGF) (157–159). These cytokines attract fibroblasts to sites of injury and up-regulate fibroblast activity. These cytokines interact synergistically in a complex cascade of events to induce fibroblast proliferation and form scar, irreversibly altering the structure of the lung.

Damage to the initially injured area is the result of free radicals on the fiber and is aggravated by asbestos-activated macrophages under oxidative stress that release free radicals (160). Mossman provided convincing evidence of this by fitting rats with a "minipump" that infused a "long-life" version of catalase and superoxide dismutase in rats that had received asbestos in the airways. BAL from these treated animals showed fewer total cells and neutrophils, as well as lesser levels of lung protein and hydroxyproline (161). This respiratory burst damages tissue and sustains the inflammatory process by direct cytotoxicity and peroxidation of cell membranes (162,163). Additional destructive substances come from macrophage release of plasminogen activator (164), a protease that converts plasminogen to plasmin and degrades interstitial matrix glycoproteins.

The chronic and progressive inflammation and injury produced by asbestos fibers continues from the time of exposure, through the subclinical phase, to the time when clinical disease is identifiable. During the latency period, before the overt clinical manifestation of the disease is detected by routine clinical tests, inflammation and injury is progressive and involves an increasingly greater number of macrophages and fibroblasts with the formation of scar. This may eventually progress to clinically recognizable asbestosis. Figure 17.4 shows the different histologic manifestations of asbestosis.

### Combined Mechanisms Producing Interstitial Lung Disease

Donaldson has presented a detailed model for the way that the "ideal" inorganic dust particle is handled in the lung (165). In this model, particles are deposited in the terminal bronchiole or into the proximal alveoli. At that point, they are opsonized, a factor that may importantly alter how they are processed, and begin to interact with epithelial cells and with macrophages. Interaction with macrophages results in mediator release (including oxidants, proteases, arachidonic acid metabolites, and different cytokines) and a stimulus toward further interaction with epithelial cells. Inflammation develops, and macrophage and epithelial cell death occur. At this time the particles are transferred into the interstitium and interact and stimulate these interstitial macrophages and fibroblasts toward interstitial inflammation and an influx of further stimulated cells. From here, further cellular proliferation and fibroblast deposition of extracellular matrix are stimulated. The end result is the fibrotic process termed pneumoconiosis.

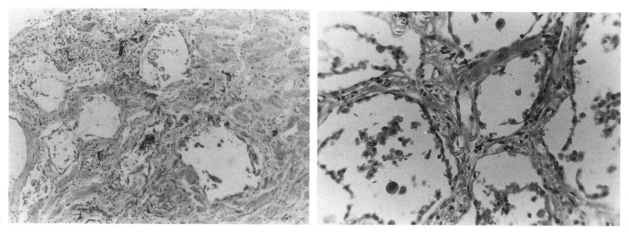

**FIG. 17.4. A:** Histologic findings of advanced asbestosis. The alveoli are nearly obliterated, and there is a tremendous amount of interstitial thickening attributable to dust-induced fibrosis. The fibrosis is advanced, with relatively little interstitial cellular infiltrate. **B:** Mild interstitial inflammation and fibrosis. In both illustrations, the appearance is that of idiopathic pulmonary fibrosis and can be identified only by the presence of asbestos fibers.

## Primary Pulmonary Hypertension

Primary pulmonary hypertension (PPH), also called pulmonary hypertension of unexplained cause (166), most often occurs in women in their third and fourth decades. PPH is reasonably defined as a mean pulmonary artery pressure exceeding 26 mm Hg (but in advanced clinical situations approaching or even exceeding mean systemic arterial pressure), in the presence of normal precapillary pulmonary pressure (i.e. the pulmonary wedge pressure is normal). Although potential secondary causes of pulmonary hypertension may be recognized in an individual patient, these are not of a sufficient severity to explain the elevated pulmonary artery pressures. Although this case definition may appear straightforward, primary pulmonary hypertension may ocur in an individual with coexisting lung disease, where one might expect pulmonary hypertension to be the result of the lung disease (167). This disease is most often diagnosed in its full-blown status (when little evidence of the initial explanation for the development of this illness is present) when the manifestations of right sided heart failure become the defining characteristics. Rubin has recently detailed the diagnostic criteria for this disease (168). Histologic features are shown in Figure 17.5.

Precapillary pulmonary hypertension with clinical and pathologic features similar to PPH can also occur with connective tissue disease, anorexic drug usage, HIV infection and hepatic cirrhosis with portal hypertension (vascular changes found in the pulmonary arteries are identical and described as "plexogenic arteriopathy") with resultant pruning of the peripheral vascular tree and obliterative lesions in the precapillary vessels. In this group of illnesses, the characteristic defect is endothelial cell proliferation (not an important aspect of pulmonary hypertension due to chronic obstructive lung disease or interstitial lung disease) that can be documented by identification of antibodies against a vascular endothelial growth factor (VEGF) receptor (169). This receptor is critical for the development of an intact vasculature. There are two genes for this receptor in the human embryo. Disruption of the first gene results in the inability of the endothelial cells to differentiate with ensuing embryo death, while disruption of the second gene allows for endothelial cell development, but with resulting thin-walled blood vessels that are incompatible with life (170, 171). Effective levels of VEGF likely play an important role in PPH.

One of the major unanswered questions in pulmonary vascular research is why conditions as diverse as those previously described result in the same vascular abnormalities. This finding indicates there probably is a genetic predisposition that is a prerequisite for the development of this type of severe progressive vasculopathy. In support of this idea, some cases of PPH have been recognized as being familial about 6 % of the time (172). The gene responsible for this abnormality has recently been localized and a family member diagnosed through genetic testing (173). In addition, there is an increased frequency of Raynaud's phenomenon and antinuclear antibody in many with PPH, but only few patients with PPH have evidence of specific markers of autoimmune disease (174), although it is sometimes difficult to separate those with PPH from those with connective tissue disease and pulmonary hypertension. There is additional work showing HLA-DR3, HLA-DR52, and HLA-DQ7 alleles to be associated with PPH (175,176). The recognition of a relationship between HLA-DQ7 and PPH may be important as this antigen shares a susceptibility allele with antiphospholipid antibody production. It is not known whether this is solely a marker of coagulation function and a hypercoagulable state or a direct link between the immune system and PPH (177).

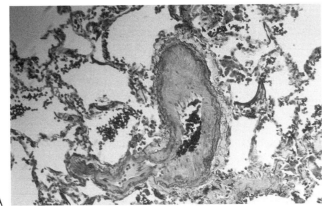

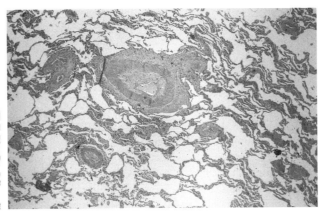

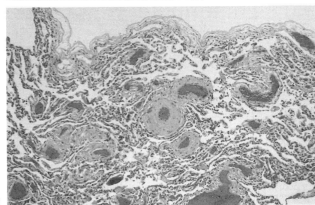

**FIG. 17.5.** Vascular changes in primary pulmonary hypertension. The term *plexogenic* refers to an aneurysmal dilation of the blood vessel wall with the development of vascular channels lined by endothelial cells. This gives a septate appearance to the blood vessels on cross-section. **A:** In this example of a lung stained with Movat's stain, this relatively smaller blood vessel shows a narrow lumen with intimal thickening with fibrous tissue. This is outlined by elastic fibers present in the media. **B:** In this example of pulmonary hypertension stained with hematoxylin and eosin, there is intimal and medial thickening in a small artery. **C:** This represents hematoxylin and eosin staining of the small arteries in pulmonary hypertension. These vessels are altered by intimal thickening and medial hypertrophy, and the pleura is also seen. This amount of thickening in blood vessels located peripherally is abnormal.

There are a series of recognized defects in the blood vessels of patients with PPH. Voelkel has presented a convincing review describing the importance of inflammatory mediators and immunologically mediated mechanisms that partially explain how some of these vascular changes might develop. Inflammation has been recognized as an important aspect of the development of this process, as mediators of angiogenesis (such as tryptase, a product of mast cells), increased levels of leukotrienes, interleukins, and platelet derived growth factor messenger RNA (a factor necessary for the induction of VEGF), and accumulations of macrophages and T and B lymphocytes in areas surrounding hypertrophic capillaries occur (178).

There is increasing amounts of data to suggest that the endothelial cells that multiply in the vessels are of monoclonal origin, implying that a certain cell population descends from one single cell, unlike the vascular changes that develop in secondary pulmonary hypertension (179). Whether this monoclonality is the same for other types of plexiform arteriopathy is not clear. This provides a view of the possibly "malignant" aspects of this disease, and raises important questions regarding the potential approaches to therapy of this disease.

By case-control study methodology, diet drug therapy with fenfluramine and its derivatives were found to be a risk factor in primary pulmonary hypertension development. When associated with drug use, this illness more often occurs with a duration of drug use exceeding 1 year, however, PPH has been reported with less than a month of therapy (180). Although PPH is rare and thought to occur in only 1 of 500,000 persons per year, this rate may increase 30 times with anorexic drug use (181). How this happens is unclear; however, there is speculation regarding an important role for the platelet and release of excessive amounts of platelet-containing serotonin (a pulmonary vessel constricting agent) induced by these drugs. Similar features of intimal proliferation and fibrosis develop in the veins and cardiac muscles of patients with carcinoid syndrome. Alternatively, a direct anorexic drug effect through potassium channel blockade (as was thought when primary pulmonary hypertension was recognized with use of the drug aminorex) has been proposed (182,183).

There appear to be important vascular defects in the blood vessels of those with pulmonary hypertension attributable to a variety of changes (not identical in all cases of this illness [184]). These include medial smooth muscle hypertrophy, intimal thickening, excessive activity of the enzyme serine elastase in the vascular wall resulting in fragmentation of the internal elastic lamina (185), thrombosis *in situ* (typically involving the small veins and arteries), and plexiform changes. Under pathologic conditions, there is a surge in the production of vasoconstrictor, proatherogenic, and growth promoting factors.

Data from a number of laboratories have supported the concept of altered eicosanoid metabolism and a role for arachidonic acid metabolites in the development of the vascular lesions in PPH (186,187). Progressive damage and distortion of the intimal wall allows for increased interactions between the circulating cells and endothelial and vascular smooth muscle cells, perpetuating the injury cycle. Perhaps the two most relevant metabolites are thromboxane $A_2$ ($TXA_2$) and prostacyclin ($PGI_2$). $TXA_2$ is produced in platelets and macrophages and is a potent agonist for platelet aggregation and vasoconstriction and may serve as a cofactor for smooth muscle growth. $PGI_2$ generated by the vascular endothelial cells acts as a inhibitor of platelet function, is a potent vasodilator, and blocks DNA synthesis in vascular smooth muscle cells. Not surprisingly, $PGI_2$ has been used as a therapeutic agent for PPH, but its usefulness has been limited by its short half-life (188).

Two important factors produced by the vascular endothelial cells are endothelium-derived relaxing factor nitric oxide (NO) and endothelium-derived vasoconstrictor peptide endothelin-1 (ET-1). NO is generated through the action of nitric oxide synthase (NOS). There are diminished amounts of NO and excessive amounts of ET-1 in the pulmonary vascular endothelial cells in patients with PPH (189,190). ET-1 exists as "big ET-1" and as its metabolite (ET-1), an active peptide that is a potent vasoconstrictor and mitogenic peptide. These forms are converted by the action of endothelin-converting enzyme (ECE), which exists as isoforms ECE-1 and ECE-2. In the lungs of patients with pulmonary hypertension, staining for NOS was no different from the vessels in control lungs, however, when ECE-1 staining was compared with control vessels, there was intense staining for this enzyme in the blood vessels from the lungs of those with PPH, and less intense staining in those with secondary hypertension (but still more than in the controls) (191).

There remain questions regarding the initiating lesions, how the identified mechanisms interact, and whether other avenues to develop the disease exist, including a better understanding of the uncontrolled growth of endothelial cells. At present, there is a clinical perspective that the imbalance between thromboxane (relative excess) and prostacyclin (relative deficit) can be treated with the continuous infusion of prostacyclin. This appears to be an effective, but relatively cumbersome, mode of therapy (192).

## CONCLUSIONS

There is great potential for pulmonary injury while the mechanisms appear to be complex and involve a different number of cells and a host of mediators. There appear to be dominant mediators in each of the diseases, but it remains unclear how the injury leads to the development of dominant cellular processes and specific manifestations. In many instances, intervening in the release or binding of a dominant mediator can dramatically affect the whole process. Future therapeutic plans need to address the importance of these dominant mediators and cells and focus on blunting their effects.

## REFERENCES

1. Brain JD. Lung macrophages: how many kinds are there? What do they do? *Am Rev Respir Dis* 1988;137:507–509.
2. Crapo JD, Barry BE, Gehr P, et al. Cell number and cell characteristics of the normal human lung. *Am Rev Respir Dis* 1982;125:332–337.
3. Banks DE, Morgan JE, deShazo RD, et al. Reliability of cell counts and protein determinations in serial bronchoalveolar lavage procedures performed on healthy volunteers. *Am J Med Sci* 1990;300:275–282.
4. VanFurth R, Cohn Z. The origin and kinetics of mononuclear phagocytes. *J Exp Med* 1968;128:415.
5. Bowden DH, Adamson IYR. Role of monocytes and interstitial cells in the generation of alveolar macrophages. *Lab Invest* 1980;42:511–517.
6. Castranova V, Bowman L, Reasor M, et al. The response of rat alveolar macrophages to chronic inhalation of coal and/or diesel dust. *Environ Res* 1985;36:405–419.
7. Robinson GR III, Canto RG, Reynolds HY. Host defense mechanisms in respiratory infection. *Immunol Allergy Clin* 1993;13:1–25.
8. Stein M, Keshav S. The versatility of macrophages. *Clin Exp Allergy* 1992;22:19–27.
9. Wright JR. Immunomodulatory function of surfactant. *Physiol Rev* 1997;77:931–962.
10. Kaltreider HB. Macrophages, lymphocytes, and antibody- and cell-mediated immunity. In: Murray J, Nadel J, eds. *Textbook of respiratory medicine.* 2nd ed. Philadelphia: WB Saunders, 1994:370–401.
11. Leijh PCJ, VanFurth R, VanZwet TL, et al. Requirement of extracellular complement and immunoglobulin for intracellular killing of microorganisms by human monocytes. *J Clin Invest* 1979;63:772.
12. Langermans JAM, Hazenbos WLW, VanFurth R. Antimicrobial functions of mononuclear phagocytes. *J Immunol Methods* 1994;174:185–194.
13. Stahl PD. The macrophage mannose receptor: current status. *Am J Respir Cell Mol Biol* 1990;2:317–318.
14. Ezekowitz RA, Sastry K, Bailly P, Warner A. Molecular characterization of the human macrophage mannose receptor demonstration of multiple carbohydrate recognition-like domains and phagocytosis in Cos-1 cells. *J Exp Med* 1990;172:1785–1794.
15. Schlesinger LS. Macrophage phagocytosis of virulent but not attenuated strains of *Mycobacterium tuberculosis* is mediated by mannose receptors in addition to complement receptors. *J Immunol* 1993;150:2920–2930.
16. Rehm SR, Gross GN, Pierce AK. Early bacterial clearance from murine lungs. *J Clin Invest* 1980;66:194–199.
17. Nash TW, Libby DM, Horwitz MA. IFN-gamma activated human alveolar macrophages inhibit intracellular multiplication of *Legionella pneumophila. J Immunol* 1988;140:3978–3981.
18. Wright S, Detmers P, Jong M, Meyer B. Interferon-gamma depresses binding of ligand by C3 and C3bi receptors on cultured human monocytes, an effect reversed by fibronectin. *J Exp Med* 1986;163:1245–1269.
19. Gyetko MR, Toews G. Immunology of the aging lung. *Clin Chest Med* 1993;14:379–391.
20. Oppenheim JJ, Ruscetti FW. Cytokines. In: Stites DP, Terr AI, Parslow TG, eds. *Medical immunology.* 9th ed. Stamford, CT: Appleton & Lange, 1997:146–168.
21. Nathan CF. Secretory products of macrophages. *J Clin Invest* 1987;79:319–326.
22. Hunninghake GW, Gadek JE, Lawley TV, Crystal RG. Mechanisms of neutrophil accumulation in the lungs of patients with idiopathic pulmonary fibrosis. *J Clin Invest* 1981;68:259–269.
23. Hunninghake GW, Garrett KL, Richerson HB, et al. Pathogenesis of granulomatous lung diseases. *Am Rev Respir Dis* 1984;130:476–496.
24. Streiter RM, Chensue SW, Basha MA, et al. Human alveolar macrophage gene expression of interleukin-8 by tumor necrosis factor-alpha, lipopolysaccharide, and interleukin-1 beta. *Am J Respir Cell Mol Biol* 1990;2:321–326.
25. Streiter RM, Phan SH, Showell HJ, et al. Monokine-induced neutrophil chemotactic factor gene expression in human fibroblasts. *J Biol Chem* 1989;264:10621–10626.
26. Tonnel AB, Gosset P, Molet S, et al. Interactions between endothelial cells and effector cells in allergic inflammation. *Ann N Y Acad Sci* 1996;796:9–20.

27. Standiford TJ, Kunkel SL, Basha MA, et al. Interleukin-8 gene expression by pulmonary epithelial cell line. *J Clin Invest* 1990;86:1945–1953.

28. Hunninghake GW, Gadek JE, Fales HM, et al. Human alveolar macrophage-derived chemotactic factor for neutrophils. *J Clin Invest* 1980;66:473–483.

29. Balter MS, Toews GB, Peters-Golden M. Different patterns of arachidonate metabolism in autologous human blood monocytes and alveolar macrophages. *J Immunol* 1989;142:602–608.

30. Rizzato G. Clinical impact of bone and calcium metabolism changes in sarcoidosis. *Thorax* 1998;53:425–429.

31. Robinson B, McLemore T, Crystal R. gamma interferon is spontaneously produced by alveolar macrophages and lung T lymphocytes in patients with pulmonary sarcoidosis. *J Clin Invest* 1985;72:1488–1495.

32. Shapiro SD. Elastolytic metalloproteinases produced by human mononuclear phagocytes: potential roles in destructive lung disease. *Am J Respir Crit Care Med* 1994;150:S160–S164.

33. Willenbrock F, Murphy G. Structure-function relationships in tissue inhibitors of metalloproteinases. *Am J Respir Crit Care Med* 1994;150: S165–S170.

34. Liu L, Mul FPJ, Kuijpers TW, et al. Neutrophil transmigration across monolayers of endothelial cells and airway epithelial cells is regulated by different mechanisms. *Ann N Y Acad Sci* 1996;796:21–29.

35. Hamacher J, Schaberg T. Adhesion molecules in lung diseases. *Lung* 1994;172:189–213.

36. Goldstein IM, Shak S. Host defenses in the lung: neutrophils, complement, and other humoral mediators. In: Murray J, Nadel J, eds. *Textbook of respiratory medicine*. 2nd ed. Philadelphia: WB Saunders, 1994:402–418.

37. Talbott GA, Sharar SR, Harlan JM, et al. Leukocyte-endothelial interactions and organ injury: the role of adhesion molecules. *New Horiz* 1994;2:545–554.

38. Sibille Y, Reynolds HY. Macrophages and polymorphonuclear neutrophils in lung defense and injury. *Am Rev Respir Dis* 1990;141: 471–501.

39. Ricevuti G. Host tissue damage by phagocytes. *Ann N Y Acad Sci* 1997;832:426–448.

40. Bowden DH, Adamson IYR. The pulmonary interstitial cell as immediate precursor of the alveolar macrophage. *Am J Pathol* 1972;78: 521–536.

41. Weissler JC, Lyons RC, Lipscomb MF, Toews G. Human pulmonary macrophages. *Am Rev Respir Dis* 1986;133:473–477.

42. Holt PG, Schon-Hegrad MA, Oliver J, et al. A contiguous network of dendritic antigen-presenting cells within the respiratory epithelium. *Int Arch Allergy Appl Immunol* 1990;91:155–159.

43. Steinman RM. The dendritic cell system and its role in immunogenicity. *Annu Rev Immunol* 1991;9:271–296.

44. Havenith CE, Breedijk AJ, Hoefsmit EC. Effect of bacillus Calmette-Guerin inoculation on numbers of dendritic cells in bronchoalveolar lavages of rats. *Immunobiology* 1992;184:336–347.

45. McWilliam AS, Nelson DJ, Holt PG. Rapid dendritic cell recruitment is a hallmark of the acute inflammatory response at mucosal surfaces. *J Exp Med* 1994;179:1331–1336.

46. Nicod LP, Lipscomb MF, Weissler JC, et al. Mononuclear cells in human lung parenchyma: characterization of a potent accessory cell not obtained by bronchoalveolar lavage. *Am Rev Respir Dis* 1987; 136:818.

47. Romagnani S. Biology of human T$_H$1 and T$_H$2 cells. *J Clin Immunol* 1995;15:121–129.

48. Maestrelli P, O'Heir RE, Tsai JJ, et al. Antigen-induced neutrophil chemotactic factor derived from cloned human T lymphocytes. *Immunology* 1988;65:605–609.

49. Shelhamer JH, ed. Airway inflammation. *Ann Intern Med* 1995;123: 288–304.

50. O' Byrne PM, Dolovich J, Hargreave FE. Late asthmatic responses. *Am Rev Respir Dis* 1987;136:740–751.

51. Drazen JM, Turino G. Progress at the interface of inflammation and asthma: workshop report. *Am J Respir Crit Care Med* 1995;152: 385–424.

52. Fabbri LM, Ciaccia A. Investigative bronchoscopy in asthma and other airways diseases. *Eur Respir J* 1992;5:8–11.

53. Pin I, Gibson PG, Kolendowicz R, et al. Use of induced sputum cell counts to investigate airway inflammation in asthma. *Thorax* 1992;47: 25–29.

54. Fahy JV, Liu J, Wong H, et al. Analysis of cellular and biochemical constituents in induced sputum after allergen challenge: a method for studying allergic airway inflammation. *J Allergy Clin Immunol* 1994; 93:1031–1039.

55. Burrows B, Martinez FD, Halonen M, et al. Association of asthma with serum IgE levels and skin test reactivity to allergens. *N Engl J Med* 1989;320:271.

56. National Heart, Lung, and Blood Institute. Guidelines for the diagnosis and management of asthma. National asthma education and prevention program. Expert panel report 2: clinical practice guidelines. NIH publication no. 97-4051. Bethesda: National Institutes of Health, April, 1997.

57. Dunnill MS. The pathology of asthma, with special reference to changes in the bronchial mucosa. *J Clin Pathol* 1960;13:27–33.

58. Fabbri LM, Danieli D, Crescioli S, et al. Fatal asthma in a subject sensitized to toluene diisocyanate. *Am Rev Respir Dis* 1988;137: 1494–1498.

59. Saetta M, Di Stefano A, Maestrelli P, et al. Airway mucosal inflammation in occupational asthma induced by toluene diisocyanate. *Am Rev Respir Dis* 1992;145:160–168.

60. Laitinen LA, Heino M, Laitinen A, et al. Damage of the airway epithelium and bronchial reactivity in patients with asthma. *Am Rev Respir Dis* 1985;131:599–606.

61. Nakamura H, Abe S, Shibata Y, et al. Elevated levels of cytokeratin 19 in the bronchoalveolar lavage fluid of patients with chronic airway inflammatory diseases—a specific marker for bronchial epithelial injury. *Am J Respir Crit Care Med* 1997;155:1217–1221.

62. Polito AJ, Proud D. Epithelial cells as regulators of airway inflammation. *J Allergy Clin Immunol* 1998;102:714–718.

63. Saetta M, Fabbri LM, Danieli D, et al. Pathology of bronchial asthma and animal models of asthma. *Eur Respir J* 1989;2[Suppl 6]:477–482.

64. Beasley R, Roche WR, Roberts JA, et al. Cellular events in the bronchi in mild asthma and after bronchial provocation. *Am Rev Respir Dis* 1989;139:806–817.

65. Saetta M, Di Stefano A, Maestrelli P, et al. Activated T-lymphocytes and macrophages in bronchial mucosa of subjects with chronic bronchitis. *Am Rev Respir Dis* 1993;147:301–306.

66. Saetta M, Maestrelli P, Di Stefano A, et al. Effect of cessation of exposure to toluene diisocyanate (TDI) in bronchial mucosa of subjects with TDI-induced asthma. *Am Rev Respir Dis* 1992;145:169–174.

67. Saetta M, Maestrelli P, Mapp CE, et al. Airway remodeling in isocyanate induced asthma. *Am J Respir Crit Care Med* 1995;151: 489–494.

68. Roche WR. Fibroblasts and asthma. *Clin Exp Allergy* 1991;21: 545–548.

69. Humbert M, Durham SR, Ying S, et al. IL-4 and IL-5 and protein in bronchial biopsies from patients with atopic and nonatopic asthma: evidence against "intrinsic" asthma being a distinct immunopathologic entity. *Am J Respir Crit Care Med* 1996;154:1497–1504.

70. Walker C, Bode E, Boer L, et al. Allergic and intrinsic asthmatics have distinct patterns of T-cell activation and cytokine production in peripheral blood and BAL. *Am Rev Respir Dis* 1992;148:109–115.

71. Virchow JC Jr, Kroegel C, Walker C, et al. Inflammatory determinants of asthma severity: mediator and cellular changes in bronchoalveolar lavage fluid of patients with severe asthma. *J Allergy Clin Immunol* 1996;98:S27–S40.

72. Lindblad JH, Farr RS. The incidence of positive intradermal reactions and the demonstration of skin sensitizing antibody to extracts of ragweed and dust in humans without any history of rhinitis or asthma. *J Allergy* 1961;32:392.

73. Thien FCK, Leung RCC, Czarny D, et al. Indoor allergens and IgE-mediated respiratory illness. *Immunol Allergy Clin* 1994;14:567–590.

74. Montanaro A, Bardana EJ Jr. Mechanisms of allergic asthma. *Immunol Allergy Clin* 1992;12:291–305.

75. Harding CV. Cellular and molecular aspects of antigen processing and the function of class II MHC molecules. *Am J Respir Cell Mol Biol* 1993;8:461–467.

76. Robinson DS, Hamid Q, Bentley A, et al. Activation of CD4$^+$ cells, increased T$_H$2-type cytokine mRNA expression, and eosinophil recruitment in bronchoalveolar lavage after allergen inhalation challenge in patients with atopic asthma. *J Allergy Clin Immunol* 1993;92: 313–324.

77. Robinson DS, Hamid Q, Sun Ying, et al. Prednisone treatment in bronchial asthma: clinical improvement is accompanied by reduction in bronchoalveolar lavage eosinophilia and modulation of n-4, n-5 and IFN-gamma cytokine gene expression. *Am Rev Respir Dis* 1993;148: 401–406.

78. Corrigan CJ, Kay AB. CD4+ T-lymphocyte activation in acute severe asthma. Relationship to disease severity and atopic status. *Am Rev Respir Dis* 1990;141:970–977.

79. Corrigan CJ, Haczku A, Gemou-Engesaeth V, et al. CD4 T-lymphocyte activation in asthma is accompanied by increased serum concentration of interleukin-5. Effect of glucocorticoid therapy. *Am Rev Respir Dis* 1993;147:540–547.

80. Bradding P, Feather IH, Howarth PH, et al. Interleukin-4 is localized to and released by human mast cells. *J Exp Med* 1992;176:1381–1386.

81. Kay AB, Corrigan CJ, Frew AJ. The role of cellular immunology in asthma. *Eur Respir J* 1991;4:105s–112s.

82. Azzawi M, Bradley B, Jeffrey PK, et al. Identification of activated T lymphocytes and eosinophils in bronchial biopsies in stable atopic asthma. *Am Rev Respir Dis* 1990;142:1407–1413.

83. Bradley BL, Azzawi M, Jacobson M, et al. Eosinophils, T-lymphocytes, mast cells, neutrophils and macrophages in bronchial biopsy specimens from atopic subjects with asthma: comparison with biopsy specimens from atopic subjects without asthma and normal control subjects and relationship to bronchial hyperresponsiveness. *J Allergy Clin Immunol* 1991;88:661–674.

84. Bentley AM, Maestrelli P, Saetta M, et al. Activated T-lymphocytes and eosinophils in the bronchial mucosa in isocyanate-induced asthma. *J Allergy Clin Immunol* 1992;89:821–829.

85. Bentley AM, Menz G, Storz C, et al. Identification of T-lymphocytes, macrophages, and activated eosinophils in the bronchial mucosa in intrinsic asthma: relationship to symptoms and bronchial responsiveness. *Am Rev Respir Dis* 1992;146:500–506.

86. Walker PR, Fellowes R, Hecht EM, et al. Characterization of streptococcal antigen-specific CD8+ II; MHC class I-restricted T cell clones that down-regulate in vitro antibody synthesis. *J Immunol* 1991;147: 3370–3380.

87. Kita O, Weiler D, Sur S, et al. IL-5 is the predominant eosinophil-active cytokine in the antigen-induced pulmonary late-phase reaction. *Am Rev Respir Dis* 1993;147:901–907.

88. Hamid Q, Azzawi M, Ying S, et al. Expression of mRNA for interleukin-5 in mucosal bronchial biopsies from asthma. *J Clin Invest* 1991;87:1541–1546.

89. Shi H-Z, Deng J-M, Xu H, et al. Effect of inhaled Interleukin-4 on airway hyperresponsiveness in asthmatics. *Am J Respir Crit Care Med* 1998;157:1818–1821.

90. Weller PF. Human eosinophils. *J Allergy Clin Immunol* 1997;100: 283–287.

91. Viksman MY, Liu MC, Bickel CA, et al. Phenotypic analysis of alveolar macrophages and monocytes in allergic airway inflammation. *Am J Respir Crit Care Med* 1997;155:858–863.

92. Gant W, Cluzel M, Shakoor Z, et al. Alveolar macrophage accessory cell function in bronchial asthma. *Am Rev Respir Dis* 1992;146: 900–904.

93. Busse WW. Leukotrienes and inflammation. *Am J Respir Crit Care Med* 1998;157:S210–S213.

94. Lamblin C, Gosset P, Tillie-Leblond I, et al. Bronchial neutrophilia in patients with noninfectious status asthmaticus. *Am J Respir Crit Care Med* 1998;157:394–402.

95. Richardson JB. Nerve supply to the lungs. *Am Rev Respir Dis* 1979; 119:785–802.

96. Lantz RC, Dey R. Mechanisms of nonallergic asthma. *Immunol Allergy Clin* 1992;12:307–327.

97. Kaliner M, Shelhammer J, Davis PB, et al. Autonomic nervous system abnormalities and allergy. *Ann Intern Med* 1982;96:349.

98. Barnes PJ. Neuroeffector mechanisms: the interface between inflammation and neuronal interface. *J Allergy Clin Immunol* 1996;98: S73–83.

99. Richardson JB, Ferguson CC. Neuromuscular structure and function in the airways. *Fed Proc* 1979;38:202.

100. Barnes PJ. Endogenous catecholamines and asthma. *J Allergy Clin Immunol* 1986;77:791–795.

101. Cerrina J, Ladurie ML, Labat C, et al. Comparison of human bronchial muscle responses to histamine in vivo with histamine and isoproterenol antagonists in vitro. *Am Rev Respir Dis* 1986;134:57–61.

102. Barnes PJ. Modulation of neurotransmission in airways. *Physiol Res* 1993;52:521–528.

103. Barnes PJ, Baraniuk J, Belvisi MG. Neuropeptides in the respiratory tract. *Am Rev Respir Dis* 1991;144:1187–1198.

104. Ollerenshaw S, Jarvis D, Woolcock A, et al. Absence of immunoreactive vasoactive intestinal peptide in tissue from the lungs of patients with asthma. *N Engl J Med* 1989;320:1244.

105. Mak JCW, Barnes PJ. Autoradiographic localization of calcitonin gene-related peptide binding sites in human and guinea-pig lung. *Peptides* 1988;9:957–964.

106. Dey RD, Hoffpauir J, Said SI. Colocalization of vasoactive intestinal peptide and substance P containing nerves in cat bronchi. *Neuroscience* 1988;24:275.

107. Kuo H-P, Rhode JAL, Tokuyama K, et al. Capsaicin and other sensory neuropeptide stimulation of goblet cell secretion in guinea pig trachea. *J Physiol* 1990;4313:629–641.

108. Ollerenshaw S, Jarvis D, Sullivan CE, et al. Substance P immunoreactive nerves in airways from asthmatics and nonasthmatics. *Eur Respir J* 1991;4:673–682.

109. Frossard N, Rhoden KJ, Barnes PJ. Influence of epithelium on guinea-pig airway responses to tachykinins: role of endopeptidase and cyclooxygenase. *J Pharmacol Exp Ther* 1989;248:292–298.

110. Matsuse T, Thomson RJ, Chen X-R, et al. Capsaicin inhibits airway hyperresponsiveness but not lipoxygenase activity or eosinophilia after repeated aerosolized antigen in guinea pigs. *Am Rev Respir Dis* 1991; 144:368–372.

111. Lotvall JO, Hui KP, Lofdahl C-G, et al. Capsaicin pretreatment does not inhibit allergen-induced airway microvascular leakage in guinea-pig. *Allergy* 1991;4:673–682.

112. Nieber K, Baumgarten CR, Rathsack R, et al. Substance P and beta-endorphin-like immunoreactivity in lavage fluids of subjects with and without allergic asthma. *J Allergy Clin Immunol* 1992;90:646–652.

113. Holt PG. Initiation and modulation of immune reactions in the lung. In: Walters EH, duBois RM, eds. *Immunology and management of interstitial lung diseases*. London: Chapman & Hall, 1995:1–18.

114. Roth MD, Golub SH. Human pulmonary macrophages utilize prostaglandins and transforming factor beta (1) to suppress lymphocyte activation. *J Leukoc Biol* 1993;53:366–371.

115. Moore SA, Streiter RM, Rolfe MW, et al. Expression and regulation of human alveolar macrophage-derived interleukin-1 receptor antagonist. *Am J Respir Cell Mol Biol* 1992;6:569–572.

116. Aubas P, Cosso B, Godard PH, et al. Decreased suppressor cell activity of alveolar macrophages in bronchial asthma. *Am Rev Respir Dis* 1984;130:875–878.

117. Thepen T, McMenamin C, Girn B, et al. Regulation of IgE production in presensitized animals: in vitro elimination of alveolar macrophages preferentially increases IgE responses to inhaled allergen. *Clin Exp Allergy* 1992;22:1107–1114.

118. Banks DE, Parker JE, eds. *Occupational lung diseases: an international perspective*. London: Arnold Publishing, 1998.

119. Hughes JM, Jones RN, Gilson JC, et al. Determinants of progression in sandblaster's silicosis. *Ann Occup Hyg* 1982;26:710–716.

120. Silicosis and Silicate Disease Committee. Diseases associated with exposure to silica and nonfibrous silicate minerals. *Arch Pathol Lab Med* 1988;112:673–720.

121. Sébastien P. La biométrologie des fibres inhalées. PhD thesis, 1982, Paris XII University, France.

122. Honda K, Kimura A, Dong R-P, et al. Immunogenetic analysis of silicosis in Japan. *Am J Respir Cell Mol Biol* 1993;8:106–111.

123. Rihs HP, Lipps P, May-Taube K, et al. Immunogenetic studies on HLA-DR in German coal miners with and without coal workers' pneumoconiosis. *Lung* 1994;172:347–354.

124. Eden K, Seebach HV. Atypical dust-induced pneumoconiosis in SPF rats. *Virchows Arch (Pathol Anat)* 1976;372:1–9.

125. Kreiss K, Greenberg L, Kogut S, et al. Hard-rock mining exposures affect smokers and nonsmokers differently. *Am Rev Respir Dis* 1989;139:1487–1493.

126. Lapp NL, Castranova V. How silicosis and coal workers' pneumoconiosis develops—a cellular assessment. In: *Occupational medicine: state of the art reviews*. Philadelphia: Hanley & Belfus, 1993:35–65.

127. Allison A, Harrington J, Birbeck M. An examination of the cytotoxic effects of silica on macrophages. *J Exp Med* 1966;124:141–154.

128. Bowden D, Adamson L. The role of cell injury and the continuing inflammatory response in the generation of silicotic pulmonary fibrosis. *J Pathol* 1981;144:149–161.

129. Iyer R, Hamilton RF, Li L, et al. Silica-induced apoptosis mediated via scavenger receptor in human alveolar macrophages. *Toxicol Appl Pharm* 1996;141:84–92.

130. Vanhee D, Gosset P, Boitelle A, et al. Cytokines and cytokine network in silicosis and coal workers' pneumoconiosis. *Eur Respir J* 1995;8:834–842.

131. Vallyathan V, Xianglin S, Dalal N, et al. Generation of free radicals from freshly fractured silica dust. *Am Rev Respir Dis* 1988;138:1213–1219.

132. Ghio AJ, Kennedy TP, Schapira RM, et al. Hypothesis: is lung disease after silicate inhalation caused by oxidant generation? *Lancet* 1990;336:967–969.

133. Chen J, Armstrong LC, Liu S, et al. Silica increases cytosolic free calcium ion concentration of alveolar macrophages in vitro. *Toxicol Appl Pharm* 1991;111:211–220.

134. Rojanasakul Y, Wang L, Malanga CJ, et al. Altered calcium homeostasis and cell injury in silica-exposed alveolar macrophages. *J Cell Physiol* 1993;154:310–316.

135. Schmidt J, Oliver C, Lepe-Zuniga J, et al. Silica-stimulated monocytes release fibroblast proliferation factors identical to interleukin 1. A potential role for interleukin 1 in the pathogenesis of silicosis. *J Clin Invest* 1984;73:1462–1472.

136. Oghiso Y, Kubota Y. Enhanced interleukin 1 production by alveolar macrophages in Ia-positive lung cells in silica-exposed rats. *Microbiol Immunol* 1986;30:1189–1198.

137. Piquet P, Collart MA, Grau J, et al. Requirement of tumour necrosis factor for development of silica-induced pulmonary fibrosis. *Nature* 1990;344:245–247.

138. Mohr C, Gemsa D, Graebner C, et al. Systemic macrophage stimulation in rats with silicosis: enhanced release of tumor necrosis factor-alpha from alveolar and peritoneal macrophages. *Am J Respir Cell Mol Biol* 1991;5:395–402.

139. Williams AO, Flanders KC, Saffiotti U. Immunohistochemical localization of transforming growth factor-beta 1 in rats with experimental silicosis, alveolar type II hyperplasia, and lung cancer. *Am J Pathol* 1993;142:1831–1840.

140. Rom WN, Bitterman PB, Rennard SI, et al. Characterization of the lower respiratory tract inflammation of nonsmoking individuals with interstitial lung disease associated with chronic inhalation of inorganic dust. *Am Rev Respir Dis* 1987;136:1429–1434.

141. Lukacs NW, Kunkel SL, Allen R, et al. Stimulus and cell-specific expression of C-X-C and C-C chemokines by pulmonary stromal cell populations. *Am J Physiol* 1995;268:1856–1861.

142. Driscoll KE, Howard BW, Carter JM, et al. Alpha-quartz induced chemokine expression by rat lung epithelial cells: effects of in vivo and in vitro particle exposure. *Am J Pathol* 1996;149:1627–1637.

143. Piquet P, Vesin C. Treatment by human recombinant soluble TNF receptor of pulmonary fibrosis induced by bleomycin or silica in mice. *Eur Respir J* 1994;7:515–518.

144. Davis G, Hill-Eubanks L, Pfeiffer L, et al. Reduced silicosis in C3H/HeJ-LPSd mice: an implied role for cytokine production deficiency. *Am Rev Respir Dis* 1992;145:A325(abst).

145. Jagirdar J, Begin R, Dufresne A, et al. Transforming growth factor-β in silicosis. *Am J Respir Crit Care Med* 1996;154:1076–1081.

146. Adamis Z, Timlar T. Studies on the effect of quartz, bentonite, and coal dust mixtures on macrophages in vitro. *Br J Exp Pathol* 1978;59:411–419.

147. Dalal NS, Suryan MM, Vallyathan V, et al. Detection of reactive free radicals in fresh coal mine dusts and their implication for pulmonary injury. *Ann Occup Hyg* 1989;33:79–84.

148. Castranova V, Bowman L, Reasor M, et al. The response of rat alveolar macrophages to chronic inhalation of coal dust and/or diesel inhalation. *Environ Res* 1985;36:405–419.

149. Adamson IYR, Bowden DH. Adaptive responses of the pulmonary macrophagic system to carbon: II. Morphologic studies. *Lab Invest* 1978;38:430–438.

150. Ray SC, King EJ, Harrison CV. The action of small amounts of quartz and large amounts of coal and graphite on the lungs of rats. *Br J Indust Med* 1951;8:68–73.

151. Lapp NL, Lewis D, Schwegler-Berry D, et al. Bronchoalveolar lavage in asymptomatic coal miners. In: Franz RL, Ramadi RV, eds. *Third symposium of respiratory dusts in the mineral industry.* Littleton, CO: Society of Mining, Metallurgy, and Exploration, Inc.1991:159–169.

152. Wagner JC, Burns J, Munday DE, et al. Presence of fibronectin in pneumoconiotic lesions. *Thorax* 1982;37:54–56.

153. Wallaert B, Lassalle P, Fortin F, et al. Superoxide anion generation by alveolar inflammatory cells in simple pneumoconiosis and in progressive massive fibrosis of non-smoking coal miners. *Am Rev Respir Dis* 1990;141:129–133.

154. Borm PJA, Henderson PT. Symposium on the health effects of occupational exposures to inorganic dusts. *Exp Lung Res* 1990;16:1–3.

155. Rom WN, Travis WD, Brody AR. Cellular and molecular basis of the asbestos-related diseases. *Am Rev Respir Dis* 1991;143:408–422.

156. Bégin R, Cantin A, Berthiaume Y, et al. Clinical features to stage alveolitis in asbestos workers. *Am J Indust Med* 1985;8:521–536.

157. Bégin R, Cantin A, Massé S. Recent advances in the clinical assessment and pathogenesis of the mineral dust pneumoconiosis. *Eur Respir J* 1989;2:988–1001.

158. Rom WN, Travis WD, Brody AR. Cellular and molecular basis of the asbestos-related diseases. *Am Rev Respir Dis* 1991;143:408–422.

159. Bégin R, Ostiguy R, Fillion R, et al. Recent advances in the early diagnosis of asbestosis. *Semin Roentgenol* 1992;27:121–139.

160. Gilmour P, Beswick PH, Donaldson K. Detection of surface free radical activity of respirable industrial fibers using supercoiled plasmid DNA. *Carcinogenesis* 1995;16:2973–2979.

161. Mossman BT, Marsh JP, Sesko A, et al. Inhibition of lung injury, inflammation and interstitial pulmonary fibrosis by polyethylene glyco-conjugated catalase in a rapid inhalation model of asbestosis. *Am Rev Respir Dis* 1990;141:1266–1271.

162. Kamp DW, Graceppa P, Pryor WA, et al. The role of free radicals in asbestos-induced diseases. *Free Radic Biol Med* 1992;12:293–315.

163. Mossman BT, Marsh JP, Sesko A, et al. Inhibition of lung injury, inflammation, and interstitial pulmonary fibrosis by polyethylene-conjugated catalase in a rapid inhalation model of asbestosis. *Am Rev Respir Dis* 1990;141:1266–1271.

164. Cantin A, Allard C, Bégin R. Increased alveolar plasminogen activator in early asbestosis. *Am Rev Respir Dis* 1989;139:604–609.

165. Donaldson K. Mechanisms of pneumoconiosis. In: Banks DE, Parker JE, eds. *Occupational lung diseases: an international perspective.* London: Arnold Publishing, 1998:139–160.

166. Hatano S, Strasser T, eds. *Primary pulmonary hypertension: report of the committee.* Geneva: World Health Organization, 1975.

167. The International Primary Pulmonary Hypertension study group. The International Primary Pulmonary Hypertension Study. *Chest* 1994;105:37S–41S.

168. Rubin LJ. Current concepts: primary pulmonary hypertension. *N Engl J Med* 1997;336:111–117.

169. Tuder RM, Groves B, Badesch DB, et al. Exuberant endothelial cell growth and elements of inflammation are present in plexiform lesions of pulmonary hypertension. *Am J Pathol* 1995;144:275–285.

170. Shalaby F, Ho J, Stanford WL, et al. A requirement for flk 1 in primitive and definitive hematopoiesis and vasculogenesis. *Cell* 1997;99:981–990.

171. Millauer B, Wizigmann-Voos S, Schnurch H, et al. High affinity VEGF binding and development expression suggest flk-1 as a major regulator of vasculogenesis and angiogenesis. *Cell* 1993;72:835–846.

172. Rich S, Dantzker DR, Ayres S, et al. Primary pulmonary hypertension: a national prospective study. *Ann Intern Med* 1987;216–223.

173. Nichols CW, Koller DL, Slovis B, et al. Localization of the gene for familial primary pulmonary hypertension to gene 2q 31-32. *Nat Genet* 1997;15:277–280.

174. Rich S, Kieras K, Hart K, et al. Antinuclear antibodies in primary pulmonary hypertension. *J Am Coll Cardiol* 1986;18:1307–1311.

175. Barst RJ, Flaster ER, Menon A, et al. Evidence for the association of unexplained pulmonary hypertension in children with the major histocompatibility complex and outcome. *Circulation* 1992;85:249–258.

176. Morse JH, Zhang Y, Fotinon M, et al. Primary pulmonary hypertension (PPH) is associated with HLA-DQ7 (DBQ1*0301) in Caucasians. *Circulation* 1994;90:1–149.

177. Barst RJ, Loyd JE. Genetics and immunogenetic aspects of primary pulmonary hypertension. *Chest* 1998;114:231S–236S.

178. Voelkel NF, Cool C, Lee SD, et al. Primary pulmonary hypertension between inflammation and cancer. *Chest* 1998;114:225S–230S.

179. Lee S-D, Shroyer KR, Markham NE, et al. Monoclonal endothelial cell proliferation is present in primary but not secondary pulmonary hypertension. *J Clin Invest* 1998;101:927–934.

180. Mark EJ, Patalas ED, Chang HT, et al. Fatal pulmonary hypertension associated with short-term use of fenfluramine and phentermine. *N Engl J Med* 1997;337:602–606.

181. Abenhaim J, Moride Y, Brenot F, et al. Appetite-suppresant drugs and the risk of primary pulmonary hypertension. *N Engl J Med* 1996;335: 609–616.

182. Hervé P, Launay J-M, Scrobohaci M-L, et al. Increased serotonin in primary pulmonary hypertension. *Am J Med* 1995;99:249–255.

183. Michelakis ED, Archer SL, Huang JMC, et al. Anorexic agents inhibit potassium current in pulmonary artery smooth muscle. *Am J Respir Crit Care Med* 1995;151[Suppl]:A725.

184. Loyd JE, Atkinson JB, Pietra GG, et al. Heterogeneity of pathologic lesions in familial primary pulmonary hypertension. *Am Rev Respir Dis* 1988;138:952–957.

185. Rabinovitch M. Elastase and the pathobiology of unexplained pulmonary hypertension. *Chest* 1998;114:213S–224S.

186. Barst RJ, Rubin LJ, Long WA, et al. A comparison of continuous intravenous epoprostenol (prostacyclin) with conventional therapy in primary pulmonary hypertension. *N Engl J Med* 1997;327:70–75.

187. Christman BW. Lipid mediator dysregulation in primary pulmonary hypertension. *Chest* 1998;114:213S–224S.

188. Ko FN. Low-affinity thromboxane receptor mediates proliferation in cultured vascular smooth muscle cells of rats. *Arterioscler Thromb Vasc Biol* 1997;17:1274–1282.

189. Giaid A, Yanagisawa M, Langleben D, et al. Expression of endothelin-1 in the lungs of patients with pulmonary hypertension. *N Engl J Med* 1993;328:1732–1739.

190. Giaid A, Saleh D. Reduced expression of endothelial nitric oxide synthase in the lungs of patients with pulmonary hypertension. *N Engl J Med* 1995;333:214–221.

191. Giaid A. Nitric oxide and endothelin-1 in pulmonary hypertension. *Chest* 1998;114:208S–212S.

192. Barst RJ, Rubin LJ, McGoon D, et al. Survival in primary pulmonary hypertension with continuous intravenous prostacyclin (epoprostenol): results of a randomized trial. *Ann Intern Med* 1994;121:409–415.

*Textbook of the Autoimmune Diseases,*
Edited by R. G. Lahita, N. Chiorazzi, and W. H. Reeves,
Lippincott Williams & Wilkins, Philadelphia © 2000.

# CHAPTER 18

# Renal Autoimmunity

Michael G. Robson and Mark J. Walport

The diseases that are discussed in the following sections are widely thought to be autoimmune in origin. A full discussion of the evidence for this is beyond the scope of this chapter, but in general terms, it is based on the presence of immune deposits and cells of the immune system in renal biopsies; the presence of immunologic abnormalities in the blood (*e.g.* reduced complement levels, or complement activation products); a response to immunosuppressive treatment; and animal models with similar histologic features that are initiated by immunologic insults. Our limited understanding of the cause of these processes means that treatment has included systemic immunosuppression with its associated side effects. It is is hoped that a better understanding of the pathogenesis of these diseases will lead to therapy that is more specific, more effective, and less toxic.

Several important autoimmune diseases affecting the kidney have been excluded from this chapter because they affect other organs in the body and are discussed elsewhere in this book. These include antiglomerular basement membrane disease, small vessel vasculitides, systemic lupus erythematosus (SLE), and cryoglobulinemia. Most primary renal diseases that are thought to be autoimmune in origin affect the glomerulus. Consequently, this chapter is largely concerned with glomerular diseases. The topics discussed include IgA nephropathy, membranous nephropathy (MN), idiopathic nephrotic syndrome [minimal change nephropathy (MCN) and focal segmental glomerulosclerosis (FSGS)], mesangio-capillary glomerulonephritis (MCGN), and postinfectious glomerulonephritis. There is also an account of acute tubulointerstitial nephritis.

It is difficult to be sure of the frequency of the diseases discussed in this chapter. They can only be diagnosed histologically, and therefore an estimate of their frequency depends on the local indications for performing a renal biopsy. Many are rare diseases, and the collection of reliable information depends on collaborative databases. The Italian registry of renal biopsies published their findings over a 7-year period, during which almost 14,000 native renal biopsies were performed. The frequency and distribution of the primary glomerular diseases varied little over this period (1). The incidence of primary glomerular diseases for 1993 are shown in Table 18.1. Poststreptococcal glomerulonephritis (PSGN) has a much higher incidence in other parts of the world.

Glomerular disease manifests with a restricted number of clinical features. These include proteinuria (if severe, then leading to the nephrotic syndrome), hematuria (microscopic or macroscopic), hypertension, and renal impairment. These are largely nonspecific, and although they may point to the glomerulus as the cause of the problem, they do not help in defining the specific disease. The nephrotic syndrome, with proteinuria exceeding 3.5 g per day, may occur in any of the diseases discussed in this chapter. Several physiologic and metabolic abnormalities accompany the nephrotic state, and these have been reviewed elsewhere (2). Important features include edema, abnormalities of the coagulation system, and abnormalities of plasma lipids, with raised total cholesterol and triglyceride levels. There is an increased incidence of deep vein thrombosis and pulmonary embolus, although it is rare for a patient to have a fatal pulmonary embolus. Renal vein thrombosis is also more common and is especially associated with membranous nephropathy.

A particular combination of clinical features and the age of the patient may make one disease more likely than another. Weighing these probabilities may be an intellectually challenging exercise, but in practical terms, a renal biopsy is almost invariably indicated when glomerular disease is suspected. The exception is the childhood nephrotic syndrome, as discussed in the section on minimal change disease and focal segmental glomerulosclerosis. An important decision for a patient with suspected glomerular disease is when to do a renal biopsy. Table 18.2 gives some guidelines about when a biopsy should be considered. These are based on the probability of finding a treatable disease.

M.G. Robson and M. J. Walport: Division of Medicine, Imperial College School of Science, Technology, and Medicine, Hammersmith Hospital, London W12 ONN, United Kingdom.

**TABLE 18.1.** *Incidence of glomerular diseases in 1993*

| Disease | Incidence per million population |
|---|---|
| IgA nephropathy | 8.4 |
| Membranous glomerulonephritis | 4.9 |
| Focal segmental glomerulosclerosis | 2.3 |
| Minimal change disease | 1.6 |
| Mesangiocapillary glomerulonephritis | 1.4 |
| Poststreptococcal glomerulonephritis | 0.7 |

From Schena FP. Survey of the Italian registry of renal biopsies. Frequency of the renal diseases for 7 consecutive years. *Nephrol Dial Transplant* 1997;12:418–426.

We offer a section on prognosis for each of the diseases discussed in this chapter. There is a large amount of literature examining the factors that affect the prognosis for each of these diseases. Authors have all come to the same conclusion, regardless of the specific diagnosis: proteinuria, renal impairment, hypertension, and tubulointerstitial fibrosis are poor prognostic indicators. This amounts to saying that a more damaged kidney has a worse outlook than a less damaged one. A review by d'Amico in 1992 considered these features in a variety of diseases and confirmed that these prognostic indicators are universally applicable (3).

## IMMUNOGLOBULIN A NEPHROPATHY

Mesangial deposits of IgA are found in a number of diseases. Henoch–Schönlein purpura is a systemic disease discussed elsewhere in this book and produces morphologic changes in the kidney indistinguishable from those found in primary IgA nephropathy. Hepatic cirrhosis may be associated with IgA deposits along with microscopic hematuria and proteinuria. The glomerular disease associated with cirrhosis is generally benign, allowing preservation of renal function. Deposition of any class of immunoglobulin may occur in SLE, and IgA is no exception. The diagnosis of primary IgA nephropathy affecting only the kidney, the subject of the remainder of this section, requires the exclusion of these other diseases.

**TABLE 18.2.** *Indications for a renal biopsy*

Possible indications for a renal biopsy

1. Unexplained acute or chronic renal impairment (with prerenal and postrenal causes excluded)
2. Mildly abnormal proteinuria (0.2–2 g per day) with microscopic hematuria and/or renal impairment
3. Moderate to severe proteinuria (>2 g per day), regardless of hematuria or renal impairment
4. Microscopic hematuria and renal impairment

Not indications for renal biopsy

1. Isolated microscopic hematuria with normal renal function
2. Mildly abnormal proteinuria (0.2–2 g per day) with normal renal function and no hematuria

Primary IgA nephropathy is thought to result from the deposition of IgA from the circulation into the mesangium. Patients often have elevated serum IgA levels, usually of the IgA1 subclass (4,5), corresponding to IgA1 deposits in the kidney. However, elevated IgA1 is not sufficient for the development of IgA nephropathy, as shown by patients with IgA1 myeloma who do not have mesangial deposits. Some patients with IgA nephropathy have increased numbers of IgA-producing lymphocytes in tonsillar tissue (6), but other investigators have not seen evidence of increased salivary IgA (5), and it also seems unlikely that tonsillar lymphocytes contribute significantly to serum IgA. Bone marrow plasma cells are a more likely source of increased IgA, and an increase in IgA-producing cells has been found in patients with IgA nephropathy, and it was restricted to the IgA1 subclass (7).

### Clinical Presentation

Table 18.3 summarizes the presenting clinical features in IgA nephropathy from a number of large series from different parts of the world (8–21). Only series that included more than a hundred patients and that documented all of the clinical features at presentation have been included. The studies from Europe and Australia described an unequal sex distribution with around 70% to 80% of patients being male. In contrast, the four Asian studies found a more even distribution with 42% to 58% being male. Patients typically presented as young adults of 25 to 35 years old. Macroscopic hematuria was an initial feature in 17% to 76% of cases. Microscopic hematuria occurred in 68% to 100% of cases. Hypertension was present in 9% to 43%, and abnormal renal function in 10% to 37% when assessed by creatinine clearance or glomerular filtration rate. Nearly all patients had proteinuria at presentation. In the series that have commented on mild proteinuria, some degree of abnormal proteinuria was present in 58% to 98%. The nephrotic syndrome was an uncommon presentation, occurring in 4% to 13%. Rarely, patients present with an acute nephritic syndrome, reported in four of the series at 1.5% to 10%.

Raised serum IgA levels are described in 21% to 71% of cases. An upper respiratory tract infection preceding the diagnosis of IgA nephropathy was found in 13% to 80% of cases, and other infections occurred in up to 25% of cases (10). However, in most of these series, the interval between the infection and diagnosis was not stated, and respiratory tract infections are common in the general population. Although there seems little doubt that infection is associated with the onset of IgA nephropathy, it is difficult to be sure of the true strength of the association. Another feature that has been observed but was not regularly reported in the series in Table 18.3 is loin pain. One study reported that this occurred in 36% of patients (21).

### Diagnosis

IgA nephropathy is the most common primary glomerular disease and may be suspected on the clinical grounds dis-

**TABLE 18.3A.** *IgA nephropathy: clinical presentation*

| Study | Location | N | Mean age | Male (%) | Hematuria (%) | | Proteinuria (%) | | High blood pressure (%) | Renal function impaired (%) |
| | | | | | Macro | Micro | Total | Nephrotic | | |
|---|---|---|---|---|---|---|---|---|---|---|
| Gärtner[8] | Europe | 153 | 30 | 80 | 36 | 94 | 88 | 12 | 42 | 29[a] |
| Rodicio[9] | Europe | 140 | NA | 70 | 76 | NA | NA | NA | NA | NA |
| Frimat[10] | Europe | 210 | 36 | 82 | 42 | 80 | 76 | NA | 31 | NA |
| Johnston[11] | Europe | 253 | 30 | 77 | NA | 77.6 | NA | 13 | 27 | 20 |
| Droz[12] | Europe | 182 | 25 | 68 | 44.5 | NA | 98 | 10 | NA | NA |
| D'Amico[13] | Europe | 374 | 30 | 70 | 50 | NA | NA | 7 | 36 | 24 |
| Mustonen[14] | Europe | 143 | 40 | 65 | 26 | NA | 77 | 5 | 32 | 32[a] |
| Bogenschütz[15] | Europe | 239 | 33 | 74 | NA | NA | NA | NA | 31 | NA |
| Almartine[16] | Europe | 182 | 28 | 79 | 27 | NA | 58 | 3 | 9 | 2 |
| Nakamoto[17] | Asia | 205 | 27.5 | 54 | 17 | 68 | NA | 13 | 30 | 23[a] |
| Kobayashi[18] | Asia | 166 | 31 | 42 | 17 | 85 | 79 | 4 | 13 | 37[a] |
| Taguchi[19] | Asia | 357 | 29 | 52 | 33 | 89 | 92 | 8 | 15 | 6 |
| Shirai[20] | Asia | 100 | 27 | 58 | 19 | NA | NA | NA | 18 | 10[a] |
| Nicholls[21] | Aust | 244 | 32 | 73 | 43 | 100 | NA | 5 | 43 | 36 |

[a] Assessed by creatinine clearance or glomerular filtration rate.

cussed earlier. Microscopic hematuria without proteinuria is unusual in IgA nephropathy, and alternatives such as thin basement membrane disease should be considered in patients with normal renal function (22). The serum IgA level may be raised, but this is not a sensitive or specific diagnostic feature. A definite diagnosis depends on the presence of characteristic histologic features in a renal biopsy (Fig. 18.1). A histologic classification of the changes seen on light microscopy has been accepted by the World Health Organization (23). Stage I consists of very mild mesangial hypercellularity, and stage II has proliferative changes in less than 50% of glomeruli. In stages I and II, tubulointerstitial changes are absent. In stage III, there is diffuse mesangial proliferation and expansion. There may also be occasional adhesions, crescents, and interstitial infiltrates. In stage IV, there is widespread mesangial proliferation and glomerulosclerosis. Adhesions and crescents are more common in stage IV than in stage III, as is tubulointerstitial inflammation and atrophy. Stage V is said to be present when these changes are severe and more than 50% of crescents are present. IgA is the dom-

inant deposit on immunofluorescence (Fig. 18.2) and occurs in association with C3. It is found in the mesangium and may also be found in the capillary wall. IgG occurs in 50% to 70% of cases, and IgM in 31% to 66% (24). C1q and C4 are rarely detected.

### Prognosis

IgA nephropathy was formerly referred to as "benign recurrent hematuria." However, the course is far from benign in a proportion of patients. Whereas some maintain stable renal function, others have a slowly progressive course. Table 18.4 summarizes the prognosis in a number of large series with a mean follow-up of more than 3 years (10,11,15,16,21, 25–28). Most patients in the series summarized were untreated, and if they did receive treatment, it was unlikely to have significantly altered the outcome, based on the evidence presented later. This means that these series can be taken as

**TABLE 18.3B.** *IgA nephropathy: clinical presentation*

| Study | Number | History Respiratory Infection (%) | Nephritic (%) | Increased Serum IgA (%) |
|---|---|---|---|---|
| Gärtner[8] | 153 | 32 | NA | 33 |
| Rodicio[9] | 140 | 80 | 4 | 50 |
| Frimat[10] | 210 | 35 | NA | NA |
| Droz[12] | 182 | NA | NA | 45 |
| D'Amico[13] | 374 | NA | NA | 38 |
| Mustonen[14] | 143 | NA | 1.5 | 48 |
| Almartine[16] | 182 | NA | 3 | NA |
| Nakamoto[17] | 205 | 13 | NA | NA |
| Kobayashi[18] | 166 | NA | NA | 71 |
| Taguchi[19] | 357 | NA | 10 | NA |
| Shirai[20] | 100 | 27 | NA | 23 |
| Nicholls[21] | 244 | NA | NA | 21 |

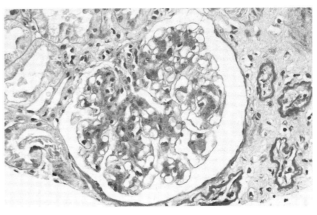

**FIG. 18.1.** Diffuse mesangial hypercellularity and an increased mesangial matrix in a case of IgA nephropathy. See color plate 2.

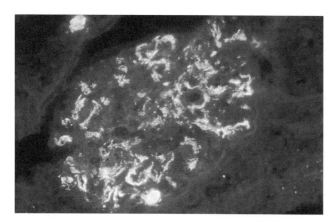

**FIG. 18.2.** Immunofluorescence for IgA shows widespread mesangial deposition in a case of IgA nephropathy. See color plate 3.

representing the prognosis in untreated IgA nephropathy. The studies suggest that, at 10 years after diagnosis, 6% to 20% of patients reach end-stage renal failure. A large amount of literature describes prognostic factors in IgA nephropathy. However, the factors affecting outcome are no different from those that apply to glomerular diseases in general.

Two factors do deserve special mention: macroscopic hematuria and angiotensin-converting enzyme (ACE) polymorphisms. It has been suggested that the presence of macroscopic hematuria confers a relatively benign prognosis (13). However, other studies contradict this, and in one large series, urinary erythrocyte count correlated with crescent formation and with progression of renal failure (21). Three studies showed that the presence of a deletion polymorphism of the ACE gene is associated with progression of IgA nephropathy. This polymorphism results in higher ACE and angiotensin II levels. The largest series retrospectively analyzed 100 patients with IgA nephropathy (29). Patients homozygous for the deletion allele presented at an earlier age, required dialysis younger, and had a faster rate of decline of renal function. Another series divided 53 patients into two groups with stable or deteriorating renal function (30). Forty-three percent of the latter group were homozygous for the

deletion allele, compared with 7% of the former. Patients homozygous for the deletion allele also had a decrease in proteinuria in response to ACE inhibitor therapy. Another report included 48 patients and found that the mean slope of the reciprocal creatinine (a measure of rate of decline of renal function) was lower in those that did not have a deletion allele compared with those with one or two alleles (31).

## Treatment

Table 18.5 summarizes randomized controlled trials of treatment for IgA nephropathy. The various therapeutic approaches are described in the following sections.

### Steroids

A crossover trial of oral prednisolone or placebo given for 3 months included 10 pediatric patients (32). Follow-up did not extend beyond the end of the short treatment period, and no difference in proteinuria, hematuria, or serum creatinine was seen. The first of two randomized controlled trials of steroid treatment for IgA nephropathy included 34 patients with IgA disease and nephrotic syndrome (33). Over a mean follow-up period of 38 months, there was no difference in renal function between treated and control patients. However, the investigators suggest that steroid treatment is warranted in nephrotic IgA disease with mild histologic changes, because 6 of 7 treated patients had remission of the nephrotic syndrome. However, in the untreated group, there were only 4 patients (of whom 2 remitted) with an equivalent histologic grading. The numbers are too small to draw any conclusions about whether the remissions in the treated group were caused by the steroids.

A later trial enrolling 86 adults with proteinuria of 1 to 3.5 g/day and a serum creatinine concentration of less than 133 µmol/L did suggest a benefit from treatment with steroids (34). Treatment comprised a 6-month course of oral prednisolone, with intravenous methylprednisolone being given for the first 3 days of months 1, 3, and 5. After a median follow-up of 4 years, there was a reduction in proteinuria due to treatment, and 21% of the treatment group had a

**TABLE 18.4.** *IgA nephropathy: prognosis*

| Study | Location | N | Mean follow-up after biopsy (years) | Reaching end-stage renal failure or death (%) | Renal function impaired (not end-stage) (%) | Number followed for 10 years after biopsy | 10-year renal death (%) |
|---|---|---|---|---|---|---|---|
| Rekola[27] | Europe | 191 | 7.3 | 10 | 45[a] | NA | NA |
| Johnston[11] | Europe | 20 | NA | NA | NA | 20 | 17 |
| Frimat[10] | Europe | 210 | 5.6 | 20 | NA | NA | NA |
| D'Amico[25] | Europe | 267 | 3.5 | 14.6 | 38 | NA | NA |
| Nicholls[21] | Australia | 217 | 5 | 9 | 18 | 33 | 13 |
| Woo[28] | Asia | 151 | 4.2 | 5 | 9 | 14 | 9 |
| Bogenschütz[15] | Europe | 239 | 4.9 | NA | NA | NA | NA |
| Almartine[16] | Europe | 282 | 8 | 6 | 18 | 101 | 6 |
| Noel[26] | Europe | 84 | NA | NA | NA | 84 | 15 |

[a] Assessed by glomerular filtration rate or creatinine clearance.

**TABLE 18.5.** *IgA nephropathy: randomized controlled trials of treatment*

| Treatment | Study | N | Follow-up (months) | Effect on outcome |
|---|---|---|---|---|
| Intravenous and oral steroids | Pozzi[34] | 86 | 48 | Less proteinuria and preserved renal function |
| Oral steroids (in nephrotics) | Lai[33] | 34 | 38 | None |
| Oral steroids and azathioprine | Yoshikawa[35] | 78 | 24 | Less proteinuria and glomerular sclerosis |
| Chlorambucil or azathioprine | Lagrue[36] | 23[a] | 24 | None |
| Dipyridamole + aspirin | Chan[37] | 38 | 33.2 | None |
| Cyclophosphamide + warfarin + dipyridamole | Woo[38] | 48 | 68 | Less proteinuria and renal function preserved |
| Cyclosporine | Lai[39] | 19 | 6 | None |
| Fish oil | Donadio[40] | 101 | 24 | Preservation of renal function |
| Fosinopril | Maschio[41] | 39 | 4 | Less proteinuria |

[a] 5 = chlorambucil, 8 = azathioprine, 10 = placebo.

50% or more increase in serum creatinine, compared with 33% of the placebo group.

### Steroids with Cytotoxic Drugs

A randomized controlled trial compared oral prednisolone and azathioprine to placebo in 78 pediatric patients (35). All patients received heparin or warfarin and dipyridamole as additional treatment. Patients were treated for 2 years, and evaluation included a repeat renal biopsy at the end of the study. Patients given prednisolone and azathioprine had less proteinuria, glomerulosclerosis, and mesangial IgA than the placebo group at the end of the treatment period. However, no difference was demonstrated in creatinine clearance, and the dose of prednisolone (2 mg/kg, decreasing over 3 months to 1 mg/kg and maintained at this dose for 21 months) was high and potentially toxic.

### Cytotoxic, Antiplatelet, and Anticoagulant Drugs

In one study, azathioprine or chlorambucil was given to 8 and 5 patients, respectively (36). There were 10 patients in the control group. Neither drug was effective compared with placebo. Aspirin and dipyridamole were ineffective in a study of 38 patients (37). The combination of cyclophosphamide, warfarin, and dipyridamole was used in 24 patients (38). After a follow-up of 68 months, the treated group had less proteinuria compared with an unchanged proteinuria level in the untreated group. Creatinine clearance rate was also unchanged (and had fallen from a mean of 109 mL/minute to 79 mL/minute in the control group). Although the difference is not large, this study does suggest a benefit. This study showed a slow rate of progression in the control group, with only one patient with IgA nephropathy reaching advanced renal failure (creatinine clearance of 13 mL/minute). This reflects the fact that the population is a group identified by a screening program of young adults. Nineteen patients were treated with cyclosporin for 12 weeks and followed for another 3 months. No benefit was shown, but follow-up was probably too short to allow any conclusions (39).

### Fish Oil

A randomized trial of fish oil included 101 patients with proteinuria greater than 1 g per 24 hours, or a creatinine level that had risen by 25% in the previous 6 months (40). Treatment consisted of 1.87 g of eicosapentenoic acid and 1.36 g docosahexanoic acid daily. The primary end point was an increase in serum creatinine of 50% or more at 2 years. This occurred in 33% of the placebo group and 6% of the treated group. During an average follow-up of 3 years, 27% of the placebo group died or developed end-stage renal failure, compared with 9% in the treated group. The frequency of end-stage renal failure in the placebo group was significantly higher than occurred in the studies listed in Table 18.3. This may reflect the entry requirements of a rising serum creatinine or significant proteinuria. Surprisingly, there was no significant difference in changes in proteinuria between the two groups. Despite this finding, the study provides definite evidence in favor of treatment with fish oils. There were no adverse reactions in the treated group although some patients complained of the fishy aftertaste.

### Angiotensin-Converting Enzyme Inhibitors

A prospective study of the ACE inhibitor fosinopril was performed in 39 normotensive patients with IgA nephropathy (41). Fosinopril or placebo were given for 4 months, and patients then crossed over to the other arm of the study for 4 months, after a 1-month break. There was a significant reduction in proteinuria with fosinopril in this short-term trial. This study did not examine the long-term effect of ACE inhibitors on renal function. A retrospective analysis of hypertensive patients with IgA nephropathy receiving ACE inhibitors or other antihypertensive treatment did suggest a slower decline in renal function in the former group (42).

## MEMBRANOUS NEPHROPATHY

Membranous nephropathy has been associated with a variety of diseases. The overall prevalence of secondary forms of membranous nephropathy has varied from 17% to 42%, as reviewed by Glassock (43). More than 85% of cases were associated with drugs, neoplasia, lupus, or infections. Other associations included sickle cell disease and thyroiditis. The most frequently implicated drugs are gold, penicillamine, and nonsteroidal antiinflammatories. Hepatitis B is the most commonly associated infection. In these cases of secondary membranous nephropathy, the clinical presentation includes features of the primary disease, and treatment and prognosis are determined by the underlying disorder.

Several animal models of membranous nephropathy have provided insights into possible mechanisms of the disease, of which the best characterized is the rat model known as Heymann nephritis (44). In this model, subepithelial deposits and glomerular basement membrane thickening occurs in response to immunization with a tubular antigen fraction (FxA1) containing a glycoprotein (GP330) that is also present on glomerular epithelial cells. It is thought that antibody binds to the antigen on glomerular podocytes and these complexes condense and become associated with the glomerular basement membrane. In humans, GP330 is present on tubular cells but not in the glomerulus. Other glomerular or exogenous antigens are presumably involved in the pathogenesis of the human disease. Several studies support a role for complement in this model. Complement depletion with cobra venom factor and depletion of C6 using an antibody abrogated disease (45,46), as did treatment with a complement inhibitor (47). In contrast to these findings, C6-deficient rats develop disease to the same degree as normal rats (48). One study emphasized a role for CD8-positive T cells, because depletion abrogated disease (49). Further evidence for an immune cause comes from the particularly strong association of idiopathic membranous nephropathy with human leukocyte antigen (HLA) DR3 in Caucasian populations (50).

The remainder of this section of the chapter concerns idiopathic membranous nephropathy only.

## Clinical Presentation

The presenting clinical features from several large series of unselected patients with idiopathic membranous nephropathy is shown in Table 18.6 (51–65). They are drawn from populations in different parts of the world. These series agreed on a male predominance (51% to 84%) and a mean age of presentation of 36 to 51 years. The nephrotic syndrome was present in 54% to 93%, with almost 100% of patients having significant proteinuria. Microscopic hematuria was present in 28% to 66% of adults, and although macroscopic hematuria was described, it was rare. Hypertension was present in 10% to 55% of adult cases. The frequency of renal impairment at presentation depends on the method of assessment. Two studies that measured creatinine clearance or glomerular filtration rate are marked with an asterisk (Table 18.6). These found frequencies of 42% and 46% for renal impairment. This may have been partly because of intravascular volume depletion resulting from the nephrotic syndrome. One series reported the clinical features of 50 children with membranous nephropathy and found a similar male predominance (76%) and frequency of nephrotic syndrome (62%) (53). However, microscopic hematuria was more common in children than in adults (85%), and hypertension was less common (1%).

## Diagnosis

There are no blood tests that help in the diagnosis. A renal biopsy is the definitive test. If membranous nephropathy is shown by the renal histology, secondary causes must be excluded. With light microscopy, the capillary loop basement

**TABLE 18.6.** *Membranous nephropathy: clinical presentation*

| Study | Origin | N | Male (%) | Mean age | Nephrotic (%) | Hematuria (%) Micro | Hematuria (%) Macro | High blood pressure (%) | Impaired renal function (%) |
|---|---|---|---|---|---|---|---|---|---|
| Honkanen[52] | Europe | 67 | 70 | 39 | 82 | 28 | 1 | 27 | 7 |
| Pereides[56] | Europe | 37 | 81 | NA | 76 | NA | NA | 20 | NA |
| Habib[53] | Europe | 50 | 76 | P | 62 | 85 | 0 | 1 | 4 |
| Whermann[59] | Europe | 334 | 66 | 43 | 73 | NA | NA | 37 | NA |
| Ramzy[57] | Europe | 35 | 51 | 39 | 74 | 54 | 9 | 37 | 46[a] |
| Zuchelli[65] | Europe | 205 | 64 | 50 | 74 | 54 | 1 | 23 | 9 |
| MacTier[55] | Europe | 44 | 84 | 42 | 93 | 66 | 5 | 45 | 6 |
| Noel[64] | Europe | 116 | 52 | 38 | 76 | 55 | 0 | 15 | 6 |
| Shieppati[58] | USA | 100 | 68 | 51 | 63 | NA | NA | 55 | NA |
| Hopper[54] | USA | 100 | 65 | 43 | 90 | NA | NA | 20 | 42[a] |
| Gluck[61] | USA | 38 | 58 | 44 | 92 | 42 | 0 | 47 | 18 |
| Erwin[62] | USA | 48 | 70 | 49 | 85 | NA | NA | 33 | 8 |
| Kida[63] | Japan | 104 | 62 | 40 | 60 | NA | NA | NA | NA |
| Abe[51] | Japan | 89 | 52 | 39 | 75 | 49 | 0 | 25 | 6 |
| Murphy[60] | Austral | 39 | 55 | 36 | 54 | 33 | 0 | 40 | 18 |

P, pediatric group (all <15 yr).
[a] Assessed by creatinine clearance or glomerular filtration rate.

membrane appears thickened and any glomerular hypercellularity is minimal (Fig. 18.3). The histologic pattern has been classified in five stages (66). Stage 1 appears normal on light microscopy with small subepithelial deposits visible on electron microscopy. Stage 2 shows capillary wall thickening with large deposits and spike formation (Fig. 18.4). In stage 3, the capillary wall has become thickened and split, with large deposits merging with spikes. In stage 4, the glomerular basement membrane is irregular and thick with vacuolation, and deposits have become smaller and may be absent. Stage 5 is said to be present when deposits are absent and the glomerular basement membrane is largely normal on light microscopy but appears delicate with some lucent areas. These stages are thought to represent a progression of disease, based on evidence from animal models and from patients who have had more than one biopsy. Deposits of IgG and C3 are found along the capillary loops. Other deposits that are present with a variable frequency include IgA, IgM, Clq, and C4.

Histologic features of secondary forms of membranous nephropathy are similar to those of idiopathic membranous nephropathy. However, several features may point to SLE as a primary cause. Mesangial deposits are almost invariably present in lupus but rare in idiopathic MN (15%). Subedothelial deposits are rarely present in idiopathic MN (3%) but are present in 82% of cases of overt lupus membranous nephritis (67). Heavy deposits of IgA, IgM, and C1q also suggest lupus membranous nephritis, although these deposits may all occur with idiopathic MN.

## Prognosis

Several series have reported the prognosis of unselected patients with untreated membranous nephropathy (55,58,64, 68–71) (Table 18.7). These are series from units in which no patients were treated during the course of the study, or they comprise the control group from a randomized trial. One study is particularly important in that it was prospective and

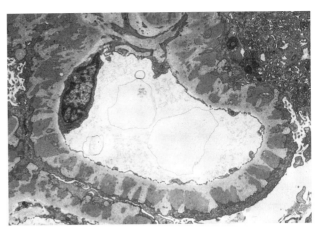

**FIG. 18.4.** Electron microscopic appearance of stage II membranous nephropathy. The basement membrane is thickened, with prominent spikes separating the subepithelial deposits.

recent, reflecting modern standards of supportive care (58). Series in which treated patients were excluded have not been included, because they are potentially biased. Overall, these studies show that 8% to 35% of patients with membranous nephropathy die or develop end-stage renal failure, 11% to 38% develop significant renal impairment (not on dialysis), and 11% to 40% enter complete remission. The wide variability in outcome may represent different types of membranous nephropathy in different locations. Given the number of different causes of secondary MN, it seems likely that different antigens are involved in the disease in different populations. This may result in the variety of clinical courses.

## Treatment

The variation in clinical course has resulted in much controversy regarding treatment. One study used the relatively good outcome of their prospective series of untreated patients as justification for continuing a no-treatment policy (58). Table 18.8 summarizes the randomized, controlled trials that have been performed in membranous nephropathy.

### Steroids

Of the three significantly sized, controlled trials of oral steroids, two showed no difference between controls and treated patients. These were the Canadian study (158 patients), and the Medical Research Council study (103 patients) (68,69). A third study suggested a benefit. This was the U.S. study of 72 patients (71). After a mean follow-up of 23 months, 1 of 34 in the treatment group had a creatinine level of more than 440 μmol/L, compared with 10 of 38 in the placebo group. There was no difference in the rate of remission from proteinuria. The reasons for the different results are not entirely clear. It may be because of different types of membranous nephropathy among different populations. However, the lack of agreement between the Canadian and

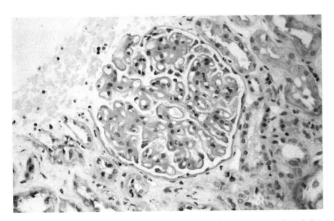

**FIG. 18.3.** Membranous nephropathy is characterized by generalized thickening of the glomerular capillary wall but no increase in cellularity. See color plate 4.

**TABLE 18.7.** *Membranous nephropathy: long-term outcome in untreated, unselected patients*

| Study | Origin | N | Follow-up (months) | End-stage renal failure or death (%) | Impaired renal function (%) | Complete remission (%) |
|---|---|---|---|---|---|---|
| MacTier[55] | Europe | 37 | 64 | 35 | 19 | 30 |
| Noel[64] | Europe | 116 | 54 | 15 | 9.5 | 23.5 |
| Cameron[69a] | Europe | 51 | 36 | 29 | 29 | 14 |
| Ponticelli[70] | Europe | 39 | 60 | 10 | 38 | 40 |
| Cattran[68a] | N. America | 60 | 48 | 8 | NA | 32 |
| U.S. study[71a] | N. America | 38 | 23 | 18 | 11 | 11 |
| Shieppati[58] | N. America | 100 | 52 | 16 | 16 | 35 |

[a] Data from the placebo group of a randomized trial.

U.S. studies makes this less likely. Overall, the evidence does not support the use of oral steroids alone for MN. A description of the Italian Collaborative Group's study comparing intravenous and oral steroids with the combination of chlorambucil and steroids is described in a following section (74).

### Cytotoxic Drugs

Two randomized trials have been performed. One found no difference with oral cyclophosphamide in a study of 22 patients and had a short follow-up of 12 months (72). A randomized trial of 41 patients allocated 11 patients to treatment with azathioprine, 16 to chlorambucil, and 14 to placebo (36). The follow-up period was short at 2 years, and outcome was assessed in terms of proteinuria without looking at renal function. None of the azathioprine treated patients entered remission, but 56% of the chlorambucil-treated patients did (compared with 14% of the placebo group).

### Steroids with Cytotoxic Drugs

A small, randomized trial of prednisolone and azathioprine in 14 patients was conducted by the Medical Research Council (73). This study did not show treatment to have any benefit, although follow-up was only for 6 months. The study by the Italian Collaborative Group in 1989 did suggest that MN was amenable to treatment (70). Inclusion criteria were the presence of the nephrotic syndrome and a creatinine concentration of less than 1.7 mg/dL. The treatment regimen has become known as the *Ponticelli regimen*. It consisted of three intravenous doses of methylprednisolone: 1 g on the first 3 days of each of months 1, 3, and 5. For the remainder of months 1, 3, and 5, patients took prednisolone (0.4 mg/kg/day), and for months 2, 4, and 6, patients had chlorambucil (0.2 mg/kg/day). Sixty-seven percent of the treatment group had complete or partial remission from proteinuria (compared with 23% of the control group). There was also evidence of preservation of renal function, with 49% of controls increasing their creatinine by 50% or more, compared with 10% of the treated group. Another study by this group in 1992 compared the Ponticelli regimen with steroids alone (three doses of methylprednisolone: 1 g at the start of months 1, 3, and 5, with 0.4 mg/kg of oral methylprednisolone on other days) (74). There was no difference in rate of decline of renal function, and at year 4, there was no difference in rate of remission from proteinuria. However, the remission was faster with chlorambucil. This regimen of steroids alone may be preferred, unless symptoms of the nephrotic syndrome make a fast remission necessary.

**TABLE 18.8.** *Membranous nephropathy: randomized controlled trials of treatment*

| Treatment | Study | N | Follow-up (months) | Effect on outcome |
|---|---|---|---|---|
| Oral steroids | MRC[69] | 103 | 36 | None |
| Oral steroids | Canadian[68] | 158 | 48 | None |
| Oral steroids | U.S. collaborative[71] | 72 | 23 | Preservation of function |
| Oral cyclophosphamide | Donadio[72] | 22 | 21 | None |
| Chlorambucil or azathioprine[a] | Lagrue[36] | 41 | 24 | Less proteinuria with chlorambucil |
| Prednisolone and azathioprine | MRC[73] | 14 | 6 | None |
| Oral and IV steroids with chlorambucil | Ponticelli[70] | 81 | 60 | Preservation of function and remission of proteinuria |
| IV and oral steroids with or without chlorambucil | Ponticelli[74] | 92 | 54 | Faster remission with chlorambucil but no other difference |
| Steriods versus IV cyclophosphamide and steroids[b] | Falk[75] | 26 | 29 | None |

[a] 16 = chlorambucil, 11 = azathioprine, 14 = placebo.
[b] In patients with severely impaired or deteriorating renal function or symptomatic nephrotic syndrome.

The Italian studies excluded patients with more than moderate renal impairment. In contrast, another included only patients with deteriorating or advanced renal impairment (creatinine doubled or creatinine clearance halved in preceding 2 years, or above 2 mg/dL) or symptomatic nephrotic syndrome (75). Twenty-six patients were randomized to treatment with steroids alone or steroids combined with intravenous cyclophosphamide. There was no significant difference between the two groups.

## IDIOPATHIC NEPHROTIC SYNDROME: MINIMAL CHANGE NEPHROPATHY AND FOCAL SEGMENTAL GLOMERULOSCLEROSIS

Several lines of evidence suggest that minimal change nephropathy (MCN) and focal segmental glomerulosclerosis (FSGS) are different histologic stages of the same pathologic process. In FSGS, a proportion of glomeruli are not sclerosed, and one study compared nonsclerotic glomeruli in patients with FSGS and MCN using electron microscopy. Identical features are seen in the glomeruli in both conditions (76). There are many examples of patients who show MCN on an initial biopsy and FSGS on a subsequent one. One study found that 45% of 33 children presenting with frequently relapsing MCN converted to FSGS within 4.5 years (77). MCN and FSGS are often referred to together as idiopathic nephrotic syndrome. Proteinuria in these conditions is thought to result from the loss of negative charge on the glomerular filtration barrier (78). A number of immunologic abnormalities have been described in MCN or FSGS, including an increase in circulating CD8-positive T cells (79), a decreased in T-cell responsiveness to nonspecific mitogens (80), and a decrease in serum IgG levels and in vitro B-cell IgG production (81). However, the T-cell hyporesponsiveness was also found in other conditions causing the nephrotic syndrome, and the IgG abnormalities resolved with resolution of the nephrotic syndrome, suggesting that these were secondary phenomena.

Several observations support the role of a circulating factor in causing the observed proteinuria. When a woman with minimal change disease gave birth on two occasions, the children had transient proteinuria, perhaps because of a circulating factor transmitted across the placenta from the mother (82). Conversely, when two kidneys were transplanted from a patient who died with the nephrotic syndrome resulting from minimal change disease, the proteinuria did not persist in the recipients (83). Serum from patients with FSGS was tested on in vitro assay of glomerular permeability. It was found that serum from transplanted patients with recurrence gave a high permeability in this assay, and this decreased after plasma exchange (84). Proteinuria was also seen to decrease after plasma exchange in these patients. Immunoabsorption (i.e., removal of predominantly IgG form the plasma) also decreased proteinuria in patients with FSGS (85), and when the eluted protein was injected into rats, they developed proteinuria. This suggests that the circulating factor may be an antibody, and the finding supports an immune pathogenesis.

Focal segmental glomerulosclerosis can be a nonspecific finding associated with many other renal diseases, and diagnosis of idiopathic FSGS depends on a lack of evidence for any of these other conditions. A proportion of glomeruli also show similar changes in adults over the age of 40, especially if there is obesity. The autopsy findings of 22 obese patients were reviewed, and 6 were found to have FSGS (86). Although the numbers were small, the presence of FSGS did not appear to correlate with hypertension or atherosclerosis. The subjects with FSGS did have higher cholesterol and triglyceride levels than obese subjects without FSGS. A number of features suggested that this is a different disease process from idiopathic FSGS. The distribution does not favor the corticomedullary junction, and the characteristic visceral epithelial cell hyperplasia is lacking.

### Clinical Presentation in Children

In 1978, the International Study of Kidney Disease in Children (ISKDC) included 521 children with the nephrotic syndrome (87). MCN was present in 76.4%, and 6.9% had FSGS. The presenting clinical features of these two groups are shown in Table 18.9 with data from other series of children with MCN or FSGS (88–92). These studies showed a male predominance of 53% to 69% for FSGS and MCN. Children with MCN had a mean age at presentation of 3 to 4 years, and children with FSGS were usually between 4.5 and 7.5 years old. Most had features of the nephrotic syndrome. The frequency of other clinical features in FSGS and MCN in these series are shown in Table 18.9. Four of the five studies on FSGS showed that hypertension is more common than in MCN (35% to 48% versus 6% to 21%). The fifth study described an unusually low incidence for hypertension in FSGS (4%). Microscopic hematuria was more common at presentation in FSGS (27% to 57% versus 13% to 36% in MCN), as was renal impairment (24% to 48% versus 10% to 32%). Selective proteinuria was less common in FSGS than MCN at 13% (versus 53% to 93%). Despite these differences, the degree of overlap in the presenting features means that the clinical picture cannot reliably differentiate these two histologic entities. However, this does not affect the initial management.

### Clinical Presentation in Adults

Some adult series of minimal change disease, summarized in Table 18.10, show a male predominance (93–95) and others a female predominance (96,97). These adult series do agree on a mean age of onset of 30 to 40 years. In four of five these series, nephrotic syndrome was an inclusion criteria. It seems that MCN in adults nearly always presents with nephrotic-range proteinuria. However, because patients may be less likely to be biopsied with subnephrotic-range proteinuria and normal renal function, it is difficult to be sure of this.

**TABLE 18.9.** *Idiopathic nephrotic syndrome: clinical presentation in children*

| Study | N | Mean age | Male (%) | High blood pressure (%) | Microscopic hematuria (%) | Impaired renal function (%) | Selective proteinuria (%) | Nephrotic syndrome |
|---|---|---|---|---|---|---|---|---|
| Minimal change | | | | | | | | |
| ISKDC 78[87] | 398 | 3 | 60 | 21 | 23 | 32 | 53 | 100 |
| Habib[89] | 209 | 4 | 72 | 6 | 36 | 10 | 93 | 100 |
| White[92] | 111 | 3 | 69 | 9 | 13 | 19 | 80 | 100 |
| Focal segmental glomerulosclerosis | | | | | | | | |
| ISKDC 78[87] | 36 | 6 | 69 | 48 | 48 | 41 | 13 | 76 |
| SWPNSG[88] | 75 | 7.7 | 61 | 36 | 57 | 48 | NA | 100 |
| Habib[89] | 47 | 4.5 | 66 | 4 | 50 | NA | NA | 100 |
| Arbus[91] | 51 | 5 | 53 | 35 | 27 | 24 | NA | 100 |
| Cattran[90] | 38 | 5.5 | 55 | 40 | 32 | NA | NA | 76 |

Compared with childhood minimal change disease, hypertension was more common (20% to 47% in four of five series), and microscopic hematuria was equally common at 15% to 33%. Renal dysfunction was present in 43% to 66% of patients in the studies that measured creatinine clearance or glomerular filtration rate. The four studies that reported clinical features in adults with FSGS agreed on a male predominance of 56% to 64% (90,98–101). The mean age was 34 to 40 years. Nephrotic syndrome was present in 55% to 75% of patients in three series and was an inclusion criteria for the other. This suggests that subnephrotic proteinuria may be more common in FSGS than MCN. Renal dysfunction was present in 47% to 62%. Microscopic hematuria and hypertension were present in 29% to 83% and 36% to 53% of patients, respectively. One report described concurrent groups of adults and children and found that nephrotic syndrome was more common in children (76% versus 55%), but there were no differences in other presenting features (90). Another report of a combined series of 28 adults and 12 children did not give the presenting clinical features separately (99).

## Diagnosis

Minimal change disease and FSGS are histologic diagnoses and can only be made with certainty by a renal biopsy. In childhood, it is usual practice in the absence of atypical features to treat the nephrotic syndrome with steroids without a renal biopsy. Atypical features such as hypocomplementemia would make MCN or FSGS unlikely and MCGN or postinfectious nephritis more likely.

Although hypertension is not uncommon in MCN or FSGS, severe hypertension may suggest an alternative diagnosis and necessitate a renal biopsy. Children younger than 1 and older than 12 years are also unusually diagnosed with MCN or FSGS, and a biopsy should be considered. A study including 368 steroid-responsive patients showed that 92% of these steroid responders had MCN (102). Thus, a diagnosis of minimal change disease can be made with reasonable certainty from the response to steroids. However, MCN cannot be excluded by a lack of response to steroids. In the previously mentioned study, 25% of nonresponders (28% of the whole group were nonresponders) had MCN. It is usual prac-

**TABLE 18.10.** *Idiopathic nephrotic syndrome: clinical presentation in adults*

| Study | N | Mean age | Male (%) | High blood pressure (%) | Microscopic Hematuria (%) | Impaired renal function (%) | Nephrotic syndrome (%) |
|---|---|---|---|---|---|---|---|
| Minimal change | | | | | | | |
| Hopper[93] | 29 | 31 | 55 | 45 | NA | 43[a] | 100 |
| Nolasco[94] | 89 | 42 | 57 | 30 | 28 | 66[a] | 100 |
| Korbet[96] | 40 | 410 | 33 | 20 | 21 | 17 | 100 |
| Mak[97] | 51 | 37 | 42 | 47 | 33 | 57[a] | 97.5 |
| Fujimoto[95] | 33 | 28 | 67 | 9 | 15 | 15 | 100 |
| Focal segmental glomerulosclerosis | | | | | | | |
| Banfi[98] | 59 | 35 | 60 | 36 | 51 | NA | 100 |
| Cameron[99] | 40[b] | 21 | 56 | 36 | 83 | 47[a] | 75 |
| Cattran[90,101] | 55 | 34 | 64 | 53 | 29 | NA | 55 |
| Rydel[100] | 81 | 40 | 58 | 49 | 37 | 62[a] | 74 |

[a] Assessed by creatinine clearance or glomerular filtration rate.
[b] Twelve children and 28 adults, not analyzed separately.

tice to perform a diagnostic renal biopsy in any adult with an unexplained nephrotic syndrome.

Glomeruli are usually normal on light microscopy in minimal change disease. However, on electron microscopy the characteristic finding is epithelial cell foot process fusion. There may be a variable degree of mesangial hypercellularity, and in some series, patients have been classified separately when this is marked. There are examples of children changing between the classes of minimal change disease, diffuse mesangial hypercellularity, and FSGS, and these are considered to be different parts of the spectrum of a single disease process. In FSGS, a variable number of glomeruli are affected. Focal lesions begin as adhesions between peripheral capillary loops with hyaline material present. These lesions first affect one segment of the glomerulus, as shown in Figure 18.5, and then progress to cover the whole glomerular tuft. Because of the focal nature of the changes, they may be missed when only a small number of glomeruli are obtained in the biopsy. The changes are most prominent in juxtamedullary glomeruli. Tubular atrophy and interstitial fibrosis are often associated. Immunostaining of glomeruli in minimal change disease is usually negative, although the sclerotic lesions of FSGS contain IgM and C3.

**Prognosis for Children**

Idiopathic nephrotic syndrome typically runs a remitting and relapsing course in children. Depending on the response to steroids, patients are classified as steroid responders or nonresponders. One series of 181 patients with minimal change disease found that 14% did not respond to treatment with steroids (89), whereas another found that 7% of 373 did not respond (103). Steroid-responsive patients may be further

divided into frequent and infrequent relapsers. The number of children having a single episode of the nephrotic syndrome is between 3% and 30%. The ISKDC (104) found that 28% of 218 children who were steroid responsive had only one episode in 2 years. Another group estimated that 30% of 152 steroid-responsive patients had only one episode, with a minimum follow-up of 13 years (105). A third series found that 31% of 111 steroid-responsive patients had a single episode after 1 to 10 years (89). In contrast to these findings, another study found that only 3% of 63 children with biopsy-proved steroid-responsive minimal change disease had a single episode (106). All these series came from specialist centers and may have been affected by referral biases. A fifth series included every child with the nephrotic syndrome in Finland in a 10-year period (107). Twenty-four percent of 94 patients with steroid-responsive nephrotic syndrome had only one episode. MCN was present in 78 of 82 biopsies from these 94 patients. In one study, an attempt was made to predict the subsequent clinical course from the initial clinical and histopathologic features (104). However, the only factor found to be predictive was the initial relapse rate. The long-term outcome of childhood idiopathic nephrotic syndrome has been described for different groups according to the response to steroids or the histologic type (Table 18.11).

**Steroid-Responsive Minimal Change Nephropathy**

What is the natural history of the relapsing course in steroid-responsive children? The most detailed analysis is provided by Lewis et al. (106). This group found that, even after 5 years without a relapse, approximately 25% of patients would relapse over the next 5 years. The risk of relapse was inversely proportional to the time since the last relapse. There was no point at which a patient could be considered "cured" and free from the possibility of relapse. This was vividly demonstrated by two patients who relapsed after 11 and 14 years of remission. Two other studies suggested that eventually a large proportion of patients enter sustained remission. One found that, after more than 13 years, none of the 100 steroid-responsive patients for whom the information was available had relapsed in the past 4 years (105). Another found that, after 5 to 14 years, 74 of 94 steroid responsive patients had been relapse free for at least 3 years (107).

Besides the question of frequency of sustained remission, there is widespread agreement that children with steroid-responsive MCN have a favorable long-term prognosis (89,92,103,105–107). A summary of the follow-up studies in this group are shown in Table 18.11. These show that a small number of patients die or develop end-stage renal failure, but most survive with normal renal function. Only 1 of 94 patients followed for 5 to 14 years with steroid-responsive idiopathic nephrotic syndrome (of which 78 had biopsy-proved MCN) died, and this death was unrelated to the renal disease (107). One hundred and fifty-two patients with steroid-responsive MCN were followed for a minimum of 13 years, and 11 had died (4 unrelated to the disease) (105). Sixty-three

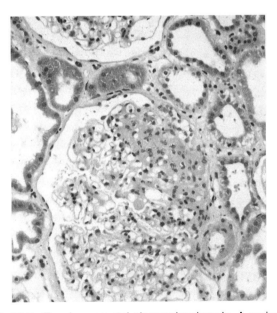

**FIG. 18.5.** Focal segmental glomerulosclerosis. A region of sclerosis is present in the upper right quadrant of the glomerulus, with obliteration of capillary lumens. See color plate 5.

**TABLE 18.11.** *Idiopathic nephrotic syndrome: prognosis in children*

| Study | N | Mean or range of follow-up (years) | Dead or end-stage renal failure (%) | Impaired renal function (%) |
|---|---|---|---|---|
| Steroid-sensitive minimal change | | | | |
| ISKDC 84[103] | 346 | 5–15 | 1.5 | NA |
| White[92] | 93 | NA | 4 | 0 |
| Habib[89] | 152 | 1–10 | 4 | 0 |
| Lewis[106] | 63 | 14 | 3 | 0 |
| Trompeter[105] | 152 | >13 | 7 | 0 |
| Koskimies[107] | 94[a] | 5–14 | 1 | 0 |
| Steroid-resistant minimal change | | | | |
| ISKDC 84[103] | 27 | 5–15 | 18.5 | 0 |
| Habib[89] | 29 | 1–10 | 27.5 | 0 |
| Steroid-resistant idiopathic nephrotic syndrome | | | | |
| Enfants Malade[108] | 84[b] | 5–25 | 44 | 6 |
| Focal segmental glomerulosclerosis—overall | | | | |
| Cameron[99] | 12 | 9.5 | 75 | 17 |
| SWPNSG[88] | 75 | 4.9 | 21 | 23 |
| Habib[89] | 47 | 1–18 | 32 | 6 |
| Arbus[91] | 51 | 10 | 33 | NA |
| Ingulli[109] | 66 | 8.4 | 70 | NA |
| Cattran[90] | 38 | 12 | 34 | 11 |
| Mongneau[110] | 25 | 20 | 44 | 0 |
| Steroid-sensitive focal segmental glomerulosclerosis | | | | |
| Habib[89] | 15 | 1–18 | 0 | 0 |
| Arbus[91] | 26 | 10 | 19 | 0 |
| SWPNSG[88] | 16 | 5.8 | 12.5 | 25 |
| Cattran[90] | 16 | 9.5 | 0 | 0 |

[a] Seventy-eight of 84 biopsies were MCN.
[b] Thirty-Four with FSGS, 33 with MCN, and 17 with diffuse mesangial hypercellularity.

patients were followed for 10 to 21 years, and 2 had died (106). The ISKDC (1984) included 346 patients with steroid-responsive minimal change disease (103). After between 5 and 15 years, 5 had died (4 of those who died were frequent relapsers). Another study found that 4 of 93 patients had died after an unspecified follow-up length (3 of these were frequent relapsers), and another series observed 6 deaths among 152 patients at 1 to 10 years (89,92). The worse outcome for frequent relapsers reflects the fact that most deaths result from infection or other complications of the nephrotic syndrome.

### Steroid-Resistant Minimal Change Nephropathy

Steroid-resistant MCN carries a worse prognosis than steroid-responsive cases. ISKDC (1984) also included 27 patients with steroid-resistant MCN (103). Compared with the steroid-responsive group, a much higher proportion (5 of 27) had died or developed end-stage renal failure after 5 to 15 years. Another analysis of steroid-resistant MCN found that 8 of 29 patients did not survive at 1 to 10 years (89).

### Steroid-Resistant Idiopathic Nephrotic Syndrome

The Enfants Malades Hospital series of steroid-resistant patients included 33 patients with MCN, 34 with FSGS and 17 with diffuse mesangial proliferation, who were followed for 5 to 25 years (108). Forty-four percent developed end-stage renal failure, 6% developed chronic renal failure, 10% continued to have proteinuria, and 40% entered complete or partial remission. There was no difference in the frequency of renal failure between patients with FSGS or MCN.

### Focal Segmental Glomerulosclerosis

Seven series have described the outcome for children with FSGS (88–91,99,109,110). These are shown in Table 18.11, and 21% to 75% of cases ended in death or end-stage renal failure. The proportion with impaired renal function (not end stage) is variable. It has been suggested that there is a worse outcome in black and Hispanic children, with one report finding that 78% reached end-stage renal failure compared with 33% of white children (109). However, only 12 white children were included in this comparison. There are conflicting data about whether the outcome is better for children with FSGS who respond to steroids. Most of these patients would not have a renal biopsy according to current practice. One report found no deaths or chronic renal failure in 15 patients at 1 to 18 years of follow-up (89). In agreement with this, none of 16 children responding to steroids developed renal insufficiency, but of 18 nonresponders, 12 developed end-stage renal failure and 3 chronic renal insufficiency (90).

However, The Southwest Pediatric Nephrology Study Group found that steroid responsiveness did not improve the outcome, with 2 of 16 steroid responders dead or at end-stage renal failure and another 4 with renal impairment at 5.8 years (88). Another study described 19 steroid-responsive patients followed for 10 years, with none developing renal failure or dying after a mean of 10.6 years (91). However, 7 other patients in this series initially responded to steroids and subsequently became unresponsive. Five of these had developed end-stage renal failure. Of the whole group who initially responded to steroids, 5 of 26 developed end-stage renal failure. As with minimal change disease, children responding to steroids may subsequently relapse, as occurred in 12 of 16 cases in one study (90).

To summarize the outcome in children, steroid-responsive MCN has a good prognosis, with all survivors having normal renal function. However, there are fatalities, and it should be remembered that the nephrotic syndrome is a dangerous condition. The overall group of steroid-resistant patients has a poor prognosis regardless of the underlying histology. There are conflicting data on the outcome for patients with FSGS who respond to steroids.

### Prognosis in Adults

The number of steroid-responsive adults with MCN having a single episode of proteinuria was 24% in two studies, with mean periods of follow-up of 12.9 and 17.5 years (94,97). A third study found that 35.5% of patients had a single episode, with a mean follow-up of 63 months (96). As in children, the disease runs a relapsing and remitting course. The long-term outcome of adult-onset minimal change disease is shown in Table 18.12 (93–97). Between 2% and 17% of patients died, and in two series, none of the survivors had significant renal impairment. In a third series, 3 of 51 patients had renal failure, but one presented in renal failure, and the other two resulted from cyclosporine and renovascular disease, respectively (97). The number of adults with steroid-resistant MCN in these series were too small to draw conclusions about the outcome in this group.

Treatment of adult FSGS is controversial. As with MCN, adults with FSGS who attain a remission in response to treatment may follow a relapsing course. Fourteen of 36 adults who responded to treatment had one or more relapses (98). Another series described 3 of 12 adults who responded to steroids and subsequently relapsed (90). Table 18.12 shows the long-term outcome for adult FSGS in four series (90,98–100). Between 25% and 56% of patients developed end-stage renal failure or died. A further 13% to 21% developed impaired renal function. In one study, the outcome for children and adults with FSGS was similar (90), although another found that more children developed end-stage renal failure (99).

### Treatment of Children

Prednisolone is usually given at an initial dose of 60 mg/kg/m$^2$ per day until remission and then reduced to 40 mg on alternate days for 4 weeks (111). This differs from the ISKDC regimen, which used a 4-week course at the starting dose of 60 mg/kg/m$^2$, regardless of when remission occurred (102). The Arbeitgemenshaft group, based on a randomized trial enlisting 61 patients, suggested that, if the dose is reduced as soon as remission occurs, there is a higher relapse rate and an equivalent total dose to those given an obligatory 4 weeks at the starting dose (112). A proportion of patients may be cured after the treatment of a single episode, as described in the section on prognosis, but most have one or more relapses. These are treated in the same way as the initial episode, and frequent relapsers may need to remain on a maintenance dose of oral steroids. A number of relapses remit without treatment. One study of 32 patients found that 23% of relapses in frequent relapsers and 10% of relapses in steroid-dependent patients remitted spontaneously (113). Seventy-nine percent of these remissions occurred within 14 days. The investigators suggested that a delay of 10 days or so before treatment may decrease the total steroid dose. There are no definite rules on when to consider alternative drugs, but they are generally used when side effects from steroids occur or relapses are particularly symptomatic or dangerous.

**TABLE 18.12.** *Idiopathic nephrotic syndrome: prognosis in adults*

| Study | N | Mean follow-up (years) | Dead or end-stage renal failure (%) | Impaired renal function (%) |
|---|---|---|---|---|
| Minimal change | | | | |
| Hopper[93] | 29 | 5.8 | 13 | 0 |
| Nolasco[94] | 89 | 7.5 | 17 | 0 |
| Mak[97] | 51 | 14.1 | 2 | 5.6[a] |
| Korbet[96] | 40 | 4.3 | 10 | NA |
| Focal segmental glomerulosclerosis | | | | |
| Cameron[99] | 28 | 9.5 | 43 | 21 |
| Banfi[98] | 59 | 6 | 56 | 19 |
| Rydel[100] | 81 | 5.1 | 25 | 14 |
| Cattran[90] | 55 | 11 | 42 | 13 |

[a] See text.

A summary of randomized trials of treatment other than steroids is given in Table 18.13. Cyclophosphamide has been effective in frequently relapsing steroid-responsive patients (114). ISKDC (1974) randomized 53 frequently relapsing patients to treatment with cyclophosphamide or no treatment. The relapse rate over the subsequent 22 months was 48%, compared with 88% for the control group. An earlier, smaller, randomized study also showed a benefit (115). After 1 year, only 2 of 10 patients treated with cyclophosphamide had relapsed, compared with 9 of 10 controls. Levamisole was used in a randomized trial of 61 patients (116). Fourteen treated patients has remissions, compared with 4 patients in the control group.

A renal biopsy is needed if the nephrotic syndrome does not respond to steroids. Ninety-four percent of children who have responded by 8 weeks will have done so by 4 weeks (102), and a lack of response by 4 weeks is considered to indicate steroid resistance (111). However, if the histologic diagnosis is FSGS, the response to treatment may take more than 3 months (90). If renal biopsy confirms the diagnosis of FSGS or MCN, there are a number of treatment options. ISKDC (1974) assessed cyclophosphamide in a small series of 14 children with steroid-resistant MCN, defined as a lack of response after 8 weeks (114). Five of 7 given cyclophosphamide, compared with 4 of 7 continuing on steroids, responded to treatment, suggesting that many patients will eventually respond to steroids if treatment is continued. The number of patients with other histologic diagnoses included in this study was too small to draw any conclusions.

Children with FSGS may have a delayed response to steroids, and the median time to response was 3 months in one report (90). Cytotoxic drugs may be used when the disease is considered steroid resistant. An uncontrolled series of children with steroid-resistant FSGS were given a high-dose steroid regimen of intravenous methylprednisolone and oral prednisolone, with chlorambucil or cyclophosphamide added

if there was no response (117). After a mean follow-up of 6 years, 3 of 32 patients had end-stage renal failure, 5 had renal impairment, and 21 complete remission. These results suggest a benefit of treatment but the findings need to be confirmed in a controlled trial. An ISKDC study tested cyclophosphamide in 37 patients with steroid-resistant FSGS and found it to be ineffective (118).

Cyclosporine is another therapeutic option. Forty-one patients (24 adults and 17 children) with steroid-resistant idiopathic nephrotic syndrome (28 with FSGS and 12 with MCN) were given cyclosporine or placebo (119). Sixty percent of cyclosporine-treated patients responded with a decrease in proteinuria, compared with 16% of controls. In another randomized trial, 12 children with steroid-resistant FSGS were treated with cyclosporine and 12 with placebo for 6 months, and there was less proteinuria in the cyclosporine-treated group (120). Neither of these studies reported an effect on renal function, although the lengths of treatment were short.

### Treatment of Adults

Between 80% and 97% of adults with MCN respond to steroids, but the response to steroids is slower than in children (94–97,121). These studies showed that patients continued to respond for up to 5 months, and therefore adults should be given a longer course of steroids than children. As with children, some adults may have only a single episode of proteinuria, whereas others have a relapsing course. The treatment of frequent relapsers and steroid-resistant patients with other immunosuppressive drugs is not based on randomized trials in adults, with the exception of the trial of cyclosporine described earlier (119). It is largely based on the evidence from studies of children.

There are no controlled trials of steroid treatment in adult FSGS. Two retrospective series have suggested that treatment may be beneficial. Fifteen of 28 patients with the nephrotic syndrome who were untreated reached end-stage renal failure, compared with 5 of 17 who were given steroids. Three of the 28 developed renal impairment (not end-stage), compared with 4 of the 17 (90). Another study found that 6 of 20 treated patients with the nephrotic syndrome developed end-stage renal failure, compared with 9 of 20 untreated patients (100). The mean duration of steroid therapy in these patients was 5 to 6 months. A further series in which all patients were treated with steroids or cytotoxic drugs found that 60% entered sustained remission, but only 28% of these had done so after 2 months of treatment (98). Treatment of adult FSGS remains controversial, but if a course of therapy is begun, sufficient time must be allowed for a response.

### MESANGIOCAPILLARY GLOMERULONEPHRITIS

MCGN has been divided into three types based histologic features. Type I MCGN is the most common and often occurs in association with a systemic disease. These include infec-

**TABLE 18.13.** *Idiopathic nephrotic syndrome: randomized, controlled trials of treatment other than steroids*

| Treatment | Study | N | Effect on outcome |
|---|---|---|---|
| **Steroid-responsive frequent relapsers** | | | |
| Cyclophosphamide | ISKDC 74[114] | 53 | Less relapses |
| Cyclophosphamide | Barrett[115] | 20 | Less relapses |
| Levamisole | BAPN[116] | 61 | Less relapses |
| **Steroid-resistant minimal change** | | | |
| Cyclophosphamide | ISKDC 74[114] | 14 | None |
| **Steroid-resistant idiopathic nephrotic syndrome** | | | |
| Cyclosporine | Ponticelli[119a] | 41 | Less proteinuria |
| **Steroid-resistant focal segmental glomerulosclerosis** | | | |
| Cyclosporine | Lieberman[120] | 25 | Less proteinuria |
| Cyclophosphamide | ISKDC 96[118] | 60 | No benefit |

[a] Twenty-eight with FSGS, 13 with MCN; 24 adults, 17 children (all other studies were in children).

tions (*e.g.* streptococcal, staphylococcal, tuberculosis, malaria, hepatitis B, hepatitis C), autoimmune disease (*e.g.*, SLE, type II cryoglobulinemia), myeloproliferative disease (*e.g.*, lymphoma, leukemia, myeloma, light chain nephropathy), sickle cell disease, carcinomas, and sarcoid. These secondary causes are discussed by Rennke (122). Most show histologic features of type I disease with subendothelial deposits. There may be histologic features specific to the primary disease. For example, the presence of IgG, IgM, and IgA supports a diagnosis of SLE. Fibrillary deposits on electron microscopy suggest mixed cryoglobulins (associated with hepatitis C or not). Although many of these secondary cases are probably caused by immune complexes (deposited or formed *in situ*), it has not been possible to identify antigens from infectious agents or malignancies.

The cause of MCGN remains obscure. There is a strong association with the presence of C3 nephritic factors. These are autoantibodies causing stabilization of C3 convertases and uncontrolled activation of the complement pathway. The relation of these nephritic factors and the hypocomplementemia to the pathogenesis of the glomerulonephritis remains to be elucidated (123). It seems likely that the complement abnormalities are central to the pathogenesis of disease, because dogs that are genetically deficient in C3 develop a histologically similar glomerulonephritis (124), as do factor H–deficient pigs (125). Moreover, a proportion of humans deficient in factor H develop gomerulonephritis. On light microscopy, the morphology has features that are similar to those seen in MCGN. However, the character and location of deposits were highly variable in these patients (123). The remainder of this section of the chapter is concerned with idiopathic MCGN.

## Clinical Features

Table 18.14 summarizes the initial clinical features observed in several series of MCGN. These have been divided into those that combine types I and II (126–134) and those that report findings in type II (135–137) or type I (138) alone.

Idiopathic MCGN is a disease of children and young adults. The series that gave a mean age for type I or type II alone showed that type I occurs at around 26 years and type II at 11 to 17 years. The data for the sex ratio has not been included in the table, but no consistent disparity between male and female frequency was found. Type I and type II disease can begin with the whole spectrum of presentation that occur in glomerular disease. Macroscopic hematuria occurred in 0% to 60%, acute nephritic syndrome in 7% to 38%, nephrotic syndrome in 12% to 82%, microscopic hematuria in 40% to 100%, abnormal creatinine in 10% to 59%, and hypertension in 23% to 60%. Abnormal proteinuria was almost invariable. The wide range of frequencies of these features in different series probably reflects the small numbers

**TABLE 18.14.** *Mesangiocapillary glomerulonephritis: clinical presentation*

| Study | Type | N | Mean age | Male (%) | Nephritic (%) | Nephrotic syndrome (%) | Hematuria (%) Macro | Micro | Impaired renal function (%) | High blood pressure (%) |
|---|---|---|---|---|---|---|---|---|---|---|
| Type I and II | | | | | | | | | | |
| Davis[127] | I | 13 | P | 52[a] | NA | 55 | 52 | 100 | 23 | 41 |
| | II | | 14 | | | | | | | |
| di Belgiojoso[126] | I | 10 | 29 | 59 | 25 | 51 | 5 | 86 | 38 | 38 |
| | II | | 111 | | | | | | | |
| Swainson[128] | I | 17 | NA | 42 | 15 | 68 | NA | NA | NA | NA |
| | II | | 23 | | | | | | | |
| Donadio[129] | I | 51 | 26.5 | 65 | 20 | 80 | 15 | 100 | 38 | 37 |
| | II | | 9 | 12 | 67 | | | | | |
| Madenalakis[130] | I + II | 22 | 26 | 50 | NA | 64 | 0 | 100 | | 32 |
| Cameron[131] | I | 104 | 26 | 49 | 20 | 50 | 25 | 88 | 59 | 31 |
| | II | | 35 | 17 | | | | | | |
| Schwertz[134] | I + III | 33 | P | 46 | NA | 54 | 20 | 60 | NA | 30 |
| | II | | 17 | | | | | | | |
| Habib[132,133] | I | 84 | P | 46 | NA | 82 | 42 | 63 | 30 | 23 |
| | II | | 44 | | 45 | | | | | |
| Type II alone | | | | | | | | | | |
| Lamb[137] | | 10 | 11 | 30 | NA | 30 | 60 | 40 | 10 | 60 |
| Antoine[136] | | 34 | 16 | 65 | 38 | 12 | 30 | NA | NA | NA |
| Chan[135] | | 46 | A | 61 | 7 | 70 | 0 | NA | 43 | 52 |
| Type I alone | | | | | | | | | | |
| Magil[138] | | 46 | NA | 50 | 6.5 | 72 | NA | NA | 35 | 43 |

A, adult population; P, pediatric population
[a] Types I and II not separated.

included and a variation in the underlying cause of these "idiopathic" cases.

Two studies allowed comparison of the clinical features of type I and type II disease, and besides age, no significant differences were found (129,131). Another study compared presenting features in children with type I or II disease and did not find any differences (besides serum complement) (133). A fourth series reported that macroscopic hematuria was more common in type II disease; it was found in 6 of 17 patients, compared with 4 of 33 with type I or III disease (134). Two studies compared the clinical features of adults and children. The study of patients with type I and type II disease found that adults had less macroscopic hematuria (10% versus 29%), more hypertension (42% versus 24%), and more renal impairment (73% versus 51%) than children (131). The other study also found a raised creatinine level to be more common in adults with type I disease (56% versus 24%) (138).

Hypocomplementemia is strongly associated with MCGN. Table 18.15 shows studies that have documented the frequency of complement abnormalities in MCGN (126–135, 138,139). These series agreed that a C3 nephritic factor was more common in type II than in type I disease, occurring in 64% compared with 21% of cases in one study (131) and 88% compared with 42% in another (134). Consistent with this increased frequency of C3 convertase-stabilizing autoantibody, a low C3 concentration occurs more often in type II disease than in type I, being found in 59% to 100% of patients with type II and 25% to 71% of patients with type I. One series found a low C4 level to be more common in type I (as expected for an immune complex disease) (133), but another series found little difference (131). Patients with type II disease and very low levels of C3 may also have low levels of factor B (139). In contrast, patients with type III disease and

severely depressed C3 levels may also have low C5, C6, C7, or C9 levels, demonstrating terminal pathway activation. In this study, the activity of C3 nephritic factors were not measured directly. However, the patterns of complement activation suggested a C3 nephritic factor stabilizing the alternative pathway C3 convertase in type II disease and a nephritic factor activating the terminal pathway and presumably stabilizing the alternative pathway C5 convertase enzyme in type III disease. Type I MCGN produced patterns of complement activation corresponding to alternative or terminal pathway activation.

A condition known as partial lipodystrophy, characterized by lipodystrophy affecting the face, trunk, and upper limbs, is associated with MCGN type II. In one study it occurred in 5 of 35 patients with MCGN type II (131), and in another study of 44 patients, it was present in 4 (133). Patients have been described with partial lipodystrophy who have C3 nephritic factor and hypocomplementemia in the absence of MCGN. The distribution of lipodystrophy may be explained by the presence of adipocytes producing the alternative pathway factor D and other components. Adipocyte lysis then occurs because of activation of the alternative complement pathway (140).

### Diagnosis

None of the clinical features is specific, although MCGN can be suspected in a child or young adult presenting with features suggesting glomerular disease and hypocomplementemia. Other possible diagnoses associated with hypocomplementemia include poststreptococcal glomerulonephritis and SLE. MCGN is a histologic diagnosis that can only be made with certainty by a renal biopsy. It is characterized by mesangial hypercellularity and matrix expansion with glomerular capillary thickening (Fig. 18.6). The hypercellularity results from mesangial proliferation and infiltrating monocytes and neutrophils. The capillary wall thickening is caused by incorporation of mesangial matrix and infiltrating cells, and the wall may have a double contoured appearance.

**TABLE 18.15.** *Mesangiocapillary glomerulonephritis: frequency of complement abnormalities*

| Study | Type | Low C3 (%) | Low C4 (%) | C3 nephritic factor (%) |
|---|---|---|---|---|
| Davis[127] | I + II | 78 | NA | NA |
| di Belgiojoso[126] | I + II | 61 | 30 | NA |
| Swainson[128] | I + II | 40 | 27 | 40 |
| Donadio[129] | I | 71 | 5[a] | NA |
| | II | 100 | | |
| Madenalakis[130] | I + II | 92 | NA | NA |
| Cameron[131] | I | 36 | 22 | 21 |
| | II | 66 | 15 | 64 |
| Habib[132,133] | I | 25 | 50 | NA |
| | II | 96 | 15 | |
| Chan[135] | I | 35 | NA | NA |
| Schwertz[134] | I | NA | NA | 42 |
| | II | | | 88 |
| Varade[139] | I | 68 | NA | NA |
| | II | 82 | | |
| | III | 84 | | |
| Magil[138] | II | 59 | NA | NA |

[a] Type I and II are not separated.

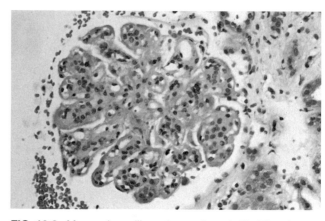

**FIG. 18.6.** Mesangiocapillary glomerulonephritis. The glomerulus is hypercellular, with an increased mesangial matrix, and the capillary wall is thickened. See color plate 6.

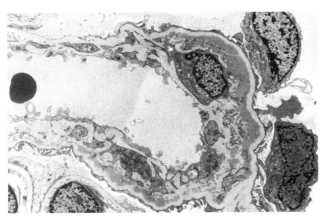

**FIG. 18.7.** Electron microscopic appearance of type I mesangiocapillary glomerulonephritis. The capillary shows large, subendothelial deposits and mesangial cell interposition.

On light microscopy, it may not be possible to differentiate type I and II disease. The former is characterized by subendothelial deposits that are seen on electron microscopy (Fig. 18.7). The latter is characterized by dense intramembranous deposits. In type II disease, these deposits are also found in tubular basement membranes, Bowman's capsule, and peritubular capillaries. These may be visible on light microscopy, but electron microscopy often is required. In types I and II, mesangial and subepithelial deposits may also be found. When these subepithelial deposits are pronounced and are interspersed by projections of basement membrane, it is called type III disease. In type I, immunofluorescence shows granular C3 in the capillary wall, outlining the glomerulus. This pattern may be associated with IgG and less often with IgM, IgA, C1q, or C4. In type II disease, a similar distribution of C3 is found, and it may also be present in the mesangium. Immunoglobulins and other complement components are less often found than in type I disease.

**Prognosis**

Table 18.16 shows a number series that describe prognosis. They include series of type I and II combined (126,130–132, 134,141) and types I (138,142) or II (135,137,143) alone. Some series are pediatric, and some are adult. They all concur that the outlook for this disease is bleak. A large proportion of patients (23% to 59%) die or develop end-stage renal failure during the follow-up period of these studies (3 to 10 years). Another 8% to 30% develop significant renal impairment (not end-stage disease). Two studies allowed a comparison of the outcome in type I and type II disease and did not find any differences (131,133). A third study found that patients with type II disease had a worse outlook, with 76% dead or with end-stage renal failure after a mean follow-up of 134 months, compared with 51% with type I or III (134). Two studies compared the outcomes for pediatric and adult populations; one considered type I and type II disease (131), and the other looked at type I disease alone (138). Both found that

children do better early on, but by 10 to 15 years (131) or 4 years (138), there is no difference.

**Treatment**

A summary of randomized trials is shown in Table 18.17. The ISKDC (144) studied 80 children with MCGN. Fifty-nine had type I, 14 had type II, and 7 had atypical disease. The primary outcome was an increase in creatinine level of 30% or 35 μmol/l. Treatment failure defined in this way occurred in 40% of the treated group, compared with 55% of the control group, over a mean duration of treatment of 41 months. This trial appears to give fairly convincing basis for steroid treatment. However, interpretation of the results is complicated by the fact that the control group had a significantly longer duration of disease before study entry than the treatment group (18.1 months versus 8.9 months). Another small trial of oral steroids in 18 patients suggested a benefit, with 4 placebo-treated patients reaching end-stage renal failure after 6.5 years, compared with none of the steroid treated group (145).

A trial of dipyridamole and aspirin, including 40 patients with type I disease, demonstrated preservation of renal function (141). Glomerular filtration rate was better maintained in the treatment group, and at 62 months, only 3 of 21 treated patients had entered end-stage renal failure, compared with 9 of 19 in the placebo group at 33 months. However, on further follow-up, a second analysis of this trial suggested there was no difference between the groups (146). Another controlled trial of aspirin and dipyridamole including 19 patients (3 with type II disease) showed less proteinuria in the treated group but no difference in renal function. However, this trial was unusual in that all patients in treated and untreated groups had stable renal function over the 36 months' duration of the study (147). A controlled trial of cyclophosphamide, dipyridamole, and warfarin in 47 patients with type I and 12 patients with type II disease did not show a benefit (148). In conclusion, there is no firm evidence to support any form of specific treatment for idiopathic MCGN.

**GLOMERULONEPHRITIS ASSOCIATED WITH INFECTION**

There are many ways in which infection may affect the kidney. This section is not concerned with cases in which the kidney itself is infected or in which a systemic disease affecting the kidney (e.g., hemolytic uremic syndrome, cryoglobulinemia, amyloidosis) is initiated by an infection. Many of these systemic diseases are discussed elsewhere in this book. This section focuses on PSGN, because it is the most common and best described infection-related glomerulonephritis. Glomerulonephritis associated with bacterial endocarditis is discussed, because it is frequently associated with serious infectious disease. Before considering these two diseases, a few points are made about other infection-related syndromes.

**TABLE 18.16.** *Mesangiocapillary glomerulonephritis: prognosis*

| Study | Number | | | Mean follow-up (months) | Dead or end-stage renal failure (%) | Impaired renal function (%) |
|---|---|---|---|---|---|---|
| | I | Total | II | | | |
| di Belgiojoso[126] | 101 | | 11 | 60 | 23 | 20 |
| Habib[133] | 84 | | 44 | 60 | 30 | 8 |
| Donadio[129] | 51 | | 9 | 60 | 42 | 30 |
| Cameron[131] | 69 | | 35 | 96 | 41 | 19 |
| Schwertz[134] | 33 | | 17 | 134 | 60 | 8 |
| Magil[138] | 46 | | 0 | 47 | 48[a] | 48[a] |
| Madenalakis[130] | NA[b] | 22 | NA | 97 | 70 | 20 |
| Schmitt[142] | 220 | | 0 | 50 | 48.6 | 24.6 |
| Vargas[143] | 0 | | 19 | 33 | 42 | 21 |
| Lamb[137] | 0 | | 10 | 120 | 40 | 10 |
| Chan[135] | 0 | | 46 | 60 | 59 | 13 |

[a] End-stage renal failure and renal impairment combined.
[b] I and II are not separated.

Other sections of this chapter discuss secondary causes of specific glomerular diseases that are often idiopathic. These include membranous glomerulonephritis and MCGN, which may both be associated with viral or bacterial infections. A full list of these secondary causes, including infective ones, is included in the appropriate section. Visceral abscesses are mentioned elsewhere in this chapter as a cause of MCGN, but a wide variety of other histologic patterns have been described. These include proliferative glomerulonephritis, mesangial proliferative glomerulonephritis, and membranous glomerulonephritis. *Staphylococcus aureus* is the most commonly implicated organism (149,150). There is no specific treatment besides that for the underlying infection. An immune complex glomerulonephritis has been described with malarial infection. *Plasmodium malariae* is associated with a nephrotic syndrome in children. A variety of histologic appearances have been described, but the most common is capillary wall thickening progressing to glomerular sclerosis. *P. malariae* antigens IgG, IgM, and C3 may be found on immunofluorescence assay. *Plasmodium falciparum* may cause renal failure because of hemolysis and hemoglobinuria, but a proliferative immune complex glomerulonephritis has also been described (151). A glomerulopathy resembling focal segmental glomerulosclerosis has been associated with human immunodeficiency virus (HIV) infection, although a causative link between the virus and the glomerulopathy has not been established with certainty. The remainder of this section concerns PSGN, with a short account of glomerulonephritis associated with endocarditis.

### Poststreptococcal Glomerulonephritis

PSGN is the prototypic postinfectious nephritis occurring after cutaneous or upper respiratory tract infection with particular serotypes of group A β-hemolytic streptococci. It is characterized histologically by endocapillary proliferation resulting in an increased number of cells in the glomerular tuft. It is assumed that the disease results from immunologic cross-reactivity with a streptococcal antigen or from an immune reaction to a streptococcal antigen deposited in the kidney. However, the search for a nephritogenic antigen has been elusive, and none of the proposed candidates has been definitely implicated in the pathogenesis (152,153).

PSGN has become rare in economically advanced countries, possibly because of standards of hygiene or changing patterns of bacterial resistance. However, among children in certain parts of the world, such as Venezuela and Singapore, acute glomerulonephritis has a poststreptococcal cause. Some regions have reported regular epidemics. These are typically areas that are overcrowded and have poor living

**TABLE 18.17.** *Mesangiocapillary glomerulonephritis: randomized, controlled trials of treatment*

| Treatment | Study | Number | | | Follow-up (months) | Effect of treatment |
|---|---|---|---|---|---|---|
| | | I | Total | II | | |
| Cyclophosphamide + dipyrimadole + coumadin | Cattran[148] | 47 | 59 | 12 | 18 | None |
| Oral steroids | Tarshish[144] | 59 | 80[a] | 14 | 41 | Less renal failure |
| Oral steroids | Mota-Hernandez[145] | 17 | 18 | 1 | 29 | Less renal failure |
| Aspirin + dipyridamole | Zäuner[147] | 16 | 9 | 3 | 36 | Less proteinuria |
| Aspirin + dipyridamole | Donadio[141] | 40 | 40 | 0 | 84 | Less renal failure[b] |
| Chlorambucil or azathioprine[c] | Lagrue[36] | NA | 43[d] | NA | 24 | None |

[a] Seven were untypable.
[b] See text.
[c] 16 = chlorambucil, 18 azatioprine, 9 = placebo.
[d] I and II were not differentiated.

**TABLE 18.18.** *Infection preceding poststreptococcal glomerulonephritis*

| Study | History of respiratory infection (%) | History of skin infection (%) | Raised ASO titer (%) | Cultures with *Streptococcus* isolated (%) | | |
|---|---|---|---|---|---|---|
| | | | | Throat | Skin | Both |
| Poon-King[155] | 12 | 74 | NA | 47 | 75 | 41 |
| Rodríguez-Iturbe[156] | 27 | 10 | 50 | NA | NA | NA |

conditions. The Red Lake Indian reservation in Minnesota reported outbreaks in 1953 and 1966 (154). In Trinidad, there were outbreaks in 1952, 1958, 1964, 1967, and 1971 (155).

### Clinical Features

PSGN is characteristically associated with streptococcal infection of the skin or the upper respiratory tract (Table 18.18). In a study of a large outbreak in Trinidad, 74% of 598 patients had a history of skin infection, compared with 12% with a history of respiratory infection (155). In this report, 279 of 598 patients had positive throat cultures for group A streptococci, 332 of 443 skin cultures were positive, and 182 persons were positive for both. Another large series found that a history of respiratory infection was more common than skin, being elicited in 27% compared with 10% (156). Raised antistreptolysin O titers were identified in 50%. Glomerulonephritis usually develops 2 weeks after a respiratory infection, but the latent period is longer after a cutaneous infection, occurring up to 5 weeks later. Particular serotypes are associated with glomerulonephritis (M types 1, 2, 4, 12, 18, 24, 55, 57, and 60).

The clinical features of PSGN have been described in the two series referred to earlier (155,156). These are summarized in Table 18.19 and are largely in agreement with each other. There was an equal sex incidence in the Trinidad series, but a male predominance of 60% in the Venezuelan study. The peak age was 6 to 8 years, with a small proportion of each series being adults; 9.5% were older than 14 in the Trinidad series, and 3% were older than 20 years in the Venezuelan study. Nearly all patients had edema and microscopic hematuria. Between 25% and 60% had macroscopic hematuria, and 80% to 90% were hypertensive at presentation. Approximately 50% had a raised serum creatinine concentration. The nephrotic syndrome and rapidly progressive glomerulonephritis were described but rare. Hypocomplementemia was a common finding. The Venezuelan group found a low C3 or CH50 level in 94% (156). Similarly, a low C3 level was found at presentation in 96% of the Trinidad

series (155), and a third study observed a low C3 level in 79% (157). In addition to hypocomplementemia, cryoglobulins were found in 66% of cases, and a positive rheumatoid factor was identified in almost 50% (158).

Four studies have shown that asymptomatic cases of PSGN are more common than symptomatic ones. Two hundred and forty-eight children infected with group A streptococci were followed prospectively, and renal biopsies were performed on those who developed urinary abnormalities or depressed serum complement (159). Twenty children developed decreased serum complement and abnormal urinalysis, and 19 remained asymptomatic. Nineteen of these 20 children had evidence of PSGN on light microscopy, and IgG and complement deposits were found in 15 of 20. Another study found, among 91 siblings of 20 index cases, 19 had biopsy-proved disease (160). This status had been clinically suspected by the parents in only 3 cases. The second Redlake outbreak, associated with type 49 *Streptococcus* occurred in 1965 (154). Twenty-five cases were recorded (21 were biopsy confirmed). Of these, 6 presented clinically, 9 were obtained from a screening program involving 100 children, and 10 were found by contact tracing index cases. One hundred and forty-one first-degree relatives of 22 index cases were studied (161). Serologic evidence of Streptococcal infection was present in 128. Fifteen cases of PSGN were found, and 12 were asymptomatic. In this series, the diagnosis was clinical and not confirmed by biopsy. This latter study, as well as demonstrating the predominance of asymptomatic cases, demonstrates that host factors are important in determining which relatives will develop glomerulonephritis after infection with a potentially nephritogenic serotype.

### Diagnosis

PSGN is suggested by the presence of the clinical features previously described. In particular, a low C3 level suggests PSGN, MCGN, lupus, or cryoglobulinemia. If the nephrotic syndrome is present, then PSGN is unlikely. The diagnosis can only be established with absolute certainty by a renal

**TABLE 18.19.** *Poststreptococcal glomerulonephritis: clinical features*

| Study | N | Mean age | Male (%) | Edema (%) | Hematuria (%) | | High blood pressure (%) | Renal function impaired (%) | Low C3 or CH50 (%) |
|---|---|---|---|---|---|---|---|---|---|
| | | | | | Macro | Micro | | | |
| Poon-King[155] | 598 | 6 | 49 | 100 | 25 | 92 | 83 | 50 | 94 |
| Rodríguez-Iturbe[156] | 384 | 8 | 59 | 91 | 60 | 100 | 90 | NA | 96 |

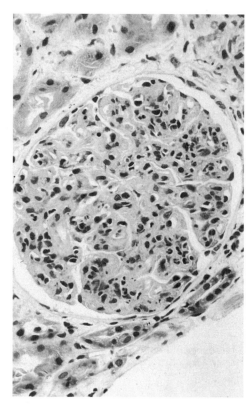

**FIG. 18.8.** Poststreptococcal glomerulonephritis. The glomerular tuft is expanded and hypercellular, with mononuclear cells and neutrophils in the capillaries. See color plate 7.

biopsy and the question becomes one of when a biopsy is necessary. When the acute nephritic syndrome develops with subnephrotic proteinuria and a low C3 concentration after a streptococcal infection, there is little doubt about the diagnosis. However, a biopsy may be indicated in less clear-cut cases. On light microscopy, a proliferation of mesangial and endothelial cells is seen with an infiltrate of inflammatory cells, including neutrophils (Fig. 18.8). This infiltrate includes monocytes and T cells (162). Immunofluorescence shows C3, usually accompanied by IgG and IgM. Three distinct patterns of immunofluorescence have been described (163). The "starry sky" pattern has deposits in the capillary wall and the mesangium. The "mesangial" pattern shows lumpy deposits in the mesangium, and the "garland" pattern has IgG and C3 outlining the glomerular capillaries. On electron microscopy, deposits are seen in subendothelial, subepithelial and intramembranous locations.

### Prognosis

There is general agreement that the short-term prognosis for PSGN is excellent, with almost all patients regaining normal renal function. Three patients died of pulmonary edema in the series of 598 from Trinidad (155). Four died acutely of pulmonary edema in the Venezuelan study, and one had a cerebral hemorrhage resulting from hypertension (156). The early prognosis for adults may be less benign, although it is not as

well described. One study described 126 patients, of which 89 were older than 14 years (157). Nine patients had died of the effects of uremia within 6 months of onset, and seven were older than 14 years.

The question of long-term prognosis is more controversial and summarized in Table 18.20. The first report of the long-term outcome came from a follow-up of the first Redlake epidemic of 1953 (164). Sixty-one patients were examined after 10 years. This careful study was performed by admitting patients overnight for urine collections and comparing all parameters with those of a concurrent control population. None of the subjects showed a creatinine clearance rate below the reference range, and there was no difference in the creatinine clearance of the test group compared with the control group. Eighteen percent of the postnephritic patients had urinary abnormalities but this frequency was similar to that of the control group. These abnormalities were often transient and not repeatable. However, in contrast, other series have shown that a proportion of patients develop chronic renal impairment or end-stage renal failure. The Venezuelan group found that 2 patients of 71 developed end-stage renal failure, and 9 (12.6%) had evidence of renal impairment (measured by creatinine clearance) after 11 to 12 years (165). A report from Trinidad found that only 1 patient of 534 developed end-stage renal failure after 12 to 17 years, with 9 (2%) of patients having raised serum creatinine levels (166). Only 1 of 60 patients developed end-stage renal failure in another study (167). However, at least 20% had a decreased inulin clearance. This must be seen as a minimum estimate, because not all of the subjects had this measurement performed. With the exception of the Redlake series, these studies suggest that fewer than 2% of children will develop end-stage renal failure and that 10% to 20% will develop impaired renal function.

There are limited data regarding the long-term prognosis of adults with PSGN, but three studies are informative. Eighty-nine of 126 patients were older than 14 years of age in one series with a follow-up continuing for 2 to 15 years (157). Four of 126 patients developed end-stage renal failure, and 26 (21%) developed a decreased inulin clearance or raised serum creatinine levels. The outcomes for adults and children were not analyzed separately. Two series looked at the outcome in adults only. One found that 5 of 57 patients had died after 2 to 14 years (168). However, four deaths were unrelated to renal failure, with the fifth occurring after renal transplantation. One of the 4 patients who died and 2 others had raised serum creatinine levels. The other series found that 3 of 51 patients reached end-stage renal failure after 2 to 13 years (169). Eight other patients had a raised serum creatinine levels. The first two of these reports suggests a similar outcome in adults compared with children. However, the third suggests that the prognosis is worse.

### Treatment

Apart from antibiotic treatment if there is evidence of continued infection, there is no specific treatment for PSGN.

**TABLE 18.20.** *Poststreptococcal glomerulonephritis: prognosis*

| Study | N | Age group | Mean or range of follow-up (years) | End-stage renal failure or death (%) | Renal function Impaired (%) |
|---|---|---|---|---|---|
| Perlman[164] | 61 | Pediatric | 10 | 0 | 0[a] |
| Garcia[165] | 71 | Pediatric | 11–12 | 1.4 | 12.6[a] |
| Potter[166] | 534 | Pediatric | 12–17 | 0.2 | 2 |
| Travis[167] | 60 | Pediatric | 3–10 | 2 | 20[a] |
| Baldwin[157] | 126 | Mixed[b] | 2–15 | 3 | 21[a] |
| Lien[168] | 57 | Adult | 7 | 9[c] | 4 |
| Vogel[169] | 51 | Adult | 2–13 | 6 | 17 |

[a] Creatinine or inulin clearance measured.
[b] 89 >14 years; 37 <14 years.
[c] Four of five were deaths unrelated to renal failure.

Treatment is supportive, with attention to fluid balance and use of diuretics and antihypertensive drugs as required. Dialysis occasionally is necessary. Prophylactic antibiotic treatment should be considered for contacts of patients with PSGN and for populations during an epidemic.

## Glomerulonephritis Associated with Bacterial Endocarditis

The largest study of glomerulonephritis associated with bacterial endocarditis comprises a series of 107 postmortems of patients with endocarditis in which 24 cases of glomerulonephritis were found (170); 22.4% of these patients had glomerular disease. Nine other cases were identified from renal biopsy results.

### Clinical Features

Clinical data were available for 30 patients. Twenty-seven had microscopic hematuria, 2 had macroscopic hematuria, and all had proteinuria (2 were in the nephrotic range). Twenty-two had raised serum creatinine levels, and 6 required dialysis (all had diffuse proliferative histologic changes). Four died on dialysis, one remained on dialysis, and one developed progressive renal failure, eventually requiring long-term dialysis. *Staphylococcus aureus* was responsible for 47% of cases with glomerulonephritis. Rheumatoid factor was positive in 8 of 16 measurements, and the C3 level was low in 6 of 10.

### Diagnosis and Treatment

A renal biopsy is required to make the diagnosis, although it may be suspected with abnormal urinalysis. It may be difficult to know whether a patient with endocarditis and renal failure has glomerulonephritis, because patients with endocarditis have a number of other possible causes of renal failure, including acute tubular necrosis due to sepsis, nephrotoxic drugs, and cardiovascular compromise. In most of these situations, renal biopsy is not likely to show a treatable disease, and it is probably not indicated, providing that the diagnosis of endocarditis is certain. Histology in this series showed a wide variety of changes, with variable crescent for-

mation, glomerular sclerosis, and interstitial nephritis. Eight of 10 samples that underwent electron microscopic review showed deposits, but there was no clear pattern, with mesangial, subendothelial, or intramembranous deposits found in different cases. Similarly, immunofluorescence showed a variety of patterns of deposition of IgG, C3, IgM, and IgA.

There is no specific treatment besides that for endocarditis.

## TUBULOINTERSTITIAL NEPHRITIS

Interstitial inflammation of the kidney may occur as part of a systemic disease such as vasculitis or lupus that primarily affects the glomerulus. There are reports of systemic diseases associated with predominantly tubulointerstitial renal lesions, in the absence of significant glomerular damage. Examples include SLE, Sjögren's syndrome, and sarcoidosis. The latter results in a granulomatous pattern of injury. A number of reports of tubulointerstitial nephritis associated with uveitis exist, and this entity has been called the renal-ocular syndrome (171). Many of these multisystem diseases are discussed elsewhere and are outside the scope of this chapter.

After excluding these systemic diseases, cases of interstitial nephritis may be placed into three broad etiologic groups: those caused by infection, those caused by drugs, and those that are idiopathic. Many drugs and infectious agents have been implicated and are listed in Table 18.21. In a series of 27 patients, 15 of the cases were associated with drugs, 9 were related to infection, and 3 were idiopathic (172). In another series of 30 cases, drugs were implicated in 13 cases and possibly were involved in another 8 (173). Most cases are thought to be a hypersensitivity reaction to drugs.

Several different classes of drugs have been implicated as causing interstitial nephritis, with β-lactam antibiotics and nonsteroidal antiinflammatory drugs being the most common. Other classes of drugs implicated include other antibiotics and analgesics, diuretics, and anticonvulsants. Several animal models demonstrate immunologic mechanisms that may cause interstitial inflammation. Disease has been initiated by antibodies to the tubular basement membrane in a variety of species (174). However, these antibodies are rarely seen in human disease. Interstitial inflammation is also a feature of Heymann nephritis, the rat model of membranous

**TABLE 18.21.** *Examples of drugs and infections causing interstitial nephritis*

| β-lactam antibiotics | Nonsteroidal antiinflammatory drugs |
|---|---|
| Ampicillin | Mefenamic acid |
| Methicillin | Diclofenac |
| Penicillin G | Ibuprofen |
| | Poroxicam |
| Other antibiotics | Diuretics |
| Rifampacin | Thiazides |
| Cotrimoxazole | Triamterene |
| Vancomycin | Frusemide |
| Ciprofloxacin | |
| Anticonvulsants | Miscellaneous drugs |
| Phenytoin | Cimetidine |
| Carbamazepine | Allopurinol |
| Valproate | Phenindione |
| | Captopril |
| | Acyclovir |
| Bacteria | Other Infections |
| Streptococci | Leptospirosis |
| *Brucella* | Hantavirus |
| *Legionella* | Cytomegalovirus |
| Tuberculosis | Epstein–Barr virus |
| Yersinia | Toxoplasma |

**TABLE 18.22.** *Interstitial nephritis: clinical presentation*

| Feature | Laberke[173] | Buyson[172] | Galpin[177a] |
|---|---|---|---|
| Number | 30 | 27 | 14 |
| Age (years) | 41 | 49 | 51 |
| Male (%) | 47 | 59 | 93 |
| Renal impairment (%) | 100 | 96 | 100 |
| Microhematuria (%) | 63 | 48 | 93 |
| Macrohematuria (%) | 3 | 15 | 21 |
| High blood pressure (%) | 0 | 15 | NA |
| ESR raised (%) | 100 | NA | NA |
| Fever (%) | 93 | 33 | 100 |
| Loin pain (%) | 37 | 15 | NA |
| Gastrointestinal symptoms (%) | 43 | 30 | NA |
| Glycosuria (%) | 13 | NA | NA |
| Rash (%) | 10 | 26 | 29 |
| Eosinophilia (%) | 17 | 37 | 100 |
| Eosinophiluria (%) | NA | NA | 100 |
| Pyuria (%) | NA | 67 | 100 |
| Proteinuria (%) | 10 | 70 | 36 |

[a] All methicillin-related cases.

glomerulonephritis, in which animals are immunized with a fraction of tubular antigen (44). This is described in the section on membranous nephropathy. Other models have emphasized a role for cell-mediated immune mechanisms (175,176).

### Clinical Features

Most investigators agree on the clinical features that may be present in interstitial nephritis, and the fact that none of them are specific for the disease. However, there are few reports of substantial series of patients with acute interstitial nephritis that allow an estimate of the relative frequency of these clinical features. Two of the largest series comprise 27 and 30 cases, respectively (172,173). A smaller series consisted of 14 cases, all of which were caused by methicillin (177). The clinical features in these three series are shown in Table 18.22. The disease manifested at all ages, with a mean of 40 to 50 years. One series comprised almost exclusively men, but the other two series had a more even sex distribution. Almost all patients had raised creatinine levels, with most patients being described as having acute renal failure. A raised erythrocyte sedimentation rate and fever were common, although one series had a lower frequency of fever (33%) than the other two (93% and 100%). Most patients had microscopic hematuria (48% to 93%), and macroscopic hematuria was uncommon. Proteinuria and rash were also uncommon features. Loin pain was present in 15% to 37% and gastrointestinal symptoms in 30% to 43%.

One series described eosinophilia and eosinophiluria as occurring in 100% of cases (177). Another did not assess eosinophiluria but found eosinophilia in only 17% (173). The third found eosinophilia in 37% (172). These findings may be related to the time of assessment, with eosinophilia occurring only at a certain point in the disease course, or it may be more common in cases of interstitial nephritis due to methicillin. Despite this variation, eosinophilia and eosinophiluria support the diagnosis of interstitial nephritis when present, although their absence does not exclude the diagnosis.

### Diagnosis

None of the previously described clinical features is specific, although the disease may be suspected in a patient with renal failure, fever, signs of an acute phase response, eosinophilia, and microscopic hematuria. The diagnosis may only be proved histologically. The characteristic finding on renal biopsy is an interstitial mononuclear cell infiltrate, which may be diffuse or patchy (Fig. 18.9). These mononuclear cells are predominantly lymphocytes. Macrophages and neutrophils are also present to a lesser degree. There may also be flattening of the tubular epithelium, and the lymphocytes may disrupt the epithelial cells (so-called tubulitis). A variable degree of interstitial edema and fibrosis may also be present. There may also be a scant cellular infiltrate in acute tubular necrosis, but the predominance of the tubular changes over the cellular infiltrate differentiates this condition. Glomeruli may show ischemic changes but are otherwise normal on light and electron microscopy. An exception to this may be found in cases related to nonsteroidal antiinflammatory drugs, which may cause minimal change disease and interstitial nephritis.

Immunofluorescent findings are usually unremarkable. However, a minority of cases show strong linear IgG and C3 depositions along the tubular basement membrane. This occurred in 1 of 30 patients in one series (173) and 2 of 43 in another (178). Both of the patients in the latter study also had circulating antibodies to the tubular basement membrane.

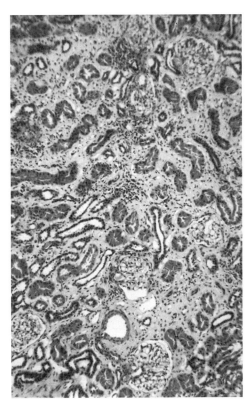

**FIG. 18.9.** Tubulointerstitial nephritis. Mononuclear cells diffusely infiltrate the interstitium. See color plate 8.

## Prognosis

Most patients have improved renal function over a period of 2 or 3 months, and acute interstitial nephritis is often considered to have a favorable prognosis. However, approximately 50% of patients are left with a degree of chronic renal impairment (Table 18.23). A small proportion have end-stage renal failure shortly after the acute episode (7% in one series [173]), and an unknown proportion of those with chronic renal impairment may eventually progress to end-stage renal failure.

## Treatment

There is no treatment of proved benefit apart from stopping a drug that is thought to be responsible. Steroids are often prescribed, but the evidence for their use comes from case reports and uncontrolled, retrospective series. Eight of 14

**TABLE 18.23.** *Interstitial nephritis: prognosis*

| Study | N | End-stage renal failure (%) | Renal impairment (%) | Mean or range of follow-up months (%) |
|---|---|---|---|---|
| Laberke[173] | 30 | 7 | 53 | 9–30 |
| Galpin[177] | 14 | 0 | 50 | NA |
| Buyson[172] | 27 | 0 | 41 | 18 |

patients received prednisolone in the one series (177). Six had returned to their previous baseline serum creatinine levels after a mean of 9 days. Conversely, 2 of the untreated 6 patients returned to their previous creatinine levels after a mean of 54 days. Seven of of 9 patients were treated with steroids, and all regained normal function (179). Of 2 patients who were not treated, 1 regained normal function slowly, and the other developed chronic renal impairment. Another report found that all 10 patients treated with steroids appeared to respond, with 6 regaining normal renal function (172). Overall, the evidence supports the use of steroids. One series used oral steroids only (177), but the other two series began treatment with 3 days of intravenous methylprednisolone (172,179).

## ACKNOWLEDGMENT

We are grateful to Dr. H. T. Cook, who provided the photomicrographs.

## REFERENCES

1. Schena FP. Survey of the Italian registry of renal biopsies. Frequency of the renal diseases for 7 consecutive years. *Nephrol Dial Transplant* 1997;12:418–426.
2. Cameron JS. The nephrotic syndrome: management, complications, and pathophysiology. In: Davison AM, Cameron JS, Grunfeld J-P, et al, eds. *Oxford textbook of clinical nephrology.* 2nd ed. Oxford: Oxford University Press, 1998:461–492.
3. D'Amico G. Influence of clinical and histological features on actuarial renal survival in adult patients with idiopathic IgA nephropathy, membranous nephropathy, and membranoproliferative glomerulonephritis: survey of the recent literature. *Am J Kidney Dis* 1992;20: 15–23.
4. Hiki Y, Saitoh M, Kobayashi Y. Serum IgA class anti-IgA class anti-IgA antibody in IgA nephropathy. *Nephron* 1991;59:552–560.
5. Layward L, Allen AC, Hattersley JM, Harper SJ, Feehally J. Elevation of IgA in IgA nephropathy is localized in the serum and not saliva and is restricted to the IgA1 subclass. *Nephrol Dial Transplant* 1993;8: 25–28.
6. Bene MC, Hurault De Ligny B, Kessler M, Faure GC. Confirmation of tonsillar anomalies in IgA nephropathy: a multicenter study. *Nephron* 1991;58:425–428.
7. van den Wall Bake AW, Daha MR, Haaijman JJ, et al. Elevated production of polymeric and monomeric IgA1 by the bone marrow in IgA nephropathy. *Kidney Int* 1989;35:1400–1404.
8. Gärtner H-V, Hönlein F, Traub U, Bohle A. IgA nephropathy (IgA-IgG nephropathy/IgA nephritis)—a disease entity? *Virchows Arch A* 1979;385:1–27.
9. Rodicio JL. Idiopathic IgA nephropathy. *Kidney Int* 1984;25:717–729.
10. Frimat L, Briançon S, Hestin D, et al. IgA nephropathy: prognostic classification of end-stage renal failure. *Nephrol Dial Transplant* 1997;12:2569–2575.
11. Johnston PA, Brown JS, Braumholtz DA, Davison AM. Clinicopathological correlations and long-term follow-up of 253 United Kingdom patients with IgA nephropathy: a report from the MRC glomerulonephritis registry. *Q J Med* 1992;84:619–27.
12. Droz D. Natural history of primary glomerulonephritis with mesangial deposits of IgA. *Contrib Nephrol* 1976;2:150–7.
13. D'Amico G, Imbasciati E, Di Belgioioso GB, et al. Idiopathic mesangial IgA nephropathy. *Medicine (Baltimore)* 1985;64:49–60.
14. Mustonen J, Pasternack A, Helin H, Nikkila M. Clinicopathologic correlations in a series of 143 patients with IgA glomerulonephritis. *Am J Nephrol* 1985;5:150–157.
15. Bogenschütz O, Bohle A, Batz C, et al. IgA nephritis: on the importance of morphological and clinical parameters in the long-term prognosis of 239 patients. *Am J Nephrol* 1990;10:137–147.

16. Almartine E, Sabatier J, Guerin C, et al. Prognostic factors in mesangial IgA glomerulonephritis: an extensive study with univariate and multivariate analysis. *Am J Kidney Dis* 1991;17:12–19.

17. Nakamoto Y, Asana Y, Dohi K, et al. Primary IgA glomerulonephritis and Schonlein-Henoch purpura nephritis: clinicopathological and immunohistological characteristics. *Q J Med* 1978;188:495–516.

18. Kobayashi Y, Tateno S, Hiki Y, Shigematsu H. IgA nephropathy: prognostic significance of proteinuria and histological alterations. *Nephron* 1983;34:146–153.

19. Taguchi T, von Bassewitz DB, Takebayashi S, Harada T. A comparative study of IgA Nephritis in Japan and Germany: an approach to its geopathology. *Pathol Res Pract* 1987;182:358–367.

20. Shirai T, Yasuhiko Y, Sato M, Yoshiki T, Tetsuo I. IgA nephropathy: Clinicopathology and immunopathology. *Contrib Nephrol* 1978;9:88–100.

21. Nicholls KM, Fairley KF, Dowling JP, Kincaid-Smith P. The clinical cause of mesangial IgA associated nephropathy in adults. *Q J Med* 1984;210:227–50.

22. Tiebosch AT, Frederik PM, van Breda Vriesman PJ, et al. Thin-basement-membrane nephropathy in adults with persistent hematuria. *N Engl J Med* 1989;320:14–18.

23. Churg J, Sobin LH. *Renal disease: classification and atlas of glomerular disease.* New York: Igaku-Shoin, 1982.

24. Schena FP. IgA nephropathies. In: Davison AM, Cameron JS, Grunfeld J-P, et al, eds. *Oxford textbook of clinical nephrology.* 2nd ed. Oxford: Oxford University Press, 1998:537–570.

25. D'Amico G, Minetti L, Ponticelli C, et al. Prognostic indicators in idiopathic mesangial IgA nephropathy. *Q J Med* 1986;59:363–378.

26. Noel LH, Droz D, Gascon M, Berger J. Primary IgA nephropathy: from the first described cases to the present. *Semin Nephrol* 1987;7:351–354.

27. Rekola S, Bergstrand A, Bucht H. Deterioration in GFR in IgA nephropathy as measured by $^{51}$Cr-EDTA clearance. *Kidney Int* 1991;40:1050–1054.

28. Woo KT, Edmondson RPS, Wu AYT, et al. The natural history of IgA nephritis in Singapore. *Clin Nephrol* 1986;25:15–21.

29. Harden PN, Geddes C, Rowe PA, et al. Polymorphisms in angiotensin-converting-enzyme gene and progression of IgA nephropathy. *Lancet* 1995;345:1540–1542.

30. Yoshida H, Mitarai T, Kawamura T, et al. Role of the deletion of polymorphism of the angiotensin converting enzyme gene in the progression and therapeutic responsiveness of IgA nephropathy. *J Clin Invest* 1995;96:2162–2169.

31. Yorioka T, Suehiro T, Yasuoka N, et al. Polymorphism of the angiotensin converting enzyme gene and clinical aspects of IgA nephropathy. *Clin Nephrol* 1995;44:80–85.

32. Welch TR, Fryer C, Shely E, et al. Double-blind, controlled trial of short-term prednisone therapy in immunoglobulin A glomerulonephritis. *J Pediatr* 1992;121:474–477.

33. Lai KN, Lai FM, Ho CP, Chan KW. Corticosteroid therapy in IgA nephropathy with nephrotic syndrome: a long-term controlled trial. *Clin Nephrol* 1986;26:174–180.

34. Pozzi C, Bolasco PG, Fogazzi GB, et al. Corticosteroids in IgA nephropathy: a randomised controlled trial. *Lancet* 1999;353:883–887.

35. Yoshikawa N, Ito H, Sakai T, et al. A controlled trial of combined therapy for newly diagnosed severe childhood IgA nephropathy. The Japanese Pediatric IgA Nephropathy Treatment Study Group. *J Am Soc Nephrol* 1999;10:101–109.

36. Lagrue G, Bernard D, Bariety J, et al. Traitment par le chlorambucil et l'azathioprine dans les glomérulonéphrites primitives. *J Urol Nephrol* 1975;9:655–672.

37. Chan MK, Kwan SY, Chan KW, Yeung CK. Controlled trial of antiplatelet agents in mesangial IgA glomerulonephritis. *Am J Kidney Dis* 1987;5:417–421.

38. Woo KT, Edmonson RPS, Yap HK, et al. Effects of triple therapy on the progression of mesangial proliferative glomerulonephritis. *Clin Nephrol* 1987;27:56–64.

39. Lai KN, Lai FM, Li PK, Vallance-Owen J. Cyclosporin treatment of IgA nephropathy: a short term controlled trial. *Br Med J* 1987;295:1165–1168.

40. Donadio JV, Bergstrahl EJ, Offord KP, et al. A controlled trial of fish oil in IgA nephropathy. *N Engl J Med* 1994;331:1194–1199.

41. Maschio G, Cagnoli L, Claroni F, et al. ACE inhibition reduces proteinuria in normotensive patients with IgA nephropathy: a multicentre, randomised, placebo-controlled study. *Nephrol Dial Transplant* 1994;9:265–269.

42. Cattran DC, Greenwood C, Ritchie S. Long-term benefits of angiotensin-converting enzyme inhibitor therapy in patients with severe immunoglobulin A nephropathy: a comparison to patients receiving treatment with other antihypertensive agents and to patients receiving no therapy. *Am J Kidney Dis* 1994;23:247–254.

43. Glassock RJ. Secondary membranous glomerulonephritis. *Nephrol Dial Transplant* 1992;7[Suppl 1]:64–71.

44. Heymann N, Knutec EP, Wilson SGF, et al. Experimental autoimmune renal disease in rats. *Ann N Y Acad Sci* 1965;124:310–326.

45. Salant DJ, Belok S, Madaio MP, Couser WG. A new role for complement in experimental membranous nephropathy in rats. *J Clin Invest* 1980;66:1339–1350.

46. Baker PJ, Ochi RF, Schulze M, et al. Depletion of C6 prevents development of proteinuria in experimental membranous nephropathy in rats. *Am J Pathol* 1989;135:185–194.

47. Couser WG, Johnson RJ, Young BA, et al. The effects of soluble recombinant complement receptor 1 on complement-mediated experimental glomerulonephritis. *J Am Soc Nephrol* 1995;5:1888–1894.

48. Leenaerts PL, Hall BM, Van Damme BJ, Daha MR, Vanrenterghem YF. Active Heymann nephritis in complement component C6 deficient rats. *Kidney Int* 1995;47:1604–1614.

49. Penny MJ, Boyd RA, Hall BM. Permanent CD8($^+$) T cell depletion prevents proteinuria in active Heymann nephritis. *J Exp Med* 1998;188:1775–1784.

50. Klouda PT, Manos J, Acheson EJ, et al. Strong association between idiopathic membranous nephropathy and HLA-DRW3. *Lancet* 1979;2:770–771.

51. Abe S, Amagasaki Y, Konishi K, Kato E, Iyori S, Sakaguchi H. Idiopathic membranous glomerulonephritis: aspects of geographical differences. *J Clin Pathol* 1986;39:1193–1198.

52. Honkanen E. Survival in idiopathic membranous glomerulonephritis. *Clin Nephrol* 1986;25:122–128.

53. Habib R, Kleinknecht C, Gubler M. Extramembranous glomerulonephritis in children: report of 50 cases. *J Pediatr* 1973;82:754–766.

54. Hopper J, Trew PA, Biava CG. Membranous nephropathy: its relative benignity in women. *Nephron* 1981;29:18–24.

55. MacTier R, Boulton-Jones RM, Payton CD, McLay A. The natural history of membranous nephropathy in the West of Scotland. *Q J Med* 1986;232:793–802.

56. Pereides AM, Malasit P, Morley AR, et al. Idiopathic membranous nephropathy. *Q J Med* 1977;182:163–177.

57. Ramzy MH, Cameron JS, Turner DR, et al. The long-term outcome of idiopathic membranous nephropathy. *Clin Nephrol* 1981;16:13–19.

58. Schieppati A, Mosconi L, Perna A, et al. Prognosis of untreated patients with idiopathic membranous nephropathy. *N Engl J Med* 1993;329:85–89.

59. Wehrmann M, Bohle A, Bogenschütz O, et al. Long term prognosis of chronic idiopathic membranous glomerulonephritis. *Clin Nephrol* 1989;31:67–76.

60. Murphy BF, Fairley KF, Kincaid-Smith PS. Idiopathic membranous glomerulonephritis: long-term follow-up in 139 cases. *Clin Nephrol* 1988;30:175–181.

61. Gluck MC, Gallo G, Lowenstein J, Baldwin DS. Membranous glomerulonephritis: evolution of clinical and pathological features. *Ann Intern Med* 1973;78:1–12.

62. Erwin DT, Donadio JV, Holley KE. The clinical course of idiopathic membranous nephropathy. *Mayo Clin Proc* 1973;48:697–712.

63. Kida H, Asamoto T, Yokoyama H, et al. Long-term prognosis of membranous nephropathy. *Clin Nephrol* 1986;25:64–69.

64. Noel LH, Zanetti M, Droz D, Barbanel C. Long term prognosis of idiopathic membranous glomerulonephritis. *Am J Med* 1979;66:82–90.

65. Zuchelli P, Pasquali S. In: Davison AM, Cameron JS, Grunfeld J-P, et al, eds. *Oxford textbook of clinical nephrology,* vol 1. Oxford: Oxford University Press, 1998:571–590.

66. Zollinger HU, Mihatsh MJ. *Epimembranous glomerulonephritis. Renal pathology in biopsy.* Berlin: Springer-Verlag, 1978:261–278.

67. Jennette JC, Newman WJ, Diaz-Buxo JA. Pathological differentiation between lupus and non lupus membranous glomerulonephritis. *Kidney Int* 1987;24:377–385.

68. Cattran DC, Delmore T, Roscoe J, et al. A randomised controlled trial of prednisone in patients with idiopathic membranous nephropathy. *N Engl J Med* 1989;320:210–215.

69. Cameron JS, Healy MJR, Adu D. The Medical Research Council trial of short-term high-dose alternate day prednisolone in idiopathic membranous nephropathy with nephrotic syndrome in adults. *Q J Med* 1990;274:133–156.

70. Ponticelli C, Zuchelli P, Passerini P, et al. A randomised trial of methylprednisolone and chlorambucil in idiopathic membranous nephropathy. *N Engl J Med* 1989;320:8–13.

71. Collaborative Study of the Adult Idiopathic Nephrotic Syndrome. A controlled trial of short-term prednisone therapy in adults with membranous nephropathy. *N Engl J Med* 1979;301:1301–1306.

72. Donadio JV, Holley K, Anderson CF, Taylor WF. Controlled trial of cyclophosphamide in idiopathic membranous nephropathy. *Kidney Int* 1974;6:431–439.

73. Report by Medical Research Council Working Party. Controlled trial of azathioprine and prednisone in chronic renal disease. *Br Med J* 1971;2:239–241.

74. Ponticelli C, Zuchelli P, Passerini P, Cesana B. Methylprednisolone plus chlorambucil as compared with methylprednisolone alone for the treatment of idiopathic membranous nephropathy. *N Engl J Med* 1992;327:599–603.

75. Falk RJ, Hogan SL, Muller JE, Jenette C. Treatment of progressive membranous glomerulopathy: a randomised trial comparing cyclophosphamide and corticosteroids with corticosteroids alone. *Ann Intern Med* 1992;116:438–445.

76. Yoshikawa N, Cameron AH, White RHR. Ultrastructure of the non-sclerotic glomeruli in childhood nephrotic syndrome. *J Pathol* 1982;136:133–147.

77. Tejani A. Morphological transition in minimal change nephrotic syndrome. *Nephron* 1985;39:157–159.

78. Kitano Y, Yoshikawa N, Nakamura H. Glomerular anionic sites in minimal change nephrotic syndrome and focal segmental glomerulosclerosis. *Clin Nephrol* 1993;40:199–204.

79. Fiser RT, Arnold WC, Charlton RK, et al. T-lymphocyte subsets in nephrotic syndrome. *Kidney Int* 1991;40:913–916.

80. Taube D, Brown Z, Williams DG. Impaired lymphocyte and suppressor cell function in minimal change nephropathy, membranous nephropathy and focal glomerulosclerosis. *Clin Nephrol* 1984;22:176–182.

81. Heslan JM, Lautie JP, Intrator L, et al. Impaired IgG synthesis in patients with the nephrotic syndrome. *Clin Nephrol* 1982;18:144–147.

82. Lagrue G, Branellec A, Niaudet P, et al. [Transmission of nephrotic syndrome to two neonates: spontaneous regression]. *Presse Med* 1991;20:255–257.

83. Ali AA, Wilson E, Moorhead JF, et al. Minimal-change glomerular nephritis: normal kidneys in an abnormal environment? *Transplantation* 1994;58:849–852.

84. Savin VJ, Sharma R, Sharma M, et al. Circulating factor associated with increased glomerular permeability to albumin in recurrent focal segmental glomerulosclerosis [see comments]. *N Engl J Med* 1996;334:878–883.

85. Dantal J, Bigot E, Bogers W, et al. Effect of plasma protein adsorption on protein excretion in kidney-transplant recipients with recurrent nephrotic syndrome [see comments]. *N Engl J Med* 1994;330:7–14.

86. Verani RR. Obesity-associated focal segmental glomerulosclerosis: pathological features of the lesion and relationship with cardiomegaly and hyperlipidaemia. *Am J Kidney Dis* 1992;20:629–634.

87. International Study of Kidney Disease in Children. Nephrotic syndrome in children: prediction of histopathology from clinical and laboratory characteristics at time of diagnosis. *Kidney Int* 1978;13:159–165.

88. Report of the Southwest Pediatric Nephrology Study Group. Focal segmental glomerulosclerosis in children with idiopathic nephrotic syndrome. *Kidney Int* 1985;27:442–449.

89. Habib R, Kleinknecht C. The primary nephrotic syndrome of childhood: classification and clinicopathological study of 406 cases. In: Sommers SC, ed. *Pathology annual*, vol 6. New York: Appleton-Century-Crofts, 1971:417–474.

90. Cattran DC, Rao P. Long-term outcome in children and adults with classic focal segmental glomerulosclerosis. *Am J Kidney Dis* 1998;32:72–79.

91. Arbus GS, Poucell S, Bacheyie GS, Baumal R. Focal segmental glomerulosclerosis with idiopathic nephrotic syndrome: three types of clinical response. *J Pediatr* 1982;101:40–45.

92. White RHR, Glasgow EF, Mills RJ. Clinicopathological study of nephrotic syndrome in children. *Lancet* 1970;1:1353–1359.

93. Hopper J, Ryan P, Lee JC, Rosenau W. Lipoid nephrosis in 31 adult patients: renal biopsy study by light, electron, and fluorescence microscopy with experience in treatment. *Medicine (Baltimore)* 1970;49:321–341.

94. Nolasco F, Cameron JS, Heywood EF, et al. Adult-onset minimal change nephrotic syndrome: a long-term follow-up. *Kidney Int* 1986;29:1215–1223.

95. Fujimoto S, Yamamoto Y, Hisanaga S, et al. Minimal change nephrotic syndrome in adults: response to corticosteroid therapy and frequency of relapse. *Am J Kidney Dis* 1991;17:687–692.

96. Korbet SM, Schwartz MM, Lewis EJ. Minimal-change glomerulopathy of adulthood. *Am J Nephrol* 1988;8:291–297.

97. Mak SK, Short CD, Mallick NP. Long-term outcome of adult-onset minimal-change nephropathy. *Nephrol Dial Transplant* 1996;11:2192–2201.

98. Banfi G, Moriggi M, Sabadini E, et al. The impact of prolonged immunosuppression on the outcome of idiopathic focal segmental glomerulosclerosis with nephrotic syndrome in adults: a collaborative retrospective study. *Clin Nephrol* 1991;36:53–59.

99. Cameron JS, Turner DR, Ogg CS, et al. The long-term prognosis of patients with focal segmental glomerulosclerosis. *Clin Nephrol* 1978;10:213–218.

100. Rydel JJ, Korbet SM, Borok RZ, Schwartz MM. Focal segmental glomerular sclerosis in adults: presentation, course, and response to treatment. *Am J Kidney Dis* 1995;25:534–542.

101. Pei Y, Cattran D, Delmore T, et al. Evidence suggesting under-treatment in adults with idiopathic focal segmental glomerulosclerosis. *Am J Med* 1987;82:938–944.

102. International Study of Kidney Disease in Children. The primary nephrotic syndrome in children: identification of patients with minimal change nephrotic syndrome from initial response to prednisone. *J Pediatr* 1981;98:561–564.

103. International Study of Kidney Disease in Children. Minimal change nephrotic syndrome in children: deaths during the first 5 to 15 years' observation. *Pediatrics* 1984;73:497–501.

104. International Study of Kidney Disease in Children. Early identification of frequent relapsers among children with minimal change nephrotic syndrome. *J Pediatr* 1982;101:514–518.

105. Trompeter RS, Hicks J, LLoyd BW, et al. long-term outcome for children with minimal change nephrotic syndrome. *Lancet* 1985;1:366–370.

106. Lewis MA, Baildom EM, Davis N, et al. Nephrotic syndrome: from toddlers to twenties. *Lancet* 1989;1:255–259.

107. Koskimies O, Vilska J, Rapola J, Hallman N. Long-term outcome of primary nephrotic syndrome. *Arch Dis Child* 1982;57:544–548.

108. Broyer M, Meyrier A, Niaudet P, Habib R. Minimal changes and focal segmental glomerulosclerosis. In: Davison AM, Cameron JS, Grunfeld J-P, et al, eds. *Oxford textbook of clinical nephrology*. 2nd ed. Oxford: Oxford University Press, 1998:493–535.

109. Ingulli E, Tejani A. Racial differences in the incidence and renal outcome of idiopathic focal segmental glomerulosclerosis in children. *Pediatr Nephrol* 1991;5:393–397.

110. Mongeau JG, Robitaille PO, Clermont MJ, et al. Focal segmental glomerulosclerosis (FSG) 20 years later: from toddler to grown up. *Clin Nephrol* 1993;40:1–6.

111. Report of a workshop by the British Association for Paediatric Nephrology and Research Unit, Royal College of Physicians: consensus statement on management and audit potential for steroid responsive nephrotic syndrome. *Arch Dis Child* 1994;70:151–157.

112. Arbeitgemeinschaft für Paediatrische Nephrologie. Short versus standard prednisone therapy for initial treatment of idiopathic nephrotic syndrome in children. *Lancet* 1988;1:380–383.

113. Wingen AM, Müller-Wieffel DE, Shärer K. Spontaneous remissions in frequently relapsing and steroid dependent nephrotic syndrome. *Clin Nephrol* 1985;23:35–40.

114. International Study of Kidney Disease in Children. Prospective, controlled trial of cyclophosphamide therapy in children with the nephrotic syndrome. *Lancet* 1974;2:423–427.

115. Barratt TM, Soothill JF. Controlled trial of cyclophosphamide in steroid-sensitive relapsing nephrotic syndrome of childhood. *Lancet* 1970;2:479–482.

116. British Association for Paediatric Nephrology. Levamisole for corticosteroid-dependent nephrotic syndrome in childhood. *Lancet* 1991;337:1555–1557.

117. Tune BM, Kirpekar R, Sibley RK, et al. Intravenous methylprednisolone and oral alkylating agent therapy of prednisone-resistant pediatric focal segmental glomerulosclerosis: a long-term follow-up. *Clin Nephrol* 1995;43:84–88.

118. Tarshish P, Tobin JN, Bernstein J, Edelmann CM Jr. Cyclophosphamide does not benefit patients with focal segmental glomerulosclerosis: a report of the International Study of Kidney Disease in Children. *Pediatr Nephrol* 1996;10:590–593.

119. Ponticelli C, Rizzoni G, Edefonti A, et al. A randomised trial of cyclosporin in steroid resistant idiopathic nephrotic syndrome. *Kidney Int* 1993;43:1377–1384.

120. Lieberman KV, Tejani A. A randomized double-blind placebo-controlled trial of cyclosporine in steroid-resistant idiopathic focal segmental glomerulosclerosis in children. *J Am Soc Nephrol* 1996;7:56–63.

121. Nair RB, Date A, Kirubakaran MG, Shastry JCM. Minimal-change nephrotic syndrome in adults treated with alternate-day steroids. *Nephron* 1987;47:209–210.

122. Rennke HG. Secondary membranoproliferative glomerulonephritis. *Kidney Int* 1995;47:643–656.

123. West CD. Nephritic factors predispose to chronic glomerulonephritis. *Am J Kidney Dis* 1994;24:956–963.

124. Cork LC, Morris JM, Olson JL, et al. Membranoproliferative glomerulonephritis in dogs with a genetically determined deficiency of the third component of complement. *Clin Immunol Immunolpathol* 1991;60:455–470.

125. Jansen JH, Hogasen K, Mollnes TE. Extensive complement activation in hereditary porcine membranoproliferative glomerulonephritis type II (porcine dense deposit disease). *Am J Pathol* 1988;143:1356–1365.

126. di Belgiojoso GB, Tarantino A, Colasanti G, et al. The prognostic value of some clinical and histopathological parameters in membranoproliferative glomerulonephritis. Report of 112 cases. *Nephron* 1977;19:250–258.

127. Davis AE, Schneeberger EE, Grupe WE, McCluskey RT. Membranoproliferative glomerulonephritis (MPGN type I) and dense deposit disease (DDD) in children. *Clin Nephrol* 1978;9:184–193.

128. Swainson CP, Robson JS, Thomson D, MacDonald M. Mesangiocapillary glomerulonephritis: a long-term study of 40 cases. *J Pathol* 1983;141:449–468.

129. Donadio JV, Slack TK, Holley KE, Ilstrup DM. Idiopathic membranoproliferative (mesangiocapillary) glomerulonephritis: a clinicopathological study. *Mayo Clin Proc* 1979;54:141–150.

130. Madelanakis N, Mendoza N, Pirani CL, Pollack VE. Lobular glomerulonephritis and membranoproliferative glomerulonephritis. *Medicine* 1971;50:319–355.

131. Cameron JS, Turner DR, Heaton J, et al. Idiopathic mesangiocapillary glomerulonephritis: comparison of types I and II in children and adults and long-term prognosis. *Am J Med* 1983;74:175–192.

132. Habib R, Kleinknecht C, Gubler MC, Levy M. Idiopathic membranoproliferative glomerulonephritis in children: report of 105 cases. *Clin Nephrol* 1973;1:194–214.

133. Habib R, Gubler M, Loirat C, et al. Dense deposit disease: a variant of membranoproliferative glomerulonephritis. *Kidney Int* 1975;7:204–215.

134. Schwertz R, de Jong R, Gretz N, et al. Outcome of idiopathic membranoproliferative glomerulonephritis in children. Arbeitsgemeinschaft Padiatrische Nephrologie. *Acta Paediatr* 1996;85:308–312.

135. Chan MK, Chan KW, Chan PCK, et al. Adult-onset mesangiocapillary glomerulonephritis: a disease with a poor prognosis. *Q J Med* 1989;267:599–607.

136. Antoine B, Faye C. The clinical course associated with dense deposits in the kidney basement membranes. *Kidney Int* 1972;1:420–427.

137. Lamb V, Tisher CG, McCoy RC, Robinson RR. Membranoproliferative glomerulonephritis with dense intramembranous alterations: a clinicopathological study. *Lab Invest* 1977;36:609–617.

138. Magil AB, Price JDE, Bower G, et al. Membranoproliferative glomerulonephritis type 1: comparison of natural history in children and adults. *Clin Nephrol* 1979;11:239–244.

139. Varade WS, Forristal J, West CD. Patterns of complement activation in idiopathic membranoproliferative glomerulonephritis, types I, II, and III. *Am J Kidney Dis* 1990;16:196–206.

140. Mathieson PW, Würzner R, Oliveira DBG, et al. Complement-mediated adipocyte lysis by nephritic factor sera. *J Exp Med* 1993;177:1827–1831.

141. Donadio JV, Anderson CF, Mitchell JC, et al. Membranoproliferative glomerulonephritis: a prospective clinical trial of platelet-inhibitor therapy. *N Engl J Med* 1984;310:1421–1426.

142. Schmitt H, Bohle A, Reineke T, et al. Long-term prognosis of membranoproliferative glomerulonephritis type I. Significance of clinical and morphological parameters: an investigation of 220 cases. *Nephron* 1990;55:242–250.

143. Vargas R, Thomson KJ, Wilson D, et al. Mesangiocapillary glomerulonephritis with dense "deposits" in the basement membranes of the kidney. *Clin Nephrol* 1976;5:73–82.

144. Tarshish P, Bernstein J, Tobin JN, Edelmann CM. Treatment of mesangiocapillary glomerulonephritis with alternate-day prednisone—a report of the International Study of Kidney Disease in Children. *Pediatr Nephrol* 1991;6:123–130.

145. Mota-Hernandez F, Gordilla-Paniagua G, Munoz-Arizpe R, et al. Prednisone versus placebo in membranoproliferative glomerulonephritis: long-term clinicopathological correlations. *Int J Pediatr Nephrol* 1985;6:25–28.

146. Donadio JV, Offord KP. Reassessment of treatment results in membranoproliferative glomerulonephritis, with emphasis on life-table analysis. *Am J Kidney Dis* 1989;14:445–451.

147. Zäuner I, Böhler J, Braun N, et al. Effect of aspirin and dipyridamole on proteinuria in idiopathic membranoproliferative glomerulonephritis: a multicentre prospective clinical trial. *Nephrol Dial Transplant* 1994;9:619–622.

148. Cattran DC, Cardella CJ, Roscoe JM, et al. Results of a controlled drug trial in membranoproliferative glomerulonephritis. *Kidney Int* 1985;27:436–441.

149. Beaufils M, Morel-Maroger L, Sraer JD, et al. Acute renal failure of glomerular origin complicating visceral abscesses. *N Engl J Med* 1976;295:185–189.

150. Beaufils M. Glomerular disease complicating abdominal sepsis. *Kidney Int* 1981;19:609–618.

151. Boonpucknavik V, Sitprija V. Renal disease in acute *Plasmodium falciparum* infection in man. *Kidney Int* 1979;16:44–52.

152. Lange K, Seligson G, Cronin W. Evidence for the in situ origin of poststreptococcal glomerulonephritis: glomerular localization of endostreptosin and the clinical significance of the subsequent antibody response. *Clin Nephrol* 1983;19:3–10.

153. Yoshimoto M, Hosoi S, Fujisawa S, et al. High levels of antibodies to streptococcal cell membrane antigens specifically bound to monoclonal antibodies in acute poststreptococcal glomerulonephritis. *J Clin Microbiol* 1987;25:680–684.

154. Anthony BF, Kaplan EL, Chapman SS, et al. Epidemic acute nephritis with reappearance of type-49 streptococcus. *Lancet* 1967;2:787–780.

155. Poon-King T, Potter EV, Svartman M, et al. Epidemic acute nephritis with reappearance of M-type 55 streptococci in Trinidad. *Lancet* 1973;1:475–479.

156. Rodríguez-Iturbe B, Garcia R, Rubio L, et al. Epidemic glomerulonephritis in Maracaibo: evidence for progression to chronicity. *Clin Nephrol* 1976;5:197–206.

157. Baldwin DS, Gluck MC, Schacht RG, Gallo G. The long-term course of post-streptococcal glomerulonephritis. *Ann Intern Med* 1974;80:342–358.

158. Rodríguez-Iturbe B. Epidemic post-streptococcal glomerulonephritis. *Kidney Int* 1984;25:129–136.

159. Sagel I, Treser G, Ty A, et al. Occurrence and nature of glomerular lesions after group A streptococci infections in children. *Ann Intern Med* 1973;79:492–499.

160. Dodge WF, Spargo BH, Travis LB. Occurrence of acute glomerulonephritis in sibling contacts of children with sporadic acute glomerulonephritis. *Pediatrics* 1967;40:1028–1030.

161. Rodríguez-Iturbe B, Rubio L, García R. Attack rate of post-streptococcal nephritis in families. *Lancet* 1981;1:401–403.

162. Parra G, Platt JL, Falk RJ, et al. Cell populations and membrane attack complex in glomeruli of patients with post-streptococcal glomerulonephritis: identification using monoclonal antibodies by indirect immunofluorescence. *Clin Immunol Immunopathol* 1984;33:324–332.

163. Sorger K. The garland type of post-infectious glomerulonephritis: morphological characteristics and follow-up studies. *Clin Nephol* 1983;17:114–128.

164. Perlman LV, Herdman RC, Kleinman H, Vernier RL. Post-streptococcal glomerulonephritis. *JAMA* 1965;194:63–70.

165. García R, Rubio L, Rodríguez-Iturbe B. Long-term prognosis of epidemic poststreptococcal glomerulonephritis in Maracaibo: follow-up studies 11–12 years after the acute episode. *Clin Nephrol* 1981;15:291–298.

166. Potter EV, Lipshultz LA, Abidh S, et al. Twelve to seventeen year follow-up of patients with post-streptococcal acute glomerulonephritis in Trinidad. *N Engl J Med* 1982;307:725–729.

167. Travis LB, Dodge WF, Beathard GA, et al. Acute glomerulonephritis in children: a review of the natural history with emphasis on prognosis. *Clin Nephrol* 1973;1:169–181.

168. Lien JWK, Mathew TH, Meadows R. Acute post-streptococcal glomerulonephritis in adults: a long-term study. *Q J Med* 1979;189:99–111.

169. Vogl W, Renke M, Mayer-Eichberger D, et al. Long-term prognosis for endocapillary glomerulonephritis of post-streptococcal type in children and adults. *Nephron* 1986;44:58–65.

170. Neugarten J, Galio GR, Baldwin DS. Glomerulonephritis in bacterial endocarditis. *Am J Kidney Dis* 1984;3:371–379.

171. Steinman TI, Silva P. Acute interstitial nephritis and iritis. Renal-ocular syndrome. *Am J Med* 1984;77:189–191.

172. Buysen JGM, Houthoff HJ, Krediet RT, Arisz L. Acute interstitial nephritis: a clinical and morphological study in 27 patients. *Nephrol Dial Transplant* 1990;5:94–99.

173. Laberke HG, Bohle A. Acute interstitial nephritis: correlations between clinical and morphological findings. *Clin Nephrol* 1980;14:263–273.

174. Wilson CB. Study of the immunopathogenesis of tubulointerstitial nephritis using model systems. *Kidney Int* 1989;35:938–953.

175. Bannister KM, Ulich TR, Wilson CB. Induction, characterization, and cell transfer of autoimmune tubulointerstitial nephritis. *Kidney Int* 1987;32:642–651.

176. Neilson EG, McCafferty E, Feldman A, et al. Spontaneous interstitial nephritis in kdkd mice. I. An experimental model of autoimmune renal disease. *J Immunol* 1984;133:2560–1565.

177. Galpin JE, Shinaberger JH, Stanley TM, et al. Acute interstitial nephritis due to methicillin. *Am J Med* 1978;65:756–765.

178. Droz D, Kleinknect D. Acute Interstitial Nephritis. In: Davison AM, Cameron JS, Grunfeld J-P, et al, eds. *Oxford textbook of clinical nephrology.* 2nd ed. Oxford: Oxford University Press, 1998:1634–1648.

179. Pusey CD, Saltissi D, Bloodworth L, et al. Drug associated acute interstitial nephritis: clinical and pathological features and the response to high dose steroid therapy. *Q J Med* 1983;206:194–211.

*Textbook of the Autoimmune Diseases,*
Edited by R. G. Lahita, N. Chiorazzi, and W. H. Reeves,
Lippincott Williams & Wilkins, Philadelphia © 2000.

# CHAPTER 19

# Autoimmune Nervous System Disease

Robin L. Brey, Richard J. Barohn, and Anthony A. Amato

## APPROACH TO THE PATIENT

A number of diseases that either primarily or exclusively affect the nervous system have an autoimmune basis. In this chapter, we review the major autoimmune disorders of the central and peripheral nervous system with emphasis on clinical presentation and immunologic basis, diagnostic approach, and therapy. Autoimmune diseases of muscle and myasthenia gravis are covered in Chapter 22.

The major consideration in approaching a patient with possible autoimmune nervous system disease is to decide whether the nervous system manifestations are restricted to the nervous system or whether they are part of a more systemic disease process. Next, the symptoms should be categorized by the anatomic regions of the nervous system that are affected, such as the peripheral nerve, neuromuscular junction, nerve root, spinal cord, or brain. As with other autoimmune diseases, a specific diagnosis is essential for planning treatment. Therapeutic options are rather specific for some autoimmune nervous system diseases. For others, options are limited to nonspecific immunosuppressive therapies.

The central nervous system (CNS) is immune privileged but only to a relative degree. Under normal circumstances, the blood-brain barrier blocks the entrance of large numbers of most immune effector cells into the CNS. Activated T lymphocytes enter the under normal conditions, possibly to perform a surveillance function (1,2). If they are not specific for exposed CNS antigens, they do not remain (3). The blood-brain barrier may be altered, however, by the release of cytokines, such as tumor necrosis factor-$\alpha$ (TNF-$\alpha$) which is produced in response to systemic infection (4,5). The intercellular adhesion molecule-1 (ICAM-1) is unregulated on

R. L. Brey: Department of Medicine, Division of Neurology, University of Texas Health Sciences Center, San Antonio, Texas 78284-7883.

R. J. Barohn: Department of Neurology, University of Texas Southwest Medical Center at Dallas, Dallas, Texas 75390-8897.

A. A. Amato: Department of Neurology, Harvard Medical School, Boston, Massachusetts 02115; Department of Neurology, Brigham and Women's Hospital, Boston, Massachusetts 02115.

brain endothelial cells by TNF-$\alpha$ and probably plays a role in the influx of activated T lymphocytes and other effector cells into the CNS (6). Cytokines secreted by activated T lymphocytes and macrophages can upregulate the expression of major histocompatibility antigen (MHC) class I molecules (TNF-$\alpha$ acting synergistically with interferon-$\gamma$ [IFN-$\gamma$]) and MHC class II molecules on brain endothelial cells, microglial cells, and astrocytes (7). This could initiate or help perpetuate a CNS-directed immune response. Finally, some of the cytokines secreted by lymphocytes and macrophages during an immune response (interleukin-1 [IL-1], IFN-$\gamma$, and TNF-$\alpha$) can be directly toxic to CNS tissue (8).

These and other advances in the past few years have furthered our understanding of both normal and pathogenic immune system functioning within the nervous system and have underscored the development of new effective and specific treatment options for diseases like multiple sclerosis (MS).

## AUTOIMMUNE NEUROPATHY

### Acute Inflammatory Demyelinating Polyradiculoneuropathy

#### Clinical Presentation

Guillain–Barré syndrome (GBS), or acute inflammatory demyelinating polyradiculoneuropathy, is associated with rapidly evolving weakness, sensory loss, and areflexia (9–11). GBS is the most common cause of acute generalized weakness, with an incidence of 1 to 2 per 100,000 population (12), and it can occur at any age. In many patients, there is an antecedent infection that is usually viral. *Campylobacter jejuni* enteritis precedes GBS in 15% to 38% of patients and is the most common antecedent bacterial infection (13–16). GBS has been reported in human immunodeficiency virus (HIV)-infected patients, but it is not clear whether HIV infection is a predisposing factor (17). Other viral precipitants are Epstein–Barr virus (mononucleosis or hepatitis) and cytomegalovirus (18). In addition, antecedent events that have been associated with GBS include immunizations (19), surgery (20), epidural anesthesia (21), and concurrent illnesses, such as Hodgkin's disease (22,23).

Initial symptoms are usually ascending numbness and tingling of the extremities, followed by weakness involving proximal and distal muscles. Aching pain in the extremities and back is common. Deep tendon reflexes are diminished or absent. More than half of patients reach a nadir by 2 weeks, 80% by 3 weeks, and 90% by 4 weeks (24). The tempo of progression is variable, and some patients can become flaccid and ventilator dependent in a few days. In addition to the classic presentation of GBS, variants have been described (25–29). These are listed in Table 19.1.

The syndrome described by Fisher (25) consists of ophthalmoplegia, ataxia, and areflexia and was the first recognized GBS variant. These patients do not have weakness, but the spinal fluid protein is elevated. Patients with otherwise typical GBS who also have ophthalmoplegia do not have the Miller-Fisher syndrome. A syndrome mimicking an acute spinal cord lesion can occur with back pain, bilateral lower extremity numbness, weakness, and areflexia, sparing the arms (26). Other regional variants include pharyngocervicobrachial weakness with ptosis (mimicking botulism), ptosis without ophthalmoplegia, and facial diplegia or sixth nerve palsies with paresthesias (26–28). Pure sensory and autonomic variants have also been reported (9,29).

An axonal variant is characterized by rapidly progressive weakness with prolonged paralysis and respiratory failure over a few days (27). The axonal variant is more often associated with antecedent *C. jejuni* enteritis and has a poor prognosis (13). The largest number of cases of the pure motor axonal form comes from northern China, although there have been descriptions from other countries as well (18,30,31). This variant has been labeled *acute motor axonal neuropathy* (32). Four cases of an acute motor-sensory axonal neuropathy have been reported, also from China (33). These cases were also associated with *C. jejuni* infection. Thus, it appears that infection with *C. jejuni* can initiate an immune attack against peripheral nerves that produces GBS, possibly by the mechanism of molecular mimicry. These patients may be more likely to develop a pure axonal or pure motor presentation with a poor prognosis. Evidence of *C. jejuni* infection,

however, can occur in cases of the otherwise typical demyelinating motor-sensory form.

Identifying the mechanisms responsible for the immune-mediated neuropathies, including GBS, remain a difficult challenge. It is not yet clear how T-cell–mediated processes lead to axonal destruction and myelin degradation or the principal immunogenic epitopes of peripheral nerve antigens. Much of the evidence that GBS is immunologically mediated is derived from comparisons with the animal model of experimental allergic neuritis (34). In this model, animals immunized with peripheral nerve develop ataxia and paralysis about 2 weeks after injection. As in GBS, pathologic studies show a marked cellular infiltration of the peripheral nerves by lymphocytes and macrophages with segmental demyelination, and the cerebrospinal fluid (CSF) shows an albuminocytologic dissociation. A basic protein of peripheral nerve myelin, P2 protein (35), can also induce experimental allergic neuritis. Most of the evidence indicates that experimental allergic neuritis is a cell-mediated disease because it can be passively transferred to naive rats by lymphocytes from sensitized animals. The role of circulating antibodies is not as clear, although some investigators have passively transferred the disease from serum (36).

One group has been able to demonstrate complement-fixing antibodies to peripheral nerve myelin in the serum of GBS patients (37). The titer of antiperipheral nerve myelin antibody declined with clinical improvement and correlated with the appearance of terminal complement complexes in the serum, CSF, and nerve (38). Antibodies to various gangliosides ($GM_1$, $GM_{1b}$, $GD_{1b}$, and others) have also been documented in several series of GBS patients (39,40–42). Studies have shown that many of these patients have evidence of *C. jejuni* infection (43,44). In one of these studies, 25% of all GBS patients had $GM_1$ antibodies, and 52% of patients with *C. jejuni* infection had these antibodies (44). *C. jejuni* has $GM_1$-like oligosaccharides on its surface that may cross-react with $GM_1$, explaining why an antibody directed against the bacteria may also produce a neuropathy (43).

Most patients with GBS recover; however, 10% to 23% require mechanical ventilation, 7% to 22% have residual defects, 3% to 10% relapse, and 2% to 5% die (44). According to Ropper et al. (9,10), only about 15% have complete recovery with no residual symptoms or signs (9,10). Age older than 60 years, low-amplitude compound motor action potentials, and prior *C. jejuni* infection are all poor prognostic indicators (45).

A monophasic course occurs in 95% of patients. Minor "relapses," in which patients may show signs of slight deterioration during the recovery phase, are uncommon. In the French plasmapheresis study, relapses occurred in 1% of the control group (46). Sometimes, however, what a physician or patient interprets as a relapse is actually a long plateau phase showing little signs of improvement on a day-to-day basis. True relapsing GBS, in which a patient recovers and then deteriorates months or years later, occurs in only about 5% of cases (47).

**TABLE 19.1.** *Guillain–Barré syndrome variants*

Miller–Fisher syndrome: ophthalmoplegia, ataxia, areflexia
Areflexic paraparesis with back pain (resembles cord lesion)
Pharyngeal, cervical, and brachial weakness (resembles botulism)
Ptosis without ophthalmoplegia
Facial diplegia with paresthesia
Sixth nerve palsy with paresthesia
Pure axonal
   Rapidly progressive weakness
   Prolonged paralysis and respiratory failure
   Associated with *Campylobacter jejuni*
   Often pure motor
Pure motor
Pure sensory
Pure autonomic

## Diagnostic Approach

A diagnosis of GBS is supported by CSF with elevated protein and minimal, if any, lymphocytic pleocytosis (albuminocyto-logic disassociation) after the first week. Early electrophysio-logic features include low-amplitude or prolonged compound motor action potentials and prolonged or absent F waves, indicating a predilection for the nerve roots and terminals (48,49). Later, slowed conduction velocities with temporal dispersion and conduction block can be demonstrated. Autopsy studies and nerve biopsies demonstrate lymphocyte and macrophage infiltration of nerves with demyelination (50).

Asbury and Cornblath (Table 19.2) (51) have proposed diagnostic criteria for GBS. The diagnosis rests on the clinical presentation and CSF findings. Nerve conduction studies can also help support the diagnosis. Because many patients do not have antibodies to gangliosides, these tests should probably not be ordered routinely. A notable exception is in the case of the Miller-Fisher variant syndrome. Most patients with the Miller-Fisher syndrome have serum $GQ_{1b}$ antibodies (52,53). One explanation for this is that high levels of $GQ_{1b}$ have been noted in cranial nerves III, IV, and VI. These antibodies, for which an assay is now commercially available, appear to be specific for the Miller-Fisher syndrome and have not been reported in GBS or other clinical variants.

## Therapy

The most important component of treatment is supportive care. Patients need to be monitored closely for respiratory and autonomic instability. Plasma exchange, involving 200 to 250 mL/kg of plasma over 7 to 10 days, has been shown to be an effective therapy in two large multicenter studies (44,54). In both the North American and French trials, the time on a respirator and the time to independent walking was shorter in the plasmapheresis-treated groups. The major criticism of these trials was the lack of a control group (sham plasma-

pheresis). A Dutch study reported intravenous immunoglob-ulin (IVIG) to be as effective as plasma exchange (55). Since then, the Plasma Exchange/Sandoglobulin Guillain–Barré Study Group conducted a multicenter trial comparing plasma exchange monotherapy, IVIG monotherapy, and plasma exchange followed by IVIG. They found that combined treatment produced no significant difference in patient outcomes compared with either therapy given alone (56). (Table 19.3). This study also showed that plasma exchange and IVIG treatments were equally effective in GBS.

Anecdotal reports suggest that IVIG may be associated with a higher incidence of relapse compared with plasma exchange (57,58). Relapses can also occur, however, after plasmapheresis or without treatment (54,59).

Both plasma exchange and IVIG have strengths and weaknesses as therapies. Both are equally effective; but in older, hemodynamically unstable patients, IVIG may be a better choice. In addition, at hospitals where plasma exchange is not available, IVIG is an ideal choice because the patient does not have to be transferred to another facility. Both therapies are equally expensive.

Corticosteroids are probably not of benefit in the treatment of GBS (60–62). Studies evaluating pulse methylpred-nisolone (63,64) had conflicting results. Further corticosteroid trials in GBS are planned, but until they have been completed, their use is not recommended for patients with this syndrome.

## Chronic Inflammatory Demyelinating Polyradiculoneuropathy

### Clinical Presentation

Chronic inflammatory demyelinating polyradiculoneuropathy (CIDP) represents a significant number of all initially undiagnosed acquired neuropathies (65,66). Diagnosis is important because CIDP is treatable with various immunomodulating

**TABLE 19.2.** *Diagnostic criteria for Guillain–Barré syndrome*

| Required | Supportive | Features casting doubt | Exclusionary |
|---|---|---|---|
| Progressive weakness of more than one limb | Progression for less than 4 weeks; symmetric weakness | Marked asymmetry | Other causes (toxins, botulism, porphyria, diphtheria) |
| Areflexia or hyporeflexia | Sensory symptoms or signs | Onset with or persistence of bladder or bowel dysfunction | |
| | Cranial nerve involvement, especially 7th cranial nerve | More than 50 lymphocytes/mm³ in CSF | |
| | Autonomic dysfunction | Polyneuropathies in CSF | |
| | CSF protein elevation; CSF cell count <20/mm³ | Sensory level | |
| | Electrophysiologic features of demyelination | | |
| | Recovery | | |

CSF, cerebrospinal fluid.
Adapted from Asbury AK, Cornblath DR. Assessment of current diagnostic criteria for Guillain–Barré syndrome. *Ann Neurol* 1990;27(Suppl):S21–S24, with permission.

**TABLE 19.3.** *Trial results of treatment of Guillain–Barré syndrome*

|  | Plasma exchange | Intravenous immunoglobulin | Both treatments |
|---|---|---|---|
| No. of patients | 121 | 130 | 128 |
| Days to walk unaided | 49 | 51 | 40 |
| Patients unable to walk unaided after 48 weeks (%) | 16.7 | 16.5 | 13.7 |
| Median days to hospital discharge | 63 | 53 | 51 |
| Median days to stop artificial ventilation | 29 | 26 | 18 |
| Deaths (%) | 4.1 | 4.6 | 6.3 |

From Plasma Exchange/Sandoglobulin Guillain–Barré Syndrome Trial Group. Randomized trial of plasma exchange, intravenous immunoglobulin, and combined treatments in Guillain–Barré syndrome. *Lancet* 1997;349:225–230, with permission.

therapies. CIDP occurs at any age. To fulfill diagnostic criteria for CIDP (65,67), weakness must be present for at least 2 months. Weakness can vary in severity but is symmetric and involves proximal and distal muscles of the upper and lower extremities. Facial and neck flexor weakness can occur. Rarely, extraocular and respiratory muscles are involved. Sensory complaints usually consist of numbness and tingling. Many patients describe a loss of balance. Deep tendon reflexes are usually depressed or absent.

The evidence for an immune-mediated pathogenesis in CIDP is much less abundant compared with the acute counterpart, GBS. Inflammatory cell infiltration and demyelination with remyelination are not seen in sural biopsies from most patients (65). However, immunostaining for T cells in nerve biopsies has been shown to yield a much higher incidence of inflammatory cell infiltration (68,69). Because inflammation and demyelination are not constant features of all CIDP patients, it may be more reasonable to use the term *Austin–Dyck syndrome* (after the two neurologists most responsible for defining this illness) to refer to these patients (65).

Preceding infections are not as common with CIDP as with GBS. There are some data suggesting a role for preceding respiratory (70,71) and *C. jejuni* (42) infection. The relationship of infections to CIDP is not as well substantiated as it is for GBS.

### Diagnostic Approach

CSF showing typical albuminocytologic dissociation supports a diagnosis of CIDP. Nerve conduction studies are suggestive of demyelination with prolonged distal latencies, slowed conduction velocities, and prolonged or absent F waves in the presence of conduction block or temporal dispersion (Fig. 19.1). Nerve biopsy may reveal thinly myelinated nerve fibers with Schwann's cell process proliferation ("onion bulbs") and rarely inflammatory cell in the endoneurium (Fig. 19.2). However, no feature on nerve biopsy is pathognomonic for CIDP. In fact, in one large series of CIDP cases, demyelination was seen in only 48% of cases; whereas 21% had axonopathy, 13% had mixed demyelinating and axonal features, and 18% were normal (65). In addition, only 11% had evidence of inflammatory infiltrates.

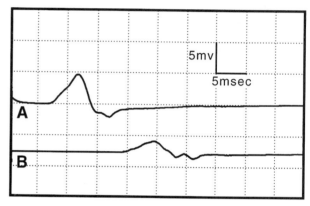

**FIG. 19.1.** Median motor nerve conduction study of a patient with chronic inflammatory polyradicoloneuropathy. **A:** Stimulation at wrist. **B:** Stimulation at elbow. Recording electrode for parts A and B is over thenar muscle group. There is a prolonged distal latency at the wrist of 6.9 msec (normal, <4.5 msec) and a slow conduction velocity between the wrist and elbow with 61% amplitude drop, indicating focal demyelination between the stimulation sites.

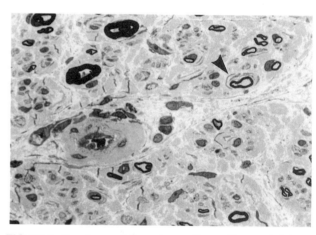

**FIG. 19.2.** Sural nerve biopsy in a patient with chronic inflammatory polyradicoloneuropathy. A few mononuclear inflammatory cells surround the endoneurial blood vessel. There is a decrease in the number of large myelinated fibers. Some thinly myelinated fibers have excessive Schwann's cell process proliferation ("onion bulbs") (*arrowhead*) (toluidine blue stain). (From Brey RL, Barohn RJ, Tami JA. Neuroimmunology: clinical and therapeutic approach. *Neurologist* 1996;2:25–52, with permission.)

In a typical CIDP patient with an elevated CSF protein and an electrophysiologic study meeting demyelinating criteria, a sural nerve biopsy may not be necessary. This is especially true when the nerve cannot be processed in a laboratory that has expertise in handling peripheral nerve tissue. If the CSF or electrophysiology are not supportive of the diagnosis in a patient who clinically resembles CIDP, a sural nerve biopsy should be performed. Sural nerve biopsy may also be helpful in excluding other causes in atypical cases.

Few blood tests are required in patients with typical CIDP. All patients with suspected CIDP should be checked for serum paraprotein. If a paraprotein is present, a search for malignancy (lymphoma, osteosclerotic myeloma) should be undertaken (72). Some authors recommend performing an assay for activity directed against myelin-associated glycoprotein, an immunoglobulin M (IgM) paraprotein. Rarely, anti–myelin-associated glycoprotein (anti-MAG) antibodies can be seen, even in the absence of a serum paraprotein (73). The presence of anti-MAG antibodies suggests that the CIDP patient may be more refractory to therapy (see later); however, the treatment approach is not altered. Therefore, there is no practical need to obtain either antiganglioside or anti-MAG antibody measurements in CIDP because, even if positive, they do not alter therapy.

### Diagnostic Criteria

Barohn et al. (74) initially proposed diagnostic criteria in 1989 that required mandatory inclusion and exclusion features and categorized cases as *definite, probable,* and *possible* based on how many laboratory features supported the diagnosis (Table 19.4) (70).

In a patient with definite CIDP, all three laboratory features supporting the diagnosis are present; in probable, two of three support the diagnosis; and in possible, one of three do (75). The criteria are valuable for research purposes; however, they can also be used in routine patient management. Patients who meet the mandatory inclusion and exclusion criteria but who fall in the probable or possible groups should still be treated. A presumptive diagnosis of CIDP can be made even if the electrophysiologic study, nerve biopsy, or even CSF does not have features fulfilling demyelinating criteria. Potentially beneficial therapy should not be withheld from these patients even if the nerve conduction studies do not fall in the demyelinating range and even if the nerve biopsy shows an axonal process without inflammation.

### Clinical Variants

In addition to so-called idiopathic CIDP, this neuropathy can occur in the setting of a variety of other disorders (Table 19.5). These are termed *CIDP with concurrent illness* (74,76–78) and include patients who have clinical or laboratory evidence of CNS demyelination, which is called *MS–CIDP overlap syndrome* (79,80).

**TABLE 19.4.** *Diagnostic criteria for chronic inflammatory demyelinating polyneuropathy*

I. *Mandatory clinical features*
  A. Progression of muscle weakness in proximal and distal muscles of upper and lower extremities for 2 months
  B. Areflexia or hyporeflexia
II. *Major laboratory features*
  A. Evidence of demyelination on nerve conduction studies
  B. Cerebrospinal fluid (CSF) studies
    1. CSF protein >45 mg/dL
    2. Cell count <10/mm³
  C. Nerve biopsy features
    1. Nerve biopsy with predominant features of demyelination that include segmental demyelination, remyelination, onion-bulb formation, and inflammation
III. *Mandatory exclusion criteria (patients must be devoid of these features)*
  A. Clinical features of a hereditary neuropathy or history of exposure
  B. Laboratory evidence from blood, urine, or CSF examination of a potential cause of the neuropathy other than chronic inflammatory demyelinating polyneuropathy (CIDP)
  C. Evidence on nerve biopsy of a potential cause of neuropathy other than CIDP
  D. Electrodiagnostic features of neuromuscular transmission defect, myopathy, or anterior horn cell disease
IV. *Diagnostic categories (must meet all mandatory exclusion criteria)*
  A. Definite CIDP
    1. Mandatory clinical features
    2. All major laboratory features
  B. Probable CIDP
    1. Mandatory clinical features
    2. Two of three major laboratory features
  C. Possible CIDP
    1. Mandatory clinical features
    2. One of three major laboratory features

Patients with CIDP who have a monoclonal gammopathy of uncertain significance, by definition, have no underlying malignancy (e.g., lymphoma, osteosclerotic myeloma) to account for the paraprotein. As outlined previously, treatment of these patients should be similar to that of patients with CIDP without paraproteins.

**TABLE 19.5.** *Chronic inflammatory demyelinating polyneuropathy with concurrent illness*

Human immunodeficiency virus infection
Monoclonal gammopathy
Chronic active hepatitis
Inflammatory bowel disease
Connective tissue disease
Bone marrow and organ transplantation
Lymphoma
Hereditary neuropathy
Diabetes mellitus
Thyrotoxicosis
Nephrotic syndrome
Central nervous system demyelination

Pure sensory and axonal variants of CIDP have been reported, and both apparently respond to immunosuppressive therapy (29,81–83). These patients do not meet the diagnostic criteria for CIDP, and the existence of these variants is somewhat controversial.

Patients who have a subacute progression of weakness between 4 and 8 weeks, intermediate between GBS and CIDP, have been reported. This variant has been labeled *subacute demyelinating polyneuropathy* (84). Treatment can be the same as that employed for CIDP, although it is interesting that three of the patients reported by Hughes et al. (84) had spontaneous recoveries, suggesting their disease may be more similar to GBS.

### Therapy

Randomized controlled trials have confirmed that steroids (85), plasma exchange (86,87), and IVIG (88) are all beneficial in patients with CIDP. Prednisone is the initial treatment of choice for patients with CIDP. When their strength has returned to normal or improvement reaches a plateau (usually within 3 to 6 months), prednisone should be slowly tapered by 5 mg every 2 to 3 weeks. A few patients can eventually be tapered completely off the prednisone; however, relapse is common (65). In patients who relapse during prednisone taper, IVIG or azathioprine can be added. In the single controlled study of azathioprine in CIDP, however, the drug was no more effective than placebo (89).

IVIG has been introduced for the treatment of CIDP. Although early studies showed variable results (90–92), two important more recent studies showed convincingly that IVIG has a role in the treatment of CIDP (88,93). Dyck et al. (93) compared plasma exchange to IVIG in 20 patients with CIDP and found both therapies to be equally effective. Hahn et al. (88) reported 30 patients who received IVIG or an intravenous placebo in a randomized, double-blind, cross-over study. The dose of IVIG was 2 g/kg given over 5 days. Nineteen of the 30 patients improved on IVIG (9 chronic progressive and 10 relapsing CIDP), and disease worsened in all patients when they were on placebo. The improvement was seen both on neurologic disability scale scores and nerve conduction studies. Eight of 9 patients with chronic progressive CIDP improved to normal function and maintained this level with the single 5-day course of IVIG; 5 of these patients were maintained on small doses of oral prednisone.

Plasma exchange has been shown to be more effective than sham pheresis for CIDP in two important studies (86,87). Plasma exchange is typically employed if patients are severely weak or if they relapse on prednisone. Five to 10 treatments are usually performed over 1 to 4 weeks at the initiation of therapy. Unlike the situation in GBS, however, there is no benchmark goal of how much total fluid to remove. We do not routinely repeat plasma exchange at fixed intervals, but instead use repeated courses of five or six treatments as needed if the patient deteriorates again. When we initiate plasma exchange in a patient who is already on prednisone but who has worsened, we usually increase the steroid dose or add a second oral immunosuppressive agent. Otherwise, the patient may relapse after the effect of the plasma exchange has worn off (usually in 4 to 8 weeks).

In the single controlled study of azathioprine in CIDP, the drug was no more effective than placebo (94). Azathioprine is still occasionally employed as second-line therapy in patients who relapse on prednisone therapy, however, especially if IVIG cannot be used. Cyclosporine (95,96) and, less often, cyclophosphamide can be used as third-line oral therapies in difficult cases. There have been several small reports describing benefit in patients with CIDP from treatment with either IFN-α (97,98) or IFN-β (99). An open-label study of IFN-α treatment in 16 patients followed for 6 weeks found improvement in 56% (100). Although encouraging, further studies involving placebo control, larger patient members, and a longer follow-up period are needed.

In our retrospective series, more than 90% of patients with CIDP initially improved with immunosuppressive treatment; however, the relapse rate was high, approaching 50% (74). Only 30% of patients in this series achieved a complete remission off medication, and two of the patients (3.3%) died (74). Thus, it appears that the longer patients are followed, the more likely it is they will relapse (74). In the series of Dyck et al. (101), 64% of patients had improved or had achieved remission and were able to return to work, 8% were ambulatory but unable to work, 11% were bedridden or wheelchair bound, and 11% died of the disease. Gorson et al. (102) found that, overall, 66% of their patients responded to one of the three main therapies for CIDP (prednisone, plasma exchange, or IVIG). These three retrospective series found no factors predictive of a poor response.

Two recent prospective studies may provide more reliable numbers regarding patient response to treatment. In the controlled trial of IVIG in CIDP patients performed by Hahn et al. (88), 63% (19 of 32) responded. Patients with an acute relapse or with disease duration of 1 year or less were more likely to respond. In a separate study by this same group, 80% of patients (12 of 15) who received plasma exchange responded (87).

## PERIPHERAL NERVE VASCULITIS

### Clinical Presentation

Peripheral neuropathy caused by vasculitis is characterized by inflammation and necrosis of blood vessel walls in peripheral nerves, resulting in ischemia in the distribution of damaged vessels. The vasculitides have been classified according to the type and size of the blood vessel involved, with an emphasis on primary (i.e., polyarteritis nodosa, Wegener's granulomatosis) versus secondary (i.e., associations with connective tissue disease, infection, drugs, or malignancy) (103). Peripheral neuropathy may complicate systemic vasculitis and can be the presenting manifestation (104). In addition, nonsystemic or isolated peripheral nerve vasculitis can occur (105).

Systemic necrotizing vasculitis is a potentially life-threatening group of disorders affecting multiple organ systems (104). These vasculitides classically involve small and medium-sized arteries. Polyarteritis nodosa is the most common of the necrotizing vasculitides. It involves the kidneys, bowels, liver, skin, and muscle. Importantly, the pulmonary circulation is spared. Peripheral nerve involvement occurs in up to half of patients. Hepatitis B antigenemia and immune complexes are found in about 30% of cases. Abdominal angiography can demonstrate vasculitis involvement of renal, hepatic, and visceral blood vessels. Churg–Strauss syndrome, or allergic angiitis and granulomatosis, is a rare condition with prominent involvement of the pulmonary system. Prominent eosinophilic infiltration of blood vessels is seen. The frequency of peripheral nerve involvement is similar to that observed in polyarteritis nodosa. Wegener's granulomatosis affects the upper and lower respiratory track and is accompanied by glomerulonephritis. Peripheral nervous system involvement is evident in about 20% of cases. The lack of an asthma history and peripheral eosinophilia can distinguish Wegener's granulomatosis from Churg–Strauss syndrome. Peripheral nerve vasculitis may complicate connective tissue diseases, most commonly seen in patients with rheumatoid arthritis, but can also be present in patients with systemic lupus erythematosus and Sjögren's syndrome (106).

Isolated peripheral vasculitis, or nonsystemic vasculitic neuropathy, involves small and medium-sized arteries of the epineurium and perineurium (104,105). The clinical presentation and histologic features are similar to systemic vasculitis with the exception of sparing of other organs. However, constitutional symptoms of fever, malaise, weight loss, and nonspecific arthralgias can occur in both isolated and systemic vasculitis (106). Patients with clinical manifestations restricted to the peripheral nerves have better prognoses than do patients with systemic vasculitis (104).

The pattern of neuropathic involvement depends on the duration and extent of the ischemically induced damage. Burning pain and dysesthesias in the distribution of involved nerves occur in 70% to 80% of patients. Usually, both motor and sensory nerves are affected, although rarely, patients have only sensory loss. True, multiple mononeuropathy with deficits restricted to the multiple individual peripheral nerves occurs in only 10% to 15% of patients (107). An overlapping multiple mononeuropathy obscuring individual nerve involvement occurs much more commonly in about 50% to 60% of patients. Because of the multiple and overlapping nerve involvement, it may be difficult to distinguish individual neuropathies, although examination may reveal asymmetries between the limbs. About 20% to 30% of patients with a diffuse overlapping neuropathy may present with a distal, symmetric "stocking-glove" motor-sensory neuropathy.

A leukocytoclastic reaction has often been considered the most likely mechanism of vessel damage in polyarteritis nodosa. In this model, circulating antigen–antibody complexes are deposited in blood vessel walls, activating the complement cascade and releasing chemotactic factors that recruit polymorphonuclear leukocytes. In a quantitative immunohistochemical analysis of 22 nerve biopsy specimens from patients with peripheral nerve vasculitis resulting from polyarteritis nodosa, however, neither polymorphonuclear leukocytes nor the cellular debris of a leukocytoclastic reaction was seen (108). Most cells in the vascular infiltrates were T cells (mostly cytotoxic CD8 cytotoxic or suppressor) and macrophages; B cells were uncommon. Although immunoglobulins and membrane attack complex deposits were found in most specimens, the paucity of B cells and polymorphonuclear leukocytes suggests that humoral mechanism may not have initiated the primary immunologic process. Instead, the immunoglobulin and complement could have been trapped in the cell-infiltrated blood vessel walls. Most of the evidence from this study implicated a T-cell–mediated cytotoxic process as the primary mechanism of vessel injury.

### Diagnostic Approach

All patients suspected of vasculitis should be evaluated for an underlying systemic vasculitis. Laboratory evaluations should include erythrocyte sedimentation rate, antinuclear antibody titer, rheumatoid factor, serum protein or immunoelectrophoresis, complement levels, quantitative immunoglobulins, hepatitis B serology, and eosinophil count. In addition, routine complete blood count, urinalysis, and renal and liver functions should be obtained for underlying systemic involvement. Electrophysiologic studies may demonstrate an asymmetric axonopathy. Nerve conduction studies can also be useful in determining the appropriate nerves to biopsy. The sural nerve is most commonly resected. The yield of biopsy can be increased by resecting the superficial peroneal nerve and the underlying peroneus brevis muscle (109). Even in so-called isolated peripheral nervous system vasculitis, involvement of blood vessels supplying muscle can be demonstrated. Characteristic findings on nerve and muscle biopsy include both perivascular and transmural inflammatory cell infiltration with necrosis of the blood vessel wall (Fig. 19.3).

### Therapy

No prospective, randomized, controlled trials have been undertaken to study therapy for vasculitis involving the peripheral nervous system. Most patients, however, respond to the combination of cyclophosphamide and corticosteroids (104). Treatment should be initiated with oral cyclophosphamide at a dose of 2 mg/kg per day in combination with prednisone, 1.5 mg/kg per day. Prednisone is given as a single morning daily dose for 2 to 4 weeks. After improvement is evident, an alternate-day regimen can be used. Cyclophosphamide is generally maintained for at least 1 year.

Because isolated peripheral nervous system vasculitis may be more benign than systemic vasculitis, a trial of steroids alone or a shorter course of cyclophosphamide may be indicated in some cases.

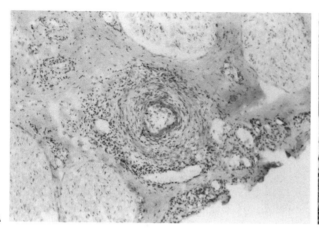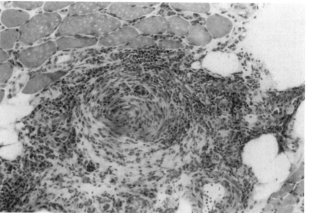

A

B

**FIG. 19.3.** Nerve **(A)** and muscle **(B)** biopsies from a patient with vasculitis. **A:** Superficial peroneal nerve biopsy shows epineurial blood vessel with intense perivascular, transmural, mononuclear cell infiltration. The vessel lies between several nerve fascicles (hematoxylin and eosin stain). **B:** Peroneus brevis muscle biopsy shows vasculitis in perimysial vessel (hematoxylin and eosin stain). **B** from Brey RL, Barohn RJ, Tami JA. Neuroimmunology: clinical and therapeutic approach. *Neurologist* 1996;2:25–52, with permission.)

## OTHER IMMUNE-MEDIATED PERIPHERAL NEUROPATHIES

### Monoclonal Gammopathies

About 10% of patients with idiopathic peripheral neuropathies have a monoclonal gammopathy, compared with 2.5% of patients with peripheral neuropathies as a result of other disease (110). Serum protein electrophoresis is not sensitive enough to detect a small monoclonal protein, and therefore serum immunoelectrophoresis or immunofixation, should be performed in patients in whom a myeloproliferative disorder is suspected. Although a variety of diseases have been associated with monoclonal gammopathies (110,111), in most patients, no underlying disease is found at presentation. The term *monoclonal gammopathy of undetermined significance* has replaced the term *benign monoclonal gammopathy,* however, because 20% of patients initially classified as having monoclonal gammopathies of undetermined significance eventually develop malignant disorders with long-term follow-up (112,113). Some (65) but not all (114–116) authorities suggest that monoclonal gammopathies of undetermined significance and peripheral neuropathies, especially the IgG and IgA groups, may be a variant of CIDP because electrophysiologic features and response to treatment are remarkably similar. The pathogenic significance of the monoclonal proteins in the development of peripheral neuropathy is unclear. Antibodies directed against MAG are present in half of patients with IgM monoclonal gammopathies and peripheral neuropathies (117). However, what role, if any, these antibodies have in the pathogenesis of the peripheral neuropathies is unknown. Patients with a monoclonal protein, neuropathy, and significant weakness are treated similarly to those with CIDP (see earlier).

Most patients with monoclonal proteins and CIDP have the same response to therapy as CIDP patients without parapro-

teins. Patients with IgM paraproteins, particularly those that are anti-MAG antibodies, may be more resistant to therapy (114,116,118,119). Much of these data, however, are based on studies of patients with monoclonal protein-associated polyneuropathies, not patients meeting the diagnostic criteria for CIDP. Retrospective studies comparing patients with CIDP and a paraprotein to those without found no differences among patients with IgM, IgG, or IgA gammopathies (120,121). Some authors advocate treating neuropathy patients who have IgM paraproteins with chemotherapeutic agents such as chlorambucil or cyclophosphamide (122–124). IVIG appeared beneficial in two small open studies of neuropathy patients with IgM gammopathy (125,126), whereas a small, controlled trial (119) found a much more modest response. A controlled study comparing IVIG and IFN-α treatment in patients with IgM gammopathy found little benefit from IVIG, whereas there was improvement in 80% of the IFN-treated group (127). There have been no prospective studies addressing treatment of patients with CIDP and monoclonal gammopathies of undetermined significance; it is reasonable to take the same therapeutic approach that is used for patients with CIDP.

### Multifocal Demyelinating Motor Neuropathy

A group of predominantly male patients between 20 and 40 years of age with multifocal demyelinating motor neuropathy can develop a neuropathy resembling the lower motor neuron form of motor neuron disease (128–130). Initially, there is weakness of one hand, which is slowly progressive over months or years, spreading asymmetrically to the other hand and ankles. Some patients have vague sensory symptoms, but the sensory examination is usually normal. On electrophysiologic testing, these patients usually have focal conduction block, temporal dispersion, and slowing in multiple motor nerves with normal sensory studies (131). Sensory nerve biopsy is often normal. The presence of IgM antibodies to $GM_1$ ganglioside have been demonstrated in some (128) but not all (129,132) patients with multifocal conduction block. The significance of ganglioside antibodies in these patients is not known (133). $GM_1$ ganglioside antibodies in lower titers have also been reported to occur in GBS, typical amyotrophic lateral sclerosis, and various other neurologic diseases as well as in control subjects (132,134). This may simply reflect an epiphenomenon of nerve damage (133).

Aggressive immunosuppressive therapy with intravenous cyclophosphamide in large doses (3 $g/m^2$) has reportedly resulted in improvement in some patients with multifocal conduction block (128,132,135). Prednisone alone has generally been ineffective. Therapy with monthly cycles of intravenous cyclophosphamide at doses of 1 $g/m^2$ followed by plasmapheresis (136) may be beneficial. The first line of treatment in multifocal demyelinating motor neuropathy cases is IVIG (129,137).

A variant of multifocal demyelinating motor neuropathy has been described with sensory involvement. This has been called *multifocal acquired demyelinating sensory and motor neuropathy* or the *Lewis–Sumner syndrome* (138). Patients present with mononeuritis multiplex and distal weakness and sensory loss confined to individual nerves in the hands or feet. This syndrome probably falls somewhere in the spectrum between CIDP and multifocal demyelinating motor neuropathy. It responds to IVIG, and at least half of patients respond to prednisone (138).

## AUTOIMMUNE PARANEOPLASTIC SYNDROMES INVOLVING BRAIN AND PERIPHERAL NERVE

Paraneoplastic effects of cancer are disorders that occur in patients with recognized or occult cancer resulting from remote effects of cancer on distant organs. Although cancer-induced metabolic or nutritional disorders may also lead to nervous system dysfunction, several characteristic paraneoplastic nervous system syndromes appear to have an autoimmune basis: subacute cerebellar degeneration, limbic and brainstem encephalitis with or without sensory neuropathy, myoclonus–opsoclonus syndrome, stiff-person's syndrome, Isaacs' syndrome, and the Lambert–Eaton myasthenic syndrome (LEMS) (139–144). The clinical presentation and diagnostic approach for each of these is considered separately in this section. Therapy is similar for all and is discussed at the end of the section.

Paraneoplastic syndromes are not common. They affect only 5% to 6% of patients with cancer; when they do occur, however, they often lead to significant neurologic morbidity even if the primary malignancy is treated (145). Malignancy may not be manifested for many years after diagnosis of the neurologic disorder (140,145,146). Therefore, one important caveat for all patients who present with one of these potentially paraneoplastic neurologic syndromes is that a thorough search for malignancy is important, particularly if the patient harbors neoplasm-associated antibodies (141–142).

The availability of antibody testing by Western blot and immunohistochemical analysis of serum and spinal fluid has provided a relatively sensitive and specific tool for the diagnosis of some of these syndromes (Table 19.6) (140,147). Some antibodies have been linked closely with specific neoplasms; therefore, their presence can guide the evaluation for underlying cancer. Some patients with paraneoplastic neurologic syndromes, however, have negative serologic tests (148), and these patients do not appear to differ clinically from those who have positive tests. Computed tomography has not proved useful diagnostically in patients with paraneoplastic nervous system syndromes. Magnetic resonance imaging (MRI) is not considered helpful in making the diagnosis of paraneoplastic subacute cerebellar degeneration (149), but it may be very helpful in the early diagnosis of paraneoplastic limbic encephalitis, myelopathy, and opsoclonus (reviewed in 150).

Although the precise pathogenesis of nervous system paraneoplastic syndromes is not known, it is assumed that they stem from an immune response to determinants that are shared between tumor and nervous system cells (142). Interestingly, detectable tumor burden is often lower in patients with paraneoplastic syndromes. This suggests that

**TABLE 19.6.** *Autoantibodies associated with paraneoplastic syndromes affecting the nervous system*

| Autoantibody | Associated neoplasms | Associated neurologic syndrome |
|---|---|---|
| Anti-Yo (type I antineuronal antibodies) | Lung, breast, ovary, fallopian tube cancer; lung adenocarcinoma; Hodgkin's lymphoma | Subacute cerebellar degeneration |
| Anti-Hu (type IIa antineuronal antibodies) | Small cell lung cancer, neuroblastoma, rhabdosarcoma, seminoma, prostate cancer | Encephalomyelitis with sensory and autonomic neuropathy |
| Anti-Ri (type IIb antineuronal antibodies) | Breast, fallopian tube, small cell lung cancer in adults; neuroblastoma in children | Ataxia with ocular dysmotility |
| Anti–glutamic acid decarboxylase antibodies | Hodgkin's lymphoma; thymoma; small cell lung, pharynx, colon, breast cancer | Stiff-person syndrome |
| Anti–potassium-sensitive channel antibodies | Thymoma, Hodgkin's lymphoma, plasmacytoma, lung cancer | Isaacs' syndrome |
| Anti–calcium-gated channel antibodies | Any malignancy, most commonly small cell lung; renal and hematologic malignancies | Lambert–Eaton myasthenic syndrome |

the immune response against tumor is an appropriate response against foreign antigen and that it is also directed against nontumor self tissues. The presence of some specific paraneoplastic autoantibodies has been associated with tumor regression or even remission (151). Unfortunately, in many instances, irreversible damage is done to CNS tissues within weeks of the onset of symptoms. Because the damage primarily involves neurons that cannot regenerate, the neurologic disorders are permanent. The presence of some paraneoplastic autoantibodies, especially in low titer, has been associated with tumor regression or even remission in the absence of a neurologic syndrome (142,151).

The antigens against which some paraneoplastic autoantibodies are directed are known, and the genes encoding for them have even been cloned. In most cases, the function of the known protein is not known (142). The immune response directed against tumor and nervous system tissue often has both a humoral and cell-mediated (cytotoxic) component. This may help explain the difficulty researchers have had in developing an animal model for the paraneoplastic nervous system syndromes. In human brain, paraneoplastic autoantibodies are localized intracellularly. Animals passively or actively immunized with these antibodies have binding to nervous system tissues but do not appear to develop neurologic disease, with the exception of the voltage-dependent calcium-channel antibody that causes LEMS (142).

It is possible that crucial epitopes have not been represented in these animal experiments, or that essential cytotoxic T-cell responses have not been activated by such an approach. Two broad groups of pathogenic mechanisms have been suggested by Vershcuuren and Dalmau (152). In one group, neoplastic cells synthesize antibodies that may damage the peripheral nervous system (e.g., antibodies against $GM_1$ ganglioside). In the other, the expression of neuronal antigens by a tumor contributes to breaking immune tolerance for these proteins. If the antigen is located on the cell surface (such as voltage-gated calcium channels in Lambert–Eaton syndrome or voltage-gated potassium channels in Isaacs' syndrome), the peripheral nervous system is most commonly involved, and treatment with immune-modulating therapies or removal of the tumor may be effective. If the antigen is located intracellularly, however, as is the case in most CNS syndromes, resolution is rarely seen with treatment.

## Subacute Cerebellar Degeneration

### Clinical Presentation

Paraneoplastic subacute cerebellar degeneration is most commonly associated with cancers of the lung, ovary, and breast but is also seen with fallopian tube cancer, adenocarcinoma of the lung, and Hodgkin's disease (148). In about half of patients, however, no tumor is ever found. Clinically, this disorder appears as a severe pancerebellar syndrome that arises over weeks to months. Severe truncal and appendicular ataxia, tremor, postural instability, nystagmus, and dysarthria

characterize this. Within a few months, the disease reaches its peak and stabilizes (142).

### Diagnostic Approach

This syndrome is associated with anti-Yo (also called type I antineuronal) (Table 19.6) antibodies detected by Western blot analysis, and the staining of Purkinje's (153) and tumor cells (154) using immunohistochemical techniques. One positron-emission tomography study revealed hypometabolism in all areas of the neuraxis (147). Rare remissions are seen even if the underlying cancer is successfully treated. It is associated pathologically with extensive Purkinje's cell loss and deep cerebellar nuclear infiltrates. Lymphocytic pleocytosis and intrathecal oligoclonal antibody production are common (155). Although imaging studies are not helpful in the diagnosis of this syndrome, brain MRI studies are important to exclude structural causes of the neurologic disorder, including metastases.

## Limbic and Brainstem Encephalitis and Peripheral or Autonomic Neuropathy

### Clinical Presentation

Paraneoplastic encephalomyelitis and sensory and autonomic neuropathy either alone or in combination are most commonly associated with small cell lung cancer, neuroblastoma, rhabdosarcoma, seminoma, and prostate cancer (142,156, 157). Clinically, symptoms begin suddenly and evolve rapidly.

More than half of patients have sensory symptoms at onset (158). The sensory loss is due to a dorsal root gangliopathy and may present as an isolated syndrome with evidence of CNS signs (157,159,160). Both hands and feet are affected over weeks to months, often asymmetrically. Severe ataxia and proprioceptive deficits resulting from damage to dorsal root ganglia are usually present (161).

In the remainder of patients, symptoms may begin in a variety of ways, including limbic encephalopathy (which may mimic Korsakoff's syndrome), cerebellar symptoms, myelopathy, a brainstem syndrome, or a pure autonomic neuropathy (162,163). More than three fourths of patients ultimately have signs and symptoms in more than one area of the central or peripheral nervous system (158). The neurologic syndrome is usually severely disabling and may be fatal, but it may also be indolent in patients with isolated sensory neuropathy (159).

### Diagnostic Approach

Limbic and brainstem encephalitis and peripheral or autonomic neuropathy are associated with anti-Hu (also called type IIa antineuronal) antibodies detected by Western blot analysis (157,158). They can also be detected using preparations of central and peripheral nervous system neurons, adenohypothesis, adrenal cortex, retina, and tumor cell nuclei using immunohistochemical techniques (164). Spinal fluid studies reveal a mild pleocytosis early on, a slightly elevated total protein (usually less than 100 mg/dL), and an increase of total IgG with evidence of intrathecal IgG synthesis and anti-Hu antibodies (165). In the series reported by Dalmau and Posner (164), the median survival of patients with anti-Hu paraneoplastic syndromes was only 7 months, less than the median survival for the general population with small cell lung cancer (164). There have been cases, however, of prolonged survival and even spontaneous tumor regression in patients with subacute sensory neuropathy and anti-Hu antibodies (151). MRI may be useful in the diagnosis of some patients with some variants of this syndrome. The characteristic features are an increase in T2-weighted signal without gadolinium enhancement in the appropriate anatomic location and clinical setting (150). As with the other paraneoplastic neurologic syndromes, brain MRI studies serve to exclude other structural causes, especially in patients without a known primary malignancy.

## Opsoclonus–Myoclonus Syndrome

### Clinical Presentation

Paraneoplastic ataxia and myoclonus with ocular dysmotility are most commonly associated with breast, fallopian tube, and small cell lung cancers in adults and with neuroblastoma in children. Clinically, mild to severe ataxia and a disturbance of ocular motility, usually opsoclonus ("dancing eyes"), is seen (149,166,167). The onset of symptoms is usually rapid, with symptoms reaching their peak in weeks to months (168). Although symptoms may improve with treatment of the underlying tumor, most patients have some degree of permanent residual deficit.

### Diagnostic Approach

Paraneoplastic ataxia–opsoclonus syndrome is associated with anti-Ri (also known as type IIb antineuronal) (Table 19.6) antibodies detected by Western blot analysis and staining of CNS neuron, retina, and tumor cell nuclei using immunohistochemical techniques, except in cases associated with neuroblastoma (149,168). Spinal fluid studies are remarkable for a mild pleocytosis, a mildly elevated protein level, and the presence of anti-Ri antibodies. Pathologically, the nervous system exhibits severe Purkinje's cell loss and perivascular and interstitial inflammatory infiltrates involving the brainstem (169).

## STIFF-PERSON SYNDROME

### Clinical Presentation

Stiff-person syndrome is a rare disorder characterized by progressive rigidity, stiffness, and intermittent spasms of axial and occasionally extremity muscles (170). Autoantibodies directed against glutamic acid decarboxylase are present in 60% of patients (170). Loss of function of γ-aminobutyric acid (GABA)-mediated inhibition of central motor neurons may lead to hyperactivity. There are reports of stiff-person syndrome associated with Hodgkin's lymphoma (171–173), thymoma (173,174), small cell lung cancer (143), and cancers of the pharynx (175), colon (176) and breast (173,176).

### Diagnostic Approach

Antibodies are directed against a nonglutamic decarboxylase 125-kd to 130-kd synaptic protein in some patients with presumed paraneoplastic stiff-person syndrome (173,176).

## ISAACS' SYNDROME

### Clinical Presentation

Neuromyotonia, or Isaacs' syndrome, is a disorder of peripheral nerve hyperexcitability resulting in continuous muscle fiber activity (144,177). Patients present with diffuse muscle stiffness, cramps, and spasms. Some have an associated motor-sensory polyneuropathy that can resemble acute or chronic inflammatory demyelinating neuropathy. Paraneoplastic neuromyotonia has been described in association with lung cancer (178–180), thymoma (181,182), plasmacytoma (183), and Hodgkin's disease (184).

### Diagnostic Approach

Nerve conduction velocities can be normal or demonstrate electrophysiologic features of demyelination. Repetitive after-discharges may occasionally occur after motor nerve stimulation. Electromyography reveals neuromyotonic and myokymic discharges. In primary autoimmune neuromyotonia, antibodies against voltage-gated potassium channels on peripheral nerves have been reported (185,186). Inactivation of these channels prolongs action-potential duration, resulting in hyperexcitability of the motor nerves. Voltage-gated potassium channels are found in high concentration in lymphoid cells (184). Antibodies against these channels could arise through molecular mimicry that could cross-react with voltage-gated potassium channels on peripheral nerve (177,184).

## LAMBERT–EATON MYASTHENIC SYNDROME

### Clinical Presentation

LEMS is an acquired autoimmune disorder of neuromuscular junction transmission in which the defect is in the presynaptic nerve terminal (187). Anderson and colleagues (188) in 1953 first described a small cell carcinoma patient and weakness. However, Lambert, Eaton, and Rooke (189) and then Eaton and Lambert (190) were responsible for defining the syndrome, including the electrophysiologic abnormalities seen on routine electromyography. Elmqvist and Lambert (191) then found that the neuromuscular junction defect was caused by an inadequate presynaptic release of acetylcholine.

LEMS is characterized by fatigability and weakness in a limb-girdle distribution (192). The weakness is first noticed in the hip girdle and later spreads to the shoulders. Unlike the situation in myasthenia gravis, patients may note that the weakness is worse soon after awakening and better later in the day. Although exercise can transiently improve strength, persistent exertion causes fatigue. Also in contrast to myasthenia gravis patients, cranial nerve and respiratory involvement is less common. Up to half of patients have mild degrees of ptosis, diplopia, dysphagia, and dysarthria (192). Patients also have autonomic involvement, including dry mouth and eyes, impotence, difficulty focusing vision, and orthostasis (192). Some patients complain of myalgias or paresthesias. On examination, in addition to the limb-girdle pattern of weakness, patients may have poorly reactive pupils and usually are hyporeflexic or areflexic. Although strength is reduced at rest, sometimes improvement can be demonstrated after a few seconds of voluntary contraction.

A malignancy is present in about half of patients with LEMS (192). The tumor is usually a small cell carcinoma of the lung, but other malignancies, such as renal cell carcinoma and hematologic tumors, occur. LEMS can be the presenting manifestation of a small cell carcinoma and can precede the detection of the tumor by months. Overall, LEMS is more common in men, with a male-to-female ratio of 4.7:1. Seventy percent of men and only 25% of women have a malignancy. Patients with nonneoplastic LEMS may have an associated autoimmune disease such as hyperthyroidism or hypothyroidism, Sjögren's syndrome, celiac disease, vitiligo, or myasthenia gravis. Nonneoplastic LEMS can occur at any age.

An immune-mediated basis for LEMS was suspected when the disease was passively transferred from the purified IgG of patients to mice (193). At about the same time, it was shown that the number of voltage-sensitive calcium channels is reduced in the motor nerve terminal (194). A number of investigators subsequently provided data to support that the LEMS IgG is directed at the voltage-gated calcium channel (195–200). A deficiency of voltage-gated calcium channels in turn inhibits the influx of calcium into the motor nerve terminal. As a result, there are decreased quantities of acetylcholine vesicles released with each action potential that reaches the nerve terminal. All LEMS patients have IgG that inhibits calcium flux in small cell lung cancer cell lines (198). An assay has been developed in which the antibodies from LEMS patients bind to calcium-channel–ω-conotoxin complexes from small cell lung carcinoma or neuroblastoma cells (118,199). The various conotoxin ligands can be used to assay for antibodies to either N-type or P/Q-type calcium channels.

### Diagnostic Approach

The diagnosis of LEMS is based on the electromyographic findings of the nerve conduction and repetitive stimulation studies. Edrophonium administration may lead to mild improvement in strength but is not helpful in the diagnosis.

Serologic assays for antibodies to voltage-gated calcium channels may be helpful as well.

The classic electrophysiologic triad of LEMS includes low-amplitude compound motor action potentials that increases dramatically after brief exercise; decremental response at low rates of repetitive stimulation (2 to 5 Hz); and incremental response at high rates of repetitive stimulation (tetanic stimulation at 20 to 50 Hz) (Fig. 19.4) (200).

The clue that LEMS may be present in a given patient often first comes in the electromyography laboratory when diffusely small-amplitude compound motor action potentials are found in the process of performing routine motor nerve conduction studies. If this abnormality is found, a screening test for LEMS is usually performed. The screening test involves performing a single nerve stimulation and recording the compound motor action potentials after the patient has exercised the muscle being tested against resistance for 10 seconds (201). There is a dramatic, often more than 100% increase in the compound motor action potentials amplitude and area. This occurs because both brief exercise and tetanic stimulation normally produce an influx of calcium into the nerve terminal, which increases quantal release and overcomes the underlying defect in LEMS. The LEMS screen is highly specific for this disorder. In one study, the screen was abnormal more frequently than an incremental response to repetitive stimulation at 20 Hz in patients with LEMS (201).

Even if the LEMS screen is dramatically positive, repetitive stimulation at slow and fast rates are usually performed. LEMS is a relatively uncommon disorder. Most busy neurophysiology laboratories evaluate one new patient with LEMS for every 100 new patients with myasthenia gravis. Thus, it is important to try to document the full classic electromyographic triad for LEMS to ensure the diagnosis.

Slow rates of repetitive stimulation (2 to 5 Hz) generally show a decremental response (more than 10%). At slow rates of stimulation, in which there is more than 200 msec between stimuli, calcium does not have time to accumulate at the nerve terminal; therefore, facilitation does not occur. At high rates of repetitive stimulation (20 to 50 Hz), in which there is 50 to 20 msec between stimuli, calcium accumulates at the nerve terminal, and facilitation occurs (brief exercise produces facilitation in the LEMS screen test by the same mechanism). A positive incremental response is not diagnosed unless there is at least a 100% increment between the first and last response. In addition, increments of as much as 40% can occur normally (202). Most LEMS patients facilitate well in excess of 100%.

Single-fiber electromyography shows increased jitter in LEMS, but this finding does not differentiate LEMS from myasthenia gravis. If the classic nerve conduction study and repetitive stimulation abnormalities of LEMS are not present, there is no reason to perform single-fiber electromyographic studies.

Assays for calcium-channel—binding antibodies have become commercially available. LEMS patients demonstrate both P/Q-type and N-type calcium-channel antibodies in serum. The P/Q-type antibodies are more often present

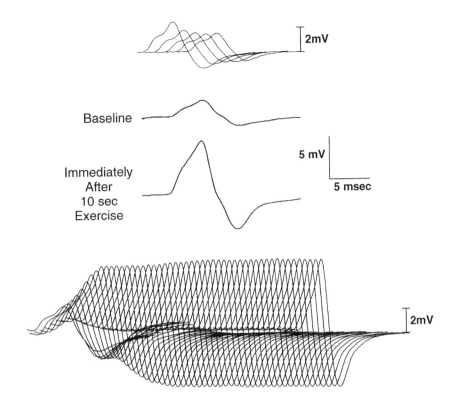

**FIG. 19.4.** Electrophysiologic testing in a patient with Lambert–Eaton syndrome. **A:** Repetitive stimulation of the ulnar nerve at a slow rate of 2 Hz. There is a 42% decrement. **B:** Brief exercise test shows a 220% increment between the baseline and after 10 seconds of exercise. **C:** Repetitive stimulation of the ulnar nerve at a high stimulation rate of 50 Hz. There is a 196% amplitude increment. (From Katz JS, Wolfe GI, Bryan WW, et al. Acetylcholine receptor antibodies in the Lambert-Eaton myasthenic syndrome. *Neurology* 1998;50:470–475, with permission.)

because the P/Q-type calcium channels are involved in acetylcholine vesicle release at the neuromuscular junction, while N-type calcium channels are involved in cerebrocortical, cerebellar, spinal, and autonomic transmission (203). Data from investigators at the Mayo Clinic indicated that P/Q-type calcium channel antibodies were detected in 100% of LEMS with lung cancer and in 91% of patients with LEMS without lung cancer. This compares with N-type calcium-channel antibody positivity in 74% of patients with LEMS who have cancer and in 40% of these patients who do not have cancer (204). These data are supported by findings from investigators at Oxford Universtiy, in the United Kingdom (205).

Both the classic electrophysiologic findings and the abnormal serologic studies are equally important in diagnosing LEMS. As with the acetylcholine receptor antibody assay in myasthenia gravis, occasionally LEMS patients may be P/Q-type calcium-channel antibody negative, making the electrophysiologic findings the key to the correct diagnoses in these rare cases (206). Interestingly, some patients can have antibodies to both acetylcholine receptor and calcium-channel antibodies. It is controversial whether these patients have a true "overlap" disease or LEMS or whether production of acetylcholine receptor antibodies is an autoimmune epiphenomenon (206).

**Therapy**

Treatment of all paraneoplastic syndromes should be directed at the underlying neoplasm (207). Plasmapheresis, corticosteroids, or other immunosuppressive medications should be considered in patients who have neurologic deficits that are severely disabling, who have progressive disease at the time of diagnosis, or in whom an underlying tumor cannot be found (160,208). Serum anti-Yo, anti-Hu, and anti-Ri titers are lowered with treatment; however, CSF levels usually remain unaffected (140,147). Plasmapheresis could theoretically blunt the immune response to tumor while leaving the autoimmune injury to the nervous system unchecked.

The treatment of patients with LEMS deserves special comment. In patients with neoplastic LEMS, as with other paraneoplastic disorders, the therapy is initially directed at the tumor. If the tumor responds to chemotherapy or radiation therapy, symptoms may improve (209). Some neoplastic patients, however, also need specific therapy for LEMS.

Anticholinesterase drugs are of limited benefit; however, a trial of pyridostigmine should be attempted, and the drug can be continued if it has some minor effect.

Ideally, drugs that increase the release of acetylcholine vesicles should be tried. Guanidine hydrochloride is the oldest drug in this group and has been beneficial in some patients with LEMS (210,211). The side effects of guanidine are prohibitive in most patients, however, and include bone marrow depression, renal failure, gastrointestinal distress, ataxia, hypotension, paresthesias, confusion, dry skin, and atrial fibrillation.

3,4-Diaminopyridine (3,4-DAP) increases the duration of the presynaptic action potential by blocking the outward potassium efflux. This then indirectly prolongs the activation of the voltage-gated calcium channels and increases calcium entry in nerve terminals. In clinical trials, 3,4-DAP both improved strength and compounded motor action potential amplitudes in LEMS patients (212–214). Doses of up to 25 mg are given four time daily. have been used. Most patients tolerated the drug except for minor side effects. Unfortunately, 3,4-DAP is only available as an investigational agent and thus is not an option for patients not enrolled in a study.

Once the autoimmune nature of LEMS was suspected, various immunosuppressive approaches were attempted. Newsom-Davis and Murray (215) reported that plasmapheresis, corticosteroids, and azathioprine can be effective in both neoplastic and nonneoplastic LEMS patients. In their study, plasmapheresis had a peak effect in 2 weeks, and the benefit had disappeared by 6 weeks. Several patients developed sustained remissions on immunosuppressive medications.

A single case report from the University of Pennsylvania described the effectiveness of IVIG in LEMS (216). Subsequently, this same group published their series of six patients treated with IVIG (217). Four of the patients had cancer. Five of the six became stronger subjectively and objectively with IVIG, including two men with small cell lung cancer and one woman with breast cancer. The improvement lasted 4 to 10 weeks. One patient (without cancer) became stronger after the initial infusion but did not respond to subsequent treatment. Interestingly, electrophysiologic evidence of improvement could be documented in only one patient.

We tried IVIG in a nonneoplastic 30-year-old woman with LEMS. Despite initial subjective improvement, it had no objective clinical or electrophysiologic benefit. Subsequently, a course of oral prednisone (100 mg/d for 1 month; then 100 mg every other day) resulted in a dramatic and sustained improvement. In general, the regimens and doses for the immunosuppressive therapies used to treat myasthenia gravis patients can be used for patients with LEMS.

## MULTIPLE SCLEROSIS

### Clinical Presentation

MS is one of the most common diseases of the CNS and primarily affects young adults. Although many CSF and brain imaging tests exist and are important in the evaluation of a patient with suspected MS, the gold standard for the diagnosis of this disorder is clinical. MS is defined as a disease that is characterized by multiple exacerbation resulting from lesions affecting CNS white matter that are separated in both space (e.g., different parts of the CNS) and time. Diagnostic criteria for MS have been devised (218) and are listed in Table 19.7.

Women develop MS two to three times more frequently than men (219–221). About 10% of patients with the diagnosis of MS have an affected family member (222); however, the inheritance pattern is multigenic, with a higher concordance in monozygotic than dizygotic twins (222,223). Several MHC antigen haplotypes are associated with MS and an animal model, experimental allergic encephalomyelitis. In humans with HLA-DR2, the DRB1, B7, CW1, and DQW1 haplotypes are all more common than in the general population (224). MS patients may have a history of family members affected with other autoimmune disorders, such as myasthenia gravis or autoimmune thyroiditis. Other autoimmune disorders may also be present in patients with MS.

Epidemiologic studies suggest that there is an increased risk for developing MS in people whose early life was spent in northern latitudes (225). Conversely, a move from northern to southern latitudes before the age of 12 years appears to decrease the risk for MS. Some evidence exists that infection

**TABLE 19.7.** *Adaptation of the Poser criteria for the diagnosis of multiple sclerosis*

| Clinical and laboratory findings | Poser criteria |
|---|---|
| Two attacks; clinical evidence of two lesions | Clinically definite multiple sclerosis |
| Two attacks; clinical evidence of one lesion | A. Clinically probable multiple sclerosis if brain magnetic resonance imaging (MRI) does not show typical white-matter lesions |
| | B. Clinically definite multiple sclerosis if brain MRI shows typical white-matter lesions |
| One attack; clinical evidence of one lesion | A. Not diagnostic if brain MRI does not show typical white-matter lesions |
| | B. Clinically probable multiple sclerosis if brain MRI shows evolving typical white-matter lesions |
| One attack; clinical evidence of one lesion plus oligoclonal bands in the cerebrospinal fluid | A. Not diagnostic if brain MRI does not show typical white-matter lesions |
| | B. Laboratory-supported definite multiple sclerosis if brain MRI shows evolving typical white-matter lesions |

Adapted from Poser CH, Paty DW, Scheinberg L, et al. New diagnostic criteria for multiple sclerosis: guidelines for research protocols. *Ann Neurol* 1983;13:227–231, with permission.

may be an important precipitating factor in the development of MS (226,227). An increased frequency of respiratory viral infection has been noted before an MS exacerbation, for example (226–228). Thus, the development of clinically symptomatic MS in a given patient appears to depend on a constellation of predisposing factors. Genetic, hormonal, infectious, and environmental factors all probably play a role in the manifestation of symptomatic disease.

Almost any type of CNS sign or symptom can occur in patients with MS. Disturbances of sensation, gait, and vision (monocular visual loss) are the most common symptoms at the time of diagnosis. Although there is no sign or symptom that is diagnostic of MS, in a patient with the appropriate demographic features, the following should prompt a consideration of MS in the differential diagnosis: optic neuritis; intranuclear ophthalmoplegia (especially if bilateral); unusual sensory symptoms; and Lhermitte's phenomenon in the absence of cervical trauma.

The disease course is relapsing–remitting in about 60% of patients, relapsing–progressive in 25%, and chronically progressive in 15% (221). The amount of disability in an individual patient can be highly variable, however. About 40% of patients have initial attacks that render them nonambulatory and may not recover. About 15% to 20% of patients have a benign form of MS and never develop permanent disability (220). On average, the relapse rate is 0.5 to 1 exacerbation per year (reviewed in 219). The relapse rate declines during pregnancy, especially in the third trimester, and increases in the first 3 postpartum months, before returning to the prepregnancy relapse rate (229). Favorable prognostic factors within the first 2 years of diagnosis include female gender, relapsing–remitting course, optic or sensory symptoms, young age at onset, and few exacerbations in the first 2 years (230).

A number of disorders can mimic MS (Table 19.8). Clues that should lead to some doubt of the diagnosis include absence of eye findings; absence of remissions; localized disease; atypical clinical features, such as prominent cortical involvement; absence of CSF abnormalities; and absence of brain MRI abnormalities.

The clinical symptoms of MS appear to result from an inflammatory response in the CNS during which the myelin sheath and oligodendrocytes are immunologically injured

**TABLE 19.8.** *Disorders that can mimic multiple sclerosis*

Collagen vascular disease, such as systemic lupus erythematosus and Sjögren's syndrome
Vasculitis of the central nervous system
Central nervous system sarcoidosis
Neurosyphilis
Paraneoplastic syndromes ("remote effects of cancer")
Combined systems degeneration (vitamin $B_{12}$ deficiency)
Spinocerebellar degeneration
Chronic infection of the central nervous system
Structural lesions of the central nervous system
Primary psychiatric disorder

(231,232). Immunization with myelin basic protein and adoptive transfer of myelin basic protein-specific T-cell clones are both effective in producing demyelinating lesions in experimental animals. These are pathologically similar to those seen in human MS (233). Animal models suggest that CNS antigen-specific T-helper lymphocytes (possibly directed against myelin basic protein) enter the brain and incite an immune response. This would be consistent with the high intrathecal production of oligoclonal IgG, but despite active search, an autoantigen in humans has yet to be identified.

The precise mechanism of myelin destruction is not clear. Studies of lymphocyte trafficking into the CNS in animal models suggest that there is a delay of several days from the time cells enter the CNS to the occurrence of demyelination (2,234). This supports the role of secreted factors, such as cytokines in myelin destruction. IFN-$\gamma$ induces the expression of class II antigen presentation in CNS cells (235,236) and increases symptoms in MS patients (237). Increased levels of other cytokines, such as IL-1, IL-6, and TNF-$\alpha$, probably contribute to demyelination and inflammation (238,239). High levels of proinflammatory cytokines have been correlated with MS exacerbations in several studies (240,241). This would support the role of the CD4$^+$ T lymphocytes in active myelin destruction. Abnormalities in other T-lymphocyte populations, such as CD8 cytotoxic cells, or those with $\gamma$ and $\delta$ T-cell receptor chains, may be important as well (242,243).

Data from a neuropathologic study suggest that in early-stage MS lesions, the oligodendrocytes probably survive the immunologic insult and can rapidly and completely remyelinate, whereas in late-state MS lesions, few oligodendrocytes remain and, therefore, remyelination cannot occur (244). This would be consistent with the notion that increased disease burden could lead to increased long-term disability.

### Diagnostic Approach

The diagnosis of MS is clinically based, requiring that signs and symptoms referable to CNS white-matter systems be disseminated in space and time (Table 19.7) (218). Both CSF and brain MRI studies are also important and help exclude other disease processes and increase the diagnostic accuracy in patients with suspected MS.

Characteristic CSF abnormalities include unique CSF oligoclonal IgG bands (two or more IgG bands found in CSF on electrophoresis studies that are not also present in serum) and a demonstration of increased IgG synthesis within the CSF compartment (245–247). These abnormalities indicate an immune response within the CNS and are sensitive, but not specific, in MS (247,248). Oligoclonal bands and other evidence for immune system activation within the CNS can be seen in many other disease processes, including those thought to have autoimmune-mediated CNS manifestations, such as systemic lupus erythematosus and Sjögren's syndrome, and those with an infectious cause, such as HIV-1 infection. The presence of unique oligoclonal bands suggests that antibodies to CNS antigens may play an important role in the disease process in MS. The presence of blood-brain barrier damage, as measured by the CSF-to-albumin ratio, and CSF cell counts exceeding 50 cells/μL cast doubt on the diagnosis of MS (249).

Brain MRI has a sensitivity of greater than 95% in patients with clinically definite MS (250,251). Characteristically, multiple periventricular white-matter lesions are seen (Fig. 19.5). Brain MRI has given us important information about the natural history of MS. New lesions develop up to 10 times more frequently than does clinical relapse (252–255). The presence of gadolinium-enhancing lesions is more common at the time of clinical relapse (256–258).

Quantitative measurement of brain MRI lesions at the time of initial presentation may predict the rate of subsequent lesion load increase, progression to MS, and disability outcome at 2 to 5 years (259–262). For example, patients with monosymptomatic disease with a lesion burden of at least 1.2 cc on brain MRI have a 90% chance of progressing to clinically definite MS over a 5-year period (263). In addition, MRI scanning has been used successfully to monitor therapeutic interventions in clinical trials (264,265). Interestingly, cross-sectional studies show little correlation between disability and lesion load (266), possibly because of the presence of lesions in clinically silent brain areas and the fact that pathologically heterogeneous lesions are not distinguishable on conventional magnetic imaging (267). New techniques, such as the analysis of T2-weighted decay curves (268), magnetization transfer imaging (269,270), and magnetic resonance spectroscopy (256,271,272), which discriminate between demyelination and axonal loss, may provide further insight into the pathology and clinical importance of brain MRI lesions. These newer techniques are especially promising in light of the evidence that early axonal damage may occur in MS and may be related to a worse prognosis (273).

*Therapy*

Glucocorticoids have been used to treat MS exacerbations for many years, although the data from most studies suggest their use does not change the natural history of the disease (274). The Optic Neuritis Treatment Trial did demonstrate, however, that treatment with intravenous methylprednisolone followed by oral prednisone after a bout of optic neuritis delays the development of clinically definite MS for up to 24 months (275). Other broad-based immunosuppressant therapies have failed to alter the disease course and have been associated with serious side effects (reviewed in 276). Low-dose (7.5 mg), weekly oral methotrexate may provide moderate benefit to MS patients with chronic progressive disease (277). The initial enthusiasm for the use of intravenous cyclophosphamide in patients with chronic progressive MS has dampened with subsequent experience. Newer treatment strategies have been aimed primarily at decreasing inflammation and suppressing the immune response in a more restricted way (278,279). The actual repair of CNS damage is a desirable therapeutic goal (279,280), but few practical options are available at this point to accomplish this.

Three drugs that have been demonstrated to alter the natural history of the disease progression have been approved to treat relapsing–remitting MS: IFN-β1b, IFN-β1a, and glatiramer acetate (281–283). IFN-β acts as an immune modulator and can reduce T-cell migration, leukocyte proliferation, and antigen presentation and modulate cytokine production (284). IFN-β1b, given subcutaneously every other day at a dose of 8 million units, has been shown to lower the frequency of all MS attacks by one third and serious attacks by one half at 2 years of follow-up (281). The mean MRI lesion burden at 2 years decreased 0.1% in the treated group and increased 20% in patients who received placebo. As of the 5-year follow-up, these treatment differences were maintained (285). Another preparation, IFN-β1a, also slowed the disability progression rate and decreased the annual exacerbation rate over 2 years by one third (282). The MRI lesion burden was lower in treated patients than in those receiving placebo; however, by 2 years, this difference was no longer significant. IFN-β1a can be given subcutaneously once a week at a dose of 6 million units (286).

Glatiramer acetate (previously known as copolymer 1) has been shown to suppress experimental allergic encephalomyelitis in several species, apparently because of cross-reactivity to myelin basic protein and an inhibition of the cell-mediated response to this and other myelin antigens (287). Treatment of patients who have chronic progressive MS with glatiramer acetate does not appear to be substantially better

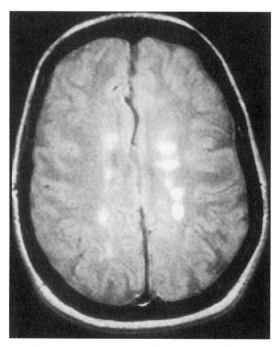

**FIG. 19.5.** Cranial magnetic resonance imaging scan of a patient with multiple sclerosis. T2-weighted image showing multiple deep periventricular white-matter lesions. (Courtesy of John Carter, M.D.)

than that with placebo (288). In a 2-year placebo-controlled study of glatiramer acetate in patients with relapsing–remitting MS, however, the 2-year relapse rate was 29% lower in treated patients than in those receiving placebo (289). In a 6-month extension of this trial, these treatment differences were maintained, and 41.6% of patients on placebo, as compared with 21.6% of patients receiving glatiramer acetate, had significant clinical worsening (290). No information about differences in MRI lesion burden is available from this trial because this was not studied. Glatiramer acetate may be given subcutaneously at a dose of 20 mg/d.

All three drugs are associated with injection-site reactions and influenza-like symptoms. The decision regarding which drug to use in a given patient must be individualized (281,288,291). Because IFN-β1b may have a greater effect on MRI lesion burden, this may be a better first choice for patients with active disease and high lesion burden (265). The convenience of once-weekly dosing with IFN-β1b is a significant factor in therapeutic decision making for many patients, however. Some patients treated with IFN-β1b develop neutralizing antibodies at low titer during treatment. These tend to fluctuate with time, and the relationship between the titer and clinical course is not well understood. In some patients, however, the presence of neutralizing antibodies appears to diminish the efficacy of this immunotherapy (292). Currently, the presence of neutralizing antibodies is not an indication to stop IFN-β1b treatment unless it is accompanied by loss of therapeutic efficacy. Neutralizing antibodies to IFN-β1b probably also cross-react with IFN-β1a. Thus, if treatment is stopped for loss of efficacy in the face of neutralizing antibodies, it is reasonable to switch to glatiramer acetate.

## TRANSVERSE MYELITIS

### Clinical Presentation

Transverse myelopathy is a clinical syndrome characterized by the rapid onset of spinal cord dysfunction, usually involving the thoracic spinal cord (293). The disorder appears abruptly, usually with severe back pain and occasionally fever and malaise. Weakness and paresthesias in the lower extremities evolve over a 12- to 24-hour period, sometimes associated with radicular pain. Occasionally, the disorder is painless. In the most severe form, complete paralysis and loss of sensation and autonomic function are present below the highest level of the lesion. In less severe forms, the disease may be patchier. A hemicord syndrome (Brown–Séquard syndrome) is sometimes present and includes loss of motor function and vibration sensation on the same side and loss of pain and temperature sensation on the opposite side. The spinal cord signs may ascend for hours to 1 or 2 weeks before they stabilize (293). In from 50% to as many as 80% of patients, there is a history of an antecedent infection or an immunization (294). Transverse myelopathy is also a rare complication of systemic lupus erythematosus (295).

### Diagnostic Approach

MRI of the spinal cord is the most important diagnostic procedure in a patient with suspected transverse myelopathy. Typical findings are normal or hypointense signals on T1-weighted imaging with an increased signal intensity on T2-weighted imaging in one of several patterns: focal segmental cord lesion; continuous lesion from conus to midcord; or discrete lesions scattered throughout the entire cord (294). These may enhance with gadolinium but do not always enhance. In one series, half of patients with clinical transverse myelitis had normal cord MRI studies (293). Computed tomography (CT) scanning of the spinal cord is usually not helpful. CSF studies may be normal, but they usually show a pleocytosis of 50 to 100 cells and an elevated protein level (293). Somatosensory evoked potential studies are usually abnormal, whereas brainstem and visual evoked potentials are nearly always normal in a patient with transverse myelopathy. Good prognostic factors include focal cord abnormalities or a normal MRI study (293). There is a low risk for developing recurrent demyelinating disease, and the predictors of recurrence are not well documented.

### Therapy

Few data are available regarding treatment of patients with transverse myelopathy. A study in children described good success with high-dose methylprednisolone therapy (296). Several studies in patients with systemic lupus erythematous and transverse myelopathy suggest that pulse cyclophosphamide and high-dose methylprednisolone may both be effective in hastening recovery (297).

## OPTIC NEURITIS

### Clinical Presentation

Optic neuritis is partial or complete loss of vision in one or both eyes as a result of an optic nerve lesion of unknown cause (298). If a cause is known or highly suspected, it is preferable to describe the clinical condition as *optic neuropathy* resulting from, for example, syphilis or MS. *Retrobulbar neuritis* refers to a lesion that is located in the posterior two thirds of the optic nerve (299). The term *papillitis* refers to a lesion in the anterior part of the optic nerve. When the lesion is located posteriorly, the fundoscopic examination is usually normal early, whereas with an anterior location, a fundoscopic abnormality indistinguishable from acute papilledema is usually present (Fig. 19.6) (298,299). One clinical differentiating feature between optic neuritis and papilledema from increased intracranial pressure is that visual acuity is decreased early in patients with optic neuritis and much later in patients with disease resulting from increased intracranial pressure (300). Pain on moving the eye is common, especially in the first few days of the illness. If the patient has retrobulbar neuritis, the opthalmoscopic examination is usually normal for the first 2 to 3 weeks. After

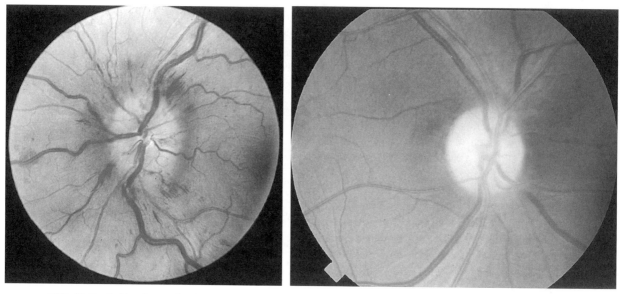

**FIG. 19.6. A:** Fundoscopic pictures from a patient with papillitis due to an episode of acute optic neuritis. **B:** Optic atrophy after resolution of the acute episode. (Courtesy of John Carter, M.D.)

this, disc pallor or more severe optic atrophy may be evident (298,300).

The visual loss in optic neuritis usually includes a central scotoma and loss of color vision. Visual loss occurs over hours to several days and almost always recovers to some degree within several weeks. Blindness rarely occurs (298). Although most patients with a diagnosis of MS have optic nerve involvement, optic neuritis does not always go on to MS. In the Optic Neuritis Treatment Trial, only 30% of patients developed clinically definite MS over a follow-up period of 5 years (301). In other studies, the risk for MS after a bout of optic neuritis has been as high as 40% (302,303). Predictors for the development of MS in patients with idiopathic optic neuritis include the presence of asymptomatic lesions in central white matter on brain MRI studies (31) and oligoclonal bands in the CSF (301,304,305). As many as 16% of patients with an isolated optic neuritis and a normal brain MRI scan, however, may go on to develop MS over a 5-year period; therefore, some caution is advised when discussing prognosis with the patient (301).

In a study of prognostic factors in childhood optic neuritis, 26% of patients had developed MS after 40 years of follow-up. A history of an antecedent viral illness in the 2 weeks before onset of the optic neuritis appears to lower the risk for MS (306).

### Diagnostic Approach

Brain MRI studies and CSF evaluation are indicated for all patients who present with idiopathic optic neuritis. Both are important to evaluate for alternative causes of optic neuritis and to help assess the risk for MS (304). A thorough neurologic history and examination and an ophthalmologic exam-

ination are also an essential part of the diagnostic workup of patients with suspected idiopathic optic neuritis.

### Therapy

The Optic Neuritis Treatment Trial examined the efficacy of a regime of pulse intravenous methylprednisolone (250 mg every 6 hours for 3 days) followed by oral prednisone (1 mg/kg per day for 11 days) or oral prednisone (1 mg/kg per day for 14 days) to oral placebo as a treatment for optic neuritis (307). After 2 years of follow-up, the group receiving intravenous methylprednisolone had a reduced rate of new MS attacks compared with the other two groups (305). This benefit was lost by the third year of follow-up, and by 5 years, about 30% of patients in all groups developed clinically definite MS (301). The benefit seen in the first 2 years is thought to result from a relatively long-term protective effect of therapy and not chance or a confounding variable. The mechanism of this protective effect is not entirely certain but may be caused by effects on cerebrovascular endothelium and stabilization of the blood-brain barrier. The recommended treatment for optic neuritis (with or without concomitant MS) is intravenous methylprednisolone followed by a short course of oral prednisone at the dose used in the Optic Neuritis Treatment Trial.

## NEUROMYELITIS OPTICA (DEVIC'S SYNDROME)

### Clinical Presentation

Neuromyelitis optica is a clinical syndrome characterized by the acute onset of optic nerve and spinal cord demyelination in a monophasic or multiphasic course (308). The literature has varied regarding how long a time interval between the two is allowable if a multiphasic course is seen. In some reports, the optic nerve and spinal cord involvement occurred years apart; whereas in others, an interval of 8 weeks or less was considered mandatory for diagnosis (reviewed in 308). Originally, neuromyelitis optica was thought to be distinct clinically and pathologically from MS, Schilder's disease, and acute disseminated encephalomyelitis (309–311). More recently, neuromyelitis optica has been assumed to represent a variant of MS in some cases, and a monophasic or multiphasic demyelinating illness in others (308). Some authors have concluded that there are sufficient distinguishing features to consider neuromyelitis optica a distinct syndrome (308,312,313).

The characteristic clinical features and prognosis for recovery may be different in adult and pediatric populations (312,313). One study of neuromyelitis optica in children that used an 8-week interval between the occurrence of optic nerve and spinal cord involvement found that the average age of onset was 7 years and that all patients had an antecedent viral illness (312). The optic neuritis was bilateral in eight of nine children, and disc edema was seen in all affected eyes. Visual loss ranged from 20/30 to no light perception. The course of transverse myelitis was similar in all patients. All had lower extremity weakness, paresthesias, and hyperreflexia. Six had bladder involvement, eight were nonambulatory, and one was able to walk only with assistance. The course was characterized by a rapid visual and neurologic recovery. All children were walking by 2 weeks into their illness. All children were treated with oral corticosteroids, but a standardized protocol was not followed. Most patients were followed for over 5 years and were without recurrent disease at that time point.

In a literature review including patients of all ages and using an 8-week interval between multiple phases, the clinical features of bilateral optic nerve involvement and viral prodrome were also commonly seen. Seventy percent had improved neurologic outcome, 14% had a poor outcome, and 16% died in the acute stages. Predictors of a poor outcome were older age at disease onset, marked CSF pleocytosis, and severe myelitis. Forty-two percent had a recurrence of demyelinating disease after complete recovery suggestive of MS. Fifty-eight percent of patients had a self-limited monophasic illness.

In contrast, another study of 12 adults that allowed a much longer time window between optic nerve and spinal cord disease found little recovery in any patients and a possible specific etiology in three patients (one with lupus, one with mixed connective tissue disease, and one with pulmonary tuberculosis) (313). Clinical features of the 9 patients without a specific etiology included nonwhite race, a nonremitting character of the neurologic disease, the lack of typical CSF immunologic abnormalities, and the lack of abnormalities on brain MRI studies. These features lead the authors to conclude that this group of patients had an immune-mediated disorder that was distinct from MS.

In summary, neuromyelitis optica is sometimes the heralding clinical presentation of MS. In many patients, however, especially in the younger age range, it appears to be a distinct clinical entity that is associated with a good prognosis and a low risk for progression to MS. This is particularly true when an antecedent infection is present and the time period between the optic nerve and spinal cord involvement is short. Occasionally, patients with connective tissue diseases or tuberculosis can develop a clinical syndrome that is consistent with the diagnosis of neuromyelitis optica. Neuromyelitis optica is not usually the presenting clinical feature in these disorders, however.

### Diagnostic Approach

The evaluation of a patient with suspected neuromyelitis optica should include MRI of the brain and spinal cord. Cord compression or some other anatomic abnormality must be excluded. Spinal cord involvement can be extensive and usually involves the lower cervical and thoracic cord (308). In most patients, brain MRI studies are normal. The presence of any abnormalities should increase the suspicion for MS (312,313). Spinal fluid studies commonly reveal a pleocytosis (usually less than 100 cells/mm$^3$) and elevated protein levels (usually less than 100 mg/dL), but oligoclonal bands are seldom present (308,312). There does not appear to be any benefit in additional studies for collagen vascular disease unless other signs or symptoms are present (313).

### Therapy

No data are available regarding treatment of this distinct syndrome. The use of high-dose intravenous methylprednisolone, similar to what would be used for a bout of optic neuritis or an MS attack, appears prudent. If extensive spinal cord involvement is present, pulse cyclophosphamide would be reasonable as well.

### REFERENCES

1. Male D. Immunology of brain endothelium and the blood brain barrier. In: MWB Bradbury, ed. *Physiology and pharmacology of the blood brain barrier.* Berlin: Springer Verlag, 1992;397–415.
2. Hickey WF. Migration of hematogenous cells through the blood-brain barrier and the initiation of CNS inflammation. *Brain Pathol* 1991;1: 97–105.
3. Male DK, Pryce G, Hughes CCW, et al. Lymphocyte migration into brain modelled in vitro; control by lymphocyte activation cytokines and antigen. *Cell Immunol* 1990;127:1–11.
4. Sinha AA, Lopez MT, McDevitt HO. Autoimmune diseases: the failure of self tolerance. *Science* 1990;248:1380–1393.
5. Wekerle H, Engelhardt B, Risau W, et al. Interactions of T lymphocytes with cerebral endothelial cells in vitro. *Brain Pathol* 1991;1:107–114.
6. Rothlein R, Barton RW, Winquist R. The role of intercellular adhesion molecule-1 (ICAM-1) in the inflammatory response. In: Cochrane CG, Gimbrone MA Jr, eds. *Cellular and molecular mechanisms in inflammation.* New York: Academic Press, 1991;171–180.
7. Engelhardt B, Conley FK, Butcher EC. Cell adhesion molecules on vessels during inflammation in the mouse central nervous system. *J Neuroimmunol* 1994;51:199–208.

8. Ellison MD, Merchant RE. Appearance of cytokine-associated central nervous system myelin damage coincides temporally with serum tumor necrosis factor induction after recombinant interleukin-2 infusion in rats. *J Neuroimmunol* 1991;33:245–251.

9. Ropper AH, Wijdicks EFM, Truax BT. *Guillain-Barré syndrome.* Philadelphia: F.A. Davis, 1991.

10. Ropper AH. The Guillain-Barré Syndrome. *N Engl J Med* 1992;326: 1130–1136.

11. Parry GJ. *Guillain-Barré syndrome.* New York: Thieme Medical Publishers, 1993.

12. Alter M. The epidemiology of Guillain-Barré Syndrome. *Ann Neurol* 1990;27[Suppl]:S7–S12.

13. Griffin JW, Ho TW. The Guillain-Barré syndrome at 75: the Campylobacter connection. *Ann Neurol* 1993;34:125–127.

14. Rees JH, Soudain SE, Gregson NA, et al. *Campylobacter jejuni* infection and Guillain-Barré syndrome. *N Engl J Med* 1995;333: 1415–1417.

15. Bolton CF. The changing concepts of Guillain-Barré syndrome. *N Engl J Med* 1995;333:1415–1417.

16. Yuki N, Takahashi M, Tagawa Y, et al. Association of *Campylobacter jejuni* serotype with antiganglioside antibody in Guillain-Barré syndrome and Fisher's syndrome. *Ann Neurol* 1997;42:28–33.

17. Cornblath DR, McArthur JC, Kennedy PG, et al. Inflammatory demyelinating peripheral neuropathies associated with human T-cell lymphotropic virus type III infection. *Ann Neurol* 1987;21:32–40.

18. Ramos-Alvarez M, Bessudo L, Sabin A. Paralytic syndromes associated with non-inflammatory cytoplasmic or nuclear neuronopathy: acute paralytic disease in Mexican children, neuropathologically distinguishable from Landry-Guillain-Barré syndrome. *JAMA* 1969;207: 1481–1492.

19. Schonberger LB, Hurwitz ES, Katona P, et al. Guillain-Barré syndrome: its epidemiology and associations with influenza vaccination. *Ann Neurol* 1981;9[Suppl]:31.

20. Arnason BG, Asbury AK. Idiopathic polyneuritis after surgery. *Arch Neurol* 1968;18:500–507.

21. Steiner I, Argov Z, Cahan C, et al. Guillain-Barré syndrome after epidural anesthesia: direct nerve root damage may trigger disease. *Neurology* 1985;35:1473.

22. Cameron DG, Howell DA, Hutchinson JL. Acute peripheral neuropathy in Hodgkin's disease: report of a fatal case with histologic features of allergic neuritis. *Neurology* 1958;8:575.

23. Lisak RP, Mitchell M, Zweiman B, et al. Guillain-Barré syndrome and Hodgkin's disease: three cases with immunological studies. *Ann Neurol* 1977;1:72.

24. Fisher CM. An unusual variant of acute idiopathic polyneuritis (syndrome of ophthalmoplegia, ataxia, and areflexia). *N Engl J Med* 1956; 255:57–65.

25. Fisher CM. An unusual variant of acute idiopathic polyneuritis (syndrome of ophthalmoplegia, ataxia, and areflexia). *N Engl J Med* 1956; 255:57–65.

26. Ropper AH. Unusual clinical variants and signs in Guillain-Barré syndrome. *Arch Neurol* 1986;43:1150–1152.

27. Feasby TE, Gilbert JJ, Brown WF, et al. An acute axonal form of Guillain-Barré polyneuropathy. *Brain* 1986;109:1115–1126.

28. Ropper AH. Further regional variants of acute immune polyneuropathy. *Arch Neurol* 1994;51:671–675.

29. Simmons Z, Tivakaran S. Acquired demyelinating polyneuropathy presenting as a pure clinical sensory syndrome. *Muscle Nerve* 1996;19: 1174–1176.

30. Valencio L, Najera E, Perez Gallardo F, et al. Outbreak of paralytic illness of unknown etiology in Albacete, Spain. *Am J Epidemiol* 1971; 94:450–456.

31. Jackson CE, Barohn RJ, Mendell JR. Acute paralytic syndrome in three American men: comparison with Chinese cases. *Arch Neurol* 1993;50:732–735.

32. McKhann GM, Cornblath DR, Griffin JW, et al. Acute motor axonal neuropathy: a frequent cause of acute flaccid paralysis in China. *Ann Neurol* 1993;33:333–342.

33. Griffin JW, Li CY, Ho TW, et al. Pathology of the motor-sensory axonal Guillain-Barré syndrome. *Ann Neurol* 1996;39:17–28.

34. Waksman BH, Adams RD. Allergic neuritis: experimental disease rabbits induced by the injection of peripheral nervous tissue and adjuvants. *J Exp Med* 1955;102:213–236.

35. Kadlubowski M, Hucher RAC. Identification of the neuritogen for experimental allergic neuritis. *Nature* 1979;277:140–141.

36. Hahn AF, Gilbert JJ, Feasby RE. Passive transfer of demyelination by experimental allergic neuritis serum. *Acta Neuropathol* 1980;49: 169–176.

37. Koske CL, Gratz E, Sutherland J, et al. Clinical correlation with anti-peripheral-nerve myelin antibodies in Guillain-Barré syndrome. *Ann Neurol* 1986;19:575–577.

38. Koske CL. Characterization of complement-fixing antibodies to peripheral nerve myelin in Guillain-Barré syndrome. *Ann Neurol* 1990;27[Suppl]:S44–S47.

39. Hartung HP, Pollard JD, Harvey GK, et al. Immunopathogenesis and treatment of the Guillain-Barré syndrome: part 1 and part 2. *Muscle Nerve* 1995;18:137–153, 154–164.

40. Vriesendorp FJ, Mishu B, Blaser MJ, et al. Serum antibodies to GM1, GD1b, peripheral nerve myelin, and *Campylobacter jejuni* in patients with Guillain-Barré syndrome and controls: correlation and prognosis. *Ann Neurol* 1993;34:130–135.

41. Ilyas AA, Willison HG, Quarles RH, et al. Serum antibodies to gangliosides in Guillain-Barré syndrome. *Ann Neurol* 1988;23:440–447.

42. van der Meché FGA, van Doorn PA. Guillain-Barré syndrome and chronic inflammatory demyelinating polyneuropathy: immune mechanisms and update on current therapies. *Ann Neurol* 1995;37[Suppl 1]:S14–S31.

43. Oomes PG, Jacobs BC, Hazenberg MP, et al. Anti-GM1 IgG antibodies and *Campylobacter* bacteria in Guillain-Barré syndrome: evidence of molecular mimicry. *Ann Neurol* 1995;38:170–175.

44. Rees JH, Gregson NA, Hughes RA. Anti-ganglioside GM1 antibodies in Guillain-Barré syndrome and their relationship to *Campylobacter jejuni* infection. *Ann Neurol* 1995;38:809–816.

45. McKhann GM, Griffin JW, Cornblath DR, et al., and the Guillain-Barré Study Group. Plasmapheresis and Guillain-Barré syndrome: analysis of prognostic factors and the effect of plasmapheresis. *Ann Neurol* 1988;23:347–353.

46. Guillain-Barré Syndrome Study Group. Plasmapheresis and acute Guillain-Barré Syndrome. *Neurology* 1985;35:1096–1104.

47. Wijdicks EFM, Ropper AH. Acute relapsing Guillain-Barré syndrome after long asymptomatic intervals. *Arch Neurol* 1990;47:82–84.

48. Albers JW, Donofrio PD, McGonagle TK. Sequential electrodiagnostic abnormalities in acute inflammatory demyelinating polyradiculoneuropathy. *Muscle Nerve* 1985;8:528–539.

49. Cornblath DR, Mellits ED, Griffin JW, et al., and the Guillain-Barré Study Group. Motor conduction studies in Guillain-Barré syndrome: description and prognostic value. *Ann Neurol* 1988;23:354–359.

50. Asbury AK, Arnason BG, Adams RD. The inflammatory lesion in idiopathic polyneuritis: its role in pathogenesis. *Medicine* 1969;48: 173–215.

51. Asbury AK, Cornblath DR. Assessment of current diagnostic criteria for Guillain-Barré syndrome. *Ann Neurol* 1990;27[Suppl]:S21–S24.

52. Willison HJ, Veitch J, Paterson G, et al. Miller Fisher syndrome is associated with serum antibodies to GQ1b ganglioside. *J Neurol Neurosurg Psychiatry* 1993;56:204–206.

53. Yuki N, Sato S, Tsuji S, et al. Frequent presence of anti-GQ1b antibody in Fisher's syndrome. *Neurology* 1993;43:414–417.

54. French Cooperative Group on Plasma Exchange in Guillain-Barré syndrome. Efficiency of plasma exchange in Guillain-Barré syndrome: role of replacement fluids. *Ann Neurol* 1987;22:753–761.

55. van der Meche FGA, Schmitz PIM, and the Dutch Guillain-Barré Study Group. A randomized trial comparing intravenous immune globulin and plasma exchange in Guillain-Barré syndrome. *N Engl J Med* 1992;326:1123–1129.

56. Plasma Exchange/Sandoglobulin Guillain Barré Syndrome Trial Group. Randomized trial of plasma exchange, intravenous immunoglobulin, and combined treatments in Guillain Barré Syndrome. *Lancet* 1997;349:225–230.

57. Irani DN, Cornblath DR, Chaudhry V, et al. Relapse in Guillain-Barré syndrome after treatment with human immune globulin. *Neurology* 1993;43:857–858.

58. Castro LHM, Ropper AH. Human immune globulin in Guillain-Barré syndrome: worsening during and after treatment. *Neurology* 1993; 43:1034–1036.

59. Ropper AH, Albers JW, Addison R. Limited relapse in Guillain-Barré syndrome after plasma exchange. *Arch Neurol* 1988;45:314–315.

60. Loffel NB, Rossi LN, Mumenthaler M, et al. The Landry-Guillain-Barré syndrome: complications, prognosis, and natural history in 123 cases. *J Neurol Sci* 1977;33:71–79.
61. Goodall JD, Kosmidis JC, Geddes AM. Effect of corticosteroids on the course of Guillain-Barré syndrome. *Lancet* 1974;1:524–526.
62. Hughes RAC, Newsom-Davis J, Perkin GD, et al. Controlled trial of prednisolone in acute polyneuropathy. *Lancet* 1978;2:750–753.
63. Guillain-Barre Syndrome Steroid Trial Group. Double-blind trial of intravenous methylprednisolone in Guillain-Barre syndrome. *Lancet* 1993;341:586–590.
64. Dutch Guillain-Barre Study Group. Treatment of Guillain-Barre syndrome with high-dose immune globulins combines with methylprednisolone: a pilot study. *Ann Neurol* 1994;35:749–752.
65. Barohn RJ, Kissel JT, Warmolts JR, et al. Chronic inflammatory demyelinating polyradiculoneuropathy: clinical characteristics, course, and recommendations for diagnostic criteria. *Arch Neurol* 1989;46:878–884.
66. Dyck PJ, Lais AC, Ohta M, et al. Chronic inflammatory demyelinating polyradiculoneuropathy. *Mayo Clin Proc* 1975;50:621–637.
67. Ad Hoc Subcommittee of the American Academy of Neurology AIDS Task Force. Research criteria for diagnosis of chronic inflammatory demyelinating polyneuropathy (CIDP). *Neurology* 1991;41:617–618.
68. Cornblath DR, Griffin DE, Welch D, et al. Quantitative analysis of endoneurial T-cells in human sural nerve biopsies. *J Neuroimmunol* 1990;26:113–118.
69. Matsummuro K, Izumo S, Umehara F, et al. Chronic inflammatory demyelinating polyneuropathy: histological and immunopathological studies on biopsied sural nerves. *J Neurol Sci* 1994;127:170–178.
70. Prineas JW, McLeod JG. Chronic relapsing polyneuritis. *J Neurol Sci* 1976;27:427–458.
71. Steck AJ. Inflammatory neuropathy: pathogenesis and clinical features. *Curr Opin Neurol Neurosurg* 1992;5:633–637.
72. Kissel JT, Mendell JR. Neuropathies associated with monoclonal gammopathies. Neuromusc Disord 1995;6:3–18.
73. Nobile-Orazio E, Latov N, Hays AP, et al. Neuropathy and anti-MAG antibodies without detectable serum M-protein. *Neurology* 1984;34:218–221.
74. Barohn RJ, Kissel JT, Warmolts JR, et al. Chronic inflammatory demyelinating polyradiculoneuropathy: clinical characteristics, course, and recommendations for diagnostic criteria. *Arch Neurol* 1989;46:878–884.
75. Mendell JR. Chronic inflammatory demyelinating polyradiculoneuropathy. *Annu Rev Med* 1993;44:211–219.
76. Romanick-Schmiedl S, Kiprov D, Chalmers AC, et al. Extraneural manifestations of chronic inflammatory demyelinating polyradiculoneuropathy. *Am J Med* 1990;89:531–534.
77. Stewart JD, McKelvey R, Durcan L, et al. Chronic inflammatory demyelinating polyneuropathy (CIDP) in diabetics. *J Neurol Sci* 1996;142:59–64.
78. Amato AA, Barohn RJ, Sahenk Z, et al. Polyneuropathy complicating bone marrow and solid organ transplantation. *Neurology* 1993;43:1513–1518.
79. Mendell JR, Kolkin S, Kissel JT, et al. Evidence for central nervous system demyelination in chronic inflammatory demyelinating polyradiculoneuropathy. *Neurology* 1987;37:1291–1294.
80. Thomas PK, Walker RWH, Rudge P, et al. Chronic demyelinating peripheral neuropathy associated with multifocal central nervous system demyelination. *Brain* 1987;110:53–76.
81. Oh SJ, Joy JL, Sunwoo IN, et al. A case of chronic sensory demyelinating neuropathy responding to immunotherapies. *Muscle Nerve* 1992;15:255–256.
82. Chroni E, Hall SM, Hughes RAC. Chronic relapsing axonal neuropathy: a first case report. *Ann Neurol* 1995;37:112–115.
83. Uncini A, Sabatelli M, Mignogna T, et al. Chronic progressive steroid responsive axonal polyneuropathy: a CIDP variant or a primary axonal disorder? *Muscle Nerve* 1996;19:365–371.
84. Hughes R, Sanders E, Hall S, et al. Subacute idiopathic demyelinating polyradiculoneuropathy. *Arch Neurol* 1992;49:612–616.
85. Dyck PJ, O'Brien PC, Oviatt KF, et al. Prednisone improves chronic inflammatory demyelinating polyradiculoneuropathy more than no treatment. *Ann Neurol* 1982;11:136–141.
86. Dyck PJ, Daube J, O'Brien P, et al. Plasma exchange in chronic inflammatory demyelinating polyradiculoneuropathy. *N Engl J Med* 1986;314:461–465.
87. Hahn AF, Bolton CF, Pillay N, et al. Plasma-exchange therapy in chronic inflammatory demyelinating polyneuropathy: a double-blind, sham-controlled, cross-over study. *Brain* 1996;119:1055–1066.
88. Hahn AF, Bolton CF, Zochodne D, et al. Intravenous immunoglobulin treatment in chronic inflammatory demyelinating polyneuropathy: a double-blind, placebo-controlled, cross-over study. *Brain* 1996;119:1067–1077.
89. Dyck PJ, O'Brien P, Swanson C, et al. Combined azathioprine and prednisone in chronic inflammatory demyelinating polyneuropathy. *Neurology* 1985;35:1173–1176.
90. van Doorn PA, Brand A, Strengers PFW, et al. High-dose intravenous immunoglobulin treatment in chronic inflammatory demyelinating polyneuropathy: a double-blind, placebo-controlled crossover study. *Neurology* 1990;40:209–212.
91. van Doorn PA, Vermeulen M, Brand A, et al. Intravenous immunoglobulin treatment in patients with chronic inflammatory demyelinating polyneuropathy: clinical and laboratory characteristics associated with improvement. *Arch Neurol* 1991;48:217–220.
92. Vermeulen M, van Doorn PA, Brand A, et al. Intravenous immunoglobulin treatment in patients with chronic inflammatory demyelinating polyneuropathy: a double-blind, placebo-controlled study. *J Neurol Neurosurg Psychiatry* 1993;56:36–39.
93. Dyck PJ, Litchy WJ, Kratz KM, et al. A plasma exchange versus immune globulin infusion trial in chronic inflammatory demyelinating polyradiculoneuropathy. *Ann Neurol* 1994;36:838–845.
94. Dyck PJ, O'Brien P, Swanson C, et al. Combined azathioprine and prednisone in chronic inflammatory demyelinating polyneuropathy. *Neurology* 1985;35:1173–1176.
95. Kolkin S, Nahman NS, Mendell JR. Chronic nephrotoxicity complicating cyclosporine treatment of chronic inflammatory demyelinating polyradiculoneuropathy. *Neurology* 1987;37:147–149.
96. Mahattanakul WO, Crawford T, Griffin JW, et al. Treatment of chronic inflammatory demyelinating polyneuropathy with cyclosporin-A. *J Neurol Neurosurg Psychiatry* 1996;60:186–187.
97. Sabatelli M, Mignogna T, Lippi G, et al. Interferon-alpha may benefit steroid unresponsive chronic inflammatory demyelinating polyneuropathy. *J Neurol Neurosurg Psychiatry* 1995;58:638–639.
98. Gorson KC, Allam G, Simovic D, et al. Improvement following interferon-alpha 2A in chronic inflammatory demyelinating polyneuropathy. *Neurology* 1997;48:777–780.
99. Choudhary PP, Thopson N, Hughes RAC. Improvement following interferon-beta in chronic inflammatory demyelinating polyneuropathy. *J Neurol* 1995;242:252–253.
100. Gorson KC, Ropper AH, Clark BD, et al. Treatment of chronic inflammatory demyelinating polyneuropathy with interferon-α 2a. *Neurology* 1998;50:84-87.
101. Dyck PJ, Lais AC, Ohta M, et al. Chronic inflammatory demyelinating polyradiculoneuropathy. *Mayo Clin Proc* 1975;50:621–637.
102. Gorson KC, Allam G, Ropper AH. Chronic inflammatory demyelinating polyneuropathy: clinical features and response to treatment in 67 consecutive patients with and without a monoclonal gammopathy. *Neurology* 1997;48:321–328.
103. Tervaert JWC, Kallenberg C. Neurologic manifestations of systemic vasculitides. *Neurol Aspects Rheum Dis* 1993;19:913–940.
104. Kissel JT, Mendell JR. Vasculitic neuropathy. *Neurol Clin* 1992;10:761–781.
105. Dyck PJ, Benstead TJ, Conn DL, et al. Nonsystemic vasculitic neuropathy. *Brain* 1987;110:843–853.
106. Olney RK. Neuropathies in connective tissue disease. *Muscle Nerve* 1992;15:531–542.
107. Kissel JT, Slivka AP, Warmolts JR, et al. The clinical spectrum of necrotizing angiopathy of the peripheral nervous system. *Ann Neurol* 1985;18:251–257.
108. Kissel JT, Riethman JL, Omerza J, et al. Peripheral nerve vasculitis: immune characterization of the vascular lesions. *Ann Neurol* 1989;25:291–297.
109. Said G. Necrotizing peripheral nerve vasculitis. *Neurol Clin* 1977;15:835–48.
110. Kelly JJ Jr, Kyle RA, Miles JM, et al. The spectrum of peripheral neuropathy in myeloma. *Neurology* 1981;31:24–31.
111. Kelly JJ, Kyle RA, Miles JM, et al. Osteosclerotic myeloma and peripheral neuropathy. *Neurology* 1983;33:202–210.
112. Kyle RA. "Benign" monoclonal gammopathy: a misnomer? *JAMA* 1984;251:1849–1854.

113. Kyle RA, Garton JP. The spectrum of IgM monoclonal gammopathy in 430 cases. *Mayo Clin Proc* 1987;62:719–731.

114. Yeung KB, Thomas PK, King RHM, et al. The clinical spectrum of peripheral neuropathies associated with benign monoclonal IgM, IgG and IgA paraproteinaemia. *J Neurol* 1991;238:383–391.

115. Gosselin S, Kyle RA, Dyck PJ. Neuropathy associated with monoclonal gammopathies of undetermined significance. *Ann Neurol* 1991;30:54–61.

116. Dyck PJ, Low PA, Windebank AJ, et al. Plasma exchange in polyneuropathy associated with monoclonal gammopathy of undetermined significance. *N Engl J Med* 1991;325:1482–1486.

117. Bosch EP, Smith BE. Peripheral neuropathies associated with monoclonal proteins. *Med Clin North Am* 1993;77:125–139.

118. Notermans NC, Wokke JHJ, van den Berg LH, et al. Chronic idiopathic axonal polyneuropathy comparison of patients with and without monoclonal gammopathy. *Brain* 1996;119:421–427.

119. Dalakas MC, Quarles RH, Farrer RG, et al. A controlled study of intravenous immunoglobulin in demyelinating neuropathy with IgM gammopathy. *Ann Neurol* 1996;40:792–795.

120. Simmons Z, Albers JW, Bromberg MB, et al. Presentation and initial clinical course in patients with chronic inflammatory demyelinating polyradiculoneuropathy: comparison of patients without and with monoclonal gammopathy. *Neurology* 1993;43:2202–2209.

121. Simmons Z, Albers JW, Bromberg MB, et al. Long-term followup of patients with chronic inflammatory demyelinating polyradiculoneuropathy, without and with monoclonal gammopathy. *Brain* 1995;118:359–368.

122. Latov N, Sherman WH, Hays AP. Peripheral neuropathy and anti-MAG antibodies. *CRC Crit Rev Neurobiol* 1988;3:301–332.

123. Nobile-Orazio E, Baldini L, Barbieri S, et al. Treatment of patients with neuropathy and anti-MAG M-proteins. *Ann Neurol* 1988;24:93–97.

124. Blume G, Pestronk A, Goodnough LT. Anti-MAG antibody-associated polyneuropathies: improvement following immunotherapy with monthly plasma exchange and IV cyclophosphamide. *Neurology* 1995;45:1577–1580.

125. Cook D, Dalakas M, Galdi A, et al. High-dose intravenous immunoglobulin in the treatment of demyelinating neuropathy associated with monoclonal gammopathy. *Neurology* 1990;40:212–214.

126. Leger JM, Younes-Chennoufi AB, Chassandro B, et al. Human immunoglobulin treatment of multifocal motor neuropathy and polyneuropathy associated with monoclonal gammopathy. *J Neurol Neurosurg Psychiatry* 1994;57[Suppl]:46–49.

127. Mariette X, Chastang C, Clavelou P, et al. A randomised clinical trial comparing interferon-α and intravenous immunoglobulin in polyneuropathy associated with monoclonal IgM. *J Neurol Neurosurg Psychiatry* 1997;63:28–34.

128. Pestronk A, Cornblath DR, Ilyas AA, et al. A treatable multifocal motor neuropathy with Antibodies to GM1 ganglioside. *Ann Neurol* 1988;24:73–78.

129. Parry GJ. Motor neuropathy with multifocal conduction block. *Semin Neurol* 1993;13:269–275.

130. Parry GJP, Clarke S. Multifocal acquired demyelinating neuropathy masquerading as motor neuron disease. *Muscle Nerve* 1988;11:103–107.

131. Katz JS, Wolfe GI, Bryan WW, et al. Electrophysiologic findings in multifocal motor neuropathy. *Neurology* 1997;88:7009–7727.

132. Tan E, Lynn J, Amato AA, et al. Immunosuppressive treatment of motor neuron syndromes: attempts to distinguish a treatable disorder. *Arch Neurol* 1994;51:194–200.

133. Parry GJP. Antiganglioside antibodies do not necessarily play a role in multifocal motor neuropathy. *Muscle Nerve* 1994;17:97–99.

134. Sadiq SA, Thomas FP, Kilidireas K, et al. The spectrum of neurologic disease associated with anti-GM1 antibodies. *Neurology* 1990;40:1067–1072.

135. Feldman EL, Bromberg MB, Albers JW, et al. Immunosuppressive treatment in multifocal motor neuropathy. *Ann Neurol* 1991;30:397–401.

136. Pestronk A, Lopate G, Kornberg AJ, et al. Distal lower motor neuron syndrome with high-titer serum IgG anti-GM1 antibodies: improvement following immunotherapy with monthly plasma exchange and intravenous cyclophosphamide. *Neurology* 1994;44:2027–2031.

137. Chaudhry V, Corse Am, Cornblath DR, et al. Multifocal motor neuropathy: response to human immune globulin. Ann Neurol 1993;33:237–242.

138. Saperstein DS, Amato AA, Katz JS, et al. Multifocal sensory and motor neuropathy differs from multifocal motor neuropathy. *Muscle Nerve* 1998;21:1589(abst).

139. Hammack JE, Kimmel DW, O'Neill BP, et al. Paraneoplastic cerebellar degeneration: a clinical comparison of patients with and without Purkinje cell cytoplasmic antibodies. *Mayo Clin Proc* 1990;65:1423–1431.

140. Moll JWB, Henzen-Logmans SC, Splinter TAW, et al. Diagnostic value of anti-neuronal antibodies for paraneoplastic disorders of the nervous system. *J Neurol Neurosurg Psychiatry* 1990;53:940–943.

141. Henson RA, Urich H. Cancer and the nervous system: the neurological manifestations of systemic disease. Oxford, UK: Blackwell Scientific, 1982.

142. Posner JB, Dalmau J. Paraneoplastic syndrome. *Curr Opin Immunol* 1997;9:723–729.

143. Bateman DE, Weller RD, Kennedy P. Stiffman syndrome: a rare neoplastic disorder? *J Neurol Neurosurg Psychiatry* 1995;53:695–696.

144. Isaacs H. A syndrome of continuous muscle-fibre activity. *J Neurol Neurosurg Psychiatry* 196;24:319–325.

145. Croft PB, Wilkinson M. The incidence of carcinomatous neuromyopathy in patients with various types of carcinoma. *Brain* 1965;88:427–434.

146. Peterson K, Rosenblum MK, Kotanides H, et al. Paraneoplastic cerebellar degeneration. I. A clinical analysis of 55 anti-Yo antibody-positive patients. *Neurology* 1992;42:1931–1937.

147. Anderson NE, Posner JB, Sidtis JJ, et al. The metabolic anatomy of paraneoplastic cerebellar degeneration. *Ann Neurol* 1988;23:533–540.

148. Hammack J, Kotanides H, Rosenblum MK, et al. Paraneoplastic cerebellar degeneration. II. Clinical and immunologic findings in 21 patients with Hodgkin's disease. *Neurology* 1992;42:1938–1943.

149. Luque FA, Furneaux HM, Ferziger LR, et al. Anti-Ri: an antibody associated with paraneoplastic opsoclonus and breast cancer. *Ann Neurol* 1991;29:241–251.

150. Glantz MJ, Biran H, Myers ME, et al. The radiographic diagnosis and treatment of paraneoplastic central nervous system disease. *Cancer* 1994;73:168–175.

151. Darnell RB, DeAngelis LM. Regression of small-cell lung carcinoma in patients with paraneoplastic neuronal antibodies. *Lancet* 1993;341:21–22.

152. Vershcuuren J, Dalmau J. Paraneoplastic neurologic disorders. In: Antel J, Birnbaum G, Hartung H-P, eds. *Clinical neuroimmunology.* Malden, MA: Blackwell Scientific, 1998:148–171.

153. Tomimoto H, Brengman JM, Yanagihara T. Paraneoplastic cerebellar degeneration with a circulating antibody against neurons and nonneuronal cells. *Acta Neuropathol* 1993;86:206–211.

154. Sakai K, Negami T, Yoskioka A, et al. The expression of a cerebellar degeneration-associated neural antigen in human tumor line cells. *Neurology* 1992;42:361–366.

155. Posner JB. Paraneoplastic cerebellar degeneration. *Can J Neurol Sci* 1993;20[Suppl 3]:S117–S122.

156. Graus F, Elkon KB, Cordon-Cardo C, et al. Sensory neuronopathy and small-cell lung cancer: antineuronal antibody that also reacts with the tumor. *Am J Med* 1986;80:45–52.

157. Graus F, Cordon-Cardo C, Posner JB. Neuronal antinuclear antibody in sensory neuronopathy from lung cancer. *Neurology* 1985;35:538–543.

158. Dalmau J, Graus F, Rosenblum MK, et al. Anti-Hu associated paraneoplastic encephalomyelitis/sensory neuronopathy: a clinical study of 71 patients. *Medicine* 1992;71:59–72.

159. Graus F, Bonaventura I, Uchuya M, et al. Indolent anti-Hu-associated paraneoplastic sensory neuropathy. *Neurology* 1994;44:2258–2261.

160. Oh SJ, Dropcho EJ, Claussen GC. Anti-Hu-associated paraneoplastic sensory neuronopathy responding to early aggressive immunotherapy: report of two cases and review of literature. *Muscle Nerve* 1997;20:1576–1582.

161. O'Leary CP, Willison HJ. Autoimmune ataxic neuropathies (sensory ganglionopathies). *Curr Opin Neurol* 1997;10:366–370.

162. Voltz RD, Posner JB, Dalmau J, et al. Paraneoplastic encephalomyelitis: an update of the effects of the anti-Hu immune response on the nervous system and tumour. *J Neurol Neurosurg Psychiatry* 1997;63:133–136.

163. Voltz R, Dalmau J, Posner JB, et al. T-cell receptor analysis in anti-Hu associated paraneoplastic encephalomyelitis. *Neurology* 1998;51:1146–1150.

164. Dalmau J, Posner JB. Neurologic paraneoplastic antibodies (anti-Yo; anti-Hu; anti-Ri): the case for a nomenclature based on antibody and antigen specificity. *Neurology* 1994;44:2241–2246.

165. Posner JB. The anti-Hu syndrome: a model paraneoplastic disorder. *Recent Results Cancer Res* 1994;135:77–90.

166. Averbuch-Heller L, Remler B. Opsoclonus. *Semin Neurol* 1996;16: 21–26.

167. Escudero D, Barnadas A, Codina M, et al. Anti-Ri-associated paraneoplastic neurologic disorder without opsoclonus in a patient with breast cancer. *Neurology* 1993;43:1605–1606.

168. Pranzatelli MR. The immunopharmacology of the opsoclonus-myoclonus syndrome. *Clin Neuropharmacol* 1996;19:1–47.

169. Hormigo A, Dalmau J, Rosenblum MK, et al. Immunological and pathological study of anti-Ri-associated encephalopathy. *Ann Neurol* 1994;36:896–902.

170. Solimena M, Folli F, Aparisi R, et al. Autoantibodies to GABA-ergic neurons and pancreatic beta cells in stiffman syndrome. *N Engl J Med* 1990;322:1555–1560.

171. Ferrari P, Federico M, Grimaldi LME, et al. Stiffman syndrome in a patient with Hodgkin's disease: an unusual paraneoplastic syndrome. *Haematologica* 1990;75:570–572.

172. Vedanarayanan V, Boylan KB, George T, et al. "Tetanus-like" syndrome associated with Hodgkin's lymphoma: a new paraneoplastic syndrome. *Muscle Nerve* 1991;14:913.

173. Grimaldi LME, Martino G, Bragghi S, et al. Heterogeneity of autoantibodies in stiffman syndrome. *Ann Neurol* 1993;34:57–64.

174. Nicholas AP, Chatterjee A, Arnold MM, et al. Stiff-persons syndrome associated with thymoma and subsequent myasthenia gravis. *Muscle Nerve* 1997;20:493–498.

175. Masson C, Prier S, Benoit C, et al. Amnesie, syndrome de l'homme raide: manifestations revelatrices d'une encephalomyelite paraneoplastique. *Ann Med Intern* 1987;138:502.

176. Folli F, Solimena M, Cofiel R, et al. Autoantibodies to a 128 kd synaptic protein in three women with stiffman syndrome and breast cancer. *N Engl J Med* 1993;328:546–551.

177. Newsom-Davis J, Mills KR. Immunological associations of acquired neuromyotonia (Isaacs' syndrome). *Brain* 1993;116:453–469.

178. Partenan VSJ, Soininen H, Saksa M, et al. Electromyographic and nerve conduction findings in a patient with neuromyotonia, normocalcemic tetany and small-cell lung cancer. *Acta Neurol Scand* 1980;61:216–218.

179. Walsh JC. Neuromyotonia: an unusual presentation of intrathoracic malignancy. *J Neurol Nerosurg Psychiatry* 1976;39:1086–1091.

180. Waerness E. Neuromyotonia and bronchial carcinoma. *Electromyogr Clin Neurophysiol* 1974;14:527–529.

181. Garcia-Merino A, Cabello A, Mora JS, et al. Continuous muscle fiber activity, peripheral neuropathy, and thymoma. *Ann Neurol* 1991;29: 215–219.

182. Halbach M, Homberg V, Freund H-J. Neuromuscular, autonomic, and central cholinergic hyperactivity associated with thymoma, and acetylcholine receptor-binding antibody. *J Neurol* 1987;234:433.

183. Zifko U, Drlicek M, Machacek E, et al. Syndrome of continuous muscle fiber activity and plasmacytoma with IgM paraproteinemia. *Neurology* 1994;44:560–561.

184. Caress JB, Abend WK, Preseton DC, et al. A case of Hodgkin's lymphoma producing neuromyotonia. *Neurology* 1997;49:258–259.

185. Shilito P, Molenaar PC, Vincent A, et al. Acquired neuromyotonia: evidence for autoantibodies directed against K+ channels of peripheral nerves. *Ann Neurol* 1995;38:714–722.

186. Hart IK, Waters C, Vincent A, et al. Autoantibodies detected to expressed K+ channels are implicated in neuromyotonia. *Ann Neurol* 1997;41:238–246.

187. Engel AG. Myasthenia SYndromes. In: Engel AG, Franzini-Armstrong C, eds. *Myology*, 2nd ed. New York: McGraw-Hill, 1994: 1798–1835.

188. Anderson HJ, Churchill-Davidson HC, Richardson AT. Bronchial neoplasm with myasthenia: prolonged apnea after administration of succinylcholine. *Lancet* 1953;2:1291–1293.

189. Lambert EH, Eaton LM, Rooke ED. Defect of neuromuscular conduction associated with malignant neoplasms. *Am J Physiol* 1956;187: 612–613.

190. Eaton LM, Lambert EH. Electromyography and electric stimulation of nerve in diseases with motor units: observations on myasthenic syndrome associated with malignant tumors. *JAMA* 1957;163:1117.

191. Elmqvist D, Lambert EH. Detailed analysis of neuromuscular transmission in a patient with the myasthenic syndrome sometimes associated with bronchogenic carcinoma. *Mayo Clin Proc* 1968;43:689–713.

192. O'Neill JH, Murray NMF, Newsom-Davis J. The Lambert-Eaton myasthenic syndrome: a review of 50 cases. *Brain* 1988;111:577–596.

193. Lang B, Newsom-Davis J, Wray D, et al. Autoimmune etiology for myasthenic (Eaton-Lambert) syndrome. *Lancet* 1981;2:224–226.

194. Fukunga H, Engel AG, Osame M, et al. Paucity and disorganization of presynaptic membrane active zones in the Lambert-Eaton myasthenic syndrome. *Muscle Nerve* 1982;5:686–697.

195. Kim YI, Neher E. IgG from patients with Lambert-Eaton syndrome blocks voltage-dependent calcium channels. *Science* 1988;239: 405–408.

196. Lang B, Vincent A, Murray NMF, et al. Lambert-Eaton myasthenic syndrome: immunoglobulin G inhibition of Ca2+ flux in tumor cells correlates with disease severity. *Ann Neurol* 1989;25:265–271.

197. Sher E, Gotti C, Canal N, et al. Specificity of calcium channel autoantibodies in Lambert-Eaton myasthenic syndrome. *Lancet* 1989;2: 640–643.

198. Lang B, Vincent A, Murray NMF, et al. Lambert-Eaton myasthenic syndrome: immunoglobulin G inhibition of Ca++ flux in tumor cells correlates with disease severity. *Ann Neurol* 1989;25:265–271.

199. Lennon VA, Lambert EH. Autoantibodies bind solubilized calcium-channel-ω-conotoxin complexes from small cell lung carcinoma: a diagnostic aid for Lambert-Eaton myasthenic syndrome. *Mayo Clin Proc* 1989;64:1498–1504.

200. Leys K, Lang B, Johnston I, et al. Calcium channel autoantibodies in the Lambert-Eaton myasthenic syndrome. *Ann Neurol* 1991;29: 307–314.

201. Tim RW, Sanders DB. Repetitive nerve stimulation studies in the Lambert-Eaton myasthenic syndrome. *Muscle Nerve* 1994;17:995–1001.

202. Oh SJ. Diverse electrophysiological spectrum of the Lambert-Eaton myasthenic syndrome. *Muscle Nerve* 1989;12:464–469.

203. Lennon VA. Serologic profile of myasthenia gravis and destruction from the Lambert-Eaton myasthenic syndrome. *Neurology* 1997;48 [Suppl 5]:S23–S27.

204. Lennon VA, Kryzer TJ, Grieswann GE, et al. Calcium channel antibodies in Lambert-Eaton myasthenic syndrome and other paraneoplastic syndromes. *N Engl J Med* 1995;332:1467–1474.

205. Motomura M, Lang B, Johnston I, et al. Incidence of serum anti-P/Q type and anti-N-type calcium channel autoantibodies in the Lambert-Eaton myasthenic syndrome. *J Neurol Sci* 1997;147:35–42.

206. Katz JS, Wolfe GI, Bryan WW, et al. Acetylcholine receptor antibodies in the Lambert-Eaton myasthenic syndrome. *Neurology* 1998;50: 470–475.

207. Jenkyn LR, Brooks PL, Forcier RJ, et al. Remission of the Lambert-Eaton syndrome and small cell anaplastic carcinoma of the lung induced by chemotherapy and radiotherapy. *Cancer* 1980;46:1123–1127.

208. Newsom-Davis J, Murray NMF. Plasma exchange and immunosuppressive drug treatment in the Lambert-Eaton myasthenic syndrome. *Neurology* 1984;34:480–485.

209. Jenkyn LR, Brooks PL, Forcier RJ, et al. Remission of the Lambert-Eaton syndrome and small cell anaplastic carcinoma of the lung induced by chemotherapy and radiotherapy. *Cancer* 1980;46: 1123–1127.

210. Cherington M. Guanidine and germine in Lambert-Eaton syndrome. *Neurology* 1976;26:944–946.

211. Oh SJ, Kim DS, Head TC, et al. Low-dose guanidine and pyridostigmine: relatively safe and effective long-term symptomatic therapy in Lambert-Eaton myasthenic syndrome. *Muscle Nerve* 1997;20: 1146–1152.

212. McEvoy KM, Windebank AJ, Daube JR, et al. 3,4-Diaminopyridine in the treatment of Lambert-Eaton myasthenic syndrome. *N Engl J Med* 1989;321:1567–1571.

213. Sanders DB, Howard JF Jr, Massey JM. 3,4-Diaminopyridine in Lambet-Eaton myasthenic syndrome and myasthenia gravis. *Ann N Y Acad Sci* 1993;681:588–590.

214. Saperstein DS, Herbelin L, Bryan WW, et al. 3,4-Diaminopyridine in the treatment of Lambert-Eaton myasthenic syndrome. *J Child Neurol* 1998;13:134–135.

215. Newsom-Davis J, Murray NMF. Plasma exchange and immunosuppressive drug treatment in the Lambert-Eaton myasthenic syndrome. *Neurology* 1984;34:480–485.

216. Bird SJ. Clinical and electrophysiologic improvement in Lambert-Eaton syndrome with intravenous immunoglobulin therapy. *Neurology* 1992;42:1422–1423.

217. Rich MM, Teener JW, Bird SJ. Treatment of Lambert-Eaton syndrome with intravenous immunoglobulin. *Muscle Nerve* 1997;20:614–615.

218. Poser CH, Paty DW, Scheinberg L, et al. New diagnostic criteria for multiple sclerosis: guidelines for research protocols. *Ann Neurol* 1983;13:227–231.

219. Weinshenker BG. Natural history of multiple sclerosis. *Ann Neurol* 1994;36:56–511.

220. Weinshenker BG, Bass B, Rice GPA, et al. The natural history of multiple sclerosis: a geographically-based study. I. Clinical course and disability. *Brain* 1989;112:133–146.

221. McAlpine D, Compston ND, Acheson ED. *Multiple sclerosis: a reappraisal,* 2nd ed. London: Churchill Livingstone, 1972:214.

222. Ebers GC, Sadovnick AD. The role of genetic factors in multiple sclerosis susceptibility. *J Neuroimmunol* 1994;54:1–17.

223. Ebers GC. Genetics and multiple sclerosis: an overview. *Ann Neurol* 1994;36:S12–S14.

224. Hillert J. Human leukocyte antigen studies in multiple sclerosis. *Ann Neurol* 1994;36:S15–S17.

225. Kurtzke JF, Kurland LT. The epidemiology of neurologic disease. In: Baker AB, ed. *Clinical neurology.* Philadelphia: Harper & Row, 1983:1–143.

226. Sibley WA, Bamford CR, Clark K. Triggering factors in multiple sclerosis. In: Poser CM, Paty DW, Scheinberg L, et al., eds. *The diagnosis of multiple sclerosis.* New York: Thieme-Stratton, 1984:14–24.

227. Sibley WA, Bamford CR, Clark K. Clinical viral infections and multiple sclerosis. *Lancet* 1985;1:1313–1315.

228. Panitch HS. Influence of infection on exacerbations of multiple sclerosis. *Ann Neurol* 1994;36:S25–S28.

229. Confavreux C, Hutchinson M, Hours MM, et al. Rate of pregnancy-related relapse in multiple sclerosis. Pregnancy in Multiple Sclerosis Group. *N Engl J Med* 1998;339:285–291.

230. Weinshenker BG, Rice GPA, Noseworthy JH, et al. The natural history of multiple sclerosis: a geographically based study. 3. Multivariate analysis of predictive factors and models of outcome. *Brain* 1991;114:1045–1056.

231. Lassmann H, Suchanek G, Ozawa K. Histopathology and the blood-cerebrospinal fluid barrier in multiple sclerosis. *Ann Neurol* 1994; 36:S42–S46.

232. Prineas JW. The neuropathology of multiple sclerosis. In: Koetsier JC, ed. *Handbook of clinical neurology,* vol 47: demyelinating diseases. Amsterdam: Elsevier, 1985:213–257.

233. Wekerle H. Experimental autoimmune encephalomyelitis as a model for immune mediated CNS disease. *Curr Opin Neurobiol* 1993;3:779–784.

234. Raine CS. The immunology of the multiple sclerosis lesion. *Ann Neurol* 1994;36:561–572.

235. Traugott U. On the immunopathology of multiple sclerosis lesions. *Ital J Neurol Sci* 1992;13(9 Suppl 2):37–45.

236. McFarland HF. Immunology of multiple sclerosis. *Ann N Y Acad Sci* 1988;540:99–105.

237. Panitch HS, Haley AS, Hirsh RL, et al. Exacerbation of MS in patients treated with gamma IFN. *Lancet* 1987;1:893–895.

238. Mosmann TR, Hesland J-M, Guilbert LJ. Cytokines and functions of T-helper cell subsets. In: Romagnani S, Mosmann TR, Abbas AK, eds. *New advances of cytokines.* New York: Raven, 1992;69–76.

239. Hauser SL, Doolittle TH, Lincoln R, et al. Cytokine accumulations in CSF of MS patients: frequent detection of IL-1 and TNF but not IL-6. *Neurology* 1990;40:1735–1739.

240. Beck J, Rondot P, Catinot L, et al. Increased production of interferon gamma and tumor necrosis factor proceeds clinical manifestations in multiple sclerosis: do cytokines trigger off exacerbations? *Acta Neurol Scand* 1988;78:318–323.

241. Rudick RA, Ransohoff RM. Cytokine secretion by multiple sclerosis monocytes: relationship to disease activity. *Arch Neurol* 1992;49:265–270.

242. Hafler DA, Weiner HL. T cells in multiple sclerosis and inflammatory central nervous system diseases. *Immunol Rev* 1987;100:307–332.

243. Arnason BGW, Antel JP. Suppressor cell function in multiple sclerosis. *Ann Immunol* (Paris) 1978;129C:159–170.

244. Bruck W, Schmied M, Suchanek G, et al. Oligodendrocytes in the early course of multiple sclerosis. *Ann Neurol* 1994;35:65–73.

245. Knight JA. Advances in the analysis of cerebrospinal fluid. *Ann Clin Lab Sci* 1997;27:93–104.

246. Walsh MJ, Tourtellotte WW. The cerebrospinal fluid in multiple sclerosis. In: Hallpike JF, Adams CWM, Tourtellotte WW, eds. *Multiple sclerosis.* Baltimore: Williams & Wilkins, 1983:275–358.

247. Kostulas V, Link H, Lefvert AK. Oligoclonal IgG bands in cerebrospinal fluid principles for demonstration and interpretation based on findings in 1114 neurological patients. *Arch Neurol* 1987;44:1041–1044.

248. McLean BN, Luxton RW, Thompson EJ. A study of immunoglobulin G in the cerebrospinal fluid of 1007 patients with suspected neurological disease using isoelectric focusing and the log IgG index. *Brain* 1990;113:1269–1289.

249. Fredrikson S. CSF-Abnormalities and MS diagnosis. *International MS Journal* 1994;1:69–71.

250. Ormerod IEC, Miller DH, McDonald WI, et al. The role of MRI in the assessment of MS and isolated neurological lesions: a quantitative study. *Brain* 1987;110:1579–1616.

251. Filippi M, Horsfield MA, Hajnal JV, et al. Quantitative assessment of magnetic resonance imaging lesion load in multiple sclerosis. 1998:1:88–93.

252. Isaac C, Li DKB, Genton M, et al. Multiple sclerosis: a serial study using MRI in relapsing patients. *Neurology* 1988;38:1511–1515.

253. Willoughby EW, Grochowski, Li DKB, et al. Serial MR scanning in patients with MS: a second prospective study in relapsing patients. *Ann Neurol* 1989;25:43–49.

254. Truyen L, Gheuhens J, Parizel PM, et al. Long term follow-up of MS by standardized, non-contrast-enhanced MRI. *J Neurol Sci* 1991;106:35–40.

255. Riahi F, Zijdenbos A, Narayanan S, et al. Improved correlation between scores on the expanded disability status scale and cerebral lesion load in relapsing-remitting multiple sclerosis: results of the application of new imaging methods. *Brain* 1998;121[Pt 7]:1305–1312.

256. Hawkins CP, Munro PMG, Landon DN, et al. Duration and selectivity of blood-brain barrier breakdown in chronic relapsing experimental allergic encephalomyelitis. *Brain* 1990;113:365–378.

257. Katz D, Taubenberger JK, Cannella B, et al. Correlation between MRI and lesion development in chronic active MS. *Ann Neurol* 1993;34:661–669.

258. McFarland HF, Frank JA, Albert PS, et al. Using gadolinium-enhanced magnetic resonance imaging lesions to monitor disease activity in multiple sclerosis. *Ann Neurol* 1992;32:758–766.

259. Filippi M, Horsfield MA, Morrissey SP, et al. Quantitative brain MRI lesion load predicts the course of clinically isolated syndromes suggestive of multiple sclerosis. *Neurology* 1994;44:635–641.

260. Morrissey SP, Miller DH, Kendall BE, et al. The significance of brain MRI abnormalities at presentation with clinically isolated syndromes suggestive of MS. *Brain* 1993;116:135–146.

261. Lee KH, Hashimoto SA, Hooge JP, et al. MR imaging of the head in the diagnosis of MS: A prospective 2-year follow-up with comparison of clinical evaluation, evoked potentials, oligoclonal banding, and CT. *Neurology* 1991;41:657–660.

262. Khoury SJ, Guttmann CRG, Orav EJ, et al. Longitudinal MRI in multiple sclerosis: correlation between disability and lesion burden. *Neurology* 1994;44:2120–2124.

263. Paty DW, Li DKB, the UBC MS/MRI Study Group, and the IFNB Multiple Sclerosis Study Group. Interferon beta-1b is effective in relapsing-remitting multiple sclerosis. II. MRI analysis results of a multicenter, randomized, double-blind, placebo-controlled trial. *Neurology* 1993;43:662–667.

264. Wiebe S, Lee DH, Kzrlik SJ, et al. Serial cranial and spinal cord magnetic resonance imaging in multiple sclerosis. *Ann Neurol* 1992;32:643–650.

265. Paty OW, Li DKB, the UBC MS/MRI Study Group, and the IFNB Multiple Sclerosis Study Group. Interferon beta 1-b is effective in relapsing-remitting multiple sclerosis. *Neurology* 1993;43:662–667.

266. Li DKB, Mayo J, Fache S, et al. Lack of correlation between clinical manifestations and lesions of MS as seen by NMR. *Neurology* 1984;34[Suppl 1]:136.

267. Miller DH. Magnetic resonance in monitoring the treatment of multiple sclerosis. *Ann Neurol* 1994;36:S91–S94.

268. Barnes D, Munro PMG, Youl BD. The longstanding MS lesion: a quantitative MRI and electron microscopic study. *Brain* 1991;114:1271–1280.

269. Dousset V, Grossman RI, Ramer KN, et al. Experimental allergic encephalomyelitis and MS: lesion characterization with magnetization transfer imaging. *Radiology* 1992;182:483–491.

270. Grossman RI. Magnetization transfer in multiple sclerosis. *Ann Neurol* 1994;36:S97–S99.

271. Davie CA, Hawkins CP, Barker GJ, et al. Serial proton MR spectroscopy in acute MS. *Brain* 1994;117:49–58.

272. Arnold DL, Riess GT, Matthews PM, et al. Use of proton magnetic resonance spectroscopy for monitoring disease progression in multiple sclerosis. *Ann Neurol* 1994;36:76–82.

273. Trapp BD, Peterson J, Ransohoff RM, et al. Axonal transection in the lesions of multiple sclerosis. *N Engl J Med* 1998;338:278–285.

274. Troiano R, Cook SC, Dowling PC. Steroid therapy in multiple sclerosis: point of view. *Arch Neurol* 1987;44:803–807.

275. Beck RW, Cleary PA, Trobe JD, et al. The effect of corticosteroid for acute optic neuritis on the subsequent development of multiple sclerosis. *N Engl J Med* 1993;329:1764–1769.

276. Whitaker JN. Rationale for immunotherapy in multiple sclerosis. *Ann Neurol* 1994;36:S103–S107.

277. Goodkin DE, Rudick RA, VanderBrug Medendorp S, et al. Low dose (7.5 mg) oral methotrexate reduces the rate of progression multiple sclerosis. *Ann Neurol* 1995;37:30–40.

278. Steinman L. The development of rational strategies for selective immunotherapy against autoimmune demyelinating disease. *Adv Immunol* 1991;49:357–379.

279. Bashir K, Whitaker JN. Current immunotherapy in multiple sclerosis. *Immunol Cell Biol* 1998;76:55–64.

280. Rodriguez M, Lennon VA. Immunoglobulins promote remyelination in the central nervous system. *Ann Neurol* 1990;27:12–17.

281. Interferon-beta Multiple Sclerosis Study Group. Interferon beta-1b is effective in relapsing-remitting multiple sclerosis. I. Clinical results of a multicenter, randomized, double-blind, placebo-controlled trial. *Neurology* 1993;43:655–661.

282. Jacobs L, Cookfair D, Rudick R, et al., and the Multiple Sclerosis Collaborative Research Group. Results of a phase III trial of intramuscular beta interferon as treatment for multiple sclerosis. *Ann Neurol* 1994;36:259.

283. Bornstein MB, Miller A, Teitelbaum D, et al. Multiple sclerosis: trial of a synthetic polypeptide. *Ann Neurol* 1982;11:317–319.

284. Yong VW, Chabot S, Stuve O, et al. Interferon beta in the treatment of multiple sclerosis. *Neurology* 1998;51:682–689.

285. IFNB Multiple Sclerosis Study Group, University of British Columbia MS/MRI Analysis Group. Interferon beta-1b in the treatment of multiple sclerosis: final outcome of the randomized controlled trial. *Neurology* 1995;37:611–619.

286. Jacobs LD, Cookfair DL, Rudick RA, et al. Intramuscular interferon beta-1a for disease progression in relapsing multiple sclerosis. *Ann Neurol* 1996;39:285–294.

287. Webb C, Teitelbaum D, Arnon R, et al. IN vivo and in vitro immunological cross-reactions between basic encephalitogen and synthetic basic polypeptides capable of suppressing experimental allergic encephalomyelitis. *Eur J Immunol* 1973;3:279–286.

288. Bornstein MB, Miler A, Slagle S, et al. A placebo-controlled, double-blind, randomized, two-center, pilot trial of Cp 1 in chronic progressive multiple sclerosis. *Neurology* 1991;41:533–539.

289. Johnson KP, Brooks BR, Cohen JA, et al. Copolymer 1 reduces relapse rate and improves disability in relapsing-remitting multiple sclerosis: results of a phase III multicenter, double-blind, placebo-controlled trial. *Neurology* 1995;45:1268–1276.

290. Johnson KP, Brooks BR, Cohen JA, et al. Extended use of glatiramer acetate (Copaxone) is well tolerated and maintains its clinical effect on multiple sclerosis relapse rate and degree of disability. *Neurology* 1998;50:701–708.

291. Neilley LK, Goodin DS, Goodkin DE, et al. Side effect profile of interferon beta-1b in MS: results of an open label trial. *Neurology* 1996; 46:552–554.

292. IFNB Multiple Sclerosis Study Group, University of British Columbia MS/MRI Analysis Group. Neutralizing antibodies during treatment of multiple sclerosis with interferon beta-1b: experience during the first three years. *Neurology* 1996;47:889–894.

293. Al Deeb SM, Yaqub BA, Bruyn GW, et al. Acute transverse myelitis: a localized form of postinfectious encephalomyelitis. *Brain* 1997;120 [Pt 7]:1115–1122.

294. Pradhan S, Gupta RK, Ghost D. Parainfectious myelitis: three distinct clinico-imagiological patterns with prognostic implications. *Acta Neurol Scand* 1997;95:241–247.

295. Chan KF, Boey ML. Transverse myelopathy in SLE: clinical features and functional outcomes. *Lupus* 1996;5:294–299.

296. Sebire G, Hollenberg H, Meyer L, et al. High dose methylprednisolone in severe acute transverse myelopathy. *Arch Dis Child* 1997;76: 167–168.

297. Mok CC, Lau CS, Chan EY, et al. Acute transverse myelopathy in systemic lupus erythematosus: clinical presentation, treatment, and outcome. *J Rheumatol* 1998;25:467–473.

298. Optic Neuritis Study Group. The clinical profile of acute optic neuritis: experience of the Optic Neuritis Treatment Trial. *Arch Ophthalmol* 1991;109:1673–1678.

299. Brain WR. Some varieties of acute optic and retrobulbar neuritis. *Trans Ophthalmol Soc UK* 1934;54:221–232.

300. O'Sullivan EP, Kennard C. Ocular manifestations of neurological disease. *Curr Opin Neurol* 1998;11:25–29.

301. Anonymous. The 5-year risk of MS after optic neuritis: experience of the optic neuritis treatment trial. Optic Neuritis Study Group. *Neurology* 1997;49:1404–1413.

302. Sandberg-Wollheim M, Bynke H, Cronqvist S, et al. A long-term prospective study of optic neuritis: evaluation of risk factors. *Ann Neurol* 1990;27:386–393.

303. Rizzo JF, Lessell S. Risk of developing multiple sclerosis after uncomplicated optic neuritis: a long-term prospective study. *Neurology* 1988;38:185–190.

304. Tumani H, Tourtellotte WW, Peter JB, et al. Acute optic neuritis: combined immunological markers and magnetic resonance imaging predict subsequent development of multiple sclerosis. The Optic Neuritis Study Group. *J Neurol Sci* 1998;155:44–49.

305. Beck RW, Cleary PA, Trobe JD, et al. The effect of corticosteroids for acute optic neuritis on the subsequent development of multiple sclerosis. *N Engl J Med* 1993;329:1764–1769.

306. Lucchinetti CF, Kiers L, O'Duffy A, et al. Risk factors for developing multiple sclerosis after childhood optic neuritis. *Neurology* 1997;49: 1413–1418.

307. Cleary PA, Beck RW, Anderson MM, et al. Design, methods and conduct of the Optic Neuritis Treatment Trial. *Control Clin Trials* 1993;14:123–142.

308. Whitham RH, Brey RL. Neuromyelitis optica: two new cases and review of the literature. *J Clin Neuro-ophthalmol* 1985;5:263–269.

309. Balser BH. Neuromyelitis optica. *Brain* 1936;59:353–365.

310. Hassin GB. Neuropticmyelitis versus multiple sclerosis: a pathologic study. *Arch Neurol Psychiatr* 1937;37:1083–1099.

311. Kohut H, Richter RB. Neuro-optic myelitis: a clinicopathological study of two related cases. *J Nerv Ment Dis* 1945;101:99–114.

312. Jeffery AR, Buncic JR. Pediatric Devic's neuromyelitis optica. *J Pediatr Ophthalmol Strabismus* 1996;33:223–229.

313. O'Riordan JI, Gallagher HL, Thompson AJ, et al. Clinical, CSF, and MRI findings in Devic's neuromyelitis optica. *J Neurol Neurosurg Psychiatry* 1996;60:382–387.

*Textbook of the Autoimmune Diseases,*
Edited by R. G. Lahita, N. Chiorazzi, and W. H. Reeves,
Lippincott Williams & Wilkins, Philadelphia © 2000.

# CHAPTER 20

# Autoimmune Endocrine Disorders

Kevan C. Herold and David H. Sarne

## AUTOIMMUNE DISEASE OF THE PITUITARY GLAND: HYPOPHYSITIS

### Description

Lymphocytic hypophysitis is thought to represent autoimmune destruction of the pituitary. The disorder is uncommon, and its true incidence and prevalence are unknown. There is a markedly higher rate of occurrence in women; only 10% to 20% of cases have been reported in men (1). Unlike autoimmune disease of most other endocrine glands, the diagnosis has usually depended on biopsy or surgical specimens and has often only been made at autopsy. Many reported cases have appeared as isolated case reports, and original series are generally small and accumulated over a number of years (1).

The pathologic findings are those of an inflammatory process with infiltration of lymphocytes and plasma cells (1,2). Infiltration with neutrophils, eosinophils, and macrophages may also be noted. These are associated with focal or diffuse areas of destruction. Although changes may be limited to the anterior pituitary, stalk and posterior pituitary involvement may also occur. Immunocytochemistry may indicate the isolated absence of corticotrophs (1). Unlike studies in other autoimmune endocrine disorders, investigators have not identified expression of major histocompatibility complex (MHC) class II antigens on the pituitary stalks from patients with lymphocytic hypophysitis.

### Mechanisms of Disease

Cases of lymphocytic hypophysitis are usually isolated, without a family history of the disorder. Individual patients have been noted to have HLA-B8, HLA-DR4, or HLA-DR5 anti-

gens, but a clear association between these markers and susceptibility to the disease has not been shown (1).

Although the autoimmune nature of the disease has been suspected since it was first described, the mechanisms of disease and the specific antigens involved have remained unclear. Most studies have focused on the role of autoantibodies in the disease. Injections of human pituitary homogenates with Freund's adjuvant has produced diffuse mononuclear infiltration of the pituitary in mice and rabbits (3). Of note, the disease in rats was more pronounced in pregnant and lactating female rats (4).

Older studies have described the presence of antipituitary antibodies detected by immunofluorescence in only a few patients (5). The association with pregnancy has been explained by the presence of antibodies to lactotropes, but in a study in which these antibodies were found in 19 of 297 patients with autoimmune disease, none of the positive patients had pituitary disease (6). An antibody to a corticotroph antigen has been described in a patient with isolated adrenocorticotropic hormone (ACTH) deficiency (7). In Japanese patients with isolated ACTH deficiency, 70% have been found to have an antibody reacting to an antigen expressed on a pituitary cell line, AtT20 (8).

One study using immunoblotting showed autoantibodies reactive with 49-kd cytosolic extracts from human autopsy pituitary tissue in 70% of patients with biopsy-proven lymphocytic hypophysitis and in 50% of patients with clinically suspected lymphocytic hypophysitis (9). Reactivity was found to extracts of a similar weight from a number of other tissues but not skeletal muscle. Pro-opiomelanocortin (POMC), the precursor of ACTH, is processed in many tissues, except muscle; thus, the lack of tissue specificity does not preclude the relevance of this antigen. Of note, a positive response was also found in 42% of patients with Addison's disease but in only 14% of patients with thyroid autoimmune disease (9). It is not known whether the response in patients with Addison's is to a different antigen of similar molecular weight or to the same antigen.

K. C. Herold: Department of Medicine, Columbia University, College of Physicians and Surgeons, New York, New York 10032; Columbia Presbyterian Medical Center, New York, New York 10032.

D. H. Sarne: Department of Medicine, University of Illinois at Chicago, Chicago, Illinois 60612; Department of Medicine, University of Illinois at Chicago Medical Center, Chicago, Illinois 60612.

## Presentation and Diagnosis

Hypophysitis most commonly occurs in women in late pregnancy or in the postpartum period. The symptoms at presentation are usually those of a pituitary mass lesion with headache and visual field abnormalities. In other cases, there may be no manifestations of a mass, and patients may present with only symptoms of hormonal insufficiency. Deficiencies of anterior pituitary hormones usually predominate, with ACTH deficiency being most common (60% to 70% of patients) (1,2,9). Patients less commonly have stalk or posterior pituitary involvement presenting as diabetes insipidus (15% to 20% of patients) (1,2,9). Hypophysitis has recurred spontaneously, but in other patients, it has not recurred, even with subsequent pregnancies (1).

In the acute disorder, the lesion cannot be distinguished from a pituitary neoplasm by computed tomography or magnetic resonance imaging. In many cases, pituitary tumors have been suspected, and only examination of the surgical specimen has confirmed the actual diagnosis (1,2,9). The differential diagnosis also includes other inflammatory and infiltrating conditions, including sarcoidosis, eosinophilic granuloma, tuberculosis, granulomatous hypophysitis, and syphilis. In the past, many cases were correctly diagnosed only at autopsy because, late in the disease, the pituitary may atrophy. Many patients diagnosed in the past with Sheehan's syndrome likely actually had lymphocytic hypophysitis. After resolution, patients may be left with a partial or empty sella (1,9).

Prolactin levels may be either low or high, and prolactin elevation is especially common in cases associated with pregnancy when prolactin levels are normally elevated. Patients with low prolactin levels secondary to pituitary destruction may present with failure to lactate. In cases not associated with pregnancy, prolactin elevation may be secondary to interference with dopaminergic inhibition or the direct release of prolactin from injured lactotropes.

## Approach to the Patient

The diagnosis should be suspected in women presenting with symptoms suggestive of a mass lesion in late pregnancy or the postpartum period or in patients with similar symptoms and other autoimmune endocrine disorders. Given the inability to exclude the presence of a neoplasm, it remains controversial whether a biopsy or surgical procedure is always warranted to confirm the diagnosis. Certainly, in women presenting in late pregnancy or the early postpartum period, close observation or an empiric trial of glucocorticoid therapy may be warranted.

Patients may recover normal endocrine function or be left with single or multiple hormonal deficiencies (1,2,9). Isolated ACTH deficiency is the most common single deficiency, but patients have been reported with isolated thyroid-stimulating hormone (TSH) deficiency and selective loss of gonadotropins (1,2,9).

Patients with this disorder frequently (20% to 25%) have been found to have other autoimmune disorders as well. Disorders specifically associated have included autoimmune thyroid disease (both hypothyroidism and Graves' disease), adrenalitis, atrophic gastritis, and parathyroiditis (1,9).

## Treatment

Therapy in these patients may be directed at different aspects of this disorder, relieving the mass effect, treating the underlying disorder, or managing pituitary hypofunction. Because most deaths with this disorder have been attributed to untreated adrenal insufficiency, glucocorticoid replacement using stress doses is essential in the acute setting. The roles of the two major primary therapies, glucocorticoids and surgery, remain unclear in the acute setting. Some reviews have suggested that glucocorticoids are not effective in treating the mass effect or the underlying disorder, whereas other reports indicate a marked beneficial response with glucocorticoids (1,2,9). Some series that suggested glucocorticoids are ineffective have included patients who were receiving only replacement steroids. Some series have excluded patients without surgical confirmation of the diagnosis, making interpretation of the efficacy of medical therapy only problematic. In patients treated surgically, improvements have occurred with a significant delay after the surgery and may actually be related to spontaneous resolution rather than the surgery itself. In some patients, the surgery itself may lead to destruction or removal of the normal pituitary and the development of hypopituitarism. Bromocriptine has been used in some patients, but its benefits apart from reducing elevated prolactin levels are not clear (1,2). Reports of patients treated with radiation therapy are extremely rare, and its benefit remains unproved.

Long-term treatment is directed at hormonal therapy, usually with glucocorticoid replacement for ACTH deficiency and thyroid hormone for TSH deficiency (dosages are discussed later). Cyclic estrogen or testosterone is also replaced unless fertility is desired, in which case gonadotropin therapy is required. Permanent diabetes insipidus is usually treated with 1-deamino(8-D-arginine) vasopressin (DDAVP). Because resolution of some or all of the deficient hormones is not uncommon, patients initially begun on treatment should be tested later to avoid unnecessary treatment. In addition, coexisting primary autoimmune disorders may also necessitate hormone replacement therapy.

## AUTOIMMUNE THYROID DISEASES

The thyroid is the most common site of autoimmune endocrine disease. The three major clinical entities are Graves' disease, chronic autoimmune thyroiditis (Hashimoto's thyroiditis), and painless thyroiditis. Although these are discussed as distinct disorders, affected patients may manifest overlapping clinical features, share immunologic and pathologic abnormalities, and have family members with a different form of immune thyroid disease. Other, less common thyroid disorders with an immune basis include transient hypothyroidism secondary to blocking antibodies, subacute thyroiditis (de Quervain's disease), and hypothyroidism secondary to hypophysitis (see earlier).

## Graves' Disease

### Description and Prevalence

Graves' disease is the most common cause of thyrotoxicosis between the ages of 20 and 50 years. In women, reports of the annual incidence range from 15 to 80 per 100,000 per year, with a rate as high as 200 per 100,000 in Japan (10–12). Survey data from the Wickham study indicate a prevalence of about 3% (11). Incidence and prevalence rates in men are about one tenth those in women. It is more frequently found in regions of iodine sufficiency where toxic nodular disease is less common (10,13).

Pathologic findings within the thyroid gland in this disorder include lymphocytic infiltration of the thyroid in addition to follicular cell hyperplasia (14). Most of the lymphocytes are T cells (15). Aggregates of B cells forming germinal centers may also be found within affected glands.

### Mechanisms of Disease

#### Genetic Factors

A genetic predilection has long been recognized, reflected by an increased incidence in family members and increased concordance rates for monozygotic twins (7%) (16,17). Multiple associations with Graves' disease and MHC class I and class II HLA alleles have been reported; HLA-B8 was among the first associations with the disease (18,19). The MHC region of human chromosome 6 encodes the DP, DQ, and DR antigens as well as other immune modifiers, including tumor necrosis factor-α (TNF-α), and complement proteins. Both the HLA-DR and HLA-DQ loci encode heterodimers made up of an α and β chain, which bind peptides for presentation to CD4+ T cells. The MHC class II alleles are polymorphic; the regions of polymorphism are found in the outer domains of the molecules. The three-dimensional configuration and other properties of the MHC molecules may alter T-cell repertoire development, tolerance to autoantigens, and responses to tissue antigens by virtue of their ability to bind and present peptides.

The strongest association in whites is with DR3, but of note, up to half of patients lack this marker (16,19). HLA-DQA1*0501 (20,21) has been found to be independently associated in some studies, whereas in others, this apparent linkage has been found to be the result of linkage disequilibrium with DR3 (19). Different results have been found in other ethnic groups, and inconsistencies have been noted for all. Although some reports have suggested an association with cytotoxic T-lymphocyte antigen 4 (CTLA-4) polymorphisms on chromosome 2q33 (22), this has not been confirmed in other studies (23). One study of more than 300 subjects from 48 families with 142 affected patients failed to establish linkage with autoimmune thyroid disease for any of the candidate genes, CTLA-4, T-cell–receptor V genes (14q11 and 7q35), or the immunoglobulin gene complex on 15q11 (24).

### Humoral Immunity

Thyroid-stimulating immunoglobulin (TSI) is the direct cause of the hyperthyroidism and goiter formation in patients with Graves' disease. These antibodies were first detected in an animal model as a long-acting thyroid stimulator distinct from TSH in the serum of some patients with Graves' disease (10). Later work proved that these were immunoglobulin G (IgG) directed against the TSH receptor (10). Studies using recombinant receptor showed that most of these antibodies are directed against the extracellular domains but that some are directed against the transmembrane portions of the receptor (25–27).

Antibody binding to the receptor increases cyclic adenosine monophosphate production and iodine uptake and stimulates cell growth (10,28). These antibodies are detected in bioassays in up to 95% of patients presenting with Graves' disease (10) (Table 20.1). The failure to find such antibodies in the serum of all affected may be a result of local production of immunoglobulins. Both the IgG subclass and the light-chain component of the antibody may be restricted, suggesting that the immunoglobulin responses are of limited heterogeneity (34,35). These antibodies also compete with TSH for its receptor and may be detected in assays of TSH-binding inhibition (TSH-binding inhibitory immunoglobulin) (10).

During treatment with antithyroid drugs or after thyroid surgery, antibody titers frequently fall (10,36). The persistence of antibodies in patients receiving medical therapy is associated with a greater likelihood of relapse (36). In addition, transplacental passage of high levels of stimulating antibodies may cause transient disease in the fetus or newborn (37).

TSH-receptor–blocking antibodies also compete with TSH for binding to the TSH receptor but do not stimulate its activation. Such antibodies also occur in some patients with Graves' disease, and patients may have both forms circulating simultaneously (10,37). In some cases, they may result in transient hypothyroidism alternating with thyrotoxicosis. Such fluctuations have also been observed in a few children with neonatal Graves' disease (37).

**TABLE 20.1.** *Autoantigens identified in human autoimmune thyroid diseases*

| Antigen | Reference No. |
|---|---|
| Heat shock protein | 29 |
| Flavoprotein subunit of mitochondrial succinate dehydrogenase (formerly unidentified 64-kd protein) | 30 |
| Sodium iodide transporter | 31 |
| Thyroglobulin | 32 |
| Thyroid peroxidase (formerly microsomal antigen) | 33 |
| Thyroid-stimulating hormone receptor | 33 |

Antithyroid peroxidase (TPO, formerly antimicrosomal antibody) and anti-Tg antibodies are also frequently observed in patients with Graves' disease. In contrast to the TSH-receptor antibodies, these tend to be polyclonal in origin (38). They are thought to be markers for autoimmune thyroid disease but not to be pathogenic (10). Antibodies to the sodium iodide symporter have also been detected in patients with Graves' disease (31,39,40). At this time, their role in the pathogenesis of the disease is uncertain.

### Cellular Immunity

Lymphadenopathy, splenomegaly, and hyperplasia of the thymus have been noted in patients with active disease. Activated T cells are found within both the thyroid and circulating in blood of Graves' disease patients. These include cells reactive with both thyroid antigens and other antigens (41). Within the thyroid, CD4$^+$ T cells predominate, whereas peripheral levels of CD8$^+$ T cells are reduced (42). In some reports, stimulation *in vitro* of lymphocytes derived from the thyroid leads to production of cytokines in a T$_H$2 pattern (more interleukin-4 [IL-4], IL-5, and IL-10) (43), whereas others have reported a T$_H$1 pattern (increased interferon-γ [IFN-γ]) (44). Elevated levels of circulating lymphokines, including IL-1, IL-4, IL-5, IL-8, IL-10, and IFN-γ, have been reported in patients with active disease (43,45).

Unlike thyroiditis, no true animal model of Graves' disease has yet been developed. When thyroid tissue from Graves' disease patients was transplanted into scid mice, antibodies to the human TSH receptor were detectable in the mice, and thyroid hormone levels increased transiently (31). The lymphocytic infiltrates, however, tended to regress over time. Immunization with recombinant TSH receptor produced animals with antibody-mediated hyperthyroidism, but they lacked both intrathyroidal lymphocytic infiltrates and ophthalmopathy (46).

Despite advances in the measurements of the thyroid receptor antibodies and an understanding of alterations in the cellular immune system of Graves' disease patients, the mechanisms that lead to the development of this disease in genetically susceptible patients remains unknown. Proposed mechanisms of pathogenesis have included failure of immune suppression either systemically or locally within the thyroid, cross-reactivity to antigens similar to the TSH receptor (including infection with viruses or *Yersinia enterocolitica*), unregulated production of antiidiotypic antibodies, injury leading to exposure of cryptic autoantigens, and cytokine stimulation leading to expression of MHC class II molecules on thyroid epithelial cells, which could present self antigens.

The higher prevalence in women and the usual onset after the age of puberty have been attributed to a direct influence of estrogens, but the specific mechanism for this effect is not clear. An association between stressful life events and the onset of Graves' disease has frequently been noted. It has been speculated that alterations in circulating cortisol and catecholamines may alter immune responses and thus trigger the onset of the disease.

### Immunology of Graves' Ophthalmopathy and Dermopathy

Although some have argued that these are separate but closely related disorders, it is generally accepted that the ophthalmopathy (or orbitopathy) and dermopathy are manifestations of the same disorder producing goiter and hyperthyroidism. The activated immune system is thought to react to antigens identical to or highly similar to those present in the thyroid.

The retroorbital and dermal fibroblasts are the likely targets of the immune attack. Evidence has suggested that the retroorbital fibroblasts may express the TSH receptor and thus provide a target for the immune response (47–49). Some retroorbital muscles have been shown to express MHC class II antigens similar to those observed on thyroid follicular cells (50).

Locally activated lymphocytes secrete cytokines, such as IL-1α, IFN-γ, and TNF-α (51,52). These cytokines stimulate the fibroblasts to produce glycosaminoglycans, which accumulate in the extracellular matrix, producing proptosis, extraocular muscle dysfunction, and dermopathy. Cytokine stimulation of heat shock proteins, intercellular adhesion molecules (53), and MHC class II expression may also further stimulate a localized immune response.

Some reports have described antibodies in the sera of patients with ophthalmopathy that reacted with orbital tissues and, more specifically, a 64-kd protein (30). This protein has now been identified as a subunit of mitochondrial succinate dehydrogenase (30). These antibodies are found in two thirds of patients with active established ophthalmopathy, 30% of patients with stable, long-standing ophthalmopathy, 30% of Graves' disease patients without clinically evident ophthalmopathy, but less than 10% of healthy subjects. These antibodies are now thought to be nonpathogenic but rather markers for the autoimmune damage to the eye muscles.

### Presentation and Diagnosis

Typical symptoms of thyroid hormone excess include weight loss, increased appetite, weakness, fatigue, nervousness, tremor, tachycardia, palpitations, heat intolerance, sleep disturbance, and hyperdefecation (54). Women may have oligomenorrhea, and men may develop gynecomastia. Uncommon symptoms include periodic paralysis, diarrhea, and abdominal pain. Common physical findings include goiter, a hyperdynamic precordium, onycholysis, hyperreflexia, tremor, and proximal muscle weakness. Sinus tachycardia is common, whereas atrial fibrillation is found in only 10% of patients, with an increased incidence in older patients. Typical eye findings include stare, lid lag, proptosis, inflammation, and increased muscle insertions. Dermopathy (pretibial myxedema) and thyroid acropachy are much less common. Some patients may have lymphadenopathy and splenomegaly.

In elderly patients, there may be a paucity of symptoms and physical findings. Laboratory abnormalities include elevations of ferritin, sex hormone–binding globulin, and alkaline phosphatase and reduced levels of cholesterol and triglycerides. Hypercalcemia occurs in about 10% of patients.

The interaction between the TSH-receptor antibodies and the extracellular domains of the receptor stimulate thyroid growth, iodine uptake, and the formation and release of thyroid hormone. Most of the manifestations of the disease are a direct result of these elevated hormone levels. The production and secretion of TSH by the pituitary is markedly suppressed; using current assays, serum TSH levels rapidly become undetectable in most patients with thyrotoxicosis. Both serum thyroxine ($T_4$) and triiodothyronine ($T_3$) levels are usually elevated. In some patients, the total $T_4$ is normal, and an estimate of free $T_4$ is needed to confirm the diagnosis. In some patients, only $T_3$ or only free $T_3$ is elevated ($T_3$ toxicosis).

Clinically evident eye disease occurs in about one third of Graves' disease patients, but when sensitive detection methods are used, abnormalities can be found in up to 90% (55). Typically, the eye disease and thyrotoxicosis present together, but the eye disease may precede overt thyrotoxicosis or occur later (55). When the eye disease is the first manifestation (euthyroid Graves' disease), evidence of thyroid autonomy is often demonstrable. Typical manifestations include enlargement of the extraocular muscles, injection of the conjunctival vessels, chemosis, and proptosis. Less common and more troubling manifestations include extraocular muscle dysfunction producing diplopia, exposure keratitis, and compression of the optic nerve leading to alterations in color perception and acuity and to permanent loss of vision. Other manifestations of the immune process include dermopathy (usually on the anterior shin) and thyroid acropachy.

Patients with thyrotoxicosis from Graves' disease have an elevated radioactive iodine uptake, as compared with a reduced value in patients with thyroiditis or ingesting exogenous thyroid hormone. Marked enlargement of the thyroid gland is also more common with Graves' disease, as is a predominance of $T_3$. The presence of ophthalmopathy is suggestive but not diagnostic of Graves' disease. The presence of a nodular goiter may indicate thyrotoxicosis secondary to an area of autonomous production, but some patients may have Graves' disease in a preexisting nodular gland. In Graves' disease, the TSH should be extremely low or undetectable. The presence of a normal or elevated TSH in a patient with elevated hormone levels and clinical thyrotoxicosis is indicative of a TSH-secreting pituitary tumor, resistance to thyroid hormone, or antibody interference creating a spuriously elevated TSH value. Measurement of TSI is usually not necessary but may be appropriate in selected cases.

During pregnancy, active Graves' disease may improve, especially during the second and third trimesters, and then become worse postpartum (56,57). Women who were previously in remission from Graves' disease may experience recurrence postpartum (56,57). Transplacental passage of antibodies in a minority of cases leads to neonatal Graves' disease, and rarely, affected infants have evidence of Graves' disease in utero (37,56). Depending on the activity, affinity, and titers of the antibodies, infants born to mothers with Graves' disease may be thyrotoxic, hypothyroid, or both (37).

Patients with Graves' disease have an increased incidence of myasthenia gravis and vitiligo. Other immunologic disorders that occur with an increased frequency in these patients include type 1 diabetes mellitus (T1DM), Addison's disease, and premature ovarian failure.

### Treatment

The major treatment options for Graves' disease remain antithyroid drugs, radioactive iodine, and surgery. These therapy options are briefly reviewed later. Because radioactive iodine is frequently used in patients failing antithyroid drug therapy, it is ultimately the most frequently used treatment in North America. The role of surgery has been declining, but it may be optimal in selected patients. β-Blockers are frequently used to treat symptoms early in the treatment course. Short-term use of inorganic iodine or the iodine-containing oral cholecystographic agents to block hormone release rapidly may be useful in acutely ill patients but require a delay of several weeks before radioactive iodine can be used for definitive therapy.

The antithyroid drugs used in North America are propylthiouracil (PTU) and methimazole (Tapazole, MMI). Typical starting doses are 100 mg three times a day for PTU or 30 mg once a day for methimazole. These drugs prevent the synthesis of thyroid hormone by blocking the incorporation of iodine into thyroglobulin. The drugs may have an inhibitory effect on lymphocytes, especially at the higher concentrations found within the thyroid gland, but this is not thought to be their major mechanism of action. Doses are adjusted to achieve euthyroidism, and therapy is maintained for 12 to 18 months, at which time the drug is usually withdrawn to determine whether remission has been attained. The persistence of an elevated TSH-receptor antibody predicts a greater likelihood of relapse, whereas shrinkage of the gland on therapy and a disappearance of the antibody are predictive of long-term remission (36). Overall, long-term remission is achieved in only 30% to 50% of those treated with these agents. Over time, there is an increasing risk for hypothyroidism, and patients should have their TSH level checked annually.

It has been suggested that the addition of thyroid hormone to suppress the gland and reduce antigenic stimulation might enhance the efficacy of these drugs. Although the addition of thyroid hormone to an antithyroid drug regimen was reported to reduce markedly the risk for relapse in one Japanese study (58), others have been unable to reproduce this finding (59–61); hence, routine use of thyroid hormone cannot be recommended. In some patients, however, thyroid hormone is needed to prevent symptomatic hypothyroidism during treatment. Few patients are truly resistant to these drugs, and most failures to achieve control relate to not increasing the dose in a patient who is not responding or to a patient who is not taking the drugs as prescribed. Although often feared, few patients have to discontinue the drugs as a result of the uncommon occurrence of severe neutropenia (two cases per 1000 patients) or hepatotoxicity. When these occur, they usually resolve on discontinuance of the drug. Although the patterns of liver disease differ (hepatitis with PTU and cholestasis with methimazole), the substitution of one for the other after the development of neutropenia results in a rapid, severe recurrence.

Radioactive iodine ($^{131}$I) may be used as initial therapy, although in very elderly or ill patients, many prefer trying several weeks to months of antithyroid drug therapy first. Because iodine crosses the placenta and is also concentrated in milk, therapy with $^{131}$I is absolutely contraindicated during pregnancy and lactation. Some physicians prefer to administer set doses, which may range from as little as 5 mCi to as much as 18 mCi, whereas others administer a dose based on an estimate of the gland size and the radioactive iodine uptake. As a general rule, the larger the gland and the lower the dose administered, the greater the chance that the therapy will not be successful. Larger doses are also required in patients who were previously treated with antithyroid drugs. A few patients have local discomfort, but the therapy is usually well tolerated and free of immediate side effects. The major consequence of the therapy is the development of permanent hypothyroidism, which ultimately occurs in more than 90% of those treated. With larger doses, this may occur as early as 4 to 6 weeks and usually occurs within the first 6 months. With smaller doses, patients may initially appear to achieve euthyroidism, only to develop hypothyroidism some years later. All Graves' disease patients treated with $^{131}$I who do not become hypothyroid within the first year should have their TSH level measured annually.

Surgical therapy for Graves' disease is usually a subtotal thyroidectomy done under general anesthesia. Patients should first be treated medically to reduce the risk for arrhythmia during anesthesia or thyroid storm. If operation is required during pregnancy, it is preferably performed during the second trimester. Complications of recurrent laryngeal nerve injury or hypoparathyroidism should be infrequent for this condition when the procedure is performed by an experienced surgeon. The recurrence rate is about 10%, with about 30% developing permanent hypothyroidism. Some patients may only develop transient hypothyroidism initially. As with the other forms of therapy, patients who achieve euthyroidism remain at lifetime risk for hypothyroidism and need to have their TSH monitored annually.

Most patients with ophthalmopathy require no specific treatment or only local therapy with artificial tears and patching. More severe inflammatory changes, acute diplopia, or progressive ophthalmopathy may be treated with oral or intravenous steroids. Progressive ophthalmopathy with optic nerve compression requires radiotherapy or orbital decompression. Stable diplopia or problems with excessive expo-sure of the conjunctiva are treated with surgery on the extraocular muscles or eyelids, respectively.

Perhaps the greatest controversy in the treatment of Graves' disease is the relationship between the choice of therapy and the progression of ophthalmopathy. Theoretically, it is argued that the release of antigen after $^{131}$I might exacerbate the eye disease, whereas the reduced antigen load after surgery or on drug therapy would improve it. Studies implicating $^{131}$I in the progression of ophthalmopathy have generally shown only mild changes and have usually chosen a comparison group treated with steroids, which would tend to ameliorate active ophthalmopathy (62). Other objections to these studies have included a failure to consider the natural history of the eye disease and a failure to initiate therapy with thyroid hormone rapidly to prevent the development of hypothyroidism, which may itself exacerbate the eye disease (63). Other studies have shown no association between therapy and the progression of eye disease. A few investigators have argued that any remaining antigen may exacerbate the eye disease; in patients with progressive eye disease, these investigators have advocated surgical removal of the thyroid combined with radioactive iodine to ablate the thyroid, as is done after thyroid cancer surgery. There are only anecdotal reports and no published trials on the usefulness of this approach.

## Hashimoto's Thyroiditis

### Description, Incidence, and Prevalence

In women, survey data based on elevated TSH values from the Wickham study indicate an incidence of Hashimoto's thyroiditis of 3.5 per 1000 population per year and a rate for men of 0.8 per 1000 population (11). The incidence increases with age, rising to 14 per 1000 women older than 60 years of age and 9 per 1000 in men older than 60 years of age. Similar rates for women and men older than 60 years of age were found in the Framingham study, with a prevalence of 14% and 6%, respectively (64). Although some differences between reports may represent ethnic variation, studies may also differ in the criteria used for diagnosis. Like Graves' disease, autoimmune thyroiditis usually does not present until after the onset of puberty. In regions of iodine sufficiency, it is the most common cause of hypothyroidism. Focal areas of thyroiditis are found in 40% of women and 20% of men (65).

Pathologic findings in the earlier phases of the disorder include lymphocytic infiltration and fibrosis as well as follicular cell hyperplasia (14). Follicular cells with increased mitochondria (Hürthle's or oncocytic cells) are common (14). These may form aggregates, which can be confused with Hürthle cell neoplasms, except that the aggregates do not have a capsule. Aggregates of lymphocytes forming follicles are also found within affected glands. In some patients, fibrosis and cell atrophy predominate. The atrophic form of the disease may be an end point of increased destruction but has also been considered by some to be a distinct entity (66). Atrophy and hypothyroidism may also be noted in patients with TSH-blocking antibodies (67).

### Mechanisms of Disease

#### Genetic Factors

As with Graves' disease, a genetic predilection has long been recognized, with an increased incidence of both autoimmune thyroiditis and Graves' disease in family members. There is a significant but weak association with DR3 (19,68). Associations with DR4 and DR5 have also been reported (19). Different results have been reported with other ethnic groups, and the associations are not particularly robust. An increased incidence of thyroiditis has been noted in patients with the chromosomal disorders of Down syndrome (69) and gonadal dysgenesis (Turner's syndrome).

#### Humoral Immunity

Autoantibodies directed against thyroglobulin (anti-Tg) were first identified in patients with thyroiditis in the 1950s (32). Previously determined by hemagglutination assays, these are now commonly measured in either enzyme-linked immunosorbent assays (ELISA) or radioimmunoassays (RIA) (32). Anti-Tg are usually IgG that does not fix complement (39). Unlike anti–TSH-receptor antibodies, they are polyclonal in that the IgG subclass and light-chain type are less restricted (32). Naturally occurring antibodies are directed against a number of nonlinear epitopes of the thyroglobulin molecule. These antibodies may serve as a marker for the autoimmune process rather than playing a major role in pathogenesis. They have been reported to be present in up to 30% of healthy subjects, although the epitope pattern of this antibody in healthy subjects may be broader than those associated with autoimmune thyroid disease. Anti-Tg is detected in 70% to 80% of patients with autoimmune thyroiditis. In experimental models, anti-Tg titers did not correlate with the severity of the disease, and the ability to transfer disease is usually dependent on cytotoxic lymphocytes (see later). Transplacental passage of anti-Tg has not been shown to induce neonatal hypothyroidism.

Antibodies against TPO were originally detected as antibodies directed against a cytosolic component of thyroid cells and were called *antimicrosomal antibodies* (70). TPO is normally expressed only at the apical portion (facing the follicular lumen) of thyroid epithelial cells. Antibodies were initially recognized by immunofluorescence after binding to unfixed thyroid tissue. Most measurements have been performed by hemagglutination (71), although more sensitive ELISA and RIA methods are available. Like anti-TG, they are polyclonal in that the IgG subclass is not restricted, but unlike anti-Tg, the epitopes of the naturally occurring antibodies are widely divergent and recognize a variety of both liner and conformational epitopes (72). Studies suggest restriction of the use of certain variable regions of the heavy and light chains (73). Anti-TPO is detected in the serum of nearly all patients with autoimmune thyroiditis but has been reported in up to 30% of healthy subjects, with the frequency increasing with age. As with anti-Tg, it remains unclear whether anti-TPO is solely a marker of the autoimmune process or has a role in pathogenesis. Antibodies binding to intact TPO may inhibit its function and thus contribute to decreased thyroid hormone production (74).

TSH-receptor antibodies are found in 10% to 20% of patients with autoimmune thyroiditis. Those that inhibit TSH binding may contribute to the development of hypothyroidism and the atrophic form of autoimmune thyroiditis. Only a small minority of patients with the features of autoimmune thyroiditis, however, can be shown to be hypothyroid only as a result of TSH inhibition. As in Graves' disease, antibodies to the sodium iodide symporter have also been detected in patients with autoimmune thyroiditis. At this time, their role in the pathogenesis of the disease is uncertain. An increased incidence of autoantibodies against heat shock proteins has also been noted (29), but the role of these antibodies also remains uncertain.

#### Cellular Immunity

In autoimmune thyroiditis patients, both circulating and intrathyroidal T cells are stimulated by thyroglobulin and TPO. Some studies have suggested that only a limited repertoire of the variable region gene of the T-cell antigen receptor gene is used by antigen reactive cells (75,76), whereas other studies have not found evidence of such a restricted response. There is an increase in the production of $T_H1$ cytokines (19). Autoimmune thyroiditis has occurred in recipients of allogenic stem cells (77).

Several studies have suggested a role for FaS/FasL pathway of apoptosis in thyroid cell destruction (78–82). FasL is expressed by activated T cells and at immune privileged sites such as the lens of the eye and the testis. Production of IL-1 by inflammatory cells in the thyroid is believed to result in expression of Fas by thyroid cells (79,81). Thus, the death of these cells may actually represent "suicide" resulting from activation of the Fas/FasL pathway on these cells.

A number of animal models of chronic thyroiditis have been useful in delineating mechanisms of the disease. The spontaneous occurrence of thyroiditis has been noted in lines of mice, rats, and chickens (83–85). Experimental autoimmune thyroid (EAT) disease can readily be introduced into immunocompetent animals by the injection of thyroglobulin combined with an adjuvant (86). EAT can also be induced with immunization with portions of the TSH receptor (87). In contrast, it is difficult to produce EAT by injecting TPO. In studies using transgenic mice, those expressing the DR3 gene (*HLA-DRB1*0301*) were susceptible to EAT with immunization with human or murine thyroglobulin, whereas those expressing the DR2 gene (*HLA-DRB1*1502*) were resistant to the development of EAT (88). The development of EAT has also been blocked *in vivo* by use of an antibody against the CD40 ligand (gp39) (89).

In animals with EAT, antibodies directed against thyroid antigens are found, and both circulating and intrathyroidal T lymphocytes can be shown to be reactive to thyroid antigens. A lymphocytic infiltration of the thyroid is also typical (83). Cytotoxic T cells have been shown to be effective in transferring thyroiditis, whereas autoantibodies alone do not (90). Direct perfusion of large amounts of antibodies, however, can induce follicular cell destruction. The iodine content of the thyroid appears to play a role in the pathogenesis because injections of poorly iodinated thyroglobulin do not induce thyroiditis (91), whereas increased iodine in the diet increases the incidence of spontaneous thyroiditis in some mice and the obese strain (OS) chicken (85,92,93). CD8$^+$ cells appear to not be required for the disease because mice lacking CD8$^+$ cells develop EAT after thyroglobulin immunization (94). There are, however, a number of differences between EAT and Hashimoto's thyroiditis. In some strains, there is no sex difference in the incidence of thyroiditis. Destruction of follicular cells and the development of fibrosis does not usually occur. In most models, the animals do not develop goiter or hypothyroidism, although hypothyroidism does occur in the OS chicken. Clinical studies have shown a restricted repertoire of intrathyroidal lymphocytes, suggesting a limited number of target antigens (95). Mice with large deletions of the T-cell repertoire, however, have also been found to be susceptible to EAT (96,97).

### Presentation and Diagnosis

Progressive immune destruction of the thyroid follicular cells reduces the production of thyroid hormone. There is also reduced hormone synthesis as a result of a defect in the organification of iodine, which can be demonstrated using the perchlorate discharge test. The reduction in thyroid hormone production leads to enhanced secretion of TSH, which stimulates thyroid cell growth, iodine uptake, and thyroid hormone production. Depending on the capacity of the thyroid to respond to TSH, patients may remain symptom free with normal circulating levels of thyroid hormone. Such patients may maintain a goiter with normal TSH, a goiter with an elevated TSH, or a thyroid of apparently normal size with an elevated TSH. A few patients may have an episode of hyperthyroidism (hashitoxicosis). With progressive destruction, patients develop low thyroid hormone levels and frank symptoms of thyroid hormone deficiency accompanied by an elevated TSH. In the later stages of the disease, destruction of the gland results in atrophy of the thyroid.

Typical symptoms of hypothyroidism include weight gain, fatigue, cold intolerance, and constipation. Women may note menometrorrhagia, infertility, and galactorrhea. Some patients may note entrapment neuropathies. Uncommon symptoms include psychosis and precocious puberty. Physical findings include cold and dry skin, bradycardia, low-pitched voice, and a delayed relaxation phase on reflex testing. If a goiter is present, it may be firm with fine irregularities; nodules may be noted in up to one third of patients. Typical laboratory abnormalities include anemia and elevations of cholesterol, triglycerides, and creatinine phosphokinase. Prolactin may be elevated, and the pituitary may be enlarged.

Patients with Hashimoto's thyroiditis have an increased incidence of pernicious anemia and Addison's disease. Other immunologic disorders that occur with an increased frequency in these patients include rheumatoid arthritis, Sjögren's syndrome, and systemic lupus erythematosus.

The precise relationship between autoimmune thyroiditis and primary lymphoma of the thyroid gland remains unclear. Most patients with lymphoma of the thyroid gland have positive antithyroid antibodies (98). Many patients have histologic features of Hashimoto's thyroiditis noted in the tissue surrounding the tumor. The entity should be suspected in older patients with a rapidly enlarging goiter and local symptoms.

### Approach to the Patient and Treatment

#### Symptomatic Hypothyroidism

Oral replacement with thyroid hormone has been available to treat symptomatic hypothyroidism for more than 100 years. Synthetic preparations of T$_4$ are among the most commonly prescribed drugs. Although available, fixed combinations with T$_3$ are not usually required. Daily, oral doses of the hormone are usually well tolerated. Therapy is adjusted to maintain the serum TSH level within the normal range.

With a complete loss of endogenous function, replacement doses average 112 µg in younger adults and 0.088 µg in the elderly. Increased hormone requirements are seen with pregnancy, in patients with malabsorption disorders, and with drugs that increase thyroid hormone metabolism.

Some patients with residual function demonstrate autonomy and readily develop symptomatic thyrotoxicosis if placed on full replacement therapy. Initiation of therapy in patients with ischemic coronary artery disease may precipitate symptoms, exacerbate preexisting angina, and even lead to myocardial infarction. In such patients, medical or surgical therapy may be required to allow full replacement. Rapid initiation of therapy is uncommonly associated with development of congestive heart failure, acute psychosis, or pseudotumor cerebri. There is no evidence that maintenance thyroid hormone therapy leads to osteoporosis or increases the fracture risk.

#### Subclinical Hypothyroidism and Euthyroid Goiter Associated With Antithyroid Antibodies

In contrast to the treatment of frank, symptomatic hypothyroidism, the treatment of subclinical hypothyroidism and euthyroid goiter remains controversial. Even the diagnostic criteria vary because some authors limit the disorder to patients with an elevated TSH that is less than 10 µU/mL, whereas others use any elevated TSH associated with normal thyroid hormone levels. One argument favoring treatment is the possibility of improvements in unrecognized symptoms or subtle dysfunction. In several small, placebo-controlled studies, treatment of subclinical hypothyroidism led to a statistically significant improvement in how patients felt, although not all patients benefited (99,100). In a number of studies, treatment of such patients has significantly improved lipid status, cardiac function, or nerve function, but none of these has been found consistently (101,102).

The second argument favoring treatment is the risk for progression to frank, symptomatic hypothyroidism. During 20 years of follow-up in the Wickham study, the annual incidence of developing hypothyroidism was 2% if antibodies were positive with a normal TSH, 3% if only the TSH was elevated, and 4% if TSH was elevated and the antibodies were positive (11).

## Painless or Postpartum Thyroiditis

### Description, Incidence, and Prevalence

Painless or postpartum thyroiditis has also been called *silent*, *transient*, or *lymphocytic thyroiditis*. The postpartum form of this disorder has been reported to occur after as few as 1% and as many as 23% of all pregnancies (56,57). The rate may be as high as 30% in women with anti-TPO antibodies (103,104). The incidence of the spontaneous occurrence of this syndrome in women and men is not known, but in patients presenting with thyrotoxicosis, it has been found to be the cause in 5% to 20%. In women with T1DM, the frequency of postpartum thyroiditis is higher and has been reported in up to 50% (105). The course in these patients is also different, with 30% developing permanent hypothyroidism. Postpartum thyroiditis also occurs with increased frequency in women who had achieved a previous remission of Graves' disease. Thyroiditis may occur during treatment with amiodarone (106) or IFN (107,108), and patients with hepatitis C are much more likely to develop thyroiditis with IFN than those with hepatitis B (108).

Pathologic findings during the acute disorder include an intense lymphocytic infiltrate with plasma cells. Germinal centers may be seen but are less common than in Hashimoto's thyroiditis, and oncocytic cells are uncommon. There is a marked distortion of the normal thyroid follicular architecture. After recovery, biopsy specimens are normal or show only mild lymphocytic infiltration.

### Mechanisms of Disease

The postpartum form is associated with HLA-DR3 and HLA-DR5 (104). Anti-TPO and anti-Tg antibodies are found in most affected patients, although the titers may not be very high. TSI is positive in less than one fourth of affected patients.

The postpartum form has been attributed to a "rebound" immune response after pregnancy, during which immune re-

activity is modulated. Injury to the follicular cells is likely the result of cellular and antibody-mediated damage. The resultant leak of thyroid hormones leads to suppression of TSH, which further reduces the activity of the cells. The abrupt onset of cellular damage and the recovery of normal function in most patients distinguishes this from the chronic changes seen in Hashimoto's thyroiditis, with the accompanying development of fibrosis and permanent dysfunction.

### Presentation and Diagnosis

The disorder characteristically is biphasic, with an initial period of thyrotoxicosis followed by a period of transient hypothyroidism and then resolution to a euthyroid state. Either the thyrotoxic or hypothyroid phase may be mild, asymptomatic, or not noted at all. In the postpartum form, about half of women have transient thyrotoxicosis only, one fourth have the thyrotoxic phase followed by a hypothyroid phase, and one fourth have only transient hypothyroidism (56,57). In the postpartum form, recurrence is common in subsequent pregnancies.

The thyrotoxic phase is characterized by symptoms of thyrotoxicosis, with no goiter or a small, painless, diffuse goiter; the absence of fever; and a normal or minimally elevated erythrocyte sedimentation rate. During the thyrotoxic phase, TSH is suppressed, $T_4$ and $T_3$ levels are proportionately elevated, the radioactive iodine uptake is low, the urinary iodine excretion is mildly elevated, and the serum thyroglobulin is high-normal or elevated. Ophthalmopathy does not usually occur. This phase is self-limited, typically persisting for only 2 to 4 months. In the postpartum form, thyrotoxicosis may begin within a few weeks of delivery or up to 10 to 12 months later. Typical features that distinguish other disorders from silent thyroiditis include: a larger goiter, higher $T_3$ levels and increased radioactive iodine uptake in patients with Graves' disease; and toxic, nodular goiters; as well as ophthalmopathy and an elevated TSI with Graves' disease; a low thyroglobulin and no goiter in patients ingesting exogenous thyroid hormone; an elevated TSH with increased radioactive iodine uptake in patients with thyroid hormone resistance or TSH-secreting adenoma and pain, fever, and an elevated erythrocyte sedimentation rate in patients with subacute thyroiditis.

Hypothyroidism ensues when the amount of hormone leaking from the gland is not able to maintain a normal level. In the postpartum form of this disorder, hypothyroidism follows the thyrotoxic phase in about one fourth of women, and another one fourth only have transient hypothyroidism (56,57). The severity and duration of this phase is highly variable and may last up to 1 year. Soon after the resolution of thyrotoxicosis, the persistence of a suppressed TSH may be misinterpreted as secondary to pituitary destruction, especially in a postpartum woman in whom Sheehan's syndrome or hypophysitis may be suspected. The correct diagnosis is supported by the presence of anti-Tg and anti-TPO, the lack of other hormonal deficiencies, and the transient nature of the TSH suppression. Over time, the TSH begins to rise, followed by an increase in the radioactive iodine uptake and the thyroid hormone values (56,57). Most patients recover, but permanent hypothyroidism is seen in about 10% of patients. Patients remain at risk for permanent hypothyroidism in future years.

### Approach to the Patient and Treatment

Because the thyrotoxic phase is transient and represents the discharge of preformed thyroid hormone, treatment is usually limited to symptomatic therapy with β-blockers. Neither radioactive iodine nor antithyroid drugs are useful during the thyrotoxic phase. Thyroid hormone should be used during the hypothyroid phase if the patient has symptoms. If the treatment dose is given to normalize the TSH, therapy should be reevaluated at 1 year, progressively reducing the $T_4$ dose because the hypothyroidism is usually transient. Attempts at prevention in women at risk as a result of a previous history or the presence of antibodies have not been successful. Oral glucocorticoids have been used to treat painless thyroiditis associated with amiodarone.

## Transient Hypothyroidism Secondary to Blocking Antibodies

Inhibitory antibodies are a rare cause of transient hypothyroidism and account for less than 10% of cases of hypothyroidism in infants (109). The incidence is higher in Japan than in North America. Because the cause of this disorder in infants is transplacental passage of the blocking antibodies, mothers of affected infants also have the antibody present. The mothers typically have a previous history of Graves' disease, but some had been diagnosed as having Hashimoto's thyroiditis or were not known to have a thyroid disorder.

Blocking antibodies uncommonly may produce transient hypothyroidism in patients with Graves' disease. These antibodies have also been reported to be associated with the early development of hypothyroidism after radioactive iodine therapy for Graves' disease, but the frequency of this is unclear (110).

Infants are typically diagnosed by neonatal screening programs. The disorder is self-limited, resolving over several months. Patients are treated with thyroid hormone for neonatal hypothyroidism; therapy is then withdrawn at a later date to document the presence of normal thyroid function.

## Subacute (de Quervain's) Thyroiditis

### Description, Incidence, and Prevalence

Subacute, or de Quervain's, thyroiditis is also known as *granulomatous* or *giant cell thyroiditis*. The incidence of the spontaneous occurrence of this syndrome in women and men is not known, but in patients presenting with thyrotoxicosis, it has been found to be the cause in up to 20%. It is more common in women and uncommon in children before the age of puberty. An increased incidence in the summer has also been reported.

### Mechanisms of Disease

An association with HLA-B35 has been reported (111). The inflammatory changes are thought to be a response to a preceding viral illness. Given the transient nature of signs of thyroid autoimmunity as well as the transient nature of the illness, it is thought that many of the manifestations of autoimmunity are secondary rather than primary.

Anti-TPO and anti-Tg are positive in only 10% of affected patients. TSI is usually absent. TSH-blocking antibodies have been noted to be more common in patients who have a prolonged hypothyroid phase (112). Antibodies directed against thyroid antigens tend to disappear after the acute episode. IL-6 levels are increased during the acute episode. An increased antibody titer to one of a number of viruses, including mumps, measles, and adenoviruses, has been noted in affected patients (113–115). Both circulating and intrathyroidal lymphocytes respond to thyroid antigens.

### Approach to the Patient and Diagnosis

Patients may have a history of an antecedent upper respiratory infection. Typical symptoms of thyrotoxicosis, including palpitations, nervousness, and tremor, may occur, or there may be no symptoms of thyrotoxicosis. The classic presentation includes fever, pain, and neck tenderness, which may radiate to the neck or jaw. Pain and tenderness may be focal and may later spread to other areas of the thyroid. Systemic symptoms include myalgias and fatigue. The erythrocyte sedimentation rate is usually markedly elevated, and granulocytosis is common. TSH is suppressed, and the radioiodine uptake is low. The thyrotoxic phase usually only lasts for 2 to 3 months, but pain and tenderness may persist for up to a year. Long-term recurrences are uncommon. As with silent thyroiditis, a hypothyroid phase may follow the thyrotoxic phase; this occurs in about one fourth of patients. Few patients develop permanent hypothyroidism.

Pain and systemic symptoms serve to differentiate this disorder from painless thyroiditis. The low uptake and the local and systemic symptoms differentiate this disorder from Graves' disease, although some Graves' disease patients with large, rapidly growing goiters complain of thyroidal pain. Patients with a local infection or suppurative thyroiditis are usually euthyroid and usually have evidence of a more severe, systemic illness. Acute hemorrhage into a preexisting, autonomously functioning nodule may produce pain and a suppressed TSH.

Pathologic features during the thyrotoxic phase include infiltration with lymphocytes and histiocytes and disruption of the follicular architecture. Abnormalities may be focal. Giant cells are typically noted. After recovery, the gland is normal or has minimal fibrosis.

## Treatment

Salicylates or other nonsteroidal antiinflammatory agents can be used to relieve pain and systemic symptoms in some patients. In patients who fail to respond, corticosteroid therapy is usually effective within 2 to 3 days. The disease may recur if the steroid therapy is discontinued in less than 4 to 8 weeks. If needed, β-blockers can be used to treat the cardiac manifestations of the thyrotoxicosis.

## AUTOIMMUNE DISEASE OF THE ADRENAL GLAND

### Description

Autoimmune destruction of the adrenal gland or idiopathic adrenal atrophy is the most common cause of primary adrenal failure in North America. Addison's disease is the eponym associated with primary adrenal gland failure and is often used as a synonym for autoimmune adrenal failure. It typically presents in women in their 20s and 30s. In many patients, it occurs as part of a polyglandular endocrine disorder, whereas in about half of patients, it occurs as an isolated autoimmune endocrine disorder (116). The incidence is unknown. One survey found a prevalence of 93 per 1 million population, with 40% having autoimmune disease and 27% being unclassified (117). Overall, autoimmune adrenal disease is thought to account for about two thirds of cases of primary adrenal disease in North America.

The pathologic findings in the adrenal are those of an inflammatory process with infiltration of lymphocytes and plasma cells. By the time of diagnosis, fibrosis is present. Germinal centers are rarely seen. Antibody binding to cortical cells may be detected by immunohistochemistry. Late in the disorder, the adrenal cortex is completely destroyed.

### Mechanisms of Disease

#### Genetic Factors

Although a positive family history is found in half the patients with autoimmune adrenal disease associated with a polyglandular syndrome, it is noted in less than one third with isolated autoimmune adrenal disease. In many studies, patients have been noted to have an increased frequency of HLA-B8, HLA-DR3, HLA-DR4, or HLA-DR5 MHC alleles (18). HLA-DR3 has been specifically associated with clinically isolated autoimmune adrenal disease (118). Specific antigens associated with autoimmune adrenal disease include DPB1*0101, DQA*0501, DQB1*0201, and DRB1*0301 (20). A specific arginine substitution in DQA1*0501 has also been linked with autoimmune adrenal disease (119). Unlike other endocrine cells, adrenocortical cells normally express MHC class II antigens. The significance of these markers and the mechanism whereby they confer susceptibility to the disease have not been determined.

### Humoral Immune Factors

Earlier studies demonstrated that affected patients have a high incidence of antibodies to adrenal cortical cells, as demonstrated by complement fixation or immunofluorescence (120). Autoantibodies are found in 60% to 75% of patients with autoimmune adrenal disease and are more common with the polyglandular syndrome (121). In individual patients, titers decline with time. More recent studies have demonstrated that these autoantibodies are directed at specific cytochrome P450 enzymes involved in steroidogenesis. Antibodies to 17α-hydroxylase (P450C17), 21α-hydroxylase (P450C21), and the side-chain cleavage enzyme (P450scc) have all been identified (122,123) (Fig. 20.1). Early reports gave inconsistent results suggesting cross-reactivity between the antigens and leaving doubts about which forms were true autoantigens. More recent studies, using recombinant proteins and immune precipitation and absorption experiments, have clearly shown the presence of specific antibodies to each antigen (122). In addition, sera reacting only with P450C17 have been shown specifically not to stain the zona glomerulosa when antibodies to that protein are absent and the others are present (122).

Studies have clarified the targets of these antibodies in autoimmune adrenal disease (Fig. 20.1). In patients with type 1 autoimmune polyglandular syndrome (APS), Peterson et al. (122) found that 33 out of 46 (72%) reacted to at least one of the three proteins. Seven reacted to only P450C17, three reacted to only P450C21, and two reacted to only P450scc. Fourteen reacted to two of the three proteins, and seven reacted to all three. In those with clinical Addison's disease, a positive reaction was noted in 85%, whereas only 39% of those without Addison's disease reacted positively. No patient had reactivity to 11β-hydroxylase, aromatase, 3β-hydroxysteroid dehydrogenase, or adrenodoxin.

In a pair of studies by Betterle et al., the presence of sera reacting with P450C21 was more highly predictive of functional abnormalities and progression to clinical autoimmune adrenal disease in children (124) than in adults (125). At the initial evaluation, 6 of the 10 (60%) children, but only 12 of the 67 (25%) adults, who were antibody positive had evidence of subclinical adrenal dysfunction. Clinical disease developed in 9 of 10 positive children in a mean of 31 months, whereas it developed in only 14 of 67 positive adults during a mean follow-up of 45 months. Over time, the prevalence of autoantibodies declines (126).

Although these antibodies may inhibit enzyme activity *in vitro,* it is unclear whether they have any pathologic role. In addition, although the antigens are all intracellular, it is possible that the autoantibodies can penetrate the cells to produce injury. Conversely, it may only be after cellular injury that they become available to stimulate autoantibody production. Importantly, prospective clinical studies have shown that many apparently healthy subjects with adrenocortical autoantibodies may have diminished adrenocortical hormone reserve (125). Although some have suggested that these pa-

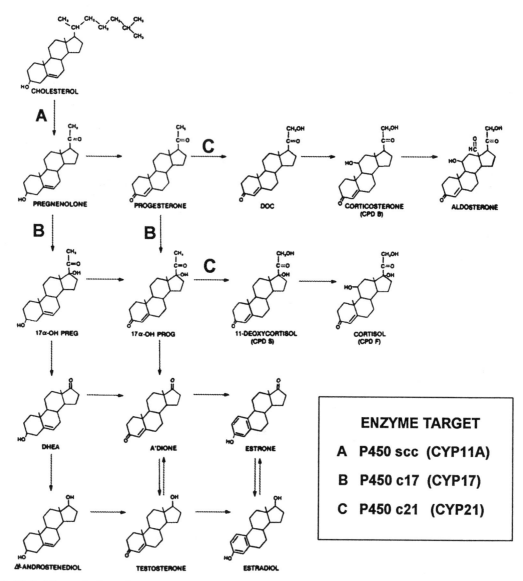

**FIG. 20.1.** Biosynthetic pathways of steroid hormones in the adrenal and enzymatic targets of autoantibodies. Three identified targets of autoantibodies are the enzymes P450 scc, P450 c17, and P450 c21.

tients may also have ACTH-blocking autoantibodies (127), these have not been consistently demonstrated in patients with autoimmune adrenal disease.

Some patients with autoimmune adrenal disease (25% of women, 5% of men) also have antibodies that interact with ovarian, testicular, or placental tissue. In women with these antibodies, premature ovarian failure is also more common. In one study of patients with type 1 APS, all patients with ovarian failure had antibodies reactive to P450C17 or P450scc (122).

### Cellular Immune Factors

Lymphocytes from affected patients proliferate in response to extracts of adrenal tissue and produce factors that inhibit the migration of leukocytes (128). In mice immunized with adrenal extracts, transfer of spleen cells led to autoantibody production and adrenal infiltrates in the recipients, but they did not develop adrenal insufficiency.

### Presentation and Diagnosis

Adrenal insufficiency disorder may present with acute adrenal crisis in the setting of an intercurrent illness or with symptoms of chronic adrenal insufficiency. The major symptom of acute insufficiency is postural hypotension. Other acute symptoms include fever, hypotension, abdominal pain, and altered consciousness. Chronic symptoms include anorexia, nausea, weight loss, fatigue, weakness, abdominal pain, diarrhea, and orthostatic hypotension. Hyperpigmentation of the skin and mucous membranes may be seen with chronic primary insufficiency. Galactorrhea may occur.

Laboratory abnormalities include an elevated blood urea nitrogen level, metabolic acidosis, hyponatremia, and hyperkalemia. Secondary adrenal insufficiency also causes hyponatremia, but not hyperkalemia. Hypoglycemia and hypercalcemia may occur but are uncommon. Hematologic abnormalities include anemia, neutropenia, and eosinophilia.

Other disorders may cause adrenal destruction. For example, adrenal hemorrhage may occur in the setting of anticoagulation therapy, in postoperative or postpartum patients, or in patients with sepsis (129). Acute destruction with sepsis is classically associated with meningococcemia (Waterhouse–Friderichsen syndrome), but it has also been reported with many organisms, including gram-positive bacteria.

In North America, tuberculosis accounts for less than 20% of cases, but worldwide, it is still the most common cause of primary adrenal insufficiency. In North America and the United Kingdom, these patients are usually older than those presenting with the autoimmune disease and usually have other evidence of the disease (130). In addition, the adrenals are usually large and contain calcifications, whereas with autoimmune disease, they are usually small or normal in size and noncalcified. Adrenal insufficiency may also be the result of destruction from fungal disease (histoplasmosis) or infiltrative disorders (amyloid or sarcoidosis). Cancers frequently metastasize to the adrenal glands but rarely cause adrenal insufficiency (131). Diffuse involvement with lymphoma or leukemia has been associated with sufficient destruction to produce adrenal insufficiency, as have rare cases of lung or breast cancer. Primary adrenal disease has been associated with the acquired immunodeficiency syndrome (AIDS) (132). In some cases, this has been attributed to adrenal hemorrhage, primary lymphoma involving the adrenal gland, or other infections. Whether the AIDS virus can directly cause adrenal insufficiency remains controversial. Adrenal insufficiency is also seen with the X-linked disorders adrenoleukodystrophy and adrenomyeloneuropathy (133,134). Both are caused by mutations in a transport protein required for peroxisomal transport of long-chain fatty acids, the accumulation of which results in demyelinating disease and adrenocortical destruction

### Approach to the Patient

If acute adrenal insufficiency is suspected, a blood sample should be drawn for cortisol, but therapy should be initiated with 100 mg of hydrocortisone intravenously, followed by 100 mg every 8 hours until the diagnosis is confirmed (or excluded) or the crisis has passed. In severely ill patients, a cortisol level of less than 20 µg/dL is suggestive but not diagnostic of autoimmune adrenal disease.

An isolated elevation of plasma renin may be the earliest evidence of autoimmune adrenal disease (135). The demonstration of an elevated ACTH level with a low cortisol level, or of a cortisol level of less than 20 µg/dL that fails to rise to more than 20 µg/dL after the administration of 250 µg of synthetic ACTH (cosyntropin), confirms the diagnosis of primary adrenal insufficiency. The presence of autoantibodies is suggestive of autoimmune adrenal disease, but an imaging study of the adrenals should still be performed because positive antibodies have been seen in patients with adrenal tumors or infection. Specific measurements of levels of long-chain fatty acids are required to make the diagnosis of adrenomyeloneuropathy; these should especially be considered in boys or men presenting with adrenal insufficiency in their teens or 20s and in young, antibody-negative women with a family history of neurologic disorders resembling multiple sclerosis.

Patients with autoimmune adrenal destruction frequently have other autoimmune disorders as well. The most common are primary hypothyroidism, vitiligo, Graves' disease, premature ovarian failure, and pernicious anemia (136).

### Treatment

Therapy involves replacement of the deficient glucocorticoid and mineralocorticoid. Liberal salt intake should be encouraged, especially when increased perspiration is expected (e.g., from exercise, increased heat). Patients should be well educated about their disease and how to adjust the dose of replacement steroids for intercurrent illnesses. They should have parenteral steroids available for emergencies and should wear a MedicAlert bracelet or necklace.

Glucocorticoids are usually given as a single dose of prednisone or one or more daily doses of the shorter-acting hydrocortisone or cortisone acetate. Prednisone is given orally in a dose of 5 to 7.5 mg, which may be given at bedtime or in the morning and supplemented with afternoon hydrocortisone if needed for symptoms. Hydrocortisone is given orally in a dose of 15 to 20 mg in the early morning, with 5 to 10 mg in the early afternoon if needed for symptoms. Cortisone acetate is given orally in a dose of 25 mg in the early morning, with 12.5 mg in the early afternoon if needed for symptoms. A single, oral dose of 0.5 mg of dexamethasone may also be used, but the risk of giving an excessive dose is greater with this potent glucocorticoid. Administration of glucocorticoids in the late evening may be associated with sleep disturbance, but the use of short-acting glucocorticoids alone in the morning may lead to increased ACTH levels and increased pigmentation. An increase in dose may be needed in patients treated with medications that increase hepatic metabolism, such as rifampin, phenytoin, and phenobarbital, and during the third trimester of pregnancy. Patients should increase their doses during mild, febrile illnesses; this can usually be accomplished by a doubling of the maintenance dose and the addition of an afternoon dose. Parenteral therapy is required for patients unable to take oral medication and in those with major illnesses or surgery.

Mineralocorticoid therapy is usually given orally as fludrocortisone in a dose of 0.05 to 0.2 mg/d. Some female patients find they need to decrease the dose for a few days around the time of menstruation to avoid symptoms of excess fluid retention.

Supine and standing blood pressure and pulse, serum potassium, and plasma renin activity are used to evaluate the dose of mineralocorticoid therapy. Replacement of glucocorticoids may be evaluated by clinical symptoms and the morning ACTH level. The development of cushingoid features or a suppressed morning ACTH value indicates excessive replacement.

## HYPOPARATHYROIDISM

### Description

Autoimmune hypoparathyroidism refers to hypoparathyroidism occurring without an identified cause. It is thought to represent an autoimmune attack of the parathyroid glands. Most commonly, the disease occurs in association with other autoimmune endocrine disease, particularly as part of the type 1 APS (see later). Hypoparathyroidism may also occur sporadically in adults, primarily in women, and often together with autoimmune thyroiditis.

### Mechanisms of Disease

Autoantibodies to the extracellular domain of the calcium-sensing receptor have been identified in patients with acquired hypoparathyroidism, 68% of whom had type 1 APS (137). The role of these antibodies in disease is not certain because these investigators were unable to demonstrate an antagonistic effect of the autoantibodies on signaling through the receptor. Nonetheless, these studies identify the calcium-sensing receptor as an important autoantigen in hypoparathyroidism and raise the possibility that a cell-mediated or humoral immune response to this antigen may lead to clinical disease.

### Presentation and Diagnosis

Hypocalcemia without an appropriate increase in parathyroid hormone (PTH) level is the cardinal feature of primary hypoparathyroidism. The symptoms of hypocalcemia are a result of enhanced neuromuscular excitability, but the severity of symptoms varies considerably (138). In acute hypocalcemia, most patients have symptoms of circumoral numbness, paresthesias of the distal extremities, or muscle cramping. Constitutional symptoms may also include fatigue, anxiety, and depression. In more severe cases, carpopedal spasm, laryngospasm, and focal or generalized seizures may occur. Clinical signs of neuromuscular irritability include Chvostek's sign (ipsilateral spasm of the facial muscles after tapping the facial nerve) and Trousseau's sign (carpal spasm induced by pressure ischemia of nerves in the upper arm during inflation of a sphygmomanometer above systolic blood pressure). A clinically important sign of hypocalcemia is prolongation of the QT interval on electrocardiogram. Chronic hypocalcemia frequently results in changes in epidermal tissues, including dry skin, coarse hair, and brittle nails. Dental and enamel hypoplasia may occur if hypocalcemia is present during childhood. Calcification of the basal ganglia is an important sign of chronic hypocalcemia, which is easily visualized on a computed tomography scan of the head.

### Approach to the Patient

The diagnosis of hypoparathyroidism may be confirmed by the presence of hypocalcemia, hyperphosphatemia, and low levels of PTH. In addition to the autoimmune disease, other, nonimmunologic conditions may cause hypoparathyroidism or hypocalcemia in young patients (Table 20.2) (137).

Of note is resistance to PTH characteristic of type 1a pseudohypoparathyroidism, because there may be resistance to other hormones leading to hypothyroidism and hypogonadism (139). Thus, the combination of these endocrine deficiencies may be mistaken for APS. The distinction may be made, however, by finding elevated levels of stimulating hormones in the resistance syndromes and low to undetectable levels in the autoimmune diseases. In addition, patients with pseudohypoparathyroidism may show the phenotype of Albright's hereditary osteodystrophy, including round facies, short stature, obesity, brachydactyly, heterotopic subcutaneous ossification, and bony exostoses.

### Treatment

Hypocalcemic crises manifest by tetany, laryngospasm, or seizures require prompt treatment. Calcium gluconate (0.2 mg/kg in up to 10 to 20 mL of 10% solution) may be infused over several minutes. An infusion of 15 mg/kg of calcium gluconate raises the serum calcium level by 2 to 3 mg/dL. Continuous infusions of calcium may be needed to maintain

**TABLE 20.2.** *Differential diagnosis of hypocalcemia*

Causes of hypoparathyroidism

  DiGeorge's syndrome
  Familial isolated hypoparathyroidism
  Associated with familial nephrosis, nerve deafness, lymphedema, mitral valve prolapse, brachydactyly
  Pseudohypoparathyroidism
  Hemochromatosis
  Wilson's disease
  Metastatic disease
  Tuberculosis
  Amyloidosis
  After neck irradiation
  Syphilis
  Magnesium deficiency

Other causes of hypocalcemia

  Vitamin D–dependent rickets
  Vitamin D–resistant rickets, type II
  Hyperphosphatemia (eg, with rhabdomyolysis or tumor lysis)
  Pancreatitis
  After treatment with calcitonin or mithramycin
  Citrated blood
  Respiratory alkalosis

calcium levels after acute treatment. For a 70-kg patient, 11 ampules of 10% calcium gluconate in normal saline or dextrose may be infused over 8 to 10 hours.

Chronic therapy for hypoparathyroidism includes oral calcium and vitamin D. The goal of therapy is maintain the calcium level between 8 and 9 mg/dL. The lower range of normal calcium level is preferred because at this level, the symptoms of hypocalcemia are prevented, as is progression of cataracts, but hypercalciuria is uncommon. In hypoparathyroidism, administration of 1,25-dihydroxyvitamin D is the most rational therapy because it bypasses the block in 1-hydroxylation caused by the absence of PTH effects on the kidney. The cost of this preparation, however, is high, and therefore, vitamin D, which is inexpensive, is used as well. Apart from its theoretical disadvantages, vitamin D has the added problem of being very lipophilic and having a long half-life. Therefore, hypercalcemia resulting from excessive administration of vitamin D can be severe and long-lasting. Calcium salt (1000 to 2000 g of elemental calcium) is generally also needed to maintain normocalcemia. Calcium salts are available as carbonate, citrate, lactate, gluconate, and glubionate. The carbonate salt contains the greatest percentage of calcium and is generally the preferred form. In patients with a deficiency of gastric acid, the citrated form may be particularly useful.

## TYPE 1 DIABETES MELLITUS

### Description

T1DM is caused by autoimmune destruction of the β cells in the islets of Langerhans (140–142). T1DM is the second most common chronic disease of childhood. It is estimated that more than 500,000 patients of all ages are affected in the United States (143). The annual incidence is about 30,000 new cases per year. Classically, the disease is recognized as the cause of diabetes in patients younger than 20 years of age, but more recent observations have changed concepts about the prevalence of the disease at different ages. As many as 9% of patients who develop diabetes after the age of 20 years may have T1DM (144). Patients with this latent form of autoimmune disease are more likely to require insulin therapy than are those without signs of autoimmunity. The incidence of T1DM shows wide geographic variation. For example, in Allegheny County, Pennsylvania, the incidence of disease among whites younger than 15 years of age between 1965 to 1989 was 17.3, whereas in Finland and Sardinia, Italy, the incidence exceeds 35 and 30 cases per 100,000, respectively (143). These genetic factors are retained by populations that move to other geographic locations (145).

The disease reaches peak incidence at 12 years of age, and a smaller rise in incidence occurs at 6 years of age, but the disease may occur even before the first year of life. However, not all diabetes diagnosed in childhood develops on an autoimmune basis. About 10% of African-American patients with onset of diabetes in youth have a form of diabetes that

differs from classic insulin-dependent diabetes (146). These patients are more commonly obese than patients with classic insulin-dependent diabetes. These patients retain β-cell function long after diagnosis and do not have the same autoimmune manifestations as those with classic T1DM.

The incidence of T1DM has been found to be increasing among certain groups. In Finland and Sweden, the incidence of T1DM was reported to rise by 3.4% and 3.7%, respectively, in 1990 (147). These observations of increasing incidence, the lack of concordance among identical twins (the concordance rate is less than 50%), and environmental influences on expression of diabetes among laboratory animals suggest that environmental agents may be important precipitators of T1DM. Of note, however, is that the periodic expression of disease may not reflect the mechanisms involved in its pathogenesis but the occurrence of acute precipitating events that result in clinical decompensation and expression of disease because studies of immune markers, described later, have indicated that the disease develops over a period of years (142).

In human disease, isolated reports have provided evidence for β-cell destruction by viruses. In one case, a coxsackievirus isolated from the pancreas of a child who died with diabetic ketoacidosis was able to transfer diabetes to mice (148). Studies of seroconversion have also implicated coxsackievirus and mumps in the disease (142,149). Congenital rubella syndrome leads to diabetes in 10% to 20% of offspring, and these patients frequently have islet cell surface autoantibodies (see later) (150,151). Viral infections, such as with encephalomyocarditis virus and coxsackievirus B, meningovirus 2T, and reovirus types 1 and 3, can cause diabetes in animals (152). In addition, the diabetes in some of these models depends on immune mechanisms that may be analogous to human disease (149).

Other environmental agents, including early diet, have been implicated in the cause of T1DM (153,154). Ecologically controlled and case-controlled studies have found that there is an inverse relationship between rates of breast-feeding and development of T1DM. This risk, however, is confined to patients carrying a high-risk HLA genotype (155). Patients with T1DM have immunity to cow-milk albumin with antibodies to an 17–amino acid albumin peptide that cross-react with a β-cell surface protein (156). Others, however, have failed to confirm unusual reactivity to cow-milk proteins in peripheral blood cells from human subjects (157).

### Mechanisms of Disease

#### Genetic Factors

The lifetime risks for T1DM for first-degree relatives of T1DM patients are 3% for parents, 7% for siblings, and 5% for children (158). In humans, two chromosomal regions show closest association with and linkage to T1DM (159). These include the MHC on chromosome 6p21 (insulin-dependent diabetes mellitus type 1) and the insulin gene region on chromosome 11p15 (IDDM2) (Table 20.3).

The association of T1DM with genes in the MHC region is strong; in several studies, the mean lod scores are more than 10. Among whites, HLA-DR3 and HLA-DR4 alleles confer increased susceptibility to T1DM, and as many as 94% of white T1DM patients carry these alleles (160–162). The strength of the association with the MHC is reflected by comparing the risk for T1DM in HLA-nonidentical siblings (1.2%) to the age-corrected empirical risk of T1DM in HLA-identical siblings (15.5%). Studies of North American white patients with these alleles, however, showed that the association is closer to the DQ region of the MHC. In fact, Todd et al. (163) found that the absence of an aspartic acid at position 57 of the DQ β chain best explained susceptibility to T1DM. Interestingly, an analogous finding exists in the unique I-Ag7 class II allele of the nonobese diabetic (NOD) mouse, a murine model of the disease (164). Thus, DQ haplotypes lacking aspartic acid, such as DQ*0201 (DQw2) and DQ*0302 (DQw8), are associated with increased risk, whereas alleles with aspartic acid, such as DQ*0602 (Dqw1.2) and DQ*0102, are protective. The phenotype of protective alleles is dominant (162). More recent data have shown unusual binding properties of the MHC alleles of T1DM in humans and the NOD mouse. Thus, the diabetes-associated alleles and I-Ag7 are "unstable" and fail to bind peptides in a conventional manner (165,166). This has lead to the suggestion that failure to bind and present self antigens to developing T cells may preclude negative selection of autoreactive T cells in the thymus.

Upstream variable-number tandem repeat sequences (VNTRs) are found in the human insulin gene. An association of these VNTRs with T1DM has been found and is reproducible in several ethnic groups (158). Although the association with this locus is strong, its functional significance is not known. It is possible that the size variation of the VNTR at the 5' end could have a direct effect on insulin gene

regulation. More recently, investigators have postulated an effect of this polymorphism on thymic expression of insulin, which may affect the peripheral repertoire of T cells that are autoreactive with insulin, a known antigen in T1DM (167).

Other regions have also been found to be linked to the disease (Table 20.3). For example, a genome-wide scan has identified linkage with at least three other genes on chromosomes 11q, 6q, and 18 (158,168–170). In general, the strength of the associations with these other loci are weaker than with the MHC and insulin genes, and studies of the association are not consistent with different study populations. Some of the regions are of particular interest, however, because they may include important immune-response genes (e.g., CTLA-4 or IL-1).

### Humoral Immunity

Autoantibodies reactive with islet cell antigens (islet cell antibodies [ICA]) may be found in most patients (84%) with newly diagnosed T1DM (Table 20.4) (171). In general, in both human and animal model studies, these immunoglobulins do not directly cause disease, although some serologic factors have been shown to have functional activity (178). Despite the absence of direct causation, the autoantibodies are of significance for at least four reasons.

First, detection of these autoantibodies in the serum of diabetic and prediabetic patients has defined the natural history of the disease (142). Studies of discordant twins and triplets who later develop diabetes have shown that autoimmunity may be present for years before disease is clinically apparent and at a time when only subtle abnormalities of insulin secretion can be detected. The antigens recognized by the autoantibodies have more recently identified the natural progression of disease. The three most predictive antibodies—antiinsulin, anti-GAD65, and anti-1A-4/ICA512—appear sequentially, suggesting an evolution of the disease process (146) (G. Eisenbarth, personnel communication). Studies of autoantibodies have furthered the notion that the disease in humans develops over a period of about three years.

Second, these autoantibodies have identified antigens important to the pathogenesis of disease (Table 20.3). The antigen glutamic acid decarboxylase (GAD65) was originally found through the search for the antigen recognized by anti-

TABLE 20.3. *Genetic loci associated with human type 1 diabetes mellitus*

| Locus | Marker | Chromosomal location |
| --- | --- | --- |
| IDDM1 | MHC | 6p21.3 |
| IDDM2 | TH/INS | 11p15 |
| IDDM3 | D15S107 | 15q26 |
| IDDM4 | FGF3 | 11q13 |
| IDDM5 | ESR | 6q25 |
| IDDM6 | D18S64 | 18q |
| IDDM7 | D2S152 | 2q31 |
| IDDM8 | D6S446 | 6q27 |
| IDDM9 | D3S1578 | 3q21-25 |
| IDDM10 | D10S193 | 10cen |
| IDDM11 | D14S67 | 14q24-31 |
| IDDM12 | CTLA-4 | 2q33 |
| IDDM13 | D2S164 | 2q34 |
| IDDM14 | — | 6p |
| IDDM15 | D6S283 | 6q21 |

TABLE 20.4. *Autoantigens identified in type 1 diabetes mellitus*

| Antigen | Reference No. |
| --- | --- |
| Insulin B chain[a] | 172 |
| IA-2/ICA512[a] | 173 |
| IA-2β/phogrin | 174 |
| GAD65[a] | 175 |
| ICA69 | 176 |
| Imogen | 177 |

[a] Autoantibodies against these antigens are most predictive of type 1 diabetes mellitus.

bodies reactive with a 64-kd islet cell membrane protein that was identified in the serum of patients and BB/W rats, a rat model of T1DM (179–181). Autoantibodies to GAD65 are seen overall in 70% of newly diagnosed diabetic children and in 4.1% of control children (171). In the NOD mouse, loss of tolerance to GAD65 has been found to correlate with development of disease (182,183). Restoration of tolerance to GAD65 through a number of different means, including intrathymic, intravenous injection or oral feeding, can prevent T1DM and even its recurrence in islets transplanted into diabetic animals (184–187). Insulin B chain is also the target of autoantibodies, particularly in young patients (146). Insulin autoantibodies have been found in 56% of newly diagnosed patients and in 2.8% of control children (171). As described later, this antigen is also recognized by pathogenic T cells and even T-cell clones in animal models of the disease. Finally, autoantibodies have identified other islet antigens, such as ICA512, GAD65, and others, that may be important T-cell antigens.

Third, immunoglobulin-producing B cells are required for the disease pathogenesis. In the NOD mouse, diabetes does not occur in the absence of B cells (188,189). The precise role of the cells in antigen presentation and T-cell activation is under investigation. B cells may serve as antigen-presenting cells and can also provide necessary costimulatory signals for T-cell activation. It is likely that their role is early in the disease because, in animal models, diabetes can be adoptively transferred in the absence of B cells or immunoglobulin (190).

Finally, detection of circulating autoantibodies is useful for prediction of future disease in patients at high risk and possibly in the general population. In children younger than 10 years of age with ICA, the probability of developing T1DM over 5 years is 75% (Fig. 20.2) (191). In the general population, when combined with associated high-risk HLA genotypes, the presence of ICA has a positive predictive value of 18%. The presence of any two biochemically defined autoantibodies (e.g., antiinsulin and anti-GAD65) with high-risk HLA genes has a positive predictive value of 9% but has a specificity of more than 99% (171). Further predictive ac-

curacy may be obtained by adding sensitive measures of β-cell function. In first-degree relatives of diabetic patients, this model of ICA, anti-insulin autoantibodies (IAA), and intravenous glucose tolerance test (IVGTT) can identify a group of relatives in whom the risk for diabetes is 72% at 3 years of follow-up and more than 90% at 4 years (192).

### Cellular Immune Responses

Studies in animal models of human T1DM have demonstrated a central role for cellular immune mechanisms in causing β-cell destruction. Depletion or inactivation of T cells prevents disease in the NOD mouse, BB/w rat, murine diabetes induced with multiple low doses of streptozotocin, as well as in some viral models (190,193,194). Both CD4$^+$ and CD8$^+$ T cells appear to be involved, although different cells may be needed at different stages of the disease (195,196). For example, adoptive transfer of diabetes in NOD mice is most efficient with both CD4$^+$ and CD8$^+$ splenocytes, but transgenic mice expressing exclusively a TCR from a CD4$^+$ diabetogenic T-cell clone from the NOD mouse can also develop disease (197). In addition, CD8$^+$ transgenic cells can trigger diabetes in the absence of other T- or B-cell specificities but do so more efficiently with the assistance of CD4$^+$ B-cell reactive T cells (198). The absence of insulitis in class I deficient β2m-NOD mice suggests a role for CD8$^+$ cells early in the disease history and a role for CD4$^+$ cells at a later stage consistent with the predominance of CD4$^+$ cells in the insulitis of diabetic NOD mice (199–201). Several diabetogenic T-cell clones have been isolated from NOD mice. A number of these clones are reactive with insulin, and GAD65 has also been shown to be the target of diabetogenic T cells from the NOD mouse (202). Only a few islet antigen reactive T-cell clones have been isolated from patients with diabetes is small. One clone, isolated from the peripheral blood of a patient with diabetes, reacts with an insulin-secretory granule (203).

In general, T$_H$1 cells are present in the diabetogenic lesions, and some of the factors produced by these cells (IFN-γ and TNF-α) may have direct toxic effects on β cells

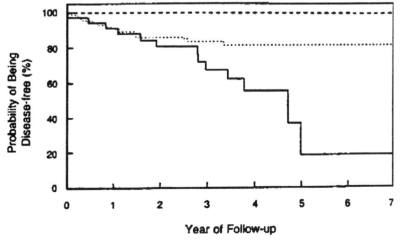

**FIG. 20.2.** Probability of remaining free of insulin-dependent diabetes mellitus in relatives of patients with type 1 diabetes mellitus (T1DM), according to islet cell antibody status and age at initial testing. Relatives negative for islet cell antibodies (*dashed line*), relatives positive for antibodies and older than 10 years old at initial testing (*dotted line*), and relatives positive for antibodies and younger than 10 years old at initial testing (*solid line*) are shown. Nondiabetic relatives of probands with T1DM who are in the first two decades of life, are members of multiplex pedigrees, and have increased titers of islet cell autoantibodies are the most likely to contract T1DM (From Riley WJ, Maclaren N, Krischer J, et al. A prospective study of the development of diabetes in relatives of patients with insulin-dependent diabetes. *N Engl J Med* 1990;323: 1157, with permission.)

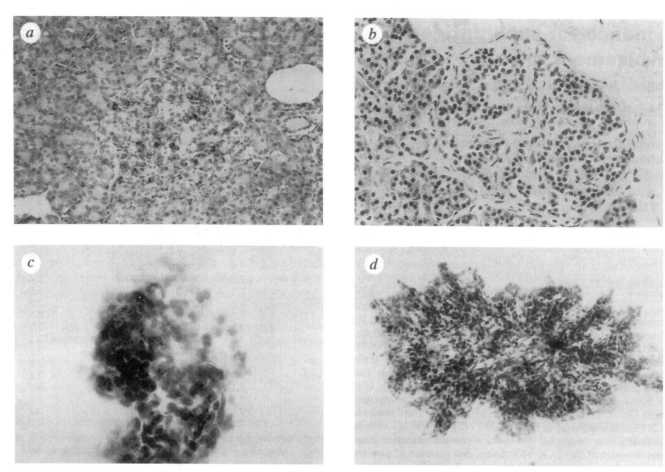

**FIG. 20.3.** Insulitis in humans. Pancreas from a 12-year-old boy who died at clinical presentation of T1DM, 1 month after onset of symptoms. **A:** A few insulin-secreting β cells are identified by immunoperoxidase staining (orange-brown). **B:** Some islets had a fibrotic ribbon-like appearance and were partially or totally devoid of insulin-secreting cells. The T-cell infiltrate was abundantly CD4⁺ **(C)** and scarcely CD8⁺ **(D)** (From Conrad B, Weldmann E, Trucco G, et al. Evidence for superantigen involvement in insulin-dependent diabetes mellitus aetiology. *Nature* 1994;371:351, with permission). See color plate 9.

(204–206) (Fig. 21.3). The requirements for these factors is unclear, however, because T$_H$2 cells can also cause disease in NOD.scid mice (207). By crossing *lpr* with NOD mice, it has been suggested that Fas/FasL interactions are needed for β-cell death (208). In other studies, direct lysis involving perforin release from CD8⁺ T cells is also required for diabetes (209). Activation of diabetogenic T cells appears to involve CD28 costimulation through complex, as yet undefined, mechanisms. Blockade of B7-2/CD28 interactions with hCTLA4Ig prevents disease in the NOD mouse, but other costimulatory molecules are also involved because CD28 knockout mice develop accelerated disease, and blockade of CD40 but not of CD28 prevents insulitis as well as diabetes (210,211).

## Approach to the Patient

### Clinical Presentation

In its classic form, T1DM presents as ketoacidosis. The clinical manifestations include polyuria, polydipsia, weight loss, volume depletion, hyperosmolality, and hyperglycemia. These manifestations reflect the consequences of insulin deficiency, hyperglycemia, and stimulation of counterregulatory hormones, including inappropriate glucagon excess. The latter augments hepatic gluconeogenesis and ketogenesis, leading to a high-anion-gap acidosis. The reader is referred elsewhere for a complete discussion of the manifestations and pathophysiology of diabetic ketoacidosis (212). Of note, the presence of ketoacidosis, although generally thought to indicate an absolute deficiency of insulin, is not pathognomonic of T1DM. In certain settings, such as maturity-onset diabetes of black youth, and in cases of type 2 diabetes that does not remain insulin dependent, ketoacidosis can occur (146).

Before ketoacidosis, the presentation of T1DM may be more subtle, including hyperglycemia or glycosuria alone. In 1997, the criteria for diagnosis of diabetes mellitus were modified based on correlations between fasting blood glucose levels and responses during an oral glucose tolerance test and relationships between the risk for long-term complications of diabetes and levels of fasting glucose (Table 20.5) (213). The

**TABLE 20.5.** *Diagnostic criteria for diabetes mellitus*

| Criteria (one of the following is sufficient for diagnosis) | Comment |
| --- | --- |
| Symptoms of diabetes plus casual plasma glucose concentration ≥200 mg/dL (11.1 mmol/L). | *Casual* is defined as any time of day without regard to time since last meal. The classic symptoms of diabetes include polyuria, polydipsia, and weight loss. |
| Fasting plasma glucose ≥126 mg/dL | *Fasting* is defined as no caloric intake for at least 8 hours. |
| Two-hour plasma glucose ≥200 mg/dL during an oral glucose tolerance test | The test should be performed using a glucose load containing the equivalent of 75-mg anhydrous glucose dissolved in water. |

most significant modification was the diagnostic criterion of a fasting plasma glucose level of 126 mg/dl or more after an 8-hour fast. In most instances of T1DM, however, these criteria are far exceeded, and the diagnosis is not in question.

The deficiency of insulin production at the time of diagnosis of T1DM is not absolute (214,215). Even among patients who have been diabetic for more than 5 years, a small percentage (11%) retain substantial insulin-secretory capacity. In addition, in younger patients after treatment of the metabolic decompensation of ketoacidosis, a clinical remission may ensue. During this period, insulin requirements may decrease, or the patient may not require insulin to maintain normoglycemia. The remission period, however, is invariably transient, and insulin dependency returns after weeks to months. In general, residual β-cell function continues for longer periods of time in adults than in younger patients with T1DM, but there is a gradual decline in β-cell function over the first few years of disease (216). After 5 years of disease, stimulated C-peptide levels are generally undetectable in adolescents and undetectable in most adults. Thus, the progressive loss of insulin-secretory function and ultimate (after 5 years) dependence on insulin treatment for avoidance of ketoacidosis is the most reliable diagnostic criterion for T1DM (217).

A common diagnostic problem in children is the incidental discovery of hyperglycemia or glycosuria during a routine blood or urine test (218,219). Transient hyperglycemia has been described in up to 0.46% of children in one children's hospital and in 0.013% of children in an outpatient practice. Among these children, 32% developed T1DM over an 18-month period when hyperglycemia was discovered in the absence of a serious illness, but only 2.3% developed T1DM when hyperglycemia was discovered during a serious illness. Islet cell antibodies and insulin autoantibodies had a 100% positive predictive value for T1DM; the negative predictive value was 96% for ICA and 98% for insulin autoantibodies. A stimulated insulin release during an intravenous glucose test had the highest overall accuracy of prediction. No child whose stimulated insulin release was above the fifth percentile developed T1DM (219).

## Diagnosis

In most cases, there is little reason to confirm the presence of autoimmune diabetes by measuring islet cell or other au-

toantibodies. The need for insulin treatment of children is apparent at diagnosis because of the degree of hyperglycemia, the extent of weight loss, or the present of ketoacidosis. Because of recent evidence that insulin treatment itself may have a beneficial effect on the natural history of T1DM, however, in cases in which the clinical symptoms may be milder, there may be value in identifying the autoimmune disease, initiating insulin treatment, and differentiating these patients from those with non–insulin-dependent diabetes mellitus in whom oral hypoglycemic therapy might be preferred (192,220).

## Treatment

### Established Type 1 Diabetes Mellitus

Diet, insulin, and exercise are the mainstays of treatment of T1DM. The goals of diet therapy may be summarized as follows:

- Maintenance of blood glucose levels to as near normal as possible by balancing food intake with insulin and activity levels
- Provision of adequate calories for maintaining or attaining reasonable weights for adults, normal growth and development rates for children and adolescents, increased metabolic needs during pregnancy and lactation, or recovery from catabolic illnesses (221,222)

*Reasonable* weight is defined as the weight the patient and health care provider acknowledge as achievable and maintainable, both short-term and long-term. In general, the distribution of calories is 50% to 60% carbohydrate and 10% to 20% protein, with the remainder (less than 30%) as fat. The liberalization of the amount of carbohydrate in the diet is a relatively recent recommendation and is still controversial because increased carbohydrates may result in increased triglyceride concentrations (223). Because 80% of mortality from diabetes is a result of macrovascular disease, a focus of nutritional management has been to reduce this risk.

Insulin injections are required to prevent development of ketoacidosis and maintain life in T1DM. Most patients are now treated with formulations of human insulin produced by recombinant DNA technology. This has reduced the frequency of insulin allergy and the production of insulin antibodies in patients during treatment. Insulin antibodies can reduce the peak concentration of free insulin in plasma, but a direct relationship between insulin antibodies and daily insulin dose has not been found (224).

The goals of insulin treatment are to maintain the plasma glucose at near-normal levels while minimizing the frequency of hypoglycemia. A long-standing debate on the benefits of tight (i.e., near-normal) glucose control was brought to a close by the results of the Diabetes Control and Complications Trial (DCCT) (225). This trial showed that intensive treatment of T1DM can slow the development and progression of long-term complications of the disease. In the DCCT trial, this was most clearly shown for eye disease, but limited results from the DCCT trial and other trials supported the notion that other complications are also favorably affected by strict control of glucose levels. However, there was also an inverse relationship between the frequency of severe hypoglycemic episodes and the control of glucose level, as reflected by the glycosylated hemoglobin level. This outcome is not surprising because in T1DM, there is a functional impairment in the response of glucagon-producing α cells and in catecholamine production, which results in impaired glucose counterregulation in response to insulin-induced hypoglycemia (226). The basis for these abnormalities remains unclear, but the impairments are functional and not anatomic. Nonetheless, the frequent occurrence of hypoglycemia remains the major limiting factor in achieving normal glucose control because with current therapy, insulin delivery only approximates normal physiology (227).

A number of different regimens for insulin delivery are now in use (Table 20.6). At a minimum, patients with T1DM who are consuming three meals (often with two or three snacks) each day may receive an injection of mixtures of intermediate- and short-acting insulin before breakfast and dinner each day. Closer regulation of glucose levels may be possible, however, with other regimens involving more frequent injections of insulin; and this is preferable, based on the DCCT experience (225). For example, by administering short-acting insulin with each meal and an intermediate- or long-acting insulin once or twice each day, the postmeal glucose excursion can be controlled, overnight insulin requirements met, and the fasting blood sugar controlled. Rather than repeated subcutaneous injections, insulin may also be delivered by a continuous subcutaneous infusion (CSII), in which insulin is infused by a pump into a subcutaneous site through a catheter that remains in place for 2 to 3 days. Many patients are able to achieve goals of strict control with this approach. Recently, an insulin analog (LysPro) has been introduced in which the amino acids proline and lysine, which normally occupy B28 and B29, are reversed (229). This insulin has a rapid onset and a duration of action that is shorter than that of regular insulin. A clinical advantage of reduced nocturnal hypoglycemia has been demonstrated with use of this insulin, but the shorter kinetics may limit its use when action is needed for as long as 4 to 6 hours.

Exercise is an important adjunct to diet and insulin therapy. Peripheral insulin disposal is increased in exercising muscle, and the beneficial effects of aerobic exercise on cardiovascular fitness is of particular value because of the heightened risk for cardiovascular disease. The reader is referred elsewhere for a more detailed discussion of use of exercise regimens in the treatment of T1DM (230).

Measuring glucose levels is essential to modify insulin regimens individually to achieve optimal glucose control. A large number of hand-held meters, based primarily on measurement of glucose by glucose oxidase, are available for use by patients. The frequency with which measurements need to be done varies with individual patients, but the results of these tests may be used to make fine adjustments in insulin doses. An important development in clinical management of diabetes has been the measurement of glycosylated hemoglobin (hemoglobin A1) levels, which reflects average blood sugar levels over the half-life of red blood cells, or about 60 days. The glycosylated hemoglobins (hemoglobin A1a, A1b, and A1c) are formed by the nonenzymatic condensation of glucose with the amino-terminal group of the β-chains of hemoglobin, a Schiff base reaction, and an Amadori reaction to form a stable ketamine (231). The amount of glycosylation is dependent on the concentration of glucose and the length of time to which the hemoglobin is exposed to glucose (232).

### Immunotherapy

The recognition of T1DM as an autoimmune disease has prompted trials of immunosuppression as a treatment for the disease. The initial effects of cyclosporine treatment begun at the time of clinical presentation on the natural history of T1DM were promising; there was a significant increase in the number of patients with non–insulin-requiring remissions toward the end of the first year after diagnosis (233,234). Despite the short-term effects of cyclosporine, all patients eventually showed metabolic deterioration (235). Other immune-suppressive agents, such as azathioprine and prednisone, have been shown to have beneficial effects on the natural history of the disease (236); however, the failure of these drugs to induce a permanent remission and their toxicities has led to a decline in their use. Recognition that T1DM develops over about 3 years and that its clinical presentation occurs only after a loss of most insulin-producing cells has prompted some to abandon immune-suppressive treatment at

**TABLE 20.6.** *Pharmacokinetics of commonly used insulin preparations*

| Insulin[a] | Onset | Peak action | Duration |
|---|---|---|---|
| Short-acting | | | |
| Lispro | 15 min | 60 min | <5 h |
| Regular | 30 min | 2–4 h | 6 h |
| Intermediate-acting | | | |
| NPH or Lente | 1.5–3 h | 8–10 h | 16–24 h |
| Long-acting | | | |
| Ultralente | | Broad peak: 7–15 h | 24–36 h |

[a] All are human insulins, except Lispro.

the time of diagnosis. Nonetheless, the fact that β-cell destruction is not complete at the time of diagnosis raises the possibility for immune intervention even at diagnosis if a safe approach that can arrest an ongoing immune response were available (214).

### Prophylaxis

Clinical and experimental data suggest that insulin treatment can modify the natural history of T1DM. In prediabetic NOD mice, parenteral and oral insulin have been shown to prevent development of diabetes (184,185). Keller et al. (192) identified first-degree relatives of patients with T1DM who were at high risk for disease based on high titers of IAA and ICA and diminished first-phase insulin response to intravenous glucose, all of whom had normal oral tolerance to glucose. Some of these patients were treated with subcutaneous insulin, and all were followed for up to 7 years. Four of five patients who received insulin did not develop T1DM over the observation period, whereas all seven patients who declined treatment developed diabetes over a 4-year observation period. Even at the time of clinical presentation, Shah et al. (220) were able to show that treatment of patients with an intensive insulin regimen resulted in improved β-cell function at the end of 1 year, as compared with control patients who received standard treatment. An important implication of this work for clinical practice is that there is little reason to discontinue insulin treatment even during the period of clinical remission (i.e., honeymoon) that frequently occurs shortly after the clinical presentation of disease.

### Pancreas and Islet Transplantation

Insulin treatment is necessary for the remainder of the patient's life. Replacement of the destroyed tissue remains the obvious cure for the disease, and successful pancreas transplantation can reverse even chronic complications. Pancreas transplantation at the time of renal transplantation for end-stage renal disease has become common (237). Whole- or partial-organ transplantation successfully restores normal glucose levels. The graft survival rate for pancreas allografts after 1 year is about 74%. Clinical studies suggest that prevention of the recurrence of diabetic renal disease and other complications, and even restoration of counterregulatory responses to hypoglycemia, may be benefits of pancreas transplantation (238–240). A troubling issue is the likelihood of recurrent autoimmune disease within the transplanted islets of Langerhans. In two reported cases, insulitis was identified in a failed pancreas allograft, whereas the exocrine pancreas was free of infiltrates (241).

Rather than whole-organ transplantation, successful islet transplantation remains a treatment goal. The ability of islet transplantation to restore normal glucose levels has been clearly shown in cases of autotransplantation after pancreatectomy, in which as few as 265,000 islets can provide normal glucose profiles (242). The results with islet allotransplantation have been generally disappointing, and overall, the likelihood of insulin independence after 1 year is about 8% (243). Success rates have improved, however, with some groups reporting insulin independence for more than 5 years after islet transplantation. In patients who have prolonged islet allograft survival, glucose control is at least as good as in those intensively treated in the DCCT trial and, more importantly, in the absence of significant hypoglycemia (244).

## INSULIN AUTOIMMUNE SYNDROME

### Description

Autoantibodies to human insulin have been described in healthy patients before the onset of type 1 diabetes, in patients with polyendocrine autoimmune disease, and even in 2% of healthy blood donors (172,245,246). These autoantibodies, however, are generally of low titer and do not cause symptoms. The insulin autoimmune syndrome (IAS) is characterized by fasting hypoglycemia, high concentration of total serum immunoreactive insulin, and the presence of autoantibodies to human insulin. The syndrome was first described by Hirata et al. in 1970 (247). The incidence of the syndrome is particularly high among East Asians, and in Japan, it represents one of the major causes of hypoglycemia. In Western countries, about 22 cases have been reported.

### Mechanisms of Disease

The strong ethnic differences in the incidence of the disease has led investigators to search for genes within the MHC that regulate responsiveness to human insulin. Indeed, DR4 is the dominant phenotype among patients with IAS (248). It has been shown that specific DR4 genotypes are associated with T-cell proliferative responses when autologous antigen-presenting cells are exposed to human insulin (249). In most cases, the autoantibodies are polyclonal, but they are generally more homogenous than those found in insulin-treated patients. In a few isolated cases, particularly among whites, monoclonal autoantibodies are seen. Particular amino acid substitutions in the DR4B1 chain have been reported to affect the clonality of the autoantibody response.

### Presentation and Diagnosis

In patients with IAS, the buffering effect of insulin antibodies leads to glucose intolerance after an oral glucose load and delayed hypoglycemia (247,250). The availability of the secreted hormone to receptors in the liver and peripheral tissues is decreased during its secretion after glucose administration, and there is a lack of a prompt hypoglycemic response after insulin administration. The half-life of injected insulin is significantly prolonged, and the release of insulin from the circulating autoantibody pool is a function of mass action and not a response to changes in blood glucose levels. As insulin is released from the bound pool, a delayed decline in glucose levels occurs; thus, patients consistently have late hypoglycemia after carbohydrate ingestion or exogenous insulin administration but not after prolonged fasting.

## Approach to the Patient

Insulin levels, measured by RIA, in patients with IAS are falsely high, generally more than 1000 pmol/L. A large percentage of the insulin, however, is antibody bound. The levels of circulating C-peptide are variable but are often not suppressed. This syndrome may be distinguished from other forms of clinical hypoglycemia by the extraordinarily high insulin levels and high percentage of insulin binding. It is important differential diagnosis is hypoglycemia from an insulin-binding monoclonal gammopathy, which has been described in multiple myeloma (251).

In several of the reported cases, an association with other autoimmune disorders has been noted; these have included rheumatoid arthritis and Graves' disease. In others, however, nonautoimmune diseases, such as alcoholic cirrhosis or malaria, have been associated (252,253). In some cases, the appearance of insulin autoantibodies is associated with administration of sulfidryl-containing drugs, such as methimazole, α-mercaptopropionylglycine, carbimazole, and penicillamine.

## Treatment

In most cases, only supportive treatment, such as glucose monitoring and adjustments in diet, is needed, and spontaneous remission has occurred within 6 months (254). In other cases, supportive treatment has been insufficient to control hypoglycemia, and plasmapheresis, together with immunosuppression with prednisone, has been used. This has resulted in clinical remission, including restoration of glucose and insulin tolerance and decrease in insulin autoantibody levels.

## TYPE B INSULIN RESISTANCE

### Description

Certain cases of severe insulin resistance result from the development of autoantibodies that bind the insulin receptor and block binding of insulin (255). This is a rare disorder and falls within the syndromes of insulin resistance that also include obesity, acanthosis nigricans, ovarian hyperandrogenism, and hypertension. Most patients, in addition, have evidence of systemic autoimmune diseases, such as systemic lupus erythematosus, primary biliary cirrhosis, and others (256).

### Mechanism

The stimulus for production of antireceptor antibodies is unknown.

### Presentation and Diagnosis

Patients are identified by the development of diabetes that is refractory to treatment with insulin. Often, doses of insulin in excess of 5000 U/d are used in attempt to control the hyperglycemia. The hyperglycemia correlates with reduced insulin binding to receptors because of the presence of the blocking antibodies.

The clinical course of the disease is dynamic. Hyperglycemia frequently evolves into a hypoglycemic phase (257). In this phase, there is enhanced binding of insulin to receptors for reasons that are not clear. The development of this phase is related to acquired agonistic characteristics of autoantibodies. The clinical course does not remain stable; there may be alternating periods of insulin-resistant diabetes, remission, and hypoglycemia.

### Approach to the Patient

In clinically suspected cases, insulin binding to its receptor can be measured *in vitro* by competition of insulin binding to receptors on IM-9 lymphocytes (257).

### Treatment

Few treatment options are available. Glucocorticoids, immunosuppressive agents, and plasmapheresis have been used. Hypoglycemia is unpredictable and is a particularly difficult clinical problem (255,256). It may require use of glucagon as well as parenteral glucose to maintain glucose levels. In isolated cases, hypoglycemia has been associated with the demise of the patient.

## POLYGLANDULAR AUTOIMMUNE ENDOCRINE DISEASE

### Description

The coexistence of endocrinopathies involving more than one gland was recognized in the early part of the 20th century, but it was not until 1980 that these syndromes were categorized based on predominant patterns of organ involvement (258–260). These syndromes are relatively rare and affect men and women with equal frequency, which is unusual because other autoimmune diseases are generally more prevalent in women.

Three syndromes have been described (Table 20.7). Type 1 APS involves parathyroid and adrenal glands as well as chronic mucocutaneous candidiasis and dystrophy of dental enamel and nails, alopecia, vitiligo, and keratopathy [autoimmune polyendocrinopathy-candidiasis-ectodermal dystrophy (APECED)]. The sequence of syndrome manifestations is characteristic. APECED usually presents in infancy with recurrent candidiasis (Fig. 20.4). Hypoparathyroidism, the most common endocrinologic manifestation of the syndrome, is seen in about 80% of patients. It also presents early in childhood, generally before 10 years of age. Adrenocortical insufficiency develops later, often not until the end of the sec-

**TABLE 20.7.** *Symptoms of autoimmune polyglandular syndromes*

Type I

Hypoparathyroidism
Adrenal insufficiency
Chronic mucocutaneous candidiasis
Hypogonadism
Pernicious anemia (juvenile onset)
Ungual dystrophy, tympanic membrane calcification
Alopecia
Vitiligo
Chronic active hepatitis
Malabsorption
Anterior hypophysitis
Sjögren's syndrome

Type II

Adrenal insufficiency
Thyroiditis
Diabetes mellitus
Vitiligo
Alopecia
Hypogonadism
Pernicious anemia (adult onset)
Myasthenia gravis

Type III

Thyroiditis
Diabetes mellitus
Pernicious anemia
Myasthenia gravis or other nonendocrine autoimmune
  disorder

ond decade. Other endocrine deficiencies are also seen, including autoimmune diabetes, gonadal failure, and anterior hypophysitis. Most patients have 3 to 5 manifestations of the disease, but they may have a delayed onset, and specific disease states may not appear until the fifth decade of life (261).

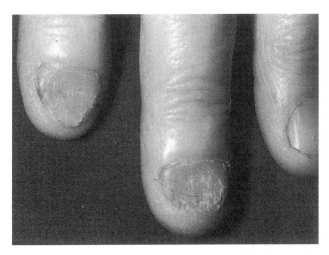

**FIG. 20.4.** Mucocutaneous candidiasis. This illustration shows cutaneous candidiasis in a 6-year-old girl who also had mucosal lesions. (From Levene GM, Goodamali SK. *Diagnostic picture tests in dermatology.* London: Wolfe Medical Publications, 1986:106, with permission.) See color plate 10.

Type 2 APS is defined as the association of adrenal insufficiency with autoimmune thyroid disease or T1DM. Hashimoto's thyroiditis and Graves' disease are the most common thyroid diseases. This syndrome occurs later in life, most commonly in adults between the ages of 20 and 40 years, and is more common in women. T1DM in this syndrome may occur after 20 years of age, whereas sporadic T1DM is more commonly a disease of children. Most commonly, adrenal insufficiency is the initial endocrine deficiency. Like the manifestations of type 1 APS, the manifestations of type 2 need not occur simultaneously; there may be a delay in presentation of features by as much as 20 years. In addition to the endocrine deficiencies, pernicious anemia and myasthenia gravis may occur in a small proportion of adult patients.

Type 3 APS has also been defined. This syndrome refers to the development of autoimmune thyroid disease with two other autoimmune disorders, including T1DM, pernicious anemia, or a nonendocrine organ-specific disorder, such as myasthenia gravis, but in the absence of Addison's disease (262).

Prominent features of each of these autoimmune diseases include inflammatory cells within the affected organs and the production of autoantibodies that recognize the affected tissue.

## Mechanisms of Disease

### Genetic Determinants

The APECED syndrome is inherited as an autosomal dominant trait. Earlier studies mapped the syndrome to chromosome 21 and to genes outside the MHC region. Two groups have identified mutations of a gene designated autoimmune regulator (*AIRE*), which encodes two zinc-finger motifs suggestive of a transcription factor in studies carried out in Finnish, German, and Swiss APECED patients (263,264). At least seven mutations of this gene have been reported to account for the development of the syndrome. It is uncertain, however, whether this gene is directly or indirectly involved in the development of the disease, and which developmental processes are regulated by *AIRE*. Of note, *AIRE* is expressed in fetal liver and thymus and lymph node, important locations for development of the immunologic repertoire.

Type 2 APS has different genetic determinants (265,266). This disorder has been associated with genes within the MHC complex. The HLA-A1/B8 haplotype is found with increased frequency in these patients, but most likely, this association reflects linkage disequilibrium with DR3, DR4, or both. The relative risk for Addison's disease is 26.5 in patients who are heterozygous for HLA-DR3 and HLA-DR4. Although further analysis of the MHC class II region in T1DM has identified DQ loci that are strongly linked to disease, a similar analysis has not been done in type 2 APS.

### Humoral Immunity

The antiadrenal autoantibodies discussed previously are found in about 65% of patients with nontuberculous Addison's disease. Most patients have antibodies against the enzyme 21-hydroxylase as well as other steroidogenic enzymes, including two different cytochrome P450 enzymes (267–271). Other autoantibodies reactive with steroid secreting tissue can be found as well.

### Cellular Immunity

The role of cell-mediated responses in the pathogenesis of these diseases is not well understood. Individual endocrine syndromes can be induced in animals by immunization with homogenates of the glands (e.g., adrenal), suggesting that cell-mediated responses are able to cause destruction of the endocrine glands. Spontaneous polyendocrine disease is also found in certain animal models of T1DM. For example, NOD mice develop mild sialitis and thyroiditis, although hypothyroidism is not seen. Thyroiditis also occurs spontaneously in the BB/W rat. Development of both diseases is not likely to reflect simply immune responses to shared antigens because induction of tolerance to diabetes by intrathymic injection of islets into young BB/W rats protects only against diabetes, not against thyroiditis. An interesting murine model of polyglandular endocrinopathies has been developed and studied. Organ-specific immune diseases can be induced by depleting certain T-cell subpopulations. For example, treatment of mice with cyclosporine between birth and 2 weeks of age results in development of gastritis and oophoritis in BALB/c mice, and oophoritis can be induced in normal mice by neonatal thymectomy (272,273). The autoimmune disease can be prevented by splenic T cells from normal syngeneic mice. The disease is exacerbated by removal of the thymus after the cyclosporine treatment. These models raise the interesting possibility that a failure of negative selection in the thymus underlies polyglandular autoimmunity.

### Presentation and Diagnosis

Type 1 APS frequently presents in infancy with recurrent mucocutaneous candidiasis. There may be periods of remissions and exacerbations, but overall, there is progression of the candidal infections over time. In most patients, the infections involve the skin, nails, and oral and perianal mucosa, but the entire gastrointestinal tract can be involved, resulting in bacterial overgrowth, chronic diarrhea, and hemorrhage.

The development of hypoparathyroidism is manifest by hypocalcemia, the clinical manifestations of which were discussed previously. The onset of adrenocortical insufficiency may be more difficult to detect because many of the symptoms are constitutional; these may include fatigue, weakness, orthostatic hypotension, weight loss, and anorexia. The development of hyperpigmentation of the skin and mucosal surfaces is specific for primary adrenal insufficiency and high ACTH levels. Hair loss, particularly in androgen-dependent areas, is commonly seen in older women. Laboratory abnormalities may support the suspicion of adrenal insufficiency. These include hyponatremia, hyperkalemia, acidosis, hypo-

glycemia, lymphocytosis, and mild eosinophilia (274). An important clue to the development of adrenocortical insufficiency in a patient with hypoparathyroidism is the correction of hypocalcemia because adrenal insufficiency itself may lead to hypercalcemia. In general, the clinical spectrum of type 1 APS is broad, and all patients need lifelong follow-up for the detection of new components of the disease (261).

Manifestations of type 2 APS begin at an older age than those of type 1 APS. Addison's disease is often the first manifestation, and the syndrome is frequently not diagnosed until 20 to 40 years of age. As in type 1 APS, the other manifestations of this syndrome, including thyroiditis and T1DM, may occur concurrently or be delayed, and the development of one of the disorders has been reported into the seventh decade. The clinical manifestations of these endocrinopathies were discussed earlier.

### Approach to the Patient

The diagnosis of adrenal insufficiency and autoimmune thyroid disease were discussed previously. Hypocalcemia occurring in the presence of candidiasis or the described ectodermal manifestations listed earlier should suggest the presence of autoimmune hypoparathyroidism and type 1 APS. Confirmation of hypoparathyroidism may be obtained by measurement of serum PTH level.

### Treatment

Replacement therapies for each of the specific disorders were discussed previously.

### REFERENCES

1. Thodou E, Asa SL, Kontogeorgos G, et al. Clinical case seminar. Lymphocytic hypophysitis: clinicopathological findings. *J Clin Endocrinol Metab* 1995;80:2302–2311.
2. Feigenbaum S, Martin M, Wilson C, et al. Lymphocytic adenohypophysitis: a pituitary mass lesion occurring in pregnancy. *Am J Obstet Gynecol* 1991;164:1549–1555.
3. Levine S. Allergic adrenalitis and adenohypophysitis: further observations on production and passive transfer. *Endocrinology* 1969;84:469–475.
4. Klein I, Kraus KE, Martines AJ, et al. Evidence for cellular mediated immunity in an animal model of autoimmune pituitary disease. *Endocr Res Commun* 1982;9:145–153.
5. Mayfield R, Levine JH, Gordon L, et al. Lymphoid adenohypophysitis presenting as a pituitary tumor. *Am J Med* 1980;69:619–623.
6. Bottazzo GF, Pouplard A, Florin-Christian A, et al. Autoantibodies to prolactin-secreting cells of human pituitary. *Lancet* 1998;2:97–101.
7. Sauter N, Toni R, McLaughlin C, et al. Isolated adrenocorticotropin deficiency associated with an autoantibody to a corticotroph antigen that is not adrenocorticotropin or other proopiomelanocortin-derived peptides. *J Clin Endocrinol Metab* 1990;70:1391–1397.
8. Sugiura M, Hashimoto A, Shizawa M, et al. Detection of antibodies to anterior pituitary cell surface membrane with insulin dependent diabetes mellitus and adrenocorticotropic hormone deficiency. *Diabetes Res* 1987;4:63–66.
9. Crock PA. Cytosolic autoantigens in lymphocytic hypophysitis. *J Clin Endocrinol Metab* 1998;83:609–618.
10. McIver B, Morris JC. The pathogenesis of Graves' disease. *Endocrinol Metabol Clin North Am* 1998;27:73–89.

11. Vanderpump M, Tunbridge W, French J, et al. The incidence of thyroid disorders in the community: a twenty-year follow-up of the Whickham Survey. *Clin Endocrinol* 1995;43:55–68.

12. Jacobson DL, Gange SJ, Rose NR, et al. Epidemiology and estimated population burden of selected autoimmune diseases in the United States. *Clin Immunol Immunopathol* 1997;84:223–243.

13. Laurberg P, Pedersen KM, Hreidarsson A, et al. Iodine intake and the pattern of thyroid disorders: a comparative epidemiological study of thyroid abnormalities in the elderly in Iceland and the Jutland, Denmark. *J Clin Endocrinol Metab* 1998;83:765–769.

14. Livolsi V. The pathology of autoimmune thyroid disease: a review. *Thyroid* 1994;4:333–339.

15. Martin A, Goldsmith NK, Friedman EW, et al. Intrathyroidal accumulation of T cell phenotypes in autoimmune thyroid disease. *Autoimmunity* 1990;6:269–281.

16. Brix TH, Kyvik KO, Hegedus L. What is the evidence of genetic factors in the etiology of Graves' disease? A brief review. *Thyroid* 1998;8:627–634.

17. Brix TH, Christensen K, Holm NV, et al. A population-based study of Graves' disease in Danish twins. *Clin Endocrinol* 1998;48:397–400.

18. Farid NR, Bear J. The human major histocompatibility complex and endocrine disease. *Endocr Rev* 1981;2:50–86.

19. Baker JR Jr. Autoimmune endocrine disease. *JAMA* 1997;278:1931–1937.

20. Badenhoop K, Walfish PG, Rau H, et al. Susceptibility and resistance alleles of human leukocyte antigen (HLA) DQA1 and HLA DQB1 are shared in endocrine autoimmune disease. *J Clin Endocrinol Metab* 1995;80:2112–2117.

21. Lavard L, Madsen HO, Perrild H, et al. HLA class II associations in juvenile Graves' disease: indication of a strong protective role of the DRB1*0701,DQA1*0201 haplotype. *Tissue Antigens* 1997;50:639–641.

22. Djilali-Saiah I, Larger E, Harfouch-Hammoud E, et al. No major role for the CTLA-4 gene in the association of autoimmune thyroid disease with IDDM. *Diabetes* 1998;47:125–127.

23. Awata T, Kurihara S, Iitaka M, et al. Association of CTLA-4 gene A-G polymorphism (IDDM12 locus) with acute-onset and insulin-depleted IDDM as well as autoimmune thyroid disease (Graves' disease and Hashimoto's thyroiditis) in the Japanese population. *Diabetes* 1998;47:128–129.

24. Barbesino G, Tomer Y, Concepcion E, et al. The International Consortium for the Genetics of Autoimmune Thyroid Disease. Linkage analysis of candidate genes in autoimmune thyroid disease. 1. Selected immunoregulatory genes. *J Clin Endocrinol Metab* 1998;83:1580–1584.

25. Da Costa CR, Johnstone AP. Production of the thyrotrophin receptor extracellular domain as a glycosylphosphatidylinositol-anchored membrane protein and its interaction with thyrotrophin and autoantibodies. *J Biol Chem* 1998;273:11874–11880.

26. Valse H, Graves P, Magnusson R, et al. Human autoantibodies to the thyrotropin receptor: recognition of linear, folded, and glycosylated recombinant extracellular domain. *J Clin Endocrinol Metab* 1995;80:46–53.

27. Rapoport B, McLachlan S, Kakinuma A, et al. Critical relationship between autoantibody recognition and thyrotropin receptor maturation as reflected in the acquisition of complex carbohydrate. *J Clin Endocrinol Metab* 1996;81:2525–2533.

28. Saito T, Endo T, Kawaguchi A, et al. Increased expression of the $Na^+/I^-$ symporter in cultured human thyroid cells exposed to thyrotropin and in Graves' thyroid tissue. *J Clin Endocrinol Metab* 1997;82:3331–3336.

29. Appetecchia M, Castelli M, Delpino A. Anti-heat shock proteins autoantibodies in autoimmune thyroiditis: preliminary study. *J Exp Clin Cancer Res* 1997;16:395–400.

30. Kubota S, Gunji K, Ackrell BAC, et al. The 64-kilodalton eye muscle protein is the flavoprotein subunit of mitochondrial succinate dehydrogenase: the corresponding serum antibodies are good markers of an immune-mediated damage to the eye muscle in patients with Graves' hyperthyroidism. *J Clin Endocrinol Metab* 1998;83:443–447.

31. Morris JC, Bergert ER, Bryant WP. Binding of immunoglobulin G from patients with autoimmune thyroid disease to rat sodium-iodide symporter peptides: evidence for the iodide transporter as an autoantigen. *Thyroid* 1997;7:527–534.

32. Tomer Y. Anti-thyroglobulin autoantibodies in autoimmune thyroid diseases: cross-reactive or pathogenic? *Clin Immunol Immunopathol* 1997;82:3–11.

33. McKenzie JM, Zakarija M. Antibodies in autoimmune thyroid disease. In: Braverman L, Utiger R, eds. *The thyroid: a fundamental and clinical text,* 7th ed. Philadelphia: JB Lippincott, 1996:416–446.

34. Zakarija M. Immunochemical characterization of the thyroid-stimulating antibody (TSAB) of Graves' disease: evidence for restricted heterogeneity. *J Clin Lab Immunol* 1983;10:77–85.

35. Weetman AP, Yateman ME, Ealey PA, et al. Thyroid-stimulating antibody activity between different immunoglobulin G subclasses. *J Clin Invest* 1990;86:723–727.

36. Michelangeli V, Poon C, Taft J, et al. The prognostic value of thyrotropin receptor antibody measurement in the early stages of treatment of Graves' disease with antithyroid drugs. *Thyroid* 1998;8:119–124.

37. Zakarija M, McKenzie JM, Hoffman W. Prediction and therapy of intrauterine and late-onset neonatal hyperthyroidism. *J Clin Endocrinol Metab* 1986;62:368–371.

38. Weetman AP, Black CM, Cohen SB, et al. Affinity purification of IgG subclasses and the distribution of thyroid autoantibody reactivity in Hashimoto's thyroiditis. *Scand J Immunol* 1989;30:73–82.

39. Ajjan RA, Findlay JC, Metcalfe RA, et al. The modulation of the human sodium iodine symporter activity by Graves' disease sera. *J Clin Endocrinol Metab* 1998;83:1217–1221.

40. Raspe E, Costagliola S, Ruf J, et al. Identification of the thyroid $Na^+/I^-$ cotransporter as a potential autoantigen in thyroid autoimmune disease. *Eur J Endocrinol* 1995;132:399–405.

41. Dayan C, Londei M, Corcoran A, et al. Autoantigen recognition by thyroid-infiltrating T cells in Graves disease. *Proc Natl Acad Sci U S A* 1991;88:7415–7419.

42. Sridama V, Pacini F, DeGroot LJ. Decreased suppressor T-lymphocytes in autoimmune thyroid diseases detected by monoclonal antibodies. *J Clin Endocrinol Metab* 1982;54:316–319.

43. Roura-Mir C, Catalfamo M, Sospedra M, et al. Single-cell analysis of intrathyroidal lymphocytes shows differential cytokine expression in Hashimoto's and Graves' disease. *Eur J Immunol* 1997;27:3290–3302.

44. Fisfalen ME, Soltani K, Kaplan E, et al. Evaluating the role of Th0 and Th1 clones in autoimmune thyroid disease by use of Hu-SCID chimeras. *Clin Immunol Immunopathol* 1997;85:253–264.

45. Hidaka Y, Okumura M, Shimaoka Y, et al. Increased serum concentration of interleukin-5 in patients with Graves' disease and Hashimoto's thyroiditis. *Thyroid* 1998;8:235–239.

46. Shimojo N, Kohno Y, Yamaguchi K-I. Induction of Graves-like disease in mice by immunization with fibroblasts transfected with the thyrotropin receptor and a class II molecule. *Proc Natl Acad Sci U S A* 1996;93:11074–11079.

47. Bahn RS, Dutton CM, Joba W, et al. Thyrotropin receptor expression in cultured Graves' orbital preadipocyte fibroblasts is stimulated by thyrotropin. *Thyroid* 1998;8:193–196.

48. Ludgate M, Crisp M, Lane C, et al. The thyrotropin receptor in thyroid eye disease. *Thyroid* 1998;8:411–413.

49. Bahn RS, Dutton CM, Natt N, et al. Thyrotropin receptor expression in Graves' orbital adipose/connective tissues: potential autoantigen in Graves' ophthalmopathy. *J Clin Endocrinol Metab* 1998;83:998–1002.

50. Gunji K, Kubota S, Swanson J, et al. Role of the eye muscles in thyroid eye disease: identification of the principal autoantigens. *Thyroid* 1998;8:553–556.

51. Natt N, Bahn RS. Cytokines in the evolution of Graves' ophthalmopathy. *Autoimmunity* 1997;26:129–136.

52. Bahn RS. Cytokines in thyroid eye disease: potential for anticytokine therapy. *Thyroid* 1998;8:415–418.

53. De Bellis A, DI Martino S, Fiordelisi F, et al. Soluble intercellular adhesion molecule-1 (sICAM-1) concentrations in Graves' disease patients followed up for the development of ophthalmopathy. *J Clin Endocrinol Metab* 1997;83:1222–1225.

54. Dabon-Almirante CLM, Surks MI. Clinical and laboratory diagnosis of thyrotoxicosis. *Endocrinol Metab Clin North Am* 1998;27:25–35.

55. Perros P, Kendal-Taylor P. Natural history of thyroid eye disease. *Thyroid* 1998;8:423–425.

56. Mestman JH. Hyperthyroidism in pregnancy. *Endocrinol Metabol Clin North Am* 1998;27:127–149.

57. Amino N, Tada H, Hidaka Y. Autoimmune thyroid disease and pregnancy. *J Endocrinol Invest* 1996;19:59–70.

58. Hashizume K, Ichikawa K, Sakurai A, et al. Administration of thyroxine in treated Graves' disease. *N Engl J Med* 1991;324:947–953.

59. Pujol P, Osman A, Grabar S, et al. TSH suppression combined with carbimazole for Graves' disease: effect on remission and relapse rates. *Clin Endocrinol* 1998;48:635–640.

60. Rittmaster R, Abbott EC, Douglas R, et al. Effect of methimazole, with or without L-thyroxine, on remission rates in Graves' disease. *J Clin Endocrinol Metab* 1998;83:814–818.

61. McIver B, Rae P, Beckett G, et al. Lack of effect of thyroxine in patients with Graves' hyperthyroidism who are treated with an antithyroid drug. *N Engl J Med* 1996;334:220–224.

62. Bartalena L, Marcocci C, Bogazzik F, et al. Relation between therapy for hyperthyroidism and the course of Graves' ophthalmopathy. *N Engl J Med* 1998;338:73–78.

63. Manso PG, Furlanetto RP, Wolosker AMB, et al. Prospective and controlled study of ophthalmopathy after tadioiodine therapy for Graves' hyperthyroidism. *Thyroid* 1998;8:49–52.

64. Sawin CT, Castelli WP, Hershman JM, et al. The aging thyroid: thyroid deficiency in the Framingham study. *Arch Intern Med* 1985; 145:1386–1388.

65. Okayasu I, Hara Y, Nakamura K, et al. Racial and age-related differences in incidence and severity of focal autoimmune thyroiditis. *Am J Clin Pathol* 1994;101:698–702.

66. Bogner U, Hegedus L, Finke R, et al. Thyroid cytotoxic antibodies in atrophic and goitrous autoimmune thyroiditis. *Eur J Endocrinol* 1995; 132:69–74.

67. Konishi J, Iida Y, Endo K, et al. Inhibition of thyrotropin-induced adenosine 3'5'-monophosphate increase by immunoglobulins from patients with primary myxedema. *J Clin Endocrinol Metab* 1983;57: 544–549.

68. Shi Y, Zou M, Robb D, et al. Typing for major histocompatibility complex class II antigens in thyroid tissue blocks: association of Hashimoto's thyroiditis with HLA-DQA0301 and DQB0201 alleles. *J Clin Endocrinol Metab* 1992;75:943–946.

69. Nicholson LB, Wong F, Ewins D, et al. Susceptibility to autoimmune thyroiditis in Down's syndrome is associated with the major histocompatibility class II DQA 0301 allele. *Clin Endocrinol* 1994;41: 381–383.

70. Czarnocka B, Ruf J, Ferrand M, et al. Purification of the human thyroid peroxidase and its identification as the microsomal antigen involved in autoimmune thyroid diseases. *Fed Euro Bio Soc* 1985;190: 147–152.

71. Amino N, Hagen S, Yamada N, et al. Measurement of circulating thyroid microsomal antibodies by the tanned red cell haemagglutination technique: Its usefulness in the diagnosis of autoimmune thyroid diseases. *Clin Endocrinol* 1976;5:115–125.

72. Hamada N, Jaeduck N, Portmann L, et al. Antibodies against denatured and reduced thyroid microsomal antigen in autoimmune thyroid disease. *J Clin Endocrinol Metab* 1987;64:230–238.

73. McIntosh RS, Asghar MS, Kemp EH, et al. Analysis of immunoglobulin G kappa antithyroid peroxidase antibodies from different tissues in Hashimoto's thyroiditis. *J Clin Endocrinol Metab* 1997;82: 3818–3825.

74. Okamoto Y, Hamada N, Saito H, et al. Thyroid peroxidase activity-inhibiting immunoglobulins in patients with autoimmune thyroid disease. *J Clin Endocrinol Metab* 1989;68:730–734.

75. Brostoff S, Howell M. Short analytical review T cell receptors, immunoregulation, and autoimmunity. *Clin Immunol Immunopathol* 1992;62:1–7.

76. McIntosh RS, Watson PF, Weetman AP. Analysis of the T cell receptor V alpha repertoire in Hashimoto's thyroiditis: evidence for the restricted accumulation of CD8+ T cells in the absence of CD4+ T cell restriction. *J Clin Endocrinol Metab* 1997;82:1140–1146.

77. Karthaus M, Gabrysiak T, Brabant G, et al. Immune thyroiditis after transplantation of allogeneic CD34+ selected peripheral blood cells. *Bone Marrow Transplant* 1997;20:697–699.

78. Shimaoka Y, Hidaka Y, Okumura M, et al. Serum concentration of soluble Fas in patients with autoimmune thyroid diseases. *Thyroid* 1998; 8:43–47.

79. Giordano C, Stassi G, De Maria R, et al. Potential involvement of Fas and its ligand in the pathogenesis of Hashimoto's thyroiditis. *Science* 1997;275:960–963.

80. Mitsiades N, Poulaki V, Kotoula V, et al. Fas/Fas ligand up-regulation and Bcl-2 down-regulation may be significant in the pathogenesis of Hashimoto's thyroiditis. *J Clin Endocrinol Metab* 1998;83: 2199–2203.

81. Arscott PL, Baker JR Jr. Apoptosis and thyroiditis. *Clin Immunol Immunopathol* 1998;87:207–217.

82. Hammond LJ, Lowdell MW, Cerrano PG, et al. Analysis of apoptosis in relation to tissue destruction associated with Hashimoto's autoimmune thyroiditis. *J Pathol* 1997;182:138–144.

83. Dietrich HM, Oliveira-dos-Santos AJ, Wick G. Development of spontaneous autoimmune thyroiditis in Obese strain (OS) chickens. *Vet Immunol Immunopathol* 1997;57:141–146.

84. Damotte D, Colomb E, Cailleau C, et al. Analysis of susceptibility on NOD mice to spontaneous and experimentally induced thyroiditis. *Eur J Immunol* 1997;27:2854–2862.

85. Rose NR, Saboori AM, Rasooly L, et al. The role of iodine in autoimmune thyroiditis. *Crit Rev Immunol* 1997;17:511–517.

86. Wan Q, McCormick DJ, David CS, et al. Thyroglobulin peptides of specific primary hormonogenic sites can generate cytotoxic T cells and serve as target autoantigens in experimental autoimmune thyroiditis. *Clin Immunol Immunopathol* 1998;86:110–114.

87. Costagliola S, Rodien P, Many MC, et al. Genetic immunization against the human thyrotropin receptor causes thyroiditis and allows production of monoclonal antibodies recognizing the native receptor. *J Immunol* 1998;160:1458–1465.

88. Kong Y-CM, Lomo LC, Motte RW, et al. HLA-DRB1 polymorphism determines susceptibility to autoimmune thyroiditis in transgenic mice: Definitive association with HLA-DRB1*0301 (DR3) gene. *J Exp Med* 1996;184:1167–1172.

89. Carayanniotis G, Masters SR, Noelle RJ. Suppression of murine thyroiditis via blockade of the CD40-CD40L interaction. *Immunology* 1997;90:421–426.

90. Costagliola S, Many MC, Stalmans-Falys M. Transfer of thyroiditis, with syngeneic spleen cells sensitized with the human thyrotropin receptor, to naive BALB/c and NOD mice. *Endocrinology* 1996;137: 4637–4643.

91. Champion B, Rayner D, Byfield G, et al. Critical role of iodination for T cell recognition of thyroglobulin in experimental murine thyroid autoimmunity. *J Immunol* 1987;139:3665–3670.

92. Ebner SA, Lueprasitsakul W, Alex S, et al. Iodine content of rat thyroglobulin affects its antigenicity in inducing lymphocytic thyroiditis in the BB/Wor rat. *Autoimmunity* 1992;13:209–214.

93. Sundick RS, Herdengen D, Brown TR, et al. The incorporation of dietary iodine into thyroglobulin increases its immunogenicity. *Endocrinology* 1987;120:2078–2084.

94. Sugihara S, Fujiwara H, Shearer G. Autoimmune thyroiditis induced in mice depleted of particular T cell subsets. *J Immunol* 1993;150: 683–694.

95. Matsuoka N, Unger P, Ben-Nun A, et al. Thyroglobulin-induced murine thyroiditis assessed by intrathyroidal T cell receptor sequencing. *J Immunol* 1994;152:2562–2568.

96. Lomo LC, Zhang F, McCormick DJ, et al. Flexibility of the thyroiditogenic T cell repertoire for murine autoimmune thyroiditis in DC8-deficient (beta2m -/-) and T cell receptor Vbeta(c) congenic mice. *Autoimmunity* 1998;27:127–133.

97. Alimi E, Huang S, Brazillet MP, et al. Experimental autoimmune thyroiditis (EAT) in mice lacking the IFN-gamma receptor gene. *Eur J Immunol* 1998;28:201–208.

98. Pedersen RK, Pedersen NT. Primary non-Hodgkin's lymphoma of the thyroid gland: a population based study. *Histopathology* 1996;28: 25–32.

99. Cooper D, Halpern R, Wood L, et al. L-thyroxine therapy in subclinical hypothyroidism. *Ann Intern Med* 1984;101:18–24.

100. Nystrom K, Caidahl K, Fager G, et al. A double-blind cross-over 12-month study of L-thyroxine treatment of women with 'subclinical' hypothyroidism. *Clin Endocrinol* 1988;29:63–76.

101. Arem R, Patsch W. Lipoprotein and apolipoprotein levels in subclinical hypothyroidism. *Arch Intern Med* 1990;150:2097–2100.

102. Forfar J, Wathen C, Todd W, et al. Left ventricular performance in subclinical hypothyroidism. *Q J Med* 1985;224:857–865.

103. Freeman R, Rosen H, Thysen B. Incidence of thyroid dysfunction in an unselected postpartum population. *Arch Intern Med* 1986;146: 1361–1364.

104. Tachi J, Amino N, Tamaki H, et al. Long term follow-up and HLA association in patients with postpartum hypothyroidism. *J Clin Endocrinol Metab* 1988;66:480–484.

105. Alvarez-Marfany M, Roman S, Drexler A, et al. Long-term prospective study of postpartum thyroid dysfunction in women with insulin dependent diabetes mellitus. *J Clin Endocrinol Metab* 1994;79:10–16.

106. Harjai K, Licata A. Effects of amiodarone on thyroid function. *Ann Intern Med* 1997;126:63–73.

107. Koh L, Greenspan F, Yeo P. Interferon-alpha induced thyroid dysfunction: three clinical presentations and a review of the literature. *Thyroid* 1997;7:891–896.

108. Fernandez-Soto L, Gonzalez A, Escobar-Jimenez F, et al. Increased risk of autoimmune thyroid disease in hepatitis C vs hepatitis B before, during, and after discontinuing interferon therapy. *Arch Intern Med* 1998;158:1445–1448.

109. Iseki M, Shimizu M, Oikawa T, et al. Sequential serum measurements of thyrotropin binding inhibitor immunoglobulin G in transient familial neonatal hypothyroidism. *J Clin Endocrinol Metab* 1983;57:384–387.

110. Chiovato L, Fiore E, Vitti P, et al. Outcome of thyroid function in Graves' patients treated with radioiodine: role of thyroid-stimulating and thyrotropin-blocking antibodies and of radioiodine-induced thyroid damage. *J Clin Endocrinol Metab* 1998;83:40–46.

111. Nyulassy S, Hnilica P, Buc M, et al. Subacute (de Quervain's) thyroiditis: association with HLA-Bw35 antigen and abnormalities of the complement system, immunoglobulins and other serum proteins. *J Clin Endocrinol Metab* 1977;45:270–274.

112. Tamai H, Nozaki T, Mukuta T, et al. The incidence of thyroid stimulating blocking antibodies during the hypothyroid phase in patients with subacute thyroiditis. *J Clin Endocrinol Metab* 1991;73:245–250.

113. McArthur A. Subacute giant cell thyroiditis associated with mumps. *Med J Aust* 1964;1:116–117.

114. Hintze G, Fortelius P, Railo J. Epidemic thyroiditis. *Acta Endocrinol* 1964;45:381–401.

115. Swann N. Acute thyroiditis five cases associated with adenovirus infection. *Metabolism* 1964;13:908–910.

116. Betterle C, Volpato M. Adrenal and ovarian autoimmunity. *Eur J Endocrinol* 1998;138:16–25.

117. Willis AC, Vince FP. The prevalence of Addison's disease in Coventry, UK. *Postgrad Med J* 1997;73:286–288.

118. Maclaren N, Riley W. Inherited susceptibility to autoimmune Addison's disease is linked to human leukocyte antigens-DR3 and/or DR4, except when associated with type I autoimmune polyglandular syndrome. *J Clin Endocrinol Metab* 1986;62:455–459.

119. Donner H, Braun J, Seidl C, et al. Codon 17 polymorphism of the cytotoxic T lymphocyte antigen 4 gene in Hashimoto's thyroiditis and Addison's disease. *J Clin Endocrinol Metab* 1997;82:4130–4132.

120. Weetman AP. Autoantigens in Addison's disease and associated syndromes. *Clin Exp Immunol* 1997;107:227–229.

121. Tanaka H, Perez MS, Powell M, et al. Steroid 21-hydroxylase autoantibodies: Measurements with a new immunoprecipitation assay. *J Clin Endocrinol Metab* 1997;82:1440–1446.

122. Peterson P, Uibo R, Peranen J, et al. Immunoprecipitation of steroidogenic enzyme autoantigens with autoimmune polyglandular syndrome type I (APS I) sera: further evidence for independent humoral immunity to P450c17 and P450c21. *Clin Exp Immunol* 1997;107:335–340.

123. Volpato M, Prentice L, Chen S, et al. A study of the epitopes on steroid 21-hydroxylase recognized by autoantibodies in patients with or without Addison's disease. *Clin Exp Immunol* 1998;111:422–428.

124. Betterle C, Volpato M, Rees Smith B, et al. II. Adrenal cortex and steroid 21-hydroxylase autoantibodies in children with organ-specific autoimmune diseases: markers of high progression to clinical Addison's disease. *J Clin Endocrinol Metab* 1997;82:939–942.

125. Betterle C, Volpato M, Rees Smith B, et al. I. Adrenal cortex and steroid 21-hydroxylase autoantibodies in adult patients with organ-specific autoimmune diseases: markers of low progression to clinical Addison's disease. *J Clin Endocrinol Metab* 1997;82:932–938.

126. Falorni A, Laureti S, Nikoshkov A, et al. 21-Hydroxylase autoantibodies in adult patients with endocrine autoimmune diseases are highly specific for Addison's disease. *Clin Exp Immunol* 1997;107:341–346.

127. Wulffraat N, Hemmo A, Drexhage A, et al. Immunoglobulins of patients with idiopathic Addison's disease block the in vitro action of adrenocorticotropin. *J Clin Endocrinol Metab* 1989;69:231–238.

128. Winqvist O, Soderbergh A, Kampe O. The autoimmune basis of adrenocortical destruction in Addison disease. *Mol Med Today* 1996;2:282–289.

129. Rao HR, Vagnucci A. The clinical profile and management of bilateral massive adrenal hemorrhage. *Adv Endocrinol Metab* 1992;3:227–235.

130. Vita J, Silverberg S, Goland R, et al. Clinical clues to the cause of Addison's disease. *Am J Med* 1985;78:461–466.

131. Seidenwurm D, Elmer E, Kaplan L, et al. Metastases to the adrenal glands and the development of Addison's disease. *Cancer* 1984;54:552–557.

132. Sellmeyer D, Grunfeld C. Endocrine and metabolic disturbances in human immunodeficiency virus infection and the acquired immune deficiency syndrome. *Endocr Rev* 1996;17:518–532.

133. Aubourg P. The expanding world of primary adrenal insufficiencies. *Eur J Endocrinol* 1997;137:10–12.

134. Korenke G, Roth C, Krasemann E, et al. Viability of endocrinological dysfunction in 55 patients with X-linked adrenoleucodystrophy: clinical, laboratory and genetic findings. *Eur J Endocrinol* 1997;137:40–47.

135. Saenger P, Levine LS, Irvine WJ, et al. Progressive adrenal failure in polyglandular autoimmune disease. *J Clin Endocrinol Metab* 1982;54:863–867.

136. Zelissen PM, Bast EJ, Croughs RJ. Associated autoimmunity in Addison's disease. *J Autoimmunol* 1995;8:121.

137. Li Y, Song Y-H, Rais N, et al. Autoantibodies to the extracellular domain of the calcium sensing receptor in patients with acquired hypoparathyroidism. *J Clin Invest* 1996;97:910–914.

138. Downs R, Levine M. Hypoparathyroidism and other causes of hypocalcemia. In: Becker K, Bilezikian J, Bremner W, et al. eds. *Principles and practice of endocrinology and metabolism*, 1st ed. Philadelphia: JB Lippincott, 1990:447–456.

139. Chase L, Melson G, Aurbach G. Pseudohypoparathyroidism: defective excretion of $3',5'$ cAMP in response to parathyroid hormone. *J Clin Invest* 1969;48:1832–1844.

140. Atkinson MA, Maclaren NK. The pathogenesis of insulin-dependent diabetes mellitus. *N Engl J Med* 1994;331:1428–1436.

141. Castaño L, Eisenbarth GS. Type-I diabetes: a chronic autoimmune disease of human, mouse, and rat. *Annu Rev Immunol* 1990;8:647–680.

142. Eisenbarth G. Type I diabetes mellitus: a chronic autoimmune disease. *N Engl J Med* 1986;314:1360–1368.

143. LaPorte R, Matsushima K, Chang Y-F. Prevalence and incidence of insulin-dependent diabetes. *Diabetes in America* 1995;37–46.

144. Niskanen L, Tuomi T, Karjalainen J, et al. GAD antibodies in NIDDM. *Diabetes Care* 1995;18:1557–1563.

145. Mutone S, Fonte M, Studuto S, et al. Incidence of insulin-dependent diabetes mellitus among Sardinian-heritage children born in Lazio region, Italy. *Lancet* 1997;349:160–162.

146. Winter W, Maclaren N, Riley WJ, et al. Maturity-onset diabetes of youth in black Americans. *N Engl J Med* 1987;316:285–291.

147. Diabetes Epidemiology Research Investigational Group. Secular trends in incidence of childhood IDDM in 10 countries. *Diabetes* 1990;39:858–864.

148. Yoon J-W, Austin M, Onodera T, et al. Isolation of a virus from the pancreas of a child with diabetic ketoacidosis. *N Engl J Med* 1998;300:1173–1179.

149. Helmke K, Otten A, Willems W. Islet cell antibodies in children with mumps infection. *Lancet* 1980;2:211–212.

150. Ginsberg-Fellner F, Witt M, Fedun B, et al. Diabetes mellitus and autoimmunity in patients with the congenital rubella syndrome. *Rev Infect Dis* 1985;[Suppl 1]:S170–S176.

151. McEvoy RC, Fedun B, Cooper L, et al. Children at high risk of diabetes mellitus: New York studies of families with diabetes and of children with congenital rubella syndrome. *Adv Exp Med Biol* 1988;246:221.

152. Yoon J-W. A new look at viruses in type 1 diabetes. *Diabetes Metab Rev* 1995;11:83–107.

153. Verge C, Howard N, Irwig L, et al. Environmental factors in childhood IDDM: a population-based, case control study. *Diabetes Care* 1994;17:1381–1389.

154. Akerbloom H, Vaarala O. Cow milk proteins, autoimmunity and type 1 diabetes. *Exp Clin Endocrinol Diabetes* 1997;105:83–85.

155. Kostraba J, Cruickshanks K, Lawler-Heavner J, et al. Early exposure to cow's milk and solid foods in infancy, genetic predisposition, and risk of IDDM. *Diabetes* 1993;42:288–295.

156. Karjalainen J, Martin J, Knip M, et al. A bovine albumin peptide as a possible trigger of insulin-dependent diabetes mellitus. *N Engl J Med* 1992; 327:302–307.

157. Atkinson MA, Bowman MA, Kao K, et al. Lack of immune responsiveness to bovine serum albumin in insulin-dependent diabetes. *N Engl J Med* 1993;329:1853–1858.

158. Todd JA, Farall M. Panning for gold: genome-wide scanning for linkage in type 1 diabetes. *Hum Mol Genet* 1996;5:1443.

159. Davies J, Kawaguchi Y, Bennett S, et al. A genome-wide search for human type 1 diabetes susceptibility genes. *Nature* 1994;371:130–136.

160. Nepom G. Immunogenetics of HLA-associated diseases. *Concepts Immunopathol* 1988;5:80–105.

161. Bach FH, Rich SS, Barbosa R, et al. Insulin-dependent diabetes-associated HLA-D region encoded determinants. *Hum Immunol* 1985;12:59–64.

162. Baisch JM, Weeks T, Giles R, et al. Analysis of HLA-DQ genotypes and susceptibility in insulin-dependent diabetes mellitus. *N Engl J Med* 1990;322:1836–1841.

163. Todd JA, Bell JI, McDevitt H. HLA-DQB gene contributes to susceptibility and resistance to insulin-dependent diabetes mellitus. *Nature* 1987;329:599–604.

164. Wicker L, Todd JA, Peterson L. Genetic control of autoimmune diabetes in the NOD mouse. *Annu Rev Immunol* 1995;13:179–200.

165. Kanagawa O, Shimizu J, Unanue ER. The role of I-Ag7 beta chain in peptide binding and antigen recognition by T cells. *Int Immunol* 1997;9:1523–1526.

166. Carrasco-Marin E, Shimizu J, Kanagawa O, et al. The class II MHC I-Ag7 molecules from non-obese diabetic mice are poor peptide binders. *J Immunol* 1996;156:450–458.

167. Pugliese A, Zeller M, Fernandez A, et al. The insulin gene is transcribed in the human thymus and transcription levels correlated with allelic variation in the INS VNTR-IDDM2 susceptibility locus for type 1 diabetes. *Nat Genet* 1997;15:293–297.

168. Todd JA, Bain SC. A practical approach to identification of susceptibility genes for IDDM. *Diabetes* 1992;41:1029–1034.

169. Todd JA, Acha-Orbea H, Bell JI, et al. A molecular basis for MHC class II-associated autoimmunity. *Science* 1988;240:1003–1009.

170. Morahan G, Huang D, Tait BD, et al. Markers on distal chromosome 2q linked to insulin-dependent diabetes mellitus. *Science* 1996;272:1808–1810.

171. Hagopian W, Sanjeevi C, Kockum I, et al. Glutamate decarboxylase-, insulin-, and islet cell-autoantibodies and HLA typing to detect diabetes in a general population-based study of Swedish children. *J Clin Invest* 1995;95:1505–1511.

172. Palmer JP, Asplin C, Clemons P, et al. Insulin antibodies in insulin-dependent diabetics before insulin treatment. *Science* 1983;222:1337–1339.

173. Rabin D, Pleasic S, Shapiro H, et al. Islet cell antigen 512 is a diabetes-specific islet autoantigen related to protein tyrosine phosphatases. *J Immunol* 1994;152:3183–3188.

174. Hawkes K, Wasmeier C, Christie MR, et al. Identification of the 37k-antigen in insulin-dependent diabetes as a tyrosine phosphatase-like protein (phogrin) related to IA-2. *Diabetes* 1996;45:1187–1192.

175. Baekkeskov S, Aanstoot H-J, Christgau S. Identification of the 64K autoantigen in insulin-dependent diabetes as the GABA-synthesizing enzyme glutamic acid decarboxylase. *Nature* 1990;347:151–156.

176. Pietropaolo M, Castaño L, Babu S, et al. Islet cell autoantigen 69 kD (ICA69): molecular cloning and characterization of a novel diabetes-associated autoantigen. *J Clin Invest* 1993;92:359–371.

177. Arden SD, Roep BO, Neophytou PI, et al. Imogen 38: a novel 38-kD islet mitochondrial autoantigen recognized by T cells from a newly diagnosed type 1 diabetic patient. *J Clin Invest* 1996;97:551–561.

178. Johnson J, Crider B, McCorkle K, et al. Inhibition of glucose transport into rat islet cells by immunoglobulins from patients with new-onset insulin-dependent diabetes mellitus. *N Engl J Med* 1990;322:653–659.

179. Baekkeskov S, Aanstoot H-J, Christgau S, et al. Identification of the 64K autoantigen in insulin-dependent diabetes as the GABA-synthesizing enzyme glutamic acid decarboxylase. *Nature* 1990;347:151–156.

180. Hagopian W, Michelsen B, Karlsen AE. Autoantibodies in IDDM primarily recognize the 65,000-Mr rather than the 67,000-Mr isoform of glutamic acid decarboxylase. *Diabetes* 1993;42:631–636.

181. Kaufman DL, Erlander MG, Clare-Salzler M, et al. Autoimmunity to two forms of glutamate decarboxylase in insulin-dependent diabetes mellitus. *J Clin Invest* 1992;89:283–292.

182. Tisch R, Yang X, Singer SM, et al. Immune response to glutamic acid decarboxylase correlates with insulitis in non-obese diabetic mice. *Nature* 1993;366:72–75.

183. Kaufman DL, Clare-Salzler M, Tian J, et al. Spontaneous loss of T-cell tolerance to glutamic acid decarboxylase in murine insulin-dependent diabetes. *Nature* 1993;366:69–72.

184. Zhang ZJ, Davidson L, Eisenbarth G, et al. Suppression of diabetes in nonobese diabetic mice by oral administration of porcine insulin. *Proc Natl Acad Sci U S A* 1991;88:10252–10256.

185. Atkinson MA, Maclaren NK, Luchetta R. Insulitis and diabetes in NOD mice reduced by prophylactic insulin therapy. *Diabetes* 1990;39:933–937.

186. Ma S-W, Zhao D-L, Yin Z-Q, et al. Transgenic plants expressing autoantigens fed to mice to induce oral immune tolerance. *Nat Med* 1997;3:793.

187. Tian J, Clare-Salzler M, Herschenfeld A, et al. Modulating autoimmune responses to GAD inhibits disease progression and prolongs islet graft survival in diabetes-prone mice. *Nat Med* 1996;2:1348–1353.

188. Noorchashm H, Noorchashm N, Kern J, et al. B-cells are required for the initiation of insulitis and sialitis in nonobese diabetic mice. *Diabetes* 1997;46:941–946.

189. Serreze DV, Chapman HD, Varnum DS, et al. B lymphocytes are essential for the initiation of T cell-mediated autoimmune diabetes: analysis of a new "speed congenic" stock of NOD.*Igμ^null* mice. *J Exp Med* 1996;184:2049–2053.

190. Miller BJ, Appel MC, O'Neil JJ, et al. Both the Lyt-2+ and L3T4+ T cell subsets are required for the transfer of diabetes in nonobese diabetic mice. *J Immunol* 1988;140:52–58.

191. Riley WJ, Maclaren N, Krischer J, et al. A prospective study of the development of diabetes in relatives of patients with insulin-dependent diabetes. *N Engl J Med* 1990;323:1167–1172.

192. Keller R, Eisenbarth G, Jackson R. Insulin prophylaxis in individuals at high risk of type 1 diabetes. *Lancet* 1993;341:927–928.

193. Shizuru JA, Taylor-Edwards C, Banks BA, et al. Immunotherapy of the nonobese diabetic mouse: treatment with an antibody to T-helper lymphocytes. *Science* 1988;240:659–662.

194. Gold DP, Bellgrau D. Identification of a limited T-cell receptor β chain variable region repertoire associated with diabetes in the BB rat. *Proc Natl Acad Sci U S A* 1991;88:9888–9991.

195. Wicker LS, Miller BJ, Coker LZ, et al. Genetic control of diabetes and insulitis in the nonobese diabetic (NOD) mouse. *J Exp Med* 1987;165:1639–1654.

196. Conrad B, Weldmann E, Trucco G, et al. Evidence for superantigen involvement in insulin-dependent diabetes mellitus aetiology. *Nature* 1994;371:351–355.

197. Katz JD, Wang B, Haskins K, et al. Following a diabetogenic T cell from genesis through pathogenesis. *Cell* 1993;74:1089–1100.

198. Verdaguer J, Schmidt D, Amrani A, et al. Spontaneous autoimmune diabetes in monoclonal T cell nonobese diabetic mice. *J Exp Med* 1997;186:1663–1676.

199. Wicker LS, Leiter EH, Todd JA, et al. β2-Microglobulin-deficient NOD mice do not develop insulitis or diabetes. *Diabetes* 1994;43:500–504.

200. Serreze DV, Leiter EH, Christianson GJ, et al. Major histocompatibility complex class I-deficient NOD-B2m^null mice are diabetes and insulitis resistant. *Diabetes* 1994;43:505–509.

201. Christianson SW, Shultz LD, Leiter EH. Adoptive transfer of diabetes into immunodeficient NOD-*scid/scid* mice: relative contributions of CD4+ and CD8+ T-cells from diabetic versus prediabetic NOD.NON-*Thy-1^a* donors. *Diabetes* 1993;42:44–55.

202. Wegmann DR, Norbury-Glaser M, Daniel D. Insulin-specific T cells are a predominant component of islet infiltrates in pre-diabetic NOD mice. *Eur J Immunol* 1994;24:1853–1857.

203. Roep BO, Kallan AA, Hasenbos WL, et al. T-cell reactivity to 38 kD insulin-secretory-granule protein in patients with recent-onset type 1 diabetes. *Lancet* 1991;337:1439–1441.

204. Herold KC, Vezys V, Sun Q, et al. Regulation of cytokine production during development of autoimmune diabetes induced with multiple low doses of streptozotocin. *J Immunol* 1996;156:3521–3527.

205. Zipris D, Greiner D, Malkani S, et al. Cytokine gene expression in islets and thyroids of BB rats, IFN-gamma and IL-12p40 mRNA increase with age in both diabetic and insulin treated nondiabetic BB rats. *J Immunol* 1996;156:1315–1321.

206. Fox CJ, Danska JS. IL-4 expression at the onset of islet inflammation predicts nondestructive insulitis in nonobese diabetic mice. *J Immunol* 1997;158:2414–2424.

207. Katz JD, Benoist C, Mathis D. T helper cell subsets in insulin-dependent diabetes. *Science* 1995;268:1185–1188.

208. Chervonsky AV, Wang Y, Wong FS, et al. The role of Fas in autoimmune diabetes. *Cell* 1997;89:17–24.

209. Kagi D, Odermatt B, Seiler P, et al. Reduced incidence and delayed onset of diabetes in perforin-deficient nonobese diabetic mice. *J Exp Med* 1998;186:989–997.

210. Lenschow DJ, Ho SC, Sattar H, et al. Differential effects of anti-B7-1 and anti-B7-2 monoclonal antibody treatment on the development of diabetes in the nonobese diabetic mouse. *J Exp Med* 1995;181:1145.

211. Lenschow DJ, Herold KC, Rhee L, et al. CD28/B7 regulation of Th1 and Th2 subsets in the development of autoimmune diabetes. *Immunity* 1996;5:285–293.

212. Shulman G, Barrett E, Sherwin RS. Integrated fuel metabolism. In: Porte D Jr, Sherwin RS, eds. *Ellenberg and Rifkin's diabetes mellitus,* 5th ed. Stamford, CT: Appleton & Lange, 1997:1–18.

213. The expert committee on the diagnosis and classification of diabetes mellitus: report of the Expert Committee on the Diagnosis and Classification of Diabetes Mellitus. *Diabetes Care* 1997;20:1183–1197.

214. O'Meara N, Sturis J, Herold KC, et al. Alterations in the patters of insulin secretion before and after diagnosis of IDDM. *Diabetes Care* 1995;18:568–571.

215. The DCCT Research Group. Effects of age, duration and treatment of insulin-dependent diabetes mellitus on residual beta-cell function. *J Clin Endocrinol Metab* 1987;65:30–36.

216. Karjalainen J, Salmela P, Ilonen J, et al. A comparison of childhood and adult type 1 diabetes mellitus. *N Engl J Med* 1989;320:881–886.

217. Madsbad S, Faber O, Binder C, et al. Prevalence of residual beta-cell function in insulin-dependent diabetics in relation to age at onset and duration of diabetes. *Diabetes* 1978;27 [Suppl 1]:262–264.

218. Bhisitkul D, Morrow A, Vinik A, et al. Prevalence of stress hyperglycemia among patients attending a pediatric emergency department. *J Pediatr* 1994;124:547–551.

219. Herskowitz-Dumont R, Wolsdorf J, Jackson R, et al. Distinction between transient hyperglycemia and early insulin-dependent diabetes mellitus in childhood. *J Pediatr* 1993;123:347–354.

220. Shah S, Malone J, Simpson N. A randomized trail of intensive insulin therapy in newly diagnosed insulin-dependent diabetes mellitus. *N Engl J Med* 1989;320:550–554.

221. Bierman K, Albrink M, Arky R. Principles of nutrition and dietary recommendations for patients with diabetes mellitus. 1971;20:633–645.

222. American Diabetes Association. Nutrition recommendations and principles for people with diabetes mellitus. *Diabetes Care* 1996;19 [Suppl 1]:S16–S19.

223. Stone D, Connor W. The prolonged effects of a low-cholesterol, high carbohydrate diet upon serum lipids in diabetic patients. *Diabetes* 1963;12:127–134.

224. Walford S, Allison S, Reeves W. The effects of insulin-antibodies on insulin dose and diabetic control. *Diabetologia* 1982;22:106–110.

225. The Diabetes Control and Complications Trial Research Group. The effects of intensive treatment of diabetes on the development and progression of long-term complications in insulin-dependent diabetes mellitus. *N Engl J Med* 1993;329:977–986.

226. Cryer P. Glucose counterregulation in man. *Diabetes* 1981;30:261.

227. Cryer P, Binder C, Bolli G, et al. Hypoglycemia in IDDM. *Diabetes* 1989;38:1193–1199.

228. Hirsch I, Farkas-Hirsch R, Skyler J. Intensive insulin therapy for treatment of type 1 diabetes. *Diabetes Care* 1990;13:1265–1283.

229. Holleman F, Hoekstra J. Insulin Lispro. *N Engl J Med* 1997;337:176–183.

230. Shi Z, Wasserman D, Vranic M. Metabolic implications of exercise and physical fitness in physiology and diabetes. In: Porte D, Jr., Sherwin RS, eds. *Ellenberg and Rifkin's diabetes mellitus,* 5th ed. Stamford, CT: Appleton & Lange, 1997:653–688.

231. Bunn H, Haney D, Kamin S. The biosynthesis of human hemoglobin A1c. *J Clin Invest* 1976;57:1652–1659.

232. Koenig R, Peterson C, Jones R. Correlation of glucose regulation and hemoglobin A1c. *N Engl J Med* 1976;295:417–420.

233. Stiller CR, Dupré J, Gent M, et al. Effects of cyclosporine immunosuppression in insulin-dependent diabetes mellitus of recent onset. *Science* 1984;223:1362–1367.

234. Bougnères P, Carel JC, Castano L, et al. Factors associated with early remission of type 1 diabetes in children treated with cyclosporine. *N Engl J Med* 1988;318:663–670.

235. Bougnères P, Landais P, Boisson C, et al. Limited duration of remission of insulin dependency in children with recent overt type 1 diabetes treated with low-dose cyclosporin. *Diabetes* 1990;39:1264–1272.

236. Silverstein J, Maclaren N, Riley WJ, et al. Immunosuppression with azathioprine and prednisone in recent-onset insulin-dependent diabetes mellitus. *N Engl J Med* 1988;319:599–604.

237. Sutherland DE. State of the art in pancreas transplantation. *Transpl Proc* 1994;26:316–320.

238. Kendall DM, Rooney DP, Smets YFC, et al. Pancreas transplantation restores epinephrine response and symptom recognition during hypoglycemia in patients with long-standing type 1 diabetes and autonomic neuropathy. *Diabetes* 1997;46:249–257.

239. Bilous RW, Mauer SM, Sutherland DE, et al. The effects of pancreas transplantation on the glomerular structure of renal allografts in patients with insulin-dependent diabetes. *N Engl J Med* 1989;321:80–85.

240. Fioreto P, Steffes MW, Sutherland DE, et al. Reversal of lesions of diabetic nephropathy after pancreas transplantation. *N Engl J Med* 1998;339:69–75.

241. Tydén G, Reinholt FP, Sundkvist G, et al. Recurrence of autoimmune diabetes mellitus in recipients of cadaveric pancreatic grafts. *N Engl J Med* 1996;335:860–863.

242. Pyzdrowski KL, Kendall KM, Halter JB, et al. Preserved insulin secretion and insulin independence in recipients of islet autografts. *N Engl J Med* 1992;327:220–226.

243. Sutherland DE. Pancreas and islet cell transplantation: now and then. *Transpl Proc* 1996;28:2131–2133.

244. Alejandro R, Lehmann R, Ricordi C, et al. Long-term function (6 years) of islet allografts in type 1 diabetes. *Diabetes* 1997;46:1983–1989.

245. Sodoyez J, Sodoyez-Goffaux F, Koch M, et al. Clonally restricted insulin autoantibodies in a cohort of 2200 healthy blood donors. *Diabetologia* 1990;33:719–725.

246. Dozio N, Scavini M, Beretta A, et al. Imaging of the buffering effect of insulin antibodies in the autoimmune hypoglycemic syndrome. *J Clin Endocrinol Metab* 1998;83:643–647.

247. Hirata Y, Ishizu H, Ouchi H, et al. Insulin autoimmunity in a case of spontaneous hypoglycemia. *J Jap Diabetes Soc* 1970;13:312–316.

248. Uchigata Y, Omori Y, Nieda M, et al. HLA-DR4 genotype and insulin-processing in insulin autoimmune syndrome. *Lancet* 1992;340:1467.

249. Uchigata Y, Tokunaga K, Nepom G, et al. Differential immunogenetic determinants of polyclonal insulin autoimmune syndrome (Hirata's disease) and monoclonal insulin autoimmune syndrome. *Diabetes* 1995;44:1227–1232.

250. Goldman J, Baldwin D, Rubenstein A, et al. Characterization of circulating insulin and proinsulin binding antibodies in autoimmune hypoglycemia. *J Clin Invest* 1979;63:1050–1059.

251. Redmon B, Pyzdrowski KL, Elson M, et al. Hypoglycemia due to an insulin-binding monoclonal antibody in multiple myeloma. *N Engl J Med* 1992;326:994–998.

252. Wong S, Ng W, Thai A. Case report: autoimmune insulin syndrome in a Chinese female with Graves' disease. *Ann Acad Med Singapore* 1996;25:882–885.

253. Shah P, Mares D, Fineberg E, et al. Insulin autoimmune syndrome as a cause of spontaneous hypoglycemia in alcoholic cirrhosis. *Gastroenterology* 1995;109:1673–1676.

254. Trenn G, Eysselein V, Mellinghoff V, et al. Clinical and biochemical aspects of the insulin autoimmune syndrome (IAIS). *Klin Wochenschr* 1986;64:929–934.

255. Moller D, Flier J. Insulin resistance: mechanisms, syndromes, and implications. *N Engl J Med* 1991;325:938–948.

256. Taylor SI, Barbetti F, Accili D, et al. Syndromes of autoimmunity and hypoglycemia: autoantibodies directed against insulin and its receptor. *Endocrinol Metab Clin North Am* 1989;18:123–143.

257. Flier J, Bar RS, Muggeo M, et al. The evolving clinical course of patients with insulin receptor autoantibodies: spontaneous remission or receptor proliferation with hypoglycemia. *J Clin Endocrinol Metab* 1978;47:985–995.

258. Schmidt M. Eine biglandulare erkrankung (Nebennieren und schilddrusse) bei morbus Addisonii. *Verh Beutsch Ges Pathol Ges* 1926;21:212–215.

259. Neufeld M, Maclaren N, Blizzard R. Two types of autoimmune Addison's disease associated with different polyglandular autoimmune (PGA) syndromes. *Metabolism* 1981;60:355–362.

260. Muir A, Maclaren N. Autoimmune diseases of the adrenal glands, parathyroid glands, gonads, and hypothalamic-pituitary axis. *Endocrinol Metab Clin North Am* 1991;20:619–644.

261. Ahonen P, Myllarniemi S, Sipila I, Perheentupa J. Clinical variation of autoimmune polyendocrinopathy-candidiasis-ectodermal dystrophy (APECED) in a series of 68 patients. *N Engl J Med* 1990;322: 1829–1836.

262. Baker J. Autoimmune endocrine disease. *JAMA* 1999;278:1931–1937.

263. The Finnish-German APECED Consortium. An autoimmune disease, APECED, caused by mutations in a novel gene featuring two PHD-type zinc-finger domains. *Nat Genet* 1997;17:399–403.

264. Nagamine K, Peterson P, Scot H, et al. Positional cloning of the APECED gene. *Nat Genet* 1997;17:393–398.

265. Betterle C, Volpato M, Greggio A, et al. Type 2 polyglandular autoimmune disease (Schmidt's syndrome). *J Pediatr Endocrinol Metab* 1996;9[Suppl 1]:113–123.

266. Huang W, Connor E, Dela Rosa T, et al. Although DR3-DQB1*0201 may be associated with multiple component diseases of the autoimmune polyglandular syndromes, the human leukocyte antigen DR4-DQB1*0302 haplotype is implicated only in B-cell autoimmunity. *J Clin Endocrinol Metab* 1996;81:2559–2563.

267. Chen S, Sawicka J, Betterle C, et al. Autoantibodies to steroidogenic enzymes in autoimmune polyglandular syndrome, Addison's disease, and premature ovarian failure. *J Clin Endocrinol Metab* 1995;81: 1871–1876.

268. Husebye E, Gebre-Medhin G, Tuomi T, et al. Autoantibodies against aromatic L-amino acid decarboxylase in autoimmune polyendocrine syndrome type 1. *J Clin Endocrinol Metab* 1997;82:147–150.

269. Winqvist O, Gebre-Medhin G, Gustafsson K, et al. Identification of the main gonadal autoantigens in patients with adrenal insufficiency and associated ovarian failure. *J Clin Endocrinol Metab* 1995;80: 1717–1723.

270. Winqvist O, Karlsson F, Kampe O. 21-Hydroxylase, a major autoantigen in idiopathic Addison's disease. *Lancet* 1992;339:1559–1562.

271. Chen S, Sawicka J, Betterle C, et al. Autoantibodies to steroidogenic enzymes in autoimmune polyglandular syndrome, Addison's disease, and premature ovarian failure. *J Clin Endocrinol Metab* 1998;81: 1871–1876.

272. Sakaguchi S, Sakaguchi N. Organ-specific autoimmune disease induced in mice by elimination of T cell subsets. *J Immunol* 1989; 142:471–480.

273. Sakaguchi S, Takahashi T, Nishizuka Y. Study on cellular events in post-thymectomy autoimmune oophoritis in mice. *J Exp Med* 1982; 156:1577–1586.

274. Oelkers W. Adrenal insufficiency. *N Engl J Med* 1996;335: 1206–1212.

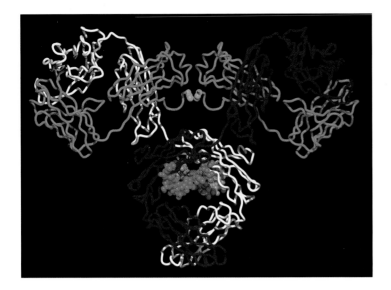

**COLOR PLATE 1.** Ribbon diagram of the x-ray crystallographic structure of the human (Mcg) IgG1 immunoglobulin. One of the heavy chains is represented in magenta and the other in white. Both light chains are in blue. The carbohydrate moieties in the Fc region are denoted as green and orange space-filling spheres. Each heavy chain is folded into four immunoglobulin domains and each light chain into two domains. The antigen-binding sites are positioned at the tips of each arm of the Y-shaped structure and are composed of CDR1, CDR2, and CDR3 loops of the variable portion of the heavy chain and the CDR1, CDR2, and CDR3 loops of the variable portion of the light chain. (Courtesy of Drs. A. Edmundson and P. Ramsland, Oklahoma Medical Research Foundation, Oklahoma City, OK.) See Fig. 2.2 on page 13.

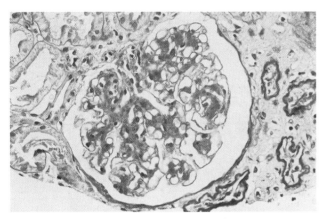

**COLOR PLATE 2.** Diffuse mesangial hypercellularity and an increased mesangial matrix in a case of IgA nephropathy. See Fig. 18.1 on page 325.

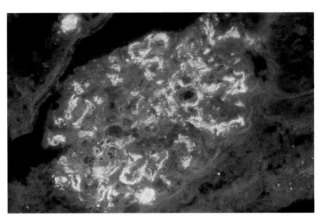

**COLOR PLATE 3.** Immunofluorescence for IgA shows widespread mesangial deposition in a case of IgA nephropathy. See Fig. 18.2 on page 326.

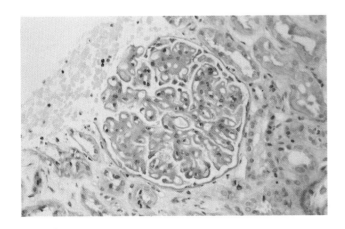

**COLOR PLATE 4.** Membranous nephropathy is characterized by generalized thickening of the glomerular capillary wall but no increase in cellularity. See Fig. 18.3 on page 329.

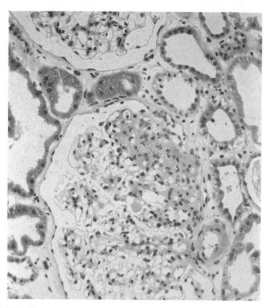

**COLOR PLATE 5.** Focal segmental glomerulosclerosis. A region of sclerosis is present in the upper right quadrant of the glomerulus, with obliteration of capillary lumens. See Fig. 18.5 on page 333.

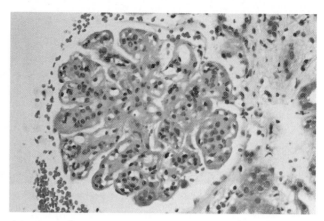

**COLOR PLATE 6.** Mesangiocapillary glomerulonephritis. The glomerulus is hypercellular, with an increased mesangial matrix, and the capillary wall is thickened. See Fig. 18.6 on page 338.

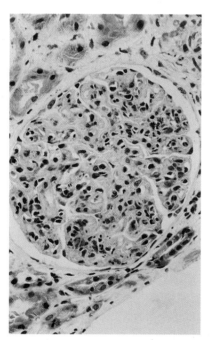

**COLOR PLATE 7.** Poststreptococcal glomerulonephritis. The glomerular tuft is expanded and hypercellular, with mononuclear cells and neutrophils in the capillaries. See Fig. 18.8 on page 342.

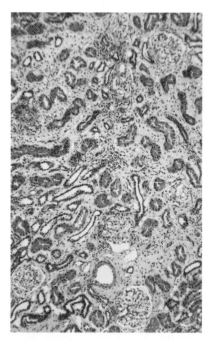

**COLOR PLATE 8.** Tubulointerstitial nephritis. Mononuclear cells diffusely infiltrate the interstitium. See Fig. 18.9 on page 345.

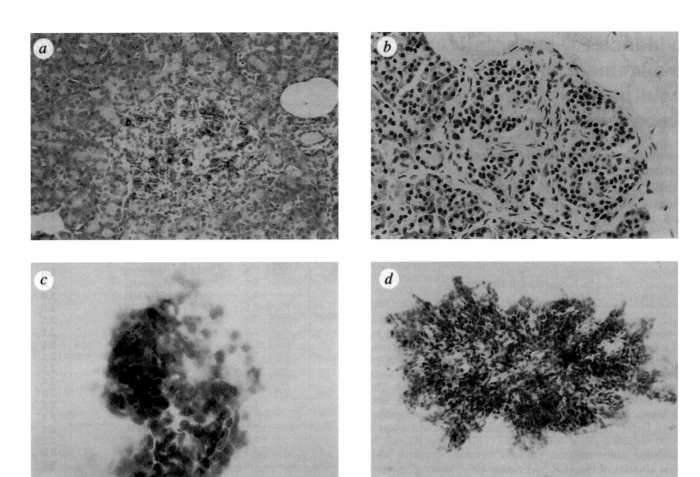

**COLOR PLATE 9.** Insulitis in humans. Pancreas from a 12-year-old boy who died at clinical presentation of T1DM, 1 month after onset of symptoms. **A:** A few insulin-secreting β cells are identified by immunoperoxidase staining (orange-brown). **B:** Some islets had a fibrotic ribbon-like appearance and were partially or totally devoid of insulin-secreting cells. The T-cell infiltrate was abundantly CD4+ **(C)** and scarcely CD8+ **(D)** (From Conrad B, Weldmann E, Trucco G, et al. Evidence for superantigen involvement in insulin-dependent diabetes mellitus aetiology. *Nature* 1994;371:351, with permission.) See Fig. 20.3 on page 394.

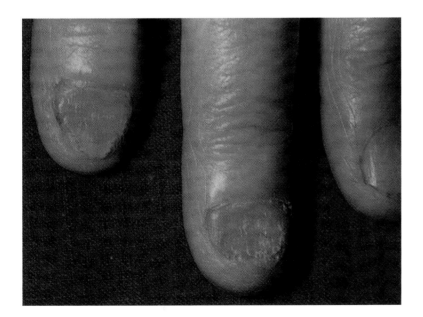

**COLOR PLATE 10.** Mucocutaneous candidiasis. This illustration shows cutaneous candidiasis in a 6-year-old girl who also had mucosal lesions. (From Levene GM, Goodamali SK. *Diagnostic picture tests in dermatology.* London: Wolfe Medical Publications, 1986:106, with permission.) See Fig. 20.4 on page 399.

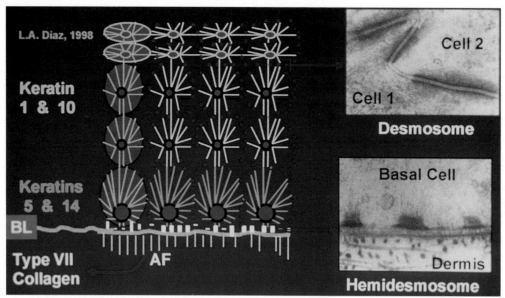

**COLOR PLATE 11.** Diagrammatic representation of the epidermis, the dermoepidermal junction, and the dermis. Shown are the structures relevant in the pathogenesis of blister formation. The epidermis is primarily made up of keratinocytes that, at the level of the basal cell layer, contain keratins 5 and 14 as part of their cytoskeleton. Above the basal cell layer, keratinocytes express keratins 1 and 10. Individual keratinocytes are attached to each other by organelles called *desmosomes* that are shown as red dots at the cell–cell junctions. The upper right panel is an electron micrograph showing the ultrastructure of the desmosome. The intracytoplasmic desmosomal plaque, which appears as two dark parallel bands, functions as the membrane attachment site for the keratin filaments. The desmosomal core is contiguous with the epidermal ICS. The hemidesmosome, shown in the electron micrograph in the lower right panel and diagrammatically as white rectangles in the lower pole of the basal cell, are organelles that anchor the keratinocyte to the basement membrane. Similar to the desmosome, the hemidesmosome contains an intracytoplasmic electron-dense plaque that attaches the keratin filaments to the plasma membrane. Below the basement membrane are the anchoring fibers (AF), which are composed of collagen VII. Components of the desmosome are targeted by the immune system in patients with pemphigus vulgaris, pemphigus foliaceus, and paraneoplastic pemphigus; whereas, antigens associated with the hemidesmosome are the major targets of autoantibodies produced by patients with bullous pemphigoid, herpes gestationis, cicatricial pemphigoid, and linear immunoglobulin A disease. See Fig. 21.1 on page 408.

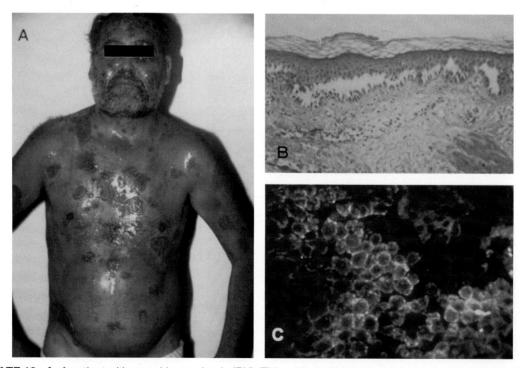

**COLOR PLATE 12.  A:** A patient with pemphigus vulgaris (PV). This patient exhibits the typical superficial blisters that, after erosion, leave large areas of denuded skin. Similar lesions are observed in the oral cavity. **B:** Histologic examination of the skin of patients with PV shows classic intraepidermal blisters, which form as a result of cell–cell detachment in the layer immediately above the basal keratinocytes. The basal cells remain attached to the dermis, producing the "tombstone" appearance. **C:** Direct immunofluorescence of lesional epidermis in patients with PV shows the typical surface staining of keratinocytes. The same autoantibodies can be detected in the serum, producing titers that roughly correlate with the activity and extent of the disease. See Fig. 21.2 on page 409.

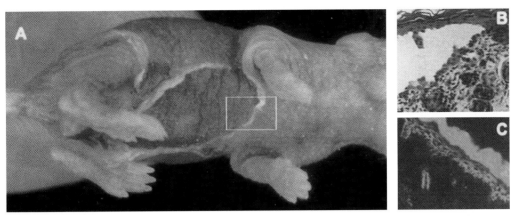

**COLOR PLATE 13.** The mouse model of pemphigus vulgaris (PV) was developed in 1982. In these studies, immunoglobulin G purified from the sera of patients with active PV was injected intraperitoneally into neonatal BALB/c mice. **A:** These animals developed superficial blisters and erosions within 24 hours after injection. **B:** Histologic examination of these lesions shows classic suprabasilar acantholysis. **C:** Direct immunofluorescence of perilesional skin of these animals shows human autoantibodies bound to the surface of keratinocytes. These passive transfer studies demonstrated for the first time that pemphigus autoantibodies are indeed pathogenic. See Fig. 21.3 on page 411.

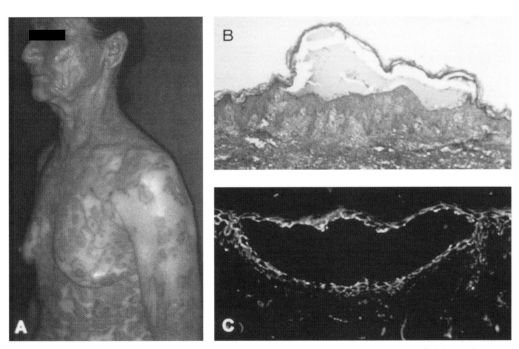

**COLOR PLATE 14.** Pemphigus foliaceus (PF). **A:** The distribution of superficial erosions and blisters in a patient with endemic PF (fogo selvagem). **B:** Histologic examination of skin lesions in PF shows a typical subcorneal vesicle that is formed as a result of detachment of keratinocytes in the upper layers of the epidermis. **C:** Direct IF of a skin biopsy from a patient with PF shows immunoglobulin G (IgG) autoantibodies bound to the surface of keratinocytes. This biopsy also shows an intraepidermal blister cavity. The serum of PF patients contains antiepidermal autoantibodies in titers that roughly correlate to activity and extent of disease. The autoantibodies belong to the IgG class and are predominantly of the IgG4 subclass. See Fig. 21.4 on page 414.

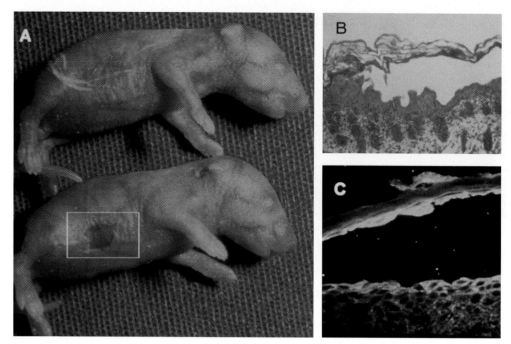

**COLOR PLATE 15.** The mouse model of pemphigus foliaceus (PF) was developed in 1985. Neonatal BALB/c mice were passively transferred with the IgG fraction from the sera of patients with either the endemic or nonendemic forms of PF. **A:** The injected animals developed superficial blisters and erosions. **B:** A biopsy taken from lesional skin of these animals shows subcorneal vesicles. **C:** Direct immunofluorescence of the skin lesions shows human autoantibodies bound to the surface of keratinocytes. A subcorneal vesicle is also observed. This study provided direct evidence that the autoantibodies in endemic and nonendemic PF are pathogenic. See Fig. 21.5 on page 415.

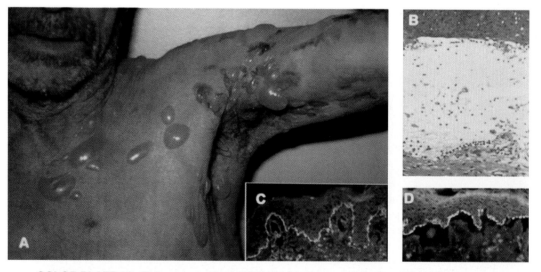

**COLOR PLATE 16.** Bullous pemphigoid (BP). **A:** A bullous eruption located on flexure areas of the skin is observed in typical cases of BP. These vesicobullous lesions are tense, and Nikolsky's sign is negative. **B:** Histologic examination of a biopsy taken from a BP lesion shows a typical subepidermal blister. **C:** Direct immunofluorescence (IF) analysis of perilesional skin shows linear deposition of immunoglobulin G at the dermoepidermal junction. Most BP patients also show C3 bound to the dermoepidermal junction. **D:** Indirect IF performed on salt split skin shows binding of BP autoantibodies to the roof of the split. This finding is typical of BP. The autoantibodies in BP are directed against hemidesmosomal antigens. See Fig. 21.6 on page 416.

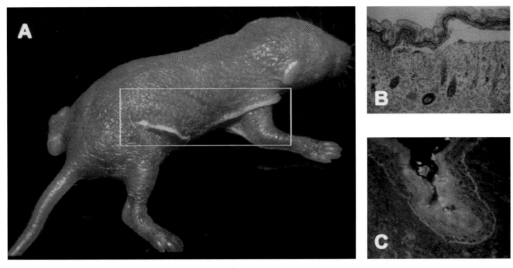

**COLOR PLATE 17.** The animal model of BP was developed in 1993. **A:** Rabbits were immunized with recombinant forms of murine BP180. The immunoglobulin G fraction from this rabbit antimurine BP180 antigen was passively transferred into neonatal BALB/c mice by either an intraperitoneal or subcutaneous route. Neonatal mice injected with this antibody develop a blistering eruption within 24 hours. **B:** Skin biopsy samples taken from lesional skin in these animals show typical subepidermal blistering with an intense neutrophilic infiltrate in the upper dermis. **C:** Direct immunofluorescence studies of perilesional skin of these animals show rabbit anti-BP180 antibodies bound in a linear fashion to the dermoepidermal junction. Blister formation in these animal models is dependent on complement activation and neutrophilic infiltration. See Fig. 21.7 on page 418.

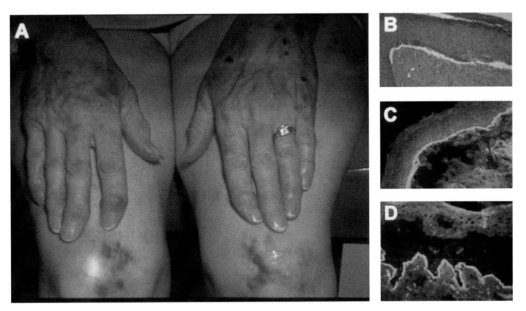

**COLOR PLATE 18.** Epidermolysis bullosa acquisita (EBA). **A:** Classic blistering eruption in a patient with EBA. The blisters are located on sites of trauma; in this case, the knees and knuckles. **B:** Histologic examination of a skin biopsy shows a subepidermal blister. **C:** Direct immunofluorescence (IF) studies of perilesional skin of these patients show a thick linear staining of the dermoepidermal junction. **D:** Indirect IF analysis performed on salt split skin shows autoantibodies bound to the floor of the split. EBA autoantibodies bind collagen type VII. See Fig. 21.8 on page 422.

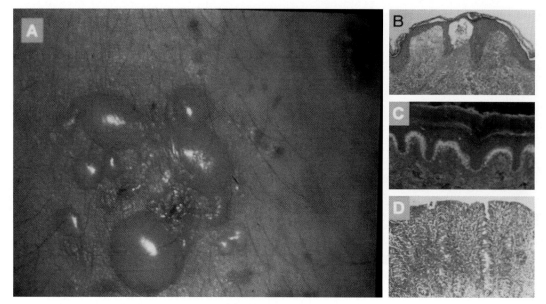

**COLOR PLATE 19.** Dermatitis herpetiformis (DH). **A:** This pruritic blistering disorder is characterized by clusters of herpetic-like blisters located on extensor surfaces of the body. **B:** Histologic examination of a skin lesion shows typical subepidermal blisters with collections of neutrophils at the tips of the dermal papillae. **C:** Typically, patients with DH show a granular deposition of immunoglobulin A along the dermoepidermal junction. **D:** Most patients with DH show an associated villus atrophy of the intestinal mucosa. These features link DH to gluten sensitive enteropathy (GSE). In GSE, however, patients do not have any skin lesions. The common feature between DH and GSE is that both diseases respond to a gluten-free diet. At present, the immunopathologic mechanisms responsible for blister formation in DH are unknown. See Fig. 21.9 on page 423.

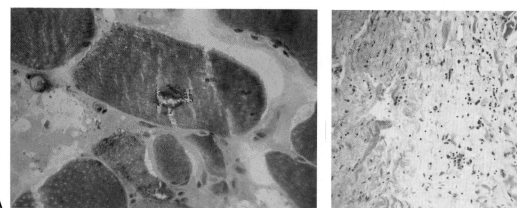
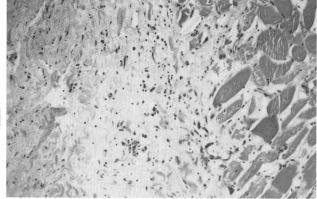

**COLOR PLATE 20.** Histopathology of inflammatory myopathies. **A:** Inclusion body myositis (trichrome stain), demonstrating rimmed vacuoles within two myofibers (Courtesy of Drs. Frederick Miller and Lori Love). See Fig. 22.1C on page 433. **B:** Eosinophilic myositis: endomysial eosinophilic infiltration of myofibers from a patient with eosinophilia myalgia syndrome (Courtesy of Dr. Lori Love). See Fig. 22.1F on page 433.

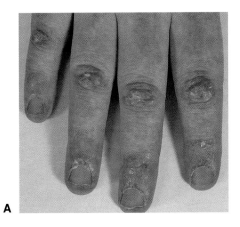

A

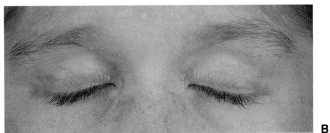

B

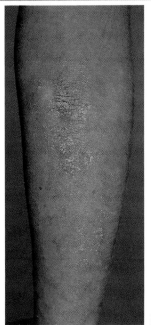

D

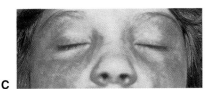

C

**COLOR PLATE 21.** Cutaneous manifestations of juvenile dermatomyositis. **A:** Gottron's papules over the extensor surfaces of the hands, with periungual erythema and cuticular overgrowth, and periungual nail-fold capillary abnormalities. See Fig. 22.3A on page 444. **B:** Heliotrope rash over the eyelids, which is characteristic of dermatomyositis. See Fig. 22.3B on page 444. **C:** Heliotrope over the eyelids with associated periorbital edema and malar erythema sparing the nasolabial fold. (Courtesy of Dr. David Sherry.) See Fig. 22.3C on page 444. **D:** Linear extensor erythema on the extensor tendons of the forearm. See Fig. 22.3D on page 444.

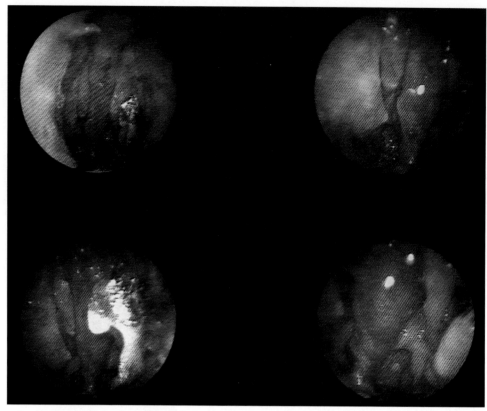

**COLOR PLATE 22.** Intranasal view of massive necrosis and atrophic rhinitis in a patient with Wegener's granulomatosis. See Fig. 24.1 on page 502.

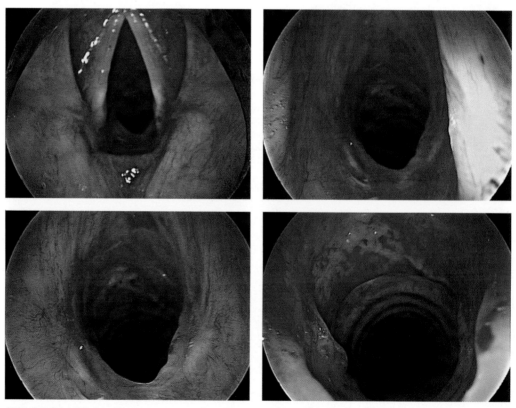

**COLOR PLATE 23.** Moderate subglottic stenosis without significant inflammation in a 17-year-old girl with Wegener's granulomatosis. See Fig. 24.2 on page 503.

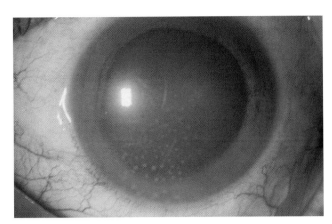

**COLOR PLATE 24.** Keratic precipitates in the inferior half of the cornea. See Fig. 25.2 on page 522.

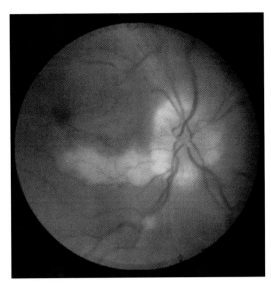

**COLOR PLATE 25.** Sheathing in a major retinal vessel. See Fig. 25.6 on page 528.

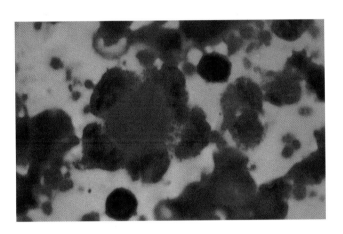

**COLOR PLATE 26.** The lupus erythematosus (LE) cell has phagocytosed several other cell nuclei coated with autoantibody. It was the first indication of autoimmunity. See Fig. 26.1 on page 539.

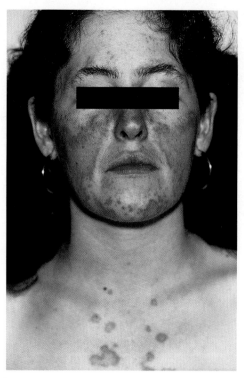

**COLOR PLATE 27.** Female patient with a malar rash. See Fig. 26.2 on page 541.

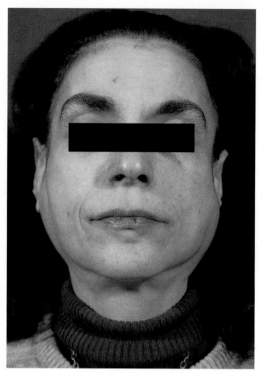

**COLOR PLATE 28.** A patient with parotid enlargement as a result of primary Sjögren's syndrome. See Fig. 29.1 on page 572.

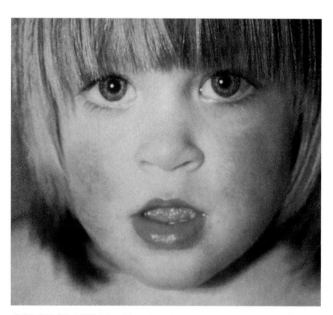

**COLOR PLATE 29.** Classic "slapped cheeks" of a child with erythema infectiosum, or fifth disease, caused by parvovirus B19. A lacy macular erythematous eruption is also present on the trunk but is not in focus. (From Feder HM Jr. Fifth disease. *N Engl J Med* 1994;331:1062, with permission.) See Fig. 37.1 on page 694.

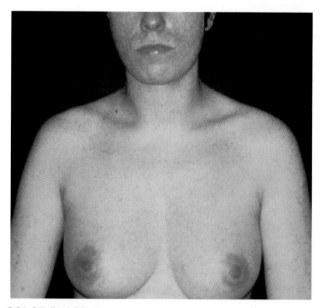

**COLOR PLATE 30.** The morbilliform rash of rubella infection. (From Naides SJ. Viral arthritis. In: Klippel JH, Dieppe PA, eds. *Rheumatology.* 2nd ed. London: CV Mosby, 1998:6.6.3.) See Fig. 37.2 on page 696.

*Textbook of the Autoimmune Diseases,*
Edited by R. G. Lahita, N. Chiorazzi, and W. H. Reeves,
Lippincott Williams & Wilkins, Philadelphia © 2000.

# CHAPTER 21

# Autoimmune Diseases of the Skin

Manish J. Gharia, Janet A. Fairley, Mong-Shang Lin, Zhi Liu,
George J. Giudice, and Luis A. Diaz

Blistering of the skin is a striking sign of disease that has long drawn the attention of clinicians and researchers. This sign of cutaneous injury is the hallmark of a group of autoantibody-mediated diseases of the skin that includes pemphigus vulgaris (PV), pemphigus foliaceus (PF), and bullous pemphigoid (BP). Blister formation, however, is not a pathognomonic sign of autoimmunity because it can also be observed in genodermatoses, in which the immune system does not play a relevant role. It is also important to recognize that other dermatologic disorders, such as contact dermatitis, infectious processes, (e.g., herpes simplex virus, varicella zoster virus), or skin necrosis, can also lead to vesicle and bullae formation. In these conditions, blister formation is a secondary event, thereby differentiating this latter group from the autoimmune bullous disorders.

## OVERVIEW

To provide a basis for understanding the mechanisms of autoimmune blister formation, we include in this chapter a brief overview of the cutaneous molecular structures that are involved in the pathogenesis of the diseases that are described in detail later in this chapter.

### Cutaneous Molecular Structures Relevant to Blister Formation

The epidermis is a stratified epithelium made up predominantly of keratinocytes. The basal cell layer overlies the der-

mis and is separated from it by a basement membrane. The stratum spinosum is composed of several cell layers of differentiating keratinocytes located above the basal layer. Above the stratum spinosum is the granular layer, which is composed of flattened cells containing inclusions called *keratohyaline granules*. The stratum corneum is the outermost, anucleate cell layer of the epidermis and provides the major barrier function of the skin.

As shown in Fig. 21.1, keratinocytes of all epidermal layers possess a cytoskeleton made of keratin intermediate filaments that link the nucleus with organelles of the cell periphery, that is, the desmosomes and hemidesmosomes. The intermediate filaments of the basal cell layer are composed of keratins 5 and 14, whereas those of the suprabasal cells are made up of keratins 1 and 10. The desmosome is an adhesive organelle that attaches neighboring keratinocytes; the hemidesmosome functions in anchoring the basal cell to the basement membrane. Two cells form the desmosome, each providing an identical half of this organelle. The structure thus formed contains two parallel intracellular plaques, into which the keratin filaments insert, and the desmosomal core, which spans the narrow epidermal intercellular space (ICS). The molecular components of the desmosome have been well defined and include the proteins of the plaque, such as desmoplakins 1 and 2, plakoglobin, envoplakin, plakophilin, and keratocalmin. The desmosomal core contains transmembrane glycoproteins that belong to the cadherin family of cell adhesion molecules. These desmosomal cadherins include desmoglein 1 (Dsg-1), 2, and 3 and desmocollins 1, 2, and 3. The desmogleins and desmocollins possess an extracellular domain that is involved in homophilic adhesive interactions with molecules of neighboring cells.

The hemidesmosome is an organelle that attaches basal cells to the dermis. The hemidesmosome comprises a bilayered intracellular plaque, which is the site of insertion of keratin filaments. The hemidesmosomal plaque contains one of the major BP antigens, named BP230 (BPAg1), and plectin. The transmembrane components of the hemidesmosome in-

M. J. Gharia: Department of Dermatology, Medical College of Wisconsin, Milwaukee, Wisconsin 53226; Department of Dermatology, Froedtert Memorial Lutheran Hospital, Milwaukee, Wisconsin 53226.

J. A. Fairley: Department of Dermatology, Medical College of Wisconsin, Milwaukee, Wisconsin 53226; Department of Dermatology, Zablocki VA Medical Center, Milwaukee Wisconsin 53226.

M.-S. Lin and L. A. Diaz: Department of Dermatology, University of North Carolina at Chapel Hill, Chapel Hill, North Carolina 27599.

Z. Liu: Department of Dermatology, Medical College of Wisconsin, Milwaukee, Wisconsin 53226.

G. J. Giudice: Departments of Dermatology and Biochemistry, Medical College of Wisconsin, Milwaukee, Wisconsin 53226.

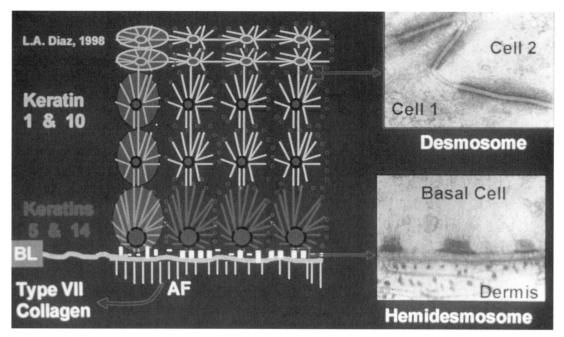

**FIG. 21.1.** Diagrammatic representation of the epidermis, the dermoepidermal junction, and the dermis. Shown are the structures relevant in the pathogenesis of blister formation. The epidermis is primarily made up of keratinocytes that, at the level of the basal cell layer, contain keratins 5 and 14 as part of their cytoskeleton. Above the basal cell layer, keratinocytes express keratins 1 and 10. Individual keratinocytes are attached to each other by organelles called *desmosomes* that are shown as red dots at the cell–cell junctions. The upper right panel is an electron micrograph showing the ultrastructure of the desmosome. The intracytoplasmic desmosomal plaque, which appears as two dark parallel bands, functions as the membrane attachment site for the keratin filaments. The desmosomal core is contiguous with the epidermal ICS. The hemidesmosome, shown in the electron micrograph in the lower right panel and diagrammatically as white rectangles in the lower pole of the basal cell, are organelles that anchor the keratinocyte to the basement membrane. Similar to the desmosome, the hemidesmosome contains an intracytoplasmic electron-dense plaque that attaches the keratin filaments to the plasma membrane. Below the basement membrane are the anchoring fibers (AF), which are composed of collagen VII. Components of the desmosome are targeted by the immune system in patients with pemphigus vulgaris, pemphigus foliaceus, and paraneoplastic pemphigus; whereas, antigens associated with the hemidesmosome are the major targets of autoantibodies produced by patients with bullous pemphigoid, herpes gestationis, cicatricial pemphigoid, and linear immunoglobulin A disease. See color plate 11.

clude a second BP antigen, named BP180 (BPAg2 or collagen XVII), and the $\alpha_6\beta_4$ integrin. Anchoring fibers, made up of collagen VII, are located in the papillary dermis, subjacent to the hemidesmosome. Other molecules of the dermoepidermal junction that are relevant in the pathogenesis of blister formation are the laminin isoforms that are localized in the lamina lucida.

## Dual Mechanisms of Blister Formation: Genetic and Autoimmune

Advances in elucidating the mechanisms of disease in a variety of genetic and autoimmune blistering disorders have been impressive. The cloning of cutaneous structural molecules has been facilitated by the use of autoantibodies from patients with autoimmune blistering disorders. Similarly, sequence analysis of cutaneous antigens has facilitated the studies on the mechanisms of blister formation in several autoimmune diseases mediated by autoantibodies, such as mapping of epitopes recognized by patients' autoantibodies and T cells.

Interestingly, for many structural proteins of the skin, mutations lead to bullous genodermatoses, whereas sensitization to these same proteins later in life results in acquired autoimmune bullous disorders. An example of this is mutation in and autoimmunity to BP180 (collagen XVII). Mutations in BP180 lead to a junctional form of epidermolysis bullosa termed *generalized atrophic benign epidermolysis bullosa,* which results in blistering and erosions of the skin. Acquired autoimmunity to the same protein results in the autoimmune blistering disorder of BP. A similar situation is true for type VII collagen (mutation: dystrophic epidermolysis bullosa; autoimmunity: acquired epidermolysis bullosa) and laminin 5 (mutation: junctional epidermolysis bullosa; autoimmunity: antiepiligrin cicatricial pemphigoid [CP]). In contrast, although mutations in the keratins lead to bullous genodermatoses (epidermolytic hyperkeratosis: mutation of keratin 1 or 10; epidermolysis bullosa simplex: mutation of keratin 5 or 14), no autoimmune disorders to keratins have been described. Likewise, there are certain autoimmune disorders in which no human mutations of the involved antigen have yet been described. The diseases in this group include PV (Dsg-3 antigen) and PF (Dsg-1 antigen).

## Cutaneous Autoimmune Diseases

The cutaneous autoimmune disorders can be divided into two categories: organ-specific and non–organ-specific. The autoimmune bullous disorders are prototypical organ-specific autoimmune diseases. In these diseases, immunologic injury of the skin leads to the loss of integrity of this organ, which is manifested as blister formation. In the non–organ-specific autoimmune diseases, the skin is one of many immunologic targets. Systemic lupus erythematosus (SLE), a disease that may show prominent skin involvement, is an example of a non–organ-specific autoimmune disease.

The focus of this chapter is to describe the diseases of the skin in which there is strong evidence that the disorders are autoimmune in nature. We describe the clinical and histologic presentation as well as the pathogenic mechanisms that may be operating in each disease. Included are mechanisms of autoimmune injury of the skin, the cellular mechanisms of autoantibody formation, and the possible etiologic agents.

## PEMPHIGUS VULGARIS

### Disease Description

PV is an autoimmune blistering disease characterized by flaccid bullae appearing on normal skin and mucosae (1). Hippocrates coined the term *pemphigoid fever* nearly 2400 years ago to describe the disease, but it was not until 1760 that De-Sauvages used the term *pemphigus* to describe a chronic blistering disorder. The nomenclature of PV was introduced by the Austrian Von Hebra in the mid-1800s. The classic intraepidermal vesicles of PV, the hallmark of this disease, were clearly defined by Civatte in 1943 (2). Finally, in 1964, Beutner and Jordon found that PV patients possess antiepidermal autoantibodies by immunofluorescence (IF) techniques (3).

PV may occur at any age but most commonly presents in the fourth to sixth decades of life. It is a rare disease with worldwide incidence rates reported between 1 and 5 cases per 100,000 per year in the general population. PV is the most common and most severe form of pemphigus in the United States, constituting more than 80% of the reported cases (4–6).

The disease is clinically characterized by flaccid, extremely fragile, noninflammatory bullae that generally arise on normal-appearing skin (Fig. 21.2A). These lesions tend to coalesce and rupture, resulting in large denuded areas of skin

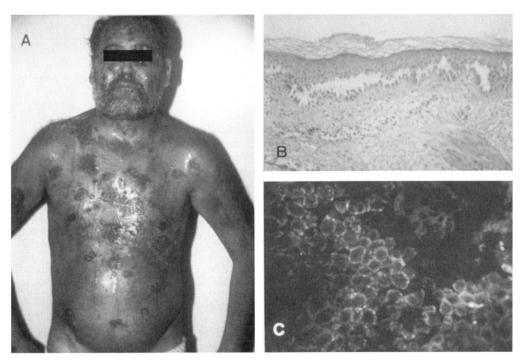

**FIG. 21.2. A:** A patient with pemphigus vulgaris (PV). This patient exhibits the typical superficial blisters that, after erosion, leave large areas of denuded skin. Similar lesions are observed in the oral cavity. **B:** Histologic examination of the skin of patients with PV shows classic intraepidermal blisters, which form as a result of cell–cell detachment in the layer immediately above the basal keratinocytes. The basal cells remain attached to the dermis, producing the "tombstone" appearance. **C:** Direct immunofluorescence of lesional epidermis in patients with PV shows the typical surface staining of keratinocytes. The same autoantibodies can be detected in the serum, producing titers that roughly correlate with the activity and extent of the disease. See color plate 12.

that often heal poorly. Healing occurs without scarring, although postinflammatory hyperpigmentation may be present. When friction or pressure is applied to perilesional skin, the epidermis is easily separated from the underlying dermis (Nikolsky's sign) (1). About 50% to 60% of patients present initially with lesions confined to the oral mucosa, although any surface with squamous epithelial tissue, such as the nasal, esophageal, and rectal mucosae or the conjunctiva, may be involved. Although some cases remain localized to the mucosa, PV generally progresses over a period of months to involve the glabrous skin. Lesions can be localized to areas such as the face, neck, axilla, and groin, or they may be generalized. About 10% to 15% of patients initially present with only skin lesions, but most of these patients go on to develop mucous membrane involvement (7).

The clinical differential diagnosis of PV with oral involvement includes BP, erosive lichen planus, erythema multiforme, paraneoplastic pemphigus, SLE, Behçet's disease, herpes simplex stomatitis, and aphthous stomatitis.

## Pathology

Detachment of epidermal cells, termed *acantholysis,* which leads to intraepidermal blister formation is the histopathologic hallmark of all forms of pemphigus (Fig. 21.2B). In PV, this process tends to be localized just above the basal cell layer of the epidermis. The earliest change seen by light microscopy is intercellular edema that gradually increases to produce widening of the epidermal ICS and progression to frank cell–cell detachment. The suprabasal acantholysis in PV occurs between the basal and spinous layers of the epidermis. The basal cells remain attached to the dermis but are detached laterally, producing an appearance described as a "row of tombstones" (1,2). At the ultrastructural level, the epidermal changes seen in PV include dissolution of the desmosomal plaque and perinuclear retraction of the tonofilaments (8,9).

Inflammation is absent in early lesions of PV; however, in rare cases, spongiosis associated with a dermal infiltrate of eosinophils (eosinophilic spongiosis) can precede the appearance of blisters (10). As bullae develop, a cellular infiltrate made up primarily of eosinophils can be observed around the upper dermal vessels, between the basal cells, and within the blister cavities. In older lesions, a mixed inflammatory infiltrate of plasma cells and eosinophils is often seen. The eosinophilic infiltration that occurs in PV lesions is not fully explained.

## Autoimmune Features

### Humoral Immune Response

The classic "honeycomb" staining pattern of the epidermal ICS produced by PV autoantibodies by indirect IF on stratified epithelium substrates was first described by Beutner and Jordon in 1964 (3). They also noted that these antiepidermal autoantibodies were detected bound to the ICS of perilesional

epidermis by direct IF (Fig. 21.2C). Thus, these studies provided the first evidence that PV autoantibodies may be involved in the pathogenesis of PV.

Several key clinical and experimental findings indicate that PV autoantibodies are pathogenic. These include the consistent demonstration by direct IF of PV autoantibodies bound to the epidermal ICS of lesional and perilesional skin of patients (11); the general correlation between autoantibody titers in patients' sera and disease severity; the presence of a neonatal form of PV in neonates born to mothers with PV, probably resulting from passive transfer of maternal autoantibody to the baby (12–14); and the demonstration that PV autoantibodies induce cell detachment, *in vitro* in skin organ cultures (15–17) and primary epidermal cell cultures (18,19) and *in vivo* by passive transfer of PV immunoglobulin G (IgG) into experimental animals (20).

The strongest evidence that PV autoantibodies were indeed pathogenic was provided by the development of the mouse model of PV (20) (Fig. 21.3). In this experimental mouse model, purified IgG from the sera of PV patients, when given in sufficient doses by intradermal or intraperitoneal injections, induces an epidermal disease in neonatal BALB/c mice that duplicates the human counterpart clinically, histologically, and immunologically. Effective doses of PV IgG trigger blisters and erosions in these animals within 24 hours after the injection. The severity of the disease depends on the total dose of IgG administered, which, in turn, affects the titer of the autoantibodies detected in the mouse serum by indirect IF. The ultrastructural changes in the epidermis of these mice, such as early widening of the ICS, splitting of desmosomes with perinuclear retraction of tonofilaments, and intact basal cell–dermis attachment, duplicated those reported in human PV (21). These studies convincingly demonstrate the pathogenic role of PV autoantibodies in the development of epidermal lesions of PV.

After the pathogenicity of the PV autoantibodies had been demonstrated, efforts were made to identify the epidermal antigens recognized by these autoantibodies. Stanley et al. (22) demonstrated that one third of PV patients' sera recognize a 130-kd glycoprotein from epidermal extracts by immunoblotting techniques. Similarly, using more sensitive immunoprecipitation techniques, they showed that most PV sera recognized the 130-kd antigen. The PV antigen was later shown to be a desmosomal glycoprotein. Amagai et al. (23) further extended their studies on the 130-kd PV antigen by cloning the cDNA from a keratinocyte cDNA expression library. Sequence analysis revealed that the PV antigen belonged to a unique subgroup of the cadherin family of $Ca^{2+}$-dependent cell adhesion molecules. This subfamily, also known as *desmosomal cadherins,* includes Dsg-1, Dsg-2, and Dsg-3 and the desmocollins.

Dsg-3 is the antigen recognized by PV autoantibodies, whereas Dsg-1 is the PF antigen. Both Dsg-1 and Dsg-3 are transmembrane desmosomal core glycoproteins (24). The epitopes recognized by PV autoantibodies on Dsg-3 are located on the ectodomain of this molecule (25–27) and are

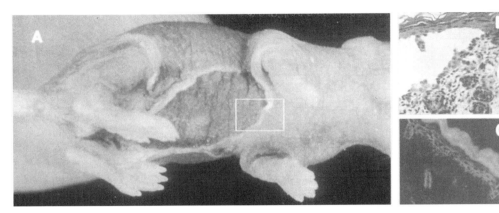

**FIG. 21.3.** The mouse model of pemphigus vulgaris (PV) was developed in 1982. In these studies, immunoglobulin G purified from the sera of patients with active PV was injected intraperitoneally into neonatal BALB/c mice. **A:** These animals developed superficial blisters and erosions within 24 hours after injection. **B:** Histologic examination of these lesions shows classic suprabasilar acantholysis. **C:** Direct immunofluorescence of perilesional skin of these animals shows human autoantibodies bound to the surface of keratinocytes. These passive transfer studies demonstrated for the first time that pemphigus autoantibodies are indeed pathogenic. See color plate 13.

conformational and calcium dependent (28). This was demonstrated by affinity chromatography procedures in which the ectodomain of Dsg-3 that was generated in the baculovirus expression system was immobilized and used to remove anti–Dsg-3 autoantibodies from PV serum. The affinity-purified PV autoantibodies were shown to be pathogenic by passive transfer experiments in the mouse model (26,27). These findings demonstrated that the pathogenic PV autoantibodies are directed against the ectodomain of Dsg-3.

### Genetic Features

Genetic factors appear to play an important role in the development of PV. PV occurs in all ethnic and racial groups, but the disease frequency is higher in those patients with a Jewish background. HLA-A26, HLA-B38, SC21, and HLA-DR4 have been detected in Ashkenazi Jews with PV, whereas HLA-DRw6 was found in non-Ashkenazi Jews. These markers were present in greater than 95% of PV patients (29–31). It was reported that 92% of Ashkenazi Jewish PV patients expressed the HLA-DR4 and HLA-DQw3 haplotype (most were HLA-DR4 and HLA-DQw8 positive) (32). From these patients, 75% expressed the extended haplotypes: HLA-B38, SC21, DR4 and HLA-B35, SC31, DR4. A potential susceptibility gene was mapped to the DR4, DQw8 region and appears to be inherited as a dominant trait.

Other studies (33–35) appear to confirm the relevance of HLA alleles in the Dsg-3 presentation to T-cell clones by antigen-presenting cells. These results indicate that the expression of certain HLA-DR alleles in PV patients may relate to the activation of autoimmune T lymphocytes. It is possible that antigen-presenting cells of patients expressing these HLA genetic types are likely to present Dsg-3 breakdown fragments to self-reactive T cells. These activated auto-

immune T cells may further regulate the production of anti–Dsg-3 autoantibodies.

Yamashina et al. (36,37) reported that Japanese PV patients expressed HLA-DRB1*0406 and HLA-DRB1*1401 as two dominant major histocompatibility complex (MHC) class II alleles in the development of this disease. This result, although different from previous reports, further suggests that different ethnic groups of PV patients may use other MHC class II alleles as genetic predisposition factors for this autoimmune disease.

### Cellular Immune Response

Although the relevance of anti–Dsg-3 autoantibodies in PV has been well defined, the cellular mechanisms involved in autoantibody formation, that is, T-cell and B-cell interactions, are mostly unknown. It is known that antibody production by B cells requires the participation of T-helper ($T_H$) cells in T-cell–dependent antibody responses. During an antigen-driven activation of T cells, they are induced to secrete lymphokines that are crucial in antibody production and immunoglobulin isotype switching by B cells. Because PV is an autoimmune disease mediated by autoantibodies, it is postulated that T lymphocytes participate in the pathogenesis of this disorder in the stages leading to the production of pathogenic autoantibodies.

Some preliminary *in vitro* studies have demonstrated decreased interleukin production and decreased interleukin receptor expression in phytohemagglutinin-stimulated peripheral blood lymphocytes from PV patients (38). There was also some correlation between this observed abnormality in lymphocyte function and the autoantibody titers and disease severity in these study patients. These findings led the investigators to hypothesize that PV patients may have a defect in the secretion of interleukin-2 (IL-2) and the expression of the receptor, resulting in excessive suppressor activity of either monocytes or T cells. Alternatively, it has been proposed that because suppressor T cells are thought to play an accessory role in the suppression of autoreactive B cells, a defect in suppressor T-cell function might account in part for defective cell-mediated immunity of autoantibody production in PV patients (39).

Wucherpfennig et al. (33) have shown that T cells from PV patients proliferate when stimulated with several Dsg-3 peptides. In these studies, the immunoreactive Dsg-3 peptides were predicted by their affinity to the region of the hypervariable of the β chain of the MHC class II alleles frequently found in PV patients, that is, HLA-DRB1*0402 and DRB1*1401. These investigators found that the Dsg-3 peptide comprising residues 190 to 204 has the strongest stimulatory effect on PV T cells. These epitope-specific T cells secreted IL-4 and IL-10, two key $T_H2$ cytokines found in $T_H2$-type immune responses.

Our own studies (34) have demonstrated that autoimmune T cells from PV patients specifically respond to three peptides covering different regions of the extracellular domains of Dsg-3, providing further evidence that self-reactive T cells play a role in the initiation of this disease. The T-cell autoimmune responses to these three immunoreactive Dsg-3 segments are specific to PV patients because T cells obtained from other patient groups, such as BP, psoriasis, SLE, epidermolysis bullosa acquisita (EBA) patients, as well as healthy subjects, do not react with these Dsg-3 peptides. Furthermore, in this study, we clearly showed that the Dsg-3–responsive T cells are of the $CD4^+$ T-cell lineage. Although $CD8^+$ T cells isolated from these PV patients proliferated to mitogen and IL-2, they remained unresponsive to these Dsg-3 peptides. Moreover, Dsg-3–specific T-cell lines and clones developed from these PV patients were shown to express a $CD4^+$ memory T-cell phenotype. On stimulation, these cell lines and clones secreted a $T_H2$-like cytokine profile. It is hypothesized that the $T_H2$-like cytokine profile produced by autoimmune PV T lymphocytes may modulate the secretion of IgG4 anti–Dsg-3 antibodies. Interestingly, we found that the Dsg-3 T-cell responses are restricted to HLA-DR, but not to HLA-DQ or HLA-DP, of the MHC class II molecules.

### Mechanisms of Pemphigus Vulgaris Acantholysis

The molecular mechanisms involved in the induction of epidermal injury by PV autoantibodies are still somewhat unclear. Although direct binding of PV autoantibodies to Dsg-3 may interfere with its function and thereby cause acantholysis, investigators have also proposed roles for complement and proteases in the development of PV lesions. It is well documented that C3, as well as C1q, C4, factor B, and properdin, are detected in the same epidermal areas where PV autoantibodies are bound (40). Most studies, however, indicate that although complement may enhance blister formation in PV, it is not necessary for lesion development. Both F(ab')2 and the Fab fragments of PV IgG are capable of inducing typical acantholytic lesions in the passive transfer mouse model. In addition, mice depleted of complement by cobra venom treatment and C5-deficient mice develop disease with the same degree of severity as those animals with an intact complement system that were injected with PV IgG (41).

Other investigators have suggested a possible role for plasminogen activator (PA) or other proteases in the pathogenesis of PV (17,18,42). An increase in protease activity and synthesis of PA was noted in the supernatants of skin organ cultures treated with PV autoantibodies, suggesting that these enzymes may participate in the formation of PV skin lesions. Also, it was shown that the protease inhibitor aprotinin (Trasylol, Cal Biochem, La Jolla, CA, U.S.A.) blocked acantholysis induced by PV autoantibodies in the mouse transfer model, supporting the hypothesis of a possible role of proteases in the disease process (43). However, pretreatment with dexamethasone, which is an inhibitor of PA synthesis, did not prevent the onset and progression of acantholysis in mice when passively transferred with PV autoantibodies despite the fact that epidermal PA activity was abolished (44).

Analysis of cultured keratinocytes that have been incubated with PV IgG suggests that activation of the signal transduction process may be involved in the acantholytic process (45,46). Transient intracellular increases in phospholipase C and inositol 1,4,5-triphosphate production, an influx of calcium, and a concomitant formation of 1,2-diacylglycerol, which is an endogenous activator of protein kinase C (PKC), are seen in these keratinocytes. It is known that PKC activation is a major step in the signal transduction pathways of cells undergoing growth and differentiation. It was also shown that the intracellular events described in cells treated with PV IgG are associated with translocation of PKC isoforms from the cytosolic portion of the cell to the cytoskeleton of the keratinocytes. It was further shown that these cultured keratinocytes had abnormal keratin cytoskeletons. These studies, however, did not correlate PV IgG-induced intracellular signaling with cell detachment assays.

### Diagnosis and Treatment

The diagnosis of PV is made by clinically recognizing the features previously described and through histopathologic and immunopathologic studies. Lesional biopsy reveals the typical suprabasilar acantholysis within the epidermis. Indirect IF of the patient's serum shows the presence of autoantibodies to the epidermal ICS in more than 90% of patients. PV autoantibodies are also detected bound to the epidermal ICS by direct IF of perilesional skin biopsies.

Therapy for PV is aimed at decreasing the overall circulating autoantibodies in a patient's serum. Before the advent of steroids and antibiotics, more than half of patients died within 1 year of diagnosis from dehydration, electrolyte imbalances, malnutrition, or sepsis. Death rates dropped to 5% to 35% since the introduction of glucocorticosteroids alone (47). Currently, mortality rates are about 10% over 5 years, as a result of the introduction of immunosuppressive therapy (48). Although steroids have been the first-line drug of choice since their introduction in the 1950s, their long-term use has been associated with numerous side effects, including diabetes mellitus, hypertension, osteoporosis, cataracts, gastrointestinal bleeding, central nervous system toxicity, myopathy, and infections. The incidence of aseptic necrosis of the femoral head has been found to be lower in patients receiving prednisone than prednisolone, prompting the recommendation to use the former.

In a few patients initially, with PV that is recalcitrant to prednisone alone, and in patients suffering from the adverse effects of long-term steroid use, adjuvant immunosuppressive medications, such as cyclophosphamide (Cytoxan), azathioprine (Imuran), and methotrexate are used. These medications are used for long-term control of PV and require several weeks to exert their effect; therefore, they should not be used to treat the acute phase of the disease. Other drugs, such as parenteral gold, have been used as steroid-sparing agents in PV as well; however, the potential side effects have limited their use. Oral gold has been argued to be a more effective form with less toxic side effects. Plasmapheresis, a process of removing autoantibodies from the patient's circulation, has been of some short-term benefit in controlling PV (49); however, a rebound rise in autoantibody titers is seen in patients who are not concurrently receiving adequate immunosuppressive medications. Several other agents, including dapsone, cyclosporine, and etretinate, have been reported through uncontrolled studies to be helpful as adjuvant treatments in PV.

The prognosis associated with PV has improved markedly with these therapies, as previously mentioned. Factors such as later age of onset, greater extent of disease, glucocorticosteroid-resistant disease, and rapidly progressive disease before treatment all negatively effect the outcome of PV. Sepsis, involving predominantly *Staphylococcus aureus,* has been the most common cause of death in patients taking steroids.

## PEMPHIGUS FOLIACEUS

### Disease Description

Subcorneal blisters and pathogenic antiepidermal autoantibodies characterize the nonendemic and endemic forms of PF (50,51). Although PF occurs worldwide, an endemic form known as *fogo selvagem* (FS) is found in subtropical regions of rural Brazil (52). Clusters of cases of an endemic FS-like disease have also been reported in other parts of Latin America (51–53) and Tunisia (54,55).

The endemic and nonendemic forms of PF share similar clinical, histologic, and immunologic features (56). Clinically, the primary lesion in PF is a superficial vesicle that ruptures easily, leaving denuded areas of skin (Fig. 21.4A). The lesions are localized in the seborrheic areas of the face and trunk. The scalp is often involved and may exhibit verrucous plaques. After a few weeks or months of evolution, the disease may spread to involve large areas of the body and ultimately produce a characteristic confluence of superficial erosions with exudative crusting known as an *exfoliative erythroderma.* Mucosal blisters and erosions are not observed in these patients, one feature that clinically distinguishes PF from PV. There are rare cases of fulminant PF in which the patient develops a rampant widespread bullous eruption within a short period of time. These severe cases require hospitalization of the patient to prevent dehydration, electrolyte imbalances, and superimposed infections. During active disease, Nikolsky's sign (removal of perilesional epidermis when shearing forces are applied) is a typical finding in FS patients.

In the localized variant of PF, round or oval keratotic plaques with a yellow-brown surface are distributed within the seborrheic areas of the face and trunk. This form of PF has been mistakenly termed *Senear–Usher syndrome* because of its close resemblance to SLE. These patients, however, have no evidence of SLE on skin biopsy or serologic studies. These lesions can also progress to become generalized, producing multiple keratotic plaques and nodular lesions.

Most FS cases in Brazil originate in endemic areas irrigated by tributaries of the major river of central Brazil. These areas tend to be agriculturally developing regions heavily infested with a variety of biting insects. A case-controlled epidemiologic study (57) and entomologic study (58) indicate that exposure to one of these insects, the black fly (family Simuliidae), may be a relevant etiologic factor of FS. Patients developing FS, however, are exposed to many other factors in their native environment; hence, elucidating a single cause is a formidable task.

### Pathology

The Brazilian dermatologist Vieira (59) first described the classic histologic features of PF in 1937. He noted that, unlike PV, in which blistering occurs directly above the basal layer of the epidermis, PF blister formation occurs at the level of the stratum granulosum.

The chief histologic feature of both endemic and nonendemic forms of PF is the presence of vesicles located in the subcorneal region of the epidermis (60). The acantholytic process occurs immediately above, within, or below cells of the stratum granulosum (Fig. 21.4B). Although light microscopy reveals acantholysis only in the subcorneal layer, electron microscopy reveals acantholysis affecting keratinocytes in all layers of the epidermis (61). The cell detachment is visible, with electron microscopy, on the lateral surfaces of cells of the basal cell layer and extends outward toward the stratum spinosum and granulosum. The cell detachment is complete at the level of the granular cell layer. The stratum corneum forms the roof of the vesicle, and stratum spinosum forms the floor.

Some of the vesicles in PF skin lesions may occasionally be filled with neutrophils. In rare situations, eosinophilic

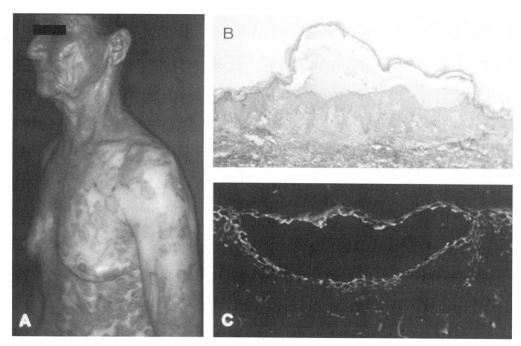

**FIG. 21.4.** Pemphigus foliaceus (PF). **A:** The distribution of superficial erosions and blisters in a patient with endemic PF (fogo selvagem). **B:** Histologic examination of skin lesions in PF shows a typical subcorneal vesicle that is formed as a result of detachment of keratinocytes in the upper layers of the epidermis. **C:** Direct IF of a skin biopsy from a patient with PF shows immunoglobulin G (IgG) autoantibodies bound to the surface of keratinocytes. This biopsy also shows an intraepidermal blister cavity. The serum of PF patients contains antiepidermal autoantibodies in titers that roughly correlate to activity and extent of disease. The autoantibodies belong to the IgG class and are predominantly of the IgG4 subclass. See color plate 14.

spongiosis may be present in some biopsy specimens. In cases in which eosinophilic spongiosis is detected in biopsy specimens from patients showing infiltrated plaques, the term *pemphigus herpetiformis* has been applied (62).

## Autoimmune Features

### Humoral Immune Response

In 1964, Beutner and Jordon (63) first reported the presence of circulating antibodies to the epidermal ICS of the skin in the sera of pemphigus patients, thus demonstrating that pemphigus is an autoimmune disease. Later, Beutner et al. (64) extended these studies to include FS (Fig. 21.4C).

The pathogenicity of FS autoantibodies has been demonstrated by passive-transfer experiments as well (65,66) (Fig. 21.5). In these studies, the IgG fraction from the serum of FS patients was able to induce blistering within 24 hours, when injected intraperitoneally into neonatal BALB/c mice. Histologic examination of lesional skin of these animals revealed typical acantholytic blisters located in the granular cell layer of the epidermis, as seen in human PF. Direct IF examination of the mouse skin showed deposits of human IgG autoantibodies and mouse C3 in the ICS. Indirect IF testing of the mouse serum showed circulating human autoantibodies in titers that correlated with the epidermal disease seen in the animals. Additionally, we demonstrated that the autoanti-

body response in FS was predominantly IgG4 and that the IgG4 from the sera of these patients was also pathogenic (67). Whole IgG, as well as the F(ab)2 and Fab fragments, was shown to be pathogenic (68,69). These studies suggested that the autoantibody injury induced by PF autoantibodies was complement independent and perhaps the result of impairment of the adhesive function of the epidermal PF antigen.

PF autoantibodies specifically recognize Dsg-1, a 160-kd desmosomal core glycoprotein (70–72). Dsg-1 has been cloned, sequenced, and shown to be a transmembrane glycoprotein belonging to the cadherin family of cell adhesion molecules (73,74). The extracellular domain of Dsg-1 contains calcium-dependent epitopes that are specifically recognized by pathogenic PF autoantibodies (75–78). This was demonstrated using affinity chromatography, in which a recombinant form of Dsg-1 was immobilized to immunoadsorb pathogenic autoantibodies from PF sera (77). The affinity-purified anti–Dsg-1 autoantibodies were pathogenic in the mouse transfer model (27).

### Genetic Factors

Strong epidemiologic evidence suggests that FS is precipitated by an environmental factor in genetically predisposed patients (57,58). Since the nonendemic form of PF is rare, HLA studies in these patients have been reported sporadi-

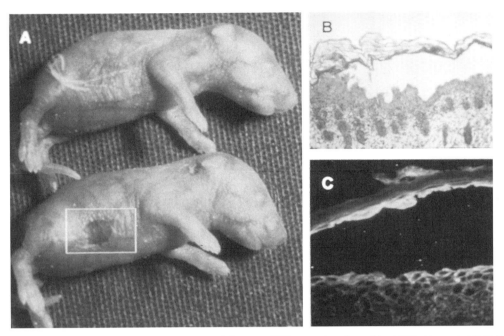

**FIG. 21.5.** The mouse model of pemphigus foliaceus (PF) was developed in 1985. Neonatal BALB/c mice were passively transferred with the IgG fraction from the sera of patients with either the endemic or nonendemic forms of PF. **A:** The injected animals developed superficial blisters and erosions. **B:** A biopsy taken from lesional skin of these animals shows subcorneal vesicles. **C:** Direct immunofluorescence of the skin lesions shows human autoantibodies bound to the surface of keratinocytes. A subcorneal vesicle is also observed. This study provided direct evidence that the autoantibodies in endemic and nonendemic PF are pathogenic. See color plate 15.

cally. In FS, however, there have been several studies documenting the familial nature of the disease and the increased frequency of certain HLA alleles in these patients (79). In a series of 2686 FS patients, 18% were familial cases, and 93% of these familial cases represented genetically related family members (80). Studies demonstrated that Amerindian populations of Brazil, with a high prevalence of FS, express certain HLA-DRB1 alleles, such as DRB1*0201, 0404, 1402, and 1406, with a relative risk as high as 14. These alleles share the same amino acid sequence (residues 67 to 74) at the third hypervariable region of the *DRB1* gene, that is, the sequence LLEQRRAA (81,82). This "shared epitope," which was originally proposed as a relevant epitope in rheumatoid arthritis (83), may also confer susceptibility in patients with FS.

### Cellular Immune Response

From the autoantibody passive-transfer model experiments, it is clear that, similar to PV, PF is an autoantibody-mediated disease. We hypothesize, therefore, that T cells from PF patients may participate in the development and progression of this disease. We have investigated the responses of T cells from 10 FS patients to recombinant Dsg-1 generated in the baculovirus expression system (84). We showed that T cells from all but 1 FS patient treated with a high dose of corticosteroid 24 hours before the experiment proliferated when incubated with recombinant Dsg-1. T cells from 6 of these pa-

tients reacted with Dsg-1–glutathione-S-transferase fusion proteins corresponding to 60 amino acids of the EC1 domain of Dsg-1, and 7 responded to segments located on the EC2, EC4, and EC5 domains of this molecule. T cells from other control groups, such as patients with SLE (n = 1), patients with psoriasis (n = 2), and healthy subjects (n = 7) did not respond to these Dsg-1 proteins, therefore suggesting that FS T cells specifically respond to Dsg-1 and may play a role in the pathogenesis of this disease.

Finally, using Dsg-1 synthetic peptides that were predicted to associate with the HLA-DRB1*0404 alleles (commonly found in FS patients), we tested the reactivity of FS T cells. We found that a 15–amino acid peptide located on the EC1 domain of Dsg-1 elicited the strongest stimulatory response. These findings suggest that multiple T-cell epitopes located on the ectodomain of Dsg-1 are involved in the autoimmune reaction of FS. Further characterization of these self-reactive T cells may help to elucidate the pathogenic role of T lymphocytes in FS.

### Diagnosis and Therapy

FS may be differentiated from nonendemic PF by the epidemiologic features mentioned previously. The absence of oral lesions distinguishes both forms of PF from PV. Histologic examination can aid in distinguishing early stages of PF from other bullous diseases. Subcorneal vesicles favor the diagnosis of PF, whereas suprabasilar vesicles are more diagnostic of PV, when viewed by light microscopy. Furthermore, direct IF studies of patients' skin biopsy specimens show deposits of IgG in the ICS, and indirect IF examination of patients' sera reveals circulating PF autoantibodies. FS autoantibodies are disease specific, and the titers correlate roughly with extent and activity of the disease. The IF staining pattern produced by PF and PV sera on squamous epithelium is indistinguishable.

PF can also be distinguished from other blistering disorders, such as BP, in that Nikolsky's sign is negative and the serologic studies reveal different autoantibody systems. In BP, the sera possess autoantibodies that bind the basement membrane zone (BMZ), producing a linear staining pattern by indirect IF.

The aforementioned immunoprecipitation and enzyme-linked immunosorbent assay (ELISA) techniques employing recombinant forms of Dsg-1 are sensitive and accurate in detecting autoantibodies in the sera of PF patients. These tests also roughly correlate the activity and extent of disease with the titers of autoantibodies in the patients' sera. However, they are not yet widely available.

Suppressing the immune response with systemic corticosteroids is the first line of therapy for all forms of pemphigus. Before the use of steroids, fewer than 10% of FS patients went into spontaneous remission, and 40% died within the first 2 years (59). About half of patients presented with a chronic disease characterized by periodic exacerbations, eventually leading to death. With the use of steroids, the mortality rate has dropped to less than 10%. Other immunosuppressive agents, such as azathioprine and cyclophosphamide, have been used

in association with steroids with good results (51,56). Plasmapheresis is a less commonly used modality that acutely drops the titer of autoantibodies in the patients' sera; however, adequate immunosuppressive agents must be used in conjunction, or a rebound rise in titer will occur. Deaths most commonly occur today as a result of delay in treatment or as a result of complications of therapy, such as infection.

## BULLOUS PEMPHIGOID

### Disease Description

Lever (85) first described BP as an entity distinct from PV and PF in 1953. The characteristic clinical appearance of tense bullae occurring on inflamed skin and the histologic features of subepidermal vesicles with neutrophilic dermal infiltrates were the key differentiating factors. In 1967, Jordon et al. (86) demonstrated, using IF techniques, that the sera of BP patients possess antiskin autoantibodies that bind the BMZ of the skin in a linear fashion. Skin biopsies from perilesional skin of these patients consistently showed IgG and C3 bound along the BMZ by direct IF.

BP most commonly occurs after the age of 60 years, has no gender or racial predilection, and has a worldwide distribution. Although the exact incidence and prevalence of BP is unknown, it is estimated that about 5 to 10 new cases are seen yearly in large medical referral centers in the United States.

Clinically, patients present with tense, fluid-filled blisters on normal or erythematous skin (Fig. 21.6A). In contrast to the various forms of pemphigus, which are characterized by intraepidermal blisters that are easily ruptured, BP lesions occur

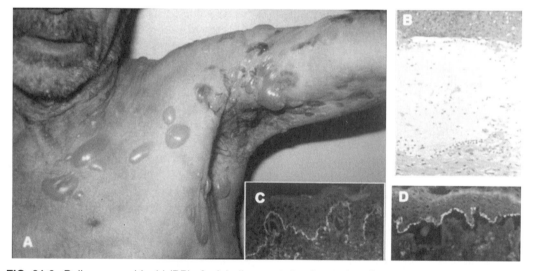

**FIG. 21.6.** Bullous pemphigoid (BP). **A:** A bullous eruption located on flexure areas of the skin is observed in typical cases of BP. These vesicobullous lesions are tense, and Nikolsky's sign is negative. **B:** Histologic examination of a biopsy taken from a BP lesion shows a typical subepidermal blister. **C:** Direct immunofluorescence (IF) analysis of perilesional skin shows linear deposition of immunoglobulin G at the dermoepidermal junction. Most BP patients also show C3 bound to the dermoepidermal junction. **D:** Indirect IF performed on salt split skin shows binding of BP autoantibodies to the roof of the split. This finding is typical of BP. The autoantibodies in BP are directed against hemidesmosomal antigens. See color plate 16.

at the dermoepidermal junction, and the blisters are often intact. Blisters may vary in size from vesicles measuring a few millimeters to large bullae. When the blister ruptures, an area of denuded skin remains that tends not to spread to surrounding skin. If the erosions remain free of infection, they heal rapidly (over several days) without scarring. The healed areas typically show postinflammatory hyperpigmentation, which resolves over a longer period of time. Patients may alternatively present with only erythematous macules and papules, typical of an eczematous dermatitis, with urticarial plaques, or even simply with generalized pruritus without any skin findings. Unlike plain urticaria, the large hivelike plaques seen in the urticarial phase of BP remain for longer than 24 hours, and blisters can develop within these lesions.

Up to 40% of BP patients exhibit oral lesions at some time during the course of the disease (87); however, it is rare for oral lesions to be the presenting sign in BP. BP mucosal lesions are not as severe as mucosal lesions seen in PV. Also of note, although BP lesions can occur on any skin surface, these lesions tend to develop in areas with relatively higher concentrations of BP antigen (as determined by indirect IF), including the flexural areas, such as the groin, axillae, and extremities (88).

## Pathology

Light microscopy of BP typically shows separation of the epidermis from the dermis with a variable inflammatory infiltrate in the upper dermis (Fig. 21.6B). In early lesions, the infiltrate is a mixture of lymphocytes and eosinophils in a perivascular location. In clinically more inflamed lesions, there may also be an increase in the histologic degree of inflammation with a more intense inflammatory infiltration, and eosinophils may be present in the blister cavity (89). In the cell-rich variant of BP, there may be eosinophilic abscesses in the papillary tips. Electron microscopic examination of BP lesions reveals cleavage at the level of the lamina lucida (90).

## Autoimmune Features

### Humoral Autoimmune Response

A milestone immunologic finding in BP was the discovery of anti-BMZ autoantibodies in the serum of BP patients by indirect IF in 1967 (86). The same BP autoantibodies produce a linear staining of the BMZ of perilesional skin by direct IF (91). IgG and, less frequently, IgA and IgM are detected (Fig. 21.6C). It has been reported that from 45% to 90% of patients have linear IgG deposits, and 80% to 100% had linear C3 (92). Circulating IgG anti-BMZ antibodies are detectable in about 70% of patient's sera by indirect IF. The IgG4 subclass is the most common IgG isotype found. About 10% of patients have neither tissue-bound nor circulating antibodies but do have detectable complement deposition at the BMZ, suggesting that complement fixing antibodies are or were present at the BMZ. Unlike PV and PF, there is no correlation between autoantibody titer and disease activity in BP (93).

Activation of the complement cascade is important to the pathogenesis of BP. The deposition of C3 along the BMZ of lesional skin biopsies on direct IF is well documented (92,94). Other components of the alternative and classic pathways have also been identified at the BMZ. The activation of complement, along with the release of cytokines, works to recruit more inflammatory cells to the BMZ. Some of the chemoattractants found in the BMZ include C5a fragments, leukotriene B4 (95), various interleukins and tumor necrosis factors, and interferon-γ (96–99). The inflammatory infiltrate includes eosinophils (100–102), neutrophils (101–103), lymphocytes (104), and mast cells (101,105,106). Degranulated eosinophils have been localized by electron microscopy to the epidermal side of the basal lamina in perilesional skin. Mast cells found in BP lesions also exhibit morphologic changes suggesting degranulation.

Several granular proteins from these inflammatory cells have been noted in perilesional skin, including eosinophil cationic protein (101,102), eosinophil major basic protein (102), and neutrophil-derived myeloperoxidase (107). Granulocyte proteinases, including plasmin, collagenase, elastase, and gelatinase, and products of the oxidative pathway, such as free radicals, have also been detected in the BMZ and are implicated in blister formation (107–110). These observations support the hypothesis that inflammatory cells and mediators are probably involved in the disruption of the BMZ in BP patients.

Most of the serum of BP patients recognizes two hemidesmosomal polypeptides, a 230-kd intracellular protein and a 180-kd transmembrane protein (111,112). These polypeptides are also referred to as BP230 (BPAG1) and BP180 (BPAG2 or type XVII collagen) and are specific markers of the hemidesmosomal unit. BP230 is an intracellular protein localized to the hemidesmosomal plaque (113), whereas BP180 has an amino-terminal domain that localizes to the hemidesmosomal plaque and a carboxy-terminal domain that projects into the lamina lucida of the BMZ. Both antigens have been cloned and characterized at the molecular level (114–116). The gene coding for BP230 has been mapped to chromosome 6 and is a member of the plakin family of proteins that includes desmoplakins I and II, plectin, periplakin, and envoplakin (117,118). BP180 has been mapped to chromosome 10 (119). The extracellular portion of BP180 consists of 15 collagen domains of lengths varying from 15 to 242 amino acids that are separated by short noncollagenous regions (115,120). Epitope mapping studies have revealed four major epitopes (designated MCW-0 through MCW-3) that are recognized by the autoantibodies of most BP patients (121,122). These epitopes are tightly clustered within a 45–amino acid stretch of the noncollagenous (NC16A) domain of BP180.

Early studies using passive transfer of BP IgG into experimental animals were unsuccessful (123,124). In these studies, IgG fractions known to have high titers of BP autoantibodies were injected into either neonatal mice or monkeys. No skin lesions were produced with these methods, nor were

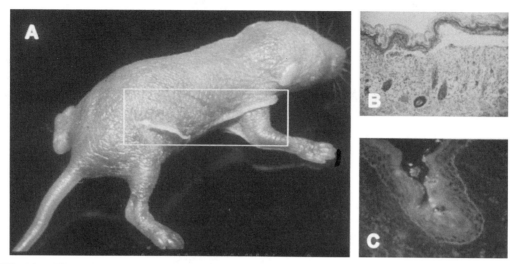

**FIG. 21.7.** The animal model of BP was developed in 1993. **A:** Rabbits were immunized with recombinant forms of murine BP180. The immunoglobulin G fraction from this rabbit antimurine BP180 antigen was passively transferred into neonatal BALB/c mice by either an intraperitoneal or subcutaneous route. Neonatal mice injected with this antibody develop a blistering eruption within 24 hours. **B:** Skin biopsy samples taken from lesional skin in these animals show typical subepidermal blistering with an intense neutrophilic infiltrate in the upper dermis. **C:** Direct immunofluorescence studies of perilesional skin of these animals show rabbit anti-BP180 antibodies bound in a linear fashion to the dermoepidermal junction. Blister formation in these animal models is dependent on complement activation and neutrophilic infiltration. See color plate 17.

BP autoantibodies bound *in vivo* to the skin of the injected animals, suggesting that the pathogenic autoantibodies do not cross-react with the homologous antigen of the recipient animal. More recently, it has been shown that the murine BP180 ectodomain has low homology with human BP180 in the region of major BP-associated epitope, MCW-1 (122,125). Recombinant forms of murine BP180 encompassing the protein stretch homologous with MCW-1 were generated in a bacterial expression system and used to produce polyclonal antimurine BP180 antibodies in rabbits. These rabbit antibodies were then purified and injected intraperitoneally and intradermally into mice. Injected animals developed subepidermal blistering that duplicated the features of human BP at the clinical and histologic levels (Fig. 21.7) (125).

We further demonstrated that complement activation was necessary for blister formation. This fact was demonstrated by the following observations: mice depleted of complement (either genetically or by pretreatment with cobra venom factor) did not develop blisters after the injection of pathogenic rabbit BP autoantibodies; fragments of the pathogenic IgG lacking the Fc portion, which is essential for complement activation, did not induce disease in injected animals; and C5a fragments injected with the pathogenic IgG were able to induce disease in complement-deficient mice (126). The animal model was also used to show that neutrophils are crucial to the pathogenesis of disease because neutrophil-depleted mice did not develop disease when injected with antimurine BP180 antibodies (127). Furthermore, gelatinase B–deficient mice are resistant to the pathogenic activity of antimurine BP180 IgG (128). We also have obtained evidence that neutrophil elastase plays a crucial role in antibody-mediated

subepidermal blistering in this mouse model (129). In addition to demonstrating the necessity of complement and neutrophils in blister formation, it is anticipated that future experiments using this mouse model system will aid in further elucidating the pathophysiology of BP.

### Immunogenetics

Immunogenetic studies in BP have yielded inconsistent findings. Three HLA studies involving American, Japanese, and British BP patients showed no significant association between the disease and the HLA-A, HLA-B, HLA-C, and HLA-DR loci (130–132). Another study of French BP patients revealed a marked increase in the HLA-DR5 haplotype (133). One study demonstrated that the frequency of the expression of HLA-DQB1*0301 is greatly increased in patients with BP and ocular CP (134), suggesting that this allele may confer susceptibility to these subepithelial autoimmune diseases. Furthermore, a preliminary investigation conducted by Büdinger et al. (135) pointed out that the immune responses of BP180-specific T lymphocytes were restricted to the expression of HLA-DQB1*0301, strongly supporting that this MHC class II allele may be involved in the precipitation of BP.

### Cellular Immune Response

The role of T lymphocytes in the pathogenesis of BP is unclear. A report by Rico et al. (136) showed that peripheral blood mononuclear cells from patients with BP have an increased frequency of response to synthetic amphipathic peptides derived from the BP230 antigen; however, these studies were preliminary. More recently, using the recombinant fusion proteins encompassing the BP180 ectodomain to assess the proliferative responses of T lymphocytes from BP patients, we have successfully obtained BP180-specific T-cell clones from BP patients. These BP T-cell clones respond to a 28–amino acid peptide within the NC16A region of BP180. Further analyses revealed that these T cells express a CD4$^+$T-cell–receptor-$\alpha\beta$ memory T-cell phenotype and secrete a T$_H$2-like cytokine profile (137). Additional studies on the function of these T cells may elucidate the role of T cells in the autoimmune responses of BP patients.

### Diagnosis and Treatment

The diagnosis of BP is made from clinical, histologic, and immunologic criteria. Anti-BMZ autoantibodies associated with BP can be detected by direct IF, indirect IF, and immunoelectron microscopy. Direct IF is routinely performed using perilesional or urticarial unblistered skin. The antigen specificity of these autoantibodies can be further characterized by immunoblotting and ELISA using either epidermal extracts or recombinant proteins encompassing segments of either the BP180 or BP230 antigens.

The mainstays of diagnosis are the direct and indirect IF findings described earlier. Several other diseases, however, such as CP, EBA, herpes gestationis (HG), and bullous SLE, are also characterized by the linear deposition of IgG and C3 at the BMZ. Clinical information and further laboratory investigation may be necessary to distinguish these disorders. The use of salt-split skin as a tissue substrate for indirect IF can aid in differentiating certain of these diseases. Incubation of human skin in 1.0 M NaCl splits the tissue at the level of the lamina lucida, resulting in the physical separation of epidermal and dermal antigens. BP and HG autoantibodies bind the roof of salt-split skin (epidermal side) (Fig. 21.6D), whereas EBA and SLE autoantibodies preferentially bind the floor of the split (dermal side).

Using a recombinant form of BP180 that contains the MCW-1 epitope, our laboratory has developed an ELISA-based protocol for detecting reactivity of BP sera (138). This highly specific method was used to test serum of 50 BP patients for reactivity to BP180. Of these patients, 94% showed reactivity to the recombinant antigen, whereas no specific reactivity was seen in 107 controls. This sensitive and specific assay is being developed in our laboratory for diagnostic purposes.

As with other bullous diseases, therapy for BP remains nonspecific. The mainstay of therapy is to modulate the patient's immune system using glucocorticoids. Most BP patients have a favorable, rapid response to this systemic therapy, but adjuvant therapy is sometimes needed for recalcitrant cases. Azathioprine and cyclophosphamide have been the most commonly used agents in addition to steroids. There has also been some success with dapsone in some cases. Other agents, such as tetracycline and nicotinamide, have been proposed as alternative therapies for BP, although these are generally most useful in mild cases (130–141).

An initial course of systemic steroids can produce prolonged clinical remission in as many as 75% of patients. Although the risk for fatality if the disease is untreated is low, the risk to debilitated and elderly patients in the active phase of the disease can be significant.

## CICATRICIAL PEMPHIGOID

### Disease Description

CP is a heterogeneous disorder, the unifying characteristic of which is scarring mucosal lesions (142–144). The mucosal surfaces, including the oral mucosa, oropharynx, nasopharynx, esophagus, conjunctiva, and genitalia, are most commonly involved in this disorder. Morbidity associated with CP is related chiefly to blindness that can result from corneal involvement and scarring caused by recurrent lesions in the eyes. The three criteria needed to diagnose CP are scarring mucosal blisters or erosions; subepithelial blisters with intact basal cell layer and variable inflammatory cell infiltrate; and direct IF of perilesional mucosa revealing linear deposits of either IgG or IgA and C3 along the BMZ.

### Pathology

CP shares many histologic features with BP; therefore, it can be difficult to differentiate these two diseases by histology. Both show separation at the dermoepidermal junction. Scarring can be a clue to the diagnosis of CP.

### Autoimmune Features

BP and CP also share several immunologic features. Most CP patients possess autoantibodies that react with the BP180 antigen and to a lesser extent with the BP230 antigen using immunoblotting procedures (145,146). At least two characteristics, however, distinguish the two entities immunologically. First, only a small number of CP patients have circulating anti-BMZ autoantibodies by indirect IF, and of those that do, the titers are often very low. Second, a subset of CP sera show reactivity to laminin-5 (epiligrin), a matrix protein located in the lamina lucida of the BMZ (147,148). The anti–laminin-5 autoantibodies in these patients may be pathogenic because rabbit anti–laminin-5 IgG is pathogenic when passively transferred to neonatal mice. These animals develop subepidermal blisters. These blisters were also induced by the anti–laminin-5 in C5-deficient mice and in mast cell–deficient neonatal mice. This finding suggests that, unlike the murine model of BP, complement activation and mast cell degranulation may not be relevant in the formation of subepidermal blisters in this anti–laminin-5 CP mouse model (149).

### Treatment

CP is a chronic disease, and treatment is tailored to the areas involved. Patients with limited oral mucosal or pharyngeal involvement should be treated with either topical, intralesional, or short bursts of oral steroids. Dapsone has been useful in some of these patients. Cases with severe involvement of the eyes, larynx, or esophagus should be treated aggressively with systemic steroids and other immunosuppressive agents, such as cyclophosphamide or azathioprine. Clinical remission has been reported to occur 2 years after the onset of therapy.

## HERPES GESTATIONIS

### Disease Description

HG, a subepidermal blistering disease also known as *pemphigoid gestationis,* is a nonviral autoimmune disorder occurring in gravid women late in pregnancy or shortly after delivery. HG is characterized by urticarial plaques that evolve into vesicles and bullae starting in the periumbilical area in most patients. Although the most common time of onset is the second or third trimester of pregnancy, flares around the time of delivery are not unusual, and HG may recur with future pregnancies or with the use of oral contraceptives (150). Lesions usually resolve within weeks or months of parturition. Patients can be treated with short courses of system corticosteroids during flares, but because the disease is typically limited to pregnancy, no long-term therapy is necessary. A genetic correlation has been noted in HG patients. There appears to be a significantly increased incidence of HLA-B8 and the HLA-DR3 and HLA-DR4 haplotypes among patients (151,152).

### History

Histologic examination of lesional skin reveals subepidermal blisters. An inflammatory infiltrate of mononuclear cells and eosinophils may be present. Differentiation from BP may not be possible by histology.

### Autoimmune Features

Direct IF examination of most HG patients shows deposition of C3 at the BMZ. A linear deposition of IgG is observed in about 30% to 40% of patients. Routine indirect IF examination of the serum of most HG patients is usually negative; however, the same sera show circulating complement-fixing antibodies in 85% to 100% of patients using complement IF techniques. These complement-fixing anti-BMZ autoantibodies were previously known as the *HG factor* (153–155).

HG autoantibodies typically belong to the IgG1 or IgG3 subclass (156,157), which can be transferred passively *in utero* to the newborn and produce transient disease (158,159). We have demonstrated that more than 84% of HG patients' sera recognize the ectodomain of the BP180 peptide using immunoblotting techniques (159a).

Investigators have begun to define the role played by autoimmune T lymphocytes in the initiation and progression of HG. Our research group found that T cells from two HG patients specifically respond to peptides encompassing the NC16A region of the BP180 antigen (160). The neonate born to one of the HG patients was shown to have circulating anti-BP180 autoantibodies; however, the T cells from the neonate did not proliferate when exposed to any of the stimulatory NC16A peptides. This result suggests that the autoantibodies in the neonatal serum were of maternal origin and that the neonate did not develop HG autoimmunity. Further characterization of the BP180-responsive T-cell clones developed from one HG patient revealed that these cells are CD4+ T-cell–receptor-αβ memory T-cells secreting a $T_H1$-like cytokine profile. The $T_H1$ cytokine profile of these T cells may modulate the production of IgG1 anti-BP180 antibodies in HG patients. Moreover, we found that T cells and autoantibodies from this HG patient also recognize a common 14–amino acid epitope, MCW-1. These results suggest that self-reactive T and B cells in this HG patient may establish T-cell–B-cell interactions through the MCW-1 epitope. This information may help to elucidate the pathogenic mechanisms involved in the development of HG.

### Therapy

Use of steroids is the first line of treatment of HG. The disease is usually self-limited and remits shortly after delivery.

## LINEAR IMMUNOGLOBULIN A DISEASE

### Disease Description

Linear IgA disease (LAD) was originally thought to be a variant of dermatitis herpetiformis (DH) based on shared clinical and histologic features (161). Chorzelski et al. (162) first distinguished LAD from DH in 1979, while attempting to differentiate typical DH with granular IgA deposits at the BMZ from atypical DH with linear IgA antibody deposits at the BMZ. These atypical cases of DH or atypical blistering disorders resembling BP were sorted out into LAD by showing that the sera of these patients produced a linear staining of the BMZ with IgA autoantibodies.

The clinical features of LAD can vary, but the classic skin findings are tense blisters occurring on normal or erythematous skin at the periphery of annular patches resembling a cluster of jewels or a string of pearls. Lesions can sometimes be generalized but commonly are localized to the perineum, perioral region, or extremities. In adults, the mucous membranes are often involved, including the mouth (37%), genitals (25%), and conjunctiva (20%). These lesions may heal with scar formation. Ocular involvement is common and can be asymptomatic; thus, careful examination by an ophthalmologist is recommended for all patients with LAD. The ocular findings are indistinguishable from those of CP, with changes in the canthal regions, conjunctiva, eyelashes, and secondary corneal opacification (163,164).

LAD is a rare disease, with reported incidence of 0.52 and 0.22 cases per 1 million people annually in France (165) and Germany (166), respectively. The disease can occur at any age, although typically the disease has a bimodal distribution, with most cases occurring before the age of 5 years and in the fifth decade. The early-onset form is termed *chronic bullous disease of childhood.*

LAD can be further differentiated from DH and other bullous diseases based on the lack of gluten sensitivity associated with the disease and the absence of a strong HLA correlation. Furthermore, the serum of DH patients is usually negative by indirect IF using salt-split skin but can yield positive results for antiendomysial antibodies (167). In LAD, however, the serum is positive by this technique, revealing IgA anti-BMZ autoantibodies (168).

The cause of LAD remains unclear, although in a minority of patients, it may be triggered by medications (169). These include antibiotics, such as vancomycin, cefamandole, and ampicillin, and other drugs, such as captopril, diclofenac, and somatostatin.

## Pathology

Biopsy specimens of lesional skin show epidermal–dermal separation with a prominent inflammatory infiltrate within the upper dermis. These inflammatory cells are composed of either eosinophils or neutrophils. Neutrophils may form microabscesses in the papillary ridges.

Direct IF of perilesional skin or mucosa shows linear deposits of IgA along the BMZ. Occasionally, deposits of C3 or IgG can also be seen at the BMZ. The serum of these patients contains low titers of anti-BMZ IgA autoantibodies. The sensitivity of the indirect IF technique may be increased by using salt-split skin as a substrate (168). The reactivity of circulating antibodies with salt-split skin is variable, with visible reaction to both the epidermal and dermal sides of the split. This variability in immunoglobulin deposition is also observed by immunoelectron microscopy.

## Autoimmune Features

The major antigen recognized by LAD autoantibodies is a 97-kd protein located on the epidermal side of salt-split skin (170). The antigen has been localized to the lamina lucida region of the BMZ, and Zone et al. (171) have shown that part of the 97-kd antigen is identical to a region of the extracellular domain of BP180 (171). This indicates that BP180 may participate in the autoimmune response in LAD.

The pathogenesis of LAD is unclear. Passive-transfer animal models to study its pathogenesis have been limited by the low circulating antibody titers found in LAD. In conclusion, LAD is an autoimmune blistering disease characterized by an IgA humoral autoimmune response against the BP180 antigen. This suggests that LAD may represent a unique subset of an IgA BP-like disease.

## Treatment

Dapsone and sulfapyridine are highly effective medications in the treatment of LAD in both children and adults. Im-

provement can be seen shortly after the initiation of therapy. Prednisone can be added to the therapy if there is no response with sulfones. Mucosal lesions are generally more resistant to therapy. In these cases, the addition of strong topical steroids may be helpful.

## EPIDERMOLYSIS BULLOSA ACQUISITA

### Disease Description

EBA is a rare, chronic subepidermal blistering disorder that is characterized by vesicles and blisters distributed in areas of trauma, most prominently on the dorsal surfaces of the hands and feet (Fig. 21.8A). Mucous membrane involvement can also be seen. The skin is fragile and easily eroded with trauma, and the lesions heal slowly, often with milia formation. Chronic involvement leads to loss of the fingernails and toenails. In addition to this classic presentation, a second inflammatory form has also been described in which tense blisters and erosions develop in the flexural areas. The inflammatory type shows less skin fragility and tends to heal without scarring or nail involvement (172). Clinically, this inflammatory form may be indistinguishable from BP. A number of patients have been described that evolve from the inflammatory type to the more typical chronic mechanobullous form. Finally, rare patients may present with a mucosal scarring disorder that has features identical to CP.

### Histology

Histologically, lesional skin shows subepidermal blisters, with the roof of the blister formed by intact epidermis (Fig. 21.8B). A variable inflammatory infiltrate composed of lymphocytes, neutrophils, and occasionally eosinophils may be seen in the upper dermis. The degree of inflammatory infiltrate may correlate with the intensity of inflammation that is seen clinically. Histologically, the noninflammatory type resembles porphyria cutanea tarda, whereas the inflammatory type may be difficult to distinguish from BP.

### Autoimmune Features

Direct IF analysis of perilesional skin shows linear deposition of IgG. Other immunoreactants, such as IgM, IgA, and C3, are variably seen (Fig. 21.8C). By indirect IF, the serum of about 25% to 50% of patients stains the BMZ, producing a linear pattern that resembles BP. In EBA, the circulating antibodies stain the floor of the salt-split skin, whereas BP autoantibodies typically stain the roof of the split (Fig. 21.8D). The utility of this method to differentiate EBA from BP is limited by the fact that not all patients have detectable circulating autoantibodies (173).

Ultrastructural studies are the most reliable method for separating EBA from BP; lesional skin reveals that the split in EBA is below the lamina densa, whereas in BP, it is above the lamina densa at the level of the lamina lucida. Immunoelectron

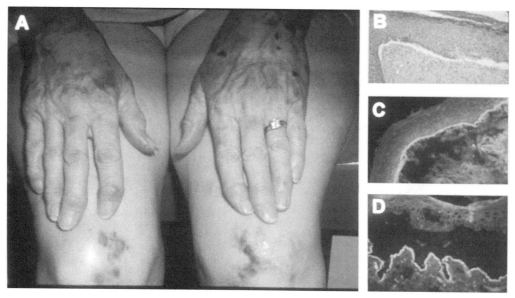

**FIG. 21.8.** Epidermolysis bullosa acquisita (EBA). **A:** Classic blistering eruption in a patient with EBA. The blisters are located on sites of trauma; in this case, the knees and knuckles. **B:** Histologic examination of a skin biopsy shows a subepidermal blister. **C:** Direct immunofluorescence (IF) studies of perilesional skin of these patients show a thick linear staining of the dermoepidermal junction. **D:** Indirect IF analysis performed on salt split skin shows autoantibodies bound to the floor of the split. EBA autoantibodies bind collagen type VII. See color plate 18.

microscopic studies localize the immunoreactants in EBA in the sublamina densa zone of the BMZ. The anti-BMZ autoantibodies in EBA patients bind the NC1 domain of type VII collagen, the major component of dermal anchoring fibrils (174). Type VII collagen has a globular glycosylated domain that lies within the lamina densa and a collagenous tail that extends into the sublamina densa fibrillar region. Type VII collagen interacts with both fibronectin and laminin-5, suggesting that as a result of the molecular interactions, type VII collagen plays a crucial role in epidermal–dermal adherence.

The pathogenicity of the antigen-specific autoantibodies in EBA is not as well established as in PV, PF, and BP. *In vitro* organ culture studies have shown that EBA autoantibodies can fix complement to the BMZ and promote adherence of neutrophils to this region of the skin. Passive-transfer experiments using EBA autoantibodies injected into neonatal mice, however, are unable to replicate the disease in these animals (175). Although passive transfer results in binding of autoantibodies to the BMZ of the skin of these animals, no clinical blisters can be detected. Further experimental work is needed to clarify the role of EBA autoantibodies in the pathogenesis of the disease.

**Therapy**

EBA tends to be chronic, with few remissions, and it is extremely difficult to treat. As with other autoimmune blistering disorders, the first line of treatment is suppression of the immune system with corticosteroids, which may be supplemented with other immunosuppressive agents. Other agents

that have been used in the treatment of EBA include cyclophosphamide, cyclosporine, dapsone, and colchicine. EBA can be recalcitrant to treatment, leading to long-term disability and scarring.

**DERMATITIS HERPETIFORMIS**

**Disease Description**

The characteristic lesion in DH is a small, pruritic, papulovesicular lesion on erythematous skin (176) (Fig. 21.9A). Lesions are grouped similar to lesions seen in herpes but are not associated with an infectious process. DH most commonly produces symmetric involvement of the elbows, extensor forearms, buttocks, and knees. Oral lesions are rare.

Lesions can occur at any age, with a predominance of cases occurring in the fourth decade of life and with an increased prevalence in men compared with women (1.5:1) (177), although many other autoimmune diseases show a female predominance. DH is rare in African Americans (178) and is more common in those of British or northern European descent. The true worldwide incidence and prevalence is unknown as a result of what appears to be an ethnic variability in its incidence. Prevalence rates of 10.4 per 100,000 and 39.2 per 100,000 have been reported in Finland (179) and central Sweden (180), respectively. Within the United States, the highest prevalence rate reported is 11.2 cases per 100,000, reported in Utah in 1987 (181). Environmental and genetic factors appear to be important in the distribution of the disease. Gluten and iodide intake are two relevant factors that may determine the prevalence of DH within a genetically homogenous population (179). DH shows a strong association with certain HLA alleles: HLA-B8 (60%), HLA-DR3 (95%), and HLA-DQw2 (100%) (182).

A gluten-sensitive enteropathy with patchy areas of villous atrophy and mild intestinal wall inflammation is found in most patients with DH (183). This form of enteropathy tends to be less severe than that seen in ordinary gluten-sensitive disease, with fewer than 20% of DH patients showing any symptoms of malabsorption. Development of intestinal lymphomas has been reported in a number of DH patients (184).

## Pathology

Biopsy specimens for histologic evaluation should be taken from erythematous, mildly indurated skin rather than tense vesicles. Infiltration with neutrophils is the initial inflammatory event seen within the dermal papillae, along with a lymphohistiocytic perivascular infiltrate (Fig. 21.9B) (185). This progresses to necrotic-appearing dermal papillae, secondary microabscess formation, and fibrin deposition. These microabscesses may coalesce to form tense bullae, which can be clinically indistinguishable from BP. A biopsy taken from these bullae may show eosinophils among the inflammatory infiltrate, making the biopsy appear more like BP, hence the need for specimens of early nonvesicular lesions. Bowel

biopsy specimens show villous atrophy similar to that seen in celiac sprue (Fig. 21.9D).

## Autoimmune Features

Cormane (186) first described the cutaneous immunopathologic findings in DH in 1967. Perilesional and normal skin of DH patients shows granular deposition of IgA and C3 along the BMZ (187) (Fig. 21.9C). Granular deposition of IgA at the dermal papillae can be detected in more than 85% of patients when tested by direct IF and is the single best criterion for the diagnosis of DH. Biopsy specimens for direct IF should be taken from normal-appearing skin immediately adjacent to an area of inflammation.

Indirect IF analysis of the sera of DH patients can detect circulating IgA antiendomysium antibodies (an intermyofibril substance antigen) on esophageal smooth muscle substrate. A significant correlation has been found between IgA antiendomysial antibodies (IgA-EmA) and the severity of gluten-induced intestinal villous atrophy. Detectable titers of IgA-EmA are specific and are found in about 70% of patients with DH (167). IgA-EmA antibodies disappear completely 1 year after strict adherence to a gluten-free diet and repair of the intestinal lining. Studies suggest that the target of antiendomysial antibodies is tissue transglutaminase (188).

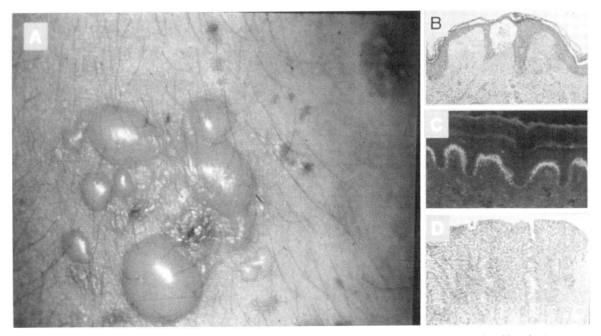

**FIG. 21.9.** Dermatitis herpetiformis (DH). **A:** This pruritic blistering disorder is characterized by clusters of herpetic-like blisters located on extensor surfaces of the body. **B:** Histologic examination of a skin lesion shows typical subepidermal blisters with collections of neutrophils at the tips of the dermal papillae. **C:** Typically, patients with DH show a granular deposition of immunoglobulin A along the dermoepidermal junction. **D:** Most patients with DH show an associated villus atrophy of the intestinal mucosa. These features link DH to gluten sensitive enteropathy (GSE). In GSE, however, patients do not have any skin lesions. The common feature between DH and GSE is that both diseases respond to a gluten-free diet. At present, the immunopathologic mechanisms responsible for blister formation in DH are unknown. See color plate 19.

## Diagnosis and Treatment

The clinical characteristics, histopathology, and immunopathology are the three well-accepted criteria for the diagnosis of DH (167,189).

With sulfone therapy, the lesions of DH are usually well controlled, with itching, burning, and new lesion formation control established within 12 to 24 hours of administration. Dapsone has been found to be more effective than sulfapyridine; however, dapsone is associated with a dose-dependent hemolytic anemia and methemoglobinemia, and patients must be closely monitored while receiving this medication. Patients receiving either therapy should be evaluated for glucose-6-phosphate dehydrogenase deficiency (G6PD) before starting therapy because of the profound hemolytic anemia caused by sulfone medications in G6PD-deficient patients. Patients of African, Asian, or Mediterranean descent are more likely to have G6PD deficiency. Other, less common side effects of these therapies include peripheral motor neuropathy, paresthesias, weakness, agranulocytosis, aplastic anemia, sulfone syndrome (fever, malaise, exfoliative dermatitis, lymphadenopathy, and hemolytic anemia) (190), and hypersensitivity hepatitis (191).

Strict adherence to a gluten-free diet for at least 6 months allows most patients to decrease the amount of sulfones being taken, but adherence to the diet must be continued indefinitely (192). Lesions recur in 1 to 3 weeks if gluten is consumed. Gluten is present in all grains except rice and corn as well as in many other foods. Gluten-free foods are commercially available; however, most patients find strict compliance with this regimen difficult. A small subgroup of DH patients who are not gluten sensitive do not benefit from dietary changes. Intake of excessive inorganic iodide has also been associated with exacerbations of DH. Brocq first discovered the association between iodine and DH in 1881. The mechanism by which iodine causes flares of DH remains unclear, but limiting intake has helped control disease in some patients.

## ACKNOWLEDGMENTS

This work was supported by research grants from the National Institutes of Health (RO1-AR32599, R37-AR32081, R01-AR40410, R29-AI40768 and T32-AR07577) and by a Merit Review Award from the Department of Veterans Affairs. Dr. Lin is the recipient of the Almay Research Fellowship, Division of Revlon Consumer Products Corporation, awarded through the Dermatology Foundation.

## REFERENCES

1. Lever WF. (1965). Pemphigus vulgaris. In: Curtis AC, ed. *Pemphigus and pemphigoid*, 1st ed. Springfield, IL: Charles C Thomas, 1965.
2. Civatte A. Diagnostic histopathologique de la dermatite polymorphe douloureseou maladie de During-Brocq. *Ann Dermatol Syph* (8th series) 1943;3:1–30.
3. Beutner EH, Jordon RE. Demonstration of skin antibodies in sera of patients with pemphigus vulgaris by indirect immunofluorescent staining. *Proc Soc Exp Biol Med* 1964;117:505–510.
4. Pisanti S, Sharav Y, Kaufman E, et al. Pemphigus vulgaris: incidence in Jews of different ethnic groups, according to age, sex and initial lesion. *Oral Surg* 1974;38:382–387.
5. Hietanen J, Salo OP (1982). Pemphigus: an epidemiological study of patients treated in Finnish hospitals between 1969 and 1978. *Acta Derm Venereol* 1982;62:491–496.
6. Simon DG, Kutchoff D, Kaslow RA, et al. Pemphigus in Hartford County, Connecticut, from 1972 to 1977. *Arch Dermatol* 1980;116:1035–1037.
7. Meurer M, Millns JL, Rogers RS, et al. Oral pemphigus vulgaris. *Arch Dermatol* 1977;113:1520.
8. Wilgram GF, Caufield JB, Lever WF. An electron microscopic study of acantholysis in pemphigus vulgaris. *J Invest Dermatol* 1961;36:373–382.
9. Hashimoto K, Lever WF. An ultrastructural study of cell junctions in pemphigus vulgaris. *Arch Dermatol* 1970;101:287–298.
10. Santi CG, Maruta CW, Aoki V, et al., and the Cooperative Group on Fogo Selvagem Research. Pemphigus herpetiform is rare clinical expression of nonendemic pemphigus foliaceus, fogo selvagem, and pemphigus vulgaris. *J Am Acad Dermatol* 1996;34, 40–46.
11. Beutner EH, Lever WF, Witebsky E, et al. Autoantibodies in pemphigus vulgaris. *JAMA* 1965;192:682–688.
12. Green D, Maize JC. Maternal pemphigus vulgaris with in vivo bound antibodies in the stillborn fetus. *J Am Acad Dermatol* 1982;7:388–392.
13. Mocada B, Kettelsen S, Hernandez-Moctezuma JL, et al. Neonatal pemphigus vulgaris: role of passively transferred pemphigus antibodies. *Br J Dermatol* 1982;115:316–319.
14. Goldberg NS, DeFeo C, Kirshenbaum N. Pemphigus vulgaris and pregnancy: risk factors and recommendations. *J Am Acad Dermatol* 1993;28:877–879.
15. Barnett ML, Beutner EH, Chorzelski TP. Organ culture studies of pemphigus antibodies. II. Ultrastructural comparison between acantholytic in vitro and human pemphigus lesions. *J Invest Dermatol* 1977;68:265–271.
16. Barnett ML. Effect of pemphigus antibodies on desmosomal structure in vitro. *J Invest Dermatol* 1978;70:141–142.
17. Schlitz JR, Michel B, Papa R. Appearance of "pemphigus acantholytic factor" in human skin cultured with pemphigus antibody. *J Invest Dermatol* 1979;73:575–581.
18. Hashimoto K, Shafron KH, Webber DS, et al. Anti-cell surface pemphigus autoantibody stimulates plasminogen activator activity of human epidermal cells: a proposed mechanism for the loss of epidermal cohesion and blister formation. *J Exp Med* 1983;157:259–272.
19. Woo TY, Hogan VA, Patel HP, et al. Specificity and inhibition of the epidermal cell detachment induced by pemphigus IgG in vitro. *J Invest Dermatol* 1983;81:115–121.
20. Anhalt GJ, Labib RS, Voorhees JJ, et al. Induction of pemphigus in neonatal mice by passive transfer of IgG from patients with the disease. *N Engl J Med* 1982;306:1189–1196.
21. Takahashi Y, Mutasim DF, Patel HP, et al. Experimentally induced pemphigus vulgaris in neonatal BALB/c mice: a time course study of clinical, immunologic, ultrastructural, and cytochemical changes. *J Invest Dermatol* 1985;84:41–46.
22. Stanley JR, Yaar M, Hawley-Nelson P, et al. Pemphigus antibodies identify a cell surface glycoprotein synthesized by human and mouse keratinocytes. *J Clin Invest* 1982;70:281–288.
23. Amagai M, Klaus-Kovtun V, Stanley JR. Autoantibodies against a novel epithelial cadherin in pemphigus vulgaris, a disease of cell adhesion. *Cell* 1991;67:869–877.
24. Buxton RS, Cowin P, Franke WW, et al. Nomenclature of the desmosomal cadherins. *J Cell Biol* 1993;121:481–483.
25. Amagai M, Karpati S, Prussick R, et al. Autoantibodies against the amino-terminal cadherin-like binding domain of pemphigus vulgaris antigen are pathogenic. *J Clin Invest* 1992;90:919–926.
26. Amagai M, Hashimoto T, Green KJ, et al. Absorption of pathogenic autoantibodies by the extracellular domain of pemphigus vulgaris antigen (Dsg3) produced by baculovirus. *J Clin Invest* 1994;94:57–67.
27. Ding X, Diaz LA, Fairley JA, et al. The anti-desmoglein 1 autoantibodies in pemphigus vulgaris sera are pathogenic. *J Invest Dermatol* 1999;112:739–744.
28. Eyre RW, Stanley JR. Human autoantibodies against a desmosomal protein complex with a calcium-sensitive epitope are characteristic of pemphigus foliaceus patients. *J Exp Med* 1987;160:1719–1724.
29. Scharf SJ, Freidmann A, Brautbar C, et al. HLA class II allelic variation and susceptibility to pemphigus vulgaris. *Proc Natl Acad Sci USA* 1988;85:3504–3508.

30. Sinha AA, Brautbar C, Szafer F, et al. A newly characterized HLA-DQB allele associated with pemphigus vulgaris. *Science* 1988;239: 1026–1029.

31. Szafer F, Brautbar C, Tzfoni E, et al. Detection of disease-specific restriction fragment length polymorphism in pemphigus vulgaris linked to the DQw1 and DQw3 alleles of the HLA-D region. *Proc Natl Acad Sci U S A* 1988;84:6542–6545.

32. Ahmed AR, Wagner R, Khatri K, et al. (1991). Major histocompatibility complex haplotypes and class II genes I non-Jewish patients with pemphigus vulgaris. *Proc Natl Acad Sci U S A* 1991;88:7658–7662.

33. Wucherpfennig KW, Yu B, Bhol K, et al. Structural basis for major histocompatibility complex (MHC)-linked susceptibility to autoimmunity: charged residues of a single MHC binding pocket confer selective presentation of self-peptides in pemphigus vulgaris. *Proc Natl Acad Sci U S A* 1995;92:11935–11939.

34. Lin MS, Swartz SJ, Lopez A, et al. Development and characterization of T cell lines responding to desmoglein-3. *J Clin Invest* 1997;99:31–40.

35. Hertl M, Amagai M, Sundaram H, et al. Recognition of desmoglein 3 by autoreactive T cells in pemphigus vulgaris patients and normals. *J Invest Dermatol* 1998;110:62–66.

36. Yamashina Y, Miyagawa S, Kawatsu T, et al. Polymorphisms of HLA class II genes in Japanese patients with pemphigus vulgaris. *Tissue Antigens* 1998;52:74–77.

37. Miyagawa S, Higashimine I, Iida T, et al. HLA-DRB1*04 and DRB1*14 alleles are associated with susceptibility to pemphigus among Japanese. *J Invest Dermatol* 1998;109:615–618.

38. Kermani-Arab V, Hirji K, Ahmed AR, et al. Deficiency of interleukin-2 production and interleukin-2 receptor expression on peripheral blood leukocytes after phytohemagglutinin stimulation in pemphigus. *J Invest Dermatol* 1984;83:101–104.

39. King AJ, Schwartz SA, Lopatin DE, et al. Suppressor cell function is preserved in pemphigus and pemphigoid. *J Invest Dermatol* 1982;79: 183–185.

40. Jordon RE, Schroeter AL, Rogers III RS, et al. Classical and alternate pathway activation of complement in pemphigus vulgaris lesions. *J Invest Dermatol* 1974;63:256–259.

41. Mascaro JM Jr, España A, Liu Z, et al. Mechanisms of acantholysis in pemphigus vulgaris: role of IgG valence. *Clin Immunol Immunopathol* 1997;85:90–96.

42. Lotti T, Bonan P, Cannarozzo G, et al. (1988). In vivo studies on the involvement of urokinase in pemphigus ancantholysis. *J Invest Dermatol* 1988;91:372–373.

43. Spillman DH, Magnin PH, Roquel L, et al. Aprotinin inhibition of experimental pemphigus in Balb/c mice following passive transfer of pemphigus foliaceus serum. *Clin Exp Dermatol* 1988;13:321–327.

44. Anhalt GJ, Patel HP, Labib RS, et al. Dexamethasone inhibits plasminogen activator activity in experimental pemphigus in vivo but does not block acantholysis. *J Immunol* 1986;136:113–117.

45. Esaki C, Seishima M, Yamada T, et al. Pharmacologic evidence for involvement of phospholipase C in pemphigus IgG induced inositol 1,4,5-triphosphate generation, intracellular calcium increase, and plasminogen activator secretion in DJM-1 cells, a squamous cell carcinoma line. *J Invest Dermatol* 1995;105:329–333.

46. Osada K, Seishima M, Kitajima Y. Pemphigus IgG activates and translocates protein kinsae C from the cytosol to the particulate/cytoskelton fractions in human keratinocytes. *J Invest Dermatol* 1997; 108:482–487.

47. Rosenberg FR, Sanders S, Nelson CT. Pemphigus: a 20 year review of 107 patients treated with corticosteroids. *Arch Dermatol* 1976;112: 962–970.

48. Bystryn JP, Steiman NM. The adjuvant therapy of pemphigus: an update. *Arch Dermatol* 1996;132:203–212.

49. Roujeu JC, Andre C, Joneau FM, et al. Plasma exchange in pemphigus. *Arch Dermatol* 1983;119:215–221.

50. Reference deleted.

51. Castro RM, Roscoe JT, Sampaio SA. Brazilian pemphigus foliaceus. *Clin Dermatol* 1983;1:22–41.

52. Diaz LA, Sampaio SAP, Rivitti EA, et al. Endemic pemphigus foliaceus (fogo selvagem). II. Current and historical epidemiologic studies. *J Invest Dermatol* 1989;92:4–12.

53. Robledo MA, Prada S, Jaramillo D, et al. South-American pemphigus foliaceus: study of an epidemic in E Barge and Nechi, Colombia 1982 to 1986. *Br J Dermatol* 1988;118:737–744.

54. Bastuji-Garin S, Souissi R, Blum L, et al. Comparative epidemiology of pemphigus in Tunisia and France: unusual incidence of pemphigus foliaceus in young Tunisian women. *J Invest Dermatol* 1995;104:302–305.

55. Morini JP, Jomaa B, Gorgi Y, et al. Pemphigus foliaceus in young women: an endemic focus in the Sousee area of Tunisia. *Arch Dermatol* 1995;129:69–73.

56. Diaz LA, Sampaio SAP, Rivitti EA, et al. Endemic pemphigus foliaceus (fogo selvagem). I. Clinical features and immunopathology. *J Am Acad Dermatol* 1989;20:657–669.

57. Lombardi C, Borges PC, Chaul, et al. Environmental risk factors in endemic pemphigus foliaceus (fogo salvagem). *J Invest Dermatol* 1992; 198:847–850.

58. Eaton DP, Diaz LA, Hans-Filho G, et al. Comparison of the black fly species (Diptera: Simuliidae) on an Amerindian reservation with a high prevalence of fogo selvagem to neighboring disease-free sites in the state of Mato Grosso do Sul, Brazil. *J Med Entomol* 1998;35:120–131.

59. Vieira JP. Novas contribuicoes ao estudo do penfigo foliaceo (fogo selvagem) no estado de Sao Paulo, Brazil. *Empresa Grafica da Revista dos Tribunais*, 1940.

60. Furtado TA. Histopathology of pemphigus foliaceus. *Arch Dermatol* 1959;80:66–71.

61. Sotto MN, Shimuzu SH, Costa JM, et al. South American pemphigus foliaceus: electron microscopy and immunoelectron localization of bound immunoglobulin in the skin and oral mucosa. *Br J Dermatol* 1980;102:521–527.

62. Santi CG, Maruta CW, Aoki, et al. Pemphigus herpetiform is rare clinical expression of nonendemic pemphigus foliaceus, fogo selvagem, and pemphigus vulgaris. *J Am Acad Dermatol* 1996;34:40–46.

63. Beutner EH, Jordon RE. Demonstration of skin antibodies in sera of patients with pemphigus vulgaris by indirect immunofluorescent staining. *Proc Soc Exp Biol Med* 1964;117:505–510.

64. Beutner EH, Prigenzi LS, Hale W, et al. (1968). Immunofluorescent studies of autoantibodies to intercellular areas of epithelia in Brazilian pemphigus foliaceus. *Proc Soc Exp Biol Med* 1968;127:81–86.

65. Roscoe JT, Diaz LA, Sampaio SAP. Brazilian pemphigus foliaceus autoantibodies are pathogenic to BALB/c mice by passive transfer. *J Invest Dermatol* 1985;85:538–541.

66. Futamura S, Martins CR, Rivitti EA, et al. Ultrastructural studies of acantholysis induced in vivo by passive transfer of IgG from endemic pemphigus foliaceus (fogo selvagem). *J Invest Dermatol* 1989;93:480–485.

67. Rock B, Martins CR, Theofilopoulos AN, et al. The pathogenic effect of IgG4 autoantibodies in endemic pemphigus foliaceus (endemic pemphigus foliaceus). *N Engl J Med* 1989;320:1463–1469.

68. Rock B, Labib RS, Diaz LA (1990). Monovalent Fab′ immunoglobulin fragments from endemic pemphigus foliaceus autoantibodies reproduce the human disease in neonatal BALB/c mice. *J Clin Invest* 1990;85:296–299.

69. España A, Diaz LA, Mascaro JM Jr, et al. Mechanisms of acantholysis in pemphigus foliaceus. *Clin Immunol Immunopathol* 1997;85:83–87.

67. Koulu L, Kusumi A, Steinberg MS, et al. Human autoantibodies against a desmosomal core protein in pemphigus foliaceus. *J Exp Med* 1984;160:1509–1518.

71. Stanley JR, Klaus-Kovtun V, Sampaio SAP. Antigenic specificity of fogo selvagem autoantibodies is similar to North American pemphigus foliaceus and distinct from pemphigus vulgaris. *J Invest Dermatol* 1986;87:197–201.

72. Allen EM, Giudice GJ, Diaz LA. Subclass reactivity of pemphigus foliaceus autoantibodies with recombinant human desmoglein. *J Invest Dermatol* 1993;100:685–691.

73. Koch PJ, Goldschmidt MD, Walsh MJ, et al. Complete amino acid sequence of the epidermal desmoglein precursor polypeptide and identification of a second type of desmoglein gene. *Eur J Cell Biol* 1991;55: 200–208.

74. Buxton RS, Cowin P, Franke WW, et al. Nomenclature of the desmosomal cadherins. *J Cell Biol* 1993;121:481–483.

75. Olague-Alcala M, Giudice GJ, Diaz LA. Pemphigus foliaceus sera recognize an N-terminal fragment of bovine desmoglein-1. *J Invest Dermatol* 1994;102:882–885.

76. Emery DJ, Diaz LA, Fairley JA, et al. (1995). Pemphigus foliaceus and pemphigus vulgaris react with the extracellular domain of desmoglein-1. *J Invest Dermatol* 1995;104:322–328.

77. Amagai M, Hashimoto T, Green KJ, et al. (1995). Antigen-specific immunoadsorption of pathogenic autoantibodies in pemphigus foliaceus. *J Invest Dermatol* 1995;104:895–901.

78. Reference deleted.
79. Petzl-Erler ML, Santamaria J. Are HLA class II genes controlling susceptibility and resistance to Brazilian pemphigus foliaceus (fogo selvagem)? *Tissue Antigens* 1989;33:408–411.
80. Auad A. Penfigo foliaceo sul-Americano no estado de goias rev patol trop 1972;1:293–346.
81. Moraes ME, Lazaro A, Fernandez-Vina M, et al. HLA class I and class II alleles in Brazilian Terena Indians. *Hum Immunol* 1995;44:61.
82. Moraes ME, Fernandez-Vina M, Lazaro A, et al. An epitope in the third hypervariable region of the DRB1 gene is involved in the susceptibility to endemic pemphigus foliaceus (fogo selvagem) in three different Brazilian populations. *Tissue Antigens* 1997;49:35–40.
83. Gregersen PK, Silver J, Winchester RJ. The shared epitope hypothesis: an approach to understanding the molecular genetics of susceptibility to rheumatoid arthritis. *Arthritis Rheum* 1987;30:1205–1212.
84. Lin MS, Swartz SJ, Lopez A, et al. Characterization of desmoglein-1 epitopes recognized by T cells from patients with fogo selvagem. *J Invest Dermatol* 1997;108:544.
85. Lever WF. Pemphigus. *Medicine* 1953;32:1–123.
86. Jordon RE, Beutner EH, Witebsky E, et al. Basement membrane zone antibodies in bullous pemphigoid. *JAMA* 1967;200:751–756.
87. Hodge L, Marsden RA, Black MM, et al. Bullous pemphigoid: the frequency of mucosal involvement and concurrent malignancy related to indirect immunofluorescence findings. *Br J Dermatol* 1981;105:65–69.
88. Hadi SM, Barnetson RSC, Gawkrodger DJ, et al. Clinical histological, and immunological studies in 50 patients with bullous pemphigoid, *Dermatologica* 1988;176:6–17.
89. Baba J, Sonozaki H, Seki K, et al. An eosinophil chemotactic factor present in blister fluids of bullous pemphigoid patients. *J Immunol* 1976;116:112–116.
90. Lever WF, Schaumberg-Lever G. *Histopathology of the skin,* 7th ed. Philadelphia: JB Lippincott, 1990:125–130.
91. Ahmed AR, Maize JC, Provost TT. Bullous pemphigoid: clinical and immunologic follow-up after successful therapy. *Arch Dermatol* 1977;113:1043–1046.
92. Diaz-Perez JL, Jordon RE. The complement system in bullous pemphigoid. *Clin Immunol Immunopathol* 1976;5:360–370.
93. Sams WM, Jordon RE. Correlation of pemphigoid and pemphigus antibody titers with activity of disease. *Br J Dermatol* 1971;84:7–13.
94. Provost TT, Tomasi TB. Evidence for complement activation via the alternate pathway in skin diseases: herpes gestationis, systemic lupus erythematosus and bullous pemphigoid. *J Clin Invest* 1973;52:1779–1787.
95. Kawana S, Ueno A, Nishiyama S. Increased levels of immunoreactive leukotriene B4 in blister fluid of bullous pemphigoid patients and effects of a selective 5-lipoxygenase inhibitor on experimental skin lesions. *Acta Derm Venereol* (Stockh) 1990;70:281–285.
96. Grando SA, Glukhenky BT, Drannik GN, et al. Mediators of inflammation in blister fluids from patients with pemphigus vulgaris and bullous pemphigoid. *Arch Dermatol* 1989;125:925–930.
97. Endo H, Iwamoto I, Fujita M, et al. Increased immunoreactive interleukin-5 levels in blister fluids of bullous pemphigoid. *Arch Dermatol Res* 1992;284:312–314.
98. Tamaki K, So K, Furuya T, et al. Cytokine profile of patients with bullous pemphigoid. *Br J Dermatol* 1994;130:128–129.
99. Zillikens D, Ambach A, Schuessler M, et al. The interleukin-2 receptor in lesions and serum of bullous pemphigoid. *Arch Dermatol Res* 1992;284:141–145.
100. Nishioka K, Hashimoto K, Katayama I, et al. Eosinophilic spongiosis in bullous pemphigoid. *Arch Dermatol* 1984;120:1166–1168.
101. Maynard B, Peters MS, Butterfield JH, et al. Bullous pemphigoid: eosinophil, neutrophil and mast degranulation in lesional tissue. *J Invest Dermatol* 1990;94:533.
102. Wintroub BU, Dvorak AM, Mihm MC, et al. Bullous pemphigoid: cytotoxic eosinophil degranulation and release of eosinophil major basic protein. *J Invest Dermatol* 1981;76:310–311.
103. Czech W, Schaller J, Schopf E, et al. Granulocyte activation in bullous diseases: release of granular proteins in bullous pemphigoid and pemphigus vulgaris. *J Am Acad Dermatol* 1993;29:210–215.
104. Nestor MS, Cochran AJ, Ahmed AR. Mononuclear cell infiltrates in bullous disease. *J Invest Dermatol* 1987;88:172–175.
105. Dvorak AM, Mihm MC, Osage JE, et al. Bullous pemphigoid, an ultrastructural study of the inflammatory response: eosinophil, basophil, and mast cell granule changes in multiple biopsies from one patient. *J Invest Dermatol* 1982;78:91–101.
106. Wintroub BU, Mihm MC Jr, Goetzl EJ, et al. Morphologic and functional evidence for release of mast-cell products in bullous pemphigoid. *N Engl J Med* 1978;298:417–421.
107. Oikarinen AI, Zone JJ, Ahmed AR, et al. Demonstration of collagenase and elastase activities in the blister fluids from bullous skin diseases: comparison between dermatitis herpetiformis and bullous pemphigoid. *J Invest Dermatol* 1983;81:261–266.
108. Gissler HM, Simon MM, Kramer MD. Enhanced association of plasminogen/plasmin with lesional epidermis of bullous pemphigoid. *Br J Dermatol* 1992;127:272–277.
109. Kramer MD, Reinartz J. The autoimmune blistering skin disease bullous pemphigoid: the presence of plasmin/alpha 2-antiplasmin complexes in skin blister fluid indicates plasmin generation in lesional skin. *J Clin Invest* 1993;92:978–983.
110. Ståhle-Bäckdahl M, Inoue M, Giudice GJ, et al. 92-kD Gelatinase is produced by eosinophils at the site of blister formation in bullous pemphigoid and cleaves the extracellular domain of recombinant 180-kD bullous pemphigoid autoantigen. *J Clin Invest* 1994;93:2022–2030.
111. Stanley JR, Hawley-Nelson P, Yuspa SH, et al. Characterization of bullous pemphigoid antigen: a unique basement membrane protein of stratified squamous epithelia. *Cell* 1981;24:897–903.
112. Labib RS, Anhalt GJ, Patel HP, et al. Molecular heterogeneity of bullous pemphigoid antigens as detected by immunoblotting. *J Immunol* 1986;136:1231–1235.
113. Tanaka T, Korman NJ, Shimizu H, et al. Production of rabbit antibodies against carboxy-terminal epitopes encoded by bullous pemphigoid cDNA. *J Invest Dermatol* 1990;94:617–623.
114. Diaz LA, Ratrie III H, Saunders WS, et al. Isolation of a human epidermal cDNA corresponding to the 180 kD autoantigen recognized by bullous pemphigoid and herpes gestationis: immunolocalization of this protein to the hemidesmosome. *J Clin Invest* 1990;86:1088–1094.
115. Giudice GJ, Emery DJ, Diaz LA. Cloning and primary structural analysis of bullous pemphigoid autoantigen, BP 180. *J Invest Dermatol* 1992;99:243–250.
116. Stanley JR, Tanaka T, Mueller S, et al. Isolation of complementary DNA for bullous pemphigoid antigen by use of patients' autoantibodies. *J Clin Invest* 1988;82:1864–1870.
117. Tanaka T, Parry DAD, Klaus-Kovtun V, et al. Comparison of molecularly cloned bullous pemphigoid antigen to desmoplakin 1 confirms that they define a new family of cell adhesion junction plaque proteins. *J Biol Chem* 1991;266:12555–12559.
118. Green KJ, Virata ML, Elgart GW, et al. Comparative structural analysis of desmoplakin, bullous antigen and plectin: members of a new gene family involved in organization of intermediate filaments. *Int J Macromol* 1992;14:145–153.
119. Li K, Sawamura D, Giudice GJ, et al. Genomic organization of collagenous domains and chromosomal assignment of human 180-kD bullous pemphigoid antigen (BP AG2), a novel collagen of stratified squamous epithelium. *J Biol Chem* 1991;266:24064–24069.
120. Giudice GJ, Squiquera HL, Elias PM, et al. Identification of two collagen domains within the bullous pemphigoid autoantigen, BP180. *J Clin Invest* 1991;87:734–738.
121. Giudice GJ, Emery DJ, Zelickson BD, et al. Bullous pemphigoid and herpes gestationis autoantibodies recognize a common non-collagenous site on the BP180 ectodomain. *J Immunol* 1993;151:5742–5750.
122. Zillikens D, Rose PA, Balding SD, et al. Tight clustering of extracellular BP180 epitopes recognized by bullous pemphigoid autoantibodies. *J Invest Dermatol* 1997;109:573–579.
123. Sams WM Jr, Gleich GJ. Failure to transfer bullous pemphigoid with serum from patients. *Proc Soc Exp Biol Med* 1971;136:1027–1031.
124. Anhalt GJ, Diaz LA. Animal models for bullous pemphigoid. *Clin Dermatol* 1987;5:117–125.
125. Liu Z, Diaz LA, Troy JL, et al. A passive transfer model of the organspecific autoimmune disease, bullous pemphigoid, using antibodies generated against the hemidesmosomal antigen, BP 180. *J Clin Invest* 1993;92:2480–2488.
126. Liu Z, Giudice GJ, Swartz SJ, et al. The role of complement in experimental bullous pemphigoid. *J Clin Invest* 1995;95:1539–1544.
127. Liu Z, Giudice GJ, Zhou X, et al. A major role of neutrophils in experimental bullous pemphigoid. *J Clin Invest* 1997;100:1256–1263.
128. Liu Z, Shipley JM, Vu TH, et al. Gelatinase B-deficient mice are resistant to experimental BP. *J Exp Med 188* 1998;188:475–482.
129. Liu Z, Zhou X, Twining SS, et al. Neutrophil elastase plays a critical role in experimental bullous pemphigoid. *J Clin Invest* (in press).

130. Hashimoto K, Miki Y, Nakata S, et al. HLA antigens in bullous pemphigoid among Japanese. *Arch Dermatol* 1979;115:96–97.

131. Ahmed AR, Konqui A, Park MS, et al. DR antigens in bullous pemphigoid. *Arch Dermatol* 1984;120:795.

132. Venning VA, Taylor JC, Ting A, et al. HLA type in bullous pemphigoid, cicatricial pemphigoid and linear IgA disease. *Clin Exp Dermatol* 1989;14:283–285.

133. Seignate J, Guillot B, Guilhou JJ, et al. Probable association between HLA-DR5 and bullous pemphigoid. *Tissue Antigens* 1987;30:190–191.

134. Delgado JC, Turbay D, Yunis EJ, et al. A common major histocompatibility complex class II allele HLA-DQB1*0301 is present in clinical variants of pemphigoid. *Proc Natl Acad Sci USA* 1996;93:8569–8571.

135. Büdinger L, Borradori L, Yee C, et al. Autoreactive CD4+ T-cell responses to the extracellular domain (ECD) of bullous pemphigoid antigen 2 in BP patients. *J Invest Dermatol* 1998;110:499.

136. Rico MJ, Streilein RD, Hall RP III. Peripheral blood mononuclear cells from patients with bullous pemphigoid have an increased frequency of response to synthetic peptides encoded by BPAG1. *J Invest Dermatol* 1994;103:73–77.

137. Lin MS, Swartz SJ, Giudice GJ, et al. Development and characterization of BP180-specific T cells from patients with bullous pemphigoid. *J Invest Dermatol* 1998;110:483.

138. Zillikens D, Mascaro JM Jr, Rose PA, et al. (1997). A highly sensitive enzyme-linked immunosorbent assay for the detection of circulating anti-BP180 autoantibodies in patients with bullous pemphigoid. *J Invest Dermatol* 1997;109:679–683.

139. Person JR, Rogers RS. Bullous pemphigoid responding to sulfapyridine and sulfones. *Arch Dermatol* 1977;113:610–615.

140. Berk MA, Lorincz AL. The treatment of bullous pemphigoid with tetracycline and niacinamide. *Arch Dermatol* 1986;122:670–674.

141. Kolbach DN, Remme JJ, Bos WH, et al. Bullous pemphigoid successfully controlled by tetracycline and nicotinamide. *Br J Dermatol* 1995;133:88–90.

142. Foster CS. Cicatricial pemphigoid. *Trans Am Ophthalmol Soc* 1986;84:527–660.

143. Chan LS, Yancy KB, Hammerberg C, et al. Immune mediated subepithelial blistering diseases of mucus membranes. *Arch Dermatol* 1993;129:448–455.

144. Eversole LR. Immunopathology of oral mucosal ulcerative, desquamative, and bullous diseases. *Oral Surg Oral Med Oral Pathol* 1994;77:555–571.

145. Bernard P, Prost C, Durepaire N, et al. The major cicatricial pemphigoid antigen is a 180-kD protein that shows immunologic cross-reactivities with the bullous pemphigoid antigen. *J Invest Dermatol* 1992;99:174–179.

146. Balding SD, Prost C, Diaz LA, et al. Cicatricial pemphigoid autoantibodies react with multiple sites on the BP 180 extracellular domain. *J Invest Dermatol* 1996;106:141–146.

147. Domloge-Hultsch N, Gammon WR, Briggaman RA, et al. Epiligrin, the major human keratinocyte integrin ligand, is a target in both an acquired autoimmune and an inherited subepidermal blistering skin diseases. *J Clin Invest* 1992;90:1628–1633.

148. Domloge-Hultsch N, Anhalt GJ, Gammon WR, et al. Antiepiligrin cicatricial pemphigoid: a subepithelial bullous disorder. *Arch Dermatol* 1994;130:1521–1529.

149. Lazarova Z, Yee C, Darling T, et al. Passive transfer of antilaminin 5 antibodies induces subepidermal blisters in neonatal mice. *J Clin Invest* 1996;98:1509–1518.

150. Shornick JK, Bangert JL, Freeman RG, et al. (1983). Herpes gestationis: clinical and histologic features of twenty-eight cases. *J Am Acad Dermatol* 1983;8:214–224.

151. Shornick JK, Stastny P, Gilliam JN. High frequency of histocompatibility antigens HLA-DR3 and HLA-DR4 in herpes gestationis. *J Clin Invest* 1981;68:553–555.

152. Shornick JK, Jenkins RE, Artlett CM, et al. Class II MHC typing in pemphigoid gestationis. *Clin Exp Dermatol* 1995;20:123–126.

153. Provost TT, Tomasi TB. Evidence for complement activation via the alternate pathway in skin disease: herpes gestations, systemic lupus erythematosus and bullous pemphigoid. *J Clin Invest* 1973;52:1779–1787.

154. Jordon RE, Heine KG, Tappeiner G, et al. (1976). The immunopathology of herpes gestation: immunofluorescent studies and characterization of the "HG factor." *J Clin Invest* 1976;57:1426–1433.

155. Katz SI, Hertz KC, Yaoita H. Herpes gestationis: immunopathology and characterization of the HG factor. *J Clin Invest* 1976;57:1434–1441.

156. Carruthers JA, Ewins AR. Herpes gestationis: studies on the binding characteristics, activity, and pathogenetic significance of the complement-fixing factor. *Clin Exp Immunol* 1978;31:38–44.

157. Kelly SE, Cerio R, Bhogal BS, et al. The distribution of IgG subclasses in pemphigoid gestationis: PG factor is an IgG1 autoantibody. *J Invest Dermatol* 1989;92:695–698.

158. Chorzelski TP, Jablonska S, Beutner EH, et al. Herpes gestationis with identical lesions in the newborn: passive transfer of the disease. *Arch Dermatol* 1976;112:1129–1131.

159. Katz A, Minto JO, Toole JW, et al. Immunopathologic study of herpes gestationis in mother and baby. *Arch Dermatol* 1977;113:1069–1072.

159a.Lin MS, Gharia M, Fu CL, et al. Molecular mapping of the major epitopes of BP180 recognized by herpes gestationis autoantibodies. *Clinical Immunology* 1999;92:285–292.

160. Lin MS, Gharia MA, Swartz SJ, et al. Identification and characterization of epitopes recognized by T lymphocytes and autoantibodies from patients with herpes gestationis. *J Immunol* 1999;162:4991–4997.

161. Katz SI, Strober W. The pathogenesis of dermatitis herpetiformis. *J Invest Dermatol* 1978;70:63.

162. Chorzelski T, Jablonska S. Linear IgA dermatosis of childhood (chronic bullous disease of childhood). *Br J Dermatol* 1979;101:535.

163. Aultbrinker EA, Starr MB, Donnenfeld ED. Linear IgA disease: the ocular manifestations. *Ophthalmology* 1988;95:340–343.

164. Kelly SE, Frith PA, Millard PR, et al. A clinicopathological study of mucosal involvement in linear IgA disease. *Br J Dermatol* 1988;119:161–170.

165. Bernard P, Valliant L, Labeile B, et al. Incidence and distribution of subepidermal autoimmune bullous skin diseases in three French regions. *Arch Dermatol* 1995;131:48–52.

166. Zillikens D, Wever S, Roth A, et al. Incidence of autoimmune subepidermal blistering dermatoses in a region of central Germany. *Arch Dermatol* 1995;131:957–958.

167. Beutner EH, Chorzelski TP, Kumar V, et al. Sensitivity and specificity of IgA-class antiendomysial antibodies for dermatitis herpetiformis and findings relevant to their pathogenic significance. *J Am Acad Dermatol* 1986;15:464–473.

168. Willsteed E, Bhogal BS, Black MM. Use of 1M NaCl split skin in the indirect immunofluorescence of the linear IgA bullous dermatoses. *J Cutan Pathol* 1990;17:144–148.

169. Whitworth JM, Thomas I, Peltz SA, et al. Vancomycin-induced linear IgA bullous dermatosis (LABD). *J Am Acad Dermatol* 1996;34:890–891.

170. Zone JJ, Taylor TB, Kadunce DP, et al. Identification of the cutaneous basement membrane zone antigen and isolation of antibody in linear immunoglobulin A bullous dermatosis. *J Clin Invest* 1990;85:812–820.

171. Zone JJ, Taylor TB, Meyer LJ, et al. The 97 kDa linear IgA disease antigen is identical to a portion of the extracellular domain of the 180 kDa bullous pemphigoid antigen, BPAg2. *J Invest Dermatol* 1998;110:207–210.

172. Gammon WR, Briggaman RA, Wheeler CE Jr. Epidermolysis bullosa acquisita presenting as an inflammatory bullous disease. *J Am Acad Dermatol* 1982;7:382–387.

173. Gammon WR, Kowalewski C, Chorzelski TP, et al. Direct immunofluorescence studies of sodium chloride-separated skin in the differential diagnosis of bullous pemphigoid and epidermolysis bullosa acquisita. *J Am Acad Dermatol* 1990;22:664–670.

174. Woodley DT, Briggaman RA, O'Keefe EJ, et al. Identification of the skin basement-membrane autoantibodies in epidermolysis bullosa acquisita. *N Engl J Med* 1984;310:1007–1013.

175. Borradori L, Caldwell JB, Briggaman RA, et al. Passive transfer of autoantibodies from a patient with mutilating epidermolysis bullosa acquisita induces specific alterations in the skin of neonatal mice. *Arch Dermatol* 1985;131:590–595.

176. Alexander J. Dermatitis herpetiformis. In: Rook A, ed. *Major problems in dermatology.* Vol. 4. Philadelphia: WB Saunders, 1975:11–30.

177. Wyatt E, Shuster S, Marks J. A postal survey of patients with dermatitis herpetiformis. *Br J Dermatol* 1971;85:511.

178. Hall R, Clark R, Ward F. Dermatitis herpetiformis in two American blacks: HLA type and clinical characteristics. *J Am Acad Dermatol* 1990;22:436.

179. Reunala T, Lokki J. Dermatitis herpetiformis in Finland. *Acta Dermatovener* (Stockholm) 1978;58:505.

180. Moi H. Incidence and prevalence of dermatitis herpetiformis in a country in central Sweden, with comments on the course of the disease and IgA deposits as diagnostic criterion. *Acta Derm Venereol* (Stockholm) 1984;64:144.

181. Smith JB, Tulloch JE, Meyer LJ, Zone JJ. The incidence and prevalence of dermatitis herpetiformis in Utah. *Arch Dermatol* 1992;128: 1608–1610.

182. Hall RP, Otley C. Immunogenetics of dermatitis herpetiformis. *Semin Dermatol* 1991;10:240–245.

183. Marks J, Shuster S, Watson A. Small-bowel changes in dermatitis herpetiformis, *Lancet* 1966;2:1280.

184. Gawkrodger DJ, Barnetson RSC. Dermatitis herpetiformis and lymphoma. *Lancet* 1982;2:987.

185. Reitamo S, Reunala T, Konttinen Y, et al. Inflammatory cells, IgA, C3, fibrin and fibronectin in skin lesions in dermatitis herpetiformis. *Br J Dermatol* 1981;105:167.

186. Cormane R. Immunofluorescent studies of the skin in lupus erythematosus and other diseases. *Pathologica Eur* 1967;2:170.

187. Katz SI, Hall RP III, Lawley TJ, et al. Dermatitis herpetiformis: the skin and the gut. *Ann Intern Med* 1980;93:857–874.

188. Dieterich W, Ehnis T, Bauer M, et al. Identification of tissue transglutaminase as the autoantigen of celiac disease. *Nat Med* 1997; 3:797.

189. Smith EP, Zone JJ. Dermatitis herpetiformis and linear IgA bullous dermatosis. *Dermatol Clin* 1993;11:511–526.

190. Millikan LE, Harrell ER. Drug reactions to the sulfones. *Arch Dermatol* 1970;102:220.

191. Johnson DA, Cattau EL Jr, Kuritsky JN, et al. Liver involvement in the sulfone syndrome. *Ann Intern Med* 1986;146:875.

192. Garioch JJ, Lewis HM, Sargent SA, et al. Twenty-five years' experience of a gluten-free diet in the treatment of dermatitis herpetiformis. *Br J Dermatol* 1994;131:541–545.

*Textbook of the Autoimmune Diseases,*
Edited by R. G. Lahita, N. Chiorazzi, and W. H. Reeves,
Published by Lippincott Williams & Wilkins, Philadelphia 2000.

# CHAPTER 22

# Muscle Diseases

Lisa G. Rider and Ira N. Targoff

## APPROACH TO THE PATIENT

The idiopathic inflammatory myopathies (IIMs) (Table 22.1) are autoimmune conditions that primarily manifest in the muscle, and myositis (muscle inflammation) is the major autoimmune manifestation in the muscle. Some forms of IIM, including polymyositis (PM) and dermatomyositis (DM), are systemic diseases that also have extramuscular manifestations. Localized forms of IIM, such as focal or orbital myositis, involve only particular muscles. IIMs may be part of overlap syndromes with other connective tissue diseases (CTDs). Some autoimmune systemic diseases, such as vasculitis or systemic lupus erythematosus (SLE), can lead to myositis indistinguishable from that of primary IIMs. Conditions primarily affecting other organs, such as Sjögren's syndrome, can sometimes result in autoimmune muscle disease through vasculitis. Other organ-specific autoimmune conditions, such as autoimmune thyroid disease, can result in pathophysiologic changes affecting the muscle, even mimicking IIMs, without actual autoimmune muscle injury. This chapter discusses the IIMs and myasthenia gravis (MG), a condition that can lead to weakness through autoimmunity to a muscle structure, the acetylcholine receptor (AChR). Other autoimmune diseases affecting the muscle are discussed elsewhere in this book.

Most of the IIMs discussed here primarily involve the skeletal, voluntary muscle. Some may also involve the cardiac muscle, but less often. Extramuscular manifestations may be a result of the consequences of skeletal muscle involvement, such as dysphagia in inclusion body myositis (IBM), or, in systemic autoimmune IIMs, may represent autoimmunity to other tissues, such as the interstitial lung disease of PM or DM.

## Clinical Features Suggesting Muscle Involvement in Autoimmune Disease

### Presentation

The possibility of autoimmune muscle disease should be considered in most cases in which myopathy is recognized on clinical or laboratory grounds. When other known causes of myopathy are excluded (infectious, noninflammatory, genetic, neurologic, endocrinologic, metabolic, drug-associated, or toxic) (Table 22.2) or features of autoimmunity are found, the IIMs are likely. A specific form of IIM, such as PM or DM, is sometimes first suspected because of a characteristic extramuscular feature of that condition. For example, the heliotrope or Gottron's papules of DM often develops before clinical weakness. Fever, interstitial lung disease (ILD), arthritis, and Raynaud's phenomenon are other extramuscular features that may be the focus of presenting symptoms for PM or DM or overlap myositis and can be helpful in discriminating IIM from other myopathies.

In the evaluation of patients with myopathy, it is important in taking a history to distinguish a feeling of generalized weakness or fatigue from true muscle weakness or loss of muscle power. The former is much more common because it is a nonspecific manifestation of many diseases, and it can be misinterpreted as muscle weakness. Perhaps more often, patients may go for long periods without diagnosis when muscle weakness is misinterpreted as fatigue. Weakness can also occasionally be misperceived as shortness of breath, although true shortness of breath may also occur as a result of weakness of the intercostal muscles, muscle deconditioning, or primary lung involvement.

The pattern of weakness that is characteristic of the IIMs, particularly PM and DM, is proximal muscle weakness,

L. G. Rider: Laboratory of Molecular and Developmental Immunology, Division of Monoclonal Antibodies, Center for Biologics Evaluation and Research, U.S. Food and Drug Administration, Bethesda, Maryland 20892.

I. N. Targoff: Department of Medicine, University of Oklahoma, Oklahoma City, Oklahoma 73104; Oklahoma Medical Research Foundation, Oklahoma City, Oklahoma 73104; and Department of Medicine, Veterans Affairs Medical Center, Oklahoma City, Oklahoma 73104.

The opinions expressed in this chapter are the authors' and do not necessarily represent the positions of the U.S. Food and Drug Administration or the Center for Biologics Evaluation and Research.

**TABLE 22.1.** *Classification of the idiopathic inflammatory myopathies in adults and children*

| Type | Description |
|------|-------------|
| I | Polymyositis |
| II | Dermatomyositis |
| III | Overlap myositis |
| IV | Inclusion body myositis |
| V | Idiopathic inflammatory myopathy associated with malignancy |
| VI | Focal myositis |
| VII | Proliferative myositis |
| VIII | Orbital myositis |
| IX | Eosinophilic myositis |
| X | Granulomatous myositis |

which differs from that of the typical neuropathic disease, such as peripheral neuropathy or cerebrovascular accident. Patients with proximal muscle weakness in the lower extremities often have difficulty standing from a chair or squatting position, climbing stairs, getting out of a car, running, or even walking. Myopathic involvement of the upper extremities may cause difficulty reaching, lifting, washing the hair, hanging clothes in closets, working overhead, or performing similar activities. Activities involving distal muscles, such as grip, heel and toe stand, or buttoning, would be relatively preserved. Sensory abnormalities are not seen in primary autoimmune myopathies but can be seen in certain systemic autoimmune diseases that can involve the muscle, such as vasculitis.

Individual syndromes may not always follow these patterns completely. For example, IBM often involves the distal muscles as well as the proximal muscles, or it may involve certain muscle groups (quadriceps, forearm flexors) and not others in a region. Distal muscle involvement in IBM may represent a component of neuropathic as well as myopathic involvement, and routine electromyography (EMG) can also sometimes suggest neuropathy (1). Focal and orbital myositis present with localized inflammation. Weakness may also present in atypical ways; for example, dysphagia may be the presenting feature of PM or IBM (2).

MG presents differently because the autoimmune response is specifically directed at the AChR of the neuromuscular junction, and the rest of the muscle is spared. The resulting characteristic pattern of weakness differs in distribution and variability compared with the weakness of PM and DM. MG commonly involves the eyelids and extraocular muscles and sometimes is confined to this area. Most other IIMs (except for orbital myositis) rarely affect these muscles. MG does not necessarily follow the proximal muscle weakness of IIM. The weakness of MG usually worsens as the day goes on and worsens with repeated efforts. Thus, the features of MG, which are direct consequences of its pathophysiology, distinguish MG clinically from IIM. In approaching a patient with muscle weakness, recognition of a myopathic or a myasthenic pattern of weakness provides the impetus for pursuing the investigations that can establish the diagnoses of specific conditions.

In the IIMs, myalgias may be common (50%) but are usually not the main presenting feature. Because myalgias are less common with dystrophy than with IIM, the symptom can focus the evaluation toward making that diagnosis (3). Myalgias are not usually as troublesome a symptom as weakness and tend not to be disabling. Marked myalgia may be an indication of rhabdomyolysis or muscle infection. Myalgia related to cramping may occur as a result of metabolic myopathies (such as inherited enzyme defects) or metabolic disturbances (such as hypokalemia or hypocalcemia). Cramping and fasciculations are not expected in IIMs.

### Examination

Physical examination is needed to establish the presence of muscle weakness as well as the pattern of involvement and its severity. Direct manual muscle strength testing is an important part of this evaluation for adults and children older than 5 years of age, comparing sides and proximal versus distal muscles. A common method of quantitation is the Medical Research Council scale, as follows: normal, 5; abnormal but with strength against resistance, 4; strength against gravity but not resistance, 3; unable to lift but able to move, 2; contraction without movement, 1; and absence of contraction, 0. Activities are observed, such as walking, climbing steps, standing from a chair, getting onto the examination table, lifting the leg or head from the table, and sitting from supine; functional assessments such as these are particularly important for children younger than 5 years of age who cannot perform manual muscle testing.

The remainder of the neurologic examination, including cranial nerve testing, evaluation of reflexes, and assessment of sensation, is important for excluding neuropathies and looking for the ocular signs of MG. The presence of fasciculations raises suspicion of amyotrophic lateral sclerosis (ALS). A general physical assessment evaluates whether extramuscular manifestations of disease are present, such as cutaneous features of DM, other CTD, arthritis, endocrine diseases, or signs of malignancy.

### Laboratory Evaluation and Diagnosis of Autoimmune Muscle Diseases

#### Enzymes

Autoimmune injury to muscle fibers often releases cytoplasmic muscle enzymes into the circulation, resulting in elevated serum levels. Processes that lead to necrosis of muscle, such as the cellular infiltration seen in PM, are most likely to lead to enzyme elevations, whereas those that result solely in atrophy, such as corticosteroid-related myopathy, usually do not. Neuropathies that lead to muscle atrophy typically do not cause enzyme elevations, but modest elevations may be seen in some, such as ALS (4).

Levels of creatine kinase (CK; formerly creatine phosphokinase), aldolase, lactate dehydrogenase (LDH), and

**TABLE 22.2.** *Differential diagnosis of idiopathic inflammatory myopathies*

I. Inflammatory myopathies (myositis)
  A. Infectious myositis
    1. Viruses
      a. Retroviruses
        i. Human immunodeficiency virus
        ii. Human T-cell leukemia virus type 1
      b. Picornaviruses (enteroviruses)
        i. Echovirus
        ii. Coxsackievirus
      c. Other viruses
        i. Influenza
        ii. Hepatitis B or C
        iii. Others (Epstein–Barr virus, cytomegalovirus, adenovirus, parvovirus)
    2. Bacteria
      a. Pyomyositis
      b. Lyme myositis
      c. Other (tuberculosis, mycoplasmosis, leprosy, group A streptococcus, etc.)
    3. Protozoa: toxoplasmosis, American trypanosomiasis, leishmania
    4. Parasites: trichinosis, cysticercosis
    5. Fungi: candidal infection

II. Noninflammatory myopathies
  A. Dystrophies
    1. Limb-girdle
    2. Fascioscapulohumeral
    3. Dystrophinopathies (Duchenne's, Becker's, carrier state)
    4. Merosin deficiency
    5. Congenital muscular dystrophy
  B. Congenital myopathies
    1. Congenital myopathies (nemaline rod, central core, etc.)
    2. Mitochondrial myopathies (some forms)
  C. Metabolic
    1. Myophosphorylase deficiency (McArdle's disease)
    2. Phosphofructokinase deficiency
    3. Myoadenylate deaminase deficiency
    4. Acid maltase deficiency
    5. Lipid storage diseases
      a. Carnitine deficiency
      b. Carnitine palmitoyl transferase deficiency
    6. Carcinomatous myopathy
    7. Acute rhabdomyolysis
  D. Myopathies in rheumatic diseases
    1. Muscle vasculitis in polyarteritis nodosa, Wegener's granulomatosis, rheumatoid arthritis, Sjögren's syndrome, Kawasaki disease, Behçet's disease

    2. Noninflammatory myopathy in scleroderma
    3. Myopathy and weakness in rheumatoid arthritis
    4. Polymyalgia rheumatica

III. Neurologic disorders
  A. Motor neuron diseases
  B. Myasthenia gravis or Eaton–Lambert syndrome
  C. Guillain–Barré syndrome

IV. Endocrine and metabolic disorders
  A. Thyroid
    1. Hypothyroidism
    2. Hyperthyroidism
  B. Hypercortisolism
    1. Endogenous
    2. Steroid myopathy
  C. Parathyroid
    1. Hyperparathyroidism
    2. Hypoparathyroidism
  D. Metabolic
    1. Hypocalcemia
    2. Hypokalemia
  E. Diabetes and neurologic complications
  F. Malnutrition

V. Drug-associated myopathies
  A. D-Penicillamine
  B. Cimetidine
  C. L-Tryptophan (eosinophilia–myalgia syndrome)
  D. Colchicine
  E. Chloroquine, hydroxychloroquine
  F. Lipid-lowering agents
    1. Lovastatin
    2. Clofibrate
    3. Gemfibrozil
    4. Niacin
  G. Cyclosporine
  H. Alcohol
  I. Ipecac, emetine
  J. Vincristine
  K. Aminocaproic acid
  L. Carbimazole, propylthiouracil
  M. Nonsteroidal antiinflammatory drugs
  N. Zidovudine
  O. Drugs of abuse (cocaine, amphetamines, heroin, phencyclidine, barbiturates)
  P. Anesthetics
  Q. Psychotropics
  R. Diuretics (hypokalemia)
  S. Corticosteroids

From Targoff IN. Polymyositis and dermatomyositis. In: Maddison PJ, Isenberg DA, Woo P, Glass DN, eds. *The Oxford Textbook of Rheumatology,* 2nd ed. Oxford, England: Oxford University Press, 1998:1249–1287, with permission.

transaminases (aspartate aminotransferase [AST] and alanine aminotransferase [ALT]) are usually elevated after muscle injury (5–8). CK is the enzyme most useful in the detection of muscle injury in adults because of its sensitivity and specificity. It can be elevated after even small degrees of muscle injury, including unaccustomed exertion by a normal person (9,10). It is sensitive enough that it can be elevated without the patient realizing that weakness is present, or in the

absence of clinical weakness. Elevated CK is useful in directing the clinician to consider myopathy as a cause of weakness or other muscle symptoms. A patient presenting with extramuscular features (ILD, DM rash) or with nonspecific complaints may have an elevated CK as the only manifestation of muscle disease. In PM and DM, the CK may be elevated before an exacerbation of muscle weakness, thereby serving as a warning of impending clinical relapse.

Some healthy people have CK levels above the normal range. Infrequently, there is an unrecognized muscle defect, as may occur in, for example, some female carriers of Duchenne's dystrophy (11,12). More often, no abnormality can be found. The normal range of CK levels is higher for African Americans than for white Americans (8,13) and higher for men than for women. When the CK is elevated in a healthy person, other muscle enzymes, including aldolase, are usually in the normal range. Most of these elevations of CK are below 1000 IU. When the CK is above the normal range, it is important to compare the result to previous test results to establish whether this value is abnormal for the patient.

The CK isoenzymes are of limited usefulness in IIMs. For example, in PM, the CK-MB may rise as high as expected in cardiac injury, without necessarily indicating cardiac damage (14). The CK-MB content of regenerating muscle, which can be found in some IIMs, is greater than that of normal skeletal muscle, and regenerating skeletal muscle myoblasts are thought to be the source of the increased CK-MB in IIM. The utility of newer markers of cardiac muscle, such as troponin-T and I, in the biochemical detection of cardiac muscle injury in IIM remains to be proved (15).

Some patients with active IIM do not have elevated CK levels (16,17). About 95% of patients have elevations of CK at some point in the disease course (18,19), but some may not have elevations of CK during all periods of disease activity. Some studies have found the frequency of CK elevation at presentation to be as low as 68% (20). Active IIM without CK elevation is more common later in the course of disease. Possible explanations for this include reduced muscle mass late in disease, CK inhibitors that interfere with functional assays of CK, as demonstrated in PM (21), and unknown causes. Normal CK levels may be more common in DM and in myositis associated with CTD (22). In other circumstances, in the absence of CTD overlap, low CK in active myositis was a poor prognostic sign in some studies (16). A few patients continue to have CK elevations without obvious ongoing muscle injury, but such enzyme elevations should be a cause for concern and investigated thoroughly (23). On the other hand, normalization of CK level with corticosteroid treatment does not always indicate response. The goal of treatment of IIMs is restoration of strength. Changes in CK can be helpful guides but cannot replace strength or other functional assessment.

Some patients with active IIM but normal CK have elevation of other enzymes. When this is found, it is important to exclude other sources of the enzyme elevations because these enzymes are also distributed in liver, lung, and other tissues. After this is accomplished, these enzymes may also be valuable in detecting and following the clinical course of IIM. In particular, aldolase is often elevated in patients who have active myositis with normal CK levels. This has been associated with scleroderma and eosinophilia–myalgia syndrome (EMS) (24). Patients with asymptomatic muscle disease leading to transaminase elevation may be suspected of having liver disease (25). Some investigators have suggested that the ALT does not rise in muscle injury, but several studies have contradicted this (26).

Other serum biochemical markers of muscle, such as myoglobin, may be elevated in PM and DM and may vary with disease activity. The urinary creatine is also elevated in myopathies or any condition that leads to muscle atrophy. It is less specific for active disease, more cumbersome to quantitate, and less readily available and thus is rarely used.

Patients with MG do not have muscle inflammation or direct injury or necrosis of muscle fibers and so do not have muscle enzyme release. Muscle enzyme levels can therefore serve to differentiate MG from IIM or other myopathies.

### Electromyography

In patients with suspected IIM, EMG is a useful step in helping to establish the diagnosis, although results of EMG are not diagnostic for a particular IIM. It can help document weakness if physical examination is equivocal, and it is particularly helpful in distinguishing myopathies from neuropathies. It can therefore serve as support for pursuing more invasive studies, such as muscle biopsy. The EMG findings that support myopathy include short-duration, low-amplitude (myopathic) motor unit action potentials, early recruitment with full interference, increased insertional irritability, and normal nerve conduction (27). Increased polyphasic potentials can be seen. In active myositis (PM, DM, IBM), other signs of spontaneous activity are common, including fibrillations and positive sharp waves that are thought to be indicative of denervation. Complex repetitive discharges are seen in about one third of cases of active myositis.

EMG can also support the diagnosis of MG by showing decremental responses by repetitive nerve stimulation testing. The more sophisticated single-fiber EMG studies are among the most sensitive tests for MG and can be useful when other studies are negative.

### Muscle Biopsy

The muscle biopsy can give the most specific information regarding the diagnosis of IIM and other forms of autoimmune muscle disease. It is not typically used to confirm a diagnosis of MG. Many patients with evidence of myopathy require a biopsy for definitive diagnosis. In some cases, a diagnosis can be established without a muscle biopsy, such as by the presence of a characteristic DM rash or a myositis-specific autoantibody. If any question about the diagnosis remains after evaluation of a patient with suspected myositis, however, muscle biopsy is advisable. The biopsy can demonstrate the expected findings of IIM, such as perivascular or endomysial inflammation, degeneration, and regeneration (Fig. 22.1) and is valuable for exclusion of certain other conditions (Table 22.2). Analysis of muscle biopsies includes routine histologic evaluation, special stains for fiber type and macrophages, enzyme histochemistry to screen for inherited enzyme defects such as myophosphorylase (Table 22.2), and electron microscopy

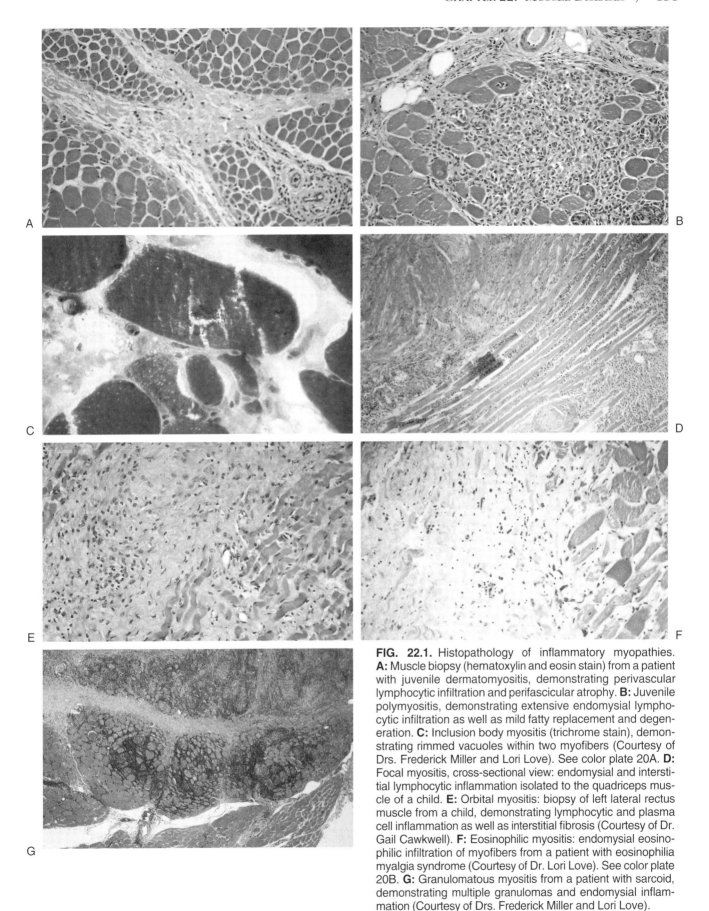

**FIG. 22.1.** Histopathology of inflammatory myopathies. **A:** Muscle biopsy (hematoxylin and eosin stain) from a patient with juvenile dermatomyositis, demonstrating perivascular lymphocytic infiltration and perifascicular atrophy. **B:** Juvenile polymyositis, demonstrating extensive endomysial lymphocytic infiltration as well as mild fatty replacement and degeneration. **C:** Inclusion body myositis (trichrome stain), demonstrating rimmed vacuoles within two myofibers (Courtesy of Drs. Frederick Miller and Lori Love). See color plate 20A. **D:** Focal myositis, cross-sectional view: endomysial and interstitial lymphocytic inflammation isolated to the quadriceps muscle of a child. **E:** Orbital myositis: biopsy of left lateral rectus muscle from a child, demonstrating lymphocytic and plasma cell inflammation as well as interstitial fibrosis (Courtesy of Dr. Gail Cawkwell). **F:** Eosinophilic myositis: endomysial eosinophilic infiltration of myofibers from a patient with eosinophilia myalgia syndrome (Courtesy of Dr. Lori Love). See color plate 20B. **G:** Granulomatous myositis from a patient with sarcoid, demonstrating multiple granulomas and endomysial inflammation (Courtesy of Drs. Frederick Miller and Lori Love).

when certain conditions such as mitochondrial myopathy or IBM are suspected on the basis of light microscopy.

Because the traditional open-biopsy is invasive, leaves a significant scar, and cannot be repeated easily, studies have looked at the possibility of using needle biopsy (28). The needle biopsy provides a much smaller specimen that may be difficult to orient histologically and that may be inadequate for functional studies, but several samples can be obtained through a single small incision, by redirecting the needle. This is often adequate for routine diagnosis of IIM.

Muscle biopsy is occasionally normal and often is nondiagnostic in IIM. Normal muscle biopsy in IIM is often attributed to biopsy of an uninvolved portion of muscle as a result of patchy involvement by the inflammatory process. Thus, selection of the biopsy site is important. The quadriceps is most often used, but the deltoid or other proximal muscles can be used alternatively if there is more evidence of involvement there. Severely atrophied muscle should be avoided to document early pathologic changes, and muscle recently studied by EMG should be avoided because the needles can cause artifact. Modern imaging techniques, discussed later, particularly muscle magnetic resonance imaging (MRI) scans, have greater precision for defining a biopsy site. Use of such techniques is especially helpful when an initial biopsy is negative.

### Serologic Studies

As with other autoimmune diseases, some forms of autoimmune muscle disease are associated with autoantibodies in the serum. In systemic conditions, such as PM and DM, antinuclear and anticytoplasmic autoantibodies are common. In patients with evidence of myopathy, clinical testing for serum autoantibodies can be diagnostically useful in assessing for the possibility of autoimmune muscle disease. The antinuclear antibody (ANA) test is the most sensitive of the clinically available autoantibody tests for IIM, present in 60% to 80% of PM and DM patients. The low specificity of the test for IIM, however, means that it cannot be used to help establish the diagnosis. The ANA is positive in 5% of healthy subjects, usually in low titer. A variety of ANA patterns may be seen, including nuclear speckled, homogeneous, nucleolar, and cytoplasmic, and therefore the pattern is not helpful in itself. A cytoplasmic pattern, however, should suggest further testing for specific autoantibodies.

Certain autoantibodies to cellular antigens have been more closely associated with myositis (myositis-specific autoantibodies [MSA] and myositis-associated autoantibodies [MAA]), which can be more helpful in establishing a diagnosis of IIM when present (Table 22.3) (29,30). The presence of an MSA is specific for myositis in that almost all

**TABLE 22.3.** *Autoantibodies in polymyositis and dermatomyositis*

| Antibody | Antigen | PM/DM (%) | Myositis subgroup[a] |
|---|---|---|---|
| I. Myositis-specific antibodies | | 30–40 | |
| Antisynthetase | Aminoacyl-tRNA synthetases | 25–30 | Antisynthetase syndrome[b] |
| Anti-Jo-1 | Histidyl-tRNA synthetase | 18–20 | |
| Anti-PL-7 | Threonyl-tRNA synthetase | <3 | |
| Anti-PL-12 | Alanyl-tRNA synthetase/tRNA[ala] | <3 | |
| Anti-OJ | Isoleucyl-tRNA synthetase | <2 | |
| Anti-EJ | Glycyl-tRNA synthetase | <2 | |
| Anti-KS | Asparaginyl-tRNA synthetase | <1 | |
| Anti-SRP | Signal recognition particle | 4 | PM (severe, resistant) |
| Anti-Mi-2 | Nuclear helicase | 8 | DM |
| II. Myositis-associated antibodies | | | |
| Anti-PM-Scl | Nuclear–nucleolar protein complex | 8 | PM/DM–scleroderma overlap |
| Anti-U1RNP | U1 small nuclear ribonucleoprotein | 12 | PM/DM–overlap syndromes |
| Anti-U2RNP | U2 small nuclear ribonucleoprotein | <2 | PM–scleroderma overlap |
| Anti-Ku | DNA-binding protein dimer | <2 | PM–scleroderma or systemic lupus erythematosus (SLE) |
| Anti-Ro/SSA | RNA protein particle | 10 | SLE; Sjögren's overlap |
| Anti-La/SSB | RNA protein | 5–7 | SLE; Sjögren's overlap |
| III. Myositis specificity not yet established | | | |
| Anti-MJ | 135-kd nuclear protein | Not determined | Juvenile DM |
| Antinuclear pore complex | | <2 | French Canadian |
| Anti-56 kd | Component of nuclear ribonucleoproteins | 85–90 | All |
| Anti-U5RNP | U5 small nuclear ribonucleoprotein | <2 | PM |

PM, polymyositis; DM, dermatomyositis.

[a] The most characteristic subgroup is shown, but most may occur in others.

[b] Some antisynthetases are less myositis specific (anti-PL-12, anti-KS).

From Targoff IN. Polymyositis and dermatomyositis. In: Maddison PJ, Isenberg DA, Woo P, Glass DA, eds. *The Oxford Textbook of Rheumatology,* 2nd ed. Oxford, England: Oxford University Press, 1998: 1249–1287, with permission.

patients who have an MSA have myositis or a CTD syndrome that includes myositis. None of the autoantibodies that are considered specific for myositis is sensitive for myositis. The most common is anti–Jo-1, present in about 20% of patients with IIMs. MAA are found in some patients with myositis as part of their condition (IIM or overlapping CTD) but are also found in patients without evidence of myositis. Because of their strong association with characteristic overlap syndromes, however, the presence of some MAA, such as anti–U1RNP or anti–PM-Scl, is also helpful for the diagnosis. Other autoantibodies that can be found in myositis, such as anti-Ro, can increase the likelihood of CTD but are less helpful than MSA for diagnosis. A significant percentage of patients with IIM, including most patients with IBM, have no evidence of ANA or autoantibodies to cellular antigens (31,32). Therefore, absence of these autoantibodies is not helpful for excluding IIM from diagnostic consideration.

In MG, most patients have specific autoantibodies to the AChR. These are specific for MG and 85% sensitive and are thus helpful for diagnosis, as discussed in the section on MG.

### Muscle Imaging

Occasionally, after evaluating a patient with suspected myopathy, a diagnosis of an IIM continues to be elusive. For example, the CK, EMG, or muscle biopsy may be normal, and specific autoantibodies may not be present. When myositis is suspected but cannot be established by other methods, MRI or ultrasound may be helpful because they are capable of detecting evidence of edema of the muscle, suggesting active inflammation as well as atrophy and fatty infiltration (33,34). MRI may help to pinpoint the location of inflammation, thereby directing the biopsy to an involved site. Edema by MRI gives increased signal on the fat-suppressed T2-weighted or short tau inversion recovery (STIR) images. MRI has the advantage of greater precision and clarity of the image, whereas ultrasound is less expensive.

In addition to its diagnostic role, MRI can play a role in treatment decisions in established disease. The level of disease activity may remain unclear after clinical assessment and enzyme tests. MRI using fat-suppressive techniques may show persistent edema when other parameters of disease activity have normalized and is therefore more sensitive (35). MRI also demonstrates muscle atrophy and fatty infiltration of muscle on T1-weighted images, as measures of disease damage.

Magnetic resonance spectroscopy (MRS) has also been used to provide information about the muscle in myositis, although it is less widely available. It can be even more sensitive than MRI. For example, MRS may be abnormal in patients with DM rashes who have normal muscle strength and serum muscle enzymes (36). The significance of such abnormalities is not fully understood, and MRS is therefore less often used at this time.

### Differential Diagnosis

Noninflammatory myopathies can sometimes be difficult to exclude, especially when there is evidence of myopathy on biopsy without a specific diagnosis. Also, inflammatory reaction can sometimes be seen in certain dystrophies, as, for example, in fascioscapulohumeral muscular dystrophy (37). Genetic tests are available for common forms of several muscular dystrophies, including Duchenne's, Becker's, myotonic dystrophy, and others. Some mitochondrial myopathies can cause isolated myopathy, although other features of mitochondrial syndromes are often present, such as ophthalmoplegia (38). The finding by biopsy of ragged red fibers is helpful in suggesting mitochondrial myopathy, which can be pursued further by electron microscopy. Confirmation can be obtained by testing mitochondrial functional activity or by genetic testing. Metabolic myopathies can also sometimes present with a picture resembling PM, including chronic progressive weakness (39). If suggestive signs are present, such as exercise intolerance, cramping, or family history, a forearm ischemic exercise test can be performed for additional support. The biopsy can provide confirmation by histochemistry for specific enzymes.

MG can cause extremity weakness with normal sensation, and if there is a suggestive history, further testing should be performed, including an edrophonium test as discussed below. Commonly, MG causes extraocular muscle weakness and ptosis, which are not expected in PM. Occasionally, motor neuron diseases can be confused with PM because sensory findings are absent and elevations of CK can occur (4). Prominent fasciculations are seen, the distribution of weakness is not proximal, and signs of myopathy are absent by EMG or biopsy.

Several endocrine or metabolic abnormalities can cause weakness or myopathy, with or without CK elevation. Hypothyroidism can cause myopathy and CK elevation, whereas Cushing's syndrome or steroid administration causes a myopathy in which CK is usually normal. Several common infections, such as toxoplasmosis (40,41), human immunodeficiency virus (HIV), human T-cell leukemia virus type 1 (HTLV-1), and enteroviruses, can cause myopathies (Table 22.2). Toxoplasmosis titers have been reported to be elevated in many cases of apparently idiopathic PM (42), without other evidence of active toxoplasmosis as the cause of the myopathy. Immune-mediated myositis can occasionally be seen in patients with HIV infection, without actual muscle fiber infection with HIV (43). A mitochondrial myopathy can also be induced by zidovudine (44). HTLV-1 can also be associated with a myositis (45–47), often in association with myelopathy.

The medication and environmental exposure history should be reviewed in all patients, looking for potential drug-induced or toxic causes. D-Penicillamine can cause a picture identical to that of PM, even associated with anti–Jo-1 in at least one case (48). Other drugs can cause a rhabdomyolysis or toxic myopathy picture. Among these are several cholesterol-lowering agents, including lovastatin and some of the other 3-hydroxy-3-methylglutaryl coenzyme A (HMG CoA) reductase inhibitors, especially in combination with fibrates (49) or cyclosporine. Vacuolar myopathies may be seen with colchicine (50) and chloroquine (51). Alcohol can also cause a chronic myopathy that can resemble PM (52).

## AUTOIMMUNE MANIFESTATIONS

### Idiopathic Inflammatory Myopathy

#### Introduction

##### Clinicopathologic Subsets of Idiopathic Inflammatory Myopathy

As implied by the name, the IIMs share the features of inflammatory muscle injury of unknown etiology. Most are thought to be autoimmune in pathogenesis, although the relative importance of autoimmunity in IBM is uncertain. The IIMs are heterogeneous clinically, and several classification systems have been proposed to define more homogeneous groups. The most widely used clinicopathologic classifications are based on that of Bohan and Peter (53), who separated adult PM, adult DM, myositis with malignancy, juvenile myositis, and myositis in overlap syndromes with other CTDs. Emphasis has been on recognizing the broader class of inflammatory myopathies, including IBM (54), as well as rare forms, including focal, orbital, granulomatous, and eosinophilic myositis (Table 22.1). Each form is discussed separately later.

By definition, DM is distinguished from PM by the presence of the characteristic DM rash, and for many years after the description of PM in 1863, and DM in 1887, they were the only forms of IIM recognized. Their myositis component was generally considered to be similar, until more recent studies demonstrated major pathogenetic differences between PM and DM. In children, there is a much higher proportion of DM than PM or IBM. Juvenile DM (JDM) has distinctive features when compared with the typical adult DM, the most striking of which are the more prominent vasculopathy and the development of dystrophic calcification. Studies now indicate a role for vasculopathy in the pathogenesis of DM in both adults and children.

A link between malignancy and IIM was first reported in 1916, and associated malignancy was later thought to be quite common. More recently, however, large population studies clarified the association of DM and malignancy as involving a small percentage of patients (55,56). These patients are usually considered in a separate subgroup. It is still uncertain whether there is a true increased frequency of malignancy in PM. Patients with a new diagnosis of IIM should be assessed for their risk for malignancy and some should have additional testing, as discussed later.

It was not until the 1960s that IBM was described and not until the past 10 to 15 years that it was recognized to be comparable in frequency to PM and DM, especially in elderly patients.

#### Autoantibody Classification

Clinical features are usually used to define the subgroups of IIMs because the cause is unknown. MSAs and some MAAs can also define complementary subsets of IIM, which differ in the presence of certain clinical features, responses to therapy, prognoses, and the HLA type from the overall myositis population (31). Autoantibody subsets incorporate patients in the clinicopathologic subsets of PM, DM, juvenile myositis, and CTD-related myositis. IBM and rarer forms of myositis are not usually associated with MSA and MAA.

Anti–Jo-1, the most common MSA, is directed at histidyl-tRNA synthetase, one of the aminoacyl-tRNA synthetases that catalyze the binding of an amino acid to its cognate tRNA during protein synthesis. At least five other antisynthetase autoantibodies, directed at other aminoacyl-tRNA synthetases, have been described in patients with myositis (29) (Table 22.3). There is a separate enzyme for each amino acid, and patients with antisynthetases (about 30% of myositis patients) each have antibodies to only a single synthetase, with rare exceptions. One exception is that patients with antiisoleucyl-tRNA synthetase (anti-OJ), which is part of a multienzyme complex of synthetases, may have autoantibodies to other synthetases in the complex (57). The clinical syndrome associated with each of the different antisynthetase autoantibodies is remarkably similar, and includes myositis, ILD, arthritis, Raynaud's, and other features (Table 22.4) (31,58). The ILD can become severe,

**TABLE 22.4.** *Features of 47 patients with antisynthetase autoantibodies*

| Feature | Affected Patients (%) |
| --- | --- |
| Myositis | 100 |
| Arthritis or arthralgia | 94 |
| Interstitial lung disease | 89 |
| Raynaud's phenomenon | 62 |
| Fever | 87 |
| Mechanic's hands | 71 |
| Myalgia | 84 |
| Dermatomyositis | 54 |
| Flares during taper | 60 |
| Anti-Ro/SSA | 25 |
| HLA-DR3 | 73 |
| Mortality | 21 |
| Female-to-male ratio | 2.7 |

Adapted from Targoff IN. Polymyositis and dermatomyositis. In: Maddison PJ, Isenberg DA, Woo P, Glass DA, eds. *The Oxford Textbook of Rheumatology,* 2nd ed. Oxford, England: Oxford University Press, 1998:1249–1287, with permission.

Additional data from Love LA, Leff RL, Fraser DD, et al. A new approach to the classification of idiopathic inflammatory myopathy: myositis-specific autoantibodies define useful homogenous patient groups. *Medicine* 1991;70:360–374.

acute, or fatal (59) and can be the major clinical problem (58,60). The arthritis can sometimes be inflammatory and deforming (61).

Some of the antisynthetases, anti–Jo-1, anti–PL-7, and anti-EJ, are more myositis specific in that almost all patients with the antibodies have myositis. Anti–PL-12, anti-KS, and anti-OJ have often been found in patients without myositis who have other features of the syndrome (usually ILD), but myositis is still present in most cases seen in the United States (62). Anti–Mi-2, directed at a component of a nuclear histone deacetylase complex, is also specific for myositis but occurs almost exclusively in DM rather than PM. The typical features of the antisynthetase syndrome are not increased in anti–Mi-2–positive patients. In contrast, anti-SRP, which is directed at one or more components of the signal recognition particle involved in translocation of newly synthesized proteins to the endoplasmic reticulum, is found almost exclusively in PM. It is often associated with a distinctive clinical picture marked by acute onset of severe myositis that is often resistant to treatment, and it frequently recurs as treatment is withdrawn. In some cases, necrosis with a paucity of inflammation has been seen.

MAAs may also identify subgroups of myositis. Often, these are overlap syndromes, such as mixed CTD associated with anti-U1RNP or the scleroderma–myositis overlap syndrome associated with anti–PM-Scl, as discussed later.

*Criteria for Diagnosis of Idiopathic Inflammatory Myopathy*

The most commonly used criteria for diagnosis of PM or DM were proposed in 1975 by Bohan and Peter (53) (Table 22.5). These criteria helped to standardize subsequent studies and clarify our concept of the diseases. Although these criteria remain useful, they were not designed to include IBM or the less common forms of IIM, and they do not take advantage of newer diagnostic modalities, including the MSA and MAA or the use of MRI. Another set of criteria for PM or DM was proposed by Tanimoto et al. (3) based on statistical study of a group of patients with myositis, compared with those with other neurologic or dermatologic conditions. Table 22.5 shows proposed modifications to the Bohan and Peter criteria designed to include newer modalities such as MSA and MRI (63). These criteria would classify patients as having an IIM, and other criteria would be used to identify the specific clinicopathologic subset.

Consensus criteria for IBM have been proposed (64) (Table 22.6), although the sensitivity and specificity of the criteria have not been studied. IBM shows both distinctive clinical features, as compared with PM and DM, and characteristic pathologic findings. To establish the diagnosis with certainty, histopathologic criteria are required. Some patients appear to have clinical IBM even though the biopsy does not show these findings. These newer criteria allow for the diagnosis of possible IBM in such instances.

**TABLE 22.5.** *Traditional and proposed modified Bohan and Peter criteria for the diagnosis of idiopathic inflammatory myopathy*

Traditional criteria
1. Symmetric proximal muscle weakness (by physical examination)
2. Elevation of serum skeletal muscle enzymes, particularly creatine phosphokinase, and often aldolase, serum glutamic oxaloacetate, and pyruvate transaminases and lactate dehydrogenase
3. Electromyographic triad of (a) short, small, polyphasic motor-unit potentials; (b) fibrillations, positive sharp waves, insertional irritability; and (c) bizarre, high-frequency repetitive discharges
4. Muscle biopsy abnormalities of degeneration, regeneration, necrosis, phagocytosis, and an interstitial mononuclear infiltrate
5. Typical skin rash of dermatomyositis, including a heliotrope rash, Gottron's sign, and Gottron's papules

Any 2 criteria = possible PM/DM
Any 3 criteria = probable PM/DM
Any 4 criteria = definite PM/DM

Patients with PM/DM who satisfy criterion 5 are considered to have DM.

Proposed revised criteria
1. Symmetric proximal muscle weakness
2. Elevation of the serum levels of enzymes, including creatine kinase (CK), but also aldolase, aspartate aminotransferase (AST), alanine aminotransferase (ALT), and lactic dehydrogenase
3. Abnormal electromyogram with myopathic motor-unit potentials, fibrillations, positive sharp waves, and increased insertional irritability
4. Muscle biopsy features of inflammatory infiltration and either degeneration–regeneration or perifascicular atrophy
5. Any one of the myositis-specific autoantibodies (antisynthetase, anti-Mi-2, or anti-SRP)
6. Typical skin rash of dermatomyositis that includes Gottron's sign, Gottron's papules, or heliotrope rash

Any 2 criteria = possible IIM
Any 3 criteria = probable IIM
Any 4 criteria = definite IIM

Patients with IIM who satisfy criterion 6 may be subclassified as having dermatomyositis. Those who satisfy the proposed criteria for inclusion body myositis (64) may be subclassified as having inclusion body myositis.
Results of magnetic resonance imaging that are consistent with muscle inflammation may be substituted for either criterion 1 or criterion 2.
The application of these criteria assumes that known infectious, toxic, metabolic, dystrophic, or endocrine myopathies have been excluded by appropriate evaluations.
Symmetry is intended to denote bilateral involvement, but not necessarily equal involvement.

PM, polymyositis; DM, dermatomyositis; IIM, idiopathic inflammatory myopathy.
Adapted from Bohan A, Peter JB. Polymyositis and dermatomyositis: parts 1 and 2. *N Engl J Med* 1975;292:344–347, 403–407; and Targoff IN, Miller FW, Medsger TA Jr, et al. Classification criteria for the idiopathic inflammatory myopathies. *Curr Opin Rheumatol* 1997;9:527–535, with permission.

**TABLE 22.6.** *Proposed diagnostic criteria for inclusion body myositis*

I. Characteristic Features: inclusion criteria
  A. Clinical features
    1. Duration of illness >6 months
    2. Age of onset >30 years old
    3. Muscle weakness: must affect proximal and distal muscles of arms and legs, and patient must exhibit at least one of the following features:
      a. Finger flexor weakness
      b. Wrist flexor weakness greater than wrist extensor weakness
      c. Quadriceps muscle weakness
  B. Laboratory features
    1. Serum creatine kinase less than 12 times normal
    2. Muscle biopsy
      a. Inflammatory myopathy characterized by mononuclear cell invasion of nonnecrotic muscle fibers
      b. Vacuolated muscle fibers
      c. Either:
        i. Intracellular amyloid deposits (must use fluorescent method of identification before excluding the presence of amyloid), or
        ii. Fifteen- to 18-nm tubulofilaments by electron microscopy
    3. Electromyography must be consistent with features of an inflammatory myopathy (long duration potentials do not exclude)
  C. Family history: For diagnosis of familial inclusion body myositis, as opposed to inclusion body myopathy, the inflammatory component must be documented.
II. Associated disorders
  A. An associated autoimmune condition does not exclude the diagnosis.
III. Diagnostic criteria
  A. Definite inclusion body myositis
    1. All muscle biopsy features, including invasion of nonnecrotic fibers by mononuclear cells, vacuolated muscle fibers, and intracellular amyloid deposits or tubulofilaments
    None of the other laboratory or clinical features are mandatory if muscle biopsy features are diagnostic.
  B. Possible inclusion body myositis
    1. Inflammation by biopsy without other pathologic features
    2. Satisfies criteria A.1., A.2., A.3., B.1., and B.3.

Griggs RC, Askanas V, DiMauro S, et al. Inclusion body myositis and myopathies. *Ann Neurol* 1995;38:705–713, with permission.

## Epidemiology

PM, DM, and IBM are uncommon disorders, and clinically significant forms of other IIMs are rare. The annual incidence of PM and DM together in adults is between 1 and 9 cases per 1 million, and the prevalence is about 10-fold more (55,65,66). A study of IIM including IBM in the 1984 to 1993 time period in Sweden found a similar (7.6 per 1 million) incidence (67). There is a suggestion in studies of an increase in incidence over time that might be the result of improved diagnosis (65). In adults, studies differ regarding the relative frequency of PM and DM (20,31), but PM is probably more common, depending on the population studied and the definitions used.

Love et al. (31) found that 79 of 212 IIM patients (37.3%) had adult primary DM without cancer or overlap. In addition, DM was diagnosed in 13 of the 36 patients with overlap myositis in the group (39%) and in 10 of the 13 patients with cancer-associated myositis. Thus, 48% had DM, compared with 40% with PM and 12% with IBM. In contrast, 51% of the 224 patients (excluding IBM) studied by Arnett et al. (32) had primary PM, and only 23% had primary DM (32). About 15% to 30% of adult IIM patients have IBM, but it is often underdiagnosed. PM and DM are more common in women (68) with a female-to-male ratio of about 2:1 overall and 5:1 during childbearing years, whereas IBM is more common in men, with a male-to-female ratio of 2:1. PM and DM are more common in African Americans than in whites. PM and DM are seen in all geographic areas, and local clusters are rare. Antibody-defined subgroups have shown seasonal variation in onset, with onset of anti–Jo-1 myositis occurring more often in April and that of anti-SRP more often in November (69).

## Etiologic Considerations

The cause of IIM is unknown. As with many other autoimmune diseases, it is believed that one or more environmental triggers act in a genetically susceptible host. It is likely that the heterogeneous clinical syndromes recognized under the rubric of IIM have heterogeneous etiologic factors. Syndromes similar to PM can be induced by D-penicillamine treatment (70), HIV infection (71), coxsackievirus infection, or toxoplasmosis (40,41). The characteristic rash of DM suggests a more homogeneous condition, but heterogeneity is likely in DM as well, with some patients having associated malignancy and differences in MSA profiles. The relationship of JDM to adult DM is not yet known. Also, whether amyopathic DM (rash without myositis) or severe vasculopathy with cutaneous ulceration or gastrointestinal perforation represent distinct conditions is uncertain.

Infections are suspected as being an initiating factor in some cases of idiopathic muscle disease (72). Picornaviruses, retroviruses, and others can induce an IIM-like picture in animal models and muscle disease in humans and have been suspected of inducing other autoimmune conditions. Coxsackievirus has been suspected of causing a portion of idiopathic cases (73). Studies have not consistently demonstrated persistent infection with coxsackievirus or other viruses or infections in most cases. Most studies to look for such evidence, using the polymerase chain reaction with rigorous methodology, have been negative (74–76). This does not exclude a role for viruses or unidentified agents in initiating the autoimmune response.

Other environmental factors have also been suspected. Autoimmune myositis resembling idiopathic disease has occurred after D-penicillamine (70). Myositis has occurred after toxin exposure, such as the ciguatera toxin. Several cases of PM or DM in patients with silicone breast implants have been identified, and the significance of this association is under study (77). Myositis has also followed bovine collagen injection, but whether there is a relationship is unknown (78).

The frequent association of autoantibodies with PM and DM supports the significance of autoimmunity in the pathogenesis of these conditions. Other evidence of the involvement of autoimmunity includes the inflammatory pathology, the response to corticosteroids and immunosuppressives, and the clinical association with other CTDs. In PM, cell-mediated attack on muscle fibers appears to play a predominant role in immune muscle injury, whereas in DM, humorally mediated injury to the small muscle blood vessels appears to be the major factor, with resultant ischemic muscle injury (54).

The significance of autoimmunity in IBM is less clear. In the sporadic form of IBM, inflammation is a much more prominent feature than in the inherited form. There is evidence that cytotoxic T cells can surround and invade muscle fibers in IBM, indicating that autoimmune damage occurs. Several factors, however, including the similarity of histopathology to the inherited form of IBM, the finding of degenerative features in IBM muscle similar to that in Alzheimer's disease brain, and the limited response to immunosuppressive treatment, have led to the hypothesis that a degenerative process is the primary problem (79).

Genetics is also an important etiologic factor in PM, DM, and sporadic IBM. Major histocompatibility complex (MHC) class II is the major immunogenetic risk factor for IIM, demonstrating an increase in PM and DM (45%) over controls (23%) in white, African-American, and Hispanic patients, with an association with DRB1*0301 (32). DRB1*0301 is also the major genetic risk factor for IBM (80). MHC class II polymorphisms also have clear associations with production of several of the MSAs and MAAs, including an increase in DR3 with anti–Jo-1 in white patients (31,32); increased DQA1*0501 or DQA1*0401 with anti–Jo-1 (32); increased DR3 with anti–PM-Scl (75% to 100% versus 22% to 23.5%) (81,82); and increased DR7 with anti–Mi-2 (83). It is rare to see cases of PM or DM in first-degree relatives. DRB1*0301 is the common genetic risk factor for sporadic and familial forms, but homozygosity of the DQA locus is an additional risk factor unique to familial IIM (84). It is more common than expected for relatives of PM or DM patients to have autoimmune diseases, suggesting genetic predisposition to autoimmunity in general (85).

### Adult Polymyositis

Patients with adult PM have onset of illness after 18 years of age and satisfy criteria for adult IIM in the absence of heliotrope or Gottron's papules. They also have other forms of IIM excluded clinically (no associated CTD or malignancy) and histologically (no IBM, eosinophilic myositis, or granulomatous myositis). Adult PM is diagnosed when the onset of IIM occurs in an adult and other forms of IIM have been excluded both clinically (e.g., by the absence of the DM rash, an associated CTD, or a malignancy) and histologically

(e.g., by the absence of signs of IBM, eosinophilic myositis, granulomatous myositis, or other forms).

Immunohistochemical studies of PM muscle have revealed much about the mechanisms of muscle injury (54,86–88). The main feature is an antigen-directed T-cell–mediated attack on muscle fibers. Typically, there is prominence of inflammatory infiltrates in the endomysial areas, with abundant activated T cells. Although CD4+ T cells are common, there is an increase in CD8+ cells toward the endomysial area. Cytotoxic CD8+ T cells surround and invade non-necrotic muscle fibers (macrophages infiltrate necrotic fibers). There are similar findings in IBM, but not in DM. T-cell–receptor gene rearrangement and restriction of V gene use is seen, more in the endomysial areas (89,90), along with evidence of clonal expansion (91,92), supporting an antigen-directed response; however, the antigen involved is unknown. Additionally, MHC class I, normally absent on muscle fibers, is expressed on muscle in PM, especially those fibers invaded by T cells (93). MHC class II can also be expressed (94). Perforin is expressed in the T cells in the muscle infiltrates and may be important in mediating fiber injury (95). In PM, but not DM, the perforin is often collected in the part of the T-cell adjacent to the muscle fiber. Further supporting evidence for cell-mediated pathogenesis comes from studies of peripheral lymphocytes, showing activation of T lymphocytes (96), sensitization of lymphocytes to muscle (97), and abnormalities of lymphocyte responsiveness (98).

Studies of cytokines in muscle have been somewhat conflicting (99,100) but generally do not show consistently high expression of proinflammatory cytokines. Interleukin-1 (IL-1) and some TNF-α have been seen in DM. Elevated levels of inhibitors of inflammatory cytokines have been found in the serum (101), possibly indicating a role. Chemokines have been observed in the muscle and may be involved in enhancing the inflammatory process (102). The DM-related features of vessel injury, such as capillary loss, complement deposition, and perifascicular atrophy, are typically absent in PM.

### Clinical Presentation

*Myositis* Most patients present with a symmetric proximal muscle weakness typical of myopathies, with distal weakness usually less severe than proximal weakness. The peak onset is between 40 and 60 years of age. Both upper and lower extremities are involved, typically lower extremities first. Facial muscles are usually spared, but chewing can be affected. Onset is typically over weeks to months, although it may vary from a slowly progressive form to an acute, explosive onset. Myalgias can occur and tend to be more severe with more acute onset. Respiratory muscle weakness can occur, becoming clinically significant in about 5% of patients. In the most severe cases of respiratory muscle involvement, assisted ventilation is required and is an indication for urgent treatment. Pharyngeal and upper esophageal muscle weakness can develop, with resultant dysphagia. Patients with dysphagia are at increased risk for aspiration.

*Extramuscular Features* PM can also have primary manifestations outside the muscles (Fig. 22.2). Systemic manifestations can occur, including fatigue and weight loss. Fever can occur during exacerbations and is much more common in patients with antisynthetase autoantibodies or as part of CTD syndromes.

Involvement of other organ systems can also occur. Cardiac abnormalities are common but are clinically significant in only a minority of patients. Only a small proportion of patients [3% in one series (18)] have myocardial involvement serious enough to cause congestive heart failure, with inflammation similar to that of skeletal muscle (103). Arrhythmias or conduction disturbances are much more common, but these are generally mild. Palpitations are relatively more common in PM (57%) than in DM (19%)(31).

ILD, seen in 10% to 30% of cases, is a cause of significant morbidity and mortality. It is clinically similar to other forms of ILD, with restrictive pulmonary function tests and a reticu-

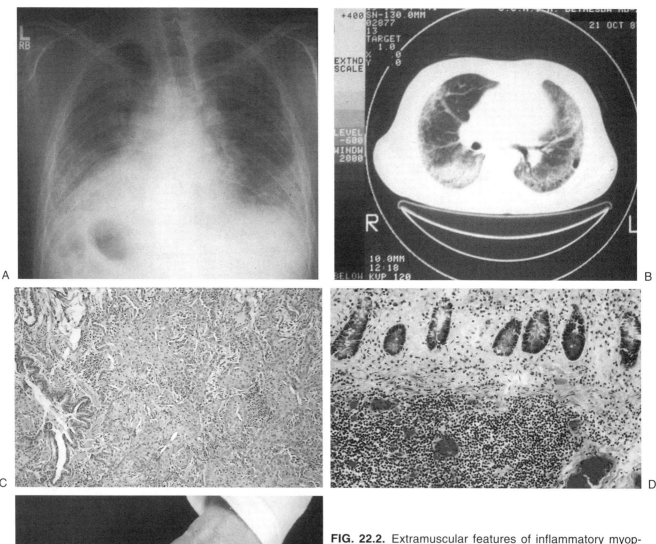

**FIG. 22.2.** Extramuscular features of inflammatory myopathies. **A:** Chest radiograph. **B:** Computed tomography scan from a dermatomyositis patient with anti–Jo-1 autoantibodies, demonstrating interstitial lung disease and alveolar changes (Courtesy of Dr. Frederick Miller). **C:** Lung biopsy from a teenage girl with anti–PL-12 autoantibody, demonstrating organizing pneumonitis in the alveolus and dense interstitial neutrophilic inflammation resulting from aspiration. **D:** Small bowel biopsy from a patient with juvenile dermatomyositis and gastrointestinal ulceration, demonstrating lymphocytic inflammation in the muscularis mucosa and a small blood vessel with thrombosis. **E:** Deforming Jaccoud's arthropathy and sclerodactyly in a woman with juvenile-onset dermatomyositis and anti–PM-Scl autoantibodies.

lonodular pattern by radiograph. Some patients present with ILD, only to have myositis revealed by an elevated CK. ILD in PM is strongly associated with antisynthetase autoantibodies and can also be seen in other CTD-overlap syndromes with myositis. Bronchiolitis obliterans organizing pneumonia can be seen and has a relatively good prognosis (104). Other histologic patterns found include usual interstitial pneumonitis, cellular interstitial pneumonia, and diffuse alveolar damage (105). Primary ILD may be difficult to distinguish from interstitial disease developing in treated PM patients as a result of opportunistic infections or hypersensitivity pneumonitis.

Some cases of dysphagia are caused by cricopharyngeal muscle dysfunction, which may persist after treatment and has been treated with cricopharyngeal myotomy with success (106). Esophageal dysmotility unrelated to myositis, similar to that seen in scleroderma, can also occur (107).

*Laboratory Tests*  The CK level in PM is usually elevated in active PM (80% to 90%). Elevations of more than 1000 IU are routine, elevations of more than 10-fold the upper limit of normal are common, and elevations more than 100-fold normal are not unusual. The CK level is more consistently elevated in PM than in DM (8) at presentation or recurrence. The average CK levels are higher for PM than for IBM. For an individual followed over time, the CK level tends to correlate with activity of disease. Other muscle-associated enzymes, including LDH, transaminases, and aldolase, are also usually elevated in PM. These are most useful clinically when elevated despite a normal CK. Serum myoglobin is also elevated in most PM and DM patients and correlates well with disease activity but is less often used.

The erythrocyte sedimentation rate (ESR) and C-reactive protein may be elevated but can be normal in active disease and do not correlate well with disease activity. An elevated ESR, however, supports a diagnosis of PM over noninflammatory myopathies. Complement is usually normal (except in deficiency states). Immunoglobulin level can be elevated, especially in those with overlap or CTD syndromes.

As noted, PM patients have a high frequency of ANAs and other autoantibodies, including MSA and MAA. The most common single MSA in PM is anti–Jo-1, which is more common in PM than in DM in most studies (32) (Table 22.3). Although antibody to the signal recognition particle (anti-SRP) occurs almost exclusively in PM, it is relatively rare, present in only 4% of myositis cases overall (108). Anti–PM-Scl may occur in PM alone but more often occurs in an overlap syndrome.

### Diagnostic Approach

PM should be suspected in any patient who presents with the new onset of proximal muscle weakness in adulthood without evidence of neuropathy or sensory abnormalities, especially when the CK is elevated or there are signs of systemic inflammatory disease (e.g., fever, weight loss) or CTD (e.g., positive ANA, arthritis). Most such patients should then have EMG testing. EMG detects evidence of myopathy in 90% of

PM patients but should be done in several areas to maximize sensitivity. EMG helps to establish the presence of myopathy and exclude neuropathy. The typical findings expected in PM were described previously. Most patients then require a muscle biopsy. Occasionally, the diagnosis can be established by other means, such as the confirmed presence of an MSA with a typical clinical picture and EMG (such a patient would satisfy the modified criteria). If the EMG is normal, but clinical suspicion of PM remains strong as a result of the clinical picture and elevated CK, a muscle biopsy would still be indicated. MRI of the thigh muscles may then be useful to provide evidence of muscle disease and inflammation and to identify an active area to biopsy. This would be especially true if a first biopsy is also negative or equivocal, and the diagnosis remains in doubt.

The muscle biopsy in PM should demonstrate evidence of inflammation, with an inflammatory infiltrate characterized by lymphocytes, plasma cells, macrophages, and sometimes other cells. These infiltrates are usually endomysial, within the fascicle, rather than predominating in the perimysial or perifascicular area (109). Inflammation may be absent in up to 25% of cases, presumably because the site of active involvement was missed. Other typical findings in PM include necrosis of individual fibers, with degeneration, and phagocytosis. There is also regeneration, with basophilia and large internal nuclei. Evidence of other conditions should not be found.

### Therapy

Most patients with a diagnosis of PM require treatment to prevent significant disability and in some cases mortality. In PM and DM, the chances of full recovery of strength fall if treatment is significantly delayed. Corticosteroids are generally accepted as the mainstay of treatment in PM, with response that is sometimes dramatic, although double-blind trials have not been done. Therapy is usually initiated at high doses, with at least 60 mg/d of prednisone or equivalent in divided doses. Patients with poor prognostic factors (dysphagia, respiratory muscle weakness, or severe weakness) are often treated first with a pulse methylprednisolone regimen, such as 1 g/d for 3 days. Alternate-day oral steroids should not be used to induce remission.

It is important to give an adequate course of high-dose steroids to suppress the myositis completely, usually 1 to 2 months (110). Once response begins, the dose may be consolidated in steps to a single daily dose. Patients who have a good response should then undergo a slow reduction in the dose to a maintenance level of 5 to 10 mg/d of prednisone (10 to 20 mg every other day). A commonly used tapering regimen, usually in the range of 25% per month (i.e., larger milligram reductions from larger doses), reduces the dose by almost half in 2 months and achieves a maintenance dose after about 6 months. As the dose is reduced, careful observation for recurrence is essential, as is continued monitoring for side effects. As a result of the prolonged course of high-dose steroids, adequate calcium and vitamin D intake should be ensured. Aseptic necrosis and opportunistic infections may occur.

If the patient fails to respond or has an inadequate response, it is important to be sure the diagnosis has been adequately established. One cause for apparent treatment-resistant PM is unrecognized IBM, which usually responds less well and may not be recognized on the first biopsy. Another possible cause is steroid myopathy, especially when the CK remains normal, or myopathy resulting from other medications. If the patient has had prolonged disease before beginning treatment and muscle atrophy is present, there may be permanent loss of strength, although some improvement usually occurs if the disease was active when treatment was started. The possibility of an associated malignancy should also be considered, although this is more commonly an issue in DM. Some cases of pure adult PM are truly refractory to steroid treatment or only partially responsive, and the addition of another medication should be considered. Such inadequate responsiveness is more frequent in association with anti-SRP autoantibodies.

A rise in CK may be a warning of impending exacerbation, but other causes of CK elevation must be considered (e.g., trauma, endocrine, drug, or toxin). If it is concluded that an exacerbation of PM has occurred, it is usually necessary to increase the prednisone to a dose higher than that which last controlled activity, but a full repeat course is usually not necessary. Addition of an immunosuppressive agent should also be considered for steroid-sparing effect to limit side effects. There is some experimental support for the routine use of an immunosuppressive agent at the initiation of therapy (111).

When an immunosuppressive agent is needed, either azathioprine or methotrexate is typically used first. Various studies indicate that these agents are effective in 35% to 75% of cases (112). There is some data suggesting better results with methotrexate, with better responses in men than women and better responses in patients with antisynthetase autoantibodies (113). Methotrexate is most often used by the oral route, as in rheumatoid arthritis, in single weekly doses starting at 7.5 to 10 mg/wk and increasing as required up to 20 mg/wk. Higher doses were often used in early studies (112), up to 50 mg/wk, and are sometimes used today for resistant cases. Such doses should be administered parenterally, often intravenously to avoid intramuscular injections when following CK levels. The liver enzymes monitored during methotrexate treatment may be elevated as a result of the muscle injury. Evidence of long-term benefit of azathioprine in PM was provided by a controlled trial comparing azathioprine plus prednisone with prednisone alone (111). Azathioprine is usually given in doses of 1.5 to 3 mg/kg/d, most often 100 to 150 mg/d. The usual time to peak benefit is greater than 3 months, which is longer than that of methotrexate. Careful monitoring for bone marrow suppression is necessary. Azathioprine has been associated with an increased risk for malignancy, but this risk appears to be small.

If use of methotrexate or azathioprine alone is not effective, a combination of the two may be helpful. In one study, up to 150 mg/d of azathioprine with up to 22.5 to 25 mg/wk of methotrexate given orally, along with maintenance-dose prednisone, led to improvement in about half of patients whose previous treatment was ineffective (114). This combination was more often effective than high-dose intravenous methotrexate with leucovorin rescue, although that treatment also helped some treatment-resistant patients.

Other medications have also been used to treat persistent myositis. Cyclosporine can be used in PM when therapy with azathioprine and/or methotrexate has been unsuccessful, or as an alternative agent. Early reports used it at high dosages, but there is a recent tendency to limit it to 5 mg/kg per day. Tacrolimus (FK-506) has also been used anecdotally with some success (115).

Intravenous immunoglobulin (IVIG) infusions, 2 g/kg per month administered over 2 to 5 days, have been used to treat PM. Controlled studies in PM comparable to those in DM are not yet available, but there are numerous reports of success (116). The frequency of side effects is low, but the high cost limits its use. The duration of response is variable, but most patients relapse if repeated infusion is not given. Trials of 3 to 9 months are sometimes given. IVIG is most useful in patients who are having exacerbation or are severely refractory. The mechanism of action in PM is uncertain; suggested mechanisms include antiidiotypes or other immunomodulatory activities, or treatment of unrecognized infection. It may be different from the mechanism in DM.

An early study of daily oral cyclophosphamide for treatment of myositis was discouraging, as was a later study of monthly intravenous pulse treatment. Effectiveness was limited, and serious adverse effects occurred, although there are reports of benefits in individual cases. This remains an option for refractory or life-threatening cases. There have been reports of success with cyclophosphamide intravenously or orally in treating severe ILD in PM (117), and it is commonly employed for this purpose. Intensive immunosuppression, especially when high doses of steroids are combined with cytotoxic agents, carries a risk for *Pneumocystis carinii* pneumonia (118,119), and prophylaxis may be considered with such regimens.

Plasmapheresis has been used in PM (120), with reports of success in individual cases or series, but a blinded, controlled study found no benefit (121). The possibility of benefit for subgroups or to enhance other treatments has not been excluded (122). As a last resort, total-body irradiation has occasionally been used (123), but it has not had consistent success (124).

Physical therapy and rehabilitation have an important role in achieving an optimal outcome (125,126). Range-of-motion exercise is helpful to avoid contractures, but resistive exercises are usually discouraged during acute periods with severely inflamed muscles. After the inflammation is controlled and the patient is stable, active exercise can be slowly and cautiously begun to help in recovery of strength, even if some degree of disease activity remains (125,127).

## Adult Dermatomyositis

DM is defined by the presence of the characteristic cutaneous manifestations, including Gottron's papules or heliotrope rash, in a patient with persistent myositis. Cancer-associated myositis should be excluded, as discussed later, which accounts for about 20% to 25% of adult DM cases. A subgroup of patients with typical cutaneous features of DM has no clinical evidence of myositis for prolonged periods ("amyopathic DM" or "DM sine myositis").

The cause of DM is unknown, as discussed previously. The pathogenetic process in the typical case of DM appears to differ from that in most PM patients based on examination of biopsy specimens. Rather than evidence of T-cell–mediated attack on muscle fibers, there is evidence of humoral attack on intramuscular small blood vessels. The inflammatory infiltrate is more concentrated in the perivascular and perimysial areas, with predominance of B cells and $CD4^+$ T cells. Later, perifascicular atrophy develops, which is relatively specific for IIM, especially DM. There is deposition of the membrane attack complex of complement in the muscle vessels, not seen in PM. Signs of endothelial injury, such as tubuloreticular inclusions, can be seen by electron microscopy. Capillary loss can be demonstrated by quantitative measures. The pathologic appearance also suggests ischemic injury. These changes in the vessels can precede the myopathic, inflammatory change, suggesting that the vasculature is the primary target. A similar process may be involved in the pathogenesis of cutaneous features because perivascular inflammation and deposition of the membrane attack complex has been identified in small vessels in the skin (128,129).

### Clinical Presentation

The myositis of DM is clinically indistinguishable from that of PM, although symmetric proximal muscle weakness may have a more rapid onset in some cases. Cutaneous features of DM often precede the myositis, most commonly by a few weeks, although simultaneous onset is also common. DM differs from IBM clinically in its pattern of muscle weakness and skin findings, the latter being absent in IBM.

Gottron's papules are erythematous, sometimes scaly papules or plaques occurring over the extensor surfaces of the fingers, usually at the metacarpophalangeal and proximal interphalangeal joints (Fig. 22.3). An erythematous area, over a similar distribution or over the extensor surfaces of the elbows or knees, or the medial malleolus, has been referred to as *Gottron's sign.* A violaceous aspect to the erythema is common. Atrophy and telangiectasia may occur associated with this. Gottron's papules are considered highly specific for DM, and Gottron's sign less specific. Gottron's lesions are found in 70% to 80% of DM patients. A similar erythema, which may be raised and scaly, extends out between the joint surfaces in a linear fashion (*linear extensor erythema*). The heliotrope sign is a violaceous, purplish color in the eyelid and surrounding areas and may be associated with periorbital

edema. Occurrence of this sign in 30% to 60% of DM patients can be helpful diagnostically, especially when it occurs in conjunction with Gottron's lesions or findings of myopathy, but a similar appearance may occur in SLE or with allergies. An erythematous, violaceous rash can also occur elsewhere. Typical is the upper chest, back, and shoulders in a "shawl" pattern, and in the V of the neck, suggesting a photosensitive distribution. It can also be exacerbated by sun exposure, but the photosensitivity is not as pronounced as that of SLE. Poikiloderma (alternating hypopigmentation and hyperpigmentation with telangiectasia and atrophy) may be associated with DM rashes. Scalp involvement is common, resembling psoriasis. Other skin findings are also associated with DM rather than PM and appear to reflect part of the DM pathophysiologic process. These findings include periungual nailfold capillary changes similar to those seen in scleroderma, calcinosis, and cutaneous ulcerations. These are discussed in more detail in the JDM section below.

### Diagnostic Approach

The evaluation and diagnostic studies for the myositis of DM are similar to that of PM. If the cutaneous features are typical, it may not be necessary to do a muscle biopsy. Often, at least an EMG is done to confirm the clinical impression of myositis. The exclusions discussed under PM should still be considered, including assessment of thyroid function and medication review (Table 22.2). If there is evidence of myositis and the typical features of Gottron's lesions or heliotrope are not seen, or if there is any uncertainty about the diagnosis, a muscle biopsy should be performed. The appearance of the skin in DM can be specific when fully developed, especially the combination of typical Gottron's lesions and heliotrope, along with nailfold capillary changes. To consider a patient to have amyopathic DM, the skin lesions should be present for at least 2 years without muscle involvement. Muscle involvement may rarely first appear later than this.

A biopsy of the erythematous or poikilodermatous lesions of the trunk or extremities is sometimes helpful in excluding other conditions, especially if the more specific features of the rash are not present or if there is no muscle involvement. The histologic findings resemble those of SLE, with vacuolar degeneration of the basal cell layer and mild inflammation at the dermoepidermal junction or upper dermis. Mucin is often present, whereas immunoglobulin deposition is usually absent (129).

Other laboratory findings in DM are similar to those in PM. CK elevation may be less consistently observed. The ANA is frequently positive in primary DM [62% of cases of primary DM (31)], but the most common specific antibodies are different. Patients with anti–Jo-1 are less likely to have DM than PM, but patients with other antisynthetases are more likely to have DM than PM. Anti-SRP is generally not seen in DM. Anti–Mi-2, which is almost exclusively seen in DM, is found in 15% to 20% of cases of adult DM in the United States and may be higher in Central America and other populations. Anti–Mi-2

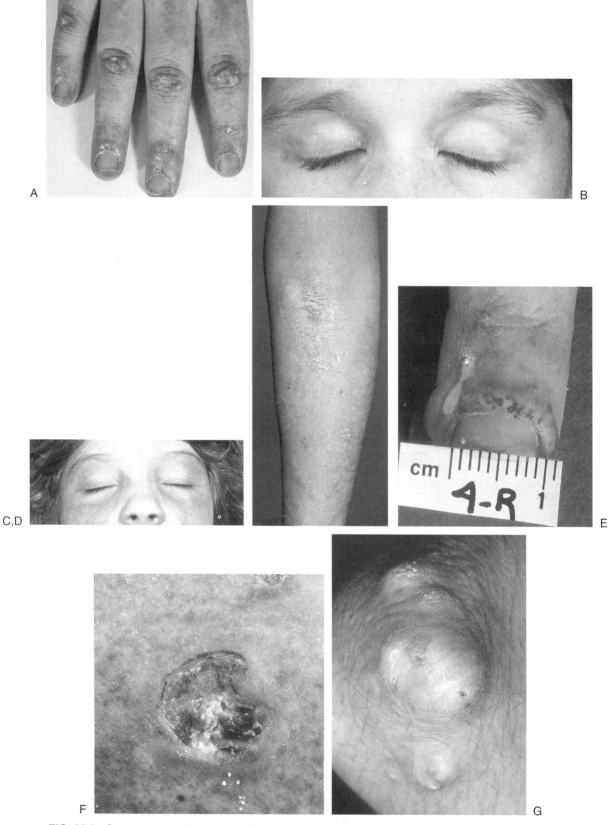

**FIG. 22.3.** Cutaneous manifestations of juvenile dermatomyositis. **A:** Gottron's papules over the extensor surfaces of the hands, with periungual erythema and cuticular overgrowth, and periungual nail-fold capillary abnormalities. See color plate 21A. **B:** Heliotrope rash over the eyelids, which is characteristic of dermatomyositis. See color plate 21B. **C:** Heliotrope over the eyelids with associated periorbital edema and malar erythema sparing the nasolabial folds. (Courtesy of Dr. David Sherry). See color plate 21C. **D:** Linear extensor erythema on the extensor tendons of the forearm. See color plate 21D. **E:** Periungual capillary dilation, tortuosity, and dropout, with cuticular hypertrophy. **F:** Cutaneous ulceration. **G:** Calcinosis over the knee.

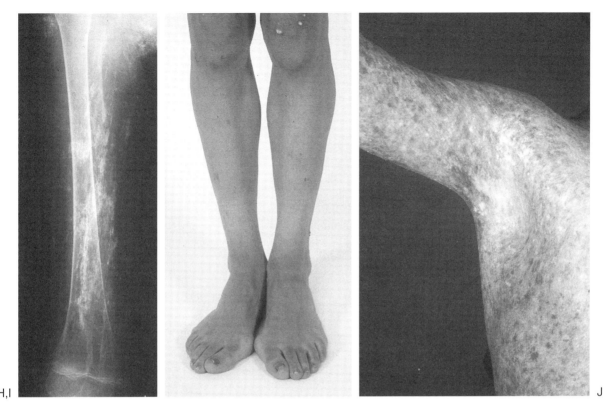

**FIG. 22.3.** *(Continued.)* **H:** Radiograph of intermuscular fascial plane calcinosis and severe osteoporosis. **I:** Generalized lipodystrophy, with loss of subcutaneous fat, skin hyperpigmentation, and muscle hypertrophy. **J:** Poikiloderma vasculare atrophicans, with admixture of hyperpigmentation and hypopigmentation, telangiectasia, and atrophy.

autoantibodies are associated with the V and shawl sign rashes as well as cuticular overgrowth in DM patients (31).

*Therapy*

The therapy of the myositis of DM is similar to that of PM. A double-blind, placebo-controlled, 3-month study of monthly IVIG infusions in 15 patients with treatment-resistant DM found a statistically significant improvement in treated patients compared with those receiving placebo, with 9 of 12 treatment courses (including crossovers) and no placebo courses resulting in major improvement (130). Reduction in complement deposition in muscle vessels was documented by biopsy, and other studies have suggested that blocking deposition of activated complement is a major mechanism of action of IVIG in DM (131). This provides added support for its use in this condition. The skin lesions of DM often respond to treatment of the myositis, but the rashes sometimes persist or recur with taper. Some evidence supports the use of hydroxychloroquine for resistant cutaneous DM (132), along with sun protection. Topical steroids may provide benefit for the pruritus associated with the rash.

For severe rashes, treatment with prednisone and immunosuppressive agents for the skin lesions alone may sometimes be considered. Low-dose weekly oral methotrexate has been used for refractory DM rash with some success (133). Cuta-

neous ulcerations, which occasionally occur in adults, may respond to IVIG (134). For amyopathic DM, it is important to watch for signs of myositis, so that systemic treatment can be instituted promptly if it develops. Treatment of other cutaneous manifestations is discussed under "Juvenile Dermatomyositis."

*Juvenile Dermatomyositis*

*Incidence and Epidemiology*

The incidence of JDM has been estimated in several epidemiologic registry studies and has been reported in the range of 1.5 to 1.9 cases per 1 million population in the United Kingdom, Canada, and Japan (135–137). The incidence in Finland is slightly higher, at 4 cases per 1 million population, which may be related to the broader surveillance methods used in that study (138). There is a bimodal age of onset during childhood, with an overall mean of 6.9 to 9.1 years in the United States and other countries (135,137,139–141). Girls are affected 1.4 to 2.7 times as frequently as boys; in the United Kingdom, affected girls outnumbered boys by five times (135–137,139,141). Two U.S. registries demonstrated similar ethnic distributions: 69% to 74% white, 14% to 15% African American, 5% to 7% Hispanic, 3% to 7% Asian American, 0% to 2.3% Native American, and 5% to 6.5% racially mixed patients (139,140).

Similar to adult DM, JDM is an illness characterized by chronic muscle and cutaneous inflammation, primarily in a perivascular distribution and is thought to result from a combination of genetic and environmental factors. Cases of familial JDM and IIM and the high frequency of autoimmune disease in families of JDM patients provide clinical support for the contribution of genetic factors in the etiology of JDM (84,142). The primary immunogenetic risk factor in white patients is the HLA haplotype DRB1*0301 DQA1*0501, as in adult IIM (143). Polymorphisms for HLA DM are possible additional immunogenetic risk factors (144).

Several reports of geographic clustering of JDM patients, as well as some reports of a seasonal predilection for JDM during the summer months, support a role for environmental risk factors in the etiology of JDM (135,139,145). The onset of JDM has been associated with a variety of infectious illnesses, which have included coxsackievirus, toxoplasmosis, group A streptococcus, parvovirus, influenza, hepatitis B, and *Borrelia* and *Leishmania* species (reviewed in 146). Cases of JDM have also occurred after exposure to vaccines, carticaine, and growth hormone, as well as after excessive or unusual sun exposure (146). A rigorous case-controlled epidemiologic study, however, did not support a role for coxsackievirus, toxoplasmosis, herpes simplex virus, or other environmental factors in the onset of JDM (139). Some studies detected coxsackievirus or parvovirus within the muscle biopsies of affected patients, whereas others have not (reviewed in 146). Molecular mimicry may also be a factor for some etiopathogenic agents, as suggested by the homology of the streptococcal M5 protein to skeletal muscle myosin and enhanced immune responses to the homologous peptide regions in patients who develop JDM after group A streptococcal infections (147).

Of 165 North American children with IIM systematically screened for autoantibodies, 11% have an MSA, and 8% have an MAA (146). From this study and review of the literature, 13 children have been identified with an antisynthetase autoantibody (Jo-1, PL-12, and PL-7), 4 children with anti-SRP, and 22 children with anti–Mi-2 autoantibody (146,148). Unlike adults with anti-SRP, there is no gender predisposition in the children. Anti-MJ, a newly recognized autoantibody of unknown specificity, has been identified in the sera of 17% of 80 juvenile IIM patients screened (149), and anti–U5-RNP has been identified in one child with JDM (150). Neither of these autoantibodies has been adequately tested to know yet if they are MSAs.

### Clinical Presentation

The clinical manifestations of JDM at illness onset have been evaluated in two large registries in the United States and Japan (Table 22.7) (151,152). Many clinical manifestations of JDM are similar to those of adult DM and are not rediscussed in this section. Certain clinical manifestations, however, are much more common or have been better defined in JDM than adult DM, including some cutaneous manifesta-

**TABLE 22.7.** *Clinical features of juvenile dermatomyositis at diagnosis*

| Symptom | Affected Patients (%) |
|---|---|
| Rash | 100 |
|   Facial rash | 98 |
|   Truncal rash | 84 |
|   Photosensitivity | 40 |
|   Pruritus | 32 |
| Weakness | 84–100 |
| Myalgia or muscle pain | 66–73 |
| Gait disturbance | 74 |
| Fever | 38–65 |
| Arthralgia | 46 |
| Dysphagia | 40–44 |
| Hoarseness | 43 |
| Abdominal pain | 37 |
| Arthritis | 35 |
| Calcinosis | 4–23 |
| Melena | 13 |
| Raynaud's phenomenon | 12 |

From Pachman LM, Hayford JR, Chung A, et al. Juvenile dermatomyositis at diagnosis: clinical characteristics of 79 children. *J Rheumatol* 1998;25:1198–1204; and Kobayashi S, Higuchi K, Tamaki H, et al. Characteristics of juvenile dermatomyositis in Japan. *Acta Paediatr Jap* 1997;39:257–262, with permission.

tions, lipodystrophy, gastrointestinal ulcerations, and osteoporosis, and these are detailed here. Additional unusual clinical manifestations described in JDM patients, including retinal cytoid bodies (153), motor-sensory peripheral neuropathy (154), pancreatitis (155), testicular vasculitis (156), and cerebral involvement (154,157), have resulted from a vasculopathy of these target organs. DM without clinically evident muscle involvement has also been reported in three children (reviewed in 146). Children presenting exclusively with cutaneous changes of DM may develop muscle involvement as late as 3 years after initial symptom onset (158).

Cutaneous ulcerations are characteristic of JDM, although they affect less than 10% of patients and have also rarely been described in association with adult DM (154,159–161). The pathologic changes associated with these lesions include denudation of the epidermis and dermal necrosis, accompanied by mononuclear perivascular infiltrates, thrombotic endarteropathy, or mucopolysaccharide accumulation in the dermis (154,161). In one series, cutaneous ulcerations were predictive of a severe illness course, characterized by persistent muscle weakness, poor responses to corticosteroid therapy, and extensive calcinosis (160). Two additional studies found patients with cutaneous ulcerations to have severe illness at disease onset but did not find ulcerative changes to be predictive of disease course or the development of calcinosis (159,162).

Periungual nailfold capillary abnormalities have been observed in 46% to 100% of patients (163–165). Nailfold capillary changes correlate with global disease activity and are hypothesized to parallel the vasculopathy occurring in muscle (163). In serial studies, the earliest changes include thrombosis and hemorrhage of periungual vessels, followed by capillary loss; giant capillary loops and "bushy" capillary formation reflect capillary regeneration and occur later in the illness course (163,165). Severe nailfold capillary changes that do not return to normal have correlated with persistent illness courses, cutaneous ulcerations or the development of calcinosis (164,165).

An additional cutaneous manifestation that is characteristic of JDM but rarely observed in adult DM is calcinosis, or dystrophic calcification of the skin, subcutaneous tissue, or muscle fascia (160). Calcinosis is reported in about 30% of patients with JDM (159,166). Dystrophic calcification is observed most commonly at least 2 years after illness onset, but as many as 23% of children have detectable lesions within 6 months of diagnosis (151). Calcinosis has several different clinical forms, including hard plaques or nodules, seen in 33% of affected patients; large tumorous deposits overlying the proximal muscles, observed in 20%; deposits in the intermuscular fascial planes, seen in 16%; severe exoskeleton after diffuse cutaneous vasculitis and erythroderma, seen in 10%; and combinations of these varieties, observed in 21% (160). Patients with tumorous deposits often develop accompanying ulceration, and patients with tumorous, fascial plane, and exoskeleton forms often develop severe limitation of movement of the involved muscles or contiguous joints (160). Superinfection of the lesions with *Staphylococcus aureus* is a common complication and is associated with depressed neutrophil chemotaxis and elevated serum immunoglobulin E (IgE) levels in affected patients (167). Spontaneous resolution of calcification, which is unpredictable but often occurs when patients increase mobility at the time that disease is clinically inactive, results from extrusion of calcium salt through the skin or internal resorption (160). The development of dystrophic calcification has been associated with a delay in diagnosis and inadequate treatment with high-dose corticosteroid therapy (151,160, 168). Calcinosis is seen more frequently in patients with lower ANA titers as well as in patients who have a polycyclic or unremitting illness course (159).

An increasingly recognized manifestation of JDM is lipodystrophy, the loss of fat deposits either focally, in areas of previous panniculitis, partially, or totally (169,170). Partial or total lipodystrophy may be seen in up to 20% of JDM patients (170); these patients, as those with other forms of lipodystrophy, often develop a syndrome of severe insulin resistance, including acanthosis nigricans, which may be accompanied by steatosis, hyperlipidemia, hypertension, polycystic ovaries, and hyperpigmentation and hypertrichosis resulting from hyperandrogenism (169–171). Lipodystrophy may be detected by body fat measurements. Separate from lipodystrophy, up to half of JDM patients develop isolated insulin resistance, particularly those patients who fail to achieve remission or who develop calcinosis (171).

Dysphagia caused by esophageal dysmotility and intestinal malabsorption are common gastrointestinal manifestations of JDM (172). Gastrointestinal ulceration is an additional manifestation resulting from endarteropathy and vasculitis of the bowel wall vessels, which may involve any segment of the alimentary tract (154,161,173). Observed in less than 10% of patients, it is one of the most serious symptoms and can lead to pneumatosis intestinalis, gastrointestinal perforation, bowel necrosis, and even death (154,161,173,174).

Reduced bone mass in children with JDM has been well-documented, often resulting in bone fractures (175,176). The cause appears to be multifactorial, related to decreased calcium absorption, particularly in the active phase of disease when patients have decreased mobility and receive glucocorticoid therapy, and to decreased osteoblast activity (175,176). Bone turnover is also increased in patients with severe calcinosis (177).

The clinical presentation of children with antisynthetase autoantibodies is similar that to adults, although "mechanic's hands" are seen less frequently (178,179). Children with anti-SRP have severe necrotizing PM, often of acute onset, but do not have cardiac involvement (146,179). Children with anti–Mi-2 autoantibodies do not appear clinically distinguished from those JDM patients who do not have MSA (179,180). Patients with anti-MJ autoantibodies frequently have arthritis, dysphagia, and calcinosis (149).

### Diagnostic Approach

The differential diagnosis for JDM should be considered in the initial evaluation of a child with myopathy or photosensitive skin rashes (Table 22.2). Regarding the Bohan and Peter (53) criteria for myositis, 84% to 100% of children with JDM have muscle weakness at the time of diagnosis, 90% have elevation of any single muscle enzyme, 81% to 92% of children tested have characteristic EMG changes, and 80% to 92% have muscle biopsy findings supporting a diagnosis (151,152). Only 64% to 70% of children with JDM have elevation of the serum CK level at the time of diagnosis. Other serum muscle enzymes, including aldolase, LDH, and the transaminases, are elevated in 50% to 94% of patients (151,152).

In routine clinical care, muscle biopsy is often not performed if the rash is characteristic and the child meets probable or definite criteria for myositis based on other test results. The muscle biopsy characteristically demonstrates perivascular lymphocytic inflammation in the perimysial and endomysial vessels as well as evidence of endarteropathy of the small arteries, veins, and capillaries with thromboses and necrosis of the endothelium, resulting in muscle infarction and perifascicular atrophy (154,161). Immunoglobulin, complement split products, and the membrane attack complex are deposited intravascularly in affected blood vessels, suggesting a role for complement in mediating vessel injury in JDM (181). The presence of vasculopathy or myonecrosis on initial muscle biopsy correlates with a chronic or relapsing course (161,182).

Serial evaluation of muscle strength and function, cutaneous assessment, and evaluation of affected extramuscular target organs are important in the long-term clinical care of JDM patients. Children younger than 5 years of age are not able to undergo formal manual muscle strength testing, and it is particularly important in this age group, as well as for older children, to assess muscle function and endurance using functional assessment tests, such as has been developed in a preliminarily validated instrument known as the Childhood Myositis Assessment Scale (183). The inability to detect all aspects of both active and chronic illness using these assessments has led to the development of a variety of blood laboratory tests and magnetic MRI scans of muscle as adjunctive measures in assessing JDM disease activity (184).

After the initial diagnosis has been established, serum CK is not a valuable marker in the serial evaluation of disease activity in JDM because it does not correlate with global disease activity and does not predict disease flare (185–187). LDH and aldolase correlate better with global disease activity, whereas LDH and AST are most useful in the detection of a flare (185,186). Other serum muscle metabolites, including CK-MB and creatine, may be more valuable in assessing disease activity in JDM than traditional serum muscle enzymes, and serum creatinine correlates with disease damage (185).

Because serum muscle enzymes are insensitive measures of JDM disease activity and do not assess extramuscular involvement, a number of immunologic activation markers have also been studied. Most of these are used for research purposes, although some are beginning to be used in the routine clinical care of patients. The von Willebrand factor VIII–related antigen correlates with active disease and appears to be a marker of JDM vasculopathy but is elevated in only 35% to 50% of patients (187). Neopterin, which is derived from interferon-γ–activated monocytes, correlates with global disease activity, muscle strength, and the presence of macrophages in affected muscle and is elevated in most patients with active disease (188,189). Elevated percentages of B lymphocytes and CD4+ T cells are seen in active JDM, and changes correlate with the level of disease activity (190).

Fat-suppressed T2-weighted or STIR thigh muscle MRI scans are valuable in detecting muscle edema corresponding to muscle inflammation and vasculopathy, whereas T1-weighted images have been helpful in detecting fibrosis or fatty replacement, which occurs in chronic disease when muscle is damaged (191–193) (Fig. 22.4). Changes on STIR or T2-weighted fat-suppressed images occur most commonly in the gluteus, adductors, and quadriceps muscles, whereas changes on T1-weighted images are more frequently observed posteriorly and medially (191,192). MRI may be useful in helping to establish a diagnosis of JDM, particularly when muscle biopsy is not performed, in selecting an active site of inflammation for biopsy, and in the serial evaluation of JDM patients. STIR or T2-weighted images correlate with global disease activity,

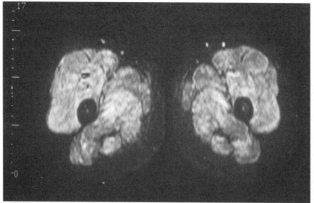

A

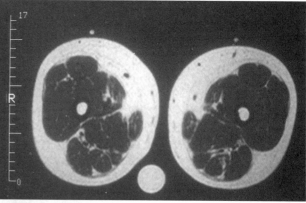

B

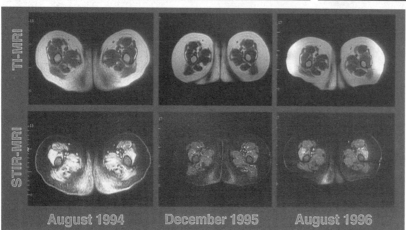

C

FIG. 22.4. Magnetic resonance imaging (MRI) of idiopathic inflammatory myopathies. **A:** Short tau inversion recovery (STIR) image from a patient with juvenile dermatomyositis demonstrating edema in muscles, representing active inflammation, which is shown as bright areas. **B:** T1-weighted image from the same patient, with mild muscle atrophy and fatty replacement. **C:** Serial MRI images from a patient with juvenile dermatomyositis. Edema on STIR images, represented by bright areas, improves over time, whereas muscle atrophy, on T1-weighted images, increases over time.

muscle strength, and serum muscle enzymes. MRI appears to be more sensitive than other measures of disease activity, such as serum muscle enzymes, in that T2-weighted fat-suppressed images continue to demonstrate abnormalities after muscle enzymes have normalized (191,192). Children should rest before undergoing MRI because exercise within 60 minutes of the scan can lead to acute changes on STIR images that mimic active inflammation (193).

*Therapy*

Therapeutic approaches to JDM have been extensively reviewed, and further details can be found in the literature (146). General approaches to the treatment of JDM are provided in Table 22.8, although therapy must be individualized to the patient, taking into account disease severity, prognostic risk factors, and risks for and history of adverse events from medications.

Daily corticosteroid therapy has been the mainstay of treatment for JDM and has reduced mortality from 40% in the era before steroid therapy to less than 3% (194). Additional first-line therapies in the management of JDM include photoprotection, use of topical steroids and hydroxychloroquine for cutaneous manifestations, incorporation of physical therapy and rehabilitation throughout the illness course, and the administration of calcium and vitamin D in patients receiving corticosteroids with inadequate dietary intake (Table 22.8).

Second-line agents should be considered in steroid-refractory patients, in patients with unacceptable corticosteroid toxicity, and as part of initial therapy in patients with risk factors for poor prognosis. Risk factors for poor prognosis include severe disease activity, ulceration, calcification, severe dysphagia, interstitial lung disease, certain MSAs (such as antiaminoacyl-tRNA synthetase and anti–SRP autoantibodies), vasculopathy on biopsy, and delay to treatment (31, 159–161,172,178,179,194). Patients not responding well to therapy should also undergo a thorough review of myopathic and photosensitizing agents that may be contributing to the persistence of symptoms (195–197). In addition to use in refractory patients, intravenous pulse methylprednisolone therapy should be considered in all moderately to severely ill patients at illness onset in an attempt to reduce the long-term exposure to corticosteroids. Patients with acute, life-threatening complications, such as severe dysphagia, gastrointestinal ulceration or malabsorption, or myocarditis, may also benefit from pulse methylprednisolone therapy (Table 22.8) (195).

Generally, when therapy in addition to corticosteroids is contemplated, methotrexate is preferred in children as the initial second-line agent (Table 22.8). Treatment benefit is apparent within 4 to 8 weeks after dose optimization. Methotrexate is usually well tolerated in children and may also be effective for treating cutaneous disease (133). IVIG has a role in the treatment of JDM and possibly JPM, particularly in an acute setting in patients who are seriously ill or at high risk for infection, because of its rapid onset of action

and lack of immunosuppression. IVIG may be useful as a short-term agent in JDM, particularly in treating severe cutaneous disease or in treating certain subsets of patients with infectious triggers. Its expense, limited supply, and the frequent occurrence of tachyphylaxis often prohibit its long-term use. Adverse effects from IVIG therapy are not uncommon. Infusion-related toxicities, including headache, fever, nausea, and hypotension, can be modulated by slowing the rate of infusion; premedicating with methylprednisolone, acetaminophen, or diphenhydramine; or switching manufacturers. Other potential side effects include aseptic meningitis, thromboembolic events resulting from increased serum viscosity, and the potential for transmission of infectious agents (198,199).

Cyclosporine shows promise as a steroid-sparing agent in steroid-refractory patients. Cyclosporine metabolism is age dependent, with increased dosage requirements in younger children because of increased drug clearance (200). Reports have documented benefit from cyclosporine in treating DM rashes (201,202). Frequent side effects, including mild decrease in glomerular filtration rate, hypertension, hirsutism, osteoporosis, and myopathy, may prohibit its long-term use in many patients (Table 22.8). Azathioprine is usually reserved for more refractory patients because the onset to peak treatment effect is often 2 to 4 months, because it has a relatively high incidence of gastrointestinal intolerance and leukopenia, and because of concerns for its oncogenic potential, although response rates appear comparable to methotrexate (Table 22.8). For patients with extremely recalcitrant or life-threatening disease, combination therapies including azathioprine, as well as cyclophosphamide, chlorambucil, and apheresis, may be used (Table 22.8). Anecdotally, cyclophosphamide may be useful in the treatment of ulcerative disease (D. Sherry, R. Rennebohm, L. Rider, unpublished observation).

Because no controlled studies have been conducted for the treatment of calcinosis, all suggested therapies remain unproved. Treatment of underlying disease activity is important in the prevention of new deposition (160). Colchicine has been effective in reducing the acute inflammation associated with new lesions (203). In severe situations, surgical removal is recommended; calcinosis may recur after surgery, but this is less likely if disease activity is low and the surgeon is experienced (204).

Although data on long-term outcome are limited, use of current treatment approaches for JDM have resulted in about one third of patients recovering from illness within 2 years without clinical relapse, one third developing a relapsing illness course, and one third experiencing continuously active disease without long-term improvement (159,162,166). Calcinosis has been observed in 29% of JDM patients (159,166). About 15% to 20% of patients have residual weakness or functional disability, and intolerance of aerobic exercise is seen in a large percentage of clinically inactive patients (166,205).

**TABLE 22.8.** *Summary of current treatment approaches for juvenile dermatomyositis and polymyositis*

| Medication | Recommended regimen[a] | Comments |
|---|---|---|
| **Primary therapies** | | |
| Prednisone | Administer 1–2 mg/kg/d PO, often in divided doses for 4–8 wks; gradually tapered but maintained until all serum muscle enzymes normal. Average course is 2 years, although mild cases require lower doses and shorter duration of treatment. | Daily prednisone is the mainstay of treatment for JDM and is responsible for reducing mortality from 40% in era before usage to 3% currently (146). Morbidity from corticosteroid treatment includes bone loss, growth failure, avascular necrosis, cushingoid features, and cataracts (166,395). |
| Sunscreens, sun avoidance, topical corticosteroids | Sunscreens protective of ultraviolet A and B light; topical steroids: mild potency for facial rash, often moderate to high potency for rashes on extremities that do not respond. | These measures are often helpful for treating photosensitive rashes and cutaneous disease associated with JDM. |
| Hydroxychloroquine | Administer ≤6 mg/kg/d PO divided b.i.d. | Hydroxychloroquine is useful for treating cutaneous disease but may also decrease daily steroid requirement and have an effect on muscle disease activity (396). Monitoring for retinal toxicity is required. Photosensitive rashes developing during therapy may resolve with dose modification. |
| Physical therapy, rehabilitation | Initial therapy: range of motion; after stabilization, progress to isometric and isotonic exercises; resistive exercises and aerobic program in final stages; assistive devices, speech therapy and swallowing instruction often helpful | No controlled studies are available to document benefit, but these approaches likely improve functional outcome (125,397). |
| Calcium, vitamin D | Daily requirements of calcium: children 1–5 y, 800 mg/d; 6–10 y, 1200 mg/d; 11–24 y, 1500 mg/d; vitamin D ≥400 IU/d | Daily intake through diet or supplementation is recommended for children receiving long-term daily corticosteroids to prevent osteoporosis (398). |
| **Secondary therapies** | | |
| Pulse methylprednisolone | 30 mg/kg IV, up to 1 g, ×3 pulses. Repeat as needed, including as often as several times weekly with concurrent low-dose daily prednisone. | From one randomized and four open-label studies, overall response is 88% in 44 JDM patients at ≥48 mo follow-up (146,399). This approach may spare daily prednisone dose, provide better absorption of steroid, aid in rapid control of disease activity, and be valuable in acute, life-threatening situations, such as severe dysphagia and myocarditis. Corticosteroid-related side effects may be reduced. Prospective studies are needed to determine whether it reduces frequency of calcinosis. |
| Methotrexate | Administer 0.4–1 mg/kg (10–30 mg/m²) weekly PO, SC, or IV, not IM. | When administered methotrexate in combination with prednisone, 21% of 38 corticosteroid-resistant patients improved and 53% attained remission in open-label studies (146,400,401). Response is apparent within 4–8 weeks, once dose is optimized. This drug may be effective for skin disease, but is also a photosensitizing agent. The patient is at risk for opportunistic infections and possibly for lymphoma when methotrexate is used in combination with steroids (260). |
| Intravenous gammaglobulin (IVIG) | Administer 1 g/kg/dose IV for 2 days, monthly for ≥3 months. | Of 54 steroid refractory or toxic patients, 63% improved strength in open-label studies at mean follow-up of 12.8 mo. Of 30 evaluable patients, 30% normalized strength; 64% of 30 patients improved rash, and 29% of 14 patients resolved rash. Calcinosis was noted to improve or resolve in 8 (reviewed in 146). Clinical effect should occur within 3 months. Several patients |

**TABLE 22.8.** *Continued*

| Medication | Recommended regimen[a] | Comments |
|---|---|---|
| | | experienced tachyphylaxis or only short-term benefit, with clinical relapse on discontinuation (402). Benefits include rapid onset of action, lack of immunosuppression, and effectiveness for skin disease. IVIG is potentially useful in these settings, for short-term treatment, or for treating certain subsets associated with infectious triggers (403). Disadvantages include expense, potential for transmitting infectious agents, and short supply. |
| Cyclosporine | Administer 2.5–7.5 mg/kg/d PO divided b.i.d. to maintain trough blood level at ≤300 ng/mL. | Of 37 JIIM patients refractory to corticosteroids or cytotoxic therapy treated in open-label studies, 86% improved muscle strength and enzymes at a mean follow-up of 25 mo (146,404–406). Prednisone dose was reduced in 94% and discontinued in 38%. Clearance is increased in younger children; Neoral may have more predictable absorption. Potential side effects include decreased creatinine clearance, hypertension, hirsutism, myopathy, and osteoporosis (407). |
| Azathioprine | Administer 1–2 mg/kg/d PO, increasing to a maximum of 3–5 mg/kg/d, monitoring white blood count. | Of 10 JDM patients refractory to steroids, 22% improved, and 60% achieved remission in open-label or retrospective studies (146). Peak treatment effect is ≥3 mo. This drug carries a small but documented risk for malignancy, leukopenia, and opportunistic infections in combination with corticosteroids. |
| Experimental therapy | Combination therapy of the above agents includes cyclophosphamide, 500–1000 mg/m² IV monthly or 10–15 mg/kg weekly for life-threatening disease; chlorambucil; apheresis | These agents may be necessary for life-threatening manifestations or for patients with severe, recalcitrant disease refractory to the above treatments. Cyclophosphamide is possibly useful for cutaneous and gastrointestinal ulceration associated with JDM; experience in treating muscle disease activity is mixed (146,408). |

JDM, juvenile dermatomyositis; JPM, juvenile polymyositis; JIIM, juvenile idiopathic inflammatory myopathy.

[a] These are general guidelines. Therapy for all patients needs to be individualized based on disease severity, irreversible disease damage, risk factors for poor prognosis, and history of and risk factors for adverse events.

Adapted from Rider LG, Miller FW. Classification and treatment of the juvenile idiopathic inflammatory myopathies. *Rheum Dis Clin North Am* 1997;23:619–655, with permission.

### *Juvenile Polymyositis*

#### *Incidence and Epidemiology*

The incidence of juvenile polymyositis (JPM) is 1.5 to 16 times less than that of JDM (135,140,206), and for this reason, much less is known about JPM. The mean age of onset is 9.4 years, and girls are affected up to six times as frequently as boys (140,206).

The major immunogenetic risk factor is HLA DRB1*0301 DQA1*0501, the same as for JDM and the adult forms of the disease (207). Many infectious agents that may trigger the onset of JDM have also been associated with the onset of JPM. In addition, HTLV-1, trichinosis, and *Wuchereria bancrofti* have also been temporally associated with the onset of JPM (reviewed in (146)). Among noninfectious agents, D-penicillamine, growth hormone, and bone marrow transplantation (graft-versus-host myositis) can trigger JPM (146).

A second form of PM that occurs during childhood is infantile PM, in which the onset of myositis occurs during the first year of life and in which IIM changes on biopsy are characteristic. Of 10 reported cases, 6 are girls, and the average age of onset is 2 months of age (range, birth to 11 months of age) (208–213). For those children presenting at birth, it has been postulated that a maternal *in utero* infection may be an etiologic agent (209,213).

#### *Clinical Presentation*

The most common initial symptom of JPM is weakness, which occurs in 67% to 88% of affected children and often involves both proximal and distal muscles (159,206). Associated muscle pain and tenderness are less common than in JDM. Fatigue is more common in JPM than in JDM. JPM patients have findings of dysphagia, rheumatic complaints, muscle atrophy, and joint contractures similar to those seen in JDM (206). Periungual capillaries are generally without associated telangiectasia, in contrast to JDM (206).

Infantile PM characteristically presents with generalized hypotonia, severe muscle weakness that is more prominent proximally and axially, delayed gross motor developmental milestones, and occasionally a weak cry or difficulty swallowing. Some infants presenting at birth have decreased fetal movements *in utero* (208–213).

### Diagnostic Approach

Overall, approaches to the diagnosis of JPM are similar to those discussed previously for JDM. It is especially important in evaluating patients for JPM to perform a muscle biopsy to exclude other myopathies (Table 22.2). Immunologic activation markers studied in JDM have not been systematically evaluated in JPM.

For patients with infantile PM, CK may be normal but most often is elevated by several hundred to thousand units. Muscle biopsy demonstrating characteristic changes of IIM is an essential part of the diagnostic evaluation to exclude various forms of congenital muscular dystrophy, including Walker–Warburg syndrome, Fukuyama's syndrome, muscle–eye–brain disease, and congenital merosin deficiency. Congenital muscular dystrophy may also demonstrate focal inflammation on biopsy, although dystrophic features are prominent; the presence of merosin staining of muscle can be helpful in excluding muscular dystrophy (214).

### Therapy

Therapeutic approaches to JPM are similar to JDM (Table 22.8). JPM patients most often have a chronic, unremitting illness course (159) and often require the use of second-line therapies.

For infantile PM, prednisone is the mainstay of therapy. Children usually have a clinical response, demonstrated by improved strength and decreased serum muscle enzymes, but corticosteroid therapy is often required for years. Residual muscle weakness that is often severe, muscle atrophy, joint contractures, and continued gross motor delays have been observed in long-term follow-up of most of these patients (208–213).

### Myositis in Connective Tissue Diseases

It is common for patients with IIM to have manifestations associated with other CTD, including SLE, systemic sclerosis, or Sjögren's syndrome. Patients who have myositis that is indistinguishable from PM may satisfy criteria for a second CTD. Because these conditions are defined clinically, sharp distinctions cannot be made. Specific autoantibodies, to the extent that they have recognized clinical associations, can sometimes help to clarify such mixed pictures. PM is more common than DM in most cases in which myositis overlaps with another CTD. PM or DM sometimes occurs in patients

with other autoimmune diseases, with uncertain relationship other than a predisposition to autoimmunity, which may be the result of HLA or other genetic factors. Among these conditions are primary biliary cirrhosis, inflammatory bowel disease, MG, thyroid disease, and insulin-dependent diabetes mellitus.

### Overlap Myositis in Children

Overlap myositis, in which patients meet diagnostic criteria for myositis and another CTD, has been observed in 6% of juvenile IIM patients, contrasted to 17% of adult IIM patients (146). The most common form of overlap myositis in childhood is mixed CTD (MCTD), in which children with high-titer U1-RNP autoantibodies develop myositis in association with SLE, systemic sclerosis, juvenile rheumatoid arthritis, or Sjögren's syndrome (215–217). About 20% to 90% of children develop myositis as part of MCTD. Patients range in age from 4 to 16 years, and boys appear to be affected more commonly than girls (216).

Overlap myositis has also been reported in children in association with several forms of primary vasculitis, including polyarteritis nodosa, Kawasaki disease, Behçet's disease, and Wegener's granulomatosis (218–221). Myositis has also been observed less commonly in children with systemic-onset juvenile rheumatoid arthritis, celiac disease, idiopathic thrombocytopenia purpura, and psoriasis (159,222–225).

### Clinical Presentation

Patients with overlap myositis syndromes have been thought to have milder and more treatment-responsive myositis than those with primary adult PM. One study, however, found that SLE-associated myositis was as severe as primary PM (226). The myositis is also similar in CK elevations and requirement for treatment. The CK did not correlate well with strength or functional outcome. CK has been found to be lower in CTDs in general, without myositis. Patients with overlap syndromes are more likely to be female, to have features of systemic illness, and to have a positive ANA.

Patients with SLE overlap syndromes that include myositis commonly have anti–U1-RNP autoantibodies. When this autoantibody is present without anti-Sm or an MSA or other MAA, in association with features of SLE, myositis, and scleroderma, MCTD can be diagnosed. Puffy fingers (dactylitis), Raynaud's phenomenon, esophageal dysmotility, and sometimes sclerodactyly associated with systemic sclerosis are common. Features of SLE can include arthritis, serositis, and rash, but renal involvement is unusual. The myositis in MCTD has also been thought to be more responsive than isolated PM, but there is individual variation. In children, MCTD-associated myositis is often prominent early in the disease course. Proximal muscle weakness in the absence of DM rashes is observed, although DM rashes are present in up to 15% of these children (216,217). Myalgias and muscle tenderness are uncommon.

Scleroderma can have a bland, noninflammatory myopathy as part of the disease, which can lead to some muscle weakness. The CK is usually not elevated. Significant CK elevation should lead to suspicion of inflammatory myopathy, and evaluation for PM and DM should be performed. This form of overlap is not unusual.

Myositis in association with primary vasculitis is characterized by myalgias, calf pain, muscle tenderness, and distal lower extremity involvement (218,220–222). Symptoms of the primary vasculitis are prominent, including fever, and DM rashes are absent. In myositis associated with Kawasaki disease, celiac disease, and idiopathic thrombocytopenic purpura, muscle involvement may be severe, involving primarily proximal muscles or both proximal and distal muscles (219,223,224). The onset of myositis in Kawasaki disease is 2 days to 2 weeks into the course of the illness. Dysphagia and dysphonia have been reported in association with the myositis of Kawasaki disease.

The myositis-associated overlap syndromes associated with certain MAAs have also been defined. Patients with anti–PM-Scl often have overlap features of scleroderma and myositis (82,227), sometimes called *scleromyositis* (228), and may have DM cutaneous features. Inflammatory arthritis is sometimes a prominent part of this syndrome. The scleroderma is usually limited in cutaneous involvement. ILD or esophageal involvement can occur, but renal and cardiac disease are uncommon. Calcinosis and mechanic's hands can occur. The myositis is usually mild and easily responsive to prednisone. Forty-three children with anti–PM-Scl autoantibodies have been reported or screened positive, and they have clinical features similar to those of adults with these autoantibodies (reviewed in 146).

Overlap syndromes involving SLE, scleroderma, and myositis have also been associated with some patients with anti-Ku, or rarely with specific antibodies to non-U1 snRNPs. Eleven children with anti-Ku autoantibodies who have myositis overlapping with scleroderma or SLE have been reported or screened positive (reviewed in 146). Anti–U2-RNP and anti–U3-RNP autoantibodies have been reported in two children with scleroderma–myositis overlap syndromes (229).

*Diagnostic Approach*

The presence of other CTD features is often helpful in establishing the diagnosis. Evidence of proximal muscle weakness, elevated CK, and another CTD can lead to strong suspicion of myositis. Evaluation, as discussed for PM, with EMG and muscle biopsy is still useful. Muscle biopsy can sometimes reveal important findings, such as unsuspected vasculitis. In such overlap syndromes, it is still important to exclude other conditions, such as thyroid disease. It is less likely that malignancy is associated than in pure DM.

The presence of CTD features is a reason to be more thorough in searching for autoantibodies. Serologic evaluation is important and more likely to be helpful in overlap patients. Such patients can sometimes present diagnostic dilemmas,

having atypical clinical pictures. Testing should begin with ANA and include testing for MAA, MSA, and autoantibodies associated with the overlapping condition.

Serum muscle enzymes are elevated in 44% to 68% of children with MCTD (215–217). EMG abnormalities are characteristic of IIM and are abnormal in 25% to 38% of children with symptomatic MCTD (216,217). Muscle biopsy changes are identical to other IIMs and are seen in 20% to 63% of children with symptomatic MCTD (216). Several children with no muscle symptomatology had vasculitis and skeletal muscle inflammation at autopsy.

In the vasculitides, CK and other muscle enzymes are moderately to markedly elevated (218,220,221). EMG, when performed, shows changes characteristic of IIM (219). Muscle biopsy findings are notable for leukocytoclastic vasculitis (218,220), although in Kawasaki disease and Wegener's granulomatosis, the biopsy specimen demonstrates endomysial and perivascular mononuclear cell infiltration and fiber necrosis (219,221).

In one patient with systemic-onset juvenile rheumatoid arthritis, muscle MRI was useful in defining the extent of myositis (222).

*Therapy*

When the inflammatory myositis in patients with CTD is significant, it should be treated as outlined earlier for PM. Patients with scleroderma who have documented inflammatory muscle involvement usually require treatment, but not those with scleroderma myopathy. In some patients with predominance of other CTD manifestations, the myositis is incidentally discovered through enzyme elevation, and there is no or minimally detectable weakness. If myositis is then found by EMG or biopsy, it should usually be treated because muscle injury may cause irreversible damage. Starting treatment with moderate (30 to 40 mg/d) rather than high doses of prednisone would be reasonable in this circumstance, with more rapid taper if successful. Treatment of the associated CTD may be more urgent, and treatment decisions may be directed at that condition.

Therapeutic data on children with myositis in association with MCTD are limited. Daily prednisone therapy of 2 months' to 8 years' duration is most commonly used, and myositis often responds to steroid treatment.

Patients with myositis in association with vasculitis require high-dose daily prednisone therapy. Responses are good, but in polyarteritis, clinical relapses are common, and chronic steroid therapy is required (218,220). Myositis in Wegener's granulomatosis responds to a combination of prednisone and cyclophosphamide (221). Myositis in Kawasaki disease responds to high-dose aspirin therapy and resolves within 2 to 6 months without recurrence (219). Myositis associated with idiopathic thrombocytopenic purpura and celiac disease responds to high-dose prednisone therapy (223,224).

### Inclusion Body Myositis

IBM is thought to be the most common myopathy beginning after 50 years of age (230), representing 15% to 28% of cases of IIM. It has important clinical and pathologic differences from PM and DM. IBM muscle shows rimmed vacuoles and eosinophilic cytoplasmic and nuclear inclusions that are not seen in other IIMs. It has been separated into a hereditary form of inclusion body myopathy that shows similar characteristic features, but without significant inflammation (231), and the sporadic form of IBM, which may show varying levels of inflammation. The hereditary form is heterogeneous, including several different syndromes with different genetics (230). The sporadic form is more common in men.

The same pathologic features of PM that suggest antigen-directed, T-cell–mediated attack on muscle fibers is seen in IBM, with CD8$^+$ cells surrounding and invading nonnecrotic muscle fibers (109). The infiltrating T cells do not show as much evidence of clonal expansion as in PM (232). Inflammation appears to be more prominent in the earlier stages of the disease. Some biopsy specimens taken from patients with sporadic IBM show less inflammation and more of the inclusions and vacuoles, which may represent a later stage of the process and may be seen after treatment (233).

Many of the proteins that accumulate in the brain in Alzheimer's disease have been found in the IBM muscle, including β-amyloid deposits, ubiquitin, prion protein, pre–senilin-1, apolipoprotein E, and others (79,230,234–237). The cytoplasmic inclusions have paired helical filaments that appear to have ubiquitin and hyperphosphorylated tau (238) resembling those seen in Alzheimer's disease. These findings suggest that IBM may be a degenerative disease with mechanisms similar to Alzheimer's disease (79,239). Mitochondrial abnormalities are also seen in IBM and may contribute to its pathogenesis (240). If the inflammatory process is not the major mechanism of injury, that would explain the poor response to treatment. Some investigators, however, have noted the higher frequency of inflammatory than degenerative findings in the early stages of disease (241), suggesting that the inflammation may play a role in muscle injury. The fact that there can be some benefits to treatment in some cases does not exclude a degenerative process as the primary problem.

The onset of sporadic IBM has been reported in five boys and one girl between 9 and 18 years of age (146,242,243). One boy had IBM in association with scleroderma and Klinefelter's syndrome. Two children developed IBM after a mumps infection. Two families with hereditary inclusion body myopathy have been described in which one or more members had onset of clinical symptoms in early childhood (244,245).

### Clinical Presentation

IBM typically presents with slowly developing weakness. Both proximal and distal weakness can occur, with distal weakness much more common than in PM and DM (31). Asymmetric involvement is also more common. There is prominence of involvement of the quadriceps (246) and of the forearm muscles (especially finger flexors, but wrist extensors can also be involved). The face is usually spared, but dysphagia is common and can be the presenting feature (247). Falling is a common problem in IBM, apparently because of the particular pattern of involvement.

The CK level is usually elevated but is typically less elevated than in PM and generally remains less than 1000 IU (246). Autoantibodies, including ANAs, can be seen more often than in the normal population (248) but are much less frequent than in patients with PM (31). Specific autoantibodies associated with CTDs are unusual, and MSAs do not occur. A small proportion of patients have coexistence of autoimmune conditions (248) or malignancies, and the significance of these associations is uncertain.

### Diagnostic Approach

IBM should be suspected whenever there is a new onset of myopathy in patients older than 50 years of age or when the typical features of slowly progressive myopathy with distal involvement are seen. Anterior thigh atrophy or unexpected falling can also be clues. IBM should be considered if a patient with PM does not respond to treatment as expected. The evaluation should be similar to that of PM (Table 22.6), starting with EMG, which usually shows findings similar to those of PM, except that the routine EMG may have more neuropathic features, with more high-amplitude polyphasic potentials and in some instances abnormal nerve conduction studies. A neurogenic component of IBM has been suggested in some studies, but its significance is uncertain (1,230,249).

The characteristic histologic features of rimmed vacuoles and eosinophilic cytoplasmic and nuclear inclusions must be demonstrated to establish the diagnosis with certainty. The rimmed vacuoles and inclusions are best seen with trichrome stain. If these are not evident by light microscopy when IBM is suspected, staining for amyloid and, if possible, phosphorylated tau or ubiquitin may help to establish the diagnosis (230,250). Becker's muscular dystrophy should also be considered in childhood or familial cases of distal myopathy with rimmed vacuoles; absence of dystrophin on muscle biopsy can be confirmatory (251). The inclusions should be studied by electron microscopy to confirm that they contain the typical microtubular filaments.

It is not unusual for the first muscle biopsy to show no sign of IBM in patients who later show definite IBM on repeat biopsies. In such cases, the initial diagnosis is commonly PM because the findings of inflammation, necrosis, and regeneration are consistent when the vacuoles and inclusions are absent. This may relate to the progressive accumulation of these structures, making them more evident in later stages (233). Patients with treatment-resistant PM should have a repeat biopsy if the clinical picture is consistent with IBM. Treatment-resistant PM patients as a group have clinical similarities to IBM patients, even if they do not ultimately show IBM by biopsy (252). If patients have a clinical picture suggestive of IBM but no histologic features of IBM, they could be classified as having possible IBM (Table 22.6).

*Therapy*

The treatment of IBM is controversial (253). Treatment is not as successful in IBM as in PM. It is unusual to see significant recovery of strength, and return to normal is not seen. Some studies, however, have shown that treatment can reduce the rate of deterioration (254,255). Patients with more inflammation and less atrophy are more likely to respond. Treatment is usually begun with high-dose prednisone at 40 to 60 mg/d, and immunosuppressive therapy is commonly added either for steroid-sparing effect or because of ineffectiveness of prednisone alone. The use of methotrexate with prednisone (255) and methotrexate with azathioprine (254) has shown benefit in some patients. Alternate-day treatment with prednisone has also been used (230).

Studies of IVIG have been conflicting. In a controlled trial of 19 patients (256), a trend toward improvement was found in several strength measures, many of which did not reach statistical significance. Improvement was lost after crossover. Most of the gains were minor, but improvement was considered functionally important in 28%. Others suggested that greater benefit is achieved by a second course 2 weeks after the first (230). Anabolic steroids have been used for symptomatic treatment in men (230). Given the reduced level of expected response, the advanced age of many patients at diagnosis, the slower pace of progression, and the common requirement for immunosuppressives, decisions regarding treatment of IBM must be made on an individual basis. The question of whether to treat, and the regimen and intensity to be used, must be decided with consideration of the patient's age and general medical condition and the specifics of the individual case.

*Cancer-Associated Myositis*

The association of some cases of IIM with malignancy has long been appreciated, but the nature of the relationship remains unknown. Cancers have been found to occur before, simultaneously with, or after DM is diagnosed, and any type of cancer may be found. Cancers that occur within 2 years of the diagnosis of PM or DM are considered to be related. In those with greater temporal separation, confidence in a pathogenetic relationship would be less, but studies differ regarding whether they would be included. The proportion of patients with DM who have malignancy varies greatly among studies, from 6% to 43% (257), possibly reflecting inclusion criteria.

It has been difficult to establish the presence of a true association rather than chance occurrence of two diseases. The large population study of Sigurgeirsson et al. (55) in Sweden found an increased frequency of malignancy in both adult PM (9%) and DM (15%), with an increase in the death rate from malignancy in DM. The relative risk was 2.4 for men and 3.4

for women. Other studies have been generally consistent in showing a stronger effect in DM than in PM, with a frequency of 15% to 20% in DM, and were supported by a meta-analysis (56).

In children, cancer-associated myositis is relatively uncommon compared with that in adults, but it has been reported in 12 children with (JDM) and in 4 children with JPM (146,258). Paraneoplastic myositis has a mean age of onset of 10.5 years (range, 3.8 to 17 years) in children and is more common in boys than girls (ratio, 4:1). The most common malignancies reported in association are lymphoma, reported in seven children, and leukemia, reported in five. One of these had myelodysplastic syndrome before the development of acute nonlymphyocytic leukemia (259). Neuroblastoma, hepatocellular carcinoma, ovarian dysgerminoma, and chromophobe adenoma of the pituitary have been described in single reports in association with juvenile myositis. Most often, the myositis precedes the onset of malignancy by up to 4 years. No risk factors for the development of cancer were identified in most of the cases. One child, however, developed an Epstein–Barr virus–associated lymphoma 5 months after receiving high-dose methotrexate therapy (260). A second child had congenital agammaglobulinemia, which carries an increased risk of malignancy (261).

*Clinical Presentation*

It is suspected in some cases that the myositis develops as a paraneoplastic syndrome, and there are some cases in which the clinical course supports this, such as by remission with removal of the tumor, resistance to treatment until removal of the tumor, or exacerbation of DM with recurrence of tumor. This was found in only 22% of one series (262). In other cases, despite a temporal association of diagnosis, there is no such paraneoplastic picture.

Any tumor can occur in association with DM, and numerous co-occurrences have been reported. Types of associated malignancies parallel the frequency seen in the overall population. In the United States and Europe, breast cancer is common (55), and nasopharyngeal cancer has been common in DM in Asian populations (263). Ovarian cancer, on the other hand, appears to be overrepresented in DM patients (55,264), with a relative risk of 16.7 within 5 years of diagnosis. Some cases have a paraneoplastic course. Some associated ovarian cancers were difficult to diagnose despite specifically directed testing, with diagnosis only after metastasis occurred (265–267). The diagnosis of ovarian cancer is often made only after metastasis occurs. Cancer, including ovarian cancer, has occurred in association with amyopathic DM (268), and the risk is generally considered at least as great.

The myositis itself is not distinctive, but resistance to treatment may suggest a paraneoplastic picture. Evidence of CTD is less common, as is the presence of autoantibodies. Some have suggested that vasculitis or vasculopathic manifestations are more common with malignancy, including cutaneous necrosis.

The clinical presentation of children with cancer-associated myositis is often characterized by atypical features. All children had rapid onset of severe muscle weakness, which included both proximal and distal myopathy. Some patients had atypical rashes for JDM, including extensive rashes on the legs and trunk, alopecia, and generalized or facial edema. Most childhood cases are associated with hepatomegaly, splenomegaly, an abdominal mass, or lymphadenopathy. Daily fevers or weight loss were reported in several children. One patient developed severe shoulder girdle muscle atrophy over a 1-month period (reviewed in 146).

### Diagnostic Approach

In adults, a thorough general history and physical should be performed to look for signs of malignancy, including testing stool for occult blood, and mammography and gynecologic examination with Papanicolaou's smear in women. Routine laboratory testing should also be performed. Any abnormalities should be thoroughly evaluated. In adult women, additional testing for ovarian cancer is recommended, including pelvic computed tomography (CT) or ultrasound. Some advocate CA-125 testing (267). There is disagreement about the extent to which additional testing for malignancy should be performed in patients with newly diagnosed DM. One approach would be to pursue further testing (barium or endoscopic gastrointestinal studies and CT scans of the chest and abdomen) for patients at higher risk for malignancy, including those with DM who are older than 45 years of age with no CTD features or specific autoantibodies. Any patient with unexplained treatment resistance, prominent cutaneous necrosis, or unexplained weight loss despite steroids should also be further evaluated. Repeat evaluation after 1 and 2 years may be indicated. Evaluation for recurrent malignancy is needed if a patient with a treated malignancy develops PM or DM (or has a PM or DM flare).

In children, the physical examination findings of adenopathy, organomegaly, or a palpable mass may lead to evaluation with CT scans or radiographs, which can provide a diagnosis (269,270). Bone marrow, lymph node, or target-organ biopsy have established the diagnosis of malignancy in other cases (reviewed in 146).

### Therapy

Myositis that is known to be associated with malignancy should be treated because it may respond even if the malignancy cannot be resected or cured. Treatment is similar to that for PM and DM, described earlier. If the diagnoses are made concurrently and chemotherapy is to be given for the malignancy, separate treatment for the myositis may be held pending the result.

Of the 14 children for which follow-up information has been reported, 7 died of their malignancy despite oncologic treatment. In 8 patients, the myositis followed a paraneoplastic course, in that improvement of muscle strength and enzymes occurred with treatment of the underlying cancer, and flare in myositis disease activity occurred simultaneously with a relapse of the tumor. Of interest, steroid therapy alone improved the myositis in 6 patients (146).

### Focal Myositis

Focal myositis, an inflammatory pseudotumor of muscle, is a rare entity, with less than 100 reported cases. Most reports are in adults ranging in age from 19 to 72 years without any gender predominance (271,272). Focal myositis has also been reported in 10 boys and 6 girls aged 6 to 18 years (reviewed in 146, 273, and 274).

Most often, no inciting cause is identified. In selected cases, trauma or excessive physical activity of the involved muscle has been reported before the onset of clinical symptoms (271). One child developed myositis of the sternocleidomastoid after an episode of pharyngitis (275). Viruses, however, were not identified in the muscle biopsy specimens of patients with focal myositis using polymerase chain reaction (276), and serologic evaluation for infectious causes, including parasites, has been negative in many reports. There is no family history of myositis or muscle disease, but in some patients, a family history of other autoimmune diseases is positive (277).

### Clinical Presentation

Focal myositis usually presents as an enlarging mass within the affected muscle, which is often painful or tender to palpation. It is unattached to the subcutaneous tissue and enlarges rapidly, over a period of weeks (271,272). Focal myositis involving certain muscles may demonstrate symptoms related to the site of involvement; myositis of the sternocleidomastoid may present with torticollis (278) or pseudothrombophlebitis (279), and myositis limited to the esophagus presents with dysphagia (280). Systemic manifestations are usually absent, although fever, weight loss, arthritis, or joint flexion contractures have been reported in some cases (279,281). The most common sites of involvement are the thighs and calves (271), followed by the neck (278,279,282). Cases have been reported involving the arm, back, rectus abdominal muscle (272), lumbrical muscle of the hand (274), tongue and perioral muscles (283,284), temporal muscle (285), and upper eyelid (286).

Several reports have described a progression of classic focal myositis into generalized PM (281) or SLE (287). Although these patients are systemically ill and have elevated serum muscle enzymes and ESRs, these abnormalities are not predictive of progression to generalized PM because other patients with these findings have myositis remaining in a focal form (275,279). A form of PM limited to the quadriceps muscles, resulting in severe muscle atrophy, has also been described (288). Classic focal myositis has been reported in association with MCTD (279), Behçet's disease (289), and Hodgkin's lymphoma as a paraneoplastic myositis (290).

*Diagnostic Approach*

Most patients have normal CK, aldolase, and ESR (271,272). EMG shows changes suggestive of myositis (271) but may be normal (291). T2-weighted MRI scans show edema of the involved muscle, and MRI is useful in serial evaluation (271).

The differential diagnosis includes rhabdomyosarcoma, PM, proliferative myositis, myositis ossificans, and pseudosarcomatous fasciitis (271,272,281). Biopsy is helpful in distinguishing focal myositis from these conditions, demonstrating endomysial and perimysial inflammation, muscle necrosis, and regeneration (272); the inflammatory cells are predominantly CD4+ lymphocytes and macrophages (292).

*Therapy*

Except for those patients progressing to PM, prognosis is favorable, with spontaneous resolution within 6 months in most cases (271,278,279,282,291). Treatment by surgical excision may also cure this condition (272,274,280). Treatment with prednisone or nonsteroidal antiinflammatory drugs (NSAIDs) has aided resolution in several reports (279,285,286). Relapsing episodes involving different muscles have been reported in several patients (277). Patients who develop PM after focal myositis usually improve with prednisone treatment.

**Proliferative Myositis**

Proliferative myositis is a rare pseudosarcomatous muscular lesion characterized by a proliferation of giant cells and fibroblasts in the perimysium, epimysium, and fascia, which has been reported in about 60 patients. In adults, the median age of onset is 50 years, ranging from 22 to 88 years of age. There is no gender predilection (293,294). Most adults are white in racial background. Proliferative myositis is also reported in children; cases range in age from 2.5 months to 13 years. Boys are affected more frequently than girls (146,295).

Most often, no predisposing cause is identified. A history of acute mechanical trauma or ongoing soft tissue injury is occasionally identified, including falling episodes, blunt trauma, and sports injuries (293).

*Clinical Presentation*

Similar to focal myositis, proliferative myositis generally presents clinically as a firm, palpable, discrete nodule or mass several centimeters in diameter. Pain or tenderness may be associated. The lesion is characterized by rapid growth, with most patients coming to medical attention within 2 weeks of developing the mass, and the remainder within 5 weeks (293–295). Sites of involvement have included muscles of the shoulder, arm, thigh, calf, trunk, head, and neck, with upper extremities and trunk involved most often (293–295).

*Diagnostic Approach*

Ultrasound examination defines the mass in the involved muscle delimited by thick hypoechoic septa (296). CT demonstrates a homogenous mass surrounded by a hypodense rim (297). The clear demarcation and lack of invasion of adjacent tissue distinguish this from a malignancy. MRI demonstrates high signal intensity on T2-weighted images in a focal distribution (298).

Several conditions are important to exclude, including malignant tumors such as rhabdomyosarcoma, fibrosarcoma, and neuroblastoma; desmoid tumors; malignant fibrous histiocytoma and reticulohistiocytoma; myositis ossificans; and nodular fasciitis (293–295). Proliferative myositis may exist in association with proliferative fasciitis (299). Surgical biopsy is, therefore, crucial in establishing the diagnosis of proliferative myositis. Histologically, characteristic elements include groups of giant cells, which may be mistaken for ganglion cells; polygonal spindle cells; and typical mitotic figures in giant cells and fibroblasts. Secondary muscle atrophy or focal ischemic necrosis may be present (293,295,297). Immunohistochemistry is helpful in identifying the giant cells as originating from myofibroblasts and in distinguishing them from sarcomas (295).

*Therapy*

The lesions of proliferative myositis resolve spontaneously without recurrence (296). Surgical excision is also curative (293–295). Treatment with a short course of prednisone has also been reported to be of benefit (297).

**Orbital Myositis**

One form of focal myositis is orbital myositis, in which chronic muscle inflammation is limited to one or more extraocular muscles. Orbital myositis may also be seen in association with other CTDs as a form of overlap myositis, including in combination with SLE, Crohn's disease, scleroderma, and giant cell myocarditis (300–303). For isolated cases of orbital myositis, the mean age of onset is 37 years, as determined in one metaanalysis, with patients ranging in age from 3 to 84 years (304). Many patients with orbital myositis are young to middle age, and it has been reported in at least 32 children (reviewed in 146). Females are affected twice as frequently as males (304). In the largest reported series of 75 patients, 33 were white, 24 Hispanic, and 18 African American (305).

No predisposing factors have been identified in most reports, and there is no family history of myositis or autoimmune disease in these patients. Several cases have been reported in which orbital myositis is temporally associated with an infection, particularly upper respiratory infections, herpes zoster virus infection, and Lyme disease (306–308). One case has been observed after influenza vaccination (309).

## Clinical Presentation

Orbital myositis characteristically presents with orbital pain worsened by eye movement and may be either acute or subacute in onset. Diplopia, proptosis, conjunctival injection, chemosis, periorbital edema, and globe retraction with narrowing of the palpebral fissure in the presence of normal visual acuity are commonly associated symptoms (310,311). Only 20% of patients have no limitation in eye muscle movement (305). When onset is acute, the affected muscle is either restricted in movement or paretic. In the subacute or recurrent presentations, similar to thyroid eye disease, limitation of gaze is opposite of the action of the affected muscle because of fibrosis (310). The frequency of extraocular muscle involvement is medial rectus (43%), superior rectus (19%), lateral rectus (17%), superior oblique (9%), inferior rectus (7%), and inferior oblique (5%) (305). The associated tendinous insertion was also affected in most patients (312). Most patients have bilateral muscle involvement, and about 10% of patients have three or four affected extraocular muscles (313,314).

## Diagnostic Approach

The primary conditions that are important to distinguish from orbital myositis include thyroid eye disease; ocular myopathies, particularly mitochondrial disorders and ocular dystrophies; and orbital pseudotumors localized to another site in the orbit. Orbital cellulitis, orbital neoplasms and metastases, MG, arteriovenous malformations and fistulae, trochleitis, Tolosa–Hunt syndrome, and cavernous sinus thrombosis are also included in the differential diagnosis (304,306).

Thyroid eye disease is the disorder most commonly mistaken for orbital myositis because both disorders have impaired muscle movement. In thyroid eye disease, in contrast to orbital myositis, onset is slow, eye movement is painless, vision may be affected, and lid lag and lid retraction are characteristic. Ptosis, which is associated with orbital myositis, is not observed in thyroid eye disease (304,306). The inferior rectus is the most frequently involved muscle, whereas it is the least frequently involved in orbital myositis (304). EMG and imaging studies of the orbit, discussed later, may also help in distinguishing these conditions. Finally, whereas orbital myositis responds rapidly and often completely to corticosteroid therapy, thyroid eye disease responds more slowly and variably to treatment with steroids (304,306).

In orbital myositis, the ESR is often elevated, and ANA is usually negative; there has been no documentation of sarcoplasmic muscle enzymes in these patients (315). EMG and orbital imaging are helpful in the diagnostic evaluation of orbital symptoms. EMG of the extraocular muscles using coaxial needle electrodes demonstrates myopathic changes in orbital myositis, including spontaneous myogenic activity and polyphasic action potentials. It is these latter features of the EMG that can be helpful in distinguishing orbital myositis from other ocular myopathies, thyroid eye disease, and MG, although EMG is most useful in distinguishing orbital myositis from other nonmyogenic ocular diseases (316).

CT and orbital ultrasound are the imaging procedures of choice (304). In orbital myositis, CT demonstrates swelling of the muscle and tendon insertion, with irregularity resulting from extension into the periorbital fat, as well as enhancement with contrast. This is in distinction to dysthyroid eye disease, in which the extraocular muscle enlargement produces a regular muscle border and no tendon involvement (311,313,314). Orbital tumors or metastases generally produce extraocular muscle enlargement as well as another orbital mass or bony involvement. Vascular lesions, such as carotid–cavernous fistulae and arteriovenous malformations, usually demonstrate uniform enlargement of the extraocular muscles as a result of vascular congestion; an enlarged superior ophthalmic vein or cavernous sinus dilation on the CT scan is an additional diagnostic feature of these conditions (304). Orbital ultrasound shows enlargement of the muscle belly on B-scan imaging, with reduced reflectivity on the A scan; thyroid eye disease would show normal or increased reflectivity on scanning (304,311). Fat-suppressed MRI and the use of gadolinium have improved the resolution of MRI for orbital myositis (317).

Extraocular muscle biopsy is reserved for patients in whom imaging studies cannot exclude a tumor or patients who are refractory to initial therapy. The pathology is similar to that of peripheral myositis, with infiltration of lymphocytes, plasma cells, and occasionally polymorphonuclear leukocytes or eosinophils surrounding muscle fibers. The orbital fat is also affected. Muscle fibrosis is present in chronic cases. The pathology is indistinguishable from thyroid eye disease, except for involvement of the orbital fat and long-term fibrotic changes, which are seen specifically in orbital myositis (304).

## Therapy

The primary therapy for orbital myositis is oral corticosteroids; response is generally rapid, within days to weeks, and therapy is continued with a tapering schedule up to several weeks or months (304,305). NSAIDs are an alternative initial therapy (312,318). Despite treatment with either steroids or NSAIDs, recurrent episodes develop in 15% to 70% of patients (304,312,318). Risk factors for recurrent disease include involvement of horizontal, rather than vertical, extraocular muscles and involvement of more than one muscle, as well as male gender, delay to diagnosis, and lack of response to initial therapy with corticosteroids or NSAIDs (312). For treatment of recurrent disease or in corticosteroid-refractory cases, orbital radiation has been employed with initial success, but with follow-up of more than 4 years, treatment failure is universal (304,318). Methotrexate has also been used in refractory cases and has been noted to improve disease activity in 70% of a series of six patients with a follow-up of 3 to 24 months and to induce remission in half of these patients (319). Cyclosporine has been reported to be successful in one patient with steroid-refractory disease; follow-up was relatively short at 5 months (320). In patients with recurrent or chronic disease, permanent ocular motility deficits and proptosis are common sequelae (321). Use of botulinum A toxin provided symptomatic relief for most patients in one series (322).

### Eosinophilic Myositis Syndromes

The eosinophilic myositis syndromes, which are characterized by eosinophilic inflammation of muscle and often accompanied by peripheral eosinophilia, include several distinct clinicopathologic entities dominated either by myositis or fasciitis (Table 22.9). Three forms of eosinophilic myositis exist: eosinophilic PM, which is accompanied by endomysial eosinophilic inflammation; eosinophilic perimyositis, in which the eosinophilic infiltrate is localized to the fascia and perimysium of muscle; and focal eosinophilic myositis, in which the inflammation is localized to one particular muscle group (244,323). The myositis associated with idiopathic hypereosinophilic syndrome is often indistinguishable from eosinophilic PM, accompanied by systemic clinical manifestations (324). Affected patients with these illnesses have ranged in age from 5 to 70 years, with a predilection for men to be affected more often than women in a ratio of 2:1 (323). Two cases of focal eosinophilic myositis and one case of eosinophilic PM have been reported in children (reviewed in 146).

Eosinophilic myositis has also been observed as part of syndromes dominated by fasciitis, including eosinophilic fasciitis (Shulman's syndrome) and EMS (24,325,326).

Often, no inciting agent is identified in the eosinophilic myositides, although tranilast and alcohol ingestion have been reported in association with the onset of eosinophilic PM, and consumption of L-tryptophan triggers the onset of EMS (24,323,327,328). Local physical trauma, including horseback riding, has been associated with the onset of focal eosinophilic myositis.

### Clinical Presentation

Eosinophilic PM and idiopathic hypereosinophilic syndrome are characterized by an acute or subacute onset of myalgias or muscle tenderness and proximal muscle weakness, often accompanied by peripheral edema or swelling. Patients frequently develop a systemic illness, which may include cardiac involvement (myocarditis, pericarditis, arrhythmias, endocardial fibrosis, or heart failure), Raynaud's phenomenon, arthritis, eosinophilic pneumonia, and peripheral neuropathy (244,323,324,329). In eosinophilic perimyositis, muscle pain and tenderness, predominantly in the lower limbs, are the primary clinical features. Muscle weakness and systemic manifestations are absent. Joint flexion contractures and a prodromal febrile illness have been reported (244,330). Cutaneous manifestations, including Gottron's papules, subcutaneous induration, erythema, and angioedema, accom-

pany eosinophilic PM or perimyositis in 38% of patients (331). Focal eosinophilic myositis presents with painless or painful swelling of the involved muscle. Involvement of the chest wall, neck, upper extremity, and facial muscles predominates (244,323).

In eosinophilic fasciitis (Shulman's syndrome), fasciitis is the primary clinical manifestation, including swelling and tenderness of the skin, followed by indurative changes resulting in the skin becoming bound down to the fascia; joint flexion contractures often result. Myositis and morphea may accompany the fasciitis (325,326,332). In terms of the myositis, proximal and distal muscle weakness, accompanied by pain with muscle contraction, may be seen. The myositis may also be asymptomatic (325,326). In EMS, myalgias and fasciitis are universally present; myopathy and muscle tenderness with documented eosinophilic myositis are seen in more than half of the cases (24). Systemic manifestations, including paresthesias and neuropathies, weight loss, pulmonary involvement, arthritis, fever, alopecia, and xerostomia, are common.

### Diagnostic Approach

In eosinophilic myositis, eosinophilia is seen in up to 80% of patients, and the ESR is also elevated as frequently. Serum muscle enzymes, including CK and aldolase, are markedly elevated in eosinophilic PM but are often normal in the other forms of eosinophilic myositis and fasciitis, even in the presence of muscle involvement. ANAs and rheumatoid factor are positive in less than 30% of patients with eosinophilic PM (244,323). The EMG is usually myogenic in eosinophilic PM focal myositis and, less frequently, in eosinophilic perimyositis and fasciitis (323,333). Muscle biopsy findings in eosinophilic PM and focal myositis are characterized by an inflammatory infiltrate of the endomysial muscle fibers in which eosinophils predominate, with accompanying necrosis, degeneration, and fiber size variation; perimysial inflammation may also be present (244,323,329). In eosinophilic perimyositis, the eosinophilic infiltrate is in the perimysium and fascia; fiber necrosis is rare, and muscle fibers are normal (330). In eosinophilic fasciitis, inflammation predominates in the fascia, although endomysial and perimysial inflammation is also present when muscle involvement occurs, whereas in EMS, muscle involvement is exclusively perimysial (24).

Several other conditions resulting in eosinophilic inflammation of muscle should be excluded as part of the evaluation. These include parasitic infections (*Taenia solium* and *Trichinella, Sarcocystis* and *Ascaris* species); fungal infections (actinomycosis); primary vasculitides, including Churg–Strauss syndrome and polyarteritis nodosa; hyperimmunoglobulin E; and malignancies, such as eosinophilic leukemia, Kimura's disease, and histocytosis X, which cause eosinophilic muscle masses (244,323,324,334,335). Becker's muscular dystrophy has been reported to present as eosinophilic PM in infancy (336). Muscle biopsy pathology, combined with serologies, cultures, and special stains for parasites,

**TABLE 22.9.** *Classification of the eosinophilic myositis syndromes*

| | Eosinophilic polymyositis, hypereosinophilic syndrome | Eosinophilic perimyositis | Focal eosinophilic myositis | Eosinophilic fasciitis (Shulman's syndrome) | Eosinophilia–myalgia syndrome |
|---|---|---|---|---|---|
| Involvement | Endomysium, perimysium | Perimysium, fascia | Endomysium of involved muscle | Fascia—primary, endomysium, perimysium | Fascia—primary, perimysium |
| Muscle tropism | Proximal muscles | Lower limbs | One muscle: upper extremity, chest wall, neck, facial predominate | Extremities underlying fasciitis | Extremities underlying fasciitis |
| Muscle symptoms | Proximal weakness, myalgias, tenderness, edema | Muscle pain, tenderness | Painless or painful swelling of involved muscle | Asymptomatic or proximal and distal weakness, muscle pain with contraction | Myalgias, proximal and distal weakness, muscle tenderness |
| Systemic manifestations | Cardiac, Raynaud's, arthritis, pneumonia, neuropathy, cutaneous | Joint flexion contractures, preceding febrile illness, cutaneous | None | Fasciitis—primary | Fasciitis, paresthesias, neuropathy, weight loss, fever, pulmonary, arthritis, alopecia, xerostomia |
| Laboratory studies | Increased CK, aldolase, increased ESR, eosinophilia, positive ANA, RF; EMG myogenic | Eosinophilia, ESR possibly elevated, aldolase possibly elevated | Eosinophilia, increased ESR, aldolase possibly elevated | Eosinophilia, increased ESR, aldolase possibly elevated | Eosinophilia, increased ESR, aldolase, LDH elevated |
| Response to therapy | High-dose prednisone, leukopheresis | Prednisone, NSAIDs; none | Prednisone, surgery | Prednisone, NSAIDs, azathioprine | Prednisone |
| Prognosis | Chronic or relapsing course | Relapsing course or remission | Relapsing course or remission | Relapsing course or remission | Remission, discontinue L-tryptophan |

CK, creatine kinase; ESR, erythrocyte sedimentation rate; ANA, antinuclear antibody; RF, rheumatoid factor; EMG, electromyogram; NSAIDs, nonsteroidal antiinflammatory drugs; LDH, lactate dehydrogenase.

From Hall FC, Krausz T, Walport MJ. Idiopathic eosinophilic myositis. *QJM* 1995;88:581–586; and Pickering MC, Walport MJ. Eosinophilic myopathic syndromes. *Curr Opin Rheumatol* 1998;10:504–510.

is helpful in distinguishing these from the idiopathic eosinophilic syndromes.

### Therapy

Corticosteroids, in doses of 20 to 100 mg/d, are the most effective therapy for all forms of eosinophilic myositis, resulting in improvement or resolution in 90% of patients (323). Eosinophilic PM requires prolonged therapy with higher steroid doses. Leukopheresis was required in one case of hypereosinophilic syndrome (337), and surgical fasciotomies for compartment syndromes were required in one case of eosinophilic PM (338). NSAIDs are beneficial in mild episodes of eosinophilic perimyositis, although spontaneous resolution may also occur (328,330). Azathioprine may be beneficial as an adjunctive agent in eosinophilic fasciitis (325). Removal of an inciting environmental agent, drug or toxin, is important (24,327).

Eosinophilic PM and fasciitis are often characterized by chronic continuous or relapsing illness courses (323,325,329,332). Focal myositis and perimyositis have relapsing illness courses or, after therapy, may enter a prolonged remission (244,323,330).

### Granulomatous Myositis

Idiopathic granulomatous myositis, characterized by the presence of epithelioid cellular granulomas and giant cells on muscle biopsy, is an extremely rare clinicopathologic subset of myositis represented by only several dozen published reports. Females are affected more frequently than males, in a ratio of 4:1 to 7:1 (339,340). Illness onset occurs from 27 to 76 years of age, although two teenage patients have also been reported (146,339).

### Clinical Presentation

Granulomatous myositis most often presents as a slowly progressive, chronic myopathy, preferentially affecting the proximal and axial musculature of the upper and lower extremities. Distal muscles, particularly of the forearms and hands, may be exclusively involved, and facial weakness has been reported (339–342). Myalgias, dysphagia, dysphonia, and joint flexion contractures are commonly associated symptoms (340,343,344). Patients generally do not have cutaneous manifestations of DM or motor-sensory deficits that occur in sarcoidosis (343).

### Diagnostic Approach

Idiopathic granulomatous myositis must be distinguished from a number of illnesses in which granulomas are seen in the muscle biopsy (Table 22.10), including CTDs, infections, malignancies, and intramuscular injections of aluminum-material contained in certain vaccines. Characteristic clinical features for these illnesses and laboratory testing, including

**TABLE 22.10.** *Differential diagnosis of granulomatous myositis*

Connective tissue and autoimmune diseases
  Sarcoid (Besnier–Boeck–Schaumann disease)
  Rheumatoid arthritis
  Crohn's disease
  Wegener's granulomatosis
  Churg–Strauss syndrome
  Giant cell arteritis
  Myasthenia gravis
Infections
  Mycobacteria: tuberculosis
  Bacteria: brucellosis
  Fungi: histoplasmosis, sporotrichosis
  Parasites: toxoplasmosis, onchocerciasis
  Protozoa: pneumocystis
  Treponema: syphilis
Carcinoma
Intramuscular vaccinations containing aluminum (DPT)

Data from references 344, 345, 347, 348, and 409–413.

cultures, infectious serologies, and special stains of the muscle biopsy for infectious organisms, can aid in distinguishing the idiopathic form of granulomatous myositis from these illnesses. The most common illness mimicking idiopathic granulomatous myositis, which often can be the most difficult to distinguish, is sarcoidosis. Chronic myositis is the most common form of sarcoid myopathy, and symptoms can be identical to those of idiopathic granulomatous myositis; other manifestations of sarcoidosis are generally present, including elevated levels of angiotensin-converting enzyme (345).

In idiopathic granulomatous myositis, serum muscle enzymes, including CK and aldolase, are typically elevated. ESR and serum immunoglobulins may be elevated, and eosinophilia may occur (340). MSAs and MAAs can be present and are helpful in distinguishing the idiopathic variety from other CTDs and infectious illnesses (343). EMG usually demonstrates myopathic features. MRI, ultrasound, and scintigraphy (technetium and gallium) have been useful techniques to determine the distribution of lesions and to select a region to biopsy (346).

Granulomas, consisting of epithelioid, infiltrating mononuclear cells and multinucleated giant cells of the Langhans variety, are characteristically present on muscle biopsy (340,342). The infiltrating inflammatory cells consist of CD4$^+$ T lymphocytes and macrophages (343). Degeneration, regeneration, and fiber size variation, common to other forms of IIM, are also frequent biopsy findings (340,341). Idiopathic granulomatous myositis is indistinguishable from sarcoid myopathy on muscle biopsy; adjunctive clinical features and biopsies of other affected tissues can distinguish these entities (340,342).

### Therapy

From the little written about the therapy of idiopathic granulomatous myositis, prednisone is the primary agent used

(339,342). The use of adjunctive agents, including azathioprine and methotrexate, have been helpful in refractory cases (344). Infectious granulomatous myopathies respond to therapy directed against the specific etiopathologic agent (347,348).

## Autoimmune Myasthenia Gravis

MG is a disease caused by autoimmunity to the AChR, resulting in muscle weakness as a result of impaired transmission across the neuromuscular junction. The disease is usually described as having a peak incidence in women in their 20s and 30s, and predominantly in men in the older age groups (349). In one study, however, MG increased in both men and women older than 50 years of age, with a larger increase in men, so that the prevalence in men and women older than 50 years of age was about equal (350). The overall prevalence is 14.2 per 100,000 population. The prevalence and average age have increased over time, which is attributed to longer survival as a result of better treatments. A higher frequency is found in African Americans than in whites.

The pathophysiologic abnormalities and disease manifestations result from the effects of autoantibody to the nicotinic AChR at the motor end plate (351). There is abundant evidence for this, reviewed by Drachman (352), who described five criteria indicating that MG is an antibody-mediated autoimmune disease: the presence of specific antibody, reaction with the antigen at the site of pathology, experimental reproduction by passive transfer, reproduction by active immunization, and clinical improvement with reduction of antibody (352). Antibody binding to the AChR is found by radioimmunoassay in about 85% of patients (see later). Even in cases that are seronegative in the clinical assay, evidence of immunoglobulin reacting with and affecting the AChR can often be demonstrated. There is also evidence that the antibody binds to the AChR *in vivo*. IgG deposition near the AChR can be detected (353,354), as can terminal components of complement, supporting the pathologic significance of this humoral attack (355). The anti-AChR from MG patients leads to disease manifestations in mice after passive transfer (356). Clinically, neonatal myasthenia may be an example of this in humans. Immunization with the AChR can produce MG in several species, which is faithful in many respects to human MG (experimental autoimmune MG). Finally, removing the antibody, as by plasmapheresis, leads to clinical improvement in the disease. The clinically measured titer of antibody, however, does not necessarily correlate with severity (357).

The AChR is a large protein of six subunits in the postsynaptic membrane at the neuromuscular junction (352). There are two α-subunits, and when they bind acetylcholine, the cation channel opens, resulting in an end-plate potential. This sets off the action potential, which leads to contraction. The number of functional AChRs in the end plate is reduced in MG (358), decreasing the amplitude of the end-plate potential, and it may not be sufficient for an action potential. When the amount of acetylcholine released is reduced by repeated stimulation, this occurs increasingly, leading to the observed fatigue effect.

Reduction of AChRs has been shown to be an effect of the autoantibody. Turnover of the AChR occurs normally, with production increased when transmission is reduced. The antibody cross-links the AChRs, which results in increased rate of loss because of "accelerated endocytosis" with resultant degradation (359,360). There are also destructive effects of the antibody on the AChR, mediated by complement. Damage is seen microscopically to the junctional folds of the postsynaptic membrane, with evidence of complement deposition (353,354,361). There is some evidence of foci of inflammation in the area of the neuromuscular junction, as would be expected with the complement activation (362). In addition, there is evidence of a functional reduction by blockade of the AChR by antibody.

The acetylcholine-binding α-subunit is the major antigen. It has a "major immunogenic region" to which a substantial proportion of antibody is directed, although there is heterogeneity in the actual epitopes recognized. This is further reflected in differences in antibody effects. Patients may differ in the extent to which their antibodies result in blocking or cross-linking (modulation). Patient antibodies may also differ in the other subunits they recognize and in the extent to which they recognize the fetal form, which has been associated with neonatal MG (363).

There is a clear association of MG with the thymus (364). About 70% of MG patients have lymphoid follicular hyperplasia with germinal center formation, and 10% have thymomas; there is commonly clinical improvement of MG with removal of an abnormal thymus. Thymus changes are not seen in experimentally induced MG, supporting a primary role for the thymus in etiologic mechanisms of MG. Several other observations are consistent, including the finding of AChRs on thymic "myoid" cells (365); the close proximity of these cells to immunologically active cells, including dendritic cells in the thymus; and the demonstration of AChR-specific T cells in the thymus, which are more abundant in MG than normally (364). The T cells are believed to promote anti-AChR production, but there is no indication of T-cell cytotoxicity against the muscle or junctional membrane. The exact role of the thymus remains to be fully defined.

The etiology is otherwise unknown. As in other autoimmune diseases, an environmental factor in a genetically susceptible host has been postulated. Infection has been suspected, and potential sites of similarity between infectious agents and the AChR have been noted (366). Genetic associations at HLA (including B8-DR3) have been found. D-Penicillamine can occasionally induce autoimmune MG. This differs from the more common drug effects that interfere with neuromuscular junction transmission (Table 22.11) and demonstrates the potential role of environmental factors.

Antibody to another antigen at the neuromuscular junction, the voltage-gated calcium channel (362), is found in another condition, Lambert–Eaton myasthenic syndrome (LEMS). The pathology in this disease occurs in the presynaptic area

**TABLE 22.11.** *Drugs that induce neuromuscular disorders, which exacerbate myasthenia gravis*

Antibiotics
   Neomycin, kanamycin, streptomycin, gentamycin, tobramycin, amikacin, polymyxin B, tetracyclines, clindamycin, erythromycin, ampicillin
Cardiovascular drugs
   β-blockers, quinidine, procainamide, verapamil, lidocaine
Anticonvulsants
   Diphenylhydantoin, trimethadione, mephenytoin
Central nervous system agents
   Lithium, chlorpromazine, promethazine, morphine, related narcotics, barbiturate anesthetics
Antirheumatic agents
   D-Penicillamine, chloroquine, prednisone, ketoprofen, colchicine
Other drugs
   Cisplatinum, carnitine, bretylium, emetine, lactate, magnesium, citrate anticoagulant, contrast agents

Adapted from Argov Z, Wirguin I. Drugs and the neuromuscular junction. In: Lisak RP, ed. *Handbook of Myasthenia Gravis and Myasthenic Syndromes.* New York: Marcel Dekker, 1994:310–311; and Verma P, Oger J. Treatment of acquired autoimmune myasthenia gravis: a topic review. *Can J Neurol Sci* 1992;19:360–375, with permission.

at the nerve terminal. There is a depletion of active zone particles in the nerve terminal, with reduction in the amount of acetylcholine released with each impulse. The main action of the antibody appears to be blockade, without evidence of complement deposition or inflammation. LEMS has distinctive clinical features compared with MG. There is variation in weakness, but in a different pattern than that of MG (worse in the morning), and a difference in distribution of weakness, with more proximal lower extremity and less extraocular muscle involvement. This condition is commonly associated with nonthymus malignancies, such as small cell lung cancer.

### Children

The two primary forms of autoimmune MG occurring during childhood are transient neonatal MG and juvenile MG. Rare congenital myasthenic syndromes, with clinical myasthenic symptoms resulting in altered neuromuscular transmission, also have onset during infancy and childhood, but they are not autoimmune diseases and therefore are not discussed here.

Transient neonatal MG occurs in an average of 21% of first-born infants of myasthenic mothers and 40% in subsequent siblings (367). There is no gender or race predilection. The pathogenesis of transient neonatal MG remains unclear and is not simply explained by the transplacental passage of maternal autoantibodies resulting in clinical illness in the neonate. Some studies report higher titers of AChR antibodies in affected compared with unaffected neonates, but this has not been confirmed in other reports; maternal AChR antibody titer may correlate with disease severity in the neonate (368). Production of AChR antibodies by the neonate has been reported by some groups (369). The presence of anti-

bodies that block the function of the AChR also correlates with the severity of clinical manifestations in the neonate, and their lower frequency of transplacental passage in unaffected compared with affected infants may partly explain variability in the transmission and severity in neonates (363). A concordance of HLA alleles (DRB1*03) between mothers and affected infants may also contribute to the pathogenesis of neonatal MG (370).

Juvenile MG, like adult MG, is an acquired autoimmune disorder affecting the neuromuscular junction and is mediated by AChR autoantibodies. The onset of juvenile MG is generally after 12 months of age, with peak ages of onset during childhood of 1 to 4 years and 11 to 16 years (371). Almost 20% of all cases of MG have their onset in childhood (372). Girls are affected at least twice as frequently as boys (371,373). Similar to adult MG, other autoimmune diseases, particularly Graves' disease, have been reported in association. Thymoma is rare in children, but thymic hyperplasia is common and associated with elevated AChR antibody titers (373). Coexisting neoplasm has been documented in two children with neuroblastoma and one with leukemia (371,372).

### Clinical Presentation

Weakness is the major symptom of MG because it occurs in many myopathies and neurologic conditions. The onset of MG can be precipitated by drugs that can have an exacerbating effect on MG, but sometimes no triggering factor is identified. MG is distinctive for the variation in weakness and its distribution. MG weakness characteristically is worsened with repeated efforts (fatiguability) and is improved with rest. It typically varies over the course of the day, is improved in the morning or after resting, and is worse at the end of the day. Symptoms most commonly begin with ocular involvement, usually ptosis, diplopia or both, representing involvement of the eyelids and extraocular muscles. Eye closure can be weak. Most patients who do not start with ocular involvement develop it within the next few years. This distribution is in marked contrast to IIMs (other than orbital myositis), in which ocular muscle involvement is unusual. In contrast to several other conditions causing lid and eye weakness (third nerve problems, Horner's syndrome, botulism), MG does not affect the pupils (374). Fatiguability can be demonstrated in the eyelid muscles by attempting to hold the upward gaze and seeing progressively worsening ptosis. Ptosis usually affects both eyes, but the eyes are often affected to different degrees (375). Other eye movements can also fatigue. Pseudointernuclear ophthalmoplegia can be seen on lateral gaze (weakness of adductor, nystagmus of abductor) but is not specific for MG (374).

In about 15% of patients, symptoms remain isolated to the ocular muscles (375). This figure may be higher outside of referral centers (350). More often, patients develop involvement of other muscles, with bulbar and other facial muscles, and generalized involvement, including limb muscles and diaphragm muscles. MG is not associated with sensory abnormalities. Weakness in the face can affect facial expression, including the smile, giving the appearance of a snarl. Patients may have changes in speech, or weakness in chewing. Some patients assist their chewing with their hand. Oropharyngeal muscle weakness can cause dysphagia. Nasal regurgitation can occur. Generalized weakness can affect the limbs, usually upper more than lower; the neck; or the diaphragm. Weakness of muscles of respiration can lead to respiratory failure, which can come on rapidly and can be life-threatening (myasthenic crisis). Reduced pulmonary function or worsening strength elsewhere should raise suspicion of possible impending crisis. Respiration can also be compromised by airway blockage as a result of pharyngeal weakness and by dysphagia leading to aspiration.

### Children

Transient neonatal MG has its clinical onset within 3 days of life in the neonate. Symptoms include generalized hypotonia and poor sucking, which are almost universally present, as well as weak cry (60% to 70%), flat and mask-like facies (37% to 60%), swallowing difficulty (50% to 71%), ptosis (15%), and local or generalized weakness (367,371). Respiratory distress may be mild or may result in mechanical ventilation in severe cases (30%) (367). Atypical forms of the disease have these clinical manifestations in association with arthrogryposis of multiple joints as well as hydramnios and decreased fetal movement (367,371).

Juvenile MG presents with ptosis as the primary complaint, and ocular myasthenia is present in 70% to 80% of children (373). Generalized weakness is observed in 15% to 50% of these children and can be variable, with the presence of fatigability and primarily proximal muscle weakness. Bulbar symptoms, with swallowing difficulties and resultant aspiration, also occur variably (371).

### Diagnostic Approach

The clinical diagnosis of MG begins by eliciting the typical clinical features of weakness in the typical distribution, with fatiguability. Several tests can be used to establish and support the diagnosis when there is a consistent clinical picture, including the edrophonium test, EMG with repetitive nerve stimulation, single-fiber EMG, and tests for autoantibodies. The combination of clinical picture and diagnostic tests allows a diagnosis in most cases, but some cases can remain difficult.

### Edrophonium Test

Acetylcholinesterase inhibitors slow the degradation of acetylcholine, increasing stimulation of available AChR and improving weakness. Testing for this response is useful diagnostically and is commonly the first step. Intravenous edrophonium (Tensilon) is particularly useful for this purpose because its effect is rapid (1 minute or less). It also has a short duration of action

(5 to 10 minutes). A specific finding of weakness is identified, such as significant ptosis or extraocular weakness, and observed for change after injection. A test dose is given first (e.g., 0.1 mL) to observe for unusual sensitivity, such as bradycardia or cholinergic symptoms. If no side effects develop, 3 to 4 mg of additional drug may be given (0.3 to 0.4 mL), with observation for change in the finding within 1 minute, and repeated once if none is seen (total maximum dose, 10 mg). Intramuscular neostigmine can also be used, which has a slower onset but longer duration of action, which may make examination for response easier. The test is not completely specific for MG. Some patients with ALS or other conditions may show some degree of response. It is also not completely sensitive, and sometimes the results are equivocal. The ease, immediacy, and low cost of the test are advantages. The potential for significant side effects is a drawback; atropine should be available, and caution should be used in patients with cardiac disease, lung disease, or the elderly.

### Anti-AChR Autoantibodies

Anti-AChR autoantibodies have high specificity for MG. A small proportion of patients with LEMS can test positive, as can some patients with SLE. Thus, demonstration of serum anti-AChR in substantial titer in a patient with a consistent clinical picture can establish the diagnosis of MG. EMG is probably not necessary in these patients. The confidence that such a specific test can confer makes it worthwhile to perform even in patients with a typical clinical picture and a positive edrophonium test.

The antibody is routinely measured clinically by radioimmunoassay using human AChR as antigen, bound to radiolabeled α-bungarotoxin, which binds specifically and tightly to the AChR. It is negative in about 10% to 20% of MG cases overall. It is more likely to be negative in patients with isolated ocular MG (up to 30%) but can be negative even in generalized MG (5% to 10%). There are various possible explanations for MG in the absence of clinically detectable anti-AChR. The antibody may be present but not detected, as suggested by passive transfer experiments. Some patients have detectable anti-AChR by other methods, such as methods looking for blocking or modulating effects on AChR (357). The antigen used in the radioimmunoassay may be lacking certain relevant epitopes. Also, if it is predominantly IgM, anti-AChR may not be detected. Other theorized possibilities include loss from the serum as a result of deposition in tissues, or antibodies to other neuromuscular junction structures (357).

In neonates with transient MG, serum AChR antibodies are elevated in affected and unaffected infants born to mothers with MG and are not helpful in predicting who will develop symptoms. A gradual decrease in antibody titer, however, correlates with clinical improvement in affected neonates (367). In juvenile MG, AChR antibodies rise in titer with age and are elevated in 25% of MG patients younger than 5 years of age but in 80% to 100% of older children

(371). As in adults, children with thymic hyperplasia are all seropositive for AChR antibodies (376).

Antistriational antibodies (anti-StrA) also occur in MG, which react with contractile structures in skeletal muscle. They are usually detected by indirect immunofluorescence on muscle and are heterogeneous in specificity. They are usually found in older patients and have been associated with thymoma. Anti-StrA were found in 6% of patients younger than 40 years of age, 55% of MG in patients older than 60 years of age, and 80% to 90% of patients with thymoma (377). They may be useful for identifying a risk for thymoma in otherwise low-risk groups. Some specific anti-StrA antibodies, including antibodies to titin and to the ryanodine receptor (sarcoplasmic reticulum calcium-release channel protein) have been strongly associated with thymoma. The pathophysiologic significance of these is not yet clear.

### Electromyography

Routine EMG and nerve conduction studies can be useful in excluding other neuropathies and myopathies. The most useful test on EMG is the repetitive nerve stimulation test (352,375,378). In MG, repetitive stimulation at a low rate, usually 3 stimulations per second, results in a progressive reduction in amplitude of the action potential. This reflects a successive reduction in the number of fibers participating, as a consequence of the expected reduction of acetylcholine released, as noted previously. The sensitivity of this test is reduced when involvement is limited, as in ocular MG, but it is not 100% even in generalized MG. Testing multiple muscles can increase the sensitivity, and proximal muscles may be more likely to test positive. Single-fiber EMG is abnormal in more than 90% of MG patients and thus is the most sensitive test in MG overall, but the findings are not specific for MG (375,378).

### Other Tests

Because of the association with thymoma and thymus abnormalities, it is important to obtain imaging studies of the thymus (CT or MRI) in all patients with MG. There is a higher than usual rate of thyroid disease, such as Graves' disease, in patients with MG, and thyroid disease is among the conditions that should be excluded in establishing the diagnosis of MG due to muscle and eye effects in both conditions. Thus, all patients with suspected or proven MG should have thyroid function tests. Numerous autoimmune diseases have been found in association with MG, such as SLE. If MG is diagnosed but does not explain the patient's entire clinical picture, further testing should be pursued.

### Differential Diagnosis

The diagnosis of MG is more difficult when the disease is limited to the ocular muscles because of the lower sensitivity of the tests discussed, or when it presents atypically, for example, without any ocular involvement, because it is less likely to be considered. Among the conditions to consider are mitochondrial myopathies that involve both extraocular muscles and limb muscles. Signs of myopathy and abnormalities on biopsy (ragged red fibers) are seen in mitochondrial myopathies, and genetic abnormalities can often be demonstrated. ALS can sometimes be difficult to distinguish, especially from MG without eye involvement, or in ALS patients who respond to edrophonium. The progressive nature of ALS eventually becomes evident with the development of associated fasciculations, atrophy, and hyperreflexia. LEMS can cause variable weakness and occasional anti-AChR, but the presence of LEMS-specific antibodies can help distinguish it. PM can be considered, especially if eye signs are absent and ANAs are positive, but in PM, anti-AChRs are negative, and the myositis should be revealed by muscle enzymes, EMG, and muscle biopsy. For ocular MG, other conditions that affect the extraocular muscles or cause ptosis should also be considered, including thyroid eye disease, orbital myositis, and botulism.

### Therapy

Therapeutic approaches to MG are primarily empiric, based on retrospective or open-label experiences. The mainstay of therapy for ocular MG and first-line therapy for severe, generalized MG is anticholinesterase drugs. These drugs inhibit the hydrolysis of acetylcholine at the neuromuscular junction, thereby enhancing neuromuscular transmission (379,380). Pyridostigmine and neostigmine can be used either alone or in combination, although MG in most patients is well controlled with pyridostigmine. The low, variable bioavailability of these agents requires tailoring the dose and schedule to the individual patient (379,380). Treatment with anticholinesterases is primarily restricted by dose-limiting muscarinic and nicotinic side effects, manifest as miosis, bronchial and nasal secretions, abdominal cramps, salivation, increased urination, and bradycardia for the former, and as muscle cramps, fasciculations, and increased weakness for the latter (380). Because of these side effects, responses to therapy are generally incomplete (379). Patients also become refractory to their therapeutic effects over several years of use (379).

Corticosteroids, particularly prednisone, are the mainstay of immunosuppressive therapy for MG and are indicated for severe, generalized MG or for ocular MG refractory to anticholinesterases. Steroids decrease synthesis of AChR antibodies and induce apoptosis of cortical thymocytes (379). About 60% to 80% of MG patients experience partial or complete remissions with corticosteroid therapy. The latency for improvement is several months, and patients can be maintained on alternate-day therapy (379,381). Azathioprine is used in patients who are steroid dependent, in those who experience intolerable side effects, and as initial immunosuppressive therapy when corticosteroids are contraindicated. Therapeutic effects are not evident for 2 to 8 months and may not be maximal for 12 to 24 months (375). Clinical improvement with azathioprine ranges from 44% to 80% (381–383). Patients demonstrating better responses to azathioprine are men older than 35 years of age, who have a shorter disease duration (less than 10 years), have lower AChR antibody titers, and test negative for HLA-DRB1*03 (381,383,384). Therapy with azathioprine is long-term, with relapses occurring after therapy is discontinued (384).

Cyclosporine is generally used after corticosteroid and azathioprine therapy, in patients with suboptimal responses, or when toxicity limits treatment. Its use is supported by efficacy demonstrated in a double-blind, placebo-controlled trial in which patients receiving cyclosporine significantly improved muscle strength, reduced AChR antibody titer, and decreased corticosteroid dose compared with the placebo group. In this study, as well as in open-label studies, 50% to 80% of patients demonstrated clinical improvement on cyclosporine therapy (381,385,386). Responses are observed 2 weeks to 4 months after initiating therapy. The toxicity observed in most treated patients, including rising serum creatinine levels, hypertension, hypertrichosis, and gingival hyperplasia, preclude its use as a first-line immunosuppressive agent (381,385,386).

Because plasma exchange produces rapid short-term improvement in MG yet carries a risk for serious adverse events, such as cardiovascular events, infection, and electrolyte disturbances, it is primarily used as short-term therapy to stabilize patients experiencing myasthenic crisis in preparation for thymectomy and other operations or as an intermediate therapy while waiting for another immunosuppressive agent to take effect (381). Plasma exchange is effective in lowering AChR antibody titer, and the onset of effect is rapid, usually after the third treatment, and short-lived, lasting 6 to 8 weeks (375,379).

IVIG is indicated for myasthenic disease exacerbation, as an alternative to plasma exchange. Support for the efficacy of IVIG, administered at 0.4 g/kg intravenously over 5 days monthly, has been demonstrated in open-label studies, with an overall improvement of 70% (387). One randomized trial of IVIG compared with plasma exchange demonstrated similar efficacy for both treatments but better tolerability of IVIG (388). Clinical improvement from IVIG therapy occurs within 1 week of treatment, and responses are sustained for 2 to 3 months, often allowing for the reduction of other immunosuppressive therapies (381). The expense, short supply, and need for ongoing treatment preclude its use in long-term management.

Thymectomy is indicated for removing a thymoma associated with MG, but it is also useful as a therapeutic modality with refractory disease, including for ocular MG. Thymectomy increases the frequency of remissions and results in decreased antibody titer (379). In two large retrospective series, the greatest benefit was observed in patients with moderate to severe MG unresponsive to other therapies (389,390). Performance of an extended cervicomediastinal procedure with complete removal of the thymus, rather than a conventional transsternal thymectomy, is associated with a more than two-fold rate of improvement after surgery (390). Female sex, African-American race, and the use of preoperative plasmapheresis are associated with less improvement after surgery (390). Preoperative treatment with methylprednisolone or IVIG reduces the risk for myasthenic crisis postoperatively (379). Responses to thymectomy in open-label studies range from 24% to 100% over the course of a decade; clinical response is apparent 6 months to 1 year after surgery and peaks at 3 years (379,390).

In terms of the general management of MG, certain drugs are contraindicated because of their potential to induce myasthenia, exacerbate existing MG, or result in postoperative respiratory depression (Table 22.11) (379,380). Most of these agents cause presynaptic or postsynaptic blockade of the neuromuscular junction. A few agents, however, including D-penicillamine, chloroquine, and possibly lithium, induce immune-mediated MG (380). Because aminoglycosides, tetracyclines, ampicillin, and clindamycin all exacerbate MG, they should not be used to treat infectious episodes in these patients. Penicillins and cephalosporins are safe antibiotics for MG patients (379).

About 8% to 27% of MG patients experience a myasthenic crisis during the course of their illness, resulting in mechanical ventilation (391). The most common causes of myasthenic crisis include postsurgical respiratory depression, muscle weakness from illness exacerbation, respiratory tract infections, and cholinergic agent overdosage (379,391). For patients with myasthenic crisis, intravenous methylprednisolone pulses, alone or in combination with pyridostigmine, are as effective as plasma exchange (391). In the 1990s, with the prompt use of mechanical ventilation, crisis has resulted in a mortality rate of 5% to 13%, primarily resulting from cardiac arrhythmias and aspiration pneumonia (391).

Management of transient neonatal MG requires management of the delivery at a tertiary care facility. The administration of antenatal plasmapheresis and prednisone therapy may benefit mothers with a history of recurrent pregnancies in which their newborns were severely affected (392). In 20% of infants, symptoms are mild, and administration of frequent, small, oral feedings with close observation for 1 week is adequate. For most infants, symptoms are moderate to severe. Treatment with neostigmine methylsulfate, 0.05 mg/kg, administered by intramuscular, subcutaneous, or nasogastric routes, is necessary. Pyridostigmine bromide, 0.2 to 2 mg/kg, is an alternative anticholinesterase with fewer muscarinic side effects (367,371). Gavage feedings and ventilatory assistance are also often required. The average duration of therapy is 4 weeks (367). Severe, refractory cases may be treated with exchange transfusion, which improves strength (393). Prognosis of transient neonatal MG is excellent, with normal neuromuscular function and development in almost all cases (394). In infants with arthrogryposis, the severity of joint contractures may improve, but they are permanent (371).

Therapeutic approaches to juvenile MG are similar to those to adult MG. Cholinesterase inhibitors are the mainstay of therapy for children with only ocular symptoms, and prednisone is used in the lowest doses and shortest durations possible for more generalized disease (371). Thymectomy is primarily performed in postpubertal children, rather than young children, because of the unknown effect of the thymus on the development of immunocompetence; clinical response to thymectomy is similar in children and adults (373). Azathioprine may be used in children with refractory disease. Like adults, plasmapheresis is used in the management of myasthenic crises or acute respiratory deterioration, or presurgically (371). Complete remission is seen in 25% of children, and about 20% have no response to therapy; 2% of children died in one large series (373).

## ACKNOWLEDGMENTS

The authors thank Elizabeth Adams, Frederick Miller, Patricia Rohan, and Maria Villalba for their critical review of the manuscript and helpful comments.

## REFERENCES

1. Lindberg C, Oldfors A, Hedström A: Inclusion body myositis: peripheral nerve involvement. Combined morphological and electrophysiological studies on peripheral nerves. *J Neurol Sci* 1990;99:327–338.
2. Riminton DS, Chambers ST, Parkin PJ, et al. Inclusion body myositis presenting solely as dysphagia. *Neurology* 1993;43:1241–1243.
3. Tanimoto K, Nakano K, Kano S, et al. Classification criteria for polymyositis and dermatomyositis. *J Rheumatol* 1995;22:668–674.
4. Harrington TM, Cohen MD, Bartleson JD, et al. Elevation of creatine kinase in amyotrophic lateral sclerosis: potential confusion with polymyositis. *Arthritis Rheum* 1983;26:201–205.
5. Bohlmeyer TJ, Wu AHB, Perryman MB. Evaluation of laboratory tests as a guide to diagnosis and therapy of myositis. *Rheum Dis Clin North Am* 1994;20:845–856.
6. Targoff IN. Laboratory manifestations of polymyositis/dermatomyositis. *Clin Dermatol* 1988;6:76–92.
7. Wolf PL. Abnormalities in serum enzymes in skeletal muscle diseases. *Am J Clin Pathol* 1991;95:293–296.
8. Rider LG, Miller FW. Laboratory evaluation of the inflammatory myopathies. *Clin Diagn Lab Immunol* 1995;2:1–9.
9. King SW, Statland BE, Savory J. The effect of a short burst of exercise on activity values of enzymes in sera of healthy young men. *Clin Chim Acta* 1976;72:211–218.
10. Kosano H, Kinoshita T, Nagata N, et al. Change in concentrations of myogenic components of serum during 93 h of strenuous physical exercise. *Clin Chem* 1986;32:346–348.
11. Gruemer H-D, Prior T. Carrier detection in Duchenne muscular dystrophy: a review of current issues and approaches. *Clin Chim Acta* 1987;162:1–18.
12. Hoffman EP, Clemens PR. HyperCKemic, proximal muscular dystrophies and the dystrophin membrane cytoskeleton, including dystrophinopathies, sarcoglycanopathies, and merosinopathies. *Curr Opin Rheumatol* 1996;8:528–538.
13. Black HR, Quallich H, Gareleck CB. Racial differences in serum creatine kinase levels. *Am J Med* 1986;81:479–487.
14. Larca LJ, Coppola JT, Honig S. Creatine kinase MB isoenzyme in dermatomyositis: a non-cardiac source. *Ann Intern Med* 1981;94:341–343.
15. Bodor GS, Survant L, Voss EM, et al. Cardiac troponin T composition in normal and regenerating human skeletal muscle. *Clin Chem* 1997; 43:476–484.
16. Fudman EJ, Schnitzer TJ. Dermatomyositis without creatine kinase elevation: a poor prognostic sign. *Am J Med* 1986;80:329–332.
17. Gran JT, Myklebust G, Johansen S. Adult idiopathic polymyositis without elevation of creatine kinase: case report and review of the literature. *Scand J Rheumatol* 1993;22:94–96.
18. Bohan A, Peter JB, Bowman RL, et al. A computer-assisted analysis of 153 patients with polymyositis and dermatomyositis. *Medicine* 1977;56:255–286.
19. Hochberg MC, Feldman D, Stevens MB. Adult onset polymyositis/dermatomyositis: an analysis of clinical and laboratory features and survival in 76 patients with a review of the literature. *Semin Arthritis Rheum* 1986;15:168–178.
20. Tymms KE, Webb J. Dermatopolymyositis and other connective tissue diseases: a review of 105 cases. *J Rheumatol* 1985;12:1140–1148.
21. Kagen LJ, Aram S. Creatine kinase activity inhibitor in sera from patients with muscle disease. *Arthritis Rheum* 1987;30:213–217.
22. Wei N, Pavlidis N, Tsokos G, et al. Clinical significance of low creatine phosphokinase values in patients with connective tissue diseases. *JAMA* 1981;246:1921–1923.
23. Oddis CV, Medsger TA Jr. Relationship between serum creatine kinase level and corticosteroid therapy in polymyositis-dermatomyositis. *J Rheumatol* 1988;15:807–811.
24. Kaufman LD, Seidman RJ, Gruber BL. L-Tryptophan-associated eosinophilic perimyositis, neuritis, and fasciitis: a clinicopathologic and laboratory study of 25 patients. *Medicine* 1990;69:187–199.
25. Helfgott SM, Karlson E, Beckman E. Misinterpretation of serum transaminase elevation in "occult" myositis. *Am J Med* 1993;95: 447–449.
26. Munsat TL, Baloh R, Pearson CM, et al. Serum enzyme alterations in neuromuscular disorders. *JAMA* 1973;226:1536–1543.
27. Bertorini TE. Electromyography in polymyositis and dermatomyositis (PM/DM). In: Dalakas MC, ed. *Polymyositis and Dermatomyositis*. Boston: Butterworths, 1988:217.
28. Haddad MG, West RL, Treadwell EL, et al. Diagnosis of inflammatory myopathy by percutaneous needle biopsy with demonstration of the focal nature of myositis. *Am J Clin Pathol* 1994;101:661–664.
29. Targoff IN. Immune manifestations of inflammatory muscle disease. *Rheum Dis Clin North Am* 1994;20:857–880.
30. Mimori T. Structures targeted by the immune system in myositis. *Curr Opin Rheumatol* 1996;8:521–527.
31. Love LA, Leff RL, Fraser DD, et al. A new approach to the classification of idiopathic inflammatory myopathy: myositis-specific autoantibodies define useful homogeneous patient groups. *Medicine* 1991;70: 360–374.
32. Arnett FC, Targoff IN, Mimori T, et al. Interrelationship of major histocompatibility complex class II alleles and autoantibodies in four ethnic groups with various forms of myositis. *Arthritis Rheum* 1996;39: 1507–1518.
33. Reimers CD, Finkenstaedt M. Muscle imaging in inflammatory myopathies. *Curr Opin Rheumatol* 1997;9:476–485.
34. Adams EM, Chow CK, Premkumar A, et al. The idiopathic inflammatory myopathies: spectrum of MR imaging findings. *Radiographics* 1995;15:563–574.
35. Park JH, Vital TL, Ryder NM, et al. Magnetic resonance imaging and P-31 magnetic resonance spectroscopy provide unique quantitative data useful in the longitudinal management of patients with dermatomyositis. *Arthritis Rheum* 1994;37:736–746.
36. Park JH, Olsen NJ, King L Jr, et al. Use of magnetic resonance imaging and P-31 magnetic resonance spectroscopy to detect and quantify muscle dysfunction in the amyopathic and myopathic variants of dermatomyositis. *Arthritis Rheum* 1995;38:68–77.
37. Arahata K, Ishihara T, Fukunaga H, et al. Inflammatory response in facioscapulohumeral muscular dystrophy (FSHD): immunocytochemical and genetic analyses. *Muscle Nerve* 1995;[Suppl 2]:S56–S66.
38. Zeviani M, Amati P, Savoia A. Mitochondrial myopathies. *Curr Opin Rheumatol* 1994;6:599–567.
39. Higgs JB, Blaivas M, Albers JW. McArdle's disease presenting as treatment resistant polymyositis. *J Rheumatol* 1989;16:1588–1591.
40. Cuturic M, Hayat GR, Vogler CA, et al. Toxoplasmic polymyositis revisited: case report and review of literature. *Neuromuscul Disord* 1997;7:390–396.
41. Montoya JG, Jordan R, Lingamneni S, et al. Toxoplasmic myocarditis and polymyositis in patients with acute acquired toxoplasmosis diagnosed during life. *Clin Infect Dis* 1997;24:676–683.
42. Magid SK, Kagen LJ. Serologic evidence for acute toxoplasmosis in polymyositis-dermatomyositis: increased frequency of specific antitoxoplasma IgM antibodies. *Am J Med* 1983;75:313–320.
43. Illa I, Nath A, Dalakas M. Immunocytochemical and virological characteristics of HIV-associated inflammatory myopathies: similarities with seronegative polymyositis. *Ann Neurol* 1991;29:474–481.

44. Dalakas MC, Illa I, Pezeshkpour GH, et al. Mitochondrial myopathy caused by long-term zidovudine therapy. *N Engl J Med* 1990;322:1098–1105.

45. Leon-Monzon M, Illa I, Dalakas MC. Polymyositis in patients infected with human T-cell leukemia virus type I: the role of the virus in the cause of the disease. *Ann Neurol* 1994;36:643–649.

46. Dalakas MC. Retroviruses and inflammatory myopathies in humans and primates. *Bailliere's Clin Neurol* 1993;2:659–691.

47. Higuchi I, Montemayor ES, Izumo S, et al. Immunohistochemical characteristics of polymyositis in patients with HTLV-I-associated myelopathy and HTLV-I carriers. *Muscle Nerve* 1993;16:472–476.

48. Jenkins EA, Hull RG, Thomas AL. D-Penicillamine and polymyositis: the significance of the anti-Jo-1 antibody. *Br J Rheumatol* 1993;32:1109–1110.

49. Pierce LR, Wysowski DK, Gross TP. Myopathy and rhabdomyolysis associated with lovastatin-gemfibrozil combination therapy. *JAMA* 1990;264:71–75.

50. Kuncl RW, Duncan G, Watson D, et al. Colchicine myopathy and neuropathy. *N Engl J Med* 1987;316:1562–1568.

51. Estes ML, Ewing-Wilson D, Chou SM, et al. Chloroquine neuromyotoxicity: clinical and pathologic perspective. *Am J Med* 1987;82:447–455.

52. Charness ME, Simon RP, Greenberg DA. Ethanol and the nervous system. *N Engl J Med* 1989;321:442–454.

53. Bohan A, Peter JB. Polymyositis and dermatomyositis: parts 1 and 2. *N Engl J Med* 1975;292:344–347, 3403–3407.

54. Dalakas MC. Polymyositis, dermatomyositis and inclusion-body myositis [see comments]. *N Engl J Med* 1991;325:1487–1498.

55. Sigurgeirsson B, Lindelof B, Edhag O, et al. Risk of cancer in patients with dermatomyositis or polymyositis: a population-based study. *N Engl J Med* 1992;326:363–367.

56. Zantos D, Zhang Y, Felson D. The overall and temporal association of cancer with polymyositis and dermatomyositis. *J Rheumatol* 1994;21:1855–1859.

57. Targoff IN, Trieu EP, Miller FW. Reaction of anti-OJ autoantibodies with components of the multi-enzyme complex of aminoacyl-tRNA synthetases in addition to isoleucyl-tRNA synthetase. *J Clin Invest* 1993;91:2556–2564.

58. Marguerie C, Bunn CC, Beynon HLC, et al. Polymyositis, pulmonary fibrosis and autoantibodies to aminoacyl-tRNA synthetase enzymes. *Q J Med* 1990;77:1019–1038.

59. Clawson K, Oddis CV. Adult respiratory distress syndrome in polymyositis patients with the anti-Jo-1 antibody. *Arthritis Rheum* 1995;38:1519–1523.

60. Clements PJ, Lachenbruch PA, Seibold JR, et al. Skin thickness score in systemic sclerosis: an assessment of interobserver variability in 3 independent studies. *J Rheumatol* 1993;20:1892–1896.

61. Oddis CV, Medsger TA Jr, Cooperstein LA. A subluxing arthropathy associated with the anti-Jo-1 antibody in polymyositis/dermatomyositis. *Arthritis Rheum* 1990;33:1640–1645.

62. Friedman AW, Targoff IN, Arnett FC. Interstitial lung disease with autoantibodies against aminoacyl-tRNA synthetases in the absence of clinically apparent myositis. *Semin Arthritis Rheum* 1996;26:459–467.

63. Targoff IN, Miller FW, Medsger TA Jr, et al. Classification criteria for the idiopathic inflammatory myopathies. *Curr Opin Rheumatol* 1997;9:527–535.

64. Griggs RC, Askanas V, DiMauro S, et al. Inclusion body myositis and myopathies. *Ann Neurol* 1995;38:705–713.

65. Oddis CV, Conte CG, Steen VD, et al. Incidence of polymyositis-dermatomyositis: a 20-year study of hospital diagnosed cases in Allegheny County, PA 1963–1982. *J Rheumatol* 1990;17:1329–1334.

66. Ahlstrom G, Gunnarsson LG, Leissner P, et al. Epidemiology of neuromuscular diseases, including the postpolio sequelae, in a Swedish county. *Neuroepidemiology* 1993;12:262–269.

67. Weitoft T. Occurrence of polymyositis in the county of Gavleborg, Sweden. *Scand J Rheumatol* 1997;26:104–106.

68. Cronin ME, Plotz PH. Idiopathic inflammatory myopathies. *Rheum Dis Clin North Am* 1990;16:655–665.

69. Leff RL, Burgess SH, Miller FW, et al. Distinct seasonal patterns in the onset of adult idiopathic inflammatory myopathy in patients with anti-Jo-1 and anti-signal recognition particle autoantibodies. *Arthritis Rheum* 1991;34:1391–1396.

70. Carroll GJ, Will RK, Peter JB, et al. Penicillamine induced polymyositis and dermatomyositis. *J Rheumatol* 1987;14:995–1001.

71. Espinoza LR, Aguilar JL, Espinoza CG, et al. Characteristics and pathogenesis of myositis in human immunodeficiency virus infection: distinction from azidothymidine-induced myopathy. *Rheum Dis Clin North Am* 1991;17:117–129.

72. Ytterberg SR. Infectious agents associated with myopathies. *Curr Opin Rheumatol* 1996;8:507–513.

73. Christensen ML, Pachman LM, Schneiderman R, et al. Prevalence of coxsackie B virus antibodies in patients with juvenile dermatomyositis. *Arthritis Rheum* 1986;29:1365–1370.

74. Leff RL, Love LA, Miller FW, et al. Viruses in idiopathic inflammatory myopathies: absence of candidate viral genomes in muscle. *Lancet* 1992;339:1192–1195.

75. Pachman LM, Litt DL, Rowley AH, et al. Lack of detection of enteroviral RNA or bacterial DNA in magnetic resonance imaging-directed muscle biopsies from twenty children with active untreated juvenile dermatomyositis. *Arthritis Rheum* 1995;38:1513–1518.

76. Leon-Monzon M, Dalakas MC. Absence of persistent infection with enteroviruses in muscles of patients with inflammatory myopathies. *Ann Neurol* 1992;32:219–222.

77. Love LA, Weiner SR, Vasey FB, et al. Clinical and immunogenetic features of women who develop myositis after silicone implants (MASI). *Arthritis Rheum* 1992;35:S46(abst).

78. Cukier J, Beauchamp RA, Spindler JS, et al. Association between bovine collagen dermal implants and a dermatomyositis or a polymyositis-like syndrome. *Ann Intern Med* 1993;118:920–928.

79. Askanas V, Engel WK. New advances in the understanding of sporadic inclusion-body myositis and hereditary inclusion-body myopathies. *Curr Opin Rheumatol* 1995;7:486–496.

80. Garlepp MJ, Laing B, Zilko PJ, et al. HLA associations with inclusion body myositis. *Clin Exp Immunol* 1994;98:40–45.

81. Genth E, Mierau R, Genetzky P, et al. Immunogenetic associations of scleroderma-related antinuclear antibodies. *Arthritis Rheum* 1990;33:657–665.

82. Oddis CV, Okano Y, Rudert WA, et al. Serum autoantibody to the nucleolar antigen PM-Scl: clinical and immunogenetic associations. *Arthritis Rheum* 1992;35:1211–1217.

83. Mierau R, Dick T, Bartz-Bazzanella P, et al. Strong association of dermatomyositis-specific Mi-2 autoantibodies with a tryptophan at position 9 of the HLA-DR beta chain. *Arthritis Rheum* 1996;39:868–876.

84. Rider LG, Gurley RC, Pandey JP, et al. Clinical, serologic, and immunogenetic features of familial idiopathic inflammatory myopathy. *Arthritis Rheum* 1998;41:710–719.

85. Ginn LR, Lin JP, Plotz PH, et al. Familial autoimmunity in pedigrees of idiopathic inflammatory myopathy patients suggests common genetic risk factors for many autoimmune diseases. *Arthritis Rheum* 1998;41:400–405.

86. Arahata K, Engel AG: Monoclonal antibody analysis of mononuclear cells in myopathies. I. Quantitation of subsets according to diagnosis and sites of accumulation and demonstration and counts of muscle fibers invaded by T cells. *Ann Neurol* 1984;16:193–208.

87. Dalakas MC. Immunopathogenesis of inflammatory myopathies. *Ann Neurol* 1995;37[Suppl 1]:S74–S86.

88. Hohlfeld R, Engel AG, Goebels N, et al. Cellular immune mechanisms in inflammatory myopathies. *Curr Opin Rheumatol* 1997;9:520–526.

89. O'Hanlon TP, Dalakas MC, Plotz PH, et al. Predominant TCR-alpha beta variable and joining gene expression by muscle-infiltrating lymphocytes in the idiopathic inflammatory myopathies. *J Immunol* 1994;152:2569–2576.

90. Lindberg C, Oldfors A, Tarkowski A. Restricted use of T cell receptor V genes in endomysial infiltrates of patients with inflammatory myopathies. *Eur J Immunol* 1994;24:2659–2663.

91. Bender A, Ernst N, Iglesias A, et al. T cell receptor repertoire in polymyositis: clonal expansion of autoaggressive CD8+ T cells. *J Exp Med* 1995;181:1863–1868.

92. Pluschke G, Rüegg D, Hohlfeld R, et al. Autoaggressive myocytotoxic T lymphocytes expressing an unusual gamma/delta T cell receptor. *J Exp Med* 1992;176:1785–1789.

93. Emslie-Smith AM, Arahata K, Engel AG. Major histocompatibility complex class I antigen expression, immunolocalization of interferon subtypes, and T cell-mediated cytotoxicity in myopathies. *Hum Pathol* 1989;20:224–231.

94. Kalovidouris AE. Mechanisms of inflammation and histopathology in inflammatory myopathy. *Rheum Dis Clin North Am* 1994;20:881–898.

95. Goebels N, Michaelis D, Engelhardt M, et al. Differential expression of perforin in muscle-infiltrating T cells in polymyositis and dermatomyositis. *J Clin Invest* 1996;97:2905–2910.

96. Miller FW, Love LA, Barbieri SA, et al. Lymphocyte activation markers in idiopathic myositis: changes with disease activity and differences among clinical and autoantibody subgroups. *Clin Exp Immunol* 1990;81:373–379.

97. Kalovidouris AE, Pourmand R, Passo MH, et al. Proliferative response of peripheral blood mononuclear cells to autologous and allogeneic muscle in patients with polymyositis/dermatomyositis. *Arthritis Rheum* 1989;32:446–453.

98. Plotz PH, Dalakas M, Leff RL, et al. Current concepts in the idiopathic inflammatory myopathies: polymyositis, dermatomyositis, and related disorders. *Ann Intern Med* 1989;111:143–157.

99. Tews DS, Goebel HH. Cytokine expression profile in idiopathic inflammatory myopathies. *J Neuropathol Exp Neurol* 1996;55:342–347.

100. Lundberg I, Brengman JM, Engel AG. Analysis of cytokine expression in muscle in inflammatory myopathies, Duchenne dystrophy, and non-weak controls. *J Neuroimmunol* 1995;63:9–16.

101. Gabay C, Gay-Croisier F, Roux-Lombard P, et al. Elevated serum levels of interleukin-1 receptor antagonist in polymyositis/dermatomyositis: a biologic marker of disease activity with a possible role in the lack of acute-phase protein response. *Arthritis Rheum* 1994;37:1744–1751.

102. Adams EM, Kirkley J, Eidelman G, et al. The predominance of beta (CC) chemokine transcripts in idiopathic inflammatory muscle diseases. *Proc Assoc Am Physicians* 1997;109:275–285.

103. Denbow CE, Lie JT, Tancredi RG, et al. Cardiac involvement in polymyositis: a clinicopathologic study of 20 autopsied patients. *Arthritis Rheum* 1979;22:1088–1092.

104. Hsue YT, Paulus HE, Coulson WF. Bronchiolitis obliterans organizing pneumonia in polymyositis: a case report with longterm survival. *J Rheumatol* 1993;20:877–879.

105. Tazelaar HD, Viggiano RW, Pickersgill J, et al. Interstitial lung disease in polymyositis and dermatomyositis. *Am Rev Respir Dis* 1990; 141:727–733.

106. Kagen LJ, Hochman RB, Strong EW. Cricopharyngeal obstruction in inflammatory myopathy (polymyositis/dermatomyositis): report of three cases and review of the literature. *Arthritis Rheum* 1985;28:630–636.

107. de Merieux P, Verity MA, Clements PJ, et al. Esophageal abnormalities and dysphagia in polymyositis and dermatomyositis. *Arthritis Rheum* 1983;26:961–968.

108. Targoff IN, Johnson AE, Miller FW. Antibody to signal recognition particle in polymyositis. *Arthritis Rheum* 1990;33:1361–1370.

109. Engel AG, Arahata K. Mononuclear cells in myopathies: quantitation of functionally distinct subsets, recognition of antigen-specific cell-mediated cytotoxicity in some diseases, and implications for the pathogenesis of the different inflammatory myopathies. *Hum Pathol* 1986; 17:704–721.

110. Oddis CV, Medsger TA Jr. Current management of polymyositis and dermatomyositis. *Drugs* 1989;37:382–390.

111. Bunch TW. Prednisone and azathioprine for polymyositis: long-term followup. *Arthritis Rheum* 1981;24:45–48.

112. Metzger AL, Bohan A, Goldberg LS, et al. Polymyositis and dermatomyositis: combined methotrexate and corticosteroid therapy. *Ann Intern Med* 1974;81:182–189.

113. Joffe MM, Love LA, Leff RL, et al. Drug therapy of the idiopathic inflammatory myopathies: predictors of response to prednisone, azathioprine, and methotrexate and a comparison of their efficacy. *Am J Med* 1993;94:379–387.

114. Villalba L, Hicks JE, Adams EM, et al. Treatment of refractory myositis: a randomized crossover study of two new cytotoxic regimens. *Arthritis Rheum* 1998;41:392–399.

115. Oddis CV, Sciurba FC, Elmagd KA, Starzl TE. Tacrolimus in refractory polymyositis with lung disease. *Lancet* 1999;353:1762–1763.

116. Cherin P, Herson S, Wechsler B, et al. Efficacy of intravenous gamma-globulin therapy in chronic refractory polymyositis and dermatomyositis: an open study with 20 adult patients. *Am J Med* 1991;91:162–168.

117. al-Janadi M, Smith CD, Karsh J. Cyclophosphamide treatment of interstitial pulmonary fibrosis in polymyositis/dermatomyositis [see Comments]. *J Rheumatol* 1989;16:1592–1596.

118. Kadoya A, Okada J, Iikuni Y, et al. Risk factors for Pneumocystis carinii pneumonia in patients with polymyositis/dermatomyositis or systemic lupus erythematosus. *J Rheumatol* 1996;23:1186–1188.

119. Bachelez H, Schremmer B, Cadranel J, et al. Fulminant Pneumocystis carinii pneumonia in 4 patients with dermatomyositis. *Arch Intern Med* 1997;157:1501–1503.

120. Cherin P, Auperin I, Bussel A, et al. Plasma exchange in polymyositis and dermatomyositis: a multicenter study of 57 cases. *Clin Exp Rheumatol* 1995;13:270–271.

121. Miller FW, Leitman SF, Cronin ME, et al. Controlled trial of plasma exchange and leukapheresis in polymyositis and dermatomyositis. *N Engl J Med* 1992;326:1380–1384.

122. Herson S, Cherin P, Coutellier A. The association of plasma exchange synchronized with intravenous gamma globulin therapy in severe intractable polymyositis. *J Rheumatol* 1992;19:828–829.

123. Dalakas MC, Engel WK. Total body irradiation in the treatment of intractable polymyositis and dermatomyositis. In: Dalakas MC, ed. *Polymyositis and dermatomyositis*. Boston: Butterworths, 1988:281.

124. Cherin P, Herson S, Coutellier A, et al. Failure of total body irradiation in polymyositis: report of three cases. *Br J Rheumatol* 1992;31:282–283.

125. Hicks JE. The role of rehabilitation in the management of myopathies. *Curr Opin Rheumatol* 1998;10:548–555.

126. Hicks JE. Comprehensive rehabilitative management of patients with polymyositis and dermatomyositis. In: Dalakas MC, ed. *Polymyositis and dermatomyositis*. Boston: Butterworths, 1988:293.

127. Hicks JE, Miller F, Plotz P, et al. Isometric exercise increases strength and does not produce sustained creatinine phosphokinase increases in a patient with polymyositis. *J Rheumatol* 1993;20:1399–1401.

128. Crowson AN, Magro CM. The role of microvascular injury in the pathogenesis of cutaneous lesions of dermatomyositis. *Hum Pathol* 1996;27:15–19.

129. Magro CM, Crowson AN. The immunofluorescent profile of dermatomyositis: a comparative study with lupus erythematosus. *J Cutan Pathol* 1997;24:543–552.

130. Dalakas MC, Illa I, Dambrosia JM, et al. A controlled trial of high-dose intravenous immune globulin infusions as treatment for dermatomyositis. *N Engl J Med* 1993;329:1993–2000.

131. Basta M, Dalakas MC. High-dose intravenous immunoglobulin exerts its beneficial effect in patients with dermatomyositis by blocking endomysial deposition of activated complement fragments. *J Clin Invest* 1994;94:1729–1735.

132. Woo TY, Callen JP, Voorhees JJ, et al. Cutaneous lesions of dermatomyositis are improved by hydroxychloroquine. *J Am Acad Dermatol* 1984;10:592–600.

133. Zieglschmid-Adams ME, Pandya AG, Cohen SB, et al. Treatment of dermatomyositis with methotrexate. *J Am Acad Dermatol* 1995;32: 754–757.

134. Peake MF, Perkins P, Elston DM, et al. Cutaneous ulcers of refractory adult dermatomyositis responsive to intravenous immunoglobulin. *Cutis* 1998;62:89–93.

135. Symmons DP, Sills JA, Davis SM. The incidence of juvenile dermatomyositis: results from a nation-wide study. *Br J Rheumatol* 1995; 34:732–736.

136. Fujikawa S, Okuni M. A nationwide surveillance study of rheumatic diseases among Japanese children. *Acta Paediatr Jap* 1997;39:242–244.

137. Symmons DPM, Jones M, Osborne J, et al., for the British Pediatric Rheumatology Group National Diagnostic Index. Pediatric rheumatology in the United Kingdom: data from the British Pediatric Rheumatology Group National Diagnostic Register. *J Rheumatol* 1996;23: 1975–1980.

138. Kaipiainen-Seppanen O, Savolainen A. Incidence of chronic juvenile rheumatic diseases in Finland during 1980–1990. *Clin Exp Rheumatol* 1996;14:441–444.

139. Pachman LM, Hayford JR, Hochberg MC, et al. New-onset juvenile dermatomyositis: comparisons with a healthy cohort and children with juvenile rheumatoid arthritis. *Arthritis Rheum* 1997;40:1526–1533.

140. Rider LG, Okada S, Sherry DD, et al. Epidemiologic features and environmental exposures associated with illness onset in juvenile idiopathic inflammatory myopathy. *Arthritis Rheum* 1995;38[Suppl]:S362(abst).

141. Hiketa T, Matsumoto Y, Ohashi M, et al. Juvenile dermatomyositis: a statistical study of 114 patients with dermatomyositis. *J Dermatol* 1992;19:470–476.

142. Rider LG, Wallace CA, Sherry DD, et al. Autoimmune diseases in family members of children with idiopathic inflammatory myopathies. *Arthritis Rheum* 1994;37[Suppl]:S403.

143. Reed AM, Pachman L, Ober C. Molecular genetic studies of major histocompatibility complex genes in children with juvenile dermatomyositis: increased risk associated with HLA-DQA1*0501. *Hum Immunol* 1991;32:235–240.

144. West JE, Reed AM. Analysis of HLA-DM polymorphisms in juvenile dermatomyositis patients. *Hum Immunol* 1999;60:255–258.

145. Reed AM, Diegelj M, Kredich D, et al. Geographic clustering of juvenile dermatomyositis subjects. *Arthritis Rheum* 1998;41[Suppl]:S265.

146. Rider LG, Miller FW. Classification and treatment of the juvenile idiopathic inflammatory myopathies. *Rheum Dis Clin North Am* 1997;23: 619–655.

147. Albani S, Costouros N, Massa M, et al. Identification of cross-reactive epitopes on human skeletal myosin and streptococcal M5 protein in patients with juvenile dermatomyositis. *Arthritis Rheum* 1997; 49[Suppl]:S140.

148. Espada G, Confalone-Gregorian M, Ortiz Z, et al. Serum autoantibodies in juvenile idiopathic inflammatory myopathies in a cohort of Argentine patients. *Arthritis Rheum* 1997;40[Suppl]:S140.

149. Oddis CV, Fertig N, Goel A, et al. Clinical and serological characterization of the anti-MJ antibody in childhood myositis. *Arthritis Rheum* 1997;40[Suppl]:S139.

150. Rider LG, Targoff IN, Leff RL, et al. Association of autoantibodies to the U5-Ribonucleoprotein (U5-RNP) with idiopathic inflammatory myopathy. *Arthritis Rheum* 1994;37:S242(abst).

151. Pachman LM, Hayford JR, Chung A, et al. Juvenile dermatomyositis at diagnosis: clinical characteristics of 79 children. *J Rheumatol* 1998; 25:1198–1204.

152. Kobayashi S, Higuchi K, Tamaki H, et al. Characteristics of juvenile dermatomyositis in Japan. *Acta Paediatr Jap* 1997;39:257–262.

153. Fruman LS, Ragsdale CB, Sullivan DB, et al. Retinopathy in juvenile dermatomyositis. *J Pediatr* 1976;88:267–269.

154. Banker BQ, Victor M. Dermatomyositis (systemic angiopathy) of childhood. *Medicine* 1966;45:261–289.

155. See Y, Martin K, Rooney M, et al. Severe juvenile dermatomyositis complicated by pancreatitis. *Br J Rheumatol* 1997;36:912–916.

156. Jalleh RP, Swift RI, Sundaresan M, et al. Necrotising testicular vasculitis associated with dermatomyositis. *Br J Urol* 1990;66:660.

157. Jimenez C, Rowe PC, Keene D. Cardiac and central nervous system vasculitis in a child with dermatomyositis. *J Child Neurol* 1994;9:297–300.

158. Stonecipher MR, Jorizzo JL, White WL, et al. Cutaneous changes of dermatomyositis in patients with normal muscle enzymes: dermatomyositis sine myositis? *J Am Acad Dermatol* 1993;28:951–956.

159. Rider LG, Okada S, Sherry DD, et al. Presentations and disease courses of juvenile idiopathic inflammatory myopathy. *Arthritis Rheum* 1995;38[Suppl]:S362(abst).

160. Bowyer SL, Blane CE, Sullivan DB, et al. Childhood dermatomyositis: factors predicting functional outcome and development of dystrophic calcification. *J Pediatr* 1983;103:882–888.

161. Crowe WE, Bove KE, Levinson JE, et al. Clinical and pathogenetic implications of histopathology in childhood polydermatomyositis. *Arthritis Rheum* 1982;25:126–139.

162. Spencer CH, Hanson V, Singsen BH, et al. Course of treated juvenile dermatomyositis. *J Pediatr* 1984;105:399–408.

163. Pachman LM, Mendez E, Kanuru R, et al. Nailfold capillary studies in 50 untreated children with juvenile dermatomyositis. *Arthritis Rheum* 1998;41[Suppl]:S265.

164. Spencer-Green G, Crowe WE, Levinson JE. Nailfold capillary abnormalities and clinical outcome in childhood dermatomyositis. *Arthritis Rheum* 1982;25:954–958.

165. Silver RM, Maricq HR. Childhood dermatomyositis: serial microvascular studies. *Pediatrics* 1989;83:278–283.

166. Huber AM, Lang B, LeBlanc CMA, et al. Multicentre study of outcome in juvenile dermatomyositis. *Arthritis Rheum* 1998;41[Suppl]:S264.

167. Moore EC, Cohen F, Douglas SD, et al. Staphylococcal infections in childhood dermatomyositis: association with the development of calcinosis, raised IgE concentrations and granulocyte chemotactic defect. *Ann Rheum Dis* 1992;51:378–383.

168. Pachman LM, Callen AM, Hayford J, et al. Juvenile dermatomyositis: decreased calcinosis with intermittent high-dose intravenous methylprednisolone therapy. *Arthritis Rheum* 1994;37[Suppl]:S429.

169. Kavanagh GM, Colaco B, Kennedy CTC. Juvenile dermatomyositis associated with partial lipoatrophy. *J Am Acad Dermatol* 1993;28: 348–351.

170. Huemer C, Kitson H, Malleson PN, et al. Lipodystrophy in juvenile dermatomyositis patients: evaluation of clinical and metabolic abnormalities. *Arthritis Rheum* 1997;40[Suppl]:S140.

171. Adams BS, Cemeeroglu AP, Haftel HM, et al. Prevalence of insulin resistance in juvenile dermatomyositis. *Arthritis Rheum* 1996;39[Suppl]:S192.

172. Taieb A, Guichard C, Salamon R, et al. Prognosis in juvenile dermatopolymyositis: a cooperative retrospective study of 70 cases. *Pediatr Dermatol* 1985;2:275–281.

173. Schullinger JN, Jacobs JC, Berdon WE. Diagnosis and management of gastrointestinal perforations in childhood dermatomyositis with particular reference to perforations of the duodenum. *J Pediatr Surg* 1985;20:521–524.

174. Oliveros MA, Herbst JJ, Lester PD, et al. Pneumatosis intestinalis in childhood dermatomyositis. *Pediatrics* 1973;52:711–712.

175. Reed A, Haugen M, Pachman LM, et al. Abnormalities in serum osteocalcin values in children with chronic rheumatic diseases. *J Pediatr* 1990;116:574–580.

176. Perez MD, Abrams SA, Koenning G, et al. Mineral metabolism in children with dermatomyositis. *J Rheumatol* 1994;21:2364–2369.

177. Murphy E, Freaney R, Bresnihan B, et al. Evidence for increased bone turnover in patients with dystrophic calcification. *Arthritis Rheum* 1996;39[Suppl]:S97(abst).

178. Rider LG, Targoff IN, Taylor-Albert ES, et al. Anti-Jo-1 autoantibodies define a clinically homogeneous subset of childhood idiopathic inflammatory myopathy. *Arthritis Rheum* 1995;38:S362(abst).

179. Rider LG, Miller FW, Targoff IN, et al. A broadened spectrum of juvenile myositis: myositis-specific autoantibodies in children. *Arthritis Rheum* 1994;37:1534–1538.

180. Feldman BM, Reichlin M, Laxer RM, et al. Clinical significance of specific autoantibodies in juvenile dermatomyositis. *J Rheumatol* 1996;23:1794–1797.

181. Kissel JT, Mendell JR, Rammohan KW. Microvasculature deposition of complement membrane attack complex in dermatomyositis. *N Engl J Med* 1986;314:329–334.

182. Calore EE, Cavaliere MJ, Perez NM. Muscle pathology in juvenile dermatomyositis. *Sao Paulo Med J* 1997;115:1555–1559.

183. Lovell DJ, Lindsley CB, Rennebohm RH. Development of validated disease activity and damage indices for the juvenile idiopathic inflammatory myopathies. II. The Childhood Myositis Assessment Scale (CMAS): a quantitative tool for the evaluation of muscle function. The Juvenile Dermatomyositis Disease Activity Collaborative Study Group. *Arthritis Rheum* 1999;42:2213–2219.

184. Rider LG. Assessment of disease activity and its sequelae in children and adults with myositis. *Curr Opin Rheumatol* 1996;8:495–506.

185. Rider L, Prasad K, Feldman B, et al., for the JDM Disease Activity Collaborative Study Group. Relationships among laboratory tests and global disease activity assessments in juvenile dermatomyositis. *Arthritis Rheum* 1996;39[Suppl]:S191(abst).

186. Guzman J, Petty RE, Malleson PN. Monitoring disease activity in juvenile dermatomyositis: the role of von Willebrand factor and muscle enzymes. *J Rheumatol* 1994;21:739–743.

187. Pachman LM, Dilling D, Litt D, et al. Sequential studies of neopterin, von Willebrand factor antigen, creatine kinase and aldolase in juvenile dermatomyositis: correlates of disease activity? *Arthritis Rheum* 1993;36:S257(abst).

188. De Benedetti F, De Amici M, Aramini L, et al. Correlation of serum neopterin concentrations with disease activity in juvenile dermatomyositis. *Arch Dis Child* 1993;69:232–235.

189. Pachman LM, Maduzia L, Liotta M, et al. Serum neopterin correlates with increased macrophages (CD14⁺) in MRI directed muscle biopsies in active juvenile dermatomyositis. *Arthritis Rheum* 1996;39[Suppl]: S191(abst).

190. Eisenstein DM, O'Gorman MRG, Pachman LM. Correlations between change in disease activity and changes in peripheral blood lymphocyte subsets in patients with juvenile dermatomyositis. *J Rheumatol* 1997;24:1830–1832.

191. Hernandez RJ, Sullivan DB, Chenevert TL, et al. MR imaging in children with dermatomyositis: musculoskeletal findings and correlation with clinical and laboratory findings. *AJR Am J Roentgenol* 1993;161: 359–366.

192. Summers RM, Brune AM, Choyke PL, et al. Juvenile idiopathic inflammatory myopathy: exercise-induced changes in muscle at short inversion time inversion-recovery MR imaging. *Radiology* 1998;209:191–196.

193. Pachman LM, Crawford S, Morrello F, et al. MRI directed muscle biopsy for assessment of juvenile dermatomyositis response to therapy: comparison of initial and follow-up biopsies using a histological rating scale evaluating disease severity/chronicity. *Arthritis Rheum* 1996;39[Suppl]:S191(abst).

194. Van Rossum MA, Hiemstra I, Prieur AM, et al. Juvenile dermato/polymyositis: a retrospective analysis of 33 cases with special focus on initial CPK levels. *Clin Exp Rheumatol* 1994;12:339–342.

195. Adams EM, Plotz PH. The treatment of myositis: how to approach resistant disease. *Rheum Dis Clin North Am* 1995;21:179–202.

196. Le Quintrec JS, Le Quintrec JL. Drug-induced myopathies. *Bailliere's Clin Rheumatol* 1991;5:21–38.

197. Gould JW, Mercurio MG, Elmets CA. Cutaneous photosensitizing diseases induced by exogenous agents. *J Am Acad Dermatol* 1995;33: 551–573.

198. Sekul EA, Cupler EJ, Dalakas MC. Aseptic meningitis associated with high-dose intravenous immunoglobulin therapy: frequency and risk factors. *Ann Intern Med* 1994;121:259–262.

199. Dalakas MC. High-dose intravenous immunoglobulin and serum viscosity: risk of precipitating thromboembolic events. *Neurology* 1994; 44:223–226.

200. Hoyer PF. Complications of cyclosporin therapy. *Contrib Nephrol* 1995;114:111–123.

201. Heckmatt J, Hasson N, Saunders C, et al. Cyclosporin in juvenile dermatomyositis. *Lancet* 1989;1:1063–1066.

202. Pistoia V, Buoncompagni A, Scribanis R, et al. Cyclosporin A in the treatment of juvenile chronic arthritis and childhood polymyositis-dermatomyositis: results of a preliminary study. *Clin Exp Rheumatol* 1993;11:203–208.

203. Taborn J, Bole GG, Thompson GR. Colchicine suppression of local and systemic inflammation due to calcinosis universalis in chronic dermatomyositis. *Ann Intern Med* 1978;89:648–649.

204. Shearin JC, Pickrell K. Surgical treatment of subcutaneous calcifications of polymyositis or dermatomyositis. *Ann Plast Surg* 1980;5:381–385.

205. Hicks J, Drinkard B, Jain M, et al. Aerobic capacity in juvenile dermatomyositis and normal juvenile subjects. *Arthritis Rheum* 1997; 40:S140(abst).

206. Hanissian AS, Masi AT, Pitner SE, et al. Polymyositis and dermatomyositis in children: an epidemiologic and clinical comparative analysis. *J Rheumatol* 1982;9:390–394.

207. Rider L, Okada S, Reed A, et al., for the Childhood Myositis Heterogeneity Study Group. Immunogenetic risk factors for juvenile idiopathic inflammatory myopathy. *Arthritis Rheum* 1996;39[Suppl]:S309.

208. Serratrice G, Schiano A, Pellissier JF, et al. Les expressions anatomo-cliniques des polymyosites chez l'enfant: Vingt-trois cas. *Ann Pediatr (Paris)* 1989;36:237–243.

209. Roddy SM, Ashwal S, Peckham N, et al. Infantile myositis: a case diagnosed in the neonatal period. *Pediatr Neurol* 1986;2:241–244.

210. Tutuncuoglu S, Tekgul H, Demirtas E, et al. Infantile polymyositis with normal serum creatine kinase level. *Brain Dev* 1997;19:63–65.

211. Tomelleri G, Orrico D, DeGrandis D, et al. Polimiosite infatile: Descrizione di un caso. *Riv Neurobiol* 1979;25:170–177.

212. Nagai T, Hasegawa T, Saito N, et al. Infantile polymyositis: a case report. *Brain Dev* 1992;14:167–169.

213. Thompson CE. Infantile myositis. *Dev Med Child Neurol* 1982;24: 307–313.

214. Pegoraro E, Mancias P, Swerdlow SH, et al. Congenital muscular dystrophy with primary laminin alpha2 (merosin) deficiency presenting as inflammatory myopathy. *Ann Neurol* 1996;40:782–791.

215. Tiddens HA, van der Net JJ, de Graeff-Meeder ER, et al. Juvenile-onset mixed connective tissue disease: longitudinal follow-up. *J Pediatr* 1993;122:191–197.

216. Kotajima L, Aotsuka S, Sumiya M, et al. Clinical features of patients with juvenile onset mixed connective tissue disease: analysis of data collected in a nationwide collaborative study in Japan. *J Rheumatol* 1996;23:1088–1094.

217. Yokota S. Mixed connective tissue disease in childhood. *Acta Paediatr Jap* 1993;35:472–479.

218. Magilavy DB, Petty RE, Cassidy JT, et al. A syndrome of childhood polyarteritis. *J Pediatr* 1977;91:25–30.

219. Gama C, Breeden K, Miller R. Myositis in Kawasaki disease. *Pediatr Neurol* 1990;6:135–136.

220. Lang BA, Laxer RM, Thorner P, et al. Pediatric onset of Behçet's syndrome with myositis: case report and literature review illustrating unusual features. *Arthritis Rheum* 1990;33:418–425.

221. Shuhart DT, Torretti DJ, Maksimak JF, et al. Acute myositis as an unusual presentation of Wegener's granulomatosis. *Arch Pediatr Adolesc Med* 1994;148:875–876.

222. Miller ML, Levinson L, Pachman LM, et al. Abnormal muscle MRI in a patient with systemic juvenile arthritis. *Pediatr Radiol* 1995; 25[Suppl 1]:S107–S108.

223. Cooper C, Fairris G, Cotton DW, et al. Dermatomyositis associated with idiopathic thrombocytopenia. *Dermatologica* 1986;172:173–176.

224. Buderus S, Wagner N, Lentze MJ. Concurrence of celiac disease and juvenile dermatomyositis: result of a specific immunogenetic susceptibility? *J Pediatr Gastroenterol Nutr* 1997;25:101–103.

225. Reed AM, Kredich DW, Schanberg LE. Seldom recognized cutaneous manifestations of juvenile dermatomyositis. *Arthritis Rheum* 1996; 39[Suppl]:S190(abst).

226. Garton MJ, Isenberg DA. Clinical features of lupus myositis versus idiopathic myositis: a review of 30 cases. *Br J Rheumatol* 1997;36: 1067–1074.

227. Marguerie C, Bunn CC, Copier J, et al. The clinical and immunogenetic features of patients with autoantibodies to the nucleolar antigen PM-Scl. *Medicine* 1992;71:327–336.

228. Hausmanowa-Petrusewicz I, Kowalska-Oledzka E, Miller FW, et al. Clinical, serologic, and immunogenetic features in Polish patients with idiopathic inflammatory myopathies. *Arthritis Rheum* 1997;40: 1257–1266.

229. Goel A, Fertig N, Oddis CV, et al. Serum autoantibodies in idiopathic inflammatory myopathy of childhood. *Arthritis Rheum* 1996; 39[Suppl]:S191(abst).

230. Askanas V, Engel WK. Sporadic inclusion-body myositis and hereditary inclusion-body myopathies: current concepts of diagnosis and pathogenesis. *Curr Opin Rheumatol* 1998;10:530–542.

231. Askanas V: New developments in hereditary inclusion body myopathies. *Ann Neurol* 1997;41:421–422.

232. O'Hanlon TP, Dalakas MC, Plotz PH, et al. The alpha beta T-cell receptor repertoire in inclusion body myositis: diverse patterns of gene expression by muscle-infiltrating lymphocytes. *J Autoimmun* 1994;7:321–333.

233. Barohn RJ, Amato AA, Sahenk Z, et al. Inclusion body myositis: explanation for poor response to immunosuppressive therapy. *Neurology* 1995;45:1302–1304.

234. Mendell JR, Sahenk Z, Gales T, et al. Amyloid filaments in inclusion body myositis: novel findings provide insight into nature of filaments. *Arch Neurol* 1991;48:1229–1234.

235. Bilak M, Askanas V, Engel WK. Strong immunoreactivity of alpha1-antichymotrypsin co-localizes with beta-amyloid protein and ubiquitin in vacuolated muscle fibers of inclusion-body myositis. *Acta Neuropathol* 1993;85:378–382.

236. Sarkozi E, Askanas V, Engel WK. Abnormal accumulation of prion protein mRNA in muscle fibers of patients with sporadic inclusion-body myositis and hereditary inclusion-body myopathy. *Am J Pathol* 1994;145:1280–1284.

237. Askanas V, Engel WK, Yang CC, et al. Light and electron microscopic immunolocalization of presenilin 1 in abnormal muscle fibers of patients with sporadic inclusion-body myositis and autosomal-recessive inclusion-body myopathy. *Am J Pathol* 1998;152:889–895.

238. Askanas V, Engel WK, Bilak M, et al. Twisted tubulofilaments of inclusion body myositis muscle resemble paired helical filaments of Alzheimer brain and contain hyperphosphorylated tau. *Am J Pathol* 1994;144:177–187.

239. Askanas V, Engel WK. Sporadic inclusion-body myositis and hereditary inclusion-body myopathies: diseases of oxidative stress and aging? *Arch Neurol* 1998;55:915–920.

240. Santorelli FM, Sciacco M, Tanji K, et al. Multiple mitochondrial DNA deletions in sporadic inclusion body myositis: a study of 56 patients. *Ann Neurol* 1996;39:789–795.

241. Pruitt JN, Showalter CJ, Engel AG. Sporadic inclusion body myositis: counts of different types of abnormal fibers. *Ann Neurol* 1996;39: 139–143.

242. Serratrice G, Pellissier JF, Pouget J, Figarella-Branger D: Formes cliniques des myosites a inclusions: 12 cas. *Rev Neurol (Paris)* 1989;145: 781–788.

243. Chou SM. Inclusion body myositis: a chronic persistent mumps myositis? *Hum Pathol* 1986;17:765–777.

244. Pickering MC, Walport MJ. Eosinophilic myopathic syndromes. *Curr Opin Rheumatol* 1998;10:504-510.

245. Cole AJ, Kuzniecky R, Karpati G, et al. Familial myopathy with changes resembling inclusion body myositis and periventricular leucoencephalopathy: a new syndrome. *Brain* 1988;111:1025–1037.

246. Lotz BP, Engel AG, Nishino H, et al. Inclusion body myositis: observations in 40 patients. *Brain* 1989;112:727–747.

247. Shapiro J, DeGirolami U, Martin S, et al. Inflammatory myopathy causing pharyngeal dysphagia: a new entity. *Ann Otol Rhinol Laryngol* 1996;105:331–335.

248. Koffman BM, Rugiero M, Dalakas MC. Immune-mediated conditions and antibodies associated with sporadic inclusion body myositis. *Muscle Nerve* 1998;21:115–117.

249. Luciano CA, Dalakas MC. Inclusion body myositis: no evidence for a neurogenic component. *Neurology* 1997;48:29–33.

250. Askanas V, Serdaroglu P, Engel WK, et al. Immunocytochemical localization of ubiquitin in inclusion body myositis allows its light-microscopic distinction from polymyositis. *Neurology* 1992; 42:460–461.
251. de Visser M, Bakker E, Defesche JC, et al. An unusual variant of Becker muscular dystrophy. *Ann Neurol* 1990;27:578–581.
252. Amato AA, Gronseth GS, Jackson CE, et al. Inclusion body myositis: clinical and pathological boundaries. *Ann Neurol* 1996;40:581–586.
253. Barohn RJ. The therapeutic dilemma of inclusion body myositis. *Neurology* 1997;48:567–568.
254. Leff RL, Miller FW, Hicks JE, et al. The treatment of inclusion body myositis: a retrospective review and a randomized, prospective trial of immunosuppressive therapy. *Medicine* 1993;72:225–235.
255. Sayers ME, Chou SM, Calabrese LH. Inclusion body myositis: analysis of 32 cases. *J Rheumatol* 1992;19:1385–1389.
256. Dalakas MC, Sonies B, Dambrosia J, et al. Treatment of inclusion-body myositis with IVIg: a double-blind, placebo-controlled study. *Neurology* 1997;48:712–716.
257. Bernard P, Bonnetblanc JM. Dermatomyositis and malignancy. *J Invest Dermatol* 1993;100:128S–132S.
258. Anzai S, Katagiri K, Sato T, et al. Dermatomyositis associated with primary intramuscular B cell lymphoma. *J Dermatol* 1997;24:649–653.
259. Stary J, Havelka S, Hrodek O, et al. Syndrome of secondary polymyositis with leukemia. *Acta Univers Carol [Med]* 1991;37:16–20.
260. Bittar B, Rose CD. Early development of Hodgkin's lymphoma in association with the use of methotrexate for the treatment of dermatomyositis. *Ann Rheum Dis* 1995;54:607–608.
261. Page AR, Hansen AE, Good RA. Occurrence of leukemia and lymphoma in patients with agammaglobulinemia. *Blood* 1963;21:197–206.
262. Bonnetblanc JM, Bernard P, Fayol J. Dermatomyositis and malignancy: a multicenter cooperative study. *Dermatologica* 1990;180:212–216.
263. Hu WJ, Chen DL, Min HQ. Study of 45 cases of nasopharyngeal carcinoma with dermatomyositis. *Am J Clin Oncol* 1996;19:35–38.
264. Davis MD, Ahmed I. Ovarian malignancy in patients with dermatomyositis and polymyositis: a retrospective analysis of fourteen cases. *J Am Acad Dermatol* 1997;37:730–733.
265. Cox NH, Lawrence CM, Langtry JA, et al. Dermatomyositis: disease associations and an evaluation of screening investigations for malignancy. *Arch Dermatol* 1990;126:61–65.
266. Whitmore SE, Rosenshein NB, Provost TT. Ovarian cancer in patients with dermatomyositis. *Medicine* 1994;73:153–160.
267. Whitmore SE, Anhalt GJ, Provost TT, et al. Serum CA-125 screening for ovarian cancer in patients with dermatomyositis. *Gynecol Oncol* 1997;65:241–244.
268. Whitmore SE, Watson R, Rosenshein NB, et al. Dermatomyositis sine myositis: association with malignancy. *J Rheumatol* 1996;23:101–105.
269. Leaute-Labreze C, Perel Y, Taieb A. Childhood dermatomyositis associated with hepatocarcinoma. *N Engl J Med* 1995;333:1083.
270. Sunde H. Dermatomyositis in children. *Acta Paediatr* 1949;37:287–308.
271. Flaisler F, Blin D, Asencio G, et al. Focal myositis: a localized form of polymyositis? *J Rheumatol* 1993;20:1414–1416.
272. Heffner RR Jr, Armbrustmacher VW, Earle KM. Focal myositis. *Cancer* 1977;40:301–306.
273. Maynie M, Robert H, Eloit S, et al. Myosite focal chez l'enfant: A propos d'un cas. *Rev Chir Orthop* 1997;83:382–386.
274. Maguire JK, Milford LW, Pitcock JA. Focal myositis in the hand. *J Hand Surg* 1988;13A:140–142.
275. Isaacson G, Chan KH, Heffner RR Jr. Focal myositis: a new cause for the pediatric neck mass. *Arch Otolaryngol Head Neck Surg* 1991;117:103–105.
276. Toti P, Romano L, Villanova M, et al. Focal myositis: a polymerase chain reaction analysis for a viral etiology. *Hum Pathol* 1997; 28:111–113.
277. Garcia-Consuegra J, Morales C, Gonzalez J, et al. Relapsing focal myositis: a case report. *Clin Exp Rheumatol* 1995;13:395–397.
278. Josephson GD, de Blasi H, McCormick S, et al. Focal myositis of the sternocleidomastoid muscle: a case report and review of the literature. *Am J Otolaryngol* 1996;17:215–217.
279. Rivest C, Miller FW, Love LA, et al. Focal myositis presenting as pseudothrombophlebitis of the neck in a patient with mixed connective tissue disease. *Arthritis Rheum* 1996;39:1254–1258.
280. Chiang IP, Wang J, Tsang YM, et al. Focal myositis of esophagus: a distinct inflammatory pseudotumor mimicking esophageal malignancy. *Am J Gastroenterol* 1997;92:174–175.
281. Heffner RR, Barron SA. Polymyositis beginning as a focal process. *Arch Neurol* 1981;38:439–442.
282. Shapiro MJ, Applebaum H, Besser AS. Cervical focal myositis in a child. *J Pediatr Surg* 1986;21:375–376.
283. Ellis GL, Brannon RB. Focal myositis of the perioral musculature. *Oral Surg* 1979;48:337–341.
284. Azuma T, Komori A, Nagayama M. Focal myositis of the tongue. *J Oral Maxillofac Surg* 1987;45:953–955.
285. Naumann M, Toyka KV, Goebel HH, et al. Focal myositis of the temporal muscle. *Muscle Nerve* 1993;16:1374–1376.
286. Lim KL, Robson K, Powell RJ. Focal myositis: an unusual cause of bilateral upper eyelid swelling. *Postgrad Med J* 1993;69:876–878.
287. Borysiewica LK, Camilleri JP, Jessop JD, et al. Focal myositis mimicking acute psoas abscess: an unusual presentation of systemic lupus erythematosus. *Br Med J* 1997;314:805–808.
288. Konagaya Y, Konagaya M, Mano Y. Quadriceps myositis. *Intern Med* 1992;31:926–929.
289. Hamza M. Localized myositis in a case of Behçet's disease. *Rev Rhum Mal Osteoartic* 1987;54:438.
290. Naschitz JE, Yeshurun D, Dryefuss U, et al. Localized nodular myositis: a paraneoplastic phenomenon. *Clin Rheumatol* 1992;11:427–431.
291. Shibuya S, Wakayama Y, Murahashi M. Benign adult-onset focal myositis confined to the calf muscles. *Muscle Nerve* 1998;21:260.
292. Caldwell CJ, Swash M, Van der Walt JD, et al. Focal myositis: a clinicopathological study. *Neuromuscul Disord* 1995;5:317–321.
293. Enzinger FM, Dulcey F. Proliferative myositis: report of thirty-three cases. *Cancer* 1967;20:2213–2223.
294. Kern WH. Proliferative myositis; a pseudosarcomatous reaction to injury. *Arch Pathol* 1960;69:209–216.
295. Meis JM, Enzinger FM. Proliferative fasciitis and myositis of childhood. *Am J Surg Pathol* 1992;16:364–372.
296. Sarteschi M, Ciatti S, Sabo C, et al. Proliferative myositis: rare pseudotumorous lesion. *J Ultrasound Med* 1997;16:771–773.
297. Jacobs JC. Aspiration cytology of proliferative myositis: a case report. *Acta Cytol* 1995;39:535–538.
298. Pollock L, Fullilove S, Shaw DG, et al. Proliferative myositis in a child: a case report. *J Bone Joint Surg Am* 1995;77:132–135.
299. Meister P, Konrad EA, Buckmann FW. Nodular fasciitis and proliferative myositis as variants of one disease entity. *Invest Cell Pathol* 1979;2:277–281.
300. Squires RH, Zwiener RJ, Kennedy RH. Orbital myositis and Crohn's disease. *J Pediatr Gastroenterol Nutr* 1992;15:448–451.
301. Arnett FC, Michels RG. Inflammatory ocular myopathy in systemic sclerosis (scleroderma). *Arch Intern Med* 1973;132:740–743.
302. Serop S, Vianna RNG, Claeys M, et al. Orbital myositis secondary to systemic lupus erythematosus. *Acta Ophthalmol* 1994;72:520–523.
303. Leib ML, Odel JG, Cooney MJ. Orbital polymyositis and giant cell myocarditis. *Ophthalmology* 1994;101:950–954.
304. Scott IU, Siatkowski RM. Idiopathic orbital myositis. *Curr Opin Rheumatol* 1997;9:504–512.
305. Siatkowski RM, Capo H, Byrne SF, et al. Clinical and echographic findings in idiopathic orbital myositis. *Am J Ophthalmol* 1994;118:343–350.
306. Casteels I, De Bleecker C, Demaerel P, et al. Orbital myositis following an upper respiratory tract infection: contribution of high resolution CT and MRI. *JBR-BTR* 1991;74:45–47.
307. Volpe NJ, Shore JW. Orbital myositis associated with herpes zoster. *Arch Ophthalmol* 1991;109:471–472.
308. Seidenberg KB, Leib ML. Orbital myositis with Lyme disease. *Am J Ophthalmol* 1990;109:13–16.
309. Thurairajan G, Hope-Ross MW, Situnayake RD, et al. Polyarthropathy, orbital myositis and posterior scleritis: an unusual adverse reaction to influenza vaccine. *Br J Rheumatol* 1997;36:120–123.
310. Kennerdell JS, Dresner SC. The nonspecific orbital inflammatory syndromes. *Surv Ophthalmol* 1984;29:93–103.
311. Moorman CM, Elston JS. Acute orbital myositis. *Eye* 1995;9:96–101.
312. Mannor GE, Rose GE, Moseley IF, et al. Outcome of orbital myositis: clinical features associated with recurrence. *Ophthalmology* 1997;104:409–414.
313. Dresner SC, Rothfus WE, Slamovits TL, et al. Computed tomography of orbital myositis. *AJR Am J Roentgenol* 1984;143:671–674.
314. Slavin ML, Glaser JS. Idiopathic orbital myositis: report of six cases. *Arch Ophthalmol* 1982;100:1261–1265.

315. Hankey GJ, Silbert PL, Edis RH, et al. Orbital myositis: a study of six cases. *Aust N Z J Med* 1987;17:585–591.

316. Huber A. Ocular electromyography. *Bull Soc Belge Ophtalmol* 1989;237:425–441.

317. Hardman JA, Hlapin SFS, Mars S, et al. MRI of idiopathic orbital inflammatory syndrome using fat saturation and Gd-DTPA. *Neuroradiology* 1995;37:475–478.

318. Mombaerts I, Koornneef L. Current status in the treatment of orbital myositis. *Ophthalmology* 1997;104:402–408.

319. Shah SS, Lowder CY, Schmitt MA, et al. Low-dose methotrexate therapy for ocular inflammatory disease. *Ophthalmology* 1992;99:1419–1423.

320. Sancehz-Roman J, Varela-Aguilar JM, Bravo-Ferrer J, et al. Idiopathic orbital myositis treatment with cyclosporin. *Ann Rheum Dis* 1993;52:84–85.

321. Weinstein GS, Dresner SC, Slamovits TL, et al. Acute and subacute orbital myositis. *Am J Ophthalmol* 1983;96:209–217.

322. Bessant DA, Lee JP. Management of strabismus due to orbital myositis. *Eye* 1995;9:558–563.

323. Kaufman LD, Kephart GM, Seidman RJ, et al. The spectrum of eosinophilic myositis: clinical and immunopathogenic studies of three patients, and review of the literature. *Arthritis Rheum* 1993;36:1014–1024.

324. Layzer RB, Shearn MA, Satya-Murti S. Eosinophilic polymyositis. *Ann Neurol* 1977;1:65–71.

325. Bjelle A, Henriksson KG, Hofer PA. Polymyositis in eosinophilic fasciitis. *Eur Neurol* 1980;19:128–137.

326. Schumacher HR. A scleroderma-like syndrome with fasciitis, myositis, and eosinophilia. *Ann Intern Med* 1976;84:49–50.

327. Arase S, Kato S, Nakanishi H, et al. Eosinophilic polymyositis induced by tranilast. *J Dermatol* 1990;17:182–186.

328. Sladek GD, Vasey FB, Sieger B, et al. Relapsing eosinophilic myositis. *J Rheumatol* 1983;10:467–470.

329. Kumamoto T, Fujimoto S, Nagao S, et al. Clinicopathologic characteristics of polymyositis patients with numerous tissue eosinophils. *Acta Neurol Scand* 1996;94:110–114.

330. Serratrice G, Pellissier JF, Cros D, et al. Relapsing eosinophilic perimyositis. *J Rheumatol* 1980;7:199–205.

331. Trueb RM, Pericin M, Winzeler B, et al. Eosinophilic myositis/perimyositis: frequency and spectrum of cutaneous manifestations. *J Am Acad Dermatol* 1997;37:385–391.

332. Miller JJ. The fasciitis-morphea complex in children. *Am J Dis Child* 1992;146:733–736.

333. Serratrice G, Pellissier JF, Roux H, et al. Fasciitis, perimyositis, myositis, polymyositis, and eosinophilia. *Muscle Nerve* 1990;13:385–395.

334. Van den Enden E, Praet M, Joos R, et al. Eosinophilic myositis resulting from sarcocystosis. *J Trop Med Hyg* 1995;98:273–276.

335. Symmans WA, Beresford CH, Bruton D, et al. Cyclic eosinophilic myositis and hyperimmunoglobulin-E. *Ann Intern Med* 1986;104:26–32.

336. Weinstock A, Green C, Cohen BH, et al. Becker muscular dystrophy presenting as eosinophilic inflammatory myopathy in an infant. *J Child Neurol* 1997;12:146–147.

337. Ellman L, Miller L, Rappeport J. Leukopheresis therapy of a hyperiosinophilic disorder. *JAMA* 1974;230:1004–1005.

338. Murray-Leslie CF, Quinnell RC, Powell RJ, et al. Relapsing eosinophilic myositis causing acute muscle compartment syndrome. *Br J Rheumatol* 1998;32:426–427.

339. Lynch PG, Bansal DV. Granulomatous polymyositis. *J Neurol Sci* 1973;18:1–9.

340. Jerusalem F, Imbach P. Granulomatose myositis und muskelsarkoidose: Klinische und bioptisch-histologische Diagnose. *Deutsche Med Wochenschr* 1970;23:2184–2190.

341. Hewlett RH, Brownell B. Granulomatous myopathy: its relationship to sarcoidosis and polymyositis. *J Neurol Neurosurg Psychiatry* 1975;38:1090–1099.

342. Schimrigk K, Uldall B. The disease of Besnier-Boeck-Schaumann and granulomatous polymyositis. *Eur Neurol* 1968;1:137–157.

343. Takanashi T, Suzuki Y, Yoshino Y, et al. Granulomatous myositis: pathologic re-evaluation by immunohistochemical analysis of infiltrating mononuclear cells. *J Neurol Sci* 1997;145:41–47.

344. Simmonds NJ, Hoffbrand BI. Contracturing granulomatous myositis: a separate entity. *J Neurol Neurosurg Psychiatry* 1990;53:998–1000.

345. Jamal MM, Cilursu AM, Hoffman EL. Sarcoidosis presenting as acute myositis: report and review of the literature. *J Rheumatol* 1988;15:1868–1871.

346. Kobayashi H, Kotoura Y, Sakahara H, et al. Solitary muscular sarcoidosis: CT, MRI and scintigraphic characteristics. *Skeletal Radiol* 1994;23:293–295.

347. Halverson PB, Lahiri S, Wojno WC, et al. Sporotrichal arthritis presenting as granulomatous myositis. *Arthritis Rheum* 1985;28:1425–1429.

348. Kim JH, Wallerstein S, Thoe M. Myopathy in tuberculosis: two presumptive cases and a review of the literature. *Mil Med* 1997;3:221–224.

349. Richman DP, Agius MA. Myasthenia gravis: pathogenesis and treatment. *Semin Neurol* 1994;14:106–110.

350. Phillips LH. The epidemiology of myasthenia gravis. *Neurol Clin North Am* 1994;12:263–271.

351. Patrick J, Lindstrom J. Autoimmune response to the acetylcholine receptor. *Science* 1973;180:871–872.

352. Drachman DB. Myasthenia gravis. *N Engl J Med* 1994;330:1797–1810.

353. Sahashi K, Engel AG, Linstrom JM, et al. Ultrastructural localization of immune complexes (IgG and C3) at the end-plate in experimental autoimmune myasthenia gravis. *J Neuropathol Exp Neurol* 1978;37:212–223.

354. Engel AG, Lambert EH, Howard FM. Immune complexes (IgG and C3) at the motor end-plate in myasthenia gravis: ultrastructural and light microscopic localization and electrophysiologic correlations. *Mayo Clin Proc* 1977;52:267–280.

355. Sahashi K, Engel AG, Lambert EH, et al. Ultrastructural localization of the terminal and lytic ninth complement component (C9) at the motor end-plate in myasthenia gravis. *J Neuropathol Exp Neurol* 1980;39:160–172.

356. Toyka KV, Drachman DB, Griffin DE, et al. Myasthenia gravis: study of humoral immune mechanisms by passive transfer to mice. *N Engl J Med* 1977;296:125–131.

357. Lewis RA, Selwa JF, Lisak RP. Myasthenia gravis: immunological mechanisms and immunotherapy. *Ann Neurol* 1995;37[Suppl 1]:S51–S62.

358. Fambrough DM, Drachman DB, Satyamurti S. Neuromuscular junction in myasthenia gravis: decreased acetylcholine receptors. *Science* 1973;182:293–295.

359. Drachman DB, Angus CW, Adams RN, et al. Myasthenic antibodies cross-link acetylcholine receptors to accelerate degradation. *N Engl J Med* 1978;298:1116–1122.

360. Stanley EF, Drachman DB. Effect of myasthenic immunoglobulin on acetylcholine receptors of intact mammalian neuromuscular junctions. *Science* 1978;200:1285–1287.

361. Engel AG, Sahashi K, Fumagalli G. The immunopathology of acquired myasthenia gravis. *Ann N Y Acad Sci* 1981;377:158–174.

362. Maselli RA. Pathophysiology of myasthenia gravis and Lambert-Eaton syndrome. *Neurol Clin North Am* 1994;12:285–304.

363. Eymard B, Vernet-der Garabedian B, Berrih-Aknin S, et al. Anti-acetylcholine receptor antibodies in neonatal myasthenia gravis: heterogeneity and pathogenic significance. *J Autoimmun* 1991;4:185–195.

364. Hohlfeld R, Wekerle H. The thymus in myasthenia gravis. *Neurol Clin North Am* 1994;12:331–342.

365. Kao I, Drachman DB. Thymic muscle cells bear acetylcholine receptors: possible relation to myasthenia gravis. *Science* 1977;195:74–75.

366. Schwimmbeck PL, Dyrberg T, Drachman DB, et al. Molecular mimicry and myasthenia gravis: an autoantigenic site of the acetylcholine receptor alpha-subunit that has biologic activity and reacts immunochemically with herpes simplex virus. *J Clin Invest* 1989;84:1174–1180.

367. Papazian O. Transient neonatal myasthenia gravis. *J Child Neurol* 1992;7:135–141.

368. Morel E, Eymard B, Vernet-der Garagedian B, et al. Neonatal myasthenia gravis: a new clinical and immunologic appraisal on 30 cases. *Neurology* 1988;38:138–142.

369. Pilkington C, Lefvert AK, Rook GAW. Neonatal myasthenia gravis and the role of agalactosyl IgG. *Autoimmunity* 1995;21:131–135.

370. Papazian O, Cullen RF Jr, Duenas D. HLA typing in females with generalized autoimmune myasthenia gravis and their offspring. *Ann Neurol* 1991;30:501.

371. Nigro MA. Myasthenia gravis in infancy and childhood. In: Lisak RP, ed. *Handbook of myasthenia gravis and myasthenic syndromes*. New York: Marcel Dekker, 1994:63.

372. Szobor A, Mattyus A, Molnar J. Myasthenia gravis in childhood and adolescence: report on 209 patients and review of the literature. *Acta Paediatr Hung* 1989;29:299–312.

373. Wong V, Hawkins BR, Yu YL. Myasthenia gravis in Hong Kong Chinese. 2. Paediatric disease. *Acta Neurol Scand* 1992;86:68–72.

374. Hopkins LC. Clinical features of myasthenia gravis. *Neurol Clin North Am* 1994;12:243–261.
375. Massey JM. Acquired myasthenia gravis. *Neurol Clin* 1997;15:577–595.
376. Afifi AK, Bell WE. Tests for juvenile myasthenia gravis: comparative diagnostic yield and prediction of outcome. *J Child Neurol* 1993;8:403–411.
377. Reyes H. Striational autoantibodies. In: Peter JB, Shoenfeld Y, eds. *Autoantibodies.* Amsterdam: Elsevier Science, 1996:805.
378. Howard JF Jr, Sanders DB, Massey JM. The electrodiagnosis of myasthenia gravis and the Lambert-Eaton myasthenic syndrome. *Neurol Clin North Am* 1994;12:305–330.
379. Verma P, Oger J. Treatment of acquired autoimmune myasthenia gravis: a topic review. *Can J Neurol Sci* 1992;19:360–375.
380. Argov Z, Wirguin I. Drugs and the neuromuscular junction: pharmacotherapy of transmission disorders and drug-induced myasthenic syndromes. In: Lisak RP, ed. *Handbook of myasthenia gravis and myasthenic syndromes.* New York: Marcel Dekker, 1994:295.
381. Chaudhry V, Cornblath DR. Immunosuppressive therapy for myasthenia gravis. In: Lisak RP, ed. *Handbook of myasthenia gravis and myasthenic syndromes.* New York: Marcel Dekker, 1994:341.
382. Witte AS, Cornblath DR, Parry GJ, et al. Azathioprine in the treatment of myasthenia gravis. *Ann Neurol* 1984;15:602.
383. Matell G. Immunosuppressive drugs: azathioprine in the treatment of myasthenia gravis. *Ann N Y Acad Sci* 1987;505:588.
384. Mertens HG, Hertel G, Reuther P, et al. Effect of immunosuppressive drugs (azathioprine). *Ann N Y Acad Sci* 1981;377:691–699.
385. Tindall RS, Phillips JT, Rollins JA, et al. A clinical therapeutic trial of cyclosporine in myasthenia gravis. *Ann N Y Acad Sci* 1993;681:539–551.
386. Schalke B, Kappos L, Dommasch D, et al. Cyclosporin A treatment of myasthenia gravis: initial results of a double blind trial of cyclosporin A versus azathioprine. *Ann N Y Acad Sci* 1988;505:872.
387. Arsura EL, Bick A, Brunner NG, et al. High dose intravenous immunoglobulin in the management of myasthenia gravis. *Arch Intern Med* 1986;146:1365–1368.
388. Gajdos P, Chevret S, Clair B, et al., for the Myasthenia Gravis Clinical Study Group. Clinical trial of plasma exchange and high-dose intravenous immunoglobulin in myasthenia gravis. *Ann Neurol* 1997;41:789–796.
389. Busch C, Machens A, Pichlmeier U, et al. Long-term outcome and quality of life after thymectomy for myasthenia gravis. *Ann Surg* 1996;224:225–232.
390. Bulkley GB, Bass KN, Stephenson GR, et al. Extended cervicomediastinal thymectomy in the integrated management of myasthenia gravis. *Ann Surg* 1997;226:324–335.
391. Berrouschot J, Baumann I, Kalischewski P, et al. Therapy of myasthenic crisis. *Crit Care Med* 1997;25:1228–1235.
392. Carr SR, Gilchrist JM, Abuelo DN, et al. Treatment of antenatal myasthenia gravis. *Obstet Gynecol* 1991;78:485–489.
393. Pasternak JF, Hageman J, Adams MA, et al. Exchange transfusion in neonatal myasthenia. *J Pediatr* 1981;99:644–645.
394. Ahlsten G, Lefvert AK, Osterman PO, et al. Follow-up study of muscle function in children of mothers with myasthenia gravis during pregnancy. *J Child Neurol* 1992;7:264–269.
395. Goans RE, Weiss GH, Abrams SA, et al. Calcium tracer kinetics show decreased irreversible flow to bone in glucocorticoid treated patients. *Calcif Tissue Int* 1995;56:533–535.
396. Olson NY, Lindsley CB. Immunoglobulin E levels and disease manifestations in childhood dermatomyositis. *Arthritis Rheum* 1989;32:S151.
397. Emery HM, Bowyer SL, Sisung CE. Rehabilitation of the child with a rheumatic disease. *Pediatr Clin North Am* 1995;42:1263–1283.
398. American College of Rheumatology Taskforce on Osteoporosis Guidelines. Recommendations for the prevention and treatment of glucocorticoid-induced osteoporosis. *Arthritis Rheum* 1996;39:1791–1801.
399. Huppertz HI, Frosch M, Kuhn C, et al., for the JDM Collaborative Study Group. Treatment of juvenile dermatomyositis with high-dose oral steroids or with steroid-pulse-therapy plus low-dose oral steroids. *Arthritis Rheum* 1998;41[Suppl]:S264.
400. Hariacek M, Miller LC, Tucker LB, et al. Long-term follow-up of children receiving methotrexate for recalcitrant dermatomyositis. *Arthritis Rheum* 1995;38[Suppl]:S231.
401. Miller LC, Sisson BA, Tucker LB, et al. Methotrexate treatment of recalcitrant childhood dermatomyositis. *Arthritis Rheum* 1992;35:1143–1149.
402. Tsai MJ, Lai CC, Lin SC, et al. Intravenous immunoglobulin therapy in juvenile dermatomyositis. *Acta Paediatr Sin* 1977;38:111–115.
403. Finkel TH, Torok TJ, Ferguson PJ, et al. Chronic parvovirus B19 infection and systemic necrotising vasculitis: opportunistic infection or aetiological agent? *Lancet* 1994;343:1255–1258.
404. Reiff A, Rawlings DJ, Shaham B, et al. Preliminary evidence for cyclosporin A as an alternative in the treatment of recalcitrant juvenile rheumatoid arthritis and juvenile dermatomyositis. *J Rheumatol* 1997;24:2436–2443.
405. Gattinara M, Lomater C, Gerloni V, et al. Cyclosporin in pediatric rheumatology: a seven years experience. *Acta Univers Carol [Med]* 1994;40:105–108.
406. Zeller V, Cohen P, Prieur AM, et al. Cyclosporin A therapy in refractory juvenile dermatomyositis: experience and longterm followup of 6 cases. *J Rheumatol* 1996;23:1424–1427.
407. Larner AJ, Sturman SG, Hawkins JB, et al. Myopathy with ragged red fibres following renal transplantation: possible role of cyclosporin-induced hypomagnesaemia. *Acta Neuropathol (Berl)* 1994;88:189–192.
408. Dau PC, Bennington JL. Plasmapheresis in childhood dermatomyositis. *J Pediatr* 1981;98:237–240.
409. Pascuzzi RM, Roos KL, Phillips LH. Granulomatous inflammatory myopathy associated with myasthenia gravis: a case report and review of the literature. *Arch Neurol* 1986;43:621–623.
410. Mrak RE: Muscle granulomas following intramuscular injection. *Muscle Nerve* 1982;5:637–639.
411. Neumann H, Baum C. Granulomatose und eosinophile myositis durch Onchozerca Volvulus. *Pathologe* 1985;6:101–107.
412. Bofill D, Gomez A, Vilanova MA, et al. Miositis granulomatosa brucelar: revision de la literaturea a propositio de un caso. *Med Clin (Barc)* 1982;78:450–452.
413. Pearl GS, Sieger B. Granulomatous *Pneumocystis carinii* myositis presenting as an intramuscular mass. *Clin Infect Dis* 1996;22:577–578.

*Textbook of the Autoimmune Diseases,*
Edited by R. G. Lahita, N. Chiorazzi, and W. H. Reeves,
Lippincott Williams & Wilkins, Philadelphia © 2000.

# CHAPTER 23

# Reproductive Autoimmunity

Harry H. Hatasaka and D. Ware Branch

## ENDOMETRIOSIS AND AUTOIMMUNITY

### Approach to the Patient

Endometriosis is defined as the presence of ectopic endometrial glands and stroma. About one half of affected women experience dysmenorrhea, and a small proportion develop extensive distortion of pelvic anatomy as a result of endometriosis-induced adhesions. The most common site of endometriosis is the ovary, followed by implants on the peritoneum of the cul-de-sac, broad ligaments, and bladder. Endometriosis affects about 5% to 20% of women of reproductive age (1), but the prevalence has been higher (20% to 77%) among women with infertility (2), suggesting an association. Whereas endometriosis-induced adhesions are a definitive source of infertility because of interference with the physical opportunity of ovulation and fertilization, even endometriosis not associated with adhesions has been linked to infertility (3,4). Factors such as prostaglandins and inflammatory cytokines have been isolated in abnormal amounts from the peritoneal fluid (PF) of women with endometriosis and may contribute to subfecundity (5–10). PF from women with endometriosis added to *in vitro* preparations appears to interfere with the fertilization process, perhaps by altering sperm function (11). Other postulated infertility effects of an abnormal peritoneal environment in endometriosis are disruption of ovulation, luteolysis, impaired tubal function, altered ovum maturation, and abnormal implantation.

Current clinical classification systems for endometriosis do not offer prognostic information regarding fecundity, pain, or the natural history of the condition (12). Other aspects of endometriosis also remain enigmatic. Whether the finding of minimal and mild endometriosis should even be considered a disease is still debatable, because serial laparo-

scopic studies in baboons indicate that visible endometriosis implants can be intermittent (13–15).

The cause of endometriosis remains unknown, although retrograde menstruation leading to transplantation of viable endometrial implants has been the most enduring association (16,17). The identification of endometriosis in such diverse locations as lung, pleura, brain, and its occasional presence in men belies the possibility that all endometriosis is associated solely with retrograde menstruation (18,19). Nevertheless, it appears that menstrual function is prerequisite in female subjects for the development of endometriosis (20). Lymphatic and hematologic spread as well as induction and celomic metaplasia have been postulated as initiating events (21). Endometriosis has been identified in all races and socioeconomic environments. A genetic component is suspected because the familial incidence has generally been observed to be elevated. A woman who has a first-degree relative affected by endometriosis has an approximately sevenfold increased chance of developing endometriosis over the general population risk (22). An international linkage study of affected sib-sib pairs is attempting to identify genetic markers associated with endometriosis (23).

With the cause of endometriosis unresolved, the possibility that immunologic abnormalities could permit the implantation and progression of the condition was proposed (24). Some investigators have proposed that endometriosis is a true autoimmune disease in the sense that it represents the induction of a protective immune response against self tissue resulting in pathologic consequences (25).

Before considering a pathogenic autoimmune mechanism for endometriosis, it is still not confirmed that endometriosis is an autoimmune disease. It could be that the activation of peritoneal macrophages and the resultant elaboration of a myriad of measurable cytokines reflect the natural mechanisms for clearing the inevitable cyclic menstrual debris without assigning causation to an abnormal immune system.

The predominant hypothesis to explain the immunologic origin of endometriosis incorporates the concept whereby macrophages process ectopic endometrial tissue for presen-

H. H. Hatasaka: Department of Obstetrics and Gynecology, University of Utah, Salt Lake City, Utah 84132; Department of Endocrinology, Utah Center for Reproductive Medicine, University of Utah School of Medicine, Salt Lake City, Utah 84132.

D. W. Branch: Department of Obstetrics and Gynecology, University of Utah, Salt Lake City, Utah 84132.

tation as antigen to T cells, leading to differentiation of the T cells (26). Immune dysregulation prevents the normal clearance of ectopic endometrium by T-cell subsets and natural killer (NK) cells. A peritoneal inflammatory response is maintained, allowing the expression of cytokines involved in promoting implantation, differentiation, and growth of endometriosis (27–29). The hypothesis extends to account for the manifestations of endometriosis such as pain, adhesions, and infertility by postulating the activation of the humoral arm of the immune system and implicating immune cellular products as causing these manifestations (30–32). Antibodies against endometriosis-specific antigens are thought to contribute to the inflammatory response and therefore to the clinical signs and symptoms. Such an autoimmune process leading to endometriosis appears to involve alterations of the cellular and humoral immune systems that are interdependent (26,33–35).

If true, the hypothesis must account for some fundamental challenges, including explaining how retrograde endometrium or other progenitor cells can be caused to implant and differentiate into ectopic glands and stroma; explaining why some women get endometriosis whereas others do not, despite the near universal presence of retrograde menstruation (36); clarifying why normally positioned (eutopic) endometrium escapes the immunologic consequences proposed to promote the growth of ectopic endometrium; and defining the essential immunologic mechanisms involved in achieving the initiation and maintenance of endometriosis.

## Historical Evolution and Substantiation of the Hypothesis

Weed and Arquembourg (24) first proposed an autoimmune basis for endometriosis when they observed that complement was present by immunofluorescence in nearly all midcycle normal uterine endometrial epithelium in endometriosis subjects but absent in fertile controls. The presence of the complement component C3 in the endometrium was interpreted to represent residual damage from an autoimmune process but was thought to be reversible if the inciting endometrial antigen was eliminated by the removal of endometrial tissue or by prolonged ovarian suppression.

### Peritoneal Fluid Characteristics in Endometriosis

Following the intriguing finding about complement, work began to assess the immunologic environment in women with endometriosis. Discrepant findings regarding PF volumes were reported. Some studies found increased mean PF volumes compared with controls (5,6,37,38), but others did not (7,39,40).

The cellular constituents of the PF were assessed by several groups attempting to demonstrate differences between women with endometriosis and those without. PF normally contains substantial numbers of leukocytes (0.5 to 2.0 $\times$ $10^6$/mL), composed of more than 85% macrophages. But in infertile women with endometriosis, increased numbers of

peritoneal macrophages were observed. Total volumes of PF and total cell counts were higher in infertile endometriosis subjects than controls (5,6). Some studies used a variety of assays that suggested the peritoneal macrophages of women with endometriosis appeared to be activated compared with macrophages from women without endometriosis (41,42). The secretory products of activated macrophages were also assayed in the PF, and some products such as prostaglandin $E_2$ and $F_{2\alpha}$ and acid phosphatase were elevated in women with endometriosis (6). However, other investigators were unable to identify increased prostanoids in the PF of women with endometriosis (37,40).

To build evidence for involvement of the immune system in the genesis of endometriosis, other descriptive studies concentrated on identifying general markers of altered immunity, detecting complement and immunoglobulin deposition in endometrium, and ascertaining the presence of antiendometrial antibodies in the PF or serum of women with endometriosis.

### General Immune Markers in Endometriosis

Although it is debatable whether general immune markers such as altered serum immunoglobulin concentrations, depressed complement concentrations, polyclonal B-cell activation, and increased inflammation are prerequisites for autoimmune states, they are often present in these conditions. There is discrepancy in the literature about whether general markers of immunologic function are different in women with endometriosis compared with those without. Serum leukocyte counts and differentials, complement component levels and circulating immunoglobulins were studied and were not found to differ between the two groups (33,43). Another group found immunoglobulins to be elevated in the serum of women with endometriosis (44), whereas others observed general immune markers including some serum immunoglobulins to be moderately decreased in endometriosis patients (38). Another study of infertile women with endometriosis identified an increase in serum IgG only (25).

### Complement Components in Endometriosis

There is a similar lack of agreement in the literature regarding complement components. Some studies have found elevations (6,43), others found decreased concentrations (38), and yet another study found no differences (33) of complement components between the sera of endometriosis subjects and controls. Complement component studies of the PF of women with endometriosis have also recorded discrepant findings.

Because complement and immunoglobulin deposition in affected tissues had been suggested to be a criterion for autoimmunity (45), complement components were measured in the eutopic endometrium of women with endometriosis. Weed and Arquembourg described the localization of complement in the endometrium of women affected with endometriosis (24). However, a subsequent study was unable to identify C3 or C4 in the endometrium of all women with endometriosis (only 66%), whereas 75% of controls without endometriosis had C3 or C4 in the uterine endometrium (46). Kreiner et al. (47) found elevated IgG deposition in the endometrium of endometriosis subjects but could not distinguish these specimens from those of women with a history of pelvic inflammatory disease. This demonstrated that the IgG deposition was not specific for endometriosis. IgG and IgA deposition in endometrium was also reported by Saiffudin et al. (44), but these findings could not be correlated with infertility. Later, it was shown that complement component C3 is produced in normal human epithelial endometrium cells (48), calling into question the specificity of complement deposition within eutopic endometrium as a criterion for endometriosis.

### Antiendometrial Antibodies

Concomitantly, work began on assessing whether antiendometrial antibodies could be detected in the sera, PF, and cervicovaginal secretions from endometriosis patients (33,43,47,49–55). In one of the initial studies, antibody titers to whole ovary, to an ovarian component, and to endometriosis tissue were measured by passive hemagglutination and immunofluorescence. When compared with normal nonpregnant females, antiovarian and antiendometrial autoantibody levels were higher in the sera of endometriosis patients. The stage of endometriosis, however, did not correlate with the antibody titers (49). Meek et al. (38) demonstrated increased serum antiendometrial antibodies in infertile endometriosis patients compared with fertile control women who lacked pelvic pathology using an immunodiffusion assay, although not when using an immunofluorescence assay. Antibody differences were not found between their cervicovaginal secretions.

Mathur et al. described specific reactivity of IgG from the PF and sera of endometriosis subjects against carefully prepared endometrial antigens from control and endometriosis subjects. They criticized the indiscriminate use of endometrial antigens in previous studies. The researchers concluded that the presence of IgG endometrial antibodies may represent true endometrial autoimmunity in patients with endometriosis, whereas IgA and IgM endometrial antibodies may indicate possible subclinical infections in women with endometriosis (52). This study joined several others that identified increased antiendometrial antibodies in serum from endometriosis subjects (33,43,47,49,50–54). Wild et al. (50) determined that the sensitivity and specificity of an indirect immunofluorescence assay for endometrial antibodies exposed to an endometrial carcinoma cell line were 83% and 79%, respectively, for distinguishing the serum of women with endometriosis. This presented the possibility of a diagnostic test from serum for endometriosis. However, contradictory findings were registered by Garza et al., who unlike others (27,38) were unable to detect elevated endometrial antibody titers from PF from endometriosis patients (54).

Others attempted to determine whether there are differences between amounts of immunoglobulins within the endometria of endometriosis patients compared with women without endometriosis. At least two groups found immunoglobulins to be more concentrated within the endometrium of endometriosis subjects compared with controls (44,49), but this observation was not universal (56).

Microbial invasion of the endometrium has been hypothesized to alter the tissue structure such that the eutopic endometrium of endometriosis patients differs from that in women without endometriosis and could potentially induce the formation of antiendometrial antibodies (55). Why such antiendometrial antibodies would not prevent the implantation of endometriosis is enigmatic.

There has been a concerted effort in the literature to identify specific antiendometrial antibodies. However, there has been disagreement regarding the existence and reproducibility of measuring antiendometrial antibodies (57,58). Different investigators have used a host of approaches, including immunodiffusion (6,38), immunofluorescence (38), hemagglutination (49,52,54), immunohistochemistry (51,59), enzyme-linked immunosorbent assay (ELISA) (60), and Western blotting (61). The lack of standardization of the various assays as pointed out by Switchenko et al. has been problematic. They repeated the techniques of a number of other studies that used an assortments of assays to identify antiendometrial antibodies in endometriosis but were unable to reproduce the earlier findings (57).

### The Humoral Immune System in Endometriosis

Besides autoantibodies to endometrium, a host of other autoantibodies were assayed in women with endometriosis in an attempt to advance the case for endometriosis as an autoimmune disease. Some studies identified abnormally high prevalence rates of autoantibodies from the sera of endometriosis patients compared with controls (25,49,62,63). Confino et al. examined autoantibody levels in the PF of endometriosis subjects and determined that there may be abnormal concentrations of IgG antiphospholipid and antihistone antibodies (64).

Gleicher et al. (25) measured concentrations of IgG and IgM autoantibodies to 16 antigens and reported that approximately two thirds of 59 laparoscopically staged endometriosis patients had lupus anticoagulant, abnormal levels of autoantibodies, or both. They speculated that these antibodies contributed to the unexplained characteristics of the disease such as infertility (35). They suggested that the antibodies represented polyclonal B-cell activation, an occasional manifestation of autoimmune disorders (65). Together with presumed tissue damage, multiorgan involvement, response to the immunotherapeutic agent danazol, genetic and female propensities, and the purported concurrence with other autoimmune disorders (66), the group identified endometriosis as a strong candidate to be an autoimmune disease. The investigators cited reports of decreased oocyte fertilization rates, decreased pregnancy rates, and increased miscarriage rates with endometriosis (67,68) as evidence of multiorgan involvement with tissue damage. They acknowledged that confirmation must await direct demonstration of tissue damage by specific autoantibodies.

Kennedy et al. emphasized that elevated autoantibody levels may merely represent a normal secondary response to ectopic endometrium and that they do not establish a cause and effect relationship with endometriosis. Correlations have not been established between autoantibody findings and the incidence or severity of endometriosis (35). In general terms, Gleicher (35) surmised that, if broad antibody profiling is pursued, approximately 95% of women with endometriosis would have abnormalities compared with 35% in controls.

### Involvement of the Cellular Immune System

Another camp of investigators felt that humoral autoimmunity was not likely in patients with mild endometriosis (69). Work therefore continued investigating the possibility of abnormal regulation of the systemic cellular immune system as a contributing source of endometriosis. A cellular immune response (i.e., localized perivascular lymphocytic infiltration) was compared between monkeys with and without endometriosis when challenged with autologous antigens from normal peritoneum and from eutopic and ectopic endometrium (70). Only the two sources of endometrium, when injected into monkeys with spontaneous endometriosis resulted in diminished cellular immune responses. The hypothesis was entertained that deficient cellular immune responses lead to the inability to obliterate ectopic endometrium, thereby allowing endometriosis to gain a foothold. These animal studies were extended to human studies of the cellular immune response in women with endometriosis. Steele et al. (33) found that circulating lymphocytes obtained from women with moderate to severe endometriosis demonstrated a diminished cytolytic effect on target endometrial cells compared with the lymphocytes from control women. This finding approached statistical significance. Other stimulation tests of the lymphocytes from subjects and controls were otherwise normal, indicating a possible specific deficiency of cellular immunity toward endometrial antigens among women with endometriosis.

Further support for cellular immune-mediated involvement in endometriosis came from the work of others (71–73). Vigano et al. tested the cytotoxic effect of lymphocytes from the serum of endometriosis and control subjects on three target cell populations: stromal and epithelial endometrial cells and an erythroleukemic cell line considered to be a universal NK target. This study postulated that diminished cytotoxic responses by lymphocytes from women with endometriosis may be caused by a general immune phenomenon reflecting a specific altered NK subpopulation activity rather than a nonspecific lymphocytic response. Only the stromal cell assay showed a significant reduction in cytolysis from the serum of endometriosis subjects over controls. This sug-

gested that a general impairment of NK function does not exist in endometriosis; rather, there is a more specific deficiency in cell-mediated cytotoxicity. The investigators speculated that the stromal component is involved in cell adhesion and therefore it is logical that diminished stromal cytolysis may contribute toward the establishment of ectopic endometrium.

Braun et al. found that, whereas peritoneal macrophages from women with endometriosis suppress endometrial cell proliferation, peripheral monocytes from these women do just the opposite in vitro. In contrast, the peripheral monocytes in normal fertile women suppress endometrial cell proliferation. The stimulatory effect of peripheral monocytes can be diminished when endometriosis patients are treated with danazol (73).

The ability to classify subpopulations of leukocytes using monoclonal antibodies against cell surface antigens allowed more specific analysis of the cell types involved in endometriosis compared with previous morphologic means. Three major populations of lymphocytes have been identified: T, B, and NK cells. NK cells, total leukocytes, helper T cells, and macrophages were all elevated in the PF of infertile women with stage I and II endometriosis when compared with the PF of populations of fertile controls and women with unexplained infertility. Although it was previously thought that more than 85% of PF leukocytes were macrophages, 30% to 40% are actually lymphocytes, and a large proportion of the later are cytotoxic.

One group observed differences in leukocyte populations within the endometrium of endometriosis subjects compared with controls (74). They also found that treatment with danazol could alter the proportions of these endometrial immune cells. Immune cell populations, however, do not differ between the sera of these same study populations (75–78). One possible explanation for this discrepancy between endometrial and peripheral blood immune cell distribution is that NK cells found in the uterus are generally of the $CD56^+/CD16^-$ phenotype, which differs from the predominant peripheral blood NK phenotypes. Uterine NK cells are regulated by sex steroids, and their endometrial content increases during the secretory phase, whereas NK cells in the peripheral blood remain more constant across the menstrual cycle, during which they represent 10% to 15% of the mononuclear population. NK cells are not human leukocyte antigen (HLA) restricted and require no prior sensitization for their activity. Their main function is to protect against tumors and viruses.

Abnormal NK cell function became a prime suspect in contributing to diminished antiendometrial lymphocytotoxicity when Oosterlynck et al. (77) found that the endometrial cytotoxicity can be prevented by treating the effector cells with the NK-specific anti-Leu-11b monoclonal antibody. Using this assay, the degree of depression of cytotoxicity correlated with the stage of endometriosis. Their findings confirmed that a generalized NK abnormality does not exist in endometriosis because mitogen stimulation testing of these lymphocytes was normal. Heterologous NK cells also demonstrated reduced cytotoxicity against the endometrium of women with endometriosis. The investigators concluded that the decreased cytotoxicity observed for endometrial cells in women with endometriosis is largely caused by a defect in NK activity but that there is also sizable resistance of the endometrium to NK cytotoxicity (79).

Other factors besides NK cell defects may be involved in the pathogenesis of endometriosis. One variable may be the ambient estrogen milieu, because NK activity in one report was shown to have an inverse correlation with estradiol concentration (80). Kanzaki et al. (81) observed that the serum from women with endometriosis decreased NK activity *in vitro,* thereby supporting a possible effect of external signaling on diminished NK activity.

Other studies also implicated abnormally diminished NK cell function as a possible factor in the pathogenesis of endometriosis (80,82,83). However, D'Hooghe et al. (84) pointed out the difficulty in interpreting the studies that assess endometrial cytotoxicity due in part to the high spontaneous release of $^{51}Cr$ by target cells even in the absence of effector cells during assay. This lowers the signal to noise ratio and calls into question those studies that found only low cytotoxicity. Meticulous attention to assay technique is required. Further issues that have clouded the abnormal NK cell hypothesis include the fact that NK activity is variable even in normal donors.

Fundamentally, abnormally diminished NK cell function as the cause of endometriosis is not consistent with the PF inflammatory environment that features activated macrophages (85) and increased interleukin-1 (IL-1) (9) and tumor necrosis factor-α (TNF-α) (31), which are expected to increase NK activity. Moreover, NK cell–mediated lysis of target cells was found to be normal using the peripheral blood leukocytes of women with laparoscopically demonstrated stage I and II endometriosis but diminished for stages III and IV. This implies that NK functional deficiency is unlikely to be involved in the cause of endometriosis (86). Ho et al. also detected diminished NK activity in the peripheral blood and PF of women with stage III and IV endometriosis. However, no differences were found in the proportion of NK cells in blood or PF between endometriosis patients and controls. It was concluded that the decreased NK cytotoxicity in PF of women with endometriosis was caused by to a functional NK cell defect rather than a quantitative defect of NK cells (87). However, even the finding of decreased NK activity associated with higher stages of endometriosis has been challenged (84), and others have found normal NK activity in the peripheral blood of women with endometriosis (71,72,88,89) and baboons with endometriosis (90).

Some have wondered why malignancies and infections are not more common if NK cell activity is truly suppressed in endometriosis. There is some epidemiologic evidence that several malignancies (e.g., breast, ovarian, hematopoietic) may be more common for women with endometriosis (91). Among other possibilities, this could be caused by diminished surveillance by abnormal NK cells.

Other NK-like T-cell populations have been proposed to be cytotoxic effector cells against endometrial cells (92), because the cytotoxicity of endometrial cells *in vitro* appears to be controlled in part by the major histocompatibility complex (MHC) antigen expression of the cells. Presence of the HLA-B7 allele on eutopic or ectopic endometrial cells confers resistance to lysis by T lymphocytes. Ectopic endometrial cells can modulate the expression of these MHC class I molecules. Treatment with interferon-γ (IFN-γ) upregulates MHC class I molecule expression and imparts resistance to cell lysis. What regulates the expression of these molecules is unknown, but even if ectopic endometrium is sensitive to lysis, the likelihood of lysis is low, because the quantity of activated cytotoxic T cells in the peritoneal cavity in endometriosis is limited. The contribution of dysregulated endometrial cells, resistant to lysis by cytotoxic T cells as a potential etiologic mechanism for endometriosis is unlikely.

Functional abnormalities have been described for all of the immune cell populations, including NK cells, T cells, B cells, monocytes, and macrophages (34). However, a primary cellular immune etiologic abnormality has not been confirmed.

### Hypothesizing Abnormal Intercellular Signaling in the Pathogenesis of Endometriosis

Investigators began to examine the notion that ectopic endometrium may be foreign to the immune system precipitating abnormal immunologic reactions that allow the subsequent establishment of endometriosis. Because it was learned that retrograde menstruation occurs in nearly all women (36) and that the effluvium contains viable cells (93), the ectopic menstrual effluvium may implant and incite a local inflammatory response leading to the recruitment and differentiation of peritoneal macrophages (29). Evidence had accumulated that increased inflammatory reactions occur in the peritoneal cavity of women with endometriosis (5,7,8,85,94) and are associated with activation of macrophage function (41). Endometriosis cells *in vitro* under inflammatory conditions can secrete substances that can attract macrophages such as granulocyte-macrophage colony-stimulating factor, monocyte chemotactic protein-1, RANTES ("regulated on activation, normally T-cell expressed and secreted"), and complement component 3 (29,48,95,96).

The hypothesis considering ectopic endometrium as the inciting element for the development of endometriosis is not cleanly supported by the literature. Dunselman et al. (97) measured a number of acute phase reactant molecules (e.g., C-reactive protein, α₁-antitrypsin, acid α₁-glycoprotein, α₂-macroglobulin, haptoglobin, C3, C4, IgG, IgA, IgM) in PF and serum of endometriosis patients compared with women without endometriosis. The concentrations of these markers of acute-phase reaction in PF depended on their molecular weights and were not selectively secreted in persons with endometriosis at a significantly elevated rate. Values of the proteins change according to the phase of the menstrual cycle. The investigators concluded that endometriosis does not cause marked peritoneal inflammatory changes.

## Abnormal Peritoneal Macrophage Function

Without the establishment of a cause and effect relationship to support the hypothesis that ectopic endometrium triggers an inflammatory response that attracts and activates macrophages, the question is a chicken or egg dilemma. Perhaps just the opposite occurs, whereby a primary abnormality of peritoneal macrophage function leads to secretion of growth factors resulting in the implantation, growth, and differentiation of ectopic endometrium (27,98). A postulated role for peritoneal macrophages as an early pathogenic element in endometriosis is depicted in Figure 23.1.

The work of Haney et al. (5) in infertile women with endometriosis showed that increases in macrophage numbers were linked with endometriosis. Halme et al. (27) also observed the numbers, size, and antigen expression of PF macrophages in endometriosis subjects were all increased compared with a control population. However, others (76,98) found that the increase in macrophage numbers may not be specific for endometriosis but may be attributed to infertility in general. A rabbit model of induced endometriosis could not demonstrate the recruitment and activation of macrophages (99), but this finding may reflect species differences, because rabbits do not exhibit spontaneous endometriosis.

Nevertheless, others continue to argue that activated peritoneal macrophages may contribute to the pathogenesis of endometriosis. A substantial body of literature has attempted to delineate competence factors (i.e., substances that allow cells to respond to mitogens) and progression factors that could promote the development of endometriosis (28) (Table 23.1). One group used [H³]thymidine incorporation into mouse endometrial stromal cells to assess the effects of macrophage-conditioned medium and other potential growth factors. They concluded that macrophage-conditioned medium appears

**TABLE 23.1.** *Growth factors in the fibroblast*

| Competence factor | Progression factor |
|---|---|
| Serum | Endometrial growth factor |
| Platelet-derived growth factor | Somatomedin C |
| Fibroblast growth factor | Insulin |
| Macrophage-derived growth factor | Platelet-poor plasma |

From Olive et al. *Am J Obstet Gynecol* 1991;164:953-958, with permission.

to function as a competence growth factor and that estrogen (in appropriate concentrations) functions as a progression growth factor (28).

Comprehensive reviews of growth factors and cytokines and their roles in the physiology of human endometrium have been published (100–103). A number of these substances are of potential relevance to the genesis of and infertility associated with endometriosis. For example, a growing list of products secreted by activated peritoneal macrophages has accumulated, and hypotheses about their growth and progression functions regarding endometriosis have been generated.

### Biochemical Substances in Abnormal Amounts in Endometriosis

Angiogenic factors such as fibroblast growth factor, angiogenin, IL-8 (104), transforming growth factor-α, and epidermal growth factor are derived from PF mononuclear cells and from endometriosis cells (105). In PF and follicular fluid, they have been correlated with the presence, but not necessarily the grade, of endometriosis. They may be involved in the outgrowth and progression of lesions (106–108).

PF macrophage-derived growth factor (MDGF) activity from peritoneal macrophages was compared between fertile and infertile women with endometriosis *in vitro*. Macrophages from 28% of the normal women exhibited MDGF activity compared with 68% of the macrophages from the infertile women with endometriosis. This was significant and may explain the ability for endometriosis to implant and differentiate in the peritoneal cavity (27,32,109).

Because fibronectin has been associated with pulmonary fibrosis, cell migration, wound healing, phagocytosis, cell adhesion, and cell differentiation, Kauma et al. (30) pursued the possibility that increased peritoneal fibronectin production may lead to the pelvic adhesion formation often seen in endometriosis. Fibronectin is a macrophage product found to be secreted from peritoneal macrophages of endometriosis subjects *in vitro* at approximately three times the rate of macrophages extracted from PF of control women. However, mean PF fibronectin concentrations were found to be 30% lower from endometriosis subjects than from the controls.

TNF-α is a product of activated leukocytes and monocytes with a variety of effects including cytotoxicity to gametes. It augments adhesion of stromal cells to mesothelium in culture (107,110), and it could theoretically play a role in the patho-

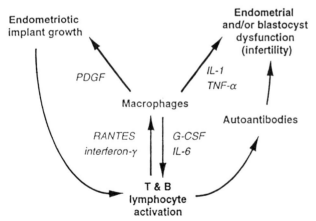

**FIG. 23.1.** Postulated central role of peritoneal macrophages in the pathogenesis of endometriosis. *PDGF*, platelet-derived growth factor; *IL-1*, interleukin-1; *TNF-α*, tumor necrosis factor-α; *G-CSF*, granulocyte colony-stimulating factor; *IL-6*, interleukin-6. (From Khorram O, Taylor RN, Ryan IP, Schall TJ, Landers DV. Peritoneal fluid concentrations of the cytokine RANTES correlate with the severity of endometriosis. *Am J Obstet Gynecol* 1993;169:1545–1549.)

genesis of endometriosis. *In vitro* release and PF concentrations of TNF-α from macrophages derived from women with infertility and endometriosis were elevated compared with those of controls. TNF-α concentrations also correlated with the amount of peritoneal adhesions in these women (31).

A role for epidermal growth factor in the growth and maintenance of endometriosis has been suggested (107,111,112). Another macrophage secretory product, platelet-derived growth factor has been proposed to contribute to the proliferation of endometrial stroma (32,107,112). Likewise, granulocyte-macrophage colony stimulating factor has been localized to eutopic and ectopic endometrial cells. It is involved in the migration, proliferation, and activation of endometrial and peritoneal macrophages (95).

Interleukins and their metabolites have been examined in the PF of women with endometriosis by several investigators. Most authorities (113) have identified IL-1, IL-5, and IL-6 in PF. IL-1 has an inhibitory role regarding stromal cell proliferation (107), suggesting a role in limiting the establishment of endometriosis. Other properties of IL-1 have paradoxically been hypothesized to play a role in endometriosis associated infertility (9).

Similarly, IL-6 is a multifunctional cytokine coupled to many immunologic, proliferative, and neoplastic processes. It is considered an inflammatory cytokine that helps to mediate cell responses to immune cell secretory products, but it is a normal constituent of PF that appears to inhibit stromal cell growth (114). No concentration differences could be detected in one study between endometriosis subjects and controls (115). However, others identified a possible defect in the production of IL-6 by endometrial stromal cells of women with endometriosis, as well as diminished IL-6 receptor quantities and diminished soluble receptor in the PF (116,117). This finding has left open the possibility that altered IL-6 responsiveness of the stromal cells within endometriosis implants contributes to the growth aberrancies of endometriosis.

IL-8 is another pleiotropic chemokine product of activated macrophages. It has chemoattractant effects for inflammatory cells as well as angiogenic and growth promoting properties (118). It was elevated in the PF of endometriosis subjects (119).

IFN-γ inhibits endometrial cell proliferation *in vitro* (120). It is secreted by resident leukocytes that are more prevalent in ectopic endometrium and therefore could play a regulatory role in preventing endometriosis (121), but its concentration could not be correlated with the severity of endometriosis (29). However, a 60-kd heat shock protein (HSP60) was found more commonly in the PF of women with endometriosis than controls and correlated with the finding of IFN-γ. HSP60 locally activates macrophages, T lymphocytes, and cytokine release (122).

RANTES is a cytokine involved in macrophage recruitment and activation. It has been found to correlate with the severity of endometriosis (29). Insulin-like growth factor types 1 and 2 were identified in PF and found to be mitogenic for endometrial stromal cells (123).

Endometriotic cells produce monocyte chemotactic and activating protein-1 in response to IL-1β and TNF-α in culture (96). This protein may help explain the greater chemotactic activity for neutrophils and macrophages observed by one group throughout the menstrual cycle in the endometrium of patients with endometriosis compared with controls (124).

Besides cytokines and growth factors, other biochemical abnormalities have been investigated in endometriosis. Aromatase, the enzyme responsible for converting androgens to estrogens is normally not expressed in endometrial and myometrial tissue. However, it is found to be expressed in ectopic endometrial tissue, suggesting a difference in ectopic endometrium or the result of complex interactions of intercellular or intracellular signaling (19). Its presence potentially links abnormalities of the immune system with the long-held clinical observation of a role for estrogen in the proliferation of endometriosis.

### Cellular Sources of Altered Cytokine Production in Endometriosis

Rana et al. (119) made the point that the source of elevated cytokine levels in the PF of women with endometriosis, such as endometrial stromal or glandular cells, macrophages, or peritoneal mesothelial cells, remains unclear, because all of these cells have the ability to produce cytokines. Their work suggested that at least the elevated cytokine concentrations of IL-8 and TNF-α in the midluteal PF of women with endometriosis are most likely to be secreted by the activated peritoneal macrophages. In peripheral blood, leukocytes have been shown to differ in their production of some cytokines, depending on whether they are from women with or without endometriosis (125).

Many other inflammatory cell products such as prostaglandins and proteolytic enzymes have also been measured in elevated concentrations in the PF of women with endometriosis compared with controls (126). However, a large body of work has been unable to confirm elevated concentrations of cytokines and inflammatory cell products in the PF of women with endometriosis (76,113,116,127).

Hill sought to place what had been learned about the complex cytokine environment in endometriosis into the context of the known cytokine cascade (128). Normally, activated macrophages secrete the inflammatory cytokines IL-1 and TNF-α. IL-1 stimulates IL-2 release from T lymphocytes, which induces release of IFN-γ by other T cells. NK cell activity is not antigen specific but is triggered by IL-1, IL-2, IFN-γ, and TNF-α. Unfortunately, the complex pleiotropic interactions and sources of the cytokines and the inherent difficulty in their measurements do not render a clear-cut biochemical mechanism for the origin or the manifestations of endometriosis. However, Hammond et al. (107) summarized the findings regarding the potential roles of growth factors and cytokines in the pathogenesis of endometriosis. At the very least, the varied functions of these substances secreted by peritoneal macrophages and endometrial cells offer all of the necessary mechanisms to promote the implantation and proliferation of ectopic endometrium in the peritoneal cavity. Nevertheless, the chicken or the egg dilemma persists. Does endometriosis cause increased cytokine levels geared at limiting the proliferation of endometriosis (119), or does abnormal cytokine function allow the proliferation of endometriosis?

## Diagnostic Approach

### Is Endometriosis an Autoimmune Condition?

Arguments have been advanced that endometriosis probably is an autoimmune entity based on circumstantial similarities shared with other autoimmune disorders. Endometriosis occurs most frequently in females, and there is a heritable propensity. Both associations lack specificity. The lack of endometrium in males does not allow gender to be a valid association. Most autoimmune disorders can be linked with specific HLA haplotypes, but no such associations have not been identified for endometriosis (129,130).

Monkeys exposed to an immunotoxin or irradiated systemically subsequently had a higher chance of developing endometriosis, giving credence to an important role of the immune system in the development of the condition (131,132). However, no specific inciting agent has been identified that may lead to polyclonal activation in endometriosis, and polyclonal activation has not been documented consistently in the condition.

Other common associations of autoimmune disorders have not been documented for endometriosis, such as a consistent histologic finding of lymphocytic infiltration within implants (24,133). Autoimmune diseases tend to demonstrated a clustering of associated autoimmune conditions among patients and families (65). Such a correlation however, has not been consistently observed with endometriosis (55).

If endometriosis is an autoimmune disease, abnormal proportions of T-cell subsets may be anticipated in peripheral blood and PF (134). Some groups have found abnormal T-cell proportions (29,87,89), but others have been unable to demonstrate such a finding (35,134). In the presence of active autoimmune disease, serum complement is often reduced. One report observed a reduction in complement in the serum of women with endometriosis (24), but others could not replicate the finding (33,43).

Drawing from other autoimmune diseases, if endometriosis is an autoimmune disease, it would be logical to expect significant alterations its manifestations if treated with immunosuppressive agents. D'Hooghe et al. (135) treated a total of 16 baboons having spontaneous ($n = 5$) or induced endometriosis (by peritoneal seeding of menstrual endometrium; $n = 7$) or no endometriosis ($n = 4$) with methylprednisolone and azathioprine for 3 months. Equal numbers of untreated baboons were studied in each category. Laparoscopies were performed in all subjects after 3 months and then in 8 baboons with induced endometriosis at 7 months and in 9 of the baboons with spontaneous disease at 12 months. Animals without endometriosis did not develop endometriosis while being immunosuppressed. Progression of endometriosis lesions was observed only in baboons who had spontaneous endometriosis while being immunosuppressed. Unlike the findings for some known autoimmune conditions, this study did not find significant overall improvement in endometriosis with immunosuppressive treatment; rather possible progression occurred.

Short-term immunosuppression does not appear to cause endometriosis in baboons, calling into question the hypothesis that the normal immune system guards against the development of the condition (135). Epidemiologic and mechanistic correlates for autoimmunity have not provided a firm case for endometriosis as an autoimmune disease.

### Limitations of the Literature

The experimental literature concerning endometriosis is difficult to interpret, and in most cases, studies are incomparable because of a number of inconsistencies. A dependable clinical definition of endometriosis is sorely needed to offer fair comparisons within the endometriosis literature. Not only do endometriosis study populations differ, but control populations are inconsistent. There has been no agreement about whether to require or include fertile or infertile subjects, pelvic pain or pain-free subjects, or adhesions or laparoscopic confirmation of the condition. Many of the studies suffer from other serious design flaws such as small study sizes.

Laboratory methodologies for determining such entities as antiendometrial and other autoantibodies have not been standardized. Even the timing of biopsies and procurement of fluid specimens for study have generally varied across the menstrual cycle. These variables can render important differences in results and interpretation, depending on the end points being studied. For example, activation of PF macrophages has been observed to progress throughout the normal menstrual cycle.

There has been a lack of a clear direction for research endeavors attempting to determine whether there is an autoimmune component involving endometriosis. Most studies have examined end points (e.g., circulating autoantibodies, cytokine concentrations, immune cell proportions) that are clouded by confounding factors without properly controlling for these factors. In general, the endometriosis literature concerning immunologic concerns has offered little confidence for reproducibility of results.

With the immunologic basis of endometriosis in question, current classification schemes for endometriosis cannot differentiate autoimmune from nonautoimmune endometriosis subclassifications. There are no validated immunologic assays that can assess a presumptive autoimmune component for endometriosis. There are no reliable assays, immunologic or otherwise, to diagnose the condition. The diagnosis remains based on the histologic confirmation of ectopic endometrial glands and stroma that generally requires laparoscopic surgery to obtain. History and physical examination can only provide presumptive evidence of endometriosis.

## Treatment

Some research has examined the effects of some endometriosis treatments on the subsequent concentrations of inflammatory cytokines and the effects of resultant PF on the mouse embryo toxicity assay. TNF and IL-1 was measured in PF of endometriosis, control and treated endometriosis subjects (136). Concentrations significantly higher than controls were found in endometriosis, whereas extremely low levels were observed in the PF of endometriosis subjects treated with danazol or a gonadotropin-releasing hormone (GnRH) agonist. The mouse embryo toxicity of the PF decreased concurrent with treatment. Subsequent embryo degeneration, however, remained greater with PF from treated endometriosis patients over controls, and some other toxic substances therefore were not measured. Another group (137) used the serum from short-term (3-day) glucocorticoid-treated endometriosis patients (stage I or II) on a two-cell mouse embryo assay. They found the serum from endometriosis patients is embryotoxic compared with controls, but toxicity decreases significantly 12 days after a 3-day steroid treatment.

GnRH therapy for women with endometriosis was shown to increase INF-γ and decrease IL-6 in PF (138). Other symptomatic treatment for endometriosis (i.e., nonsteroidal antiinflammatories and danazol) have also been found to elicit changes in immune cell function in women with endometriosis (139,140). Accordingly, some of the clinical treatments commonly used for endometriosis may alter some immune cell products and offer some substantiation for a role of the immune system in the maintenance of the disease. However, with the exceptions of danazol and antiinflammatory treatment, no clinical trials with adequate power of any other immunomodulatory treatment have shown convincing beneficial clinical effects for diminishing the dysmenorrhea attributed to endometriosis. Immunomodulatory treatments for endometriosis have not consistently increased pregnancy rates in the face of endometriosis-related infertility.

## Summary

The hypothesis that endometriosis is an autoimmune disease with its cause based within the abnormal regulation of the immune system is appealing. Experimental support for the premise, however, remains inadequate. The postulates of Witebsky to identify an immunologic basis of disease include demonstration of antibody production against an identical antigen in an animal model and the isolation or characterization of that antigen (141). Neither of these postulates have yet been met for endometriosis (38).

A number of plausible hypotheses directed at a potential autoimmune cause for endometriosis have emerged (Table 23.2). Abnormal function of components of the cellular and humoral immune systems have been implicated. Functional deficits of immune cells of a variety of phenotypes have been described. Likewise, abnormal concentrations of a multitude of substances, such as prostanoids, enzymes, cytokines, and

**TABLE 23.2.** *Immune-related pathogenic hypotheses for endometriosis*

- Enhanced immune system activation with a loss of immune tolerance to self antigens (142)
- Deficient cellular immunity causing insufficient eradication of ectopic endometrium and causing these products to be immunogenic (33, 70, 77, 143)
- Abnormal macrophage function leading to the development and maintenance of endometriosis (69)
- Endometriosis as a typical idiopathic autoimmune disease characterized by the classic hallmarks of autoimmune disorders (25)
- Ectopic endometrium (outside of the immunologically privileged uterus) triggers an autoimmune response, including a proliferation of autoantibodies that account for the clinical signs and symptoms of endometriosis (26, 35).
- Infections within eutopic endometrium render the tissue antigenic and may trigger an autoimmune cascade leading to endometriosis (55).
- Dysregulation of cytokine economy may contribute to the pathogenesis of endometriosis (114, 144).

growth factors have been detected, and their elaborate and sometimes detailed potential involvement in the pathogenesis of endometriosis have been postulated, but cause and effect relationships have not been established.

Evidence for involvement of the immune system in endometriosis ranges from circumstantial involvement to specific hypothesized mechanisms at the cellular level. However, virtually all avenues of investigation have been obscured by conflicting data. This has resulted in no small measure from discrepancies in laboratory techniques, study designs, and interpretation. Future investigations into the immunologic basis of endometriosis would do well to heed eight guidelines set forth by Hill and D'Hooghe (26):

1. Employ proper study power.
2. Use laparoscopically defined study and control groups, and include fertile and infertile subjects in all study groups.
3. Target tissues should be clearly defined (i.e., standardized eutopic and ectopic endometrium).
4. Specificity of target tissues should be confirmed using other control tissues.
5. Use standardized assay techniques.
6. When antibody-mediated studies are done, the presence of endogenous immunoglobulin should be controlled for in endogenous tissues.
7. Control for spontaneous $^{51}$Cr release in cytotoxic assays.
8. Strict attention should be directed to appropriate statistical analysis.

Even if abnormal immune function is not etiologic, as Hill (26) suggested, altered immune function may still be involved in the maintenance, proliferation and sequelae of endometriosis. It appears that research endeavors have reached a crossroads. Substantial numbers of complex immune mechanisms could be involved in the cause of endometriosis. However, to guide future research direction, many of the studies will need to be repeated using the strict guidelines listed earlier. Ultimately, the mysteries of the involvement of the immune system in endometriosis may best yield to a reverse genetic approach to ascertain defects at the molecular level (23).

## AUTOIMMUNE ORCHITIS

Orchitis is characterized histologically by the finding of inflammatory infiltrates throughout the testis, where normally there are no lymphocytes. Orchitis can compromise the steroidogenic and spermatogenic functions of the testes, potentially leading to azoospermia and the need for androgen replacement therapy. A related problem has been autoimmunity to sperm that has definitively been shown to lead to fertilization impediments (145).

Orchitis has been attributed to infectious, traumatic events, and autoimmune origins. Mumps infections, especially postpurbertally, frequently (25%) lead to clinical unilateral or bilateral orchitis that may then result in testicular atrophy or infertility in 60%. Testicular trauma may also trigger some cases of autoimmune orchitis (146–148). However, the unequivocal existence of isolated autoimmune orchitis has been controversial, because testicular inflammatory infiltrates have yet to be differentiated based on cause (149). Antisperm antibodies (ASAs) do not appear to be the primary pathogenetic instigator of mumps orchitis (150,151), traumatic orchitis (147), or autoimmune orchitis (152); rather, they may be a consequence of orchitis.

Evidence for an autoimmune origin of orchitis comes primarily from multiple animal models of induced experimental autoimmune orchitis (EAO). There are also idiopathic inflammatory testicular conditions described in men with autoimmune orchitis histology comparable to animal EAO but without conclusive evidence of immune complexes (153). The most compelling evidence for the existence of clinically relevant autoimmune orchitis in humans is the well-recognized orchitis associated with autoimmune polyendocrinopathy syndromes (154).

### Background

Testicular autoantigens can be classified as aspermatogenic or testis specific. The testis-specific type are organ-specific autoantigens that are orchitogenic. Orchitogenic antigens have not been characterized. Aspermatogenic refers to a subtype of autoantigen expressed only by germ cells that elicit an immune response that causes diminished sperm production and damage of germ cells. Spermatozoa and some of their haploid precursors are known to be autoantigenic. It appears however that the expression of their autoantigens postdates the early lymphocyte interactions that confer immunologic tolerance of self antigens. It is not until puberty that new antigenic expression takes place on maturing spermatozoa thereby rendering them foreign to the immune system. Mechanisms must be maintained to isolate the spermatozoa and precursor cells from immunologic recognition. The testis is thought to be an immunologically privileged site because heterologous tissue transplanted within the testis is not rejected immediately (155).

The anatomic pathway that spermatozoa follow after exiting the seminiferous tubules where they are produced is called the excurrent duct system. It includes a straight tubule region that is adjacent to the rete testis. From there, sperm enter the efferent ducts and continue into the epididymis, where they are stored and final maturational changes occur. Ejaculation forces sperm through the vas deferens and the urethra. Beyond the seminiferous tubules, the epithelial junctions are less tight, rendering sperm more susceptible to immunologic attack. Throughout this pathway, CD8+ cells are observed in the mucosa (where they may play a role in immunosuppression), and CD4+ lymphocytes are found in the connective tissue between the ducts (156). Other immunocompetent cells, including macrophages, also reside along the course of the excurrent duct system.

A major anatomic and physiologic mechanism for isolating the testis immunologically is the blood–testis barrier. Tight junctions form between and over the apical regions of the supporting Sertoli cells of the seminiferous tubules (157) to preclude the influx of immune cells and antibodies into the lumina, where the mature germ cells are released. Immune cells are normal residents within the interstitial tissue between the seminiferous tubules and often in semen but not inside the tubules (158). The testis possesses the conditions to be an immunocompetent organ.

It is unknown whether all self antigens remain sequestered within the blood–testis barrier in normal men (154). Some autoantigens in specific locations appear to be accessible to immune cells and antibodies. Mechanisms other than the blood–testis barrier are also required to prevent autoimmune orchitis.

Local testicular immunoregulatory factors may play a role in providing immunologic tolerance for spermatozoa (159). Although no lymphocytes reside within the germinal compartment of the testis, the Leydig cell-containing interstitial tissue has macrophages. Certain clinical situations, such as severe obstruction with oligospermia or azoospermia, manifest interstitial tissue containing a predominance of CD8+ (suppressor/cytotoxic) lymphocytes, but in other situations, such as vasectomy in which there has been trauma to the excurrent duct system, CD4+ (helper/inducer) lymphocytes are more common (160). This suggests local immune regulation. A number of cytokines known to regulate lymphocyte-mitogen interactions have been identified within the testis (161). Sertoli cells have been reported to produce immunosuppressive molecules (162).

Tolerance mechanisms may also involve systemic regulation at the level of T cells. For example, thymectomy of normal mice within 3 days of birth places the mice at risk for autoimmune orchitis (163). However, normal T cells infused systemically into these thymectomized mice can abrogate the risk of autoimmune orchitis (164). When vasectomy is added to early thymectomy, the risk of autoimmune orchitis increases dramatically from approximately 25% to over 90% suggesting that local and systemic mechanisms are important in maintaining tolerance. Nevertheless, mechanisms of immune tolerance to maintain normal functioning of the human male reproductive tract remain incompletely understood.

## Hypotheses for the Initiation of Autoimmune Orchitis

There are a number of murine experimental autoimmune orchitis models in use to help define pathophysiologic mechanisms (154). The two major experimental tactics to produce EAO are immunization using testicular or sperm antigens in conjunction with adjuvant and specifically timed modifications of the immune system. Evidence from EAO models supports the possible roles for cell-mediated and humoral immunity in producing the condition.

## Cellular Immune System in Experimental Autoimmune Orchitis

Experiments that alter the thymus or T-cell production (e.g., use of the immunosuppressive agent cyclosporin A, viral infections, ionizing radiation) can cause various autoimmune diseases in mice, including orchitis (165). This indicates that there are T-cell and thymus controlling effects on tolerance to pathogenic self-reactive T cells. The essential immune cell conferring adoptively transferred EAO is the CD4$^+$ T cell (166). When CD4$^+$ T cells are removed, adoptive transfer of EAO is inhibited. CD4$^+$ T cells only recognize antigens when the peptide antigens are associated with class Ia or II MHC on antigen-presenting cells. The antigen-presenting cells must have access to testicular antigens for adoptively transferred EAO to occur. Tung found that the one location where class Ia MHC macrophages are detected is the straight tubule region of the testis, which corresponds with where passive EAO always begins histologically. This is also a region of the testis that lacks tight junctional complexes in the seminiferous tubules. The opportunity for initiation of passive EAO is present (154).

An elegant set of experiments demonstrated that testis or mature sperm-specific antigen-derived T-cell clones produced from crude tissue preparations can adoptively be transferred into normal syngeneic mice and lead to autoimmune orchitis (153). A specific role of the cell-mediated immune system in EAO has been confirmed. The mechanism was further characterized by implicating the T$_H$1 CD4$^+$ T-cell subset as the essential T cell in the transfer of EAO. On activation, these T cells produce IL-2, TNF, and INF-$\gamma$ and are associated with the delayed hypersensitivity form of immune reaction. Antibodies to TNF abrogate the development of EAO, indicating an essential role for this cytokine. The EAO induced in these experiments had a common histologic pattern independent of the particular clone transferred. Clones were derived from mature spermatozoa or testicular tissue. This finding demonstrates a close pathogenetic relationship between autoantigenic determinants from testicular tissue and mature spermatozoa.

A CD4$^+$ T-cell line has also been isolated that can prevent the induction of autoimmune orchitis when passively transferred, further supporting a role for systemic cellular regulation (167). Other work has demonstrated the existence of pathogenic but normally nonfunctional T cells in the spleens of adult mice (168). It appears that regulatory T cells normally suppress the activity of the pathogenic T cells, but if the regulation fails, autoimmune disease of the gonads could ensue. Several mechanisms have been proposed whereby pathogenic T cells can predominate (169). First, alterations such as early thymectomy could deplete regulatory T cells. Second, during the neonatal time frame, populations of pathogenic autoreactive T cells could amplify. Third, the mechanism of molecular mimicry of orchitic or oophoritogenic T-cell peptides by unrelated peptides could activate T cells that cause gonadal autoimmune disease.

Another possibility for the development of autoimmune orchitis involves abnormal expression of HLA-DR. This molecule is expressed on various immune cells and is involved in antigen presentation. HLA-DR has been found to be expressed by epithelial cells within the male reproductive tract (170), and aberrant expression could potentially lead to T-cell activation and autoimmune orchitis.

## Humoral Immune System in Experimental Autoimmune Orchitis

Tung et al. formulated a working hypothesis about how EAO may begin that involves the humoral immune system. Besides the possibility of germ cell antigens permeating through the weak junctions of the straight tubule region where they can initiate a CD4$^+$ T-cell response, an autoimmune response has inexplicably been observed in the seminiferous tubule region as well. In EAO, IFN-$\gamma$ can be used to upregulate the expression of Ia MHC molecules on the interstitial macrophages in the region. Thereafter, Tung hypothesizes that germ cell antigens located outside the blood–testis barrier, such as basal lamina antigens, preleptotene spermatocytes, and Sertoli cells, may complex with the Ia$^+$ macrophages to initiate an antibody response. The antibodies could then be passively transferred to the luminal compartment of the tubules across the blood–testis barrier, causing disruption of the barrier and germ cells. There is evidence of immune complexes infiltrating the peritubular spaces in EAO (154) but not the luminal compartments.

ASAs alone in humans are insufficient to elicit orchitis, as evidenced by the frequent clinical finding of vasectomy-induced ASAs in the absence of orchitis. Yule et al. demonstrated that sperm-specific T-cell clones can initiate EAO, thereby showing that germ cell immunity alone can lead to EAO through a cellular mechanism without the involvement necessarily of antibodies (153). Immune deposits themselves are unable to initiate EAO (171).

There is stronger evidence of a cellular or cytokine-mediated mechanism of autoimmune orchitis than an antibody-initiated mechanism. The complexity of the interactions between antibodies and antigens and the development of orchitis, vasitis, and epididymitis is highlighted by the observation that orchitis, vasitis, and epididymitis in mice appear to be immunogenetically distinct manifestations (172). Although antibodies are known to bind to testicular antigens during the evolution of autoimmune orchitis, their roles remain enigmatic.

### Potential Causes of Antisperm Antibodies

The presence of ASAs has been classified as primary when the apparent cause is inflammatory, infectious, or idiopathic and as secondary when the cause appears to be obstruction of the tract (173). Although unsettled, the development of ASAs has been ascribed to defective immunoregulation, mechanical breeches of the blood–testis barrier, or other overwhelming inoculations of sperm antigens leading to sensitization. The epididymis appears to contain mature sperm with autoantigen concentrations exceeding those within the testis. The epididymis has been implicated as the more likely site than the testis for initiation of the ASAs independent of the proximal cause (174).

A clear pattern of risk factors for the development of ASAs has not emerged. Hendry reported that testis biopsies from infertile men with unilateral testicular obstruction often exhibit normal spermatogenesis despite having ASAs and oligospermia and only rarely manifest focal orchitis (175,176). Similarly, Hinting et al. observed an association between unilateral testis obstruction from a variety of causes and the development of ASAs (177). Testicular torsion, trauma, cancer, varicocele, orchitis, cryptorchidism, and surgical biopsies and vasectomies have all been variably associated with ASAs and infertility (178). The associations however have been tenuous in many of these circumstances. A multivariate analysis found that the presence of ASAs is associated with vas reversal procedures but not other manipulations of the cord such as varicocele and hernia repairs (145). Infection including sexually transmitted disease, orchitis, and epididymitis were also associated with subsequent ASAs (177,145). For example, an association of infection with *Chlamydia trachomatis* and the presence of ASAs has been described (179,180). Trauma causing testicular atrophy does not necessarily induce ASAs (181). Presumably, trauma that compromises the blood flow to a testis without significant blood–testis barrier interruption could lead to atrophy without the inducement of autoimmunity against testicular or sperm antigens. Unfortunately, it is not possible to predict which individuals, given the risk factors described, will develop ASAs.

One of the most pertinent clinical associations has been the presence of ASAs after vasectomy for men who subsequently would like more children. Early studies in mice indicated that vasectomy can induce ASAs and anitesticular antibodies (182). In humans, vasectomy has been associated with the subsequent development of ASAs in approximately 50% to 80% of men (183), but antitesticular antibodies and testicular atrophy have not been consistently observed. Even men who develop ASAs after vasectomy are often able to father more children after vasectomy reversal, but fertility appears to decline as a function of time since the vasectomy. This decline in fecundity has been ascribed to an increased prevalence of ASAs with time. Fortunately, postvasectomy spermatogenesis is generally spared.

### Potential Mechanisms of Sperm Autoimmunity Causing Subfecundity

Several mechanisms for ASAs leading to subfecundity have been described. Cytotoxic sperm antibodies have been associated with diminished fertilization of zona-free hamster eggs (184) and mature human oocytes during *in vitro* fertilization (185). It appears that IgA or IgG or both isotypes together can decrease sperm binding to salt-stored human zona pellucida, whereas both isotypes must be associated to decrease sperm penetration using zona-free hamster oocytes (186). In the setting of ASAs in men with infertility, the number of sperm bound to the zona pellucida (ZP) also predicts whether fertilization is likely to occur (187).

There may be a particular dose-dependent effect of IgG ASAs in inhibiting the fusion of sperm and oolemma (188). Diminished sperm motility and survival has also been attributed to ASAs (189,190). Impaired embryo cleavage has been linked to the presence of ASAs (191). Sperm capacitation and acrosome reaction may be altered by the presence of ASAs on spermatozoa (192). One study observed that intact acrosomes were significantly diminished in men with sperm autoimmunity, especially with cytotoxic and IgA antibodies in seminal plasma. The investigators hypothesized that the increased exposure to acrosome membrane antigens may lead to immunologic subfecundity (193).

Diminished mucus penetration by sperm with ASAs has been described (194). This was confirmed by indirect immunobead testing using serum from male and female partners of infertile couples (195). However, not all couples with serum ASAs demonstrated abnormal mucus penetration. There is evidence to support an elevated presence of ASAs in men who develop testicular cancer, which may explain their predilection for oligospermia and azoospermia (196). Altogether, there is no pathognomonic ASA isotype composition that reliably predicts male factor infertility.

### Clinical Presentation

Presentations of autoimmunity of the male reproductive tract are generally asymptomatic. However, there are occasional reports of acute orchitis thought to be of autoimmune origin (197,198). These have been associated with recurrent episodes of acute scrotal swelling and pain. There may be fever and inguinal lymphadenopathy. Unilateral and bilateral presentations have been described. Most often, there is a history of autoimmune disease in patients presenting with autoimmune orchitis. Orchitis may be the initial presenting complaint for some men who develop multisystem autoimmune diseases. Some cases of autoimmune orchitis may exhibit testicular enlargement first and atrophy thereafter.

Infertility is one the most common presentations of otherwise asymptomatic men presumed to have reproductive impairment from autoimmune sources. Occasionally, men may present with the effects of testicular failure caused by an autoimmune process. These manifestations are often insidious in onset in the postpubertal male and include the effects of androgen deprivation such as diminished sexual hair growth, decreased libido, gynecomastia, osteoporosis, and decreased aggressive behavior. Testes are often less than 15 mL in volume.

## Methods of Assessing Antisperm Antibodies

The first report of an abnormality in a clinical test associated with ASAs was the detection of shaking movements of spermatozoa when allowed to contact cervical mucus (199). Currently, however, documentation that sperm motility abnormalities during postcoital testing predict the presence of ASAs has been inconsistent. Numerous tests have been developed to detect ASAs (200). Autoantibodies to sperm can be detected in seminal plasma and serum in males (145) and in serum and cervical mucus in female partners. The clinical significance of female partner serum and cervical mucus ASAs to infertility is debated (200).

Despite its labor intensity, the immunobead test (IBT) has gained popularity. Advantages of the IBT include its ability to localize the binding sites to head, midpiece, or tail and its ability to assess individually the isotypes of the immunoglobulins. It appears that immunoglobulins bound to sperm head most accurately predict the inability of the sperm to fertilize oocytes (187). The IBT can also be used to perform direct and indirect testing, and it reacts with agglutinating and cytotoxic ASAs, unlike the tray agglutination test that screens for agglutinating antibodies only.

## Semen Analysis Parameters Associated with Antisperm Antibodies

Efforts have been made to identify any semen analysis parameters that could predict the presence of ASA. Low sperm concentration, motility, and volume have not consistently been associated with ASAs (145). Abnormal lateral head movement has been associated with ASAs, and it predicted *in vitro* fertilization failure or success in one study (187). Another study by the same group indicated that sperm motility parameters varied not according to antibody localization or isotype but possibly according to the composition of the extracellular media (i.e., seminal plasma, serum, or Tyrode's solution) (201). Cookson et al., in a retrospective multivariate study of routine semen analysis parameters and ASAs, found a general diminution in motility with concentrations of more than 20 million/mL in men who exhibited ASAs. However, these parameters proved to have inadequate positive and negative predictive values to serve as a screening method for ASAs (202). A typical semen analysis profile for samples exposed to ASAs has not been elucidated. However, ASAs should be suspected when sperm agglutination, diminished sperm viability, or low motility are observed.

## Diagnostic Approach

### The Acute Scrotum

When there is an acute, painful presentation, the differential diagnosis should include testicular torsion, trauma, infection, epididymitis, and orchitis. A history of prostatitis and urinary tract infections generally precedes epididymitis. Vasculitis from autoimmune disease may cause inflammation and infarction of testicular tissue. Polyarteritis nodosa and Henoch-Schönlein purpura have been associated with testicular vasculitis. Torsion often presents similarly to autoimmune orchitis with recurrent episodes, fever, and pyuria.

Examination may reveal a tender and often enlarged testicle. The sedimentation rate and complement levels can be helpful when autoimmune vasculitis is suspected. There are no specific serologic markers for autoimmune orchitis, and efforts to diagnose specific known autoimmune diseases should be undertaken. Culturing seminal fluid and urine is important. When there is epididymo-orchitis, urinalysis may reveal pyuria. With an acute scrotal presentation, color-flow Doppler imaging (203) and nuclear imaging generally reveal increased perfusion to the testis and hemiscrotum when there is orchitis, whereas absent flow and ischemic photon deficiency are the rule when there is torsion.

Antigonadal antibodies have been demonstrated by immunohistochemistry to various cells, including Leydig cells (204). However, most testis autoantigens come from the haploid germ cells. The antigens do not develop until puberty after induction of tolerance to self tissue has occurred (154). Unfortunately, circulating specific antigonadal assays are not predictive for a diagnosis of autoimmune orchitis. Likewise, ASA assays are not specific or sensitive markers of autoimmune orchitis. Ultimately, the diagnosis requires testicular biopsy. Tumors, granulomatous disease, vasculitis, infection, and orchitis are differentiated in this manner.

### Infertility

When couples present with infertility, semen analysis should be routine. If orchitis has affected both testicles, there may be oligospermia or azoospermia, depending on the extent of the damage. Fluctuating semen analysis values can be seen in men undergoing concurrent bouts of autoimmune-related orchitis. In this circumstance, multiple-sample cryopreservation would be prudent in anticipation of eventual testicular failure. Although these samples may be suboptimal because of ASAs or pyospermia, the availability of intracytoplasmic sperm injection with its utility for even severe oligospermia dictates consideration of sperm cryopreservation.

When there is azoospermia in men suspected of having had autoimmune orchitis, serum follicle-stimulating hormone (FSH) and total testosterone concentrations are measured. If the values are normal with no evidence of testicular failure, a testicular biopsy can be performed to confirm the diagnosis of orchitis and to determine whether there will be viable, motile sperm sufficient for intracytoplasmic sperm injection (ICSI). Some urologists feel that, when hormonal parameters are normal, a preliminary biopsy is unnecessary and that usable spermatozoa can be anticipated at the time of the actual *in vitro* fertilization with ICSI procedures. Another strategy we prefer is to cryopreserve any spermatozoa obtained at the preliminary biopsy, which are thawed at the time of the *in vitro* fertilization procedure. If adequate spermatozoa are available to proceed with ICSI, a second testicular biopsy is unnecessary.

### Testicular Failure

The diagnosis of postpubertal male hypogonadism usually can be made by the history of autoimmune orchitis with subsequent manifestations of diminished androgens. Testicular volumes tend to be less than 15 mL. Low serum measurements of total testosterone confirm the diagnosis along with elevated FSH determinations. Eventually, as Leydig cell compromise occurs, the luteinizing hormone (LH) level rises as well. Careful consideration should be given to eliminating other causes of primary and secondary hypogonadism, because other causes such as central nervous system lesions can be morbid.

## Therapy

### Acute Autoimmune Orchitis

With acute presentations of testicular pain, initial antibiotic therapy for presumptive bacterial infection is justified while cultures are pending and the remainder of the evaluation is completed. When the biopsy reveals autoimmune vasculitis or orchitis, glucocorticoid therapy generally brings relief rapidly. Glucocorticoid therapy is usually maintained for 6 months for those who respond rapidly.

### Infertility

Treatment of infertility focuses on ASAs. The split ejaculate technique has been used in an attempt to isolate only the most viable and motile first fraction to minimize ASA exposure in the inseminate. Meinertz, however, showed that there were no differences in bound ASAs between fractions 1 or 2 or whole ejaculates from men with ASAs who had undergone vasovasostomy (205).

Various sperm preparations have also been employed in an attempt to remove antibodies attached to spermatozoa. Although there has been some success in altering the distribution of ASA binding, a reliable means of increasing pregnancy rates through intrauterine insemination sperm preparation has not yet been described (206).

The use of the immunosuppressive agent cyclosporin A for 6 months for male infertility associated with ASAs resulted in three eventual conceptions among 9 men who had a mean duration of infertility of 8.3 years. ASA titers, however, did not correlate with the pregnancy outcomes (207).

A number of immunosuppressive glucocorticoid regimens have also been used for infertile men with ASAs (208–212). The regimens have met with mixed results. For instance, cyclic intermediate-dose steroid therapy (20 mg taken orally twice daily on cycle days 1 to 10 and then 10 mg daily days 11 and 12) has resulted in lowered ASA titers in seminal plasma but not serum. Using this regimen, pregnancy rates were significantly higher (cumulative pregnancy rates of 39.4%) when swim-up prepared intrauterine inseminations were used compared with timed intercourse (4.8%) in women undergoing superovulation (213). This concurred with the findings of a previous study using the same steroid regimen (211), but another study of this regimen could not establish a benefit (212). Potential risks of glucocorticoid therapy include osteoporosis, aseptic necrosis of the femoral heads, cataract formation, flushing, peptic ulcers, hypertension, and Cushing's syndrome (214). Side effects with the intermediate-dose protocol appear to be in the range of 3% without serious effects (213), although others have warned that the risks may not justify such therapy (212). The use of a low dose prednisolone program (5 mg orally daily for 3 to 6 months) may be less risky and has been shown to improve sperm motility, hypoosmotic swelling, and possibly pregnancy rates (215).

An innovative treatment approach has been initiated in which magnetized microspheres coated with specific monoclonal antibodies to murine immunoglobulins are incubated with murine antihuman immunoglobulins. The microspheres are then incubated with sperm exposed to ASAs. The microspheres are then separated out magnetically. In theory, only sperm with attached ASA will be culled out, leaving an antibody-free sperm population for insemination. The process, however, has not yielded high proportions of antibody-free spermatozoa (216).

ICSI has been used for men with severe sperm autoimmunity, resulting in the encouraging early findings of normal fertilization and embryo development (217,218). Although limited by the need for expensive gonadotropin oocyte recruitment and oocyte retrieval associated with *in vitro* fertilization, ICSI appears to adequately bypass physicomechanical barriers to fertilization caused by ASAs.

### Testicular Failure

No specific therapy has proven beneficial for reestablishing spermatogenesis in the face of hypogonadism. Testosterone replacement therapy is generally given as intramuscular testosterone cypionate or enanthate (200 mg every 2 weeks). This base dose has been satisfactory for most men. Scrotal transdermal patches became available for testosterone replacement, and subcutaneous implants and sublingual tablets are under development.

## Summary

As reviewed by Tung (219), establishment of autoimmunity for all organ-specific conditions involves a T-cell response to the target self peptide antigen, demonstration of histopathology of the organ, serum autoantibodies to the organ, and binding of specific autoantibodies to the target antigens permitting the possibility of alteration of the physiologic function of the organ. In men, these conditions have not been completely demonstrated. An argument for an autoimmune origin of orchitis is its association with systemic autoimmunity (197) or syndromes marked by autoimmunity of other endocrine organs (220). A case history has also been reported in which ASAs were linked to infertility and a polyglandular autoimmune syndrome (221). Unfortunately, the molecular genetics of autoimmune orchitis have not been delineated in the human.

Circumstantial associations have been reported in an attempt to link serum autoantibodies to male autoimmune reproductive problems. One study found a correlation between ASAs and some other autoimmune antibodies—antithyroglobulin, thyroid peroxidase, and antinuclear antibodies—indicating at least the possibility of a more global autoimmune process (222). Likewise, El-Roeiy et al. examined an autoimmune panel (IgG, IgM, and IgA) of seven phospholipids, four histone subfractions, four polynucleotides, and total immunoglobulin levels in conjunction with ASAs. They concluded that there may be a cross-reactivity between ASAs and other autoantibodies (especially antiphospholipid antibodies). They further speculated that this may represent polyclonal B-cell activation mimicking some other autoimmune diseases (223). Others were unable to find an association between ASAs and antiphospholipid antibodies or HLA tissue typing (224).

Autoimmune orchitis of the testis can be produced experimentally by a number of models in animals. The induced lesions exhibit inflammatory infiltrates, including immune complexes and granulomas within the testis, epididymis, and vas deferens. Similar lesions have been described in infertile men, suggesting the possibility of human autoimmune orchitis (169). However, a T-cell response in humans, specific serum autoantibodies, and their relevant binding to testis antigens have yet to be documented conclusively. Serum antibodies to sperm antigens and direct binding to spermatozoa has been substantiated with possible effects on alteration of sperm function, but the role of autoantibodies in orchitis is unknown. The presence of ASAs does not contribute to the diagnosis of orchitis, nor does the histologic diagnosis of orchitis mean there will be ASAs. An orchitogenic antigen remains to be documented and immune complexes containing such testicular autoantigens in the presence of a testicular inflammatory response will be required before a convincing case for autoimmune orchitis can be established. Definitive evidence of autoimmune orchitis will require the identification of immune complexes containing testicular autoantigens along with the presence of an inflammatory response.

## PREMATURE OVARIAN FAILURE

### Approach to the Patient

Premature ovarian failure (POF) is defined as a clinical condition of ovarian compromise leading to the elevation of gonadotropins, amenorrhea, and hypoestrogenism before the age of 40. It occurs in approximately 1% of women (226). Known causes include genetic sources such as Turner's syndrome, irradiation and chemotherapy, ovarian trauma and surgery, enzyme deficiencies precluding appropriate steroidogenesis, galactosemia, cell signaling defects, and idiopathic sources. Autoimmunity has also convincingly been shown to be a cause of some cases of POF when associated with Addison's disease and autoimmune polyglandular syndrome (APS) or when there are documented gonadotropin autoantibodies associated with myasthenia gravis (227–232). An autoimmune cause has also been suspected in up to 20% of idiopathic cases of POF (233).

Evidence indicating a role of autoimmunity in otherwise unexplained (idiopathic) POF includes the finding of increased proportions of antiovarian antibodies (AOAs) compared with controls, as well as reports of ovarian leukocyte infiltration and perhaps altered subsets of T cells. Others have observed waxing and waning or even the spontaneous recovery of ovarian function as an indicator of possible autoimmune involvement in the condition (234–235). Perhaps the strongest evidence of an autoimmune cause for some women with POF is its association with other organ-specific autoimmune disorders (236–239). Humoral and cellular and genetic autoimmune mechanisms have been proposed as well (237,240–243), but a distinct mechanism has not been elucidated.

### Clinical Presentation

Generally, women with POF have experienced a normal age at menarche with normal menstrual periods thereafter (236). Approximately two thirds of these women manifest POF between the ages of 26 to 34 (238). Approximately 4% of women with POF have a family history of the disease (244–246). Of women with primary amenorrhea, 10% to 28% have POF, whereas 4% to 18% of women with secondary amenorrhea are found to have POF (247).

Secondary amenorrhea is the most common presentation, but other women with POF may present first with infertility, oligomenorrhea, or vasomotor symptoms (in about one half). Cases of POF have also been described that were first brought to medical attention because of the sequelae of cystic enlargement of the ovaries, possibly caused by the elevated gonadotropins of POF and subsequent asynchronous follicular development (248,249). This increases the chance that POF may manifest with ovarian torsion and dysfunctional uterine bleeding, presumably because of disordered folliculogenesis with resultant aberrant sex steroid secretion (238). Other cases of oophoritis have been incidental histologic findings at the time of oophorectomy (238). Another interesting possible presentation of autoimmune oophoritis reported in one case was amenorrhea associated with a persistent corpus luteum producing luteal-phase progesterone concentrations (250). It seems paradoxical that follicular growth is often seen in women with POF (with hypoestrogenemia), but one explanation could involve the propensity for T-cell infiltration to affect maturing follicles selectively (241). This could allow some follicular growth, whereas these dysfunctional follicles may be unable to produce adequate estrogen (251).

The manifestations of POF vary widely, and the natural history of the condition remains poorly understood. Although there is a general correlation between the age of menopause of women and their daughters, the same relationship has not yet been documented for women with POF. Fecundity is initially normal for many women who eventually develop POF, but there then appears to be a period of reduced fecundity as the pathologic process begins. The widespread use of basal FSH determinations for women presenting with previously unexplained infertility has shown that approximately 20% demonstrate diminished ovarian reserve. Ultimately, women with POF appear to have smaller than average family sizes (238).

The presence of POF is frequently associated with other autoimmune diseases. Approximately 15% of women with POF have other autoimmune conditions (252), with autoimmune thyroid disease being the most frequent (9% to 14%) (252–254). Other autoimmune conditions reported in association with POF have been rheumatoid arthritis in about 1% and even less frequently, vitiligo, insulin-dependent diabetes mellitus, systemic lupus erythematosus, Crohn's disease, and myasthenia gravis.

Only about 2% of women with POF develop idiopathic Addison's disease apart from the autoimmune polyglandular syndromes seen in approximately 3% of POF patients. However, in one study of 50 women with POF, 18% had associated Addison's disease (239). It is known that POF can be present before the development of Addison's disease and *vice versa* (239). Typically, Addison's disease manifests several years after POF but has been reported as late as 14 years after the diagnosis of POF (255).

Even adhering to a strict definition for POF, an occasional woman ovulates and conceives (256). Spontaneous resumption of follicular activity and pregnancies in POF patients may be most common in women suspected of an autoimmune source, although the frequency of resumption of follicular activity is low and unpredictable (247,254,257). One report indicated that as many as 10% of women may go on to conceive even after the diagnosis of POF is made (246).

## Postulated Mechanisms of Autoimmune Premature Ovarian Failure

There has been concern that advanced reproductive technologies could lead to the induction of pathogenic antiovarian antibodies by the associated hormonal stimulation (258) or by enhanced presentation of ovarian antigens to the immune system by the physical trauma of follicular aspiration (259,260). However, convincing evidence for this hypothesis has been lacking (261,262). Even if trauma induces AOAs, the antibodies may not be etiologic for POF. The fact that numerous women with POF have not been found to have serum AOAs argues that such antibodies may not be necessary to initiate the pathologic process.

Antibodies are, however, critical in the pathogenesis of POF associated with the autoimmune polyglandular syndromes involving Addison's disease. Originally, a group of antibodies were detected in patients with autoimmune Addison's disease that cross-reacted with other steroid-producing organs such as ovary, testis, and placenta and were called steroid cell antibodies (SCAs). In a specific subset of women with POF, those with APS type 1 (characterized by autoimmune adrenal insufficiency, chronic hypoparathyroidism, and chronic candidiasis usually manifesting in childhood), the target antigens have been identified to be 17α-hydroxylase and side-chain cleavage enzyme (254). Both are essential enzymes in the steroidogenic pathway and are the specific targets of the SCAs. These antibodies represent adequate markers of autoimmune POF, especially when there is adrenal insufficiency in common with POF, and approximately 60% to 80% have SCAs (239). The concomitant presence of SCAs and POF has not always been identified such that the presence of SCAs may precede the onset of clinical POF or be an epiphenomenon of POF. Type II APS involves Addison's disease, thyroid autoimmune disease, or insulin-dependent diabetes mellitus and arises mainly in women in their fourth decade of life. Between 5% and 10% of such women are affected by POF (228), whereas 58% of women with type 1 APS have POF (263). SCAs have been detected in 20% to 40% of patients with the type II APS (232).

A case for a cell-mediated immune mechanism in the cause of idiopathic POF has been made. In murine models, helper T cells specific for the zona pellucida 3 protein can induce oophoritis when transferred to recipients (240), whereas antizona pellucida antibodies alone do not initiate oophoritis (264). Rabinowe et al. (237) described increased peripheral T-cell activation in women with POF, as evidenced by an increase in the T-cell subset HLA-DR (Ia+). Low circulating estrogen, however, may lead in part to this observation (265). Another study supported a cellular mechanism by showing increased secretion of leukocyte migration inhibitory factor from the peripheral lymphocytes of some women with POF on exposure to crude ovarian protein preparations (266). Moreover, these researchers found lower than normal proportions of NK cells, presenting the possibility that B cells could proliferate in a relatively unchecked manner and potentially produce AOA. One study (267) found increased numbers of B cells in women with POF that appeared to correlate with the presence of autoantibodies. However, this finding has not been corroborated (268). The literature also has no consensus regarding alterations of the helper-suppressor T-cell ratio in POF to further advance a role for cellular autoimmunity (267,269).

Hill et al. found evidence that there may be ectopic expression of MHC class II antigen expression from the granulosa cells of some women with POF (243). This response can be enhanced by the addition of IFN-γ to granulosa cells in culture. Ovarian lymphocytes recruited in response to viral infection could therefore in theory induce abnormal HLA-DR expression on granulosa cells. These autoantigens, when presented to helper T lymphocytes, could play a role in initiating autoimmune responses involved in POF (270). Because it has also been demonstrated that the use of FSH and human chorionic gonadotropin *in vitro* can synergize with IFN-γ within the ovary to enhance HLA-DR antigen expression, there was theoretical concern that the use of gonadotropins in women with autoimmune POF may exacerbate the condition (270). This concern did not materialize in a study of neonatal thymectomized mice treated with gonadotropin stimulation (271) and has not been reported in studies of human ovulation induction in women with POF.

Postthymectomy autoimmune oophoritis in certain mouse strains shares similar histologic appearance and immune characteristics to its human counterpart and may manifest a model to help decipher the autoimmune mechanisms in the future (272,273). A possible human counterpart is the condition of ataxia-telangiectasia, which is associated with thymic aplasia or hypoplasia, POF, and ovarian fibrosis (274). However, in general, other conditions used to establish POF in animal models do not share similarities with clinical POF in humans. The one known mechanism of autoimmune POF involves steroid cell antibodies, but other potential autoimmune mechanisms will require more substantiation.

## Diagnostic Approach

### Physical Examination

Although variable, POF usually has signs of hypoestrogenism such as atrophic vaginitis and a paucity of cervical mucus. The ovaries of women with long-standing POF on average tend to be smaller than age-matched controls, but ovaries enlarged because of dysfunctional follicular cysts are common at presentation in about 50% of young women with POF (238). Oophoritis and steroidogenic enzyme deficiencies can also present with ovarian enlargement. A concerted effort should also be made to identify signs of associated endocrinopathies such as goiter, skin pigmentation abnormalities, and malar rash.

### Laboratory Evaluation

#### Hormonal Assessment

Even before the clinical criteria for POF are met, an elevated basal FSH level in regularly cycling women with serum estradiol, LH, and progesterone concentrations in the normal ranges may presage early POF (275). The FSH-LH ratio tends to be elevated early in the course. Before a diagnosis is confirmed, multiple measurements should be obtained before the diagnosis is proposed. It is wise to require FSH concentrations in excess of 40 IU/L before acknowledging this important diagnosis. Bannatyne et al. reported some cases of women with normal serum FSH measurements despite histologic confirmation of ovarian leukocyte infiltration consistent with an autoimmune oophoritis (238). Low estradiol concentrations are not necessary to make the diagnosis of POF in the face of elevated FSH concentrations.

#### Histologic Evidence of Autoimmune Oophoritis

Full-thickness ovarian biopsy has been considered the definitive method of confirming a diagnosis of POF. Technically, the diagnosis depends on finding the absence of follicles, whereas the presence of primordial and immature follicles constitutes the resistant ovary syndrome (247,276). However, a uniformly agreed on histologic definition has not been formulated for autoimmune POF. Accepted histologic features for POF have differed, but there are some common features in the literature, including the preservation of primordial follicles (238,241).

Bannatyne et al. reported 12 cases in which various stages of autoimmune oophoritis were confirmed histologically, although clinical POF or antiovarian antibodies were not necessarily present. Eleven of the cases had lymphoplasmacytic infiltrates. In all cases, primordial follicles were spared, but infiltration of follicular structures increased in intensity with progressive maturation through the corpus luteum stage. Although the investigators designated a case as autoimmune when there was evidence of a folliculotropic inflammation, they also observed the frequent inflammatory involvement of extrafollicular structures (i.e., hilar or medullary, perivascular, and perineural). One fourth of the cases displayed "follicular dysplasia," and one case exhibited granulomatous oophoritis. The investigators called for early ovarian biopsy and tissue antibody evaluation in women suspected of having POF with the hope that timely diagnosis and intervention may prove beneficial (238).

However, histologic evidence of autoimmune oophoritis is infrequent in idiopathic POF. By 1991, Tung and Lu identified only 29 cumulative cases in the literature, and many also had Addison's disease (277). Ovarian biopsy is invasive, is expensive, and poses a risk for periovarian adhesion formation. Laparoscopic ovarian biopsies tend to be inadequate, but even when there is a full-thickness biopsy obtained at laparotomy, the absence of detectable follicles does not guarantee the cessation of ovulation and fertility. The routine deployment of ovarian biopsy in women with POF is also not indicated, because even the detection of an apparent autoimmune oophoritis it not clinically helpful because there are no validated, reliable treatments for those desiring childbearing. Hoek et al. make the argument that, because of its rarity, even the finding of lymphocytic oophoritis in women with POF (without concomitant adrenal autoimmunity) does not support an autoimmune pathogenesis of POF (254). The diagnosis of POF needs to be made on a clinical rather than a histologic basis.

### Antiovarian Autoantibodies

There have been numerous efforts attempting to characterize antiovarian antibodies as potential markers or etiologic agents for POF. Antibodies against various components of the ovary have been sought including gonadotropin receptors, steroid-producing cells, steroidogenic enzymes, ova, and thecal, interstitial, and granulosa cells and corpora lutea (230,238,240,278–284). Among AOA-positive POF subjects, consistent specific ovarian antigens have not been discovered (252,283).

Two general classes of AOAs are recognized. The first are the steroid cell antibodies discussed in relation with the autoimmune polyglandular syndromes known to be causes of autoimmune POF. The second category of antibodies are less specific, representing nonsteroid cell antibodies. High proportions of women with POF have been found to have these serum AOAs by ELISA (285,286), but the ELISAs used have cross-reacted to a high degree with fallopian tube antigens, and there has been a general inability to correlate these antibodies with the cause and clinical course of POF (233, 287,288). For instance, antiovarian antibodies have been isolated in women with known iatrogenic causes of POF and in women with 45,X gonadal dysgenesis (233).

Overall, there has been tremendous variability in identifying antiovarian antibodies. Efforts have been confounded by various assays, cutoffs, antigens, antibodies, subject populations, and the lack of controls for such potentially confounding variables as menstrual cycle timing of sample collections and subject ages. This has been particularly true for non-SCA antiovarian antibodies.

Several basic techniques have been used to identify AOAs. The most common techniques have been immunofluorescence, and ELISA. Wide ranges of antibody positivity have been reported especially with immunofluorescence. A direct comparison of the two methods among the same patient populations revealed a poor correlation (288). Further evaluation by immunoblotting revealed the lack of common binding patterns (288). Both of these findings cast doubt on the specificity of AOA as markers for autoimmune POF.

Commercially available kits have not been consistent in identifying AOAs (289). Some assays for antiovarian antibodies continue to hold promise (262) to yield a clinically useful marker for the diagnosis of POF.

Although there is general overlap between the finding of AOAs with other potential markers of autoimmune POF, including HLA typing, nonovarian autoantibodies, and associated autoimmune disease, clear-cut relationships have not been elaborated. The duration of amenorrhea and a history of previous physical trauma have not been well correlated with AOAs (262). The finding of AOAs can be evanescent over time and does not appear to adequately reflect disease activity (232,239,269,286). The clinical significance of positive AOA measurements remain unknown (254,286), and the routine measurement of AOAs for idiopathic POF is not indicated.

### Nonovarian Autoantibodies

Blumenfeld et al. proposed that the finding of some nonovarian autoantibodies and abnormal complement levels can isolate candidates among women with POF for the use of ovulation induction (289). Confirmation through clinical trials is needed. Moreover, other investigations of panels of nonspecific autoantibodies and their markers have not consistently identified a reliable marker for autoimmune-induced POF (239,266,287).

## HLA Typing

Although known autoimmune endocrinopathies have been associated with specific HLA-DR haplotypes, none has been definitively associated with POF (290,291).

## Ultrasound Detection of Ovarian Follicles

Follicular activity in women with clinical POF has been documented in more than 40% of 65 women with karyotypically normal POF by ultrasound (292,293). In a different study, 50% of women diagnosed with POF had evidence of follicular function (i.e., serum estradiol of more than 50 pg/mL), and 16% showed evidence of ovulation (i.e., serum progesterone of more than 3 ng/mL) spontaneously during a median of 4 months of observation (256). However, biopsies of antral follicles indicated that more than one half were inappropriately luteinized Graafian follicles, which may contribute to why pregnancies are seen only rarely. This may help explain why ultrasonographic follicular assessment has not proved predictive of future pregnancies. Like AOAs, routine ultrasound screening for POF is not diagnostic and does not change clinical management.

## Recommended Laboratory Evaluation for Premature Ovarian Failure

One comprehensive autoimmune evaluation has been recommended by one group for idiopathic POF that includes AOAs, anti-FSH/LH receptors antibodies, HLA haplotyping, and cell-mediated immunologic assessments against gonadal tissue (239). Unfortunately, most of these tests, while they would add to the suspicion of autoimmune POF, are not routinely available, are expensive, and have not yet demonstrated diagnostic, prognostic, or therapeutic utility. These tests are not recommended routinely for idiopathic POF.

In a study of 119 karyotypically normal women with POF, a panel of screening tests for associated autoimmune conditions demonstrated that screening for hypothyroidism and diabetes with TSH, free thyroxine, and fasting serum glucose levels were worthwhile. Other testing for pernicious anemia, hypoparathyroidism, and adrenal insufficiency can be deferred until clinically indicated (294).

Suggested laboratory evaluation for POF includes

- Serial gonadotropin measurements
- Complete blood cell count and urinalysis
- Karyotyping (the finding of Y chromosome dictates prophylactic gonadectomy)
- Nonspecific autoimmunity screens: sedimentation rate, rheumatoid factor, and antinuclear antibody titer
- Levels of TSH, free thyroxine, and fasting serum glucose
- Screens for associated endocrinopathies as indicated: antithyroid antibodies, ACTH stimulation testing, and an electrolyte panel for suspected Addison's disease

An autoimmune basis for POF should be suspected clinically in women having normal chromosomes whose POF is accompanied by the history of other autoimmune findings (e.g., thyroid disease, vitiligo, adrenal insufficiency, hypoparathyroidism, pernicious anemia, rheumatoid arthritis, a strong family history of autoimmune disorders). Bear in mind that even cases of POF in women with these associated autoimmune conditions may not necessarily demonstrate AOA positivity or histologic evidence of ovarian lymphocyte infiltration (295). There remain no recommended specific tests for suspected autoimmune POF with the exception of steroid cell antibodies in women with POF associated with Addison's disease.

In reviewing the modified Witebsky criteria for a possible autoimmune cause for POF as defined by Rose and Bona (296), Wheatcroft and Weetman (252) found that only one of eight criteria is completely fulfilled. There is an association with other autoimmune diseases in the same individual or family. Autoimmune POF is unlikely to comprise a large proportion of ideopathic cases, and this helps to justify withholding routine, extensive autoimmune testing for women with idiopathic POF.

## Therapy

Treatment takes into account whether a woman affected by POF desires childbearing. If not, hormone replacement therapy is indicated to diminish the risks of osteoporosis and cardiovascular disease and to ameliorate any vasomotor symptoms.

A reliable, reproducible, noninvasive, and practical method of ascertaining autoimmune-associated POF is needed before therapeutic measures can be rigorously studied or instituted. Nonetheless, empiric fertility treatments have been reported for idiopathic POF.

### Hormone Replacement Therapy

Alper found that 6 (7.5%) of a cohort of 80 women with POF conceived (235). Two conceived spontaneously, 2 were on conjugated estrogens, and the other 2 were on oral contraceptives. Whereas many of the reported pregnancies in POF have been associated with the use of estrogen therapy, there is no compelling evidence that the hormone replacement is therapeutic regarding pregnancy. Most women with POF are necessarily prescribed hormone replacement and the reported conceptions appear to be coincidental.

### Suppression of Ovarian Activity

Following the report of a pregnancy in a woman with POF after she had used oral contraceptives (297), Nelson and Merriam postulated that oral contraceptives could reduce granulosa-theca cell activity, which may reduce the presence of trigger antigens (251). This could allow remission of the autoimmune response. Unfortunately, a clinical trial using gonadotropin-releasing hormone agonist suppression to achieve the same end in women with POF did not demonstrate a higher pregnancy rate (298).

### Ovulation Induction

One pilot study found that the use of gonadotropin therapy for women suspected of autoimmune POF may have a higher ovulation and subsequent pregnancy rate (299). However, ovulation induction for POF has generally been disappointing. Kim et al. attempted to prime with cyclic estrogen-progestin therapy followed by ovulation induction but achieved no pregnancies among women with primary POF but 9.2% in those with secondary POF (286).

Some have warned that there is a theoretical risk of gonadotropin therapy in women with autoimmune POF. The gonadotropins could potentially increase the risk of ovarian autoantigen formation by synergizing with IFN-γ to induce abnormal HLA-DR autoantigens on granulosa cells, thereby promoting a cellular autoimmune response (270).

### Immunosuppression

The use of immunosuppressive therapy has been associated with the resumption of regular menses and with pregnancies (253,300–303). However, such reports have been uncommon, inconsistent, and uncontrolled so that the routine clinical use of immunosuppressive agents has not been validated. Danazol has been reported to have immunomodulatory and gonadotropin-suppressing effects when used for endometriosis. However, a controlled trial of 800 mg of daily oral danazol for women with spontaneous POF and normal karyotypes failed to demonstrate efficacy in inducing ovulation over estrogen and progestin replacement therapy (304). Little experience with azathioprine or plasmapheresis has been reported (238).

A combination approach featuring gonadotropin-releasing hormone agonist, high-dose gonadotropin and corticosteroid therapy resulted in a 40% pregnancy rate within three attempts among 15 infertile women with POF. All 15 women were selected by being positive for at least one of a panel of some 19 nonspecific autoimmune variables (289). Although encouraging, the utility of this approach is difficult to ascertain, because as with other studies of therapy for POF, the true diagnosis of autoimmune POF has been unclear, presenting a large risk for selection bias. Confirmation of a high pregnancy rate using this approach is awaited.

### Ovum and Embryo Donation

Although expensive and emotionally unacceptable to some, the use of donated embryos and ova carry the most promise of overcoming the infertility associated with POF. Success in the 50% range per attempt are realistic, and although not formally reported, it is logical to anticipate that autoimmunity affecting ovarian follicle development should not reduce delivery rates using donated ova or embryos.

### Follow-up

Women with autoimmune POF will be at risk of developing other serious sequelae of autoimmune organ failure, including hypothyroidism and adrenal failure. Because the onset of Addison's disease can be insidious, vigilance is prudent for symptoms of fatigue and weakness, weight loss, nausea, anorexia, abdominal pain, and salt craving. Increased skin pigmentation can also result. Because of the well-defined sequelae of estrogen deficiency (293), appropriate hormone replacement therapy should be emphasized for appropriate candidates, and regular, expectant monitoring should be arranged.

### REFERENCES

1. Vercellini P, Crosignani PG. Epidemiology of endometriosis. In: Brosens IA, Donnez J, eds. *The current status of endometriosis: research and management.* London: Parthenon, 1993:111–130.
2. Koninckx PR, Meuleman C, Demeyere S, et al. Suggestive evidence that pelvic endometriosis is a progressive disease, whereas deeply infiltrating endometriosis is associated with pelvic pain. *Fertil Steril* 1991;55:759–765.
3. Seibel MM. Minimal pelvic endometriosis and infertility. *Semin Reprod Endocrinol* 1985;3:307–311.
4. Marcoux S, Maheux R, Bérubé S, Canadian Collaborative Group on Endometriosis. Laparoscopic surgery in infertile women with minimal or mild endometriosis. *N Engl J Med* 1997;337:217–222.
5. Haney AF, Muscato JJ, Weinberg JB. Peritoneal fluid cell populations in infertility populations. *Fertil Steril* 1981;35:696–698.
6. Badawy SZA, Cuenca V, Marshall L, et al. Cellular components in peritoneal fluid in infertile patients with and without endometriosis. *Fertil Steril* 1984;42:704–708.
7. DeLeon FD, Vijayakumar R, Brown M, et al. Peritoneal fluid volume, estrogen, progesterone, prostaglandin and epidermal growth factor concentrations in patients with and without endometriosis. *Obstet Gynecol* 1986;68:189–194.
8. Syrop CH, Halme J. Peritoneal fluid environment and infertility. *Fertil Steril* 1987;48:1–9.
9. Fakih H, Baggett B, Holtz G, et al. Interleukin-1: a possible role in the infertility associated with endometriosis. *Fertil Steril* 1987;47:213–217.
10. Weinberg JB, Haney AF, Xu FJ, et al. Peritoneal fluid and plasma levels of human macrophage colony-stimulating factor in relation to peritoneal fluid macrophage content. *Blood* 1991;78:513–516.
11. Aeby TC, Huang T, Nakayama RT. The effect of peritoneal fluid from patients with endometriosis on human sperm function in vitro. *Am J Obstet Gynecol* 1996;174:1779–1785.
12. Schenken RS. Endometriosis classification for infertility. *Acta Obstet Gynecol Scand* 159:41–44.
13. D'Hooghe TM, Bambra CS, Isahakia M, Koninckx PR. Evolution of spontaneous endometriosis in the baboon *(Papio anubis, Papio cynocephalus)* over a 12 month period. *Fertil Steril* 1992;58:409–412.
14. Evers JLH. Endometriosis does not exist; all women have endometriosis. *Hum Reprod* 1994;9:2206–2208.
15. Koninckx PR, Oosterlynck D, D'Hooghe T, et al. Deeply infiltrating endometriosis is a disease whereas mild endometriosis could be considered a nondisease. *Ann N Y Acad Sci* 1994;734:333–341.
16. Sampson JA. Peritoneal endometriosis due to menstrual dissemination of endometrial tissue into the pelvic cavity. *Am J Obstet Gynecol* 1927;14:422–469.
17. D'Hooghe TM, Bambra CS, Suleman MA, et al. Development of a model of retrograde menstruation in baboons *(Papio anubis).* *Fertil Steril* 1994;62:635–638.
18. Ridley JG, Edwards K. Experimental endometriosis in the human. *Am J Obstet Gynecol* 1985;76:783–789.
19. Noble LS, Simpson ER, Johns A, Bulun SE. Aromatase expression in endometriosis. *J Clin Endocrinol Metab* 1996;81:174–179.
20. Dmowski WP, Radwanska E. Current concepts on pathology, histogenesis and etiology of endometriosis. *Acta Obstet Gynecol Scand* Suppl 1984;(S)123:29–33.
21. Witz CA, Schenken R. Pathogenesis. *Semin Reprod Endocrinol* 1997;15:199–208.
22. Simpson JL. Genes and chromosomes that cause female infertility. *Fertil Steril* 1985;44:725–739.
23. Kennedy S. Is there a genetic basis to endometriosis? *Semin Reprod Endocrinol* 1997;15:309–318.
24. Weed JC, Arquembourg PC. Endometriosis: can it produce an autoimmune response resulting in infertility? *Clin Obstet Gynecol* 1980;23:885–893.
25. Gleicher N, El-Roeiy A, Confino E, Friberg J. Is endometriosis an autoimmune disease? *Obstet Gynecol* 1987;70:115–122.
26. Hill JA. Immunology and endometriosis: Fact, artifact or epiphenomenon? *Obstet Gynecol Clin North Am* 1997;24:291–306.
27. Halme J, Becker S, Haskill S. Altered maturation and function of peritoneal macrophages: possible role in the pathogenesis of endometriosis. *Am J Obstet Gynecol* 1987;156:783–789.
28. Olive DL, Montoya I, Riehl RM, Schenken RS. Macrophage-conditioned media enhance endometrial stromal cell proliferation in vitro. *Am J Obstet Gynecol* 1991;164:953–958.
29. Khorram O, Taylor RN, Ryan IP, Schall TJ, Landers DV. Peritoneal fluid concentrations of the cytokine RANTES correlate with the severity of endometriosis. *Am J Obstet Gynecol* 1993;169:1545–1549.
30. Kauma S, Clark MR, White C, Halme J. Production of fibronectin by peritoneal macrophages and concentration of fibronectin in peritoneal fluid from patients with or without endometriosis. *Obstet Gynecol* 1988;72:13–18.
31. Halme J. Release of tumor necrosis factor-α by human peritoneal macrophages in vivo and in vitro. *Am J Obstet Gynecol* 1989;161:1718–1725.
32. Surrey ES, Halme J. Effect of peritoneal fluid from endometriosis patients on endometrial stomal cell proliferation in vitro. *Obstet Gynecol* 1990;76:792–797.
33. Steele RW, Dmowski WP, Mormer DJ. Immunologic aspects of human endometriosis. *Am J Reprod Immunol* 1984;6:33–36.
34. Dmowski WP, Gebel HM, Braun DP. The role of cell-mediated immunity in pathogenesis of endometriosis. *Acta Obstet Gynecol Scand* Suppl 1994;159:7–14.
35. Gleicher N. The role of humoral immunity in endometriosis. *Acta Obstet Gynecol Scand* Suppl 1994;159:15–17.
36. Kruitwagen RFPM, Poels LG, Willemsen WNP, et al. Endometrial epithelial cells in peritoneal fluid during the early follicular phase. *Fertil Steril* 1991;55:297–303.

37. Chaco KJ, Chacho MS, Andersen PJ, Scommegna A. Peritoneal fluid in patients with and without endometriosis: prostanoids and macrophages and their effect on the sperm penetration assay. *Am J Obstet Gynecol* 1986;154:1290–1299.

38. Meek SC, Hodge DD, Musich JR. Autoimmunity in infertile patients with endometriosis. *Am J Obstet Gynecol* 1988;158:1365–1373.

39. Halme J, Becker S, Hammond MG, Raj S. Pelvic macrophages in normal and infertile women: the role of patent tubes. *Am J Obstet Gynecol* 1982;142:890–895.

40. Rezai N, Ghondgaonkar RB, Zacur HA, et al. Cul-de-sac fluid in women with endometriosis: fluid volume, protein and prostanoid concentration during the periovulatory period—days 13–18. *Fertil Steril* 1987;48:29–32.

41. Halme J, Becker S, Hammond MG, Raj MHG, Raj S. Increased activation of pelvic macrophages in infertile women with mild endometriosis. *Am J Obstet Gynecol* 1983;145:333–337.

42. Halme J, Hammond MG, Hulka JF, et al. Retrograde menstruation in healthy women and in patients with endometriosis. *Obstet Gynecol* 1984;64:151–154.

43. Badawy SZA, Cuenca V, Stitzel A, et al. Autoimmune phenomena in infertile patients with endometriosis. *Obstet Gynecol* 1984;63:271–275.

44. Saiffudin A, Buckley CH, Fox H. Immunoglobulin content of the endometrium in women with endometriosis. *Int J Gynecol Pathol* 1983;2:255–263.

45. Spitzer RE. Immunology and clinical importance of the complement system of man. *Adv Pediatr* 1977;27:43.

46. Bartosik D, Viscarell RR, Damjanow I. Endometriosis as an autoimmune disease. *Fertil Steril* 1984;41:21S.

47. Kreiner D, Gromowitz FB, Richardson DA, Kenigsberg D. Endometrial immunofluorescence associated with endometriosis and pelvic inflammatory disease. *Fertil Steril* 1986;46:243–246.

48. Isaacson KB, Galman M, Coutifaris C, Lyttle CR. Endometrial synthesis and secretion of complement component-3 by patients with and without endometriosis. *Fertil Steril* 1990;836–841.

49. Mathur S, Peress MR, Williamson HO, et al. Autoimmunity to endometrium and ovary in endometriosis. *Clin Exp Immunol* 1982;50:259–266.

50. Fernéndez-Shaw S, Hicks BR, Yudkin PL, et al. Antiendometrial and antiendothelial auto-antibodies in women with endometriosis. *Hum Reprod* 1993;8:310–315.

51. Wild RA Shivers CA. Antiendometrial antibodies in patients with endometriosis. *Am J Reprod Immunol Microbiol* 1985;8:84–86.

52. Chihal HJ, Mathur S, Holtz GL, Williamson HO. An endometrial antibody assay in the clinical diagnosis and management of endometriosis. *Fertil Steril* 1986;46:408–411.

53. Mathur S, Garza DE, Smith LF. Endometrial autoantigens eliciting immunoglobulin (Ig) G, IgA, and IgM responses in endometriosis. *Fertil Steril* 1990;54:56–63.

54. Garza D, Mathur S, Dowd MM, et al. Antigenic differences between the endometrium of *women* with and without endometriosis. *J Reprod Med* 1991;36:177–182.

55. Odukoya OA, Wheatcroft N, Weetman AP, Cooke ID. The prevalence of endometrial immunoglobulin G antibodies in patients with endometriosis. *Hum Reprod* 1995;10:1214–1219.

56. Bartosik D. Immunologic aspects of endometriosis. *Semin Reprod Endocrinol* 1985;3:329–337.

57. Switchenko AC, Kauffman RS, Becker M. Are there antiendometrial antibodies in sera of women with endometriosis? *Fertil Steril* 1991;56:235–241.

58. Wild RA, Shivers CA, Medders D. Detection of antiendometrial antibodies in patients with endometriosis: methodological issues. *Fertil Steril* 1992;58:518–521.

59. Kennedy SH, Sargent IL, Starkey PM, et al. Localization of antiendometrial antibody binding in women with endometriosis using a double-labelling immunohistochemical method. *Br J Obstet Gynaecol* 1990;97:671–674.

60. Kennedy SH, Starkey PM, Sargent IL, et al. Antiendometrial antibodies in endometriosis measured by an enzyme-linked immunosorbent assay before and after treatment with danazol and nafarelin. *Obstet Gynecol* 1990;75:914–918.

61. Mathur S, Chihall HJ, Homm RJ, et al. Endometrial antigens involved in the autoimmunity of endometriosis. *Fertil Steril* 1988;50:860–863.

62. Kennedy SH, Nunn B, Cederholm-Williams SA, Barlow DH. Cardiolipin antibody levels in endometriosis and systemic lupus erythematosus. *Fertil Steril* 1989;52:1061–1062.

63. Taylor PV, Maloney MD, Campbell JM, et al. Autoreactivity in women with endometriosis. *Br J Obstet Gynaecol* 1991;98:680–684.

64. Confino E, Harlow L, Gleicher N. Peritoneal fluid and serum autoantibody levels in patients with endometriosis. *Fertil Steril* 1990;53:242–245.

65. Roitt I. *Essential immunology.* Malden, MA: Blackwell Scientific Publications, 1997.

66. Grimes DA, Lebolt SC, Grimes KR, Wingo PA. Systemic lupus erythematosus and reproductive function: a case control study. *Am J Obstet Gynecol* 1985;153:179–186.

67. Yovich JL, Yovich JM, Tuvik AI, et al. In vitro fertilization for endometriosis. *Lancet* 1985;2:723.

68. Wheeler JM, Johnson BM, Malinak LR. The relationship of endometriosis to spontaneous abortion. *Fertil Steril* 1983;39:656–660.

69. Halme J, Mathur S. Local autoimmunity in mild endometriosis. *Int J Fertil* 1987;32:309–311.

70. Dmowski WP, Steele RN, Baker GF. Deficient cellular immunity in endometriosis. *Am J Obstet Gynecol* 1981;141:377–383.

71. Vigano P, Vercellini P, DiBlasio AM, et al. Deficient antiendometrium lymphocyte-mediated cytotoxicity in patients with endometriosis. *Fertil Steril* 1991;56:894–899.

72. Melioli G, Semino C, Semino A, et al. Recombinant interleukin-2 corrects in vitro the immunological defect of endometriosis. Am J Reprod Immunol 1993;30:218–227.

73. Braun DP, Muriana A, Gebel H, et al. Monocyte-mediated enhancement of endometrial cell proliferation in women with endometriosis. *Fertil Steril* 1994;61:78–84.

74. Ota H, Igarashi S, Tanaka T. Expression of gamma delta T cells and adhesion molecules in endometriotic tissue in patients with endometriosis and adenomyosis. *Am J Reprod Immunol* 1996;35:477–482.

75. Gleicher N, Dmowski WP, Siegel I, et al. Lymphocyte subsets in endometriosis. *Obstet Gynecol* 1984;63:463–466.

76. Hill JA, Faris HMP, Schiff I, Anderson DJ. Characterization of leukocyte subpopulations in the peritoneal fluid of women with endometriosis. *Fertil Steril* 1988;50:216–222.

77. Oosterlynck DJ, Cornillie FJ, Waer M, et al. Women with endometriosis show a defect in natural killer activity resulting in a decreased cytotoxicity to autologous endometrium. *Fertil Steril* 1991;56:45–51.

78. Mettler L, Volkow NI, Kulakow VI, et al. Lymphocyte subsets in the endometrium of patients with endometriosis throughout the menstrual cycle. *Am J Reprod Immunol* 1996;36:342–348.

79. Oosterlynck DJ, Meuleman C, Waer M, et al. The natural killer activity of peritoneal fluid lymphocytes is decreased in women with endometriosis. *Fertil Steril* 1992;58:290–295.

80. Garzetti GG, Ciavattini A, Provinciali M, et al. Natural killer cell activity in endometriosis: correlation between serum estradiol levels and cytotoxicity. *Obstet Gynecol* 1993;81:665–668.

81. Kanzaki H, Sheng-Wang HS, Kariya M, Mori T. Suppression of natural killer cell activity by sera from patients with endometriosis. *Am J Obstet Gynecol* 1992;167:257–261.

82. Tanaka E, Sendo F, Kawagoe S, Hiroe M. Decreased natural killer cell activity in women with endometriosis. *Gynecol Obstet Invest* 1992;34:27–30.

83. Iwasaki K, Makino T, Maruyama T, et al. Leukocyte subpopulations and natural killer activity in endometriosis. *Int J Fertil Menopausal Stud* 1993;38:229–234.

84. D'Hooghe TM, Hill JA. Killer cell activity, statistics, and endometriosis [Letter]. *Fertil Steril* 1995;64:226–228.

85. Olive DL, Haney AF, Weinberg JB. The nature of the intraperitoneal exudate associated with infertility: peritoneal fluid and serum lysozyme activity. *Fertil Steril* 1987;48:802–806.

86. Wilson TJ, Hertzog PJ, Angus D, et al. Decreased natural killer cell activity in endometriosis patients: relationship to disease pathogenesis. *Fertil Steril* 1994;62:1086–1088.

87. Oosterlynck DJ, Meuleman C, Lacquet FA, et al. Flow cytometry analysis of lymphocyte subpopulation in peritoneal fluid of women with endometriosis. *Am J Reprod Immunol* 1994;31:25–31.

88. Hirata J, Kikuchi Y, Imaizumi E, et al. Endometriotic tissues produce immunosuppressive factors. *Gynecol Obstet Invest* 1994;37:43–47.

89. Ho H-N, Chao K-H, Chen H-F, et al. Peritoneal natural killer cytotoxicity and CD25$^+$CD3$^+$ lymphocyte subpopulation are decreased in

women with stage III–IV endometriosis. *Hum Reprod* 1995;10: 2671–2675.

90. D'Hooghe TM, Scheerlinck J-PY, Koninckx PR, et al. Anti-endometrial lymphocytotoxicity and natural killer cell activity in baboons (*Papio anubis* and *Papio cynocephalus*) with endometriosis. *Hum Reprod* 1995;10:558–562.

91. Brinton LA, Gridley G, Persson I, et al. Cancer risk after a hospital discharge diagnosis of endometriosis. *Am J Obstet Gynecol* 1997;176: 572–579.

92. Semino C, Semino A, Pietra G, et al. Role of major histocompatibility complex class I expression and natural killer-like T cells in the genetic control of endometriosis. *Fertil Steril* 1995;64:909–916.

93. Halme J, Becker S, Wing R. Accentuated cyclic activation of peritoneal macrophages in patients with endometriosis. *Am J Obstet Gynecol* 1984;148:85–90.

94. Fazleabas AT, Khan-Dawood FS, Dawood MJ. Protein, progesterone, and protease inhibitors in uterine and peritoneal fluids of women with endometriosis. *Fertil Steril* 1987;47:218–224.

95. Sharpe-Timms KL, Bruno PL, et al. Immunohistochemical localization of granulocyte-macrophage colony-stimulating factor in matched endometriosis and endometrial tissues. *Am J Obstet Gynecol* 1994;171: 740–745.

96. Akoum A, Lemay A, Brunet C, Hérbert J, Groupe d'Investigation en Gynécologie. Cytokine-induced secretion of monocyte chemotactic protein-1 by human endometriotic cells in culture. *Am J Obstet Gynecol* 1995;172:594–600.

97. Dunselman GAJ, Boukaert PX, Evans JL. The acute-phase response in endometriosis of women. *J Reprod Fertil* 1988;83:803–808.

98. Olive DL, Weinberg JB, Haney AF. Peritoneal macrophages and infertility: the association between cell number and pelvic pathology. *Fertil Steril* 1985;44:772–777.

99. Johnson JV, Rozek MM, Moreno AC, et al. Surgically induced endometriosis does not alter peritoneal factors in the rabbit model. *Fertil Steril* 1991;56:343–348.

100. Giudice LC. Growth factors and growth modulators in human uterine endometrium: their potential relevance to reproductive medicine. *Fertil Steril* 1994;61:1–17.

101. Smith SK. Growth factors in the human endometrium. *Hum Reprod* 1994;9:936–946.

102. Tabibzadeh SS. Human endometrium: an active site of cytokine production and action. *Endocr Rev* 1991;12:272–290.

103. Tabibzadeh S. Cytokines and the hypothalamic-pituitary-ovarian-endometrial axis. *Hum Reprod* 1994;9:947–967.

104. Ryan IP, Tseng JF, Schriock ED, et al. Interleukin-8 concentrations are elevated in peritoneal fluid of women with endometriosis. *Fertil Steril* 1995;63:929–932.

105. Haining RE, Cameron IT, van Papendorp C, et al. Epidermal growth factor in human endometrium: proliferative effects in culture and immunocytochemical localization in normal and endometriotic tissues. *Hum Reprod* 1991;6:1220–1225.

106. Oosterlynck DJ, Meuleman C, Sobis H, et al. Angiogenic activity of peritoneal fluid from women with endometriosis. *Fertil Steril* 1993;59: 778–782.

107. Hammond MG, Oh S-T, Anner J, et al. The effect of growth factors on the proliferation of human endometrial stromal cells in culture. *Am J Obstet Gynecol* 1993;168:1131–1138.

108. Nisolle M, Casanas-Roux F, Anaf V, et al. Morphometric study of the stromal vascularization in peritoneal endometriosis. *Fertil Steril* 1993;59:681–684.

109. Halme J, White C, Kauma S, et al. Peritoneal macrophages from patients with endometriosis release growth factors activity in vitro. *J Clin Endocrinol Metab* 1988;66:1044–1049.

110. Zhang R, Wild RA, Ojago JM. Effect of tumor necrosis factor-α on adhesion of human endometrial stromal cells to peritoneal mesothelial cells: an in vitro system. *Fertil Steril* 1993;59:1196–1201.

111. Melega C, Balducci M, Bulletti C, et al. Tissue factors influencing growth and maintenance of endometriosis. *Ann N Y Acad Sci* 1991; 622:256–265.

112. Chegini N, Rossi MJ, Masterson BJ. Platelet-derived growth factor (PDGF), epidermal growth factor (EGF), and EGF and PDGF β-receptors in human endometrial tissue: localization and in vitro action. *Endocrinology* 1992;130:2373–2385.

113. Koyama N, Matsuura K, Okamura H. Cytokines in the peritoneal fluid of patients with endometriosis. *Int J Gynecol Obstet* 1993;43:45–50.

114. Zarmakoupis PN, Rier SE, Maroulis GB, Becker JL. Inhibition of human endometrial stromal cell proliferation by interleukin 6. *Hum Reprod* 1995;10:2395–2399.

115. Buyalos RP, Funari VA, Azziz R, et al. Elevated interleukin-6 levels in peritoneal fluid of patients with pelvic pathology. *Fertil Steril* 1992;58:302–306.

116. Rier SE, Parsons AK, Becker JL. Altered interleukin-6 production by peritoneal leukocytes from patients with endometriosis. *Fertil Steril* 1994;61:294–299.

117. Rier SE, Zarmakioupis PN, Hu X, Becker JL. Dysregulation of interleukin-6 responses in ectopic endometrial stromal cells: correlation with decreased soluble receptor levels in peritoneal fluid of women with endometriosis. *J Clin Endocrinol Metab* 1995;80:1431–1437.

118. Luster AD. Chemokines-chemotactic cytokines that mediate inflammation. *N Engl J Med* 1998;338:437–445.

119. Rana N, Braun DP, House R, et al. Basal and stimulated secretion of cytokines by peritoneal macrophages in women with endometriosis. *Fertil Steril* 1996;65:925–930.

120. Tabibzadeh SS, Satyaswaroop PG, Rao PN. Antiendometrial epithelial cells in vitro: potential local growth modulatory role in endometriosis. *J Clin Endocrinol Metab* 1988;67:131–132.

121. Klein NA, Pérgola GM, Rao-Tekmal R, et al. Enhanced expression of resident leukocyte interferon-γ mRNA in endometriosis. *Am J Reprod Immunol* 1993;30:74–81.

122. Kligman I, Grifo JA, Withkin SS. Expression of the 60 kDa heat shock protein in peritoneal fluids from women with endometriosis: implications for endometriosis-associated infertility. *Hum Reprod* 1996;11: 2736–2738.

123. Giudice LC, Dsupin BA, Gargosky SE, et al. The insulin-like growth factor system in human peritoneal fluid: its effects on endometrial stromal cells and its potential relevance to endometriosis. *J Clin Endocrinol Metab* 1994;79:1284–1293.

124. Leiva MC, Hasty LA, Lyttle CR. Inflammatory changes of the endometrium in patients with minimal-to-moderate endometriosis. *Fertil Steril* 1994;62:967–972.

125. Braun DP, Gebel H, House R, et al. Spontaneous and induced synthesis of cytokines by peripheral blood monocytes in patients with endometriosis. *Fertil Steril* 1996;65:1125–1129.

126. Rock JA, Hurst BS. Clinical significance of prostanoid concentration in women with endometriosis. *Prog Clin Biol Res* 1990;323:61–80.

127. Keenan JA, Chen TT, Chadwell NL, et al. IL-6 beta, TNF-alpha, and IL-2 in peritoneal fluid and macrophage-conditioned media of women with endometriosis. *Am J Reprod Immunol* 1995;34:381–385.

128. Hill JA. Immunology and endometriosis. *Fertil Steril* 1992;58: 262–264.

129. Simpson JL, Malinak LR, Elias S, et al. HLA associations in endometriosis. *Am J Obstet Gynecol* 1984;148:395–397.

130. Maxwell C, Kilpatrick DC, Haning R, Smith SK. No HLA-DR specificity is associated with endometriosis. *Tissue Antigens* 1989;34: 145–147.

131. Wood DH, Yochmowitz MG, Salmaon YL, et al. Proton irradiation and endometriosis. *Aviat Space Environ Med* 1983;54:718–724.

132. Rier SE, Martin DC, Bowman RE, et al. Endometriosis in rhesus monkeys (*Macaca mulatta*) following chronic exposure to 2,3,7,8-tetrachlorodibenzo-p-dioxin. *Fundam Appl Toxicol* 1993;21:433–441.

133. Fernβndez-Shaw S, Clarke MT, Hicks B, et al. Bone marrow derived cell populations in uterine and ectopic endometrium. *Hum Reprod* 1995;10:2285–2289.

134. Badawy SZ, Cuenca V, Stitzel A, Tice D. Immune rosettes of T and B lymphocytes in infertile women with endometriosis. *J Reprod Med* 1987;32:194–197.

135. D'Hooghe TM, Bambra CS, Raeymaekers BM, et al. The effects of immunosuppression on development and progression of endometriosis in baboons (*Papio anubis*). *Fertil Steril* 1995;64:172–178.

136. Taketani Y, Kuo T-M, Mizuno M. Comparison of cytokine levels and embryo toxicity in peritoneal fluid in infertile women with untreated or treated endometriosis. *Am J Obstet Gynecol* 1992;167:265–270.

137. Simón C, Gómez E, Mir A, et al. Glucocorticoid treatment decreases sera embryotoxicity in endometriosis patients. *Fertil Steril* 1992;58: 284–289.

138. Ho H-N, Wu M, Chao K, et al. Decrease in interferon gamma production and impairment of T-lymphocyte proliferation in peritoneal fluid of women with endometriosis. *Am J Obstet Gynecol* 1996;175: 1236–1241.

139. El-Roeiy A, Dmowski WP, Gleicher N, et al. Danazol but not GnRH agonists suppresses autoantibodies in endometriosis. *Fertil Steril* 1988; 50:864–871.

140. Braun DP, Gebel H, Rotman C, et al. The development of cytotoxicity in peritoneal macrophages from women with endometriosis. *Fertil Steril* 1992;57:1203–1210.

141. Witebsky E. Historical roots of present concepts of immunopathology. In: Grabar P, Miescher P, eds. *Immunopathology.* Basel: Schwabe, 1959.

142. Homm RJ, Mathur S. Autoimmune factors in endometriosis: cause or effect? *Semin Reprod Endocrinol* 1988;6:279–285.

143. Gilmore SM, Aksel S, Hoff C, Peterson RDA. In vitro lymphocyte activity in women with endometriosis—an altered immune response? *Fertil Steril* 1992;58:1148–1152.

144. Rier SE, Yeaman DR. Immune aspects of endometriosis: relevance of the uterine mucosal immune system. *Semin Reprod Endocrinol* 1997;15:209–220.

145. Gubin DA, Dmochowski R, Kutteh WH. Multivariant analysis of men from infertile couples with and without antisperm antibodies. *Am J Reprod Immunol* 1998;39:157–160.

146. Sakamoto Y, Matsumoto T, Mizunoe Y, et al. Testicular injury induces cell-mediated autoimmune response to testis. *J Urol* 1995;153: 1316–1320.

147. Sakamoto Y, Matsumoto T, Kumazawa J. Cell-mediated autoimmune response to testis induced by bilateral testicular injury can be suppressed by cyclosporin A. *J Urol* 1998;159:1735–1740.

148. Suominen JJ. Sympathetic auto-immune orchitis. *Andrologia* 1995;27:213–216.

149. Tung KS, Lu CY. Immunologic basis of reproductive failure. In: Kraus FT, Damjanov I, Kaufman N, eds. *Pathology of reproductive failure.* New York: Williams & Wilkins, 1991:33:308–333.

150. Andrada JA, von der Walde F, Hoschoian JC, et al. Immunological studies in patients with mumps orchitis. *Andrologia* 1977;9:207–215.

151. Shulman A, Shohat B, Gillis D, et al. Mumps orchitis among soldiers: frequency, effect on sperm quality and sperm antibodies. *Fertil Steril* 1992;57:1344–1346.

152. Tung KS, Ellis LE, Childs GV, Dufau M. The dark mink: a model of male infertility. *Endocrinology* 1984;114:922–929.

153. Yule TD, Tung KSK. Experimental autoimmune orchitis induced by testis and sperm antigen-specific T cell clones: an important pathogenic cytokine is tumor necrosis factor. *Endocrinology* 1993;133: 1098–1107.

154. Tung KSK. Regulation of testicular autoimmune disease. In: Desjardins C, Ewing LL, eds. *Cell and molecular biology of the testis.* New York: Oxford University Press, 1993.

155. Head JR, Neaves WB, Billingham RE. Immune privilege in the testis. I. Basic parameters of allograft survival. *Transplantation* 1983;36: 423–431.

156. Ritchie AWS, Hargreave TB, James K, Chisholm GD. Intra-epithelial lymphocytes in the normal epididymis: a mechanism for tolerance to sperm auto-antigens. *Br J Urol* 1984;56:79–83.

157. Pelletier RM, Byers SW. The blood-testis barrier and Sertoli cell junctions: structural considerations. *Microsc Res Tech* 1992;20:3–33.

158. El-Demiry MIM, Hargreave TB, Busuttil A, et al. Lymphocyte subpopulations in the male genital tract. *Br J Urol* 1985;57:769–774.

159. Pollanen P, von Euler M, Soder O. Testicular immunoregulatory factors. *J Reprod Immunol* 1990;18:51–76.

160. El-Demiry MIM, Hargreave TB, Busuttil A, et al. Immunocompetent cells in human testis in health and disease. *Fertil Steril* 1987;48: 470–479.

161. Hedger MP, Qin JX, Roberson DM, de Kretser DM. Intragonadal regulation of immune system functions. *Reprod Fertil Dev* 1990;2: 263–280.

162. De Cesaris P, Filippini A, Cervelli C, et al. Immunosuppressive molecules produced by Sertoli cells cultured in vitro: biological effects on lymphocytes. *Biochem Biophys Res Commun* 1992;186:1639–1646.

163. Taguchi O, Nishizuka Y. Experimental autoimmune orchitis after neonatal thymectomy in the mouse. *Clin Exp Immunol* 1981;46: 425–434.

164. Taguchi O, Nishizuka Y. Self-tolerance and localized autoimmunity: mouse models of autoimmune disease that suggest that tissue-specific suppressor T cells are involved in tolerance. *J Exp Med* 1987;165: 146–156.

165. Sakaguchi N, Sakaguchi S. Causes and mechanism of autoimmune disease: cyclosporin A as a probe for the investigation. *J Invest Dermatol* 1992;98:60S–76S.

166. Mahi-Brown CA, Tung KSK. Activation requirements of donor T cells and host T cell recruitment in adoptive transfer of murine experimental autoimmune orchitis (EAO). *Cell Immunol* 1989;124:368–379.

167. Itoh M, Mukasa A, Tokunaga Y, et al. Suppression of efferent limb of testicular autoimmune response by a regulatory CD4+ T cell line in mice. *Clin Exp Immunol* 1992;87:455–460.

168. Sakaguchi N, Sakaguchi S. Thymus and autoimmunity: capacity of the normal thymus to produce self-reactive T cells and conditions required for their induction of autoimmune disease. *J Exp Med* 1990;172: 537–545.

169. Tung KSK, Teuscher C. Mechanisms of autoimmune disease in the testis and ovary. *Hum Reprod Update* 1995;1:35–50.

170. Pudney JA, Anderson DJ. Organization of immunocompetent cells and their function in the male reproductive tract. In: Griffin PD, Johnson PM, eds. *Local immunity in reproductive tract tissues.* Oxford: Oxford University Press, 1993:131–145.

171. Yule TD, Montoya GD, Russell LD, et al. Autoantigenic germ cells exist outside the blood testis barrier. *J Immunol* 1988;141;1161–1167.

172. Roper RJ, Doerge RW, Call SB, et al. Autoimmune orchitis, epididymitis, and vasitis are immunogenetically distinct lesions. *Am J Pathol* 1998;152:1337–1345.

173. Hendry WF. The significance of antisperm antibodies: measurement and management. *Clin Endocrinol* 1992;36:219–221.

174. Pollanen P, Cooper TG. Immunology of the testicular excurrent ducts. *J Reprod Immunol* 1994;26:167–216.

175. Hendry WF. Clinical significance of unilateral testicular obstruction in subfertile males. *Br J Urol* 1986;58:709–714.

176. Hendry WF, Levison DA, Parkinson MC, et al. Testicular obstruction: clinicopathological studies. *Ann R Coll Surg Engl* 1990;72:396–407.

177. Hinting A, Soebadi DM, Santoso RI. Evaluation of the immunological cause of male infertility. *Andrologia* 1996;28:123–126.

178. Turek PJ, Lipshultz LI. Immunologic infertility. *Urol Clin North Am* 1994;21:447–468.

179. Witkin SS, Jeremias J, Grifo JA, Ledger WJ. Detection of *Chlamydia trachomatis* in semen by the polymerase chain reaction in male members of infertile couples. *Am J Obstet Gynecol* 1993;168:1457–1462.

180. Witkin SS, Kligman I, Bongiovanni AM. Relationship between an asymptomatic male genital tract exposure to *Chlamydia trachomatis* and an autoimmune response to spermatozoa. *Hum Reprod* 1995;10: 2952–2955.

181. Kukadia AN, Ercole CJ, Gleich P, et al. Testicular trauma: potential impact on reproductive function. *J Urol* 1996;156:1643–1646.

182. Isahakia M, Alexander NJ. Vasectomy-induced autoimmunity: antisperm and antinuclear autoimmune monoclonal antibodies. *Am J Reprod Immunol* 1984;5:117–124.

183. Haas GG Jr. Antibody mediated causes of male infertility. *Urol Clin North Am* 1987;14:539–550.

184. Abdel-Latif A, Mathur S, Rust PF, et al. Cytotoxic sperm antibodies inhibit sperm penetration of zona-free hamster eggs. *Fertil Steril* 1986;45:542–649.

185. Mathur S, Mathur RS, Holtz GL, et al. Cytotoxic sperm antibodies and in vitro fertilization of mature oocytes: a preliminary report. *J In Vitro Fert Embryo Transf* 1987;4:177–180.

186. Zouari R, De-Almeida M. Effect of sperm-associated antibodies on human sperm ability to bind to zona pellucida and to penetrate zona-free hamster oocytes. *J Reprod Immunol* 1993;24:175–186.

187. Zouari R, De-Almeida M, Rodrigues D, Jouannet P. Localization of antibodies on spermatozoa and sperm movement characteristics are good predictors of in vitro fertilization success in cases of male autoimmune infertility. *Fertil Steril* 1993;59:606–612.

188. Wolf JP, De-Almeida M, Ducot B, et al. High levels of sperm-associated antibodies impair human sperm-oolemma interaction after subzonal insemination. *Fertil Steril* 1995;63:584–590.

189. Isojima S, Li T, Ashitaka Y. Immunological analysis of sperm immobilizing factor found in sera of women with unexplained sterility. *Am J Obstet Gynecol* 1968;101:677–683.

190. Mathur S, Rosenlund C, Carlton M, et al. Studies on sperm survival and motility in the presence of cytotoxic sperm antibodies. *Am J Reprod Immunol Microbiol* 1988;17:41–47.

191. Naz RJ. Effects of antisperm antibodies on early cleavage of fertilized ova. *Biol Reprod* 1992;46:130–139.

192. Zouari R, De-Almeida M, Feneux D. Effect of sperm-associated antibodies on the dynamics of sperm movement and on the acrosome reaction of human spermatozoa. *J Reprod Immunol* 1992;22:59–72.

193. Harrison S, Hull G, Pillai S. Sperm acrosome status and sperm antibodies in infertility. *J Urol* 1998;159:1554–1558.
194. Haas GG Jr. The inhibitory effect of sperm associated immunoglobulins on cervical mucus penetration. *Fertil Steril* 1986;46:334–337.
195. Busacca M, Fusi F, Brigante C, et al. Evaluation of antisperm antibodies in infertile couples with immunobead test: prevalence and prognostic value. *Acta Eur Fertil* 1989;20:77–82.
196. Guazzieri S, Lembo A, Ferro G, et al. Sperm antibodies and infertility in patients with testicular cancer. *Urology* 1985;26:139–142.
197. Pannek J, Haupt G. Orchitis due to vasculitis in autoimmune diseases. *Scand J Rheumatol* 1997;26:151–154.
198. Teichman JM, Mattrey RF, Demby AM, Schmidt JD. Polyarteritis nodosa presenting as acute orchitis: a case report and review of the literature. *J Urol* 1993;149:1139–1140.
199. Kremer J, Jager S. The sperm-cervical mucus contact test: a preliminary report. *Fertil Steril* 1976;27:335–340.
200. Ohl DA, Naz RK. Infertility due to antisperm antibodies. *Urology* 1995;46:591–602.
201. De Almeida M, Zouari R, Jouannet P, Feneux D. In-vitro effects of anti-sperm antibodies on human sperm movement. *Hum Reprod* 1991;6:405–410.
202. Cookson MS, Witt MA, Kimball KT, et al. Can semen analysis predict the presence of antisperm antibodies in patients with primary infertility? *World J Urol* 1995;13:318–322.
203. Herbener TE. Ultrasound in the assessment of the acute scrotum. *J Clin Ultrasound* 1996;24:405–421.
204. Elder M, Maclaren N, Riley W. Gonadal autoantibodies in patients with hypogonadism and/or Addison's disease. *J Clin Endocrinol Metab* 1981;1137–1142.
205. Meinertz H. Antisperm antibodies in split ejaculates. *Am J Reprod Immunol* 1991;26:110–113.
206. Byrd W, Kutteh WH, Carr BR. Treatment of antibody-associated sperm with media containing high serum content: a prospective trial of fertility involving men with high antisperm antibodies following intrauterine insemination. *Am J Reprod Immunol* 1994;31:84–90.
207. Bouloux PM, Wass JA, Parslow JM, et al. Effect of cyclosporin A in male autoimmune infertility. *Fertil Steril* 1986;46:81–85.
208. Shulman JF, Shulman S. Methylprednisolone treatment of immunologic infertility in the male. *Fertil Steril* 1982;38:591–599.
209. Alexander NJ, Sampson JH, Fulgham DL. Pregnancy rates in patients treated for antisperm antibodies with prednisone. *Int J Fertil* 1983;28:63–67.
210. Haas GG Jr, Manganiello P. A double blind, placebo controlled study of the use of methylprednisolone in infertile men with sperm-associated immunoglobulins. *Fertil Steril* 1987;47:295–301.
211. Hendry WF, Hughes L, Scammel G, et al. Comparison of prednisolone and placebo in subfertile men with antibodies to spermatozoa. *Lancet* 1990;335:85–88.
212. Bals-Pratsch M, Dorn M, Karbowski B, et al. Cyclic corticosteroid immunosuppression is unsuccessful in the treatment of sperm antibody-related male infertility: a controlled study. *Hum Reprod* 1992;7:99–104.
213. Robinson JN, Forman RG, Nicholson SC, et al. A comparison of intrauterine insemination in superovulated cycles to intercourse in couples where the male is receiving steroids for the treatment of autoimmune infertility. *Fertil Steril* 1995;63:1260–1266.
214. Hendry WF. Bilateral aseptic necrosis of femoral heads following intermittent high dose steroid therapy [Letter]. *Fertil Steril* 1982;38:120.
215. Omu AE, al-Qattan F, Abdul Hamada B. Effect of low dose continuous corticosteroid therapy in men with antisperm antibodies on spermatozoal quality and conception rate. *Eur J Obstet Gynecol Reprod Biol* 1996;69:129–134.
216. Vigano P, Fusi FM, Brigante C, et al. Immunomagnetic separation of antibody-labelled from antibody-free human spermatozoa as a treatment for immunologic infertility: a preliminary report. *Andrologia* 1991;23:367–371.
217. Bourne H, Richings N, Harari O, et al. The use of intracytoplasmic sperm injection for the treatment of severe and extreme male infertility. *Reprod Fertil Dev* 1995;7:237–245.
218. Mercan R, Oehninger S, Muasher SJ, et al. Impact of fertilization history and semen parameters on ICSI outcome. *J Assist Reprod Genet* 1998;15:39–45.
219. Tung KS. Elucidation of autoimmune disease mechanism based on testicular and ovarian autoimmune disease models. *Horm Metab Res* 1995;27:539–543.
220. LaBarbra AR, Miller MM, Ober C, Rebar RW. Autoimmune etiology in premature ovarian failure. *Am J Reprod Immunol Microbiol* 1988;16:115–122.
221. Tsatsoulis A, Shalet SM. Antisperm antibodies in the polyglandular autoimmune (PGA) syndrome type I: response to cyclical steroid therapy. *Clin Endocrinol (Oxf)* 1991;35:299–303.
222. Paschke R, Bertelsbeck DS, Tsalimalma K, Nieschlag E. Association of sperm antibodies with other autoantibodies in infertile men. *Am J Reprod Immunol* 1994;32:88–94.
223. El-Roeiy A, Valesnini G, Friberg J, et al. Autoantibodies and common idiotypes in men and women with sperm antibodies. *Am J Obstet Gynecol* 1988;158:596–603.
224. Coulam CB, Stern JJ. Evaluation of immunological infertility. *Am J Reprod Immunol* 1992;27:130-135.
225. Salomon F, Saremaslani P, Jakob M, Hedinger CE. Immune complex orchitis in infertile men: immunoelectron microscopy of abnormal basement membrane structures. *Lab Invest* 1982;47:555–567.
226. Coulam CB, Adamson SC, Annegers JF. Incidence of premature ovarian failure. *Obstet Gynecol* 1986;67:604–606.
227. Irvine WJ, Chan MMW, Scarth L, et al. Immunological aspects of premature ovarian failure associated with idiopathic Addison's disease. *Lancet* 1968;2:883–887.
228. Neufeld M, Maclaren NK, Blizzard RM. Two types of autoimmune Addison's disease associated with different polyglandular autoimmune (PGA) syndromes. *Medicine (Baltimore)* 1981;60:355–362.
229. Elder M, MacLaren N, Riley W. Gonadal autoantibodies in patients with hypogonadism and/or Addison's disease. *J Clin Endocrinol Metab* 1981;52:1137–1142.
230. Kuki S, Morgan RL, Tucci JR. Myasthenia gravis and premature ovarian failure. *Arch Intern Med* 1981;141:1230–1232.
231. Chiauzzi V, Cigorraga S, Escobar ME, et al. Inhibition of follicle-stimulating hormone receptor binding by circulating immunoglobulins. *J Clin Endocrinol Metab* 1982;54:1221–1228.
232. Ahonen P, Miettinen A, Perheentupa J. Adrenal and steroidal cell antibodies in patients with autoimmune polyglandular disease type I and risk of adrenocortical and ovarian failure. *J Clin Endocrinol Metab* 1987;64:494–500.
233. Wheatcroft NJ, Toogood AA, Li TC, Cooke ID, Weetman AP. Detection of antibodies to ovarian antigens in women with premature ovarian failure. *Clin Exp Immunol* 1994 96:122–128.
234. Rebar RW, Erickson GF, Yen SS. Idiopathic premature ovarian failure: clinical and endocrine characteristics. *Fertil Steril* 1982;37:35–41.
235. Alper MM, Jolly EE, Garner PR. Pregnancies after premature ovarian failure. *Obstet Gynecol* 1986;67[Suppl 3]:59S–62S.
236. Alper MM, Garner PR. Premature ovarian failure: its relationship to autoimmune disease. *Obstet Gynecol* 1985;55:27–30.
237. Rabinowe SL, Ravnikar VA, Dib SA, et al. Premature menopause: monoclonal antibody defined T lymphocyte abnormalities and anti-ovarian antibodies. *Fertil Steril* 1989;51:450–454.
238. Bannatyne P, Russell P, Sherman R. Autoimmune oophoritis: a clinicopathologic assessment of 12 cases. *Int J Gynecol Pathol* 1990;9:191–207.
239. Bitterly C, Ross A, Dallas-Pia S, et al. Premature ovarian failure: autoimmunity and natural history. *Clin Endocrinol (Oxf)* 1993;39:35–43.
240. Rhim SH, Millar SE, Robey F, et al. Autoimmune disease of the ovary induced by a ZP3 peptide from the mouse zona pellucida. *J Clin Invest* 1992;89:28–35.
241. Sedmak DD, Hart WR, Tubbs RR. Autoimmune oophoritis a histopathologic study of involved ovaries with immunologic characterization of the mononuclear cell infiltrate. *Int J Gynecol Pathol* 1987;6:73–81.
242. Walfish PG, Gottesman IS, Shewchuk AB, et al. Association of premature ovarian failure with HLA antigens. *Tissue Antigens* 1983;21:168–169.
243. Hill JA, Welch WR, Faris HM, Anderson DJ. Induction of class II major histocompatibility complex antigen expression in human granulosa cells by interferon gamma: a potential mechanism contributing to autoimmune ovarian failure. *Am J Obstet Gynecol* 1990;162:534–540.

244. Mattison DR, Evans MI, Schwimmer WB, et al. Familial premature ovarian failure. *Am J Hum Genet* 1984;36:1341–1348.

245. Krauss CM, Turksoy RN, Atkins L, et al. Familial premature ovarian failure due to an interstitial deletion of the long arm of the X chromosome. *N Engl J Med* 1987;317:125–131.

246. Rebar RW, Connolly HV. Clinical features of young women with hypergonadotropic amenorrhea. *Fertil Steril* 1990;53:804–810.

247. Aiman J, Smentek C. Premature ovarian failure. *Obstet Gynecol* 1985; 66:9–14.

248. Biscotti CV, Hart WR, Lucas JG. Cystic ovarian enlargement resulting from autoimmune oophoritis. *Obstet Gynecol* 1989;74:492–495.

249. Lonsdale RN, Roberts PF, Trowell JE. Autoimmune oophoritis associated with polycystic ovaries. *Histopathology* 1991;19:77–81.

250. Friedman CI, Gurgen-Varol F, Lucas J, Neff J. Persistent progesterone production associated with autoimmune oophoritis. A case report. *J Reprod Med* 1987;32:293–296.

251. Nelson LM, Merriam GR. Premature ovarian failure. *Am J Obstet Gynecol* 1990;3:874–876.

252. Wheatcroft NJ, Weetman AP. Is premature ovarian failure an autoimmune disease? *Autoimmunity* 1997c;25:157–165.

253. LaBarbera AR, Miller MM, Ober C, Rebar RW. Autoimmune etiology in premature ovarian failure. *Am J Reprod Immunol Microbiol* 1988; 16:115–122.

254. Hoek A, Schoemaker J, Drexhage HA. Premature ovarian failure and ovarian autoimmunity. *Endocr Rev* 1997;18:107–134.

255. Turkington RW, Lebovitz HE. Extra-adrenal endocrine deficiencies in Addison's disease. *Am J Med* 1967;43:499–507.

256. Nelson LM, Anasti JN, Kimzey LM, et al. Development of luteinized graafian follicles in patients with karyotypically normal spontaneous premature ovarian failure. *J Clin Endocrinol Metab* 1994;79: 1470–1475.

257. Tan SL, Hague WM, Becker F, Jacobs HS. Autoimmune premature ovarian failure with polyendocrinopathy and spontaneous recovery of ovarian follicular activity. *Fertil Steril* 1986;45:421–424.

258. Moncayo R, Moncayo H, Dapunt O. Immunological risks of IVF [Letter]. *Lancet* 1990;1:180.

259. Barbarino-Monnier P, Gobert B, Guillet-Rosso F, et al. Antiovary antibodies, repeated attempts, and outcome of in vitro fertilization. *Fertil Steril* 1991;56:928–932.

260. Gobert R, Barbarino-Monnier P, Guillet-May F, et al. Antiovary antibodies after attempts at human in vitro fertilization induced by follicular puncture rather than hormonal stimulation. *J Reprod Fertil* 1992;96:213–218.

261. Geva E, Vardinon N, Lessing JB, et al. Organ-specific autoantibodies are possible markers for reproductive failure: a prospective study in an in-vitro fertilization-embryo transfer programme. *Hum Reprod* 1996; 11:1627–1631.

262. Fénichel P, Sosset C, Barbarino-Monnier P, et al. Prevalence, specificity and significance of ovarian antibodies during spontaneous premature ovarian failure. *Hum Reprod* 1997;12:2623–2628.

263. Ahonen P, Koskimies S, Lokki M-L, et al. The expression of autoimmune polyglandular disease type I appears associated with several HLA-A antigens but not with HLA-DR. *J Clin Endocrinol Metab* 1988;66:1151–1157.

264. Lou Y, Ang J, Thai H, et al. A zona pellucida 3 peptide vaccine induces antibodies and reversible infertility without ovarian pathology. *J Immunol* 1995;155:2715–2720.

265. Ho PC, Tang GWK, Lawton JW. Lymphocyte subsets and serum immunoglobulins in patients with premature ovarian failure before and after oestrogen replacement. *Hum Reprod* 1993;8:714–716.

266. Pekonen F, Siegberg R, Makinen T, et al. Immunological disturbances in patients with premature ovarian failure. *Clin Endocrinol* 1986;25: 1–6.

267. Ho PC, Tang WK, Fu KH, et al. Immunologic studies in patients with premature ovarian failure. *Obstet Gynecol* 1988;71:622–626.

268. Hoek A, van Kasteren Y, de Haan-Meulman M, et al. Analysis of peripheral blood lymphocyte subsets, NK cells, and delayed type hypersensitivity skin test in patients with premature ovarian failure. *Am J Reprod Immunol* 1995;33:495–502.

269. Mignot MH, Drexhage HA, Kleingeld M, et al. Premature ovarian failure. II. Considerations of cellular immunity defects. *Eur J Obstet Gynecol Reprod Biol* 1989;30:67–72.

270. Tidey GF, Nelson LM, Phillips TM, Stillman RJ. Gonadotropins enhance HLA-DR antigen expression human human granulosa cells. *Am J Obstet Gynecol* 1992;167:1768–1773.

271. Nair S, Mastorakos G, Raj S, Nelson LM. Murine experimental autoimmune oophoritis develops independently of gonadotropin stimulation and is primarily localized in the stroma and theca. *Am J Reprod Immunol* 1995;34:132–139.

272. Miyake T, Taguchi O, Ikeda H, et al. Acute oocyte loss in experimental autoimmune oophoritis as a possible model of premature ovarian failure. *Am J Obstet Gynecol* 1988;158:186–192.

273. Kalantaridou SN, Nelson LM. Autoimmune premature ovarian failure: of mice and women. *JAMA* 1998;53:18–20.

274. Pallor AS. Ataxia-telangiectasia. *Neurol Clin* 1987;5:447–449.

275. Ahmed NA, Lenton EA, Salt C, Ward AM, Cooke ID. The significance of elevated basal follicle stimulating hormone in regularly menstruating infertile women. *Hum Reprod* 1994;9:245–252.

276. Kinch RAH, Plunkett ER, Smout MS, Carr DH. Primary ovarian failure: a clinicopathological and cytogenetic study. *Am J Obstet Gynecol* 1965;91:630–641.

277. Tung KSK, Lu CY. Immunologic basis of reproductive failure. In: Krans FT, Danijanov I, Kaufman N, eds. *Pathology of reproductive failure.* Baltimore: Williams & Wilkins, 1991:308–333.

278. de Moraes-Ruehsen M, Blizzard RM, Garcia-Bunnuel R, Jones GS. Autoimmunity and ovarian failure. *Am J Obstet Gynecol* 1972;112: 693–703.

279. Sotsiou F, Bottazzo GF, Doniach D. Immunofluorescence studies on autoantibodies to steroid-producing cells and to germline cells in endocrine disease and infertility. *Clin Exp Immunol* 1980;39:97–111.

280. Coulam CB, Kempers RD, Randall RV. Premature ovarian failure: evidence for the autoimmune mechanism. *Fertil Steril* 1981;36:238–240.

281. Tang VW, Faiman C. Premature ovarian failure: a search for circulating factors against gonadotropin receptors. *Am J Obstet Gynecol* 1983;146:816–821.

282. Moncayo H, Moncayo R, Benz R, et al. Ovarian failure and autoimmunity. Detection of autoantibodies directed against both the unoccupied luteinizing hormone/human chorionic gonadotropin receptor and the hormone-receptor complex of bovine corpus luteum. *J Clin Invest* 1989;84:1957–1965.

283. Anasti JN, Flack MR, Froehlich J, Nelson LM. The use of human recombinant gonadotropin receptors to search for immunoglobulin G-mediated premature ovarian failure. *J Clin Endocrinol Metab* 1995;80: 324–328.

284. Chen S, Sawicka J, Bitterly C, et al. Autoantibodies to steroidogenic enzymes in autoimmune polyglandular syndrome, Addison's disease, and premature ovarian failure. *J Clin Endocrinol Metab* 1996;81: 1871–1876.

285. Luborsky JL, Visintin I, Boyers S, et al. Ovarian antibodies detected by immobilized antigen immunoassay in patients with premature ovarian failure. *J Clin Endocrinol Metab* 1990;70:69–75.

286. Kim JG, Moon SY, Chang YS, Lee JY. Autoimmune premature ovarian failure. *J Obstet Gynaecol* 1995;21:59–66.

287. Wheatcroft NJ, Rogeres CA, Metcalfe RA, et al. Is subclinical ovarian failure an autoimmune disease? *Hum Reprod* 1997a;12:244–249.

288. Wheatcroft NJ, Salt C, Milford-Ward A, et al. Identification of ovarian antibodies by immunofluorescence, enzyme-linked immunosorbent assay or immunoblotting in premature ovarian failure. *Hum Reprod* 1997;12:2617–2622.

289. Blumenfeld Z, Halachmi S, Peretz BA, et al. Premature ovarian failure—the prognostic application of autoimmunity on conception after ovulation induction. *Fertil Steril* 1993;59:750–755.

290. Anasti JN, Adams S, Kimzey LM, et al. Karyotypically normal spontaneous premature ovarian failure: evaluation of association with the class II major histocompatibility complex. *J Clin Endocrinol Metab* 1994;78:722–723.

291. Jaroudi KA, Arora M, Sheth KV, et al. Human leukocyte antigen typing and associated abnormalities in premature ovarian failure. *Hum Reprod* 1994;9:2006–2009.

292. Mehta A, Matwijiw I, Lyons EA, Faiman C. Non invasive diagnosis of resistant ovary syndrome by ultrasonography. *Fertil Steril* 1992;57: 56–61.

293. Conway GS, Kaltsas G, Patel A, et al. Characterization of idiopathic premature ovarian failure. *Fertil Steril* 1996;65:337–341.

294. Kim TJ, Anasti JN, Flack MR, et al. Routine endocrine screening for patients with karyotypically normal spontaneous premature ovarian failure. *Obstet Gynecol* 1997;89:777–779.

295. Fox H. Review article: the pathology of premature ovarian failure. *J Pathol* 1992;167:357–363.

296. Rose NR, Bona C. Defining criteria for autoimmune diseases (Witebsky?s postulates revisited). *Immunol Today* 1993;14:426–430.

297. Check JH, Chase JS, Spence M. Pregnancy in premature ovarian failure after therapy with oral contraceptives despite resistance to previous human menopausal gonadotropin therapy. *Am J Obstet Gynecol* 1989;160:114–115.

298. Nelson LM, Kimzey LM, White BJ, Merriam GR. Gonadotropin suppression for the treatment of karyotypically normal spontaneous premature ovarian failure: a controlled trial. *Fertil Steril* 1992;57:50–55.

299. Check JH, Chase JS. Ovulation induction in hypergonadotropic amenorrhea with estrogen and human menopausal gonadotropin therapy. *Fertil Steril* 1984;42:919–922.

300. Rabinowe SL, Berger MJ, Welch WR, Dluhy RG. Lymphocyte dysfunction in autoimmune oophoritis: resumption of menses with corticosteroids. *Am J Med* 1986;81:347–350.

301. Finer N, Fogelman I, Bottazzo GF. Pregnancy in a women with premature ovarian failure. *Postgrad Med J* 1985;61:1079–1080.

302. Cowchock FS, McCabe JL, Montgomery BB. Pregnancy after corticosteroid administration in premature ovarian failure (polyglandular endocrinopathy syndrome). *Am J Obstet Gynecol* 1988;158:118–119.

303. Corenblum B, Rowe T, Taylor PJ. High doses, short term glucocorticoids for the treatment of infertility resulting from premature ovarian failure. *Fertil Steril* 1993;59:988–991.

304. Anasti JN, Kimzey LM, Defensor RA, et al. A controlled study of danazol for the treatment of karyotypically normal spontaneous premature ovarian failure. *Fertil Steril* 1994;62:726–730.

*Textbook of the Autoimmune Diseases,*
Edited by R. G. Lahita, N. Chiorazzi, and W. H. Reeves,
Lippincott Williams & Wilkins, Philadelphia © 2000.

# CHAPTER 24

# Autoimmune Disorders in Otolaryngology

## Robert S. Lebovics

The head and neck include numerous anatomic structures and organs, many of which are targeted in diseases of autoimmunity. This complex anatomy, including that of the ears (with the inner ear complex), nose, and mouth, paranasal sinuses, pharynx, larynx, thyroid gland, and lower aerodigestive tract, functions in a complex mechanism providing for normal homeostasis. Many different autoimmune disorders can secondarily target specific areas within the head and neck in addition to primary disease in various organs.

An understanding of basic anatomy and normal physiology of the multitude of organ systems involved in local immunity is a prerequisite to the diagnosis and treatment of all immunologically mediated disease throughout the head and neck. This chapter considers various target organs, individually and as part of systemic disease, as they produce different disease states.

### WEGENER'S GRANULOMATOSIS

Probably the most common midline destructive disease affecting the head and neck is Wegener's granulomatosis. This disorder is a necrotizing granulomatous vasculitis that classically involves the upper respiratory tract including the nose and paranasal sinuses, followed by involvement of the lungs and kidneys. The hallmark of the disease is a primary small vessel arteritis. Disease that only involves the lungs or sinuses is by definition "limited" Wegener's granulomatosis.

Approximately 90% of the patients with Wegener's granulomatosis have or will have disease within the sinonasal tract. Findings include nasal obstruction, sinusitis, epistaxis, and severe crusting. Pain and secondary infection requiring mechanical debridements with sinus surgery are common in patients with Wegener's granulomatosis. Dacryocystitis can occur, such that patients often require reconstruction of the

R. S. Lebovics: Department of Otolaryngology, Mount Sinai School of Medicine, New York, New York 10027; Department of Surgery, Cabrini Hospital and Medical Center, New York, New York 10003.

lacrimal system to control epiphora and pus within the lacrimal system (1–3).

The nasal septum frequently is destroyed as part of the disease process, and external cosmetic deformities manifested by the so-called saddle-nose deformity are common findings in many patients (Fig. 24.1). Middle ear effusions are also frequent findings and usually result from inflammation in the nasopharynx affecting eustachian tube function. These ears frequently need ventilating tubes to be placed to maintain drainage and aeration.

Approximately 16% of patients with Wegener's granulomatosis develop subglottic stenosis of the larynx. This is manifested by a decreased exercise tolerance, inspiratory stridor, and decreased energy levels. Pulmonary function testing shows a narrowing of the extrathoracic tracheal airway loop. Other pathology includes skin lesions in various sites, while even mucosal lesions of the mouth can occur (1,4).

Histologically, Wegener's granulomatosis is characterized by a necrotizing vasculitis. Multinucleated giant cells, histiocytes, and granulomas are classically seen. However, various infections can also cause tissue necrosis with granuloma formation, but special stains can exclude fungal and acid-fast infections (2–4).

The cause and pathogenesis of Wegener's granulomatosis remain unknown at this time, although several hypotheses have been postulated. It is now believed that the disease is caused by some inhaled particles or allergens that trigger an upper airway inflammatory process in appropriately susceptible individuals. Certain clusters of patients have also been determined to exist, although the epidemiologic reasons for this are unclear.

The cytoplasmic form of antineutrophil cytoplasmic antibody (C-ANCA) is thought to be associated with Wegener's granulomatosis. This antibody is directed against the neutral protein serinase, which is found in the secondary granules of neutrophils. Protinease 3 is a proteolytic enzyme that reacts to C-ANCA. Whether this process is primary or secondary to the vasculitic process is unknown, and the possibility of an epiphenomenon needs to be considered (1).

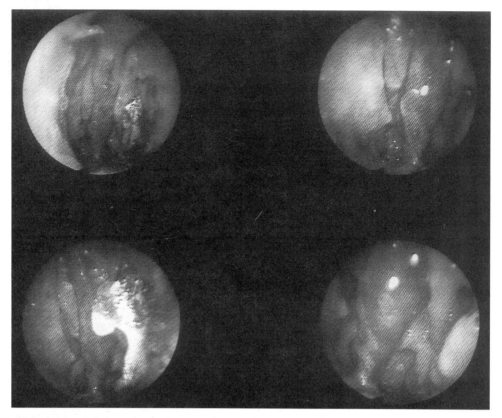

**FIG. 24.1.** Intranasal view of massive septal necrosis and atrophic rhinitis in a patient with Wegener's granulomatosis. See color plate 22.

Treatment in Wegener's granulomatosis is directed at the affected organ systems with systemic immunosuppression. In full-blown disease involving the sinuses, lungs, and kidneys, prednisone, and cyclophosphamide are the mainstays of treatment. In more limited forms of disease, particularly that involving the nose and sinuses only, the possibility of a less toxic medication such methotrexate has been proposed. Other drugs have included azathioprine, interleukin-10, and FK506, and procedures such as plasmapheresis have been advocated in treatment of the disease, with various degrees of success. The use of sulfamethoxazole-trimethoprim has been suggested as treatment for limited disease, although well-controlled studies demonstrating efficacy are not available.

Treatment of Wegener's granulomatosis within the sinonasal tract is usually for symptomatic relief and reestablishment of drainage of tissue severely damaged by mucosal inflammation. Severe crusting requiring mechanical debridements and regular cleaning of the nose is often seen. For patients in remission from their underlying disease, techniques of open rhinoplasty and functional nasal reconstruction exist, with good results obtained. I use only autologous materials and avoid any type of foreign-body prosthesis for the cosmetic repair of the nose.

The laryngeal stenosis associated with Wegener's can be severe and life threatening and often requires tracheotomy (Fig. 24.2). Techniques of open repair and endoscopic submucosal injections of a glucocorticoid have been advocated,

and most patients with tracheotomies can be decannulated successfully (4–7).

Granulomatous vasculitis or Wegener's granulomatosis needs to be differentiated from histologically similar lesions within the nose and oral cavity. Diseases such as the so-called lethal midline granuloma are known as the idiopathic midline destructive diseases and are different from Wegener's granulomatosis. These diseases most likely represent a spectrum of lymphoma, with an angiocentric T-cell type being the most common form of midline destruction. These lesions can be differentiated by immunohistochemistry. Treatment after staging usually requires radiation with or without concomitant chemotherapy.

## SARCOIDOSIS

Sarcoidosis is a disease of unknown cause and is characterized by noncaseating granulomas, particularly in the lungs. This disease is more common among African Americans than Caucasians and frequently occurs in the third or fourth decade of life.

Sarcoid granulomas present in the lungs and commonly occur in the cervical and mediastinal lymph nodes. Systemic symptoms can include weight loss, arthralgias, fevers, and sinus symptoms. Head and neck manifestations occur in approximately 15% of patients, with cervical lymphadenopathy being the most common presentation. Laryngeal dis-

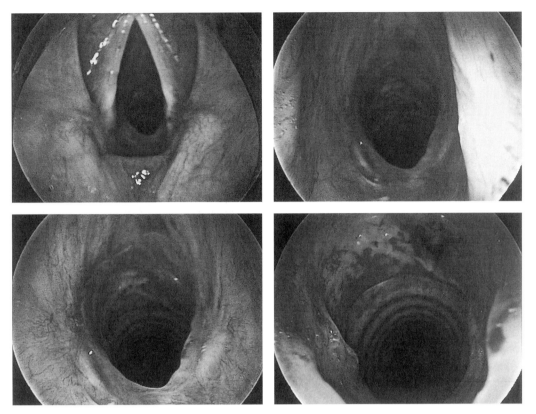

**FIG. 24.2.** Moderate subglottic stenosis without significant inflammation in a 17-year-old girl with Wegener's granulomatosis. See color plate 23.

ease is usually seen in the subglottic space. However, uveitis and lacrimal disease are common findings in sarcoidosis. Parotid swelling and involvement may occur, with or without facial nerve involvement. Sarcoid may also manifest primarily within the nasal cavity on the nasal septum or within the turbinates. The maxillary sinus is frequently a location for active granulomatous inflammation.

The diagnosis of sarcoid includes blood tests demonstrating elevated calcium levels and increased levels of angiotensin-converting enzymes. The hallmark of diagnosis, however, is histologic documentation of noncaseating granulomas. T-cell–mediated cytokine production has been implicated in the cause of sarcoid (8–10).

Sarcoid is usually treatable with oral prednisone. Secondary treatment of disease in the head and neck is directed to affected organ systems, such as exenteration of infected sinuses, debridement and cleaning of obstructed nasal cavities, and ventilating the middle ear space.

## AUTOIMMUNE DEAFNESS

In 1979, Brian McCabe described immunologically mediated mechanisms of hearing loss for the first time (11). Although this occurrence still leaves much to be characterized and defined, immune mechanisms have been shown to contribute to certain cases of sensorineural hearing loss. As part of the clinical evaluation of sensorineural hearing loss, particularly that which is sudden in onset, screening studies of the immune system are in order. The exact antigens involved in autoimmune sensorineural hearing loss are still not defined. However, selected laboratories have isolated inner ear antigens and have developed assays to measure serum antibodies against these inner cochlear antigens (12–15).

In general, it is believed that the inner ear is immunocompetent and that systemic immune disease can produce immune-mediated inner ear disease. However, the natural history of autoimmune inner ear disease is unknown. Immunologic disorders of the inner ear can be separated into those originating within the inner ear or secondary to disorders originating from outside the ear (Table 24.1). Primary inner ear disease can result from autoimmunity or a host defense against infections or tumors. Autoimmune inner ear disease probably exists, although specifics are unclear. Theoretically antibodies to inner ear antigens may react primarily within the cochlea or cross-react with antigens in distant organs (16,17).

Secondary inner ear disease can result from direct or indirect effects of systemic illness. Autoantibodies originating from other organs may cross-react with inner ear antigens, causing an immune complex reaction, with localized inflammation and destruction leading to sensorineural hearing loss (18–21).

**TABLE 24.1.** *Immunologically based ear disease*

| Location | Disease |
|---|---|
| External ear | Relapsing polychondritis |
| | Eczema |
| | Darrier's disease |
| Middle ear | Acute otitis media |
| | Chronic otitis media with effusion |
| | Otosclerosis |
| | Tympanosclerosis |
| Inner ear | |
|   Primary (originates in the inner ear | Ménière's disease |
| | Autoimmune hearing loss (due to inner ear antigens) |
| | Host defense against tumor or infection |
|   Secondary (originates outside the ear and targets inner ear organs) | Behçet's disease |
| | Cogan's syndrome |
| | Vascular insufficiency (secondary to vasculitis) |
| | Immune complexes trapped in stria vascularis |

### Diagnosis of Immune Inner Ear Disease

The clinical features of immune-mediated inner ear disease may help to differentiate it from other disorders. The most common age reported has been in the third to sixth decade, with pediatric cases being relatively uncommon. As with most autoimmune diseases, a female preponderance has been reported for cases of inner ear disease. Whether other autoimmune diseases, such as rheumatoid arthritis or systemic lupus erythematosus, may contribute to inner ear disease is not clear.

Findings in patients usually show that the middle ears and external auditory canals are normal. Exceptions include diseases such as systemic vasculitis (i.e., Wegener's granulomatosis), in which there may be active disease in the middle or inner ear, or diseases such as relapsing polychondritis where the outer ear may be affected.

Probably the other most important issue that is apparent to the clinician is bilaterality. Infections, tumors, trauma, and even localized vascular insults are often unilateral, but immune hearing loss may be bilateral. Audiometric configurations vary; however, pure tone thresholds can produce an upward-sloping or downward-sloping pattern. Symmetric presentations in bilateral disease are common. Speech discrimination testing is often quite poor, and the pattern of hearing loss, particularly in terms of speech discrimination scores, may mimic that seen in syphilis. It is also important to exclude by history any use of ototoxic medications. Vertigo is rare in these patients, and tinnitus does occur occasionally (20,22–25).

### Laboratory Evaluation of Immune Hearing Loss

Laboratory tests generally are divided into two types, those that are antigen specific or antigen nonspecific. Antigen-specific serologic testing uses homologous inner ear tissues that are thought to contain the active antigens and therefore search for cellular or humoral activity as direct evidence of immunoreactivity. Antigen-nonspecific tests do not use inner ear tissues and search for soluble circulating immune complexes as indirect evidence of immune activity.

Antigen-specific cellular immune tests include lymphocyte transformation tests and migration inhibition tests. The underlying assumption is that circulating lymphocytes are activated against the hypothetical inner ear antigens. Antigen-specific humoral immune tests include indirect immunofluorescence, Western blot assays, and enzyme-linked immunoabsorbent assay testing. Antigen-nonspecific tests include cryoprecipitation, complement system autoantibodies (specifically C1q), and rheumatoid factors. The acute-phase reaction components such as erythrocyte sedimentation rate and C-reactive proteins may correlate with disease activity but usually are nonspecific. However, they may have value as a general screening device for autoimmune hearing loss (26,28).

The lymphocyte transformation testing or Western blot assay against specific inner ear antigens is the best way of confirming the diagnosis of autoimmune hearing loss. Because few laboratories have the capabilities of doing these assays, an appropriate site has to be found and sera sent. Most of these laboratories require inclusion of clinical data and audiometric evaluations, and results usually take several weeks to process. The usefulness of the assay in acute situations is therefore minimal.

### Treatment of Autoimmune Hearing Loss

If the clinician suspects an autoimmune cause for hearing loss, empirical treatment with steroids is invaluable. In my experience, cases of autoimmune hearing loss that have been subsequently confirmed with serologic evidence have responded fairly rapidly to glucocorticoids. Pure tone thresholds and speech discrimination scores improve significantly within 3 to 5 days. Doses of prednisone starting in the range of 60 mg per day for 3 to 4 days and rapidly tapered over 10 days may achieve good results. The use of cytotoxic drugs (e.g., cyclophosphamide) is theoretically sound. However, because of the potential for severe complications of such treatment, their use is not recommended except for extreme cases in which there is serologic evidence of an inner ear antibody and an impending otologic catastrophe.

Contraindications to steroids are numerous. Before a physician gives steroids for autoimmune disease of the ear, secondary steps need to be considered. General contraindications include pregnancy, known peptic ulcer disease, a history of tuberculosis, and uncontrolled diabetes. There are many side effects associated with systemic glucocorticoids, the classic ones being increased appetite, weight gain, insomnia, susceptibility to infection, and Cushing's syndrome. Complications of cytotoxic drugs, particularly cyclophosphamide, include marrow suppression, sterility, hemorrhagic cystitis, and bladder carcinoma. There is also an increased risk of lymphoma. Occasionally, methotrexate is given, particularly in younger patients, to limit the long-term effects of drug therapy (29).

As in other autoimmune diseases, plasmapheresis has been proposed and tried, and there are anecdotal reports of success. Plasmapheresis is time consuming and expensive, and not all clinical facilities are equipped to perform this procedure. Blood filtering several times a week for 2 to 4 weeks may have value, but definitive data are not available (30,31).

## Systemic Diseases That May Produce Hearing Loss

There are myriad autoimmune and connective tissue disorders that have associations with sensorineural hearing loss. Many laboratory tests may help differentiate all these conditions. Often, there is a blurring of distinctions. Cogan's syndrome illustrates this problem, because it is a systemic immune disease that involves the inner ear in addition to the eye. Interstitial keratitis is present in addition to severe hearing loss. Cogan's syndrome often responds well to oral glucocorticoids (32).

Other diseases that are known to affect the ear include polyarteritis nodosa and Takayasu's arteritis. Rheumatoid arthritis, systemic lupus erythematosus, relapsing polychondritis, Sjögren's syndrome, and Behçet's disease have all been implicated in producing otologic symptoms. Hematologic disorders such as autoimmune thrombocytopenic purpura and Hashimoto's thyroiditis, ulcerative colitis, sarcoidosis, and Wegener's granulomatosis also have associated otologic symptoms, particularly hearing loss. The latter more commonly result in eustachian tube dysfunction, nasopharyngeal inflammation, or granulomas (33–37).

### Ménière's Disease

Prosper Ménière first described the syndrome that bears his name in 1861. The disorder is characterized by recurring attacks of vertigo, sensorineural hearing loss, and tinnitus. In some patients, a fluctuating sense of fullness in the ear is also present. The syndrome, however, is arbitrarily defined today as fluctuating hearing loss with vertigo or tinnitus in the affected ear. The attacks usually are unpredictable but are superimposed over a general deterioration in the neural hearing base of the involved ear. Generally the lower frequencies are involved initially, and over time the ipsilateral peripheral vestibular system may also become involved.

The pathologic hallmark of this disorder is endolymphatic hydrops, which essentially is an overaccumulation of endolymph within the endolymphatic sac. Temporal bone sections in patients with Ménière's syndrome demonstrate this finding in association with an overaccumulation of fluid that occurs at the expense of the perilymphatic space (38).

### Etiology

The symptoms of fluctuating hearing, tinnitus, and vertigo, associated with aural fullness define Ménière's syndrome. The cause of primary Ménière's disease is unknown. Secondary endolymphatic hydrops can be produced by certain diseases, as exemplified by syphilis. In general, obstruction of the endolymphatic duct is the basis for the development of hydrops in humans and in experimental animals. Similarly, a failure in resorption of endolymph may also cause endolymphatic hydrops. Other causes include chemical fibrosis, viral inflammation, and immunologically induced inflammation.

Special consideration has been given to autoimmune processes as a significant etiologic factor in Ménière's syndrome. The human endolymphatic sac is a primary immunocompetent structure in the inner ear that is capable of processing antigens, stimulating the synthesis of antibodies, and in general raising a cellular immune response. Circulating immune complexes have been found to be increased in patients with Ménière's disease (39). These results have been interpreted as suggesting that a type III immune complex-mediated vascular injury might be responsible for a fibrosis occurring in the endolymphatic sacs of some patients with Ménière's disease. A generalized deposition of IgG complexes has been found in these cases, with data available to suggest that immunoglobulins are deposited directly into the tissues of the endolymphatic sac. Indirect evidence also implicates autoimmunity as a cause in certain cases on the basis of positive responses to systemic glucocorticoid treatment.

Antibodies against a bovine 68-kd heat shock protein are increased in about 50% of patients with Ménière's disease (40). These heat shock proteins can be found in the inner ear. Increases have been observed in response to infection and in patients with autoimmune diseases such as systemic lupus and rheumatoid arthritis. Antibodies to these proteins may develop when an organism with its own similar protein infects a host, indicating that cross-reacting antibodies generated by a host might be the cause of injury to host tissues. Not surprisingly, such antibodies are commonly seen in patients with bilateral Ménière's disease rather than patients with unilateral disease (41).

An autoimmune cause also may be related to the familial and genetic occurrence of disease. Those with Ménière's disease have an increased incidence of specific genetically acquired human leukocyte antigens (HLAs), and some have been linked to nonspecific and otic autoimmune disease formation (42,43).

Viral infection has been implicated as another cause of damage to the endolymphatic duct and sac, resulting in Ménière's disease. Other proposed mechanisms include ischemia of the endolymphatic sac and inner ear. Although numerous factors have been implicated as possible causes of hydrops, the disorder still reflects a continued overall lack of understanding of its cause. This syndrome may be multifactorial and may represent a common anatomic end point to a variety of injuries (44,45).

### Diagnosis

Diagnosis of Ménière's disease is primarily a clinical one and requires a detailed history and careful physical examination. A classic history includes recurrent attacks of vertigo with tinnitus and hearing loss of the affected ear, associated with aural fullness. Attacks may be preceded by an aura that slowly crescendos to a loud roaring tinnitus while the hearing deteriorates. Attacks last from minutes to hours, and the long-term clinical course is highly variable. However, in most patients, vertigo eventually disappears over time, as does the tinnitus. Electronystagmography during acute vertiginous episodes may demonstrate a loss of vestibular function in the hydropic ear.

In the past (but less practical today), dehydrating agents such as glycerol were used as a measure of endolymphatic sac overload. The glycerol test consisted of the administration of a loading dose of glycerin, followed by serial audiograms over several hours. The hypothesis was that in dehydrating the patient, the endolymphatic space would also dehydrate and come into better equilibrium with the perilymph. Positive test results consisted of a statistically significant improvement in pure tone thresholds and speech discrimination scores.

Electrocochleography is probably the most valuable clinical adjunct available to the clinician. A positive test result reflects an increased negative summating potential and is thought to reflect distention of the basilar membrane in the scala tympani (46–50).

### Treatment

There is no uniformly established treatment for Ménière's disease or syndrome. The goals of therapy include control of debilitating vertigo and annoying tinnitus. The reversal of hearing loss, although ideal, is rarely a practical attainable goal. However, the vertigo is generally the most debilitating portion of the disease process.

Medical therapy is directed at the prevention of overloading the endolymphatic space. Treatment may include a low-sodium diet in addition to loop diuretics to help decrease the body's salt content. Glucocorticoids have been given with some success. In the past, carbonic anhydrase inhibitors such as acetazolamide were recommended, but their efficacy has not been established in clinical studies (51–54).

Vasodilating agents have been administered in various studies, although with minimal success. Probably the most important medical treatments are those geared toward the antivertiginous effects. These have included antiemetics, sedatives, and antidepressants, all of which have all been used with various degrees of success. Meclizine is often given as a nonsedating antihistamine that works by suppressing the vestibular system (51,53).

Surgical treatment in Ménière's syndrome is generally reserved for patients who have failed medical management and persist in having severe debilitating symptoms. The most popular procedure is the endolymphatic sac decompression. This has numerous variations, but all work on the basic principle of drilling out the mastoid and delivering the endolymphatic duct and its sac. The ultimate goal of all such surgery is the reduction of endolymph volume through increased drainage or increased absorption of fluid. Different types of sheetings and one-way tubes have been used in the past to facilitate drainage of the endolymphatic space (55,56).

As Ménière's disease represents a consequence of endolymphatic sac distention, it seemed only normal that removal of the excess fluid would alleviate symptoms. Clinical studies, however, have demonstrated that only approximately two thirds of patients have long-term significant improvements in their vertigo with sac-shunting procedures. Approximately one third of patients require follow-up surgery after their initial operations. Other surgical procedures such as the Cody tack create fistulas of the saccule at the oval window, although their efficacy is somewhat controversial.

Vestibular neurectomy with preservation of hearing is a definitive procedure for patients with vertigo that is intractable and unresponsive to more conservative approaches. Selective eighth nerve sections generally produce resolution of vertigo in approximately 90% of patients. However, hearing stabilizes in approximately only two thirds of the patients undergoing such surgery.

Another method for managing intractable vertigo is chemical vestibular ablation. Ototoxicity and vestibulotoxicity of aminoglycosides are well-recognized side effects of these antibiotics. Streptomycin and gentamicin are particularly vestibulotoxic and have been locally instilled into the middle ear as management for unilateral Ménière's disease. The chemical labyrinthectomy works primarily by ablating the vestibular response in the treated ear. In most patients, no further attacks of vertigo occur after the healing phase (57,58).

Other destructive operations exist for patients with Ménière's disease. These are generally categorized as "nonhearing" vestibular ablative procedures and are essentially labyrinthectomies. A labyrinthectomy is an effective treatment for vertigo in patients when serviceable hearing is absent or severely depressed. The natural history of Ménière's syndrome is such that, over time, most patients' tinnitus and vertigo will resolve, although with an associated sensorineural hearing deficit (59,60).

## RECURRENT AUTOIMMUNE SIALADENITIS

The differential diagnosis of recurrent parotid swelling includes autoimmune "pseudosialectasis" and Mikulicz's syndrome. If an autoimmune parotitis is associated with xerophthalmia or xerostomia, it is called sicca syndrome or primary Sjögren's disease. If sialadenitis is associated with a connective tissue disorder, it is called secondary Sjögren's.

Mikulicz's syndrome therefore is essentially a term used for all cases of recurrent parotid swelling that are not autoimmune conditions. This includes the three major categories of chronic recurrent sialadenitis, sialosis, and multinodular salivary glands.

## Autoimmune Parotid Swelling

All of the autoimmune disorders of the major salivary glands have the unifying pattern of early lymphocytic infiltration. This is followed by a thinning and fragmentation of the connective tissue in the intercalated duct walls, with destruction of the salivary gland acini. Usually larger ducts are not involved unless there is chronic severe secondary infection. There are four progressive radiographic features of autoimmune parotid swelling. These include punctate changes (with circular collections of 1 mm or less), globular disease (with collections of 1 to 2 mm), cavitary pathology, and parenchymal destruction (with no recognizable branching). The latter two stages represent the consequences of severe secondary infection.

Autoimmune parotitis usually presents unilaterally with painless swelling. Sjögren's syndrome is the second most common connective tissue disorder, predominantly occurring in women between the ages of 40 and 60 years. Findings include xerophthalmia, xerostomia, and parotid swelling. Filamentary keratitis is diagnostic of keratoconjunctivitis sicca and is a common finding. The most common connective tissue disorder associated with secondary Sjögren's syndrome is rheumatoid arthritis. Extraglandular symptoms include dry eyes, dry skin, arthralgias, and myalgias (61–63).

Certain humoral antibodies are characteristic of Sjögren's syndrome. Specifically anti-SS-A and anti-SS-B are autoantibodies seen in the primary syndrome. Rheumatoid factor and antinuclear antibodies may be present in primary and secondary disease forms. Erythrocyte sedimentation rates are often increased (61,64).

About 5% of patients with Sjögren's syndrome develop a lymphoproliferative neoplasm. The greatest risk for this is seen in patients with the primary form, constant parotid swelling, and lymphadenopathy. A decrease in serum IgM levels can suggest progression to malignant degeneration (65).

Diagnosis is often made with a lip biopsy of a minor salivary gland. This can usually be performed in an office under local anesthesia. Various staging systems exist for lymphocytic infiltration in Sjögren's syndrome and include the Greenspan, Tarply, and Chisolm scales. Treatment for Sjögren's syndrome is usually symptomatic, with oral steroids or ophthalmic steroid drops used in more severe cases (66).

## Mikulicz's Syndrome

Mikulicz's syndrome represents several clinical entities that include recurrent gland infection (i.e., sialadenitis and sialosis) and multinodular glands. Recurrent sialadenitis may present as a unilateral, swollen, painful, red, tender gland with purulent discharge. This is often easily confirmed by intraoral examination, with pus expressed from Stensen's duct on mechanical palpation. Peripheral gland ducts are usually normal.

Sialography is usually performed to demonstrate a stone or stricture and to differentiate the glandular pattern from an autoimmune process. Treatment of sialadenitis includes the removal of obstructing stones, systemic antibiotics, warm compresses, sialogogues, and hydration. In cases of recurrent infections, surgical excision may be necessary, although the scarring and inflammation present can significantly complicate the technical aspects of parotidectomy and result in injury to the facial nerve. However, the facial nerve should not be sacrificed for benign disease.

The "multinodular gland" represents a group of diseases that can produce a so-called lumpy parotid gland. About one third of patients with sarcoid have parotid involvement. Heerfordt's syndrome is sarcoid that involves the parotid gland and facial nerve with localized swelling and occasional uveitis. Approximately 25% of parotid glands contain intraparotid lymph nodes that can act as the nidus for a granulomatous disorder. These lymphoid diseases range from the foci of chronic infection to lymphomas. A computed tomography (CT) sialogram may be helpful in differentiating other causes of parotid swelling. In these cases, a fine-needle aspirate of cells can be useful in differentiating lymphoid masses from salivary gland masses. However, specific histology is needed to obtain a proper diagnosis of a salivary mass.

## ALLERGIC RHINITIS

Allergic rhinitis is included in this chapter because of the multitude of cases of immunologically mediated disease of the nose and sinus cavities. Although allergic rhinitis is not a true autoimmune disease in the classic sense, it is an IgE-mediated response to an external allergen. It is an abnormal response to a foreign antigen that is somewhat akin to an abnormal response to a self antigen—hence its inclusion in a chapter primarily on autoimmune diseases of the head and neck. Because allergic rhinitis is common, it is important to include a detailed discussion regarding its pathogenesis and pathophysiology.

The nasal cavities are the beginning of the respiratory tract. These spaces contain the erectile turbinates and are lined with ciliated respiratory epithelium whose function is involved in the exchange of air and filtration in addition to humidification and the secretion of both immunoglobulins (predominantly in the IgG and secretory IgA classes) and various proteolytic enzymes (67–69). The nose externally is subject to the same skin diseases as those affecting the face. However, the tissue surfaces within the nasal cavity and (by extension) the paranasal sinuses are more likely to be targeted by immunologically based diseases. Allergic rhinitis is a common clinical disorder, with symptoms varying from nasal obstruction to various sinus complaints, alterations in the sense of smell, and obstructive apnea.

The basic allergic reaction is discussed elsewhere in this textbook. The primary nasal reaction in response to environmental allergens is usually an immediate anaphylactic hypersensitivity reaction (i.e., Coombs type) or an allergen-specific one (i.e., an IgE-mediated response to an allergen) produced by prior exposure to an allergen. The activated IgE then reacts with its unique allergen to cause mast cell degranulation, with a subsequent release of histamines and other mediators of inflammation (70–72).

The time scale is relatively rapid, with symptoms appearing as early as 5 minutes after the antigen-antibody reaction is activated and peaking anywhere from 15 to 30 minutes later. There is a late phase of allergic inflammation that is the result of the release of polymorphonuclear cells, such as eosinophils, that occurs 3 to 6 hours after the acute phase. Detailed understanding of the prototypical allergic reaction is critical for understanding its pathogenesis, pathophysiology, and the therapeutic measures that may be considered in the clinician's office (73).

### Diagnosis

The diagnosis of inhalant allergy can usually be suspected on the basis of a complete history and physical examination. A patient may present to a clinician with complaints such as itching within the nasal mucous membranes, occasional eye involvement, and sometimes even symptoms affecting the oral cavity. A clear rhinorrhea is common in addition to sneezing and nasal obstruction. The so-called postnasal drip causing coughing and a feeling of gagging is common. Seasonal allergens are limited to the period of time in which allergens occur, but perennial allergens can be ongoing, such as allergies secondary to animal danders, dust mites, or certain types of mold and dust. Anosmia may be present in allergic rhinitis (74,75).

On physical examination, the patients may demonstrate open-mouth breathing in addition to a so-called allergic salute, manifested by repetitive wiping of the tip of the nose. In younger patients whose facial skeletons are still undergoing development, a so-called adenoid facies may be present. Periorbital edema and bluish discoloration under the inferior eyelids (so-called allergic shiners) are an additional sign of allergic disease. On close examination of the nasal mucosa (with or without nasal or sinus endoscopy), the mucosa is generally seen to be swollen and pale, and often clear mucus is seen on the turbinates and occasionally coming out of the middle meatus. Although this rhinorrhea is usually clear, secondary infection results in its discoloration. Hyperplastic respiratory tissue originating within the sinus cavity may extrude through the middle meatus and be seen clinically as polyps. The turbinates themselves may undergo polypoid degeneration not related to allergy.

Other tests that can be useful in the diagnosis of allergic rhinitis include nasal smears showing eosinophilia within the mucus. In addition to the eosinophils, mast cells and goblet cells present on such a smear are highly suggestive of an atopic cause. There is a so-called NARES syndrome, in which a nonallergic rhinitis occurs with eosinophilia. This syndrome may occasionally be found in patients who are nonatopic (76).

Skin testing, particularly against seasonal allergens that may be inhaled and are known to be prevalent in the patient's environment, is helpful in establishing a diagnosis. In some cases, the measurement of serum IgE levels may have value in defining those patients who may or may not be atopic. The demonstration of an allergen-specific IgE, however, is the best proof of an upper respiratory allergy (77). The functional size of the nasal cavity can be measured with such techniques as rhinomanometry.

Definitive testing of allergy and atopic disease in general requires careful screening and skin testing to various allergens. The classic wheal and flare response is then tallied and an allergic profile developed. *In vitro* IgE measurements are considered more specific but less sensitive than skin testing. Because this requires venipuncture alone, without risk of systemic anaphylaxis, some clinicians find this technique preferable to standard skin testing.

There are some necessary uses of *in vitro* testing for allergy, and these are required in patients who are uncooperative for intracutaneous skin pricks and patients with skin disorders such as dermatography or severe eczema. In some very atopic patients, such as those with severe allergic asthma (i.e., patients unable to be taken off treatment with drugs that suppress the wheal response), *in vitro* serum IgE testing for an allergy may be necessary. Other uses include testing for severe hypersensitivity to insects (e.g., bees) and for patients with a history of severe reaction to prior antigen administration or anaphylactic food hypersensitivities. When atypical reactions occur or skin testing is equivocal and unclear, serum IgE testing may prove diagnostic (78–82). $T_H2$-type cytokine mRNA upregulation in allergic mucosa has been shown (83–85).

In many cases of allergic rhinitis, CT scanning of the paranasal sinuses is a requirement. This helps to define the level and extent of disease in areas that are often not seen on a routine clinical examination, especially in each of the paranasal sinuses to show whether or not inflammatory or polypoid tissue is present (86–88).

### Treatment

Immunotherapy has value in the treatment of allergic rhinitis but is often needed on a long-term basis. The best way to deal with an allergic cause, if feasible, is for the patient to avoid the offending allergen. Although this goal is almost always attainable with drug allergies such as to penicillin, a person cannot always avoid breathing air contaminated with pollen. In some cases, an "allergy clean-out" of the house is encouraged by vacuuming of window shades and bed box springs and careful filter cleaning of air vents. Multiple weekly changing of bed linens is but one example used to facilitate avoidance of inciting allergens and therefore preventing the allergic response in target organs.

Unfortunately, environmental control can be difficult for many patients. For example, allergic patients are often unwilling to give up pets that carry immunogenetically potent antigens. Cat hair, dander, pelt, and saliva have all been implicated in atopically mediated rhinosinusitis. Despite intensive attempts at cleaning, animal danders may be carried in areas of the house for months, even after an animal is removed.

The so-called house dust is not a unique antigen but is a more generic term for multiple antigens. These include cockroaches, molds, pollens from in-house plants, and the house dust mite. The dust mite is a small arachnid that lives off the desquamation of human skin and usually thrives in a moist environment. Regular multiple weekly linen changes have value in treating this disorder, while commercially available chemicals such as benzyl benzoate can be applied to upholstered surfaces and carpets, followed by thorough vacuuming. This approach can kill dust mites for a long time.

Outdoor molds are usually more common from spring to the middle of the autumn but may be present in flower beds, gardens, piles of leaves, and mulch. Indoor molds may be found in places as discordant as carpets, old newspapers, old shoes, and even shower curtains and bathroom tile. Environmental control is quite difficult in the avoidance of pollen, short of living indoors continually with a highly efficient laminar flow air filtration system (89).

### Pharmacologic Treatment

First-line treatment includes antihistamines to effectively compete with $H_1$ receptor sites on target organs during the allergic response. If taken before exposure to an allergen, they are generally more effective. Their main effect is to relieve the symptoms of itching, sneezing, and rhinorrhea. Certain preparations, however, can produce the side effects of sedation, drying of mucous membranes, and even aggravating narrow-angle glaucoma. There are available non-sedating systemic antihistamines that include loratadine, brompheniramine maleate, and cetirizine, and topical forms, such as levocabastine, also exist (89–95).

Systemic decongestants help to decongest and open a clogged nasal cavity. Severe congestion within the nose can be a severely debilitating symptom to people and a major quality-of-life issue. Decongestants as a rule, however, are sympathomimetics that work by inducing vasoconstriction within the nasal turbinates. This leads to a shrinkage of the congested tissue. Care must be taken to consider possible concurrent medical conditions such as hypertension, coronary artery disease, prostatic hypertrophy, and psychiatric or mood disturbances. These groups of diseases can be adversely affected by the administration of systemic sympathomimetic medications.

Pseudoephedrine is a stereoisomer of ephedrine and is the most commonly prescribed decongestant. Phenylpropanolamine is similar to ephedrine but has less central nervous system stimulation and often can be prescribed in conjunction with mucolytics such as guaifenesin.

All of the systemic decongestants exert an α-adrenergic effect and can cause unpleasant central nervous system stimulation. Because patients on monoamine oxidase inhibitors and tricyclic antidepressants are at particular risk for central nervous system complications when these decongestants are taken systemically, they must be prescribed with extreme caution (93).

In addition to antihistamines and decongestants, other pharmacotherapy of nasal allergies includes the use of topical sprays such as cromolyn. In the immediate hypersensitivity allergic reaction, an allergen reacts with adjacent antigen-specific IgE molecules fixed to the surface of mast cells or basophils. This causes mast cell degranulations and the release of preformed and newly formed mediators of inflammation such as histamines and leukotrienes. Cromolyn stabilizes and protects mast cells from such degranulation by helping to phosphorylate the 78-kd proteins, preventing the acute and late-phase allergic reactions. Cromolyn is therefore unique in its pharmacology, in that it helps to prevent an allergic reaction rather than only providing treatment for the after-effects of allergy.

Cromolyn nasal spray is delivered topically, with treatment administered in each nostril every 4 hours while the patient is awake. Approximately 1 week is required to obtain clinical relief. However, for a topical mast cell stabilizer such as cromolyn to work, the nasal cavity must be open to facilitate its delivery. Topical nasal decongestants are occasionally prescribed to help unblock the nose and facilitate the delivery of cromolyn. Cromolyn has no intrinsic antihistamine effect, and its action is predominantly local. There is minimal systemic absorption of intranasally administered cromolyn (92,93).

### Treatment of Complicating Factors in Allergic Rhinitis

Atopic disease of the sinonasal tract, although common, is not the only cause of recurrent sneezing. Even if nasal allergy is present, other types of rhinitis may be complicating the clinical picture or may be the predominant form of disease. The clinician must continually assess the clinical status of all rhinitis patients by history, physical examination, and response to therapy and must adjust treatment regimens appropriately (Table 24.2).

If an atopic person has done well on antiallergic treatment and develops an exacerbation or new symptoms while still on treatment, the physician should consider the possibility of

**TABLE 24.2.** *Management of allergic rhinitis without secondary sinus infection*

| |
|---|
| Environmental modification—*avoid offending allergen* |
| Decongestants with antihistamines |
| Cromolyn |
| Topical glucocorticoids |
| Immunotherapy (may last up to 2 years) |

other types of rhinitis before changing the therapy. Other forms of nonallergic rhinitis include vasomotor rhinitis, which causes an excessive clear rhinorrhea that is often the result of temperature extremes, stress, or exposure to chemical irritants. Nasal obstruction, with congestion and anterior and posterior rhinorrhea, is often exacerbated as the patient assumes a recumbent position. Allergic and vasomotor rhinitis are common disorders, and it is reasonable to expect to find the two conditions occurring simultaneously in many clinical settings. In an analogous manner to allergic rhinitis, the best way to treat vasomotor rhinitis is to avoid the causative or inciting factors. After that, treatment usually involves the symptomatic relief of discomfort (96).

Infectious disorders of the sinonasal tract may certainly occur in patients with underlying atopic disease. These infections must be promptly recognized and appropriate antimicrobial treatment initiated. In certain cases, infections can alter a patient's responses to systemic immunotherapy. As a general rule, allergic immunotherapy treatments should be stopped until after an infection is resolved, particularly if a patient is febrile (97).

Rhinitis medicamentosa is caused by the excessive use of topical nasal decongestants or sprays, and this may cause a rebound congestion that complicates an underlying clinical process. It is important to stop the continuing use of these drops; otherwise, medical therapy will fail. Beta blockers and some antihypertensive medications may also contribute to nasal congestion and obstruction, requiring their removal.

Pregnancy is known to produce congestion of the nasal mucosa. Treatment of the allergic rhinitis of pregnancy should focus first on environmental controls, because antihistamines and decongestants, topical nasal steroids, immunotherapy, and cromolyn are drugs best avoided during pregnancy, particularly the first trimester.

### *Topical and Systemic Glucocorticoid Treatments for Control of Severe or Nonresponsive Allergic Rhinitis*

Systemic glucocorticoids are the most potent pharmacologic agents available to relieve the symptoms of allergic rhinitis. They are, however, not primary treatments because they do not prevent an allergic reaction but are used to reverse and ameliorate its effects. Systemic glucocorticoids can produce significant side effects. These can sometimes occur even when drugs are administered topically. Glucocorticoids lessen the effects of the acute and late-phase allergic reactions by decreasing capillary permeability and stabilizing lysosomal membranes. They may inhibit arachidonic acid metabolism and limit the production of certain cytokines.

Generally, topical glucocorticoids are used initially for treatment. There are various rapidly acting preparations, such as mometasone furoate monohydrate and fluticasone propionate. These are superior to the previously available topical steroids that usually took several days before having any type of local effect. In my experience, there has been little

risk of adrenal suppression with topical nasal steroids (92,93,98–101).

In severe or refractory cases of allergic rhinitis or allergically mediated rhinosinusitis, systemic steroids may be considered necessary. Relatively small doses using prednisone or methylprednisolone with rapidly tapering regimens over 1 or 2 weeks often constitute sufficient therapy to improve the patient's clinical status and facilitate continued treatment with antihistamines or decongestants alone. Any long-term treatment with glucocorticoids requires caution, especially because the potential side effects of these medicines can be harmful.

Some of the complications of topical nasal steroids include dryness of the nasal mucosa with secondary irritation, bleeding, and *Candida* fungal infections. Occasional crusting and septal perforations have been reported. Local irritations most often occur after delivery by fluorinated hydrocarbon propellants, but they can also occur after administration using a pump spray.

Because the topical nasal steroids act locally over the nasal mucosa, a patent nasal airway is required to allow for the proper distribution of medicine over affected tissues. Systemic or topical nasal decongestants may be required to open up the nose. Mass lesions such as large polyps and large septal deviations decrease the usefulness of these medicines by obstructing the nasal airway (99,100).

As part of the treatment, patient education must focus on the prophylactic and regular use of topical nasal steroids to prevent the possible side effects of allergically mediated disease. Although 4 to 6 weeks of topical nasal steroid treatment is common and should pose no significant harm to most patients, any long-term use of topical nasal steroids requires regular monitoring with careful examination of nasal tissues.

In certain cases, glucocorticoids have been injected directly into the nasal turbinates to relieve the symptoms of allergic rhinitis. There are, however, several documented cases of injection-induced blindness, with the mechanism thought to be a retrograde embolization from the nasal veins into the retinal circulation (102). The safe injection of steroids into the turbinate include the following actions. First, the nasal mucosa should be pretreated with a topical vasoconstrictor. Second, a corticosteroid should be used that has a small particle size, such as triamcinolone acetonide or prednisone tebutate. Technically, the injection should be placed beneath the mucosa along the anterior tip of the inferior turbinate. The steroid should then be injected gently, avoiding undue pressure.

### *Immunotherapy*

Immunotherapy, at least theoretically, provides for the possible cure of the allergically mediated, IgE antibody–antigen reaction. In general, candidates for allergic immunotherapy are patients whose symptoms are not easily controlled with medicines and are sensitive to allergens that cannot be readily avoided, particularly those in the air, and patients with severe symptoms spanning two or more allergy seasons. Most importantly, any consideration for immunotherapy requires patients who are willing to cooperate in a long-term treatment that requires discipline and patience in arriving at a satisfactory therapeutic result (103).

Immunotherapy involves the parenteral administration of antigens identified as appropriate by *in vivo* or *in vitro* testing. This is done is to stimulate the formation of allergen-specific IgG blocking antibodies that compete with IgE antibodies for target sites on mast cells or basophils.

Through an average ragweed season, for example, the patient may be exposed to a total of less than 1 µg of ragweed antigen. Immunotherapy with ragweed approaches levels of 50 to 1,000 µg of antigen per injection. Laboratory data show that chronic exposure to small doses of antigens may produce IgE, whereas large doses of parenterally administered antigens have been shown to suppress IgE formation and produce IgG-blocking antibodies. It can be further inferred from this that small initial doses of immunotherapy may actually increase the level of serum IgE. However, continued therapy at higher doses can decrease IgE production and initiate blocking IgG antibody production. The parenteral therapy, therefore, is necessary to deliver the high enough doses of antigens to stimulate formation of blocking antibodies.

Immunotherapy based on skin end point titration or *in vitro* methods is normally administered weekly until symptom response is observed. Treatment is continued on a weekly basis for 1 or 2 years, adjusted to longer periods according to responses, and then is discontinued when patients become symptom free.

### Complicating Factors Associated with Allergic Rhinitis

Intranasal polyps may be associated with allergic rhinitis, although many of these are caused by infections. Patients with nasal polyps should still be tested for underlying atopic disease (70,71,104). Although pharmacotherapy and immunotherapy may not produce total resolution of polyps in all allergic patients, such treatment can make the recurrence of polyps less likely if it is started before their surgical removal.

### Sinusitis

Most instances of recurrent sinusitis are associated with obstruction of the ostiomeatal complex in the nasal cavity from whatever cause. Mucosal edema due to allergic inflammation is an important cause. Chronic hyperplastic rhinosinusitis may also arise from repeated allergic reactions involving these target organs.

### Asthma

Although improvement in reactive bronchospasm frequently follows surgery for suppurative sinusitis or allergic sinusitis, a firm connection between reactive airway disease of the

lungs and allergic rhinosinusitis has yet to be established. These patients generally are sicker than most asthma patients. Some also have hypersensitivity to aspirin in addition to chronic polyposis and asthma. This triad, also known as Samter's triad, is one of the most difficult problems in treating allergic sinusitis and polyposis (104). Some preliminary data suggest that certain oncogenes are activated in these patients, suggesting that polyps maybe transformed over time into benign adenomas.

## ALLERGIC EMERGENCIES

Although it is rare to have an anaphylactic reaction in a clinical office, physicians must be aware and able to deal with this life-threatening emergency should it ever occur. The physician must first differentiate early anaphylaxis from vasovagal syncope, or the so-called needle reaction. If the patient is syncopal, placement in a recumbent position and the administration of oxygen is usually enough to help the patient recover.

Anaphylactic reactions may also be associated with increased secretions, nasal congestion, and hoarseness or wheezing but are uncommon findings in vasovagal episodes. Anaphylactic reactions may also produce urticarial reactions along the skin. If a true anaphylactic reaction occurs, prompt appropriate medical support is required. The patient is placed in a recumbent position; oxygen is administered by mask, and epinephrine is given by intramuscular injection. Parenteral diphenhydramine, dexamethasone, or both and airway support may be necessary.

## REFERENCES

1. Hoffman GS, Kerr GS, Leavitt RY, et al. Wegener's granulomatosis: an analysis of 158 patients. *Ann Intern Med* 1992;116:488–498.
2. Fauci AS, Haynes BF, Katz P, Wolff SM. Wegener's granulomatosis: prospective clinical and therapeutic experience with 85 patients for 21 years. *Ann Intern Med* 1983;98:76–85.
3. Sneller MC, Hoffman GS, Talar-Williams C, et al. An analysis of forty-two Wegener's granulomatosis patients treated with methotrexate and prednisone. *Arthritis Rheum* 1995;38:608–613.
4. Lebovics RS, Hoffman GS, Leavitt RY, et al. The management of subglottic stenosis in patients with Wegener's granulomatosis. *Laryngoscope* 1992;102:1341–1345.
5. Waxman J, Bose WJ. Laryngeal manifestations of Wegener's granulomatosis: case reports and review of the literature. *J Rheumatol* 1986;13:408–411.
6. McCaffrey TV. Management of subglottic stenosis in the adult. *Ann Otol Rhinol Laryngol* 1991;100:90–94.
7. McDonald TJ, Neel HB, DeRemee RA. Wegener's granulomatosis of the subglottis and the upper portion of the trachea. *Ann Otol Rhinol Laryngol* 1982;91:588–592.
8. Moller DR. Involvement of T cells and alterations in T cell receptors in sarcoidosis. *Semin Respir Infect* 1998;13:174–183.
9. Agostini C, Semenzato G. Cytokines in sarcoidosis. *Semin Respir Infect* 1998;13:184–196.
10. Kataria YP, Holter JF. Sarcoidosis: a model of granulomatous inflammation of unknown etiology associated with a hyperactive immune system. *Methods* 1996;9:268–294.
11. McCabe BF. Autoimmune sensorineural hearing loss. *Otol Rhinol Laryngol* 1979;88:585.
12. McCabe BF. Autoimmune inner ear disease: clinical varieties of presentation. In: Veldman JE, McCabe BF, eds. *Otoimmunology.* Amsterdam: Kugler, 1987:143.

13. Hughes GB, Barna BP. Autoimmune inner ear disease: fact or fantasy? *Adv Otorhinolaryngol* 1991;46:82.
14. Yamawaki M, Ariga T, Gao Y, et al. Sulfoglucuronosyl glycolipids as putative antigens for autoimmune inner ear disease. *J Neuroimmunol* 1998;84:111–116.
15. Harris JP, Ryan AF. Fundamental immune mechanisms of the brain and inner ear. *Otolaryngol Head Neck Surg* 1995;112:639–653.
16. Harris JP, Heydt J, Keithley EM, Chen MC. Immunopathology of the inner ear: an update. *Ann N Y Acad Sci* 1997;830:166–178.
17. Barna BP, Hughes GB. Autoimmune inner ear disease—a real entity? *Clin Lab Med* 1997;17:581–594.
18. Hoistad DL, Schachern PA, Paparella MM. Autoimmune sensorineural hearing loss: a human temporal bone study. *Am J Otolaryngol* 1998;19:33–39.
19. Suzuki M, Krug MS, Cheng KC, et al. Antibodies against inner-ear proteins in the sera of patients with inner-ear diseases. *ORL J Otorhinolaryngol Relat Spec* 1997;59:10–17.
20. Luetje CM. Autoimmune inner ear disease. *Otolaryngol Head Neck Surg* 1996;114:507–508.
21. Kosaka K, Yamanobe S, Tomiyama S, Yagi T. Inner ear antibodies in patients with sensorineural hearing loss. *Acta Otolaryngol Suppl (Stockh)* 1995;519:176–177.
22. Quaranta A, Scaringi A, Portalatini P, Vantaggiato D. Auditory findings in subjects with immunomediated sensorineural hearing loss. *Ann N Y Acad Sci* 1997;830:277–290.
23. Arnold W. Systemic autoimmune diseases associated with hearing loss. *Ann N Y Acad Sci* 1997;830:187–202.
24. Kataoka H, Takeda T, Nakatani H, Saito H. Sensorineural hearing loss of suspected autoimmune etiology: a report of three cases. *Auris Nasus Larynx* 1995;22:53–58.
25. Welling DB. Clinical evaluation and treatment of immune-mediated inner ear disease. *Ear Nose Throat J* 1996;75:301–305.
26. Hughes GB, Barna BP, Kinney SE, et al. Predictive value of laboratory tests in autoimmune inner ear disease. *Laryngoscope* 1986;48:251.
27. Hughes GB, Barna BP, Calabrese LH. Immune mechanisms in auditory and vestibular disease. In: Cummings CW, Fredrickson JM, Harker LA, et al, eds. *Otolaryngology—head and neck surgery.* St Louis: CV Mosby, 1986:3149.
28. Hughes GB, Barna BP, Kinney SE, et al. Clinical diagnosis of immune inner ear disease. *Laryngoscope* 1988;48:251.
29. Sismanis A, Wise CM, Johnson GD. Methotrexate management of immune-mediated cochleovestibular disorders. *Otolaryngol Head Neck Surg* 1997;116:146–152.
30. Luetje CM, Berliner KI. Plasmapheresis in autoimmune inner ear disease: long-term follow-up. *Am J Otol* 1997;18:572–576.
31. Luetje CM. Theoretical and practical implications for plasmapheresis in autoimmune inner ear disease. *Laryngoscope* 1989;99:1137.
32. Haynes BF, Pikus A, Kaiser-Kupfer M, Fauci AS. Successful treatment of sudden hearing loss in Cogan's syndrome with corticosteroids. *Arthritis Rheum* 1981;24:501.
33. Peitersen E, Carlsen BH. Hearing impairment as the initial sign of polyarteritis nodosa. *Acta Otolaryngol* 1966;61:189.
34. Brama I, Fainaru M. Inner ear involvement in Behçet's disease. *Arch Otolaryngol* 1980;106:215.
35. Damiani JM, Levine HL. Relapsing polychondritis: report of 10 cases. *Laryngoscope* 1979;89:929.
36. Hoshino T, Kato I, Kodama A, et al. Sudden deafness in relapsing polychondritis. *Acta Otolaryngol (Stockh)* 1978;86:418.
37. Karmody CS. Wegener's granulomatosis: presentation as an otologic problem. *Otolaryngol Head Neck Surg* 1978;86:573.
38. Symposium on Meniere's disease. *Otolaryngol Clin North Am* 1980;13:565–773.
39. Filipo R, Mancini P, Nostro G. Meniere's disease and autoimmunity. *Ann N Y Acad Sci* 1997;830:299–305.
40. Billings PB, Keithley EM, Harris JP. Evidence linking the 68 kilodalton antigen identified in progressive sensorineural hearing loss patient sera with heat shock protein 70. *Ann Otol Rhinol Laryngol* 1995;104:181–188.
41. Rauch SD, San Martin JE, Moscicki RA, Bloch KJ. Serum antibodies against heat shock protein 70 in Meniere's disease. *Am J Otol* 1995;16:648–652.
42. Pulec JL. The discovery of the pathogenesis of Meniere's disease. *Ear Nose Throat J* 1995;74:510–511.
43. Schuknecht HF. Meniere's disease, pathogenesis, and pathology. *Am J Otolaryngol* 1982;3:349–352.
44. Van de Heyning PH, Wuyts FL, Claes J, et al. Definition, classification and reporting of Meniere's disease and its symptoms. *Acta Otolaryngol Suppl (Stockh)* 1997;526:5–9.
45. Pollock KJ. Meniere's disease: a review of the problem. *ORL Head Neck Nurs* 1995;13:10–13.
46. Dornhoffer JL. Diagnosis of cochlear Meniere's disease with electrocochleography. *ORL J Otorhinolaryngol Relat Spec* 1998;60:301–305.
47. Orchik DJ, Shea JJ Jr., Ge NN. Summating potential and action potential ratio in Meniere's disease before and after treatment. *Am J Otol* 1998:478–482.
48. Storper IS, Spitzer JB, Scanlan M. Use of glycopyrrolate in the treatment of Meniere's disease. *Laryngoscope* 1998;108:1442–1445.
49. Claes J, Van de Heyning PH. Medical treatment of Meniere's disease: a review of literature. *Acta Otolaryngol Suppl (Stockh)* 1997;526:37–42.
50. Levine S, Margolis RH, Daly KA. Use of electrocochleography in the diagnosis of Meniere's disease. *Laryngoscope* 1998;108:993–1000.
51. Slattery WH 3rd, Fayad JN. Medical treatment of Meniere's disease. *Otolaryngol Clin North Am* 1997;30:1027–1037.
52. Saeed SR. Fortnightly review: diagnosis and treatment of Meniere's disease. *BMJ* 1998;316:368–372.
53. Grant IL, Welling DB. The treatment of hearing loss in Meniere's disease. *Otolaryngol Clin North Am* 1997;30:1123–1144.
54. Hoffer ME, Balough B, Henderson J, et al. Use of sustained release vehicles in the treatment of Meniere's disease. *Otolaryngol Clin North Am* 1997;30:1159–1166.
55. LaRouere MJ. Surgical treatment of Meniere's disease. *Otolaryngol Clin North Am* 1996;29:311–322.
56. Rivas JA. Surgical treatment of Meniere's disease. *Ear Nose Throat J* 1994;73:764–767.
57. McFeely WJ, Singleton GT, Rodriguez FJ, Antonelli PJ. Intratympanic gentamicin treatment for Meniere's disease. *Otolaryngol Head Neck Surg* 1998;118:589–596.
58. Hirsch BE, Kamerer DB. Role of chemical labyrinthectomy in the treatment of Meniere's disease. *Otolaryngol Clin North Am* 1997;30:1039–1049.
59. Van de Heyning PH, Verlooy J, Schatteman I, Wuyts FL. Selective vestibular neurectomy in Meniere's disease: a review. *Acta Otolaryngol Suppl (Stockh)* 1997;526:58–66.
60. Yazdi AK, Rutka J. Results of labyrinthectomy in the treatment of Meniere's disease and delayed endolymphatic hydrops. *J Otolaryngol* 1996;25:26–31.
61. Gerli R, Muscat C, Giansanti M et al. Quantitative assessment of salivary gland inflammatory infiltration in primary Sjögren's syndrome: its relationship to different demographic, clinical and serological features of the disorder. *Br J Rheumatol* 1997;36:969–975.
62. Fox RI. Sjogren's syndrome. Controversies and progress. *Clin Lab Med* 1997;17:431–444.
63. Fox RI, Maruyama T. Pathogenesis and treatment of Sjogren's syndrome. *Curr Opin Rheumatol* 1997;9:393–399.
64. Nakamura S, Ikebe-Hiroki A, Shinohara M, et al. An association between salivary gland disease and serological abnormalities in Sjögren's syndrome. *J Oral Pathol Med* 1997;26:426–430.
65. Jordan RC, Speight PM. Lymphoma in Sjögren's syndrome: from histopathology to molecular pathology. *Oral Surg Oral Med Oral Pathol Oral Radiol Endosc* 1996;81:308–320.
66. DiGiuseppe JA, Corio RL, Westra WH. Lymphoid infiltrates of the salivary glands: pathology, biology and clinical significance. *Curr Opin Oncol* 1996;8:232–237.
67. Bienenstock J, Befus AD. Mucosal immunology. *Immunology* 1980;41:249–270.
68. Mestecky J, McGhee JR. Immunoglobulin A (IgA): molecular and cellular interactions involved in IgA biosynthesis and immune response. *Adv Immunol* 1987;40:153–245.
69. Brandtzaeg P. Immune functions of human nasal mucosa and tonsils in health and disease. In: Bienenstock J, ed. *Immunology of the lung and upper respiratory tract.* New York: McGraw–Hill, 1984:28–95.
70. Bertrand B, Eloy P, Rombeaux P. Allergy and sinusitis. *Acta Otorhinolaryngol Belg* 1997;51:227–237.
71. Settipane GA. Nasal polyps and immunoglobulin E (IgE). *Allergy Asthma Proc* 1996;17:269–273.
72. Ingram JM. Nothing to sneeze about: allergies and allergic rhinitis. *J Ark Med Soc* 1996;93:81–86.

73. Shambaugh GE Jr. Allergy in otolaryngology—the experience of an expert. *Ear Nose Throat J* 1995;74:798–799.

74. Simola M, Malmberg H. Sense of smell in allergic and nonallergic rhinitis. *Allergy* 1998;53:190–194.

75. Apter AJ, Mott AE, Frank ME, Clive JM. Allergic rhinitis and olfactory loss. *Ann Allergy Asthma Immunol* 1995;75:311–316.

76. Sanico A, Togias A. Noninfectious nonallergic rhinitis (NINAR): considerations on possible mechanisms. *Am J Rhinol* 1998;12:65–72.

77. Mabry RL. Allergy for rhinologists. *Otolaryngol Clin North Am* 1998;31:175–187.

78. Ferguson BJ, Mabry RL. Laboratory diagnosis. *Otolaryngol Head Neck Surg* 1997;117[3 Pt 2]:S12–S26.

79. Saito H, Asakura K, Ogasawara H, et al. Topical antigen provocation increases the number of immunoreactive IL-4-, IL-5-, and IL-6-positive cells in the nasal mucosa of patients with perennial allergic rhinitis. *Int Arch Allergy Immunol* 1997;114:1:81–85.

80. Min YG, Jung HW, Kim HS, et al. Prevalence and risk factors for perennial allergic rhinitis in Korea: results of a nationwide survey. *Clin Otolaryngol* 1997;22:139–144.

81. Benninger MS. Nasal endoscopy: its role in office diagnosis. *Am J Rhinol* 1997;11:117–180.

82. Spector SL. Overview of comorbid associations of allergic rhinitis. *J Allergy Clin Immunol* 1997;99:S773–S780.

83. Bachert K, Wagenmann M, Holt-Appels G. Cytokines and adhesion molecules in allergic rhinitis. *Am J Rhinol* 1998;12:3–8.

84. Suzuki H, Takahashi Y, Wataya H, et al. Mechanism of neutrophil recruitment induced by IL-8 in chronic sinusitis. *J Allergy Clin Immunol* 1996;98:659–670.

85. Jirapongsananuruk O, Vichyanond P. Nasal cytology in the diagnosis of allergic rhinitis in children. *Ann Allergy Asthma Immunol* 1998;80:165–170.

86. Bonifazi F, Bilo MB, Antonicelli L, Bonetti MG. Rhinopharyngoscopy, computed tomography and magnetic resonance imaging. *Allergy* 1997;52[Suppl]:28–31.

87. Slavin RG. Complications of allergic rhinitis: implications for sinusitis and asthma. *J Allergy Clin Immunol* 1998;101[2 Pt 2]:S357–S360.

88. Naclerio RM, de Tineo ML. Ragweed allergic rhinitis and the paranasal sinuses: a computed tomographic study. *Arch Otolaryngol Head Neck Surg* 1997;123:193–196.

89. Fireman P. Treatment strategies designed to minimize medical complications of allergic rhinitis. *Am J Rhinol* 1997;11:95–102.

90. Thoden GR, Drews HM, Furey SA, et al. Brompheniramine maleate: a double-blind placebo-controlled comparison with terfenadine for symptoms of allergic rhinitis. *Am J Rhinol* 1998;12:293–299.

91. Acquadro MA, Montgomery WW. Treatment of chronic paranasal sinus pain with minimal sinus disease. *Ann Otol Rhinol Laryngol* 1996;105:607–614.

92. Wright DN, Huang SW. Current treatment of allergic rhinitis and sinusitis. *J Fla Med Assoc* 1996;83:389–393.

93. Kaliner M. Medical management of sinusitis. *Am J Med Sci* 1988;316:21–28.

94. Nolen TM. Sedative effects of antihistamines: safety, performance, learning, and quality of life. *Clin Ther* 1997;19:39–55.

95. Braun JJ, Alabert JP, Michel FB, et al. Adjunct effect of loratadine in the treatment of acute sinusitis in patients with allergic rhinitis. *Allergy* 1997;52:650–655.

96. Aust MR, Madsen CS, Jennings A, et al. Mucin mRNA expression in normal and vasomotor inferior turbinates. *Am J Rhinol* 1997;11:293–302.

97. Kaliner MA. Recurrent sinusitis: examining medical treatment options. *Am J Rhinol* 1997;11:123–132.

98. Stern MA, Dahl R, Nielsen LP, et al. A comparison of aqueous suspensions of budesonide nasal spray (128 μg and 256 μg once daily) and fluticasone propionate nasal spray (200 μg once daily) and the treatment of adult patients with seasonal allergic rhinitis. *Am J Rhinol* 1997;11:323–330.

99. Edwards TB. Effectiveness and safety of beclomethasone dipropionate, an intranasal corticosteroid, in the treatment of patients with allergic rhinitis. *Clin Ther* 1995;17:1032–1041.

100. Mygind N. Effects of corticosteroid therapy in non-allergic rhinosinusitis. *Acta Otolaryngol (Stockh)* 1996;116:164–166.

101. Drouin M, Yang WH, Bertrand B, et al. Once daily mometasone furoate aqueous nasal spray is as effective as twice daily beclomethasone dipropionate for treating perennial allergic rhinitis patients. *Ann Allergy Asthma Immunol* 1996;77:153–160.

102. Mabry RL. Visual loss after intranasal corticosteroid injection. *Arch Otolaryngol* 1998;107:484.

103. Mabry RL, Mabry CS. Immunotherapy for allergic fungal sinusitis: the second year. *Otolaryngol Head Neck Surg* 1997;1167:367–371.

104. Hurwitz B. Nasal Pathophysiology impacts bronchial reactivity in asthmatic patients with allergic rhinitis. *J Asthma* 1997;34:427–431.

*Textbook of the Autoimmune Diseases,*
Edited by R. G. Lahita, N. Chiorazzi, and W. H. Reeves,
Lippincott Williams & Wilkins, Philadelphia © 2000.

# CHAPTER 25

# Ocular Autoimmunity

Luiz Vicente Rizzo and Rubens Belfort, Jr.

Four classic mechanisms are employed by the immune system to avoid the development of autoimmunity: clonal selection (1,2), active suppression (3,4), immune privilege (5–7), and clonal inactivation (3,4). Because of the unique situation of the eye (an immune-privileged site, partially integrated to the central nervous system and surrounded by a mucosal surface), these mechanisms operate in a peculiar form. Negative selection (i.e., clonal selection) of putatively autoaggressive T-cell clones occurs in the thymus, and it depends on the target autoantigens found there (2). However, not all self antigens are present in the thymus in sufficient concentrations to induce deletion of the respective T cells bearing antigen receptors capable of recognizing such antigens (8–12). During ontogeny, the eye becomes a sequestered organ before the thymus is fully developed, and some ocular antigens may never reach the thymus. Consequently, T cells bearing antigen receptors capable of recognizing such antigens are not deleted (13,14).

The importance of thymic presentation of ocular antigens in terms of the development of uveitis has been confirmed by experiments showing that experimental autoimmune uveoretinitis (EAU)–susceptible rat strains do not express arrestin (S-Ag) or interphotoreceptor retinoid-binding protein in the thymus and as a result are easily induced to respond to such antigens and generate an autoimmune reaction in the eye (15). Mice that do express such antigens in the thymus and therefore undergo negative selection of T cells reacting with high affinity to these retinal antigens require doses 500- to 1,000-fold higher of protein immunization than those used in rats to develop uveitis (15). Some components of the eye, such as lens antigens, behave in a different fashion. Studies

have shown that the synthesis of lens proteins is not restricted to the eye.

The major component of the lens is a group of proteins known as crystallins. Three subsets of crystallin proteins have been described: α, β, and γ (16,17). The α-crystallin is expressed in the lens in higher concentrations than the other two subsets. It is composed by two subunits, A and B, each encoded by separate genes (16,18). The promoter for α-A-crystallin is apparently expressed exclusively in the eye (17,18). However, the promoter for α-B-crystallin is expressed in other tissues, including the heart, skeletal muscle, and thymus (16), demonstrating that the expression of this component is not exclusive to the eye. The lens capsule is not impermeable and does not constitute a barrier to the leakage of lens antigens. Crystallins can be found in the aqueous humor of normal individuals (19,20). Leakage to the anterior chamber may contribute to tolerization against lens antigens through a mechanisms known as anterior chamber–associated immune deviation (ACAID). Some lens proteins have a high degree of homology with other nonlens proteins, suggesting they may also share antigenic epitopes. Antilens antibodies are recognizable in many normal individuals (21), and their frequency and titers are greatly enhanced after extracapsular cataract surgery without pathologic implications (22). Taken together, these data suggest that the immune system had ample opportunities to recognized and respond to lens antigens and that it does so without generating an autoimmune response, as it would against any other autoantigen. In that regard, crystallins behave similar to other non–organ-specific antigens throughout the body.

Ocular-antigen–specific T cells reach the blood at a frequency of one to five precursors per million cells (23,24). Despite the presence of such autoreactive cells in the blood, most people do not develop uveitis. Part of the protection against autoreactive cells in the periphery comes from the eye being a immune-privileged site. In the eye, the anterior chamber, cornea, and retina are considered immune-privileged sites. The concept of immune privilege was first defined by Medawar, even though the phenomenon had been known for

L. V. Rizzo: Department of Immunology, Institute of Biomedical Sciences, University of São Paulo, São Paulo, Brazil 05508-900; Division of Allergy and Clinical Immunology, Clinical Hospital, University of São Paulo, São Paulo, Brazil 05508-000.

R. Belfort, Jr.: Department of Ophthalmology, Federal University of São Paulo, São Paulo, Brazil 04023-062; Department of Ophthalmology, São Paulo Hospital, São Paulo, Brazil 04023-062.

more than 50 years at the time of his observations (25). According to his theory, the lack of lymphatic drainage would restrict autoantigens of immune-privileged sites from being recognized and attacked by the immune system. Years later, it was shown that antigens placed inside the eye (an immune-privileged site) are capable of inducing an immune response (26,27), changing the concept of immune privilege. Immune-privileged sites are no longer considered inaccessible. However, because of particular local circumstances in these organs, immune responses there develop differently from the process in the rest of the body. It has been shown that FAS ligand (FASL)–expressing cells encircle the eye forming a protective barrier against the deleterious effects of activation of T lymphocytes in the eye (28). FASL has been shown to be expressed on the corneal epithelium and endothelium, iris, ciliary body, and throughout the retina. The expression of FASL in such tissues allows them to induce apoptosis of any activated T lymphocyte that expresses FAS.

Several other characteristics contribute to the immune-privileged site status of the eye. The absence of efferent lymphatic drainage and consequent drainage of lymph directly to the blood results in immune suppression (29–30). Soluble substances that can suppress the immune response are also part of the mechanisms involved in maintenance of immune privilege. Transforming growth factor-β, prostaglandin E$_2$, and neuropeptides (i.e., melanocyte-stimulating hormone-α, vasoactive intestinal peptide, and calcitonin-related gene) all contribute to the generation of a deviant immune response in places where these substances are secreted (6,31–36). In the eye, substances attached to the cellular membrane act as inhibitors of the complement cascade (37–38). Cells with suppressor activity, such as Müller cells and retinal pigment epithelial cells (RPE), play a role in modifying the response inside the eye to curtail inflammation (39–44). Another important component of immune privilege is the local tissue barrier. The eye cells from the parenchyma (RPE cells) have tight junctions. The expression of hialuronic acid on the cellular surface and reduced expression of major histocompatibility complex (MHC) class I and II complete the array of physical constituents of what is called the blood–retinal barrier (14,35,39–44).

An additional mechanism for controlling autoimmunity in the eye is the phenomenon of ACAID (26,27,45–47). In response to the introduction of antigens to the anterior chamber of the eye, a state of systemic tolerance to that antigen results. ACAID is a unique aspect of immune privilege in the eye, and it may play a role in the development of tolerance against ocular antigens (48–50).

Autoimmunity develops only if all the safeguard mechanisms described earlier and others not described in this chapter fail. In experimental models of disease, the point at which tolerance is broken and autoimmunity ensues is easily determined because disease induction is produced by active immunization with a specific target antigen. Nevertheless, it is often necessary to use one or more adjuvants to break the state of tolerance (51–54). In the case of experimental and human uveitis, a break in the blood–retinal barrier generally represents the beginning of the autoimmune process and sometimes may constitute its precipitating factor (55).

Ocular autoimmunity can be divided into two categories: external diseases affecting the cornea, conjunctiva, and adnexa and internal diseases. Diseases of the latter category have been called uveitis. Much of this chapter deals with uveitides, because these diseases are common and are the ones with special features because autoimmunity is occurring in an immune-privileged site. All endogenous uveitis contribute to 10% of severe ocular handicap cases in the United States and appear at a rate of 70,000 new cases per year, representing an important concern in ophthalmology and in public health (56–57). The concept that some endogenous uveitis may be caused by an autoimmune phenomenon was first introduced in the beginning of the century. In 1903, Uhlenhuth showed the existence of antibodies recognizing crystallin antigens (58). In 1910, Elschnig introduced the idea that autoantigens could be involved in the development of uveitis (59).

Originally, uveitis was a term used to describe an inflammatory process of the uvea that includes the iris, ciliary body, and choroid. Later, this term was used to describe any intraocular inflammation affecting the uvea and the retina, sclera, and vitreous humor. We have learned from the animal models of autoimmune uveitis that uveitogenic T cells can be elicited in the periphery by immunization with one of several retinal antigens. The diseases induced by different uveitogenic proteins share their histopathologic features and cellular mechanisms, suggesting that they also share the immunopathogenic mechanisms necessary for disease induction and progression. The existence of many retinal antigens that may act as a target for the autoimmune process in uveitis may account for the difficulty to isolate a single candidate target in human uveitis, although peripheral blood lymphocytes from patients with intermediate and posterior uveitis were shown to proliferate in response to S-Ag (60–61).

After T cells that recognize uveitogenic epitopes are activated, they migrate to the eye and initiate a cascade of events leading to the destruction of the photoreceptor layer and visual loss. Any activated T cell can penetrate the retina, but only cells recognizing pathogenic epitopes remain in the retina after 12 hours (62). These cells break the blood–retinal barrier through the secretion of various cytokines that induce expression of adhesion molecules and MHC class II molecules throughout the retina and its draining blood vessels. This breach allows the recruitment of other T cells, monocytes, and polymorphonuclear cells from the blood. In the rat and mouse models of uveitis, CD4-positive (CD4$^+$) T cells that recognize retinal antigens have been used to adoptively transfer disease to naive recipients confirming the nature of the autoimmune phenomenon (63–64). Uveitogenic cells have also been isolated from the uveitic eye in murine EAU and shown to behave in a similar fashion to those found in the periphery, suggesting that they constitute the same population at different stages of differentiation and that cells migrate from the periphery into the eye and mediate its autoimmune destruction (14,65).

In the rat model of autoimmune uveitis, the infiltrating T-lymphocyte populations change from mostly CD4$^+$ to predominately CD8$^+$ as disease progresses (66). The same dynamics in the infiltrating cell population was shown in a case of sympathetic ophthalmia in which both eyes were enucleated from a patient at different times during the course of disease. The eye enucleated early showed mainly CD4$^+$ cells, whereas the eye enucleated a year later was infiltrated mostly with CD8$^+$ cells (67). The T-cell dynamics in some human uveitis parallels that seen in the animal model.

The responses of ocular tissues in human uveitis and in the animal models seem to parallel each other. The expression of cell membrane markers is one of the earliest events seen when uveitis is induced experimentally. MHC class II molecules are expressed on many resident ocular cells, including the RPE, Müller cells, and vascular endothelial cells. Adhesion molecules are expressed as a result of experimental uveitis induction and in patients with endogenous disease (68).

As with most autoimmune diseases, strong human leukocyte antigen (HLA) associations have been observed in many types of human uveitic diseases (Table 25.1). The association with antigens from the major histocompatibility complex (56,61,69–72) suggests that the capacity to recognize certain epitopes expressed in ocular antigens or antigens that mimic such epitopes is associated with disease development. This finding also suggests that defects in clonal selection of T cells, whether it is the negative selection of autoreactive clones or the positive selection of suppressor clones, may be involved in disease development. The latter possibility was reinforced by the finding that uveitis develops in nude mice transplanted with embryonic thymi from susceptible rat strains (73). One of the strongest associations between HLA and disease occurs between birdshot retinochoroidopathy and

HLA-A29; the relative risk for this association is between 50 and 225 in Caucasians. Particularly in cases of birdshot retinochoroidopathy, most patients show peripheral blood lymphocyte proliferation to S-Ag (61), making this one of the few uveitic conditions for which a putative target antigen is known. An increased frequency of certain types of uveitis in specific ethnic groups has also been reported in the literature. Most of the associations between human uveitis and HLA are to class I antigens, despite the putative role of CD4$^+$ class II–restricted cells in the pathogenic process. This discrepancy may signify that the participation of CD8$^+$ cells is more important in humans than in the animal models as effector cells or as regulatory cells.

The availability of an animal model has been instrumental in better understanding the importance of the association between MHC haplotypes and susceptibility to disease induction (74). Murine studies have suggested that susceptibility is controlled by MHC and non-MHC genes (72,75). These studies revealed that the primary control of susceptibility is determined by MHC genes of the class II I-A subregion (equivalent to human HLA-DR), suggesting that the ability to recognize uveitogenic epitopes in the target ocular antigen plays a major part in the development of uveitis. The presence of certain H-2 haplotypes was shown to be crucial for the establishment of disease, and the genes involved were designated as "permissive" to the development of disease. Expression of I-E gene products (equivalent to the human HLA-DQ) was shown to decrease disease severity. Secondary control of susceptibility appears to be linked to non-MHC genes. Some backgrounds were shown to prevent completely the development of disease, regardless of the MHC haplotype these strains expressed. The genes involved were called "conducive" to the development of disease. Non-MHC influences on susceptibility can be caused by diverse mechanisms, including differences in hormonal responses to stress, mast cell numbers, vascular response to cytokines, and lymphokine response patterns. All these factors may play a role in susceptibility to autoimmunity. Data from the animal models suggest that genetic susceptibility to autoimmune uveitis may be linked to the ability to mount a $T_H1$-type response against the retinal antigen used to immunize the animals (75,76). However, resistance to disease has not been linked to a $T_H2$ response but rather to a "null" profile. In resistant strains, the response toward the immunizing antigen never includes any of the $T_H1$-type response characteristics (high IgG2a and interferon-$\gamma$ secretion in response to the immunizing antigen) and may or may not include $T_H2$-type response characteristics (high IgG1 production and secretion of interleukin-4 [IL-4], IL-5, and IL-10).

The diagnosis and classification of uveitis is based on the clinical history and physical examination. Uveitis can be classified in several different ways. Anatomically, it may be anterior (encompassing the anterior segment of the eye, such as the iris and ciliary body), intermediate (when involving the vitreous and pars plana), posterior (when the choroid and retina are involved), or panuveitis (when all segments are

**TABLE 25.1.** *Association between HLA and disease*

| Disease | HLA | Relative risk |
|---|---|---|
| Acute anterior uveitis | HLA-B27 (W) | 10 |
| | HLA-B8 (AA) | 5 |
| Ankylosing spondylitis | HLA-B27 (W) | 100 |
| | HLA-B7 (AA) | |
| Behçet's disease | HLA-B51 (O) | 4–6 |
| Birdshot retino-choroidopathy | HLA-A29 | 50–225 |
| Ocular-cutaneous pemphigoid | HLA-B12 (W) | 3–4 |
| Ocular histoplasmosis | HLA-B7 (W) | |
| Reiter's syndrome | HLA-B27 (W) | 40 |
| Sympathetic ophthalmia | HLA-A11 (M) | 4 |
| Vogt–Koyanagi–Harada syndrome | MT-3 (O) | 75 |

AA, African-American; M, mixed ethnicity; O, oriental; W, white Caucasian.
From Nussenblatt RB, Withcup SM, Palestine AG. *Uveitis: fundamentals and clinical practice.* 2nd ed. St. Louis: Mosby, 1996.

involved). Clinically, uveitis can be acute or chronic, unilateral or bilateral, granulomatous or nongranulomatous, and associated or not with systemic manifestations. In terms of its cause, exogenous uveitides are those in which an exogenous agent can be identified as the cause of the inflammation (such is the case in viral, bacterial, or parasitic uveitis). Uveitis is said to be endogenous when the triggering agent for the inflammatory process is unknown or when uveitis is of a well-established autoimmune nature. Uveitis may be part of a systemic syndrome affecting other organs, as is the case for the uveitis associated with ankylosing spondylitis, juvenile rheumatoid arthritis, Vogt–Koyanagi–Harada syndrome (uveoencephalitis), Behçet's disease, and sarcoidosis. Alternatively, uveitis be a single entity affecting solely the eye, as is the case of birdshot chorioretinopathy or sympathetic ophthalmia. Uveitis with autoimmune characteristics may also develop as a consequence of a known agent or entity without direct ocular involvement, as is the case in the paraneoplastic syndromes or septic shock (56).

The establishment of a putative diagnosis and the differential diagnosis is crucial, because each of the different diseases that may lead to uveitis may be treated differently. Tables 25.2 and 25.3 show the possible causes of anterior or posterior uveitis and their relative incidence in the United States. The choice of appropriate laboratory tests can improve the chances of diagnosing the nature of the uveitis. A nonselective approach to diagnostic testing is costly and inefficient, and it may even provide misleading information. Diagnostic procedures for each disease are discussed later. Briefly, for the diagnosis of autoimmune uveitis, the most useful tests are those that evaluate the acute phase response such as the erythrocyte sedimentation rate (ESR), C-reactive protein, serum immunoglobulins, and cryoglobulins. The latter are useful because mixed type cryoglobulins may be found in systemic lupus erythematous (SLE), rheumatoid arthritis, Sjögren's syndrome, polyarteritis nodosa, and sarcoidosis. Although these cryoglobulins may also be found in infectious diseases, their presence combined with the history

**TABLE 25.2.** *Differential diagnoses for anterior uveitis*

| Diagnosis | Frequency (%) |
|---|---|
| Idiopathic iridocyclitis | 12–33 |
| HLA B27+ iridocyclitis | ~3 |
| Juvenile rheumatoid arthritis | 3–5 |
| Fuchs heterochromic iridocyclitis | 2–6.5 |
| Herpes simplex virus keratouveitis | 1.5–2 |
| Intraocular lenses related to uveitis | 1–2 |
| Reiter's syndrome | 1–5 |
| Herpes zoster keratouveitis | 0.5–2 |
| Syphilis | 0.8–1.5 |
| Traumatic iridocyclitis | 0.5–1 |
| Inflammatory bowel disease | 0.3–3 |
| Glaucomatocyclitic crisis | 0.3–0.5 |
| Other | 41–63 |

Data from Nussenblatt RB, Withcup SM, Palestine AG. *Uveitis: fundamentals and clinical practice.* 2nd ed. St. Louis: Mosby, 1996.

**TABLE 25.3.** *Differential diagnoses for posterior uveitis*

| Diagnosis | Frequency (%) |
|---|---|
| Toxoplasmosis | 7–10 |
| Retinal vasculitis | 4.5–7 |
| Idiopathic | 6–7 |
| Ocular histoplasmosis | 3.5–4 |
| Toxocariasis | 2.5–3 |
| Cytomegalovirus retinitis | 2.5–4 |
| Serpiginous choroidopathy | ~2 |
| Acute retinal necrosis | ~1.5 |
| Birdshot choroidopathy | ~1.5 |
| Leukemia or lymphoma | 0.5–1.5 |
| Primary intraocular lymphoma | ~1 |
| Ocular candidiasis | ~1 |
| Tuberculous uveitis | ~0.5 |
| Systemic lupus erythematosus | ~0.5 |
| Other | 60–75 |

Data from Nussenblatt RB, Withcup SM, Palestine AG. *Uveitis: fundamentals and clinical practice.* 2nd ed. St. Louis: Mosby, 1996.

and clinical features of the patient may point toward autoimmunity. Other useful tests are those used for rheumatologic diseases, which may present initially with ocular manifestations only. The presence of rheumatoid factors, antinuclear antibodies, or lupus anticoagulant is suggestive of an autoimmune uveitis. The Kveim antigen skin test has not been used routinely because it involves a risk of hepatitis or retroviral infection, it has low specificity and sensitivity, and it is difficult to obtain the antigen. Association with HLA haplotypes is a characteristic of autoimmune uveitis, and testing for specific haplotypes is generally useful. Table 25.1 shows the most frequent associations between HLA and uveitis. Other tests that may be useful are the PPD skin test, which may become negative in sarcoidosis, and the angiotensin-converting enzyme (ACE), the result of which may be elevated in sarcoidosis.

Therapeutic choices for autoimmune uveitis are similar to those of any other autoimmune disease, except for surgical management of complications. The lack of specificity of current drugs has lead to intensive research of alternative forms of treatment some of which may become available soon to the practicing ophthalmologist. Table 25.4 summarizes the most prominent forms of immunotherapy being tested. Conventional treatment of autoimmune uveitis is discussed later.

The most frequent autoimmune diseases affecting the eye are presented here according to their anatomic and clinical characteristics. Patient management is discussed individually for each disease. However, because therapy is frequently similar, general guidelines for treatment are presented at the end of this chapter.

## EPISCLERITIS

### Clinical Characteristics

*Episcleritis* is a term used to describe any inflammation that involves episclera and Tenon's capsule without underlying

**TABLE 25.4.** *Antigen-specific immunotherapeutic approaches for autoimmune ocular diseases under development*

| Treatment | Mechanism | State of development |
|---|---|---|
| Oral tolerance | Anergy/deletion/induction of regulatory T cells | Phase I/II clinical trial |
| Anti-IL-2 receptor | Anergy/deletion of activated autoimmune cells | Phase I clinical trial |
| Anti-CD4 | Anergy/deletion of CD4+ cells | Animal models |
| Antiadhesion molecule | Inhibition of cell migration and recruitment to the inflammatory site | Request for clinical trial |
| Blocking of costimulation | Anergy/deletion of autoimmune T cells | Request for clinical trial |
| Intrathymic antigen | Deletion of autoimmune T cells | Animal models |
| Intravenous antigen | Anergy/deletion of autoimmune T cells | Animal models |
| ACAID | Immune deviation | Animal models |
| T-cell vaccination | Deletion of autoimmune T cells | Animal models |
| IL-10 | Inhibition of inflammation | Request for clinical trials |
| Anti-IL-12 | Blockade of $T_H1$ cell development | Animal models |
| IL-12 | Deletion of activated cells | Animal models |
| P40 (IL-12 homodymer) | Blockade of $T_H1$ cell development | Request for clinical trial |
| Anti-TNF | Inhibition of inflammation | Animal models |
| TNF-soluble receptor | Inhibition of inflammation | Clinical trial approved |
| Idiotypic network manipulation | Idiotypic adjustment of the autoimmune response | Animal models, except for the use of IVIG |

ACAID, anterior chamber–associated immune deviation; IVIG, intravenous immunoglobulin.

edema of the sclera. Episcleritis may be classified as diffuse (simple) or nodular. Clinically, although the redness may be intense, examination reveals that the inflammation is confined to the episcleral tissue, with the vessels of the conjunctiva remaining normal or just slightly dilated. There are no distortions of the vascular pattern. Ordinarily, the patients feel no pain nor have any ocular discharge, but there may be a prickly sensation that leads to considerable discomfort.

### Diagnosis

The diagnosis is clinical, made by external examination of the eye. Association with systemic diseases is rare.

### Patient Management

Episcleritis is a superficial disease and self-limiting, although recurrent, and unless it causes severe discomfort, it requires no treatment. Patients often demand therapy because of the distress caused by the appearance of the inflamed eye. Local steroids can reduce the inflammatory response and decrease the patient's discomfort. Systemic nonsteroidal antiinflammatory drugs are often useful and may be used instead of local steroids.

## SCLERITIS

### Clinical Characteristics

Scleritis is a more severe disease than episcleritis, in which the sclera and all its coats including the conjunctiva are involved in a destructive process that, if not treated properly, may lead to severe visual loss (Fig. 25.1). The disease may be classified anatomically as anterior, posterior, or both. It may also be classified clinically as diffuse, nodular, or necro-

tizing with inflammation or without inflammation. More than two thirds of the patients have an underlying systemic disease that must be diagnosed and treated. Scleritis may be associated with rheumatoid arthritis, Wegener's granulomatosis, polyarteritis nodosa, mixed connective tissue disease, and SLE. The disease may also be infectious, and diseases such as tuberculosis, syphilis, and herpes virus infection must be excluded before starting treatment. It may be surgically induced, which is an easy diagnosis if a careful history has been taken. It also may be caused by neoplasias.

The disease is ordinarily extremely painful, although in scleromalacia perforans, it may be painless. The pain tends to be referred to the temple and face, and it characteristically wakes the patient during the night. The disease is usually recurrent and bilateral, with an insidious onset that may involve one eye initially, and it may take several weeks to involve the fellow eye.

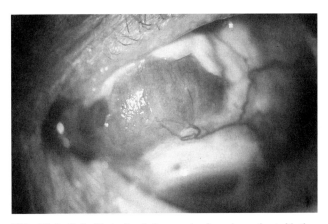

**FIG. 25.1.** Scleritis in the left eye of a female patient. Notice the extensive destruction of the sclera, edema of the peripheral tissues, and injection of the local vessels.

## Diagnosis

A careful history has to be made to determine the type of onset, associated symptoms, and diseases. A consultation with a rheumatologist is always welcome. Investigation of the hemoglobin levels, white cell count, erythrocyte sedimentation rate, C-reactive protein, serum uric acid, and serology for syphilis (a major infectious cause of scleritis) should be performed. A chest computed tomography (CT) scan is useful in diagnosing sarcoidosis. The presence of rheumatoid factor, anti-DNA, and antinuclear antibodies should be tested for if a second round of laboratory examinations is required to clarify the diagnosis. If the history suggests vasculitis, the presence of antinuclear cytoplasmic antibodies should be investigated. These should reveal the presence or absence of an underlying systemic disease, thereby determining whether the patient requires extensive immunosuppression. The presence of anterior scleritis can be deduced from the physical examination. However, the diagnosis of posterior scleritis is difficult, because its presence can only be implied from the destruction of surrounding tissues. When posterior scleritis is suspected, B-scan ultrasonography may be of help, although the results rarely help the examiner decide whether the choroid and sclera are involved together or separately.

## Patient Management

Local steroid therapy is often of no value in scleritis. Patients with diffuse, nodular anterior scleritis and their counterparts in the posterior segment sometimes respond to a nonsteroidal antiinflammatory drug (NSAID). Treatment should be tapered as soon as the eye becomes quiet. Control of the inflammatory response can be measured by the absence of pain and the degree of swelling and vascular congestion. Failure to respond to NSAID should prompt the physician to think of an early necrotizing scleritis, although occasionally nonnecrotizing scleritis does not respond to NSAID. Patients with necrotizing scleritis must be given systemic steroids at immunosuppressive doses. As soon as the disease is under control, the medication can be slowly tapered to antiinflammatory doses. At this point, combinations with NSAIDs may reduce the requirement for systemic steroids. Patients who fail to respond should be treated with combination therapy that can include cyclosporin A or cytotoxic drugs. Cyclophosphamide is the drug of choice in combination with steroids for patients with systemic vasculitis. All of these drugs have serious side effects.

Surgery for a graft replacement of the sclera should only be undertaken after the systemic disease is controlled. If a perforation requires immediate surgical treatment, pulse steroid or cytotoxic drug therapy is recommended.

## SJÖGREN'S SYNDROME

### Clinical Characteristics

Sjögren's syndrome is defined as the presence of dry mouth, dry eye, and an autoimmune disease, usually rheumatoid arthritis. Because dry mouth and dry eye (i.e., sicca symptoms) are subjective complaints, a set of specific criteria have been defined to fully characterize the disease: a low score on the Schirmer test, which consists of measuring basal and stimulated lacrimal gland production; low salivary gland production on examination by the physician; and proof of lymphocytic infiltration of the labial salivary glands (i.e., biopsy of at least four glandular lobules with an average of at least two foci of 50 or more lymphocytes per four square millimeters. The final diagnosis of Sjögren's syndrome is based on the presence of the previously described characteristics associated with the diagnosis of a systemic autoimmune disease. Patients generally report eye irritation and a foreign-body sensation, which is generally more pronounced in the late afternoon or evening. Other symptoms associated with the keratoconjunctivitis sicca (KCS) due to Sjögren's syndrome are a burning feeling, redness of the conjunctiva, photophobia, blurred vision, itching, and pain. Keratoconjunctivitis sicca is a common finding, especially in postmenopausal women, and most of these cases are not related to Sjögren's syndrome.

### Diagnosis

Slit-lamp examination of the conjunctiva reveals a diminished or absent tear meniscus. The presence of debris or mucus is also common. Fluorescein staining is also useful, and using a dry fluorescein strip to the inferior bulbar conjunctiva can indicate the wetness of the surface and stains the tear meniscus, allowing better visualization. It can also provide useful information regarding the integrity of the ocular epithelium. Fluorescein stains ulcers in the epithelium. Rose Bengal staining may also be employed. Rose Bengal dye stains degenerating epithelial cells lacking a protective mucin coating. The Schirmer test is the most commonly used test to quantify tear production. To perform the test, a standardized strip of paper is placed over the temporal lower lid margin, letting the paper absorb the liquid by capillary action. The amount of wetting of the strip is measured in millimeters after 5 minutes. Because the application of the filter strip to an unanesthetized eye itself stimulates tear production, most individuals produce at least 10 mm of tears. The Schirmer test, however, has low sensitivity and specificity and should never be considered alone as diagnostic of KCS. Other tests such as the fluorescein dilution test, the tear lysozyme and lactoferrin tests, tear osmolarity determination, conjunctival scrapings, and conjunctival impression cytology may be useful.

### Patient Management

Treatment is largely directed at providing symptomatic relief. A randomized, double-masked clinical trial, comparing the use of several immunosuppressive drugs, including cyclosporine, began in 1998 at the National Eye Institute (National Institutes of Health, Bethesda, MD, U.S.A.). A phase II/III clinical trial is underway evaluating the use of cyclosporine in KCS. Until the results of this trial are known, topically applied lubricating drops and ointments continue to be the only proven therapy the physician can offer to patients. Secretagogues agents are still under scrutiny and no reliable data is yet available on their use in KCS.

## KAWASAKI'S DISEASE

### Clinical Characteristics

Kawasaki's disease is a rare disease that induces a variety of ocular signs and symptoms. However, ocular involvement does not usually lead to serious visual disturbances. Conjunctivitis is the most common ocular manifestation of Kawasaki's disease; about 90% of the patients show some degree of conjunctival injection. Characteristically, patients have minimal or no discharge despite the bulbar injection. Acute, nongranulomatous iridocyclitis is another common feature and is observed in approximately 80% of the patients. Superficial keratitis may also be present in about one fifth of the patients. Vitreous opacification, papilledema, dilation of the retinal vessels, retinal folds, or subretinal hemorrhages have been described.

### Diagnosis

The principles of diagnosis for Kawasaki's disease are discussed elsewhere in this book. The diagnosis of Kawasaki's disease associated ocular symptoms is based on the previous knowledge that the patients bears such affliction and present at the medical office with one or more of the symptoms and signs described earlier.

### Patient Management

Severe anterior uveitis associated with Kawasaki's disease may be treated with topical corticosteroids. Most cases, however, appear to be mild, are self-limited, and resolve spontaneously.

## HLA-B27–ASSOCIATED ANTERIOR UVEITIS AND IDIOPATHIC ANTERIOR UVEITIS

### Clinical Characteristics

Disease onset is often sudden, and symptoms may persist for up to 6 weeks. Attacks are generally unilateral, although either eye may be involved at different times, and with time, some patients may develop chronic bilateral uveitis with poor visual prognosis. Clinical features of patients with anterior uveitis vary greatly whether they are HLA-B27 positive or not. The association between HLA-B27 and acute anterior uveitis has been known for more than two decades, and in the United States, approximately one half of patients with anterior uveitis alone carry the HLA-B27 haplotype, while its frequency in the normal population varies between 5% and 10%. HLA-B27+ patients tend to show earlier onset, more severe acute disease, and a contrasting, somewhat better ophthalmologic prognosis. The clinical characteristics of patients with anterior uveitis and of those with ankylosing spondylitis and Reiter's syndrome vary according to whether they are HLA-B27 positive (56,77).

### Diagnosis

Diagnosis is based on the presence of anterior uveitis that is not associated with any other systemic manifestation. HLA typing is instrumental, because HLA-B27+ patients may behave differently from those who are negative for this haplotype. Laboratory tests include acute-phase proteins that are altered, with the possible exception of transferrin. An elevated ESR is also indicative of disease. It has been described that $\alpha_1$-antitrypsin, factor B, and haptoglobin show the most significant changes when compared with control individuals or patients with traumatic uveitis (77).

### Patient Management

Patients with acute anterior uveitis without systemic disease generally respond well to topical corticosteroids. Occasionally, these patients require sub-Tenon injections of corticosteroids given every 1 to 2 weeks. The major concerns regarding this form of therapy are with possible intraocular penetration, proptosis of the globe, and fibrosis of the extraocular muscles. Transient ptosis of the upper lid may occur. The induction of glaucoma is also a concern, and repeated injections, particularly in children, may result in the same systemic side effects observed with corticoids given orally or intravenously. The use of mydriatic agents such as atropine drops is suggested because of the potential for the development of adherence (synechiae) between the iris and the lens.

## UVEITIS ASSOCIATED WITH CHILDHOOD ARTHRITIS

### Clinical Characteristics

In most patients (often young girls), the intraocular inflammation of uveitis associated with childhood arthritis (i.e., juvenile rheumatoid arthritis [JRA] and juvenile psoriatic arthritis) appears as a bilateral nongranulomatous chronic anterior uveitis. Keratic precipitates (Fig. 25.2) are usually small in size and located mainly in the inferior half of the corneal endothelium. Koeppe nodules and dense protein synechiae are typically present. Mononuclear cells infiltrate the aqueous humor and the anterior vitreous.

About 75% of the cases of ocular involvement in patients with JRA and juvenile psoriatic arthritis are bilateral. Generally, both eyes are involved simultaneously or within a month of each other. It is unusual for these patients with unilateral uveitis to develop uveitis in the second eye after more than 12 months have elapsed from the start of the ocular symptoms. Uveitis onset is usually asymptomatic, and it is detected initially by routine slit-lamp examination of patients at risk. Even during exacerbations with intense cell infiltrate in the aqueous humor, the eye remains nonsymptomatic to

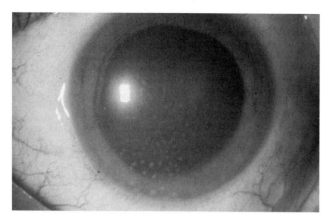

**FIG. 25.2.** Keratic precipitates in the inferior half of the cornea. See color plate 24.

the external examination. Occasionally, patients may refer to blurred vision and vitreous floaters.

Some risk factors for the development of uveitis have been recognized in children with chronic arthritis. Females are at higher risk than males, as are children who develop oligoarticular arthritis before age 6. In patients with JRA, the arthropathy tends to get better when these individuals reach adulthood, but the uveitis is sometimes progressive and leads to significant visual loss. Most cases of uveitis associated with JRA develop in children with the oligoarticular or pauciarticular form of the disease and often in children without other systemic symptoms, such as cardiac disease.

### Diagnosis

Diagnosis is made generally by slit-lamp examination, because earlier uveitis is often asymptomatic. The presence of antinuclear antibodies is often seen in patients with JRA that develop uveitis. In contrast, the presence of rheumatoid factor is considered a marker of resistance to uveitis. Children bearing the HLA-DR5 haplotype are also at higher risk to develop ocular complications, unlike patients bearing the HLA-DR4.

### Patient Management

In most patients, the uveitis can be controlled by the appropriate use of topical corticosteroids. Patients who are unresponsive to topical medication may respond to oral corticosteroid therapy. Some cases require intravenous pulse therapy. Methylprednisolone is the drug of choice in a dose of 20 to 30 mg/kg/day for up to 3 consecutive days. Systemic immunosuppressive drugs are seldom required, and they often do not work. In these cases, cyclosporine may an alternative drug, although indications are that the results are not as promising as once was thought. The use of cytotoxic and antimetabolic agents have to be weighed against important side effects in children, most notably the increased risk for the development of leukemia and lymphoma. Chlorambucil adds the prospect of sterility in male children.

## FUCHS HETEROCHROMIC CYCLITIS

### Clinical Characteristics

Fuchs uveitis was first described by Dr. Ernst Fuchs around 1906. The disease in its classic form affects young adults and is characterized by a quiet external eye and heterochromia with the involved eye lighter in color. The disease is unilateral in 90% of the cases, and peripupillary anterior iris atrophy is common. Ocular examination reveals hyaline keratic precipitates with intervening filaments. Occasionally, Koeppe or Bussaca nodules are associated with a cellular infiltrate in the vitreous. Chorioretinal scars may be seen occasionally. The disease has a long, insidious course, and the prognosis is good. The Amsler sign (i.e., hyphema after sudden reduction in the intraocular pressure during surgery) is pathognomonic. The most common complications are cataracts beginning with posterior subcapsular changes, and secondary glaucoma, which may be aggravated by the use of corticosteroids.

The cause of Fuchs heterochromic cyclitis is unknown, and the differential diagnosis includes diseases as diverse as herpesvirus infection and masquerade syndromes. A primary infectious cause may trigger an autoimmune response, leading to Fuchs heterochromic cyclitis. The association between ocular toxoplasmosis and Fuchs lends support to this hypothesis (78).

Nonclassic forms of the disease exist. These variants of the typical disease may affect individuals at any age group, a red eye may be present, and heterochromia may be reversed, with the darker eye being affected. Iris atrophy may be absent in some cases, even in the presence of significant heterochromia, and occasionally, iris atrophy may be seen in the absence of heterochromia. Some patients may show pupil irregularities due to sphincter atrophy, and peripheral anterior synechiae may also be present. Patients with the variant forms often develop cataracts. Secondary glaucoma may be present in more than 50% of the patients. Vitreous hemorrhage is common, and the incidence of corneal edema is high. Radial vessels may be seen in the iris, and rubeosis is common. Patients that develop glaucoma have a worse prognosis than all the others, but unlike individuals with the classic form of the disease, it is hard to predict the evolution of patients with the variant forms.

### Diagnosis

There are no specific laboratory tests, and the diagnosis is based on the clinical findings only. Association with HLA haplotypes has been described, but the risk factors are few. Diagnosis of Fuchs heterochromia is often made in the course of a routine examination for a patient complaining of vitreous floaters or with symptoms of cataracts. The heterochromia should be the first clue for the diagnosis, and it is often not apparent to the patient, even after the physician points it to the patient. However, individuals with variant forms may not have heterochromia, especially a patient with dark-pigmented irises. A study of more than 100 patients in Brazil showed that heterochromia was present in fewer than 40% of the patients (79).

## Patient Management

Uveitis in these patients is often mild and asymptomatic and does not require specific therapy. Occasionally, Fuchs uveitis causes some discomfort because of ciliary injection and an increase in keratic precipitates or cells, leading to an increase in floaters. These symptoms may warrant a short-term topical corticosteroid therapy. Cellular debris in the vitreous can lead to significant visual disturbance, which can increase after intracapsular cataract surgery. Occasionally, a vitrectomy may be necessary to clear the vitreous. Patients that develop glaucoma usually respond well to clinical or surgical management of glaucoma. The recommended approach for cataract treatment in these patients consists of extracapsular cataract extraction and phacoemulsification with intraocular lenses (80).

## INTERMEDIATE UVEITIS

### Clinical Characteristics

Intermediate uveitis is a common diagnosis, and it represents 8% to 22% of all cases of endogenous uveitis seen in adult patients (81–82) and 15% to 32% of all cases of uveitis in children (83–84). Cases may be unilateral, bilateral, and asymmetric. The course of disease is generally chronic, with periodic exacerbations and remissions.

Intermediate uveitis has an insidious onset, and patients with symptomatic intermediate uveitis most often complain of blurred vision. Floaters are also a common complaint of these patients. Children have a tendency to develop anterior segment inflammation, more so than adult patients. Inflammatory cells infiltrating the vitreous humor is the most consistent sign of intermediate uveitis, and vitreous humor detachment can occasionally mark the onset of disease. The cellular infiltrate in the vitreous resembles "dust" at the slit-lamp examination. Vitreous humor opacities (i.e., "snowballs") can be seen in about one third of the patients. The presence of characteristic peripheral pars plana and retina exudates establishes the diagnosis of pars planitis, a subgroup of intermediate uveitis. Children tend to present significant anterior segment inflammation and exuberant exudates that extend to the back of the crystalline lens. Cuffing of retinal vessels with obliterative vasculitis may be identified.

The most common complication is macular edema. Retinal neovascularization, glaucoma, vitreous hemorrhage, and retinal detachment may also occur.

### Diagnosis

The diagnosis is clinical, and there is no confirmatory test. Laboratory tests should be used mostly to exclude any of the diseases in the differential diagnosis list. According to the patient's age and clinical presentation, it may include multiple sclerosis, sarcoidosis, lymphoma, and infectious diseases such as syphilis, borreliosis, toxocariasis, and Lyme disease.

## Patient Management

Clinical treatment should be limited to patients with vision at or below 20/40, which is caused more often by macular edema. Some ophthalmologists recommend a more aggressive approach, treating all symptomatic patients with visual macular cysts at any level of visual acuity. Periocular injection of corticosteroids is the treatment of choice to decrease the macular edema. Children who develop a chronic macular edema often develop cystoid macular degeneration with or without a macular hole that leads to permanent visual loss. Many of these patients require repeated periocular injections often under general anesthesia, which complicates even further their care. Patients with pars planitis and visual loss due to macular edema or vitreous opacities may also be treated with cryocoagulation of the peripheral retina. In the most severe and refractory cases pars plana vitrectomy can improve vision by draining inflammatory cells. Topical steroids should be used only in cases with anterior segment inflammation, because they do little to ameliorate posterior inflammation and increase the rate of cataracts in phakic eyes. Systemic administration of corticosteroids and other immunosuppressive drugs are reserved for bilateral severe disease. The doses and choice of drugs alone or in association are described in more detail at the end of this chapter.

## SARCOIDOSIS

### Clinical Characteristics

Patients with systemic sarcoidosis have a rate of ocular involvement that varies from 25% to 75% (85–86). Despite the presence of physical findings, some of these patients have no visual symptoms. Among the symptomatic patients, most have developed systemic disease by the time visual loss occurs. Rarely, patients with uveitis later develop biopsy-confirmed extraocular sarcoidosis.

The initial presentation of sarcoidosis may be acute, subacute, or chronic. Uveitis and its complications are the most common vision-threatening manifestation of sarcoidosis. The presence of conjunctival granuloma, although it does not contribute to visual morbidity, is diagnostic. There may also be involvement of the lacrimal glands leading to tear deficiency. Inferior corneal thickening is the most common corneal finding in patients with sarcoidosis.

Patients with acute anterior uveitis complain of blurred vision, pain, photophobia, or red eyes. The ocular examination may reveal the presence of large, often pigmented, granulomatous keratic precipitates with protein and cells in the aqueous with Koeppe (pupillary margin) or Bussaca (iris surface) nodules. The formation of posterior synechiae is also common, leading to anterior synechiae and cataracts.

Chronic anterior disease usually has an insidious onset, and patients may have anterior synechiae, posterior synechiae, cataracts, and keratic precipitates in addition to aqueous inflammation. Some investigators have suggested that chronic anterior disease is more common than acute uveitis (87). Patients with panuveitis typically have posterior synechiae, retinal vasculitis, and macular edema.

The pars plana may be involved, leading to a clinical picture indistinguishable from pars planitis. Posterior segment involvement may occur in 15% to 45% of the patients, and involvement of the fundus has been associated with central nervous system involvement (88); periphlebitis is the most common posterior pole fundus lesion in sarcoidosis. Cellular infiltration of the vitreous humor is the most common manifestation of posterior segment involvement. The inflammatory cells may be dispersed in the vitreous, forming aggregates called snowballs. When these aggregates occur in chains, they are called "string of pearls" and may cast a shadow on the retina. The choroid may also be involved, and the presence of a granuloma is often associated to a retinal detachment and may exist without anterior segment inflammation. Optic nerve involvement may take many forms, with edema of the optic disc, granuloma of the optic disc, or atrophy of the nerve. Neovascularization may also occur.

Ocular involvement is a common feature of children with sarcoid arthritis. Anterior uveitis is present in 70% to 95% of the patients. Because the ocular and systemic manifestations are similar to those of patients with JRA, it is important to differentiate between the two diseases early.

### Diagnosis

The differential diagnosis of sarcoidosis consists of a significant number of diseases, which include other autoimmune diseases, infectious diseases, reactive responses to drugs, and malignancies. The intricacies of this differential diagnosis are discussed in Chapters 17 and 21. Only a small percentage of all patients with sarcoidosis present ocular signs and symptoms before the systemic manifestations of disease. In these cases, some laboratory tests may be useful. The simplest test is a chest CT scan that may reveal the typical features of pulmonary involvement. Pulmonary function test results often are normal for patients with early sarcoidosis. Serum angiotensin-converting enzyme levels are elevated in most untreated sarcoidosis patients and may be useful diagnostically in adults and children. Lysozyme is another marker that may be explored, because it is also elevated, although it is a less specific test. Some HLA haplotypes such as B13, BW15, B8, and DR3 have been associated with sarcoidosis or neurosarcoidosis.

### Patient Management

Because of the systemic characteristics of this disease, the decision to treat must be individualized, taking into account the potential for structural damage of the organs involved,

loss of function, and potential for life-threatening evolution. Patients often respond well to systemic corticosteroids. Patients with mild anterior uveitis may be treated with topical steroids and cycloplegics. If the uveitis is unresponsive to these measures, periorbital corticosteroids are indicated. Unilateral or asymmetric intermediate and posterior uveitis should be treated initially with periocular injections of corticosteroids. In the absence of systemic symptoms, systemic steroids administration should be reserved for severe cases that are unresponsive to local treatment or when the disease is bilateral and sight threatening. Systemic cytotoxic and chemotherapeutic agents may occasionally be required in patients with complications of corticosteroid therapy. The use of immunosuppressive drugs such as cyclosporin A or FK506 have not been successful in our hands.

## SYMPATHETIC OPHTHALMIA

### Clinical Characteristics

Sympathetic ophthalmia is a bilateral granulomatous panuveitis that develops in the contralateral eye after a penetrating injury involving the uvea of the other eye. The injured eye is called the exciting eye, and the fellow eye is called the sympathizing eye. Prevalence of disease varies between 0.1% and 0.2% after penetrating ocular trauma. The interval between injury and onset can be as short as 5 days or as long as 66 years. Disease onset is usually insidious, with slight pain, photophobia, and decreased vision in both eyes as the norm. Generally, the exciting eye is chronically inflamed and phthisic. The typical diagnostic feature of sympathetic ophthalmia is the presence of small yellowish white infiltrates at the level of the retinal pigmented epithelium (i.e., Dalen-Fuchs nodules). These nodules are most commonly present in the midperiphery of the fundus. Cataracts, iriditis, glaucoma, retinal detachment (Fig. 25.3), macular edema, and subretinal neovascularization may complicate the evolution of disease.

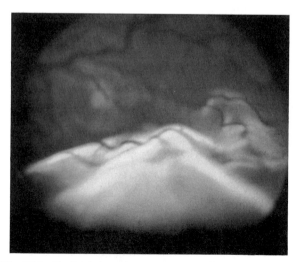

**FIG. 25.3.** Retinal detachment of the lower hemisphere of the retina.

## Diagnosis

The diagnosis is clinical, and the sole feature that differentiates sympathetic ophthalmia from idiopathic panuveitis is the history of a penetrating lesion to the exciting eye. HLA haplotypes A11, B40, DR4, DRw53, DQw3 are all associated with predisposition to develop disease (89–92).

## Patient Management

The only known preventive measure for sympathetic ophthalmia is the enucleation of the traumatized eye before disease develops in the sympathizing eye. Most experts agree that enucleation of the traumatized eye helps prevent uveitis of the sympathizing eye only if performed up to 3 weeks after injury. However, because the disease is rare, enucleation is only indicated for traumatized eyes that become blind. If disease develops, high-dose corticosteroid therapy should be instituted, starting with 1.5 mg/kg/day of oral prednisone. The dose should be gradually tapered as inflammation subsides. Topical steroids and cycloplegics may be used with systemic therapy. Refractory cases should be treated with a combination between corticosteroids and another agent. Cyclosporin A is the drug of choice. Cytotoxic and antimetabolic agents may also be used if the combination of steroids and cyclosporin A is unsuccessful. Some cases may require repeated pulse therapy with corticosteroids and or cytotoxic drugs.

## VOGT–KOYANAGI–HARADA SYNDROME

### Clinical Characteristics

Vogt–Koyanagi–Harada syndrome (VKH) is a bilateral diffuse granulomatous panuveitis with exudative bilateral retinal detachments associated with various extraocular manifestations such as meningitis, pleocytosis in the cerebrospinal fluid, hearing loss that may be transient or permanent, tinnitus, dysacusis, vitiligo, alopecia, and premature graying of the hair (i.e., poliosis). Rarely, the disease may manifest with ocular symptoms only. VKH seems to be more common in Asians (especially those with Japanese heritage), Native Americans, and in Hispanics. The most common complaint is an acute blurring of vision in both eyes. Choroidal inflammation is often multifocal and is associated with retinal detachments and changes of the underlying retinal pigmented epithelium. A chronic phase follows these acute manifestations and is characterized by depigmentation of the choroid. Depigmentation of the choroid occurs 2 to 3 months after the uveitic attack, and the fundus exhibits a characteristic orangered color that is known as "sunset glow." Vitiligo may start at this stage of disease. Recurrences are common and generally are characterized by a panuveitis. The long-term complications of VKH syndrome include cataracts, secondary glaucoma, subretinal neovascular membranes, and optic nerve atrophy.

## Diagnosis

The differential diagnosis of VKH syndrome includes other autoimmune causes of diffuse uveitis such as sympathetic ophthalmia (which should be excluded by the clinical history), uveal effusion, syphilis, Lyme disease, borreliosis, and sarcoidosis. The diagnosis is based on clinical findings, and a lumbar puncture may help, revealing pleocytosis. An echography of the globe may be useful to excluded tumors and show retinal detachments in those eyes with opaque media that do not allow direct visualization by fundoscopy. A fluorescein angiogram of the retina in the acute phase usually shows multiple punctate hyperfluorescent dots at the level of the RPE that overlie areas of choroiditis and optic disc staining.

## Patient Management

The basic principle of treatment for VKH syndrome is to suppress inflammation early and aggressively using systemic corticosteroids that may be tapered over a period of 3 to 6 months after the eye becomes quiet. The doses vary from 100 to 200 mg of prednisone daily or pulse therapy of up to 3 g of corticosteroids. Local corticosteroids and mydriatic agents should also be employed. Some investigators suggest topical steroids should be administered if the anterior uveitis is confirmed by examination, even if is asymptomatic (93,94). Other immunosuppressive agents should be employed if the disease is resistant to systemic corticosteroid therapy. Cyclosporine is the second drug of choice, used as a corticoid-sparing agent or in association with cytotoxic agents if steroid therapy fails. The doses vary between 1 and 5 mg/kg/day, aiming at a maintenance dose of 0.1 to 0.4 µg/mL of serum. Patients using of cyclosporine have always to be monitored for their renal function because of the well-known nephrotoxicity of this drug. Cyclophosphamide may be used at 1 to 2 mg/kg/day and chlorambucil at 0.05 to 0.1 mg/kg/day (maximum dose of 18 mg/day). Azathioprine is another drug that can be used in the treatment of VKH at dose of 1 to 5 mg/kg/day. A less toxic derivative of azathioprine is being tested, and results are promising.

## BIRDSHOT RETINOCHOROIDOPATHY

### Clinical Characteristics

Birdshot retinochoroidopathy is a rare disease. Unlike other uveitic diseases that typically affect younger patients, birdshot retinochoroidopathy occurs between the third and sixth decades of life. The disease is found more frequently in Caucasians of northern European extraction. The disease is usually bilateral, and patients generally complain of floaters with variable degrees of vision loss. Photophobia, difficulty in distinguishing colors, and night blindness are also reported as associated symptoms. The classic description of the disease is of a quiet nonpainful eye with minimal anterior segment inflammation, vitritis without snowballs or snowbanks (Fig. 25.4), retinal vascular leakage, and the distinctive scattered

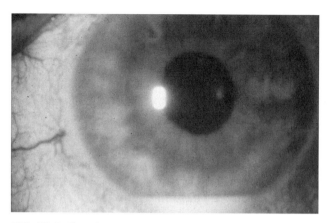

**FIG. 25.4.** Snowbanking.

cream-colored (or depigmented) spots located predominately in the nasal area of the fundus (95). A vitreous humor cellular reaction is present in all patients, but its severity varies between patients and in a same patient from one examination to the next. The clinical course of the disease is marked by exacerbations and remissions, and the prognosis is variable.

### Diagnosis

Birdshot retinochoroidopathy shares many features with several disorders such as intermediate uveitis and many other white-dot syndromes (i.e., diseases characterized by the presence of whitish lesions in the choroid, RPE, or the sensory retina). Infectious diseases that belong in the differential diagnosis are tuberculosis, syphilis, histoplasmosis, and choroidal pneumocystosis in acquired immunodeficiency syndrome (AIDS) patients. The clinical diagnosis may be helped by HLA typing, because HLA-A29 is present in 80% to 90% of all cases (97–98). HLA-A29 subtyping does not further help the diagnosis (96). A diagnostic vitrectomy may be helpful in excluding an intraocular lymphoma. Auxiliary tests such as fluorescein angiography, indocyanine green angiography, and electrophysiology may be useful.

### Patient Management

Because the number of patients with birdshot retinochoroidopathy is small and disease may resolve spontaneously, there is no consensus about the best therapeutic approach. High doses of prednisone (1 mg/kg/day) have been used with various results. Unfortunately, some patients become dependent on doses higher than 20 to 30 mg/day of corticosteroids, which causes a problem for long-term maintenance in these individuals. This is not, however, a specific characteristic of patients with birdshot retinochoroidopathy, because it also occurs in patients with sarcoidosis, VKH, sympathetic ophthalmia, and Behçet's disease who use corticosteroids for prolonged periods. Azathioprine, cyclophosphamide, and chlorambucil have all been used alone or in association without proven efficacy. The addition of

cyclosporine as a steroid-sparing agent has been reported as successful at doses from 1 to 2.5 mg/kg/day or in association with azathioprine or chlorambucil (99–100).

## BEHÇET'S DISEASE

### Clinical Characteristics

The disease was first described by Behçet, although similar syndromes were described as early as ancient Greece. The disease is found worldwide, but it has a higher incidence between the latitudes of 30° and 45° N. It is the leading cause of endogenous uveitis in Japan and Turkey, and it is one of the major causes of blindness in both countries (101,102). It is also a common entity in countries around the Mediterranean sea and in South America.

Behçet's disease is a systemic inflammatory illness characterized by intraocular nongranulomatous inflammation, oral and mucosal ulcers, skin lesions, and a variety of other disorders that affect the joints, the intestine, the epididymis, and the vascular and nervous systems. It is a episodic disease, and onset is generally sudden, followed by quiet periods that can last for months.

The ocular manifestations of Behçet's disease are often serious. In an epidemiologic survey in Japan, around 70% of the patients with Behçet's disease had some type of ocular involvement (103). The visual prognosis is particularly poor for patients who manifest posterior segment inflammation. The disease is characterized by recurrent attacks of severe ocular inflammation. Although the disease can affect the anterior and posterior segments of the eye separately, most patients have panuveitis or posterior uveitis, with only a small number (less than 10% in some reports) showing anterior segment inflammation only. Ocular disease usually develops 2 to 3 years after the initial lesions appear, which in most cases are represented by oral ulcers. In approximately 20% of the patients, ocular manifestations are the first signs of disease (104). Most patients have bilateral ocular involvement, but the interval between involvement of both eyes may be more than 5 years (56). Anterior uveitis with hypopyon (Fig. 25.5) is present in about one third of the patients. The

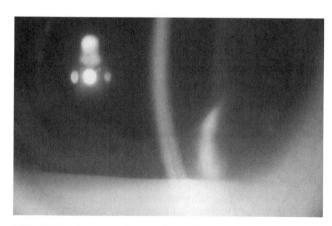

**FIG. 25.5.** Hypopyon in a patient with Behçet's disease.

hypopyon resolves spontaneously after a few hours to several days without sequelae (111–113). The hypopyon is composed mostly by neutrophils (114), and it characteristically shifts with gravity as the patient's head changes positions. Posterior synechiae, iris atrophy, and peripheral anterior synechiae may develop during the course of disease, as well as secondary glaucoma and cataract. Recurrent retinal vascular occlusions lead to severe visual loss because of the destruction these infarcts cause to the sensory retina.

Fundoscopic examination reveals venous engorgement, retinal hemorrhages, vascular sheathing, yellow-white exudates, retinal edema and infiltrates, hyperemia, and edema of the optic nerve disc. Papillitis may be associated with a vitreous inflammatory response. The posterior segment inflammation may lead to retinal and optic disc atrophy. If large areas of the retina are involved, neovascularization may occur leading to vitreous hemorrhages, vitreous contraction, and retinal detachments.

### Diagnosis

The Behçet's Disease Research Committee, organized by the Ministry of Health and Welfare of Japan in 1972 (115), proposed guidelines for the diagnosis of Behçet's disease that have been followed worldwide (Table 25.5). In 1990, the International Study Group for Behçet's Disease proposed a similar set of criteria (117). The Japanese group emphasizes the ocular findings, whereas the International Group stresses the presence of oral ulcerations (Table 25.6). In patients with the incomplete form of disease (Table 25.5) or with mild or atypical presentations, the differential diagnosis must include HLA-B27–related uveitis and sarcoidosis. There are no laboratory tests specific for Behçet's disease, although HLA-B51 is strongly associated with the disease, especially in the Japanese population. Although the International Study Group on Behçet's Disease suggests that the pathergy test be used as a major diagnostic criteria, the differences in positivity between patients in the United States and in the Mediter-

ranean, as well as suggestions that surgical cleaning of the skin before the "prick" may reduce its positivity rate, make this an unreliable test.

### Patient Management

Colchicine has been the drug of choice of many physicians in Japan at a dose of 0.5 to 1 mg/day. However, its effectiveness may vary among races. Most ophthalmologists outside Japan do not prescribe it as frequently. Various immunosuppressive agents have been used in the treatment of Behçet's disease. Azathioprine has been reported to be ineffective in restoring compromised vision but effective in preventing further attacks (118). Chlorambucil and cyclophosphamide have also been widely used, and they are thought to be efficient in preventing attacks and in maintaining good visual acuity over extended periods. Their effects on bone marrow cells, however, preclude long-term use of these drug (109). Cyclosporine has been used by many ophthalmologists as the second drug of choice, at an initial dose of 5 mg/kg/day under continuous evaluation of serum creatinine levels and, if pos-

**TABLE 25.6.** *Diagnostic criteria for Behçet's disease of the International Study Group*

| | |
|---|---|
| Recurrent oral ulceration | Aphthous ulcers or herpetiform lesions that have recurred at least 3 times in one 12-month period |
| Plus two of the following | |
| Recurrent genital ulcers | Aphthous ulceration or scarring |
| Ocular lesions | Anterior uveitis, posterior uveitis, cells infiltrating the vitreous humor, or retinal vasculitis |
| Skin lesions | Erythema nodosum, pseudofolliculitis, papulopustular lesions, acneiform nodules |
| Positive pathergy test | |

Adapted from the International Study Group for Behçet's Disease. Criteria for diagnosis of Behçet's disease.

**TABLE 25.5.** *Diagnostic criteria for Behçet's disease of the Japanese Ministry of Health and Welfare*

| Criteria | | Diagnosis | |
|---|---|---|---|
| Major | Minor | Complete type | Incomplete type |
| Recurrent oral aphthous ulcers | Arthritis | Presence of all 4 major criteria, simultaneously or at different times during the course of disease | Presence of 3 major criteria or 2 major criteria and two minor criteria, simultaneously or at different times during the course of disease |
| Erythema nodosum–like, acneiform, folliculitis, thrombo-phlebitis, cutaneous hyper-sensitivity | Epididymitis | | |
| Genital ulcers | Intestinal symptoms | | An ocular disease criterion and any other major criterion or an ocular disease criterion plus 2 minor criteria, simultaneously or at different times during the course of disease |
| Ocular disease: iridocyclitis with hypopyon, chorioretinitis | Neurologic symptoms | | |
| | Vascular symptoms | | |

Adapted from Mizushima Y, Inaba G, Mimura Y et al. *Guide for the diagnosis of Behçet's disease a report of the Behçet's Disease Research Committee, Japan, 1987.* Tokyo: Ministry of Health and Welfare, 1987.

sible, creatinine clearance. Unlike other ocular autoimmune diseases, corticosteroids are not drugs of choice, although they may be used concurrently with other drugs. An important and often forgotten aspect of therapy for patients with Behçet's disease is the treatment of ocular complications such as cystoid macular edema, glaucoma, neovascularization, vitreous hemorrhage, and cataracts.

## RETINAL VASCULITIS

### Clinical Characteristics

Patients with retinal vasculitis often complain of decreased vision. The disease may be divided clinically into three categories: nonocclusive edematous retinal vasculitis, occlusive ischemic retinal vasculitis, and retinal vasculitis with choroiditis. Most patients fall into the nonocclusive category. The disease is characterized by severe and continuous leakage from the retinal veins and capillaries that can be easily appreciated on a fluorescein angiography. The main cause of visual loss in these patients is cystoid macular edema. About one fifth of the patients fall in the occlusive ischemic category. The fundus examination of these individuals is dominated by the appearance of peripheral retinal hemorrhages and capillary nonperfusion seen in the fluorescein angiogram. A minority of the patients fall in the category associated with choroiditis.

Retinal ischemia in many patients leads to scotoma formation, and the vitritis causes floaters. Some patients may complain of distortion of color vision or metamorphopsia, especially if the macula is involved. Association with scleritis leads to pain and redness. Cellular infiltration of the vitreous is common, but even when severe, it does not impair the visualization of retinal details. Snowballs, if present, manifest inferiorly. Most patients have detachment of the posterior vitreous face. Vascular sheathing (Fig. 25.6) is characteristic of retinal vasculitis, and the peripheral vessels are involved.

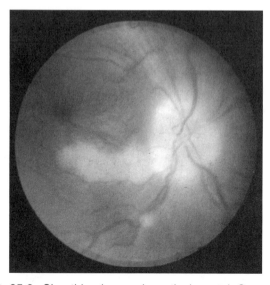

**FIG. 25.6.** Sheathing in a major retinal vessel. See color plate 25.

### Diagnosis

The differential diagnosis of idiopathic retinal vasculitis is vast. The list includes systemic autoimmune diseases as varied as SLE and Behçet's disease to allergic granulomatosis. It also includes infectious diseases caused by herpes and other viruses; rickettsial diseases' bacterial diseases such as syphilis, Lyme, and tuberculosis; diseases caused by fungi; and diseases cause by protozoa such as amebiasis and toxoplasmosis. The differential diagnosis must include primary ocular diseases such as Eales' disease and birdshot retinochoroiditis.

Because of the extensive list of diseases that may present with retinal vasculitis, a full medical history and physical examination are essential. Idiopathic disease is rare, and all effort must be made to diagnose the putative underlying disease. Serology and presence of the agent tests for the infectious diseases that may lead to retinal vasculitis are a good starting point. HLA testing may help the association with an autoimmune disease.

### Patient Management

Idiopathic retinal vasculitis or retinal vasculitis associated with autoimmune diseases often responds well to corticosteroid therapy. A schedule that has been widely used starts patients at 80 mg/day or 1 to 2 mg/kg in children for 4 days, 60 mg for 4 days, and then 40 mg/day for 1 month, with the dose adjusted thereafter according to the clinical signs of inflammation. Laser photocoagulation may be required in the management of persistent neovascularization. Surgical treatment is reserved for the severe complications that do not respond to medical treatment, such as raised intraocular pressure. It is imperative to reduce the ocular inflammation to a minimum before surgery is performed.

## SERPIGINOUS CHOROIDOPATHY

### Clinical Characteristics

Serpiginous choroiditis usually occurs in the fourth to sixth decades of life, but it may occur earlier. The disease may be bilateral or unilateral and is rarely associated to a systemic disorder. Patients complain of a decrease in central vision, metamorphopsia, or flashing scotomas. Pigmented cells in the vitreous have been reported in up to one half of the eyes examined (110). Fundus lesions classically develop first peripapillarly and spread centrifugally. The size of the lesions vary. If the patient presents with unilateral disease, there is usually evidence of inactive disease in the asymptomatic eye, and disease progression is generally asymmetric. The lesions develop deep to the retina and have a gray-white appearance with irregular, ill-defined edges. The overlying retina appears edematous and a detachment of the sensory retina may occur. Multiple areas of activity are seen, most frequently at the edges of inactive scars. As the disease progresses, these areas of activity turn into areas of chorioretinal atrophy. Skip areas of normal retina completely surrounded by disease may be seen, these are often spared as the disease progresses toward the periphery.

## Diagnosis

The diagnosis is relatively simple when a patient with the appropriate age has an acute episode of typical lesions in one eye accompanied by scars in the fellow eye. The first episode, however, is more difficult to diagnose, because the fellow eye is yet to be compromised. The differential diagnosis must include outer retinal toxoplasmosis, multifocal choroiditis and panuveitis syndrome, and acute posterior multifocal placoid pigment epitheliopathy (APMPPE).In older patients, metastatic tumors and non-Hodgkin's lymphoma may mimic some of the characteristics of serpiginous choroiditis.

The most effective complementary test is the fluorescein angiography, in which the appearance of serpiginous choroiditis is diagnostic (110–113). Indocyanine green angiography also helps to show acute lesions that fluoresce early and a progressive late staining. As the lesions resolve, the blockage diminishes. Atrophic lesions show early hypofluorescence secondary to choriocapillaries loss, and progressive hyperfluorescence develops secondary to staining at the borders of the lesions. Diffuse late staining is eventually seen. The focal clouding of the hyperfluorescent border of the lesion may be seen in eyes with early disease activity. This may be the first indication of disease reactivation and is called the Bernard sign.

## Patient Management

There is no consensus regarding the efficacy of treatment for serpiginous choroiditis. Reports of oral, periocular, or systemic corticosteroid therapy of the acute lesions have been conflicting with some investigators demonstrating a clear benefit, whereas others were unable to record any improvement linked to treatment. Treatment with cyclosporine has also produced mixed results. Although the reports are scarce, the use of antimetabolic agents alone does not seem promising. Although a large, long-term clinical trial of all possible treatments has not been done, it seems reasonable that intensive corticosteroid therapy should be reserved for the treatment of eyes with active lesions close to the fovea or the optic nerve. Oral and periocular use of corticosteroids can be use initially in unilateral disease with cellular infiltration in the vitreous or anterior chamber inflammation.

Subretinal neovascular membranes do not seem to respond well to antiinflammatory treatment, and laser photocoagulation may be required. Because neovascularization may be difficult to differentiate from acute lesions, a complete and careful angiography study should be performed before deciding on laser treatment.

## MULTIPLE SCLEROSIS

### Clinical Characteristics

Multiple sclerosis (MS) is a complex disease that involves predominantly the central nervous system and whose pathogenesis and clinical course are discussed in more detail in Chapter 31. MS may develop with one or more of an array of ocular afflictions.

Demyelination of the optic nerve leads to optic neuritis, which develops often in patients between the ages of 15 and 45 years. Females seem more prone to develop this condition. Visual loss is sudden and may progress for many days associated with pain that exacerbates with ocular movement. Examination reveals that color vision and contrast sensitivity are impaired. The optic nerve may appear normal if the neuritis is retrobulbar or swollen in an acute attack of papillitis.

Retinal vasculitis and retinitis are also common features of MS involvement of the eye. Sheathing may be present in cases of periphlebitis and chronic venous sclerosis. Periphlebitis appears as a focal white-yellow opacity with feathered margins surrounding the length of a vein. They are often located in the equator of the retina. There may be associated constriction and dilation of the veins, with an occasional retinal hemorrhage. The chronic form of sheathing appears as dense, white linear stripes along the course of a vein.

Uveitis is also common in patients with MS, although reports on its incidence vary from 2.4% to 27% of all MS patients (114–117). Peripheral uveitis is the most common manifestation, ranging from mild cellular infiltration of the vitreous to full pars planitis. The relation of uveitis activity to the course of MS exacerbations is unclear.

MS may also lead to numerous disturbances of the eye movements. The most common is internuclear ophthalmoplegia.

## Diagnosis

The most confounding feature of ocular involvement of MS is the optic neuritis. There are several possible causes for optic neuritis, such as syphilis, sarcoidosis, or a viral or postviral syndrome, as well as Behçet's disease and SLE. The diagnosis of optic neuritis and the other ocular symptoms of MS is based on clinical findings. A complete workup with serology for infectious agents and the appropriate tests to exclude sarcoidosis is indicated. Cerebrospinal fluid abnormalities of the type seen in MS are suggestive, but they also have been reported for idiopathic optic neuritis. Nuclear magnetic resonance may be useful in revealing the demyelinating lesions in the spinal cord and brain.

## Patient Management

Patients should be treated by the eye specialist in unison with the neurologist, because there are varied approaches to therapy.

## OTHER AUTOIMMUNE DISEASES WITH OCULAR INVOLVEMENT

Many other systemic diseases involve the eye to a lesser degree than the ones described previously. In such cases, ocular involvement seldom requires the attention of an ophthalmologist other than to correct possible visual defects induced by the systemic disease. Patients with myasthenia gravis often show lid ptosis, ophthalmoplegia, inability to accommodate to light changes, and an inability to converge. Patients with scleroderma often present with a hardened, thinned eyelids. The eyebrows may have an area with thinning of the hair. Patients with Goodpasture's syndrome may show hemorrhagic lesions on the basal membranes of the choroid plexus and retina similar to those observed in the eyes of patients with SLE. Patients with Horton's syndrome occasionally have an ischemic lesion of the pupils.

Because of the general nature of this book, we have chosen to present the more common ocular manifestations of autoimmunity. However, other diseases such as Cogan's syndrome, Mooren's ulcer, Theodore's superior limbic keratoconjunctivitis, lens-associated uveitis, neuroretinitis, and Posner–Schlossman syndrome may also have an autoimmune component. In-depth coverage of ocular immunologic disease is provided elsewhere (110).

## MEDICAL MANAGEMENT OF UVEITIS PATIENTS

### General Guidelines

Because all the therapeutic agents available to the treatment of ocular autoimmunity have potential side effects, the decision to treat and how to treat the patient must have guidelines. The degree of inflammation and its location is the first such parameter. The physician should evaluate the seriousness of the inflammation and determine whether there is any structural damage. If the integrity of the eye is not being threatened and the inflammation is anterior, topical steroids are the common choice. If the disease is located in the posterior pole of the eye, particularly if the macula is involved, which may lead to severe visual loss, a more aggressive approach is necessary. Before embarking on immunosuppressive treatment, any infectious cause of the ocular disease must be excluded. Another important parameter is the comfort of the patient.

Pain and photophobia are two of the most common complaints that lead a patient with ocular autoimmunity to the physician. Relieving these symptoms is an important goal of therapy because it is the physician's duty to make his patient more comfortable and because compliance to the treatment schedules that may involve drugs with very unpleasant side effects is a major problem. Making sure that the patient's complaints are addressed can improve the physician's rapport with the patient and improves the chance of achieving full compliance with the treatment. If the patient is comfortable, it will be easier to perform a better ocular examination and to obtain a better assessment of visual acuity, which determines the success of the therapeutic approach.

After the diagnosis of ocular autoimmunity is made, it is imperative to determine the physical entity that is leading to visual loss (e.g., macular edema, cataracts, neovascularization, retinal detachment). The potential for visual recovery should also guide the physician's therapeutic efforts. It would be wrong to start aggressive therapy when there is no hope for visual recovery. It is also important to remember that ocu-

lar lesions resulting from autoimmunity are slow to resolve, and it therefore takes time to evaluate the success of treatment. It is unwise to stop or alter therapy too soon. Nevertheless, the physician must define clear criteria for visual improvement, because it is as unreasonable to continue treatment if minimal criteria for success are not met in due time. An another important point to consider is whether the disease is unilateral or bilateral. Systemic treatment is often reserved for bilateral disease.

### Common Agents for the Treatment of Ocular Autoimmunity

#### Corticosteroids

Corticosteroids remain the mainstay of therapy for ocular inflammation. There are no situations, with the exception of Behçet's disease, in which corticosteroids should not be the first drug of choice, given locally or systemically. Periocular injections should be used in uniocular disease only at a dose of 20 to 40 mg in 0.5 mL of vehicle every 1 to 2 weeks. Possible side effects are described in Table 25.7. Before starting systemic corticosteroid treatment, the patient must understand the extensive list of side effects and the importance of complying with treatment, as well as the importance of reporting any and all side effects to the attending physician. The initial doses are generally between 1 and 2 mg/kg of prednisone per day. Patients with VKH are the exception, and starting doses should be 3 to 4 mg/kg/day. Therapy should be maintained until clinical improvement is observed within a reasonable amount of time, which depends on the severity of the inflammation and visual recovery. Often, if steroids do not work within 3 weeks, they are not likely to improve the patient's condition. Tapering should be achieved slowly over a period of several weeks to a dose of 15 to 20 mg/day. This range of dosage can be maintained over a significant period without important side effects. The rate of taper should be guided by clinical parameters such as recurrence or change in visual acuity. Alternate-day therapy schedules do not seem to work well in uveitis, although they are effective for other inflammatory processes. Systemic steroid therapy usually leads to a vast array of side effects (Table 25.7). Because weight gain is a significant problem, patients should be referred to a nutritionist early in therapy. Monitoring of electrolytes and glucose is mandatory.

#### Alkylating Agents

Alkylating agents are cytotoxic drugs that work by forming a covalent link between DNA strands at the level of the 7-nitrogen guanine, preventing cells from separating during division and causing them to die. Alkylating agents are thought to be more efficient than antimetabolic agents in decreasing inflammation. Cyclophosphamide is the prototype alkylating agent, and it has been used in the treatment of ocular complications of Wegener's granulomatosis, polyarteritis

**TABLE 25.7.** *Possible side effects of the most common drugs used in treating ocular inflammation*

| Drug | Side Effects |
|---|---|
| Periocular steroids | Possible intraocular penetration |
| | Propoptosis of the globe |
| | Fibrosis of the extraocular muscles |
| | Ptosis of the upper lid |
| | Glaucoma |
| Systemic steroids | Sodium and fluid retention, potassium loss |
| | Muscle weakness, osteoporosis, steroid myopathy |
| | Convulsions, moodiness, psychosis |
| | Menstrual irregularities, cushingoid state, hirsutism, diabetes, suppression of the adrenocortical-pituitary axis |
| | Nausea, increased appetite, gastrointestinal ulcers, pancreatitis |
| | Extended time for wound healing, increased sweating, bruises |
| | Cataracts, glaucoma |
| | Reactivation of chronic infections, such as herpes |
| Cyclophosphamide | Leukopenia and anemia |
| | Secondary infections |
| | Hair thinning or hair loss (may be permanent) |
| | Leukemia and lymphoma, especially in children; cutaneous origin is also common |
| Chlorambucil | Leukopenia (may be irreversible) |
| | Azospermia |
| | Hair loss |
| | Neoplasias |
| | Pulmonary fibrosis |
| Azathioprine | Medullary hypoplasia |
| | Gastrointestinal symptoms, intrahepatic cholestasis |
| | Acute pancreatitis |
| | Secondary infections |
| Methotrexate | Gastrointestinal symptoms, oral ulceration, hepatic fibrosis |
| | Alopecia |
| | Pulmonary fibrosis |
| | Increased risk of fungal infections |
| | Increased risk of neoplasias, specially in children |
| Cyclosporin A | Hypertrichosis, gum hypertrophy |
| | Nephrotoxicity |
| | Paresthesias, tremors, anorexia |

nodosa, rheumatoid arthritis, Behçet's disease, sympathetic ophthalmia, and VKH. The pharmacokinetic profiles of orally or intravenously give cyclophosphamide seem to be the same. Cytotoxic derivatives may be secreted in the breast milk. The drug interacts with allopurinol, increasing the risk of leukopenia in patients taking both drugs. A daily regimen of 0.5 to 2 mg/kg is often recommended.

Patients on cyclophosphamide therapy should have a complete blood cell count (CBC), platelet count, and urinalysis at least every week for the first 2 months and then every 2 to 4 weeks. A reasonable target is to keep at least 3500 WBC with 1500 PMN. Because of the risk for neoplasias, administration

beyond 2 years is not recommended. Unfortunately, the incidence of cancer in patients with rheumatic diseases with a cumulative dose of 50 g is 10 times higher than in patients with other diseases using cyclophosphamide.

Chlorambucil is another alkylating agent used in Behçet's disease and in some cases of JRA. Starting doses should be at 2 mg/day and increase weekly by 2 mg/day until reaching a final dose of 10 to 12 mg/day. Platelet counts should be monitored weekly throughout the treatment. The target hemogram is the same as described for cyclophosphamide.

### Antimetabolites

Antimetabolites constitute another category of cytotoxic agents that has as its standard drug azathioprine. A less toxic, equally effective, second-generation drug has been developed, and its results in transplantation patients and in patients with JRA are promising. The indications for azathioprine include Wegener's granulomatosis, SLE, scleritis, cicatricial pemphigoid, inflammatory bowel disease, JRA, sympathetic ophthalmia, birdshot retinochoroidopathy, and VKH. After oral administration, the drug is rapidly metabolized to 6-mercaptopurine and is incorporated into the DNA and RNA of active cells, leading to the generation of unreadable or false codons and inhibiting the normal metabolism of cells. The starting dose is between 1 and 3 mg/kg/day. Patients should have a CBC, urinalysis, and liver function tests every month for the first 3 months of treatment and every 3 months thereafter. The drug should be discontinued promptly if liver disease or unexplained severe abdominal pain develops.

Methotrexate is another drug in the antimetabolite category. It is a folate antagonist, indicated in the treatment of ocular complications of SLE, sympathetic ophthalmia, and rheumatoid arthritis in the presence of necrotizing scleritis. The drug is found in the blood (around 50%) bound to proteins. It can be displaced from these proteins by other drugs such as sulfonamides, salicylates, tetracycline, and chloramphenicol. Drugs that interfere with renal function increase the potential for side effects of methotrexate. The usual dose of methotrexate is 10 to 30 mg per week. Patients administered methotrexate infusions should have a CBC and platelet count before each infusion, have liver function tests every 2 to 4 months, and even a liver biopsy should be considered after each 1.5 g of methotrexate. A chest radiograph is mandatory if cough or dyspnea occurs. Immunosuppressive effects usually take more than a month to appear, and improvement in function is rare after 6 months of therapy.

### Immunomodulatory Agents

Other than the experimental immunotherapeutic approaches described in the introduction, these agents are the closest immunology has come to providing "antigen-specific" therapy. As a group, these compounds work by blocking the acquisition or functional IL-2 receptors, preventing resting T cells from becoming activated and preventing activated

B cells from upregulating the receptors and consequently proliferating. Cyclosporin A is the first drug described in this category, which has been joined by FK-506 (tacrolimus) and rapamycin.

The indications for cyclosporin A therapy include Behçet's dice, VKH, sympathetic ophthalmia, pars planitis, and birdshot retinochoroidoopathy. It is often used when a sight-threatening disease occurs in a patient unable to tolerate systemic steroids or a patient that does not respond well to steroid therapy. The initial dose varies from 1 to 5 mg/kg/day as a split dose taken twice daily with or without 10 to 30 mg/day of prednisone. Patients should be monitored for blood pressure, serum creatinine level, and blood urea nitrogen (BUN) level on each visit. We also recommend a 24-hour creatinine clearance test every 3 months and a glomerular filtration rate (GFR) assay every year together with liver function tests. A drop of 30% in GFR or a sustained increase in the creatine or BUN is a sure sign the dose must be reduced. Cyclosporin interacts with many drugs such as aminoglycosides, cimetidine, erythromycin, ketoconazole, mannitol, NSAIDs, oral contraceptives, and phenobarbital. The specific interactions are fully described elsewhere (56,57) and should be considered when deciding on a dose for each patient.

# REFERENCES

1. Nossal GJ. Negative selection of lymphocytes. *Cell* 1994;76:229–239.
2. Pardoll D, Carrera A. Thymic selection. *Curr Opin Immunol* 1992;4: 162–165.
3. Robey E, Fowlkes BJ. Selective events in T cell development. *Annu Rev Immunol* 1994;12:675–705.
4. Fowlkes BJ, Ramsdell F. T-cell tolerance. *Curr Opin Immunol* 1993; 5:873–879.
5. Streilein JW. Unraveling immune privilege [Comment]. *Science* 1995; 270:1158–1159.
6. Streilein JW. Immune privilege as the result of local tissue barriers and immunosuppressive microenvironments. *Curr Opin Immunol* 1993;5: 428–432.
7. Barker C, Billingham R. Immunological privileged sites. *Adv Immunol* 1977;25:1–54.
8. Jones DE, Diamond AG. The basis of autoimmunity: an overview. *Baillieres Clin Endocrinol Metab* 1995;9:1–24.
9. Roitt IM. The role of autoantigens in the driving of autoimmune diseases. *Immunol Ser* 1993;59:119–129.
10. Schwartz RS, Datta SK. Autoimmunity and Autoimmune diseases. In: Paul WE, ed. *Fundamental immunology*. 3rd ed. New York: Raven Press, 1995:819–866.
11. Steinman L. Escape from horror autotoxicus: pathogenesis and treatment of autoimmune disease. *Cell* 1995;80:7–10.
12. Theofilopoulos AN. The basis of autoimmunity: Part I. Mechanisms of aberrant self-recognition. *Immunol Today* 1995;16:90–98.
13. Rizzo LV, Caspi RR. Immunotolerance and prevention of ocular autoimmune disease. *Curr Eye Res* 1995;14:857–864.
14. Rizzo LV. Estudos sobre a imunonopatogenese e imunoterapia da uveite experimental autoimmune. PhD thesis, University of Sao Paulo, 1997.
15. Egwuagu CE, Charukamnoetkanok P, Gery I. Thymic expression of autoantigens correlates with resistance to autoimmune disease. *J Immunol* 1997;159:3109–3112.
16. Horwitz J. The function of alpha-crystallin. *Invest Ophthalmol Vis Sci* 1993;34:10–22.
17. Pietagorsky J. Gene expression and genetic engineering in the lens. *Invest Ophthalmol Vis Sci* 1987;28:9–16.
18. Egwuagu CE, Mahadi R, Chapelewski A, et al. Extralenticular expression of the alpha A-crystallin promoter/gamma interferon transgene. *Exp Eye Res* 1997;64:491–495.
19. D'Ermo F, Secchi AG, Segato T, et al. Immunopathology of the lens II. 86Rb efflux and protein leakage from normal lenses exposed to antilens and antiuveoretina antibodies. *Ophthalmologica* 1978;176: 230–237.
20. Sandberg HO. The alpha crystallin content of aqueous humor in cortical, nuclear and complicated cataracts. *Exp Eye Res* 22:75–84.
21. Kalil MK, Lorenzetti DW. Lens-induced inflammation. *Can J Ophthalmol* 1986;21:96.
22. Wirostko E, Spalter HF. Lens-induced uveitis. *Arch Ophthalmol* 1967;78:1.
23. Hirose S, Tanaka T, Nussenblatt RB, et al. Lymphocyte responses to retinal-specific antigens in uveitis patients and healthy subjects. *Curr Eye Res* 1988;7:393–402.
24. Hirose S, McAllister C, Mittal K, et al. A cell line and clones of lymphocytes from a healthy donor with specificity to S-antigen. *Invest Ophthalmol Vis Sci* 1988;29:1636–1641.
25. Medawar PB. Immunity to homologous grafted skin. III. The fate of skin homografts transplanted to the brain, the subcutaneous tissue, and to the anterior chamber of the eye. *Br J Exp Pathol* 1948;29:58–69.
26. Kaplan HJ, Streilein JW. Immune response to immunization via the anterior chamber of the eye. I. lymphocyte-induced immune deviation. *J Immunol* 1977;118:809–814.
27. Kaplan HJ, Streilein JW. Immune response to immunization via the anterior chamber of the eye. II. An analysis of F1 lymphocyte-induced immune deviation. *J Immunol* 1978;120:689–693.
28. Griffith TS, Brunner T, Fletcher SM, et al. Fas ligand-induced apoptosis as a mechanism of immune privilege [see comments]. *Science* 1995;270:1189–11892.
29. Jacobs MJ, van den Hoek AE, van de Putte LB, van den Berg WB. Anergy of antigen-specific T lymphocytes is a potent mechanism of intravenously induced tolerance. *Immunology* 1994;82:294–300.
30. Jacobs MJ, van den Hoek AE, van de Putte LB, van den Berg WB. Suppression of hen egg lysozyme-induced arthritis by intravenous antigen administration: no role in this for antigen-driven bystander suppression. *Clin Exp Immunol* 1994;96:36–42.
31. Wilbanks GA, Mammolenti M, Streilein JW. Studies on the induction of anterior chamber-associated immune deviation (ACAID). III. Induction of ACAID depends upon intraocular transforming growth factor-beta. *Eur J Immunol* 1992;22:165–173.
32. Wilbanks GA, Streilein JW. Fluids from immune privileged sites endow macrophages with the capacity to induce antigen-specific immune deviation via a mechanism involving transforming growth factor-beta. *Eur J Immunol* 1992;22:1031–1036.
33. Wilbanks GA, Streilein JW. Studies on the induction of anterior chamber-associated immune deviation (ACAID). 1. Evidence that an antigen-specific, ACAID-inducing, cell-associated signal exists in the peripheral blood. *J Immunol* 1991;146:2610–2617.
34. Taylor AW, Streilein JW, Cousins SW. Immunoreactive vasoactive intestinal peptide contributes to the immunosuppressive activity of normal aqueous humor. *J Immunol* 1994;153:1080–1086.
35. Streilein JW. Ocular immune privilege and the Faustian dilemma: the Proctor lecture. *Invest Ophthalmol Vis Sci* 1996;37:1940–1950.
36. Streilein JW. Immunological non-responsiveness and acquisition of tolerance in relation to immune privilege in the eye. *Eye* 1995;9 [Pt 2]: 236–240.
37. Shimada K. The complement components and their inactivators in the intraocular fluids of the guinea pig. *Invest Ophthalmol* 1970;9: 307–315.
38. Bora NS, Gobleman CL, Atkinson JP, et al. Differential expression of the complement regulatory proteins in the human eye. *Invest Ophthalmol Vis Sci* 1993;34:3579–3584.
39. Roberge FG, Caspi RR, Chan CC, Nussenblatt RB. Interactions between retinal glial cells and immune mononuclear cells. *Yen Ko Hsueh Pao* 1986;2:101–102.
40. Roberge FG, Caspi RR, Chan CC, Nussenblatt RB. Inhibition of T lymphocyte proliferation by retinal glial Muller cells: reversal of inhibition by glucocorticoids. *J Autoimmun* 1991;4:307–314.
41. Liversidge J, McKay D, Mullen G, Forrester JV. Retinal pigment epithelial cells modulate lymphocyte function at the blood-retina barrier by autocrine PGE₂ and membrane-bound mechanisms. *Cell Immunol* 1993;149:315–330.
42. Helbig H, Gurley RC, Palestine AG, Nussenblatt RB, Caspi RR. Dual effect of ciliary body cells on T lymphocyte proliferation. *Eur J Immunol* 1990;20:2457–2463.

43. Caspi RR, Roberge FG. Glial cells as suppressor cells: characterization of the inhibitory function. *J Autoimmun* 1989;2:709–722.

44. Caspi RR, Roberge FG, Nussenblatt RB. Organ-resident, nonlymphoid cells suppress proliferation of autoimmune T-helper lymphocytes. *Science* 1987;237:1029–1032.

45. Kaplan HJ, Streilein JW. Do immunologically privileged sites require a functioning spleen? *Nature* 1974;251:553–554.

46. Kaplan HJ, Streilein JW, Stevens TR. Transplantation immunology of the anterior chamber of the eye. II. Immune response to allogeneic cells. *J Immunol* 1975;115:805–810.

47. Kaplan HJ, Stevens TR, Streilein JW. Transplantation immunology of the anterior chamber of the eye. I. An intraocular graft-vs-host reaction (immunogenic anterior uveitis). *J Immunol* 1975;115:800–804.

48. Hara Y, Caspi RR, Wiggert B, et al. Analysis of an *in vitro* generated signal that induces systemic immune deviation similar to that elicited by antigen injected into the anterior chamber of the eye [published erratum appears in *J Immunol* 1992;149:4116]. *J Immunol* 1992;149:1531–1538.

49. Hara Y, Caspi RR, Wiggert B, et al. Use of ACAID to suppress interphotoreceptor retinoid binding protein-induced experimental autoimmune uveitis. *Curr Eye Res* 1992;11[Suppl I]:97–100.

50. Hara Y, Caspi RR, Wiggert B, Chan CC, Wilbanks GA, Streilein JW. Suppression of experimental autoimmune uveitis in mice by induction of anterior chamber-associated immune deviation with interphotoreceptor retinoid-binding protein. *J Immunol* 1992;148:1685–1692.

51. Mizuno K, Clark AF, Streilein JW. Induction of anterior chamber associated immune deviation in rats receiving intracameral injections of retinal S antigen. *Curr Eye Res* 1988;7:627–632.

52. Kleinau S, Lorentzen J, Klareskog L. Role of adjuvants in turning autoimmunity into autoimmune disease. *Scand J Rheumatol Suppl* 1995;101:179–181.

53. Sasaki K, Sanui H, Inomata H. Uveitis induced by various cross-reactive antigens in guinea pigs. *Ophthalmic Res* 1990;22:330–336.

54. Weiner HL, Zhang ZJ, Khoury SJ, et al. Antigen-driven peripheral immune tolerance: suppression of organ-specific autoimmune diseases by oral administration of autoantigens. *Ann N Y Acad Sci* 1991;636:227–232.

55. Wacker WB, Rao NA, Marak G Jr. Experimental sympathetic ophthalmia. In: Silverstein AM, O'Connor GR, eds. *Immunology and immunopathology of the eye.* New York: Masson, 1979:121–126.

56. Nussenblatt RB, Withcup SM, Palestine AG. *Uveitis: fundamentals and clinical practice.* 2nd ed. St Louis: Mosby, 1996.

57. Whitcup SM, Nussenblatt RB. Treatment of autoimmune uveitis. *Ann N Y Acad Sci* 1993;696:307–318.

58. Uhlenhuth PT. *Zur lehre von der unterscheidung verschiedener eiweissarten mit hilfe spezifixher sera. Fetschritf zum 60 geburstag von Robert Koch.* Fisher, Germany: Jena, 1903:49–74.

59. Elschnig A. Albrecht von Graefes Arch. *Ophthalmology* 1910;76:509–546.

60. Nussenblatt RB, Gery I, Ballintine EJ, Wacker WB. Cellular immune responsiveness of uveitis patients to retinal S-antigen. *Am J Ophthalmol* 1980;89:173–179.

61. Nussenblatt RB, Mittal KK, Ryan S, et al. Birdshot retinochoroidopathy associated with HLA-A29 antigen and immune responsiveness to retinal S-antigen. *Am J Ophthalmol* 1982;94:147–158.

62. Predengast RA, Coskuncan NM, Lutty GA, et al. T cell traffic and the pathogenesis of experimental autoimmune uveoretinitis. In: Nussenblatt RB, Whitcup SW, Caspi RR, Gery I, eds. *Advances in ocular immunology. 6th International Symposium on the Immunology and Immunopathology of the Eye 1994, Bethesda, MD.* Amsterdam: Elsevier 1994:59–62.

63. Gery I, Streilein JW. Autoimmunity in the eye and its regulation. *Curr Opin Immunol* 1994;6:938–945.

64. Nussenblatt RB, Gery I. Experimental autoimmune uveitis and its relationship to clinical ocular inflammatory disease. *J Autoimmun* 1996;9:575–585.

65. Rizzo LV, Silver P, Wiggert B, et al. Establishment and characterization of a murine CD4+ T cell line and clone that induce experimental autoimmune uveoretinitis in B10.A mice. *J Immunol* 1996;156:1654–1660.

66. Chan CC, Mochizuki M, Palestine AG, et al. Kinetics of T-lymphocyte subsets in the eyes of Lewis rats with experimental autoimmune uveitis. *Cell Immunol* 1985;96:430–434.

67. Chan CC, BenEzra D, Rodrigues MM, et al. Immunohistochemistry and electron microscopy of choroidal infiltrates and Dalen-Fuchs nodules in sympathetic ophthalmia. *Ophthalmology* 1985;92:580–590.

68. Whitcup SM, Chan CC, Li Q, Nussenblatt RB. Expression of cell adhesion molecules in posterior uveitis. *Arch Ophthalmol* 1992;110:662–666.

69. Broekhuyse RM, Kuhlmann ED, Winkens HJ. Experimental autoimmune anterior uveitis (EAAU): induction by melanin antigen and suppression by various treatments. *Pigment Cell Res* 1993;6:1–6.

70. Broekhuyse RM, Kuhlmann ED, Winkens HJ. Experimental autoimmune posterior uveitis accompanied by epithelioid cell accumulations (EAPU): a new type of experimental ocular disease induced by immunization with PEP-65, a pigment epithelial polypeptide preparation. *Exp Eye Res* 1992;55:819–829.

71. Caspi RR, Grubbs BG, Chan CC, et al. Genetic control of susceptibility to experimental autoimmune uveoretinitis in the mouse model. Concomitant regulation by MHC and non-MHC genes. *J Immunol* 1992;148:2384–2389.

72. Wetzig RP, Chan CC, Nussenblatt RB, et al. Clinical and immunopathological studies of pars planitis in a family. *Br J Ophthalmol* 1988;72:5–10.

73. Ichikawa T, Taguchi O, Takahashi T, et al. Spontaneous development of autoimmune uveoretinitis in nude mice following reconstitution with embryonic rat thymus. *Clin Exp Immunol* 1991;86:112–117.

74. Caspi RR. Immunogenetic aspects of clinical and experimental uveitis. *Reg Immunol* 1992;4:321–330.

75. Caspi RR, Silver PB, Chan CC, et al. Genetic susceptibility to experimental autoimmune uveoretinitis in the rat is associated with an elevated Th1 response. *J Immunol* 1996;157:2668–2675.

76. Sun B, Rizzo LV, Sun S-H, Caspi RR. Genetic susceptibility to experimental autoimmune uveitis involves more than a predisposition to generate a Th1-like or a Th2-like response. *J Immunol* 1997;154:6602–6611.

77. Tandon K, Sen DK, Mathur MD. Acute phase proteins in patients with idiopathic anterior uveitis. In: Usi M, Ohno S, Aoki K, eds. *Ocular immunology today.* Amsterdam: Elsevier Science Publishers, 1990:353–355.

78. Toledo de Abreu M, Belfort R Jr, Irata PS. Fuchs heterochromic cyclitis and ocular toxoplasmosis. *Am J Ophthalmol* 1982;93:739–744.

79. Silva HF, Oréfice F, Pinheiro SRA. Fuch's heterochromic cyclitis: clinical study of 132 cases. In: Belfort Jr R, Petrilli AMN, Nussenblatt R, eds. *Proceedings of the First World Uveitis Symposium.* Sao Paulo: Editora Rocca, 1989:215–222.

80. Sherwood DR, Rosenthal AR. Cataract surgery in Fuch's heterochromic iridocyclitis. *Br J Ophthalmol* 1972;76:238–240.

81. Abrahams IW, Jiang Y. Ophthalmology in China. *Arch Ophthalmol* 1973;75:685–688.

82. Smith RE, Godfrey WA, Kimura SJ. Chronic cyclitis. I. Course and visual prognosis. *Trans Am Acad Ophthalmol Otolaryngol* 1973;77:760–768.

83. Chung H, Choi DG. Clinical analysis of uveitis. *Korean J Ophthalmol* 1989;3:33–37.

84. Witmer VR, Körner G. Uveitis in Kendesalter. *Ophthalmologica* 1966;152:277–282.

85. Obenauf CD, Shaw HE, Sydnor CF, Klintworth GK. Sarcoidosis and its ophthalmic manifestations. *Am J Ophthalmol* 1978;86:648–655.

86. Siltzbach LE, James DG, Neville E, et al. Course and prognosis of sarcoidosis around the world. *Am J Med* 1974;57:847–852.

87. Karma A, Huhti E, Poukkula A. Course and outcome of ocular sarcoidosis. *Am J Ophthalmol* 1988;106:467–472.

88. Spalton DJ, Sanders MD. Fundus changes in histologically confirmed sarcoidosis. *Br J Ophthalmol* 1981;65:562–566.

89. Azen SP, Marak Jr GE, Minckler DS, et al. Sympathetic ophthalmia following laser cyclocoagulation. *Am J Ophthalmol* 1984;98:117–119.

90. Crews SJ, MacKintosh P, Barry DR, et al. HLA antigen and certain types of uveitis. *Trans Ophthalmol Soc UK* 1979;99:156–159.

91. Davis JL, Mittal KK, Freidlin V, et al. HLA association and ancestry in Vogt-Koyanagi-Harada disease and sympathetic ophthalmia. *Ophthalmology* 1990;97:1137–1142.

92. Ohno S: Immunogenetic studies on ocular diseases. In: Blodi F, ed. *The XXVth International Congress of Ophthalmology.* Rome: Kugler and Ghedini, 1986.

93. Sasamoto Y, Ohno S, Matsuda H. Studies on corticosteroid therapy in Gogt-Koyanagi-Harada disease. *Ophthalmologica* 1990;201:161–167.

94. Yamamoto T, Sasaki T, Saito HA, et al. Visual prognosis in Harada's disease: a reevaluation of massive systemic corticosteroid therapy. *Jpn J Clin Ophthalmol* 1986;40:461–464.

95. Ryan SJ, Maumenee AE. Birdshot retinochoroidopathy. *Am J Ophthalmol* 1980;89:31–45.

96. LeHoang P, Ozdemir N, Benhamou A, et al. HLA-A29.2 subtype associated with birdshot retinochoroidopathy. *Am J Ophthalmol* 1992;113:33–35.

97. Nussenblatt RB, Mittal KK, Ryan S, et al. Birdshot retinochoroidopathy associated with HLA-A29 antigen and immune responsiveness to S-Ag. *Am J Ophthalmol* 1982;94:147–158.

98. Priem HA, Kijlstra A, Noens L, et al. HLA typing in birdshot chorioretinopathy. *Am J Ophthalmol* 1988;105:182–185.

99. LeHoang P, Girard B, Deray G, et al. Cyclosporine in the treatment of birdshot retinochoroidopathy. *Transplant Proc* 1988;20[Suppl 4]:128–130.

100. Vitale AT, Rodrigues A, Foster CS. Low-dose cyclosporine therapy in the treatment of birdshot retinochoroidopathy. *Ophthalmology* 1994;101:822–831.

101. Yurdakul S, Gunaydin I, Tuzun Y, et al. The prevalence of Behçet's syndrome in a rural area in Northern Turkey. *J Rheumatol* 1988;15:820–822.

102. Mishima S, Masuda K, Izawa Y, et al. Behçte's disease in Japan: ophthalmologic aspects. *Trans Am Ophthalmol Soc* 1979;77:225–279.

103. Ministry of Health and Welfare. *A nation-wide epidemiological survey on Behçet's disease, reports 1 and 2. Report of Behçet's Disease Research Committee, Japan 1987.* Tokyo: Ministry of Health and Welfare of Japan, 1992.

104. Imai Y. Studies on prognosis and symptoms of Behçet's disease in long term observation. *Jpn J Clin Ophthalmol* 1971;25:661–694.

105. Shimizu T. Behçet's disease. *Jpn J Ophthalmol* 1974;18:291–194.

106. Shimada K, Yaoita H, Shikano S. Chemotatic activity in the aqueous humor in patients with Behçet's disease. *Jpn J Ophthalmol* 1972;16:84–92.

107. International Study Group for Behçet's disease. Criteria for diagnosis of Behçet's disease. *Lancet* 1990;335:1078–1080.

108. Yazici H, Pazarli H, Barnes CG, et al. A controlled trial of azathioprine in Behçet's syndrome. *N Engl J Med* 1990;322:281–285.

109. Godfrey WA, Epstein WV, O'Connor GR, et al. The use of chlorambucil in intractable idiopathic uveitis. *Am J Ophthalmol* 1974;78:415–428.

110. Chisholm IH, Gass JDM, Hutton WL. The late stage serpiginous (geographic) choroiditis. *Am J Ophthalmol* 1982;82:343:351.

111. Gass JDM. *Stereoscopic atlas of macular diseases: diagnosis and treatment*, vol 1. 3rd ed. St Louis, Mosby, 1987:136–144.

112. Hamilton AM, Bird AC. Geographical choroidopathy. *Br J Ophthalmol* 1974;58:784–797.

113. Hardy RA, Schatz H. Macular geographic helicoid choroidopathy. *Arch Ophthalmol* 1987;105:1237–1242.

114. Banford CR, Ganley JP, Sibley WA, Laguna JF. Uveitis, perivenous sheathing and multiple sclerosis. *Neurology* 1978;28:119–124.

115. Breger BC, Leopold IH. The incidence of uveitis in multiple sclerosis. *Am J Ophthalmol* 1966;62:540–545.

116. Hauser SL, Dawson DM, Lehrich JR, et al. Intensive immunosuppression in progressive multiple sclerosis: a randomized, three-armed study of high-dose intravenous cyclophosphamide, plasma exchange and ACTH. *N Engl J Med* 1983;308:173–180.

117. Porter R. Uveitis in association with multiple sclerosis. *Br J Ophthalmol* 1972;56:478–481.

118. Pepose JS, Holland GN, Wilhelmus KR. eds. *Ocular infection and inflammation.* St Louis: Mosby, 1995.

# The Systemic Autoimmune Diseases

*Textbook of the Autoimmune Diseases,*
Edited by R. G. Lahita, N. Chiorazzi, and W. H. Reeves,
Lippincott Williams & Wilkins, Philadelphia © 2000.

# CHAPTER 26

# Systemic Lupus Erythematosus

Robert G. Lahita

Systemic lupus erythematosus (SLE) is a complex autoimmune disease affecting numerous organs and tissues. It is characterized by the production of antibodies to components of the cell nucleus and cytoplasm, as well as a diverse array of antibodies against other tissues and cell particles (1).

SLE is primarily a disease of young women, and the peak incidence occurs between the ages of 15 and 40. During these childbearing years, the female to male ratio is 10 to 1 (2). However, The disease can begin anytime between early childhood and advanced age. In early childhood, the ratio of young girls to boys is approximately 4 to 1, but in later life, in the female to male ratio approximates 8 to 1.

Lupus varies with ethnicity. The disease is more common among African Americans, Asians, and Hispanics. The disease affects 1 of 2,000 Caucasians, whereas the prevalence among African, Asian, and Hispanic persons is approximately 1 in 250 (3,4). These numbers vary greatly, depending on the source. The Lupus Foundation of America completed a telephone marketing study, not based on standard epidemiologic procedures, which indicated that more than 2.5 million Americans might be affected by lupus (5).

As a multisystem disease, lupus can affect any or all systems of the body. SLE has a strong familial aggregation, because there is a higher frequency among first-degree relatives of patients. In extended families, the disease coexists with other autoimmune conditions such as autoimmune hemolytic anemia, thyroiditis, and idiopathic thrombocytopenic purpura and with diseases that have no known autoimmune basis such as fibromyalgia (Table 26.1).

There is a familial aspect to lupus, suggesting that it is inherited, but it is not inherited in a typical mendelian manner (6). SLE occurs in approximately 25% to 50% of monozygotic twins and 5% of dizygotic twins (7). Despite the fact that this disease can occur in families, most cases are sporadic. Numerous human leukocyte antigen (HLA) genes are associated with the disease.

## ETIOPATHOGENESIS OF LUPUS

The cause of lupus remains unknown, despite an extensive search over the past three decades for a viral, bacterial, or chemical source. The pathophysiologic aspects of this disease are extraordinarily interesting and involve the immune and other systems. The manifestations of this disease are inflammation, premature infarction of blood vessels, vasculitis, and immune complex deposition in a variety of organs (8). Perhaps the most intensively studied organ of the body is the kidney. Various forms of microscopy have found several pathologic changes, including increases of the mesangial cells and the mesangial matrix, the accumulation of inflammatory cells, basement membrane abnormalities, and immune complex deposition. These deposits within the kidney include the immunoglobulins G, M, and A and components of complement (9). On electron and light microscopy, deposits can be seen in the mesangial area and the subendothelial and subepithelial side of the basement membrane (10,11). The pathologic findings in the kidney are classified according to a variety of schemes and biopsy can predict outcome (12). The World Health Organization classification is based on the extent and location of the similar changes within the glomeruli as well as alterations of the basement membrane. A second classification is based on an activity and chronicity score. These two systems are extremely useful in that they predict outcome and provide a reason for biopsy of the kidney (13,14).

The skin lesions found in lupus can show inflammation in combination with deposition of immunoglobulins at the dermal-epidermal junction (15,16). In these skin lesions, the deposition of immunoglobulins and complement components is reminiscent of the pattern in the kidney. These immune complexes deposit in a bandlike pattern and can be seen by immunofluorescent microscopy (17,18).

R. G. Lahita: Department of Medicine, New York Medical College, Valhalla, New York 10595; Department of Rheumatology, St. Vincent's Hospital, New York, New York 10011.

**TABLE 26.1.** *Revised criteria for the diagnosis of systemic lupus erythematosus*[a]

| Criterion | Definition |
| --- | --- |
| Malar rash | Fixed erythema, flat or raised, over the malar eminence, tending to spare the nasolabial folds |
| Discoid rash | Erythematous raised patches with adherent keratotic scaling and follicular plugging; atrophic scarring may occur in older lesions |
| Photosensitivity | Skin rash as a result of unusual reaction to sunlight, by patient history or physician observation |
| Oral ulcers | Oral or nasopharyngeal ulceration, usually painless, observed by a physician |
| Arthritis | Nonerosive arthritis involving two or more peripheral joints, characterized by tenderness, swelling, or effusion |
| Serositis | a) Pleuritis: convincing history of pleuritic pain or rub heard by physician or evidence of pleural effusion<br>OR<br>b) Pericarditis: documented by electrocardiogram or rub or evidence of pericardial effusion |
| Renal disorder | a) Persistent proteinuria greater than 0.5 g per day or greater than 3+ if quantitation not performed<br>OR<br>b) Cellular casts: may be red cell, hemoglobin, granular, tubular, or mixed |
| Neurologic disorder | a) Seizures: in the absence of offending drugs or known metabolic derangement, such as uremia, ketoacidosis, or electrolyte imbalance<br>OR<br>b) Psychosis: in the absence of offending drugs or known metabolic derangement, such as uremia, ketoacidosis, or electrolyte imbalance |
| Hematologic disorder | a) Hemolytic anemia: with reticulocytosis<br>OR<br>b) Leukopenia: less than $4,000/mm^3$ total on two or more occasions<br>OR<br>c) Lymphopenia: less than $1500/mm^3$ on two or more occasions<br>OR<br>d) Thrombocytopenia: less than $100,000/mm^3$ in the absence of offending drugs |
| Immunologic disorder[b] | a) Anti-DNA: antibody to native DNA in abnormal titer<br>OR<br>b) Anti-SM: presence of antibody to SM nuclear antigen<br>OR<br>c) Positive finding of antiphospholipid antibodies based on (a) an abnormal serum level of IgG or IgM anti-cardiolipin antibodies, (b) a positive test result for lupus anticoagulant using a standard method, or (c) a false-positive serologic test for syphilis known to be positive for at least 6 months and confirmed by *Treponema pallidum* immobilization or fluorescent treponemal antibody absorption test |
| ANA | An abnormal titer of ANA by immunofluorescence or an equivalent assay at any point in time and in the absence of drugs known to be associated with "drug-induced" lupus syndrome |

[a] This classification is based on 11 criteria. For the purpose of identifying patients in clinical studies, a person must have SLE if any four or more of the 11 criteria are present, serially or simultaneously, during any interval of observation (4).

[b] The modifications to criterion number 11 were made in 1997 (6).

From Hochberg MC. Updating the American College of Rheumatology revised criteria for the classification of systemic lupus erythematosis. *Arth Rheum* 1997;40:1725, with permission.

Many other organs can be affected by lupus, and these organs usually display nonspecific inflammation because of the deposition of immune complexes. Occasionally, clots can occlude vital vessels that supply various organs, resulting in macroinfarcts or microinfarcts and subsequently in degenerative or prolific changes. The origin of these thrombi are often the result of phospholipid directed antibodies that cause a procoagulant state. There is a suggestion that antiendothelial antibodies are involved in the pathogenesis (19).

Other aspects of the disease remain unexplained, including accelerated atherosclerosis with an extraordinary risk for cardiovascular disease (20) and severe osteonecrosis (21). It is unclear whether these two associated phenomena are the result of the pathogenesis of the disease or the result of treatment with steroids.

The hallmarks of lupus are the aberrant cell populations directed against autoantigens and a plethora of different autoantibodies (22). The antibodies found in this disease are directed at host of self molecules that are found in the nucleus and the cytoplasm or cell surface (Fig. 26.1). Lupus sera also contain antibodies to histocompatibility markers and clotting factors. At any one time, a lupus patient can have high titers of antibodies to antigens found in many other well-described autoimmune diseases.

The antibodies directed against components of the cell nucleus are called antinuclear antibodies (ANAs). Patients with the disease have these antibodies (Table 26.2). There are said to be patients who are ANA negative, but these determinations are usually the result of poor substrate staining or poor interpretation (23). There are many antigens within the

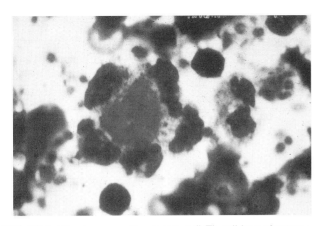

**FIG. 26.1.** The lupus erythematosus (LE) cell has phagocytosed several other cell nuclei coated with autoantibody. It was the first indication of autoimmunity. See color plate 26.

cell that can become targets for autoantibodies. Many of these autoantigens, like DNA or RNA, are highly conserved among mammalian species. The use of ANA patterns is not useful in the diagnosis of the disease (24). Only the nucleolar pattern is of some use, because it is associated with scleroderma or mixed connective tissue disease (25).

Analysis of the autoantibodies indicates that most of them are not useful in following the progress or activity of the disease. Only two antibodies, the Smith (Sm) and the antinative DNA antibody, are specific to patients with lupus (26). These two autoantibodies differ in their patterns of expression and clinical association. Although anti-DNA levels fluctuate with disease activity, anti-Sm remains constant during the course of the disease. The anti-DNA antibodies are particularly useful in following the course of renal disease in patients with lupus (27). Some antibody systems are associated with disease classification. These include antibodies to ribosomal P proteins and psychiatric disease (28), antibodies to Ro with neonatal lupus (29) and subacute cutaneous lupus (30), antibodies to phospholipid with the thrombosis of blood vessels, and antibodies to blood cells with resulting hemolytic anemia (31).

## Heredity

There are many determinants of disease activity within the immune system. SLE is associated with specific genetic abnormalities (32,33). Exogenous and endogenous factors can trigger lupus, but the predisposition to this disease is clearly inherited. However, the origin of the disease is likely to be multigenic and to involve different sets of genes in different individuals (34). On chromosome 6 in humans, there are a variety of gene markers called the major histocompatibility complex (MHC). Population-based studies indicate that susceptibility to SLE involves class II gene polymorphism. SLE is commonly associated with HLA-DR2 and HLA-DR3. The presence of these alleles confers a twofold to fivefold risk for lupus (32).

Class II genes appear to exert a more decisive influence on the production of a particular ANA (35). There are various class II specificities found within the response genes (33). Inherited complement deficiencies (MHC class III) also influence disease susceptibility in a manner that is not clear (36). Like class I and class II molecules, complement components, especially those within chromosome 6 (e.g., C4A, C4B), show striking genetic polymorphism. If there is a deficiency of C4A molecules, a common occurrence in the population, as many as 80% of patients are at high risk for developing lupus (37). SLE is also associated with inherited deficiencies of the early components of complement C1Q, C1R/S, and C2 (38). The mechanism involved in the acquisition of lupus from complement deficiency may reflect an excess amount of antigen that cannot be cleared by the complement system.

Other susceptibility factors involved in the acquisition of lupus include the immunoglobulins and T-cell receptor gene systems (39). Despite these hypotheses, known polymorphisms of the T-cell receptor have been associated with the disease. The heavy-chain allotypes of immunoglobulins have not been helpful in predicting disease susceptibility.

Developments in the area of lupus genetics are provocative. Besides MHC class II and III genes, there is some suggestion that variants of the Fcγ receptor confer distinct

**TABLE 26.2.** *Common autoantibodies in systemic lupus erythematosus and drug-induced lupus*

| Condition | Autoantibody | Positive (%) | Comments |
|---|---|---|---|
| SLE | Anti-dsDNA | 30–70 | Associated with nephritis, Marker for SLE |
| | Anti-Sm | 20–40 | Marker for SLE |
| | Anti-RNP | 40–60 | Also seen in MCTD and PSS |
| | Anti-Ro/SS-A | 10–15 | Associated with sicca syndrome, also seen in Sjögren's syndrome |
| | Anti-PCNA | 5–10 | |
| | Anti-Ku | 30–40 | Also seen in overlap syndromes |
| | Anti-lamin B | 5–10 | Also seen in autoimmune liver disease |
| | Anti-ribosomal P | 5–10 | Associated with psychosis |
| | Anti-histone | 30 | Seen in many disorders |
| | Anti-ssDNA | | Seen in many disorders |
| Drug-induced lupus | Anti-histone | 95–100 | Seen in many disorders |
| | Anti-ssDNA | | Seen in many disorders |

MCTD, mixed connective tissue disease; PSS, progressive systemic sclerosis.
From Lahita RG. The clinical presentation of SLE in the adult. In: Lahita RG, ed. *Systemic lupus erythematosis.* San Diego: Academic Press, 1999:325–336, with permission.

phagocytic properties to cells in certain patients. The absence of certain alleles provides a mechanism for the acquisition of immune complex disease. When the receptor FcγRIIa is present, a certain protective effect is obtained for African Americans who would otherwise develop severe lupus nephritis. This determination showed that lupus nephritis increased in this population when the receptor numbers decreased. Hypothetically, this increased risk of nephritis can occur because of ineffective clearance of immune complexes (40). In other carefully performed case-control studies, factors such as mannose-binding protein, interleukin-6 (IL-6), BCL-2 (encoded by the B-cell leukemia/lymphoma gene), and IL-10 (41) have been associated with lupus nephritis or SLE.

One research group suggested that autoimmunity is a mendelian dominant trait (42). Evidence for linkage of a chromosome 1q41-42 region with familial lupus exists and is based on murine studies of a similar locus (34).

### Gender Aspects

Few aspects of the disease are as impressive as the large female prevalence. Approximately 10 females are affected for every male after puberty. The reasons for this skewed sex effect is unknown. The various theories include abnormal sex hormone metabolism (43–45) and the effect of sex hormones on the immune system (46). Observations from humans (47) and animals (48) showing that sex steroids affect immune function provides the basis for the use of androgens such as dehydroepiandrosterone (DHEA) in the treatment of SLE (49–51). It is also the rationale for the avoidance of estrogen hormones in the premenopausal female.

### Murine Models

Murine lupus has been an interesting model with which to study the disease. There are several strains of inbred mice with inherited lupus-like disease. These mice display all the features that mimic human lupus, such as the production of ANA, immune complex glomerulonephritis, lymphadenopathy, and abnormal B-cell and T-cell function. All of the mouse strains differ concerning certain serologic and clinical findings, as well as the incidence of the disease between the sexes. It is apparent from studies of mice that the development of a full lupus-like syndrome requires many unlinked genes (52).

The properties of certain mice can promote anti-DNA production and alter the number and functional properties of B and T cells (53,54). In mice that have the lpr and the gld abnormalities, immunologic problems arise from mutations of apoptotic genes (55,56). The process of apoptosis, also known as programmed cell death, plays a major role in the development of the immune system in some murine models and in the establishment and maintenance of tolerance. Lpr mutations result in the absence of FAS (CD95). The FAS mutation results in the defective apoptosis of lymphocytes, and it is hypothesized that apoptosis results in the destruction of autoreactive T cells (56). Unlike human lupus, the murine strains lack

MHC class I or II markers that can be identified as susceptibility factors. One interesting aspect of the New Zealand lupus strains of mice is the low level of the proinflammatory cytokine tumor necrosis factor-α (57). This absence is important, because reconstitution of the mouse with the tumor necrosis factor results in amelioration of renal disease (58). Murine studies prove that a significant genetic background is necessary for the development of the disease (59), and in mice, most of the genes involved are not in the MHC (60).

The immunologic abnormalities in the lupus patient are curious. All cell types are involved. Immune cell disturbances promote the cellular hyperactivity that leads to hypergammaglobulinemia, increased antibody-producing cells, and heightened responses to many self and foreign antigens. There are many antigens in SLE, and the reasons for the immune responses to these antigens are not clear.

## CLINICAL MANIFESTATIONS

### Skin Manifestations

The skin is the one organ system in which lupus can manifest in many ways (Tables 26.3, 26.4, and 26.5). The most recognized manifestation in SLE is the so-called butterfly rash, which is an erythematosus, elevated, pruritic, ulcerated, and painful lesion in a malar distribution. This malar rash is found in only 30% of patients (61) (Fig. 26.2). Lupus patients may also have erythematous or bullous lesions and photosensitive rashes. One such lesion is called subacute cutaneous lupus erythematosus (SCLE) (18). This is not a distinct cutaneous

**TABLE 26.3.** *Initial manifestations of systemic lupus erythematosus*

| Manifestation | Estes and Christian[a] | Dubois et al.[b] |
|---|---|---|
| Arthritis or arthralgia | 53[c] | 46 |
| Cutaneous | | |
|   Discoid | 9 | 11 |
|   Malar rash | 9 | 8 |
|   Other skin manifestations | 1 | |
| Nephritis | 6 | 4 |
| Fever | 5 | 3 |
|   Other | 17 | 16 |
|   Serositis (pleurisy, pericarditis) | 5 | |
|   Seizures | 3 | |
|   Raynaud's phenomenon | 3 | |
|   Anemia | 2 | |
|   Thrombocytopenia | 2 | |
|   False positive syphilis test | 1 | |
|   Jaundice | 1 | |

[a] Data from Estes D, Christian CL. The natural history of systemic lupus erythematosus by prospective analysis. *Medicine* 1971;50:85–95.
[b] Data from Dubois E et al. Clinical manifestations of systemic lupus erythematosis: computer analysis of 520 cases. *JAMA* 1964;190:104.
[c] Expressed as percent.
From Lahita RG. The clinical presentation of SLE in the adult. In: Lahita RG, ed. *Systemic lupus erythematosis.* San Diego: Academic Press, 1999:325–336, with permission.

**TABLE 26.4.** *Frequency (%) of some common clinical manifestations of SLE*

| Manifestation | Estes et al. | Hochberg et al. |
|---|---|---|
| Musculoskeletal | 95 | 83 |
| Arthritis | 95 | 76 |
| Aseptic necrosis | 7 | 24 |
| Myositis | 5 | 5 |
| Cutaneous | 88 | 81 |
| Malar rash | 39 | 61 |
| Alopecia | 37 | 45 |
| Photosensitivity | n.a. | 45 |
| Dermal vasculitis | 21 | 27 |
| Raynaud's phenomenon | 21 | 44 |
| Discoid lesions | 14 | 15 |
| Rheumatoid nodules | 11 | 12 |
| Oral ulcers | 7 | 23 |
| Fever | 77 | n.a. |
| Serositis | n.a. | 63 |
| Pleurisy | 40 | 57 |
| Pericarditis | 19 | 23 |
| Peritonitis | n.a. | 8 |
| Neuropsychiatric | 59 | 55 |
| Psychosis | 37 | 16 |
| Neurosis | 5 | n.a. |
| Grand mal seizures | 13 | 26 |
| Peripheral neuropathy | 7 | 21 |
| Cranial nerve palsies | n.a. | 5 |
| Hemiparesis | n.a. | 5 |
| Renal (nephritis) | 53 | 31 |
| Nephrotic syndrome | 26 | 13 |
| Hypertension | 46 | n.a. |
| Pulmonary | n.a. | n.a. |
| Lupus pneumonia | 9 | n.a. |
| Fibrosis | 6 | n.a. |
| Cardiac | n.a. | n.a. |
| Myocarditis | 8 | n.a. |
| Sinus tachycardia | 13 | n.a. |
| Heart failure | 11 | n.a. |

Data from Estes D, Christian CL. The natural history of systemic lupus erythematosus by prospective analysis. *Medicine* 1971;50:85–95; and Hochberg MC, Perlmutter DL, White B, et al. The prevalence of self reported physician diagnosed systemic lupus erythematosus (Abstract). *Arth Rheum* 1994; 37:S302.

From Lahita RG. The clinical presentation of SLE in the adult. In: Lahita RG, ed. *Systemic lupus erythematosis.* San Diego: Academic Press, 1999:325–336, with permission.

**TABLE 26.5.** *Cutaneous changes in lupus erythematosus*

*Specific lesions*
Discoid
Subacute cutaneous
 Papulosquamous
 Annular/polycyclic
Neonatal lupus erythematosus
Malar dermatitis

*Nonspecific lesions*
•Bullous
Lupus panniculitis
Alopecia
Vasculitis
Urticaria-like vasculitis
Livedo reticularis
Raynaud's phenomenon
Photosensitivity
Oral ulcerations
Nail changes
Cutaneous mucinosis
Rheumatoid nodules

## Musculoskeletal Manifestations

One of the most common systems involved in lupus is the musculoskeletal system; arthralgia and arthritis are seen in 90% of patients initially (62). Arthritis can involve any joint of the body but typically involves the small joints of the hands, the wrists, and knees in a symmetric pattern. The arthritis can be migratory and transient or persistent and

lesion; it is nonfixed, nonscarring, and variable. The lesions of this particular skin disease occur in sun-exposed areas as a papulosquamous variant or annular lesions that can look like erythema anulare. Another form of lupus skin lesion is the discoid lesion (61). These lesions are disfiguring and begin as red papules or plaques with adherent, scaly, and poorly pigmented central areas. There is much scarring and central atrophy.

Alopecia or hair loss can be diffuse or localized. The hair tends to fall out at the time of flare, but it usually grows back. A common form of skin lesion involves the mucous membranes, and mouth ulcers, vaginal ulcers, and even erosions of the nasal septum occur. Other manifestations include purpura, nailfold and digital ulcerations, splinter hemorrhages, and Osler's nodes or Janeway's nodes (seen in endocarditis).

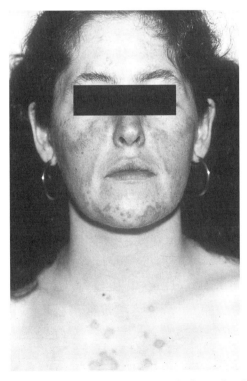

**FIG. 26.2.** Female patient with a malar rash. See color plate 27.

chronic. Soft tissue swelling is common. Microscopic analysis of the synovium usually shows some inflammation. Rarely is there erosion of bone, the presence of effusion, or any kind of contracture. A particular form of unusual joint involvement in lupus is that of Jaccoud's arthropathy, a nonerosive, deforming form. Patients with lupus complain of muscle aches and weakness, and they may have myositis (63). The creatine phosphokinase and aldolase levels can be elevated.

### Renal Manifestations

All patients with lupus have immunoglobulin deposition in the kidney (10) (Table 26.6). Patients that have lupus can have involvement of the kidneys to the exclusion of other manifestations. Patients may not notice symptoms and present with nephrotic syndrome or hematuria as their initial complaint (64). The presence of protein in the urine, casts, hematuria, or abnormal renal function test results require immediate investigation. The renal manifestations depend on the degree of deposition. The degree of kidney involvement is determined only by renal biopsy (65). The overall therapy of this manifestation depends on the histology of the lesion and the activity-chronicity index (11) (Tables 26.7 and 26.8).

### Neuropsychiatric Manifestations

Neuropsychiatric manifestations occur in more than 67% of patients with SLE (66). These manifestations are associated with active disease or exist as an isolated finding. Nervous system involvement may include that of the central nervous system, the cranial and peripheral nerves, and psychiatric abnormalities (Table 26.9). Patients with lupus often have intractable headaches, and migraine headaches are common (67). Seizures, chorea, and cerebrovascular accident–related specific antibodies such as the phospholipid antibody have been observed (68). However, other antibody systems can be found, and there are some suggestions of specificity. Peripheral neuropathies can be motor, sensory, or mixed (69). A Guillain–Barré type of neuropathy has been described in

**TABLE 26.6.** *World Health Organization classification of lupus nephritis*

| Class | Pattern | Site of Immune Complex Deposition |
|---|---|---|
| I | Normal | None |
| II | Mesangial | Mesangial only |
| III | Focal and segmental proliferative | Mesangial, subendothelial ± subepithelial |
| IV | Diffuse proliferative | Mesangial, subendothelial, ± subepithelial |
| V | Membranous | Mesangial, subepithelial |

From Appel GB, Silva FG, Pirani CL. Renal involvement in systemic lupus erythematosus (SLE): a study of 56 patients emphasizing histologic classification. *Medicine (Baltimore)* 1978;57:371, with permission.

**TABLE 26.7.** *Indices of activity and chronicity in lupus nephritis*[a]

*Activity Index (range, 0 to 24)*
Glomerular hypercellularity
Leukocyte exudation
Karyorrhexis/fibrinoid necrosis
Cellular crescents
Hyaline thrombi
Tubulointerstitial inflammation

*Chronicity Index (range, 0 to 12)*
Glomerular lesions
    Glomerular sclerosis
    Fibrous crescents
Tubulointerstitial lesions
    Tubular atrophy
    Interstitial fibrosis

[a] Individual lesions are scored 0 to 3+ (absent, mild, moderate, severe).
Indices are composite scores for individual lesions in each category of activity or chronicity.
Necrosis/karyorrhexis and cellular crescents are weighted by a factor of 2.

lupus (66). Rarer types of transverse myelitis have also been observed in patients with and without phospholipid antibodies. Organic brain syndromes of lupus are defined as states of disturbed mental function, and delirium, emotional problems, impaired memory and concentration, a variety of other neuropsychiatric manifestations can be found (70). The diagnosis of neuropsychiatric lupus is difficult and often is one of exclusion. Other possible causes must be eliminated. One helpful antibody system has been the antiribosomal P protein, which has some specificity in cases of neuropsychiatric disease (28).

**TABLE 26.8.** *Factors that may influence the prognosis of lupus nephritis*

General
  Age
  Sex
  Race
  Education
Clinical aspects of renal involvement
  Acuity of illness
  Disease duration
  Presence of hypertension
  Other organ system involvement
Renal histology
  Activity Index (disease activity and severity)
  Chronic Index (sclerosis and fibrosis)
  Location of immune deposits
  Capillary thrombosis
Immunologic/pathogenetic factors
  Type of circulating immune complexes
  Anti–double-stranded DNA antibodies
  Complement activation
  Reticuloendothelial system dysfunction
  Circulating anticoagulant
  Platelets
  Fibrinolytic abnormalities
Specific treatment

**TABLE 26.9.** *Neuropsychiatric manifestations in systemic lupus erythematosus*

*Central nervous system*
Diffuse manifestations (35%–60%)
    Organic brain syndromes
        Organic amnestic/cognitive dysfunction
        Dementia
        Altered consciousness
    Psychiatric
        Psychosis
        Organic mood/anxiety syndromes
Focal manifestations (10%–35%)
    Cranial neuropathies
    Cerebrovascular accidents/strokes
    Transverse myelitis
    Movement disorders
Seizures (15%–35%)
    Grand mal
    Focal
    Temporal lobe
    Petit mal
Other
    Headaches
    Aseptic meningitis
    Pseudotumor cerebri
    Normal pressure hydrocephalus

*Peripheral nervous system*
Peripheral neuropathies (10%–20%)
    Sensory polyneuropathy
    Mononeuritis multiplex
    Chronic, relapsing polyneuropathy
    Guillain–Barré syndrome
Other
    Autonomic neuropathy
    Myasthenia gravis
    Eaton–Lambert syndrome

The diagnosis of lupus of the central nervous system is largely clinical (71). Cerebrospinal fluid (CSF) abnormalities such as pleocytosis or high CSF protein levels are nonspecific. Electroencephalographic abnormalities are also nonspecific. Radionuclide scans employing labeled oxygen and positron emission tomography have been promising. Magnetic resonance imaging (MRI) can be helpful in finding small areas of increased signal intensity in the gray and white matter (72). The additional use of magnetic resonance angiography can indicate whether microthrombi or cerebrovasculitis is at fault. The overall significance of MRI-positive areas in the brain is not clear in most instances (69,73–76).

## Cardiac Manifestations

Cardiac involvement in lupus can vary. Most commonly, it is pericarditis (77). Serositis in lupus is common and can present as pericarditis, peritonitis, or pleurisy (78). The most common cause of death of lupus patients is atherosclerotic heart disease (79). Other forms of cardiac involvement include myocarditis, endocarditis, or severe coronary artery disease. Patients present with cardiac arrhythmia or conduc-

tion defects (80,81). Patients who present with pericarditis often have chest pain and congestive heart failure, and the physician must exclude other reasons for these symptoms. Coronary vasculitis is not common in SLE patients, but it has been reported in cases of phospholipid syndrome. Often, it is not certain whether coronary death is the result of thrombus or accelerated atherosclerosis (20). Moreover, nonbacterial verrucous vegetations (Libman–Sacks disease), described at autopsy, are seen frequently in patients with the antiphospholipid syndrome (82).

## Pulmonary Manifestations

Pulmonary lupus can manifest as pneumonitis, pulmonary hemorrhage, pulmonary embolus, pulmonary hypertension, or the so-called shrinking lung syndrome (83,84). A typical acute presentation consists of cough, fever, shortness of breath, and occasionally, hemoptysis. In all instances, the pneumonitis of SLE must be differentiated from classic infection (85). Such differentiation may require bronchoalveolar lavage, the collection and culture of sputum, or in the worst-case scenario, open lung biopsy (86–88). A common presentation is that of pleural effusion. This is more commonly observed in patients with drug-induced lupus (89). Pulmonary hemorrhage presenting with hemoptysis or as an infiltrate is uncommon (90).

Pulmonary hypertension because of the antiphospholipid antibody syndrome or occurring for unknown reasons is indistinguishable from idiopathic pulmonary hypertension (91,92). This diagnosis poses particular problems, because patients present with dyspnea, a normal chest radiograph, and a restrictive pattern on pulmonary function testing. These patients frequently have Raynaud's phenomenon. The etiopathogenesis is unknown.

## Gastrointestinal Manifestations

The gastrointestinal manifestations of systemic lupus are common, and symptoms can range from abdominal pain, anorexia, or nausea to intractable vomiting (93). The many reasons for these gastrointestinal symptoms peritonitis, vasculitis of the bowel, pancreatitis, and inflammatory bowel disease (94). In most patients, the peritoneal inflammation causes acute abdominal pain that does not resolve until the infusion of steroids. As with every other manifestation, patients can have a chronic condition of the gastrointestinal tract with ascites that resembles many other diseases. Mesenteric vasculitis generally presents with insidious lower abdominal pain that can come and go over many weeks or months (94). Angiography reveals the vasculitis (95).

Overt clinical liver disease in lupus erythematosus is not common (96). Liver enzyme elevations are associated with lupus vasculitis and with the ingestion of nonsteroidal antiinflammatory drugs or salicylates (97,98). Pancreatitis is common in SLE, and elevated amylase levels can be found (99,100).

Immunosuppression is often the therapy of choice in the control of the gastrointestinal manifestations of lupus (101).

### Reticuloendothelial Manifestations

Splenomegaly is a common finding in SLE (102). However, atrophy of the spleen from frequent infections, infarctions, or lymphoma also occurs. Large lymph nodes can be found in patients with lupus at single or multiple sites. Repeated biopsy of these lymph nodes is unnecessary, because the usual histologic finding is reactive hyperplasia. Unlike Sjögren's syndrome, there is no predisposition for hematologic malignancy. Malignancy can be the result of chemotherapy.

## LABORATORY DIAGNOSIS OF LUPUS

Many common laboratory abnormalities are apparent before complex immunologic testing results are available. These results should suggest lupus in the context of the patient's history. The most common of these laboratory abnormalities are the cytopenias: leukopenia, anemia, lymphopenia, and thrombocytopenia (102) (Table 26.10). These low cell counts can result from chronic inflammatory disease, blood loss, renal disease, drug use, or autoantibodies to a particular progenitor. Various tests such as the Coombs' test or an antibody detection method are employed to determine whether there are antibodies to cells such as platelet's or neutrophils. Most common in SLE is a generalized leukopenia, with neutrophil counts ranging between 1500 and 4000 cells/mm³ (1). Lymphocytopenia can result from specific cold or warm antibodies to lymphocytes (33). Thrombocytopenia can be associated with anemia and specific antibodies to glycoprotein (102). Thrombocytopenia is commonly found in patients with the antiphospholipid antibody syndrome.

Varieties of clotting abnormalities are reported in lupus (103). These can result from circulating procoagulant associated with the phospholipid syndrome. Lupus anticoagulants and anticardiolipin antibodies are associated with these clotting abnormalities (104). At the outset, clues to the presence of these particular antibodies are a false-positive VDRL test result and a prolonged partial thromboplastin time (105). The erythrocyte sedimentation rate can also be elevated for persons with lupus, but because it represents plasma fibrinogen levels, it is not a very accurate measure of activity.

Many serologic abnormalities are possible in lupus patients. Only three specific serologic markers are truly useful in the management of the disease activity in that changes of these markers affect the prognosis of the disease: measurement of the total hemolytic complement, anti-DNA antibody, and the antiphospholipid antibody. Many other antibodies systems are measured to support a diagnosis, including antibodies to the SM glycoprotein, the anti-RNP antibody, and the anti-Ro and anti-La antibody systems. All patients with SLE should have an ANA assay. If the test is negative, the method or substrate is usually suspect. A small group of patients may be ANA negative (23), and a patient could become serologically negative during aggressive therapy.

**TABLE 26.10.** *Frequency (%) of common laboratory manifestations of SLE*

| Manifestation | Estes et al. | Hochberg et al. |
|---|---|---|
| Hematologic | | |
| Anemia[a] | 73 | 57 |
| Leukopenia[b] | 66 | 41 |
| Thrombocytopenia[c] | 19 | 45 |
| Positive direct Coombs' test | 27 | 27 |
| Immunologic | | |
| Antinuclear antibodies | 87 | 94 |
| Hypocomplementemia[d] | n.a. | 59 |
| Rheumatoid factor | 21 | 34 |
| Hyperglobulinemia[e] | 77 | 30 |
| False positive syphilis test | 24 | 26 |
| LE cells | 78 | 71 |
| Anti-dsDNA | n.a. | 28 |
| Anti-Sm | n.a. | 17 |
| Anti-RNP | n.a. | 34 |

[a] Defined as hemoglobin <11 g/dl (Estes D, Christian CL. The natural history of systemic lupus erythematosus by prospective analysis. *Medicine* 1971;50:85–95) or hematocrit <35% (Hochberg MC, Perlmutter DL, White B, et al. The prevalence of self reported physician diagnosed systemic lupus erythematosus (Abstract). *Arth Rheum* 1994;37:S302).
[b] Defined as white blood cells <4500/mm³ (Estes D, Christian CL. The natural history of systemic lupus erythematosus by prospective analysis. *Medicine* 1971;50:85–95) or <4000/mm³ (Hochberg MC, Perlmutter DL, White B, et al. The prevalence of self reported physician diagnosed systemic lupus erythematosus (Abstract). *Arth Rheum* 1994;37:S302).
[c] Defined as platelets <100,000/mm³ (Estes D, Christian CL. The natural history of systemic lupus erythematosus by prospective analysis. *Medicine* 1971;50:85–95) or <150,000/mm³ (Hochberg MC, Perlmutter DL, White B, et al. The prevalence of self reported physician diagnosed systemic lupus erythematosus (Abstract). *Arth Rheum* 1994;37:S302).
[d] Defined as CH50 <26 units
[e] Defined as gamma globulins >1.5 g/dl (Estes D, Christian CL. The natural history of systemic lupus erythematosus by prospective analysis. *Medicine* 1971;50:85–95) or >4 g/dl (Hochberg MC, Perlmutter DL, White B, et al. The prevalence of self reported physician diagnosed systemic lupus erythematosus (Abstract). *Arth Rheum* 1994;37:S302).
n.a., not available.
From Lahita RG. The clinical presentation of SLE in the adult. In: Lahita RG, ed. *Systemic lupus erythematosis.* San Diego: Academic Press, 1999:325–336, with permission.

## DRUG-INDUCED LUPUS

Drug-induced lupus is transient and related to the ingestion of specific medicines (106). Patients with drug-induced disease manifest clinical and serologic signs and symptoms in response to the ingestion of specific agents, such as procainamide, hydralazine, and isoniazid (107). There are undoubtedly many other agents that are associated with drug-induced disease. When the offending agent is removed, the disease abates. The clinical features of drug-induced lupus are rarely severe. The symptoms are usually constitutional, such as fever, arthritis, and serositis. Central nervous system and renal disease rarely occur.

Investigations into the possible reasons for this form of autoimmune disease are important to our understanding of idiopathic lupus (108). The laboratory findings in this particular variant of lupus include the cytopenias, positive LE cells, and positive ANA and rheumatoid factor test results (106). Antibodies to single-stranded DNA are common, but antibodies to double-stranded DNA are not. In 90% of cases, antihistone antibodies are found, but they are not specific, because they are also found in the idiopathic disease. However, the serologic abnormalities can be slow to resolve in drug-induced disease. Commonly found laboratory antibodies include the antihistone 2A and 2B antibody systems (109).

## PREGNANCY AND LUPUS

The fertility rates of patients with SLE are identical to those of the general population (110). The lupus patient may conceive normally, although she may have difficulty carrying the pregnancy to term. Among SLE patients, there are greater numbers of spontaneous abortions, premature infants, and intrauterine defects (111,112). Some studies have suggested that the infant mortality is related to socioeconomic status, but it is more likely the result of factors such as activity of disease or the presence of antiphospholipid antibodies (113). Whether patients with lupus who become pregnant have flares of the disease is controversial (114), but it is generally agreed that patients who are gravely ill before conception have a greater chance of worsening their illness than those who are stable. This is particularly true of patients with renal disease (13). The definition of the lupus flare has specific importance to the pregnant female, because her physician must differentiate a lupus flare from eclampsia and preeclampsia. Both latter conditions are commonly found in pregnant patients with lupus (115).

## TREATMENT

The treatment of lupus erythematosus depends on the extent of disease, the immunologic activity, and the specific organs involved (116). The first line of treatment for this disease is nonpharmacologic and involves bed rest. Second, symptoms such as joint and muscle aches, as well of some signs of serositis, can be treated with nonsteroidal antiinflammatory agents. These drugs can have an adverse effect on renal function and may not be good for a patient with previously compromised renal function. Newer agents that inhibit cyclooxygenase-2 (COX-2) enzymes selectively have shown no greater promise with regard to the treatment of lupus arthralgia, and there is chance that the sulfur moiety on some COX-2 inhibitors may exacerbate the illness.

Corticosteroid therapy (117) is reserved for patients with organ compromise and evidence of serologic activity such as elevated anti-DNA antibodies, low total hemolytic complement, or low C3 and C4 levels (118). The dose of such agents varies with the extent of disease. In some cases, it may be necessary to use parenteral pulse steroid therapy with large doses for short periods (117). The physician should be familiar with the use of chemotherapeutic agents such as methotrexate, cyclophosphamide, and azathioprine. These agents are used for life-threatening organ involvement such as diffuse proliferative glomerulonephritis or lupus cerebritis. There are many new experimental agents (119).

## REFERENCES

1. Lahita RG. Early diagnosis of systemic lupus erythematosus in women. *J Womens Health* 1992;1:117.
2. Lash AA. Why so many women? Part 1. Systemic lupus erythematosus. *Medsurg Nurs* 1993;2:259–264.
3. Fessel WJ. Systemic lupus erythematosus in the community: incidence, prevalence, outcome, and first symptoms; the high prevalence in black women. *Arch Intern Med* 1974;134:1027–1035.
4. Hochberg MC, Perlmutter DL, White B, et al. The prevalence of self reported physician diagnosed systemic lupus erythematosus. *Arthritis Rheum* 1994;37:S302(abst).
5. Lahita RG. Special Report: adjusted lupus prevalence: results of a marketing study by the Lupus Foundation of America. *Lupus* 1995;4:450–453.
6. Hochberg MC. The application of genetic epidemiology to systemic lupus erythematosus. *J Rheumatol* 1987;14:867–869.
7. Deapen DM, Weinrib L, Langholz B. A revised estimate of twin concordance in SLE: a survey of 138 pairs. *Arthritis Rheum* 1986;29:S26(abst).
8. Mannik M. Immune complexes. In: Lahita RG, ed. *Systemic lupus erythematosus.* San Diego: Academic Press, 1999:279–292.
9. Appel GB, Silva FG, Pirani CL. Renal involvement in systemic lupus erythematosus (SLE): a study of 56 patients emphasizing histologic classification. *Medicine (Baltimore)* 1978;57:371.
10. Koffler D, Agnello V, Carr RI. Variable patterns of immunoglobulin and complement deposition in the kidneys of patients with systemic lupus erythematosus. *Am J Pathol* 1969;56:305.
11. Balow JE, Boumpas DT, Austin HA. Systemic lupus erythematosus and the kidney. In: Lahita RG, ed. *Systemic lupus erythematosus.* San Diego: Academic Press, 1999:657–686.
12. Blanco FJ, De la Mata J, Lopez-Fernandez JI, Gomez-Reino JJ. Light, immunofluorescence and electron microscopy renal biopsy findings as predictors of mortality in eighty-five Spanish patients with systemic lupus erythematosus. *Br J Rheumatol* 1994;33:260–266.
13. Krane NK, Thakur V, Wood H, Meleg-Smith S. Evaluation of lupus nephritis during pregnancy by renal biopsy. *Am J Nephrol* 1995;15:186–191.
14. Salach RH, Cash JM. Managing lupus nephritis: algorithms for conservative use of renal biopsy. *Cleve Clin J Med* 1996;63:106–115.
15. Beutner EH, Blaszczyk M, Jablonska S, et al. Preliminary, dermatologic first step criteria for lupus erythematosus and second step criteria for systemic lupus erythematosus. *Int J Dermatol* 1993;32:645–651.
16. Blaszczyk M, Jablonska S, Chorzelski TP, et al. Clinical relevance of immunologic findings in cutaneous lupus erythematosus. *Clin Dermatol* 1992;10:399–406.
17. Velthuis PJ, Kater L, van der Tweel I, et al. Immunofluorescence microscopy of healthy skin from patients with systemic lupus erythematosus: more than just the lupus band. *Ann Rheum Dis* 1992;51:720–725.
18. Gilliam J. Systemic lupus erythematosus and the skin. In: Lahita RG, ed. *Systemic lupus erythematosus.* New York: Wiley, 1987:616.
19. Brasile L, Kramer JL, Clarke JL. Identification of an autoantibody to vascular endothelial cell specific antigen in patients with systemic vasculitis. *Am J Med* 1989;87:74.
20. Tsakraklidesm VG, Blieden IC, Edwards JE. Coronary atherosclerosis and myocardial infarction associated with systemic lupus erythematosus. *Am Heart J* 1974;87:637–641.
21. Meyers MH. Avascular necrosis of the femoral head, diagnostic techniques, reliability and relevance. In: Hungerford DS, ed. *The Hip: Proceedings of the Eleventh Open Scientific Meeting of the Hip Society.* St Louis: CV Mosby, 1983:263.

22. Reeves WH, Satoh M, Richards HB. Origins of antinuclear antibodies. In: Lahita RG, ed. *Systemic lupus erythematosus*. San Diego: Academic Press, 1999:293–318.

23. Urowitz MB, Gladman DD. Antinuclear antibody negative lupus. In: Lahita RG, ed. *Systemic lupus erythematosus*. New York: Churchill Livingstone, 1992:561.

24. Worral JG, Snaith MI, Batchelor JR, Isenberg DA. SLE—a rheumatological view: analysis of the clinical features, serology and immunogenetics of 100 SLE patients during long term follow up. *Q J Med* 1990;319:330.

25. Sharp GC, Hoffman RW. Overlap syndromes: mixed connective tissue disease. In: Lahita RG, ed. *Systemic lupus erythematosus*. San Diego: Academic Press, 1999:551–574.

26. Estes D, Christian CL. The natural history of systemic lupus erythematosus by prospective analysis. *Medicine (Baltimore)* 1971;50: 85–85.

27. Jennette JC, Falk RJ. Diagnosis and management of glomerular diseases. *Med Clin North Am* 1997;81:653–677.

28. Bonfa E, Golombek SJ, Kaufman LD. Association between lupus psychosis and anti-ribosomal P protein antibodies. *N Engl J Med* 1987; 317:265–271.

29. Buyon J. Neonatal lupus syndromes. In: Lahita RG, ed. *Systemic lupus erythematosus*. San Diego: Academic Press, 1999:337–360.

30. Drosos AA, Dimou GS, Siamopoulou-Mavidou A. Subacute cutaneous lupus erythematosus in Greece: a clinical, serological and genetic study. *Ann Med Interne* 1990;421:424.

31. Asherson RA, Harris NE, Gharavi AE, Hughes GRV. Systemic lupus erythematosus, antiphospholipid antibodies, chorea and oral contraceptives. *Arthritis Rheum* 1986;29:1535–1536.

32. Arnett FC, Bias WB, Reveille JD. Genetic studies in systemic lupus erythematosus and Sjögren's syndrome. *J Autoimmunity* 1989; 403:413.

33. Reveille JD. Major histocompatibility complex class II and non-major histocompatibility complex genes in the pathogenesis of systemic lupus erythematosus. In: Lahita RG, ed. *Systemic lupus erythematosus*. San Diego: Academic Press, 1999:67–90.

34. Tsao BP, Cantor RM, Kalunian KC, et al. The genetic basis of systemic lupus erythematosus. *Proc Assoc Am Physicians* 1999;110:113–117.

35. Provost TT, Arnett F, Reichlin M. C2 deficiency, lupus erythematosus and anticytoplasmic Ro (SSA antibodies). *Arthritis Rheum* 1983;26: 1279–1282.

36. Atkinson JP, Schneider PM. Genetic susceptibility and class III complement genes. In: Lahita RG, ed. *Systemic lupus erythematosus*. San Diego: Academic Press, 1999:91–104.

37. Complement C4B null status confers risk for systemic lupus erythematosus in a Spanish population. *Eur J Immunogenet* 1999;25: 317–320.

38. Cook L, Agnello V. Complement deficiency and systemic lupus erythematosus. In: Lahita RG, ed. *Systemic lupus erythematosus*. San Diego: Academic Press, 1999:105–128.

39. Alarcon-Segovia D, Alarcon-Riquelme ME. Etiopathogenesis of systemic lupus erythematosus: a tale of three troikas. In: Lahita RG, ed. *Systemic lupus erythematosus*. San Diego: Academic Press, 1999: 55–66.

40. Salmon JE, Millard S, Schachter LA, et al. Fc gamma RIIA alleles are heritable risk factors for lupus nephritis in African Americans. *J Clin Invest* 1999;97:1348–1354.

41. Mehrian R, Quismorio FP, Strassmann G, et al. Synergistic effect between IL-10 and BCL-2 genotypes in determining susceptibility to systemic lupus erythematosus. *Arthritis Rheum* 1999;41:596–602.

42. Bias WB, Reveille JD, Beaty TH. Evidence that autoimmunity in man is a Mendelian dominant trait. *Am J Hum Genet* 1987;39:584.

43. Lahita RG, Bradlow HL, Fishman J, Kunkel HG. Estrogen metabolism in systemic lupus erythematosus: patients and family members. *Arthritis Rheum* 1982;25:843–846.

44. Lahita RG, Bradlow HL, Ginzler E, et al. Low plasma androgens in women with systemic lupus erythematosus. *Arthritis Rheum* 1987; 30:241–248.

45. Lahita RG, Bradlow HL, Kunkel HG, Fishman J. Increased oxidation of testosterone in systemic lupus erythematosus. *Arthritis Rheum* 1983;26:1517–1521.

46. Ansar Ahmed S, Penhale WJ, Talal N. Sex hormones, immune responses, and autoimmune diseases: mechanisms of sex hormone action. *Am J Pathol* 1985;121:531–551.

47. Lahita RG. Gender and age in lupus. In: Lahita RG, ed. *Systemic lupus erythematosus*. San Diego: Academic Press, 1999:129–144.

48. Roubinian JR, Talal N, Greenspan JS, et al. Effect of castration and sex hormone treatment on survival, anti-nucleic acid antibodies, and glomerulonephritis in NZB/NZW F1 mice. *J Exp Med* 1978;147:1568.

49. Lahita RG. Dehydroepiandrosterone (DHEA) and lupus erythematosus: an update [Editorial]. *Lupus* 1997;6:491–493.

50. Van VR, Engleman EG, McGuire JL. Dehydroepiandrosterone in systemic lupus erythematosus: results of a double-blind, placebo-controlled, randomized clinical trial. *Arthritis Rheum* 1995;38:1826–1831.

51. Van VR, McGuire JL. Studies of dehydroepiandrosterone (DHEA) as a therapeutic agent in systemic lupus erythematosus. *Ann Med Interne* 1996;147:290–296.

52. Theofilopoulos AN, Kono DH. Murine lupus models: gene specific and genome-wide studies. In: Lahita RG, ed. *Systemic lupus erythematosus*. San Diego: Academic Press, 1999:145–182.

53. Theofilopoulos AN, Dixon FJ. Etiopathogenesis of murine SLE. *Immunol Rev* 1981;55:179.

54. Theofilopoulos AN, Dixon FJ. Murine models of systemic lupus erythematosus. *Adv Immunol* 1985;37:269–390.

55. Fleck M, Zhou T, Tatsuta T, et al. Fas/Fas ligand signaling during gestational T cell development. *J Immunol* 1998;160:3766–3775.

56. Mountz JD, Wu J, Zhou T, Hsu HC. Cell death and longevity: implications of Fas-mediated apoptosis in T-cell senescence. *Immunol Rev* 1997;160:19–30.

57. Jacob CO. Cytokines and anti-cytokines. *Curr Opin Immunology* 1989;2:249–257.

58. Jacob CO. Tumor necrosis factor-alpha in murine autoimmune "lupus" nephritis. *Nature* 1988;331:356–358.

59. Rozzo SJ, Vyse TJ, Drake CG, Kotzin BL. Effect of genetic background on the contribution of New Zealand black loci to autoimmune lupus nephritis. *Proc Natl Acad Sci USA* 1996;93:15164–15168.

60. Sutmuller M, Ekstijn GL, Ouellette S, et al. Non-MHC genes determine the development of lupus nephritis in H-2 identical mouse. *Clin Exp Immunol* 1999;106:265–272.

61. Sontheimer RD. Systemic lupus erythematosus of the skin. In: Lahita RG, ed. *Systemic lupus erythematosus*. San Diego: Academic Press, 1999:631–656.

62. Di Cesare PE, Zuckerman JD. Articular manifestations of systemic lupus erythematosus. In: Lahita RG, ed. *Systemic lupus erythematosus*. San Diego: Academic Press, 1999:793–812.

63. Yood RA, Smith TW. Inclusion body myositis and systemic lupus erythematosus. *J Rheumatol* 1985;12:568.

64. Rothfield NF. Kidney in lupus erythematosus. *Contrib Nephrol* 1977;7:128.

65. Kashgarian M. The role of the kidney biopsy in the treatment of lupus nephritis. *Ren Fail* 1996;18:765–773.

66. Moore PM. Neuropsychiatric systemic lupus erythematosus. In: Lahita RG, ed. *Systemic lupus erythematosus*. San Diego: Academic Press, 1999:575–602.

67. Klippel JH, Zwaifler NJ. Neuropsychiatric abnormalities in systemic lupus erythematosus. *Clin Rheum Dis* 1975;1:621.

68. Calabrese LV, Stern TA. Neuropsychiatric manifestations of systemic lupus erythematosus. *Psychosomatics* 1995;36:344–359.

69. Singer J, Denburg JA. Diagnostic criteria for neuropsychiatric systemic lupus erythematosus: the results of a consensus meeting. The Ad Hoc Neuropsychiatric Lupus Workshop Group. *J Rheumatol* 1990; 17:1397.

70. McCune WJ, Golbus J. Neuropsychiatric lupus. *Rheum Dis Clin North Am* 1988;149.

71. Kohen M, Asherson RA, Gharavi AE, Lahita RG. Lupus psychosis: differentiation from the steroid-induced state. *Clin Exp Rheumatol* 1993;11:323–326.

72. West SG, Emlen W, Wener MH, Kotzin BL. Neuropsychiatric lupus erythematosus: a 10-year prospective study on the value of diagnostic tests. *Am J Med* 1995;99:153–163.

73. Sibbitt WLJ, Brooks WM, Haseler LJ, et al. Spin-spin relaxation of brain tissues in systemic lupus erythematosus. A method for increasing the sensitivity of magnetic resonance imaging for neuropsychiatric lupus. *Arthritis Rheum* 1995;38:810–818.

74. Colamussi P, Trotta F, Ricci R, et al. Brain perfusion SPECT and proton magnetic resonance spectroscopy in the evaluation of two systemic lupus erythematosus patients with mild neuropsychiatric manifestations. *Nucl Med Commun* 1997;18:269–273.

75. Otte A, Weiner SM, Peter HH, et al. Brain glucose utilization in systemic lupus erythematosus with neuropsychiatric symptoms: a controlled positron emission tomography study. *Eur J Nucl Med* 1997;24: 787–791.

76. Colamussi P, Giganti M, Cittanti C, et al. Brain single-photon emission tomography with $^{99m}$Tc-HMPAO in neuropsychiatric systemic lupus erythematosus: relations with EEG and MRI findings and clinical manifestations. *Eur J Nucl Med* 1995;22:17–24.

77. Ginzler EM. Clinical manifestations of disease activity, its measurement, and associated morbidity in systemic lupus erythematosus. *Curr Opin Rheumatol* 1991;3:780–788.

78. Petri M. Systemic lupus erythematosus and the heart. In: Lahita RG, ed. *Systemic lupus erythematosus*. San Diego: Academic Press, 1999: 687–706.

79. Stevens MB. SLE and the cardiovascular system: the heart. In: Lahita RG, ed. *Systemic lupus erythematosus*. New York: Churchill Livingstone, 1992:707.

80. Lagana B, Tubani L, Maffeo N, et al. Heart rate variability and cardiac autonomic function in systemic lupus erythematosus. *Lupus* 1996;5:49–55.

81. Laversuch CJ, Seo H, Modarres H, et al. Reduction in heart rate variability in patients with systemic lupus erythematosus. *J Rheumatol* 1997;24:1540–1544.

82. Ziporen L, Goldberg I, Arad M, et al. Libman–Sacks endocarditis in the antiphospholipid syndrome: immunopathologic findings in deformed heart valves. *Lupus* 1996;5:196–205.

83. Hunninghake G, Fauci A. Pulmonary involvement in the collagen Vascular diseases. *Am Rev Respir Dis* 1979;119:471.

84. Lawrence EC. Systemic lupus erythematosus and the lung. In: Lahita RG, ed. *Systemic lupus erythematosus*. San Diego: Academic Press, 1999:719–732.

85. Matthay RA, Schwartz MI, Petty TL. Pulmonary manifestations of SLE: review of twelve cases of acute lupus pneumonitis. *Medicine (Baltimore)* 1974;54:397.

86. Koh WH, Boey ML. Open lung biopsy in systemic lupus erythematosus patients with pulmonary disease. *Ann Acad Med Singapore* 1993;22:323–325.

87. Tsai SC, Kao CH, ChangLai SP, Lan JL, Wang SJ. The relationship of alveolar permeability and pulmonary inflammation in patients with systemic lupus erythematosus. *Kao Hsiung I Hsueh Ko Hsueh Tsa Chih* 1995;11:521–527.

88. Hsu BY, Edwards DK 3, Trambert MA. Pulmonary hemorrhage complicating systemic lupus erythematosus: role of MR imaging in diagnosis. *AJR Am J Roentgenol* 1992;158:519–520.

89. Cherin P, Delfraissy JF, Bletry O, et al. [Pleuropulmonary manifestations of systemic lupus erythematosus]. *Rev Med Interne* 1991;12: 355–362.

90. Blanche P, Krebs S, Renaud B, et al. Systemic lupus erythematosus presenting as iron deficiency anemia due to pulmonary alveolar hemorrhage. *Clin Exp Rheumatol* 1996;14:228.

91. Luchi ME, Asherson RA, Lahita RG. Primary idiopathic pulmonary hypertension complicated by pulmonary arterial thrombosis. Association with antiphospholipid antibodies. *Arthritis Rheum* 1992;35: 700–705.

92. Marchesoni A, Messina K, Carrieri P. Pulmonary hypertension and systemic lupus erythematosus. *Clin Exp Rheumatol* 1983;1:247.

93. Salomon P, Mayer L. Non-hepatic gastrointestinal manifestations of systemic lupus erythematosus. In: Lahita RG, ed. *Systemic lupus erythematosus*. New York: Churchill Livingstone, 1992:747–760.

94. Toy LS, Mayer L. Nonhepatic gastrointestinal manifestations of systemic lupus erythematosus. In: Lahita RG, ed. *Systemic lupus erythematosus*. San Diego: Academic Press, 1999:733–746.

95. Wang SJ, Lan JL, Lin WY, et al. Three-phase abdominal scintigraphy in lupus vasculitis of the gastrointestinal tract. *Clin Nucl Med* 1995;20:695–698.

96. Mackay IR. Hepatic disease and systemic lupus erythematosus: coincidence or convergence? In: Lahita RG, ed. *Systemic lupus erythematosus*. San Diego: Academic Press, 1999:747–764.

97. Bearn AG, Kunkel HG, Slater RJ. The problem of chronic liver disease in young women. *Am J Med* 1956;21:3.

98. Runyon BA, LaBreque DR, Anuras S. The spectrum of liver disease in systemic lupus erythematosus—report of 33 histologically proved cases and review of the literature. *Am J Med* 1980;69:187.

99. Baron M, Brisson ML. Pancreatitis in systemic lupus erythematosus. *Arthritis Rheum* 1982;25:1006.

100. Seifert GG, Heintz N, Ruffman A. Pancreatitis in visceral systemic lupus erythematosus. *Gastroenterologia* 1967;107:317.

101. Grimbacher B, Huber M, von Kempis J, et al. Successful treatment of gastrointestinal vasculitis due to systemic lupus erythematosus with intravenous pulse cyclophosphamide: a clinical case report and review of the literature. *Br J Rheumatol* 1998;37:1023–1028.

102. Simantov R, Laurence J, Nachman R. The cellular hematology of systemic lupus erythematosus. In: Lahita RG, ed. *Systemic lupus erythematosus*. San Diego: Academic Press, 1999:765–792.

103. Shapiro S, Long M. Hematology: Coagulation problems. In: Lahita RG, ed. *Systemic lupus erythematosus*. San Diego: Academic Press, 1999:871–886.

104. Merrill J. Pathogenesis and treatment of the antiphospholipid syndrome. In: Lahita RG, ed. *Systemic lupus erythematosus*. San Diego: Academic Press, 1999:887–908.

105. Asherson RA, Cervera R, Lie JT. The antiphospholipid syndromes. In: Lahita RG, ed. *Systemic lupus erythematosus*. San Diego: Academic Press, 1999:829–870.

106. Mongey AB, Hess EV. Drug and environmental lupus: clinical manifestations and differences. In: Lahita RG, ed. *Systemic lupus erythematosus*. San Diego: Academic Press, 1999:929–944.

107. Cush JJ, Goldings EA. Drug induced lupus: clinical spectrum and pathogenesis. *Am J Med Sci* 1985;290:36.

108. Yung RL, Richardson BC. Pathophysiology of drug induced lupus. In: Lahita RG, ed. *Systemic lupus erythematosus*. San Diego: Academic Press, 1999:909–928.

109. Rubin RL. Anti-histone antibodies. In: Lahita RG, ed. *Systemic lupus erythematosus*. San Diego: Academic Press, 1999:227–246.

110. Lockshin MC, Sammaratano L, Schwartzmann S. Lupus pregnancy. In: Lahita RG, ed. *Systemic lupus erythematosus*. San Diego: Academic Press, 1999:507–536.

111. Parke AL. Pregnancy and systemic lupus erythematosus. In: Lahita RG, ed. *Systemic lupus erythematosus*. New York: Churchill Livingstone, 1992:543.

112. Khamashta MA, Ruiz-Irastorza G, Hughes GR. Systemic lupus erythematosus flares during pregnancy. *Rheum Dis Clin North Am* 1997;23:15–30.

113. Marabani M, Zona A, Hadley D. Transverse myelitis occurring during pregnancy in a patient with systemic lupus erythematosus. *Ann Rheum Dis* 1989;48:160.

114. Lockshin MD, Reinitz E, Druzin ML. Lupus pregnancy: case-control progressive study demonstrating absence of lupus exacerbation during or after pregnancy. *Am J Med* 1984;77:893–898.

115. Jaff MR. Medical aspects of pregnancy. *Cleve Clin J Med* 1994;61: 263–271.

116. Lahita RG. The clinical presentation of systemic lupus erythematosus. In: Lahita RG, ed. *Systemic lupus erythematosus*. San Diego: Academic Press, 1999:325–336.

117. Kimberly RP. Corticosteroid use in systemic lupus erythematosus. In: Lahita RG, ed. *Systemic lupus erythematosus*. San Diego: Academic Press, 1999:945–966.

118. Davis JC, Klippel JH. Antimalarials and immunosuppressive drugs. In: Lahita RG, ed. *Systemic lupus erythematosus*. San Diego: Academic Press, 1999:967–984.

119. Van Vollenhoven RF. Unproven experimental therapies. In: Lahita RG, ed. *Systemic lupus erythematosus*. San Diego: Academic Press, 1999:985–1003.

*Textbook of the Autoimmune Diseases,*
Edited by R. G. Lahita, N. Chiorazzi, and W. H. Reeves,
Lippincott Williams & Wilkins, Philadelphia © 2000.

# CHAPTER 27

# Vasculitis

## Robert G. Lahita

Vasculitis represents inflammation of blood vessels within the body. There can be many causes of vasculitis in animals, but in humans, the cause is unknown. Diagnosis is difficult in most cases because of the insidious nature of the disease and the fact that various parts of the circulation can be affected without definitive signs or symptoms. More often than not, vasculitis is a diagnosis made indirectly. Various imaging studies are often inconclusive, and blind biopsy is likely to yield little information. Vasculitis is a definitive autoimmune syndrome.

## PATHOLOGY

Inflammation can involve some or all of a vessel wall (1). All layers can be involved, or there can be skip areas or segmental involvement. The cell types that can be involved include neutrophils, eosinophils, lymphocytes, and plasma cells (2). In certain types of vasculitis, giant cells can be the major pathologic entity and cause granulomas that are seen in giant cell arteritis, temporal arteritis, or Takayasu's disease (3). Intimal proliferation is found, as is thrombosis and fibrinoid necrosis. When this fibrinoid process goes forward in some types of vasculitis, there can be aneurysm formation and often rupture. In the granulomatous forms of vasculitis, fibrinoid necrosis is rare (4). Churg–Strauss disease or granulomatous angiitis share the pathologic and clinical features of polyarteritis nodosa (PAN) and Wegener's granulomatosis.

Immune complexes are a major component of the vasculitis syndromes. The antigenic component of these complexes is a major aspect of the vasculitic process. Some of the antigens are hepatitis C and B (in PAN or mixed cryoglobulinemia) (5,6), autoantibodies themselves (in rheumatoid vasculitis and diseases like lupus erythematosus) (7), and certain drugs (in certain forms of leukocytoclastic vasculitis) (8).

Cellular mechanisms may be the major pathogenic mechanism, as in giant cell arteritis. A granuloma forms because

of the action of T cells in the recruitment of macrophages that form a granuloma.

## Etiology

Generally infective agents are the only identifiable causes of vasculitis. Most investigators believe that immune complexes mediate these forms of vascular disease. Animal data reveal that *Mycoplasma gallisepticum* can cause cerebral angiitis (9–11). Mycoplasma, herpes zoster, cytomegalovirus, and fungal infections have at one time or another been invoked to explain cerebral vasculitis (12,13). The strongest etiologic association exists between hepatitis B or C and PAN (14). Because of retroviral activity in peripheral blood mononuclear cells isolated from patients with Kawasaki disease, another form of vasculitis of children, an infectious agent is suspected in its cause (15,16). In the case of Kawasaki disease, a lymphocytotropic virus has been implicated. In human immunodeficiency virus (HIV) infections, vasculitis is common and associated with the vascular infiltration of CD8$^+$ T cells and plasma cells (11,17–19).

There is compelling evidence that infection is not the only possible cause of vasculitis; perhaps immune complex–mediated diseases of uncertain origins are more common. Such is the case with the vasculitis associated with cancer in which the antigen-antibody complexes are tumor and antitumor (20–23). In the case of urticarial angiitis associated with complement deficiency, the IgG antibodies are directed against the component C1q. Antiendothelial cell antibodies (24) have been identified in conditions such as the phospholipid syndrome (in which vasculitis is found), Wegener's granulomatosis, microscopic polyarteritis, Kawasaki's disease, and rheumatoid arthritis (RA).

## Classification and Diagnosis

The vasculitis syndromes are usually classified according to vessel size (Table 27.1). One of the most common classifications is that of Fauci et al. (25).

R. G. Lahita: Department of Medicine, New York Medical College, Valhalla, New York 10595; Department of Rheumatology, St. Vincent's Hospital, New York, New York 10011.

**TABLE 27.1.** *Vasculitis syndromes, mechanisms of vascular damage, and general treatment approach*

| Diseases within the spectrum of vasculitis | Mechanisms of vascular damage | General treatment approach |
|---|---|---|
| Polyarteritis nodosa group of systemic necrotizing vasculitis | | |
| Classic polyarteritis nodosa | Immune complex formation, cellular immune response, infectious agents, antilysosomal antibodies | Glucocorticoids, cytotoxic therapy |
| Allergic granulomatosis of Churg–Strauss | Immune complex formation, cellular immune response, antilysosomal antibodies | Antihistamines, glucocorticoids, cytotoxic therapy |
| Systemic necrotizing vasculitis and polyangiitis "overlap syndrome" | Immune complex formation, cellular immune response, infectious agents, antilysosomal antibodies | Glucocorticoids, cytotoxic therapy |
| Hypersensitivity vasculitis | | |
| Serum sickness and serum sickness-like reactions | Immune complex formation | NSAIDs, glucocorticoids, cytotoxic therapy, plasmapheresis |
| Henoch–Schönlein purpura | Immune complex formation | Steroids |
| Essential mixed cryoglobulinemia with vasculitis | Immune complex formation, infectious agents | NSAIDs, glucocorticoids, cytotoxic therapy, plasmapheresis |
| Vasculitis associated with malignancies | Immune complex formation, tumor cell mediated, antiendothelial cell antibodies | Treat underlying malignancy, glucocorticoids |
| Vasculitis associated with collagen vascular diseases | Immune complex formation, cellular immune response, antiendothelial cell antibodies, antilysosomal antibodies | Treat collagen vascular diseases |
| Wegener's granulomatosis | Cellular immune response, antilysosomal antibodies, immune complex formation | Glucocorticoids, cytotoxic therapy |
| Lymphomatoid granulomatosis | Tumor cell-mediated | Glucocorticoids, cytotoxic therapy, combination chemotherapy |
| Giant cell arteritis | | |
| Temporal arteritis | Cellular immune response | Glucocorticoids, rarely cytotoxic therapy |
| Takayasu's arteritis | Cellular immune response | Glucocorticoids, cytotoxic therapy, angioplasty |
| Thromboangiitis obliterans (Buerger's disease) | ? Immune complex formation, ? cellular immune response | Tobacco avoidance, revascularization |
| Mucocutaneous lymph node syndrome (Kawasaki's disease) | Immune complex formation, cellular immune response, infectious agent | Gammaglobulin, salicylates |
| Miscellaneous vasculitides | | |
| HIV-associated vasculitis | Immune complex formation, infectious agent | Glucocorticoids |
| HTLV-I-associated vasculitis/arthritis syndrome | Tumor cell mediated, infectious agent | Treat the HTLV-I adult T cell leukemia syndrome |
| Cogan's syndrome | Cellular immune response | Glucocorticoids, cytotoxic therapy, cyclosporin A |
| Behçet's disease | Cellular immune response, ? immune complex formation | Colchicine, glucocorticoids, cytotoxic therapy, cyclosporin A |
| Erythema elevatum dilutinum | Immune complex formation | Dapsone |

Adapted from Fauci AS, et al. The spectrum of vasculitis: Clinical, pathologic, immunologic, and therapeutic considerations. *Ann Intern Med* 1978;89:660, with permission.

The greatest aid in the diagnosis of the disease besides tissue biopsy is the association between autoimmunity and lysosomal enzymes. Two major types of antineutrophilic antibodies (ANCAs) have been described in vasculitis (26–28). C-ANCA, directed against the neutrophil granule serine protease (proteinase 3), is detected by cytoplasmic immunofluorescence, and P-ANCA, directed against the myeloperoxidase enzyme, is detected by perinuclear staining. Cytoplasmic staining is 85% specific for Wegener's granulomatosis, whereas P-ANCA staining is typical for microscopic PAN, PAN, Churg–Strauss syndrome, or idiopathic crescentic glomerulonephritis.

An additional test that can be helpful but that needs more research is determination of the level of von Willebrand factor VIII (29). Such levels are increased in vasculitis, particularly in giant cell arteritis and polymyalgia rheumatica (PMR), but these levels are not disease specific.

The biopsy diagnosis of vasculitis really depends on the type of disease manifested. Several treatises have suggested that vasculitis can be differentiated from the phospholipid syndromes (see Chapter 34), which can have vasculitis as part of their presentation or just thrombosis. More often than not, vasculitis is not part of the disease. The critical aspect of differentiation is determining whether anticoagulation should be used or immunosuppression.

## VASCULITIC SYNDROMES

### Takayasu's Disease

Takayasu's disease is better known as pulseless disease, and it primarily affects Asian women (30,31). Most of the patients in studies of this disease were women, and the median age of onset was about 25 to 30 years. The most common symptoms are claudication and weak or absent pulses. Patients may have carotid bruits and hypertension (32). Pain over the carotid arteries (carotidynia) is common. The most likely vessels involved are the carotid, ulnar, radial, brachial, and axillary vessels. Central nervous system findings include lightheadedness to actual stroke. The clinical presentation is varied and includes joint and muscle pains, generalized weakness, and fever. Besides bruits that can be heard over the large vessels, it is common to hear cardiac murmurs such as aortic regurgitation (33).

Laboratory data for this disease are nonspecific and include findings such as an elevated erythrocyte sedimentation rate (ESR). Angiography is used to make the diagnosis. The aorta often shows long stenotic lesions, but lesions can be found in many or all large vessels (34).

Takayasu's disease is characterized by thickened and inflamed intima of blood vessels without fibrinoid degeneration. This is not found in the other arteritides such as giant cell arteritis, which is characterized by granulomatous involvement with medial necrosis and rarely with intimal involvement.

Takayasu's disease is best treated with immunosuppression. Patients often improve with modest doses of prednisone (1 mg/kg/day). If remission is not observed with prednisone, methotrexate or Cytoxan is appropriate. Patients with this disease experience frequent relapses and may require frequent courses of chemotherapy (35). The hypertension found in this syndrome should be treated aggressively. Calcium channel blockers often are helpful. Because the disease is associated with great morbidity resulting from progressive stenosis, it is helpful to control the vasospasm and platelet aggregation that can cause ischemic symptoms. Treatment of the stenotic lesions with angioplasty and stents can be useful (36).

### Giant Cell Arteritis

The diagnosis of giant cell arteritis is a pathologic one (37). The most common syndromes that result from this kind of pathology are temporal arteritis and PMR.

Temporal arteritis is a disease in which arteries of predominantly the head and neck are affected. The most common presenting complaint is headache, along with tenderness of the scalp and claudication of the jaw, although unusual

forms have been described (38). The major concern of all physicians who treat this disease is the rare involvement of the ophthalmic artery or more specifically the posterior ciliary artery, with resulting blindness. Some patients rarely have involvement of the occipital artery, which can be associated with diplopia, intermittent blindness, weight loss, and anemia. In 50% of the patients, malaise, weakness, joint pains, and muscle aches can occur that are related to coexistent PMR. Uncommon presentations of this syndrome can include fever of unknown origin, chest pain from aortitis, coma, peripheral gangrene, peripheral neuropathies, and marked anemia of unknown cause.

In this form of vasculitis, biopsy is the principal way to make the diagnosis. Most patients also have an elevated ESR, but the temporal artery biopsy is the way to confirm the diagnosis. The examiner looks for histologic evidence of giant cell arteritis. There are "skip" areas in all forms of vasculitis, which makes a perfect biopsy impossible. Only 60% of unilateral temporal biopsies are positive, and contralateral biopsy of the temporal artery may be necessary (39–41).

A diagnosis of temporal arteritis without a biopsy or when the biopsy is inconclusive is possible, and criteria for this kind of diagnosis have been established. Criteria include an elevated ESR; at least three of the following—severe headaches, PMR, tender temporal arteries, jaw claudication, and visual changes such as amaurosis fugax, blindness, or diplopia; no clinical evidence of another disease such as RA or systemic lupus erythematosus; and response to steroid therapy (42–44).

This disease is treated with high-dose corticosteroids, and the most common reason is to prevent blindness. In the absence of appropriate therapy, about 20% of patients can lose their vision. High-dose corticosteroids (60 to 80 mg/day of prednisone) are used for many weeks. Relapses are common, and the ESR provides the best method to follow the course of the disease.

PMR is another form of giant cell disease. This is a disease of the elderly, who have aching and stiffness of the torso (neck and shoulder girdle) and proximal portions of the lower extremities (pelvic or waste girdle). There is also evidence of an underlying inflammatory reaction. The symptoms that suggest the latter include malaise, loss of weight, low-grade fever, anemia, and a high ESR. These symptoms should be present for more than 4 weeks to exclude other diseases, such as viral infections, other connective tissue diseases, and malignancies.

Controversy exists about the coexistence of temporal arteritis with PMR (45). The two are found together in 16% of patients studied in the Mayo series and in as many as 50% of the patients in Scandinavian countries. The incidence of blindness in the "pure PMR" group should approximate 2% per year because of undetected temporal arteritis and because low-dose steroids are used to treat pure PMR, but this is not the case. A patient with PMR who has claudication, scalp tenderness, a high ESR, visual changes, or strokes should have a temporal artery biopsy.

In patients with pure PMR and mild disease, a trial of non-steroidal antiinflammatory drugs may be used before the institution of low-dose corticosteroids (10 to 20 mg/day). The disease can completely resolve in some patients, but recurrences are frequent.

## Wegener's Granulomatosis

Wegener's granulomatosis is a multisystem vasculitis of unknown cause that involves the upper respiratory tract, lungs, and kidneys (46,47). Other affected sites can include the eyes, skin, joints, and nervous system (48,49). The usual clinical presentation of a patient with Wegener's granulomatosis is a chronic upper respiratory tract disease that includes rhinorrhea, sinusitis, or otitis media. More than 70% of patients have pulmonary infiltrates, but only one half of these are symptomatic. Only 10% of patients have functional renal impairment at the time of diagnosis, and one third of these have disease that progresses to end-stage renal disease (50). The disease may be exacerbated by pregnancy (51).

The diagnosis requires that both vasculitis and granulomas exist in the same biopsy specimen. A biopsy of the lung can be conclusive, but an open lung biopsy has the highest yield of diagnostic tissue. Endobronchial biopsy gives a low diagnostic yield. Kidney biopsy usually is not helpful, because the observed glomerulonephritis is nonspecific.

Laboratory data include abnormal chest and sinus radiographs. There is also evidence of active urinary sediment, and the anemia of chronic disease and an elevated ESR are also found in these patients. ANCA testing helps with the diagnosis of this disease and can be used to monitor clinical activity, although the titer of antibody does not necessarily decline with treatment. Some investigators have suggested that the clinical signs and the a positive ANCA finding obviate the need for biopsy. More than 95% of patients with this disease are ANCA positive. The ANCA that is characteristic of Wegener's granulomatosis is an antiserine protease (29 kd) or C-ANCA. Antibodies to a myeloperoxidase constitute a P-ANCA that is not specific for Wegener's granulomatosis but is found in other forms of vasculitis (52,53).

Treatment of Wegener's granulomatosis requires the use of Cytoxan (Bristol-Myers Squibb Company, New York, NY, U.S.A.) (2 mg/kg) and prednisone (1 mg/kg) (54). The prednisone dose can be tapered within 6 weeks of beginning the Cytoxan therapy. In mild cases of Wegener's granulomatosis, trimethoprim–sulfamethoxazole has been used with modest success. Treatment of concomitant infections or superinfections of the upper respiratory tract and renal transplantation for patients in renal failure are additional therapeutic considerations.

## Polyarteritis Nodosa

PAN is a rare disease characterized by transmural inflammation of medium to small arteries. It is more common in men than in women although some estrogen-sensitive forms have been reported (55). The characteristic aspects of this syndrome are a wasting illness with severe hypertension and

renal dysfunction (Table 27.2). Other organs of the body, such as the gastrointestinal tract, nervous system, joints, skin, and muscle, can be involved. The signs and symptoms of such involvement are bleeding in the bowel (56), peripheral neuropathy (mononeuritis multiplex) or psychosis (57), and joint pain. More than one half of the patients with this disease are positive for hepatitis B antigen (58), and hepatitis C also has been associated with the disease (5). The symptoms of some patients may result from serum sickness, allergic reactions to drugs (59) and other toxins, amphetamine abuse, or HIV infection (18).

The diagnosis of this condition is often made with angiography, during which aneurysms are observed in the mesenteric, hepatic, and renal systems. Tissue biopsy is definitive

**TABLE 27.2.** *1990 ACR criteria for the classification of Polyartritis Nodosa*

| Criterion | Definition |
| --- | --- |
| Weight loss >4 kg | Loss of 4 kg or more of body weight since illness began, not due to dieting or other factors |
| Livedo reticularis | Mottled reticular pattern over the skin of portions of the extremities or torso |
| Testicular pain or tenderness | Pain or tenderness of the testicles, not due to infection, trauma, or other causes |
| Myalgias, weakness, or polyneuropathy | Diffuse myalgias (excluding shoulder and hip girdle) or weakness of muscles or tenderness of leg muscles |
| Mononeuropathy or polyneuropathy | Development of mononeuropathy, multiple mononeuropathies, or polyneuropathy |
| Diastolic BP >90 mmHg | Development of hypertension with the diastolic BP higher than 90 mm Hg |
| Elevated BUN or creatinine | Elevation of BUN >40 mg/dL (14.3 μmol/L) or creatinine >1.5 mg/dL (132 μmol/L), not due to dehydration or obstruction |
| Hepatitis B virus | Presence of hepatitis B surface antigen or antibody in serum |
| Arteriographic abnormality | Arteriogram showing aneurysms or occlusions of the visceral arteries, not due to arteriosclerosis, fibromuscular dysplasia, or noninflammatory causes |
| Biopsy of small- or medium-sized artery containing PMN | Histologic changes showing the presence of granulocytes or granulocytes and mononuclear leukocytes in the artery wall |

For classification purposes, a patient with vasculitis shall be said to have polyarteritis nodosa if at least three of these 10 criteria are present. The presence of any three or more criteria yields a sensitivity of 82.2% and a specificity of 86.6%. BP, blood pressure; BUN, blood urea nitrogen; PMN, polymorphonuclear neutrophils.

From Lightfoot RW, Michel BA, Bloch DA, et al. The American College of Rheumatology 1990 criteria for the classification of polyarteritis nodosa. *Arthritis Rheum* 1990;33:1088, with permission.

even when aneurysms are not observed (3). Skin and muscle often yield excellent data, or in cases of documented peripheral neuropathy, a sural nerve biopsy is extremely helpful. ANCA determinations can be helpful in the diagnosis of PAN. The type of antibody in this disease is usually of the P-ANCA variety or antimyeloperoxidase.

Treatment of PAN should involve several steps (54). First is the removal of the source of the antigen, such as an infective agent or a drug. Second, the primary disease is treated (60). Third, prednisone (1 mg/kg/day) should be given when there is no evidence of severe disseminated or systemic disease in patients who experience a hypersensitivity drug reaction. Fourth, prednisone should be tapered as soon as possible. Fifth, low-dose Cytoxan (1 to 2 mg/kg/day) is added, with or without corticosteroids, in patients with severe disseminated necrotizing vasculitis or in patients who have failed to respond to steroid therapy (61).

## Churg–Strauss Syndrome:
## Allergic Granulomatosis and Angiitis

Churg–Strauss syndrome is a form of vasculitis characterized by high levels of eosinophils and systemic vasculitis in a person with severe asthma and allergic rhinitis. The disease can vary from simple, nonsegmental parenchymal infiltrates of the lung to diffuse interstitial disease. Glucocorticoids are useful, but cytotoxic agents may be necessary in some patients (62) (Table 27.3).

## Isolated Vasculitis of the Central Nervous System

Isolated vasculitis of the central nervous system is an unusual form of vasculitis (63). It affects only the central nervous system, and it is serious and life threatening. The clinical presentation can vary from encephalitis to focal deficits that mirror that of stroke. This disease shows pathologic lesions such as Wegener's granulomatosis. The diagnosis is best made with angiography, and typical beading of the cerebral vessels is commonly observed. Magnetic resonance spectroscopy with flow studies can also be diagnostic. The treatment of CNS vasculitis is cytotoxic therapy and corticosteroids.

## Leukocytoclastic Vasculitides

Leukocytoclastic vasculitis involves small vessels and capillaries, with prominent skin manifestations (64–66) (Fig. 27.1). A variety of names have been given to the syndromes, including hypersensitivity vasculitis and allergic angiitis. The vessels involved are usually less than 0.1 mm in diameter. The classic manifestations are palpable purpura concentrated in the areas of dependency. Patients also have livedo reticularis and ulcers. There is evidence of systemic involvement in the kidneys, lungs, and gastrointestinal tract. The cause is unknown, but drugs (65), viral infections (67), and connective tissue diseases (66) are the main associated causes. In more than one half of cases, no cause is known. Corticosteroid and immunosuppressive therapy is suggested in difficult cases.

**TABLE 27.3.** *1990 ACR criteria for the classification of Churg–Strauss syndrome*

| Criterion[a] | Definition |
|---|---|
| Asthma | History of wheezing or diffuse, high-pitched rales on expiration |
| Eosinophilia | Eosinophilia >10% on white blood cell differential count |
| Mononeuropathy or polyneuropathy | Development of mononeuropathy, multiple mononeuropathies, or polyneuropathy (i.e., glove/stocking distribution) attributable to vasculitis |
| Pulmonary infiltrates nonfixed | Migratory or transitory pulmonary infiltrates on radiographs (not including fixed infiltrates), attributable to a systemic vasculitis |
| Paranasal sinus abnormality | History of acute or chronic paranasal sinus pain or tenderness or radiographic opacification of the paranasal sinuses |
| Extravascular eosinophils | Biopsy, including artery, arteriole, or venule, showing accumulations of eosinophils in extravascular areas |

[a]For classification purposes, a patient with vasculitis is said to have Churg–Strauss syndrome if at least four of these six criteria are present. The presence of four or more criteria yields a sensitivity of 85% and a specificity of 99.7%.

From Masi AT, Hunder GG, Lie JT, et al. The American College of Rheumatology 1990 criteria for the classification of Churg–Strauss syndrome (allergic granulomatosis angiitis). *Arthritis Rheum* 1990;33:1094, with permission.

Henoch–Schönlein purpura is an example of small vessel vasculitis that may affect any age group but that has different prognoses for each (64,68–72). Most commonly affected are children between the ages of 4 and 8 years. The combination of purpura and abdominal and join pains is typical for this disease. The disease usually follows an upper respiratory infection in children. Renal involvement occurs in one half of the patients. A few eventually develop severe renal disease.

All of these conditions respond to corticosteroids. In adults, the gastrointestinal and renal symptoms predominate. Biopsy of involved skin can assist in the diagnosis. The finding of fibrin, complement products, and IgA deposition in the cutaneous vessel walls is helpful.

Hypocomplementemic vasculitis typically comprises nonpruritic urticaria, low complement levels, joint pains, and renal disease (73). The syndrome responds to corticosteroids. There is a high frequency of chronic obstructive pulmonary disease reported for these patients. Kidney disease is rare.

Essential mixed cryoglobulinemia is a rare syndrome of cryoglobulins, palpable purpura, and severe glomerulonephritis (74). Other symptoms include Raynaud's phenomenon and fever. The cryoglobulin is an IgM rheumatoid factor in most cases. Hepatitis B and hepatitis C surface antigens are associated with this disease in more than one half of patients. Concentrations of liver enzymes usually are elevated, and liver disease is common. Plasmapheresis is help-

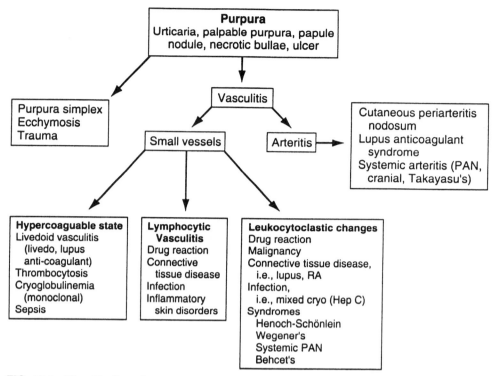

**FIG. 27.1.** Classification of cutaneous vasculitis. (From Gibson LE, Su WP. Cutaneous vasculitis. *Rheum Dis Clin North Am* 1995; 21:1097–1113, with permission.)

ful for these patients. Long-term therapy with corticosteroids and agents such as chlorambucil has been reported.

### Kawasaki's Disease

Kawasaki's disease was first described as a new syndrome in Japanese children, who presented with fever; conjunctival congestion; dry, red "strawberry lips and tongue"; erythematous palms and soles; edema of the peripheral extremities; desquamation of the fingertips; and various rashes of the trunk and cervical lymphadenopathy (75,76). The disease is also called mucocutaneous lymph node syndrome. This disease resembles scarlet fever or Stevens–Johnson syndrome. Cardiovascular complications include myocarditis, pericarditis, murmurs, coronary artery aneurysms, myocardial infarction, angina, stroke, peripheral vascular insufficiency, and gangrene (77). Gallbladder disease, hepatitis, small bowel obstruction, anemia, arthritis, meningitis (aseptic), uveitis, pyuria, and meatitis may be found. Coronary thrombosis can occur in these young children (78).

Antiendothelial cell antibodies are described in the early stages of the disease. The disease has also been associated with *Mycoplasma* infections (16). Recurrent disease has also been described in HIV patients (15).

The treatment of this disease includes intravenous immune globulin (IVIG) and aspirin. The IVIG is given over 2 hours for 4 consecutive days (400 mg/kg/day), and 100 mg of aspirin is given daily in four divided doses through day 14. The dose of aspirin is then reduced to 3 to 5 mg/kg/day.

## REFERENCES

1. McCarthy SA, Kuzu I, Gatter KC. Heterogeneity of the endothelial cell and its role in organ preference for tumor metastases. *Trends Pharmacol Sci* 1991;12:462–467.
2. Granger DM, Kubes P. The microcirculation and inflammation: modulation of leukocyte-endothelial cell adhesion. *J Leukoc Biol* 1994; 55:662.
3. Cid MC, Grau JM, Casademont J. Immunohistochemical characterization of inflammatory cells and immunological activation markers in muscle and nerve biopsy specimens from patients with systemic polyarteritis nodosa. *Arthritis Rheum* 1994;37:1055.
4. Scmitt WH, Csernol E, Kobayashi S, et al. Churg–Strauss syndrome: serum markers of lymphocyte activation and endothelial damage. *Arthritis Rheum* 1998;41:445–452.
5. Quint L, Deny P, Guillevin L. Hepatitis C virus in patients with polyarteritis nodosa: prevalence in 38 patients. *Clin Exp Rheumatol* 1991; 9:253.
6. Finkel TH, Torok TJ, Ferguson PJ. Chronic parvovirus B19 infection and systemic necrotizing vasculitis: opportunistic infections or etiological agent. *Lancet* 1994;343:1255–1258.
7. Wang SJ, Lan JL, Lin WY, et al. Three-phase abdominal scintigraphy in lupus vasculitis of the gastrointestinal tract. *Clin Nucl Med* 1995;20:695–698.
8. Gibson LE, Su WP. Cutaneous vasculitis [Review]. *Rheum Dis Clin North Am* 1990;16:309–324.
9. Gerber O, Roque C, Coyle PK. Vasculitis owing to infection. *Neurol Clin* 1997;15:903–925.
10. Lie JT. Vasculitis associated with infectious agents. *Curr Opin Rheumatol* 1996;8:26–29.
11. Mandell BF, Calabrese LH. Infections and systemic vasculitis. *Curr Opin Rheumatol* 1998;10:51–57.
12. Hosseinipour MC, Smith NH, Simpson EP, et al. Middle cerebral artery vasculitis and stroke after varicella in a young adult. *South Med J* 1998;91:1070–1072.
13. Grouhi M, Dalal I, Nisbet-Brown E, Roifman CM. Cerebral vasculitis associated with chronic mucocutaneous candidiasis. *J Pediatr* 1998; 133:571–574.

14. Jennette JC, Falk RJ, Andrassy K. Nomenclature of systemic vasculitides. *Arthritis Rheum* 1994;37:187–192.
15. Martinez-Escribano JA, Redopndo C, Galera C, et al. Recurrent Kawasaki syndrome in an adult with HIV-1 infection. *Dermatology* 1998;197:96–97.
16. Leen C, Ling S. *Mycoplasma* infection and Kawasaki disease. *Arch Dis Child* 1996;75:266–267.
17. Kleinschmidt-DeMasters BK, Mahalingam R, Shimek C, et al. Profound cerebrospinal fluid pleocytosis and Froin's syndrome secondary to widespread necrotizing vasculitis in an HIV-positive patient with varicella zoster virus encephalomyelitis. *J Neurol Sci* 1998;159:213–218.
18. Gherardi R, Belec L, Mhiri C. The spectrum of vasculitis in human immunodeficiency virus infected patients: a clinicopathological evaluation. *Arthritis Rheum* 1993;36:1164–1174.
19. Gisselbrecht M, Cohen P, Lortholary O, et al. Human immunodeficiency virus-related vasculitis: clinical presentation of and therapeutic approach to eight cases. *Ann Med Interne (Paris)* 1998;149:398–405.
20. Fortin PR. Vasculitides associated with malignancy. *Curr Opin Rheumatol* 1996;8:30–33.
21. Oh SJ. Paraneoplastic vasculitis of the peripheral nervous system. *Neurol Clin* 1997;15:849–863.
22. Wooten MD, Jasin HE. Vasculitis and lymphoproliferative diseases. *Semin Arthritis Rheum* 1996;26:564–574.
23. Sweeney S, Utzschneider R, Fraire AE. Vasculitis carcinomatosa occurring in association with adenocarcinoma of the stomach. *Ann Diagn Pathol* 1998;2:247–249.
24. Brasile L, Kramer JL, Clarke JL. Identification of an autoantibody to vascular endothelial cell specific antigen in patients with systemic vasculitis. *Am J Med* 1989;87:74.
25. Mills JA, Michel BA, Bloch DA, et al. The American College of Rheumatology 1990 criteria for the classification of Henoch-Schölein purpura. *Arthritis Rheum* 1990;33:1114–1121.
26. Tervaert JW, Stegeman CA, Kallenberg CG. Serial ANCA testing is useful in monitoring disease activity of patients with ANCA associated vasculitis. *Sarcoid Vasc Diffuse Lung Dis* 1996;13:241–245.
27. Hoffman GS, Specks U. Antineutrophil cytoplasmic antibodies. *Arthritis Rheum* 1998;41:1521–1537.
28. Nash MC, Dillon MJ. Antineutrophil cytoplasm antibodies and vasculitis. *Arch Dis Child* 1997;77:261–264.
29. Tesar V, Masek Z, Rychlik I, et al. Cytokines and adhesion molecules in renal vasculitis and lupus nephritis. *Nephrol Dial Transplant* 1998;13:1662–1667.
30. Michel BA, Arend WP, Hunder G. Clinical differentiation between giant cell (temporal) arteritis and Takayasu's arteritis. *J Rheumatol* 1996;23:106–111.
31. Wilke WS. Large vessel vasculitis (giant cell arteritis, Takayasu arteritis). *Baillieres Clin Rheumatol* 1997;11:285–313.
32. Rocci CA, Ferrera PC. Takayasu arteritis presenting as amaurosis fugax in a man. *Am J Emerg Med* 1998;16:185–187.
33. Lande A. Abdominal Takayasu's aortitis, the middle aortic syndrome and atherosclerosis: a critical review. *Int Angiol* 1998;17:1–9.
34. Matsunaga N, Hayashi K, Sakamoto I, et al. Takayasu arteritis: MR manifestations and diagnosis of acute and chronic phase. *J Magn Reson Imaging* 1998;8:406–414.
35. Langford CA, Sneller MC, Hoffman GS. Methotrexate use in systemic vasculitis. *Rheum Dis Clin North Am* 1997;23:841–853.
36. Wang YM, Mak GY, Lai KN, Lui SF. Treatment of Takayasu's aortitis with percutaneous transluminal angioplasty and wall stent—a case report. *Angiology* 1998;49:945–949.
37. Caselli RJ, Hunder GG. Giant cell (temporal) arteritis. *Neurol Clin* 1997;15:893–902.
38. Hatzis GS, Aroni KG, Kelekis DA, Boki KA. Giant cell arteritis presenting as pulseless disease of the upper extremities. *Clin Rheumatol* 1996;15:88–90.
39. Hodgkins P, Hull R. Diagnosing and managing polymyalgia rheumatica and temporal arteritis: patients starting steroids should be given advice on risk of osteoporosis. *BMJ* 1997;315:550.
40. Freeman AG. Diagnosing and managing polymyalgia and temporal arteritis: urgency in giving steroids in giant cell arteritis is still not widely appreciated. *BMJ* 1997;315:549–550.
41. Sudlow C. Diagnosing and managing polymyalgia rheumatica and temporal arteritis: sensitivity of temporal artery biopsy varies with biopsy length and sectioning strategy. *BMJ* 1997;315:549.
42. AbuRrahma AF, Thaxton L. Temporal arteritis: diagnostic and therapeutic considerations. *Am Surg* 1996;62:449–451.
43. Kachroo A, Tello C, Bais R, Panush RS. Giant cell arteritis: diagnosis and management. *Bull Rheum Dis* 1996;45:2–5.
44. Fontana PE, Gabutti L, Piffaretti JC, Marone C. Antibiotic treatment for giant cell arteritis? *Lancet* 1996;348:1630.
45. Zilko PJ. Polymyalgia rheumatica and giant cell arteritis. *Med J Aust* 1996;165:438–442.
46. Lynch JP, Hoffman GS. Wegener's granulomatosis: controversies and current concepts. *Compr Ther* 1998;24:421–440.
47. Shoenfeld Y, Tomer Y, Blank M. A new experimental model for Wegener's granulomatosis. *Isr J Med Sci* 1995;31:13–16.
48. Kelly PJ, Toker DE, Boyer P, et al. Granulomatous compressive thoracic myelopathy as the initial manifestation of Wegener's granulomatosis. *Neurology* 1998;51:1769–1770.
49. Burrell HC, McConachie NS. Pachymeningitis in Wegener's granulomatosis. *Australas Radiol* 1998;42:364–366.
50. Haubitz M, Koch KM, Brunkhorst R. Survival and vasculitis activity in patients with end-stage renal disease due to Wegener's granulomatosis. *Nephrol Dial Transplant* 1998;13:1713–1718.
51. Kumar A, Mohan A, Gupta R, et al. Relapse of Wegener's granulomatosis in the first trimester of pregnancy: a case report. *Br J Rheumatol* 1998;37:331–333.
52. Wong SN, Shah V, Dillon MJ. Antineutrophil cytoplasmic antibodies in Wegener's granulomatosis. *Arch Dis Child* 1998;79:246–250.
53. Lang SM, Astner S, Fischer R, et al. Dissociation between high anti-PR3 titers (c-ANCA) and the clinical course of disease in a case of Wegener granulomatosis. *Wien Klin Wochenschr* 1998;110:691–694.
54. Langford CA, Sneller MC. New developments in the treatment of Wegener's granulomatosis, polyarteritis nodosa, microscopic polyangiitis, and Churg–Strauss syndrome. *Curr Opin Rheumatol* 1997;9:26–30.
55. Cvancara JL, Meffert JJ, Elston DM. Estrogen-sensitive cutaneous polyarteritis nodosa: response to tamoxifen. *J Am Acad Dermatol* 1998;39:643–646.
56. Dieudonne T, Van Offel JF, De Clerck LS, Stevens WJ. A patient with fulminant systemic vasculitis type polyarteritis nodosa and negative histology of small bowel infarction. *Acta Clin Belg* 1998;53:322–324.
57. Fernandes SR, Coimbra IB, Costallat LT, et al. Uncommon features of polyarteritis nodosa: psychosis and angio-oedema. *Clin Rheumatol* 1998;17:353–356.
58. Gocke DJ, Hsu K, Morgan C. Association between polyarteritis and Australian antigen. *Lancet* 1970;2:1149.
59. Chochrad D, Langhendries JP, Stolear JC, Godin J. Isotretinoin-induced vasculitis imitating polyarteritis nodosa, with perinuclear antineutrophil cytoplasmic antibody in titers correlated with clinical symptoms. *Rev Rheum Engl Ed* 1997;64:129–131.
60. Hatama S, Kumagai H, Fujiwara M, Fujishima M. A case of microscopic polyarteritis nodosa with interstitial pneumonia successfully treated with steroid pulse therapy and immunosuppressive agents. *Ren Fail* 1998;20:737–746.
61. Harris EN. Systemic vasculitis. In: Dale DC, Federman DD, eds. *Scientific American medicine.* New York: Scientific American, 1999:1–9.
62. Lhote F, Cohen P, Guillevin L. Polyarteritis nodosa, microscopic polyangiitis and Churg–Strauss syndrome. *Lupus* 1998;7:238–258.
63. San Pedro EC, Mountz JM. CNS vasculitis in systemic lupus erythematosus complicated by antiphospholipid antibody syndrome: temporal evaluation of stroke by repeated Tc-99m HMPAO SPECT. *Clin Nucl Med* 1998;23:709–710.
64. Claudy A. Pathogenesis of leukocytoclastic vasculitis. *Eur J Dermatol* 1998;8:75–79.
65. Gavura SR, Nusinowitz S. Leukocytoclastic vasculitis associated with clarithromycin. *Ann Pharmacother* 1998;32:543–545.
66. Houck HE, Kauffman CL, Casey DL. Minocycline treatment of leukocytoclastic vasculitis associated with rheumatoid arthritis. *Arch Dermatol* 1997;133:15–16.
67. Chia JK, Bold EJ. Life-threatening leukocytoclastic vasculitis with pulmonary involvement due to echovirus 7. *Clin Infect Dis* 1998;27:1326–1327.
68. Blanco R, Martinez-Taboada VM, Rodriguez-Valverde V, et al. Henoch-Schölein purpura in adulthood and childhood. *Arthritis Rheum* 1997;40:859–864.
69. Hirayama K, Kobayashi M, Kondoh M, et al. Henoch-Schölein purpura nephritis associated with methicillin-resistant *Staphylococcus aureus* infection [Letter]. *Nephrol Dial Transplant* 1998;13:2703–2704.

70. Merrill J, Lahita RG. Henoch-Schölein Purpura remitting in pregnancy and during sex steroid therapy. *Br J Rheumatol* 1994;33:586–588.

71. Michel BA, Hunder GG, Bloch DA, Calabrese LH. Hypersensitivity vasculitis and Henoch-Schölein purpura: a comparison between the two disorders. *J Rheumatol* 1992;19:721–728.

72. Tancrede-Bohin E, Ochonisky S, Vignon-Pennamen M, et al. Schölein-Henoch purpura in adult patients. *Arch Dermatol* 1997; 133:438–442.

73. Wisnieski JJ, Naff GB. Serum IgG antibodies to C1q in hypocomplementemic urticarial vasculitis syndrome. *Arthritis Rheum* 1989; 32:1119.

74. Levo Y, Gorevic PD, Kassab HJ. Association between hepatitis B virus and essential mixed cryoglobulinemia. *N Engl J Med* 1977;296:1501.

75. Kawasaki T. Kawasaki disease. *Acta Paediatr* 1995;84:713–715.

76. Nakamura Y, Yanagawa H, Kato H, et al. Mortality among patients with a history of Kawasaki disease: the third look. The Kawasaki disease follow-up group. *Acta Paediatr Jpn* 1998;40:419–423.

77. Fruhwald FM, Luha O, Schumacher M, et al. Myocardial infarction caused by an aneurysm of the left main coronary artery without evidence of Kawasaki disease [Letter]. *Heart* 1998;80:532.

78. Tomita H, Fuse S, Chiba S. Images in cardiology: delayed appearance of coronary aneurysms in Kawasaki disease. *Heart* 1998;80:425.

*Textbook of the Autoimmune Diseases,*
Edited by R. G. Lahita, N. Chiorazzi, and W. H. Reeves,
Lippincott Williams & Wilkins, Philadelphia © 2000.

# CHAPTER 28

# Scleroderma

Margaret D. Smith

The clinician is often confused by scleroderma, a disease that has a spectrum of manifestations and a variety of therapeutic implications. The term *scleroderma* requires definition (Table 28.1). This chapter emphasizes systemic sclerosis (SSC), with mention of the localized (dermatologic) forms of the condition, such as morphea or linear scleroderma.

The American College of Rheumatology (ACR) has outlined criteria for the diagnosis of this disease. The essential clinical parameter is skin thickening proximal to the metacarpophalangeal joints (Table 28.2). Raynaud's phenomenon is such a frequent, almost universal, component of scleroderma that it is also considered in detail. SSC is the disease most worthy of the designation "collagen vascular," because its major manifestations include inappropriate excessive collagen synthesis and deposition, endothelial dysfunction, spasm, collapse, and obliteration by fibrosis.

The cause of scleroderma is unknown. However, genetic predisposition is important, and the trigger needs definition. Abnormalities involving autoimmunity and alteration of endothelial cell and fibroblast function comprise the scleroderma disorder. Ultimately, excessive deposition of collagen and matrix in a variety of tissues is the hallmark of the disease. Pathogenetic mechanisms are being slowly unraveled (Table 28.3).

## INCIDENCE AND EPIDEMIOLOGY

Population-based surveys estimate a prevalence of Raynaud's phenomenon of 4.9% to 20.1% for women and 3.8% to 13.5% for men, with the higher figures obtained from rheumatologic centers. These data are similar throughout the world (1). Familial aggregation of primary Raynaud's has been reported (2).

Scleroderma is a rare disease with a stable incidence of approximately 19 cases per 1 million persons. Put into per-

spective, scleroderma has an incidence rate that is 40% of that for systemic lupus and 6% that for rheumatoid arthritis (3). Prevalence data depend on proper diagnosis and survival rates. The prevalence rate for adults is about 240 cases per 1 million persons in the United States, with somewhat lower rates reported in Britain, Japan, and Iceland (3). Studies reveal a 5-year survival rate consistently around 85% and a 10-year survival rate of approximately 60%, with an average survival time from diagnosis of 13 years (3). The presence and severity of internal organ involvement clearly relate to survival. Pulmonary, renal, and cardiac disease are significant risk factors for mortality, especially when present within the first year of presentation (4,5). Geographic clusters have been described in a rural area in Italy (6) and among Choctaw Native Americans in southeast Oklahoma (7,8). Several human leukocyte antigen (HLA) haplotypes were prevalent in the latter population, indicating a significant genetic risk factor, but there has otherwise been no evidence of familial clustering (9) and no difference between identical and fraternal twin concordance (10). Ethnic background clearly influences the clinical and serologic features of scleroderma, with earlier and more severe pulmonary disease in the black population (11). The disease occurs much more frequently in women (female to male ratio of 3.8 to 1), with a particular increase in the childbearing years (11).

## CLINICAL PRESENTATION

Initial complaints that lead the patient to seek medical care include diffuse puffiness of the hands, carpal tunnel syndrome, Raynaud's phenomenon, and gastrointestinal symptoms, including gastroesophageal reflux. Consideration and diagnosis of the disease at an early stage can, with proper assessment and management, offset the development of significant morbidity and even mortality.

### Dermatologic Features

*Raynaud's phenomenon* was described by Maurice Raynaud in his monograph presented to the Syndenham Society in

M. D. Smith: Department of Medicine, New York Medical College, New York, New York 10011; Department of Rheumatology, St. Vincent's Hospital and Medical Center of New York, New York, New York 10011

**TABLE 28.1.** *Definition and classification of the sclerodermas*

I. Localized scleroderma: A rare dermatologic disease associated with fibrosis and manifestations limited to skin.
  A. Morphea—irregular plaques of hypopigmentation and fibrosis
  B. Linear scleroderma—longitudinal fibrosis extending into deeper tissues
II. Systemic sclerosis (SSC): Multisystem diseases, with variable risks for internal organ involvement and variation in the extent of skin disease
  A. Diffuse SSC
  B. Limited SSC (CREST = calcinosis, Raynaud's, esophageal dysfunction, sclerodactyly, telangiectasiae)
III. Overlap syndromes
  A. Diffuse or limited SSC plus typical features of one or more of the other connective tissue disorders
  B. Mixed connective tissue disease with RNP antibodies and clinical features of one or more of the following connective tissue diseases: systemic lupus, scleroderma, polymyositis, and/or rheumatoid arthritis
IV. Scleroderma-like disorders
  A. Related to industrial environmental exposure
    1. Silicon dioxide
    2. Vinyl chloride
    3. Organic solvents
    4. Amines in epoxy resins
  B. Epidemic
    1. Eosinophilia myalgia syndrome (EMS) (e.g., 1989 ingestion of contaminated L-tryptophan)
    2. Toxic oil syndrome (TOS) (e.g., 1981 ingestion of Spanish rapeseed oil denatured with aniline)
  C. Eosinophilic fasciitis (Schulman's syndrome): lack of Raynaud's, visceral involvement of microvascular disease; vigilance needed for associated hematologic disorders
  D. Other illnesses associated with fibrosis
    1. Bleomycin exposure
    2. Carcinoid
    3. Chronic graft-versus-host disease
    4. Insulin-dependent diabetes mellitus
    5. Local lipodystrophies
    6. Myeloma/paraproteinemia
    7. Phenylketonuria
    8. POEMS (plasma cell dyscrasia, polyneuropathy, organomegaly, endocrinopathy, monoclonal spikes, scleroderma-like skin changes)
    9. Porphyria cutanea tarda
    10. Progeria
    11. Werner's
V. Sine scleroderma: Internal organ involvement without skin changes

---

**TABLE 28.2.** *Criteria for the classification of systemic sclerosis (scleroderma)[a]*

A. Major criterion
  *Proximal scleroderma:* Symmetric thickening, tightening, and induration of the skin of the fingers and the skin proximal to the metacarpophalangeal or metatarsophalangeal joints. The changes may affect the entire extremity, face, neck, and trunk (thorax and abdomen).
B. Minor criteria
  1. *Sclerodactyly:* above-indicated skin changes limited to the fingers
  2. *Digital pitting scars* or loss of substance from the finger pad: depressed areas at tips of fingers or loss of digital pad tissue as a result of ischemia
  3. *Bibasilar pulmonary fibrosis:* bilateral reticular pattern of linear or lineonodular densities most pronounced in the basilar portions of the lungs on standard chest roentgenogram; may assume appearance of diffuse mottling or "honeycomb lung." These changes should not be attributable to primary lung disease.

---

[a] For the purposes of classifying patients in clinical trials, population surveys, and other studies, a person shall be said to have systemic sclerosis (scleroderma) if the one major or two or more minor criteria are present. Localized forms of scleroderma, eosinophilic fasciitis, and the various forms of pseudoscleroderma are excluded from these criteria.
From Klippel JH, ed. *Primer on the rheumatic diseases.* Atlanta: Arthritis Foundation, 1997:456, with permission.

---

**TABLE 28.3.** *Factors in the pathogenesis of the sclerodermas*

*Environmental agents*
  Particles (release cytokines from macrophages as they are phagocytosed)
    Coal
    Uranium
    Silica (rarely including silicone implants) (47)
  Drugs
    Appetite suppressants
    Pentazocine (Talwin, Sanofi Pharmaceuticals, Inc., New York, NY, U.S.A.)
    Cocaine
    Bleomycin
    Beta blockers (?)
  Foreign cells
    Maternal/fetal cell transplacental transfer resulting in chronic graft-versus-host disease (48)

*Activated T cells* (T4 in skin, T8 in lungs)
  Cytokines
    Transforming growth factor-β (TGF-β)
    Adhesion molecules
    Growth factors

*Endothelium*
  Vascular spasm (endothelin I, platelet vasoconstrictors, vasa nervorum)
  Vascular injury
    Leakage of fluid and protein
    Increased factor VIII—von Willebrand
  Vessel narrowing and fibrosis

*Activated or transformed fibroblasts*
  Gene upregulation resulting in transcription of genes encoding types I and III collagen
  Autocrine TGF-β release
  Excessive collagen and matrix production

---

1862, entitled *On Local Asphyxia and Symmetrical Gangrene of the Extremities* (12). *Definite* Raynaud's as defined by the U.K. Scleroderma Study Group comprises repeated episodes of biphasic color changes on cold exposure. *Possible* Raynaud's is defined as uniphasic color changes plus paresthesia. The color change on exposure to cold is essential to the diagnosis. In 1929, Thomas Lewis distinguished between idiopathic and secondary Raynaud's (13). To avoid confusion, LeRoy and Metsger (14) suggest the use of terms primary and secondary Raynaud's. A list of some of the causes of secondary Raynaud's can be found in Table 28.4. Cold exposure induces a contractile response of the vascular smooth muscle that can be abolished by blocking $\alpha_2$-adrenoceptors but not $\alpha_1$-adrenoceptors. It seems likely that the impairment in Raynaud's relates to a dysfunction of the $\alpha_2$-adrenergic pathways. At which level this occurs, whether at the receptor, the intracellular transduction pathway, or through another modulation of $\alpha_2$-adrenoreceptor activity is unclear (1).

Abnormal serotonin receptor activity may also be contributing to the spasm, as may increased blood viscosity and the release of vasoconstrictors from platelets and damaged endothelial cells. An imbalance of the vasoconstrictor endothelin compared with the vasodilator calcitonin gene-related peptide (CGRP) has also been reported (1).

*Primary Raynaud's* describes the condition when it is not associated with a known cause. This usually appears in late-adolescent girls who are otherwise healthy, with no evidence of autoimmune disease developing for the next 2 years after the onset of the cold-induced vasospasm. Despite the discomfort and color changes, digits are not at risk for ischemic damage. The presence of abnormal nailfold capillary loops or significant titers of autoantibodies suggests secondary Raynaud's. Nailfold capillarioscopy is accomplished with an ophthalmoscope set at 40 diopters and held a few millimeters away from the nailbed. Typical abnormal findings of irregular dropout and tortuous, dilated vessels are observed only in scleroderma and dermatomyositis.

With *Raynaud's secondary to scleroderma,* in addition to the vasospasm, a vasculopathy develops that is characterized by endothelial cell structural changes such as intimal hyperplasia with fibrosis but minimal muscular hypertrophy. Because of the vessel fibrosis, a cutaneous hypoxia exists, exaggerated by increased adhesion of cells to the damaged endothelial wall, increased demand for oxygen by the thickened skin, and increased hydrostatic pressure in the tissue. When severe, prolonged ischemia continues, digital pitting, ulceration, fissuring, and diminution of distal digits (acrolysis) and bones (osteolysis) are the result (Fig. 28.1). Secondary infection is common, and amputation is sometimes necessary (Fig. 28.2). Internal organ ischemia triggered by cold or trauma to the vessels supplying the organ (i.e., systemic Raynaud's) is also a potential complication of scleroderma. For example, cold or the manipulation of cardiac catheterization may hasten angina, and renal crisis is more likely to occur during the winter months.

*Skin thickening* usually commences with the fingers (i.e., sclerodactyly) (Fig. 28.3), and progresses in an unpredictable fashion. As shown in Table 28.2, the ACR defines the major criterion for the presence of SSC as thickening of the skin proximal to the metacarpophalangeal joints. Pruritus is com-

**TABLE 28.4.** *Causes of secondary Raynaud's phenomenon*

*Connective tissue diseases*
  Polymyositis and dermatomyositis
  Scleroderma
  Sjögren's syndrome
  Systemic lupus erythematosus
  Systemic vasculitis
  Undifferentiated connective tissue disease
*Drugs and toxins*
  Amphetamines
  Clonidine
  Ergotamines
  Vinblastine and bleomycin
  Vinyl chloride exposure
*Structural arterial disease*
  Atheroemboli
  Atherosclerosis
  Thoracic outlet syndrome
  Thromboangiitis obliterans (Buerger's disease)
*Occupational disorders*
  Hand-arm vibration syndrome
  Hypothenar hanmmer syndrome
*Hematologic diseases*
  Cold agglutinin disease
  Cryoglobulinemia
  Paraproteinemia
*Other causes*
  Hypothyroidism
  Paraneoplastic
  Frostbite
  Reflex sympathetic dystrophy

From Klippel JH, ed. *Primer on the rheumatic diseases.* Atlanta: Arthritis Foundation, 1997:268, with permission.

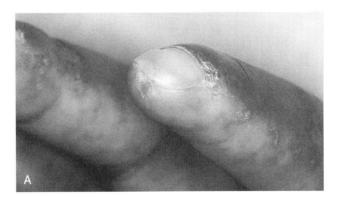

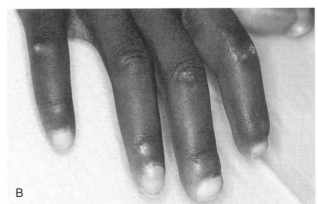

**FIG. 28.1. A, B:** Severe, prolonged ischemia with digital pitting, ulcerations, fissuring, and diminution of distal digits (acrolysis) and bones (osteolysis).

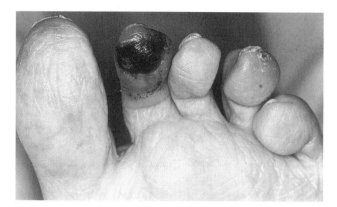

**FIG. 28.2.** Severe ischemic changes.

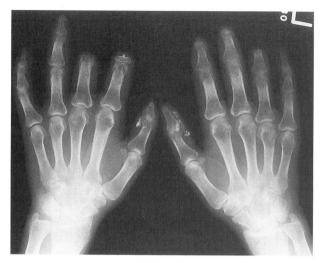

**FIG. 28.4.** Calcinosis of the fingers, with acrolysis, osteolysis, and digital amputation.

mon, and skin appendages are affected, with changes in pigmentation and hair growth. Calcinosis may result in disruption of the dermal barrier to infection and may be extruded as a white semisolid substance (Fig. 28.4). Restriction by skin tightening results in loss of joint mobility, chest expansion, and the oral opening (Fig. 28.5). Tendon friction rubs may be heard or palpated. The typical youthful appearance without wrinkling, and the "pinched" facies (Mauskopf) of later diffuse disease are easily recognized (Fig. 28.6). The risk of developing internal organ involvement is related in a parallel fashion to the aggressiveness of the skin fibrosis, with limited SSC (i.e., CREST syndrome: *c*alcinosis, *R*aynaud's phenomenon, *e*sophageal hypomotility, *s*clerodactyly, *t*elangiectasias) usually progressing at a slower pace. Spontaneous improvement in the skin can occur.

The total skin score has been useful as an objective measure of disease activity and is particularly useful in clinical trials (15). Modifications for simplicity have proven successful, using a scale of 0 (no involvement) through 3 (completely hidebound) and the number of areas (n = 17), for a maximal score of 51. Areas include the face, upper arms (two), forearms (two), hands (two), fingers (two), thighs (two), lower legs (two), and feet (two), chest/abdomen (one), and back (one).

**Pulmonary Features**

Scleroderma lung disease has taken first place in the potentially life-threatening manifestations of the disease (16).

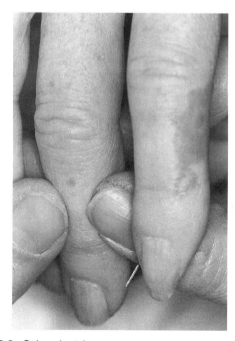

**FIG. 28.3.** Sclerodactyly.

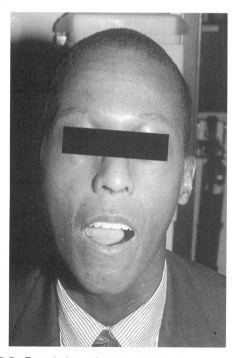

**FIG. 28.5.** Restriction of oral opening because of skin tightening.

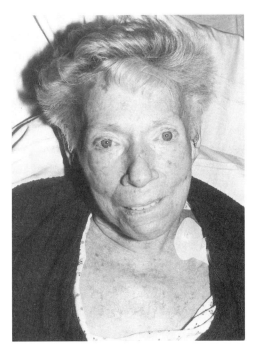

**FIG. 28.6.** Youthful appearance at 85 years of age.

Although occasionally mild and nonprogressive, this problem can result in critical situations, including severe pulmonary hypertension, interstitial fibrosis, and acute alveolar hemorrhage. Esophageal reflux may lead to aspiration pneumonitis, and traction fibrosis may result from fibrosis.

*Pulmonary hypertension* can be primary or secondary to interstitial lung disease. It is the more common pulmonary complication of limited scleroderma (i.e., CREST). The most common symptom is dyspnea, but up to one third of patients may be asymptomatic. Although clinically thought to occur in approximately 10% of these patients, pathologic (biopsy or autopsy) studies suggest that 65% demonstrate some evidence of pulmonary hypertension, which is defined physiologically as a resting pulmonary artery pressure (PAP) of greater than 25 mm Hg or an exercise PAP of greater than 30 mm Hg. Pathologic changes include intimal fibrosis and smooth muscle hyperplasia but no evidence of vasculitis (17). Measurement of the diffusing capacity for carbon dioxide (DLCO) is helpful in assessing the risk for developing this problem, and an isolated DLCO of less than 55% is predictive (18). A DLCO of less than 43% has a sensitivity of 87% in predicting pulmonary hypertension (19). Other evidence of the condition (unfortunately in the later stages) include prominent $P_2$ heart sound, prominence of the pulmonary arteries on chest radiographs, right bundle branch block, and right ventricular or atrial hypertrophy on an electrocardiogram and echocardiogram.

Organ (visceral) Raynaud's phenomenon occurring in the lungs may be the primary event leading to the development of pulmonary hypertension in scleroderma. Nitric oxide produced from arginine by endothelial cells using nitric oxide synthetase is of extreme importance in maintaining vascular tone in the lungs. It is postulated that a decreased expression of endothelial nitric oxide synthetase may be contribution to the pathogenesis. Endothelin-1 levels in the peripheral blood may be elevated, and their measurement may become important in the early recognition of the condition (20). The average 5-year survival rate from the time of diagnosis of isolated pulmonary hypertension is less than 10% (16).

*Interstitial lung disease* begins as an inflammatory condition with infiltration of lymphocytes and plasma cells into the alveolar walls and macrophages into the alveolar spaces (21). Symptoms of dyspnea on exertion and nonproductive cough are common, and bibasilar rales are often present. This complication is more likely to occur in diffuse disease. Prognosis for 5-year survival from the initial pulmonary function test abnormalities is 45% (16). Bronchoalveolar lavage (BAL) studies have demonstrated neutrophilic alveolitis with occasional increases in eosinophils and increased numbers of activated macrophages (22). The presence of neutrophilic alveolitis is usually associated with worse dyspnea and a poor prognosis if left untreated, presumably because of the development of irreversible fibrosis. Fibroblasts with smooth muscle cell differentiation (i.e., myofibroblasts) are demonstrated in scleroderma lung fluid and pathologic specimens (23).

Elevated albumin levels in the BAL fluid suggest increased vascular permeability, and increased IgG and immune complexes suggest immunologic activation. Tumor necrosis factor (TNF) and interleukin-1 (IL-1) may also be elevated in the BAL fluid and in animal models. Treating with anti-TNF-$\alpha$ (24) can abrogate lung fibrosis after exposure to silica and bleomycin. Thrombin generated by injured endothelial cells may increase vascular permeability, enhance leukocytic adherence, and act as a mitogen for the transformation of fibroblasts to myofibroblasts. Plasmin can convert latent transforming growth factor-$\beta$ to its active form (Table 28.3). Production of type 2 cytokine mRNA (IL-4 and IL-5) by CD8 T cells is associated with a decrease in lung function and may implicate these T cells in the pathogenesis of interstitial fibrosis in SSC (25).

**Renal Features**

Scleroderma renal crisis is manifested by sudden onset of accelerated hypertension or rapidly worsening renal failure in the setting of scleroderma. Moore and Sheehan first described it in 1952 (26). Presenting symptoms are variable and include headache, profound fatigue, acute neurologic symptoms or acute renal failure with typical hyperpnea secondary to acidosis, and nausea. Chronic progressive azotemia is distinctly unusual. Approximately 10% of all SSC patients, almost exclusively with diffuse SSC and especially those with a rapidly progressive course and diffuse skin thickening in the upper extremities and trunk, experience renal crisis. Seventy-five percent of the cases occur in the first 4 years after the onset of disease (27). Mortality is high, but vigorous treatment early in the course of the problem is often successful.

The role of the renin-angiotensin system in perpetuating the condition is not disputed, and extreme elevation of plasma renin is the hallmark of the disease, but other initiating factors must be present to trigger the crisis. The added factor of diminished renal blood flow from any number of sources may be important. Hypotension related to sepsis or dehydration, pericarditis secondary to scleroderma, heart failure, arrhythmia, and medications, including nonsteroidal antiinflammatory drugs, antihypertensives, and especially corticosteroids (28), have been implicated.

### Cardiac Features

Rarely does scleroderma present with cardiac manifestations, although patchy myocardial fibrosis is the rule at autopsy. A higher risk of significant myocardial disease is associated with skeletal muscle dysfunction. Clinical manifestations include arrhythmias, congestive heart failure, and rarely, pericarditis, even calcific constrictive pericarditis (29). Ventricular tachyarrhythmias portend a poor prognosis, with an increased risk of sudden death, and pericarditis is a predictor for renal crisis. Caution must be exercised in the recommendations for cardiac catheterization because severe vasospasm with ischemic damage to myocardium can result from the trauma of the procedure. Differentiation of cardiac chest pain from esophageal pain can be a problem. If possible, cardiac catheterization should be avoided. If the procedure is necessary, the ready availability of vasodilators should be emphasized.

### Muscular Features

Fatigue is the most common symptom of muscle involvement. Limited (CREST) and diffuse disease have been associated with muscle weakness. Most patients with scleroderma have myopathic symptoms, with demonstrable weakness in about 80%. This is distinguishable from the mixed connective disease or overlap syndromes, which must also be considered. A mild, self-limited course is the rule, without need for medication, but more severe disease can occur. Symptomatic myopathy may have normal creatine phosphokinase values. Studies suggest that the primary target of the damage is the vascular bed and that the myopathic process is T-cell mediated (30).

### Gastrointestinal Features

The entire scleroderma gastrointestinal tract, from mouth to anus, is subject to altered function, especially dysmotility and spasm. Most patients with either type of systemic disease are affected, especially with esophageal symptoms, most often acid reflux and dysphagia. These are frequently the initial presenting complaints. Gastrointestinal symptoms do not have a significant impact on mortality, but they are linked with considerable morbidity and are often very amenable to therapeutic intervention. Abdominal bloating, gas, diarrhea, and constipation are common. Anorectal involvement occurs in 50% and 70% of patients.

Pathologically, the small arteries are distinctly abnormal with the initial perivascular mononuclear response followed by fibroblast induced intimal sclerosis. These changes compromise the *vasa nervorum*, which may also later be compressed by collagen deposition. The muscularis propria becomes atrophic and fragmented in a patchy way, mostly in the circular muscular layer. The myopathic changes may be secondary to a primary neurogenic event (31). The final event in the progression of disease is muscle fibrosis.

Blind loop syndrome is not uncommon secondary to bacterial overgrowth from stasis. Malabsorption, including malabsorption of water-soluble vitamins such as folate and $B_6$, may result from bacterial overgrowth, reduced intestinal permeability, or lack of adequate mixing of food related to dysmotility. Wide-mouth diverticuli of the small or large intestine can be seen. *Pneumocystis cystoides* intestinalis with the possible complication of peritoneal free air can be confusing. Primary biliary cirrhosis is reportedly associated with scleroderma, but the incidence of this association is not clear.

### Neurologic Features

Abnormalities of the central, peripheral, and autonomic nervous system have been detected in scleroderma. Perhaps the most common neurologic symptom is carpal tunnel syndrome, followed by trigeminal neuralgia. Peripheral sensory neuropathy is difficult to assess in the presence of altered skin. Multiple other neurologic abnormalities have been reported, including mononeuritis, mononeuropathy multiplex, and cerebral disease (32).

The pathogenetic importance of neurologic changes in other systemic manifestations of scleroderma awaits further evaluation, with the possibility that neurogenic control of vascular tone, aggravated by endoneural fibrosis, may be a primary event in the disease process or that antineuronal antibodies may play a key role. Gastrointestinal autonomic neurologic impairment is an important feature.

## DIAGNOSTIC TESTING

Although the diagnosis of scleroderma is based on the history and physical examination, its confirmation and appropriate management depend on a variety of tests. These confirm the presence of disease, assess risks, and allow earlier, hopefully more effective, therapeutic interventions.

### Antinuclear Antibodies

Antinuclear antibodies are found in more than 95% of patients with scleroderma (33) (Table 28.5). These antibodies differ from those seen in other connective tissue disease and target intracellular molecules, including DNA topoisomerase I (Scl-70); chromosomal centromere or kinetochore proteins; RNA polymerase (RNAP) I, II, or III; and some nucleolar components.

**TABLE 28.5.** *Autoantibodies in scleroderma*

| Antibodies | Diffuse disease | Limited (CREST) disease |
|---|---|---|
| Antinuclear | 95% often speckled or nucleolar | 95% often speckled or nucleolar |
| Anticentromere | Negative | 44–98% good prognosis |
| Antitopoisomerase I (Scl-70) | 30% poor prognosis for pulmonary and peripheral vascular disease; correlates with ethnicity | Negative |
| Anti-RNAP I | 4% quite specific | Negative |
| Anti-RNAP II | Rare | Rare |
| Anti-RNAP III | 45% severe skin disease; poor prognosis for renal crisis and cardiac involvement; better prognosis for pulmonary disease | 6% |

Topoisomerase I, identified in 1979 by Douvas et al. (34), is an enzyme important in DNA replication. It catalyzes the relaxation of supercoiled DNA in the nucleoplasm. Antibodies to topoisomerase I are specific markers for SSC and rarely occur in patients with other diseases. They are only present in about 30% of scleroderma patients, but they predict a high incidence of pulmonary fibrosis and peripheral vascular disease. They do not correlate with renal or cardiac involvement (35). Kuwana et al. (11) demonstrated that serologic expression in scleroderma patients is strongly influenced by ethnic background. In comparing topoisomerase I–positive patients, they found that the frequency of lung involvement is lower in white patients than in black, Japanese, or Choctaw patients; that white patients have better survival rates than black and Japanese patients; and that pulmonary interstitial fibrosis in white patients is less progressive than that in black and Japanese patients.

RNAPs were identified in 1993 (36). RNAP I is an enzyme that synthesizes ribosomal RNA precursors in nucleoli. RNAP II is an enzyme that synthesizes the precursors of messenger RNA and most of the small nuclear RNA in the nucleoli. RNAP III is an enzyme that also synthesizes small RNAs, including ribosomal and messenger RNA, in the nucleoli. Anti-RNAP I antibodies are found in approximately 4% of SSC sera (37) and are specific. Anti-RNAP II antibodies are less specific for scleroderma but are associated with more diffuse disease. Anti-RNAP III antibodies are present in about 45% of patients with diffuse cutaneous involvement (a higher incidence than topoisomerase I) and about 6% of patients with limited (CREST) disease. Prognosis is poorer with positive anti-RNAP III, with a predictive value for severe skin disease, a higher incidence of renal crisis and cardiac disease, but a lower incidence of pulmonary involvement (37).

Anticentromere antibodies, identified in 1980 by Moroi et al. (38), react with the centromere of mitotic chromosomes, an area where two sister chromatids of replicated chromosome are tightly paired. The kinetochore is located on the surface of the chromosome in the centromere and attached by spindle microtubules at mitosis. Anticentromere antibodies interfere with centromere assembly during interphase, causing disrupted mitotic events. Anticentromere antibodies identify patients with limited (CREST) SSC (44% to 98%) and who have a less severe, more slowly progressive internal organ disease, and a more favorable prognosis, with a 92% 10-year survival rate (35).

**Pulmonary Studies**

The major mortality related to scleroderma results from pulmonary involvement in the form of pulmonary hypertension, which is more likely with the limited (CREST) form of the disease, or pulmonary fibrosis, which is more often linked with diffuse disease. In the latter case, early intervention with aggressive therapy aimed at the inflammatory response may favorably affect outcome. Assessment of pulmonary status at regular intervals, at least as a baseline and, depending on the patient, at approximately 12-month intervals, is of great importance (Table 28.6).

Of all the pulmonary function tests, the DLCO is of most importance for pulmonary hypertension and for interstitial disease. A value of less than 55% is cause for concern, and a value of less than 43% has an 87% sensitivity in predicting pulmonary hypertension (16). In addition to the DLCO, forced vital capacity, and forced expiratory volume at 1 second, the total lung capacity may be reduced in cases of diffuse interstitial disease or of chest wall restriction from skin disease.

Radiographic studies of importance include the chest film and the high-resolution computed tomography scan (HRCT). The chest x-ray film may suggest pulmonary hypertension if there is prominence of the pulmonary vessels. The presence of aspiration may be suggested by pneumonia, especially in the right middle or lower lobes. Bronchiectasis may be considered with recurrent pneumonias, productive cough, and a high sedimentation rate (ESR). Pulmonary alveolar hemorrhage, which may be life threatening, may be suggested by the sudden development of diffuse infiltrates, hypotension, anemia, and hemoptysis. With interstitial disease, there may be linear and reticular shadows or a honeycombed appearance, often with lower lobe predominance.

HRCT scan of the chest is more sensitive than plain film in assessing early interstitial disease. Patchy areas with a ground glass appearance indicate inflammatory cell infiltration, and reticular shadows indicate fibrosis.

Echocardiogram is an effective, noninvasive technique for assessing pulmonary hypertension, but it may not be sensitive to early disease. Right ventricular enlargement or dilata-

**TABLE 28.6.** *Pulmonary tests for scleroderma*

| Tests | Scleroderma | Normal |
|---|---|---|
| Forced vital capacity, forced expiratory volume at 1 second, residual volume, and total lung capacity | May be significantly decreased in interstitial disease but not in pulmonary hypertension | Normal |
| Diffusing capacity for carbon dioxide (DLCO) | <55% is significant in both types of lung involvement | Normal |
| Chest radiograph | Increased markings, often in the lower lung bases | Normal |
| High-resolution CT scan of the chest | Nonspecific linear and reticular shadows or honeycombed appearance | Clear |
| BAL | | |
| Total cells | $17.2 \pm 2.0$ | $7.8 \pm 1.4$ |
| Macrophages | $15.4 \pm 1.8$ | $7.2 \pm 1.3$ |
| Neutrophils | $1.1 \pm 0.03$ | $0.1 \pm 0.1$ |
| IgG | $1.44 \pm 0.2$ | $0.51 \pm 0.1$ |
| Albumin | $3.34 \pm 0.4$ | $1.99 \pm 0.4$ |
| Fibronectin | $306 \pm 74$ | $18 \pm 3$ |
| Immune complexes | $32.7 \pm 3.3$ | $8.9 \pm 5.6$ |

From Silver RM. Clinical problems: the lungs. *Rheum Dis Clin North Am* 1996;22:831, with permission.

tion, asymmetric septal hypertrophy, paradoxical septal motion, and color Doppler flow study abnormalities may be seen.

BAL is becoming important as a dynamic indicator of interstitial inflammation. In this study, total cells, alveolar macrophages, granulocytes (i.e., neutrophils plus eosinophils), IgG, albumin, immune complexes, and fibronectin are elevated compared with normal controls (16).

## Gastrointestinal Studies

The gastrointestinal tract may not be altered by scleroderma in a fashion that changes mortality, but limited and diffuse forms of disease result in significant morbidity. Identification of and differentiation from other conditions is important in the evaluation of the symptomatic patient.

Radiology continues to provide important data in the evaluation of gastrointestinal scleroderma. Barium swallow may detect esophageal dilatation, reflux, and strictures. Upper gastrointestinal series may demonstrate gastroparesis. In the small bowel follow-through procedure, loops of duodenum and jejunum show characteristic dilatation without stenosis. Prolonged transit and fluid retention are seen. Normally, the small bowel dilates in response to obstruction, and the valvulae separate longitudinally. With the hidebound appearance in scleroderma, there is relative decrease in the distance separating the valvulae conniventes for a given degree of small bowel dilatation (39). Barium enema may demonstrate wide-mouth diverticula or colonic dilatation.

Gastrointestinal motility studies, especially of the esophagus, are highly sensitive and specific. Abnormal study results predict esophagitis, aspiration, and Barrett's esophagus.

Endoscopy is considered standard in the periodic follow-up of the scleroderma patient to assess mucosal integrity and evaluate with biopsy for Barrett's esophagus. The frequency of repeat examinations is dictated by the clinical picture and previous pathology. Duodenal or jejunal aspirates can be obtained for culture if blind loop is suspected.

The hydrogen breath test offers a noninvasive way of evaluating for intestinal bacterial overgrowth. The patient ingests a nondigestable radiolabeled carbohydrate such as lactulose or D-xylose. Bacteria rapidly metabolize these substrates, resulting in the release of excess hydrogen or radiolabeled carbon dioxide in the patient's breath. The test result is considered abnormal if the fasting value is greater than 11 ppm (40). Malabsorption tests also may be indicated, including a complete blood cell count and serum carotene, D-xylose absorption, and vitamin level measurements.

## Renal Function Tests

Although plasma renin levels are markedly elevated in renal crisis, they may be high without a crisis and are not particularly helpful for routine monitoring of disease activity or progression. Urinalysis is important in monitoring drug therapy with D-penicillamine, which can cause a nephrotic syndrome.

Red cell smear to evaluate for schistocytes and microangiopathic hemolytic anemia is helpful in renal crisis. Mild thrombocytopenia and reticulocytosis may be seen in 40% to 45% of patients with renal crisis.

## TREATMENT OF SCLERODERMA

Despite the lack of curative treatments, proper surveillance and management of the scleroderma patient results in significant improvement in well-being, decreased morbidity, and even decreased mortality. Innovative but high-risk therapy proposed includes autologous stem cell transplantation (41). Meaningful statistical data regarding treatment outcomes must be gathered when possible to improve future therapies. The ACR Scleroderma Study Group and the U.K. Scleroderma Study Group represent the combined efforts of multiple medical centers to accomplish such a goal.

## Management of Raynaud's and Skin Problems

Maintaining core body temperature with the use of warm clothing and gloves is essential for persons with Raynaud's phenomena. The use of hand warmers carried in the pockets may be helpful. The benefits of biofeedback and behavioral therapy are variable in any individual, but worthwhile trying in many cases. Unnecessary use of vasoconstrictors, including tobacco, decongestants, caffeine, amphetamines, and ergotamines, is to be avoided. Beta blockers are said to produce hypothermia of the hands, but objective studies using Doppler and finger skin temperature fail to validate these reports, and their use is not contraindicated (1).

The benefits of sympathectomy may be short lived. The procedure is more likely to be beneficial in the secondary forms of Raynaud's, despite the fact that secondary Raynaud's is usually more refractory to therapy because of the microvascular morphologic changes that are present. Localized microsurgical digital sympathectomy may be indicated in the patient who has had some relief with temporary sympathectomy, and who has failed medical therapy (1). Experimental interventional therapies include epidural spinal cord stimulation, although data supporting its use are lacking.

Capsaicin-sensitive nerve endings are prominent in the cutaneous circulation, where they can release vasodilator neurotransmitters. The use of topical capsaicin may be helpful. Topical nitroglycerin applied at the wrists may provide some relief. The use of other direct vasodilators such as papaverine and niacin have been disappointing. Reducing blood viscosity with the addition of pentoxifylline may be of occasional benefit. Antiplatelet agents such as aspirin and piracetam may be added. The serotonin receptor antagonist ketanserin is under study, as is the vasodilator CGRP (1,42).

Other drugs that have been used in Raynaud's therapy without much success include agents that induce vasodilation or inhibit platelet aggregation such as prostanoids (e.g., iloprost, prostaglandins $E_1$ and $E_2$, prostacyclin), sympatholytic agents (e.g., reserpine, guanethidine, methyldopa—previously used intraarterially), angiotensin-converting enzyme (ACE) inhibitors (e.g., catapril, enalapril), α-adrenergic antagonists (e.g., prazosin, thymoxamine, phenoxybenzamine, phentolamine), and thrombolytic agents.

Calcium channel blockers have antiplatelet and vasodilatory effects and are the mainstay of pharmacologic therapy for Raynaud's (43). Side effects, especially ankle edema, or tolerance may limit their use. There are four classes of calcium channel antagonists; the most useful agents for vascular smooth muscle effect are the dihydropyridines, including nifedipine, amlodipine, nicardipine, isradipine, and felodipine. Decreases in the frequency and severity of vasospastic attacks have been confirmed in the treatment of Raynaud's. Approximately one third of patients do not respond to nefidipine. Benefit seems more likely in primary Raynaud's (15). The use of combined calcium channel blockers has not been studied.

## Scleroderma Skin

Attention to dryness and fissuring, with recommendations for the copious use of lubricants and moisturizers, is important to prevent secondary infection. Appropriate use of topical or systemic antibiotics is key.

Calcinosis (Fig. 28.3) is extremely difficult to treat. The use of diltiazem and colchicine has been successful in isolated cases (44,45). Intralesional steroids, Benemid and coumarin, have not been adequately assessed to recommend them. Surgical removal is not recommended, because the deposits tend to recur, and healing may be impaired in sclerodermatous skin.

Direct attempts to slow the tethering of the skin have been unsuccessful. One third of patients demonstrate improvement without treatment. Multiple agents have been tried in studies of variable reliability. Generally negative results have emerged with the use of methotrexate, aminobenzoate potassium, photophoresis, chlorambucil, 5-fluorouracil, dimethyl sulfoxide, isotretinoin, cyclosporin, interferon-α, interferon-γ, irradiation, and N-acetylcysteine (42).

D-Penicillamine, the traditional mainstay of therapy in scleroderma, has performed in a disappointing manner in a 3-year controlled study completed by the ACR Scleroderma Study Consortium. The low doses of the drug (50 mg/day) proved as effective as the usual higher dose (750 mg/day) (46). Nevertheless, data from the past have suggested that benefits other than the skin may accrue with the use of D-penicillamine, including increased survival rate and decreased frequency of renal crisis and progression of pulmonary involvement (42). The addition of supplemental $B_6$ (pyridoxine) should be remembered, as well as the need for monitoring with complete blood cell counts and urinalysis at regular intervals. The uncommon side effect of new-onset connective tissue disease such as dermatomyositis should be recognized if it occurs.

## Gastrointestinal Scleroderma

Successful treatment of gastrointestinal scleroderma can anticipated at all levels. Simple measures to combat gastroesophageal reflux include elevation of the head of the bed, avoidance of eating after the evening meal, and the ingestion of smaller, more frequent meals. Omeprazole and $H_2$ blockers have greatly reduced the need for esophageal dilatation in the treatment of stenosis secondary to chronic reflux.

Gastric emptying can be enhanced by prokinetic agents such as cisapride or octreotide. Octreotide is a synthetic octapeptide analog of somatostatin that is administered subcutaneously and that may stimulate bowel action independent of the hormone motilin. Metoclopramide can be associated with tardive dyskinesia, a most distressing and permanent side effect. Erythromycin, a macrolide antibiotic, binds to the motilin receptor and may improve the hypomotility of the gut. The blind loop syndrome related to bacterial overgrowth and associated with diarrhea can be successfully treated with antibiotics, including ciprofloxin, metronidazole, and doxycycline. With recurring cases, the antibiotics can be rotated on a biweekly schedule.

## Lung Disease

Pulmonary fibrosis is irreversible. The key to any hope for successful treatment is early intervention at the inflammatory stage of the disease. Because this complication is the leading cause of mortality in scleroderma, a great effort is underway with multicenter trials to assess objectively the benefit-risk ratio of cytotoxic agents such as cyclophosphamide. Intravenous pulse therapy and oral therapy are under study, with a more favorable long-term side effect profile observed with the pulse therapy.

Dau first reported treatment with cyclophosphamide in 1981 (47). Since then, there has been mild improvement of pulmonary function test results for some of the 84 patients reported in the literature. Improvement was correlated with the presence of active inflammatory disease (48). Final data in this regard are pending.

Pulmonary hypertension has also been treated with cyclophosphamide with some suggestion of benefit, but results are too preliminary to be definite. Although intravenous iloprost may lower mean PAP values, efficacy is not sustained when the infusions are stopped. Calcium channel blockers used early in the disease need further study. Lung transplantation should be considered at a relatively early stage so that appropriate arrangements can be made.

### Renal Crisis

The use of ACE inhibitors has resulted in a drop in mortality from renal crisis, which still remains a life-threatening complication, most often in diffuse disease. The sudden development of malignant hypertension usually is not heralded by gradually increasing blood pressure levels. The use of ACE inhibitors is not warranted in anticipation of renal crisis but should be initiated promptly when levels climb to 140/90 or more. Men, older patients, concomitant scleroderma cardiac involvement, inability to control blood pressure within 72 hours, and a pretreatment creatinine level of more than 3 mg/dL are factors that portend a poor prognosis. When normotensive patients develop renal crisis, the prognosis is extremely poor.

ACE inhibitors are still the first-line therapy. The dose of ACE inhibitor should be increased every 6 to 12 hours until the blood pressure remains in normal range. The addition of other drugs such as calcium channel blockers, hydralazine, or minoxidil may be helpful if control is not obtained in 48 hours with maximum doses of ACE inhibitors. Regardless of deteriorating renal function, ACE inhibitors should be continued. Short-acting ACE inhibitors allow more flexibility. The use of losartan, an angiotensin II receptor blocker, may be beneficial, although this is not proved. Nitroprusside is rarely needed. Temporary or permanent dialysis may be necessary and may be associated with improvement in the skin. ACE inhibitors should be continued during dialysis, although the dose just before dialysis can be deleted to avoid hypotension. If renal function has not returned in 12 to 18 months, transplantation can be considered. Renal crisis is usually a one-time event, and survivors generally do as well as other scleroderma patients (49).

### Neuromuscular Problems

Mild forms of exercise to promote muscular blood flow are beneficial. The use corticosteroids (40 to 60 mg/day), alone or with immunosuppressive medications, including methotrexate, azathioprine, and chlorambucil, may be indicated when neuromuscular involvement is severe (30). The physician must consider the risk for developing renal crisis with the use of corticosteroids (28).

### Quality of Life

Accurate assessment of the scleroderma patient must focus on the entire lifestyle, including medical, emotional, and social aspects. For example, the advisability of moving to a warmer climate may be an an important decision to be made. Coping mechanisms, vocational rehabilitation, and family issues must also be considered. Improvement in standardized evaluation protocols is providing a tool for accomplishing this goal.

## CONCLUSIONS

The proper evaluation and follow-up of the scleroderma patient is needed now more than ever. With appropriate care, their survival and quality of life are greatly enhanced.

## REFERENCES

1. Wigley FM, Flavahan NA. Raynaud's phenomenon. *Rheum Dis Clin North Am* 1996;22:797–823.
2. Freedman RR, Mayes MD. Familial aggregation of idiopathic Raynaud's disease. *Arthritis Rheum* 1996;39: 1189–1191.
3. Mayes MD. Scleroderma epidemiology. *Rheum Dis Clin North Am* 1996;22: 751–764.
4. Seibold JR. Slow progress in scleroderma? *Curr Opin Rheumatol* 1998;10: 563.
5. Altman RD, Medsger TA Jr, Bloch DA et. al. Predictors of survival in systemic sclerosis (scleroderma). *Arthritis Rheum* 1991;34:403–413.
6. Valesini G, Litta A, Bonavita MS et. al. Geographic clustering of scleroderma in a rural area in the province of Rome. *Clin Exp Rheumatol* 1993;11:41.
7. Howard R, Arnett F, Reveille J, et al. Clustering of scleroderma among Choctaw Native Americans: preliminary clinical, serological and immunogenetic studies. *Arthritis Rheum* 1992;36:S206(abst).
8. Tan FK, Howard RF, Reveille JD, et al. Case-control study of systemic sclerosis among Choctaw Native Americans in southeastern Oklahoma. *Arthritis Rheum* 1994;37:S282(abst).
9. Tuffanelli DL, Winkleman RK. Systemic sclerosis: a clinical study of 727 cases. *Arch Dermatol* 1961;84:359–371.
10. Feghali CA, Wright TM. Epidemiologic and clinical study of twins with scleroderma. *Arthritis Rheum* 1995;38:S308(abst).
11. Kuwana M, Kaburaki FC, Arnett F, et al. Influence of ethnic background on clinical and serological features in patients with systemic sclerosis and anti-topoisomerase I antibody. *Arthritis Rheum* 1999;42:465–474.
12. Raynaud M. On local asphyxia and symmetrical gangrene of the extremities. In: Barlow T, trans. Selected monographs, 121. London: Syndenham Society, 1888:1–199.
13. Lewis T. Experiments relating to the peripheral mechanism involved in spasmodic arrest of the circulation of the fingers: a variety of Raynaud's disease. *Heart* 1929;14:7–101.
14. LeRoy EC, Medsger TA Jr. Raynaud's phenomenon: a proposal for classification. *Clin Exp Rheumatol* 1992;10:485–488.

15. Seibold JR. Clinical features of systemic sclerosis. In: Klippel JH, Dieppe PA, eds. *Practical rheumatology.* London: Mosby-Wolfe Publishers, 1997:334–342.

16. Silver RM. Clinical problems: the lungs. *Rheum Dis Clin North Am* 1996;22:825–840.

17. Stupi AM, Steen VD, Owens GR, et al. Pulmonary hypertension in the CREST syndrome variant of systemic sclerosis. *Arthritis Rheum* 1986;29:515–524.

18. Steen VD, Graham D, Conte C, et al. Isolated diffusing capacity reduction in systemic sclerosis. *Arthritis Rheum* 1992;35:765–770.

19. Ungerer RG, Tashkin DP, Furst DE, et al. Prevalence and clinical correlates of pulmonary arterial hypertension in progressive systemic sclerosis. *Am J Med* 1983;75:65–74.

20. Vancheeswaran R, Magoulas T, Efrat G, et al. Circulatory endothelin I levels in systemic sclerosis subsets—a marker or fibrosis or vascular dysfunction. *J Rheumatol* 1994;21:1838–1844.

21. Harrison NK, Myers AR, Corin B, et al. Structural features of interstitial lung disease in systemic sclerosis. *Am Rev Respir Dis* 1991;144:706–713.

22. Silver RM, Miller KS, Kinsella MB, et al. Evaluation and management of systemic sclerosis lung disease using bronchoalveolar lavage. *Am J Med* 1990;88:470–475.

23. Sappino AP, Masouye I, Saurat JH, et al. Smooth muscle differentiation in systemic sclerosis fibroblastic cells. *Am J Pathol* 1990;137:585–591.

24. Piguet PF, Collart MA, Grace GE, et al. Requirement of TNF for development of silica induced pulmonary fibrosis. *Nature* 1990;334:245–247.

25. Atamas SP, Yurovsky VV, Wise R, et al. Production of type 2 cytokines by CD8$^+$ lung cells is associated with greater decline in pulmonary function in patients with systemic sclerosis. *Arthritis Rheum* 1999;42:1168–1178.

26. Moore HC, Sheehan HL. The kidney of scleroderma. *Lancet* 1952;1:68.

27. Steen VD, Medsger TA Jr, Osial TA Jr, et al. Factors predicting development of renal involvement in progressive systemic sclerosis. *Am J Med* 1984;76:779–786.

28. Steen VD, Medsger TA Jr. Case-control study of corticosteroids and other drugs that either precipitate or protect from the development of scleroderma renal crisis. *Arthritis Rheum* 1998;41:1613–1620.

29. Panchal P, Adams E, Hsieh A. Calcific constrictive pericarditis: a rare complication of CREST syndrome. *Arthritis Rheum* 1996;39:347–350.

30. Olsen NJ, King LE, Park JH. Muscle abnormalities in scleroderma. *Rheum Dis Clin North Am* 1996;22:783–796.

31. Young MA, Rose S, Reynolds JC. Gastrointestinal manifestations of scleroderma. *Rheum Dis Clin North Am* 1996;22:797–823.

32. Cerinic MM, Generini S, Pignone A, Casale R. The nervous system in systemic sclerosis (scleroderma): clinical features and pathogenetic mechanisms. *Rheum Dis Clin North Am* 1996;22:879–892.

33. Okano Y. Antinuclear antibody in systemic sclerosis (scleroderma). *Rheum Dis Clin North Am* 1996;22:709–735.

34. Douvas AS, Acten M, Tan EM. Identification of a nuclear protein (Scl-70) as a unique target of human antinuclear antibodies in scleroderma. *J Biol Chem* 1979;254:10514.

35. Steen VD, Ziegler GL, Rodnan GP, et al. Clinical and laboratory associations of anticentromere antibody in patients with systemic sclerosis. *Arthritis Rheum* 1984;27:125.

36. Okano Y, Steen VD, Medsger TA Jr. Autoantibody reactive with RNA polymerase III in systemic sclerosis. *Ann Intern Med* 1993;119:1005.

37. Reimer G, Rose KM, Scheer U, et al. Autoantibody to RNA polymerase I in scleroderma sera. *J Clin Invest* 1987;79:65.

38. Moroi Y, Peebles C, Fritzler MJ, et al. Autoantibody to centromere (kinetochore) in scleroderma sera. *Proc Natl Acad Sci USA* 1980;77:1627.

39. Horowitz AL, Meyers MA. The hide-bound small bowel of scleroderma: characteristic mucosal fold pattern. *AJR Am J Roentgenol* 1973;1:A332(abst).

40. Ulsher MH. Breath hydrogen test for carbohydrate. In: Drossman DA, ed. *Manual of gastrointestinal procedures.* 3rd ed. New York: Raven Press, 1992.

41. Martini A, Maccario R, Ravelli A, et al. Marked and sustained improvement two years after autologous stem cell transplantation in a girl with systemic sclerosis. *Arthritis Rheum* 1999;42:807–811.

42. Pope JE. Treatment of systemic sclerosis. *Rheum Dis Clin North Am* 1996;22:893–907.

43. Sturgill MG, Seiobold JR. Rational use of calcium channel blockers in Raynaud's phenomenon. *Curr Opin Rheumatol* 1998;10:584–588.

44. Palmieri G, Sebes JI, Aelion JA, et al. Treatment of calcinosis with diltiazem. *Arthritis Rheum* 1995;38:1646–1654.

45. Taborn J, Bole GG, Thompson GR. Colchicine suppression of local systemic inflammation due to calcinosis universalis in chronic dermatomyositis. *Ann Intern Med* 1978;89:648–649.

46. Clements PJ, Furst DE, Wong WK, et al. High-dose versus low-dose D-penicillamine in early diffuse systemic sclerosis. *Arthritis Rheum* 1999;42:1194–1203.

47. Dau PC, Kahaleh MB, Sagebiel RW. Plasmapheresis and immunosuppressive drug therapy in scleroderma. *Arthritis Rheum* 1981;24:1128–1136.

48. Akesson A. Cyclophosphamide therapy for scleroderma. *Curr Opin Rheumatol* 1998;10:579–583.

49. Steen VD. Scleroderma renal crisis. *Rheum Dis Clin North Am* 1996;22:861–876.

50. Hochberg MC, Perlmutter DL, Medsger TA Jr, et al. Lack of association of augmentation mammoplasty with systemic sclerosis (scleroderma). *Arthritis Rheum* 1996;39:1125–1131.

51. Nelson JL. Microchimerism and the pathogenesis of systemic sclerosis. *Curr Opin Rheumatol* 1998;10:564–571.

*Textbook of the Autoimmune Diseases,*
Edited by R. G. Lahita, N. Chiorazzi, and W. H. Reeves,
Lippincott Williams & Wilkins, Philadelphia © 2000.

# CHAPTER 29

# Sjögren's Syndrome

Robert G. Lahita

Sjögren's Syndrome is an autoimmune disease characterized by a particular form of dry eyes and dry mouth because of infiltration of the lachrymal and parotid glands by lymphocytes (1). These signs, commonly referred to as sicca symptoms, result from a systemic problem of autoimmunity characterized by antibodies to various cells and tissues and other organ involvement. Involved organs may include the lungs, skin, central and peripheral nervous systems, vagina, and kidneys. Characteristically, the mucous membranes are dry. This disease has the unusual property of being associated with a 40 times greater incidence of lymphoid malignancy throughout the life of the patient. The disease is found as a primary form (2) that is unassociated with any other disorder and as a secondary form that is associated with other illnesses such as rheumatoid arthritis, systemic lupus erythematosus (SLE), or scleroderma.

Dr. Henrik Sjögren described the initial disease triad of parotid enlargement, dry eyes, and rheumatoid arthritis in 1933 (3). This syndrome, however, was probably first mentioned in 1888 by Mikulicz (4), who found small round cell infiltrates in the parotids and lachrymal glands of a farmer, and it later in more detail by Gougerout in 1925 (5). Both reports were before Sjögren, but he is generally credited with the earliest detailed description. The first and secondary forms came later.

## EPIDEMIOLOGY

The prevalence and incidence of this disease depend on classification criteria that are not universally accepted. The criteria (6) for the diagnosis of Sjögren's syndrome are given in Table 29.1. The signs and symptoms of Sjögren's syndrome are quite general and can be seen at any one time in the general population. These include mouth dryness, dry eyes, myalgias, joint aches, fatigue, and depression. Attempts to establish

stringent criteria have met with limited success. The presence of the anti-Ro (SSA) and anti-La (SSB) antibodies, clinical sicca symptoms, and biopsy-confirmed lymphocyte infiltrates of the parotid glands have been found in 40% to 50% of primary Sjögren patients. One estimate of the incidence is 1 case per 1,250 females (7).

## PATHOGENESIS

The most common antibodies associated with this disease are the antinuclear antibodies and rheumatoid factor. Autoantibodies against SSA are found in 90% of primary patients and 40% of SLE patients. This antibody can be found in normal individuals and in patients with hematologic malignancies such as multiple myeloma. The rheumatoid factor found in patients with Sjögren's syndrome appears to have unique light-chain specificity as determined by cross-reactive idiotype studies, because unlike that found in the rheumatoid arthritis patient, the light chains of the rheumatoid factor found in the Sjögren's patient is $V_\kappa$IIIb coded by the VK325 gene segment (8).

The environmental factors associated with the Sjögren's syndrome remain unknown, but one candidate is the Epstein–Barr virus (EBV). EBV can stimulate the production of polyclonal antibodies and rheumatoid factor. EBV-induced carcinomas of the nasopharynx are associated with specific lymphocyte responses that resemble those found in primary Sjögren's syndrome.

The salivary glands are infiltrated with CD4$^+$ T cells that produce cytokines such as interleukin-2 (IL-2) and interferon-$\gamma$ (IFN-$\gamma$) and drive the inflammatory response. Moreover, there appear to be immunoglobulin gene rearrangements within B cells of this syndrome. It is unknown whether these changes contribute to the higher risk of malignancy found in these patients.

As with all of the connective tissue autoimmune diseases, there is evidence for a genetic component (9,10). In Sjögren's syndrome, the autoantibodies are associated with human leukocyte antigen (HLA) class II genes found at the HLA-

R. G. Lahita: Department of Medicine, New York Medical College, Valhalla, New York 10595; Department of Rheumatology, St. Vincent's Hospital and Medical Center, New York, New York 10011.

**TABLE 29.1.** *Criteria for diagnosis of primary and secondary Sjögren's syndrome*

---

I. Primary SS[a]
  A. Symptoms and objective signs of ocular dryness
    1. Schirmer's test: <8 mm wetting per 5 min
    2. Positive rose bengal or fluorescein staining of cornea and conjunctiva to demonstrate kerato-conjunctivitis sicca
  B. Symptoms and objective signs of dry mouth
    1. Decreased parotid flow rate using Lashley cups or other methods
    2. Abnormal biopsy of minor salivary gland (focus score of ≥2 based on average of four evaluable lobules)
  C. Evidence of a systemic autoimmune disorder
    1. Elevated rheumatoid factor >1:160
    2. Elevated antinuclear antibody 1:160
    3. Presence of anti-SS-A (Ro) or anti-SS-B (La) antibodies
II. Secondary SS
  A. Characteristic signs and symptoms of SS (described above) plus clinical features sufficient to allow a diagnosis of RA, SLE, polymyositis, or scleroderma
  B. Exclusions: sarcoidosis, preexistent lymphoma, acquired immunodeficiency disease, hepatitis, other known causes of keratitis sicca, salivary gland enlargement, or autonomic neuropathy

---

SS, Sjögren's syndrome; RA, rheumatoid arthritis; SLE, systemic lupus erythematosus.

[a] Diagnosis of definite primary SS requires the presence of item I.A.1,2; item I.B.1,2; item I.C.1 or 2; and lack of exclusions in item II. Probable SS can be diagnosed if other criteria are fulfilled but in the absence of a minor salivary gland biopsy (item I.B.2).

Modified from Fox RI, Robinson C, Curd J, et al. First international symposium on Sjögren's syndrome: suggested criteria for classification. *Scand J Rheumatol* 1986;61:28–30.

DQA1 and HLA-DQB1 loci, which have in common the presence of specific amino acid residues that are found in the second hypervariable region of the first (outermost) domain. Family studies also suggested a non–major histocompatibility complex (MHC) autosomal dominant gene that could be associated with the familial disease (11).

## CLINICAL PRESENTATION

The eyes are the major affected organ in this disease (12). Patients have immune attacks against the serous glands and neurovascular innervation. Consequently, patients lack tears or lubrication for the eyes, which usually burn and become quite dry. The patient can use artificial tears or have the lachrymal gland plugged for therapy. Patients may develop filamentary keratitides, which are tenacious mucous filaments that bind to the cornea and the conjunctiva. The patient feels as though something is constantly in the eye. Blepharitis, or irritation of the eyelids and the conjunctiva, and light sensitivity result in conjunctivitis and edema around the cornea (13). Although there are many diseases and conditions that cause keratitis, Sjögren's syndrome is one of the more perplexing.

A second disturbing aspect of this disease is involvement of the mouth, which is often dry and painful (14). Pain is not a cardinal feature; a patient with pain has a superinfection of the dry mouth. Characteristically, the patient also requires liquid to swallow food, suggesting sicca symptoms. One of the principal oral findings for patients with sicca symptoms is unrelenting severe dental caries. Several methods for the measurement of saliva content are available. More common is the need for biopsy of the salivary gland, which shows focal lymphocytic infiltrates and solidifies the diagnosis (15).

The many other sites of extraglandular involvement include the pulmonary, gastrointestinal, dermatologic, endocrine, renal, hematologic, and nervous systems (1). The nasal passages and the bronchi are often dry in these patients. In many cases, the inspissation of mucous plugs results in the trapping of secretions and auscultatory findings suggesting congestion. In other cases, pleurisy with rubs and the sounds of coarse ronchi (i.e., dry lung) are common findings. Three major pulmonary findings from studies of Sjögren patients have been interstitial pneumonitis, chronic obstructive airway disease, and diffusion decrements across the alveolar membrane (16–18).

Esophageal dysmotility in the upper third of the esophagus is common in this illness (19). The lack of saliva contributes to the complaints of an inability to swallow. Because the saliva has a major role in the neutralization of acid, its absence results in the existence and worsening of esophageal spasm. There is also evidence of subclinical pancreatic disease in some patients with the disease. The liver can also be affected in 5% to 10% of primary Sjögren's syndrome patients. Primary biliary cirrhosis patients also can have sicca symptoms, a form of secondary Sjögren's syndrome (20). Vasculitis of the skin can also be found in patients with Sjögren's syndrome (21). Hypergammaglobulinemic purpura of the lower extremities has been described in patients with high plasma levels of γ-globulin. Moreover, periungual and perioral telangiectasias have appeared in patients with this disease, suggesting the crossover of this disease with scleroderma (22,23).

Between 10% and 15% of patients with Sjögren's syndrome have clinical hypothyroidism. Antibody to thyroglobulin and thyroid microsomal antigens can be found, suggesting that Hashimoto's thyroiditis can be common in this group (24,25).

Patients with Sjögren's syndrome have problems with renal tubular acidosis (26). This may result from dysfunction of the distal nephron, and it could be related to hypergammaglobulinemia. Renal stones are also more common because of the latter defect. Glomerulonephritis is not found in patients with Sjögren's syndrome, and its presence should suggest a concurrent connective tissue disease. Patients with this disease may have interstitial nephritis and a variety of related conditions caused by agents such as nonsteroidal antiinflammatory drugs (NSAIDs) and antibiotics.

The hematologic system is significantly involved in Sjögren's syndrome (27). Patients with this condition have leukopenia, a finding common with many of the autoimmune diseases. However, patients with this syndrome exhibit increased levels of serum and urinary paraproteins, which may result from the increased occurrence of polyclonal hypergammaglobulinemia. It is common to see cryoglobulins, which are typically type II mixed cryoglobulins containing an IgM-κ monoclonal rheumatoid factor similar to that found in Waldenström's macroglobulinemia. One major aspect of hematologic pathology is the propensity for patients to get hematologic malignancies. Patients with this condition are 40 times more likely to develop lymphomas. The onset of lymphoma may be preceded by angioblastic lymphadenopathy or pseudolymphoma (Table 29.2).

In 20% of primary Sjögren's syndrome patients, investigators found central and peripheral nervous system involvement (28). Some investigators found demyelination in the brains of patients with Sjögren's syndrome and abnormal cerebrospinal fluid test results. The increases of cerebrospinal symptoms were associated with a cutaneous vasculitis. Peripheral neuropathies and mononeuritis multiplex were found in some patients with primary Sjögren's syndrome. The significance or associations of these findings with the disease are not clear (29).

## DIAGNOSIS

The signs and symptoms of this disease can overlap with those of many other connective issue diseases. The antinuclear antibody test result is generally positive in Sjögren's syndrome. The highest titered antibodies in this disease remain the SSA and SSB antibodies (30). Although these antibodies are found in many of the connective tissue diseases such as lupus, they are found in the highest titer in patients with this illness. These antibodies are generally of the IgG isotype, and there is a preference for the IgG1 subgroup. These antibodies are most commonly associated with

neonatal lupus and, in rare cases, with congenital heart block. Immunoblotting or "dissection" of these autoantibodies reveals that the SSA antibody has a 60-kd and a 52-kd molecular form (31). These proteins are associated with small cellular RNAs. The SSB antibodies reacted with a 48-kd antigen complexed with an RNA polymerase III transcript.

Direct biopsy of the parotid glands is usually unnecessary; a biopsy of the lip should be sufficient to establish the diagnosis (Fig. 39.1). The appearance and size of the specimen are important in establishing the diagnosis, because at least four evaluable salivary glands must be observed to have interpretable results. The findings of focal collections of CD4$^+$ lymphocytes and some B cells in the infiltrates are important for the diagnosis. A simple method to establish the sicca complex includes the Schirmer test, which measures tear flow in 5 minutes using paper strips placed in the lower conjunctival sac (a normal result is more than 6 mm in 5 minutes) (32). Variations of this test include everything from stimulating tears with a cotton swab in the nose to the use of chemical stimulants. Salivary function is somewhat more difficult to examine and quantitate. Sialograms may not be appropriate in someone with parotitis, and easier methods of establishing a lack of saliva include the measurement of cotton sponge weight after 3 minutes in the mouth or the decrement in sugarless candy size over a 3-minute period.

## TREATMENT

Artificial tears are the mainstays of continued lubrication of the outer eye (33). Those that are more viscous or that use of specific lubricating "planchets" require less rigorous installation. The eyes, which are continually at risk of drying, should be specially lubricated during times of unconsciousness, such as during surgery or sleep.

Artificial saliva, toothpaste, and oral gels are available for the control of caries and oral irritation. Local treatment of infections such as *Candida* and other opportunistic organisms can help oral hygiene.

**TABLE 29.2.** *The spectrum of Sjögren's syndrome*

| Benign autoimmune exocrinopathy | Pseudolymphoma | Malignant lymphoma |
|---|---|---|
| **Clinical** | | |
| Xerostomia | Lymphadenopathy | Massive lymphadenopathy |
| Xerophthalmia | Splenomegaly | Massive salivary gland enlargement |
| RA (or another systemic rheumatic disease) | Purpura | Wasting |
| | Pulmonary infiltrates | |
| | Renal infiltrates | |
| **Pathology** | | |
| Benign lymphoid infiltrates confined to glandular tissue | Atypical extraglandular lymphoid infiltrates | B-cell lymphoma |
| **Serology** | | |
| Hypergammaglobulinemia | Hypergammaglobulinemia | Hypogammaglobulinemia |
| Anti-Ro and -La(+) | Anti-Ro and -La (+) | Loss of autoantibodies |
| | Monoclonal spike | |

The natural history of Sjögren's syndrome shows progression from a benign to a malignant lymphoproliferative disease.

RA, rheumatoid arthritis.

From Talal N. Sjögren's syndrome: historical overview and clinical spectrum of disease. *Rheum Dis Clin North Am* 1992;18:507–575, with permission.

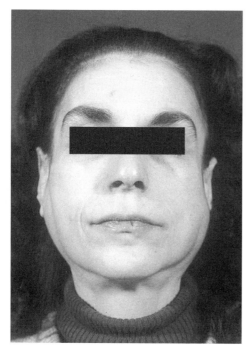

**FIG. 29.1.** A patient with parotid enlargement as a result of primary Sjögren's syndrome. See color plate 28.

Hashimoto's thyroiditis is common in this population, and patients who complain of fatigue and weight gain must be evaluated for hypothyroidism and treated. Use of agents to control myalgias and joint pains include low-dose corticosteroids, hydroxychloroquine, and NSAIDs (34). The latter agents should be used sparingly because of the possible renal consequences and gastrointestinal toxicity in this particularly vulnerable group. In the experience of some authorities, low-dose corticosteroids (5 to 10 mg/day) often provide enough immunosuppression to allow saliva and tears to normalize. Patients with vasculitis, should be treated with corticosteroids and cytotoxic agents in the usual manner.

## REFERENCES

1. Fox RI. Sjögren's syndrome. In: Kelly W, Harris EN, Ruddy S, Sledge C, eds. *Rheumatology*. Philadelphia: WB Saunders, 1997:955–968.
2. Fox RI, Howell PV, Bone RC. Primary Sjögren's syndrome: clinical and immunopathologic Features. *Semin Arthritis Rheum* 1984;14:77–105.
3. Zur kenntnis der keratoconjunctivitis sicca (Keratitis folliformis bei hypofunktion der tranendrusen). *Acta Ophthalmol* 1933;2:1.
4. Mikulicz JH. Uber eine eigenartige symmetrische Erkrankung der Tranen und Mundspeicheldrusen. *Beitr Chir Fortschr* 1892.
5. Gougerout A. Insuffisance progressive et atrophie des glandes salivaires et muqueuses de la bouche, des conjunctives (et parfois des muqueuses, nasale, laryngee, vulvarie) "Secheresse" de la bouche, des conjonctives, etc. *Bull Soc Fr Derm Syph* 1925;32:376.
6. Fox RI, Robinson CA, Curd JC. Sjögren's syndrome: proposed criteria for classification. *Arthritis Rheum* 1986;29:577–585.
7. Block KJ, Buchanan WW, Woho MJ. Sjögren's syndrome: a clinical, pathological and serological study of 62 cases. *Medicine (Baltimore)* 1956;44:187.
8. Fox RI, Kang H. The pathogenesis of Sjögren's syndrome. In: Fox RI, ed. Rheumatic disease clinics of North America, vol 18. Philadelphia: WB Saunders, 1992:18:517–538.
9. Arnett FC, Bias WB, Reveille JD. Genetic studies in systemic lupus erythematosus and Sjögren's syndrome. *J Autoimmun* 1989;2:403–413.
10. Reveille JD, Arnett F. The immunogenetics of Sjögren's syndrome. In: Fox RI, ed. Rheumatic disease clinics of North America, vol 18. Philadelphia: WB Saunders, 1992:539–550.
11. Bias WB, Reveille JD, Beaty TH. Evidence that autoimmunity in man is a mendelian dominant trait. *Am J Hum Genet* 1987;39:584.
12. Whaley K, Williamson J, Chisholm D. Sjögren's syndrome. I. Sicca components. *Q J Med* 1973;66:279–304.
13. Bridges A, Burns R. Acute iritis associated with Sjögren's syndrome and high-titer anti-SS-A/Ro and anti-SS-B/LA antibodies. Treatment with combination immunosuppressive therapy. *Arthritis Rheum* 1992;35:560–563.
14. Chisholm D, Waterhouse J, Mason D. Lymphocytic sialadenitis in the major and minor glands: a correlation in postmortem subjects. *J Clin Pathol* 1970;23:690–694.
15. Daniels TE. Labial salivary gland biopsy in Sjögren's syndrome. Assessment as diagnostic criterion in 362 suspected cases. *Arthritis Rheum* 1984;27:147–156.
16. Hunninghake G, Fauci A. Pulmonary involvement in the collagen vascular diseases. *Am Rev Respir Dis* 1979;119:471–503.
17. Newball H, Brahim S. Chronic obstructive airway disease in patients with Sjögren's syndrome. *Am Rev Respir Dis* 1977;115:295–304.
18. Segel I, Fink G, Machtey I, et al. Pulmonary abnormalities in Sjögren's syndrome. *Thorax* 1981;36:286–289.
19. Kjellen G, Fransson SG, Lindstrom F, et al. Esophageal function, radiography, and dysphagia in Sjögren's syndrome. *Dig Dis Sci* 1986;31:225–229.
20. Webb J, Whaley K, MacSween R, et al. Liver disease in rheumatoid Arthritis and Sjögren's syndrome. Prospective study using biochemical and serological markers of hepatic dysfunction. *Ann Rheum Dis* 1975;34:70–81.
21. Alexander E, Provost TT. Sjögren's syndrome: association of cutaneous vasculitis with central nervous system disease. *Arch Dermatol* 1987;123:801–810.
22. Ford AL, Kurien BT, Harley JB, Scofield RH. Anti-centromere autoantibody in a patient evolving from a lupus/Sjögren's overlap to the CREST variant of scleroderma. *J Rheumatol* 1998;25:1419–1424.
23. Caramaschi P, Biasi D, Carletto A, et al. Sjögren's syndrome with anti-centromere antibodies. *Rev Rheumatol Engl Ed* 1997;64:785–788.
24. Scofield RH. Autoimmune thyroid disease in systemic lupus erythematosus and Sjögren's syndrome. *Clin Exp Rheumatol* 1996;14:321–330.
25. Punzi L, Ostuni PA, Betterle C, et al. Thyroid gland disorders in Sjögren's syndrome. *Rev Rheumatol Engl Ed* 1996;63:809–814.
26. Eriksson P, Denneberg T, Larsson L, et al. Biochemical markers of renal disease in primary Sjögren's syndrome. *Scand J Urol Nephrol* 1995;29:383–392.
27. Kruize AA, Hene RJ, van der Heide A, et al. Long-term follow-up of Patients with Sjögren's syndrome. *Arthritis Rheum* 1996;39:297–303.
28. Alexander EL, Malinow K, Lejewski JE, et al. Primary Sjögren's syndrome with central nervous system disease mimicking multiple sclerosis. *Ann Intern Med* 1986;104:323–330.
29. Satake M, Yoshimura T, Iwaki T, et al. Anti-dorsal root ganglion neuron antibody in a case of dorsal root ganglionitis associated with Sjögren's syndrome. *J Neurol Sci* 1995;132:122–125.
30. Martinez-Lavin M, Vaughan J, Tan E. Autoantibodies and the spectrum of Sjögren's syndrome. *Ann Intern Med* 1979;91:185–190.
31. Ben-Chetrit E, Fox RI, Tan E. Dissociation of immune Responses to the SSA(Ro) 52 kd and 60 kd polypeptides in systemic lupus erythematosus and Sjögren's syndrome. *Arthritis Rheum* 1990;33:349–355.
32. Danjo Y. Diagnostic usefulness and cutoff value of Schirmer's test in the Japanese diagnostic criteria of dry eye. *Graefes Arch Clin Exp Ophthalmol* 1997;235:761–766.
33. Fox RI, Chan E, Michelson JB. Beneficial effect of artificial tears made with autologous serum in patients with keratoconjunctivitis sicca. *Arthritis Rheum* 1984;27:459–461.
34. Fox RI, Chan E, Benton L. Treatment of primary Sjögren's syndrome with hydroxychloroquine. *Am J Med* 1988;85:62–67.

*Textbook of the Autoimmune Diseases,*
Edited by R. G. Lahita, N. Chiorazzi, and W. H. Reeves,
Lippincott Williams & Wilkins, Philadelphia © 2000.

# CHAPTER 30

# Rheumatoid Arthritis

Cornelia M. Weyand and Jörg J. Goronzy

Rheumatoid arthritis (RA) is a crippling disease that affects individuals in the prime of their life. Early in the disease, pain and stiffness dominate the clinical presentation. Eventually, functional loss due to structural damage becomes the major problem. Because hands and feet are preferred targets of the disease, patients lose the ability to walk and to use their hands for daily activities. Accumulation of inflammatory cells in the synovial membrane and induction of an injury response in the joint are principal events of this disease. The inflammatory response in the synovium leads to the formation of tissue that is invasive and destructive in character. The invasion of cartilage, tendons, and bone creates irreversible tissue damage with subsequent crippling. Although diarthrodial joints are the primary targets of the disease, RA is in essence a systemic disease, and extraarticular spreading is not uncommon. Extraarticular RA has a tendency to involve peripheral nerves, muscles, lungs, and particularly the arterial walls, giving rise to rheumatoid vasculitis, which causes infarction and hemorrhage.

Manifestation of RA in major organ systems is one of the reasons for the shortened life expectancy of RA patients. The recognition that RA is not simply a disease of painful joints but is associated with disability and increased mortality has changed the therapeutic management of affected patients. To prevent irreversible tissue damage, aggressive treatment should be initiated in the early stages of the disease. This shift in therapeutic approach has created multiple challenges for clinicians caring for RA patients, but it can be expected to improve the overall outcome.

The primary cause of RA is unknown, and the disease has defied the formulation of a unifying and comprehensive pathogenetic model. Curative interventions are therefore not available. Studies of the disease have, however, benefited from the enormous progress made in understanding pathways of inflammation, tissue destruction and repair, and matrix

degradation and the mechanism of cell death. The accepted paradigm holds that RA is a multifactorial syndrome with contributions from several environmental and genetic factors in disease pathogenesis. Although the possibility remains that future studies will uncover a single and primary cause of RA, such as an infectious agent, it is more likely that more than one instigator has a place in the cause of this highly complex syndrome. Multiple inherited and acquired elements set the stage for the inflammation and modulate the chain of events that lead to tissue destruction. This concept provides the framework for the identification of molecular targets that are suitable to influence and even turn off the disease process before a seemingly programmed destruction of affected organ systems has occurred.

## INCIDENCE AND EPIDEMIOLOGY

In 1800, Landré-Beauvais (1) described a new form of polyarthritis that he felt was different from gouty arthritis. The designation of "rheumatoid arthritis" was proposed by Garrod in 1859. This recognition of RA, as opposed to ankylosing spondylitis, gout, and osteoarthritis, which are all accepted as ancient diseases, spurred the idea that RA is a syndrome of modern times. If RA has only existed for 200 years, it would lend strong support for the model that a newly emerged factor, such as a microorganism, has a critical role in pathogenesis. The theory that RA is a new disease has mostly been based on negative evidence in the medical and nonmedical literature, in paintings of medieval artists, and in paleopathologic studies. This conclusion was challenged when bony erosions were described in Native American skeletons. Skeletons found in the upper western Mississippi basin displayed symmetric erosions in small and large joints in a distribution characteristic of RA (2). These skeletons date back as far as 6,500 years, and it is therefore likely that RA existed in North America several thousand years ago. It has been proposed that the disease might have been brought to Europe after 1492, explaining the relatively recent appearance of RA in the Old World.

C. M. Weyand and J. J. Goronzy: Department of Medicine, Division of Rheumatology, Mayo Clinic and Foundation, Rochester, Minnesota 55905.

In the absence of a known primary cause of RA, epidemiologic studies have strived to identify environmental factors important in disease cause. These studies have failed to provide conclusive evidence of environmental risk factors and have not given any clues about the cause of the disease. In multiple cross-sectional population studies, the prevalence of RA has been estimated at about 1% in North American and European Caucasians older than 15 years. Consistently, females have a twofold to fourfold higher risk than males, and prevalence rates increase with age (3). Incidence rates have varied, probably because of differences in case definition. Overall, it has been estimated that 20 men and 60 women per 100,000 individuals develop RA per year. Most studies have shown increasing incidence rates with age (4,5).

The most interesting aspect of these studies has come from the observation that the incidence of RA seems to have declined over the last 30 years. Incidence rates have dropped by about 50% in several populations, including Pima Indians, a high-risk ethnic group with prevalence rates of approximately 5%. The use of oral contraceptives has been cited as one possible reason for the declining frequency of RA (4). Whether the decline in new-onset RA reflects a true change in the disease is not entirely clear. Several confounding factors have to be considered when interpreting the results of epidemiologic surveys, including shifts in the age distribution of populations and changes in the ethnic composition of populations. Central in all of these studies is the case definition of RA, which has evolved with revisions of the American College of Rheumatology criteria. It is also possible that RA is a heterogeneous syndrome consisting of multiple different entities. The mix of entities may vary among geographical areas and patient populations.

## DISEASE RISK FACTORS

### Genetics

The risk for developing RA is increased for persons with a sibling affected by the disease. However, the odds ratio for a first-degree relative of an RA patient to develop RA is only 1.6. Higher sibship concordance rates have been found when the index cases had severe disease (6), demonstrating that the estimations of familial risk strongly depend on the methods of case assessment. Familial clustering may indicate sharing of genetic factors or of environmental factors predisposing to RA. Inheritance of risk factors has been supported by twin studies documenting increased disease concordance in monozygotic compared with dizygotic twins (7). A concordance rate of 12% was found for monozygotic twin pairs, whereas dizygotic twins had disease concordance of only 4%. This provides compelling evidence for a role of genetic determinants in disease risk.

Additional evidence for genetic risk has come from the demonstration that RA is an human leukocyte antigen (HLA)–associated disease. Initial observations described an enrichment of HLA-DR4 among patients compared with healthy individuals (8). Sequence analysis of the HLA-DR region provided the information for a refinement of this association. HLA-DR4 has been found to include several variants that differ in the HLA-DRB1 locus. A set of HLA-DRB1 alleles that share a sequence stretch in a region of allelic polymorphisms have been identified as RA risk alleles (9). The shared sequence motif in these otherwise quite dissimilar alleles has been named the *shared epitope*. The importance of shared epitope–positive alleles in conferring risk to develop RA has been confirmed in multiple different populations (10,11). Frequencies of HLA-DRB1 alleles vary in different ethnic groups and geographic regions, providing an explanation for variations in the population prevalence of RA.

### Socioeconomics

Data on the influence of the socioeconomic status in RA are conflicting. Worse outcome has been associated with lack of education of U.S. male patients (12), although only a marginal effect was demonstrated in subsequent studies (13). The influences of higher levels of education and income on outcome are not specific for RA but have been demonstrated in most chronic diseases and probably reflect differences in lifestyle, coping, and self-care. Epidemiologic evidence for specific occupations predisposing persons to RA has not been forthcoming.

### Lifestyle Factors

Tobacco smoking is associated with an increased risk for RA. The best evidence has been provided by studying smoking discordant twin pairs (14). An excess risk to develop RA with an odds ratio of 12 was demonstrated in smokers.

### Gender and Sex Hormones

As in many other autoimmune diseases, the incidence of RA is increased several-fold among women, indicating a role for gender and sex hormones in conferring risk (3). A population-based case-control study explored whether disease patterns are similar or different in female and male patients with the disease (15). Although erosive disease developed earlier and more frequently in men, the rate of hand and foot arthroplasties was twofold higher for women, suggesting that the disease process is distinct in female and male patients or that differences in target organ susceptibility exist. Rheumatoid organ disease displayed different patterns in both sexes, with nodule formation and lung disease being the dominant manifestations in men and sicca syndrome in women.

A potential role of hormonal factors in RA has long been appreciated. Hench's observation that pregnancy can induce remission in RA provided the clue for the development of corticosteroids as therapeutic agents. Nulliparity and the postpartum period appear to be disease risk factors, with breast-feeding and prolactin production as possible modulators (16). Conversely, the use of oral contraceptives was found to be associated with reduced risk (17). Subsequent studies have produced conflicting results, and the issue remains unresolved. Estrogen replacement therapy in postmenopausal women does not protect against the development of RA but may have an influence on the severity of the disease.

## PATHOGENESIS

The ultimate challenge in the study of a disease is the elucidation of its cause and pathogenesis. Understanding why and how individuals develop RA holds promise for treating or preventing this crippling disorder. Even if pathogenic studies cannot identify a single primary cause in the disease process, they are ultimately valuable for the care of patients with RA. Recognition of pathogenic mechanisms can help create a clearer definition of RA as a disease entity and enhance epidemiologic and genetic studies. Characterization of pathogenic pathways can define biologic abnormalities, which would be useful in developing novel diagnostic tests. The best example of this is the study of autoantibodies, such as rheumatoid factors, which were first described in the 1940s, studied in detail in the 1950s and 1960s, and remain quintessential diagnostic tools today. It is possible that the definition of molecules involved in the disease process will provide targets for therapeutic intervention.

The cause of RA is unknown, but accumulating data support the theory that the pathogenic events in RA are highly complex and involve the contribution of multiple elements (18). There is excellent evidence for genetic susceptibility, immune reactivity, and a cascade of tissue destructive mechanisms intermingled with tissue repair responses producing the clinical picture of RA (19). It is likely that several perturbations in the generation and perpetuation of immune responses tip the balance toward pathology, with the common denominator being a breakdown in self-tolerance. Equally important are regulatory mechanisms that contribute to inflammation. Recruitment of inflammatory cells into the tissue; formation of new blood vessels; production of cytokines, growth factors, and chemokines by immune and nonimmune cells; release and regulation of free radicals, prostaglandins, leukotrienes, and kinins; degradation of cartilage and bone; and unique features of the microenvironment in the affected joint have a role in the complex events cumulating in the formation of the tissue destructive lesions of RA (20).

The emerging paradigm makes the basic assumption that all of these factors contribute, with some of them representing major contributors and others minor elements (Fig. 30.1). The relative contribution of individual factors may vary from patient to patient, a scenario that makes pathogenetic and treatment studies complicated and explains the high variability in clinical response rates to a given treatment. These dif-

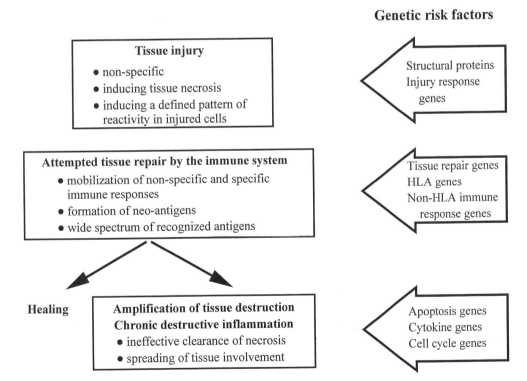

**FIG. 30.1.** Multiple-hit model for rheumatoid arthritis. The pathogenesis of rheumatoid arthritis is complex and has contributions from multiple elements, including tissue-specific factors and immune mechanisms. Many of these elements are influenced by rheumatoid arthritis susceptibility genes that, in combination, predispose for the disease. (From Weyand CM, Goronzy JJ. Pathogenesis of rheumatoid arthritis. *Med Clin North Am* 1997;81:29–55, with permission.)

ferent contributing factors should not be regarded as mutually exclusive but rather as components that come together in an additive or synergistic fashion to produce the pathology of RA. Although much evidence has been collected to imply a central position of the immune system, data on the initial trigger of the pathologic cascade remain inconclusive.

Infectious agents are prime candidates. Although biologically plausible, the experimental data for causality are at best suggestive. It is unlikely that a single microorganism is the primary cause in all patients and in all geographic regions. It is equally unlikely that a single self antigen is initiating or perpetuating the immune response, although autoreactivity may maintain the inflammation. With a more comprehensive understanding of the regulation of the immune system, it has become clear that antigen-nonspecific mechanisms are as important as the nature of the antigen in maintaining self-tolerance. The term *immune deviation* has been coined to describe more global deviations in the network of immune cells and mediators, and it is possible that biases in the immune system toward certain pathways contribute to the pathologic immune response in rheumatoid joints.

### Infections as Triggers of Rheumatoid Arthritis

Epidemiology does not support an infectious cause of RA. Specifically, neither clustering in space nor time has been convincingly described. Nevertheless, the hypothesis that a microorganism is the primary cause of RA has remained attractive. Serologic studies have been used to detect prior infection with bacterial and viral agents. These approaches have not been able to unequivocally implicate known infectious agents, including cytomegalovirus, retroviruses, mycoplasma, or mycobacteria. Elevation of antibodies against parvovirus B19 and the association of a symmetric polyarthritis with rubella infection or vaccination have been cited to suggest a role for these viruses in the disease, but subsequent studies have failed to confirm a role of these viruses in RA. Other reports have described virus-like particles in synovial lesions of RA patients, but data showing a clear correlation between disease and these particles are missing, and there are no studies exploring a causative relationship.

The best evidence supports a possible role of Epstein–Barr virus (EBV) in the pathogenesis of RA. Originally, it was observed that antibodies to EBV antigens were elevated in RA patients (21). EBV is attractive as a potential causative agent because it acts as a polyclonal activator of B cells and may provide an explanation for the production of rheumatoid factors. Sharing of an amino acid sequence in the EBV protein, GP110, and the HLA-DRB1 gene implicated in conferring the increased disease risk yielded support for a molecular mimicry mechanism (22). Recent data have renewed the interest in EBV as a trigger of rheumatoid synovitis. CD8 T cells isolated from the joints of RA patients were shown to have antigen specificity for two proteins encoded by EBV, the EBV transactivators BZLF1 and BMLF1 (23).

Besides EBV, retroviruses have been candidates as potential instigators of RA. The emergence of a symmetric pol-

yarthritis in patients infected with the human T-cell lymphotropic virus (HTLV-1) in Japan supports this notion (24). HTLV-1 proviral DNA and expression of the *tax* gene have been demonstrated in synoviocytes from infected patients with chronic proliferative synovitis (25). However, failure to incriminate exogenous retroviruses in other patient populations indicates that these findings cannot be generalized to individuals affected by RA (26).

### Loss of Self-Tolerance

The first immunologic abnormality defined in patients with RA was the production of rheumatoid factors that were autoantibodies with specificity for the Fc portion of IgG. This observation provided the basis for a disease model that assumed that RA is an autoimmune disease. Immune responsiveness is a critical part in the pathogenesis, but it remains undecided whether the primary trigger is the recognition of autoantigens, whether autorecognition results from molecular mimicry with a preceding infection, or whether autoreactivity is a secondary event reflecting the spreading of immunity to initially uninvolved antigens (Table 30.1).

The function of the immune system is not solely dictated by antigen; other factors come into play. The recognition that superantigens, which often derive from infectious organisms, can activate large proportions of T cells and B cells through alternative mechanisms has added complexity to the understanding of immune responses to bacteria and viruses. We are beginning to understand that tolerance is regulated by multiple factors, of which antigen represents only one. The fate of a T cell recognizing antigen is critically determined by costimulatory signals that dictate whether the T cell proliferates and differentiates into an effector cell, undergoes programmed cell death, or enters a state of anergy. The nature of antigen-presenting cells and the microenvironment in which an immune response occurs are therefore important components shaping the outcome of immune stimulation.

### Nature of the Immune Response in the Rheumatoid Joint

Rheumatoid lesions in the joint are composed of T cells, B cells, macrophages, and synoviocytes. There is also abundant neoangiogenesis. Histomorphology reveals that infiltrating

**TABLE 30.1.** *Immunologic abnormalities in rheumatoid arthritis*

- Upregulation of acute phase proteins
- Production of autoantibodies against IgG (rheumatoid factors) and filagrin
- Expression of CD4+CD28–deficient T cells
- Formation of ectopic lymphoid tissue in the synovial membrane
- Granuloma formation
- Formation of tissue-destructive inflammatory lesions
- Enrichment for individuals with selected (RA-associated) HLA-DRB1 alleles

inflammatory cells accumulate in the sublining tissue layers. Often they are arranged in follicular structures that morphologically and functionally resemble germinal centers (27). Germinal centers are specialized microanatomic structures resulting from antigen-driven interactions among T cells, dendritic cells, B cells, and follicular dendritic cells and are usually only present in lymphoid organs (28). They are required for the generation of high-affinity antibodies and for the selection of memory B cells in response to protein antigens. Evidence has been provided that the ectopic germinal centers in the synovium are sites of affinity maturation and may have a role in the production of autoantibodies (29). Formation of germinal centers in RA synovium lends strong support to a role of antigen specific immune responses occurring in the joint.

Other indirect evidence for the involvement of antigen recognition in synovial inflammation has come from analysis of the repertoire of T-cell receptor molecules. These studies made the basic assumption that antigen stimulation provides a survival advantage for specific T cells and leads to a redistribution of T-cell specificities in the lesions. Although most groups have reported a high degree of heterogeneity of tissue infiltrating T cells, clonal expansion of selected T cells has been a common finding (30). Generally, individual T-cell clones have been small, with identical clones expressed in different joints of the same patient but with no convincing sharing among different patients. These findings are consistent with the interpretation that some synovial T cells recognize antigen in the synovial tissue. However, more than one antigen may be involved, and different antigens may be relevant in different patients.

### Potential Autoantigens

IgG, recognized by rheumatoid factors, remains a potential candidate as the antigen inducing or amplifying RA. Molecular analysis of antibodies with rheumatoid factor specificity from RA patients has shown that rheumatoid factors are polyclonal and show evidence of somatic mutations, consistent with an antigen-driven immune response (31). Altered galactosylation in RA patients may contribute to an enhanced immunogenicity of IgG (32). Besides this ubiquitously distributed autoantigen, several matrix components of the joint have been suspected to be targets of pathologic immune responses, including type II collagen, the cartilage proteoglycan, aggrecan, and the cartilage link protein. In mice and rats, type II collagen can elicit experimental polyarthritis reminiscent of RA (33,34). Collagen-induced arthritis has been a useful model in understanding immunopathogenic aspects of polyarthritis. In particular, collagen-induced arthritis is an major histocompatibility complex (MHC)–restricted, T-cell–dependent disease. Similarly, erosive polyarthritis can be induced in selected mouse strains by immunization with aggrecan or cartilage link protein (35). The cartilage glycoprotein-39 is a joint-specific antigen that triggers an HLA-DR4–restricted T-cell response in RA patients and gives rise to chronic synovitis in an animal model (36).

### Systemic Autoimmunity

Immune abnormalities in RA are not restricted to the synovial tissue, consistent with the notion that RA is not only a joint-specific disease. Clonal expansion of T cells is found throughout the lymphoid system, including the peripheral blood (37–39). CD4 T cells undergoing clonal expansion are deficient for CD28, a molecule that is considered to be pivotal in the stimulation of T cells (40). As expected from the crucial role of CD28, CD28-deficient CD4 T cells are rare in normal individuals. In contrast, most RA patients express increased frequencies of CD28-deficient CD4 T cells. These cells are already present in very early disease in the synovial tissue and the peripheral blood. They have several unusual features, including marked oligoclonality with individual clones persisting over many years. Quite unexpectedly, these cells are functionally competent. They produce high amounts of interferon-γ and synthesize the pore-forming protein, perforin, that enables them to have cytolytic activity. They have a defect in apoptosis, which may explain their longevity *in vivo*. This defect has been associated with overexpression of the BCL-2 protein, a molecule instrumental in regulating cell death.

Evidence for a genetic component in the generation of CD28-deficient CD4 T cells has come from studies in twins. Monozygotic twins were highly concordant for the size of the CD28-deficient CD4 T-cell compartment. Most importantly, CD28-deficient CD4 T-cell clones isolated from RA patients have been found to exhibit autoreactivity directed against autologous monocytes or macrophages (40). The suspected autoantigen may be shared by different RA patients, because T-cell receptors with identical amino acid sequences have been isolated from different patients (41). In RA patients, part of the CD4 compartment is replaced by these unusual T cells that lack surface expression of the CD28 molecule. These cells have characteristics that are compatible with an autoimmune and proinflammatory commitment. The frequency of these T cells is particularly high in patients with extraarticular manifestations, consistent with their systemic distribution and activity (42).

A serendipitous observation added support to the model that generalized autorecognition can be a primary event in polyarthritis. Kouskoff et al. generated a T-cell receptor transgenic mouse with specificity of the receptor for self-MHC class II molecules (43). T cells expressing the transgenic receptor were incompletely deleted in the thymus. The animals did not develop the expected graft-versus-host disease, but T cells accumulated in the joints and caused proliferative synovitis. The restriction of the antiself response to the joint raises the possibility that synovitis may result from a generalized but compartmentalized autoproliferation. This fortuitously generated animal model displays several other features seen in RA, including bony erosion and polyclonal B-cell activation. It is not understood how a systemic autoimmune response can be controlled in the periphery but still lead to pathology in the synovial microenvironment.

## Inherited Susceptibility

Without ignoring the importance of environmental factors, the unraveling of genetic susceptibility determinants will dominate the research effort in RA in the coming decades. Clinicians are well aware of the increased risk of individuals to develop RA if they have a first-degree relative with the disease. The risk is highest for persons who have a monozygotic twin with RA. Nevertheless, genetic background alone cannot determine the outcome, as documented by a rather high frequency of discordance in identical twin pairs. RA is understood to be a complex genetic disease with rules applying similarly to those for atherosclerosis, hypertension, and diabetes (19). Unlike the classic genetic disorders in which abnormal genes are inherited in a Mendelian pattern, multiple susceptibility genes have a role in common genetic disorders. Individual disease-risk genes are usually not mutated or abnormal. They are instead functionally intact, but when they are inherited in a certain combination and on a certain genetic background, they can predispose to develop RA. The combination of multiple genes and their functional intactness can partially explain the complex inheritance pattern of the disease. A person has to inherit several of the disease-risk genes to reach a threshold on a liability scale and to develop disease.

It is also believed that individual disease risk genes do not function as independent units but instead interact against the genetic background. This phenomenon has been described as *epistasis*. In this model, synergistic effects of susceptibility factors are possible, and some predisposing genes may amplify the importance of others. However, individuals with multiple disease risk genes may be spared from disease if the contribution of individual genetic components is not supported in the context of a complex genetic background.

The best studied genetic system in RA is the HLA genes (44). Initially, it was observed that the diversity of HLA alleles among RA patients was no longer maintained; rather, most patients diagnosed with RA shared certain HLA-DR alleles. Refining of the associated genetic element gave rise to the shared epitope hypothesis (9–11). Guided by the finding that a group of HLA-DR alleles was enriched among patients, researchers attempted to define what was common among all of the RA-associated HLA-DR genes. A sequence stretch was identified that was shared by certain HLA-DR4 alleles and by HLA-DR1. This sequence stretch containing by amino acid positions 67 to 74 of the HLA-DRβ1 chain has been mapped on the HLA-DR molecule and has been found to form a pocket relevant in binding amino acid side chains of antigenic peptides embedded into the binding site of the HLA-DR dimer (45). The position of this RA associated genetic element in the HLA-DR molecule has supported the paradigm that the HLA association of RA reflects a critical role of antigen selection, binding, and presentation in the disease process. In essence, it is proposed that arthritogenic antigens exist that are preferentially bound and presented by a RA-associated HLA molecule to initiate a pathologic T-cell response.

Detailed clinical studies investigating the distribution of HLA-DR alleles in RA patients challenged the straight-forward model (44). Genotyping of a large cohort of RA patients revealed that many of these patients had inherited two RA-associated haplotypes (46). If the crucial contribution of disease associated HLA-DR molecules is related to the antigen presentation function, it is difficult to envision why patients would preferentially have two such genes. Arthritogenic peptides should be effectively presented by one haplotype only. Careful clinical evaluation led to the recognition that the dosing of two RA-associated HLA alleles correlated with the clinical pattern of disease (47). Specifically, patients with RA restricted to the joints usually expressed a single copy of the relevant HLA-DR alleles. Patients with extraarticular spreading of RA frequently typed positive for a member of the HLA-DR4 family and HLA-DR1. Patients with rheumatoid vasculitis were found to carry a combination of two RA associated HLA-DR4 subtypes, and were usually homozygous for HLA-DR B1*0401, the HLA allele with the strongest disease association. Two interpretations could explain these data.

HLA-DR molecules may regulate the progression of disease and determine the severity of RA. Alternatively, the clinical categories of RA may not simply represent stages on a severity scale but may reflect disease heterogeneity with distinct variants of RA (44). Different pathomechanisms may apply in the distinct subtypes of RA. Although a single RA-associated HLA-DR is sufficient to predispose a person to joint-restricted RA, a different dimension of HLA-related immune functions may come into play in extraarticular RA. Experimental evidence has demonstrated a role of disease-associated HLA-DR molecules beyond the selective binding and presentation of antigen to mature T cells. The composition of the repertoire of naive CD4 T cells was found to be different in RA patients compared with HLA-DR–matched healthy controls (48). These data raise the possibility that the pool of T cells in RA patients is basically different from that in non-RA individuals and that HLA molecules predispose for disease by virtue of their selection of T cells in the thymus (49).

A correlation of the clinical heterogeneity of RA with the inheritance of HLA-DRB1 gene has also been established for patients with the seronegative variant of RA (50). Patients with nonerosive, slowly progressing seronegative RA often lack RA-associated HLA-DR alleles, indicating that these molecules are not an absolute requirement for the initiation of the disease process. Among seronegative patients, the expression of HLA-DR4 was correlated with more severe disease and the requirement for more aggressive therapy. The possibility remains that HLA-DR molecules influence the disease process by amplifying pathologic events and determining disease severity. Alternatively, the disease subsets defined clinically may follow different pathologic rules with distinct roles for HLA molecules in destructive inflammation. Whatever the correct explanation, these data have implications that are important for the study of RA and the design of clinical interventions. The correlation of HLA genotypes with severe forms of RA provides the unique opportunity to predict a disease course early after onset of synovitis and could be used to target aggressive therapy to patients who need them most (Fig. 30.2). The recognition of disease phenotypes with different pathogenic events requires careful stratification of RA patients in genetic studies and in treatment trials. Molecular components targeted by new and more selective therapeutic strategies may not be shared by all patients, an important consideration in the design and evaluation of experimental trials.

The polygenic character of RA predicts that several other genetic elements besides genes in the HLA region have a role in RA (Fig. 30.1). Modern molecular techniques have provided the opportunity for genome-wide searches of disease-risk genes by linkage disequilibrium studies. Alternatively, candidate genes can be defined by an educated guess, and patient populations and multicase families can be evaluated for the presence of polymorphisms and their relation to RA. The suspected implication of the immune system in the rheumatoid process has encouraged a series of studies exploring whether molecules with critical roles in the immune response are altered in RA patients. Polymorphisms in the T-cell receptor genes as well as such in the coding and regulatory regions of cytokine genes are obvious candidates. The available data are too inconclusive to unequivocally define any of these genes as RA risk genes. Many other genes, including those involved in tissue repair, apoptosis, and the structural modeling of organ systems attacked by RA, could affect the risk of an individual to be affected by RA. It is already clear that the HLA region alone does not account for the total genetic risk in RA. It can therefore be expected that multiple new disease genes will emerge in the coming years.

## Mechanisms of Tissue Destruction in the Rheumatoid Joint

Synovial inflammation in RA is associated with the formation of a particular tissue called *pannus*. Pannus is a heterogeneous tissue composed of mesenchyme- and bone marrow–derived cells and is believed to represent the destructive unit in rheumatoid synovitis. The cellular composition and the functional properties of the pannus have attracted intense interest in the belief that this tissue may hold the key to understanding RA. This may not be the case, and pannus formation may simply represent the response pattern of the synovial membrane to an injury. The inflammatory tissue has been dissected into a lining layer composed of type A and type B synoviocytes. This lining is not separated from the subintimal tissue by a basement membrane and does not really represent an intima. In the sublining tissue, lymphocytes and macrophages accumulate, surrounded by intense neoangiogenesis. Neutrophils are rare in the synovial tissue but are plentiful in the synovial fluid. There is discussion about whether the synovial tissue at the invasive front, where it invades cartilage and bone, has a unique appearance. Cells with stellate extensions of cytoplasm have been described that appear to directly penetrate into the cartilage (51). The origin of these pannocytes, their concrete role in destruction, and, particularly their regulation remain an issue of debate.

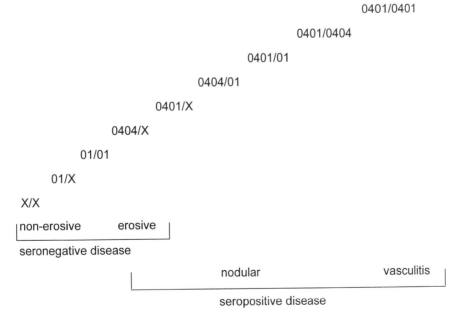

**FIG. 30.2.** Hierarchy of HLA-DRB1 alleles in determining disease severity and extraarticular manifestations. The proposed model implies that HLA-DRB1 alleles differ in their impact on disease severity and that combinations of two disease-associated alleles predispose for more severe joint disease and for extraarticular manifestations. The 0404 stands for a group of alleles, including HLA-DRB1*0404, *0405, and *0408. (From Weyand CM, McCarthy TG, Goronzy JJ. Correlation between disease phenotype and genetic heterogeneity in rheumatoid arthritis. *J Clin Invest* 1995;95:2120–2126, with permission.)

Overall, the synovial lining is a mixture of resident fibroblast-like cells and of macrophages that probably derive from the bone marrow. Efforts to distinguish matrix-producing fibroblasts from phagocytosing macrophages have not been successful. It is possible that synovial lining cells in an intensely inflamed joint acquire a hybrid status combining fibroblast and macrophage features. The most impressive change in these cells is their functional profile, which identifies them as highly activated cells. Most importantly, these cells can produce metalloproteinases, which have a central role in tissue degradation. It has been reported that they synthesize cytokines, such as interleukin-1 (IL-1) and IL-6. They have been implicated in producing matrix components such as collagen, hyaluronan, fibronectin, and laminin (52). The phenotype and functional capacity of activated synoviocytes has raised the question about whether they are "transformed." The expression of protooncogenes by synovial cells is compatible with activation and does not confirm that these cells are autonomous. Demonstration of a *P53* mutation probably is a secondary event and is not sufficient to document a transformed state of these cells (53). The capability to produce excessive proteases and cytokines by itself does not prove that these cells have become independent from regulatory control. Although rheumatoid synovitis has an aggressive and invasive character, experimental data demonstrating autonomy of synovial cells are lacking.

Besides synovial fibroblasts and macrophages, multinucleated giant cells and mast cells have been found in synovial tissue (54,55). Multinucleated giant cells contribute to cartilage destruction by acquiring chondroclast-like features. Mast cells, integrated into a network of cell-cell interactions with other immune and nonimmune cell types in the synovium, may contribute to the destructive character of the pannus.

Another important aspect of cartilage destruction in the rheumatoid joint is an adaptive response of chondrocytes. Chondrocytes undergo a change in gene expression with the induction of cytokines and metalloproteinases (56). This mechanism could initiate self-destruction of cartilage, aggravating the tissue damage induced by the inflamed synovial membrane.

The destruction of cartilage, tendons, and bones undoubtedly results from multiple pathways that possibly vary between patients, joints, and stages of disease. Stromelysin is believed to represent the most important tissue-degrading enzyme, but gelatinase and collagenase are also expressed abundantly in rheumatoid synovium. Although metalloproteinases have a central role in the destructive process, many other pathways contribute, including oxygen-derived free radicals, nitric oxide, neuropeptides, arachidonic acid metabolites, and the kinin, complement, and clotting systems. A model for cartilage invasion has been proposed by Harris, who summarizes the current knowledge on rheumatoid synovitis and the end result of cartilage and bone degradation (20). Harris suggests that the destructive unit of synovitis is created as synovial lining cells are strongly activated and T cells, B cells, and macrophages accumulate in the subsynovial layers. In this model, elastases and proteases released by neutrophils accumulate in the synovial fluid and initiate damage to the superficial regions of the cartilage. Proteoglycans are then depleted from the matrix, exposing chondrocytes to stimulatory signals and thereby inducing the expression of adhesion molecules and facilitating the attachment of pannus cells to underlying structures. Metalloproteinases are secreted and digest surrounding tissue, and the remnants are phagocytosed by macrophages.

## CLINICAL PRESENTATION AND DIAGNOSIS

RA is a chronic, progressive systemic disease that primarily manifests in diarthrodial joints. Irreversible tissue damage is induced by inflammatory lesions that accumulate in the synovial membrane but can form in many different organs. Extraarticular manifestations are rare in early disease. During the initial phase, RA patients suffer from pain and stiffness in multiple joints, often in the hands and feet, combined with functional loss. In most patients, the disease onset is insidious, with slowly developing synovitis over weeks and months. An acute onset within days is possible. Initial disease manifestations and exacerbations are noticed twice as frequently during the winter months.

### Diagnosis

RA is a clinical diagnosis. No single laboratory, radiographic, or histomorphologic test can establish the diagnosis. Diagnostic criteria have been developed by the American College of Rheumatology and have found widespread use (57) (Table 30.2) They are helpful in dissecting RA from other chronic polyarthropathies and are an essential tool in epidemiologic studies. They are of limited utility during early disease, when the pattern of clinical manifestations is often incomplete. For more progressed disease, the diagnosis is no longer difficult, but estimating the extent of disease activity and the rate of progression becomes the most challenging task.

**TABLE 30.2.** *American College of Rheumatology criteria for classification of rheumatoid arthritis*

1. Morning stiffness (lasting at least 1 hour)
2. Arthritis in three or more joint areas (soft tissue swelling or effusion observed by a physician, simultaneous involvement of joint areas: proximal interphalangeal, metacarpophalangeal, wrist, elbow, knee, ankle, metatarpophalangeal)
3. Arthritis of hand joints (swelling of wrist, metacarpophalangeal, proximal interphalangeal—at least one area)
4. Symmetric arthritis (bilateral involvement of joint areas listed in 2)
5. Rheumatoid nodules (subcutaneous nodules observed by a physician)
6. Rheumatoid factors in the serum
7. Radiographic changes (erosions or periarticular unequivocal bony calcification on hand and wrist radiographs)

## Syndrome of Early Rheumatoid Arthritis and Differential Diagnoses

Joint inflammation can occur in many different diseases. If it persists for several weeks and involves several joints, the question arises about whether the patient has developed RA. In early disease, the diagnosis of RA remains presumptive and is a matter of exclusion. In distinguishing RA from other syndromes, a multitude of findings are considered. Features suggesting the diagnosis of RA include:

- pain and swelling in the wrist, metacarpophalangeal (MCP), proximal interphalangeal (PIP), or metatarsophalangeal (MTP) joints;
- association with morning stiffness;
- loss of grip strength;
- systemic symptoms such as malaise, fatigue, or low-grade fever;
- lack of evidence for a connective tissue disease;
- anemia, slight leukocytosis, or thrombocytopenia;
- elevated erythrocyte sedimentation rate (ESR);
- lack of evidence for gout;
- demonstration of rheumatoid factors; and
- joint fluid analysis compatible with RA. It is important to realize that many of these parameters can be normal and can vary widely in individual patients.

Because synovial inflammation, even in a symmetric distribution, is a nonspecific finding, the list of differential diagnoses is extensive. A summary of polyarticular syndromes that have to be distinguished from RA early in the disease course is given in Table 30.3.

## Progressive Rheumatoid Arthritis and Complications

With the lack of a pathognomonic test for establishing the diagnosis of RA, it can be expected that some patients may have a self-limited course or may change diagnosis eventually. Whether true long-term remissions of RA exist and how frequent they are remain unresolved issues. A patient with a 1-year history of chronic synovitis probably will not experience a spontaneous resolution and should be prepared for a chronic course. A subset of RA patients may have episodes of active disease alternating with periods of clinical silence. Between 50% and 70% of affected individuals have progressive RA with a high likelihood of tissue destruction. The extent of resulting disability and the rate of disease progression vary considerably. The heterogeneity of patients in respect to the rate of disease progression and the aggressiveness of the inflammatory process is the most difficult problem in clinical management. No diagnostic tests are available to help in assigning a patient to a prognostic category and permit a rational choice of therapy. The best data are available for HLA-DRB1 allelic polymorphisms. Certain allelic combinations of HLA-DRB1 genes have been associated with more severe joint destruction and the development of extraarticular complications, and these are being explored as potential prognostic markers for clinical use.

**TABLE 30.3.** *Differential diagnosis of early synovitis*

- Fibromyalgia
- Crystal-induced synovitis (e.g., gout, calcium pyrophosphate dihydrate deposition disease)
- Connective tissue disease (e.g., systemic lupus erythematosus, scleroderma, mixed connective disease, inflammatory myopathies)
- Seronegative spondyloarthropathies (e.g., ankylosing spondylitis, Reiter's syndrome, reactive arthritis, psoriatic arthritis, enteropathic arthritis, Whipple's disease)
- Infectious arthritis and infection-associated arthritides (e.g., bacterial infection, Lyme disease, viral infections, associated synovitis [rubella, hepatitis, hepatitis C], bacterial endocarditis, human immunodeficiency virus infection)
- Vasculitis (e.g., Behçet's syndrome, Wegener's granulomatosis, Churg–Strauss syndrome, cryoglobulinemia, polychondritis)
- Osteoarthritis
- Polymyalgia rheumatica or giant cell arteritis
- Malignancies (e.g., lymphoma, hairy cell leukemia)
- Rare conditions (e.g., amyloidosis, congenital arthropathy, hypertrophic osteoarthropathy, hypereosinophilic syndrome, multicentric reticulohistiocytosis, Sweet's syndrome, pigmented villonodular synovitis)
- Arthritis of thyroid disease
- Calcific periarthritis
- Familial Mediterranean fever
- Withdrawal of corticosteroids
- Hemochromatosis
- Hemophilia
- Hyperlipoproteinemia
- Rheumatic fever
- Sarcoidosis

The common denominator of progressive RA is the destruction of ligaments, tendons, cartilage, bone, and other structures attacked by the disease. The effects and consequences vary with the anatomic region involved. The complications of established RA are therefore best described by a regional approach.

### Cervical Spine

The atlantoaxial joint is a preferred target of RA, potentially leading to serious clinical complications and mortality. As a result of destruction of bony structures and ligaments, anterior, posterior, and vertical subluxation of the atlas in relation to the axis can occur. Affected patients complain about severe neck pain with occipital radiation. They may develop slowly progressive quadriparesis with painless sensory loss in the hands. Vertical penetration of the dens can produce episodes of medullary dysfunction that are often associated with paresthesia in the shoulders or arms.

Magnetic resonance imaging (MRI) is the diagnostic test of choice and can clearly delineate the relationship between the spinal cord, the odontoid peg, the atlas, and the ligaments. Operative stabilization and craniocervical decompression may be necessary but may not relieve all symptoms. The subaxial cervical spine can also be affected with osteochondral destruction of discovertebral joints, causing subluxation with resulting pain and neurologic symptoms.

## Shoulders

Rheumatoid shoulder disease mostly is related to structural damage of the glenohumeral joint, the distal end of the clavicle, and the rotator cuff. Rotator cuff tears occur and lead to severe pain and loss of shoulder mobility. MRI is superior to other imaging modalities in assessing destruction of bones and soft tissues.

## Elbows

Loss of elbow extension is often found on clinical examination. Significant disability develops with instability of the elbow combined with shoulder, elbow, and wrist disease. Such patients have difficulty feeding and grooming themselves. Only recently has total elbow replacement emerged as a possible treatment option. Synovectomy is a reasonable choice in patients with refractory elbow disease.

## Hand and Wrist

Most activities of human beings, including the tasks of daily living, depend on the use of the hands. Loss of hand function produces profound disability. Synovitis in multiple joints of the hand and involvement of the wrist is an early and consistent finding in RA. Chronic inflammation in the MCP and PIP joints and the tendon sheets leads to typical deformities that cause much of the disability in RA patients. Ulnar deviation of the phalanges, swan-neck deformities (i.e., flexion of the distal interphalangeal [DIP] and MCP joint, hyperextension of the PIP joint), and boutonnière deformities (i.e., PIP flexion, DIP hyperextension) limit the ability to close a fist, reduce pinch function, and produce loss of strength (Fig. 30.3).

Multiple pathomechanisms are suspected to act in synergy in causing weakness of the hands. Tenosynovitis of the extensor and flexor tendon sheets document that RA is not solely

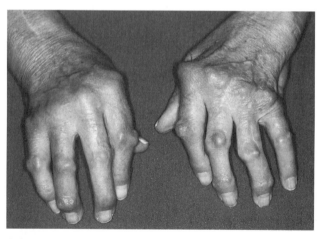

**FIG. 30.3.** Hand deformities in rheumatoid arthritis include metacarpophalangeal joint proliferative synovitis with subcutaneous tissue and muscle atrophy. There is mild ulnar deviation of the metacarpophalangeal joints, mostly of the right (dominant) hand.

a disease of joints but that it can also manifest in the synovial membrane. Tendon ruptures contribute significantly to the loss of hand function, and their prevention is an important therapeutic goal. Carpal tunnel syndrome, resulting from local pressure by the hyperplastic and edematous synovium, can be an early sign of RA and can precede clinically detectable joint disease.

## Hip

Large joint involvement is typically seen in more progressed and late disease. Cystic lesions in the femoral head, protrusion of the acetabulum, and avascular necrosis represent complications of recurrent synovitis and corticosteroid therapy.

## Knee

Knee involvement is easily detected clinically, and the knee joint is a readily accessible source of synovial fluid for diagnostic purposes. Functional consequences of persistent inflammation include extension deficit and eventually the inability to walk because of severe knee joint destruction. Recurrent synovitis can produce a popliteal or Baker's cyst. Recognition of this complication is important because rupture of these cysts with penetration of the inflamed fluid into the soft tissue of the calf causes swelling and tenderness of the lower extremity, reminiscent of acute thrombophlebitis. Ultrasound imaging is a fast and cost-effective technique to demonstrate popliteal cysts and their extension into the calf muscles.

## Ankle and Foot

Rheumatoid foot deformities include subluxation of the metatarsal heads, producing "cocking-up" of the toes. Severe and progressive RA is often complicated by the additional involvement of several compartments of the ankle joint. Destruction of the subtalar joint results in eversion of the foot with pain when walking barefoot. Tarsal tunnel syndrome can add to foot pain and difficulties with walking.

## Extraarticular Complications of Rheumatoid Arthritis

Despite a preference for the synovial membrane, RA should not be understood as a syndrome limited to the joint. Extraarticular manifestations affect an important subset of patients and are associated with a high risk of morbidity and mortality (Table 30.4). Extraarticular disease is unlikely merely a consequence of severe joint disease. Several studies have supported the concept that articular and extraarticular RA represent different dimensions of disease with shared but also unique pathomechanisms. Several organ systems can be affected by rheumatoid disease. With the diversity of target tissue structures, a broad spectrum of clinical symptoms and complications emerges.

**TABLE 30.4.** *Extraarticular manifestations of rheumatoid arthritis*

| Organ system | Manifestation |
|---|---|
| General | Rheumatoid nodule formation |
| Blood vessels | Arteritis of visceral medium-sized vessels |
| | Distal gangrene |
| | Nonhealing ulcerations |
| | Neurovascular disease (mononeuritis multiplex, peripheral neuropathy, CNS vasculitis) |
| | Coronary arteritis |
| | Palpable purpura |
| Cardiac involvement | Pericarditis |
| | Myocarditis |
| | Endocarditis |
| | Conduction defects |
| Eye | Scleritis and episcleritis |
| Hematologic disease | Anemia |
| | Large granular lymphocyte syndrome |
| | Felty's syndrome |
| Muscles | Myositis |
| Pulmonary involvement | Pleurisy |
| | Nodular lung disease |
| | Interstitial fibrosis |
| | Bronchiolitis |
| | Small airway disease (?) |
| Renal involvement | Necrotizing glomerulonephritis |
| | Amyloidosis |
| Salivary glands | Sicca syndrome |
| Skeleton | Diffuse bone loss (?) |

### Rheumatoid Nodules

About one third of all RA patients experiences the formation of rheumatoid nodules that accumulate on extensor surfaces but can evolve in most tissues. Histomorphologically, they represent granulomas with central necrosis surrounded by a palisade of histiocytes. Peripheral to the corona of activated cells, an infiltrate of lymphocytes and macrophages is frequently arranged in a perivascular distribution. The granulomatous reaction leading to the formation of nodules has been considered to indicate more aggressive disease. Nodule formation occurs in the subset of patients producing rheumatoid factors, and genetically, rheumatoid nodules have been associated with the inheritance of a double dose of MHC-risk genes.

### Sicca Syndrome

Secondary Sjögren's syndrome usually develops in patients with rheumatoid factor–positive disease. Clinical manifestations include dryness of the eyes combined with a foreign-body sensation and possibly with keratoconjunctivitis. Xerostomia leads to dysphagia and increased caries and periodontal disease. Diagnostic testing is based on the demonstration of diminished tear and saliva production and can be complemented by salivary gland biopsy. The RA-associated

sicca syndrome has to be distinguished from primary Sjögren's syndrome, which has characteristic autoantibodies, anti-Ro (SSA) and anti-La (SSB) antibodies. There is a strong preference for female RA patients to develop secondary sicca syndrome (15).

### Rheumatoid Eye Disease

Besides keratoconjunctivitis and sicca, RA can cause serious eye pathology. Inflammation of the connective tissue component of the sclera produces scleritis and episcleritis. A late complication is scleromalacia perforans, with destruction of the sclera down to the uveal tissue layers. The leading clinical symptom is intense ocular pain.

### Rheumatoid Pulmonary Disease

Pleurisy, sometimes combined with effusions, is the most frequent form of pulmonary involvement and affects more than 70% of RA patients. Clinical presentation is dominated by pleuritic chest pain. The exudate is characterized by low glucose concentrations. Clinically more significant is interstitial pneumonitis resulting in fibrosis (Fig. 30.4). Chest radiographs demonstrate bilateral diffuse interstitial pattering. Pulmonary function testing reveals a decrease in diffusion capacity. Interstitial fibrosis is predominantly a complication in male patients (15) and is possibly aggravated by smoking. High-resolution computed tomography (CT) is helpful in

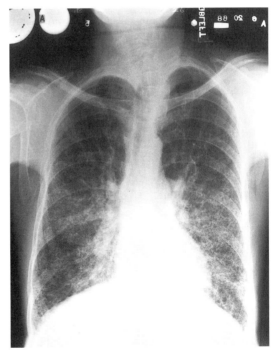

**FIG. 30.4.** Rheumatoid lung disease. Bilateral interstitial fibrosis involves the lower lung fields. The radiographic findings of rheumatoid lung disease are similar to those for idiopathic fibrosis.

judging disease activity. It is not entirely clear whether interstitial pneumonitis is a risk factor for methotrexate-related pulmonary toxicity. Pneumonitis can progress to alveolar involvement and bronchiolitis. These patients are threatened by respiratory insufficiency with fatal outcome.

The lung is a preferred tissue for rheumatoid nodule formation. Single lesions can be difficult to distinguish from bronchiogenic carcinoma. Clusters of pulmonary nodules may appear. Whether airway disease with reduced expiratory flow rate is a manifestation of RA remains unresolved. Arteritis may, in rare cases, affect the pulmonary vascular tree.

### Rheumatoid Renal Disease

In contrast to other connective tissue diseases, the kidney is rarely targeted by RA. Most renal complications are related to drug toxicity, such as the use of nonsteroidal antiinflammatory drugs (NSAIDs). D-Penicillamine and gold salts can cause a membranous nephropathy. Necrotizing glomerulitis is only found in patients with widespread arteritis.

### Rheumatoid Heart Disease

RA can also manifest in the pericardial lining. Pericarditis has been frequently reported in autopsy studies. Clinically relevant disease with impairment of left ventricular function is a complication of seropositive severe disease. Involvement of the myocardial muscles can produce myocarditis in an interstitial or granulomatous form. Conduction defects have been described and are likely related to granuloma formation. Endocardial inflammation and valvular disease may occur but are rare. The most significant cardiac complication is coronary arteritis in patients with rheumatoid vasculitis who develop acute coronary syndromes.

### Felty's Syndrome

The triad of seropositive RA, neutropenia, and splenomegaly establishes the diagnosis of Felty's syndrome. Anemia and thrombocytopenia may be present. The spleen is not always enlarged. A major concern is the increased susceptibility of these patients to infections. Patients with Felty's syndrome often have quiescent joint disease but advanced rheumatoid deformities documenting a history of aggressive disease. Many patients with Felty's syndrome have additional manifestations of rheumatoid organ involvement, particularly nodule formation and rheumatoid vasculitis.

Splenectomy cannot correct neutropenia in all patients and often has only a transient benefit. Multiple pathomechanisms, such as production of antineutrophil antibodies, splenic sequestration, and defective production of granulocytes are suspected to play a role. Neutropenic patients with infections may require granulocyte colony-simulating factor therapy.

It is not completely understood whether Felty's syndrome can be distinguished from large granular lymphocyte (LGL) syndrome with RA or both syndromes are related (59). LGLs represent oligoclonal populations of CD16$^+$CD56$^+$ natural killer cells or of CD8$^+$CD57$^+$ T cells. They infiltrate the bone marrow, and their expansion is associated with neutropenia and recurrent infections. Progression to leukemia is possible but infrequent.

### Rheumatoid Vasculitis

Rheumatoid disease manifesting as vasculitis is the quintessential form of extraarticular RA. Rheumatoid vasculitis is an inflammatory vasculopathy that affects small and medium-sized arteries. Histomorphology demonstrates perivascular inflammatory infiltrates in mild cases and fibrinoid necrosis of blood vessel walls in more severe forms. The consequences of vascular inflammation depend on the size, the site, and the extent of blood vessel involvement. Focal inflammatory lesions producing aneurysms and arterial rupture are unusual. Rather, segmental lesions affecting the entire circumference of the artery induce an arterial injury response pattern characterized by luminal occlusion with end organ infarction. Neither nature of the inflammatory lesions is well understood, nor is any information available on the preferential targeting of certain vascular beds.

Rheumatoid vasculitis best reflects the systemic nature of RA. However, clinical activity of synovitis and of extraarticular disease often do not correlate. Relatively mild symptoms of joint inflammation do not exclude active rheumatoid vasculitis. Vasculitis most frequently manifests in patients in whom the joint component is no longer the major clinical challenge. Usually, in these patients, RA has left its imprint in the form of marked deformities and production of high titers of rheumatoid factor.

Palpable purpura is a consequence of small vessel disease and generally does not pose any major clinical problems. Additional involvement of arterioles and small muscular arteries results in impaired perfusion of vital organs. The spectrum of clinical manifestations ranges from digital arteritis with gangrene of distal fingers and toes to visceral lesions. Cutaneous ulcerations manifesting with a pyoderma gangrenosum-like picture have a tendency to occur on the lower extremities. Nonhealing leg ulcers in patients with RA suggest underlying rheumatoid vasculitis but may be difficult to distinguish from atherosclerotic ulcers (Fig. 30.5). Inflammatory and noninflammatory mechanisms may function in a synergistic fashion. In most patients, therapeutic management of RA is required to permit healing. Immunodeficiency of RA patients, partially attributable to the underlying autoimmune disease and partially related to therapy, creates heightened susceptibility for infection, with the risk of systemic spreading and death.

Another preferred target for rheumatoid vasculitis is the neurovascular system. Arteritis takes the form of a distal sensory neuropathy or mononeuritis multiplex. Clinical symptoms of the distal sensory neuropathy are burning and painful feet, more so at night when the patient goes to bed. Mononeuritis multiplex is characterized by motor and sensory defi-

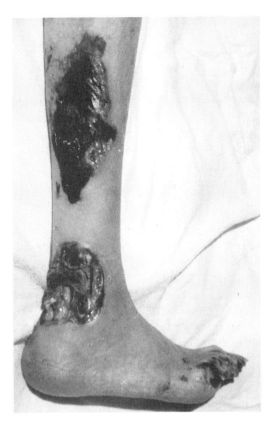

**FIG. 30.5.** Leg ulcers in rheumatoid vasculitis. The photograph shows the lower legs of a man with long-standing rheumatoid arthritis and high-titer rheumatoid factors. The extensive skin ulceration and the gangrenous toes are typical features of rheumatoid vasculitis.

ciencies identical to that seen in other vasculitides. Rheumatoid vasculitis can be detected in nerve biopsies. Central nervous system vasculitis in patients with RA is distinctly rare and identifies patients with the most severe course of the disease. It is believed that the underlying pathology is a small vessel vasculitis. Organic brain syndrome is the typical clinical picture in these individuals. Neurologic defects related to spinal cord involvement are seen in patients with rheumatoid pachymeningitis.

Case reports document that rheumatoid arteritis can essentially affect any organ system. As a general rule, the larger the affected blood vessel the poorer the prognosis. Mesenteric vasculitis with bowel infarction is a severe complication and needs to be considered in patients with long-standing advanced disease presenting with abdominal pain.

## Diagnostic Testing

RA is primarily a clinical diagnosis. A set of criteria has been developed and tested (57). These criteria stress the chronicity of joint inflammation, the symmetry of involvement, the dominance of manifestations in the wrists and hands, and the combination of polyarthritis with stiffness. Measuring of autoantibodies adds an important aspect to the diagnosis and

is helpful in distinguishing RA from other autoimmune syndromes. Because RA manifests primarily in the diarthrodial joints, imaging has a significant role in establishing the diagnosis and following the progression of the disease.

### Radiographic Imaging

The biologic end point of rheumatoid joint disease is the destruction of ligaments, cartilage, and bone. Assessment of these components can be achieved by different means. Radiographs of involved joints can demonstrate bony destruction. The major limitation of x-ray analysis is the insensitivity of this technique to alterations that have not affected bony structures. Standard x-ray techniques cannot image articular cartilage, muscles, tendons, and the medullary compartments of bone. Rheumatoid disease of these components can only be diagnosed indirectly. The presence of bony erosions indicates a disease process that must have been present for several months, if not years (Fig. 30.6). Similarly, bony destruction may progress despite successful suppression of the inflammatory reaction, limiting the use of standard radiographs in assessing disease progression.

Radiographic findings in RA include periarticular soft tissue swelling, osteopenia in a periarticular but later in a more diffuse distribution, marginal erosions produced by the invasion of the bone by pannus, and eventually cyst formation. All of these changes occur in the absence of healing reactions associated with bone repair. In early RA, radiographs of affected joints may be negative or may only show periarticular soft tissue swelling. With progression of the disease, joint space is lost and juxtaarticular osteoporosis develops. Early erosions are seen as a breakdown in the continuity of the cor-

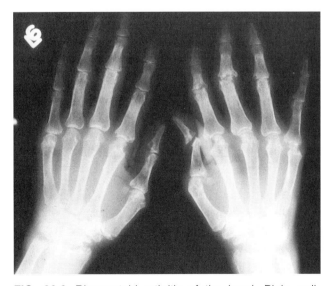

**FIG. 30.6.** Rheumatoid arthritis of the hand. Plain radiographs show diffuse osteopenia; severe erosive changes of the distal radioulnar, wrist, and intercarpal joints; and typical marginal erosions of the metacarpophalangeal and proximal interphalangeal joints.

tical line. Malalignment and subluxation strongly suggest more advanced disease.

The distribution of RA changes are also helpful in radiologic diagnosis. Almost all patients have symmetric involvement of the hands and wrists. Posteroanterior views of the hands are therefore often used to search for RA-suggestive changes. Standard posteroanterior films should be complemented by supinated-oblique views, which may be superior in demonstrating subtle erosions of the base of the proximal phalanges. Erosions of the ulnar styloid on wrist radiographs are considered to represent early changes. In more advanced disease, large subchondral erosions appear (Fig. 30.6). Metacarpal joints display ulnar drift. Subluxations of the phalanges produce swan-neck and boutonnière deformities. In general, all compartments of the wrist joints are affected and eventually bony ankylosis may occur.

The feet are involved by disease in most RA patients, and foot disease may precede hand involvement. Juxtaarticular osteoporosis and erosive destruction of the heads of the metatarsal bones are typical findings.

Rheumatoid knee disease is characterized by the loss of cartilage thickness that is best appreciated by x-ray analysis of the standing patient. The lack of new bone formation can be helpful in distinguishing RA from osteoarthritic disease, although a combination of rheumatoid knee destruction superimposed on mechanical damage is not rare. Involvement of the hip is a late event in RA. Radiographs can demonstrate the uniform loss of cartilage and the erosion of the acetabulum. Acetabular protrusion, diagnosed when the acetabular line is medial to the ilioischial line by more than 3 mm in males and more than 6 mm in females, is one of the manifestations of rheumatoid hip disease. Erosive changes of the femoral head are found at the margin between the cartilage and the bone. In contrast to osteoarthritis hip disease, RA is not associated with the formation of osteophytes or subchondral bone.

Imaging of the shoulder can demonstrate erosive changes of the humoral head, often localized in the superior lateral region adjacent to the greater tuberosity. Synovial cysts may form in the humoral head. The distal end of the clavicle is another site where bony erosions frequently occur. As a result of advanced rheumatoid synovitis, the glenohumeral joint space becomes narrowed, and the humoral head migrates medially. Upward migration of the humoral head is produced by associated rotator cuff disease.

The axial skeleton is usually spared in RA, with the exception of the cervical spine, which is involved in more than 60% of patients. Rheumatoid disease of the occipital atlantoaxial joint is of clinical relevance, because it is frequently associated with cervical myelopathy. The subaxial parts of the cervical spine are also targeted by the disease, with manifestations relating to the synovial and cartilaginous joints, the tendons, and the ligaments critical in spinal integrity. Lateral views of the cervical spine are used to demonstrate subluxations, often beginning at the C-4 level, disk destruction, and

disease of the apophyseal joints. RA of the occipital atlantoaxial joint can produce atlantoaxial subluxation with laxity or even rupture of the transverse ligament. This can be visualized on flexed lateral views of the cervical spine. Vertical subluxation progressing to vertical translocation at the C1–2 level is another complication of RA. Standard radiographs are of limited value. To delineate the exact anatomic relationships of the structures of the occipital atlantoaxial joint, MRI imaging is considered to be superior.

### Magnetic Resonance Imaging

The ability to visualize cartilage, synovial tissue, tendons, and bone marrow in addition to the bony structures qualifies MRI as the optimal technology to document rheumatoid synovitis and its consequences in affected joints and paraarticular areas. Technical difficulties and cost have prevented the routine use of MRI so far, but an increasing number of studies are beginning to demonstrate that the use of this imaging technique may be justified in selected critical scenarios. Analysis of intraarticular structures, which are invisible to conventional radiographs, could be an important aspect in early RA. It is believed that most of the joint destruction occurs in the first 2 years of disease. However, the biologic end point, the erosion of bone, consistently lags behind. This dilemma has complicated the early and aggressive management of rheumatoid synovitis. MRI demonstration of rheumatoid inflammation in the nonbony components of the joints and higher sensitivity for bony lesions could be important for the assessment of early disease. MRI can provide quantitative estimates of the amount of synovitis, a necessary tool for following treatment responses.

Because of the ability to image more than just bony structures, MRI has become the technique of choice for selected clinical problems. MRI is highly sensitive in detecting insufficiency fractures and osteonecrosis. Osteonecrosis can complicate corticosteroid treatment and, in its early stages, is often not visualized by conventional radiographs. MRI has also been recommended as the optimal approach in evaluating rotator cuff destruction. MRI has emerged as the modality of choice for the assessment of cervical spine disease.

### Ultrasound

Ultrasound evaluation has been widely used in Europe to identify effusions and to demonstrate increased mass of inflamed tendons, ligaments, and synovial membrane. It has replaced other techniques to image synovial cysts of the knee joints. Ultrasound can confirm the presence of popliteal cysts and delineate the extent to which they have dissected into the calf muscles.

### Laboratory Testing

Laboratory testing is helpful in establishing the diagnosis of RA and in monitoring disease activity as patients progress and undergo treatment. There is no pathognomonic laboratory abnormality that allows for an unequivocal diagnosis of RA. Demonstration of autoantibodies can confirm an ongoing autoimmune process in a patient with clinical signs of synovial inflammation. The systemic nature of RA is best reflected by an upregulated acute-phase response that can be useful in following patients longitudinally. Rheumatology has not made optimal use of quantifying the inflammatory reaction in the joint or the destruction of cartilage by measuring the release of mediators or destruction products in the blood. As more information accumulates on the genetics of RA, an important place for genetic testing can be foreseen in categorizing patients into subsets with different response pattern to therapeutic intervention.

### Autoantibodies

Demonstration of rheumatoid factor remains a critical component in the establishment of the diagnosis. Production of anti-IgG Fc autoantibodies distinguishes the patient with RA from other connective tissue diseases. A high titer of rheumatoid factor is believed to be associated with a poor prognosis and an increased risk for developing extraarticular manifestations. Monitoring rheumatoid factor has not been helpful in following disease activity, probably reflecting the persistence of an underlying abnormal immune response despite successful suppression of synovial inflammation. In evaluating a patient with short-term signs and symptoms of synovitis, the demonstration of rheumatoid factor in the blood provides important information for diagnosis.

Rheumatoid factors are not unique to RA; they also occur in other autoimmune diseases such as systemic lupus erythematosus, scleroderma, mixed connective tissue disease, and primary Sjögren's syndrome. Rheumatoid factor may also indicate chronic infections and hematologic malignancies. Low-titer rheumatoid factor can be found in healthy elderly individuals.

Two other autoantibodies may be highly specific for RA. Antikeratin antibodies and antiperinuclear factors are found in most RA patients, but they do not necessarily correlate with the presence of rheumatoid factor. Antikeratin antibodies are demonstrated by their ability to bind to the stratum corneum of rat esophagus epithelium. They react to filagrin, a filament associated protein with a role in the aggregation of cytokeratin filaments. Antiperinuclear factors probably bind to an identical or closely related autoantigen. They are found by staining human buccal mucosa cells, where autoantibodies bind to profilagrin contained in keratohyalin granules.

### Acute-Phase Reactants

In response to tissue injury, the body produces an acute-phase response with the upregulation of a series of proteins synthesized in the liver, including C-reactive protein, fibrinogen, and serum amyloid A. The synthesis of these acute phase proteins is regulated by cytokines, particularly IL-6, which is induced by many other proinflammatory mediators. A downstream effect of increased acute-phase protein production is an alteration of the plasma viscosity and erythrocyte motion. This is measured as an increased erythrocyte sedimentation rate (ESR). The ESR can be obtained easily and cost effectively, making this a clinically useful indicator of acute phase response. In RA, marked elevations of ESR and C-reactive protein have been reported to predict severe and erosive disease. However, the monitoring of the acute-phase response has not developed into a reliable tool in assessing treatment responses.

It can be predicted that many other markers, such as cytokines and soluble cytokine receptors, are released as a chronic immune response progresses. Data on the clinical utility of such markers compared with cheap and easy measures of increased acute-phase reaction are not available.

### Markers of Increased Connective Tissue Turnover

The longitudinal assessment of patients while undergoing therapy remains a challenge in the practice of rheumatologists. Radiographic studies are limited by their insensitivity to acute changes and the lag period between inflammation and bony destruction. It would be desirable to quantify disease activity by measuring the increased turnover of connective tissue in the joint. Multiple components of cartilage have been evaluated as possible indicators of disease activity (59). The issue is complicated by the concomitant occurrence of cartilage breakdown and repair. Active disease and healing are associated with an increased turnover. Patients with rapidly progressive erosive RA have been reported to have markedly increased levels of cartilage oligomeric protein (COMP), and it has been suggested that COMP could be a sensitive indicator of persistent synovitis (60).

## TREATMENT

RA is an incurable disease. If joint inflammation has persisted for a year, the chances of a spontaneous remission are minimal. However, the disease may take a remitting course with extended periods of minimal disease activity. Overall, the destructive power of this disease is determined by the intensity of the inflammatory response and its chronicity.

When developing a treatment plan for a patient with RA, it is important to recognize several unique features in managing this chronic progressive and destructive disorder. The patient needs to understand that there does not exist a single therapeutic intervention that can cure RA. Joint destruction starts early in the disease course, definitely before objective documentation of the underlying disease process can be obtained. After radiographs demonstrate typical bony erosions, these changes are irreversible, and after clinical examination reveals rheumatoid deformities or extraarticular manifestations, the disease has already caused substantial damage. Much progress in the management of RA patients has come from the realization that irreversible loss of articular cartilage begins early. Traditional management, including awaiting unequivocal signs of RA, necessarily missed the chance to prevent tissue destruction in the early phases of RA. It used to be standard to treat "behind" the disease. Recent years have seen a shift in therapy with the initiation of second-line agents as soon as possible, optimally within the first few months after the onset of synovitis. The concept to treat early and aggressively is widely accepted. With this concept, several aspects of RA management have gained importance:

1. How can we identify patients who are prone to experience a rapidly progressive course of RA? How can we predict which patients will develop extraarticular manifestations which account to a large degree for the mortality of the disease? Genetic markers that are independent from disease activity hold the greatest promise to be helpful in prognostic stratification of RA patients. Specifically, the inheritance of two RA-associated HLA-DRB1 alleles has been shown in retrospective studies to be strongly correlated with more severe disease. Homozygosity for HLA-DRB1*0401 has been found to accumulate in patients with rheumatoid vasculitis.

2. How reliable are clinical markers of disease activity? Can we use them to titrate medications? This aspect of RA management definitely needs further research. Acute-phase reactants and assays of functional impairment, such as the Health Assessment Questionnaire, are used but are rather limited instruments for guiding adjustments of second-line agents (61).

3. A series of drugs is available to suppress disease activity in RA. These drugs vary in their potency to slow the rate of progression associated with irreversible tissue damage. All of these drugs can cause toxicity, which is particularly important, because they need to be used over a long period. Complications of therapy are a major issue in the management of RA and are responsible for morbidity, mortality, and for reduction in life quality.

The emerging principles of treating RA are to begin therapy with a second-line agent as early as possible, to be aware of the potential side effects of the medications used, to educate the patient about the nature of the disease and the potential complications of therapy, and to assemble a team of specialist early in the disease course to monitor the progress. Experience shows that there are few generalizable principles in prescribing drugs with the potential to downregulate RA activity. To some extent, a treatment plan is individualized for each patient and has to be adapted to the speed of the disease. A comprehensive treatment plan should include a rheumatologist, an orthopedic surgeon, and a specialist experienced in occupational and physical therapy. Surgical interventions should not be considered for advanced patients only. Total joint replacements have introduced an extraordinary advance in the management of patients with end-stage joint destruction and have added a new dimension to the treatment of RA. Arthroscopic surgery and open synovectomy may have a place before irreversible joint destruction has

occurred, particularly in efforts aimed at preventing tendon ruptures in selected areas.

Treatment of RA should not be limited to pharmacologic and surgical modalities. Intensive research has demonstrated that the involvement of the patient in the design of the treatment plan is critical and that psychologic aspects of coping have an important role. Learned helplessness has been identified as a potential impediment to successful management. Thorough education about the disease, the treatment, and the adaptation to pain and functional limitations has had beneficial effects. Careful instructions in modalities of pain control, rest, exercise, and joint protection principles should be an integral part of the treatment of RA.

Choosing a pharmacologic management for RA requires the definition of goals that can be realistically achieved. In general, disease remission cannot be induced. Attainable goals include alleviating pain, slowing or arresting the progression of structural damage, preserving function, minimizing side effects, and maximizing the overall quality of life. The physician and patient need to be aware of the cost-benefit ratio for each of the therapeutic modalities applied. The stage of the disease influences the choice of treatment. After structural damage has occurred, emphasis must be put on restoring joint motion and strength. At a certain point of advanced disease, the risk associated with treatment may not be justified by the small gain, and joint replacement may be the better line of action.

## Nonsteroidal Antiinflammatory Drugs

NSAIDs are a mainstay in treating patients with inflammatory polyarthritis. They are widely used for all types of joint-related pain syndromes and are among the most prescribed medications. Their fast mode of action allows for their use for pain relief and for reducing the inflammatory response in the synovial membrane. Despite their antiinflammatory action, NSAIDs are not believed to function as a disease modifier. The synovial lesions persist and progress, and alternative therapies have to be added to influence the underlying disease process.

The therapeutic benefit of NSAIDs is sometimes accompanied by a variety of life-threatening side effects. Although there is little doubt that aspirin is effective in treating RA, the high rate of gastrointestinal side effects has led to the use of alternative NSAIDs. A long list of choices is available for clinical use. The mechanisms of action of these different NSAIDs are probably relatively similar. Plasma half-lives are different, affecting the dosing regimen. There is some indication that toxicity may vary, with salsalate having the lowest toxicity index score and indomethacin being associated with the highest toxicity index score.

The therapeutic benefits and side effects of NSAIDs are directly related to their ability to inhibit prostaglandin synthesis. Although this action reduces the inflammatory pathways in the synovial lesions, it simultaneously inhibits the production of prostaglandin $E_2$ in the gastric mucosa, leading to the most significant clinical side effects. Reduction in prostaglandin synthesis is also suspected to underlie the adverse effects in renal function. In patients with impaired renal function, the decrease in glomerular filtration rate can become relevant. Acute ischemic renal insufficiency is a feared complication of NSAID use. Acute interstitial nephritis is rare and is more likely to occur in older patients. Analgesic nephropathy is suspected to result from chronic diminishment of renal blood flow affecting the medulla. Other adverse effects include increased risk of bleeding because of alterations in platelet function.

Gastrointestinal pathology induced by NSAID use is the most frequent cause of drug-related death. Major efforts have been made to identify predisposing factors. The following parameters have been associated with increased likelihood of developing gastrointestinal side effects: age, history of previous NSAID-induced gastrointestinal side effects, disability index, NSAID dose, and concurrent use of prednisone (62). Several lines of action have been taken to minimize NSAID-associated mucosal lesions. Misoprostol, a prostaglandin E analogue, appears to be able to prevent NSAID-induced gastric ulcers, and its concomitant use may be cost effective (63). New impulses have come from the introduction of a novel class of NSAIDs designed to predominantly target cyclooxygenase-2 (64). This new class of drugs spares gastric and renal prostaglandin synthesis.

## Corticosteroids

The observation by Hench et al. that glucocorticoids suppressed disease activity in RA was a quantum leap in the therapeutic management of this disease. Corticosteroids, although associated with serious side effects, continue to hold the position of a major therapy in RA. The recognition that a natural hormone had a place in regulating inflammation created the clinical category of "steroid-responsive" diseases and supported the autoimmune hypothesis in RA pathogenesis.

Systemic corticosteroids have a fast and reliable effect in downregulating the inflammatory process in RA. They are the only therapeutic agent that can be used in cases where time is limited and an immediate effect is warranted. This scenario applies to the management of patients with life-threatening complications of the disease such as vasculitis, coronary arteritis, and rapidly progressive lung disease. Constitutional symptoms of RA, such as fever, respond within hours. When treating acutely ill RA patients, doses of 40 to 80 mg of prednisone per day are recommended. Glucocorticoid-mediated suppression of rheumatoid disease is usually not complete, but some degree of inflammation persists.

A short course of high-dose prednisone may be required to control acute disease flares associated with massive and disabling polyarthritis. Lower doses are usually given to treat less acute presentations. Doses of 10 mg of prednisone per day are efficacious in reducing synovitis and other disease manifestations. Surprisingly, small doses of prednisone, such

as 3 to 4 mg/day have a quite significant clinical effect and can be essential in improving overall life quality for the patient.

Corticosteroids are rarely given as a single agent but are usually combined with other treatment modalities. One study documented that low doses of prednisone can slow the progression of cartilage and bone destruction (65). Efforts are made to minimize the usage of corticosteroids, mainly because of the well-established toxicity profile associated with these drugs. When given over a prolonged period, corticosteroids can cause a wide spectrum of complications. Steroid myopathy may aggravate the deficit in muscle strengths preexisting in patients with chronic RA. Aseptic necrosis may produce hip or shoulder disease and may necessitate premature joint replacement. Steroid-related bone loss has triggered intense interest in preventing osteoporotic fractures. Steroids may aggravate preexisting problems, because it has been suggested that RA by itself has negative effects on bone mineral density. Several therapeutic interventions are available that can potentially preserve bone in patients treated with corticosteroids.

The American College of Rheumatology has developed and published guidelines for the evaluation of the patients before the institution of therapy and for measures to prevent and treat steroid-induced osteoporosis (66). Unless contraindicated, estrogen replacement therapy has been recommended for menopausal and postmenopausal women. Calcium (1000 mg of elemental calcium per day) should be supplemented and can be combined with vitamin D. Adjunct therapies, such as alendronate, should be considered in patients requiring chronic corticosteroid therapy with a history of osteoporosis and compression fractures.

Cardiovascular and metabolic complications of chronic corticosteroid use have attracted attention. Steroid-induced hyperlipidemia, precipitation of diabetes mellitus, and hypertension can contribute to premature coronary heart disease and may be associated with a high risk of mortality.

Intraarticular injection of corticosteroids is an integral part of managing chronic RA. Depending on the size of the joint, 10 to 40 mg of triamcinolone hexacetonide are injected. The local application of steroids permits the targeting of "problem joints" without increasing the dose of systemic therapy. A preexisting infection must be excluded before proceeding with intrasynovial therapy.

## Second-Line Agents

It is standard practice to provide a combination therapy for patients with early and advanced RA. NSAIDs and corticosteroids should be complemented by a second-line agent. Second-line agents have been demonstrated to be effective in slowing the progression of structural damage. None of these drugs can abolish rheumatoid disease. All of them have adverse effects, particularly so when given chronically (Table 30.5). Long-term studies have established that patients are better off when treated with a second-line agent. The

**TABLE 30.5.** *Effects of second-line agents*

| Drug | Dose | Skin rash | GI intolerance | Mucosal lesions | Bone marrow toxicity | Side effects |
|---|---|---|---|---|---|---|
| Hydroxychloroquine | Initially 400 mg daily, then 200 mg daily | + | + | | | Retinopathy, photosensitivity |
| Gold sodium thiomalate or aurothioglucose | Week 1: 10 mg Week 2: 25 mg, then 50 mg/week (up to 1 g total), then maintenance 50 mg/3–4 weeks | + | | + | + | Nephrotic syndrome, pneumonitis |
| Auranofin | 3–6 mg daily | + | + | | | Diarrhea |
| D-Penicillamine | Initially 125–250 mg daily, increase to 750 mg daily | + | + | + | + | Metallic taste, nephrotic syndrome, myositis, myasthenia gravis, SLE, pemphigus |
| Sulfasalazine | Initially 500 mg daily, then increase to 2,000–3,000 mg daily | + | + | + | + | |
| Azathioprine | Initially 0.5–1 mg/kg daily, then increase to 2.5 mg/kg daily | | + | + | + | |
| Cyclophosphamide | Initially 50–100 mg daily, increase to max of 2.5 mg/kg daily | | + | | + | Gonadal suppression, bladder toxicity, malignancies |
| Methotrexate | 7.5–25 mg PO weekly | | + | + | + | Liver fibrosis, cirrhosis, pneumonitis, EBV-associated lymphoproliferative disease |
| Cyclosporine | Initially 2.5 mg/kg daily | | + | | | Hypertension, nephrotoxicity, gingival hyperplasia, hypertrichosis, neurotoxicity |

EBV, Epstein–Barr virus; SLE, systemic lupus erythematosus; +, adverse effect is elicited.

choice of a particular drug depends on the aggressiveness of the disease, preexisting medical conditions, and the willingness of the patient to accept the associated toxicity risk (67). As a general rule, the exact mechanisms of action of these second-line agents in RA are not understood. They have evolved from empirical studies or were serendipitously found to be beneficial.

### Antimalarial Drugs

Therapy with hydroxychloroquine is initiated at a dose of 400 mg daily and is frequently reduced after 4 to 6 months to 200 mg daily. Benefit can be expected after 4 to 6 months of treatment. This drug is usually well tolerated and is considered to be relatively safe. Ophthalmologic monitoring is recommended to prevent the development of irreversible retinopathy. In clinical practice, hydroxychloroquine is preferred for patients with less aggressive disease.

### Sulfasalazine

The suspicion that RA was caused by bacterial infection led to the development of sulfasalazine by Nana Svartz in 1939 in Sweden. Colon bacteria split the drug into the two compo-

nents, sulfapyridine and 5-aminosalicylic acid. Which of these two metabolites is the therapeutic agent in RA patients is unknown. Therapy is initiated with a daily dose of 500 mg and increased, as tolerated, to a maximum dose of 3,000 mg. Patients with known allergic reactions to sulfa components must be excluded. There is evidence that sulfasalazine is effective within a few weeks in improving pain and joint scores (68).

Gastrointestinal side effects such as nausea and vomiting occur and limit the clinical utility. Avoidance of gastrointestinal side effects by changing the pharmacologic preparation of the drug may widen its use in RA.

### Gold Salts

Several trials have established the therapeutic effectiveness of gold salts. Disadvantages of this second-line agent include the need to inject gold sodium thiomalate and aurothioglucose. Auranofin (3 to 6 mg daily) is given orally but is less effective. Commonly recommended dosages are to start with a single injection of 10 mg to test for sensitivity. One week later, a dose of 25 mg is injected, and subsequently, doses of 25 to 50 mg are given weekly until an accumulative dose of 1 g is reached. Frequency of injections should then be reduced.

Mucocutaneous side effects presenting as mucosal ulcers and skin rashes are disturbing and are the main reason for discontinuing the drug. A nephritic syndrome can develop, and regular monitoring of the urinary sediment is necessary for early detection. Bone marrow toxicity manifests as thrombocytopenia and leukopenia. Rare complications of gold therapy include adult respiratory distress syndrome caused by a pulmonary hypersensitivity reaction, necrotizing enterocolitis, and encephalopathy.

### D-Penicillamine

The development of D-penicillamine followed, to some extent, a rational drug design. Assuming that rheumatoid factors were major mediators of pathology, attempts were made to break the disulfide bonds linking the immunoglobulin chains of rheumatoid factors. A thiol-containing derivative of cysteine, D-penicillamine, was tested for its efficacy in treating RA and was shown to have disease-suppressive effects. To avoid side effects, therapy is started with 125 mg daily and then slowly increased to a maintenance dose of 750 to 1,000 mg/day. D-Penicillamine is mainly used in patients who have failed other second-line agents. It has to be given for several months before therapeutic benefits become measurable. Side effects are partially overlapping with those known for gold salts. A metallic taste can be very disturbing to the patient and can limit the use of this drug. Mucocutaneous lesions occur, and urticarial, macular, and papular eruptions have all been described. Close monitoring for emerging proteinuria is recommended to detect the development of a membranous glomerulonephritis presenting as nephrotic syndrome. Bone marrow suppression with pancytopenia can complicate early or chronic therapy and cell counts have to be checked regularly. Rare side effects of D-penicillamine have the character of autoimmune diseases and may affect different organ systems. Inflammatory myopathy resembling dermatositis or polymyositis, myasthenia gravis, drug-induced systemic lupus erythematosus, and pemphigus are serious complications that may persist over an extended time after discontinuation of D-penicillamine.

### Methotrexate

Methotrexate has gained a unique position among the second-line agents. It is widely used to treat RA and is the first choice of many rheumatologists when initiating long-acting medication. Several features of methotrexate therapy are responsible for the preferred role of this drug. Methotrexate is given orally once per week, it is tolerated well, and there is a tendency for patients to continue taking it over several years. Therapeutic benefits are seen relatively quickly, within a few weeks after the initiation of therapy. Methotrexate is inexpensive and, because of its toxicity profile, can be combined well with other second-line agents.

Advised doses of methotrexate are 7.5 to 20 mg, given as a single weekly dose. A large proportion of patients appears to be able to tolerate this treatment regimen chronically, which is probably one of the factors explaining the wide use of this drug. Multiple trials have shown improvement in inflammation. Encouraging data have come from monitoring of radiographic evidence for structural damage. Radiographic stabilization of erosive disease and a slowing in radiographic progression have been reported (69).

Reasons for discontinuing methotrexate are most frequently related to gastrointestinal side effects, particularly mouth soreness with or without oral ulceration. Daily supplementation of 1 mg of folic acid seems to be able to reduce this side effect without subtracting from the efficacy of the drug (70). Gastrointestinal distress can be approached by switching to injection instead of oral administration. Serious adverse effects include hepatic, pulmonary, and bone marrow toxicity. With widespread use of methotrexate, reliable data have been collected on the risk of liver fibrosis or cirrhosis. Recommendations have been developed for adequate monitoring of hepatic toxicity (71). Provided that patients abstain from alcohol, the risk to develop fibrosis or cirrhosis of the liver is probably small.

Pulmonary complications in patients on methotrexate are essentially unpredictable and can occur at any time in the course of treatment. Methotrexate pneumonitis is diagnosed in individuals who present with acute onset of dyspnea, tachypnea, radiologic evidence of pulmonary infiltrates, and decreased diffusion capacity (72). Fever is a frequent finding, and eosinophilia may be present. Patients starting methotrexate need to be instructed to seek medical evaluation when they experience cough, fever, and flulike symptoms. Methotrexate pneumonitis is believed to represent a hypersensitivity reaction and is appropriately managed with corticosteroids. It has to be differentiated from infectious pneumonitis, particularly infection with *Pneumocystis carinii*. One curious side effect of methotrexate is the induction or worsening of rheumatoid nodules despite suppression of the synovial inflammation (73). The effect of methotrexate on other extraarticular manifestations is less clear.

As with all antiproliferative agents, there is concern that methotrexate may have a role in inducing malignancies. Development of lymphomas, especially those associated with EBV infection, has been described and reversibility of the lymphoma on withdrawal of methotrexate suggests a place of immunosuppression in disease pathogenesis. However, from the available data, it appears that the risk for methotrexate-induced malignancies is small (74).

### Cytotoxic Agents

Because of significant short- and long-term toxicity, cytotoxic agents have to be used with caution in the management of RA. They are usually reserved for patients with aggressive disease, complicated by extraarticular manifestations, who have failed other second-line agents or have a contraindication for taking methotrexate. Azathioprine can serve as a steroid-sparing therapy and has also been shown to improve parameters of disease activity. The major concern related to this drug is bone marrow suppression. When treating with therapeutic doses of 1.5 to 2.0 mg/kg/day, close monitoring is required, and patients should be tested for a possible deficiency of thiopurine methyltransferase, an enzyme critically involved in purine metabolism, before initiation of therapy.

Experience with cyclophosphamide has mainly been collected in patients with other rheumatic diseases, such as aggressive systemic lupus erythematosus, systemic vasculitis, and Wegener's granulomatosis. Under these conditions, cyclophosphamide can be given as intravenous pulse therapy at doses of 750 to 1,000 mg/m². Intravenous application has the advantage that measures of bladder protection can be instituted to lower the cyclophosphamide-associated risk of cystitis and bladder cancer. Intravenous pulsing is a treatment modality that provides rapid and profound immunosuppression if clinically needed. In patients with RA, pulsing is used rarely. Oral doses are usually 2 mg/kg daily. Bone marrow suppression, gonadal suppression, and induction of malignancies are the major complications of cyclophosphamide therapy, indicating that it only has a place in the management of selected patients.

Chlorambucil, an alkylating agent like cyclophosphamide, also remains a reserve drug used only when progressive, destructive disease demands a powerful immunosuppressant and other therapeutic options have failed.

### Cyclosporine

Although RA has been understood as a T-cell–dependent autoimmune disorder, therapeutic interventions targeting T-cell function have not become the mainstay of treatment. This also applies to cyclosporine, a drug that interferes with activation of T lymphocytes and has been highly successful in preventing rejection in organ transplant recipients. Several trials have documented therapeutic efficacy, but the degree of improvement remained relatively minor (75). Renal toxicity proved to be a major problem and triggered interest in low-dose regimens. When given in doses of 5 mg/kg/day, cyclosporin A can retard structural damage of joints. The best use of this drug may lie in combination therapy in which low doses can be used. Patients considered for cyclosporin A treatment should have good renal function and need to be made aware of the toxicity profile of this agent, including gingival hyperplasia, hypertrichosis, and hypertension.

### Biologic Therapy

The central contribution of immunostimulation in the pathogenesis of rheumatoid disease encourages the design of therapeutic strategies aimed at molecules with a key role in the disease lesions (Table 30.6). Increasing knowledge about the function of HLA molecules and their interaction with T-cell receptors has provided the framework for multiple experimental therapies in RA. Cytokines produced in the lesions have become targets for antiinflammatory intervention. A series of antibodies directed against mediators identified in the rheumatoid inflammation and recombinant products

**TABLE 30.6.** *Targeted immunotherapy in rheumatoid arthritis*

- Antibodies against T-cell surface markers (anti-CD5, anti-CD4, Campath-1H, anti-CD7, anti-IL-2 receptor)
- Cytokine-directed therapy (anti-TNF-α, soluble TNF receptor, IL-1RA, soluble IL-1 receptor, anti-IL-6)
- T-cell vaccination
- HLA-DR4–directed therapy
- Oral tolerance induced with type II collagen
- Adhesion molecule–directed therapy

IL, interleukin; RA, receptor agonist; TNF, tumor necrosis factor.

replacing antibodies in disrupting immunostimulation and amplification have been explored for their effects in RA patients (76). For many of these compounds, reduction in disease activity scores have been reported. Insufficient data are available to fully judge the potential of many of these compounds. Most substances tested have not had overwhelming therapeutic benefits. An exception are antibodies specific for tumor necrosis factors (TNFs) and recombinant fusion proteins of TNF-α receptors (77,78). Both approaches target TNF-α, a highly potent proinflammatory cytokine that appears to have a central role in regulating rheumatoid synovitis.

### ACKNOWLEDGMENTS

The authors thank Toni L. Higgins for secretarial assistance and Dr. E. Matteson for generously providing clinical illustrations.

### REFERENCES

1. Short CL. The antiquity of rheumatoid arthritis. *Arthritis Rheum* 1974; 17:193–205.
2. Rothschild BM, Turner KR, DeLuca MA. Symmetrical erosive peripheral polyarthritis in the late Archaic period of Alabama. *Science* 1988;241:1498–1501.
3. Hochberg MC, Spector TD. Epidemiology of rheumatoid arthritis: update. *Epidemiol Rev* 1990;12:242–252.
4. Linos A, Worthington JW, O'Fallon WM, Kurland LT. The epidemiology of rheumatoid arthritis in Rochester, Minnesota: a study of incidence, prevalence and mortality. *Am J Epidemiol* 1980;111:87–98.
5. Chan KW, Felson DT, Yood RA, Walker AM. Incidence of rheumatoid arthritis in central Massachusetts. *Arthritis Rheum* 1993;36:1691–1696.
6. Deighton CM, Roberts DF, Walker DJ. Effect of disease severity on rheumatoid arthritis concordance in same sexed siblings. *Ann Rheum Dis* 1992;51:943–945.
7. Aho K, Koskenvuo M, Tuominen J, Kaprio J. Occurrence of rheumatoid arthritis in a nationwide series of twins. *J Rheumatol* 1986;13: 899–902.
8. Stastny P. Association of the B-cell alloantigen DRw4 with rheumatoid arthritis. *N Engl J Med* 1978;298:869–871.
9. Gregersen PK, Silver J, Winchester RJ. The shared epitope hypothesis. *Arthritis Rheum* 1987;30:1205–1213.
10. Nepom GT, Nepom BS. Prediction of susceptibility to rheumatoid arthritis by human leukocyte antigen genotyping. *Rheum Dis Clin North Am* 1992;18:785–792.
11. Winchester R. The molecular basis of susceptibility to rheumatoid arthritis. *Adv Immunol* 1994;56:389–466.
12. Pincus T, Callahan LF. Formal education as a marker for increased mortality and morbidity in rheumatoid arthritis. *J Chronic Dis* 1985;38: 973–984.

13. Leigh JP, Fries JF. Education level and rheumatoid arthritis: evidence from five data centers. *J Rheumatol* 1991;18:24–34.
14. Silman AJ, Newman J, MacGregor AJ. Cigarette smoking increases the risk of rheumatoid arthritis. *Arthritis Rheum* 1996;39:732–735.
15. Weyand CM, Schmidt D, Wagner U, Goronzy JJ. The influence of sex on the phenotype of rheumatoid arthritis. *Arthritis Rheum* 1998;41: 817–822.
16. Hazes JMW, Dijkmans BAC, Vandenbroucke JP, et al. Pregnancy and the risk of developing rheumatoid arthritis. *Arthritis Rheum* 1990;33: 1770–1775.
17. Wingrave SJ, Kay CR. Reduction in incidence of rheumatoid arthritis associated with oral contraceptives. *Lancet* 1978;1:569–571.
18. Weyand CM, Goronzy JJ. The molecular basis of rheumatoid arthritis. *J Mol Med* 1997;75:772–785.
19. Weyand CM, Goronzy JJ. Pathogenesis of rheumatoid arthritis. *Med Clin North Am* 1997;81:29–55.
20. Harris ED Jr. *Rheumatoid arthritis.* Philadelphia: WB Saunders, 1997.
21. Alspaugh MA, Henle G, Lennette ET, Henle W. Elevated levels of antibodies to Epstein–Barr virus antigens in sera and synovial fluids of patients with rheumatoid arthritis. *J Clin Invest* 1981;67:1134–1140.
22. Roudier J, Petersen J, Rhodes GH, et al. Susceptibility to rheumatoid arthritis maps to a T-cell epitope shared by the HLA-Dw4 DR beta-1 chain and the Epstein–Barr virus glycoprotein gp110. *Proc Natl Acad Sci USA* 1989;86:5104–5108.
23. Scotet E, David-Ameline J, Peyrat MA, et al. T cell response to Epstein–Barr virus transactivators in chronic rheumatoid arthritis. *J Exp Med* 1996;184:1791–1800.
24. Nishioka K, Sumida T, Hasunuma T. Human T lymphotropic virus type I in arthropathy and autoimmune disorders. *Arthritis Rheum* 1996;39:1410–1418.
25. Nakajima T, Aono H, Hasunuma T, et al. Overgrowth of human synovial cells driven by the human T cell leukemia virus type I *tax* gene. *J Clin Invest* 1993;92:186–193.
26. Nelson PN, Lever AML, Bruckner FE, et al. Polymerase chain reaction fails to incriminate exogenous retroviruses HTLV-1 and HIV-1 in rheumatological diseases although a minority of sera cross react with retroviral antigens. *Ann Rheum Dis* 1994;53:749–754.
27. Kurosaka M, Ziff M. Immunoelectron microscopic study of the distribution of T cell subsets in rheumatoid synovium. *J Exp Med* 1983;158: 1191–1210.
28. Kelsoe G. Life and death in germinal centers (redux). *Immunity* 1996;4: 107–111.
29. Schroder AE, Greiner A, Seyfert C, Berek C. Differentiation of B cells in the nonlymphoid tissue of the synovial membrane of patients with rheumatoid arthritis. *Proc Natl Acad Sci USA* 1996;93:221–225.
30. Goronzy JJ, Weyand CM. T cells in rheumatoid arthritis-Paradigms and Facts. *Rheum Dis Clin North Am* 1995;21:655–674.
31. Randen I, Thompson KM, Pascual V, et al. Rheumatoid factor V genes from patients with rheumatoid arthritis are diverse and show evidence of an antigen-driven response. *Immunol Rev* 1992;128:49–71.
32. Axford JS, Mackenzie L, Lydyard PM, et al. Reduced B-cell galactosyltransferase activity in rheumatoid arthritis. *Lancet* 1987;2: 1486–1488.
33. Cremer MA, Ye XJ, Terato K, et al. Type XI collagen-induced arthritis in the Lewis rat: characterization of cellular and humoral immune responses to native types XI, V, and II collagen and constituent alpha-chains. *J Immunol* 1994;153:824–832.
34. Nabozny GH, Baisch JM, Cheng S, et al. HLA-DQ8 transgenic mice are highly susceptible to collagen-induced arthritis: a novel model for human polyarthritis. *J Exp Med* 1996;183:27–37.
35. Buzas EI, Brennan FR, Mikecz K, et al. A proteoglycan (aggrecan)-specific T cell hybridoma induces arthritis in BALB/c mice. *J Immunol* 1995;155:2679–2687.
36. Verheijden GF, Rijnders AW, Bos E, et al. Human cartilage glycoprotein-39 as a candidate autoantigen in rheumatoid arthritis. *Arthritis Rheum* 1997;40:1115–1125.
37. DerSimonian H, Sugita M, Glass DN, et al. Clonal Vα12.1+ T cell expansions in the peripheral blood of rheumatoid arthritis patients. *J Exp Med* 1993;177:1623–1631.
38. Goronzy JJ, Bartz-Bazzanella P, Hu W, et al. Dominant clonotypes in the repertoire of peripheral CD4+ T cells in rheumatoid arthritis. *J Clin Invest* 1994;94:2068–2076.
39. Fitzgerald JE, Ricalton NS, Meyer A-C, et al. Analysis of clonal CD8+ T cell expansions in normal individuals and patients with rheumatoid arthritis. *J Immunol* 1995;154:3538–3547.
40. Schmidt D, Goronzy JJ, Weyand CM. CD4+ CD7−CD28− T cells are expanded in rheumatoid arthritis and are characterized by autoreactivity. *J Clin Invest* 1996;97:2027–2037.
41. Schmidt D, Martens PB, Weyand CM, Goronzy JJ. CD4+ T cells lacking CD28− expression undergo clonal expansion and express shared T cell receptor sequences in rheumatoid arthritis. *Mol Med* 1996;2: 608–618.
42. Martens PB, Goronzy JJ, Schaid DJ, Weyand CM. Expansion of unusual CD4+ T cells in severe rheumatoid arthritis. *Arthritis Rheum* 1997;40:1106–1114.
43. Kouskoff V, Korganow A-S, Duchatelle V, et al. Organ-specific disease provoked by systemic autoimmunity. *Cell* 1996;87:811–822.
44. Weyand CM, Klimiuk PA, Goronzy JJ. Heterogeneity of rheumatoid arthritis: From phenotypes to genotypes. In: Izui S, Miescher P, eds. *Rheumatoid arthritis.* Geneva: Springer-Verlag, 1998.
45. Dessen A, Lawrence CM, Cupo S, et al. X-ray crystal structure of HLA-DR4 (DRA*0101, DRB1*0401) complexed with a peptide from human collagen II. *Immunity* 1997;7:473–481.
46. Weyand CM, Hicok KC, Conn DL, Goronzy JJ. The influence of HLA-DRB1 genes on disease severity in rheumatoid arthritis. *Ann Intern Med* 1992;117:801–806.
47. Weyand CM, Xie C, Goronzy JJ. Homozygosity for the HLA-DRB1 allele selects for extra-articular manifestations in rheumatoid arthritis. *J Clin Invest* 1992;89:2033–2039.
48. Walser-Kuntz DR, Weyand CM, Weaver AJ, et al. Mechanisms underlying the formation of the T cell receptor repertoire in rheumatoid arthritis. *Immunity* 1995;2:597–605.
49. Albani S, Keystone EC, Nelson JL, et al. Positive selection in autoimmunity: abnormal immune response to a bacterial dnaJ antigenic determinant in patients with early rheumatoid arthritis. *Nat Med* 1995;1: 448–452.
50. Weyand CM, McCarthy TG, Goronzy JJ. Correlation between disease phenotype and genetic heterogeneity in rheumatoid arthritis. *J Clin Invest* 1995;95:2120–2126.
51. Zvaifler NJ, Tsai V, Alsalameh S, von Kempis J, et al. Pannotypes: distinctive cells found in rheumatoid arthritis articular cartilage erosions. *Am J Pathol* 1997;150:1125–1138.
52. Ritchlin C, Dwyer E, Bucala R, Winchester R. Sustained and distinctive patterns of gene activation in synovial fibroblasts and whole synovial tissue obtained from inflammatory synovitis. *Scand J Immunol* 1994; 40:292.
53. Firestein GS, Echeverri F, Yeo M, Zvaifler NJ, Green DR. Somatic mutations in the p53 tumor suppressor gene in rheumatoid arthritis synovium. *Proc Natl Acad Sci USA* 1997;94:10895–10900.
54. Brinckerhoff CE, Harris ED Jr. Collagenase production by cultures containing multinucleated cells derived from synovial fibroblasts. *Arthritis Rheum* 1978;21:745–753.
55. Crisp AJ, Chapman CM, Kirkham SE, et al. Articular mastocytosis in rheumatoid arthritis. *Arthritis Rheum* 1984;27:845–851.
56. Geng Y, Valbracht J, Lotz M. Selective activation of the mitogen-activated protein kinase subgroups c-Jun NH₂ terminal kinase and p38 by IL-1 and TNF in human articular chondrocytes. *J Clin Invest* 1996;98:2425–2430.
57. Arnett FC, Edworthy SM, Bloch DA, et al. The American Rheumatism Association 1987 revised criteria for the classification of rheumatoid arthritis. *Arthritis Rheum* 1988;31:315–324.
58. Barton JC, Prasthofer EF, Egan ML, et al. Rheumatoid arthritis associated with expanded populations of granular lymphocytes. *Ann Intern Med* 1986;104:314–323.
59. Poole AR, Dieppe P. Biological markers in rheumatoid arthritis. *Semin Arthritis Rheum* 1994;23:17–31.
60. Saxne T, Glennas A, Kvien TK, et al. Release of cartilage macromolecules into the synovial fluid in patients with acute and prolonged phases of reactive arthritis. *Arthritis Rheum* 1993;36:20–25.
61. Fries JF, Ramey DR. "Arthritis specific" global health analog scales assess "generic" health related quality-of-life in patients with rheumatoid arthritis. *J Rheumatol* 1997;24:1697–1702.
62. Fries JF, Williams CA, Bloch DA, Michel BA. Nonsteroidal anti-inflammatory drug-associated gastropathy: incidence and risk factor models. *Am J Med* 1991;91:213–222.
63. Silverstein FE, Graham DY, Senior JR, et al. Misoprostol reduces serious gastrointestinal complications in patients with rheumatoid arthritis receiving nonsteroidal anti-inflammatory drugs: a randomized, double-blind, placebo-controlled trial. *Ann Intern Med* 1995;123:241–249.

64. Furst DE. Meloxicam: selective COX-2 inhibition in clinical practice. *Semin Arthritis Rheum* 1997;26[Suppl 1]:21–27.
65. Kirwan JR. The effect of glucocorticoids on joint destruction in rheumatoid arthritis: the Arthritis and Rheumatism Council Low-Dose Glucocorticoid Study Group. *N Engl J Med* 1995;333:142–146.
66. American College of Rheumatology Task Force on Osteoporosis Guidelines. Recommendations for the prevention and treatment of glucocorticoid-induced osteoporosis. *Arthritis Rheum* 1996;39:1791–1801.
67. Fries JF, Williams CA, Morfeld D, Singh G, Sibley J. Reduction in long-term disability in patients with rheumatoid arthritis by disease-modifying antirheumatic drug-based treatment strategies. *Arthritis Rheum* 1996;39:616–622.
68. Felson DT, Anderson JJ, Meenan RF. The comparative efficacy and toxicity of second-line drugs in rheumatoid arthritis: results of two meta-analyses. *Arthritis Rheum* 1990;33:1449–1461.
69. Rau R, Herborn G, Karger T, Werdier D. Retardation of radiologic progression in rheumatoid arthritis with methotrexate therapy: a controlled study. *Arthritis Rheum* 1991;34:1236–1244.
70. Morgan SL, Baggott JE, Vaughn WH, et al. The effect of folic acid supplementation on the toxicity of low-dose methotrexate in patients with rheumatoid arthritis. *Arthritis Rheum* 1990;33:9–18.
71. Kremer JM, Alacron GS, Lightfoot RW, et al. Methotrexate for rheumatoid arthritis: suggested guidelines for monitoring liver toxicity. *Arthritis Rheum* 1994;37:316–328.
72. Carroll GJ, Thomas R, Phatouros CC, et al. Incidence, prevalence and possible risk factors for pneumonitis in patients with rheumatoid arthritis receiving methotrexate. *J Rheumatol* 1994;21:51–54.
73. Kerstens PJ, Boerbooms AM, Jeurissen ME, et al. Accelerated nodulosis during low dose methotrexate therapy for rheumatoid arthritis: an analysis of ten cases. *J Rheumatol* 1992;19:867–871.
74. Kamel OW, van de Rijn M, Weiss LM, et al. Brief report: reversible lymphomas associated with Epstein–Barr virus occurring during methotrexate therapy for rheumatoid arthritis and dermatomyositis. *N Engl J Med* 1993;328:1317–1321.
75. Landewé RBM, Goei Thé HSG, van Rijthoven AWAM, et al. A randomized, double-blind, 24-week controlled study of low-dose cyclosporine versus chloroquine for early rheumatoid arthritis. *Arthritis Rheum* 1994;37:637–643.
76. Cush JJ, Kavanaugh AF. Biologic interventions in rheumatoid arthritis. *Rheum Dis Clin North Am* 1995;21:797–816.
77. Elliott MJ, Maini RN, Feldmann M, et al. Randomised double-blind comparison of chimeric monoclonal antibody to tumour necrosis factor alpha (cA2) versus placebo in rheumatoid arthritis. *Lancet* 1994;344:1105–1110.
78. Moreland LW, Baumgartner SW, Schiff MH, et al. Treatment of rheumatoid arthritis with a recombinant human tumor necrosis factor receptor (p75)-Fc fusion protein. *N Engl J Med* 1997;337:141–147.

*Textbook of the Autoimmune Diseases,*
Edited by R. G. Lahita, N. Chiorazzi, and W. H. Reeves,
Lippincott Williams & Wilkins, Philadelphia © 2000.

# CHAPTER 31

# Multiple Sclerosis

P. K. Coyle

## DEFINITION

Multiple sclerosis (MS) is a neuroimmune disorder involving the central nervous system (CNS). It affects brain and spinal cord while sparing peripheral nerves and muscle. Cardinal disease features are penetration of blood immune cells into the CNS compartment, local inflammation and immune responses, demyelination, and axon damage. MS affects young adults, with a highly variable spectrum of severity ranging from an asymptomatic pathologic process, to mild symptomatic disease, to severe disabling disease. There are two clinical patterns. Relapsing MS is characterized by acute neurologic attacks that are generally associated with some degree of recovery. Between episodes, patients appear stable. Progressive MS involves gradual development of neurologic abnormalities and slow worsening. Both forms show similar pathology, although progressive MS has more pronounced axon damage (1,2).

## HISTORICAL OVERVIEW

The first reported case of MS in the medical literature dates to 1824 and describes a young man with episodic neurologic disease and accumulating disability, who was considered to have a myelitis (3). In 1866, Vulpian used the term *sclerose en plaque dissemine* and presented three cases of typical MS to the Medical Society of Paris Hospitals (4). Charcot, in a series of lectures beginning in 1868, described the clinical features and pathology of the disease (5–7). The first definitive report in the English literature was that of William Moxon, who described eight cases of *insular sclerosis* (8). In 1884, Pierre Marie suggested this entity was the sequela of multiple different infections (9). The term *multiple sclerosis*

P. K. Coyle: Department of Neurology, Multiple Sclerosis Comprehensive Care Center, State University of New York at Stony Brook, School of Medicine, Stony Brook, New York 11794-8121; Department of Neurology, Health Sciences Center T-12, School of Medicine, State University of New York at Stony Brook, Stony Brook, New York 11794.

arose from a German description, and this ultimately replaced the earlier title of *disseminated sclerosis* (10).

## DEMOGRAPHICS

The demographics of MS are interesting (Table 31.1). One striking feature is the strong gender preference. About 70% to 75% of MS patients are women (11,12). The one exception is the primary progressive form of the disease (see later), which shows an equal sex ratio (13,14). This gender preference suggests hormonal disease influences, also supported by the observation that pregnancy influences disease activity. The clinical attack rate during the last trimester is reduced by 70% below prepregnancy baseline (15). This decrease in attacks is more than twice that achieved by the current disease-modifying therapies. Unfortunately, the relapse rate rebounds to 70% above baseline during the first 3 months postpartum. Pregnancy is an immunosuppressive state, with multiple maternal, fetal, and placental factors to explain a beneficial effect (16). Pregnancy involves high levels of estrogen and progesterone after the first trimester, both of which have multiple immunosuppressive effects. Pregnancy also involves prostaglandin and cytokine changes, production of immunoregulatory proteins such as $\alpha$-fetoprotein, and mechanisms to control maternofetal major histocompatibility complex (MHC) class II disparity. There is a lymphocyte shift from a helper T-cell subset 1 ($T_H1$) to a $T_H2$ profile, with consequent inhibition of cell-mediated immunity and enhancement of immunoglobulin responses, including blocking antibody and immune complex formation. Another supportive observation is worsening of MS symptoms shortly before or during menses (17).

MS affects young people. Most cases have their onset between 15 and 50 years of age, with a peak onset at about 28 to 30 years of age. The only exceptions are patients who begin with progressive disease, who are typically older than 35 years of age. Less than 1% of MS cases have their onset in patients younger than 10 years of age or older than 60 years of age.

**TABLE 31.1.** *Basic demographic features of multiple sclerosis*

Gender
    Female predominance (70%–75%), except in primary progressive subtype
Age
    Onset at 15–50 years of age (90%)
    Average onset at 30 years of age
    Unusual before 10 years of age or after 60 years of age (<1%)
Race
    White predominance (>90%)
    Rare in Asians, Africans, Native Americans
    Resistant groups (Innuits and Hutterites in Canada, Lapps in Finland)
Frequency
    Variable, depending on geographic location

**TABLE 31.2.** *Pathogenesis of multiple sclerosis*

Genetic factors
    Family history (20%)
    Familial risk
    Twin studies
    Polygenetic susceptibility
    Immune response genes
Environmental factors
    Infectious agents
    Other factors
        Diet
        Climate
        Toxins
Immune factors
    Lymphocytes
        T cells (CD4$^+$, CD8$^+$)
        B cells
        Natural killer cells
    Immunoglobulin or complement
    Cytokines
    Antigen-presenting cells
    Oligodenrocytes
    Astrocytes
    Endothelial cells

Another feature of MS is its racial distribution. MS is largely a disease of whites (more than 90%), with a high representation of northern European and Scandinavian populations. MS is unusual in other racial populations (Asians, Africans, Native Americans). African Americans actually show a frequency of MS between that of whites and Africans, suggesting that a mixed gene pool increases MS risk (18). MS remains exceedingly rare in certain populations who live in high-frequency areas. Examples are the Innuits and Hutterites in Canada and the Lapps in Finland. This observation also supports the role of genetic factors in MS.

Finally, the frequency of MS differs based on geographic location (see Epidemiology). Estimates suggest that at least 250,000 to 350,000 Americans have MS, and at least 1 million people are affected worldwide.

## PATHOGENESIS

Three crucial areas interact to produce MS (Table 31.2). The first involves genetics. Although most cases of MS are sporadic, 20% of patients report a relative with the disease. Some families have multiple affected members, and both relapsing and progressive MS can occur within the same family. With a positive family history, degree of consanguinity determines relative risk for MS. This risk can be 20 to 40 times greater than for someone without an affected relative. The age-adjusted risk is highest when there is a sibling with MS (3.2%), is next highest with an affected parent, especially a mother (2.1%), and is about 2% with an affected child (19). Twin studies show a higher concordance rate for monozygotic than dizygotic twins; however, concordance is no higher than 21% to 50%, even when neuroimaging and lumbar puncture are used to detect asymptomatic cases (19).

Several laboratories have searched the human genome for an MS gene without success (20–22). Within defined populations, however, certain genes increase disease susceptibility. The strongest association so far is with the human leukocyte antigen (HLA) *DRB1*1501* haplotype *DQA1*0102*

*DQB1*0602*, the DR2 extended haplotype (23). Additional genes have also been implicated. One study reported that the combination of two non-HLA cytokine genes, the interleukin-1 (IL-1) receptor antagonist allele 2$^+$ and the IL-1β allele 2$^-$, was associated with more rapid progression and more severe disease (24). These genes may be MS severity genes, and the IL-1 receptor antagonist allele 2 has been associated with disease severity in a variety of disorders (e.g., alopecia areata, psoriasis, lichen sclerosis, and ulcerative colitis).

MS is genetically heterogeneous, and multiple genes appear to contribute to development of the MS phenotype. Japanese, Chinese–Taiwanese, and Africans show a form of MS with predominant optic nerve and spinal cord involvement, similar to neuromyelitis optica. These patients have an increased frequency of the DR2-associated DRB1*1501 and DRB5*0101 alleles (25). Certain women with presumed MS and prominent visual failure have had a pathogenic mitochondrial mutation, consistent with Leber's hereditary optic neuropathy (26–28). Despite these genetic associations, no risk genes appear to be shared across all MS populations.

The second area implicated in the pathogenesis of MS involves environmental exposures. Overall, the epidemiologic data support a geographic influence on the disease (see later). Although the precise environmental factors are not defined, they are believed to be one or more ubiquitous infectious agents. Other environmental factors implicated in MS include diet (saturated versus nonsaturated fatty acids, smoked sausage), climate (sunlight exposure), and toxins (leading to oligodendrocyte or mitochondrial damage), but the data are fragmentary.

An infectious cause was postulated for MS almost from the time it was first described, and over the years, multiple pathogens have been implicated. Both viruses and bacteria are being investigated (Table 31.3). Human herpesvirus type

**TABLE 31.3.** *Infectious agents implicated in multiple sclerosis*

Viruses
  Herpesvirus
    Human herpesvirus type 6
    Epstein–Barr virus
    Others
  Retroviruses
    Human T-cell lymphotrophic virus
    Others
Bacteria
  *Chlamydia pneumoniae*
  *Borrelia burgdorferi*

6 (HHV-6) is a ubiquitous herpes virus that infects more than 90% of the adult population. There are two variants, types A and B, which show 90% to 96% homology. HHV-6 causes childhood exanthem subitum (roseola), is implicated in febrile seizures, and is implicated in focal brain and spinal cord demyelinating disease in both immunocompetent and immunocompromised hosts (29–31). Several laboratories report HHV-6 DNA, using polymerase chain reaction techniques, in CNS tissue, cerebrospinal fluid (CSF), and serum of a subset of MS patients (32–35). In a few limited pathologic cases, there has been evidence of active CNS tissue infection (36). Some MS patients show elevated serum antibody levels, including immunoglobulin M (IgM) (34). Another herpesvirus implicated in MS is Epstein–Barr virus (EBV). Virtually 100% of MS patients have evidence of EBV infection, compared with 95% of matched controls (37,38). The association of infectious agents with MS is not limited to viruses. CNS infection with *Chlamydia pneumoniae,* a bacterial agent, has been reported in a preliminary study in most patients with secondary progressive MS studied using culture, polymerase chain reaction, and antibody data (39).

The final area involved in the pathogenesis of MS is the host immune system. MS involves ongoing lesion formation within the CNS, referred to as *plaques.* These plaques involve areas of demyelination, axon damage, and gliosis, and they result from penetration of blood inflammatory cells around veins near the CSF compartment. Most plaque formation is clinically silent. It has only recently been recognized that axon damage is an important component of the MS disease process (40–42). It occurs at all time points, mirrors degree of inflammation, and leads to irreversible neurologic deficit. Although MS is often called *autoimmune,* this is not strictly accurate because there is no documented critical CNS antigen target. It is more accurate to consider MS as *immune mediated.*

The role of the immune system in MS was initially thought to involve a trimolecular complex–mediated process. Myelin peptides would bind to MHC class II molecules on antigen-presenting cells (APCs). Subsequent binding to T-cell receptors would create activated CD4+ T cells sensitized to myelin antigens. These activated blood lymphocytes would then attach to CNS endothelial cells by means of adhesion molecules, leading to local release of proteases and enzymes, such as matrix metalloproteinases; passage across the blood-brain barrier (BBB); and entry into the CNS. Subsequent local immune reactions would release cytokines and chemokines, produce migration of other blood immune cells, and activate resident CNS cells (microglia and astrocytes). This immune cascade would result in myelin damage, axon damage, and release of sequestered antigens from the CNS compartment to the systemic system, with the possibility of epitope spread and enhanced autoantigen responses.

This paradigm was based on experimental autoimmune encephalomyelitis (EAE), an autoimmune disease created in susceptible inbred animal strains by inoculation with complete Freund's adjuvant and whole CNS tissue, myelin, or myelin components (such as myelin basic protein, proteolipid protein, or myelin oligodendrocyte glycoprotein). EAE is a CD4+ T-cell–mediated disorder. It has been used to develop and test immunomodulatory therapies for MS. EAE is not a good MS model. Most animals have a monophasic disease course more consistent with acute disseminated encephalomyelitis or postinfectious encephalomyelitis. Several treatments that benefit EAE, such as interferon-γ (IFN-γ) and tumor necrosis factor (TNF) receptor, actually make MS worse.

The trimolecular complex paradigm has been questioned (43). It is not at all clear that the T cell initiates the MS disease process. An alternative explanation might involve a pathogen that either directly invades and disrupts CNS tissue or causes a systemic infection with secondary CNS involvement. Secondary mechanisms by which infectious agents could lead to immune-mediated CNS damage include molecular mimicry, superantigen induction, dual T-cell–receptor expression, neoantigen expression, immune dysregulation, and bystander damage. Another triggering event for MS might involve a toxic mechanism, causing dysfunction or death of crucial CNS cells. There is pathologic evidence that a proportion of MS patients may have a dying-back oligodendrogliopathy, with little in the way of inflammatory changes (44).

Many central issues about the role of the host immune system need to be clarified. It is not clear whether the immune response is a primary cause of MS or a secondary consequence. The crucial immune component has not been identified. It could be a cell, antibody and complement, or a soluble cytokine. Many cells other than the CD4+ T cell have been suggested to play a role in MS, including the following:

- CD8+ T cells—cells that mediate suppressor activity
- Macrophages—major components of the CNS cell infiltrates in MS, which phagocytize myelin
- Microglia—resident APCs of the CNS that are activated in MS, can process antigen, and can release cytotoxic factors, such as free radicals, excitatory amino acids, chemokines, and proinflammatory cytokines.
- Endothelial cell—BBB disruption is the earliest detectable feature in CNS lesion formation, and newer neuroimaging techniques such as magnetization transfer ratio suggest that there may be a low-grade diffuse BBB defect in early MS.
- Oligodendrocyte—This myelin-producing cell dies in a proportion of MS patients.

**TABLE 31.4.** *Putative antigen targets in multiple sclerosis*

Myelin or oligodendrocyte antigens
    Myelin basic protein
    Proteolipid protein
    Myelin oligodendrocyte glycoprotein
    $\alpha\beta$ Crystallin
    Transaldolase
    Alu peptide (7–amino acid B-cell epitope)
Nonmyelin antigens
    S-100$\beta$ protein (astrocyte)
    Glial fibrillary acidic protein
    Stress proteins
    Central nervous system pathogen

- Astrocytes—a major CNS cell type that is capable of expressing activation molecules and immune processing, promotes remyelination, and helps to maintain the BBB
- Natural killer cells—part of the innate immune response to virally infected cells.

One study reported that antibodies to myelin oligodendrocyte glycoprotein, a minor CNS myelin component, may play a significant role in MS along with complement to amplify damage (45). Cytokines are implicated in MS based on both *in vitro* and *in vivo* data (46). Proinflammatory cytokines are upregulated both systemically and within the intrathecal compartment.

No crucial antigen target is identified in MS. Although there are several possible myelin targets, there is also evidence for nonmyelin targets (Table 31.4). If MS involved infection of the CNS, with release of sequestered antigens and secondary immune responses, a single antigen target would be unlikely.

## EPIDEMIOLOGY

### Geographic Distribution

MS is not evenly distributed (Table 31.5). There are clear low-risk (less than 5 per 100,000 population), medium-risk (5 to 30 per 100,000), and high-risk zones (>30/100,000) (47). In areas where it has been studied, the equator zone is a very-low-risk area, but MS increases as one moves north and south.

### Incidence and Prevalence

As noted earlier, MS is associated with a white, northern European and Scandinavian background. Although the number of diagnosed MS patients in the United States is estimated at 250,000 to 350,000, asymptomatic cases (based on autopsy studies) may account for 25% or more of MS patients (48).

The frequency of MS has not been stable. Within geographically defined regions, there have been examples of increasing and decreasing numbers of patients. Overall, there is a sense that MS may be on the rise, independent of improved disease awareness and ascertainment.

**TABLE 31.5.** *Epidemiologic features of multiple sclerosis*

Geographic distribution
    Low-risk (<5/100,000), medium-risk (5–30/100,000), and high-risk (>30/100,000) zones
    Latitude effect
Incidence and prevalence
    Racial population
    Temporal changes
Clusters and epidemics
    Faeroe Islands
    Iceland
Migration studies
    Childhood exposure
Precipitating factors
    Infection
    Postpartum
    Immune factors
    Possibly stress

### Clusters and Epidemics

MS clusters and epidemics have been reported (49). Clusters, involving small numbers, can be difficult to establish. Epidemics, involving larger numbers, tend to be more convincing. The best documented epidemic of MS involves the Faeroe Islands, between Iceland and Great Britain (49). These islands had no known MS cases, despite sophisticated health care. During World War II (1942 to 1945), several thousand British troops were based on the Faeroes. Within 3 years, MS began to appear among the native Islanders. Although ultimately MS cases stopped, there were several waves of affected patients. It was postulated that the British introduced some external factor that was able to bring out MS in a population in which it had not been described previously.

### Migration Studies

Most migration studies of MS indicate that the lifetime risk for disease is determined by the childhood (up to 15 years of age) environment. One of the most impressive studies involved West Indies immigrants to London. They had a very low rate of MS, but their children subsequently showed a rate consistent with that of their neighbors (50).

### Environmental Factors

Certain factors can precipitate MS disease activity. Among the best documented are infections, particularly benign respiratory tract viral pathogens. At least one third of MS relapses follow viral infection (51,52). The evidence for bacterial infection being a trigger for MS relapses is not as strong, but suggestive data indicate that urinary tract infections are more common when MS patients present with clinical worsening (53).

A European study on pregnancy and MS confirmed that the 3-month postpartum period shows a 70% increase in attack rate, effectively counteracting the protection of the last trimester (15).

Certain immune factors increase MS disease activity. The best examples come from therapeutic trials that evaluated IFN-γ and TNF receptor complexed to Fc IgG fusion protein (Lenercept) (54,55). The fact that these immunotherapies were not just neutral, but actually precipitated attacks, provides important clues to the immunopathogenesis of MS. TNF receptor therapy antagonizes a proinflammatory cytokine, which should have been helpful in MS. This study emphasizes the complexity of the cytokine network.

Many believe that stress can precipitate MS disease activity, but this has been hard to document. A study using monthly magnetic resonance imaging (MRI) scans combined with self-report measures found an increase in MRI lesion activity after periods of increased stress (56).

## CLINICAL PRESENTATION

### Disease Subtype

In 1996, the National Multiple Sclerosis Society defined a standardized clinical classification of MS based on expert consensus (57) (Table 31.6). The terms *chronic progressive* and *relapsing progressive* were discarded. Although defined solely by clinical course, these subtypes carry different prognoses. It remains to be determined whether they have meaningful biologic differences. From a pragmatic viewpoint, the subtypes are important because they are the basis for testing new therapies.

Relapsing MS has clearly defined attacks (also called *relapses, exacerbations,* and *flare-ups*). About 85% of MS patients begin with relapsing disease. Attacks often have onset over days, but onset can range from minutes (mimicking a stroke) to several weeks. The attack is followed by complete recovery, or the patient may be left with residual deficits. Between relapses, the patient is clinically stable. By convention, relapses must last at least 24 to 48 hours. If they involve paroxysmal problems (lasting seconds), they must occur repetitively over several weeks. Relapses are distinguished from pseudoexacerbations, which involve temporary neurologic worsening during infection. This worsening is presumed to be related to raised body temperature, with tem-

porary failure of nerve conduction. In contrast to true relapses, deficits clear as soon as infection is under control. The degree of recovery from attacks is not uniform and has prognostic value. About 96% of first attacks show some recovery. In general, there is a trend to complete recovery from early attacks and incomplete recovery from later attacks. The timing of the next relapse also has prognostic significance. After a first attack, 25% to 40% of patients relapse within 1 year, 50% to 67% within 3 years, and more than 80% within 5 years. Over time, relapses decrease.

Progressive MS involves slow worsening, with gradual development of neurologic deficit. This usually takes months to appreciate. Temporary minor improvements, or clinical stability for up to several years, can occur. There are three forms of progressive MS. Primary progressive and progressive relapsing subtypes show gradual deterioration from the start. Primary progressive MS makes up about 10% of patients. By definition, patients never experience disease attacks. There is accumulating evidence to suggest that primary progressive MS is biologically different from the rest of MS. Patients have an older age of onset (typically older han 35 years of age) and an equal gender ratio. Most (more than 60%) present with a myelopathy (spinal cord) syndrome, characterized by atrophy and axon loss rather than inflammation and white-matter lesions. There is often little in the way of brain MRI lesion load or activity. Progressive relapsing MS is a newly described subtype and accounts for only 5% of patients. It describes disease that is progressive from the outset but goes on to include superimposed relapses.

The major progressive subtype is secondary progressive MS. Five to 15 years into the course of relapsing MS, some cases start to worsen slowly. These patients may continue to have attacks or may stop having attacks and experience slow disease progression. Based on untreated natural history data, 50% of relapsing MS cases convert to secondary progressive disease within 10 years, and close to 80% convert within 20 years (58).

In a cross-sectional MS population, the major subtypes are relapsing (55%) and secondary progressive (30%). Primary progressive (10%) and progressive relapsing (5%) subtypes are unusual.

### Symptoms and Signs

MS produces a number of problems that affect quality of life and add to the economic burden of this disease (Table 31.7). Management of these symptoms is an important component of any therapeutic MS program (see later).

The first attack is more likely to be monoregional (involving a single neurologic system, such as an optic neuritis) than polyregional (involving multiple systems, such as a combination of motor, cerebellar, and sensory features). The most common clinical signs and symptoms in the first attack are motor, sensory, or visual. Optic neuritis is the first clinical manifestation of MS in 16% to 29% of patients. In contrast, bladder and bowel dysfunction, sexual dysfunction, or cog-

---

**TABLE 31.6.** *Clinical subtypes of multiple sclerosis*

Relapsing
  85% at onset
Primary progressive
  10%
  Older age at onset
  Equal gender ratio
Progressive relapsing
  5%
Secondary progressive
  Develops in up to 80% of relapsing patients
  5–15 years after onset

**TABLE 31.7.** *Common clinical features of multiple sclerosis*

Fatigue
Depression
Cognitive loss
Sensory disturbances
    Lhermitte's sign
    Paresthesias
    Numbness
    Pain
Motor disturbances
    Spasticity
    Weakness
Bladder and bowel disturbances
Sexual dysfunction
Vision loss
Cerebellar dysfunction
    Dysmetria
    Postural or intention tremor
    Unsteady gait
Brainstem
    Diplopia
    Vertigo

nitive loss are unusual early manifestations. Over time, these areas are affected in more than half of all MS patients. Perhaps the major symptom of MS is fatigue, which is considered the single most disabling feature. Fatigue is distinct from clinical subtype, disease duration, or disease severity. At least 90% of MS patients experience significant fatigue problems at some point.

Depression is another common MS symptom. It can reflect a reactive process or can be due to disease activity. Depression often worsens during relapses. It is an important symptom to recognize because the suicide rate is increased in patients with MS (59,60). Although cognitive loss is considered a neuronal rather than white-matter feature, eventually more than 40% of patients develop cognitive problems. Dementia occurs in 10%. Cognitive loss is more common in the secondary progressive subtype and is associated with neuroimaging features (lesion load of 30 cm or greater, corpus callosum atrophy, confluent periventricular lesions, brain atrophy) (61). Psychiatric symptoms in MS are associated with temporal lobe lesions (61). Sensory disturbance is another common symptom, and most MS patients experience problems at some point.

Sensory problems in MS can be negative (numbness or rarely anesthesia) or positive (paresthesias, hyperesthesia, pain). Lhermitte's sign (an electrical sensation down the spine on flexing the neck) is suggestive of MS and is reported by one third of patients. It reflects a lesion in the posterior column of the cervical spinal cord. Any process, however, that produces a lesion in this area (such as vitamin $B_{12}$ deficiency or disc disease) can be associated with Lhermitte's sign. Pain is a common complaint in MS and can be a primary symptom (reflecting lesion damage) or a secondary symptom (reflecting a musculoskeletal consequence of neurologic impairment or disability). Trigeminal neuralgia (tic douloureux) is caused by

a brainstem lesion and in a young person is suggestive of MS. Chronic pain or burning pain problems are also common in MS.

Motor abnormalities in MS range from changes in tone, to minimal weakness, to complete paralysis. Increased tone (spasticity) can be a major problem in MS. It can produce hyperreflexia, clonus, and flexor or extensor spasms and can lead to pain problems as well as inability to ambulate.

Neurogenic bladder is another common problem in MS over time. Three distinct bladder disturbances are described. The most common is a spastic bladder with failure to store, characterized by urinary urgency and frequency. Frequent spontaneous bladder muscle contractions occur despite small urine volumes. The next most common is a dyssynergic bladder disorder, in which bladder muscle contraction is dissociated from external sphincter relaxation. The sphincter paradoxically constricts when the bladder contracts to expel urine. Patients note urgency, frequency, and multiple attempts to void limited volumes. The final and least common neurogenic bladder is a flaccid (atonic) bladder, with failure to empty. In this scenario, the bladder muscle does not contract despite excessive urine volumes. Patients present with dribbling and overflow incontinence. Bowel disturbances also occur in MS. Constipation is much more frequent than diarrhea, but both problems occur.

Sexual dysfunction is common in MS over time. In men, this involves mainly erectile dysfunction. Women note a variety of problems, including dryness, loss of sensation, and lack of desire.

Most visual problems in MS reflect optic neuritis, with monocular vision loss; nystagmus and ocular motility disturbances also affect vision. About 1% of MS patients develop uveitis (inflammation of the anterior eye) (62).

Cerebellar dysfunction involves unsteady gait, uncoordinated movements, dysarthria, extremity dysmetria, and truncal titubation. It carries a poor prognosis. Perhaps the most disabling problem is intention or postural tremor, which actually reflects both cerebellar and brainstem disease. This tremor often results in loss of arm and leg function, despite good strength.

Brainstem problems in MS include ocular motility disturbances that can result in diplopia; facial numbness, pain, or weakness; hearing loss or vertigo; difficulty with swallowing, chewing, or speaking; and tongue weakness.

### Prognosis

Life span of MS patients is mildly shortened compared with that of matched controls (49,63,64). Although MS can be a primary cause of death (e.g., when lower brainstem lesions affect vital cardiovascular or respiratory centers) or can lead to suicide, many MS deaths are related to secondary complications associated with advanced disability.

Up to 80% of patients have their ability to work adversely affected. Fifteen years into untreated disease, at least 50% of patients require an assistive device to ambulate, and 30% are wheelchair bound (12,64).

A number of prognostic clinical and laboratory features have been identified for MS (Table 31.8). Women generally do better than men. Relapsing MS has a better prognosis than progressive MS. The number, frequency, and nature of attacks, as well as the degree of recovery, all have prognostic significance. For patients who have had MS for 5 years or longer, the number of systems affected on the baseline neurologic examination, as well as the nature of the last attack (number of systems involved and degree of recovery), are important. The strongest laboratory prognostic factors are neuroimaging features, particularly in relapsing and secondary progressive disease. In particular, brain and spinal cord atrophy on MRI is emerging as the best neuroimaging correlate of disability. These features are useful to predict disease severity and guide therapeutic choices but do not always apply.

## DIAGNOSTIC TESTS

### Overview

Diagnosis of MS is important to define appropriate therapy, remove uncertainty, allow informed planning, and improve sense of well being. The misdiagnosis rate of MS is 5% to 10%. Incorrect diagnosis often reflects overinterpretation of abnormalities on brain MRI. There is also an extensive differential diagnosis to consider because a number of conditions can mimic MS. In addition to overdiagnosis, there is also underdiagnosis, particularly in women who present with transient problems attributed to stress.

The diagnosis of MS is clinical but should be supported by laboratory data (Table 31.9). Appropriate laboratory investigations help to minimize misdiagnosis and to create a prognostic profile. Basic clinical diagnostic principles were outlined by Schumacher et al. and are provided in Table 31.9 (65). In these criteria, appropriate age is considered to range from 10 to 50 years. The disease process must involve white matter, and relapsing and progressive courses are recognized. Lesions have to be disseminated in time and space, so that one cannot make a definite diagnosis at onset despite MRI and CSF abnormalities. Laboratory testing, however, does allow predictions of the risk for MS over the next few years.

The Poser Committee criteria refined the clinical criteria to take advantage of ancillary tests and to establish more formal criteria for research protocols (66). They recognized clinically definite and probable MS as well as laboratory-

**TABLE 31.8.** *Prognostic factors in multiple sclerosis[a]*

Mortality
  75% survive 25 years
  Mortality increases with disability
Morbidity
  70%–80% negative vocational impact
  50% require assistive device to walk
  30% wheelchair bound
Favorable features
  Female gender
  Early age at onset (≤35 yr)
  Relapsing subtype
  Long interval between first and second relapse
  Low relapse rate in first 2 years
  Monoregional relapses
  Visual, brainstem, or sensory relapses
  Complete recovery from relapses, minimal disability at 5 years
  Minimal number of affected systems after 5 years
  Monoregional relapses with excellent recovery, after 5 years
  MRI parameters showing little T2-weighted burden of disease, active lesions, atrophy, myelin damage
  Possibly, oligoclonal band–negative CSF
Unfavorable features
  Male gender
  Late age at onset (>35 yr)
  Progressive subtype
  Short interval between first and second relapse
  High relapse rate (>5 relapses) in first 2 years
  Polyregional relapses
  Motor, cerebellar, or bladder and bowel dysfunction relapses
  Incomplete recovery from relapses
  Moderate to severe disability after 5 years
  Large number of affected systems after 5 years
  Polyregional relapses with incomplete recovery after 5 years
  MRI parameters showing significant T2-weighted burden of disease, active lesions, atrophy, myelin damage
  Possibly, oligoclonal band–positive CSF

[a] Data are based on the pre–disease-modifying therapy period.
MRI, magnetic resonance imaging; CSF, cerebrospinal fluid

**TABLE 31.9.** *Diagnostic evaluation for multiple sclerosis*

Clinical principles
  Appropriate age
  Central nervous system white-matter process
  Lesions disseminated in time and space
  Objective abnormalities
  Consistent time course
    Attacks lasting ≥24h, spaced ≥1 mo apart
    Slow or stepwise progression ≥6 mo
  No better explanation
Laboratory
  Blood work (to exclude conditions)
    Collagen vascular disease
    Infections
    Endocrine disturbance
    Vitamin deficiency
    Sarcoidosis
    Vasculitis
    Adrenoleukodystrophy
    Mitochondrial encephalomyopathies
  Magnetic resonance imaging
    Brain
    Spinal cord
  Cerebrospinal fluid
    Oligoclonal bands
    Intrathecal immunoglobulin G production
    Other tests
  Evoked potentials
  Urodynamics

supported definite and probable MS. These criteria expand the age range from 10 to 59 years. Clinical evidence for MS requires documented abnormalities on the neurologic examination. Poser et al. added paraclinical evidence (neuroimaging, evoked potential, urodynamic abnormalities) and CSF abnormalities (presence of oligoclonal bands or intrathecal IgG production). Clinically definite MS requires two disease attacks and either two examples of clinical evidence or one example of clinical evidence accompanied by one example of paraclinical evidence. Clinically probable MS involves less rigorous combinations of attacks accompanied by clinical and paraclinical evidence. A laboratory-supported diagnosis requires abnormal CSF along with other features.

The differential diagnosis of MS includes conditions that can be screened for by appropriate blood work. Collagen vascular disorders (systemic lupus erythematosus, Sjögren's disease) can occasionally mimic MS; however, these diseases should show evidence of extraneural involvement (rash, kidney, and joint disease in the case of lupus; dry eyes and mouth in the case of Sjögren's disease). Infections such as Lyme disease, syphilis, HHV-6, and human T-cell lymphotrophic virus type 1 can occasionally masquerade as MS. Metabolic disorders (thyroid, parathyroid, adrenal gland disease) and nutritional deficiencies (vitamin $B_{12}$, folate, vitamin E) can mimic MS. Occasionally, sarcoidosis, vasculitis, primary phospholipid syndrome, and genetic disorders (adrenoleukodystrophy, cerebral autosomal dominant arteriopathy with subacute infarction and leukoencephalopathy, mitochondrial encephalomyopathies) can masquerade as MS.

The MS spectrum also has several variations. Baló's concentric sclerosis is a rare condition of young people characterized by a unique pathology: concentric bands of demyelination separated by intact myelin. Devic's syndrome (neuromyelitis optica) is a disorder that involves the spinal cord and optic nerves. Most of these patients (80%) do not have true MS; their brain MRI is normal, whereas the spinal MRI has extensive (more than three) segment lesions. CSF shows increased protein and significant pleocytosis, which is often neutrophilic. One third of patients with Devic's syndrome experience a single attack, whereas two thirds go on to relapses, with a 40% mortality rate at 5 years. Marburg disease is an acute variant of MS that results in extensive damage and significant morbidity over a short span of a few months to years. Data suggest that these patients have a post-translational modification in myelin basic protein, with extensive citrullination and poor phosphorylation of the myelin protein (67). Schilder's disease (myelinoclastic diffuse sclerosis) is a rare disorder of children that involves bilateral large hemispheral demyelinating lesions. Patients often present with visual problems and cortical blindness, seizures, headache, and vomiting. Acute disseminated encephalomyelitis (postinfectious encephalomyelitis) is a monophasic syndrome that follows infection or vaccination. Although the pathology is indistinguishable from that of acute MS, the two show a number of differences. Postinfectious encephalomyelitis is more common in children than adults and is typically a more severe

syndrome (involving depressed level of consciousness, seizures, multifocal abnormalities, bilateral optic neuritis, complete transverse myelitis). MRI tends to show bilateral extensive and symmetric lesions that involve the basal ganglia and diffusely enhance. CSF immune disturbances are less common than in MS and disappear over time.

Certain clinical features should suggest a misdiagnosis of MS. They include consistently normal examination, lack of dissemination in time and space, strongly positive family history (particularly with early age onset and unexplained non-CNS disease), lack of optic nerve or ocular motility disturbance, progressive disease beginning before 35 years of age, disease localized to a single area of the CNS, and nonsupportive brain MRI and CSF. Other atypical features include disease onset before 10 years of age or after 55 years of age, abrupt hemiparesis, prominent pain (with the exception of trigeminal neuralgia), peripheral neuropathy, nonscotomatous (altitudinal, hemianopic, or quadrantanopic) field cuts, prominent gray-matter or neuronal features (early dementia, seizures, aphasia, muscle fasciculations, extrapyramidal movement disorders), no sensory system or bladder involvement, and progressive myelopathy without bladder or bowel involvement.

## Neuroimaging

Neuroimaging of the brain (MRI) reveals abnormality in 65% of patients at initial diagnosis and in 90% to 95% of patients over time (61). Brain MRI shows 10 times more lesions than spinal MRI. In patients older than 50 years of age, however, intramedullary lesions on spinal MRI are more specific than comparable brain lesions (which can be due to vascular disease), and it is recommended that brain MRI not be used to support a diagnosis of MS in patients in this age group. Most brain MRI lesions are clinically silent, and studies estimate 5 to 10 times more new lesions than clinical attacks in patients with relapsing or secondary progressive disease. This silent lesion activity leads to an annual increase in brain MRI burden of disease of about 10% a year in untreated MS patients (61). These lesions may not be truly silent but may contribute to subtle cognitive deficits. A National Multiple Sclerosis Society panel concluded that MRI is the best current biologic marker of disease activity in relapsing and secondary progressive MS and that MRI parameters could be used as primary outcome in preliminary trials to test new therapeutic agents (61).

The classic brain MRI picture is of scattered white-matter lesions, which are hyperintense on T2-weighted scans and hypointense on T1-weighted scans. Gadolinium enhancement indicates damaged BBB, a lesion 6 weeks of age or less, and current disease activity. MRI lesion patterns that increase the probability of MS include four or more white-matter lesions at least 3 mm in size; three white-matter lesions, one of which is periventricular; lesions that are 6 mm or larger in size; ovoid lesions that are perpendicular to the ventricles; corpus callosum lesions; brainstem lesions;

and contrast-enchancing lesions with an open-ring appearance. Common lesion location areas are periventricular white matter, occipital and frontal region, brainstem, and cerebellum. Unusual lesion locations are the basal ganglia (25%) and internal capsule (11%).

MRI is useful not only for diagnosis but also for prognosis to identify extent of disease and to evaluate disease activity and response to treatment. New neuroimaging techniques (magnetic resonance spectroscopy, magnetization transfer ratio, fluid-attenuated inversion recovery, echoplanar systems) are allowing enhanced detection of abnormalities as well as identification of distinct pathologies (edema, inflammation, demyelination, remyelination, gliosis, axon loss). Standardized techniques to quantitate burden of disease are being evaluated.

## Cerebrospinal Fluid

The two essential tests for the diagnosis of MS are oligoclonal band positivity and elevated intrathecal IgG production, as measured by the IgG index or 24-hour synthesis rate. Oligoclonal bands are the most specific test but need to be run as a paired sample with blood to interpret results. Ultimately, 90% to 95% of MS patients are CSF oligoclonal band positive (68), but similar to MRI, early in the course, the positivity rate is much lower. Once positive, oligoclonal bands remain so over time. Other conditions on occasion can produce oligoclonal bands, particularly chronic infections and inflammatory conditions. The false-positive rate has been reported as high as 4%; however, MS is the major disorder associated with CSF band formation. Oligoclonal bands in MS correlate with plasma cell infiltration of meninges.

Intrathecal IgG production is not as specific for MS but does indicate an intrathecal immune disturbance. Ultimately, 70% to 90% of patients test positive for intrathecal IgG. Free light chains are another immune assay reported to be elevated in MS CSF (69).

Although myelin basic protein can be measured in CSF, it is not very helpful from a diagnostic viewpoint because assay sensitivity varies, positivity fluctuates, and positivity can reflect any destructive process, including stroke.

Other CSF features can be helpful to suggest another diagnosis. Pleocytosis (more than 50 white blood cells per cubic millimeter) and protein levels higher than 100 mg/dL are unusual in MS and should raise the possibility of another diagnosis.

## Other Laboratory Tests

Evoked potential tests can document subclinical lesions. In particular, visual evoked potentials, to detect optic nerve lesions, and somatosensory evoked potentials, to document sensory abnormalities within the spinal cord or subcortical regions, can help to document disseminated lesion involvement. Likewise, urodynamics can be used to document a neurogenic bladder.

## TREATMENT

### Symptomatic

Symptom management is an important component of MS therapy. Table 31.10 outlines a multimodality approach, which starts with identification of the patient's major problems, in rank order. Symptoms need to be considered in the

**TABLE 31.10.** *Symptom management in multiple sclerosis*

| Symptom | Management approaches |
|---|---|
| Fatigue | Exclude other conditions and medication use |
| | Sleep hygiene |
| | Programmed daily activities |
| | Energy conservation techniques |
| | Aerobic exercise program |
| | Cooling |
| | Medications |
| |    Amantadine |
| |    Pemoline |
| |    Amphetamines |
| |    Fluoxetine |
| |    Selegiline |
| |    Caffeine |
| Depression | Counseling or psychotherapy |
| | Medications |
| |    Selective serotonin reuptake inhibitors |
| |    Tricyclics |
| |    Others |
| Cognitive loss | Counseling |
| | Cognitive therapy |
| | Medications |
| Sensory disturbances | Medications |
| |    Tricyclics |
| |    Anticonvulsants |
| |    Conventional analgesics |
| | Rehabilitation therapy |
| | Biofeedback |
| | Surgery |
| Motor disturbances | Rehabilitation therapy and exercise |
| | Medications |
| |    Primary agents |
| |    Secondary agents |
| | Surgery |
| |    Baclofen pump |
| Bladder and bowel | Medication |
| | Programmed voiding |
| | Intermittent catheterization |
| | Fluids, fiber, bowel regimen |
| | Behavioral modification |
| Sexual dysfunction | Counseling |
| | Local techniques |
| | Medications |
| | Surgery |
| Vision loss | Visual aids |
| Cerebellar | Rehabilitation |
| | Medications |
| | Surgery |
| Brainstem | Local techniques |
| | Exercises |
| | Medications |
| | Surgery |

context of lifestyle, daily activities, and other conditions and factors that may influence them. Management strategies can include changes in lifestyle, physical strategies, pharmacologic therapy, and surgical therapy and are influenced by contributing factors. For example, fatigue associated with thyroid disease, anemia, use of a certain medication, or poor sleep hygiene would require that the specific associated problem be addressed. Forty minutes of aerobic exercise, three times a week, was shown not only to have significant positive physiologic effects on maximal aerobic activity, isometric strength, body fat, and blood lipid profile but also to have significant positive psychological effects on fatigue, depression, anger, social activities, emotional behavior, and recreational pursuits (70). Cooling techniques can improve fatigue. They range from sophisticated garments, to battery operated neck devices, to cold drinks and showers, to air conditioning and cool clothing. Among the drugs used to treat fatigue are amantadine (100 mg b.i.d.), pemoline (18.75 to 37.5 mg q.d. to t.i.d.), and fluoxetine (20 mg q.d. to t.i.d.).

Pain can be a major feature in MS. Treatment may involve optimizing posture, movements, and positioning; appropriate use of icing or local heat; massage and other physical therapy techniques; short-term administration of nonsteroidal antiinflammatory agents; or more invasive techniques, such as trigger-point injections, epidural steroids, or facet joint injections. Treatment for acute pain syndromes generally involves anticonvulsants (carbamazepine, phenytoin, gabapentin), baclofen, clonazepam, and surgical technique (radiofrequency rhizotomy, glycerol injection). Chronic pain management includes tricyclic antidepressants, addition of anticonvulsants, TENS units, and behavioral pain control techniques.

Practical measures to treat neurogenic bladder problems involve use of a bedside commode or urinal; following a fluid schedule; practicing timed voiding; using emptying techniques, such as tapping, crede maneuver, or straining (which should be employed every 3 hours for training purposes); use of intermittent catheterization to avoid urine volumes of more than 400 mL; and use of pads or special undergarments. Treatment of the spastic bladder involves programmed voiding, anticholinergics (tolterodine, oxybutynin, hyoscyamine, propantheline, dicyclomine, imipramine), behavioral modification techniques, and avoidance of caffeine, alcohol, and aspartame. Nocturia can respond well to nasal desmopressin acetate. Dyssynergic bladders are treated by programmed voiding, intermittent catheterization, α-blockers, $α_2$-agonists, anticholinergics, and antispasticity agents. Flaccid bladders are treated by intermittent catheterization, a combination of α-blockers and emptying techniques, or a combination of cholinergic agents and emptying techniques. Bowel management requires sufficient daily fluids (1.5 to 2 L), fiber (15 g), bulk-forming agents, and creating a regular bowel regimen. This may involve stool softeners, oral stimulants, mild laxatives, rectal suppositories, mini enemas, and anticholinergics.

Treatment of spasticity involves preventing, removing, or treating any triggering factors (such as infection or relapse), physical measures (stretching, standing, gait and bicycle training, vibration), first-line drugs (baclofen, tizanidine, diazepam), second-line drugs (gabapentin, clonidine, cyproheptadine, dantrolene, threonine), or invasive surgical techniques (intrathecal baclofen pump, botulinum toxin, phenol injection, selective posterior rhizotomy). Tremor is extraordinarily difficult to treat. Physical measures include weighted bracelets and mechanical damping devices. Drugs include carbamazepine, primidone, propranolol, ondansetron, and clonazepam. Stereotoxic surgical procedures include thalamic stimulation, with the electrode placed in the thalamic ventral intermediate nucleus. This procedure is being used principally for Parkinson's disease and essential tremor; however, there is a limited but growing experience with its use in MS patients.

Glucocorticoids are an important component of symptomatic MS management. They are not considered to be disease-modifying therapy, although pulse steroid therapy continues to be studied. Adrenocorticotropic hormone was first used in a multicenter cooperative study in 1970 and was shown over the short-term to be associated with more rapid recovery (71). Subsequently, agents such as methylprednisolone, prednisone, and dexamethasone have been used. Steroids can hasten the timeframe of recovery from an MS relapse. They do not improve the degree of recovery, nor do they have a documented effect on timing of the next attack. There is the sense that, over time, patients respond less well. Glucocorticoids have potent antiinflammatory and immunomodulatory activities. They decrease synthesis of prostaglandins, thromboxane, leukotrienes, and lipolytic and proteolytic enzymes. They decrease matrix metalloproteinase levels and increase their tissue inhibitors. They decrease expression of adhesion molecules, increase lysosomal stability, and decrease gene transcription of inducible nitric oxide synthase, cyclooxygenase, and phospholipase $A_2$. They decrease gene transcription of proinflammatory cytokines (such as IFN-γ, TNF-α, IL-1, and IL-2) and chemokines (IL-8, RANTES, MIP-1α). They decrease cell recruitment and activation, T-cell proliferation, and MHC class I expression on APCs. The most commonly used regimen is 1 g of intravenous methylprednisolone for 3 to 7 days, with or without an oral taper.

Many questions about steroid use in MS remain unknown. Studies suggest that equivalent amounts can be given orally at significant cost savings. There are also suggestive data that higher doses than are currently used may be better. The optimal parameter of glucocorticoid therapy for MS has not been established.

**Disease Modifying**

Four immunomodulatory disease-modifying therapies have been shown to benefit patients with relapsing MS; one has also been shown to benefit patients with secondary progressive MS (Table 31.11). Three of the treatments involve cytokine manipulation strategies, with parenteral administration of the antiinflammatory cytokine IFN-β. This cytokine also has antiinfection properties. The fourth agent, glatiramer acetate, has biophysical similarities to myelin basic protein and is an antigen analog (altered peptide ligand) trimolecular complex manipulation strategy.

IFN-β1b (Betaseron, Berlex Laboratories, Richmond, CA, U.S.A.) was the first drug approved for the treatment of relapsing MS. This recombinant protein has three molecular differences from human IFN-β: it is not glycosylated; there is no amino-terminal methionine; and at position 17, serine is substituted for cysteine. In the original phase III study, low-dose (1.6 mIU q.o.d.) and high-dose (8 mIU q.o.d.) IFN-β1b were studied along with placebo. The high-dose arm showed a significant decrease in clinical attacks as well as a significant effect on MRI disease parameters (burden of disease, number of active lesions). The trial ultimately reported 3- and 5-year data and was able to show a sustained (although not statistically significant) effect lasting 5 years (72–74). IFN-β1b was shown to be effective for secondary progressive MS as well, at the same high dose (8 mIU q.o.d.) that was approved for treatment of relapsing MS (75). This study had a placebo and treatment arm. Although designed as a 3-year study, at the predetermined 2-year interim, analysis treatment was so overwhelmingly superior to placebo that the study was stopped. Over 2 years, IFN-β1b slowed progression (sustained worsening on the neurologic examination) by 11.5 months. There was significant benefit on multiple clinical parameters, including relapses, severity of relapses, time to wheelchair dependence, and need to hospitalize or treat with steroids. There was a profound effect on MRI disease parameters, with an approximate 80% decrease in new lesion formation and a decrease in accumulating burden of disease. A North American study of IFN-β1b for secondary progressive MS has been completed and will report results shortly.

IFN-β1a duplicates human IFN-β. IFN-β1a (Avonex, Biogen, Inc., Cambridge, MA, U.S.A.) was the second disease-modifying therapy approved in the United States for relapsing MS (76). Approval was based on a 2-year, two-arm study that showed a significant effect on sustained worsening on the neurologic examination, relapse rate, and some MRI disease parameters. This study entered patients with less severe relapsing disease than either the IFN-β1b or glatiramer acetate studies, and later information suggested that the results are probably not extrapolatable to patients with more severe MS, at least at the current dosing schedule (77).

IFN-β1a (Rebif, Serono Laboratories, Norwell, MA, U.S.A.) is molecularly identical to Avonex. In contrast to the Avonex product, it is given subcutaneously three times a week. This drug was evaluated in 560 patients with relapsing MS who were randomized to placebo, low-dose, or high-dose arms (77). In this 2-year study, high-dose IFN-β1a significantly decreased relapses, severity of relapses, sustained worsening on the neurologic examination, and MRI disease parameters (accumulating burden of disease, number of active lesions). Of particular interest was a *post hoc* analysis of 94 relapsing patients with more severe disease. In these patients, high-dose IFN-β was required to see optimal benefit. Relapses were reduced by 60% over placebo, compared with only 40% in the low-dose IFN-β arm. Only high-dose treatment had a significant effect on proportion of relapse-free patients, median time to first relapse, reduction in moderate to severe relapses, sustained worsening on the neurologic examination, and time to sustained worsening.

Glatiramer acetate consists of random polymers of acetate salts of four synthetic amino acids: L-glutamic acid, L-alanine, L-tyrosine, and L-lysine. It was originally synthesized to study in EAE, in which the compound was found to suppress disease. These observations led to its being studied in MS. The phase III trial in relapsing MS patients showed that glatiramer acetate treatment significantly decreased relapses compared with placebo (32% in the extension study carried out to 35 months) (78,79). The proportion of patients who remained relapse free was significant in the glatiramer acetate group for the core plus extension trial data, with evidence that disease was more likely to be stable or improved at the end of the study if patients had received active drug. In the open-label continuation of this study, patients taking glatiramer acetate for 5 years have shown a low relapse rate and little sustained worsening. Glatiramer acetate was reported to have a positive effect on MRI parameters (80), but in the phase III trial, this was studied at only one center. A large European trial was specifically designed to examine MRI effects and has just been completed. It documents that the drug lessens MRI disease features.

All four disease-modifying therapies benefit relapsing MS, and high-dose IFN-β therapy also benefits secondary progressive patients. The precise mechanisms by which they act to moderate MS disease activity is not clear. IFN-β has multiple beneficial actions. It blocks cell migration across the BBB by inhibiting matrix metalloproteinase production and downreg-

**TABLE 31.11.** *Disease–modifying therapies for multiple sclerosis*

| Drug | Immunomodulatory strategy | Dosing | Disease subtypes |
|---|---|---|---|
| Interferon-β1b (Betaseron) | Cytokine | 8 mIU (250 μg) SC q.o.d. | Relapsing and secondary progressive |
| Interferon-β1a (Avonex) | Cytokine | 6–9 mIU (30 μg) IM weekly | Relapsing |
| Interferon-β1a (Rebif) | Cytokine | 6 mIU (22 μg) and 12 mIU (44 μg) SC 3× weekly | Relapsing |
| Glatiramer acetate (Copaxone) | Trimolecular complex | 20 mg SC q.d. | Relapsing |

ulating adhesion molecule expression. It also enhances functional suppressor cell activity, downregulates HLA class II expression, antagonizes proinflammatory cytokine activity, and has antiviral activity. Glatiramer acetate is believed to work by activating suppressor cells locally. These cells then migrate into the CNS and act through a bystander suppression mechanism to inhibit local immune reactions.

All the disease-modifying therapies appear safe with long-term use. The major side effects of IFN-β involve influenza-like reactions, which typically dissipate after 2 to 3 months. Simple measures to minimize these reactions involve evening dosing, dose escalation, and premedication strategies (nonsteroidal antiinflammatory agents or antipyretics). When IFN-β is injected subcutaneously, it produces skin reactions. Simple measures can be used to minimize these reactions, and they are not often a problem. IFN-β can probably worsen depression in susceptible patients; therefore, any depression must be treated appropriately. The last three major IFN-β trials, however, failed to find a significant increase in depression in the treated versus placebo group. Occasionally,

IFN-β therapy can produce laboratory disturbances in liver enzymes or blood cell counts. It is unusual to have to stop therapy for such abnormalities because they generally clear spontaneously. In extremely rare instances, autoimmune liver disease, thyroid disease, and rheumatoid arthritis have developed while taking IFN-β.

Glatiramer acetate has minimal side effects; these include mild injection-site reactions and an odd immediate postinjection systemic reaction. This latter reaction affects 10% of patients and is most often a one-time occurrence. It is a symptom complex of flushing, chest pain, palpitations, anxiety, dyspnea, and throat constriction that is transient (0.5 to 30 minutes), self-limited, and not associated with permanent sequelae. It occurs shortly after injection and is limited to patients on treatment for at least 1 month. It may reflect inadvertent intravenous glatiramer acetate injection. Patients need to be aware of this side effect, but it appears to be benign and self-limited.

A number of other disease-modifying strategies are in development (Table 31.12). They include other cytokine

**TABLE 31.12.** *Disease-modifying strategies in development for multiple sclerosis*

| | |
|---|---|
| Cytokine manipulation | Immunosuppression |
|   Antiinflammatory cytokines |   Azathioprine |
|     New agents |   Cladribine |
|     Oral interferons |   Cyclophosphamide |
|   Inhibitors of proinflammatory cytokines |   Methotrexate |
|   Shift $T_H1/T_H2$ balance |   Mitoxantrone |
| Trimolecular complex |   Sulfasalazine |
|   Antigenic peptide |   Total lymphoid irradiation |
|     Glatiramer acetate (oral) | Immunomodulation |
|     Oral tolerance |   Intravenous immune globulin |
|     Altered peptide ligands |   Plasma exchange |
|     Apoptosis inducing antigens |   Leukapheresis |
|   MHC class II | Immune reconstitution |
|     Monoclonal antibody |   Bone marrow transplantation |
|     MHC binding peptides | Antiinfection strategies |
|     MHC peptide vaccination |   Antiviral agents |
|   T-cell receptor |   Antibacterial agents |
|     T-cell vaccination (single or multiple antigens) | Hormonal strategies |
|     T-cell–receptor peptide vaccination |   Estrogens |
|     Anti–T-cell–receptor antibodies | DNA-based strategies |
|   Combination |   Antisense oligonucleotides |
|     Soluble MHC–peptide complexes |   Immunologic gene therapy |
| Target molecule interference |   DNA vaccines |
|   Adhesion molecule blockade | Combination strategies |
|   Costimulatory molecule manipulation |   Interferon-β plus glatiramer acetate |
|   Leukocyte differentiation molecules |   Disease modifying therapy plus oral agent (azathioprine, |
|     Monoclonal antibodies to diverse molecules |     methotrexate) or pulse intravenous agent (glucocorti- |
|     Immunotoxins |     coids, intravenous immunoglobulin) |
|     Mimetic peptides |   Induction therapy (intravenous immunosuppression) fol- |
| Antiinflammatory agents |     lowed by disease-modifying therapy |
|   Matrix metalloproteinase inhibitors | CNS repair strategies |
|   Selective cyclooxygenase inhibitors |   Remyelination |
|   Leukotriene inhibitors or antagonists |   Axon protection/neuroprotection |
|   Inducible nitric oxide inhibitors |   Axon regeneration |
|   Complement inhibitors | |
|   Anti-CR3 monoclonal antibodies | |
|   Desferrioxamine | |

$T_H$, helper T cell; MHC, major histocompatibility complex.

manipulation strategies as well as testing of oral IFN preparations. There are a number of trimolecular complex strategies, including oral glatiramer acetate and at least two different T-cell vaccine strategies. Target molecule strategies include the use of humanized monoclonal antibodies to adhesion molecules, to block cell migration into the CNS. Many different antiinflammatory therapies are under investigation. These therapies are noteworthy because they are antigen independent.

Immunosuppression has been used for some time in MS, without major success. Cladribine, mitoxantrone, and high-dose methotrexate with leukovorin rescue have been studied (81–84). There is an interest in examining immunosuppression as induction therapy or temporary add-on therapy in patients who are not responding well to disease-modifying therapy. Immunomodulation therapies include intravenous immune globulin (IVIG). At least one large study suggested that monthly pulse IVIG could be used as disease-modifying therapy (85). Bone marrow transplantation, to replace the entire immune system, is now being evaluated in MS.

Based on studies that report more favorable prognosis for women with MS, a strong protective effect of late pregnancy, and in vitro immunologic studies, high-dose estrogen is being evaluated in a pilot study. DNA-based strategies are not currently being tested in MS but are likely to be the subject of future studies. They are being evaluated in selected medical conditions. Drug combination strategies are under evaluation. Finally, CNS repair strategies attempt to boost remyelination, protect axons, and promote axon regeneration. These particular strategies offer the possibility of restoration of function and repair of fixed deficit.

## CONCLUSION

MS is the major immune-mediated disorder in neurology. Significant advances have been made in diagnosis, management, and understanding of the basic biology of the disease. These advances have been driven by new information on the role of the immune system in MS. Further advances are likely to occur in the areas of therapy, pathogenesis, and neuroimaging. MS is now a treatable disease. A consensus statement from the National Multiple Sclerosis Society recommends that disease-modifying therapy be considered in all MS patients with definite relapsing disease (86). Although the available disease-modifying therapies are only partial treatments, they appear to be changing the natural history of MS. They are the first wave of therapies and will be followed by other and even better approaches. The future will also bring a better understanding of disease pathogenesis, including how the immune system, environment, and genetics interact. A final area for advancement will occur in neuroimaging. A core assessment battery will allow determination of individual responses to therapy. Neuroimaging will allow identification of the heterogeneity of MS and detection of early CNS abnormalities. Information about this prototype immune-mediated disease should provide invaluable clues to understanding and treating other neuroimmune and autoimmune disorders.

## REFERENCES

1. Matthews PM, Pioro E, Narayana WS, et al. Assessment of lesion pathology in multiple sclerosis using quantitative MRI morphometry and magnetic resonance spectroscopy. *Brain* 1996;119:715–722.
2. Davie CA, Barker GJ, Thompson AJ, et al. A magnetic resonance spectroscopy of chronic cerebral white matter lesion and normal appearing white matter in multiple sclerosis. *J Neurol Neurosurg Psychiatry* 1997;63:736–742.
3. Ollivier CP. De la moelle epiniere et de ses maladies. Paris: Crevot, 1824.
4. Vulpian E. Note sur la sclerosie en plaques de la moelle epiniere. *Union Medicale Pratique Francais* 1866;30:459–465, 475–582, 541–548.
5. Charcot JM. Histologie de la sclerose en plaques. *Gazette Hopitaux* (Paris) 1868;41:554–555, 557–558, 566.
6. Charcot JM. Seance du 14 mars. *Cr Soc Biol* (Paris) 1868;20:13–14.
7. Charcot JM. Lectures on disease of the nervous system. London: New Sydenham Society Series, 1887.
8. Moxon W. Eight cases of insular sclerosis of the brain and spinal cord. *J Neurol Neurosurg Psychiatry* 1875;20:437–478.
9. Marie P. Sclerose en plaques et maladies infecteuses. *Prog Med* (Paris) 1884;12:287–289, 305–397, 349–351, 365–366.
10. Ebers G. Introduction: a historical overview. In: Paty DW, Ebers GC, eds. *Multiple sclerosis.* Philadelphia: FA Davis, 1998:1–4.
11. Duquette P, Pleines J, Girard M, et al. The increased susceptibility of women to multiple sclerosis. *Can J Neurol Sci* 1992;19:466–471.
12. Minden SL, Marder WD, Harrold LN, et al. Multiple sclerosis: a statistical portrait. Cambridge, Ma: National Multiple Sclerosis Society, ABT Associates, 1993.
13. McDonnell GV, Hawkins SA. Primary progressive multiple sclerosis: a distinct syndrome? *Mult Scler* 1996;2:137–141.
14. Thompson AJ, Polman CH, Miller DH, et al. Primary progressive multiple sclerosis. *Brain* 1997;120:1085–1096.
15. Confavreux C, Hutchinson M, Hours MM, et al., for the Pregnancy in Multiple Sclerosis Group. Rate of pregnancy-related relapse in multiple sclerosis. *N Engl J* Med 1998;339:285–291.
16. Abramsky O. Pregnancy and multiple sclerosis. *Ann Neurol* 1994;36:538–541.
17. Zorgdrager A, Dekeyser J. Menstrually related worsening of symptoms in multiple sclerosis. *J Neurol Sci* 1997;149:95–97.
18. Dupont B, Lisak RP, Jersild C. HLA antigens in black American patient with multiple sclerosis. *Transplant Proc* 1976;91:181–185.
19. Robertson NP, Compston DAS. Prognosis in multiple sclerosis: genetic factors. In: Siva A, Kesselring J, Thompson AJ, eds. *Frontiers in multiple sclerosis.* Vol 2. London: Martin Dunitz, 1999:51–61.
20. Sawcer S, Jones HB, Feakes R, et al. A genome screen reveals susceptibility loci on chromosome 6p21 and 17q22. *Nat Genet* 1996;13:464–468.
21. Multiple Sclerosis Genetics Group. A complete genomic screen for multiple sclerosis underscores a role for the major histocompatibility complex. *Nat Genet* 1996;13:469–471.
22. Ebers GC, Kukay K, Bulman DE, et al. A full genome search in multiple sclerosis. *Nat Genet* 1996;13:472–476.
23. Dyment DA, Sadovnick AD, Ebers GC. Genetics of multiple sclerosis. *Hum Mol Genet* 1997;6:1693–1698.
24. Schrijver HM, Crusius JBA, Uitdehaag BMJ, et al. Association of interleukin-1β and interleukin-1 receptor antagonist genes with disease severity in MS. *Neurology* 1999;52:595–596.
25. Kira J-I, Kanai T, Nishimura, et al. Western vs Asian types of multiple sclerosis immunogenetically and clinically distinct disorders. *Ann Neurol* 1996;40:569–574.
26. Harding AE, Sweeney MG, Miller DM, et al. Occurrence of a multiple sclerosis-like illness in women who have a Leber's hereditary optic neuropathy mitochondrial DNA mutation. *Brain* 1992;115:979–989.
27. Kellar-Wood H, Robertson NP, Goven GG, et al. Leber's optic neuropathy mitochondrial DNA mutations in multiple sclerosis. *Ann Neurol* 1994;36:109–112.

28. Riordan-Eva P, Sanders M, Goven GG, et al. The clinical features of Leber's hereditary optic neuropathy defined by the presence of a pathogenic mitochondrial mutation. *Brain* 1995;118:319–337.

29. Hall CB, Long CE, Schnabel KC, et al. Human herpesvirus 6 infection in children: a prospective study of complications and reactivations. *N Engl J Med* 1944;331:432–438.

30. Novoa LJ, Nagra RM, Nakawatase T, et al. Fulminant demyelinating encephalomyelitis associated with productive HHB-6 infection in an immunocompetent adult. *J Med Virol* 1997;52:301–308.

31. Bosi A, Zazzi M, Amantini A, et al. Fatal herpesvirus 6 encephalitis after unrelated bone marrow transplant. *Bone Marrow Transplant* 1998;22:285–288.

32. Wilborn F, Schmidt CA, Brinkmann V, et al. A potential role for human herpesvirus type of a nervous system disease. *J Neuroimmunol* 1994;49:213–214.

33. Challoner PB, Smith KT, Parket JD, et al. Plaque associated expression of human herpesvirus 6 in multiple sclerosis. *Proc Natl Acad Sci U S A* 1995;92:7440–7444.

34. Soldan SS, Berti R, Salem N, et al. Association of human herpes virus 6 (HHV-6) with multiple sclerosis: increased IgM response to HHV-6 early antigen and detection of serum HHV-6 DNA. *Nat Med* 1997;3:1394–1397.

35. Ablashi DV, Lapps W, Kaplan M, et al. Human herpesvirus 6 (HHV-6) infection in multiple sclerosis: in preliminary report. *Mult Scler* 1998;4:490–496.

36. Carrigan DR, Harrington D, Knox KK. Subacute leukoencephalitis caused by CNS infection with human herpesvirus six manifesting as acute multiple sclerosis. *Neurology* 1996;47:145–148.

37. Myhr KM, Riise T, Barrett-Connor E, et al. Altered antibody pattern to Epstein–Barr virus but not to other herpesviruses in multiple sclerosis: a population based case-control study from western Norway. *J Neurol Neurosurg Psychiatry* 1998;64:539–542.

38. Munch M, Hvas J, Christensen I, et al. A single subtype of Epstein–Barr virus in members of multiple sclerosis clusters. *Acta Neurol Scand* 1998;98:395–399.

39. Sriram S, Mitchell W, Stratton C. Multiple sclerosis associated with *Chlamydia pneumoniae* infection of the CNS. *Neurology* 1998;50:571–572.

40. Ferguson B, Matyszak MK, Esiri MM, et al. Axonal damage in acute multiple sclerosis. *Brain* 1997;120:393–399.

41. Trapp BD, Peterson J, Ransohoff RM, et al. Axonal transection in the lesions of multiple sclerosis. *N Engl J Med* 1998;338:278–285.

42. Waxman SG. Demyelinating diseases: new pathological insights, new therapeutic targets. *N Engl J Med* 1998;338:323–325.

43. Sriram S, Rodriguez M. Indictment of the microglia as the villain in MS. *Neurology* 1997;48:469–473.

44. Lucchinettii CF, Bruce W, Rodriguez M, Lassmann H. Distinct patterns of multiple sclerosis pathology indicates heterogeneity in pathogenesis. *Brain Pathol* 1996;6:259–274.

45. Genain CP, Cannella B, Hauser SL, et al. Identification of autoantibodies associated with myelin damage in multiple sclerosis. *Nat Med* 1999;5:170–175.

46. Brosnan C, Raine C. Mechanisms of immune injury in multiple sclerosis. *Brain Pathol* 1996;6:243–257.

47. Kurtzke JF. A reassessment of the distribution of multiple sclerosis: parts I and II. *Acta Neurol Scand* 1975;51:110–136, 137–157.

48. Allen IV. Asymptomatic multiple sclerosis: what does it mean? In: Siva A, Kesselring J, Thompson AT, eds. *Frontiers in multiple sclerosis.* Vol 2. London: Martin Dunitz, 1999:1–14.

49. Weinshenker BG. Epidemiology of multiple sclerosis. *Neurol Clin* 1996;14:291–398.

50. Elian M, Dean G. Multiple sclerosis among the United Kingdom-born children of immigrants from the west indies. *J Neurol Neurosurg Psychiatry* 1987;50:327–332.

51. Sibley WA, Bamford CR, Clark K. Clinical viral infections and multiple sclerosis. *Lancet* 1985;1:1313–1315.

52. Edwards S, Zvartau M, Clarke H, et al. Clinical relapses and disease activity on magnetic resonance imaging associated with viral upper respiratory tract infections in multiple sclerosis. *J Neurol Neurosurg Psychiatry* 1998;64:736–741.

53. Rapp NS, Gilroy J, Lerner AM. Role of bacterial infection in exacerbation of multiple sclerosis. *Am J Phys Med Rehabil* 1995;4:415–418.

54. Panitch HS, Hirsch RL, Schindler J, et al. Treatment of multiple sclerosis with gamma interferon: exacerbations associated with activation of the immune system. *Neurology* 1987;37:1097–1102.

55. Reder AT, Kanabudal R. Raising issues in multiple sclerosis: part II. In: Siva A, Kesselring J, Thompson AT, eds. *Frontiers in multiple sclerosis.* Vol 2. London: Martin Dunitz, 1999:260–272.

56. Mohr DC, Russo D, Reiss M, et al. Relationship of stress, psychological distress, and disease activity in multiple sclerosis patients (abst). *Ann Neurol* 1997;42:T201.

57. Lublin FD, Reingold SC, for the National Multiple Sclerosis Society (USA) Advisory Committee on Clinical Trials of New Agents in Multiple Sclerosis. Defining the clinical course of multiple sclerosis: results of an international survey. *Neurology* 1996;46:907–911.

58. Runmarker B, Andersen O. Prognostic factors in a multiple sclerosis coincidence cohort within twenty-five years of follow-up. *Brain* 1993;116:117–134.

59. Sadovnick AD, Eisen K, Ebers GC, et al. Cause of death in patients attending multiple sclerosis clinics. *Neurology* 1991;41:1193–1196.

60. Stenager EN, Stenager E, Koch-Henriksen N, et al. Suicide and multiple sclerosis: an epidemiological investigation. *J Neurol Neurosurg Psychiatry* 1992;55:542–545.

61. Miller DH, Albert PS, Barkhof F, et al. Guidelines for the use of magnetic resonance techniques in monitoring the treatment of multiple sclerosis. *Ann Neurol* 1996;39:6–16.

62. Biousse V, Trichet C, Block-Michel E, et al. Multiple sclerosis associated with uveitis in two large clinic-based series. *Neurology* 1994;52:179–181.

63. Sadovnick AD, Ebers GC. Epidemiology of multiple sclerosis: a critical overview. *Can J Neurol Sci* 1993;20:17–29.

64. Weinshenker BG. The natural history of multiple sclerosis. *Neurol Clin* 1995;13:119–146.

65. Schumacher GA, Beebe G, Kibler RF, et al. Problems of experimental trials of therapy in multiple sclerosis: report by the panel on the evaluation of experimental trials of therapy in multiple sclerosis. *Ann N Y Acad Sci* 1965;122:552–568.

66. Poser CM, Paty DW, Scheinberg L, et al. New diagnostic criteria for multiple sclerosis: guidelines for research protocols. *Ann Neurol* 1983;13:227–231.

67. Wood DD, Bilbao JM, O'Connors P, et al. Acute multiple sclerosis (Marburg type) is associated with developmentally immature myelin basic protein. *Neurology* 1996;40:18–26.

68. Rudick RA, Cookfair DL, Simonian NA, et al. Cerebrospinal fluid abnormalities in a phase III trial of Avonex (R) (IFN beta-1a) for relapsing multiple sclerosis. *J Neuroimmunol* 1999;93:8–14.

69. Rudick RA, French CA, Breton D, et al. Relative diagnostic value of cerebrospinal fluid Kappa chains in MS: comparison within other immunoglobulin tests. *Neurology* 1989;30:964–968.

70. Petajan J, Gappmaier E, White AT, et al. Impact of aerobic training in fitness and quality of life in multiple sclerosis. *Ann Neurol* 1996;39:432–441.

71. Rose AS, Kuzuma JW, Kurtzke JF, et al. Cooperative study in the evaluation of therapy in multiple sclerosis: ACTH vs placebo *Neurology* 1970;5:1–59.

72. IFNβ Multiple Sclerosis Study Group. Interferon beta-1b is effective in relapsing remitting multiple sclerosis. I. Clinical results of a multicenter, randomized, double-blind, placebo-controlled trial. *Neurology* 1993;43:655–661.

73. Paty DW, Li DKB, for the UBC MS/MRI Study Group and the IFNB Multiple Sclerosis Study Group. Interferon beta-1b is effective in relapsing-remitting multiple sclerosis. II. MRI analysis results of a multicenter, randomized, double-blind, placebo controlled trial. *Neurology* 1993;43:662–667.

74. IFNβ Multiple Sclerosis Study Group and The University of British Columbia MS/MRI Analysis Group. Interferon beta-1b in the treatment of multiple sclerosis: final outcome of the randomized controlled trial. *Neurology* 1995;45:1277–1285.

75. Knight R, Hern J, Coleman R, et al., for the European Study Group on Interferon β-1b in Secondary Progressive MS. Placebo-controlled multicentre randomized trial of interferon β-1b in treatment of secondary progressive multiple sclerosis. *Lancet* 1998;352:1491–1497.

76. Jacobs LD, Cookfair DL, Rudick RA, et al. Intramuscular interferon beta-1a for disease progression in relapsing multiple sclerosis. The Mul-

tiple Sclerosis Collaborative Research Group (MSCRG). *Ann Neurol* 1996;39:285–294.

77. PRISMS (Prevention of Relapses and Disability by Interferon β-1a Subcutaneously in Multiple Sclerosis) Study Group. Randomized double-blind placebo-controlled study of interferon β-1a in relapsing-remitting multiple sclerosis. *Lancet* 1998;352:1498–1504.

78. Johnson KP, Brooks BR, Cohen JA, et al. Copolymer 1 reduces relapse rate and improves disability in relapsing-remitting multiple sclerosis: results of a phase III multicenter, double-blind, placebo-controlled trial. *Neurology* 1995;45:1268–1276.

79. Johnson KP, Brooks BR, Cohen JA, et al., for the Copolymer 1 Multiple Sclerosis Study group. Extended use of glatiramer acetate (Copaxone) is well tolerated and maintains its clinical effect on multiple sclerosis relapse rate and degree of disability. *Neurology* 1998;50:701–708.

80. Mancardi GL, Sardanelli F, Parodi RC, et al. Effect of copolymer-1 on serial gadolinium-enhanced MRI in relapsing remitting multiple sclerosis. *Neurology* 1998;50:1127–1133.

81. Sipe JC, Romine JS, Koziol JA, et al. Cladribine in treatment of chronic progressive multiple sclerosis. *Lancet* 1994;344:9–13.

82. Edan G, Miller D, Claney M, et al. Therapeutic effect of mitoxantrone combined with methylprednisolone in multiple sclerosis: a randomized multicenter study of active disease using MRI and clinical criteria. *J Neurol Neurosurg Psychiatry* 1997;62:112–118.

83. Millefiorini E, Gasperini C, Pozzilli C, et al. Randomized, placebo-controlled trial of mitoxantrone in relapsing-remitting multiple sclerosis: 24 month clinical and MRI outcome. *J Neurol* 1997;244:153–159.

84. Conrad CA, Rowe VD. Treatment of primary and secondary progressive multiple sclerosis with high dose methotrexate and leukovorin rescue (abst). *Neurology* 1998;50:A146.

85. Fazekas F, Deisenhammer F, Strasser-Fuchs S, et al. Randomized placebo-controlled trial of monthly intravenous immunoglobulin therapy in relapsing remitting multiple sclerosis. *Lancet* 1997;349:589–593.

86. MS Disease Management Advisory Task Force. *National MS Society disease management consensus statement.* New York: National MS Society, 1998:1–8.

Textbook of the Autoimmune Diseases,
Edited by R. G. Lahita, N. Chiorazzi, and W. H. Reeves,
Lippincott Williams & Wilkins, Philadelphia © 2000.

# CHAPTER 32

# Goodpasture's Syndrome

W. Kline Bolton

In 1919, Ernest Goodpasture (1,2) described a clinical syndrome associated with pulmonary hemorrhage in patients with influenza infection. The histologic findings in these patients consisted of acute crescentic glomerulonephritis (GN). Immunofluorescence technology was not available at that time; thus, it is not clear whether those patients had antibodies directed against the glomerular basement membrane (GBM) as the cause of their GN and pulmonary hemorrhage or whether other etiologies might have been involved, such as vasculitis. The term *Goodpasture's syndrome* has since been widely used throughout the literature variously to mean pulmonary hemorrhage with some type of renal dysfunction, that is, a pulmonary renal syndrome (3). A more narrowly defined definition of Goodpasture's syndrome includes patients with pulmonary hemorrhage associated with anti-GBM antibodies, as distinct from those with GN alone resulting from anti-GBM antibodies but lacking pulmonary hemorrhage (4).

Other terminology has been used, including the lumping of all disease associated with antibody to type IV collagen as a related group (5). Type IV collagen makes up basement membranes throughout the body, including the kidney. The GBM plays a major role in glomerular filtration and plasma protein exclusion. Alterations of the GBM result in proteinuria and abnormal renal function (6).

Type IV collagen classically consists of a heterotrimer of α1 and α2 chains and is composed of a 390-nm long triple-helical collagenous rod terminated at its C-terminus by a globular noncollagenous domain (NC1) (7–9). A 30-nm long 7-S segment at the N-terminus forms tetramers with other 7-S segments, whereas the NC1 globular domains form dimers with each other. These covalently linked structures form a lattice infrastructure for other GBM molecules. Interspersed within the lattice are protein constituents, including laminin, nidogen, heparin sulfate proteoglycan, and a variety of other matrix proteins. After collagenase digestion, the hexameric noncollagenous domains remain and contain the antigen that Goodpasture's sera recognize (10–14).

In kidney, lung, eye, ear, and choroid plexus, novel collagen chains α3 to α6 are present for reasons yet to be delineated, as opposed to other basement membrane regions (15). Size and charge chromatography and gel electrophoresis can partially separate the various NC domains, and monoclonal antibodies serve further to identify the α1, α2, and novel collagen chains (16–20). The Goodpasture's epitope appears to be cryptic, contained in the α3 chain, and is discontinuous, reflecting a conformational antigen (12,17). Although most of the antibody activity in Goodpasture's syndrome appears to be directed to the NC1 of the α3 chain of type IV collagen, the assertion that this is the only chain involved in Goodpasture's syndrome or the *de novo* disease that occurs in renal transplant recipients is less certain. Nonetheless, α3 is the predominant antigen involved and accounts for limitation of disease expression to areas containing the α3 NC1 domain readily accessible to circulating antibody, that is, kidney and lung (13,21–24).

Antibody activity to other chains and GBM constituents is being documented (23,25). Studies with serum from animal models or from patients with Goodpasture's syndrome show a variety of anti-GBM antibody specificities using chains derived from recombinant proteins, column chromatography, or peptides for mapping (23,26–28). Fixation of these different antibodies to the lung and kidney results in different clinical phenotypes. The resultant clinical findings range from normal renal function with anti-GBM deposits and pulmonary hemorrhage to pulmonary hemorrhage with or without GN.

The presence or absence of pulmonary hemorrhage appears to be consequent to environmental factors rather than differences in disease pathogenesis; therefore, the distinction of pulmonary hemorrhage as a defining subset of Goodpasture's syndrome would appear impractical. Thus, it seems most reasonable to consider patients with anti-GBM antibodies deposited in the tissue as having Goodpasture's dis-

W. K. Bolton: Department of Internal of Medicine, Division of Nephrology, University of Virginia School of Medicine, Health Sciences Center, Charlottesville, Virginia 22908.

ease and those patients with GN or hemoptysis or both as having *Goodpasture's syndrome* (13). This classification would include patients with antibodies directed to α3, α4, α5, and α6 as well as the standard α1 and α2 NC1 domains and would include patients with Alport's syndrome who have a variety of antibodies directed against the GBM (29,30). Using this classification, patients with any type of antibody deposited on GBM would represent one end of the spectrum of Goodpasture's disease, whereas those with pulmonary hemorrhage and GN would represent the other end of the spectrum. In between would be the range of clinical presentations varying from asymptomatic nonconsequential deposition of any antibody directed against GBM to the presence of florid disease.

The factors involved in the phenotypic expression of different antibody deposition remain to be elucidated. Although it was originally considered that only α3 was capable of inducing florid disease with the full phenotypic spectrum of GN, it is now clear that antibodies directed against other chains of type IV collagen are capable of a similar clinical presentation, as are antibodies directed against type I collagen in terms of pulmonary symptomatology (31). It is likely that as we develop the sophistication to test patients for specific antibodies to various NC1 domains, the spectrum of disease will be broadened rather than narrowed. This should offer the opportunity for a better understanding of the pathogenetic factors involved in the development of different phenotypic expressions.

## INCIDENCE AND EPIDEMIOLOGY

Goodpasture's syndrome is a rare disease, occurring in about 0.1 to 0.5 cases per 1 million population. In our own series of renal biopsies, about 1% to 2% of patients who underwent biopsy for GN have the histologic diagnosis of Goodpasture's syndrome by the characteristic findings of antibody along the basement membrane (32). The male-to-female incidence ratio is about equal, although in some series, there is a slight male prepromdance. Although the original description by Goodpasture suggested that the disease occurred only in young male patients, it is clear now that the age of presentation can range from the first year to the ninth decade (13,33). Furthermore, there is a bimodal distribution, with a larger number of patients presenting at about 30 years of age, with a second peak at about 60 years of age (34). Occurrence of the disease is more common in white patients than in those who are African American and has a greater predilection for certain racial groups, such as the Maoris in New Zealand (35).

Goodpasture's syndrome has been described to occur throughout the year, but there appears to be an increased incidence in the spring and early summer. Localized outbreaks have been reported, possibly associated with infections or other common causes. In our series, about half of patients have had some type of pulmonary presentation consistent with upper respiratory infection or other types of infections, suggesting an association with viral or bacterial infection.

As with other autoimmune diseases, there is persuasive evidence of inherited predeposition to anti-GBM disease. There is an increased association with HLA antigen DR2, and patients with HLA-B7 in addition to DR2 have worse GN (36,37). Anti-GBM disease has been reported in identical twins and siblings as well as in members of the same family (38,39). More recently, restricted clonality and antibody response to Goodpasture's epitope have been reported, as has HLA-restricted T-cell responses in isolated clones of T cells derived from patients with Goodpasture's syndrome (40). These observations suggest a significant influence of genetic susceptibility in the phenotypic expression of Goodpasture's syndrome.

Evidence suggests that in susceptible patients, numerous environmental factors may be significant in the pathogenesis or phenotypic expression of Goodpasture's syndrome. As noted previously, a large number of the patients whom we have seen in our series have had symptoms suggesting upper respiratory or other types of infection and vague systemic findings suggestive of viral illnesses, such as fever, rash, myalgia, malaise, headache, or weight loss before the onset of GN. Exposure to a variety of toxic substances has been associated with the onset of Goodpasture's syndrome. These include petroleum-containing products, hair spray, solutions used for dry-cleaning purposes, paint and other petroleum products, and exposure to tobacco smoking (41–44). There appears to be a close correlation with the presence of pulmonary hemorrhage and active exposure to substances that can damage the endothelium of the pulmonary system, especially smoking (44). Studies in experimental animals suggest that damage to the alveolar lining by a variety of mechanisms can be associated with the phenotype of pulmonary hemorrhage in animals with preexisting circulating anti-GBM antibodies (45,46). The widespread distribution of the various substances associated with the development of Goodpasture's syndrome and the small incidence of the clinical phenotype of disease make it extremely difficult to document a cause-and-effect relationship between environmental exposure and the resultant phenotypic expression.

## PATHOGENESIS

A detailed assessment of the pathogenesis of Goodpasture's syndrome is beyond the scope of this chapter. Briefly, however, information regarding pathogenesis is derived from a host of experimental models in many different species and strains of animals. Two major models have been used during the past several decades. The first, the nephrotoxic serum nephritis model, depends on the passive administration of heterologous antibody raised against host GBM antigen (47,48). The GBM from the species of interest is isolated and used to immunize an unrelated species. When high-titer antibody is present, this antibody is harvested, purified, absorbed with red cells and serum of the recipient species, and then administered intravenously.

The clinical and histologic phases are determined by whether the recipient animal is preimmunized, by the species and strain, and by whether complement fixation is present (47,48). Multiple cytokines and chemokines have been shown to be important in the pathogenesis of the disease, as have T cells and T-cell subsets (49–52). The T-cell constitution is extremely important in the type of disease that results from nephrotoxic serum administration (51–54). In certain strains of rats, CD8$^+$ cells are key in the development of the disease, whereas in murine models, CD4$^+$ cells have been shown to be important (51,52,55). In some strains of mice, complement is essential, but in others, it is not. In rabbits and rats, complement appears to be important. Interleukin-1 (IL-1), IL-2, and tumor necrosis factor-$\alpha$ (TNF-$\alpha$) are all important in pathogenesis, as shown by blocking with antibody and administration of soluble protein-receptor antagonists to compete with cytokines (56–58). Chemokines of a variety of types, including fractalkine, MIP-1, MIP-2, MIF, and MCP-1, have also been shown to be important (54,59). It is likely that Fc receptors are crucial because mice lacking Fc receptors develop glomerular antibody deposition without GN (60–62). All of these models of nephrotoxic serum nephritis probably have only modest relevance to human disease. Disease does not occur in humans secondary to the passive administration of antibody to the GBM, either in the naive or in the preimmunized state!

The second model, which has more relevance to human disease, is that developed by Steblay (63), in which animals are immunized against GBM constituents. This is probably far closer to the human situation, whereby infection or exposure to a host of toxic agents can result in release of endogenous antigens and the autoimmune state (13). In a manner analogous to nephrotoxic serum nephritis, however, induction of Steblay autoimmune GN is highly dependent on the immunization procedure, the type of antigen used, the species and strain of animal employed, and the immune background of the animal (64–68). Both cellular and antibody immunity are involved in the pathogenesis of this model (49,50,69–74).

There are marked differences in susceptibility to disease induction and the consequent severity of the disease. Whereas the human disease is associated with predominance of antibody to $\alpha$3, disease in rats and mice is associated with antibody to other NC1 domains. Indeed, rats can be induced to develop Goodpasture's syndrome not only with dimers and monomers of $\alpha$3 isolated by column chromatography but also by recombinant $\alpha$3 NC1 as well as recombinant $\alpha$4 NC1 domain (65,75,76). Thus, the disease process, which appears histologically analogous to human disease, is probably somewhat different pathogenically.

Nonetheless, these experimental animal models provide a great deal of information about the pathogenesis of disease, including the roles of monocytes and macrophages, which appear to be pivotal, as shown by macrophage depletion with antimacrophage antiserum and phenotypic analysis of biopsies (77,78). Breaks in the GBM and Bowman's capsule appear to be essential in initiating the fibrinogen deposition and migration of macrophages into Bowman's space, with expression of neoantigens of the coagulation cascade (79–81). It is not clear whether communication from the interior of Bowman's capsules or the periglomerular infiltrate of macrophages and T cells are responsible for induction of the tubulointerstitial disease so characteristic of animal and human anti-GBM disease (78). All animal models are associated with heavy proteinuria, which has been shown to result in activation of proximal tubular cells and inside-out signaling, with consequent changes in the basement membrane and interstitium. Likewise, the peritubular and periglomerular infiltrates with mononuclear cells and elaboration of consequent cytokines probably play a role.

Finally, the antibody–ligand interaction between GBM epitopes and circulating and bound anti-GBM antibodies is probably important in the phenotypic expression of the disease. Many animal models and human examples of anti-GBM–bound antibody with minimal or no disease have been described, and severe histologic lesions in the lung without detectable antibody have likewise been described (13). It is likely that a combination of antibody and cellular immune processes are responsible for the phenotypic expression of the disease, especially in humans. The cloning and expression of the putative nephritogenic antigen, $\alpha$3(IV) NC1 recombinant protein chain, offers exciting opportunity for further examining the pathogenesis of this disease process and potential treatment (21,82–85). This chain, like the native antigen, undergoes conformational rearrangement, which varies with expression system. There are consequent differences in antibody avidity and affinity of binding, different capability for disease induction in animal models, and different specificities of antibody binding for patients' sera with Goodpasture's syndrome.

Further studies to delineate the differences in binding between mild and severe disease in relation to conformational epitopes and posttranslational modifications will likely lead to be a better understanding of the pathogenesis of this disease. This will help to clarify why strains within the same species have such significant differences in response and why the same strain of animal may differ in response. This knowledge will lead to better, more rational modes of therapy of human disease in the future. Space does not allow a full and detailed examination and analysis of these various pathogenic processes; of the intricate differences that apply to strains, species, and type of antigens involved; nor of the cytokines, chemokines, antibody isotypes, and variability in receptor–ligand interaction. These subjects are dealt with in other sections of this text in much more detail and likely apply to the autoimmune processes involved in the development of Goodpasture's syndrome both in experimental animal models and in humans.

## CLINICAL PRESENTATION

Patients with pulmonary involvement in Goodpasture's syndrome have no specific findings. Goodpasture's is one of many causes of pulmonary hemorrhage (Table 32.1), including a variety of types of GN, vasculitis, including microscopic polyangiitis, Wegener's granulomatosis, Churg–Strauss vasculitis, collagen vascular disease, and other types of vasculitis. The differential diagnosis includes infection, malignancy, and any renal syndrome associated with pulmonary hemorrhage whether or not there is an immune-mediated GN. Interestingly, with Goodpasture's syndrome, pulmonary hemorrhage can occur many years before the development of overt GN or after the GN has become apparent. Whether the pulmonary symptoms represent the deposition of antibody on the basement membrane or a preceding illness leading to the initiation of an anti-GBM immune response remains to be clarified.

**TABLE 32.1.** *Renal disease with pulmonary hemorrhage*

Blood dyscrasias
Cardiovascular
  Advanced uremia with superimposed CHF
  Mitral stenosis
  Pulmonary embolism with infarct and underlying renal
    vein thrombosis
Collagen vascular disease
  Systemic lupus erythematosus
  Progressive systemic sclerosis
  Rheumatoid arthritis
Glomerulonephritis
  Goodpasture's syndrome
  Immune complex glomerulonephritis
  Acute silicoproteinosis
  Glomerulonephritis with CHF
  D-Penicillamine toxicity, trimellitic anhydride toxicity
Hemolytic uremic syndrome
Idiopathic hemosiderosis
Infection
  Legionnaires' disease
  Necrotizing pneumonitis
  Bronchitis
  Tuberculosis
  Fungus
  Lung abscess
  Bronchiectasis
Malignancy with associated glomerulopathy
Thrombotic thrombocytopenic purpura
Vasculitis
  Polyarteritis nodosa
  Microscopic polyangiitis
  Wegener's granulomatosis
  Henoch–Schönlein purpura
  Mixed immunoglobulin M–immunoglobulin G cryoglobu-
    linemia
  Churg–Strauss syndrome
  Lymphoid granulomatosis
  Necrotizing sarcoid granulomatosis
  Hypersensitivity
  Behçet's syndrome
  Hughes–Stovin syndrome
  Giant cell arteritis
  Hypocomplementemic urticaria
  Takayasu's arteritis

CHF, congestive heart failure.

The pulmonary hemorrhage associated with Goodpasture's syndrome can range from blood-streaked sputum to massive fatal intrapulmonary hemorrhage leading to immediate death. In patients whose disease is otherwise quiescent, exposure to toxic substances, smoking, and other environmental eliciting agents including infection can precipitate pulmonary hemorrhage (44,86). Most patients present with shortness of breath and cough, sometimes with hemoptysis and occasionally with wheezing. They do not usually have chest pain such as seen with emboli, pleurisy, or other causes of pulmonary pain. The sputum shows hemosiderin-containing macrophages on microscopic examination, indicating pulmonary hemorrhage. There is increased uptake of carbon monoxide, which can be used as a test of pulmonary hemorrhage and to document episodes of pulmonary hemorrhage not associated with significant clinical pulmonary manifestations (87). Positive tests result because of bonding of carbon monoxide to blood that has been extravasated within the lung, with consequent formation of carboxy hemoglobin. Alveolar infiltrates radiating from the hilum bilaterally are frequent but nodular densities, and segmental and patchy infiltrates of nonspecific nature may also be observed. Thus, the pulmonary radiograph serves as documentation of an infiltrate but is not specific for Goodpasture's syndrome. The finding of an abnormal carbon monoxide uptake test is highly suggestive of intrapulmonary hemorrhage and in a patient with preexisting anti-GBM disease can be used as a method for following the patient for evidence of reactivation of disease.

An active urinary sediment is common with numerous dysmorphic red blood cells, red blood cell casts, and casts containing both white and red blood cells. If a sample is well prepared, correctly spun, examined fresh, and perhaps stained, evidence of nephritic activity within the urine should be seen in all cases. If a careful examination of the urine does not reveal evidence of GN, one of the other causes of pulmonary renal syndrome should be considered. Proteinuria is usually present, generally in the range of 1 to 2 g per 24 hours and not often in the nephrotic range (3.5 g or more per 24 hours), although some patients have heavy proteinuria associated with their nephritic presentation. Renal function may be entirely normal, modestly decreased, or significantly decreased. The course of the decreasing kidney function can be gradual or can be devastating and rapid over a few weeks or months (13,32,88,89). When a patient has a decrease in renal function consisting of a doubling of serum creatinine or halving of the creatinine clearance within a 3-month period or less, the patient is defined as having rapidly progressive GN (32). Goodpasture's syndrome is one of those glomerulonephritic diseases that frequently does have a rapidly progressive course. By ultrasonography, the kidneys are usually of normal size, and there is no evidence of increased echotexture, as occurs with chronic GN. Anatomic abnormalities are absent.

The clinical presentation of these patients is frequently nonspecific, with a variety of vague complaints, such as easy fatigability, malaise, myalgias, weight loss, change in appetite, and history of upper respiratory infection. Hypertension is not a usual feature, but there may be a mild increase in blood pressure consistent with the age of the patient.

A subset of patients with anti-GBM disease have the associated presence of antineutrophilic cytoplasmic antibody (ANCA) (90–93). In these patients, there is a propensity for a remitting and relapsing course of clinical signs and symptoms, patients are more likely to have a rash or more specific complaints of myalgias and arthralgias, and patients present clinically with symptoms much more like microscopic polyangiitis than pure anti-GBM disease.

Lung biopsies in patients dying from Goodpasture's syndrome or obtained from open pulmonary biopsy show evidence of consolidation. Alveoli are filled with extravasated red blood cells, fibrin, neutrophils, and macrophages. Interstitial hemorrhage between basement membranes and edema is common. Immunofluorescence examination of pulmonary tissues is extremely difficult because of intrinsic highlighting of the basement membrane. In many cases with appropriate controls, however, antibody fixed in a linear fashion along alveolar basement membranes can be observed. More often, alveoli filled with fibrin are observed (Fig. 32.1). Even in patients who do not have definite antibody present along the basement membrane in the lung, elution of tissue, and application of the eluted antibody to GBM substrate reveal *in vitro* fixation of antibody to basement membrane components. The intraalveolar hemorrhage observed with Goodpasture's syndrome is not distinctive in relationship to Wegener's granulomatosis and various other vasculitides.

The kidneys in patients with Goodpasture's syndrome are swollen and pale and frequently have petechiae on their surfaces, as seen in other types of GN. Immunofluorescence examination of tissue invariably shows smooth linear deposition of immunoglobulins, predominantly immunoglobulin G (IgG), along the GBM, Bowman's capsule, and various tubular basement membranes (Fig. 32.2A). In advanced cases, the deposits can assume a fragmented or finely granu-

lar pattern, although the linear nature is confirmed by ultrastructure that shows no evidence of immune reactants. This latter pattern most likely reflects damage to the basement membrane by proteolytic enzymes, resulting in pseudogranular staining. In more advanced cases, other immunoglobulins are deposited in the same general pattern, and complement may be present in about one third of patients. Intense staining for fibrinogen is observed in crescents (Fig. 32.2B). In severe cases, there is extravasation and insudation of immunoglobulins and complement into crescents that line Bowman's space. There are gaps in the basement membrane through which macrophages and neutrophils may be seen to migrate; formation of multinucleated giant cells, both within the glomeruli and in the interstitium; and an extremely intense mononuclear cell infiltrate in a periglomerular and interstitial pattern.

Phenotypic analysis of these infiltrates (78,94) demonstrates a preponderance of macrophages and activated macrophages with CD4 cells, fewer CD8 cells, and few B cells. In initial biopsy specimens, the crescents are cellular, with cells composed of monocytes, macrophages, polymorphs, and activated epithelial cells (Fig. 32.3). There is elaboration of basement membrane materials, collagen, and fibrosis, with associated necrosis and rapid progression to fibrocellular and obsolescent glomeruli. The glomerular tuft may be involved with mild proliferation but frequently is only minimally involved because most of the activity occurs in the development of exuberant crescents, which crush the glomerular tuft. The disease can progress from cellular crescent to total obsolescence within the period of a few weeks (Fig. 32.4).

The differential diagnosis includes any of the entities listed in Table 32.1. A careful history and physical examination, urinalysis, and serologic tests, as detailed later, plus a renal biopsy, serve to make the correct diagnosis.

A unique form of Goodpasture's syndrome occurs in some patients with Alport's syndrome after allografting for renal failure. Alport's syndrome, a hereditary, generally X-linked, but sometimes autosomal dominant syndrome, develops from multiple mutations and deletions in the gene for $\alpha5(IV)$ collagen, resulting in abnormal production of GBM (30,95). Generally, there is absence of the $\alpha5$ NC1 domain, resulting in lack of assembly of $\alpha3$, $\alpha5$, and other chains within the GBM in patients carrying the trait. It results in progressive renal dysfunction, generally in male patients, and when these patients receive an allograft that contains antigens not previously present because of disassembly, there is the potential for the development of *de novo* anti-GBM antibody against the new antigens in the allograft. Although this was originally thought to be a significant problem in transplantation, only 3% to 5% of patients actually develop *de novo* disease to the point of losing their grafts, although some 10% or so may develop circulating antibodies (30,96). Furthermore, although this was previously thought to result exclusively from antibody to $\alpha3$, it is now known that it is much more common to have antibodies to $\alpha5$ and less common to have reactivity to $\alpha3$ (29).

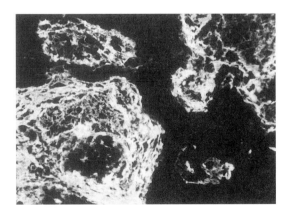

**FIG. 32.1.** Lung biopsy specimen from a 19-year-old white woman with Goodpasture's syndrome. The alveolar space is filled with fibrin-positive inflammatory debris.

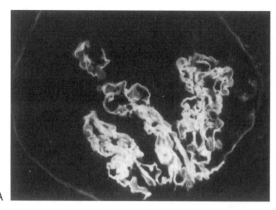
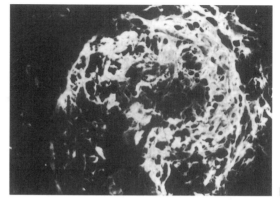

**FIG. 32.2.** Renal biopsy specimen from a 27-year-old African-American man demonstrating **(A)** linear-staining immunoglobulin G along the glomerular basement membrane and Bowman's capsule, and **(B)** intensely staining fibrin within a crescent. (From Bolton WK, Sturgill BC. Proliferative glomerulonephritis: post-infectious, non-infectious and crescentic forms. In: Tisher CC, Brenner BM, eds. *Renal pathology.* Philadelphia: JB Lippincott, 1989:156, with permission.)

This is another example of how antibodies against different chains within the GBM can be resultant of anti-GBM disease and illustrates that the spectrum of pathogenic process involving the basement membrane is much more complex than previously thought.

## DIAGNOSTIC TESTING

### Anti–Glomerular Basement Membrane Assays

The diagnosis of Goodpasture's syndrome requires documentation of anti-GBM antibodies bound to the glomeruli of the kidneys. This is usually associated with the presence of circulating anti-GBM antibodies of the IgG class, although IgA and IgM have also been reported (44,97,98). A number of assays are available for detecting the presence of circulat-

ing anti-GBM antibody. Although circulating antibodies are present in more than 90% of patients with anti-GBM disease, the sensitivity and specificity of the assays vary. Indirect immunofluorescence assays using different species of kidney substrates, such as monkey or bovine kidneys, can be falsely negative in 10% or more of test samples. Radioimmunoassays and enzyme-linked immunosorbent assays (ELISA) are much more specific and sensitive and have less than a 5% false-negative rate. There are few false-positive assays either by indirect immunofluorescence, immunoassay, or ELISA. False-positive results probably occur in 1% or less of tests that are positive. False-positive tests may occur because of antibodies directed to other constituents of type IV collagen, lack of proper control, inexperience in observer interpretation of the test, and artifactual positive assays. A variety of errors can include drying of the tissue substrate, incorrect dilution

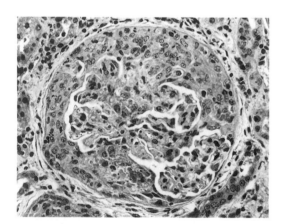

**FIG. 32.3.** Light microscopic section of kidney biopsy demonstrating cellular crescent with compression of the glomerular tuft (periodic acid–Schiff stain). (From Bolton WK, Couser WG. Intravenous pulse methylprednisolone therapy of acute crescentic rapidly progressive glomerulonephritis. *Am J Med* 1979;66:495–502, with permission.)

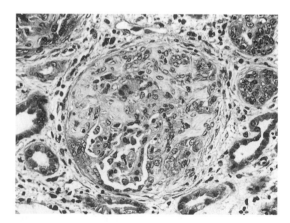

**FIG. 32.4.** Kidney section illustrating fibrocellular crescent and early glomerular obsolescence (hematoxylin and eosin stain). (From Bolton WK, Couser WG. Intravenous pulse methylprednisolone therapy of acute crescentic rapidly progressive glomerulonephritis. *Am J Med* 1979;66:495–502, with permission.)

of the serum or the secondary antibody, and other factors. When pulmonary hemorrhage and GN are related to anti-GBM antibodies, positive assays are usually observed. The chance of Goodpasture's syndrome is small if these two clinical findings are present and the assay is negative, but this has been seen in isolated cases.

Some of the problems with indirect immunofluorescence, immunoassays, and ELISA have been addressed with the use of recombinant DNA technology. The sequence for all of the type IV collagen chains has now been elaborated, and recombinant proteins have been developed from α1 through α6 for use in immunoassays, ELISA, and Western blot analysis. Different forms of recombinant protein have been studied, including those produced in bacterial hosts, miniconstructs developed in baculovirus, and protein developed in mammalian cell systems (Fig. 32.5) (21,28). These all vary in their sensitivity and specificity. It remains to be determined whether they will be more sensitive in detecting antibodies than the current assay technique using native GBM antigens in ELISA or immunoassay techniques. The specificity may well be much greater for these pure recombinant proteins for the various NC1 domains, but the utility gained by specificity may be lost by a lack of sensitivity.

### Serologic Assays

The erythrocyte sedimentation rate is usually elevated, reflecting nonspecific inflammation. Tests for antinuclear antibodies and anti-DNA should be negative.

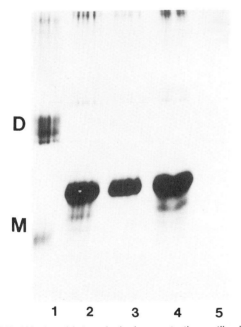

**FIG. 32.5.** Western blot analysis demonstrating antibody activity to native glomerular basement membrane monomers (*M*) and dimers (*D*) in lane 1, recombinant α3(IV) in lanes 2 and 4, and recombinant α4(IV) NC1 domain in lane 3. Recombinant proteins are larger than native protein because of the addition of protein sequences for identification and isolation. Lane 5 shows normal serum versus glomerular basement membrane.

### Circulating Antineutrophil Cytoplasmic Antibody

A variety of diseases may be associated with positive circulating ANCA (Table 32.2). Clinicians generally associate the presence of ANCA with many vasculitic syndromes (99). In the past, the coexistence of Goodpasture's syndrome and vasculitis was considered rare, and few isolated reports of this association have been made (100,101). In 1989, however, O'Donoghue (90) reported three patients with ANCA-positive serum as well as anti-GBM disease. Since then, a number of additional patients have been described with coexistent ANCA and Goodpasture's syndrome (91–93). About 20% to 30% of patients with circulating anti-GBM antibodies may have coexisting circulating ANCA at some time during the course of the disease. The ANCA may develop after anti-GBM disease has been documented or may occur before anti-GBM disease. In about three fourths of cases, the ANCA is in a perinuclear pattern, whereas it is cytoplasmic in nature in the other one fourth of patients. There is generally an inverse relationship between the titer of ANCA and that of anti-GBM antibody, with patients who have high titers of anti-GBM antibody having low ANCA titers, and *vice versa.*

### Pulmonary Function

Carbon monoxide diffusion is usually abnormal, as noted previously, and the pulmonary radiograph is nonspecific and may show evidence of pulmonary infiltrates of multiple causes that cannot be ascribed to pulmonary hemorrhage, even in patients with Goodpasture's syndrome. In the absence of pulmonary hemorrhage and in patients in the early course of their disease in whom relapse is suggested, especially after exposure to environmental stimulants, carbon monoxide diffusion tests can be used as an early diagnostic test for the occurrence of pulmonary hemorrhage.

**TABLE 32.2.** *Entities associated with circulating antineutrophil cytoplasmic antibody*

| |
| --- |
| Chronic liver disease |
| Crohn's disease |
| Felty's syndrome |
| Hemodialysis patients |
| Henoch–Schönlein purpura |
| Human immunodeficiency virus |
| Polymyositis |
| Silicosis |
| Sjögren's syndrome |
| Systemic lupus erythematosus |
| Rheumatoid arthritis |
| Ulcerative colitis |
| Other acute or chronic infection |
| Vasculitis |
|     Anti–glomerular basement membrane |
|     Churg–Strauss allergic vasculitis |
|     Microscopic polyangiitis |
|     Wegener's granulomatosis |

### Radiographic and Renal Imaging

Radiographic and renal imaging techniques are useful in confirming that pulmonary involvement is present, although they are extremely nonspecific. Renal imaging, as described previously, also provides evidence of an acute onset of renal disease, with normal renal size and absence of increased echotexture suggestive of scarring.

### Lung and Kidney Biopsy

Lung biopsy is extremely difficult to interpret, and the author considers it to be much more invasive than renal biopsy. Renal biopsy can be done expeditiously and should be performed within the first 24 hours of presentation of the patient because of the alarming rate of progression that can occur in patients with anti-GBM disease. Ultrasound-guided needle biopsy or open renal biopsy can be accomplished with rapid processing of the tissue to ascertain whether anti-GBM disease is present. It is extremely important to obtain tissue as quickly as possible because progression of the histologic changes can occur over a period of only a few weeks, and therapeutic intervention, to be successful, needs to be undertaken as soon as possible. All tissue should be examined by immunofluorescence, including antibody to all immunoglobulins, components of complement and fibrin, and κ and light chains, and by thin section with hematoxylin and eosin, periodic acid–Schiff, and silver stains. Ultrastructure analysis is also useful, especially late in the course of the disease when the issue of granular versus linear deposits may be more difficult to distinguish.

### Diagnostic Algorithm

The approach that I take to patients with pulmonary renal syndrome is described in Figure 32.6. Based on this approach, patients can be divided into those who test ANCA negative and anti-GBM positive and those who test positive for both. These are important characteristics in directing the type and intensity of therapy.

### TREATMENT

### Natural Course and Prognosis

The clinical course of Goodpasture's syndrome is frequently that of a rapidly progressive GN with a devastating decrement in renal function. Goodpasture's syndrome is often associated with life-threatening pulmonary hemorrhage, which, although usually responsive to pulse methylprednisolone and plasma exchange, may at times be extremely refractory to therapy. The prognosis is generally considered to be extremely poor (34,102,103). As diagnostic acumen and rapidity of therapy institution improves, it is apparent that there is a broader spectrum of disease, with some patients having minimal or no clinical manifestation of their anti-

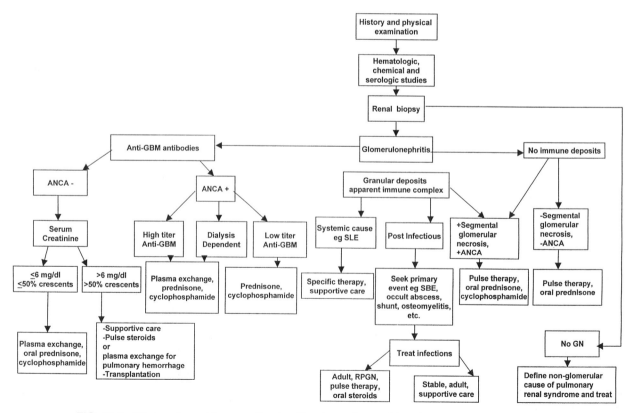

**FIG. 32.6.** Diagnostic and therapeutic algorithm for patients with pulmonary renal syndromes.

GBM disease. Nonetheless, most patients with anti-GBM disease do pursue a rapid downhill course.

Before the use of various types of aggressive immunotherapy and plasmapheresis, about 90% of patients with anti-GBM disease described in the literature progressed to death or dialysis. Only a few of these patients showed improvement, occasionally spontaneously but usually with immunosuppressive therapeutic agents (32). The documentation that these patients had circulating antibodies directed against the GBM in studies by Lerner, Dixon, and Glassock (104,105) and that antibodies to the GBM could cause disease in experimental models led to the use of plasma exchange as the preferred therapeutic approach (106–108). About half of patients treated aggressively with plasma exchange showed evidence of improvement. Few patients on dialysis or with oligoanuria responded to plasma exchange, pulse methylprednisolone, or any other type of therapy (32,106,108,109). A few isolated reports of patients with Goodpasture's syndrome who recovered spontaneously after acute renal failure requiring dialysis and with certain environmental agents provide an exception to this observation (110–112). The prognosis observed in most patients with anti-GBM disease, however, is extremely poor.

The overall prognosis also appears to be influenced by the genetic deposition of patients; those who carry HLA-B7 along with HLA-DRW2 experience a worse GN course than those without this combination (36,108). Prognosis appears also to be related to the degree of crescent formation, the intensity of the tubulointerstitial disease, and the presence and degree of scarring, glomerular sclerosis, and fibrosis present at the time of biopsy. The greater all of these histologic findings, the worse the prognosis for the patient (109,113). Finally, those patients who have advanced renal failure, with oliguria, anuria, dialysis, or serum creatinine levels higher than 5 to 6 mg/dL, rarely respond to any type of therapy.

## Influence of Positive Antineutrophilic Cytoplasmic Antibody

The clinical course for patients who have both ANCA and anti-GBM circulating antibodies is different than those patients who have only anti-GBM disease. About half of the double-positive patients require dialysis, in contrast to a much greater number of patients with anti-GBM disease. Additionally, as opposed to patients with pure Goodpasture's syndrome, a number of ANCA-positive patients have been shown to recover renal function sufficiently to allow them to discontinue dialysis. This is extremely unusual in anti-GBM disease and raises the issue of whether anti-GBM disease patients who have responded to therapy while on dialysis may have had positive ANCA as well (91,92).

There appears to be an inverse correlation between anti-GBM and ANCA titers, disease course, and response to treatment. Patients with higher ANCA titers and lower anti-GBM titers have a course suggestive of systemic microangiopathic vasculitis, with response to therapy for vasculitis and recov-

ery from dialysis. Those with high-titer anti-GBM disease have a devastating deteriorating course without return of function. In addition, patients who are double positive have a tendency for relapse, which is not often seen in patients with pure anti-GBM disease. It would appear that the spectrum of patients with anti-GBM disease needs to be broadened and subclassified into patients who are ANCA negative and positive. Patients who are ANCA positive with anti-GBM antibodies appear to have a primary vasculitic process, with secondary formation of anti-GBM disease; their clinical course and response to therapy are comparable to those in patients with ANCA-positive vasculitis. Patients with primary anti-GBM disease and low titer secondary positive ANCA have a clinical course that appears to be typical of anti-GBM disease, with the ANCA as an epiphenomenon.

## Conventional Therapy

The pulmonary hemorrhage associated with Goodpasture's syndrome responds to pulse methylprednisolone or to plasma exchange with a rapid decrease in the severity of pulmonary hemorrhage in most cases (32,108,114). I have had a few patients with pulmonary hemorrhage who have died of their pulmonary disease despite plasma exchange, pulse methylprednisolone, and cyclophosphamide. Whether they represent a different spectrum of disease or for some reason are unresponsive to the aggressive therapeutic modality employed is not clear.

As described previously, before the use of pulse methylprednisolone and plasma exchange, the mortality rate for Goodpasture's syndrome approached 90%. The presence of circulating anti-GBM antibody is an obvious indication that removal of these antibodies by plasmapheresis or immunoglobulin-sorbent columns might be beneficial to the patient. For these reasons, plasma exchange would appear to be the most rational approach to patients with anti-GBM disease. Lockwood et al. (34,106,108,115) have reported one of the world's largest experiences, including more than 100 patients with anti-GBM disease treated with plasma exchange and immunosuppression. In these series, patients with normal renal function, whether treated or not, showed improvement of renal function. Three fourths of patients with serum creatinine levels of less than 7 mg/dL improved with plasma exchange, but only 1 of 12 patients with a serum creatinine level higher than 7 mg/dL who was not on dialysis showed any improvement. None of the 58 patients on dialysis showed any improvement.

Serial measurement of anti-GBM antibody titers has shown that plasma exchange is quickly beneficial in the removal of circulating antibodies using *in vitro* tests for circulating antibody (107,114). Routine therapy consists of 14 exchanges of 4 L each over a 2-week period, along with prednisone and cyclophosphamide or azathioprine. This regimen decreases circulating antibody levels without rebound after cessation of plasma exchange. Of note, however, is the caveat that there is not a good correlation between circulating antibodies at presentation and the degree of GN, nor between the decrease in antibody titers caused by plasmapheresis and the response to therapy in patients who do not require dialysis (107,116).

This is an extremely rare and devastating disease, and unfortunately, little information from prospective randomized controlled studies is available. In a study by Johnson et al. (114), therapy with pulse methylprednisolone, as compared with immunosuppression with plasma exchange, showed no added beneficial effect of plasma exchange. Although antibody levels were reduced, the clinical outcomes between the two groups were comparable. Analysis of the data showed that the percentage of crescents on initial renal biopsy and entry serum creatinine levels correlated better with outcome than with the type of therapy used. These investigators concluded that a lower degree of crescent formation and well-preserved renal function provided a better opportunity for response to treatment than the modality of treatment assigned.

My experience and that of others on which data are available also suggest that patients with mild anti-GBM disease may respond well to therapies other than plasma exchange (117,118). This is described graphically in Figure 32.7, which illustrates the results of four series in which enough information was available to assess the impact of serum creatinine level and degree of crescent involvement (109,114,116,119). In this retrospective analysis, I assessed treatment with plasma exchange, pulse methylprednisolone, or conventional therapy (defined as no therapy or any type of immunosuppression other than plasma exchange or pulse methylprednisolone). Interestingly, patients with anti-GBM disease segregated almost completely into those with less than 50% crescents and a serum creatinine level of less than 5 mg/dL on presentation or those with more than 50% crescents and a serum creatinine level of more than 5 mg/dL. Three fourths of patients with a lower degree of crescent and lower serum creatinine levels treated with conventional therapy or pulse methylprednisolone improved, compared with all

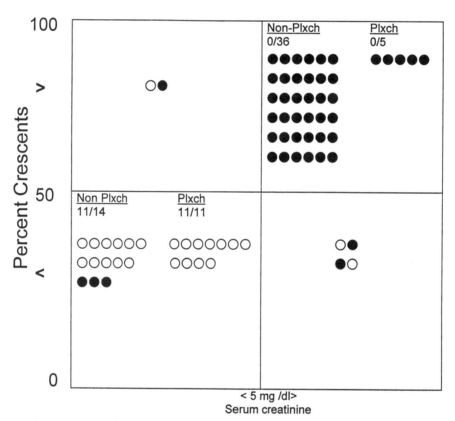

**FIG. 32.7.** Influence of renal function and percentage of crescents on prognosis in patients with Goodpasture's syndrome. *Closed circles* indicate treatment failure. *Open circles* represent the response to treatment, which includes therapy with plasma exchange (*Plxch*) and other therapies (*Non-Plxch*). Data from Bolton WK, Sturgill BC. Methylprednisolone therapy for acute crescentric rapidly progressive glomerulonephritis. *Am J Nephrol* 1989;9:368–375; Johnson JP, Moore J Jr, Austin HA III, et al. Therapy of anti-glomerular basement membrane antibody disease: analysis of prognostic significance of clinical, pathologic and treatment factors. *Medicine* 1985;64:219–227; Briggs WA, Johnson JP, Teichman S, et al. Antiglomerular basement membrane antibody-mediated glomerulonephritis and Goodpasture's syndrome. *Medicine* 1979;58:348–361; and Simpson IJ, Doak PB, Williams LC, et al. Plasma exchange in Goodpasture's syndrome. *Am J Nephrol* 1982;2:301–311. Adapted from Bolton WK. Goodpasture's syndrome. Nephrology Forum. *Kidney Int* 1996;50:1753–1766, with permission.

of the patients with plasma exchange. On the other hand, patients with a greater degree of crescent formation and higher serum creatinine levels failed to respond regardless of the type of immunosuppression or use of plasma exchange.

## Therapeutic Algorithm

Although one prospective randomized controlled study showed no beneficial effect of plasmapheresis, and other studies suggest that the spectrum of disease is important, until appropriate prospective randomized controlled studies are formed, I approach patients with pulmonary hemorrhage using the diagnostic and therapeutic stratagem outlined in Figure 32.6. Table 32.3 lists the therapeutic protocols and their various components. Essential components for the deci-

**TABLE 32.3.** *Therapeutic protocols*

A. Pulse methylprednisolone
   Volume repletion ascertained
   No diuretics 3 hr before pulse or 24 hr after
   30 mg/kg methylprednisolone given IV over 20 min
      every other day for three doses
   Single dose not to exceed 3 g
   Monitor blood pressure during and 4 hr after infusion
B. Oral prednisone, given every other day

| Dose (mg/kg)[a] | Duration of therapy (mo)[b] |
|---|---|
| 2.0 | 0.5 |
| 1.75 | 1.0 |
| 1.50 | 3.0 |
| 1.25 | 6.0 |
| 1.00 | 6.0 |
| 0.75 | 6.0 |
| 0.50 | 6.0 |
| 0.25 | 6.0 |
| 0.125 | 12.0 |
| 0.0625 | 12.0 |

C. Cyclophosphamide
   2.0 mg/kg daily for 3 mo
   1.5 mg/kg for 3 mo
   1.0 mg/kg daily for 3 mo
   0.5 mg/kg daily for 3 mo
   Decrease dose 50% for creatinine clearance ≤10
      mL/min
   Hold dose if white blood cell count ≤3500/mm$^3$, or
      platelets ≤100,000/mm$^3$
D. Plasma exchange
   4-L exchanges 5 of 7 days or every other day × 14
      exchanges minimum
   Replacement with 5% normal human serum albumin
   Fresh-frozen plasma if bleeding problems
   Always be certain cyclophosphamide is used when
      patients receive plasma exchange (immunoglobulin
      rebound suppression)

[a] Patients ≥60 years of age should receive 75% of oral prednisone dose on alternate days; for very obese patients, ideal body weight should be used.
[b] If full remission of proteinuria is achieved, with normal function for 1 month, decrease to next dose step.

sion tree are serum ANCA, serum anti-GBM assay, renal biopsy, and patient renal function.

In patients who are ANCA negative with a serum creatinine level of less than 6 mg/dL and less than 50% crescents, we employ plasmapheresis with immunosuppression. In patients with more than 50% crescents and a serum creatinine level of more than 6 mg/dL and in those who are oligoanuric or on dialysis, we treat pulmonary hemorrhage but use a short course only of plasma exchange and immunosuppression, or frequently none at all. On the other hand, if the ANCA is positive, we treat as it if the patient had vasculitis combined with anti-GBM disease. In those with maintained renal function and high-titer anti-GBM antibodies, we use plasma exchange and immunosuppression.

As noted previously, although plasma exchange probably does not have any beneficial effect on patients on dialysis, there is evidence that the dialysis dependence may resolve better in patients in whom the renal failure is secondary to vasculitis (120). Therefore, we use plasma exchange and immunosuppression for dialysis-dependent double-positive patients.

In patients with low-titer anti-GBM and ANCA positivity, we may treat the disease as if the patients have pure vasculitis, using pulse methylprednisolone or oral prednisone and cyclophosphamide. We have not used intravenous cyclophosphamide, although others have used this therapeutic modality (121,122). In the presence of a clinical course of rapidly progressive GN and this clinical picture, or if highly active histologic lesions were present on renal biopsy, plasma exchange would likely be added. When we perform plasma exchange, we routinely use albumin rather than plasma replacement, although one could argue that plasma could be beneficial in the subset of vasculitis patients, as has been described by others (123).

## Protein A Columns

Because antibodies to the GBM can be adsorbed out by protein A columns, it is possible that immunosorbent columns consisting of protein A could be used to remove anti-GBM antibodies. This approach has been used for ANCA in a few patients in pilot studies, and results have suggested an improvement in ANCA levels as well as some clinical improvement in patients. Removal of anti-GBM antibodies by this method has been reported with no benefit (124).

## Epitope-specific Immunosorbent Columns

The cloning, sequencing, and expression of recombinant proteins for α3(IV) collagen and the observation of a high prevalence of circulating antibodies in patients with Goodpasture's syndrome to α3 in preference to other NC1 domains suggest the possibility that immunosorbent columns consisting of recombinant α3 NC1 domains could be therapeutically beneficial in patients with anti-GBM disease (85). Numerous obstacles remain to the development of immunosorbent columns, but it is likely that these will be available in the near future. Problems that remain include the ability to develop and produce large enough quantities of recombinant protein, the ascertainment that the recombinant proteins are able to bind all of the circulating anti-GBM antibodies that are injurious, the utility of immunosorbent columns without undue risks for the patient, and the cost of therapy with immunosorbent columns.

Because Goodpasture's syndrome can progress at an alarmingly rapid pace and because the cost of the immunosorbent columns could be prohibitive for such a small number of patients, access to these columns in a timely and cost-effective fashion could be of considerable concern. The prospect of being able to use epitope-specific immunosorbent columns, however, provides an exciting potential in this disease process.

### Cytotoxic Agents

A variety of cytotoxic agents have been tried with minimal success in Goodpasture's syndrome. These have consisted variously of nitrogen mustard, cyclophosphamide, azathioprine, methotrexate, and others (113). Alone, they have shown little benefit, but these agents may be useful in combination with prednisone, methylprednisolone, or plasma exchange for diminishing the propensity for antibody response.

Therapeutic agents have been tested in a variety of experimental animal models of Goodpasture's syndrome, most frequently the nephrotoxic serum or autoimmune GN model (48,63,65,125,126). Immunoregulatory proteins, including IL-1–receptor antagonist, TNF-α–receptor protein, and antibodies to cell-surface adhesion molecules, as well as deoxyspergualin, CTLA-Ig (57,58,127,128), and mycophenolate mofetil (129–132), have all proved efficacious in these animal models. Although monoclonal anti–T-cell antibodies and intravenous immunoglobulin have been used with some success in the treatment of vasculitis, there is no information on these modalities for anti-GBM disease (122,123,133).

Studies of immune complex GN have suggested that CR1 recombinant protein may be useful in those diseases associated with complement activation. More recently, efforts to manipulate these cytokine systems in experimental animal models have demonstrated the key importance of the IL-4 cytokine phenotype, suggesting that the administration of the appropriate stimulatory or suppressive cytokines at the proper cycle in the development of GN, or transient gene therapy to affect cytokine balance, could be beneficial in ameliorating or halting the development of various forms of GN (134).

As in all models of GN in animals, there are marked specificities of species, strain, antigen dose, and immunization procedure necessary for the effects of note to be accomplished, and extensive examination of these techniques in cell culture and other models is necessary before they can be brought to possible human use. Nonetheless, several of these promising interventions are near therapeutic trials in humans. The next decade may well bring the advent of more specific, directed therapeutic agents without the multiplicity of complications and side effects that pertain to the broad immunosuppressive regimens currently used. Until such agents are tested and have proved beneficial, it behooves the clinician to make the diagnosis of Goodpasture's syndrome with the histologic and serologic approaches outlined here as expeditiously as possible. Perhaps in no other area of immune renal disease is expediency more important in defining the prognosis and potential response to therapy than in Goodpasture's syndrome.

### ACKNOWLEDGMENTS

The author is grateful for the secretarial assistance of C.V. Cook. This work was supported in part by PHS grant DK55801 from the NIDDKD.

### REFERENCES

1. Goodpasture EW. The significance of certain pulmonary lesions in relation to the etiology of influenza. *Am J Med Sci* 1919;158:863–870.
2. Stanton MC, Tange JD. Goodpasture's syndrome (pulmonary haemorrhage associated with glomerulonephritis). *Aust Ann Med* 1958;7: 132–144.
3. Holdsworth SR, Boyce N, Thomson NM, et al. The clinical spectrum of acute glomerulonephritis and lung haemorrhage (Goodpasture's syndrome). *Q J Med* 1985;55:75–86.
4. Cohen AH, Glassock RJ. Anti-GBM glomerulonephritis including Goodpasture's syndrome. In: Tisher CC, Brenner BM, eds. *Renal pathology*. Philadelphia: JB Lippincott, 1989:494.
5. Hudson BG. Anti-type IV collagen diseases. In: *The immunologic basis of renal disease: paradigms for the 21st century*. The American Society of Nephrology's Advances in Basic Science Conference, San Diego, Nov. 8–11, 1995.
6. Kanwar YS, Liu ZZ, Kashihara N, et al. Current status of the structural and functional basis of glomerular filtration and proteinuria. *Semin Nephrol* 1991;11:390–413.
7. Timpl R. Structure and biological activity of basement membrane proteins. *Eur J Biochem* 1988;180:487–502.
8. Timpl R, Wiedemann H, Van Delden V, et al. A network model for the organization of type IV collagen molecules in basement membranes. *Eur J Biochem* 1981;120:203–211.
9. Hudson BG, Reeders ST, Tryggvason K: Type IV collagen: structure, gene organization, and role in human diseases. *J Biol Chem* 1993;268:26033–26036.
10. Weber M, Zum Büschenfelde KHM, Köhler H. Immunological properties of the human Goodpasture target antigen. *Clin Exp Immunol* 1988;74:289–294.
11. Butkowski RJ, Wieslander J, Wisdom BJ, et al. Properties of the globular domain of type IV collagen and its relationship to the Goodpasture antigen. *J Biol Chem* 1985;260:3739–3747.
12. Saus J, Wieslander J, Langeveld JP, et al. Identification of the Goodpasture antigen as the α3(IV) chain of collagen IV. *J Biol Chem* 1988; 263:13374–13380.
13. Bolton WK. Goodpasture's syndrome. Nephrology Forum. *Kidney Int* 1996;50:1753–1766.
14. Hudson BG, Wieslander J, Wisdom BJ, et al. Goodpasture syndrome: molecular architecture and function of basement membrane antigen. *Lab Invest* 1989;61:256–269.
15. Kleppel MM, Santi PA, Cameron JD, et al. Human tissue distribution of novel basement membrane collagen. *Am J Pathol* 1989;134: 813–825.

16. Wieslander J, Bygren P, Heinegård D. Isolation of the specific glomerular basement membrane antigen involved in Goodpasture syndrome. *Proc Natl Acad Sci U S A* 1984;81:1544–1548.

17. Wieslander J, Langeveld J, Butkowski R, et al. Physical and immunochemical studies of the globular domain of type IV collagen: cryptic properties of the Goodpasture antigen. *J Biol Chem* 1985;260: 8564–8570.

18. Michael AF, Yang JY, Falk RJ, et al. Monoclonal antibodies to human renal basement membranes: heterogenic and ontogenic changes. *Kidney Int* 1983;24:74–86.

19. Pusey CD, Dash A, Kershaw MJ, et al. A single autoantigen in Goodpasture's syndrome identified by a monoclonal antibody to human glomerular basement membrane. *Lab Invest* 1987;56:23–31.

20. Ding J, Kashtan CE, Fan WW, et al. A monoclonal antibody marker for Alport syndrome identifies the Alport antigen as the α5 chain of type IV collagen. *Kidney Int* 1994;46:1504–1506.

21. Neilson EG, KallurI R, Sun MJ, et al. Specificity of Goodpasture autoantibodies for the recombinant noncollagenous domains of human type IV collagen. *J Biol Chem* 1993;268:8402–8405.

22. Bygren P, Cederholm B, Heinegåd D, et al. Non-Goodpasture anti-GBM antibodies in patients with glomerulonephritis. *Nephrol Dial Transplant* 1989;4:254–261.

23. Kefalides NA, Ohno N, Wilson CB. Heterogeneity of antibodies in Goodpasture syndrome reacting with type IV collagen. *Kidney Int* 1993;43:85–93.

24. Johnansson C, Hellmark T, Wieslander J. One major epitope in Goodpasture's syndrome (abst). *J Am Soc Nephrol* 1993;4:608.

25. Matsukura H, Butkowski RJ, Fish AJ. The Goodpasture antigen: common epitopes in the globular domains of collage IV. *Nephron* 1993;64:532–539.

26. Dehan P, Weber M, Reeders ST, et al. Anti-GBM antibodies from patients with Goodpasture syndrome react with the NC1 domain of recombinant α3(IV) and α4(IV) collagen chains (abst). *J Am Soc Nephrol* 1993;4:649.

27. Levy JB, Coulthart A, Pusey CD. Mapping B cell epitopes in Goodpasture's disease. *Am J Soc Nephrol* 1997;8:1698–1705.

28. Turner N, Forstova J, Rees AJ, et al. Production and characterization of recombinant Goodpasture antigen in insect cells. *J Biol Chem* 1994;269:17141–17145.

29. Brainwood D, Kashtan C, Gubler MC, et al. Targets of alloantibodies in Alport anti-glomerular basement membrane disease after renal transplantation. *Kidney Int* 1998;53:762–766.

30. Kashtan C, Michael AF. Alport syndrome. *Kidney Int* 1996;50: 1445–1463.

31. Kalluri R, Petrides S, Wilson CB, et al. Anti-α(IV) collagen autoantibodies associated with lung adenocarcinoma presenting as the Goodpasture syndrome. *Ann Intern Med* 1996;124:651–653.

32. Bolton WK. The role of high dose steroids in nephritic syndromes: the case for aggressive use. In: Narins RG, ed. *Controversies in nephrology and hypertension.* New York: Churchill Livingstone, 1984:421.

33. Bigler SA, Parry WM, Fitzwater DS, et al. An 11-month-old anti-glomerular basement membrane disease. *Am J Kidney Dis* 1997;30: 710–712.

34. Savage COS, Pusey CD, Bowman C, et al. Antiglomerular basement membrane antibody mediated disease in the British Isles 1980–4. *Br Med J* 1986;292:301–304.

35. Teague CA, Doak PB, Simpson IJ, et al. Goodpasture's syndrome: an analysis of 29 cases. *Kidney Int* 1978;13:492–504.

36. Rees AJ, Peters DK, Compston DAS, et al. Strong association between HLA DRW2 and antibody mediated Goodpasture's syndrome. *Lancet* 1978;1:966–968.

37. Rees AJ, Lockwood DM, Peters DK. Nephritis due to antibodies to GBM. In: Kincaid-Smith P, D'Apice AJF, Atkins RC, eds. *Progress in glomerulonephritis.* New York: John Wiley & Sons, 1979:347.

38. Simonsen H, Brun C, Thomsen OF, et al. Goodpasture's syndrome in twins. *Acta Med Scand* 1982;212:425–428.

39. D'Apice AJ, Kincaid-Smith P, Becker GH, et al. Goodpasture's syndrome in identical twins. *Ann Intern Med* 1978;88:61–62.

40. Merkel F, Kalluri R, Marx M, et al. Autoreactive T-cells in Goodpasture's syndrome recognize the N-terminal NC1 domain on α3 type IV collagen. *Kidney Int* 1996;49:1127–1133.

41. Bombassei GJ, Kaplan AA. The association between hydrocarbon exposure and anti-glomerular basement membrane antibody-mediated disease (Goodpasture's syndrome). *Am J Ind Med* 1992;21:141–153.

42. Beirne GJ, Brennan JT. Glomerulonephritis associated with hydrocarbon solvents: mediated by antiglomerular basement membrane antibody. *Arch Environ Health* 1972;25:365–369.

43. Roy AT, Brautbar N, Lee DBN. Hydrocarbons and renal failure. *Nephron* 1991;58:385–392.

44. Donaghy M, Rees AJ. Cigarette smoking and lung haemorrhage in glomerulonephritis caused by autoantibodies to glomerular basement membrane. *Lancet* 1983;2:1390–1392.

45. Queluz TH, Pawlowski I, Brunda MJ, et al. Pathogenesis of an experimental model of Goodpasture's hemorrhagic pneumonitis. *J Clin Invest* 1990;85:1507–1515.

46. Yamamoto T, Wilson CB. Binding of anti-basement membrane antibody to alveolar basement membrane after intratracheal gasoline instillation in rabbits. *Am J Pathol* 1987;126:497–505.

47. Unanue ER, Dixon FJ. Experimental glomerulonephritis. VI. The autologous phase of nephrotoxic serum nephritis. *J Exp Med* 1965;121: 715–725.

48. Unanue ER, Dixon FJ. Experimental glomerulonephritis. V. Studies on the interaction of nephrotoxic antibodies with tissues of the rat. *J Exp Med* 1965;121:697–714.

49. Bolton WK. Mechanisms of glomerular injury: injury mediated by sensitized lymphocytes. *Semin Nephrol* 1991;11:285–293.

50. Bolton WK, Benton FR, Lobo PI. Requirement of functional T-cells in the production of autoimmune glomerulotubular nephropathy in mice. *Clin Exp Immunol* 1978;33:474–477.

51. Tipping PG, Huang XR, Qi M, et al. Crescentic glomerulonephritis in CD4- and CD8-deficient mice. *Am J Pathol* 1998;152:1541–1548.

52. Kelly CJ, Frishberg Y, Gold DP. An appraisal of T cell subsets and the potential for autoimmune injury. *Kidney Int* 1998;53:1574–1584.

53. Tipping PG, Xiao RH, Berndt MC, et al. A role for P selection in complement-independent neutrophil-mediated glomerular injury. *Kidney Int* 1994;46:79–88.

54. Bolton WK. Cell mediated immunity. In: Massry SG, Glassock RG, eds. *Textbook of nephrology.* Baltimore: Lippincott Williams & Wilkins, 2000 (in press).

55. Kawasaki K, Yaoita E, Yamamoto T, et al. Depletion of CD8 positive cells in nephrotoxic serum nephritis of WKY rats. *Kidney Int* 1992; 41:1517–1526.

56. Tomosugi NI, Cashman SJ, Hay H, et al. Modulation of antibody-mediated glomerular injury in vivo by bacterial lipopolysaccharide, tumor necrosis factor, and IL-1. *J Immunol* 1989;142:3083–3090.

57. Nikolic-Paterson DJ, Lan HY, Hill PA, et al. Suppression of experimental glomerulonephritis by the interleukin-1 receptor antagonist: inhibition of intercellular adhesion molecule-1 expression. *J Am Soc Nephrol* 1994;4:1695–1700.

58. Lan HY, Nikolic-Paterson DJ, Zheng S, et al. Suppression of experimental crescentic glomerulonephritis by the interleukin-1 receptor antagonist. *Kidney Int* 1993;43:479–485.

59. Fujinaka H, Yamamoto T, Takeya M, et al. Suppression of anti-glomerular basement membrane of nephritis by administration of anti-monocyte chemoattractant protein-1 antibody in WKY rats(abst). *J Am Soc Nephrol* 1999;8:1174–1178.

60. Lynch RG. The biology and pathology of lymphocytes Fc receptors. *Am J Pathol* 1998;152:631–639.

61. Boyce NW, Holdsworth SR. Macrophage-Fc-receptor affinity: role in cellular mediation of antibody initiated glomerulonephritis. *Kidney Int* 1989;36:537–544.

62. Park SY, Ueda S, Ohno H, et al. Resistance of FC receptor-deficient mice to fatal glomerulonephritis (abst). *J Clin Invest* 1998;102: 1229–1238.

63. Steblay RW. Preliminary evidence for the production of nephritis in sheep by an autoimmune mechanism. In: Mills LC, Moyer JH, eds. *Inflammation and diseases of connective tissue.* Philadelphia: WB Saunders, 1961:272.

64. Sado Y, Naito I, Akita M, et al. Strain specific responses of inbred rats on the severity of experimental autoimmune glomerulonephritis. *J Clin Lab Immunol* 1986;19:193–199.

65. Bolton WK, May WJ, Sturgill BC. Proliferative glomerulonephritis in rats: a model for autoimmune glomerulonephritis in humans. *Kidney Int* 1994;44:294–306.

66. Lelongt B, Kashihara N, Makino H, et al. Influence of genetics on the nephritogenic potential of proteoglycans. *Am J Pathol* 1992;141: 561–569.

67. Bolton WK, May WJ, Sturgill BC, et al. Study of EHS type IV collagen lacking Goodpasture's epitope in glomerulonephritis. *Kidney Int* 1995;47:404–410.

68. Reynolds J, Mavromatidis K, Cashman S, et al. Experimental autoimmune glomerulonephritis (EAG) induced by homologous and heterologous glomerular basement membrane in two substrains of Wistar-Kyoto rat. *Nephrol Dial Transplant* 1998;13:44–52.

69. Bolton WK, Tucker FL, Sturgill BC. New avian model of experimental glomerulonephritis consistent with mediation by cellular immunity. *J Clin Invest* 1984;73:1263–1276.

70. Bolton WK, Chandra M, Tyson TM, et al. Transfer of experimental glomerulonephritis in chickens by mononuclear cells. *Kidney Int* 1980;34:598–610.

71. Reynolds J, Sallie BA, Syrganis C, et al. The role of T-helper lymphocytes in priming for experimental autoimmune glomerulonephritis in the BN rats. *J Autoimmun* 1993;6:571–585.

72. Sado Y, Naito I, Okigaki T. Transfer of anti-glomerular basement membrane antibody-induced glomerulonephritis in inbred rats with isologous antibodies from the urine of nephritic rats. *J Pathol* 1989; 158:325–332.

73. Sado Y, Kagawa M, Rauf S, et al. Isologous monoclonal antibodies can induce anti-GBM glomerulonephritis in rats. *J Pathol* 1992;168: 221–227.

74. Kalluri R, Danoff TM, Okada H, Neilson EG. Susceptibility to anti-glomerular basement membrane disease and Goodpasture's syndrome is linked to MHC class II genes and the emergence of T cell-mediated immunity in mice. *J Clin Invest* 1997;100:2263–2275.

75. Kalluri R, Gattone VH II, Noelken ME, et al. The α3 chain of type IV collagen induces autoimmune Goodpasture syndrome. *Proc Natl Acad Sci U S A* 1994;91:6201–6205.

76. Sado Y, Boutaud AA, Kagawa M, et al. Induction of anti-GBM nephritis in rats by recombinant α3(IV) NC1 and α4(IV) NC1 of type IV collagen. *Kidney Int* 1998;53:664–671.

77. Holdsworth SR, Neale TJ, Wilson CB. Abrogation of macrophage-dependent injury in experimental glomerulonephritis in the rabbit: use of an antimacrophage serum. *J Clin Invest* 1981;58:686–698.

78. Bolton WK, Innes DJ, Sturgill BC, et al. T-cells and macrophages in rapidly progressive glomerulonephritis: clinicopathologic correlations. *Kidney Int* 1987;32:869–876.

79. Nikolic-Paterson DJ, Lan HY, Atkins R. Macrophages in immune renal injury. In: Neilson EG, Couser WG, eds. *Immunologic renal diseases*. Philadelphia: Lippincott-Raven, 1997:575.

80. Lan HY, Nikolic-Paterson DJ, Mu W, et al. Local macrophage proliferation in the pathogenesis of glomerular crescent formation in rat anti-glomerular basement membrane (GBM) glomerulonephritis. *Clin Exp Immunol* 1997;110:233–240.

81. Holdsworth SR, Tipping PG. Macrophage-induced glomerular fibrin deposition in experimental glomerulonephritis in the rabbit. *J Clin Invest* 1985;76:1367–1374.

82. Kleppel MM, Ding J, Lee HK, et al. Nucleotide sequence of human basement membrane α3(IV) NC1 (the Goodpasture antigen): relationship of deduced protein sequence to other collagen chains (abst). *J Am Soc Nephrol* 1991;2:549.

83. Bolton WK, Fox P, Sneed AE, et al. Studies of experimental autoimmune glomerulonephritis (EAG in rats using recombinant (r) protein α3 col (IV) containing Goodpasture's epitope (GPEp). *J Am Soc Nephrol* 1995;6:823.

84. Morrison KE, Mariyama M, Yang-Feng TL, et al. Sequence and localization of a partial cDNA encoding the human α3 chain of type IV collagen. *Am J Hum Genet* 1991;49:545–554.

85. Boutaud AA, Kalluri R, Kahsai TZ, et al. Goodpasture syndrome: selective removal of anti-α3(IV) collagen antibodies. A potential therapeutic alternative to plasmapheresis. *Exp Nephrol* 1996;4:205–212.

86. Whitworth JA, Morel-Maroger L, Mignon F, et al. The significance of extracapillary proliferation. *Nephron* 1976;16:1–19.

87. Ewan PW, Jones HA, Rhodes CG, et al. Detection of intrapulmonary hemorrhage with carbon monoxide uptake: application in Goodpasture's syndrome. *N Engl J Med* 1976;295:1391–1396.

88. Bailey RR, Simpson IJ, Lynn KL, et al. Goodpasture's syndrome with normal renal function. *Clin Nephrol* 1981;15:211–215.

89. Zimmerman SW, Varanasi UR, Hoff B. Goodpasture's syndrome with normal renal function. *Am J Med* 1979;66:163–171.

90. O'Donoghue DJ, Short CD, Brenchley C, et al. Sequential development of systemic vasculitis and anti-neutrophil cytoplasmic antibodies complicating anti-glomerular basement membrane disease. *Clin Nephrol* 1989;32:251–255.

91. Jayne DRW, Marshall PD, Jones SJ, et al. Autoantibodies to GBM and neutrophil cytoplasm in rapidly progressive glomerulonephritis. *Kidney Int* 1990;37:965–970.

92. Bosch X, Mirapeix E, Font J, et al. Prognostic implication of anti-neutrophil cytoplasmic autoantibodies with myeloperoxidase specificity in anti-glomerular basement membrane disease. *Clin Nephrol* 1991;36: 107–113.

93. Short AK, Esnault VL, Lockwood CM. ANCA and anti-GBM antibodies in RPGN. *Adv Exp Med Biol* 1993;336:441–444.

94. Nolasco FE, Cameron JS, Hartley B, et al. Intraglomerular T cells and monocytes in nephritis: study with monoclonal antibodies. *Kidney Int* 1987;31:1160–1166.

95. Tryggvason K, Zhou J, Hostikka SL, et al. Molecular genetics of Alport syndrome. *Kidney Int* 1993;43:38–44.

96. Peten E, Pirson Y, Cosyns JP, et al. Outcome of thirty patients with Alport's syndrome after renal transplantation. *Transplantation* 1991; 52:823–826.

97. Segelmark M, Butkowski R, Wieslander J. Antigen restriction and IgG subclasses among anti-GBM autoantibodies. *Nephrol Dial Transplant* 1990;5:991–996.

98. Border WA, Baehler RW, Bhathena D, et al. IgA antibasement membrane nephritis with pulmonary hemorrhage. *Ann Intern Med* 1979; 91:21–25.

99. Wilkowski MJ, Bolton WK. Autoantibodies and other autoimmune serologic abnormalities in dialysis patients. *Semin Dial* 1995;8: 226–231.

100. Wu MJ, Rajaram R, Shelp WD, et al. Vasculitis in Goodpasture's syndrome. *Arch Pathol Lab Med* 1980;104:300–302.

101. Wahls TL, Bonsib SM, Schuster VL. Coexistent Wegener's granulomatosis and anti-glomerular basement membrane disease. *Hum Pathol* 1987;18:202–205.

102. Walker JF, Watson AJ, Garrett P, et al. Goodpasture's syndrome: 7 years' experience of two Dublin renal units. *Irish Med J* 1982;75: 328–333.

103. Strutz F, Neilson EG. The role of lymphocytes in the progression of interstitial disease. *Kidney Int* 1994;45:S106–110.

104. Lerner RA, Dixon FJ. Transfer of ovine experimental allergic glomerulonephritis (EAG) with serum. *J Exp Med* 1966;124:431–442.

105. Lerner RA, Glassock RJ, Dixon FJ. The role of anti-glomerular basement membrane antibody in the pathogenesis of human glomerulonephritis. *J Exp Med* 1967;126:989–1004.

106. Lockwood CM, Pearson TA, Rees AJ, et al. Immunosuppression and plasma exchange in the treatment of Goodpasture's syndrome. *Lancet* 1976;1:711–714.

107. Peters DK, Rees AJ, Lockwood CM, et al. Treatment and prognosis in antibasement membrane antibody-mediated nephritis. *Transplant Proc* 1982;14:513–521.

108. Rees AJ, Lockwood CM. Antiglomerular basement membrane antibody-mediated nephritis. In: Schrier RW, Gottschalk CW, eds. *Diseases of the kidney*. Boston: Little, Brown, 1988;2091–2126.

109. Bolton WK, Sturgill BC. Methylprednisolone therapy for acute crescentic rapidly progressive glomerulonephritis. *Am J Nephrol* 1989;9: 368–375.

110. Cohen LH, Wilson CB, Freeman RM. Goodpasture syndrome: recovery after severe renal insufficiency. *Arch Intern Med* 1976;136: 835–837.

111. Bernis P, Hamels J, Quoidbach A, et al. Remission of Goodpasture's syndrome after withdrawal of an unusual toxic. *Clin Nephrol* 1985;23: 312–317.

112. Strauch BS, Charney A, Doctorouff S, et al. Goodpasture syndrome with recovery after renal failure. *JAMA* 1974;229:444.

113. Glassock RJ. Clinico-pathologic spectrum and therapeutic strategies in "rapidly progressive" glomerulonephritis. *Proc Dial Transplant Forum* 1975;5:109–116.

114. Johnson JP, Moore J Jr, Austin HA III, et al. Therapy of anti-glomerular basement membrane antibody disease: analysis of prognostic significance of clinical, pathologic and treatment factors. *Medicine* 1985;64:219–227.

115. Hind CRK, Lockwood CM, Peters DK, et al. Prognosis after immunosuppression of patients with crescentic nephritis requiring dialysis. *Lancet* 1983;1:263–264.

116. Briggs WA, Johnson JP, Teichman S, et al. Antiglomerular basement membrane antibody-mediated glomerulonephritis and Goodpasture's syndrome. *Medicine* 1979;58:348–361.

117. Couser WG. Rapidly progressive glomerulonephritis: classification, pathogenetic mechanisms, and therapy. *Am J Kidney Dis* 1988;11: 449–464.

118. Bolton WK. Treatment of crescentic glomerulonephritis. *Nephrology* 1995;1:257–268.

119. Simpson IJ, Doak PB, Williams LC, et al. Plasma exchange in Goodpasture's syndrome. *Am J Nephrol* 1982;2:301–311.

120. Pusey CD, Rees AJ, Evans DJ, et al. Plasma exchange in focal necrotizing glomerulonephritis without anti-GBM antibodies. *Kidney Int* 1991;40:757–763.

121. Falk RJ, Hogan S, Carey TS, et al. Clinical course of anti-neutrophil cytoplasmic autoantibody-associated glomerulonephritis and systemic vasculitis. *Ann Intern Med* 1991;114:430–431.

122. Wilkowski MJ, Bolton WK. The kidneys. In: Leroy EC, ed. *Systemic vasculitis: the biological basis.* New York: Marcel Dekker, 1992:381.

123. Jayne DR, Davies MJ, Fox CJ, et al. Treatment of systemic vasculitis with pooled intravenous immunoglobulin. *Lancet* 1991;337: 1137–1139.

124. Esnault VLM, Testa A, Jayne DRW, et al. Influence of immunoadsorption on the removal of immunoglobulin G autoantibodies in crescentic glomerulonephritis. *Nephron* 1993;65:180–184.

125. Hammer DK, Dixon FJ. Experimental glomerulonephritis. II. Immunologic events in the pathogenesis of nephrotoxic serum nephritis in the rat. *J Exp Med* 1963;117:1019–1034.

126. Steblay RW. Animal model: experimental autoimmune anti-glomerular basement membrane glomerulonephritis in the sheep. *Am J Pathol* 1979;96:875–878.

127. Nishikawa K, Guo YJ, Miyasaka M, et al. Antibodies to intercellular adhesion molecule 1/lymphocyte function-associated antigen 1 pre- vent crescent formation in rat autoimmune glomerulonephritis. *J Exp Med* 1993;177:667–677.

128. Lan HY, Zarama M. Suppression of experimental crescentic glomerulonephritis by deoxyspergualin. *J Am Soc Nephrol* 1993;3:1765–1774.

129. Nachman PH, Dooley MA, Hogan SL, et al. Mycophenolate mofetil therapy in patients with cyclophosphamide-resistant or relapsing diffuse proliferative lupus nephritis (abst). *J Am Soc Nephrol* 1997;8:94.

130. Briggs WA, Choi M, Scheel PJ Jr, et al. Mycophenolate mofetil treatment of glomerular disease (abst). *J Am Soc Nephrol* 1997;8:83.

131. Hebert LA, Cosio FG, Bay WH, et al. Mycophenolate mofetil (Cell-Cept, MMF) therapy of systemic lupus erythematosus and ANCA vasculitis (abst). *J Am Soc Nephrol* 1997;8:87.

132. Nowack R, Göbel U, Klooker P, et al. Mycophenolate mofetil is effective for maintenance therapy of systemic vasculitis(abst). *J Am Soc Nephrol* 1994;4:1695–1700. *J Am Soc Nephrol* 1997;8:95.

133. Lockwood CM, Thiru S, Isaacs JD, et al. Long-term remission of intractable systemic vasculitis with monoclonal antibody therapy. *Lancet* 1993;341:1620–1623.

134. Kitching AR, Tipping PG, Mutch DA, et al. Interleukin-4 deficiency enhances Th1 responses and crescentic glomerulonephritis in mice. *Kidney Int* 1998;53:112–118.

135. Bolton WK, Sturgill BC. Proliferative glomerulonephritis: postinfectious, non-infectious and crescentic forms. In: Tisher CC, Brenner BM, eds. *Renal pathology.* Philadelphia: JB Lippincott, 1989: 156.

136. Bolton WK, Couser WG. Intravenous pulse methylprednisolone therapy of acute crescentic rapidly progressive glomerulonephritis. *Am J Med* 1979;66:495–502.

*Textbook of the Autoimmune Diseases,*
Edited by R. G. Lahita, N. Chiorazzi, and W. H. Reeves,
Lippincott Williams & Wilkins, Philadelphia © 2000.

# CHAPTER 33

# Interstitial Cystitis

C. Lowell Parsons and Robert L. Ochs

## CLINICAL PRESENTATION

Interstitial cystitis (IC) has been recognized as a clinical entity dating back more than 100 years. It was initially recognized only in its most severe end-stage form and as such represented less than 1% of the patients with the disease. IC is problematic in that it is defined solely by clinical symptoms and not by diagnostic tests. In many patients, however, there appears to be a disease progression, beginning with a milder intermittent version of the symptom complex and progressing gradually to the more severe or classically recognized end stage. A varied presentation of the symptom complex is one of urinary urgency, frequency, or pain associated with the urinary bladder or urethra. These symptoms are typically intermittent in nature in the early phases of the disease and progress both in severity and duration as the disease advances; this appears to occur in about 20% of patients initially afflicted with a mild case of IC.

For most patients with the syndrome, the symptoms typically mimic those of urinary tract infection, urgency and frequency, and discomfort associated with the bladder and urethra. Because they tend to be intermittent and occur with certain flare periods in the early phases of disease, in most patients, urinary tract infection is diagnosed initially and treated. Typically, the disease begins insidiously with flares that occur perimenstrually, just before the menstrual cycle, or in association with sexual intercourse. As a result, the disease is usually misdiagnosed as recurrent urinary tract infection, urethral syndrome, endometriosis, vaginitis (yeast), vulvodynia, or nonspecific pelvic pain. The gynecologic-associated symptoms of dyspareunia and the perimenstrual flare account for much of the confusion.

We reviewed clinical data on 500 patients presenting to our center with the classic symptoms of IC. We found that 75% of premenopausal patients had a history of symptoms flaring before the menstrual cycle, and 75% of sexually active people had discomfort associated with sexual intercourse either immediately or within 1 to 2 days. Thirty-one percent of subjects did not void more than one time at night, so that nocturia is not of particular importance in the earlier phases of this disease. It would appear that many patients can sleep through the milder sensory urgency present in the early to middle phases of this disease. Patients voided typically on an average of 8 to 18 times (90%) per day. Sixteen percent of patients had no pain or discomfort associated with the syndrome, and about 8% of patients had little urgency or frequency and primarily pain associated with the bladder. By expanding the older and traditional concepts of only recognizing end-stage patients, one can now suspect IC when the symptoms of urinary frequency and urgency, pain associated with the bladder or urethra, dyspareunia, pain after sex, and perimenstrual flares of symptoms are present in the absence of other obvious bladder problems. The disease is defined primarily based on this symptom complex, with the exclusion of other bladder disorders that may also have similar symptoms, such as urinary tract infection or cancer. This leaves the definition of IC as significant urinary urgency and frequency or bladder-associated pain in the absence of other defined causes.

If the preponderance of patient complaints is related to urinary urgency and frequency, patients usually have a urologic referral and evaluation. When patients have perimenstrual flare, pelvic pain, discomfort, and dyspareunia, they usually present to the gynecologist, and their disease is frequently misdiagnosed, as noted previously.

## CLINICAL DIAGNOSIS

The most useful methods to diagnose IC include a good clinical history, a physical examination, a voiding log, and urodynamic studies. Cystoscopy is not an important aspect of the diagnosis of IC, whereas the other parts of the evaluation probably result in 97% to 99% accuracy in establishing the diagnosis.

C. L. Parsons: Division of Urology, Department of Surgery, University of California, San Diego, Medical Center, San Diego, California 92103-8897.

R. L. Ochs: Precision Therapeutics, Pittsburgh, Pennsylvania 15213.

## History

A good history can result in as high as a 90% accurate diagnosis or at least strong suspicion of IC. Typically, this disease is manifested by urgency and frequency and bladder-associated pain or discomfort that presents intermittently at first, with a misdiagnosis of urinary tract infection, urethritis, vaginitis, or endometriosis. About 75% of patients complain of perimenstrual flare that occurs just before the menstrual cycle and symptoms that are aggravated by sexual intercourse, either dyspareunia or symptoms appearing 20 to 24 hours after sexual activity. Patients even complain of orgasm inducing a cascade of symptoms and discomfort. As the disease progresses, even sexual arousal provokes the symptom complex. Many patients complain of certain dietary triggers of their symptoms, such as citrus fruit, spicy foods, chocolate, tomatoes, tomato sauce, and bananas. For these flares, many patients say that increasing fluids helps relieve discomfort.

Patients frequently have a long history of urinary frequency and urgency, which they have learned to discount or consider "normal" for them and pay little attention to this unless the frequency becomes so severe that it interferes with sleep or work. More typically, they start seeing their physician when there is a flare of their symptoms associated with pain and discomfort, such as occurs perimenstrually. In the earlier phases of the disease, it tends to occur intermittently, with two or three flare cycles per year that last for about 2 to 3 days before the menstrual cycle. As the disease escalates, the symptoms appear more frequently and last for progressively longer durations. In the early phases of the disease, treating the 2- to 3-day flare cycles with antibiotics confuses the issue, and patients are frequently treated for prolonged periods of time for recurrent urinary tract infections. In male patients, there may be a similar history of urinary urgency and frequency and pain, but they may complain of pain associated with ejaculation and may be misdiagnosed as having prostatitis; alternatively, the same disease process in the bladder may also affect the prostate.

Allergies have a significant effect on this disease in as many as 40% to 50% of patients; their symptoms flare during allergy seasons. Most patients and physicians, however, are usually unaware of the seasonal variations.

## Voiding Logs

One of the most useful and inexpensive tests to note abnormalities in voiding patterns is to obtain a 1- or 2-day voiding log from the patient in which urination times and amounts are recorded. Ninety-five percent of healthy subjects void between 4 and 6 times a day, with an average of 150 to 250 mL per void. IC patients presenting with recurrent complaints typically void 8 to 20 times per day, with an average of 60 to 90 mL per void. Plotting the number of voids per day and the average volume reveals that 97% of IC patients void, on average, less than 100 mL and 97% of healthy subjects void more than that. This makes for a discriminating and sensitive test that is helpful in the diagnosis of IC (Fig. 33.1).

## Urinary Screening

All patients should be screened for other potential urologic abnormalities of the bladder that can cause similar symptoms, primarily urinary tract infection and bladder cancer. This can best be done by a combination of urinalysis to isolate those patients with hematuria (an unusual presenting problem for IC patients), a urinary cytology, and a urinary tract culture. In patients older than 40 years of age in whom there is a suspicion of potential malignancy, even though all the screening tests are negative, cystoscopy should probably be done to exclude this possibility. All men older than 40 years of age should probably undergo cystoscopy. Anyone with hematuria or a questionable or positive cytology should also be evaluated by cystoscopy.

## Urodynamics

Another useful method that is sensitive and accurate in defining the patient population with IC is urodynamics (Fig. 33.2). In our experience with the National Institutes of Health (NIH) Data Base, this test was found to be discriminating at isolating abnormal voiding patterns in that 97% of patients had significant urgency with a voiding volume of less than 100 mL (normal volume was 150 mL or more) and functional bladder capacity without anesthesia of less than 250 mL (normal was more than 400 mL). In the NIH Data Base, urodynamics was just as accurate as cystoscopy at predicting abnormalities of the bladder (1). This test is probably more useful to the clinician than endoscopy in making the diagnosis of IC.

## Cystoscopy

Cystoscopy has historically been a mainstay of the diagnosis of IC. Bladders have been examined for either Hunner's ulcer or petechial hemorrhages after overdistention. The presence of either one of these abnormalities would essentially confirm the diagnosis of IC; in fact, however, the absence of these two findings does not exclude IC. In our experience, a reliance on the endoscopic changes to make the diagnosis resulted in a missed diagnosis in as many as half of patients.

The primary role of cystoscopy should be to exclude the possibility of a bladder malignancy, and this should be done in all high-risk patients, including those with hematuria or an abnormal urinary cytology, men older than 40 years of age, and women older than 45 years of age. An office cystoscopy would be more than sufficient to exclude bladder malignancy. The bladder should not be dilated without anesthesia because dilation causes significant patient discomfort and adds nothing to the evaluation process.

The main reason to perform a cystoscopy under anesthesia in cases of hydrodistention of the bladder is not to look for glomerulations or ulcers but rather to obtain a remission of the disease. It has been known since the 1930s that about 60% of patients undergoing this type of therapy have a significant response, that is, a clinical remission that averages between 6 and 10 months (2).

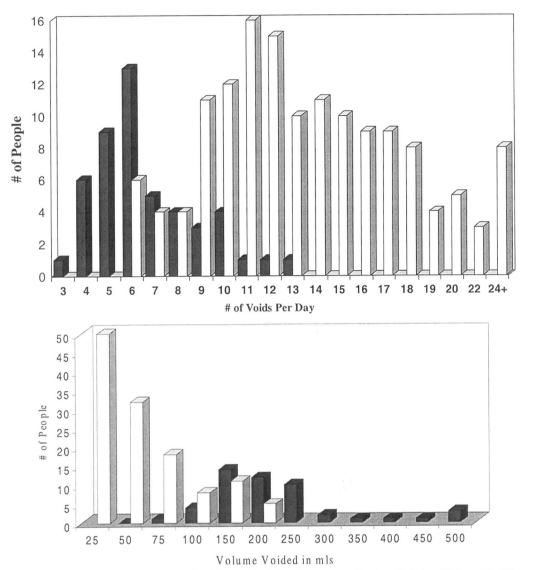

**FIG. 33.1. A:** Voids per day in normal subjects (*dark bars*) versus patients with interstitial cystitis (IC) (*light bars*). Normal subjects (*n* = 48) average 6.5 voids per day. IC patients (*n* = 145) average 16.5 voids per day. **B:** Average voided volume in IC (*light bars*) versus normal subjects (*dark bars*). Normal subjects (*n* = 48) average 270 mL. IC patients (*n* = 135) average 73 mL.

## EPIDEMIOLOGY AND NATURAL HISTORY

Reflecting its relative newness as a recognizable disease entity (symptom complex), the epidemiology and natural history of IC have, until recently, been largely undocumented. Reviews have been published by Jones and Nyberg (3) and Ho et al. (4). Pioneering work in this area has been done primarily by Koziol (5), who studied a cohort of about 565 IC patients, analyzing for risk factors, associated conditions, demographics, psychosocial factors, and the natural progression of the disease. These topics are addressed separately in the following sections.

### Prevalence and Incidence

The first documented study of the prevalence and incidence of IC was published by Oravisto et al. in 1975 (6), who doc-

umented the disease as it occurred in Finland. These investigators reported the prevalence as being 18.1 cases per 100,000 adult women in the population and the incidence as 1.2 new cases per 100,000 adult women per year. The female-to-male ratio was reported to be 10:1. This study, however, was conducted well before the diagnostic criteria for IC were standardized (7) and before IC was acknowledged as a legitimate disease entity. Later studies of the U.S. population revealed the prevalence of IC to be much higher, at 30 per 100,000 adults (male and female) in one study (8) and 501 per 100,000 adults in another study (3). In both of these studies, the female-to-male ratio was 9:1. In the latest study, Bade et al. (9) reported the prevalence of IC in the Netherlands to be 8 to 16 per 100,000 adult women. Thus, there is still a great disparity in the reported prevalence and incidence of IC, perhaps reflecting differences in the country of origin, diagnostic criteria applied, or ability to recognize the disease.

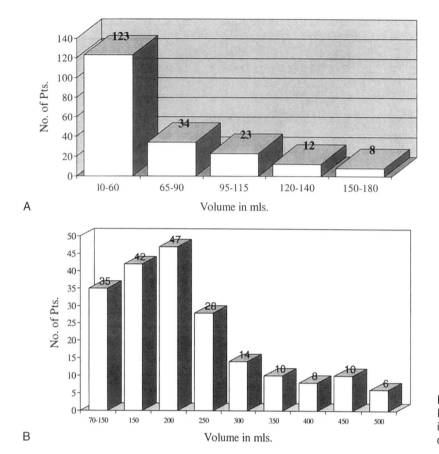

**FIG. 33.2.** Results of cystometrograms in 200 IC patients (30 men and 170 women). **A:** Voiding volume, first urge. **B:** Functional bladder capacity (mean = 250 mL).

Until recently, only patients with end-stage IC were recognized, and IC was thought to be a rare disease. Clinical studies that were done to define the incidence tended to focus on the more advanced patients who had IC. As a result, the estimates were only the minimum associated with the disease, never reflecting the maximum or actual number of patients who had the syndrome. In 1975, Oravisto et al. (6) estimated that the incidence of IC was about 10 per 100,000. As it began to be recognized that early phases of this disease existed (10), the true incidence of this disease changed dramatically. In part, the difficulty was that patients with milder and intermittent symptoms were assigned all the misdiagnoses as noted previously, that is, recurrent urinary tract infection, prostatitis, vaginitis, pelvic pain, and endometriosis. Held et al. (8) estimated an incidence that was significantly more than that estimated by Oravisto (6). More recently, Jones and Nyberg (3) produced estimates ranging up to 2.5 million women in the United States.

Perhaps a better way to obtain an accurate idea of who has this disease is to look at the patient population of women who present every year with symptoms of urgency and frequency, which is about 4% to 6% of the U.S. population (11). A fact that has been recognized since the 1960s is that most of these women actually had symptoms with negative cultures, and these investigators defined this patient population as having urethral syndrome (essentially a mild and ear-

lier version of IC) (11a). Moreover, one study (12) showed that in a trial conducted on a new antibiotic, more than half of patients entered had negative cultures. This population of slightly more than 1000 patients were studied in an outpatient setting in England. In this study, investigators used voided specimens to make the diagnosis of bladder infection. This is not acceptable in the population experiencing symptoms of urgency and frequency.

Patients with IC void with such low volumes (60 to 90 mL) that a midstream culture cannot be obtained accurately. Had this antibiotic study actually used catheterized specimens, it may well have been that 75% to 80% of the cultures would have been negative. It has been an error in logic to assume that patients who present with urgency and frequency have a bladder infection when, in fact, there have been no studies with catheterized specimens to define the actual cause of their symptoms. Consequently, if it is true that most women presenting with intermittent symptoms have early-phase IC, the true incidence of this disease is about 2% to 3% of the adult female population. It appears that men represent only about 10% of patients with the syndrome, but if these cases are being misdiagnosed as prostatitis (about 2% of male population), then it may well be that the actual sexual difference is not as great as has been believed.

The point to be emphasized is that as we learn more about the disease and its presentation and can define more accurately the cause of the symptoms, we add to our awareness of patients who actually have the disease. Historical estimates of the incidence of IC represent the minimum and not the maximum number of patients with IC.

## Risk Factors

A number of risk factors have been identified that may be either associated with the presence of IC or causative. In the study by Koziol et al. (13), the highest associated risk factor was hysterectomy (44% of the IC patient population under study). Other notable risk factors included allergies (38%) and irritable bowel syndrome (26%).

## Associated Conditions

According to Alagiri et al. (14), allergies, irritable bowel syndrome, and "sensitive skin" were the most common disease complaints in the IC patient population. Compared with healthy subjects, IC patients were 100 times more likely to have inflammatory bowel disease and 30 times more likely to have systemic lupus erythematosus. These findings compare well with those previously reported by Koziol et al. (13), in which there was a high incidence of allergic sensitivity to different foods and medications and an abnormally high percentage of IC patients with symptoms of inflammatory bowel disease.

## Demographics, Symptoms, and Natural History

Adult patients with IC are predominantly white, middle-aged women. The average age at the first sign of symptoms is 40 to 54 years, with the time from the first onset of symptoms to diagnosis averaging 2 to 5 years. The disease progresses rapidly and then stabilizes, with flares and remissions thereafter. It has been difficult to classify the IC patient population other than by the histologic criterion of whether there is ulceration in the bladder wall. About 5% to 20% of all IC patients have Hunner's ulcers, and these patients have been described as having the "classic" disease according to its first description by Hunner in 1915 (15). The remaining 80% to 95% of patients with IC do not have ulcers; these patients are referred to as having nonclassic or nonulcer IC.

It is generally accepted that the classic form of IC is associated with the most severe symptoms. Once diagnosed, patients without ulcers never go on to develop them, indicating that the distinction between ulcer and nonulcer may define different forms of the disease that do not overlap.

## Psychosocial Factors

Because of the chronic pain, sleep deprivation, and inconvenience of urinating up to 60 times per day, the psychological and social toll exacted by IC is great. Many patients are homebound, sleep deprived, and chronically depressed. Overall, the quality of life is poor, and the chronic pain involved is likened to that of a terminally ill patient with cancer.

## ETIOLOGY AND PATHOPHYSIOLOGY

Since the original description of the "elusive ulcer" of Hunner about 85 years ago, there has been slow progress in defining the etiology of IC (15,16). In part, this is because the severe form is relatively rare, making it necessary to access large numbers of patients. The many suggested causes have included chronic infection; lymphatic, neurologic, psychological, and autoimmune disorders; and vasculitis (17–24). Most of the proposed causes are hypothetical, with little data to define the role of these mechanisms. For example, Oravisto (23) had suggested that there were increased antinuclear antibodies (ANAs) in patients with IC, but they were present in very low titers. It is difficult to know what this means because there is no obvious association with systemic autoimmune phenomena in these patients. In addition, modest rises in autoantibodies may occur nonspecifically in any chronic disease, making this observation an epiphenomenon.

Several factors appear to play an etiologic role in IC. One of the more popular theories is that there is a defective bladder epithelium, with loss of the blood–urine barrier resulting in a leaky membrane (25,26). An epithelium permeable to small molecules could then explain many of the symptoms associated with the complex. Chronic leak of small molecules into the interstitium could actually induce sensory nerves to depolarize, resulting in urgency, frequency, and pain (27,28). In particular, diffusion of potassium across the membrane could trigger the sensory nerve endings (29). This latter concept is attractive because most patients do not have significant signs of inflammatory responses in their bladder muscle or serum (30), and few patients have mast cells that would explain the sensory/urgency induced from their degranulation (22,31–33).

## Inflammation

The concept that IC is primarily an inflammatory disease is probably not true. In fact, little inflammation is reported in IC biopsies, and it may be that the presence of inflammation is reactive and not causative. In addition, inflammatory mediators are rarely present in IC urine (34).

Mast cells, on the other hand, are prominent in about one third of patients and may be important in the provocation of symptoms, especially in atopic people (35–38). Animal models of mast cell stimulation also suggest that these cells may provoke abnormalities in both smooth muscle activity and epithelial permeability (39,40). Even if the mast cells are not always the primary factor in IC, it may be important to address mast cell problems relative to therapy, suggesting the need for a combination of treatments to control the disease.

## Vascular Insufficiency

Reduction of vascular perfusion may negatively affect mucosal muscle and nerve nutrition and initiate or promote a cascade that causes symptoms. Radiation impairs bladder blood supply and certainly causes the symptoms of IC. In addition, other perfusion abnormalities, such as reflex sympathetic dystrophy (41), may result in a secondary decrease in blood flow that also triggers events causing symptoms in the IC syndrome. Potassium leak into the bladder interstitial space may also result in diminished blood flow to the bladder (42–44).

### Epithelial Leak

The most popular theory concerning pathogenesis, as noted previously, is that of an epithelial leak. There have been few data to support the concept of such a leak (25), and a subsequent study was unable to confirm the initial observation that both healthy subjects and IC patients had similar findings in their tight junctions relative to ruthenium red penetration. A well-controlled study in 56 patients has provided data to support the hypothesis that the bladder surface in many patients with IC may indeed leak (26). These investigators have since developed an even more sensitive leak assay and believe that about 70% of patients with IC have a "leaky epithelium" (45,46). Other investigations have reported similar responses to potassium chloride (47,48). We propose that patients with no obvious leak may have false-negative responses to potassium chloride or another problem, such as a neurologic abnormality or inflammation. Additional support for epithelial dysfunction comes from data suggesting that fluorescein absorption is increased in IC patients over that in healthy subjects (49).

### Glycosaminoglycans: The Blood–Urine Barrier

Control of epithelial permeability in the bladder has traditionally been ascribed to tight junctions that are unique to the bladder epithelium (in the absence of physiologic data) and ion pumps (25,50–55). More recent studies, however, have provided physiologic data to suggest that the bladder surface proteoglycans or glycosaminoglycans (GAGs) may actually be a crucial component of the mechanism by which the epithelium maintains a barrier between the bladder wall and urine, the so-called blood–urine barrier (26–28).

Surface proteoglycans (GAG, mucus) appear to have multiple protective roles in the bladder, including antiadherence and regulation of transepithelial solute movement (22, 50–52). The transitional cell's external surface GAGs are capable of preventing the adherence of bacteria, crystals, proteins, and ions, a function that is lost when this layer is removed with a dilute acid or detergent (28,56–59) but restored when GAG is replaced by exogenous polysaccharides, such as heparin or pentosan polysulfate sodium (PPS; Elmiron, Alza Pharmaceuticals, Mountain View, CA, U.S.A.) (56,60,61). The oxygen atom present on the sulfate group of polysaccharides is negatively charged and has a high affinity to bond ionically with water. This results in exclusion of urinary ionic solutes by a Donnan effect (62).

When GAG is present at a surface (the bladder), it binds water molecules tightly to the oxygen of the sulfate groups in preference to calcium, barium, and even hydrogen ions (63–65). Water molecules become trapped and interposed at the boundary between the cell surface (bladder) and the environment (urine) (Fig. 33.3). This bound molecular layer of water acts as a physical barrier, such that urinary solutes, including urea and calcium (28,56), are not able to reach the underlying cell membranes, nor move across it.

Quaternary amines, on the other hand, have a high affinity for sulfated polysaccharides and displace the water bound to the oxygen groups (62,66,67). This concept is supported by the fact that when GAG chemically reacts with quaternary amines, an increased entropy results, reflecting the loss of water ordering around the sulfate groups (62,68). This interaction is the basis for the clinical use of protamine sulfate (a quaternary amine) to precipitate and inactivate the anticoagulant effects of heparin. It has been demonstrated both in animal and human models that protamine sulfate inactivates native cell surface polysaccharides, resulting in increased epithelial permeability. Such damage to the transitional cells can be reversed by the addition of a GAG, such as heparin (27,28).

Based on these concepts, it has been proposed that the surface polysaccharide is functionally defective (but not absent) in some patients with IC. The deficiency has many possible causes, including qualitative or quantitative changes in surface GAG or damage to it from urinary compounds, such as highly charged amines. It has been demonstrated that healthy subjects who have their bladder surface challenged by the quaternary amine protamine lose the impermeability of the epithelium. The permeability to urea in healthy subjects increases from 5% to 25% (27). When the blood–urine barrier is lost because of protamine treatment, most healthy subjects experience urgency, frequency, and bladder pain (the same symptoms of IC), symptoms that are reversed with a subsequent treatment with heparin. This GAG concept is additionally supported by the fact that a synthetic polysaccharide similar to heparin is effective in ameliorating the symptoms of IC (69–72).

To test the hypothesis that some patients with IC have a permeable transitional cell layer, Parsons et al. (26) measured the permeability of the normal bladder epithelium to a con-

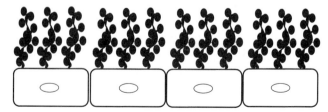

FIG. 33.3. The concept of a biofilm layer at the bladder surface schematically drawn to demonstrate the location of the trapped water at the surface. *Small dark circles* represent bound water, and *wavy lines* represent the protein backbone.

centrated solution of urea and compared this measure with that of patients with IC. Twenty-nine healthy controls absorbed about 5% of the urea, whereas 56 patients with IC absorbed 25%. Evidence from Buffington et al. (49) adds additional support to the epithelial permeability dysfunction in IC. These investigators showed that of subjects given oral fluorescein, those with IC maintained significantly higher serum levels and took longer to clear the fluorescein from their urine than did healthy subjects. They concluded that the patients were "reabsorbing" (recycling) the fluorescein from their bladders.

Based on these observations, we propose that some patients with IC do have a leaky epithelium and that the leak of urinary solute results in urgency and frequency. It may be that not all patients with IC have such leaks, but at least 70% to 90% can be shown to have them (41,42).

### Role of Urinary Potassium in Pathogenesis and Diagnosis

It has been proposed for a number of years that the urinary leak of toxic substances through a defective mucosal permeability barrier results in symptoms of urgency and pain. It is now proposed that the principal toxic substance is urinary potassium. The normal urinary potassium levels range from 20 to 150 mEq/L. The average level is about 75 mEq/L. This concentration of potassium is not only well in excess of a lethal level for mammalian cells (15 to 20 mEq) but also well in excess of levels required to depolarize sensory nerves (15 to 20 mEq/L) and induce pain and urgency. It may be that one of the most important roles for the blood–urine barrier is to prevent toxic levels of urinary potassium from diffusing into the bladder wall.

The role of the transitional epithelium in regulating potassium metabolism is summarized in Fig. 33.4. Should urinary potassium excessively leak into the bladder interstitium, another defense mechanism is proposed. The blood-rich subepithelial plexus of lymphatic and blood vessels could reabsorb this cation (73) and restore equilibrium. If the diffusion of potassium is excessive and overcomes the secondary defense mechanism, potassium could destroy these blood and lymphatic vessels, accelerating the disease process. In essence, toxic levels of urinary potassium normally present could explain both the symptoms and progression of disease when the epithelium loses its impermeability. Potassium diffusion could induce other agents, such as substance P, and perhaps upregulate pain fibers. This hypothesis may explain the lack of any significant inflammatory response in most patients with IC, either in the urine or bladder interstitium (35).

Based on these concepts, we propose that there are two important components to the paradigm of IC pathogenesis. First, the regulatory role of mucus in reducing permeability is impaired (for reasons unknown); second, once the role of mucus is impaired, the high levels of urinary potassium result in increased interstitial levels in the bladder that cause sen-

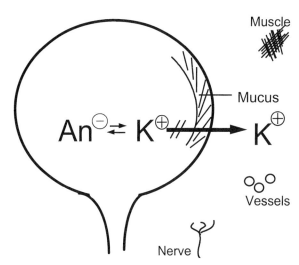

**FIG. 33.4.** The high levels of urinary potassium are more than sufficient to depolarize sensory nerves if they present themselves to the subepithelial area. Once in the subepithelial space, they can depolarize muscle or nerves or be carried away by an intact vascular supply (restoring tissue levels of potassium to normal).

sory nerves (and muscle) to depolarize, inducing pain and urgency and resulting in tissue destruction.

To test the hypothesis that potassium induces symptoms in IC, healthy subjects and subjects with a variety of bladder sensory disorders were examined for sensitivity to a solution of intravesical potassium, as noted in Table 33.1. As can be seen, IC patients reacted strongly, but healthy subjects did not. Patients with acute urinary tract infection and radiation cystitis were also found to be potassium sensitive, whereas patients with benign prostatic hyperplasia and most of those with detrusor instability were not provoked. Finally, to test the potassium hypothesis, sodium (which should not depolarize nerves) was compared with potassium; sodium chloride did not cause symptoms in the IC patients but potassium did (Table 33.2). Therefore, it would appear that potassium is a major factor in the pathogenesis of IC, and patient sensitivity to potassium chloride may be a useful diagnostic tool that is discussed in a later section.

### Mast Cells and Nerve Fibers

The role of mast cells in this disorder is not well understood. Mast cells have been reported by a number of investigators to be present in IC bladders, whereas other data suggest that they are also present in non-IC bladders (22,24,31,32,74). The central point of confusion is whether mast cells play a causative or secondary role in that they may be degranulating and producing symptoms, or, on the other hand, that they represent a response to whatever is causing IC (e.g., an epithelial leak) and be a type of defense mechanism that may ultimately become part of the problem.

Attempts have been made to quantitate mast cells (granulated and degranulated) both in the mucosa and in the subep-

**TABLE 33.1.** *Results of stimulation of sensory urgency or pain in various groups using potassium chloride*

| Group | N | % Positive[a] to KCl | p Value[b] | % Positive to $H_2O$ |
|---|---|---|---|---|
| Normals | 41 | 4 | — | 0 |
| IC (meeting NIH criteria) | 92 | 74 | <0.001[c] | 10 |
| IC (not cystoscoped) | 139 | 76 | <0.001[c] | 10 |
| Radiation cystitis[d] | 5 | 100 | 0.001 | 0 |
| BPH | 29 | 3 | 1.0 | 3 |
| Acute UTI[e] | 4 | 100 | 0.01 | 0 |
| Uninfected UTI[f] | 5 | 0 | 1.0 | 0 |
| Detrusor instability | 16 | 25 | 0.03 | 0 |

[a] At least a two-point change in visual analogue scale.
[b] Fisher's exact test was employed to compare group to controls.
[c] $\chi^2$ analysis.
[d] Data on radiation cystitis from Parsons CL, Stein PC, Bidair M, et al. Abnormal sensitivity to intravesical potassium in interstitial cystitis and radiation cystitis. *Neurourol Urodyn* 1994;13:515.
[e] Test performed when infected.
[f] Test performed when uninfected.
IC, interstitial cystitis; NIH, National Institutes of Health; BPH, benign prostatic hyperplasia; UTI, urinary tract infection.

ithelial tissues. Some investigators believe mast cells are involved, whereas others believe there is no increase of mast cells in patients with IC compared with other patient groups. Most of the control subjects studied, however, had bladder cancer and were, in fact, not "normal" (34,75,76). Nonetheless, the presence of mast cells in one third of patients may result in degranulation and symptom aggravation. Control of this degranulation (even though the cells may be a defense mechanism) may be helpful therapy in some patients and is discussed later. It is again important to emphasize the potential for multiple causes of IC. The increased presence of mast cells in a subset of patients may be important for diagnosis and therapy in the afflicted group.

As IC progresses, patients experience a steady increase in pain. A number of reports suggest an increase in nerve fibers in IC and a possible link to an increase in mast cells. These events may explain the clinical association of allergies and pain progression (5,13,74,77–80).

## AUTOIMMUNE ASPECTS

A number of reports document the existence of autoantibodies in some patients with IC (81–84), and because the disease has many of the clinical and pathologic features of autoimmune conditions, such as an episodic and remissive disease

**TABLE 33.2.** *Provocation of urgency by sodium versus potassium in interstitial cystitis*

| Treatment arm | % Urgency Na | | % Urgency K | | p Value |
|---|---|---|---|---|---|
| Control | 0/10 | (0%) | 0/11 | (0%) | — |
| Protamine | 1/10 | (10%) | 10/11 | (90%) | <0.001 |
| Heparin | 1/10 | (10%) | 5/11 | (54%) | 0.035[a] |

[a] Compares KCl after protamine to KCl after heparin.
From Parsons CL, Greenberger M, Gabal L, et al. The role of urinary potassium in the pathogenesis and diagnosis of interstitial cystitis. *J Urol* 1998;159:1862–1867, with permission.

course, infiltration with inflammatory mononuclear cells (lymphocytes, monocytes, plasma cells), and the presence of ANAs, it has been suggested that IC may be a bladder-specific autoimmune disease or a chronic inflammatory condition of the bladder involving autoimmune responses. Indeed, autoimmune phenomena could account for a number of the common clinical and pathologic features observed in the IC patient population (21,85). Support for an autoimmune causation of IC was provided in animal studies by Bullock et al. (86,87), who immunized mice with autologous bladder antigens and then observed histologic evidence of IC-like disease. Adoptive transfer of disease was observed when injecting lymphocytes from immunized animals into naive mice.

As a possible manifestation of an autoimmune response, Ochs et al. (82) characterized autoantibodies from the sera of patients with IC. Of the 96 IC patients studied initially, 38 (39%) had detectable levels of autoantibodies by immunofluorescence on HEp-2 cells (ANA slides) or Western blotting on whole-cell extracts of T24 bladder cells. None of the patients had detectable bladder tissue-specific autoantibodies. Most of the autoantibodies were against nuclear or nucleolar antigens, but an additional three autoantibodies against mitochondria and three autoantibodies against unknown cytoplasmic antigens were detected. The incidence of ANAs was somewhat higher than the value of 25% previously reported by Oravisto (23) and similar to that reported by Jokinen et al. (88), who reported that 7 of 33 (21%) IC patients had ANAs of titer 1/160 or greater, with fine-speckled nuclear staining the most common pattern. All but 4 of the 35 ANA-positive sera were exclusively of the immunoglobulin G (IgG) class. The most common ANA patterns were nucleolar and nucleoplasmic dense fine-speckled patterns. Thus far, only one of the nucleolar antibodies has been characterized. By Western blotting and cDNA cloning techniques, it was a novel 55-kD nucleolar protein never before reported to be an autoantigen (89). The dense fine-speckled nucleoplasmic pattern was also unique and characterized by staining of chromosomes in mitotic cells. The autoantigen recognized by this antibody is a 70-kD protein by Western blotting (82), and because all autoantibodies with this immunofluorescence pattern recognize the same 70-kD protein, this may be the most common autoantibody–autoantigen complex in the IC patient population.

Another distinctive autoantibody type was antimitochondria, occurring in 2.5% of IC patients. Autoantibodies to mitochondria are more commonly observed in patients with chronic liver diseases (90). The centromere pattern, found in less than 1% of IC patients, is also shared with patients who have the systemic autoimmune disease scleroderma (90,91).

Even if autoimmunity is not the direct cause of IC, there may still be a role for serum autoantibodies in IC diagnosis and treatment. For example, patients with autoantibodies may represent a separate subpopulation of the IC patient group, with a different set of symptoms and perhaps a need for different treatment modalities. The presence or absence of a particular autoantibody may indicate a better or worse prognosis. As described in the systemic autoimmune diseases (90,91), sets or profiles of specific disease-related autoantibodies may also be important in classifying different groups of IC patients. For instance, in scleroderma, autoantibodies to centromere proteins are associated with the CREST (calcinosis cutis, Raynaud's phenomenon, esophageal dysfunction, sclerodactyly, and telangiectasia) form of the disease, whereas autoantibodies to DNA topoisomerase I (so-called Scl-70) are associated with diffuse scleroderma. This degree of specificity is difficult to explain unless the pathophysiology of each of these forms of scleroderma is unique, perhaps resulting in an "antigen-driven" (91) autoimmune response to different cellular components. Thus, the different autoantibody responses may reflect subtly different forms or categories of the same disease.

Likewise, IC patients with nuclear autoantibodies, as distinct from those with nucleolar autoantibodies, may distinguish different forms of the disease. Several potential candidate autoantibody–autoantigen systems have been identified that appear to occur in more than one patient. If further work indicates that these occur in a significant number of patients and demonstrate specificity for IC, then they could prove to be useful in diagnosis. Objective laboratory findings such as these would augment what is currently a diagnosis based on clinical findings (31,81).

Although the role of autoimmunity in IC is still controversial and may be of an indirect nature, it is obvious that patients with serum autoantibodies are manifesting components of an autoimmune response that may be contributing directly or indirectly to disease progression and symptoms.

In the first case scenario, an autoimmune response could be mounted against the bladder, and autoantibodies would be pathogenic, causing direct cell death and tissue destruction. Because there is no compelling evidence for bladder-specific autoantibodies and only a portion of IC patients have autoantibodies (82), this is unlikely to be the explanation for IC in all patients. More complicated might be a case of immunologic attack on a bladder infected by viruses or bacteria. Similar to tuberculosis, the infectious agent is the actual cause of disease, but the pathology and major symptoms arise as a result of the ensuing immunologic response to what may now be altered or diseased tissue. More complicated still is the case of "molecular mimicry," in which circulating antibodies against a past or present foreign organism can cross-react with self antigens (in this case, a bladder antigen), causing inflammation and cell and tissue destruction. Lacking strong proof for bladder-specific autoantibodies, molecular mimicry as a mechanism for immune attack on the bladder is not likely.

In the second case, the autoimmune response in IC is indirect, and autoantibodies arise as a result of cell and tissue destruction caused by chronic inflammation. In this case, autoantibodies could be targeted to the bladder in an attempt to "clean up" cellular debris, and their presence would be considered an epiphenomenon as a result of the massive tissue destruction. In the presence of antibody and complement and other cytokines and chemoattractants, even more cell and tissue destruction could occur, resulting in repeating cycles of tissue destruction and inflammation. In this case, not every IC patient would necessarily have serum autoantibodies; this would depend on the individual immune response and the amount of tissue damage involved. In fact, the titers or presence of autoantibody could be a reflection of disease severity and may fluctuate during the disease course.

In the last case, the presence of autoantibodies in some IC patients may have nothing to do with the disease, being the result of another coexisting condition or disease process. This possibility seems unlikely because the incidence of autoantibodies in the IC patient population can be relatively high and the types of autoantibodies observed are, for the most part, unlike those found in well-defined autoimmune diseases (82).

## CURRENT CONCEPTS AND TREATMENT

### Therapy

A number of drugs have been employed for the treatment of IC. Most were used empirically, and only a few have been reported in controlled trials. Basically, therapy for IC can be divided into three major categories:

1. Drug therapy that alters nerve function directly or indirectly, such as narcotics, antidepressants, antihistamines, antiinflammatories, anticholinergics, antispasmodics, and analgesics.
2. Cytodestructive techniques, which destroy the umbrella cells of the bladder, causing regeneration, a new bladder surface, and a period of remission. In general, these techniques cause symptoms to flare substantially before the repair process is completed and symptoms resolve. These techniques include the use of dimethylsulfoxide (DMSO), hydrodistention, Corpactin, and silver nitrate.

3. Cytoprotective techniques, which involve the use of medications, primarily polysaccharides, that can "coat" the bladder and help reestablish or protect the bladder surface mucus. These drugs include heparin, PPS, and possibly hyaluronic acid.

When discussing therapy with the patient, it is important for the physician to emphasize that if the symptoms have been present continuously for more than a year, no particular therapy is likely to be curative. In this case, it should be considered a chronic disease that requires chronic therapy. Although the patient may have a significant remission of symptoms, there is a high risk for relapse. If patients are prepared for this eventuality, they are much less distressed when symptoms return and can cope better with their disease. The physician–patient relationship is strengthened in terms of credibility if this topic is addressed before initiating treatment. Patients readily accept this explanation and are better able to adjust to their disorder when their outlook is a realistic one.

### Antidepressant Therapy

Chronic pain and sleep loss cause depression. Thus, it is valuable to place most IC patients with moderate or worse symptoms on antidepressant medications. Tricyclic antidepressants have several modes of action that are beneficial. They cause drowsiness (aid sleep), increase pain thresholds, and elevate mood. If tricyclic antidepressants are used, start with low doses, and warn patients they will be tired for 12 to 15 hours per day for the first 2 to 3 weeks of therapy. After they become tolerant to this side effect, increase the dose, if necessary. Amitriptyline (92) or imipramine can be prescribed in doses of 25 mg (or even 10 mg) 1 hour before bedtime. The exact mechanism of action of amitriptyline is unknown, although it may block histamine-1 receptors and perhaps mast cell degranulation. More likely, the drug raises pain tolerance as a result of its antidepressant activity. If fluoxetine (Prozac, Dista Products Company, Indianapolis, IN, U.S.A.) is selected, use 20 mg per day and increase if needed to 40 mg. Sertraline (Zoloft, Pfizer Inc., New York, NY, U.S.A.) is another well-tolerated antidepressant; it can be used at 50 mg per day and increased to 100 mg if needed.

Antidepressant therapy is an important adjunct to treatment. It does not cure IC, but patients function much better with their disabling symptoms if not depressed. In essence, they "feel better" even if they still void 20 times per day. Surprisingly, many patients (about 25% to 30%) improve dramatically only with antidepressant therapy. No matter what other therapy has been initiated, we place all moderately (or more) symptomatic patients on antidepressants and stop this treatment if they improve and are being successfully managed with some other treatment (e.g., heparin or PPS).

### Dimethylsulfoxide

DMSO was approved for the treatment of IC in 1977 (93). Although no controlled clinical trials were ever conducted with DMSO, it appears to induce remission in 34% to 40% of the patients. The difficulty with DMSO is that it may induce an excellent remission with the first one to three cycles of therapy, but as the patient relapses and requires subsequent treatment, progressive resistance to its beneficial effects is usually seen.

For treatment, 50 mL of 50% dimethylsulfoxide is instilled into the bladder for 5 to 10 minutes. Longer periods are unnecessary because DMSO rapidly absorbs into the bloodstream. Instillations are performed on an outpatient basis, or the patient can be taught to perform them. We recommend that patients receive 6 to 8 weekly treatments to determine whether a therapeutic response is achieved. If the patient has moderate or worse symptoms, therapy is continued for an additional 4 to 6 months once every other week. Remember, after DMSO therapy is stopped, the patient is likely to become resistant to its use; therefore, continued use is the best regimen with this medication.

Some patients experience a flare of symptoms when DMSO is placed into the bladder. This phenomenon may be related to the ability of DMSO to degranulate mast cells and may occur primarily in patients who have significant bladder mastocytosis. More likely, the detergent activity destroys the superficial transitional cells, resulting in an increased leak of solute and more symptoms. As the epithelium heals over a span of weeks, remissions are seen. Nonetheless, DMSO may be effective treatment in these patients. Patients who experience pain with DMSO should receive 10 mL of 2% viscous lidocaine jelly (Xylocaine, Astra, Wayne, PA, U.S.A.) intravesically 15 minutes before the DMSO. If this is not successful, use an injectable narcotic or ketorolac tromethamine (Toradol, Roche Laboratories, Nutley, NJ, U.S.A.), 60 mg intramuscularly, before the intravesical instillation. The flare of symptoms associated with DMSO usually disappears over 24 hours. As these patients receive subsequent treatments, the pain tends to diminish. In most patients with moderate or worse symptoms, DMSO takes 2 to 4 months to work.

Patients may also receive indefinite therapy using DMSO. As originally reported by Stewart (93), patients have used DMSO weekly for several years without problems. DMSO has been reported to be associated with cataracts in animals; however, this complication has not been reported in humans. In patients receiving chronic therapy, some recommend slit-lamp evaluation at periodic intervals. We do not do this, however, and have never seen a problem during the more than 18 years we have used DMSO.

### Antihistamines

Antihistamines are crucial to the management of IC in patients with hay fever, sinusitis, or food allergies. Patients in good control of their IC symptoms experience symptom "breakthrough" in allergy season. Antihistamines have been tried in IC but without controlled studies. Antihistamines were chosen because of the possible role of mast cells

(76,94–96). Although most patients may not respond to antihistamines, subsets of patients appear to have major benefit, especially when combined with other therapy. Allergic people in particular benefit from hydroxyzine, 25 to 50 mg at bedtime (80). This is an extremely effective way to manage allergies when the medication is used chronically. This medication is not only an antihistamine but also, when used chronically, suppresses mast cell release of histamines and is probably the only drug that does this. Beneficial effects appear 2 to 3 months after start of treatment, and patients are urged to stay on the medication for at least 3 months to determine effectiveness. The mast cell inhibition is only seen when used chronically.

## Steroids

Because of the assumption that inflammation plays a role in IC, patients have received steroids. Badenoch (97) found significant improvement in 19 of 25 patients treated with prednisone; however, all were treated after hydrodistention under anesthesia, which may have been responsible for most of the benefit. In our experience, steroids do not ameliorate the symptoms of this complex. As with most drugs, there have been no controlled clinical trials conducted on the efficacy of steroids in the treatment of IC.

## Intravesical Oxychlorosene Sodium

Oxychlorosene sodium (Clorpactin WCS-90, Guardian Laboratories, Hauppauge, NY, U.S.A.) is a highly reactive chemical compound that is a modified derivative of hypochlorous acid in a buffered base. Its activity is dependent on the liberation of hypochlorous acid and its resulting oxidizing effects and detergency (98). It was used originally by Wishard et al. (99), who treated 20 patients with 5 weekly instillations of 0.2% Clorpactin WCS-90 under local anesthesia. Improvement was reported in 14 of the 20 patients, and follow-up was brief. Messing and Stamey (81), treating 38 patients with 0.4% oxychlorosene sodium, reported significant improvement in 72%. Ureteral reflux is a contraindication to the use of oxychlorosene sodium. It is recommended that the compound usually be used under anesthesia. This medication works in a cytodestructive fashion. It destroys the surface epithelial cells (umbrella cells) and when they regenerate, remission is seen. It may take 2 to 4 weeks for the flare of symptoms to resolve, and then remission occurs.

## Intravesical Silver Nitrate

Intravesical silver nitrate was first reported by Dodson (98). Pool (100) fashioned a treatment regimen in which bladder irrigations were begun under anesthesia with a 1:5000 concentration. This was followed subsequently by gradually increasing the concentrations on a daily basis, ultimately employing a 1% solution. Again, this was done in an uncontrolled setting in patients who had undergone dilation of the

bladder under anesthesia. Pool (100) reported good results in 89% of patients. There have been other uncontrolled studies reporting that this compound is helpful; nevertheless, it is not very widely used today. One caution in the use of silver nitrate is never to instill it into the bladder after biopsy. If there is a perforation and this solution is placed into the bladder, intraperitoneal and extraperitoneal extravasation could occur, resulting in major tissue damage. As with oxychlorosene sodium, this agent works by destroying the epithelial surface.

## Urinary Alkalinizers

Polycitra (ALZA Pharmaceuticals, Palo Alto, CA, U.S.A.) is a chelating agent that not only alkalinizes the urine but also binds potassium. Both effects may be beneficial in IC, and it is recommended that patients receive a trial of therapy for 3 to 6 months. Employing two doses a day of medication appears to be sufficient. In general, this drug should be combined with other treatments, such as heparin, PPS, or amitriptyline (Elavil, Zeneca Pharmaceuticals, Wilmington, DE, U.S.A.), to obtain the best effect. The best tolerated salt of Polycitra is potassium. Sodium bicarbonate is also recommended for chronic treatment because urinary potassium levels can be lowered by increasing the sodium, and sodium is beneficial to the bladder.

## Heparinoid Therapy

A major breakthrough in therapy is the use of heparin-like drugs (heparin, PPS), which, when effective, reverse the course of the disease (Table 33.3). Patients rarely become resistant to their use, possibly because these drugs correct the epithelial leak and halt the disease (101).

## Heparin

Heparin, when given by injection, has been reported to alleviate the symptoms of IC (102). This was not in a controlled study. Chronic systemic heparin therapy cannot be employed in most patients because it results in osteoporosis in almost 100% of patients who use it for 26 weeks or longer. In our experience, intravesical heparin has significant activity in about half of patients (101). Here, too, the data were obtained in an uncontrolled investigation. Previous controlled studies that we conducted demonstrated a placebo effect of about 20%, suggesting possible activity for heparin (63). Heparin is recommended for moderate or worse patients. The tech-

**TABLE 33.3.** *Heparinoid therapy*

| Drug | Dose | Route |
|------|------|-------|
| Heparin | 20–40,000 U/d | Intravesical and self-administered |
| Pentosan polysulfate | 100–200 mg t.i.d. | Oral |

nique uses 40,000 units of heparin in 20 mL of saline, and this solution is instilled intravesically daily, then after 3 to 4 months, it is reduced to 3 to 4 times per week. If there is no effect after 3 months, instillation is increased to 40,000 units daily. This treatment can be carried on indefinitely. It takes 3 to 12 months to begin to see improvements, but therapy should be continued at least 12 to 18 months before abandoning it. The best improvements are noted after 1 to 2 years. Long-term therapy is recommended for patients with moderate or worse disease who respond to its use. Serum prothrombin time and partial thromboplastin time are monitored for several weeks after therapy begins to exclude the formation of an unusual antibody to heparin or systemic absorption (heparin should not be absorbed across the bladder mucosa). Patients are instructed in self-catheterization so that this therapy can be performed at home.

### Pentosan Polysulfate Sodium

Parsons et al. (69) first reported the effectiveness of PPS in ameliorating the symptoms of IC. Because this agent is a sulfated polysaccharide, it could augment the bladder surface defense mechanism or detoxify agents in urine that have a capacity to attack the bladder surface, such as quaternary amines. In a controlled clinical study, symptoms were controlled in 42% of patients, compared with 20% of those taking placebo (69). This has been borne out in several subsequent studies, including a five-center trial in which 28% of patients, compared with 13% taking placebo, improved (70). In a seven-center study of 150 patients, there was a 32% patient improvement on drug versus 15% on placebo (103). Additionally, an English–Danish study also found a significant reduction of pain in patients taking this drug compared with placebo (26).

PPS is administered in an oral dose of 100 mg three times per day. In patients with moderate symptoms, it appears to have about 40% to 50% activity. In the controlled clinical trials that were done on patients with severe disease, its activity was lower. Continued use of this agent for several years leads to long-term disease control in most responders (104), and an efficacy rate of up to 74% was reported when used for 6 months or longer. This sustained response is usually not found in other therapies, except heparin. Response to therapy is first seen after 6 to 10 weeks but may take 6 to 12 months. All male and female patients with more severe disease may need 200 mg three times daily to control the disease. It takes 3 to 12 months to get a good response; therefore, the medication should be used at least 9 to 12 months before abandoning it. We see about a 60% efficacy rate when using it longer and at a larger dose.

The primary side effects of PPS are gastrointestinal and can frequently be reduced by taking the medication with a small snack or taking it out of the capsule and dissolving it in 1 oz of water. Hair loss is reported in about 3% to 4% of patients, but this is completely reversible, even when continuing to take the medication.

## REFERENCES

1. Nigro DA, Wein AJ, Foy M, et al., for the ICDB Study Group. Associations among cystoscopic and urodynamic findings for women enrolled in the Interstitial Cystitis Data Base Study. *Urology* 1997; 49[Suppl 5A]:86.
2. Bumpus HC. Interstitial cystitis. *Med Clin North Am* 1930;13:1495.
3. Jones CA, Nyberg L. Epidemiology of interstitial cystitis. *Urology* 1997;49[Suppl 5A]:2.
4. Ho N, Koziol JA, Parsons CL. Epidemiology of interstitial cystitis. In: Sant GR, ed. *Interstitial cystitis*. Philadelphia: Lippincott-Raven, 1997:9–16.
5. Koziol JA. Epidemiology of interstitial cystitis. *Urol Clin North Am* 1994;21:7–20.
6. Oravisto KJ. Epidemiology of interstitial cystitis. *Ann Chir Gynaecol Fenn* 1975;64:75–77.
7. Gillenwater JY, Wein AJ. Summary of the National Institutes of Arthritis, Diabetes, Digestive and Kidney Diseases Workshop on Interstitial Cystitis. National Institutes of Health, Bethesda, Maryland, August 28–29, 1987. *J Urol* 1988;140:203–206.
8. Held PJ, Hanno PM, Wein AJ. Epidemiology of interstitial cystitis. In: Hanno PM, ed. *Interstitial cystitis*. London: Springer-Verlag, 1990: 29–48.
9. Bade JJ, Rijcken B, Mensink HJA. Interstitial cystitis in the Netherlands: prevalence, diagnostic criteria and therapeutic preferences. *J Urol* 1995;154:2035–2038.
10. Messing E, Pauk D, Schaeffer A, et al., for the ICDB Study Group. Associations among cystoscopic findings and symptoms and physical examination findings in women enrolled in the Interstitial Cystitis Data Base (ICDB) Study. *Urology* 1997;49[Suppl 5A]:81.
11. Kass EH, Savage WD, Santamaria BAG. The significance of bacteria in preventative medicine. In: Kass EH, ed. *Progress in pyelonephritis*. Philadelphia: FA Davis, 1964:3.
11a. Hamilton-Miller JMT, Iravani A, Brumfitt W, et al. Comparative trials of cefaclor AF in uncomplicated cystitis and asymptomatic bacteriuria. *Postgrad Med J* 1992;68[Suppl 3]:S60–S67.
12. Hamilton-Miller JMT. The urethral syndrome and its management. *J Antimicrob Chemother* 1994;33[Suppl A]:63.
13. Koziol JA, Clark DC, Gittes RF, et al. The natural history of interstitial cystitis: a survey of 374 patients. *J Urol* 1993;149:465–469.
14. Alagiri M, Chottiner S, Ratner V, et al. Interstitial cystitis: unexplained associations with other chronic disease and pain syndromes. *Urology* 1997;49[Suppl 5A]:52–57.
15. Hunner GL. A rare type of bladder ulcer in women: report of cases. *Boston Med Surg J* 1915;172:660–664.
16. Hunner GL. Elusive ulcer of the bladder: further notes on a rare type of bladder ulcer with a report of 25 cases. *Am J Obstet* 1918;78:374.
17. Oravisto KJ, Alfthan OS, Jokinen EJ. Interstitial cystitis: clinical and immunological findings. *Scand J Urol Nephrol* 1970;4:37–42.
18. Hand JR. Interstitial cystitis: a report of 223 cases. *J Urol* 1949;61:291.
19. Hanash KA, Pool TL. Interstitial and hemorrhagic cystitis: viral, bacterial and fungal studies. *J Urol* 1970;104:705–706.
20. Oravisto KJ, Alfthan OS. Treatment of interstitial cystitis with immunosuppression and chloroquine derivatives. *Eur Urol.* 1976;2: 82–84.
21. Silk MR. Bladder antibodies in interstitial cystitis. *J Urol* 1970;103: 307–309.
22. Holm-Bentzen M, Lose G. Pathology and pathogenesis of interstitial cystitis. *Urology.* 1987;29[Suppl 4]:8–13.
23. Oravisto KJ. Interstitial cystitis as an autoimmune disease: a review. *Eur Urol* 1990;6:10–13.
24. Weaver RG, Dougherty TF, Natoli C. Recent concepts of interstitial cystitis. *J Urol* 1963;89:377.
25. Eldrup J, Thorup J, Nielsen SL, et al. Permeability and ultrastructure of human bladder epithelium. *Br J Urol* 1983;55:488–492.
26. Parsons CL, Lilly JD, Stein P. Epithelial dysfunction in non-bacterial cystitis (interstitial cystitis). *J Urol* 1991;145:732–735.
27. Lilly JD, Parsons CL. Bladder surface glycosaminoglycans: a human epithelial permeability barrier. *Surg Gynecol Obstet* 1990;171:493–496.
28. Parsons CL, Boychuk D, Jones S, et al. Bladder surface glycosaminoglycans: an epithelial permeability barrier. *J Urol* 1990;143:139–142.
29. Hohlbrugger G, Lentsch P. Intravesical ions, osmolality and pH influence the volume pressure response in the normal rat bladder, and this is more pronounced after DMSO exposure. *Eur Urol* 1985;11: 127–130.

30. MacDermott JP, Miller CH, Levy N, et al. Cellular immunity in interstitial cystitis. *J Urol* 1991;145:274–278.

31. Hanno P, Levin RM, Monson FC, et al. Diagnosis of interstitial cystitis. *J Urol* 1990;143:278–281.

32. Holm-Bentzen M, Jacobsen F, Nerstrom B, et al. Painful bladder disease: clinical and pathoanatomical differences in 115 patients. *J Urol* 1987;138:500.

33. Lynes WL, Flynn SD, Shortliffe LD, et al. Mast cell involvement in interstitial cystitis. *J Urol* 1987;138:746–752.

34. Lotz M, Villiger PM, Hugli T, et al. Interleukin-6 and interstitial cystitis. *J Urol* 1994;152:869–873.

35. Holm-Bentzen J, Halt T, Sondergaard I. Urinary excretion of a metabolite of histamine (1,4-methyl-imidazole-acetic-acid). *J Urol* 1986;135:187.

36. Kastrup J, Hald J, Larsen L. Histamine content and mast cell count of detrusor muscle in patients with interstitial cystitis and other types of chronic cystitis. *Br J Urol* 1983;55:495–500.

37. Sant GR. Interstitial cystitis: pathophysiology, clinical evaluation and treatment. *Ann Urol* 1989;3:172–179.

38. Sant GR, Kalaru P, Ucci AA Jr. Mucosal mast cell (MMC) contribution to bladder mastocytosis in interstitial cystitis. *J Urol* 1988;139:276A.

39. Bjorling DE, Saban MR, Zine MJ, et al. In vitro passive sensitization of guinea pig, rhesus monkey and human bladders as a model of non-infectious cystitis. *J Urol* 1994;152:1603–1608.

40. Saban R, Christensen M, Keith I, et al. Experimental model for the study of bladder mast cell degranulation and smooth muscle contraction. *Semin Urol* 1991;9:88–101.

41. Galloway N, Gabale D, Irwin P. Interstitial cystitis or reflex sympathetic dystrophy of the bladder? *Semin Urol* 1991;9:148.

42. Parsons CL, Stein PC, Bidair M, et al. Abnormal sensitivity to intravesical potassium in interstitial cystitis and radiation cystitis. *Neurourol Urodyn* 1994;13:515–520.

43. Parsons CL. Potassium sensitivity test. *Tech Urol* 1996;2:171–173.

44. Parsons CL, Greenberger M, Gabal L, et al. The role of urinary potassium in the pathogenesis and diagnosis of interstitial cystitis. *J Urol* 1998;159:1862–1867.

45. Parsons CL, Stein PC, Bidair M, et al. Abnormal sensitivity to intravesical potassium in interstitial cystitis and radiation cystitis. *Neurol Urodyn* 1994;13:515–520.

46. Parsons CL, Greenberger M, Gabal L, et al. The role of urinary potassium in the pathogenesis and diagnosis of interstitial cystitis. *J Urol* 1998;159:1862–1867.

47. Payne CK, Browning S. Graded potassium chloride testing in interstitial cystitis. *J Urol* 1996;155:438A.

48. Teichman JMH, Nielsen-Omeis BJ, McIver BD. Modified urodynamics for interstitial cystitis. *J Urol* 1996;155:433A.

49. Buffington CAT, Woodworth BE. Excretion of fluorescein in the urine of women with interstitial cystitis. *J Urol* 1997;158:786.

50. Englund SE. Observation on the migration of some labeled substances between the urinary bladder and blood in rabbits. *Acta Radiol* (Suppl) 1956;135:9–13.

51. Fellows GJ, Marshall DH. The permeability of human bladder epithelium to water and sodium. *Invest Urol* 1972;9:339–344.

52. Hicks RM. The permeability of rat transitional epithelium. *J Cell Biol* 1966;28:21–31.

53. Hicks RM, Ketterer B, Warren RC. The ultrastructure and chemistry of the luminal plasma membrane of the mammalian urinary bladder: a structure with low permeability to water and ions. *Phil Trans R Soc Lond B* 1974;268:23–38.

54. Staehelin LA, Chlapowski FJ, Bonneville MA. Luminal plasma membrane of the urinary bladder. *J Cell Biol* 1972;53:73–91.

55. Lewis SA, Diamond JM. Na$^+$ transport by rabbit urinary bladder, a tight epithelium. *J Membrane Biol* 1976;28:1–40.

56. Parsons CL, Stauffer C, Schmidt J. Bladder surface glycosaminoglycans: an efficient mechanism of environmental adaptation. *Science* 1980;208:605–607.

57. Parsons CL, Greenspan C, Mulholland SG. The primary antibacterial defense mechanism of the bladder. *Invest Urol* 1975;13:72–76.

58. Parsons CL, Greenspan C, Moore SW, et al. Role of surface mucin in primary antibacterial defense of bladder. *Urology* 1979;9:48–52.

59. Gill WB, Jones KW, Ruggiero KJ. Protective effects of heparin and other sulfated glycosaminoglycans on crystal adhesion to urothelium. *J Urol* 1982;127:152–154.

60. Hanno PM, Parsons CL, Shrom SH, et al. The protective effect of heparin in experimental bladder infection. *J Surg Res* 1978;25:324–329.

61. Parsons CL, Mulholland S, Anwar H. Antibacterial activity of bladder surface mucin duplicated by exogenous glycosaminoglycan (heparin). *Infect Immunol* 1979;24:552–557.

62. Menter JM, Hurst RE, Nakamura N, et al. Thermodynamics of mucopolysaccharide-dye binding. III. Thermodynamic and cooperativity parameters of acridine orange-heparin system. *Biopolymers* 1979;18:493–505.

63. Gryte CC, Gregor HP. Poly-(styrene sulfonic acid)-poly-(vinylidene fluoride) interpolymer ion-exchange membranes. *J Polymer Sci* 1976;14:1839–1854.

64. Gregor HP. Anticoagulant activity of sulfonate polymers and copolymers. In: Gregor HP, ed. *Polymer science and technology.* Vol 5. New York: Plenum Press, 1975:51–56.

65. Gregor HP. Fixed charge ultrafiltration membranes. In: Selegny E, ed. *Charged gels and membranes.* Part I. Dordrecht, Holland: D Reidel, 1976:235.

66. Hurst RE, Rhodes SW, Adamson PB, et al. Functional and structural characteristics of the glycosaminoglycans of the bladder luminal surface. *J Urol* 1987;138:433–437.

67. Bekturov EA, Bakauova KH, eds. *Synthetic water-soluble polymers in solution.* Basel, Switzerland: Hüthig & Wepf, 1986:38–54.

68. Hurst RE. Thermodynamics of the partition of chondroitin sulfate-hexadecylpyridinium complexes in butanol/aqueous salt biphasic solutions. *Biopolymers* 1978;17:2601–2608.

69. Parsons CL, Mulholland S. Successful therapy of interstitial cystitis with pentosanpolysulfate. *J Urol* 1987;138:513–516.

70. Mulholland SG, Hanno P, Parsons CL, et al. Pentosan polysulfate sodium for therapy of interstitial cystitis: a double-blind placebo-controlled clinical study. *Urology* 1990;35:552–558.

71. Fritjofsson A, Fall M, Juhlin R, et al. Treatment of ulcer and nonulcer interstitial cystitis with sodium pentosanpolysulfate: a multicenter trial. *J Urol* 1987;138:508.

72. Holm-Bentzen M, Jacobsen F, Nerstrom B, et al. A prospective double-blind clinically controlled multicenter trial of sodium pentosanpolysulfate in the treatment of interstitial cystitis and related painful bladder disease. *J Urol* 1987;138:503.

73. Hohlbrugger G. The vesical blood-urine barrier: a relevant and dynamic interface between renal function and nervous bladder control. *J Urol* 1995;154:6–14.

74. Hofmeister MA, He F, Ratliff TL, et al. Mast cells and nerve fibers in interstitial cystitis (IC): an algorithm for histologic diagnosis via quantitative image analysis and morphometry (QIAM). *Urology* 1997;49[Suppl 5A]:41–47.

75. Theoharides TC, Sant GR. Bladder mast cell activation in interstitial cystitis. *Semin Urol* 1991;9:74–87.

76. Larsen S, Thompson SA, Hald T, et al. Mast cells in interstitial cystitis. *Br J Urol* 1982;54:283.

77. Hofmeister MA, He F, Ratliff TL, et al. Analysis of histochemical stains in interstitial cystitis (IC): detrusor to mucosa mast cell ratio is predictive of IC. *Lab Invest* 1994;70:60A.

78. Christmas TJ, Rode J, Chapple CR, et al. Nerve fibre proliferation in interstitial cystitis. *Virchows Arch A Pathol Anat Histopathol* 1990;416:447–451.

79. Lundeberg T, Liedberg H, Nordling L, et al. Interstitial cystitis: correlation with nerve fibers, mast cells and histamine. *Br J Urol* 1993;71:427–429.

80. Theoharides T. Hydroxyzine in the treatment of interstitial cystitis. *Urol Clin North Am* 1994;21:113–119.

81. Messing EM, Stamey TA. Interstitial cystitis: early diagnosis, pathology, and treatment. *Urology* 1978;12:381–392.

82. Ochs RL, Stein TW Jr, Peebles CL, et al. Autoantibodies in interstitial cystitis. *J Urol* 1994;151:587–592.

83. Ochs RL. Autoantibodies and interstitial cystitis. *Clin Lab Med* 1997;17:571–579.

84. Ochs RL, Tan EM. Autoimmunity and interstitial cystitis. In: Sant GR, ed. *Interstitial cystitis.* Philadelphia: Lippincott-Raven, 1997:47–52.

85. Golstein MA, Manto M, Noel JC, et al. Chronic interstitial cystitis occurring during the shift between rheumatoid arthritis and lupus. *Clin Rheumatol* 1994;13:119–122.

86. Bullock AD, Becich MJ, Klutke CG, et al. Experimental autoimmune cystitis: a potential murine model for ulcerative interstitial cystitis. *J Urol* 1992;148:1951–1956.

87. Ratliff TL, Klutke CG, Hofmeister M, et al. Role of the immune response in interstitial cystitis. *Clin Immunol Immunopathol* 1995;74: 209–216.

88. Jokinen EJ, Alfthan OS, Oravisto KJ. Antitissue antibodies in interstitial cystitis. *Clin Exp Immunol* 1972;11:333–339.

89. Ochs RL, Stein TW Jr, Chan EKL, et al. cDNA cloning and characterization of a novel nucleolar protein. *Molec Biol Cell* 1996;7: 1015–1024.

90. von Mühlen CA, Tan EM. Autoantibodies in the diagnosis of systemic rheumatic diseases. *Semin Arthritis Rheum* 1995;24:323–358.

91. Tan EM. Antinuclear antibodies: diagnostic markers for autoimmune diseases and probes for cell biology. *Adv Immunol* 1989;44:93–151.

92. Hanno PM, Buehler J, Wein AJ. Use of amitriptyline in the treatment of interstitial cystitis. *J Urol* 1989;141:846–848.

93. Stewart BH, Persky L, Kiser WS. The use of dimethylsulfoxide (DMSO) in the treatment of interstitial cystitis. *J Urol* 1967;98:671.

94. Smith BH, Dehner LP. Chronic ulcerating interstitial cystitis (Hunner's ulcer). *Arch Pathol* 1972;93:76–81.

95. Bohne AW, Hodson JM, Rebuck JW, et al. An abnormal leukocyte response in interstitial cystitis. *J Urol* 1962;88:387.

96. Simmons JL. Interstitial cystitis: an explanation for the beneficial effect of an antihistamine. *J Urol* 1961;85:149.

97. Badenoch AW. Chronic interstitial cystitis. *Br J Urol* 1971;43:718.

98. Dodson AI. Hunner's ulcer of the bladder: a report of 10 cases. *Va Med Month* 1926;53:305.

99. Wishard WN, Nourse MH, Mertz JHO. Use of Clorpactin WCS90 for relief of symptoms due to interstitial cystitis. *J Urol* 1957;77:420.

100. Pool TL. Interstitial cystitis: clinical considerations and treatment. *Clin Obstet Gynecol* 1967;10:185–191.

101. Parsons CL, Housley T, Schmidt JD, et al. Treatment of interstitial cystitis with intravesical heparin. *Br J Urol* 1994;73:504–507.

102. Lose G, Frandsen B, Hojensgard JC, et al. Chronic interstitial cystitis: increased levels of eosinophil cationic protein in serum and urine and an ameliorating effect of subcutaneous heparin. *Scand J Urol Nephrol* 1983;17:159.

103. Parsons CL, Benson G, Childs SJ, et al. A quantitatively controlled method to prospectively study interstitial cystitis and which demonstrates the efficacy of pentosanpolysulfate. *J Urol* 1993;150:845–848.

104. Hanno PM. Analysis of long-term Elmiron therapy for interstitial cystitis. *Urology* 1997;49[Suppl 5A]:93–99.

*Textbook of the Autoimmune Diseases,*
Edited by R. G. Lahita, N. Chiorazzi, and W. H. Reeves,
Lippincott Williams & Wilkins, Philadelphia © 2000.

# CHAPTER 34

# The Antiphospholipid Syndromes

Ronald A. Asherson and Ricard Cervera

## INCIDENCE AND EPIDEMIOLOGY

Antiphospholipid syndrome (APS) is defined by the occurrence of venous and arterial thromboses, often multiple, and recurrent fetal losses, frequently accompanied by a moderate thrombocytopenia, in the presence of antiphospholipid antibodies (APLAs), namely lupus anticoagulant (LA), anticardiolipin antibodies (ACAs), or both (Table 34.1). Chronic biologic false-positive serologic tests for syphilis (BFP-STS) may be present in some of these patients because these tests also detect the presence of APLAs. Other autoantibodies have also been detected in many patients with an APS, such as anti-$\beta 2$ glycoprotein I (GPI) and antimitochondrial (M5 type), antiendothelial cell, antiplatelet, antierythrocyte, and antinuclear antibodies (ANAs).

APS can be found in patients having neither clinical nor laboratory evidence of another definable condition (primary APS), or it may be associated with other diseases. Systemic lupus erythematosus (SLE) is the disorder in which an APS is most commonly associated. Less frequently, it may also be encountered in other groups of patients (1).

The epidemiology of APS and of APLA is still in its infancy because of lack of clear definitions of the outcome and predictive variables, gold standards for APLA assays, and uniform definition of APS. Many studies of APLA prevalence in a wide variety of conditions and hundreds of case reports have been published, however, providing some clues for epidemiologic studies.

### General Population

Reports of the prevalence of the APLA in the general population vary widely. A prevalence of 7.5% for ACA determi-

nations in a group of Southern Californian healthy women was originally determined (2), whereas in a study of 1449 pregnant women, positive ACA tests were demonstrated in 1.79% (for immunoglobulin G [IgG] ACA) and 4.3% (for IgM ACA) (3). A subsequent study conducted in 300 people with a mean age of 70 years showed ACA detectable in 12% (compared with 2% in a younger population) (4). In addition, ACA elevations were detected in 23% of patients who tested positive for ANAs. These data suggest that ACA may also be associated with an age-related senescent immune system.

The prevalence of ACA in patients attending a routine anticoagulation clinic was found to be 19% in those being treated for thrombotic episodes and 11% in those receiving anticoagulation therapy after heart valve replacements. The highest ACA titers were evident in the younger patients scheduled for short-term anticoagulation therapy (5). A 30% prevalence of LA positivity was found in a study of patients attending another anticoagulation clinic (6). There is also some evidence that the frequency of APLA and its relationship to thrombotic events may be related to ethnic and racial differences (7,8).

### Systemic Lupus Erythematosus

SLE, either defined according to the 1982 revised American College of Rheumatology (ACR) criteria for the classification of SLE (9) or presenting with less than four of these criteria, termed "lupus-like" or "probable SLE," is the disorder in which an APS is most commonly associated. The frequency of APLA in SLE has varied from 6% to 80%, depending on the studies (1,10,11). Some of this variation may be a result of differing sensitivities of assays, selection of patients, and the bias introduced by the retrospective study design. Additionally, detection of APLA in a cross-sectional study may be influenced by the transient production of the antibody, dropping at the time of a thrombotic event or as a result of treatment. Some of the more consis-

R. A. Asherson: Rheumatic Diseases Unit, Department of Medicine, The Groot Schuur Hospital, Observatory, Cape Town, South Africa 7937.

R. Cervera: Department of Medicine, University of Barcelona, Barcelona 08036, Catalonia, Spain; Systemic Autoimmune Diseases Unit, Hospital Clinic, Barcelona 08036, Catalonia, Spain.

**TABLE 34.1.** *Main features of the antiphospholipid syndrome*

Clinical
  Venous thrombosis
  Arterial thrombosis
  Recurrent fetal loss
  Thrombocytopenia
Laboratory
  Immunoglobulin G ACAs (moderate/high levels)
  Immunoglobulin M ACAs (moderate/high levels)
  Positive lupus anticoagulant test

ACAs, anticardiolipin antibodies.

tent studies indicate that about 30% to 40% of SLE patients have APLAs, and between one third and one half of them develop an APS (1).

## Other Systemic Autoimmune Diseases

The presence of APLA has been occasionally described in patients with a variety of other systemic autoimmune diseases, including rheumatoid arthritis (12–16), systemic sclerosis (17–24), primary Sjögren's syndrome (25–28), dermatopolymyositis (14,15), psoriatic arthropathy (29), and several systemic vasculitides (Table 34.2) (30–57). Their association with thrombotic events is uncommon, however. Therefore, their presence probably simply forms part of the natural repertoire of antibody production in these patients, and they are not pathogenic.

## Infections

The APLAs may be produced as a consequence of a variety of infections. These are predominantly viral [e.g., human immunodeficiency virus (58–65), Epstein–Barr virus

**TABLE 34.2.** *Systemic autoimmune diseases with antiphospholipid antibodies*

Systemic lupus erythematosus
Rheumatoid arthritis
Systemic sclerosis
Primary Sjögren's syndrome
Dermatomyositis and polymyositis
Psoriatic arthropathy
Vasculitis
  Polyarteritis nodosa and microscopic polyarteritis
  Giant cell arteritis
  Behçet's disease
  Relapsing polychondritis
  Leukocytoclastic vasculitis
  Mesenteric inflammatory venoocclusive disease
  Capillaritis
  Other types of vasculitis

(66–68), parvovirus (69), hepatitis A, B, and C (70), rubella infection and mumps (71)], but APLA may also be seen in spirochetal conditions [e.g., syphilis (72) and Lyme disease (73)]; chronic conditions, such as tuberculosis (74) or leprosy (75); those conditions associated with an important immune response, such as infective endocarditis (76) and rheumatic fever (77–80); and protozoal infections (e.g., malaria (81) and toxoplasmosis (82) (Table 34.3). It is likely that the APLA response occurs mainly in infections with encapsulated envelope viruses. The association with thrombosis is extremely rare in these patients.

## Malignancies

A variety of malignant conditions may be accompanied by APLA (Table 34.4) (83–99). Occasionally, disappearance of APLA after surgical resection of a tumor has also been reported (83). The association of malignancy with ANA is well documented (94,95), and it is therefore not surprising that other immunologic aberrations, such as the presence of APLA, sometimes occur in these patients. However, APLA-related thromboses are less common in the course of malignancies. Three patients with thrombosis and positive LA among 192 with either lymphoplasmacytoid immunocytoma or multiple myeloma were reported in a German population (93).

## Hematologic Conditions

The APLAs have been described in a variety of nonmalignant hematologic conditions. These include idiopathic thombocytopenic purpura, sickle cell disease, and pernicious anemia. The highest frequency of APLA is found in patients with idiopathic thrombocytopenic purpura (100), and the APLAs are usually unassociated with thrombotic

**TABLE 34.3.** *Infections with antiphospholipid antibodies*

Viral
  Human immunodeficiency virus infection
  Mononucleosis
  Rubella
  Parvovirus
  Hepatitis A, B, C
  Mumps
Bacterial
  Syphilis
  Lyme disease
  Tuberculosis
  Leprosy
  Infective endocarditis
  Rheumatic fever
  *Klebsiella* species infection
Protozoal
  Malaria
  Toxoplasmosis

**TABLE 34.4.** *Malignancies with antiphospholipid antibodies*

Solid tumors
  Lung
  Colon, cecum
  Cervix
  Prostate
  Liver
  Kidney (hypernephroma)
  Thymus (thymoma)
  Esophagus
  Maxilla
  Ovary
  Breast
Hematologic
  Myeloid and lymphatic leukemias
  Polycythemia vera
  Myelofibrosis
Lymphoproliferative diseases
  Hodgkin's disease
  Non-Hodgkin's lymphoma
  Lymphosarcoma
  Cutaneous T-cell lymphoma, Sézary's syndrome
Paraproteinemias
  Monoclonal gammapathies
  Waldenström's macroglobulinemia
  Myeloma

complications. There is an unanswered question about whether patients with idiopathic thrombocytopenic purpura and APLA will later develop SLE or lupus-like disease. Another hematologic condition in which APLAs have been described is sickle cell disease (101). Once again, there does not appear to be a relationship between the finding of APLA and the thrombotic complications encountered in this condition. Two patients with the uncommon association of pernicious anemia and APLA have also been reported (102, 103).

## Drug-induced Antiphospholipid Antibodies

The administration of several drugs can result in the production of APLA. Most of these drugs are the same compounds responsible for the drug-induced lupus-like syndrome. Drugs associated with APLAs include procainamide, phenothiazines, ethosuximide, chlorothiazide, quinine and oral contraceptives (104–127).

## Other Associations

The APLAs have been occasionally described in a wide variety of other conditions, some of which are autoimmune in nature, although in most cases, their value is unknown and their clinical relevance scarce. These conditions include diabetes mellitus (128,129), autoimmune thyroid disease (130–134), inflammatory bowel diseases (135–141), dialysis (142), and Klinefelter's syndrome (143–145).

## CLINICAL PRESENTATION

The clinical picture of APS is characterized by venous and arterial thromboses, fetal losses, and thrombocytopenia. Single vessel involvement or multiple vascular occlusions may give rise to a wide variety of presentations (146–160). Any combination of vascular occlusive events may occur in the same patient, and the time interval between them varies considerably from weeks to months or even years. Rapid chronologic occlusive events, occurring over days to weeks, have been termed *catastrophic APS* (146,147).

### Large Vessel Manifestations

#### Deep Vein Thrombosis

The most frequently reported association with APLA is deep vein thrombosis (DVT). Attention to this complication was first published in 1963 (155). DVT is frequently multiple and bilateral, affecting the lower limbs particularly. Larger veins, such as the iliofemoral, subclavian, jugular, or axillary vessels, may also be involved. Superficial thrombophlebitis (148) may accompany DVT or occur independently. DVT may be complicated by chronic venous stasis ulcers affecting the area around the medial malleolus. These ulcers should be distinguished from those caused by multiple small vessel occlusions, which are characteristically starlike and situated on the lateral aspect of the lower limbs. DVT is also complicated by pulmonary embolism and infarction in one third of cases. Recurrent thromboembolism can lead to pulmonary hypertension (PHT). Venous occlusions can also affect other vessels, such as the superior vena cava (149–151), the inferior vena cava, and the renal, mesenteric, adrenal, hepatic, and renal veins, resulting in specific manifestations, such as a superior vena cava syndrome, renal vein thrombosis, hypoadrenalism or Addison's disease, Budd–Chiari syndrome, or central retinal vein occlusion (158,159).

#### Large Peripheral Arterial Occlusions

The first paper to describe in detail large peripheral arterial occlusions in SLE patients was published in 1965 (160). Livedo reticularis, chronic leg ulcers, recurring thrombophlebitis, skin infarcts, and other arterial occlusions, as well as transient ischemic attacks, also occurred in these patients, whereas several demonstrated a BFP-STS or LA. Several other reports of large arterial occlusions and gangrene in patients with SLE or lupus-like disease who demonstrated APLA at some point during the course of their illness have subsequently been published (119,154, 161,162).

### Aortic Occlusions

Several patients with an aortic arch syndrome and SLE have been reported (41,42,163,164), most of whom demonstrated APLA (42,163). Occlusions of the abdominal aorta have also been documented in patients with APLA (165,166).

## Neurologic Manifestations

Neurologic manifestations of APS are listed in Table 34.5.

### Thrombotic Infarctions

Thrombotic infarctions in APS are second only to DVT in frequency. They are often multiple and recurrent and, most commonly, affect the territory of the middle cerebral artery, with lesions occurring predominantly in the frontal and parietal lobes. The vertebrobasilar system may be affected less frequently. After a first ischemic stroke, the presence of ACA has been shown to be associated with an increased risk for recurrence of stroke over 2 years as well as of other thromboembolic events and death (167). Patients with the highest IgG ACA titers have been shown to have the shortest times to subsequent thromboocclusive events (168). Recurrent stroke and thromboocclusive events often occur in the first year in patients with APLA and an index cerebral ischemic event (169,170). The APLA-associated stroke occurs more often in younger people and is more common in women (168). The Antiphospholipid Antibodies in Stroke Study

**TABLE 34.5.** *Neurologic manifestations in the antiphospholipid syndrome*

Thrombotic infarctions
Sneddon's syndrome
Transient ischemic attacks
Multiinfarct dementia
Acute ischemic encephalopathy
Embolic stroke
Cerebral venous and dural sinus thrombosis
Psychosis
Cognitive defects
Transient global amnesia
Pseudomultiple sclerosis
Migraine and migranous stroke
Epilepsy
Movement disorders
   Chorea
   Hemiballismus
   Cerebellar ataxia
Spinal syndromes
   Transverse myelopathy
   Guillain–Barré syndrome
   Anterior spinal artery syndrome
   Lupoid sclerosis
Ophthalmic complications
   Retinal vascular occlusions
   Acute retrobulbar optic neuritis
   Ischemic optic atrophy
   Progressive optic atrophy

(APASS) Group, which published their first report in 1993 (171), found that the prevalence of ACA was significantly increased in stroke patients, compared with age- and sex-matched hospitalized nonstroke patients, and that the association of ACA with stroke was independent of other stroke risk factors. They also found that ACA was a significant risk factor in older ischemic stroke patients and were as strongly associated with stroke as hypertension. This has been confirmed by other authors (172). In an analysis of young adults with cerebral ischemia, it was found that 18% of unselected patients with focal cerebral ischemia (stroke or transient ischemic attacks [TIAs]) had APLA, which is much higher than that reported in patients of all ages (7% to 9%) (173).

### Sneddon's Syndrome

The association of livedo and ischemic stroke, accompanied on occasion by hypertension, has been known as *Sneddon's syndrome* since 1965 (174). It is, however, an infrequent cause of cerebral ischemia, accounting for only 0.26% of all cases of cerebrovascular ischemia (175). The syndrome is more frequent in women, it is usually diagnosed in the fourth or fifth decade, and there is a familial clustering in some patients. It clearly may be a manifestation of the primary APS (176), although confusion in nomenclature has occurred (177,178). Focal and segmental intimal hyperplasia and recanalization of thrombi have been seen histologically (175). Some investigators have stressed that early inflammatory reactions (endothelitis) of small arteries occur; these are followed by subendothelial cell proliferation, leading to partial or complete occlusion (179).

### Transient Ischemic Attacks

Transient cerebroocular ischemia resulting in amaurosis fugax, transient paresthesias and motor weakness, or vertigo have all been described in patients with APLA.

### Multiinfarct Dementia

Several patients with multiinfarct dementia and APLA have been reported (180–185). The pathology of the vasculopathy in these patients is noninflammatory (186). The clinical manifestations of dementia associated with APS are not different from those encountered in patients with vascular dementia of any other cause, including Binswanger's subcortical arteriosclerotic encephalopathy, cerebral amyloid angiopathy, or Alzheimer's disease (Fig. 34.1) (187).

### Acute Ischemic Encephalopathy

Acute ischemic encephalopathy has been observed and reported by several authors (188,189). Patients are acutely ill, confused, and obtunded, with an asymmetric quadriparesis, hyperreflexia, and bilateral extensor plantar responses. Seizures may also occur. These patients have been recorded

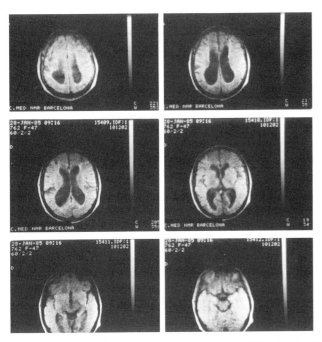

**FIG. 34.1.** Magnetic resonance imaging scan of the brain of a patient with primary antiphospholipid syndrome and multi-infarct dementia.

as having the highest ACA levels among a large series of patients (188). Plasmapheresis and immunosuppression were effective therapies in some of the patients reported (188). Small cortical hypodensities were discernible on magnetic resonance imaging (MRI) scanning in several patients. The differential diagnosis lies between acute lupus cerebritis and even steroid psychosis in patients with predominantly frontal lobe symptoms. With the unraveling of catastrophic APS, it appears likely that cerebral thrombotic microangiopathy, predominant in that condition, is the basis of acute ischemic encephalopathy, a common accompaniment of catastrophic APS.

### Embolic Stroke

Embolic stroke may arise in underlying nonbacterial thrombotic endocarditis but may also arise from dislodging of basically atherogenic plaques in the aorta (190) or carotid system. Heart valves may previously be damaged by lupus vasculitis or APLA valvulitis (191) as a result of deposition of cardiolipin, ACA, and complement on the subendothelial surface of the valves (192) or on a congenitally abnormal valve. Cerebral embolic events in patients with APLA have been reported by many investigators (193–196).

### Cerebral Venous and Dural Sinus Thrombosis

Cerebral venous sinus thrombosis (CVST), or dural sinus thrombosis, has a diverse spectrum of clinical manifestations, the most common of which is headache, accompanied by papilledema, nausea, vomiting, and visual field loss. CVST is one of the causes of the syndrome referred to as *pseudotu-*

*mor cerebri* (benign intracranial hypertension), many cases of which are idiopathic and related to disturbed cerebrospinal fluid dynamics. Several cases documenting the association between CVST and APLA have been reported (197–202).

### Psychosis

Several cases have been recorded in which APS is preceded by psychosis many years before the occurrence of thrombotic symptoms (203). Increased APLA levels have been documented in schizophrenic patients (204) and in patients with major depression (205). The role of APLA in this group of conditions is undetermined at this time.

### Cognitive Defects

It is well known that cognitive defects, including behavioral and affective disturbances, are not uncommon in SLE patients, usually ascribed to a "lupus cerebritis" (206,207). Studies have related neurologic and behavioral deficits in experimental animal models of APS to effects of APLAs. On immunofluorescence staining, immunoglobulin deposits have been observed in vessel walls of brain derived from these animals (208). Four patients with APS who presented with rapidly progressive change in mental status, confusion, memory disturbance, and emotional lability have also been reported (209); psychometric testing revealed severe impairment.

### Transient Global Amnesia

Transient global amnesia, a syndrome of sudden unexplained short-term memory loss often associated with stereotyped behavior, has been linked to APLA in one patient (210), with the investigators suggesting that APLA-linked ischemia may underlie the process.

### Pseudomultiple Sclerosis

In addition to lupoid sclerosis, in which the symptoms and serology may resemble multiple sclerosis, other patients with positive APLAs have been described in whom the distinction between the two conditions may be difficult. Several of these patients were young and had fluctuating and recurrent neurologic events with focal and visual neurologic symptoms. High signal lesions in the periventricular white matter on T2-weighted images resembled multiple sclerosis (211,212).

### Migraine and Migrainous Stroke

Headaches, often nonmigrainous in type, may precede or accompany TIA or strokes in APLA positive patients (213–223). Migraine is, however, common in SLE (213,214). Although many investigators have commented on an association between true migraine and APLA (215,216), some even suggesting that patients with APLA may be a subset of migraineurs in whom the migraine might have an immunologic basis (219), several studies have not borne out any association (222,223). The prevalence of APLA in 16 patients with migrainous stroke was found to be about 40% (224). No other immunologic disorder was present in these patients. Migraines in these patients are usually frequent, long-lasting, and severe, with a poor response to specific therapy (225,226).

### Epilepsy

Epileptiform seizures are common in SLE and may precede the appearance of other serologic or clinical evidence of the disease by many years. Pathogenesis may be related to hypertension, uremia, or electrolyte disturbances when the epilepsy is deemed secondary. It is most frequently seen concomitant with SLE activity (227), however, and it may be immunologically mediated or, as a result of ischemic vascular disease, secondary to the hypercoagulable state associated with APLA (228–230). In 1994, 221 unselected patients with SLE were studied, of whom 21 suffered from epileptic seizures not attributable to any cause other than SLE. LA was detected in 43.8% of the epileptic patients and in 20.8% of controls ($P = 0.057$). A statistically significant association was found between moderate to high titers of IgG ACA and the presence of seizures ($P = 0.02$) (231).

### Movement Disorders

#### Chorea

Chorea is an infrequent clinical manifestation of SLE (occurring in less than 4% of cases) that has been strongly linked to the presence of APLA. Its occurrence in APS has been reviewed and discussed (232–236). It does not differ from chorea encountered with rheumatic fever (Sydenham's chorea) or the inherited form (Huntington's chorea). It may antedate other manifestations or be seen during the course of APS. The chorea may appear without any obvious precipitating factors or be induced by oral contraceptives (237,238). In a review of 50 cases (232), we have found that 96% were women and that the mean age was 23 years. Only one episode of chorea occurred in 66% of the patients, whereas in 34%, it was recurrent. Oral contraceptive–induced chorea, chorea gravidarum, and postpartum chorea occurred in 2% to 6% of patients. It was seen bilaterally or unilaterally and occasionally commenced on one side, only to reappear on the other side within weeks to months. Computed tomography (CT) scans are usually normal, but infarcts outside the basal ganglia may be seen. MRI findings were reported in only 13 of the 50 cases, and infarcts in the caudate nuclei were only seen in 3 cases. Steroids, haloperidol, aspirin, and anticoagulation were used in several patients, and all patients recovered, but the time taken in recovery varied from days to a few months. Some authors (239,240) have suggested that reversible immune-mediated responses, hormonally influenced in some

patients, is the most likely pathogenesis of chorea, rather than a vascular hypothesis with thrombosis and infarction. Binding of autoantibodies to striatal interneurons may cause hypermetabolic dysfunction of these cells. Striatal hypermetabolism has in fact been demonstrated (239).

### Hemiballismus

Hemiballismus, a rare movement disorder, has been reported in an ACA-positive patient (241).

### Cerebellar Ataxia

Cerebellar ataxia may also be related to the presence of APLA (242).

### Spinal Syndromes

#### Transverse Myelopathy

Transverse myelopathy is uncommon in SLE (occurring in less than 1% of patients) and is generally associated with a poor prognosis (243). The presentation is usually acute, with paresthesia in the legs ascending to the thorax within 24 to 48 hours. Paraplegia, back pain, and loss sphincter control may follow (244,245). Several papers have stressed the occurrence of transverse myelitis with the presence of APLA (246–248). Optic neuritis may occur simultaneously with transverse myelitis, presenting with rapid visual loss accompanied by orbital pain (249).

#### Guillain–Barré Syndrome

Two patients with Guillain–Barré syndrome have been reported (250,251). It has been suggested that ACAs of the IgA isotype are associated with peak disease activity (252).

#### Anterior Spinal Artery Syndrome

Sparing of the posterior columns occurs in anterior spinal artery syndrome, and patients present with a flaccid paraplegia, sphincter disturbances, and dissociated sensory impairment. One positive-ACA patient has been reported (253).

#### Lupoid Sclerosis

Lupoid sclerosis is a rare syndrome that has been described as the association of symptoms resembling multiple sclerosis with laboratory findings suggestive of SLE. The most common neurologic finding in this condition is spastic paraplegia, and several patients have been reported (254,255).

### Ophthalmic Complications

Small vessel occlusions affecting the choroid, retina, and optic nerve result in ischemia and even infarctions. Neovascularization leads to secondary vitreous hemorrhage, traction retinal detachments, or glaucoma (256,257). Several reports have estimated retinal vascular occlusions in 8% to 12% of patients with APLA (258,259). Optic neuropathy (acute retrobulbar optic neuritis, ischemic optic atrophy, and progressive optic atrophy) has also been linked to the presence of APLA (260–262).

### Cardiac Manifestations

Cardiac manifestations of APS are listed in Table 34.6.

### *Myocardial Infarction*

Myocardial infarction (MI) in SLE is usually a result of accelerated atherosclerosis or vasculitis; since the discovery of APLA, however, it has become evident that MI is not an uncommon accompaniment of APS (263–266). Conversely, reports of APLA in patients with MI have yielded conflicting results. Although it has been reported that ACAs are common in young post-MI patients and should be regarded as markers for recurrent cardiovascular events (267), other investigators could not confirm this finding (268–270). In an analysis of 43 patients with coronary artery disease presenting when younger than 50 years of age, it was found that 67% had primary coagulation defects (271). Other authors (272) subsequently summarized all cases of MI with APLA reported up until 1993 (60 patients) and concluded that APLAs were a significant risk factor for acute MI but in selected patients only. Finnish investigators (273) found that the presence of high ACA titers is an independent risk factor for MI and cardiac death. APLAs have in fact been reported as an immunologic response to myocardial damage during acute MI. In most patients studied, titers did not vary significantly after MI. In a few cases, however, increased titers were noted weeks or months after the acute episode (usually within 3 months) (274). The presence of APLA was also related to an increased risk for subsequent MI and other thromboembolic events. MI has been reported during pregnancy and in the postpartum period (275,276). MI may also be caused by car-

**TABLE 34.6.** *Cardiac manifestations in the antiphospholipid syndrome*

Myocardial infarction
Unstable angina
Coronary bypass graft and angioplasty occlusions
Cardiomyopathy
   Acute
   Chronic
Valvular disease
   Valve thickening and deformity
   Vegetations
   Pseudoinfective endocarditis
Intracardiac thrombus
Cyanotic congenital heart disease
Complications of cardiovascular surgery

**TABLE 34.7.** *Categories of patients in which antiphospholipid antibody–associated coronary artery disease should be most suspected*

Myocardial infarction or ischemia
   Male or female patient less than 45 years old
   Patient with diagnosed autoimmune disease
   Patient with another thrombotic event, especially if arterial
   Patient of any age without other risk factors for atherosclerosis
   Normal or near-normal–appearing coronary arteries at angiography, after thrombolytic therapy
   Myocardial infarction despite concurrent therapy with warfarin or aspirin
Aortocoronary graft closure
   Occlusion of vein grafts less than 1 year after surgery
   Occlusion despite anticoagulation with warfarin and aspirin
Percutaneous transluminal coronary angioplasty
   Reocclusion of successfully dilated arteries within 3 months of angioplasty
   Reocclusion despite warfarin or aspirin therapy

diac microvasculopathy, and this has been seen in patients with the catastrophic APS (277,278). Table 34.7 summarizes the categories of patients in which APLA-associated coronary artery disease should be most suspected.

### *Unstable Angina*

This subject has also been studied, but no association between APLA positivity and either the severity of angiographic changes or an adverse clinical outcome could be found (279).

### *Coronary Bypass Graft and Angioplasty Occlusions*

Elevated ACA levels in patients who developed late bypass vein graft occlusions have been detected (280). Another study (281) reported increased IgA ACA levels in men with coronary artery disease treated with percutaneous transluminal coronary angioplasty who experience restenosis.

### *Cardiomyopathy*

Multiple small vascular occlusions ("thrombotic microvasculopathy") are responsible for both acute and chronic cardiomyopathy seen in patients with APLA, and the clinical picture is dependent on the rapidity of the process. Acute cardiac collapse (often together with respiratory decompensation) is common in patients with catastrophic APS and is one of the most common causes of death in this group of patients. Circulatory failure, as an isolated event, has also been reported (277,282), analogous to that seen with renal thrombotic microangiopathy. Chronic cardiomyopathy may be global or localized. Segmental ventricular dysfunction can supervene (283,284). Impaired left ventricular diastolic filling has also been documented in primary APS patients (285).

This has been associated with cardiomyopathy and is an early manifestation of myocardial ischemia caused by coronary arteriolar occlusions, which may lead to myocardial fibrosis and a decrease in left ventricular compliance.

### Valvular Disease

#### Valve Thickening

Valve thickening, resulting in valve dysfunction and incompetence, is common in APS; the mitral valve is most frequently affected. Several series of patients have been published demonstrating valvulopathy in patients with primary APS (286–288) as well as in those with SLE (289,290). Other investigators (291) studied patients undergoing valve replacement. There appears to be an increased frequency of elevated ACA levels in patients with valves showing fibrocalcific changes and a significant association between ACA and valve thrombus. It has been suggested that the procoagulant effect of APLA promotes valve thrombus, the organization of which results in fibrosis and calcification.

#### Vegetations

Nonbacterial vegetations may be combined with valve thickening and are thought to reflect the same pathologic process (288). Libman–Sacks endocarditis, as these lesions are named, may eventually heal with a fibrous plaque, sometimes with focal calcification and marked scarring, thickening, and deformity, leading to valve dysfunction (292). Regurgitation is common, whereas stenosis is rare. The mitral valve is mainly affected, followed by the aortic valve; the tricuspid and pulmonary valves are even less frequently affected. Usually, in APS patients, these valve lesions are not of clinical or hemodynamic significance, but in cases of extensive deformity, surgical replacement may be necessary (Fig. 34.2). Thromboembolic events constitute the major danger to the patient with Libman–Sacks endocarditis and can damage brain, kidney, and other organs. A study on valves derived from patients with SLE-related as well as primary APS showed that subendothelial immunoglobulin deposits contained APLA (293).

#### Pseudoinfective Endocarditis

SLE patients in the presteroid era often had large verrucae as a result of Libman–Sacks endocarditis, and it was not uncommon for these to become infected. Large vegetations, however, are now rare (294). The APLA-associated valvular lesions may still serve as a substrate for microbial colonization, and diagnostic and therapeutic problems may arise in patients with so-called pseudoinfective endocarditis. These patients may present with fever, splinter hemorrhages, cardiac murmurs with echocardiographic evidence of valve vegetations, moderate to high levels of APLA, and repeatedly negative blood cultures (295,296).

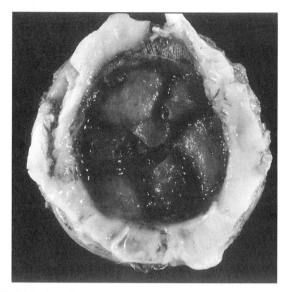

**FIG. 34.2.** Cardiac vegetations.

### Intracardiac Thrombus

Several patients with APLA have been reported who developed thrombi in the ventricular cavities (297–301). Clinically, patients may present with systemic or pulmonary embolic symptoms (e.g., TIA, stroke, pulmonary infarction), depending on the location of the thrombus (right or left ventricle). Thrombus tends to form on akinetic segments of the ventricle. Atrial thrombus may mimic atrial myxoma (302). Occasionally, clot may form on a normal mitral valve (303).

### Cyanotic Congenital Heart Disease

Three patients with cyanotic congenital heart disease and elevated ACA have been published. Two had thrombotic episodes and a BFP-STS. The three were also thrombocytopenic (304).

### Complications of Cardiovascular Surgery

A 10% prevalence of a hypercoagulable condition has been detected on screening 158 patients with cardiovascular surgical procedures, and these patients had a significantly higher incidence of early graft thrombosis (27% versus 1.6%.; $P < 0.01$) (305). Other authors (306) identified 19 patients with APLA among 1078 treated for vascular surgical problems over a 5-year period and noted that these patients tended to be female, younger, nonsmokers, and more likely to have involvement of the upper extremity than patients who were APLA negative. In a survey over a 2-year period, another group (307) found that 26% of their patients were APLA positive and that they were 1.8 times more likely to have undergone previous lower-extremity vascular surgical procedures and 5.6 times more likely to have suffered occlusion of previous reconstructions. In 1995, in a 5-year study, investigators identified 71 APLA positive patients, of whom 19 had cardiovascular surgical procedures (including lower-extremity reconstructions and fistulas, cardiac valve replacements, coronary artery bypass procedures, major amputations, carotid endarterectomies, and infrarenal aortic reconstruction) (308). Of those studied, 84.2% suffered major postoperative complications, including thrombosis of graft, strokes, MI, pulmonary emboli, and major bleeding events. APLA positivity, therefore, identifies a subset of the population who appear to be at increased risk for thrombotic complications of cardiovascular surgery.

## Pulmonary Manifestations

### Pulmonary Embolism and Infarction

Because DVT is the most common clinical manifestation of APS, it is not surprising that pulmonary embolism and infarction are the most frequent pulmonary complications seen, occurring in about one third of patients presenting with DVT. Infrequently, this may lead to thromboembolic PHT (309,310).

### Pulmonary Hypertension

Thromboembolic PHT is an uncommon complication in patients with APS (311). However, there may also be a relationship of the APLA to primary PHT (312), in which an underlying autoimmune diathesis has been suspected because of the not uncommon occurrence of positive ANA and other immunologic markers in this condition (313). In addition, it appears that many patients with SLE and PHT do not exhibit other features of APS, suggesting that the presence of the APLA in these patients may be merely a result of their high frequency in SLE (30% to 40%). There may be a real relationship between APLA and PHT (unrelated to underlying thromboembolic disease), however, perhaps related to endothelial cell damage, diminished prostacycline production, or endothelin I (314,315).

### Pulmonary Arterial Occlusions

#### Major Pulmonary Arterial Thrombosis

Only one case of major pulmonary arterial thrombosis has been reported in association with APS (316).

#### Pulmonary Microthrombosis

Pulmonary microthrombosis is also uncommon in APS, although it was originally suspected as being etiologically important in the pathogenesis of PHT in the presence of APLA (314,314,317,318).

### Adult Respiratory Distress Syndrome

Several patients with APS and adult respiratory distress syndrome (ARDS) have been reported (319,320). A high fre-

quency of ARDS in patients with catastrophic APS has also been described (147), and this often occurred in association with adrenal hypofunction, suggesting a cause-and-effect relationship.

### Intraalveolar Pulmonary Hemorrhage

Intraalveolar pulmonary hemorrhage in association with APS has been documented by several authors (317,321–325). Coexisting pulmonary pathology, such as pulmonary capillaritis, ARDS, microvascular thrombi, and bronchiolitis obliterans, was present in several patients simultaneously (Figs. 34.3 and 34.4).

### Fibrosing Alveolitis

Two documented cases of the coexistence of fibrosing alveolitis and APS have appeared (326,327).

### Postpartum Syndrome

A postpartum syndrome including spiking fevers and pleuritic chest pain associated with pleural effusion and patchy infiltration of the lungs on chest radiograph has been described in association with APS (328,329).

## Renal Manifestations

### Glomerular Capillary Thrombosis in Lupus Nephritis

Several studies have demonstrated that glomerular thrombi may be seen in 32% of biopsy specimens from patients with SLE nephritis, and this figure rises to 48% in patients with the proliferative forms of the disease (330–336). In addition, there is a striking preponderance of glomerular thrombi in patients with positive APLA, and the presence of glomerular thrombi in the initial biopsy specimen is strongly predictive

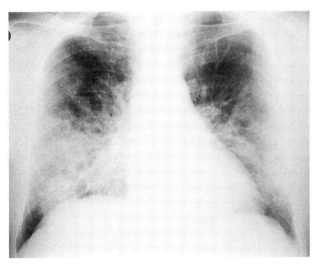

**FIG. 34.3.** Pulmonary hemorrhage.

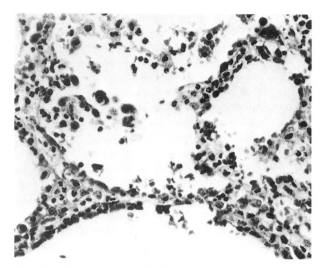

**FIG. 34.4.** Pulmonary capillaritis.

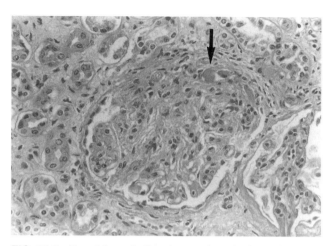

**FIG. 34.5.** Renal thrombotic microangiopathy (*arrow*).

of progression to glomerular sclerosis in subsequent specimens. Thrombosis in patients with positive APLA occurred in the absence of necrosis and subendothelial deposits, usually seen and thought to be the consequence of inflammation.

### Intrarenal Vascular Lesions (Thrombotic Microangiopathy)

Termed *noninflammatory renal microangiopathy* by some authors (337), intrarenal vascular lesions closely resemble those seen in malignant hypertension and other thrombotic microangiopathies, such as those found in patients with scleroderma, eclampsia, the thrombotic thrombocytopenic purpura (TTP) and hemolytic-uremic syndrome (HUS) group of conditions, and transplant rejection (338). The lesions may be accompanied by other features, such as microangiopathic hemolytic anemia, the presence of schistocytes, and often, moderate to severe thrombocytopenia (339). The clinical picture may be dominated by severe or malignant hypertension and renal insufficiency, requiring dialysis in some patients. Similar lesions may be seen in pregnant patients (340) or in those presenting with catastrophic APS (Fig. 34.5) (146).

### Renal Artery Occlusions

Renal artery trunk lesions have been documented in at least 13 patients with primary or SLE-related APS (331). Severe hypertension is common, and renal failure may result. Unilateral (341) or bilateral renal artery occlusions (55) have been documented. Renal infarction may develop, and at least 11 cases of this complication have been reported. It may occur as a complication of renal artery trunk "stenosis," as an *in situ* thrombosis of a branch of the main renal artery, or as an embolic event, analogous to cerebral infarction (342). Thrombosis of the infrarenal aorta may coexist (343).

### Renal Vein Thrombosis

A relationship between thrombosis of the renal veins and the APLA has been suggested despite the fact that renal vein thrombosis is not uncommon in patients with a nephrotic syndrome, regardless of cause (344). It has also been documented in the postpartum period (345) and in a fetus (346). Thrombosis of a graft renal vein coinciding with reappearance of LA has also been reported (347).

### End-Stage Renal Failure and Hemodialysis

One study analyzed 146 patients receiving dialysis for end-stage renal failure and found that ACA positivity predisposes to thrombotic events (348). Additionally, concentrations of ACA were lower in patients receiving hemodialysis than in those with SLE. The association of repeated clotting of arteriovenous grafts has also been emphasized by several authors (349–351).

### Renal Transplantation

Post–renal transplantation thrombotic complications, including thrombotic microangiopathy, have been reported in patients with APLA (352,353).

### Pregnancy and Postpartum Syndromes

Renal failure occurring during pregnancy and, in particular, the postpartum period may also be caused by thrombotic microangiopathy developing during the course of HUS. Several cases of HUS associated with APLA have appeared in the literature (354–356).

## Adrenal Manifestations

Adrenal insufficiency is being recognized increasingly within APS (357–369), and although mainly reported in the adult literature (357–359), it has also been documented in children and teenagers, the youngest being 10 years of age (360). The mechanism for development of adrenal insufficiency appears to be a combination of adrenal vein thrombosis and hemorrhagic infarction, and it is usually bilateral. It has been proposed that any rise in adrenal venous pressure (e.g., such as occurs with venous thrombosis) would result in hemorrhage into the gland (364). The adrenal blood supply of 50 to 60 small branches emanating from the three suprarenal arteries feeds into a subcapsular plexus, which drains into medullary sinusoids by relatively few venules; this is known as a *vascular dam.* In addition to this peculiar vascular arrangement, the adrenal glands are also susceptible at times of stress, when there may be up to a 7-fold increase in cortisol production as well as a great increase in vascularity of the glands themselves.

Several risk factors for adrenal hemorrhage have been identified, including severe systemic illnesses, such as heart disease or infection; previous thromboembolic disease, on the basis of a coagulopathy; and the postoperative state (364). Most patients with APLA who developed this complication were receiving anticoagulation therapy, but good control was the rule, and it was not felt that excessive anticoagulation had been responsible for the adrenal hemorrhage in most of the patients reported. Indeed, this complication also occurred in many who had not been receiving anticoagulation therapy (358).

## Hepatic Manifestations

### Budd–Chiari Syndrome

Budd–Chiari syndrome is characterized by obstruction of large hepatic veins. Hepatic congestion and liver cell necrosis result (370,371). The association with APLA was first documented in 1984 (372). Several other case reports have also appeared (373–375).

### Portal Hypertension

The existence of portal hypertension in association with APLA has been documented (376–379). Several patients reported had a combination of both portal and pulmonary hypertension (376,378). The association of primary PHT with portal hypertension resulting from hepatic cirrhosis and thromboembolism has been documented (380), and these investigators speculated whether thromboembolism associated with ACA may be a common pathway.

### Obstruction of Small Hepatic Veins (Hepatic Venoocclusive Disease)

Hepatic venoocclusive disease is characterized by nonthrombotic concentric narrowing of the lumens of small centrilobular veins by loose connective tissue and results in congestion and liver cell necrosis in the centrilobular areas (370).

Several patients with this disease and APLA have been reported. The condition is often associated with nodular hyperplasia of the liver and has also been reported in patients after bone marrow transplantation (381–383).

### Nodular Regenerative Hyperplasia

A role of APLA in the pathogenesis of nodular regenerative hyperplasia of the liver has been suggested (384). This condition may also follow hepatic venoocclusive disease or hepatic infarction, and it is commonly associated with a variety of systemic autoimmune diseases (385).

### Hepatic Infarction

Overt clinical hepatic infarction is rare but has occasionally been reported in APS (385). It appears to be somewhat common during pregnancy (386,387). It has also been reported in a postpartum patient (388).

### Hepatitis

Chronic active hepatitis as part of APS has been described in a few patients (389–393). In a study looking for hepatitis C virus (HCV) markers in patients with thrombotic disease and ACA, investigators found that these markers were absent in all patients who tested negative for ACA but were present in 16.7% of those who tested positive for ACA. They concluded that occult HCV infection was present in a significant proportion of patients with ACA-positive thrombotic disorders (394). In a series of 88 patients with APS, however, only 2 (2.2%) had anti-HCV antibodies (395). In a subsequent study, 33% of patients with chronic HCV infection had ACA positivity. IgG ACA was present in 72% of cases alone, IgM in 13%, and 10% demonstrated both isotypes. Two patients tested positive only for LA (396). A case report (397) described the development of an APS during the course of HCV infection. The patient relapsed 3 months after interferon-γ therapy, and this relapse was accompanied by further thrombotic complications.

### Alcoholic Liver Disease

In a study of 77 patients with a history of alcohol abuse, 48% had ACA elevations (IgG in 81%, IgM in 13%, and both in 6%) (395). Other investigators (398) had previously studied long-term alcoholic patients. Of those with alcoholic hepatitis or cirrhosis, 81% tested positive for APLA. Antiphosphatidylethanolamine antibodies correlated significantly with disease activity, and the isotype was IgA or IgM in 25 of 40 patients.

### Cirrhosis

It has been postulated that the decreased synthesis of clotting factors in cirrhotic patients offsets the hypercoagulable effects of ACA. One patient with cryptogenic cirrhosis of 30 years' duration, however, sustained a cerebral infarction before liver transplantation. IgG and IgM ACA levels were elevated. Titers dropped to normal after transplantation (399). ACAs of the IgM isotype have been found in up to 43% of patients with primary biliary cirrhosis (15); however, it has been suggested that this may represent a partial cross-reactivity between IgM ACA and antimitochondrial antibodies (400), probably as a result of the presence of low-affinity antibodies, which may have broad epitope specificities. Conversely, this may also be a result of nonspecific binding of the antibody in the enzyme-linked immunosorbent assay (ELISA), related to the polyclonal elevation of IgM found in this group of patients (401). Another group of investigators (402) studied 73 patients with biopsy-diagnosed cirrhosis. Nine patients (12%) were shown to have splenic thromboses. More than half of patients with thromboses were positive for LA or ACA, indicating that APLA may be an important risk factor for thrombosis in these patients. In addition, 75% of LA-positive patients were also positive for HCV, again pointing to a relationship to chronic HCV infection and production of APLA.

## Digestive Manifestations

### Esophageal Necrosis

A patient with a primary APS with thrombosed vessels at the lower end of the esophagus resulting in necrosis, septic mediastinitis, and death has been documented (403). Bleeding esophageal varices from portal vein thromboses have also been reported.

### Gastric Ulceration

Progressive gastric ulceration with necrosis in a patient presenting with severe abdominal pain was found in one patient to be caused by widespread occlusive vascular disease involving veins, small arteries, and arterioles (404).

### Small and Large Bowel Vascular Occlusions

Several cases of large bowel and intestinal infarctions in patients with APLA have been reported (405–411). Peritonitis is a relatively common accompaniment. Severe gastrointestinal hemorrhage may also result from bowel ischemia or from an atypical duodenal ulcer (412).

### Mesenteric Inflammatory Vasoocclusive Disease

One patient with an unusual form of vasculitis involving the mesenteric vessels, labeled *mesenteric inflammatory vasooc-clusive disease,* has been reported who also developed APS with DVT, thrombocytopenia, and high titers of ACA. Small bowel infarction had occurred as a result of the vasoocclusive disease (413). This condition primarily affects veins and venules of the bowel and mesentery, resulting in ischemic

injury; almost half of cases thus far described are primary or idiopathic. There is often a family history of thromboembolism in these primary cases, suggesting that an inherited hypercoagulable disorder may be present. The association of idiopathic mesenteric thrombosis and peripheral thrombosis has, in fact, been known for a long time (414).

### Inflammatory Bowel Disease

Thromboembolic disease is a well-recognized, although uncommon, complication of inflammatory bowel disease. It has been reported that the presence of APLA may be associated with thrombosis in patients with ulcerative colitis and Crohn's disease (135–141).

### Pancreatitis

Abdominal pain in patients with APS may be due to pancreatic involvement by the microangiopathy characteristic of APLA. The presentation may be acute, with abdominal pain and vomiting (415,416). Pancreatic involvement was noted in 6 of 50 patients with catastrophic APS (147). In only 1 patient, however, was the diagnosis made clinically. In 3 patients, microvascular thromboses of pancreatic vessels was noted postmortem, and in 2, pancreatic enzymes were found to be elevated.

### Cholecystitis

Two patients presenting with acute cholecystitis in the absence of gallstones have been reported in the course of catastrophic APS (387,417).

### Occlusion of Splenic Vessels

Occlusion of splenic vessels has been reported in combination with other vascular occlusions (405,418). Splenic infarction may supervene. Splenic atrophy is a rare event, even in SLE, but one such patient with long-standing SLE and ACA who developed this complication has been reported (419).

## Obstetric Manifestations

### Maternal Complications

Several reports have suggested that women with APLA are more likely to develop toxemia of pregnancy and preeclampsia (420,421) as well as the HELLP (*h*emolyis, *e*levated *l*iver enzymes, and *low p*latelets) syndrome (422). The postpartum cardiopulmonary syndrome (328,329), chorea gravidarum (232), postpartum cerebral infarct after aspirin withdrawal (423), and maternal death (424) have also been reported in patients with APLA. Clinical thrombosis, both arterial and venous, is associated with pregnancy and the postpartum period in these women; therefore pregnancy, is a challenge to both mother and baby.

### Fetal Complications

In 1989, a review of all previous clinical reports was published (425). A total of 183 patients diagnosed with APLA had 652 pregnancies. Pregnancy failure occurred in 305 at unspecified gestational age (47%); 129 ended as spontaneous abortion (20%), and 129 ended as fetal death (20%). Only 89 (13.7%) of the pregnancies resulted in the delivery of a viable infant. Viable infants, however, are not necessarily untouched by the effects of APLA. Intrauterine growth retardation is significantly more common in mothers with APLA (426,427). Increased incidence of severe early-onset pre-eclampsia and abruptio placentae may precipitate premature birth. Abnormal uterine artery flow velocity may predict poor outcome in cases of APLA (428), and elevated maternal serum α-fetoprotein levels may be harbingers of fetal death (429). The potential for transplacental passage of the procoagulant tendency (by transplacental transfer of IgG) has been reinforced by reports of neonatal stroke (430), multiple placental vascular thromboses, and disseminated neonatal thrombosis (431) in infants delivered of mothers with APLA.

## Osteoarticular Manifestations

### Avascular Necrosis of Bone

The cause of avascular necrosis (AVN) of bone in SLE patients is probably multifactorial (432), and several risk factors have been suggested, including Raynaud's phenomenon (433); glucocorticoid therapy (434), particularly in these patients developing features of Cushing's syndrome (435); and vasculitis (436). A possible link between AVN and APLA was postulated in 1983 (437,438), and this was strengthened by reports of AVN in patients with primary APS who had not been exposed to glucocorticoid therapy at all (439–441). Other investigators (442–445), however, did not find a positive relationship between AVN and APLA positivity. The relationship, therefore, remains unproved; the occurrence of AVN in primary APS patients with no other risk factors other than APLAs is possibly still linked to their effects in some way (446,447).

### Arthralgias and Arthritis

Other articular symptoms, such as arthralgias, arthritis, and even myositis, are mainly related to the connective tissue disease associated with APS. Arthritis is found only in patients with SLE-related APS, whereas arthralgias are not uncommon in primary APS. The presence of frank arthritis excludes the diagnosis of primary APS in the empiric set of criteria recently proposed (448).

## Dermatologic Manifestations

### Livedo Reticularis

Livedo reticularis is a constant violaceous reticulated skin pattern usually found on the extremities and the trunk and is due to stagnation of blood in dilated superficial capillaries and venules (449). A high prevalence was found in patients with either primary or SLE-related APS in a European multicenter study (450) and confirmed by other studies (451–453).

### Skin Ulcerations

Skin ulcerations are considered to be among the most frequent manifestations of APS (155).

### Small, Painful Leg Ulcers of Livedoid Vasculitis

Leg ulcers of livedoid vasculitis are a noninflammatory occlusion of dermal arterioles that results in superficial cutaneous ulceration and atrophic skin (454). These may later develop into large pyoderma gangrenosum–like ulcers or Kaposi's sarcoma–like nodules, Degos' disease–type ulcers, and nailfold ulcers, which develop late in the disease. Ulcers related to APS are specifically localized on the lower extremities. The association of Degos' disease (malignant atrophic papulosis), essentially a vasculopathy affecting skin, alimentary tract, and bowel, with APLA has been documented (455). Painless, small, yellowish papules occur over the trunk. Skin ulcers may be the presenting symptom of APS and may resolve with anticoagulant therapy (456). Improvement of skin lesions occurs with anticoagulant therapy. The ulcers described were painful, superficial, starlike ulcers around the ankles. They healed with white atrophic scars surrounded by a dark pigmented halo (457–461).

### Cutaneous Necrosis

Superficial skin necrosis has been reported by several investigators (462–465). Necrosing livedo reticularis of the legs has been described in a patient with pulmonary hemorrhage (466) and widespread skin necrosis and in a patient with acquired immunodeficiency syndrome and APLA (467). Widespread cutaneous necrosis is associated with massive thrombosis of small and medium-sized dermal vessels and has also been reported in primary APS (468) (Fig. 34.6), SLE (463,469), rheumatoid arthritis (470), and mycosis fungoides (471). Painful cutaneous necrosis has been observed on the cheeks and earlobes of a patient with LA (472). A case of skin necrosis occurring during warfarin sodium (Coumadin, DuPont Pharmaceuticals Company, Wilmington, DE, U.S.A.) therapy who had an acquired protein S deficiency and primary APS has been documented (473).

### Macules and Nodules

Erythematous macules and painful skin nodules occurring in APLA-positive patients have been reported. These lesions are a result of thrombotic skin disease and are located on the palms, soles, and fingers and do not disappear on the application of pressure (347,472,474,475). These painful lesions have been reported as improving with salicylate therapy

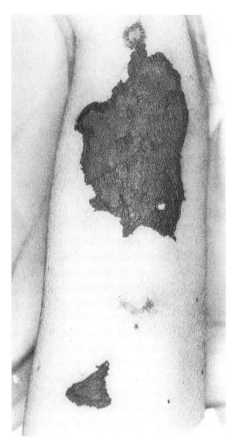

**FIG. 34.6.** Widespread cutaneous necrosis. (From Del Castillo LF, Soria C, Schoendorff C, et al. Widespread cutaneous necrosis and antiphospholipid antibodies: two episodes related to surgical manipulation and urinary tract infection. *J Am Acad Dermatol* 1997;36:872–875, with permission.)

(476). One patient with lymphocyte vasculitis, thrombosis, and ACA was also reported (477).

### Multiple Subungual Hemorrhages

Subungual hemorrhages have been reported in APS patients, in the absence of infective bacterial endocarditis and consequent to warfarin withdrawal and the appearance of catastrophic APS, the administration of oral contraceptives, pregnancy (478–480), and amaurosis fugax (481,482) (Fig. 34.7).

### Gangrene and Digital Necrosis

Cutaneous ischemic symptoms may culminate in digital gangrene and APLA-associated gangrene, particularly in patients with SLE, and this must be distinguished from vasculitis, cryoglobulinemia, and disseminated intravascular coagulation (DIC). It is one of the hallmarks of the cutaneous complication of catastrophic APS.

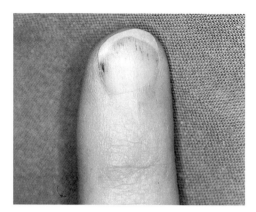

**FIG. 34.7.** Subungual splinter hemorrhages.

### Other

Other dermatologic syndromes, such as anetoderma (461, 483–485), discoid lupus erythematosus (484), intravascular coagulation, necrosis of the skin associated with cryofibrinogenemia and diabetes mellitus (486), and pyoderma gangrenosum (487,488), have also been reported in patients with APLA.

## Hematologic Manifestations

### Thrombocytopenia

Varying degrees of thrombocytopenia occur with APS in 20% to 40% of patients, and several theories have been proposed regarding why the platelet count is reduced (489). Clearly, multiple factors are involved that affect platelet antibodies or immune-mediated destruction of the reticuloendothelial system. The thrombocytopenia associated with APLA is usually moderate, ranging from 75 to 130 × 10⁹/L in most patients, and is not associated with hemorrhagic phenomena. Occasionally, however, it may be severe, and the differential diagnosis then lies between idiopathic thrombocytopenic purpura and APS. This may be difficult. Thrombotic events are unusual with very low platelet counts but have been reported with APLA (490–492).

### Coombs' Test Positivity and Hemolytic Anemia

Several studies have noted the frequent findings of a positive direct Coombs' test in patients with APLA (442,493–497). Some data suggest that the ACA may be capable of recognizing a phospholipid epitope on the surface of the red blood cell. The association of hemolytic anemia with the IgM isotype of ACA has also been demonstrated (496,497).

### Neutropenia

A significant association of IgM anticardiolipin antibody with neutropenia has also been described (497).

## Microangiopathic Syndromes

In the microangiopathic syndromes, the predominant disturbance is on small vessels, as opposed to large veins and arteries, which are predominantly involved in patients with simple APS. When predominantly small vessel vasoocclusive disease occurs, there are often difficulties in making the differential diagnosis between catastrophic APS, thrombotic microangiopathic hemolytic anemia, DIC, and HELLP syndrome.

### Catastrophic Antiphospholipid Syndrome

This term was first used in 1992 (142) to define an accelerated form of APS with consequent multiorgan failure. Previous cases had been documented under a variety of titles, including "devastating noninflammatory vasculopathy" (499), "occlusive vasculopathy" (500), and "acute disseminated coagulopathy-vasculopathy" (501). Originally, 10 patients were analyzed, and the clinical and serologic features were defined (146). A further 21 cases were reviewed in 1996 (502), and another 19 have since been added, totaling 50 patients suffering from this initially seemingly rare manifestation of APS (147).

From an analysis of these patients, all of whom demonstrated multiple occlusive events over a short period of time (days to weeks), it is clear that most in fact did not suffer from SLE or lupus-like disease but rather from primary APS. A smaller number had either rheumatoid arthritis, primary Sjögren's syndrome, or scleroderma. Precipitating factors, as in patients with simple APS, included surgical procedures (both major and minor), infections, oral contraceptive therapy, and anticoagulation withdrawal. Catastrophic APS occurred in the postpartum period in 3 patients. Multiorgan presentation and failure was the rule, and most patients with catastrophic APS ended up in intensive care units with physicians of a wide variety of specialties in attendance. Renal and pulmonary involvement predominated, with most patients showing severe renal impairment. About one third developed ARDS. Half demonstrated cerebral symptoms, and drowsiness and confusion may end in coma. Gastrointestinal, cardiac, hepatic, adrenal, and pancreatic disturbances were seen. There was an abnormally high frequency of hypoadrenalism, often together with ARDS. Unusual organ involvement, such as testes and prostate, was documented. Skin manifestations were also frequent. High levels of IgG ACA were found in more than 50% of patients, and thrombocytopenia was sometimes severe. Hemolytic anemia (26%) and evidence of DIC (30%) were evident. Death occurred in 50%. At postmortem, overwhelming evidence of microthrombotic occlusive disease of small vessels was evident ("thrombotic microangiopathy"). Many organs, including particularly the kidneys, brain, and heart, were affected by this process. A minority of patients demonstrated large vessel occlusions (veins and arteries), in contrast to patients with simple APS, and one can speculate about whether the same etiopathogenic process is

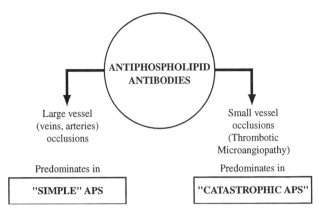

**FIG. 34.8.** Differences between simple and catastrophic antiphospholipid syndrome.

operating in this group of patients and whether the patients with catastrophic APS represent a different "subset" of patients with APS in whom the accent of the disease is on the microvasculature (Fig. 34.8).

### Thrombotic Microangiopathic Hemolytic Anemia

The link between APLA and TTP has been well documented (340,503–507). The seemingly high frequency of this association in patients with renal disease particularly is probably a result of the fact that the kidney is the organ that most frequently is resected and histologically examined. It has since been recognized that this lesion is not uncommon in other patients with APS. The presence of hypertension, renal failure, and proteinuria however, may be present alone in patients with APS, and early diagnosis and treatment lead to improved prognosis in such patients. HUS has been reported in two patients with APLA (508,509). The first patient developed the syndrome in the puerperium after termination of pregnancy for severe eclampsia and responded well to plasma exchange. The second suffered acute renal failure in the postpartum period that was associated with normocytic anemia, thrombocytopenia, and hypertension. High levels of lactic dehydrogenase and low haptoglobin levels, however, favored a hemolytic cause of the anemia. No schistocytes were found. An explanation was that reduced renal perfusion resulted in little destruction of red blood cells and platelets by the injured vessels.

### Disseminated Intravascular Coagulation

In DIC, excessive thrombin production releases this compound into the circulation. This produces widespread microvascular thrombosis. In an attempt to maintain the patency of blood vessels, excess plasmin is generated, resulting in local and systemic fibrinogenolysis. Thrombosis and hemorrhage are, therefore, the clinical manifestations of this condition. The laboratory diagnosis depends on the demonstration of thrombocytopenia, (usually severe) prolonged prothrombin time and activated partial thromboplastin time (in 70% and 50%, respectively), and low fibrinogen concentrations. High levels of free plasmin are usually measured by D-dimers. Red blood cell fragmentation (schistocytes) may be present, but not in excessive amounts such as are usually found in patients with TTP. A report was made of a high prevalence (33%) of APLA in patients with DIC secondary to a variety of conditions (510).

### HELLP Syndrome

It is well known that there is a higher frequency of preeclampsia in patients with APS (421,511). A group of preeclamptic patients have been defined with the HELLP syndrome, which may occur when the usual clinical findings to diagnose severe preeclampsia are absent. Although typically encountered during pregnancy, the HELLP syndrome may be atypical and persist into the postpartum period. Opinion is divided about whether this syndrome is a variant of preeclampsia or represents an hypercoagulable state with thrombotic microangiopathy. Reports of an association between this syndrome and APLA appeared in 1994 with a documentation of two cases (512), both of which demonstrated ACA and appeared to be refractory despite delivery, corticosteroids, and anticoagulation. The clinical course of both patients was remarkably similar, even including a macular rash that extended to the palms. Placental pathology and skin biopsy revealed diffuse deposition of fibrin with small vessel thrombi. Plasmapheresis resulted in resolution of the syndrome in these patients. It was postulated by the authors that the APLA may have contributed to the refractoriness.

## DIAGNOSTIC TESTING

### Lupus Anticoagulant Tests

The LA tests depend on the ability of some groups of APLA to prolong phospholipid-dependent *in vitro* clotting tests; these include the activated partial thromboplastin time, the Russell viper venom clotting time, the kaolin clotting time, and the prothrombin time determined using dilute thromboplastin (513). Most investigators agree that the presence of a persistently positive LA is the best marker of high risk for thrombosis and fetal loss. The main problems come from the laboratory techniques that are necessary to detect the LA activity. These rely on coagulation procedures that are subjected to a variety of conditions. The subcommittee on LA of the Scientific and Standardisation Committee of the International Society of Thrombosis and Hemostasis has elaborated a set of recommendations for the detection of LA activity (513). Platelet-free plasma obtained by double centrifugation is necessary, and confirmation by a platelet neutralization test is mandatory. To exclude deficiencies of coagulation factor, the tests should also be performed with mixtures of patient and control plasmas.

### Solid-Phase Techniques to Detect Anticardiolipin Antibodies

Solid-phase techniques include radioimmunoassay (9) and ELISA (10). Essentially, these assays involve coating plastic plates with pure cardiolipin dissolved in ethanol, then blocking nonspecific binding by incubation with fetal calf or adult bovine serum, and incubating with diluted patient test sera. Finally, antibody bound to the phospholipid is identified using $^{125}$I-labeled or enzyme-labeled antihuman antibody. These assays are the most sensitive and reliable methods for the detection and measurement of APLA. The ACA assays are more sensitive than the LA tests, have less observer error, and can be performed using stored sera.

### Serologic Tests for Syphilis

STS detect reagin, the APLA present in syphilis. In fact, the seminal description of a test for the detection of APLA dates back to 1906, when Wasserman et al. (514) developed a test for the detection, by a complement-fixation technique, of a reaction between a lipoid tissue antigen and an autoantibody (reagin) in syphilitic sera. It was later determined that an alcoholic extract of beef heart, the antigen used in most tests, contained a phospholipid, then termed *cardiolipin*. It has been known since World War II that mass screening for syphilis resulted in patients with false-positive STS who had a high incidence of autoimmune disorders, especially SLE (24). The standard STS in use today is the Venereal Disease Research Laboratory (VDRL) test, an easily quantitated slide flocculation procedure. Others frequently used include the rapid plasma reagin, circle card agglutination screen, and unheated serum reagin. All are simple, inexpensive, and well standardized; however, their sensitivity in detecting patients at risk for thrombotic events is low. Therefore, these tests should not be considered routine for the detection of APLA.

### Solid-Phase Techniques to Detect Other Antiphospholipid Antibodies

Detection of other APLAs may also be performed by means of ELISA using either pure phospholipid (phosphatidylserine, phosphatidylinositol, phosphatidic acid, phosphatidylcholine, phosphatidylethanolamine, sphingomyelin) (515) or a mixture of phospholipids (diluted in chloroform) (516) as antigens. It has been reported that the detection of antibodies against bovine thromboplastin (mixture of phospholipids) is more closely related to the detection of LA activity than that of ACA or other APLAs (516). Detection of these other APLAs, however, generally provides little additional information, and few laboratories perform these tests routinely.

### Solid-Phase Techniques to Detect Antibodies to Cofactors of the Antiphospholipid Antibodies

In 1990, three groups independently found that autoimmune ACA required a cofactor for binding to antigen (517–519).

This cofactor proved to be β2-GPI, a single-chain polypeptide consisting of 326 amino acids weighing 50 kd. β2-GPI inhibits the contact phase of the intrinsic coagulation pathway, platelet prothrombinase activity, and adenosine diphosphate–induced platelet aggregation and is one of the naturally occurring anticoagulants (along with protein C, protein S, and antithrombin III). A number of studies have shown that ACAs that are associated with infection (syphilis, tuberculosis), which are usually unassociated with thrombosis, do not react with β2-GPI but rather bind to cardiolipin alone. In contrast, autoimmune ACAs derived from patients with SLE and a history of thrombosis more frequently directly recognize β2-GPI (519). These data suggest that measurement of the subset of APLAs that bind β2-GPI directly may yield the strongest association with thrombosis. The conventional ELISA to detect ACA, however, measures both anti–β2-GPI and antibodies to cardiolipin alone. Therefore, new solid-phase techniques (ELISA) to detect antibodies to β2-GPI have been developed. Studies seem to confirm that the presence of anti-β2-GPI antibodies provides a higher positive predictive value for the development of thrombotic events (520). Conflicting results have been reported, however, concerning the risk for fetal losses and thrombocytopenia. In the near future, direct assays for measuring antibodies to other cofactors, such as prothrombin, and other phospholipid-binding proteins, such as protein C, protein S, or thrombomodulin, will be routinely available (521). Thus far, however, there is no available information on their value in predicting the risk for thrombotic events or the other manifestations of APS.

### Laboratory Tests in Seronegative Patients

Patients with typical clinical manifestations of APS can present, in some determinations, with seronegativity for LA, ACA, or both. The term *seronegative APS* has been proposed to described these patients (522). Before labeling a case as seronegative for APLA, however, several situations must be considered (523), including the following:

1. Concordance between LA and ACA is not absolute; in 20% to 30% of patients, either one may be absent (497).
2. LA may be undetectable, particularly weak LA, if a sample of plasma not correctly "platelet-free" is used (513).
3. A small proportion of IgG and IgM ACA–negative patients are positive for IgA ACA (524,525).
4. Few ACA and LA seronegative patients may occasionally have antibodies against other membrane phospholipids, such as phosphatidylserine, phosphatidylinositol, phosphatidic acid, phosphatidylcholine, or phosphatidylethanolamine (525).
5. Some patients manifest only anti–β2-GPI antibodies (520).
6. A decrease in APLA level has been observed with development of nephrotic syndrome. This has been attributed to urinary loss of IgG APLA, decrease of APLA synthesis, or increase of APLA catabolism (526).

7. The APLA (particularly the LA) titers may markedly decrease during treatment with corticosteroids (527).
8. Temporal disappearance of APLAs during the course of thrombotic events, probably as a result of their consumption, has also been described, and their determination immediately after a thrombotic episode cannot be considered definitive (528).

## TREATMENT

Elimination of APLA, particularly LA, may be accomplished by several therapeutic regimens, including high-dose steroid administration, immunosuppression (e.g., cyclophosphamide), or plasma exchange. The decrease or elimination is temporary, however, and antibodies rapidly return (within 1 to 3 weeks) on cessation of therapy. Therefore, therapy should not be primarily directed at effectively reducing the APLA levels, and the use of immunotherapy is generally not indicated, unless required for the treatment of the underlying condition (e.g., SLE) or in acute life-threatening situations, such as catastrophic APS.

Energetic attempts must be made to avoid or to treat any associated risk factors; such as hypertension, hyperlipidemia, active nephritis, smoking, and sedentarism. Care should also be taken with the administration of oral contraceptives.

### Asymptomatic Disease

Prophylaxis of arterial thrombosis in the general population is controversial, as it is in patients with APLA. A case may be made, however, for the prophylactic treatment of patients with high levels of IgG ACA or persistent LA activity with antiaggregants (aspirin, 75 to 150 mg daily), especially in those with added risk factors.

On the other hand, prophylaxis of venous thrombosis is required in patients undergoing surgical procedures (particularly hip surgery), those requiring long stays in bed, or during the puerperium. The use of low-molecular-weight subcutaneous heparin is recommended in these circumstances.

### Thrombosis

A prospective study found that in patients with a first event of venous thromboembolism treated for 6 months with oral anticoagulants, the risk for recurrence during the following 42 months is higher in those with elevated titers of ACA (529), and this agrees with previous retrospective studies in patients with primary or SLE-related APS (530–532). The predictive value of ACA increases with the antibody levels (497,529), but an increased risk for recurrence at low titers has also been found. The risk for recurrence was markedly increased in the first 6 months after discontinuation of therapy, suggesting a rebound phenomenon. Therefore, for patients who have already experienced thrombotic events, life-long treatment with anticoagulants is essential. Several important considerations need to be emphasized, including the following:

1. Anticoagulant resistance has been encountered in several of these patients, who may require up to 20 mg/day of warfarin to achieve an international normalized ratio (INR) within the therapeutic range (between 2 and 3). Although it has been proposed that the INR in patients with APLA should be kept at higher levels (between 3 and 4) (530), this recommendation awaits further prospective randomized clinical trials, such as the Warfarin in the Antiphospholipid Syndrome Project trial, to assess the risk-to-benefit ratio of a high INR.
2. Because of the common finding of fluctuating levels of the INR, frequent and regular visits to the anticoagulation clinic are recommended as well as education of patients and medical personnel regarding the dangers of noncompliance and of the taking of drugs that can interfere with the actions of warfarin and its absorption.
3. In the specific case of thrombotic stroke, in addition to the control of other risk factors, the use of newer antiplatelet agents and the role of aspirin or warfarin therapy await the results of the Warfarin Aspirin Recurrent Stroke Study and the Aspirin and Warfarin in Antiphospholipid Syndrome study (532).

### Prophylaxis for Fetal Loss

Low-dose aspirin (50 to 100 mg daily) administered from the beginning of pregnancy until just before delivery is the accepted standard for the prevention of fetal loss. This may be combined with daily subcutaneous heparin in the face of previous fetal loss using aspirin. The risk for maternal osteoporosis may be minimized by the administration of low-molecular-weight heparin, although this complication has also occasionally been encountered with this new type of heparin. Some authorities recommend moderate doses of steroids (15 to 20 mg daily) if the ACA level rises suddenly or routinely in the second trimester. Steroids should be administered with caution because of the dangers of hypertension, diabetes, and infection (533,534). Warfarin administration should be discontinued as soon as pregnancy is diagnosed because it is teratogenic.

Close monitoring of pregnancy with Doppler ultrasound techniques, to detect early placental vascular insufficiency, and delivery at the first signs of fetal distress are mandatory. Other forms of therapy, such as intravenous gammaglobulin or plasmapheresis, have been attempted with some success in patients with a particularly poor obstetric history.

### Thrombocytopenia

The thrombocytopenia that occurs during the course of APS is usually mild and does not require active intervention. In a minority of cases, however, it can be severe and refractory to prednisone therapy. Low-dose aspirin and warfarin have proved useful in some cases (535,536), but their administration may not be without risk, especially in patients with less than 20,000 platelets/mm³. In these cases, immunosuppressive therapy (e.g., azathioprine), danazol (537), or intravenous gammaglobulin may be effective. In contrast, splenectomy should be considered with caution in patients with APLA because of the increased thromboembolic risk related to post-splenectomy thrombocytosis.

### Catastrophic Antiphospholipid Syndrome

Despite the use of adequate anticoagulation with heparin, pulse steroids, and cyclophosphamide, many APS patients still suffer from repeated thrombotic events. Plasmapheresis is advised, and most patients receiving this additional therapy survive. New therapies, such as the use of defibrotide, are undergoing investigation (146,147), whereas the use of fibrinolytic therapy (e.g., streptokinase) and prostacyclin requires further evaluation. The rationale for the use of plasmapheresis is unclear, but clearing of antibodies to von Willebrand factor cleaving protease, as well as replacing plasma von Willebrand factor cleaving protease, which is deficient in patients with TTP, is a possibility (538).

### REFERENCES

1. Asherson RA, Cervera R, Piette JC, et al. The antiphospholipid syndrome: history, definition, classification, and differential diagnosis. In: Asherson RA, Cervera R, Piette JC, et al., eds. *The antiphospholipid syndrome.* Boca Raton, FL: CRC Press, 1996:3–12.
2. Kalunian KC, Peter JB, Middlekauff HR, et al. Clinical significance of a single test for anti-cardiolipin antibodies in patients with systemic lupus erythematosus. *Am J Med* 1988;85:602–608.
3. Harris EN, Spinnato JA. Should anticardiolipin tests be performed in otherwise healthy pregnant women? *Am J Obstet Gynecol* 1991; 165:1272–1277.
4. Fields RA, Toubbeh H, Searles RP, et al. The prevalence of anticardiolipin antibodies in a healthy elderly population and its association with antinuclear antibodies. *J Rheumatol* 1989;16:623–625.
5. Exner T, Koutts J. Autoimmune cardiolipin-binding antibodies in oral anticoagulant patients. *Aust N Z J Med* 1988;18:669–673.
6. Chu P, Pendry K, Blecher TE. Detection of lupus anticoagulant in patients attending an anticoagulation clinic. *Br Med J* 1988;297: 1449.
7. Jones HW, Ireland R, Senaldi G, et al. Anticardiolipin antibodies in patients from Malaysia with systemic lupus erythematosus. *Ann Rheum Dis* 1991;50:173–175.
8. Dessein PH, Gledhill RF, Rossouw DS. Systemic lupus erythematosus in black South Africans. *S Afr Med J* 1988;74:387–389.
9. Tan EM, Cohen AS, Fries JF, et al. The 1982 revised criteria for the classification of systemic lupus erythematosus. *Arthritis Rheum* 1982; 25:1271–1277.
10. Harris EN, Gharavi AE, Boey ML, et al. Anticardiolipin antibodies: detection by radioimmunoassay and association with thrombosis in systemic lupus erythematosus. *Lancet* 1983;2:1211–1214.
11. Loizou S, McCrea JD, Rudge A, et al. Measurement of anticardiolipin antibodies by an enzyme-linked immunosorbent assay (ELISA): standardization and quantitation of results. *Clin Exp Immunol* 1985; 62:738–745.
12. Keane A, Woods R, Dowding V, et al. Anticardiolipin antibodies in rheumatoid arthritis. *Br J Rheumatol* 1987;26:346–350.
13. Monteagudeo M, Montalbán J, Alvarez J, et al. Stroke and anticardiolipin antibodies in a patient with rheumatoid arthritis and large granular lymphocyte proliferation. *J Rheumatol* 1988;15:1589–1590.

14. Fort JG, Cowchock FS, Abruzzo JL, et al. Anticardiolipin antibodies in patients with rheumatic diseases. *Arthritis Rheum* 1987;30: 752–760.

15. Font J, Cervera R, López-Soto A, et al. Anticardiolipin antibodies in patients with autoimmune disease: isotype distribution and clinical associations. *Clin Rheumatol* 1989;8:475–483.

16. Buchanan RC, Wardkaw JR, Riglar AG, et al. Antiphospholipid antibodies in the connective tissue diseases: their relation to the antiphospholipid syndrome and orme fruste disease. *J Rheumatol* 1989;16: 757–761.

17. Seibold JR, Knight PJ, Peter JB. Anticardiolipin antibodies in systemic sclerosis. *Arthritis Rheum* 1986;29:1052–1053.

18. Bamberga P, Asero R, Vismara A, et al. Anticardiolipin antibodies in progressive systemic sclerosis (PSS). *Clin Exp Rheumatol* 1987;3: 387–388.

19. McHugh MJ, Reilly PA, McHugh LA, et al. Pregnancy, the menopause and anticardiolipin antibodies in rheumatoid arthritis and systemic sclerosis. *Br J Rheumatol* 1987;26[Suppl 2]:20.

20. Malia RG, Greaves M, Rowlands LM, et al. Anticardiolipin antibodies in systemic sclerosis: immunological and clinical associations. *Clin Exp Rheumatol* 1988;73:456–460.

21. Manoussakis MN, Gharave AE, Drosos AA, et al. Anticardiolipin antibodies in unselected autoimmune rheumatic disease patients. *Clin Immunol Immunopathol* 1987;44:297–307.

22. Albert J, Ekoe JH, Cunningham M, et al. Circulating anticoagulant in CREST syndrome. *Br J Rheumatol* 1984;23:20–23.

23. Guillevan L, Leroux G, Berdah J. Anticoagulant lupique et thromboses au coeur de la scleroderma. *Ann Med Interne* (Paris) 1987; 138:144.

24. Shapiro LS. Large vessel arterial thrombosis in systemic sclerosis associated with antiphospholipid antibodies. *J Rheumatol* 1990;17: 685–686.

25. Asherson RA, Fei HM, Staub HL, et al. Antiphospholipid antibodies and HLA associations in primary Sjögren's syndrome. *Ann Rheum Dis* 1992;51:499–502.

26. Jedryka-Goral A, Jagiello P, D'Cruz DP, et al. Isotype profile and clinical relevance of anticardiolipin antibodies in Sjögren's syndrome. *Ann Rheum Dis* 1992;51:889–891.

27. Pennec YL, Magadur G, Jouquan J, et al. Serial measurements of anticardiolipin antibodies in primary Sjögren's syndrome. *Clin Exp Rheumatol* 1991;9:165–167.

28. Cervera R, García-Carrasco M, Font J, et al. Antiphospholipid antibodies in primary Sjögren's syndrome: prevalence and clinical significance in a series of 80 patients. *Clin Exp Rheumatol* 1997;15: 361–365.

29. Tullett JP, Bowman CA, Greaves M. Lupus anticoagulant in psoriatic-type arthropathy. *J R Soc Med* 1989;82:505–506.

30. Norden DK, Ostrov BE, Shafritz AB, et al. Vasculitis associated with antiphospholipid syndrome. *Semin Arthritis Rheum* 1995;24: 273–281.

31. Cohney S, Savige J, Stewart MR. Lupus anticoagulant in antineutrophil cytoplasmic antibody associated polyarteritis. *Am J Nephrol* 1995;15:157–160.

32. Bleil L, Manger B, Winker TH, et al. The role of antineutrophil cytoplasm antibodies, anticardiolipin antibodies, von Willebrand factor antigens, and fibronectin for the diagnosis of systemic vasculitis. *J Rheumatol* 1991;18:1199–1206.

33. Cid MC, Cervera R, Font J, et al. Recurrent arterial thrombosis in a patient with giant cell arteritis and raised anticardiolipin antibody level. *Br J Rheumatol* 1988;27:164–166.

34. Cid MC, Cervera R, Font J, et al. Late thrombotic events in patients with temporal arteritis and anticardiolipin antibodies. *Clin Exp Rheumatol* 1990;3:359–363.

35. Pucetti L, D'Ascanio A, Marotta G, et al. Anticardiolipin antibodies (aCLAbs) in polymyalgia rheumatica-giant cell arteritis (PMR-GCA). *Clin Exp Rheumatol* 1987;5[Suppl 1]:49.

36. Aguilar JL, Espinoza LR, Kneer CH, et al. Anticardiolipin antibodies in polymyalgia rheumatica/temporal arteritis. *Arthritis Rheum* 1989;32[Suppl]:835.

37. McHugh NJ, James IE, Plant GT. Anticardiolipin and antineutrophil antibodies in giant cell arteritis. *J Rheumatol* 1990;17:916–922.

38. Yokoi K, Hosoi E, Akaike M, et al. Takayasu's arteritis associated with anticardiolipin antibodies. *Angiology* 1996;47:315–319.

39. Misra R, Aggarwal A, Chag M, et al. Raised anticardiolipin antibodies in Takayasu's arteritis. *Lancet* 1994;343:1644–1645.

40. Fain O, Mathieu A, Seror O, et al. Aortitis: a new manifestation of primary antiphospholipid syndrome. *Br J Rheumatol* 1995;34: 686–696.

41. Ferrante FM, Myerson GE, Goldman JA. Subclavian artery thrombosis mimicking the aortic arch syndrome in systemic lupus erythematosus. *Arthritis Rheum* 1982;25:1501–1504.

42. Asherson RA, Harris EN, Gharavi AE, et al. Aortic arch syndrome associated with anticardiolipin antibodies and the lupus anticoagulant [Comment on Ferrante paper]. *Arthritis Rheum* 1985;28:594–595.

43. Saxe PA, Altman RD. Takayasu's arteritis syndrome associated with systemic lupus erythematosus. *Semin Arthritis Rheum* 1992;21: 295–305.

44. Hull RG, Harris EN, Gharavi AE, et al. Anticardiolipin antibodies: occurrence in Behçet's syndrome. *Ann Rheum Dis* 1984;43:746–748.

45. Efthimiou J, Harris EN, Hughes GRV. Negative anticardiolipin antibodies and vascular complications in Behçet's syndrome. *Ann Rheum Dis* 1985;44:725–726.

46. Cervera R, Navarro M, López-Soto A, et al. Antibodies to endothelial cells in Behçet's disease: cell-binding heterogeneity and association with clinical activity. *Ann Rheum Dis* 1994;53:265–267.

47. Balsa-Criado A, González-Hernandez T, Cuesta MV, et al. Lupus anticoagulant in relapsing polychondritis. *J Rheumatol* 1990;17: 1426–1427.

48. Quéré I, Biron C, Dubois A. Lupus anticoagulant and thrombosis in relapsing polychondritis. *J Rheumatol* 1996;23:946–947.

49. Jeffery P, Asherson RA, Rees J. Recurrent deep vein thrombosis, thromboembolic pulmonary hypertension and the "primary" antiphospholipid syndrome. *Clin Exp Rheumatol* 1989;7:567–573.

50. Gül A, Inanc M, Öcal L, et al. Primary antiphospholipid syndrome associated with mesenteric inflammatory veno-occlusive disease. *Clin Rheumatol* 1996;15:207–210.

51. Weidensaul D, Vassa N, Luger A, et al. Primary antiphospholipid syndrome and microscopic polyarteritis in the puerperium: a case report. *Int Arch Allergy Immunol* 1994;103:311–316.

52. Gertner E, Lie JT. Pulmonary capillaritis, alveolar hemorrhage and recurrent microvascular thrombosis in primary antiphospholipid syndrome. *J Rheumatol* 1993;20:124–128.

53. Crausman RS, Aggenbag GA, Pluss WT, et al. Pulmonary capillaritis and alveolar hemorrhage associated with the antiphospholipid antibody syndrome. *J Rheumatol* 1995;22:554–556.

54. Lie JT, Kobayashi S, Tokano Y, et al. Systemic and cerebral vasculitis coexisting with disseminated coagulopathy and systemic lupus erythematosus associated with antiphospholipid syndrome. *J Rheumatol* 1995;22:2173–2176.

55. Ames PRJ, Cianciaruso B, Bellizzi V, et al. Bilateral renal artery occlusion in a patient with primary antiphospholipid syndrome: thrombosis, vasculitis or both. *J Rheumatol* 1992;19:1802–1806.

56. Goldberger E, Elder RC, Swartz RA, et al. Vasculitis in the antiphospholipid syndrome: a cause of ischemia responding to corticosteroids. *Arthritis Rheum* 1992;35:569–572.

57. Rocca PV, Siegel LB, Cupps TR. The concomitant expression of vasculitis and coagulopathy: synergy for marked tissue ischemia. *J Rheumatol* 1994;21:556–560.

58. Cohen AJ, Philips TM, Kesler CM. Circulating coagulation inhibitors in the acquired immunodeficiency syndrome. *Ann Intern Med* 1986; 104:175–180.

59. Bloom EJ, Abrams DI, Rodgers SG. Lupus anticoagulant in acquired immunodeficiency syndrome. *JAMA* 1986;256:491–493.

60. Canoso RT, Zon LI, Groopman JE. Anticardiolipin antibodies associated with HTLV-III infection. *Br J Haematol* 1987;65:495–498.

61. Gold J, Haubenstock A, Zalusky R. Lupus anticoagulant and AIDS. *N Engl J Med* 1986;314:1252–1253.

62. Masala C, Sorice M, Di Prime MA, et al. Anticardiolipin antibodies and *Pneumocystis carinii* pneumonia. *Ann Intern Med* 1989;110:749.

63. Haire W. The acquired immunodeficiency syndrome and lupus anticoagulant. *Ann Intern Med* 1986;105:301–302.

64. Mulhall BP, Naselli G, Whittingham S. Anticardiolipin antibodies in homosexual men: prevalence and lack of association with human immunodeficiency virus (HIV) infection. *J Clin Immunol* 1989;9: 208–213.

65. Cohen H, Mackie IJ, Anagnostopoulos M, et al. Lupus anticoagulant, anticardiolipin antibodies and human immunodeficiency virus in haemophilia. *J Clin Pathol* 1989;42:629–633.

66. Misra R, Venables PJW, Watkins RP, et al. Autoimmunity to cardiolipin in infectious mononucleosis. *Lancet* 1987;2:629.

67. Misra R, Venables PJW, Plater-Zvberk C, et al. Anticardiolipin antibodies in infectious mononucleosis react with the membrane of activated lymphocytes. *Clin Exp Immunol* 1989;75:35–40.

68. Colaco CB, Mackie IJ, Irving W, et al. Anticardiolipin antibodies in viral infections. *Lancet* 1989;1:622.

69. Dostal C, Paleckova A, Travsk YK, et al. Anticardiolipin antibodies in infectious mononucleosis. *J Rheumatol* 1991;17:1573–1574.

70. Gratacós E, Torres PJ, Vidal J, et al. Prevalence and clinical significance of anticardiolipin antibodies in pregnancies complicated by parvovirus B19 infection. *Prenat Diagn* 1995;15:1109–1113.

71. Vaarala O, Palosuo T, Kleemola M, et al. Anticardiolipin response in acute infections. *Clin Immunol Immunopathol* 1986;41:8–15.

72. Harris EN, Gharavi AE, Wasley GD, et al. Use of an enzyme-linked immunosorbent assay and of inhibition studies to distinguish between antibodies to cardiolipin from patients with syphilis or autoimmune disorders. *J Infect Dis* 1988;157:23–31.

73. Mackworth-Young CG, Harris EN, Steere AC, et al. Anticardiolipin antibodies in Lyme disease. *Arthritis Rheum* 1988;31:1052–1056.

74. Santiago MB, Cossermelli W, Tuma MF, et al. Anticardiolipin antibodies in patients with infectious diseases. *Clin Rheumatol* 1989;8:23–28.

75. Furukawa F, Kashihara-Sawami M, Imamura S, et al. Evaluation of anticardiolipin antibody and its cross reactivity in sera of patients with lepromatous leprosy. *Arch Dermatol Res* 1986;278:317–319.

76. Asherson RA, Tikly M, Staub H, et al. Infective endocarditis, rheumatoid factor, and anticardiolipin antibodies. *Ann Rheum Dis* 1990;49:107–108.

77. Asherson RA, Hughes GRV, Gledhill R, et al. Absence of antibodies to cardiolipin in patients with Huntington's chorea, Sydenhan's chorea and active rheumatic fever. *J Neurol Neurosurg Psychiatry* 1988;51:1459.

78. Diniz RE, Goldenberg J, Andrade LE, et al. Antiphospholipid antibodies in rheumatic fever chorea. *J Rheumatol* 1994;21:1367–1368.

79. Figueroa F, Berrios X, Gutiérrez M, et al. Anticardiolipin antibodies in acute rheumatic fever. *J Rheumatol* 1992;19:1175–1180.

80. Figueroa F, Berrios X, Gutiérrez M, et al. Antiphospholipid antibodies in rheumatic fever chorea. *J Rheumatol* 1994;21:1368.

81. Facer CA, Agiostradidou G. High levels of antiphospholipid antibodies in uncomplicated and severe Plasmodium falciparum and P. vivax malaria. *Clin Exp Immunol* 1994;95:304–309.

82. Barrile A, Quattrocchi P, Bonnano D, et al. Sulla presenza e sul significato degli anticorpi anticardiolipina nelle malattie infective. *Rec Progr Med* 1992;88:350–353.

83. Malnick SD, Sthoeger Z, Ahali M, et al. Anticardiolipin antibodies associated with hypernephroma. *Eur J Med* 1993;2:308–309.

84. Malnick SD, Geltner D, Shoerger Z. Anticardiolipin antibody associated with renal carcinoma. *J Rheumatol* 1995;22:2007–2008.

85. Levine SR, Diaczok IM, Deegan MJ, et al. Recurrent stroke associated with thymoma and anticardiolipin antibodies. *Arch Neurol* 1987;44:678–679.

86. Tu H, Davies RB, Davis LD. Lupus anticoagulant in a patients undergoing oral surgery. *J Oral Maxillofac Surg* 1984;42:53–59.

87. Kozlowski CL, Johnson JM, Gorst DW, et al. Lung cancer, immune thrombocytopenia and the lupus inhibitor. *Postgrad Med J* 1987;63:793–795.

88. Shaukat MN, Hughes P. Recurrent thrombosis and anticardiolipin antibodies associated with adenocarcinoma of the lung. *Postgrad Med J* 1990;66:316–318.

89. Marcus RM, Grayzel AI. A lupus antibody syndrome associated with hypernephroma. *Arthritis Rheum* 1979;22:1396–1398.

90. Schleider MA, Nachman RL, Jaffe DE, et al. A clinical study of the lupus anticoagulant. *Blood* 1976;48:499–509.

91. Duncombe AS, Dalton RG, Savidge GF. Lupus-type coagulation inhibitor in hairy cell leukaemia and resolution with splenectomy. *Br J Haematol* 1987;65:120–121.

92. Elias M, Eldor A. Thromboembolism in patients with the "lupus" type circulating anticoagulant. *Arch Intern Med* 1984;144:510–515.

93. Dührsen U, Paar D, Kölbel C, et al. Lupus anticoagulant associated syndrome in benign and malignant systemic disease-analysis of 10 observations. *Klin Wochenschr* 1987;65:818–822.

94. Zeromski JO, Gormy MK, Jarczewska K. Malignancy associated with antinuclear antibodies. *Lancet* 1972;2:1035–1036.

95. Ablin RJ. Malignancy associated with antinuclear antibodies. *Lancet* 1972;2:1253.

96. Green JA, Dawson AA, Walker W. SLE and lymphoma. *Lancet* 1978;2:753–756.

97. Boxer M, Ellman L, Carvalho A. The lupus anticoagulant. *Arthritis Rheum* 1982;19:1244–1248.

98. Mills RC, Zacharski LR, McIntyre OR. Case report: circulating anticoagulant, autoimmune hemolytic anaemia and malignant lymphoma. *Am J Med Sci* 1977;274:75–78.

99. Salem NB. Lupus antibody syndrome with intestinal lymphoma. *Arthritis Rheum* 1980;23:613–614.

100. Stasi R, Stipa E, Masi M, et al. Long-term observation of 208 adults with chronic idiopathic thrombocytopenic purpura. *Am J Med* 1995;98:436–442.

101. De Ceular K, Khamashta MA, Harris EN, et al. Antiphospholipid antibodies in homozygous sickle-cell disease. *Arthritis Rheum* 1989;32[Suppl]:144.

102. Costello C, Abdelaal M, Coomes EN. Pernicious anemia and systemic lupus erythematosus in a young woman. *J Rheumatol* 1985;12:798–799.

103. Heckerling PS, Froelich CJ, Schoda SG. Retinal vein thrombosis in a patient with pernicious anaemia and anticardiolipin. *J Rheumatol* 1989;16:1144–1146.

104. Russell AS, Ziff M. Natural antibodies to procainamide. *Clin Exp Immunol* 1968;3:901–909.

105. Blomgren SE, Condemi JJ, Bignall MC. Antinuclear antibody induced by procainamide: a prospective study. *N Engl J Med* 1969;281:64–66.

106. Galanakis DK, Newman J, Summers D. Circulating thrombin time anticoagulant in a procainamide-induced syndrome. *JAMA* 1978;239:18.

107. Bell WR, Boss GR, Wolfson JS. Circulating anticoagulant in the procainamide-induced lupus syndrome. *Arch Intern Med* 1977;137:1471–1473.

108. Mueh JR, Herbst KD, Rapaport SI. Thrombosis in patients with the lupus anticoagulant. *Ann Intern Med* 1980;92:156–159.

109. Day JH, Cherrey R, O'Hara D, et al. Incidence of procainamide-induced lupus anticoagulants. *Thromb Haemost* 1987;58:394.

110. Asherson RA, Zulman J, Hughes GRV. Pulmonary thromboembolism associated with procainamide-induced lupus syndrome and anticardiolipin antibodies. *Ann Rheum Dis* 1989;48:232–235.

111. Schlesinger P, Peterson L. Procainamide-associated lupus anticoagulants and thrombotic events. *Arthritis Rheum* 1988;31:S54.

112. Li GC, Greenberg CS, Currie MS. Procainamide induced lupus anticoagulants and thrombosis. *South Med J* 1988;81:262–264.

113. Zarrabi MH, Zucker S, Miller F, et al. Immunologic and coagulation disorders in chlorpromazine-treated patients. *Ann Intern Med* 1979;91:194–199.

114. Gharavi AE, Harris EN, Asherson RA, et al. Anticardiolipin (a-CL) isotypes: a study of their clinical relevance. *Clin Rheumatol* 1986;5:154.

115. Berglund S, Gottfries CG, Gottfries I, et al. Chlorpromazine-induced antinuclear factors. *Acta Med Scand* 1970;187:67–74.

116. Steen VD, Ramsey-Goldman R. Phenothiazine-induced systemic lupus erythematosus with superior vena cava syndrome: case report and review of the literature. *Arthritis Rheum* 1988;31:923–926.

117. Canoso RT, de Olivier RM. Chlorpromazine-induced anticardiolipin antibodies and lupus anticoagulant. *Arthritis Rheum* 1986;29[Suppl 4]:S96.

118. Rose CD, Larouche SJ, Goldsmith DP. Ethosuximide-induced digital ischaemia. *Rheum Dis* 1987;46:251.

119. Bird AG, Lendrum R, Asherson RA, et al. Disseminated intravascular coagulation, antiphospholipid antibodies and ischaemic necrosis of extremities. *Ann Rheum Dis* 1987;46:251–255.

120. Rosa-Re D, García F, Gascon J, et al. Quinine induced lupus-like syndrome and cardiolipin antibodies. *Ann Rheum Dis* 1996;55:559–560.

121. Petri M, Robinson C. Oral contraceptives and systemic lupus erythematosus. *Arthritis Rheum* 1997;40:797–803.

122. Buyon JP, Kalunian KC, Skovron ML, et al. Can women with systemic lupus erythematosus safely use exogenous estrogens? *J Clin Rheumatol* 1995;1:205–211.

123. Bruneau C, Intractor L, Sobel A, et al. Antibodies to cardiolipin and vascular complications in women taking oral contraceptives. *Arthritis Rheum* 1986;29:1294.

124. Asherson RA, Harris EN, Hughes GRV, et al. Complications of oral contraceptives and antiphospholipid antibodies. *Arthritis Rheum* 1988; 31:575–576.

125. Asherson RA, Derksen RHWM, Harris EN, et al. Chorea in systemic lupus erythematosus and "lupus-like" disease: association with antiphospholipid antibodies. *Semin Arthritis Rheum* 1987;16:253–259.

126. Asherson RA, Hughes GRV. Antiphospholipid antibodies and chorea. *J Rheumatol* 1988;15:377–379.

127. Kleiger RE, Boxer M, Ingham RE, et al. Pulmonary hypertension in patients using oral contraceptives: a report of six cases. *Chest* 1976: 69:143–147.

128. Hendra TJ, Baguley E, Harris EN, et al. Anticardiolipin antibody levels in diabetic subjects with and without coronary artery disease. *Postgrad Med J* 1989;65:140–143.

129. Manzanares JM, Conget I, Rodríguez-Villar C, et al. Antiphospholipid syndrome in a patient with type I diabetes presenting as retinal artery occlusion. *Diabetes Care* 1996;19:92–94.

130. Diez JJ, Doforno RA, Iglesias P, et al. Prevalence of anticardiolipin antibodies in autoimmune thyroid disease. *Eur J Clin Invest* 1992; 22[Suppl]:A15.

131. Diez JJ, Borbujo J. Anticardiolipin antibodies in autoimmune thyroid disease. *Clin Endocrinol* 1994;41:697–698.

132. Paggi A, Caccavo D, Ferri GM, et al. Anticardiolipin antibodies in autoimmune thyroid disease. *Clin Endocrinol* 1994;40:329–333.

133. Petri M, Karlson EW, Cooper DS, et al. Autoantibody tests in autoimmune thyroid disease: a case control study. *J Rheumatol* 1991;18: 1529–1531.

134. Stagnaro-Green A, Roman SH, Cobin RH, et al. Detection of at-risk pregnancy by means of highly sensitive assays for thyroid autoantibodies. *JAMA* 1990;264:1422–1425.

135. Vianna JL, D'Cruz D, Khamashta MA, et al. Anticardiolipin antibodies in a patient with Crohn's disease and thrombosis. *Clin Exp Rheumatol* 1992;10:165–168.

136. Chamouard P, Grunebaum L, Wiesel ML, et al. Prevalence and significance of anticardiolipin antibodies in Crohn's disease. *Dig Dis Sci* 1994;39:1501–1504.

137. Chamouard P, Duclos B, Baumann R, et al. Antiphospholipid antibodies in inflammatory bowel disease. *Dig Dis Sci* 1995;40:1525.

138. Souto JC, Borrell M, Fontcuberta J, et al. Antiphospholipid antibodies in inflammatory bowel disease. *Dig Dis Sci* 1995;40:1524–1525.

139. Hudson M, Hutton RA, Wakefield AJ, et al. Evidence for activation of coagulation in Crohn's disease. *Blood Coagul Fibrinol* 1992;3: 773–778.

140. Webberly MJ, Hart MT, Melikian V. Thromboembolism in inflammatory bowel disease: role of platelets. *Gut* 1993;34:247–251.

141. Papi C, Ciaco A, Acierno G, et al. Severe ulcerative colitis, dural sinus thrombosis and the lupus anticoagulant. *Am J Gastroenterol* 1995;80: 1514–1517.

142. Gronhagen-Riska C, Teppo A-M, Helantera A, et al. Raised concentrations of antibodies to cardiolipin in patients receiving dialysis. *Br Med J* 1990;300:1696–1697.

143. Nurchis P, Pala R, Saviono M, et al. Lupus eritematoso sistémico con síndrome antifosfolipídica in corso di síndrome di Klinefelter. *Il Reumatologo* 1988;2:49–55.

144. Durand JM, Quiles N, Kaplanski G, et al. Lupus anticoagulant and Klinefelter's syndrome. *J Rheumatol* 1993;20:920–921.

145. Bajocchi G, Sandri G, Trotta F. Anticardiolipin antibodies in Klinefelter's syndrome. *J Rheumatol* 1994;21:1370.

146. Asherson RA. The catastrophic antiphospholipid syndrome syndrome. *J Rheumatol* 1992;19:508–512.

147. Asherson RA, Cervera R, Piette JC, et al. Catastrophic antiphospholipid syndrome: clinical and laboratory features of 50 patients. *Medicine* (Baltimore) 1998;77:195–207.

148. Peck B, Hoffman GS, Franck WA. Thrombophlebitis in systemic lupus erythematosus. *JAMA* 1978;240:1728–1730,

149. Kwong T, Leonidas JC, Ilowite NT. Asymptomatic superior vena cava thrombosis and pulmonary embolism in an adolescent with SLE and antiphospholipid antibodies. *Clin Exp Rheumatol* 1994;12:215–217.

150. Tomer Y, Kessler A, Eyal A, et al. Superior vena cava occlusion in a patient with antiphospholipid antibody syndrome. *J Rheumatol* 1991;18:95–97.

151. Ravelli A, Caporali R, Montecucco C, et al. Superior vena cava thrombosis in a child with antiphospholipid syndrome. *J Rheumatol* 1992;19: 502–503.

152. Taylor LM, Chitwood RW, Dalman RL, et al. Antiphospholipid antibodies in vascular surgery patients. *Ann Surg* 1994;220:544–551.

153. Fields RA, Sibbitt WL, Troubbeh H, et al. Neuropsychiatric lupus erythematosus, cerebral infarctions and anticardiolipin antibodies. *Ann Rheum Dis* 1990;49:114–117.

154. Asherson RA, Derksen RHWM, Harris EN, et al. Large vessel occlusion and gangrene in systemic lupus erythematosus and "lupus-like" disease: a report of six cases. *J Rheumatol* 1986;13:740–747.

155. Bowie EJ, Thompson JH Jr, Pascuzzi CA, et al. Thrombosis in systemic lupus erythematosus despite circulating anticoagulants. *J Lab Clin Med* 1963;62:416–430.

156. Asherson RA, Cervera R, Gharavi AE. Antiphospholipid antibodies and the antiphospholipid syndrome. *Ann Med Interne* 1993;144: 367–376.

157. Vivancos J, López-Soto A, Font J, et al. Síndrome antifosfolípido primario: estudio clínico y biológico de 36 casos. *Med Clin* (Barc) 1994;102:561–565.

158. Provenzale JM, Ortel TL. Anatomic distribution of venous thrombosis in patients with antiphospholipid antibody: roentgenographic findings. *AJR Am J Roentgenol* 1995;165:365–368.

159. Kitchens CS. Thrombotic storm: when thrombosis begets thrombosis. *Am J Med* 1998;104:381–385.

160. Alarcón-Segovia D, Osmundson PJ. Peripheral vascular syndromes associated with systemic lupus erythematosus. *Ann Intern Med* 1965; 62:907–919.

161. Jindal BK, Martin MFR, Gayner A. Gangrene developing after minor surgery in a patient with undiagnosed systemic lupus erythematosus and lupus anticoagulant. *Ann Rheum Dis* 1983;42:347–349.

162. Hall S, Buettner H, Luthra HS. Occlusive retinal vascular disease in systemic lupus erythematosus. *J Rheumatol* 1984;11:846–850.

163. Lessof MH, Glynn LE. The pulseless syndrome. *Lancet* 1959;1: 799–801.

164. Asherson RA, Ridley MG, Khamashta MA, et al. Gangrena en el lupus eritematoso sistémico. *Piel* 1988;3:409–412.

165. Drew P, Asherson RA, Zuk RJ, et al. Aortic occlusion in systemic lupus erythematosus associated with antiphospholipid antibodies. *Ann Rheum Dis* 1987;46:612–616.

166. Ter Borg EJ, Van Der Meer J, De Wolf JTM, et al. Arterial thrombotic manifestations in young women associated with the lupus anticoagulant. *Clin Rheumatol* 1988;7:74–79.

167. Stern BJ, Brey RL. Anticardiolipin antibodies are associated with an increased risk of stroke occurrence. *Neurology* 1994;44[Suppl 2]: A327.

168. Levine SR, Brey RL, Sawaya KL, et al. Recurrent stroke and thromboocclusive events in the antiphospholipid syndrome. *Ann Neurol* 1995;38:119–124.

169. Coull BM, Goodnight SH. Antiphospholipid antibodies, prethrombotic state and stroke. *Stroke* 1990;21:1370–1374.

170. Brey RL, Hait RG, Sherman DG, et al. Antiphospholipid antibodies and cerebral ischemia in young people. *Neurology* 1990;40: 1190–1196.

171. The Antiphospholipid Antibodies in Stroke Study Group (APASS). Clinical, radiological and pathological aspects of cerebrovascular disease associated with antiphospholipid antibodies. *Stroke* 1993; 24[Suppl I]:120–123.

172. Tohgi H, Takahashi H, Kashiwaya M, et al. The anticardiolipin antibody in elderly stroke patients: Its effect on stroke types, recurrence and the coagulation-fibrinolysis system. *Acta Neurol Scand* 1994; 90:86–90.

173. Nancini P, Baruffi MC, Abbate R, et al. Lupus anticoagulant and anticardiolipin antibodies in young adults with cerebral ischemia. *Stroke* 1992;23:189–193.

174. Sneddon IB. Cerebrovascular lesions and livedo reticularis. *Br J Dermatol* 1965;77:180–185.

175. Rebollo M, Val FJ, Garijo F, et al. Livedo reticularis and cerebrovascular lesions (Sneddon's syndrome): clinical, radiological and pathological features in eight cases. *Brain* 1983;106:965–979.

176. Brey RL, Escalante A, Futrell N, et al. Cerebral thrombosis and other neurologic manifestations in the antiphospholipid syndrome. In: Asherson RA, Cervera R, Piette J-C, eds. *The antiphospholipid syndrome.* 1996:133–150.

177. Asherson RA, Mayou S, Black M, et al. Livedo reticularis, connective tissue disease, anticardiolipin antibodies and CNS complications. *Arthritis Rheum* 1987;30[Suppl 4]:S69.

178. Asherson RA, Cervera R. Sneddon's and the "primary" antiphospholipid syndrome: confusion clarified. *J Stroke Cerebrovasc Dis* 1993;3: 121–122.

179. Stockhammer G, Felber SR, Zelger B, et al. Sneddon's syndrome: diagnosis by skin biopsy and MRI in 17 patients. *Stroke* 1993;24: 685–690.

180. Jura E, Palasik W, Meurer M, et al. Sneddon's syndrome (livedo reticularis and cerebrovascular lesions) with antiphospholipid antibodies and severe dementia in a young man: a case report. *Acta Neurol Scand* 1994;39:143–146.

181. Asherson RA, Mercey D, Phillips G, et al. Recurrent stroke and multiinfarct dementia in systemic lupus erythematosus: association with antiphospholipid antibodies. *Ann Rheum Dis* 1987;46:605–611.

182. Coull BM, Bourdette DN, Goodnight SH, et al. Multiple cerebral infarctions and dementia associated with anticardiolipin antibodies. *Stroke* 1987;6:1107–1112.

183. Kushner M, Simonian Y. Lupus anticoagulants, anticardiolipin antibodies and cerebral ischemia. *Stroke* 1989;20:225–229.

184. Biller J, Mershut M, Emanuele MA. Non haemorrhagic infarction of the thalamus. *Neurology* 1984;34:1269–1270.

185. Graff-Radford NR, Eslinger PJ, Damasio AR, et al. Non haemorrhagic infarction of the thalamus: behavioural, anatomic and physiologic correlates. *Neurology* 1984;34:11–23.

186. Westerman EH, Miles JM, Backonja M, et al. Neuropathologic findings in multi-infarct dementia associated with anticardiolipin antibody. *Arthritis Rheum* 1992;35:1028–1041.

187. Scheinberg P. Dementia due to vascular disease: a multifactorial disorder. *Stroke* 1988;19:1291–1299.

188. Briley DP, Coull BM, Goodnight SH. Neurological disease associated with antiphospholipid antibodies. *Ann Neurol* 1989;25:221–227.

189. Fields RA, Sibbitt WL, Toubbeh H, et al. Neuropsychiatric lupus erythematosus, cerebral infarctions and anticardiolipin antibodies. *Ann Rheum Dis* 1990;44:114–117.

190. Tullio MD, Sacco RL, Santonio-Rugio D, et al. Increased frequency of lupus anticoagulant in stroke patients with aortic arch atheroma. *Neurology* 1995;45[Suppl 4]:A274.

191. Cervera R, Font J, Paré C, et al. Cardiac disease in systemic lupus erythematosus: prospective study of 70 patients. *Ann Rheum Dis* 1992;51:156–159.

192. Ziporen L, Goldberg I, Arad M, et al. Libman Sacks endocarditis in antiphospholipid syndrome: immunopathologic findings in deformed heart valves. *Lupus* 1996;5:196–205.

193. Young SM, Fisher M, Sigsbee A, et al. Cardiogenic brain embolism and lupus anticoagulant. *Ann Neurol* 1989;26:390–392.

194. Hart RG, Miller VT, Coull BM, et al. Cerebral infarction associated with lupus anticoagulants-preliminary report. *Stroke* 1984;15:293–298.

195. D'Alton JG, Preston DN, Bormanis J, et al. Multiple transient ischemic attacks, lupus anticoagulant and verrucous endocarditis. *Stroke* 1985;16:512–514.

196. Anderson D, Bell D, Lodge R, et al. Recurrent cerebral ischemia and mitral valve vegetation in a patient with phospholipid antibodies. *J Rheumatol* 1987;14:839–841.

197. Levine SR, Kieran S, Puzio K, et al. Cerebral venous thrombosis with lupus anticoagulant: report of two cases. *Stroke* 1987;18:801–804.

198. Lau SO, Bock GH, Edson JR, et al. Sagittal sinus thrombosis in the nephrotic syndrome. *J Pediatr* 1980;97:948–950.

199. Averback P. Primary cerebral venous thrombosis in young adults: the diverse manifestations of an unrecognised disease. *Ann Neurol* 1978; 3:81–86.

200. Provenzale JM, Loganbill HA. Dural sinus thrombosis and venous infarction associated with antiphospholipid antibodies: MR findings. *J Comput Assist Tomogr* 1994;18:719–723.

201. Mokri B, Jack CR Jr, Petty GW. Pseudotumour syndrome associated with cerebral venous sinus occlusion and antiphospholipid antibodies. *Stroke* 1993;24:469–472.

202. Khoo KBK, Long FL, Tuck RR, et al. Cerebral venous sinus thrombosis associated with the primary antiphospholipid syndrome. *Med J Aust* 1995;162:30–32.

203. Jurtz G, Muller N. The antiphospholipid syndrome and psychosis. *Am J Psychiat* 1994;151:1841–1842.

204. Sirota P, Schild K, Firer M, et al. The diversity of autoantibodies in schizophrenic patients and their first degree relatives: analysis of multiple case families. In: *Abstracts of the First International Congress of the International Society of Neuro-Immune Modulation.* Florence, Italy: International Society of Neuro-Immune Modulation, 1991:389.

205. Maes M, Meltzer H, Jacobs J, et al. Autoimmunity in depression: increased antiphospholipid autoantibodies. *Acta Psychiatry Scand* 1993;87:160–166.

206. Calabrese LV, Stern TA. Neuropsychiatric manifestations of systemic lupus erythematosus. *Psychosomatics* 1995;36:344–359.

207. Abel T, Goldman DD, Urowitz MB. Neuropsychiatric lupus. *J Rheumatol* 1980;7:325–333.

208. Ziporen L, Eilam D, Shoenfeld Y, et al. Neurologic dysfunction associated with antiphospholipid antibodies: animal models. *Neurology* 1996;46:A459.

209. Mikdashi JA, Chase C, Kay GG. Neurocognitive deficits in antiphospholipid syndrome. *Neurology* 1996;46:A359.

210. Montalbán J, Arboix A, Staub H, et al. Transient global amnesia and antiphospholipid antibodies. *Clin Exp Rheumatol* 1989;7:85–87.

211. Scott TF, Hess D, Brillman J. Antiphospholipid antibody syndrome mimicking multiple sclerosis clinically and by magnetic resonance imaging. *Arch Intern Med* 1994;154:917–920.

212. Hughes GRV. The antiphospholipid syndrome and "multiple sclerosis." *Lupus* 1999;8:89.

213. Brandt KD, Lessell S. Migrainous phenomena in systemic lupus erythematosus. *Arthritis Rheum* 1978;21:7–16.

214. Brandt KD, lessell S, Cowen AS. Cerebral disorders of vision in systemic lupus erythematosus. *Ann Intern Med* 1975;83:163–169.

215. Landi G, Galloni MV, Sabbandini MG. Recurrent ischemic attacks in young adults with the lupus anticoagulant. *Stroke* 1983;14:377–379.

216. Hogan MJ, Brunet DG, Ford PM, et al. Lupus anticoagulant, antiphospholipid antibodies and migraine. *Can J Neurol Sci* 1988;15:420–425.

217. Asherson RA, Harris EN, Gharavi AE, et al. Clinical and laboratory features associated with anticardiolipin antibodies in non-SLE patients. *Arthritis Rheum* 1985;28:77.

218. Levine SR, Welch KMA. The spectrum of neurologic disease associated with antiphospholipid antibodies (lupus anticoagulant, anticardiolipin antibodies). *Arch Neurol* 1987;44:876–883.

219. Levine SR, Joseph R, D'Andrea G, et al. Migraine and the lupus anticoagulant: case reports and review of the literature. *Cephalalgia* 1987; 7:93–99.

220. Shuaib A, Barklay L, Lee M, et al. Migraine and antiphospholipid antibodies. *Headache* 1989;29:42.

221. Hughes GR, Khamashta MA. Anticardiolipin antibodies. *Br Med J* 1989;299:1414–1415.

222. Hering R, Couturier EGM, Steiner TJR, et al. Antiphospholipid antibodies in migraine. *Cephalalgia* 1991;11:19–21.

223. Montalbán J, Cervera R, Font J, et al. Lack of association between anticardiolipin antibodies in migraine in systemic lupus erythematosus. *Neurology* 1992;42:681–682.

224. Silvestrini M, Matteis M, Troisi E, et al. Migrainous stroke and the antiphospholipid antibodies. *Eur Neurol* 1994;34:316–319.

225. Silvestrini M, Cupini M, Matteis M, et al. Migraine in patients with stroke and antiphospholipid antibodies. *Headache* 1993;33:421–426.

226. Daras M, Koppel B, Leyfermann M, et al. Anticardiolipin antibodies in migraine patients: an additional risk factor for stroke? *Neurology* 1995;45[Suppl 4]:A367.

227. Bluestein HG, Zuaifler NJ. Brain-reactive lymphocytotoxic antibodies in the serum of patients with systemic lupus erythematosus. *J Clin Invest* 1976;57:509–516.

228. Mackworth-Young CG, Hughes GRV. Epilepsy: an early symptom of systemic lupus erythematosus. *J Neurol Neurosurg Psychiatry* 1985; 48:185.

229. Inzelberg R, Korzyn AD. Lupus anticoagulant and late onset seizures. *Acta Neurol Scand* 1989;79:114–118.

230. Montalbán J, López M, Jordana R, et al. Anticuerpos antifosfolípido en la epilepsia tardía. *Rev Neurol* (Barc) 1991;19:119–121.

231. Herranz MT, Rivier G, Khamashta MA, et al. Association between antiphospholipid antibodies and epilepsy in patients with systemic lupus erythematosus. *Arthritis Rheum* 1994;37:568–571.

232. Cervera R, Asherson RA, Font J, et al. Chorea in the antiphospholipid syndrome: clinical, neurologic and immunologic characteristics of 50 patients from our clinics and the recent literature. *Medicine* (Baltimore) 1997;76:203–212.

233. Asherson RA, Derksen RHWM, Harris EN, et al. Chorea in systemic lupus erythematosus and 'lupus-like' disease: association with antiphospholipid antibodies. *Semin Arthritis Rheum* 1987;16:253–259.

234. Bouchez B, Arnott G, Hatron PY, et al. Choré et lupus érytémateux disséminé avec anticoagulant circulant: trois cas. *Rev Neurol* (Paris) 1985;141:571–574.

235. Khamashta MA, Gil A, Anciones B, et al. Chorea in systemic lupus erythematosus: association with antiphospholipid antibodies. *Ann Rheum Dis* 1988;47:681–683.
236. Hodges JR. Chorea and the lupus anticoagulant. *J Neurol Neurosurg Psychiatry* 1987;50:368–369.
237. Asherson RA, Harris EN, Gharavi AE, et al. Systemic lupus erythematosus, antiphospholipid antibodies, chorea and oral contraceptives. *Arthritis Rheum* 1986;29:1535–1536.
238. Asherson RA, Harris EN, Hughes GRV, et al. Complications of oral contraceptives and antiphospholipid antibodies. *Arthritis Rheum* 1988; 31:575.
239. Furie R, Ishikawa T, Dhawan V, et al. Alternating hemichorea in primary antiphospholipid syndrome: evidence for contralateral striatal hypermetabolism. *Neurology* 1994;44:2197–2199.
240. Sundén-Cullberg J, Tedroff J, Aquilonius S-M. Reversible chorea in primary antiphospholipid syndrome. *Movement Disorders* 1998;13: 147–149.
241. Tam L-S, Cohen MG, Li EK. Hemiballismus in systemic lupus erythematosus: possible association with antiphospholipid antibodies. *Lupus* 1995;4:67–69.
242. Singh PR, Piasaa K, Qumar A, et al. Cerebellar ataxia in systemic lupus erythematosus: three case reports. *Ann Rheum Dis* 1988;97:954–956.
243. Propper DJ, Bucknall RC. Acute transverse myelitis complicating lupus erythematosus. *Ann Rheum Dis* 1989;48:512–515.
244. Adrianakos AA, Duffy UJ, Suzuki M, et al. Transverse myelopathy in systemic lupus erythematosus: a report of three cases and a review of the literature. *Ann Intern Med* 1975;83:616–624.
245. Harisdangkul V, Doorenbos D, Subramony SH. Lupus transverse myelopathy: better outcome with early recognition and aggressive high-dose intravenous corticosteroid pulse treatment. *J Neurol* 1995;242:326–331.
246. Lavalle C, Pizarro S, Drenkard C, et al. Transverse myelitis: manifestation of systemic lupus erythematosus strongly associated with antiphospholipid antibodies. *J Rheumatol* 1990;17:34–37.
247. Chang R, Quismorio P Jr. Transverse myelopathy in systemic lupus erythematosus (SLE). *Arthritis Rheum* 1990;33[Suppl 9]:S102.
248. Smyth AE, Bruce IN, McMillan SA, et al. Transverse myelitis: a complication of systemic lupus erythematosus that is associated with the antiphospholipid syndrome. *Ulster Med J* 1996;645:91–94.
249. Oppenheimer S, Hofbrand BI. Optic neuritis and myelopathy in systemic lupus erythematosus. *Can J Neurol Sci* 1986;13:129–132.
250. Harris EN, Englert H, Derue G, et al. Antiphospholipid antibodies in acute Guillain–Barré syndrome. *Lancet* 1983;2:1361–1362.
251. Palosuo T, Vaarala O, Kinnuren E. Anticardiolipin antibodies in the Guillain–Barré syndrome. *Lancet* 1985;2:839.
252. Frampton G, Weiner JB, Cameron JS, et al. Severe Guillain–Barré syndrome: an association with IgA anticardiolipin antibodies in a series of 92 patients. *J Neuroimmunol* 1988;19:133–139.
253. Marcusse HN, Hahn J, Tan WD, et al. Anterior spinal artery syndrome in systemic lupus erythematosus. *Br J Rheumatol* 1989;28:344–346.
254. Harris EN, Gharavi AE, Mackworth-Young CG, et al. Lupoid sclerosis: a possible pathogenetic role for antiphospholipid antibodies. *Ann Rheum Dis* 1985;44:281–283.
255. Marullo S, Clauvel J-P, Intrator L, et al. Lupoid sclerosis with antiphospholipid and antimyelin antibodies. *J Rheumatol* 1993;20: 747–749.
256. Labutta RJ. Ophthalmic manifestations in the antiphospholipid syndrome. In: Asherson RA, Cervera R, Piette J-C, et al., eds. *The antiphospholipid syndrome*. Boca Raton, FL: CRC Press, 1996: 213–218.
257. Jabs DA, Fine SL, Hochberg MC, et al. Severe retinal vaso-occlusive disease in systemic lupus erythematosus. *Arch Ophthalmol* 1986;104: 558–563.
258. Asherson RA, Merry P, Acheson JF, et al. Antiphospholipid antibodies: a risk factor for occlusive ocular vascular disease in systemic lupus erythematosus and the 'primary' antiphospholipid syndrome. *Ann Rheum Dis* 1989;48:358–361.
259. Montehermoso A, Cervera R, Font J, et al. Association of antiphospholipid antibodies with retinal vascular disease in systemic lupus erythematosus. *Semin Arthritis Rheum* 1999;28:326–332.
260. Gerber SL, Cantor LB. Progressive optic atrophy and the antiphospholipid antibody syndrome. *Am J Ophthalmol* 1990;110:443–444.
261. Watts MT, Greaves M, Rennie IG, et al. Antiphospholipid antibodies in the aetiology of ischemic optic neuropathy. *Eye* 1991;5:75–79.
262. Reino S, Muñoz-Rodríguez FJ, Cervera R, et al. Optic neuropathy in the "primary" antiphospholipid syndrome: report of a case and review of the literature. *Clin Rheumatol* 1997;16:629–631.
263. Asherson RA, Cervera R. Antiphospholipid antibodies and the heart: lessons and pitfalls of the cardiologist. *Circulation* 1991;84:920–923.
264. Kaplan S, Chartash EK, Pizzarello RA, et al. Cardiac manifestations of the antiphospholipid syndrome. *Am Heart J* 1992;124:1331–1338.
265. Cervera R, Font J, Ingelmo M. Cardiac manifestations in the antiphospholipid syndrome. In: Asherson RA, Cervera R, Piette J-C, et al., eds. *The antiphospholipid syndrome*. Boca Raton, Fl: CRC Press, 1996: 151–160.
266. Asherson RA, Khamashta MA, Baguley E, et al. Myocardial infarction and antiphospholipid antibodies in SLE and related disorders. *Q J Med* 1989;73:1102–1105.
267. Hamsten A, Norberg R, Bjorkholm M, et al. Antibodies to cardiolipin in young survivors of myocardial infarction: an association with recurrent cardiovascular events. *Lancet* 1986;2:113–116.
268. Sletnes KE, Smith P, Abdelnoor M, et al. Antiphospholipid antibodies after myocardial infarction and their relation to mortality, reinfarction, and non-haemorrhagic stroke. *Lancet* 1992;339:451–453.
269. De Catarina R, Asconia A, Mazzone A, et al. Prevalence of anticardiolipin antibodies in coronary artery disease. *Am J Cardiol* 1990; 65:922–923.
270. Yilmaz E, Adalet K, Yilmaz G, et al. Importance of serum anticardiolipin antibody levels in coronary artery disease. *Clin Cardiol* 1994; 17:117–121.
271. Bick RL, Ishmail Y, Baker WF. Coagulation abnormalities in precocious coronary artery thrombosis and in patients failing coronary artery bypass grafting and percutaneous transcoronary angioplasty. *Semin Thromb Hemost* 1993;10:412–417.
272. Baker WF, Bick RL. Antiphospholipid antibodies in coronary artery disease: a review. *Semin Thromb Hemost* 1994;20:27–45.
273. Vaarala O, Mänttäri M, Manninen V, et al. Anticardiolipin antibodies and risk of myocardial infarction in a prospective cohort of middle-aged men. *Circulation* 1995;91:23–27.
274. Zuckerman E, Toubi E, Shiran A, et al. Anticardiolipin antibodies and acute myocardial infarction in non-systemic lupus erythematosus patients: a controlled prospective study. *Am J Med* 1996;171:381–386.
275. Ralling P, Exner T, Abraham R. Coronary artery vasculitis and myocardial infarction associated with antiphospholipid antibodies in a pregnant woman. *Aust N Z J Med* 1989;19:357–360.
276. Thorp JM, Chescheir NC, Fann B. Postpartum myocardial infarction in a patient with antiphospholipid syndrome. *Am J Perinatol* 1994;11: 1–3.
277. Murphy JJ, Leach IH. Findings of necropsy in the heart of a patient with anticardiolipin syndrome. *Br Heart J* 1989;62:61–64.
278. Kattwinkel N, Villaneuva AG, Labib SB, et al. Myocardial infarction caused by cardiac microvasculopathy in a patient with the primary antiphospholipid syndrome. *Ann Intern Med* 1992;116:974–976.
279. Díaz MN, Becker RC. Anticardiolipin antibodies in patients with unstable angina. *Cardiology* 1994;84:380–384.
280. Morton KE, Gavaghan TP, Krilis SA, et al. Coronary artery bypass graft failure: an autoimmune phenomenon? *Lancet* 1986;2:1353–1356.
281. Eber B, Schumacher M, Auer-Grumbach P, et al. Increased IgM anticardiolipin antibodies in patients with restenosis after percutaneous transluminal coronary angioplasty. *Am J Cardiol* 1992;69:1255–1258.
282. Brown JH, Doherty CC, Allen DC, et al. Fatal cardiac failure due to myocardial microthrombi in systemic lupus erythematosus. *Br Med J* 1988;296:1505.
283. Nihoyannopoulos P, Gómez PM, Joshi J, et al. Cardiac abnormalities in systemic lupus erythematosus: association with raised anticardiolipin antibodies. *Circulation* 1990;82:369–375.
284. Leung WH, Wong KL, Lau CP, et al. Association between antiphospholipid antibodies and cardiac abnormalities in patients with systemic lupus erythematosus. *Am J Med* 1990;89:411–419.
285. Hasnie AMA, Stoddard MF, Gleason CB, et al. Diastolic dysfunction is a feature of the antiphospholipid syndrome. *Am Heart J* 1995; 129:1009–1113.
286. Cervera R, Khamashta MA, Font J, et al. High prevalence of significant heart valve lesions in patients with the 'primary' antiphospholipid syndrome. *Lupus* 1992;1:43–47.
287. García-Torres R, Amigo M-C, De la Rosa A, et al. Valvular heart disease in primary antiphospholipid syndrome (PAPS): clinical and morphological findings. *Lupus* 1995;5:56–61.

288. Galve E, Ordi J, Barquinero J, et al. Valvular heart disease in the primary antiphospholipid syndrome. *Ann Intern Med* 1992;116:293–298.

289. Khamashta MA, Cervera R, Asherson RA, et al. Association of antibodies against phospholipids with heart valve disease in systemic lupus erythematosus. *Lancet* 1990;335:1541–1544.

290. Hojnik M, George J, Ziporen L, et al. Heart valve involvement (Libman-Sacks endocarditis) in the antiphospholipid syndrome. *Circulation* 1996;93:1579–1587.

291. Ford SE, Charrette EJP, Knight J, et al. Possible role of antiphospholipid antibodies in acquired cardiac valve deformity. *J Rheumatol* 1990;17:1449–1503.

292. Asherson RA, Hughes GRV. The expanding spectrum of Libman-Sacks endocarditis: the role of antiphospholipid antibodies. *Clin Exp Rheumatol* 1989;7:225–228.

293. Ziporen L, Goldberg I, Arad M, et al. Libman-Sacks endocarditis in the antiphospholipid syndrome: immunopathologic findings in deformed heart valves. *Lupus* 1995;5:196–205.

294. Lehman TJA, Palmeri ST, Hastings C, et al. Bacterial endocarditis complicating systemic lupus erythematosus. *J Rheumatol* 1983;10:655–658.

295. Asherson RA, Gibson DG, Evans DW, et al. Diagnostic and therapeutic problems in two patients with antiphospholipid antibodies, heart valve lesions and transient ischemic attacks. *Ann Rheum Dis* 1988;47:947–953.

296. Font J, Cervera R, Pare C, et al. Non-infective verrucous endocarditis in a patient with 'primary' antiphospholipid syndrome. *Br J Rheumatol* 1991;30:305–307.

297. Bruce D, Bateman D, Thomas R. Left ventricular thrombi in a patient with the antiphospholipid syndrome. *Br Heart J* 1995;74:202–203.

298. Baum RA, Jundt JW. Intracardiac thrombosis and antiphospholipid antibodies: a case report and review of the literature. *South Med J* 1994;87:928–932.

299. Coppock MA, Safford RE, Danielson GK. Intracardiac thrombosis, phospholipid antibodies and two-chambered right ventricle. *Br Heart J* 1988;60:455–458.

300. O'Neill D, Magaldi J, Dobkins D, et al. Dissolution of intracardiac mass lesions in the primary antiphospholipid antibody syndrome. *Arch Intern Med* 1995;155:325–327.

301. O'Hickey S, Skinner C, Beattie J. Life threatening right ventricular thrombosis in association with phospholipid antibodies. *Br Heart J* 1993;70:279–281.

302. Gertner E, Leatherman JW. Intracardiac mural thrombus mimicking atrial myxoma in the antiphospholipid syndrome. *J Rheumatol* 1992;19:1293–1298.

303. Nickele GA, Foster DA, Kenny D. Primary antiphospholipid syndrome and mitral valve thrombosis. *Am Heart J* 1994;128:1245–1247.

304. Martínez-Levín M, Fonseca C, Arugo MC, et al. Antiphospholipid syndrome in patients with cyanotic congenital heart disease. *Clin Exp Rheumatol* 1995;13:489–491.

305. Donaldson MC, Weinberg D, Belkin M, et al. Screening for hypercoagulable states in vascular surgical practice: a preliminary study. *J Vasc Surg* 1990;11:825–831.

306. Shortell CK, Ouriel K, Green RM, et al. Vascular disease in the antiphospholipid syndrome: a comparison with the patient population with atherosclerosis. *J Vasc Surg* 1992;15:158–166.

307. Taylor IM, Chitwood RW, Dalman RL, et al. Antiphospholipid antibodies in vascular surgery patients: a cross-sectional study. *Ann Surg* 1994;226:545–551.

308. Ciocca RG, Choi J, Graham AM. Antiphospholipid antibodies lead to increased risk in cardiovascular surgery. *Ann J Surg* 1995;170:198–200.

309. Asherson RA, Cervera R. Review: antiphospholipid antibodies and the lung. *J Rheumatol* 1995;22:62–66.

310. Cervera R, García-Carrasco M, Asherson RA. Pulmonary manifestations in the antiphospholipid syndrome. In: Asherson RA, Cervera R, Piette J-C, et al., eds. *The antiphospholipid syndrome.* Boca Raton, FL: CRC Press, 1996:161–167.

311. Sandoval J, Amigo M-C, Barragan R, et al. Primary antiphospholipid syndrome presenting as chronic thromboembolic pulmonary hypertension: treatment with thromboendarterectomy. *J Rheumatol* 1996;23:772–775.

312. Sato M, Okazaki H, Okamoto H, et al. Pulmonary hypertension in systemic lupus erythematosus: a report of an autopsied case. *Int Med* 1994;33:540–542.

313. Rich S, Kieras K, Hart K, et al. Antinuclear antibodies in primary pulmonary hypertension. *J Am Coll Cardiol* 1986;8:1307–1311.

314. Asherson RA, Oakley CN. Pulmonary hypertension and systemic lupus erythematosus. *J Rheumatol* 1986;13:1–5.

315. Asherson RA, Higenbottam TW, Dinh Xuan AT, et al. Pulmonary hypertension in a lupus clinic: experience with twenty four patients. *J Rheumatol* 1990;17:1292–1296

316. Luchi ME, Asherson RA, Lahita RG. Primary idiopathic pulmonary hypertension complicated by pulmonary arterial thrombosis: association with antiphospholipid antibodies. *Arthritis Rheum* 1992;35:700–705.

317. Gertner E, Lie JT. Pulmonary capillaritis, alveolar haemorrhage and recurrent microvascular thrombosis in primary antiphospholipid syndrome. *J Rheumatol* 1993;20:1224–1228.

318. Brucato A, Baudo F, Barberis M, et al. Pulmonary hypertension secondary to thrombosis of the pulmonary vessels in a patient with the primary antiphospholipid syndrome. *J Rheumatol* 1994;21:942–944.

319. Ghosh S, Walters HD, Joist JH, et al. Adult respiratory distress syndrome associated with antiphospholipid antibody syndrome. *J Rheumatol* 1993;20:1406–1408.

320. Kerr JE, Poe R, Kramer Z. Antiphospholipid antibody syndrome presenting as a refractory non-inflammatory pulmonary vasculopathy. *Chest* 1997;112:1707–1710.

321. Howe HS, Boey ML, Fong KY, et al. Pulmonary haemorrhage, pulmonary infarction and the lupus anticoagulant. *Ann Rheum Dis* 1988;47:869–872.

322. Hillerdal G, Hagg A, Licke G, et al. Intraalveolar haemorrhage in the anticardiolipin antibody syndrome. *Scand J Rheumatol* 1991;20:58–62.

323. Crausman RS, Achenbach GA, Pluss WT, et al. Pulmonary capillaritis and alveolar haemorrhage associated with the antiphospholipid syndrome. *J Rheumatol* 1995;22:554–556.

324. Schwab EP, Schumacher HR, Freundlich B, et al. Pulmonary alveolar haemorrhage in systemic lupus erythematosus. *Semin Arthritis Rheum* 1993;23:8–15.

325. Asherson RA, Greenblatt M, Churg A, et al. Recurrent alveolar haemorrhage, pulmonary capillaritis in the 'primary' antiphospholipid syndrome (in press).

326. Savin H, Huberman M, Koh E, et al. Fibrosing alveolitis associated with primary antiphospholipid syndrome. *Br J Rheumatol* 1994;33:977–980.

327. Kelion AD, Cockroft JR, Ritter JM. Antiphospholipid syndrome in a patient with rapidly progressive fibrosing alveolitis. *Postgrad Med J* 1994;71:233–235.

328. Branch DW, Kochenour NP, Rote NS, et al. New post-partum syndrome associated with antiphospholipid antibodies. *Obstet Gynecol* 1987;69:460–468.

329. Kupferminc MJ, Lee MJ, Green D, et al. Severe post-partum pulmonary, cardiac and renal syndrome associated with antiphospholipid antibodies. *Obstet Gynecol* 1994;83:806–807.

330. Asherson RA, Kant KS. Antiphospholipid antibodies and the kidney. *J Rheumatol* 1993;20:1268–1272.

331. Piette J-C, Kleinknecht D, Bach J-F. Renal manifestations in the antiphospholipid syndrome. In: Asherson RA, Cervera R, Piette J-C, et al., eds. *The antiphospholipid syndrome.* Boca Raton, FL: CRC Press, 1996:169–181.

332. Cervera R, Asherson RA. Anticuerpos antifosfolípidos e hipertensión arterial. *Hipertensión* 1994;11:79–81.

333. Frampton G, Hicks J, Cameron JS. Significance of antiphospholipid antibodies in patients with lupus nephritis. *Kidney Int* 1991;39:1225–1231.

334. Kant KS, Pollack KVE, Weiss MA, et al. Glomerular thrombosis in SLE: prevalence and significance. *Medicine* (Baltimore) 1981;60:71–86.

335. Glueck HI, Kant KS, Weiss MA, et al. Thrombosis in SLE: relation to the presence of circulatory anticoagulants. *Arch Intern Med* 1985;145:1389–1395.

336. Leaker B, Carrley KF, Dowling J, et al. Lupus nephritis: clinical and pathological correlation. *Q J Med* 1987;238:163–179.

337. Bhathena DB, Sobel BJ, Mydal SD. Non-inflammatory renal microangiopathy of systemic lupus erythematosus ("lupus vasculitis"). *Am J Nephrol* 1981;1:144–159.

338. Churg J, Goldstein MH, Bernstein J. Thrombotic angiopathy including haemolytic-uremic syndrome, thrombotic thrombocytopenic purpura

and postpartum renal failure. In: Tister CC, Brenner BM, eds. *Renal pathology with clinical and functional correlates.* Vol 2. Philadelphia: JB Lippincott, 1989:1081–1113.

339. Hughson MD, Madasdy T, McCarty GA, et al. Renal thrombotic microangiopathy in patients with systemic lupus erythematosus and the antiphospholipid syndrome. *Am J Kidney Dis* 1992;20:150–158.

340. Kinkaid-Smith P, Fairley KF, Kross M. Lupus anticoagulation associated with renal thrombotic microangiopathy and pregnancy related renal failure. *Q J Pediatr* 1988;69:795–815.

341. Asherson RA, Nobel GE, Hughes GRV. Hypertension, renal artery stenosis and the 'primary' antiphospholipid syndrome. *J Rheumatol* 1991;18:1413–1415.

342. Asherson RA, Hughes GRV, Derksen RHWM. Renal infarction associated with antiphospholipid antibodies in systemic lupus erythematosus and 'lupus-like' disease. *J Urol* 1988;140:1028.

343. Poux JM, Boudet R, Lacroix P, et al. Renal infarction and thrombosis of the infra-renal aorta in a 35-year old man with primary antiphospholipid syndrome. *Am J Kidney Dis* 1996;27:721–725.

344. Asherson RA, Lanham JG, Hull RG, et al. Renal vein thrombosis in systemic lupus erythematosus: association with the lupus anticoagulant. *Clin Exp Rheumatol* 1984;2:75–79.

345. Asherson RA, Buchanan M, Baguley E, et al. Postpartum bilateral renal vein thrombosis in the primary antiphospholipid syndrome. *J Rheumatol* 1993;20:874–876.

346. Hage ML, Liv R, Harcheschi DG, et al. Fetal renal vein thrombosis, hydrops fetalis and maternal lupus anticoagulant: a case report. *Prenat Diagn* 1994;14:873–877.

347. Liaño F, Mampaso F, Barcia-Martín F. Allograft membranous glomerulonephritis and renal vein thrombosis in a patient with lupus anticoagulation factor. *Nephrol Dial Transplant* 1988;3:684–689.

348. Gronhagen-Riska C, Teppo AM, Helentera A, et al. Raised concentration of antibodies to cardiolipin in patients receiving haemodialysis. *Br Med J* 1990;300:1696–1697.

349. Prakash R, Miller CC, Suki WM. Anticardiolipin antibody in patients on maintenance haemodialysis and its association with recurrent arteriovenous graft thrombosis. *Am J Kidney Dis* 1995;26:347–352.

350. Kirschbaum B, Mullinax F, Curry N, et al. Association between anticardiolipin antibody and frequent clotting problems in haemodialysis patients. *J Am Soc Nephrol* 1991;2:332.

351. Brunet P, Aillava M-F, San Marco M, et al. Antiphospholipids in haemodialysis patients: relationship between lupus anticoagulant and thrombosis. *Kidney Int* 1995;48:794–800.

352. Radhakrishnan J, Williams GS, Appel GB, et al. Renal transplantation in anticardiolipin antibody-positive lupus erythematosus patients. *Am J Kidney Dis* 1994;23:286–289.

353. Mondragón-Ramírez G, Bochicchio T, García-Torres R, et al. Recurrent renal thrombotic angiopathy after kidney transplantation in two patients with end-stage renal disease. *Thromb Res* 1993;72:109–117.

354. Huang JJ, Chen M-W, Sung J-M, et al. Postpartum haemolytic-uremic syndrome associated with antiphospholipid antibody. *Nephrol Dial Transplant* 1988;13:182–186.

355. Kniaz D, Eisenberg GH, Elrad H, et al. Postpartum haemolytic-uremic syndrome associated with antiphospholipid antibodies. *Am J Nephrol* 1992;12:126–133.

356. Ornstein MH, Rand JH. An association between refractory HELLP syndrome and antiphospholipid antibodies during pregnancy: a report of two cases. *J Rheumatol* 1994;21:1360–1364.

357. Asherson RA, Hughes GRV. Hypoadrenalism, Addison's disease and antiphospholipid antibodies. *J Rheumatol* 1991;18:1–3.

358. Asherson RA. Hypoadrenalism and the antiphospholipid antibodies: a new cause of idiopathic "Addison's disease." In: Bhatt HR, James VHT, Besser GM, et al., eds. *Advances in Thomas Addison's diseases.* Vol 1. *J Endocrinol* 1994;1:87–101.

359. Arnason JA, Graziano FM. Adrenal insufficiency in the antiphospholipid antibody syndrome. *Semin Arthritis Rheum* 1995;25:109-116.

360. Pelkonen P, Simell O, Rasi V, et al. Venous thrombosis associated with the lupus anticoagulant. *Ann Intern Med* 1980;92:156–159.

361. Grottolo A, Ferrari V, Mariarosa M, et al. Primary adrenal insufficiency, circulating lupus anticoagulant and anticardiolipin antibodies in a patient with multiple abortions and recurrent thrombotic episodes. *Haematologia* 1988;73:517–519.

362. Asherson RA, Hughes GRV. Recurrent deep vein thrombosis in Addison's disease in "primary" antiphospholipid syndrome. *J Rheumatol* 1989;16:378–380.

363. Carette S, Jobin F. Acute adrenal insufficiency as a manifestation of the anticardiolipin syndrome. *Ann Rheum Dis* 1989;48:430–431.

364. Rao R, Vagnucci A, Amico J. Bilateral massive adrenal haemorrhage: early recognition and treatment. *Ann Intern Med* 1989;110:227–235.

365. Marie I, Levesque H, Heron F, et al. Acute adrenal failure secondary to bilateral infarction of the adrenal glands as the first manifestation of primary antiphospholipid antibody syndrome. *Ann Rheum Dis* 1997;56:567–568.

366. Argento A, Di Benedetto RJ. ARDS and adrenal insufficiency associated with the antiphospholipid antibody syndrome. *Chest* 1998;113:1136–1138.

367. Guibal F, Rybojad M, Cordoliani F, et al. Melanoderma revealing primary antiphospholipid syndrome. *Dermatology* 1996;192:75–77.

368. Provenzale JM, Ortel TL, Nelson RC. Adrenal haemorrhages in patients with primary antiphospholipid syndrome: imaging findings. *AJR Am J Roentgenol* 1995;165:361–364.

369. Oelkers W. Adrenal insufficiency IV. *N Engl J Med* 1996;335:1206–1212.

370. Pessayre D, Larrey D. Drug induced liver injury. In: McIntyre N, Benhamou J-P, Bircher J, et al., eds. *Oxford textbook of clinical hepatology.* Oxford, England: Oxford University Press, 1991:876–902.

371. Valla D, Benhamou J-P. Disorders of the hepatic veins and venules. In: McIntyre N, Benhamou J-P, Bircher J, et al., eds. *Oxford textbook of clinical hepatology.* Oxford, England: Oxford University Press, 1991:1004–1011.

372. Pomeroy C, Knodell RG, Swain WR, et al. Budd-Chiari syndrome in a patient with the lupus anticoagulant. *Gastroenterology* 1984;86:158–161.

373. Shimizu S, Miyata M, Kamiike W, et al. Budd-Chiari syndrome combined with antiphospholipid syndrome: case report and literature review. *Vasc Surg* 1993;27:501–509.

374. Farrant JM, Judge M, Thompson RDH. Thrombotic cutaneous nodules and hepatic vein thrombosis in the anticardiolipin syndrome. *Clin Exp Dermatol* 1989;14:306–308.

375. Ouwendijk RJT, Koster JC, Wilson JHP, et al. Budd-Chiari syndrome in a young patient with anticardiolipin antibodies: need for prolonged anticoagulant treatment. *Gut* 1994;35:1004–1006.

376. Mackworth-Young CG, Gharavi AE, Boey ML, et al. Portal and pulmonary hypertension in a case of systemic lupus erythematosus: possible relationship with a clotting abnormality. *Eur J Rheumatol Inflamm* 1984;7:71–74.

377. Ordi J, Vargas V, Vilardell M, et al. Lupus anticoagulant and portal hypertension. *Am J Med* 1988;84:566–568.

378. De Clerck L, Michielsen PP, Ramael MR, et al. Portal and pulmonary vessel thrombosis associated with systemic lupus erythematosus and anticardiolipin antibodies. *J Rheumatol* 1991;18:1919–1921.

379. Takahaski C, Kumagai S, Tsubata R, et al. Portal hypertension associated with anticardiolipin antibodies in a case of systemic lupus erythematosus. *Lupus* 1995;4:232–235.

380. Mantz FA, Craige E. Portal axis thrombosis with spontaneous portacaval shunt and resultant cor pulmonale. *Arch Pathol* 1951;52:91–97.

381. Nakamura H, Uehara H, Okada T, et al. Occlusion of small hepatic veins associated with systemic lupus erythematosus with the lupus anticoagulant. *Hepatogastroenterology* 1989;36:393–397.

382. Morio S, Oh H, Hirasawa A, et al. Hepatic veno-occlusive disease in a patient with lupus anticoagulant after allogeneic bone marrow transplantation. *Bone Marrow Transplant* 1991;8:147–149.

383. Rio B, Andreu G, Nicod A, et al. Thrombocytopenia in veno-occlusive disease after bone marrow transplantation or chemotherapy. *Blood* 1986;67:1773–1776.

384. Pérez-Ruiz F, Orte-Martínez FJ, Zea-Mendoza AC, et al. Nodular regenerative hyperplasia of the liver in rheumatic diseases: report of seven cases and review of the literature. *Semin Arthritis Rheum* 1991;21:47–54.

385. Morlà RM, Ramos-Casals M, García-Carrasco M, et al. Nodular regenerative hyperplasia of the liver and antiphospholipid antibodies: report of two cases and review of the literature. *Lupus* 1999;8:160–163.

386. Mor T, Beigel Y, Inbal A, et al. Hepatic infarction in a patient with the lupus anticoagulant. *Arthritis Rheum* 1989;32:491–495.

387. Kinoshita K. Hepatic infarction during pregnancy complicated by antiphospholipid syndrome. *Am J Obstet Gynecol* 1993;169:199–202.

388. Young N, Wong KP. Antibody to cardiolipin causing hepatic infarction in a postpartum patient with systemic lupus erythematosus. *Aust Radiol* 1991;35:83–85.

389. Saeki R, Kaneko S, Terasaki S, et al. Mixed types of chronic active hepatitis and primary biliary cirrhosis associated with the antiphospholipid antibody syndrome. *Hepatogastroenterology* 1993;40:499–501.

390. Beales ILP. An acquired pseudo-Bernard-Soulier syndrome occurring with autoimmune chronic active hepatitis and anticardiolipin antibody. *Postgrad Med J* 1994;70:305–308.

391. Kesler A, Pomeranz IS, Huberman H, et al. Cerebral venous thrombosis and chronic active hepatitis as part of the antiphospholipid antibody syndrome. *Postgrad Med J* 1996;72:690–692.

392. Muñoz RP, Costago MA, Fernández-Nebro A, et al. Autoimmune hepatitis associated with the antiphospholipid syndrome (in press).

393. Reynolds TB, Edmondson HA, Peters RL, et al. Lupoid hepatitis. *Ann Intern Med* 1964;61:650–655.

394. Prieto J, Yuste JR, Beloqui O, et al. Anticardiolipin antibodies in chronic hepatitis C: implication of hepatitis C virus as the cause of the antiphospholipid syndrome. *Hepatology* 1996;23:199–204.

395. Muñoz-Rodríguez FJ, Tàssies D, et al. Prevalence of hepatitis C virus infection in patients with antiphospholipid syndrome. *J Hepatol* 1999;30:770–773.

396. Biron C, Andréani H, Blanc P, et al. Prevalence of antiphospholipid antibodies in patients with chronic liver disease related to alcohol or hepatitis C virus: correlation with liver injury. *J Lab Clin Med* 1998;131:243–250.

397. Alric L, Oskman F, Sanmarco M, et al. Association of antiphospholipid syndrome and chronic hepatitis C. *Br J Rheumatol* 1998;37:589–590.

398. Chadid A, Chadalawada KR, Morgan TR. Phospholipid antibodies in alcoholic liver disease. *Hepatology* 1994;20:1465–1471.

399. Talenti DA, Falk GW, Carey WD, et al. Anticardiolipin antibody-associated cerebral infarction in cirrhosis: clearance of anticardiolipin antibody after liver transplantation. *Am J Gastroenterol* 1994;89:785–788.

400. Meroni PL, Harris EN, Brucato A, et al. Anti-mitochondial type M5 and anti-cardiolipin antibodies in autoimmune disorders: studies on their association and cross-reactivity. *Clin Exp Immunol* 1987;67:484–491.

401. Cowchok S, Fort J, Muñoz S, et al. False positive ELISA tests for anticardiolipin antibodies in sera from patients with repeated abortions, rheumatological disorders and primary biliary cirrhosis: correlation with elevated polyclonal IgM and implications for patients with repeated abortion. *Clin Exp Immunol* 1988;73:289–294.

402. Violi F, Ferro D, Basili S, et al. Relation between lupus anticoagulant and splenic venous thrombosis in cirrhosis of liver. *Br Med J* 1994;309:239.

403. Cappell M. Oesophageal necrosis and perforation associated with the anticardiolipin antibody syndrome. *Am J Gastroenterol* 1994;89:1241–1245.

404. Kalman DR, Khan A, Romain PL, et al. Giant gastric ulceration associated with antiphospholipid antibody syndrome. *Am J Gastroenterol* 1996;91:1244–1247.

405. Asherson RA, Morgan S, Harris EN, et al. Arterial occlusion causing large bowel infarction: a reflection of clotting diathesis in SLE. *Clin Rheumatol* 1986;5:102–106.

406. Asherson RA, Mackworth-Young C, Harris EN, et al. Multiple venous and arterial thromboses associated with the lupus anticoagulant and antibodies to cardiolipin in the absence of SLE. *Rheumatol Int* 1985;5:90–93.

407. Sánchez-Guerrero J, Reyes E, Alarcón-Segovia D. Primary antiphospholipid syndrome as a cause of intestinal infarction. *J Rheumatol* 1992;19:623–625.

408. Hamilton ME. Superior mesenteric artery thrombosis associated with antiphospholipid syndrome. *West J Med* 1991;155:174–176.

409. Blanc P, Barki J, Fabre J-M, et al. Superior mesenteric vein thrombosis associated with anticardiolipin antibody without autoimmune disease. *J Lab Invest* 1995;72:137.

410. England RJA, Woodcock B, Zeiderman MR. Superior mesenteric artery thrombosis in a patient with the antiphospholipid syndrome. *Eur J Vasc Endovasc Surg* 1995;10:372–373.

411. Vahl AC, Gans ROB, Mackaay AJC, et al. Superior mesenteric artery occlusion and peripheral emboli caused by an aortic ulcer in a young patient with antiphospholipid syndrome. *Surgery* 1997;121:588–590.

412. Cappell MS, Mikhail N, Gujral N. Gastrointestinal haemorrhage and intestinal ischaemia associated with anticardiolipin antibodies. *Dig Dis Sci* 1994;39:1359–1364.

413. Gül A, Inanc M, Öcal L, et al. Primary antiphospholipid syndrome associated with mesenteric inflammatory veno-occlusive disease. *Clin Rheumatol* 1996;15:207–210.

414. North JP, Wollenman OJ Jr. Venous mesenteric occlusion in the course of migratory thrombophlebitis. *Surg Gynaecol Obstet* 1952;95:665–667.

415. Wang R, Hsieh C, Leeg L, et al. Pancreatitis related to antiphospholipid antibody syndrome in a patient with systemic lupus erythematosus. *J Rheumatol* 1992;19:1223–1225.

416. Chang K-Y, Kuoy-C, Chiuc-T, et al. Anticardiolipin antibodies associated with acute haemorrhagic pancreatitis. *Pancreas* 1993;8:654–657.

417. Date K, Shirai Y, Hatakeyama K. Antiphospholipid antibody syndrome presenting as acute acalculous cholecystitis. *Am J Gastroenterol* 1997;92:2127–2128.

418. Arnold MH, Schreiber L. Splenic and renal infarction in systemic lupus erythematosus: association with anticardiolipin antibodies. *Clin Rheumatol* 1988;7:406–410.

419. Pettersson T, Julkunen H. Asplenia in a patient with systemic lupus erythematosus and antiphospholipid antibodies. *J Rheumatol* 1992;19:115.

420. Scott RAH. Anti-cardiolipin antibodies and preeclampsia. *Br J Obstet Gynecol* 1987;94:604–605.

421. Kilpatrick DC, Maclean C, Liston WA, et al. Antiphospholipid antibody syndrome and pre-eclampsia. *Lancet* 1989;1:987–988.

422. Ornstein MH, Rand JH. An association between refractory HELLP syndrome and antiphospholipid antibodies during pregnancy: a report of 2 cases. *J Rheumatol* 1994;21:1360–1364.

423. Huong DLT, Weschler B, Edelman P, et al. Postpartum cerebral infarction associated with aspirin withdrawal in the antiphospholipid antibody syndrome. *J Rheumatol* 1993;20:1229–1232.

424. Hochfeld M, Druzin ML, Maia D, et al. Pregnancy complicated by primary antiphospholipid antibody syndrome. *Obstet Gynecol* 1994;83:804–805.

425. Triplett DA. Antiphospholipid antibodies and recurrent pregnancy loss. *Am J Reprod Immunol* 1989;20:52–67.

426. Polzin WJ, Kopelman JN, Robinson RD, et al. The association of antiphospholipid antibodies with pregnancies complicated by fetal growth restriction. *Obstet Gynecol* 1991;78:1108–1011.

427. Sletnes KE, Wisloff F, Moe N, et al. Antiphospholipid antibodies in pre-eclamptic women: relation to growth retardation and neonatal outcome. *Acta Obstet Gynecol Scand* 1992;71:112–117.

428. Caruso A, DeCarolis S, Ferrazzani F, et al. Pregnancy outcome in relationship to uterine artery flow velocity waveforms and clinical characteristics in women with antiphospholipid syndrome. *Obstet Gynecol* 1993;82:970–977.

429. Silver RM, Draper ML, Byme JLB, et al. Unexplained elevations of maternal serum alpha-fetoprotein in women with antiphospholipid antibodies: a harbinger of fetal death. *Obstet Gynecol* 1994;83:150–155.

430. Roddy SM, Giang DW. Antiphospholipid antibodies and stroke in an infant. *Pediatrics* 1991;87:933–935.

431. Tabbutt S, Groswold WR, Ogino MT, et al. Multiple thromboses in a premature infant associated with maternal phospholipid antibody syndrome. *J Perinatol* 1994;14:66–70.

432. Lioté F, Meyer O. Osteoarticular manifestations in the antiphospholipid syndrome. In: Asherson RA, Cervera R, Piette J-C, et al., eds. *The antiphospholipid syndrome.* Boca Raton, FL: CRC Press, 1996:195–200.

433. Klippel TM, Stevens MB, Zizic TM, et al. Ischemic necrosis of bone in systemic lupus erythematosus. *Medicine* (Baltimore) 1976;55:251–257.

434. Zizic TM, Marcor K, Hungerford DS, et al. Corticosteroid therapy associated with ischemic necrosis of bone in systematic lupus erythematosus. *Lancet* 1987;1:902–906.

435. Massando L, Jacobelli S, Leissner M, et al. High dose intravenous methylprednisone therapy associated with osteonecrosis in patients with systemic lupus erythematosus. *Lupus* 1992;2:401–405.

436. Zizic TM, Hungerford DS, Stevens MB. Ischemic bone necrosis in systemic lupus erythematosus. II. The early diagnosis of ischemic necrosis of bone. *Medicine* (Baltimore) 1980;59:134–142.

437. Asherson RA, Jungers P, Lioté F, et al. Ischaemic necrosis of bone associated with the "lupus anticoagulant" and antibodies to cardiolipin. *Proceedings of the XVIth International Congress of Rheumatology.* Sydney, Australia, 1983:373.

438. Asherson RA, Lioté F, Page B, et al. Avascular necrosis of bone and antiphospholipid antibodies in systemic lupus erythematosus. *J Rheumatol* 1993;20:284–288.

439. Asherson RA, Khamashta MA, Ordi-Ros J, et al. The 'primary' antiphospholipid syndrome: major clinical and serological features. *Medicine* (Baltimore) 1989;68:366–374.

440. Seleznick MJ, Silveira LH, Espinoza LR. Avascular necrosis associated with anticardiolipin antibodies. *J Rheumatol* 1991;18:1416–1417.

441. Alijotas J, Argemí M, Barquinero J. Kienbock's disease and antiphospholipid antibodies. *Clin Exp Rheumatol* 1990;8:297–298.

442. Alarcón-Segovia D, Delez$fp M, Oria CV, et al. Antiphospholipid antibodies and the antiphospholipid syndrome in systemic lupus erythematosus: a prospective analysis of 500 patients. *Medicine* (Baltimore) 1989;68:353–365.

443. Picillo U, Migliaresi S, Marciolis MR, et al. Longitudinal survey of anticardiolipin antibodies in systemic lupus erythematosus: relationship with clinical manifestations and disease activity in an Italian series. *Scand J Rheumatol* 1992;21:271–276.

444. Petri M. Musculoskeletal complication of systemic lupus erythematosus in the Hopkins Lupus Cohort: an update. *Arthritis Care Res* 1995;18:137–145.

445. Houissau FA, N'Zeusseu-Toukap A, Depresseu XG, et al. Magnetic resonance imaging-detected, avascular necrosis in systemic lupus erythematosus: lack of correlation with antiphospholipid antibodies. *Br J Rheumatol* 1998;37:448–453.

446. Nagasawa K, Ishii Y, Mayumi T, et al. Avascular necrosis of bone in systemic lupus erythematosus: possible role of haemostatic abnormalities. *Ann Rheum Dis* 1989;48:672–676.

447. Mont MA, Glueck CJ, Pacheco IH, et al. Risk factors for osteonecrosis in systemic lupus erythematosus. *J Rheumatol* 1997;24:654–662.

448. Piette JC, Wechsler B, Francàs C, et al. Systemic lupus erythematosus and the antiphospholipid syndrome: reflections about the relevance of ARA criteria. *J Rheumatol* 1992;19:1835–1837.

449. Hughes GRV. Connective tissue disease and the skin. The Prosser-White Oration 1983. *Clin Exp Dermatol* 1984;9:535–544.

450. Vianna J, Khamashta M, Ordi-Ross J, et al. Comparison of the primary and the secondary antiphospholipid syndrome. European multicentre study of 114 patients. *Am J Med* 1994;96:3–9.

451. Asherson RA, Mayou SC, Merry P, et al. The spectrum of livedo reticularis and anticardiolipin antibodies. *Br J Dermatol* 1989;120:215–221.

452. Englert HJ, Loizou S, Derue GGH, et al. Clinical and immunologic features of livedo reticularis in lupus: a case-control study. *Am J Med* 1989;87:408–410.

453. McHugh MJ, Maymo H, Skinner RP, et al. Anticardiolipin antibodies, livedo reticularis and major cerebrovascular and renal disease in systemic lupus erythematosus. *Ann Rheum Dis* 1988;47:110–115.

454. Bard JW, Winkelman RK. Livedo vasculitis-segmental hyalinizing vasculitis of the dermis. *Arch Dermatol* 1967;96:489–499.

455. Englert HJ, Hawkes CH, Boey ML, et al. Degos' disease: association with anticardiolipin antibodies and the lupus anticoagulant. *Br Med J* 1989;576:1984.

456. Tishler M, Papo J, Taron M. Skin ulcer as the presenting symptoms of primary antiphospholipid syndrome: resolution with anticoagulant therapy. *Clin Rheumatol* 1995;14:112–114.

457. Johansson EA, Niemi KH, Hustakillio KK. A peripheral vascular syndrome overlapping with systemic lupus erythematosus. *Dermatologica* 1977;155:257–267.

458. Tuffanelli DL, Dubois EL. Cutaneous manifestations of systemic lupus erythematosus. *Arch Dermatol* 1984;90:377–386.

459. Lazareth I, Picaid C, Crickx B, et al. Ulcére de jambe révélant un lupus syst$fpmique avec anticoagulant circulant. *Ann Dermatol Venereol* 1990;117:855–856.

460. Bazex A, Bazex J, Boneau B, et al. Ulcére de jambe, anticoagulant circulant et lupus erythemateux aigu disséminé. *Bull Soc Fr Derm Syph* 1976;83:350–352.

461. Cuny JF, Schmutz JL, Jeandel C, et al. Ulcére de jambe et anticoagulant circulants. *Ann Dermatol Venereol* 1986;113:825.

462. Kleiner RC, Najarian IV, Schatten S, et al. Vaso-occlusive retinopathy associated with antiphospholipid antibodies (lupus anticoagulant retinopathy). *Ophthalmology* 1989;96:896–904.

463. Francàs C, Tribout B, Boisnic S, et al. Cutaneous necrosis associated with the lupus anticoagulant. *Dermatologica* 1989;178:194–201.

464. Dessein PH, Lamparelli RD, Phillips SA, et al. Severe immune thrombocytopenia and the development of skin infarctions in a patient with an overlap syndrome. *J Rheumatol* 1989;16:1494–1496.

465. Dodd HJ, Sarkany I, O'Shaughnessy D. Widespread cutaneous necrosis associated with the lupus anticoagulant. *Clin Exp Dermatol* 1985;10:581–586.

466. Aronoff DM, Callen JP. Necrosing livedo reticularis in a patient with recurrent pulmonary haemorrhage. *J Am Acad Dermatol* 1997;37:300–302.

467. Soweid M, Hajjar RR, Hewan-Low KO, et al. Skin necrosis indicating antiphospholipid syndrome in a patient with AIDS. *South Med J* 1995;88:786–788.

468. Del Castillo LF, Soria C, Schoendorff C, et al. Widespread cutaneous necrosis and antiphospholipid antibodies: Two episodes related to surgical manipulation and urinary tract infection. *J Am Acad Dermatol* 1997;36:872–875.

469. Amster MS, Conway J, Zeid M, et al. Cutaneous necrosis resulting in protein S deficiency and increased antiphospholipid antibody in a patient with systemic lupus erythematosus. *J Am Acad Dermatol* 1993;29:853–857.

470. Wolf P, Soyer P, Auer-Grumbach P, et al. Widespread cutaneous necrosis in a patient with rheumatoid arthritis associated with anticardiolipin antibodies. *Arch Dermatol* 1991;127:1739–1740.

471. Hill VA, Whittaker SJ, Hunt BJ, et al. Cutaneous necrosis associated with the antiphospholipid syndrome and mycosis fungoides. *Br J Dermatol* 1994;130:92–96.

472. Doff HJ, Sarkany I, O'Shaughnessy D. Widespread cutaneous necrosis associated with the lupus anticoagulant. *Clin Exp Dermatol* 1985;10:581–586.

473. Wattiaux H-J, Herve R, Robert A, et al. Coumarin-induced skin necrosis associated with acquired protein S deficiency and antiphospholipid antibody syndrome. *Arthritis Rheum* 1994;37:1096–1100.

474. Grobb JJ, Bonerandi JJ. Cutaneous manifestations associated with the presence of the lupus anticoagulant: a report of two cases and review of the literature. *J Am Acad Dermatol* 1986;15:211–219.

475. Asherson RA, Cervera R. Antiphospholipid syndrome. *J Invest Dermatol* 1993;100:21S–27S.

476. Asherson RA, Jacobelli S, Rosenberg H, et al. Skin nodules and macules resembling vasculitis in the antiphospholipid syndrome. *Clin Exp Dermatol* 1992;17:166–169.

477. Renfro L, Franks AG, Grudberg M, et al. Painful nodules in a young female: antiphospholipid syndrome [Technical Note]. *Arch Dermatol* 1992;128:847.

478. Asherson RA. Subungual splinter haemorrhages: a new sign of the antiphospholipid coagulopathy? *Ann Rheum Dis* 1990;49:268.

479. Williams H, Laurent R, Gibson T. The lupus coagulation inhibitor and venous thrombosis, a report of four cases. *Clin Lab Haematol* 1980;2:139.

480. Kleiner RC, Najarian IV, Schatten S, et al. Vaso-occlusive retinopathy associated with antiphospholipid antibodies (lupus anticoagulant retinopathy). *Ophthalmology* 1989;96:896–904.

481. Digre KB, Durcan FJ, Branch DW, et al. Amaurosis fugax associated with antiphospholipid antibodies. *Ann Neurol* 1989;25:228–232.

482. Francàs C, Piette J, Saada V, et al. Multiple subungual splinter haemorrhages in the antiphospholipid syndrome: a report of 5 cases and review of the literature. *Lupus* 1994;30:123–128.

483. Disdier P, Harle J, Andrac I, et al. Primary anetoderma with the antiphospholipid syndrome. *J Am Acad Dermatol* 1994;30:133–134.

484. Ruffatti A, Veller-Fornasa C, Patrassi GM, et al. Anticardiolipin antibodies and antiphospholipid syndrome in chronic discoid lupus erythematosus. *Clin Rheumatol* 1995;14:402–404.

485. Alarcón-Segovia D, Pérez-Vásquez M, Villa A, et al. Preliminary classification criteria in the antiphospholipid syndrome with systemic lupus erythematosus. *Semin Arthritis Rheum* 1992;21:275–286.

486. Zouboulis CC, Gollnick H, Weber S, et al. Intravascular coagulation necrosis of the skin associated with cryofibrinogenemia, diabetes mellitus and cardiolipin antibodies. *J Am Acad Dermatol* 1991;25:882–888.

487. Chacek S, MacGregor-Gooch J, Halabe-Cherem J, et al. Pyoderma gangrenosum and extensive canal thrombosis associated with the antiphospholipid syndrome. *Angiology* 1998;49:157–160.

488. Schlesinger IH, Farber GA. Cutaneous ulceration resembling pyoderma gangrenosum in the primary antiphospholipid syndrome: a report of two additional cases and review of the literature. *J La State Med Soc* 1995;147:357–361.

489. Harris EN, Asherson RA, Gharavi AE, et al. Thrombocytopenia in SLE and related autoimmune disorders: association with anticardiolipin antibody. *Br J Haematol* 1985;59:227–230.

490. Dessein PH, Lamparelli DR, Philips SA, et al. Severe immune thrombocytopenia and the development of skin infarctions in a patient with an overlap syndrome. *J Rheumatol* 1989;16:1494–1496.

491. Alarcón-Segovia D, Sánchez-Guerrero J. Correction of thrombocytopenia with small dose aspirin in the primary antiphospholipid syndrome. *J Rheumatol* 1989;16:1359–1361.

492. Locht H, Lindstöm FD, Merdere A. Large vessel occlusion, cerebral infarction, and thrombocytopenia in the "primary" antiphospholipid syndrome. Response to anticoagulation. *Clin Exp Rheumatol* 1991; 9:169–172.

493. Alarcón-Segovia D. Pathogenic potential of antiphospholipid antibodies. *J Rheumatol* 1988;15:890–893.

494. Kelley RE, Gilman PB, Kovacs AG. Cerebral ischaemia in the presence of the lupus anticoagulant. *Arch Neurol* 1984;41:521–523.

495. Hazeltine M, Rauch J, Danoff D, et al. Antiphospholipid antibodies in systemic lupus erythematosus: evidence of an association with positive Coombs' and hypocomplementaemia. *J Rheumatol* 1988;15:80–86.

496. Delezé M, Oria CV, Alarcón-Segovia D. Occurrence of both hemolytic anemia and thrombocytopenic purpura (Evans' syndrome) in systemic lupus erythematosus: relationship to antiphospholipid antibodies. *J Rheumatol* 1988;15:611–615.

497. Cervera R, Font J, López-Soto A, et al. Isotype distribution if anticardiolipin antibodies in systemic lupus erythematosus: prospective analysis of a series of 100 patients. *Ann Rheum Dis* 1990;49:109–113.

498. Asherson RA, Cervera R, Font J. Multiorgan thrombotic disorders in systemic lupus erythematosus: a common link? *Lupus* 1992;1:199–203.

499. Ingram SB, Goodnight SH, Bennett RM. An unusual syndrome of devastating non-inflammatory vasculopathy associated with anticardiolipin antibodies: report of two cases. *Arthritis Rheum* 1987;30: 1167–1171.

500. Greisman SG, Thayaparan R-S, Godwin TA, et al. Occlusive vasculopathy in systemic lupus erythematosus associated with anticardiolipin antibodies. *Arch Intern Med* 1991;151:389–392.

501. Harris EN, Bos K. An acute disseminated coagulopathy-vasculopathy associated with the antiphospholipid syndrome. *Arch Intern Med* 1991;151:231–233.

502. Asherson RA, Piette J-C. The catastrophic antiphospholipid syndrome 1996: acute multi-organ failure associated with antiphospholipid antibodies. A review of 31 patients. *Lupus* 1996;5:414–417.

503. Hess DC, Sethi K, Awad E. Thrombocytopenic purpura in systemic lupus erythematosus and antiphospholipid antibodies: effective treatment with plasma exchange and immunosuppression. *J Rheumatol* 1992;19:1474–1478.

504. D'Agati V, Kunia C, Williams G, et al. Anticardiolipin antibody in renal disease: a report of three cases. *J Am Soc Nephrol* 1990;1: 777–784.

505. Becquemont L, Thervet E, Rondeau E, et al. Systemic and renal fibrinolytic activity in a patient with anticardiolipin syndrome and renal thrombotic microangiopathy. *Am J Nephrol* 1990;10:254–258.

506. Amigo MC, García M-C, García-Torres R, et al. Renal involvement in primary antiphospholipid syndrome. *J Rheumatol* 1992;19:1181–1185.

507. Jain R, Chartash E, Susin M, et al. Systemic lupus erythematosus complicated by thrombotic microangiopathy. *Semin Arthritis Rheum* 1994;24:173–182.

508. Kniaz D, Eisenberg GM, Elrad H, et al. Postpartum hemolytic-uremic syndrome associated with antiphospholipid antibodies. *Am J Nephrol* 1992;12:126–133.

509. Huang J-J, Chen M-W, Sung JM, et al. Postpartum hemolytic uremic syndrome associated with antiphospholipid antibody. *Nephrol Dial Transplant* 1998;13:182–186.

510. Karmochkine M, Mazoyer E, Marcelli A, et al. High prevalence of antiphospholipid antibodies in disseminated intravascular coagulation. *Thromb Haemost* 1996;75:971–982.

511. Branch DWS, Anders R, Digre KB, et al. The association of antiphospholipid antibodies with severe pre-eclampsia. *Obstet Gynecol* 1989; 73:J41–J45.

512. Ornstein MH, Rand JH. An association between refractory HELLP syndrome and antiphospholipid antibodies during pregnancy: a report of 2 cases. *J Rheumatol* 1994;21:1360–1364.

513. Brandt JT, Triplett DA, Alving B, et al. Criteria for the diagnosis of lupus anticoagulants: an update. *Thromb Haemost* 1995;74: 1185–1190.

514. Wasserman A, Neisser A, Bruck C. Eine serodiagnostiche reaktion bei syphilis. *Dtsch Med Wochenschr* 1906;32:745.

515. López-Soto A, Cervera R, Font J, et al. Isotype distribution and clinical significance of antibodies to cardiolipin, phosphatidic acid, phophatidylinositol and phosphatidylserine in systemic lupus erythematosus: prospective analysis of a series of 92 patients. *Clin Exp Rheumatol* 1997;15:143–149.

516. Font J, López-Soto A, Cervera R, et al. Antibodies to thromboplastin in systemic lupus erythematosus: isotype distribution and clinical significance in a series of 92 patients. *Thromb Res* 1997;86:37–48.

517. McNeil HD, Simpson RJ, Chesterman CN, et al. Antiphospholipid antibodies are directed against a complex antigen that includes a lipid-binding inhibitor of coagulation: beta-2-glycoprotein I (apolipoprotein H). *Proc Natl Acad Sci U S A* 1990;87:4120–4124.

518. Galli M, Confurius P, Maassen C, et al. Anticardiolipin antibodies (ACA) directed not to cardiolipin but to a plasma protein cofactor. *Lancet* 1990;335:1544–1547.

519. Matsuura H, Igarasha T, Fujimoto M, et al. Anticardiolipin cofactor(s) and differential diagnosis of autoimmune disease. *Lancet* 1990;336: 117–118.

520. Teixidó M, Font J, Reverter JC, et al. Anti-β2-glycoprotein I antibodies: a useful marker for the antiphospholipid syndrome. *Br J Rheumatol* 1997;36:113–116.

521. Roubey RAS. Immunology of the antiphospholipid antibody syndrome. *Arthritis Rheum* 1996;39:1444–1454.

522. Joseph J, Scopelitis E. Seronegative antiphospholipid syndrome associated with plasminogen activator inhibitor. *Lupus* 1994;3:201–203.

523. Miret C, Cervera R, Reverter JC, et al. Antiphospholipid syndrome without antiphospholipid antibodies at the time of thrombotic event: transient 'seronegative' antiphospholipid syndrome? *Clin Exp Rheumatol* 1997;15:541–544.

524. Frampton G, Winer JP, Cameron JS, et al. Severe Guillain-Barré syndrome: an association with IgA anticardiolipin antibody in a series of 92 patients. *J Neuroimmunol* 1988;19:133–139.

525. Gharavi AE, Harris EN, Asherson RA, et al. Anticardiolipin antibodies: isotype distribution and phospholipid specificity. *Ann Rheum Dis* 1987;46:1–6.

526. Pérez-Vβzquez ME, Cabiedes J, Cabral AR, et al. Decrease in serum antiphospholipid antibody levels upon development of nephrotic syndrome in patients with systemic lupus erythematosus: relationship to urinary loss of IgG and other factors. *Am J Med* 1992;92:357–363.

527. Silveira LH, Jara LJ, Espinoza LR. Transient disappearance of serum antiphospholipid antibodies can also be due to prednisone therapy. *Clin Exp Rheumatol* 1996;14:217–226.

528. Drenkard C, Sánchez-Guerrero J, Alarcón-Segovia D. Fall in antiphospholipid antibody at time of thromboocclusive episodes in systemic lupus erythematosus. *J Rheumatol* 1989;16:614–617.

529. Schulman S, Svenungsson E, Granqvist S. Anticariolipid antibodies predict early occurence of thromboembolism and death maong patients with venous thromboembolism following anticoagulant therapy. Duration of Anticoagulation Study Group. *Am J Med* 1998;104:332–338.

530. Khamashta MA, Cuadrado MJ, Mujic F, et al. The management of thrombosis in the antiphospholipid-antibody syndrome. *N Engl J Med* 1995;332:993–997.

531. Rosove MH, Brewer PM. Antiphospholipid thrombosis: clinical course after the first thrombotic event in 70 patients. *Ann Intern Med* 1992;117:303–308.

532. Hunt BJ, Khamashta MA. Management of the Hughes syndrome. *Clin Exp Rheumatol* 1996;14:115–117.

533. Balasch J, Carmona F, López-Soto A, et al. Low-dose aspirin for prevention of pregnancy losses in women with primary antiphospholipid syndrome. *Hum Reprod* 1993;8:2234–2239.

534. Lima F, Khamashta MA, Buchanan NMM, et al. A study of sixty pregnancies in patients with the antiphospholipid syndrome. *Clin Exp Rheumatol* 1996;14:131–136.

535. Alarcón-Segovia D, Sβnchez-Guerrero J. Correction of thrombocytopenia with small dose aspirin in the primary antiphospholipid syndrome. *J Rheumatol* 1989;16:1359–1361.

536. Yamazaki M, Asakura H, Matsuda T. Resolution of thrombocytopenia in a patient with lupus anticoagulant who received warfarin therapy. *Acta Haematol* 1994;92:52–53.

537. Kavanaugh A. Danazol therapy in thrombocytopenia associated with the antiphospholipid antibody syndrome. *Ann Intern Med* 1994;121: 767–768.

538. Moake JL. Moschowitz, multimers and metalloprotease [Editorial]. *N Engl J Med* 1998;339:1629–1631.

*Textbook of the Autoimmune Diseases,*
Edited by R. G. Lahita, N. Chiorazzi, and W. H. Reeves,
Lippincott Williams & Wilkins, Philadelphia © 2000.

# CHAPTER 35

# Hepatitis C–Associated Autoimmunity

Robert W. McMurray

Within the past several years, a broad spectrum of extrahepatic immune and autoimmune perturbations have been associated with HCV infection. Although causality remains to be clearly established, this chapter presents basic information regarding HCV infection, clinical presentations of HCV-associated immune and autoimmune abnormalities, HCV diagnostic testing, and potential therapeutic strategies and toxicities.

## INCIDENCE AND EPIDEMIOLOGY

Hepatitis C virus (HCV) is a linear, single-stranded RNA virus with extensive genomic variability. There are six different subtypes that have unknown significance to the development of hepatic or extrahepatic disease. A patient may be infected by more than one HCV subtype at the same time. Transmission is typically parenteral or through the exchange of bodily fluids, although the mode of transmission remains obscure in half of cases. Demographic groups at greatest risk for HCV infection include those with a history of blood transfusion, intravenous drug use, sexual promiscuity, sexual and household contacts of HCV-infected patients, or low socioeconomic status. Persistent infection occurs in 50% to 80% of those infected and may lead to the development of chronic liver disease, cirrhosis, or hepatocellular carcinoma (1–5). The prevalence of antibody to HCV in the general population of the United States is about 1.8%, corresponding to an estimated 3.9 million Americans infected with HCV. Apparently, only 25% to 30% of HCV infections are sufficiently symptomatic to gain medical attention. An estimated 8000 to 10,000 deaths each year are attributed to HCV-associated chronic liver disease (4–6).

Autoimmune perturbations in patients with HCV infection are significant (7–12). Seventy percent of HCV infected patients may have autoantibody formation, and 20% to 30% may have detectable manifestations of autoimmunity. Examination of extrahepatic immunologic abnormalities in HCV-infected patients has demonstrated antinuclear antibody (ANA) seropositivity (22%), cryoglobulinemia (36%), anti-tissue antibodies (41%), lymphocytic capillaritis of the salivary gland (49%), and rheumatoid factor seropositivity (71%) (13,14). Conversely, a number of rheumatologic-based studies have examined autoimmune disease populations for HCV infection with conflicting results. Anti-HCV antibodies were found in 26% of patients with autoimmune disorders and 36% of patients with idiopathic thrombocytopenic purpura (15). A 14% to 20% prevalence of HCV infection was detected in patients with Sjögren's syndrome (16,17). A separate study of ANA and anti-SSA/anti-SSB–positive Sjögren's syndrome patients did not, however, find anti-HCV antibodies or HCV RNA (18). Comparably, only four of 71 patients with systemic lupus erythematosus (SLE) had anti-HCV antibodies (19), and only 10% of dermatomyositis (DM) patients were believed to have had HCV infection (20). These rates are higher than, but not significantly different from, those found in the general population.

Small-scale studies (less than 50 patients) have not routinely detected HCV infection at a rate significantly different than that in control populations. Thus, HCV infection does not appear to be a common cause of autoimmunity but may be associated with autoimmune diseases in one of every 10 to 20 patients in defined populations. The importance of detecting HCV-associated autoimmunity is founded in vigilance for potential hepatic and extrahepatic manifestations; sequelae of HCV infection such as cirrhosis, hepatocellular carcinoma, and hematologic malignancy; choice of therapeutic intervention; and potential exacerbation of HCV infection by immunosuppression of autoimmune disease.

## CLINICAL PRESENTATION

An autoimmune response to HCV infection is likely multifactorial. Data suggest that resolution of HCV infection

R.W. McMurray: Department of Medicine, University of Mississippi Medical Center, Jackson, Mississippi 39216; Department of Medicine, G. V. (Sonny) Montgomery Veterans Affairs Hospital, Jackson, Mississippi 39216.

occurs in patients whose antibody response to viral antigens HVR-1 or E2/NS is brisk and that infection tends toward chronicity in patients with a delayed antibody response (21–23). In chronic infection, HCV antigenemia persists, leading to a fluctuating pattern of transaminitis in which one third of the infected population have normal liver enzymes (3–5). The immunologic response and clinical presentation of HCV infection appear to be determined by major histocompatibility complex class II genotypes (24,25). For example, patients with HLA-DR3 and chronic hepatitis had higher serum immunoglobulin and a three-fold greater frequency of severe liver disease than HLA-DR4 hepatitis patients. In contrast, chronic viral hepatitis patients with HLA-DR4 genotype had a five-fold increased incidence of concurrent immunologic disease (26).

HCV disease manifestations are probably independent of HCV subtype (27,28). HCV-initiated immune responses result in immune complexes that are deposited in liver, skin (29), or kidney (30). These complexes contain HCV antigens and antibodies, rheumatoid factor, and the third component of complement (C3) (31). The role of T cells in HCV infection has not been completely elucidated, although a more vigorous peripheral blood mononuclear cell reaction to HCV core antigen correlates with a more benign course of infection (1). HCV-infected patients have significantly elevated serum interleukin-2 (IL-2), IL-4, IL-10, and interferon-γ (IFN-γ) compared with healthy subjects; treatment with IFN-γ produces a parallel reduction in HCV RNA, IL-4, and IL-10 (32). These immune perturbations in response to HCV infection may lead to a variety of autoantibody and clinical autoimmune syndromes, as described later.

### Autoantibody Formation

Autoantibody formation occurs frequently in association with HCV infection (Table 35.1). About 10% to 30% of chronically infected HCV patients have low-titer ANA, 60% to 70% have anti–smooth muscle antibodies (anti-SMA), and 60% to 80% have positive rheumatoid factors. ANA seropositivity and hypergammaglobulinemia were more common in chronic HCV infection than in hepatitis B infection, and the increased prevalence occurred in association with HLA-DR4 (26,33,34). Anticardiolipin antibodies (ACAs) have been detected in 22% of HCV-infected patients (35), and antineu-

**TABLE 35.1.** *Autoantibodies in association with hepatitis C virus*

Cryoglobulins
Rheumatoid factor
Antinuclear antibodies
Anticardiolipin antibodies
Antineutrophil cytoplasmic antibodies
Antithyroid antibodies
Anti–smooth muscle or anti–liver-kidney-microsomal antibodies

trophil cytoplasmic antibodies have also been reported (36). Chronic HCV infection has been associated with the development of the autoimmune hepatitis (AH)–associated anti–liver-kidney-microsomal (anti-LKM) autoantibody, although the reactivity of this autoantibody may be slightly different from that of classic AH anti-LKM (37,38). Antithyroid antibodies have also been associated with HCV infection (39).

### Cryoglobulinemia

Cryoglobulinemia was the initial and most widely recognized extrahepatic manifestation of HCV infection (40,41). Cryoglobulins are antiimmunoglobulin immunoglobulins that reversibly precipitate at reduced temperatures. They occur in a variety of diseases and are grouped into two general categories: type I, consisting of a single monoclonal immunoglobulin (e.g., multiple myeloma and macroglobulinemia); and type II, consisting of more than one class of immunoglobulin. Mixed cryoglobulins usually contain immunoglobulin M (IgM) and IgG, with the IgM having rheumatoid factor activity directed against IgG molecules. This leads to immune complex formation, cryoprecipitation, and glomerulonephritis (GN) or vasculitis. Type II cryoglobulinemia has been classified as either essential or secondary to connective tissue diseases, infections, or chronic liver disease.

Cutaneous lesions are common and include palpable purpura, urticaria, and ulcers as well as arthralgias, peripheral neuropathy, hepatosplenomegaly, and lymphadenopathy (42). Mixed essential cryoglobulinemia has been associated strongly with HCV infection and presents in the classic fashion of mixed cryoglobulinemia (40,41). The cryoglobulinemic immune responses to HCV infection include purpura, urticaria, and livedo reticularis; glomerulonephritis; vasculitis; and mononeuritis multiplex (43–48). Improvement in HCV-induced cryoglobulinemic manifestations occurs during treatment with IFN-α (49) as well as treatment with glucocorticoids or cytotoxic agents (50). IFN-α therapy, however, may worsen HCV-related cryoglobulinemia (51).

### Antiphospholipid Antibody Syndrome

Several reports have emerged describing an association of ACAs and clinical thrombosis in the setting of HCV infection (35,52–54). Occult HCV infection is present in a significant number of patients with thrombotic disorders and ACAs. Conversely, ACAs are more common in HCV patients and have a strong association with thrombocytopenia, thrombosis, and portal hypertension in these patients. Markers of HCV infection were present in 17% of patients with thrombotic episodes; clinical evidence of liver disease was rare (35). Whether HCV-induced ACAs are the basis of this association is confounded by the observation that HCV increases thrombin production from the liver, resulting in an increased coagulable state (55). IFN-α had been shown to be effective in the treatment of HCV-associated ACA syndrome in reducing HCV viremia and without further evidence of thrombotic events (53), although the most appropriate treatment remains to be determined.

## Glomerulonephritis

HCV-associated GN has been documented and includes membranous, membranoproliferative, and acute proliferative glomerular disease (56–59) as well as that associated with cryoglobulinemia (40–41). HCV antibody prevalence is significantly higher in patients with GN than in those with other types of renal disease (e.g., interstitial nephritis) and in control subjects (60). Primary risk factors for HCV-related GN include a history of intravenous drug abuse or blood transfusion (57). In an investigation of 34 patients who presented with proteinuria and circulating anti-HCV antibodies, most had nephrotic syndrome; the remaining one third had nonnephrotic proteinuria and membranoproliferative or acute proliferative GN on renal biopsy. Signs of clinical liver disease were absent in most patients, and one third had normal serum transaminases (58).

Most patients with HCV-related GN have evidence of hypocomplementemia, circulating rheumatoid factors, or cryoglobulinemia. Hypocomplementemia probably results from circulating HCV immune complex deposition (59). Immune deposits, virus-like particles, and HCV RNA have been detected in the renal tissue of patients with GN (61,62). The association of autoantibodies, immune complex deposition, hypocomplementemia, cutaneous disease, and GN suggest a diagnosis of SLE (63); however, few cases have been reported of HCV coincident with SLE, and HCV infection was not detected in 14 cases of lupus nephritis (57).

Treatment with IFN-α improves proteinuria, suppresses viremia, and stabilizes renal function in HCV infection; however, patients often relapse after discontinuation of therapy (58). There may be an advantage in using plasmapheresis in the treatment of hepatitis-related GN, in combination with IFN-α or corticosteroids (64,65), but that remains to be proved. Alternatively, HCV-associated membranoproliferative GN has been treated successfully with cyclophosphamide (66).

## Vasculitis

Numerous case reports have suggested an association between HCV and vasculitis (67–79), with most cases presenting as a leukocytoclastic vasculitis secondary to an HCV-induced cryoglobulinemia. Patients with HCV-associated vasculitis may have palpable purpura, urticaria, or livedo reticularis (45). HCV RNA is detectable in the skin of patients presenting with an associated vasculitis (71,74). Mononeuritis multiplex is a common presentation of cryoglobulinemia in association with HCV infection (78); unique vasculitic presentations included pulmonary (68) and intestinal (70) vasculitis. HCV infection may be detected before the development of vasculitis, subsequent to the presentation of vasculitis, or coincident in diagnosis. Rheumatoid factor was

present in about half of the referenced cases. IFN therapy was initiated in many of these cases and may result in improvement without a decrease in cryoglobulins (76). Some cases (67,68,73) showed no improvement with IFN therapy, whereas the remainder generally had reduction in serum transaminases, cryoglobulinemia, and symptoms and signs of vasculitis. Immunosuppression with glucocorticoids or cytotoxic agents improved cryoglobulinemic manifestations in some patients (67); however, in a patient with anticytoplasmic neutrophil antibody–positive vasculitis, immunosuppression activated a latent HCV infection (79).

## Systemic Lupus Erythematosus

About 10% to 30% of chronic HCV patients have ANA seropositivity (33,34,37); conversely, the percentage of ANA-positive patients who have HCV antibodies is unknown. A study of ANA-positive patients who were anti-SSA/anti-SSB antibody positive yielded no HCV-positive patients by enzyme immunoassay (EIA), recombinant immunoblot assay (RIBA), or HCV RNA by polymerase chain reaction (PCR) (18). Abnormal serum transaminases and hepatitis occur frequently in SLE (80), suggesting that HCV may be a causative agent in some patients diagnosed with SLE.

A case of SLE associated with hepatitis B and HCV infection has been reported (81). A woman with the acute onset of SLE coincident with the diagnosis of HCV has been described whose presentation was classic for SLE, with mild hepatitis, arthritis, membranoproliferative GN, and positive ANA. HCV was diagnosed by RIBA and PCR for HCV RNA. She refused IFN therapy but responded partially to corticosteroids and cyclophosphamide, although nephrotic-range proteinuria persisted (82). A similar case report and therapeutic dilemma has been documented (83). In an investigation of HCV seropositivity in consecutive SLE patients on corticosteroids and immunosuppressive agents, Marchesoni et al. reported four patients (6% incidence rate) with HCV seropositivity, which was greater than but not significantly different from the expected incidence for the general population in their geographic area (19). Three of four patients had a history of hepatitis, but none had elevated transaminases at the time of the study. All had positive ANA, but interestingly, none had a positive rheumatoid factor. Patient genotyping was not performed. Only one false-positive HCV case (confirmed by negative RIBA and PCR) was found in this group of SLE patients. Given the association of HCV with autoantibody formation, immune complex deposition, hypocomplementemia, cutaneous lesions, and GN, HCV infection should be suspected as mimicking SLE in a patient presenting with hepatitis, a prior history of hepatitis, or risk factors for HCV infection.

## Arthralgias and Rheumatoid Arthritis

Polyarthralgias and polyarthritis have been associated with HCV infection (84,85), and HCV RNA has been isolated from synovial fluid (86). Polyarthralgias may occur during the acute stage of HCV infection and resolve despite the persistent circulating HCV RNA and anti-HCV antibodies. Alternatively, polyarthritis may occur in the setting of chronic HCV infection and liver disease. Polyarthralgias and myalgias may be a manifestation of chronic HCV infection or may be the presenting complaint (84–91). Rheumatoid arthritis (88–92) and adult-onset Still's disease (93) have been reported to occur after HCV infection.

In six patients (five men and one woman) with chronic HCV and polyarthralgias and myalgias, two had a positive rheumatoid factor, three had positive ANA without anti-DNA antibodies, five had low serum complement, and four had a cryoprecipitate (87). The high frequency of rheumatoid factor seropositivity (approaching 70%) in HCV-infected patients may make distinction of rheumatoid arthritis from the polyarthritis of HCV difficult, particularly in the setting of normal serum transaminases, as occurs in up to one third of HCV-infected patients.

It appears as though HCV arthropathy may be associated with or without erosions. Distinguishing features may include carpal tunnel syndrome and palmar tenosynovitis. The optimal treatment for HCV-associated polyarthritis has not been determined, but gold, methotrexate, prednisone, and hydroxychloroquine (84–91) have been used with modest success and minimal complications. Responses of rheumatoid arthritis or polyarthritis to IFN-α are not well documented. Although liver histology was not examined, serum transaminases were only modestly elevated and eventually reduced by rheumatoid arthritis remittive therapy with methotrexate in one HCV patient (84).

Studies have suggested that HCV infection may be present in 15% of patients meeting criteria for the diagnosis of fibromyalgia, compared to only 5% of those with rheumatoid arthritis (94). Fibromyalgia appears to be a common manifestation of HCV infection (94,95). Most fibromyalgia patients had normal serum liver enzyme concentrations and no distinguishing clinical characteristics (94).

## Polymyositis and Dermatomyositis

Polymyositis (PM) and DM are inflammatory diseases of striated skeletal muscle, the cause of which is unknown, although multiple viral causes have been implicated (96). Case reports suggest associations of PM and DM with HCV (20,97–101). Nishikai et al. (20) reported a patient who developed DM after infection with HCV, and a small-scale survey demonstrated an HCV seropositive incidence of 10% in patients with PM and DM patients, which was increased, but not significantly different, from a control group. In each case, patients exhibited proximal muscle weakness, elevated serum muscle enzymes, and hepatitis in the setting of anti-HCV antibodies; none of the reports demonstrated HCV in muscle. One report associated HCV infection with Jo-1 autoantibody–positive PM and pulmonary fibrosis (97). An association between interstitial lung disease and HCV infection has been proposed (102,103).

Although IFN-α therapy could be considered for treating PM and DM associated with HCV infection and has improved myositis in some of the referenced cases, it appears to have precipitated myositis in others (104,105). Immunosuppression with corticosteroids and cytotoxic agents has been successful in the setting of HCV-related myositis (97), but long-term sequelae of immunosuppression use in HCV infection are unknown. No causal relationship has been firmly established between HCV and PM or DM in any of these cases; however, these reports suggest that the immune response to HCV infection or HCV itself may be important in the pathogenesis of some cases of inflammatory myopathy.

## Sjögren's Syndrome

HCV has been reported to occur in 10% to 20% of patients with Sjögren's syndrome (16,17,106,107); however, others (18,108–111) have refuted this finding. It appears that primary Sjögren's syndrome, if defined as sicca syndrome in the presence of anti-SSA (anti-Ro)/anti-SSB (anti-La) autoantibodies, is only sporadically associated with HCV infection. Conversely, chronic HCV infection has been associated frequently with sialoadenitis and occasionally with sicca symptoms (112–115). It appears as though sialoadenitis in HCV infection is less severe than classic Sjögren's syndrome, associated with cryoglobulinemia and purpura, and is typically anti-SSA/anti-SSB negative (16,113–115). In delineating a causal relationship, transgenic mice expressing HCV envelope proteins developed an exocrinopathy resembling sialoadenitis (116), implicating HCV as a cause of Sjögren's syndrome.

Perhaps more important is the pathogenic overlap of the increased risk of B-cell malignancies in Sjögren's syndrome (117) and the emergence of an association between HCV infection and monoclonal gammopathies and lymphoproliferative disorders, such as low-grade, non-Hodgkin's lymphomas (118–125). In patients with HCV and cryoglobulinemia, 39% were shown to have low-grade non-Hodgkin's lymphoma by bone marrow biopsy (121). DeVita et al. (122) demonstrated HCV RNA within the lymphoma of a parotid gland. Clonal IgG rearrangements were shown to occur in all HCV-infected patients with cryoglobulinemia and in 24% of patients without cryoglobulinemia. Rheumatoid factor serum levels were increased in all patients with clonal expansion, suggesting that the expanded B-cell clones belong to the rheumatoid factor B-cell subset (123). The causal relationship of HCV-associated malignancies may be related to chronic immune stimulation caused by persistent HCV viremia resulting in benign proliferation of B cells, which may ultimately mutate into low-grade malignancies (126).

## Thyroid Disease

HCV may induce autoimmune thyroid disease (127–130), although this association has also been refuted (131–133). Although it is evident that HCV infection is associated with a high prevalence of thyroid autoantibodies (39,127–130), a significantly lower percentage have autoimmune thyroid dysfunction (39). A more striking association of autoimmune thyroid disease in the setting of HCV infection has emerged during IFN-α treatment. IFN-α therapy induced thyroid autoantibodies in HCV-infected patients and precipitated thyroid dysfunction in patients with existing autoantibodies (134–137). Exacerbation of thyroid autoimmunity may be associated with preexistent antimicrosomal antibodies (137). Discontinuation of IFN-α led to resolution of thyroid autoimmunity in most cases. IFN-α administration appears to have a deleterious effect on an already increased incidence of thyroid autoimmunity in HCV-infected patients.

## Autoimmune Hepatitis

AH is a heterogeneous, chronic, active hepatitis that occurs predominantly in young women with a Eurocaucasian-background HLA-DR3 genotype. AH is manifest clinically by modestly elevated serum liver transaminases, hepatosplenomegaly, progressive jaundice, anorexia, weakness, spider angiomas, and palmar erythema. The most common extrahepatic manifestations are arthralgias and skin rashes. AH has been characterized by hypergammaglobulinemia and autoantibodies, the absence of viral hepatitis markers, and a beneficial response to glucocorticoids. AH is commonly divided into two, and occasionally three, subsets based on serologic classifications. Type I AH is also known as *classic autoimmune* or *lupoid hepatitis* and is characterized by the presence of anti–SMA (100% of patients) and antinuclear autoantibodies (70% to 100% of patients). Type 2 AH is characterized by the presence of anti–LKM autoantibodies and the absence of ANAs. The third subset is characterized by the presence of antibodies to soluble liver antigens (SLAs), occasional anti-SMA, and the absence of ANAs (138).

A controversial but probable role for HCV infection in AH is emerging (139–144). It is likely that a subset of AH patients have hepatitis with autoimmune features secondary to HCV infection, and it has been suggested that ANA, anti-SMA, and anti-LKM are no longer specific for the diagnosis of AH (143). AH patients generally have more symptoms, are younger at time of onset (144), and have fewer lymphoid follicles and more severe inflammation and cirrhosis on liver biopsy (145) than patients with HCV-induced hepatitis.

Although it is intuitive that differentiation of HCV infection from AH would have important therapeutic implications (146), a favorable response of HCV-induced hepatitis to prednisone alone or in combination with azathioprine (147) has been reported, with only minimally increased expression of hepatic HCV RNA (148). Liver transplantation of HCV-infected patients frequently results in a 10- to 20-fold increase in HCV RNA levels after transplantation, presumably because of the effects of immunosuppression (149). There is a report of fulminant hepatic necrosis leading to death in an HCV patient with multiple sclerosis treated with cyclosporine (150). In contrast, patients with HCV-induced hepatitis or AH do not differ in response to antiviral therapy (144).

## Miscellaneous Associations

Immune and autoimmune associations with HCV infection have been considered for autoimmune hemolysis and thrombocytopenia (15,151,152), abdominal lymphadenopathy (153), Behçet's syndrome (154), myasthenia gravis (155), and idiopathic cardiomyopathy (156); these reports await further evidence and verification.

## DIAGNOSTIC TESTING

Viral antigen is detectable by PCR within 2 weeks of exposure, and serum liver transaminases rise 4 to 6 weeks after exposure. HCV may elevate liver enzymes only minimally or transiently, which is a clinical and epidemiologic problem, in that serum transaminases may be normal despite HCV infection, even in the setting of histologically proven cirrhosis (1,2). Antibody seroconversion appears subsequent to both viremia and onset of liver disease; however, antibody response is highly variable, and antibody seroconversion does not prevent chronic infection or active hepatitis (1–4). Diagnostic testing for HCV infection identifies the presence of anti-HCV antibodies in the sera of infected patients using EIA and RIBA. The sensitivity of second- and third-generation HCV EIA appears to be about 85% to 95%. False-positive results may occur in the setting of hyperglobulinemia, rheumatoid factor seropositivity, or recent influenza vaccination. Studies have shown, however, that a positive anti-HCV EIA result with two different commercial kits is virtually diagnostic. Additionally, the presence of anti-HCV antibodies by the highly sensitive and specific second- or third-generation (RIBA-2 or RIBA-3) assays in the presence of elevated serum transaminase levels is believed to be diagnostic of HCV infection. Among high-risk populations or EIA-reactive patients with elevated liver enzymes, confirmation of HCV infection by RIBA approaches 95% to 100%. The specificity of HCV RIBA appears to be unaffected by the presence of cryoglobulins. The emergence of third-generation EIA and RIBA assays has improved sensitivity slightly, but specificity is already high, approaching the gold standard of HCV RNA detection by PCR technology. Reverse transcription PCR is the most sensitive technique for the diagnosis of HCV infection. The detection and quantitation of HCV RNA has become more important as a determinant of treatment choices and therapeutic success (157–160).

Although a positive RIBA and elevated liver enzymes diagnose HCV infection, there is no reliable correlation between serum enzyme concentration and the degree of liver injury. Liver biopsy in HCV-infected patients may be useful for gauging disease severity and excluding other causes of hepatitis. Characteristic morphologic features of HCV infection include steatosis, lymphoid aggregation within the portal triads, and infiltration of the interlobular bile ducts with lymphocytes and plasma cells, in contrast to the finding in AH, in which the lymphoid aggregation is periportal (145,161,162). For clinical purposes, a positive anti-HCV

EIA in the setting of normal or abnormal liver enzyme tests followed by a confirmatory RIBA is the most common diagnostic pathway. Liver biopsy and determination of HCV RNA should be considered in atypical cases and in situations that influence therapeutic decisions.

## TREATMENT OF INFECTION WITH INTERFERON-α

The only FDA approved treatment for HCV infection is IFN-α, 3 million units three times per week for 24 or 48 weeks. Retreatment of failures is being investigated. Generally speaking, about 25% of patients do not exhibit a response to IFN, as defined by a reduction in serum liver enzyme levels and HCV RNA; 25% show a partial response to therapy but relapse when IFN administration is stopped; and 50% respond favorably. If serum transaminase levels have not normalized after 12 weeks of treatment, there appears to be no advantage to continued treatment for 24 weeks. A favorable response, defined by a near normalization of serum transaminase levels and reduction in HCV RNA, may be predicted by younger age, female sex, low body weight, and shorter duration of disease as well as minimal hepatic fibrosis, absence of cirrhosis, and low levels of circulating HCV RNA. IFN-α has been shown to reduce cryoglobulins and improve associated proteinuria, vasculitis, and neuropathy (163–167). Alternative or adjuvant therapy with amantadine or ursodeoxycholic acid is being examined (168,169).

Conversely, IFN-α has been shown to have no effect, to precipitate, or to worsen a variety of autoimmune diseases, including vasculitis, myositis, sicca syndrome, myasthenia gravis, and thyroiditis (170–174). Acute and chronic adverse side effects from IFN-α therapy may occur. Side effects occurring during the first 2 weeks of administration include fever, chills, myalgias, anorexia, and an influenza-like syndrome. Long-term administration results in leukopenia and thrombocytopenia, precipitation of autoantibodies, alopecia, lupus-like autoimmune disease, vasculitis, severe psychological disturbances, and an increased incidence of bacterial infections. The cost of a full course of self-administered IFN-α therapy, inclusive of diagnostic liver biopsy, is approximated between $5000 to $10,000 (163–167,175). A preliminary cost-effective analysis demonstrated borderline cost-effectiveness of IFN-α treatment that was within established trends of medical care in the United States (175). In patients with preexisting autoimmunity or a predisposition to autoimmunity, IFN-α therapy should be administered cautiously with close vigilance for exacerbation or precipitation of more symptoms. Clearly, immunosuppressive therapy for HCV-associated autoimmune disorders is also successful, but these patients must also be monitored closely for progressive HCV infection and liver damage (176–179).

## CONCLUSIONS

There is ample clinical evidence to suspect a role for HCV-associated autoimmunity for a broad-spectrum of autoimmune diseases (Table 35.2). Although this association may be sporadic or indicate an increased incidence of HCV infection in patients with autoimmune disease, multiple case reports document the occurrence of acute and chronic HCV infection before the development of autoimmune disease, suggesting a causal role in patients who may be predisposed to the development of autoimmunity. A role for HCV infection in the pathogenesis of mixed essential cryoglobulinemia and cryoglobulinemic GN and vasculitis is strong. An association with other autoimmune diseases may be emerging. HCV appears to trigger autoimmune responses in predisposed patients; these responses manifest as ANAs, rheumatoid factors, cryoglobulins, GN, vasculitis, sicca syndrome, polyarthritis, or myositis. HCV infection should be suspected in any autoimmune disease patient with hepatitis. In addition, characteristic clinical presentations listed in Table 35.3 should be screened for HCV infection. Chronic lymphocyte stimulation may eventually lead to a lymphoproliferative malignancy.

The optimal treatment strategy for HCV-related autoimmunity remains to be defined; therefore, treatment must be individualized with consideration given to cost factors, follow-up, relapse rate, risk for exacerbation of autoimmune disease, and unknown sequelae of immunosuppression in the setting of HCV infection. IFN-α appears to be most effective for symptomatic essential mixed cryoglobulinemia with or without GN; however, the relapse rate on discontinuation of IFN-α is high. There is only anecdotal evidence that IFN-α improves other HCV-related autoimmune diseases, but it is clear that autoimmune diseases develop during treatment of HCV infection with IFN-α. Therefore, strong consideration should be given to traditional immunosuppressive regimens

**TABLE 35.2.** *Immune manifestations of hepatitis C virus infection*

Mixed cryoglobulinemia with:
  Glomerulonephritis
  Vasculitis
  Mononeuritis multiplex
Lymphoproliferative disorders
  Monoclonal gammopathies
  Low-grade non-Hodgkin's lymphoma
Musculoskeletal manifestation
  Palmar tenosynovitis and carpal tunnel syndrome
  Polyarthralgias
  Nonerosive, progressive arthritis
  Rheumatoid arthritis
  Systemic lupus erythematosus
  Polymyositis and dermatomyositis
Glandular manifestations
  Thyroiditis
  Sialoadenitis
Autoimmune liver disease
Antiphospholipid syndrome and thrombotic disorders
Renal manifestations
  Membranoproliferative glomerulonephritis
  Membranous glomerulonephritis
  Acute proliferative glomerulonephritis
Interstitial lung disease

**TABLE 35.3.** *Clinical presentations suggestive of hepatitis C virus infection*

History of hepatitis or risk factors for hepatitis C virus infection
Palpable purpura, urticaria, or livedo reticularis
Nonerosive, nonprogressive polyarthritis with carpal tunnel syndrome or palmar tenosynovitis
Liver abnormalities in association with thrombocytopenia or thrombosis
Seronegative xerostomia or xerophthalmia
Unexplained glomerulonephritis
Interstitial lung disease
Monoclonal gammopathies
Systemic lupus erythematosus patients with hepatitis or membranoproliferative glomerulonephritis

as a result of the relatively high cost of IFN-α and its potential for exacerbating autoimmunity. Further investigations controlling for HCV risk factors, prior history of hepatitis, HCV subtype, HLA genotype, and geographic and environmental variables are required to elucidate the potential causal relationship for HCV infection in autoimmune disease.

## ACKNOWLEDGMENTS

The authors would like to thank Ms. Rose Anne Tucker of the Jackson VAMC library service for her excellent assistance in performing an extensive literature search.

## REFERENCES

1. Koziel MJ. Immunology of viral hepatitis. *Am J Med* 1996;100: 98–109.
2. Martin P. Hepatitis C genotypes: the key to pathogenicity? *Ann Int Med* 1995;122:227–228.
3. Alter MJ. To C or not to C: these are the questions. *Blood* 1995;85: 1681–1695.
4. Alter MJ, Margolis HS, Krawcynski K, et al. The natural history of community acquired hepatitis C in the United States. *N Engl J Med* 1992;327:1899–1903.
5. Seeff LB. Natural history of hepatitis C. *Hepatology* 1997;26[3 Suppl 1]: 21S–28S.
6. Alter MJ. Epidemiology of hepatitis C. *Hepatology* 1997;26[3 Suppl 1]: 62S–65S.
7. Gumber SC, Chopra S. Hepatitis C: a multifaceted disease. Review of extrahepatic manifestations. *Ann Intern Med* 1995;123:615–620.
8. Gordon SC. Extrahepatic manifestations of hepatitis C. *Dig Dis* 1996;14:157–168.
9. Hadziyannis SJ. The spectrum of extrahepatic manifestations in hepatitis C virus infection. *J Viral Hepatitis* 1997;4:9–28.
10. Wener MH, Johnson RJ, Sasso EH, et al. Hepatitis C virus and rheumatic disease. *J Rheumatol* 1996;23:953–959.
11. Bartal C, Sikuler E, Buskila D. Autoimmune phenomena and musculoskeletal manifestations in hepatitis C viral infection. *Harefuah* (Hebrew) 1997;132:639–642.
12. McMurray RW, Elbourne KE. Autoimmune associated disorders with hepatitis C viral infection. *Semin Arthritis Rheum* 1997;26:689–701.
13. Pawlotsky JM, Roudot-Thoraval F, Simmonds P, et al. Extrahepatic immunologic manifestations in chronic hepatitis C virus serotypes. *Ann Intern Med* 1995;122:169–173.
14. Dickson RC, Gaffey MJ, Ishitani MB, et al. The international autoimmune hepatitis score in chronic hepatitis C. *J Viral Hepatitis* 1997;4: 121–128.
15. Pivetti S, Novrino A, Merico F, et al. High prevalence of autoimmune phenomena in hepatitis C virus antibody positive patients with lymphoproliferative and connective tissue disorders. *Br J Hematol* 1996; 95:204–211.
16. Jorgensen C, Legouffe MC, Perney P. Sicca syndrome associated with hepatitis C virus infection. *Arthritis Rheum* 1996;39:1166–1171.
17. Garcia-Carrasco M, Ramos M, Cervera R, et al. Hepatitis C virus infection in 'primary' Sjögren's syndrome: prevalence and clinical significance in a series of 90 patients. *Ann Rheum Dis* 1997;56:173–175.
18. King PD, McMurray RW, Becherer PR. Sjögren's syndrome without mixed cryoglobulinemia is not associated with hepatitis C virus infection. *Am J Gastroenterol* 1994;89:1047–1050.
19. Marchesoni A, Battafarano N, Podico M, et al. Hepatitis C virus antibodies and systemic lupus erythematosus [Letter]. *Clin Exp Rheumatol* 1995;13:267–268.
20. Nishikai M, Miyairi M, Kosaka S. Dermatomyositis following infection with hepatitis C virus [Letter]. *J Rheumatol* 1994;21:1584–1585.
21. Zibert A, Meisel H, Kraas W, et al. Early antibody response against hypervariable region 1 is associated with acute self-limiting infections of hepatitis C virus. *Hepatology* 1997;25:1245–1249.
22. Kobayashi M, Tanaka E, Matsumoto A, et al. Antibody response to E2/NS1 hepatitis C virus protein in patients with acute hepatitis C. *J Gastroenterol Hepatol* 1997;12:73–76.
23. Allander T, Beyene A, Jacobson SH, et al. Patients infected with the same hepatitis C virus strain display different kinetics of the isolate specific antibody response. *J Infect Dis* 1997;175:26–31.
24. Hohler T, Gerken G, Notghi A, et al. MHC class II genes influence the susceptibility to chronic active hepatitis C. *J Hepatol* 1997;27: 259–264.
25. Alric L, Fort M, Izopet J, et al. Genes of the major histocompatibility complex class II influence the outcome of hepatitis C virus infection. *Gastroenterology* 1997;113:1675–1681.
26. Czaja AJ, Carpenter HA, Santrach PJ, et al. Significance of human leukocyte antigens DR3 and DR4 in chronic viral hepatitis. *Dig Dis Sci* 1995;40:2098–2106.
27. Vento S, Guella L, Concia E. Discordant manifestations of hepatitis C in monozygotic twin [Letter]. *N Engl J Med* 1995;333:1224–1225.
28. Simmonds P. Clinical relevance of hepatitis C virus genotypes. *Gut* 1997;40:291–293.
29. Sansonno D, Cornacchiulo V, Iacobelli AR, et al. Localization of hepatitis C virus antigens in liver and skin tissues of chronic hepatitis C virus-infected patients with mixed cryoglobulinemia. *Hepatology* 1995;21:305–312.
30. Sinico RA, Winerals CG, Sabadini E, et al. Identification of glomerular immune deposits in cryoglobulinemic glomerulonephritis. *Kidney Int* 1988;34:109–116.
31. Szymanski IO, Pullman JM, Underwood JM. Electron microscopic and immunochemical studies in a patient with hepatitis C virus infection and mixed cryoglobulinemia type II. *Am J Clin Pathol* 1994;102: 278–283.
32. Cacciarelli TV, Martinex OM, Gish RG, et al. Immunoregulatory cytokines in chronic hepatitis C virus infection: pre- and post-treatment with interferon alfa. *Hepatology* 1996;24:6–9.
33. Clifford BD, Donahue D, Smith L, et al. High prevalence of serological markers of autoimmunity in patients with chronic hepatitis C. *Hepatology* 1995;21:613–619.
34. Kawamoto H, Sakaguchi K, Takaki A, et al. Autoimmune responses as assessed by hypergammaglobulinemia and the presence of autoantibodies in patients with chronic hepatitis C. *Acta Med Okayama* 1993;47:305–310.
35. Prieto J, Yuste JR, Beloqui O, et al. Anticardiolipin antibodies in chronic hepatitis C: implication of hepatitis C virus as the cause of the antiphospholipid syndrome. *Hepatology* 1996;23:199–204.
36. Romani J, Puig L, de Moragas JM. Detection of anti neutrophil cytoplasmic antibodies in patients with hepatitis C virus-induced cutaneous vasculitis with mixed cryoglobulinemia. *Arch Dermatol* 1996;132: 974–975.
37. Abuaf N, Lunel F, Giral P, et al. Non-organ specific autoantibodies associated with chronic C virus hepatitis. *J Hepatol* 1993;18:359–364.
38. Muratori L, Lenzi M, Ma Y, et al. Heterogeneity of liver/kidney microsomal antibody type 1 in autoimmune hepatitis and hepatitis C virus related liver disease. *Gut* 1995;37:406–412.
39. Custro N, Montalto G, Scafidi V, et al. Prospective study on thyroid autoimmunity and dysfunction related to chronic hepatitis C and interferon therapy. *J Endocrinol Invest* 1997;20:374–380.

40. Miaiani R, Bellavita P, Fenili D. Hepatitis C virus infection in patients with essential mixed cryoglobulinemia. *Ann Intern Med* 1992;117:573–577.

41. Cacoub P, Fabiani FL, Musset L, et al. Mixed cryoglobulinemia and hepatitis C virus. *Am J Med* 1994;96:124–132.

42. Gorevic PD, Kassab HY, Levo Y, et al. Mixed cryoglobulinemia: clinical aspects and long term follow-up of 40 patients. *Am J Med* 1980;69:287–301.

43. Schwaber MJ, Zlotogorski A. Dermatologic manifestations of hepatitis C infection. *Int J Dermatol* 1997;36:251–254.

44. Dupin N, Chosidow O, Lunel F, et al. Essential mixed cryoglobulinemia: a comparative study of dermatologic manifestations in patients infected or non-infected with hepatitis C virus. *Arch Dermatol* 1995;131:1124–1127.

45. Karlsberg PL, Lee WM, Casey DL, et al. Cutaneous vasculitis and rheumatoid factor positivity as presenting signs of hepatitis C virus induced mixed cryoglobulinemia. *Arch Dermatol* 1995;131:1119–1123.

46. Johnson RJ, Willson R, Yamabe H, et al. Renal manifestations of hepatitis C virus infection. *Kidney Int* 1994;46:1255–1263.

47. Stehman-Breen C, Willson R, Alpers CE, et al. Hepatitis C associated glomerulonephritis. *Curr Opin Nephrol Hypertens* 1995;4:287–294.

48. Khella SL, Frost S, Hermann GA, et al. Hepatitis C infection, cryoglobulinemia, and vasculitic neuropathy. Treatment with interferon alfa: case report and literature review. *Neurology* 1995;45:407–411.

49. Misiani R, Bellavita P, Fenili D, et al. Interferon alfa 2a therapy in cryoglobulinemia associated with hepatitis C virus. *N Engl J Med* 1994;330:751–756.

50. Levey JM, Bjornsson B, Banner B, et al. Mixed cryoglobulinemia in chronic hepatitis C infection: a clinicopathologic analysis of 10 cases and review of recent literature. *Medicine* 1994;73:53–67.

51. Harle JR, Disdier P, Pelletier J, et al. Dramatic worsening of hepatic C virus-related cryoglobulinemia subsequent to treatment with interferon alfa [Letter]. *JAMA* 1995;274:126.

52. Violi F, Ferro D, Basili S. Hepatitis C virus, antiphospholipid antibodies, and thrombosis [Letter]. *Hepatology* 1997;25:782.

53. Malnick SD, Abend Y, Evron E, et al. HCV hepatitis associated with anticardiolipin antibody and a cerebrovascular accident: response to interferon therapy. *J Clin Gastroenterol* 1997;24:40–42.

54. Biron C, Andreani H, Blanc P, et al. Antiphospholipid antibodies in patients with chronic hepatitis C virus infection or alcoholic liver disease: preliminary results. *Ann Med Interne* 1996;147[Suppl 1]:48–49.

55. Violi F, Ferro D, Basili S, et al. Increase rate of thrombin generation in hepatitis C virus cirrhotic patients: relationships to venous thrombosis. *J Invest Med* 1995;43:550–554.

56. Rocino C, Roccaguo D, Gianino O, et al. Hepatitis C virus and membranous glomerulonephritis. *Nephron* 1991;59:319–320.

57. Yamabe H, Johnson RJ, Gretch DR, et al. Hepatitis C virus infection and membranoproliferative glomerulonephritis in Japan. *J Am Soc Nephrol* 1995;6:220–223.

58. Johnson RJ, Gretch DR, Couser WG, et al. Hepatitis-C virus-associated glomerulonephritis: effect of alpha interferon. *Kidney Int* 1994;46:1700–1704.

59. Johnson RJ, Gretch DR, Yamabe H. Membranoproliferative glomerulonephritis associated with hepatitis C virus infection. *N Engl J Med* 1993;328:465–470.

60. Garcia-Valdecasas J, Bernal C, Garcia F, et al. Epidemiology of hepatitis C virus infection in patients with renal disease. *J Am Soc Nephrol* 1994;5:186–192.

61. Horikoshi S, Okada T, Shirato I. Diffuse proliferative glomerulonephritis with hepatitis C virus-like particles in paramesangial dense deposits in a patient with chronic hepatitis C virus hepatitis. *Nephron* 1993;64:462–464.

62. Misiani R, Vicari O, Bellavita P, et al. Hepatitis C virus in renal tissue of patients with glomerulonephritis [Letter]. *Nephron* 1994;68:400.

63. Nepveu K, Libman B. Hepatitis C and another possible cause of porphyria cutanea tarda and systemic lupus erythematosus: comment on the article by Kutz and Bridges [Letter]. *Arthritis Rheum* 1996;39:352.

64. Nadir A, Smith JW, Matter B, et al. Type 2 cryoglobulinemia and hepatitis C virus: its recognition and treatment. *J Okla State Med Assoc* 1994;87:449–453.

65. Mouthon L, Deblois P, Sauvaget F, et al. Hepatitis B virus-related polyarteritis nodosa and membranous nephropathy. *Am J Nephrol* 1995;15:266–269.

66. Quigg RJ, Brathwaite M, Gardner DF. Successful cyclophosphamide treatment of cryoglobulinemic membranoproliferative glomerulonephritis associated with hepatitis C virus infection. *Am J Kidney Dis* 1995;25:798–800.

67. Revenga AF, Diaz DR, Iglesias DL, et al. Cryoglobulinemic vasculitis associated with hepatitis virus infection: a report of eight cases. *Acta Derm Venereol* 1995;75:234–236.

68. Roithinger FX, Allinger S, Kirchgatterer A, et al. A lethal course of chronic hepatitis C, glomerulonephritis, and pulmonary vasculitis unresponsive to interferon treatment. *Am J Gastroenterol* 1995;90:1006–1008.

69. Schirren CA, Zachoval R, Schirren CG, et al. A role for chronic hepatitis C virus infection in a patient with cutaneous vasculitis, cryoglobulinemia, and chronic liver disease: effective therapy with interferon-alpha. *Dig Dis Sci* 1995;40:1221–1225.

70. Gorg S, Niederstadt C, Klouche M, et al. Intestinal vasculitis and glomerulonephritis in hepatitis C-associated cryoglobulinemia [translated from German]. *Immunitat und Infektion.* 1995;23:29–31.

71. Ornstein MH, Phelps R, Kerr LD, et al. Correlation of liver and skin histopathology with serology in a patient with cutaneous vasculitis and hepatitis C infection. *South Med J* 1994;87:1174–1177.

72. Shakil AO, Di Bisceglie AM. Images in clinical medicine: vasculitis and cryoglobulinemia related to hepatitis C. *N Engl J Med* 1994;331:1624.

73. Marcellin P, Descamps V, Martinot-Peignoux M, et al. Cryoglobulinemia with vasculitis associated with hepatitis C virus infection. *Gastroenterology* 1993;104:272–277.

74. Durand JM, Kaplanski G, Richard MA, et al. Cutaneous vasculitis in a patient infected with hepatitis C virus: detection of hepatitis C virus RNA in the skin by polymerase chain reaction [Letter]. *Br J Dermatol* 1993;128:359–360.

75. Remond B, Reygagne P, Aractingi S, et al. Cutaneous vasculitis with mixed cryoglobulinemia during chronic hepatitis C [translated from French]. *Ann Dermatol Venereol* 1992;119:827–829.

76. Sepp NT, Umlauft F, Illersperger B, et al. Necrotizing vasculitis associated with hepatitis C virus infection: successful treatment of vasculitis with interferon-alpha despite persistence of mixed cryoglobulinemia. *Dermatology* 1995;191:43–45.

77. Manna R, Todaro L, Latteri M, et al. Leukocytoclastic vasculitis associated with hepatitis C virus antibodies. *Br J Rheumatol* 1997;36:124–125.

78. David WS, Peine C, Schlesinger P, et al. Non-systemic vasculitic mononeuropathy multiplex, cryoglobulinemia, and hepatitis C. *Muscle Nerve* 1996;19:1596–602.

79. Arend SM, Hagen EC, Kroes AC, et al. Activation of chronic hepatitis C virus infection by cyclophosphamide in a patient with cANCA-positive vasculitis. *Nephrol Dial Transplant* 1995;10:884–887.

80. MacKay IR. Hepatic disease and systemic lupus erythematosus. In: Lahita RG, ed. *Systemic lupus erythematosus.* New York: Churchill Livingstone, 1992:761–765.

81. Borisova VV, Krel' PE: Systemic lupus erythematosus etiologically due to the hepatitis B and C viruses [translated from Russian]. *Ter Arkh* 1992;64:92–93.

82. Bronson W, McMurray RW. Hepatitis C virus and systemic lupus erythematosus: a case report. *J Clin Rheumatol* 1997;6:153–157.

83. Albero MD, Rivera F, Merino E, et al. Hepatitis C virus infection complicating lupus nephritis. *Nephrol Dial Transplant* 1996;11:1342–1345.

84. Siegel LB, Cohn L, Nashel D. Rheumatic manifestations of hepatitis C infection. *Semin Arthritis Rheum* 1993;23:149–154.

85. Ueno Y, Kinoshito R, Kishimoto I, et al. Polyarthritis associated with hepatitis C virus infection. *Br J Rheumatol* 1994;33:289–291.

86. Ueno Y, Kinoshito R, Tsujinoue H, et al. A case of hepatitis C virus (HCV)-associated arthritis: quantitative analysis of HCV RNA of the synovial fluid and the serum [Letter]. *Br J Rheumatol* 1995;34:691–692.

87. Bon E, Cantarel A, Moulinier L, et al. Rheumatic manifestations of chronic hepatitis C and response to interferon alpha. *Rev Rhum* Edition Francaise. 1994;61:497–504.

88. Hirohata S, Inoue T, Ito K. Development of rheumatoid arthritis after chronic hepatitis caused by hepatitis C virus infection. *Intern Med* 1992;31:493–493.

89. Barkhuizen A, Bennett RM. Hepatitis C infection presenting with rheumatic manifestations. *J Rheumatol* 1997;24:1238–1239.

90. Lovy MR, Starkebaum G, Uberoi S. Hepatitis C infection presenting with rheumatic manifestations: a mimic of rheumatoid arthritis. *J Rheumatol* 1996;23:979–983.

91. Sawada T, Hirohata S, Inoue T. Development of rheumatoid arthritis after hepatitis C virus infection. *Arthritis Rheum* 1991;34:1620–1621.

92. Hirohata S, Inoue T, Ito K. Hepatitis C virus infection and rheumatoid arthritis: differential expression of anti-c100 and anti GOR antibodies [Letter]. *J Rheumatol* 1993;20:204–205.

93. Castanet J, Lacour JP, Fuzibet JG, et al. Adult Still's disease associated with hepatitis C virus infection. *J Am Acad Dermatol* 1994;31:807–808.

94. Rivera J, de Diego A, Trinchet M, et al. Fibromyalgia-associated hepatitis C virus infection. *Br J Rheumatol* 1997;36:981–985.

95. Barkhuizen A, Schoepflin G, Bennett R. Fibromyalgia: a prominent feature in patients with muskuloskeletal problems in chronic hepatitis C. A report of 12 patients. *J Clin Rheumatol* 1996;2:180–184.

96. Dalavacs MC. Polymyositis, dermatomyositis, and inclusion body myositis. *N Engl J Med* 1991;325:1487–1498.

97. Weidensaul D, Imam T, Holyst MM, et al. Polymyositis, pulmonary fibrosis, and hepatitis C. *Arthritis Rheum* 1995;38:437–439.

98. Horsmans Y, Geubel AP. Symptomatic myopathy in hepatitis C infection without interferon therapy [Letter; Comment]. *Lancet* 1995;345:1236.

99. Ueno Y, Kondo K, Kidodoro N, et al. Hepatitis C infection and polymyositis [Letter; Comment]. *Lancet* 1995;346:319–320.

100. Ferri C, La Civita L, Fazzi P, et al. Polymyositis, lung fibrosis, and cranial neuropathy in a patient with hepatitis C virus infection. *Arthritis Rheum* 1996;39:1074–1075.

101. Gomez A, Solans R, Simeon CP, et al. Dermatomyositis, hepatocarcinoma, and hepatitis C: comment on the article by Weidensaul et al [Letter]. *Arthritis Rheum* 1997;40:394–395.

102. Ferri C, La Civita L, Fazzi P, et al. Interstitial lung fibrosis and rheumatic disorders in patients with hepatitis C virus infection. *Br J Rheumatol* 1997;36:360–365.

103. Ueda T, Ohta K, Suzuki N, et al. Idiopathic pulmonary fibrosis and high prevalence of serum antibodies to hepatitis C virus. *Am Rev Respir Dis* 1992;146:266–268.

104. Iguchi H, Kishi M, Fukioka T, et al. Polymyositis after interferon beta treatment of chronic hepatitis type C. *Rinsho Shinkeigaku* 1996;26:22–24.

105. Arai H, Tanaka M, Ohta K, et al. Symptomatic myopathy associated with interferon therapy for chronic hepatitis C. *Lancet* 1995;345:582.

106. Mariette X, Zerbib M, Jaccard A, et al. Hepatitis C virus and Sjögren's syndrome. *Arthritis Rheum* 1993;36:280–281.

107. Wattiaux MJ, Jouan-Flahault C, Youinou P, et al. Association of Gougerot-Sjögren syndrome and viral hepatitis C: apropos of 6 cases. *Ann Med Interne* 1995;146:247–250.

108. Poet JL, Torolli-Serabian I, Garnier PP. Chronic hepatitis C and Sjögren's syndrome [Letter]. *J Rheumatol* 1994;21:1376–1377.

109. Marrone A, DiBisceglie AM, Fox P. Absence of hepatitis C viral infections among patients with primary Sjögren's syndrome [Letter]. *J Hepatol* 1995;22:599.

110. Barrier JH, Magadur-Joly G, Gassin M. Hepatitis C virus: an improbable etiological agent of Gougerot-Sjögren's syndrome [Letter]. *Presse Med* 1993;22:1108.

111. Vitali C, Sciuto M, Neri R, et al. Anti-hepatitis C virus antibodies in primary Sjögren's syndrome: false positive results are related to hypergammaglobulinemia [Letter]. *Clin Exp Rheumatol* 1992;10:102–104.

112. Haddad J, Deny P, Munz-Gotheil C, et al. Lymphocytic sialoadenitis of Sjögren's syndrome associated with chronic hepatitis C virus liver disease. *Lancet* 1992;339:321–323.

113. Pirisi M, Scott C, Fabris C, et al. Mild sialoadenitis: a common finding in patients with hepatitis C virus infection. *Scand J Gastroenterol* 1994;29:940–942.

114. Scott CA, Avellini C, Desman L, et al. Chronic lymphocytic sialoadenitis in HVC-related chronic liver disease: comparison of Sjögren's syndrome. *Histopathology* 1997;30:41–48.

115. Yamamoto T, Yokoyama A. Hypergammaglobulinemic purpura associated with Sjögren's syndrome and chronic C type hepatitis. *J Dermatol* 1997;24:7–11.

116. Koike K, Moriya K, Ishibashi K, et al. Sialadenitis histologically resembling Sjögren syndrome in mice transgenic for hepatitis C virus envelope genes. *Proc Nat Acad Sci U S A* 1997;94:233–236.

117. Tziofas AG, Moutsopoulous HM, Talal N. Lymphoid malignancy and monoclonal proteins. In: Talal N, Moutsopoulous HM, Kassan SS. *Sjögren's syndrome: clinical and immunological aspects*. Berlin: Springer-Verlag, 1987:129–136.

118. Mussini C, Ghini M, Mascia MT, et al. Monoclonal gammopathies and hepatitis C virus infection [Letter]. *Blood* 1995;85:1144–1145.

119. Andreone P, Gramenzi A, Cursaro C, et al. Hepatitis C virus infection and lymphoproliferative disorders [Letter]. *Blood* 1995;86:3610–3611.

120. Ferri C, Monti M, La Civita, et al. Hepatitis C virus infection in non-Hodgkin's B cell lymphoma complicating mixed cryoglobulinemia. *Eur J Clin Invest* 1994;24:781–784.

121. Pozzato G, Mazzaro C, Crovatto M, et al. Low grade malignant lymphoma, hepatitis C virus infection, and mixed cryoglobulinemia. *Blood* 1994;84:3047–3053.

122. DeVita S, Sansonno D, Dolcetti R, et al. Hepatitis C virus within a malignant lymphoma lesion in the course of type II mixed cryoglobulinemia. *Blood* 1995;86:1887–1892.

123. Franzin F, Efremov DG, Pozzato G, et al. Clonal B-cell expansions in peripheral blood of HCV-infected patients. *Br J Hematol* 1995;90:548–552.

124. Sikuler E, Shnaider A, Zilberman D, et al. Hepatitis C virus infection and extrahepatic malignancies. *J Clin Gastroenterol* 1997;24:87–89.

125. Zuckerman E, Zukerman T, Levine AM, et al. Hepatitis C virus infection in patients with B-cell non-Hodgkin lymphoma. *Ann Intern Med* 1997;127:423–428.

126. Agnello V. The aetiology of mixed cryoglobulinemia associated with hepatitis C virus infection. *Scand J Immunol* 1995;42:179–184.

127. Tran A, Quaranta JF, Beusnel C, et al. Hepatitis C virus and Hashimoto's thyroiditis. *Eur J Med* 1992;1:116–118.

128. Kawaguchi K, Okuwaki J, Takami S. A case of HCV-RNA positive liver cirrhosis with hypergammaglobulinemia and high titers of ANA, accompanied by hypothyroidism. *Nippon Shokakibyo Gakkai Zasshi* 1995;92:909–913.

129. Quaranta JF, Tran A, Regnier D, et al. High prevalence of antibodies to hepatitis C virus in patients with anti-thyroid autoantibodies (Letter). *J Hepatol* 1993;18:136–138.

130. Tran A, Quaranta JF, Banzaken S, et al. High prevalence of thyroid autoantibodies in a prospective series of patients with chronic hepatitis C before interferon therapy. *Hepatology* 1993;18:253–257.

131. Boadas J, Rodriguea-Espinosa J, Enriquez J, et al. Prevalence of thyroid autoantibodies is not increased in blood donors with hepatitis C virus infection. *J Hepatol* 1995;22:611–615.

132. Wong S, Mehta AE, Faiman C, et al. Absence of serologic evidence for hepatitis C virus infection in patients with Hashimoto's thyroiditis. *Hepatogastroenterology* 1996;43:420–421.

133. Metcalfe RA, Ball G, Kudesia G, et al. Failure to find an association between hepatitis C virus and thyroid autoimmunity. *Thyroid* 1997;7:421–424.

134. Preziati D, LaRosa L, Covini G, et al. Autoimmunity and thyroid function in patients with chronic active hepatitis treated with recombinant interferon-alpha 2a. *Eur J Endocrinol* 1995;132:587–593.

135. Imagawa A, Itoh N, Hanafusa T, et al. Autoimmune endocrine disease induced by recombinant interferon alpha therapy for chronic active type C hepatitis. *J Clin Endocrinol Met* 1995;80:922–926.

136. Nagayama Y, Ohta K, Tsuruta M, et al. Exacerbation of thyroid autoimmunity by interferon alpha treatment in patients with chronic viral hepatitis: our studies and review of the literature. *Endocr J* 1994;41:565–572.

137. Watanabe U, Hashimoto E, Hisamitsu T, et al. The risk factor for development of thyroid disease during interferon alpha therapy for chronic hepatitis C. *Am J Gastroenterol* 1994;89:399–403.

138. Boyer JL, Reuben A. Chronic hepatitis. In: Schiff L, Schiff ER, eds. *Disease of the liver*. 7th ed. Philadelphia: JB Lippincott, 1993:612–618.

139. Czaja AJ, Carpenter HA, Santrach PJ, et al. Evidence against hepatitis viruses as important causes of severe autoimmune hepatitis in the United States. *J Hepatol* 1993;18:342–352.

140. Pawlotsky JM, Deforges L, Bretagne S, et al. Hepatitis C virus infection can mimic type 1 (antinuclear antibody positive) autoimmune chronic active hepatitis. *Gut* 1993;34:S66–S68.

141. Friedman LS, Patel KP, Munoz SJ. Hepatitis C virus and autoimmune chronic active hepatitis:closing the ring. *Gastroenterology* 1992;102:1436–1438.

142. Lee WM. Where is the dividing line between autoimmune hepatitis and hepatitis C? *Gastroenterology* 1992;102:1814–1815.

143. Lenzi M. Autoimmune hepatitis and hepatitis C virus infection. *FEMS Microbiol Rev*. 1994;14:247–252.

144. Fried MW, Dragueku JO, Shindo M, et al. Clinical and serological differentiation of autoimmune and hepatitis C virus related chronic hepatitis. *Dig Dis Sci* 1993;38:631–636.

145. Bach N, Thung SN, Schaffner F. The histological features of chronic hepatitis C and autoimmune chronic hepatitis: a comparative analysis. *Hepatology* 1992;15:572–577.

146. Heintges T, Niederau C. Differentiation between autoimmune hepatitis and hepatitis C virus related liver disease. *Z Gastroenterol* 1993; 31:285–288.

147. Bellary S, Schiano T, Hartman G, et al. Chronic hepatitis with combined features of autoimmune chronic hepatitis and chronic hepatitis C: favorable response to prednisone and azathioprine. *Ann Intern Med* 1995;123:32–34.

148. Savage K, Dhillon AP, Schmilovitz-Weiss H, et al. Detection of HCV-RNA in paraffin embedded liver biopsies from patients with autoimmune hepatitis. *J Hepatol* 1995;22:27–34.

149. Chazouilleres O, Kim M, Ferrell L, et al. Quantitation of hepatic C virus RNA in liver transplant recipients. *Gastroenterology* 1994;106: 994–999.

150. Funaoka M, Kato K, Komatsu M, et al. Fulminant hepatitis caused by hepatitis C virus during treatment for multiple sclerosis. *J Gastroenterol* 1996;31:119–122.

151. Emilia G, Luppi M, Ferrari MG, et al. Hepatitis C virus-induced leukothrombocytopenia and haemolysis. *J Med Virol* 1997;53:182–184.

152. Pawlotsky JM, Bouvier M, Fromont P, et al. Hepatitis C virus infection and autoimmune thrombocytopenic purpura. *J Hepatol* 1995;23: 635–639.

153. Cassani F, Valentini P, Catela M, et al. Ultrasound-detected abdominal lymphadenopathy in chronic hepatitis C: high frequency and relationship with viremia. *J Hepatol* 1997;26:479–483.

154. Munke H, Stockmann F, Ramadon G. Possible association between Behçet's syndrome and chronic hepatitis C virus infection. *N Engl J Med* 1995;332:400–401.

155. Halfon P, Levy M, San Marco M, et al. Myasthenia gravis and hepatitis C virus infection. *J Viral Hepatitis* 1996;3:329–332.

156. Matsumori A. Molecular and immune mechanisms in the pathogenesis of cardiomyopathy: role of viruses, cytokines, and nitric oxide. *Jap Circ J* 1997;61:275–291.

157. Gretch DR. Diagnostic tests for hepatitis C. *Hepatology* 1997;26 [3 Suppl 1]:43S–47S.

158. Urdea MS, Wuestehuebe LJ, Laurenson PM, et al. Hepatitis C: diagnosis and monitoring. *Clin Chem* 1997;43:1507–1511.

159. De Medina M, Schiff ER. Hepatitis C: diagnostic assays. *Semin Liv Dis* 1995;15:33–40.

160. Monteverde A, Airoldi G, Ballare M, et al. Reliability of immunoassays for anti-HCV antibodies (ELISA and RIBA 2) in patients with essential mixed cryoglobulinemia. *Clin Exp Rheumatol* 1993;11: 609–613.

161. Czaja AJ, Carpenter HA. Sensitivity, specificity, and predictability of biopsy interpretations in chronic hepatitis. *Gastroenterology* 1993; 105:1824–1832.

162. Perrillo RP. The role of liver biopsy in hepatitis C. *Hepatology* 1997; 26[3 Suppl 1]:57S–61S.

163. Fried MW, Hoofnagle JH. Therapy of hepatitis C. *Semin Liver Dis* 1995;15:82–91.

164. Wright T, Terrault N. Interferon and hepatitis C. *N Engl J Med* 1995; 332:1509–1511.

165. Keeffe EB, Hollinger FB. Therapy of hepatitis C: consensus interferon trials. Consensus Interferon Study Group. *Hepatology* 1997;26 [3 Suppl 1]:101S–107S.

166. Davis GL, Lau JY. Factors predictive of a response to therapy of hepatitis C. *Hepatology* 1997;26[3 Suppl 1]:122S–127S.

167. Alberti A, Chemello L, Noventa F, et al. Therapy of hepatitis C: re-treatment with alpha interferon. *Hepatology* 1997;26[3 Suppl 1]: 137S–142S.

168. Smith JP. Treatment of chronic hepatitis C with amantadine. *Dig Dis Sci* 1997;42:1681–1687.

169. Clerici C, Distrutti E, Gentili G, et al. Interferon plus ursodeoxycholic acid versus interferon in the treatment of chronic C viral hepatitis. *Minerva Medica* 1997;88:219–225.

170. Ronnblom LE, Alm GV, Oberg KE. Autoimmunity after alpha-interferon therapy for malignant carcinoid tumors. *Ann Intern Med* 1991;115:178–183.

171. Unoki H, Moriyama A, Tabaru A, et al. Development of Sjögren's syndrome during treatment with recombinant human interferon alpha 2b for chronic hepatitis C. *J Gastroenterol* 1996;31:723–727.

172. Doutre MS, Baquey A, Bernard P, et al. Appearance of antiphospholipid antibodies in patients with hepatitis C treated with interferon alpha. *Ann Med Interne* 1997;148:99–100.

173. Matsuda J, Saitoh N, Gotoh M, et al. High prevalence of antiphospholipid antibodies and anti-thyroglobulin antibody in patients with hepatitis C virus infection treated with interferon alpha. *Am J Gastroenterol* 1995;90:1138–1141.

174. Uyama E, Fujiki N, Uchino M. Exacerbation of myasthenia gravis during interferon alpha treatment. *J Neurol Sci* 1996;144:221–222.

175. Koff RS. Therapy of hepatitis C: cost effective analysis. *Hepatology* 1997;26[3 Suppl 1]:152S–155S.

176. Tran A, Benzaken S, Yang G, et al. Chronic hepatitis C and autoimmunity: good response to immunosuppressive treatment. *Dig Dis Sci* 1997;42:778–780.

177. Toda G. Interferon or corticosteroid: treatment of patients with chronic hepatitis C positive for serum markers of autoimmune disease. *Intern Med* 1997;36:233–235.

178. Calleja JL, Albillos A, Cacho G, et al. Interferon and prednisone therapy in chronic hepatitis C with non-organ specific antibodies. *J Hepatol* 1996;24:308–312.

179. Thiele DL, DuCharme L, Cunningham MR, et al. Steroid therapy of chronic hepatitis: characteristics associated with response in anti-hepatitis C virus positive and negative patients. *Am J Gastroenterol* 1996;91:300–308.

*Textbook of the Autoimmune Diseases,*
Edited by R. G. Lahita, N. Chiorazzi, and W. H. Reeves,
Lippincott Williams & Wilkins, Philadelphia © 2000.

# CHAPTER 36

# Rheumatic Fever

Allan Gibofsky, Kumar Visvanathan, Suresh Kerwar, and John B. Zabriskie

Acute rheumatic fever (ARF) is a delayed, nonsuppurative sequela of a pharyngeal infection with the group A streptococcus. After the initial streptococcal pharyngitis, there is a latent period of 2 to 3 weeks. The onset of disease is usually characterized by an acute febrile illness that may manifest in one of three classic ways: (a) the patient may present with migratory arthritis predominantly involving the large joints of the body, (b) there may be concomitant clinical and laboratory signs of carditis and valvulitis, and (c) there may be involvement of the central nervous system, manifesting as Sydenham's chorea. The clinical episodes are self-limiting, but damage to the valves may be chronic and progressive, resulting in cardiac decompensation and death.

Although there has been a dramatic decline in the severity and mortality of the disease since the turn of the century, there have been reports of its resurgence in the United States (1) and elsewhere in the world, reminding us that the disease remains a public health problem. In addition, the disease continues essentially unabated in many developing countries. Estimates suggest there will be 10 to 20 million new cases per year in those countries where two thirds of the world's population lives.

## EPIDEMIOLOGY

The incidence of rheumatic fever actually began to decline long before the introduction of antibiotics into clinical practice, decreasing from 250 to 100 patients per 100,000 population from 1862 to 1962 in Denmark (2). The introduction of antibiotics in 1950 rapidly accelerated this decline, until by 1980, the incidence ranged from 0.23 to 1.88 patients per 100,000 population, primarily in children and teenagers. A notable exception

A. Gibofsky: Departments of Medicine and Public Health, Weill Medical College of Cornell University, New York, New York 10021; Department of Rheumatology, Hospital for Special Surgery, New York, New York 10021.

K. Visvanathan, J. B. Zabriskie: Laboratory of Clinical Microbiology and Immunology, Rockefeller University, New York, New York 10021; Rockefeller University Hospital, New York, New York 10021.

S. Kerwar, CV Therapeutics, Palt Alto, California 94304.

to this has been in the native Hawaiian and Mauri populations (both of Polynesian ancestry), in which the incidence continues to be 13.4 per 100,000 hospitalized children per year (3).

As reviewed by Markowitz and Gordis (4), only a few M serotypes (types 5, 14, 18, and 24) have been identified with outbreaks of RF, suggesting that certain strains of group A streptococci may be more rheumatogenic than others. In Trinidad, however, types 41 and 11 have been the most common strains isolated from the oropharynx of rheumatic patients. Finally, the report by Kaplan et al. (5) indicates that several different M types were isolated from the patients seen during an outbreak in Utah, and these strains were both mucoid and nonmucoid in character. Thus, the question of whether certain strains are more rheumatogenic than others remains unresolved. What is true, however, is that a streptococcal strain capable of causing well-documented pharyngitis is almost always potentially capable of causing rheumatic fever [although some notable exceptions have been recorded, as reviewed by Whitnack and Bisno (6)].

## PATHOGENESIS

Although there is little evidence for the direct involvement of group A streptococci in the affected tissues of ARF patients, there is a large body of epidemiologic and immunologic evidence indirectly implicating group A streptococcus in the initiation of the disease process. For example, it is well known that outbreaks of rheumatic fever closely follow epidemics of either streptococcal sore throats or scarlet fever (7). Adequate treatment of a documented streptococcal pharyngitis markedly reduces the incidence of subsequent rheumatic fever (8). Appropriate antimicrobial prophylaxis prevents the recurrence of disease in known ARF patients (9). When investigators test the sera of most ARF patients for three antistreptococcal antibodies (streptolysin "O," hyaluronidase, and streptokinase) most, have elevated antibody titers to these antigens (10) even if they do not recall an antecedent streptococcal sore throat.

A note of caution is necessary concerning documentation (either clinically or microbiologically) of an antecedent streptococcal infection. The frequency of isolation of group A streptococci from the oropharynx is extremely low, even in populations without access to antibiotics. Further, there appears to be an age-related discrepancy in the clinical documentation of an antecedent sore throat. In older children and young adults, the recollection of a streptococcal sore throat approaches 70%; in younger children, this rate approaches only 20% (1). Thus, it is important to have a high index of suspicion of ARF in children or young adults presenting with signs of arthritis or carditis even in the absence of a clinically documented sore throat.

Another intriguing, and as yet unexplained, observation has been the invariable association of rheumatic fever only with streptococcal pharyngitis. Although there have been many outbreaks of impetigo, rheumatic fever almost never occurs after infection with these strains. Potter et al. (11) reported that in Trinidad, where impetigo and rheumatic fever may occur together, the strains colonizing the skin were different from those associated with rheumatic fever and did not influence the incidence of ARF. The exception to this rule appears to be the observation by Carapetis and Currie (12), who isolated only pyoderma strains from their patients. There is a high incidence of rheumatic fever in these aboriginal patients but no evidence of throat strains being isolated.

The explanations for these observations remain obscure. It is clear that group A streptococci fall into two main classes based on differences in the C repeat regions of the M protein (Fig. 36.1). One class is clearly associated with streptococcal pharyngeal infection; the other (with some exceptions) belongs to strains commonly associated with impetigo. Thus, the particular strain of streptococcus may be crucial in initiating the disease process. The pharyngeal site of infection, with its large repository of lymphoid tissue, may also be important in the initiation of the abnormal humoral response by the host to those antigens cross-reactive with target organs (see later discussion). Finally, although impetigo strains do colonize the pharynx, they do not appear to elicit as strong an immunologic response to the M-protein moiety as do the pharyngeal strains. This may prove to be an important factor, especially in light of the known cross-reactions between various streptococcal structures and mammalian proteins.

## GROUP A STREPTOCOCCUS

Figure 36.1 is a cross-sectional drawing of a streptococcal cell. One can easily see that there a number of streptococcal antigens both on the surface of the organism and as part of the structure of the cell, many of which cross-react with mammalian tissues. Some of these antigens are discussed in more detail later.

The capsule of the group A streptococcus is composed of equimolar concentrations of *N*-acetyl glucosamine and glucuronic acid and is structurally identical to hyaluronic acid of mammalian tissues (13). Although numerous attempts to pro-

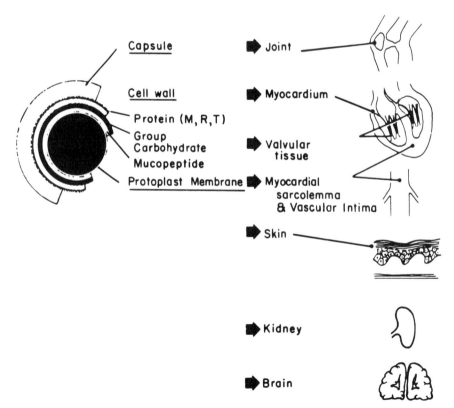

**FIG. 36.1.** Schematic representation of the various structures of the group A streptococcus. Note the wide variety of cross-reactions between its antigens and mammalian tissues.

duce antibodies to this capsule have been unsuccessful (14,15), Fillit et al. (16) were able to demonstrate high titers to hyaluronic acid using techniques designed to detect non-precipitating antibodies in the sera of animals. The data implicating the importance of this capsule in human infections has been almost nonexistent; however, Stollerman (7) has commented on the presence of a large mucoid capsule as being one of the more important characteristics of certain rheumatogenic strains.

Investigations by Lancefield and others spanning almost 70 years have established that the M-protein molecule (at least 80 distinct serologic types) is perhaps the most important virulence factor in group A streptococcal infections of humans (reviewed in reference 17). The protein is a helical coiled-coil structure that has a noncoiled variable region at its N-terminal end, which accounts for the type specificity of each M protein. This is followed by a B repeat region and a C repeat motif and finally an anchoring area that is common to many organisms (Fig. 36.2). Much of its structure bears a striking structural homology to the cardiac cytoskeletal proteins tropomyosin and myosin and to many other coil-coiled structures, such as keratin, DNA, lamin, and vimentin.

After the amino acid sequence of a number of M proteins became known, it was possible to localize those cross-reactive areas. The studies of Dale and Beachey (18) show that the part of the M protein involved in the opsonic reaction also cross-reacts with human sarcolemma antigens. Sargent et al. (19) more precisely localized this cross-reaction to the M-protein amino acid residues 164 to 197.

The evidence implicating these cross-reactions in the pathogenesis of ARF remains scant. Antibodies to myosin have been detected in the sera of ARF patients, but they are also present in a high percentage of the sera obtained from patients who had a streptococcal infection but did not subsequently develop ARF (20). The significance of this observation is unclear because myosin is an internal protein of cardiac muscle cells and therefore not easily exposed to M-protein cross-reacting antibodies.

The group-specific carbohydrate of the streptococcus is a polysaccharide chain consisting of repeating units of rhamnose capped by N-acetyl glucosamine molecules. The N-acetyl glucosamine is immunodominant and gives rise to the serologic group specificity of group A streptococci (21). The cross-reaction between group A carbohydrate and valvular glycoproteins was first described by Goldstein and Caravano (22), and the reactivity was related to the N-acetyl glucosamine moiety present in both structures. Goldstein and Caravano (22) noted that rheumatic fever sera reacted to the heart valve glycoprotein. Fillit (Rockefeller University, unpublished data, 1985) observed strong reactivity of rheumatic fever sera with purified proteoglycan material. Thus, these cross-reactions could involve the sugar moiety present in the proteoglycan portion of the glycoprotein and the carbohydrate.

It has always been assumed that group A anticarbohydrate antibodies did not play a role in phagocytosis of group A

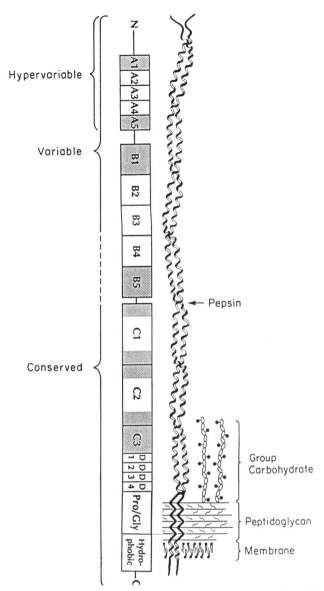

**FIG. 36.2.** Schematic drawing of the entire structure of the M protein of the group A streptococcus. Note the different regions of the molecule with the variable region at the end terminal and the B and C repeat regions as described in the diagram. (Courtesy of Dr. Vincent A. Fischetti.)

streptococci. The studies of Salvadori et al. (23), however, have demonstrated that human sera containing high titers of anti–group A carbohydrate antibody were opsonophagocytic for a number of different M-protein–specific strains, and the opsonophagocytic properties were directed to the N-acetyl glucosamine moiety of the group A carbohydrate.

The mucopeptide portion of the cell wall is the "backbone" of the organism. Rigid in structure, it is composed of repeating units of muramic acid and N-acetyl glucosamine cross-linked by peptide bridges (24). It is particularly difficult to degrade and induces a wide variety of lesions when injected into various species, including arthritis in rats (25) and myocardial granulomas in mice resembling (but not identical to) rheumatic fever Aschoff's lesions (26).

The relationship of cell wall mucopeptides to the pathogenesis of rheumatic fever remains obscure. Elevated levels of antimucopeptide antibody have been detected in the sera of patients with ARF but also in the sera of patients with rheumatoid arthritis and juvenile rheumatoid arthritis (27); its pathogenic relationship to clinical disease, however, has been difficult to establish. There is no evidence that cell wall antigens are present either in Aschoff's lesion or myocardial tissue obtained from patients with RF.

Another cell wall fragment that deserves attention is the lipoteichoic acid. Several reports have indicated that this molecule is able to induce cytokine production as well as nitric oxide synthase in macrophages. The mechanism appears to be through binding of the molecule to CD14 receptors on monocytes. Its role in rheumatic fever has yet to be ascertained (28,29).

Kingston and Glynn (30) were the first to show that animals immunized with streptococcal antigens developed antibodies in their sera that stained astrocytes. Husby et al. (31) demonstrated that sera from ARF patients with chorea exhibited antibodies that were specific for caudate cells. Absorption of the sera with streptococcal membrane antigens eliminated the reactivity with caudate cells.

Perhaps the most significant cross-reactions are with the streptococcal membrane structure. We have shown that immunization with membrane material elicits antibodies that bind to heart sections in a pattern similar to that observed with ARF sera (32). Numerous other cross-reactions between streptococcal membranes and other tissues for a more detailed discussion (32).

Most of the reactions discussed so far have been humoral in nature; however, a number of cellular studies have implicated a significant cellular response to streptococcal antigens (33). We will discuss some of these responses in more detail. For example, it was originally thought that one of the reasons for the observed cellular reactivity to streptococcal antigens was that M protein had "superantigen" properties (34). Using highly purified and recombinant M protein, it is now clear that M protein is not a superantigen. Rather, the mitogenic effects noted were most likely caused by contaminating pyrogenic exotoxin C and mitogenic factor MF in the M-protein material (35,36). Using cell proliferation assays, it has been shown that peripheral mononuclear cell populations from rheumatic fever patients have an exaggerated response to streptococcal membrane antigens compared with that of control subjects (37). Furthermore, the increased reactivity was seen only with those antigens extracted from group A streptococcal strains associated with rheumatic fever and not in antigens extracted from nephritogenic strains. In more recent studies, T-cell clones isolated from rheumatic fever heart valves were reactive to streptococcal antigens and mammalian cytoskeletal antigens, such as myosin and tropomyosin (38).

A number of streptococcal antigens and products have a direct effect on the immune system. For example, the peptidoglycan portion of the streptococcal cell wall is capable of stimulating the production of tumor necrosis factor-α (TNF-α) in normal human monocyte populations. The amount needed to induce TNF production is much higher than that observed with lipopolysaccharide (LPS). This fact, coupled with the observation that the peptidoglycan moiety and the LPS molecule bind to the same 70-kd site on monocytes (39), prompted the authors to examine these structural moieties in more detail. Although at first glance these moieties appear to be different, the rigid backbones of LPS and mucopeptide are quite similar. This similarity was also seen immunologically in that rabbit antibodies prepared against streptococcal mucopeptide blocked the production of TNF-α of human monocytes stimulated by either peptidoglycan or LPS (J.B. Zabriskie and M.S. Blake, unpublished data, 1986). Because the peptidoglycan moiety is similar in all gram-positive organisms and differs primarily in the nature of their linking peptide side chains, the cell walls of all of these organisms are potentially capable of stimulating monocytes with production of inflammatory cytokines.

Finally, clinicians must consider the exotoxins secreted by streptococci and staphylococci (40–42). These superantigens have the ability to bind nonspecifically to the major histocompatibility complex (MHC) molecule on the macrophage and the T-cell receptor. This binding results in the activation of large numbers of T cells bearing particular Vβ gene elements. As a result, cytokine expression is profoundly elevated. Furthermore, after activation, T cells bearing certain Vβ receptors are often deleted (43). These observations have led to the concept that they might be used as potential therapeutic agents in the treatment of autoimmune diseases.

## GENETICS

The concept that rheumatic fever might be the result of a host genetic predisposition has intrigued investigators for more than a century (44). It has been variously suggested that the disease gene is transmitted in an autosomal recessive fashion (45) or autosomal dominant fashion with limited penetrance (46), or that it is possibly related to the genes conferring blood group secretor status (47).

Renewed interest in the genetics of rheumatic fever occurred with the recognition that gene products of the human MHC were associated with certain clinical disease states. Using an alloserum from a multiparous donor, an increased frequency of a B-cell alloantigen was reported in several genetically distinct and ethnically diverse rheumatic fever populations and was not MHC related (48).

Most recently, studies were accomplished with a monoclonal antibody (D8/17) prepared by immunizing mice with B cells from a patient with rheumatic fever patient (49). This B-cell antigen was found to be expressed in a low number of B cells from control subjects, but the number of B cells was found to be 2 standard deviations (SD) above normal in nearly 100% of rheumatic fever patients of diverse ethnic and geographic origins. It should be noted that about 5% to 7% of unaffected people express the antigen on their B cells 1 SD above the normal range. It has been speculated but not proved that this group might represent the susceptible population from which affected patients are drawn. The antigen defined by this monoclonal antibody showed no association with or linkage to any of the known MHC haplotypes, nor was it related to B-cell activation antigens (49).

Despite many attempts, the exact nature of the antigen as defined by the D8/17 antibody remains unknown. More recent attempts (unpublished data) indicate that the antigen has a weight of 95 kd. Preliminary data suggest it is a unique protein, but the full sequence has not been determined.

These studies have been expanded to a larger number of rheumatic fever patients of diverse ethnic origins, with essentially the same results (Table 36.1). The presence or absence of elevated levels of D8/17-positive B cells in cases in which the diagnosis of rheumatic fever has been in doubt has been helpful in establishing or excluding the diagnosis.

These studies are in contrast to other reports in which an increased frequency of HLA-DR4 and HLA-DR2 has been seen in white and African-American patients with rheumatic heart disease (50). Other studies have implicated DR1 and DRW6 as susceptibility factors in South African black patients with rheumatic heart disease (51). Most recently, Guilherme et al. (52) reported an increased frequency of HLA-DR7 and DW53 in rheumatic fever patients in Brazil. These seemingly conflicting results concerning HLA antigens and rheumatic fever susceptibility prompt speculation that these reported associations might be of class II genes close to (or in linkage disequilibrium with), but not identical, to the putative rheumatic fever susceptibility gene. Alternatively, and more likely, susceptibility to ARF is polygenic, and the D8/17 antigen might be associated with only one of the genes conferring susceptibility (i.e., those of the MHC

complex encoding for DR antigens). Although the explanation remains to be determined, the presence of the D8/17 antigen appears to identify a population at special risk for contracting ARF.

**ETIOLOGIC CONSIDERATIONS**

Although a large body of evidence, both immunologic and epidemiologic, has implicated group A streptococcus in the induction of the disease process, the exact pathologic mechanisms involved in the process still remain obscure. At least three main theories have been proposed.

The first theory is concerned with the question of whether persistence of the organism is important. Despite several controversial reports, no investigators have been able to demonstrate consistently and reproducibly live organisms in rheumatic fever cardiac tissues or valves (53).

The second theory revolves around the question of whether the deposition of toxic products or stimulation by them is required. Although an attractive hypothesis, little or no experimental evidence has been obtained to support this concept. For example, Halbert et al. (54) have suggested that streptolysin O (an extracellular product of group A streptococci) is cardiotoxic and might be carried to the site by circulating complexes containing streptolysin O and antibody. Despite an intensive search for these products, however, no such complexes *in situ* have been identified (55,56).

Renewed interest in these extracellular toxins has emerged with the observation by Schlievert et al. (57) that certain streptococcal pyrogenic toxins (A and C) may act as superantigens. These antigens may stimulate large numbers of T cells through their unique interaction between MHC class II and T-cell receptors of specific Vβ types. This interaction does not involve the usual concept of antigen presentation in the context of the MHC complex. Once activated, these cells induce production of TNF, interferon-γ, and a number of interleukin moieties, thereby contributing to the initiation of pathologic damage. Furthermore, it has been suggested that in certain disease states, such as rheumatoid arthritis, autoreactive cells of specific Vβ lineage may "home" to the target organ (43). Although an attractive hypothesis, no data concerning the role of these superantigens in rheumatic fever have as yet been forthcoming.

Perhaps the best evidence to date favors the theory of an abnormal host immune response (both humoral and cellular) in the genetically susceptible person to those streptococcal antigens cross-reactive with mammalian tissues. The evidence supporting this theory may be divided into three broad categories.

1. Employing a wide variety of methods, numerous investigators have documented the presence of heart-reactive antibodies in rheumatic fever sera. The incidence of these antibodies has varied from a low of 33% to a high of 85% in various series. Although these antibodies are seen in other people (notably those with uncomplicated strepto-

**TABLE 36.1.** *Frequency of the D8/17 marker in patients with rheumatic fever and other diseases and in controls in various geographic populations*

| Population | No. of patients (positive/total) | Percentage positive |
|---|---|---|
| Rheumatic fever patients | | |
| New York (USA) | 43/45 | 93 |
| New Mexico (USA) | 30/31 | 97 |
| Utah[a] (USA) | 18/18 | 100 |
| Russia (Georgian) | 27/30 | 90 |
| Russia (Moscow) | 50/52 | 96 |
| Mexico | 35/39 | 89 |
| Chile | 45/50 | 90 |
| Control subjects | | |
| Russia | 4/78 | 5 |
| New York | 6/68 | 8 |
| Chile | 8/50 | 16 |
| Mexico | 6/72 | 8 |
| Patients with other diseases | | |
| Rheumatoid arthritis | 2/42 | 4 |
| Ischemic heart disease | 0/10 | 0 |
| Multiple sclerosis | 1/25 | 4 |
| Lupus erythematosus | 1/12 | 9 |

[a] Acute patients

coccal infections that do not go on to rheumatic fever and patients with poststreptococcal glomerulonephritis), the titers are always lower than those seen in rheumatic fever (Table 36.2) and decrease with time during the convalescent period.

An important point, both in terms of diagnosis and prognosis, has been the observation of Zabriskie et al. (56) that these heart-reactive antibody titers decline over time (56). By the end of 3 years, these titers are essentially undetectable in patients who had only a single attack (Fig. 36.3). This pattern is consistent with the well-known clinical observations that recurrences of rheumatic fever most often occur within the first 2 to 3 years after the initial attack and become rarer 5 years after an initial episode.

As illustrated in Fig. 36.4, this pattern of titers also has prognostic value. During the 2- to 5-year period after the initial attack, the titer of anti–heart-reactive antibody in this representative patient dropped to undetectable levels. With a known break in prophylaxis starting in year 6, however, at least two streptococcal infections occurred, as evidenced by the rise in anti–streptolysin O titers during that period. Of note was the concomitant rise in heart-reactive antibody titers. The final infection was followed by a clinical recurrence of classic rheumatic carditis complete with isolation of the organism, elevated heart-reactive antibodies, and acute-phase reactants 11 years after the initial attack.

2. Rheumatic fever serum also contains increased levels of antibodies to myosin and tropomyosin, compared with serum from patients with pharyngeal streptococcal infections who do not go on to develop RF. These myosin affinity purified antibodies also cross-react with M-protein moieties, suggesting that this molecule could be the antigenic stimulus for the production of myosin antibodies in these sera (20). Khanna et al. tested ARF sera against crude and later purified cardiac extracts and found that ARF sera react primarily to human cardiac tropomyosin (58).

3. Finally, as indicated previously, autoimmune antibodies are a prominent finding in another major clinical manifestation of ARF, namely chorea, and these antibodies are directed against the cells of the caudate nucleus. The titer of this antibody corresponds to clinical disease activity (31).

Although not necessarily autoimmune in nature, the presence of elevated levels of immune complexes in ARF has been well documented in the sera and joints of ARF patients (59,60). These levels, which may be as high as those seen in classic poststreptococcal glomerulonephritis, may be responsible for the immune complex vasculitis seen in ARF tissues and may provide the initial impetus for vascular damage followed by the secondary penetration of autoreactive antibodies. Support for this concept is the close clinical similarity of rheumatic fever arthritis to experimentally induced serum sickness in animals or the arthritis seen secondary to drug hypersensitivity. Deposition of host immunoglobulin and complement is also seen in the cardiac tissues of ARF patients, suggesting autoimmune deposition of immunoglobulins in or near Aschoff's lesions.

At a cellular level, there is now ample evidence for the presence of lymphocytes and macrophages at the site of pathologic damage in the heart in patients with ARF (61). The cells are predominantly CD4+ (helper) lymphocytes during acute stages of the disease (4:1). The ratio of CD4+ to CD8+ lymphocytes (2:1) more closely approximates the normal ratio in chronic valvular specimens. Most of these cells express DR antigens. A potentially important finding has been the observation that macrophage-like fibroblasts present in the diseased valves express DR antigens (62) and might be the antigen-presenting cells for the CD4+ lymphocytes. Increased cellular reactivity to streptococcal antigens has also been noted in the peripheral blood mononuclear cell preparations of ARF patients when compared with these cells isolated from nephritis patients (37). This abnormal reactivity peaks 6 months after the attack but may persist for as long as 2 years after the initial episode. Once again, the reactivity was specific only for those strains associated with ARF, suggesting an abnormal humoral and cellular response to streptococcal antigens unique to rheumatic fever–associated streptococci.

Support for the potential pathologic importance of these T cells is further strengthened by the observation that lym-

TABLE 36.2. *Heart-reactive antibody titers in the sera of patients with acute rheumatic fever as compared with uncomplicated streptococcal infections and other arthritic conditions*

| Clinical disorder | No. of patients | Serum dilutions | | | Average ASO titer |
| --- | --- | --- | --- | --- | --- |
| | | 1:5 | 1:10 | 1:20 | |
| Acute rheumatic fever (grade 1) | 34 | 4+ | 2+ | +[a] | 700 |
| Uncomplicated streptococcal infections (grade 2) | 40 | 1+ | 0 | 0 | 561 |
| APSGN | 20 | +/− | 0 | 0 | 520 |
| Rheumatoid arthritis | 10 | 0 | 0 | 0[b] | ND |
| Lupus erythematosus | 10 | 0 | 0 | 0 | ND |

[a] Serum samples obtained at onset of rheumatic fever and at a comparable time in the group with uncomplicated scarlet fever.
[b] Sera obtained during active disease.
APSGM, acute poststreptococcal glomerulonephritis; ASO, anti-streptolysin O; ND, not determined.

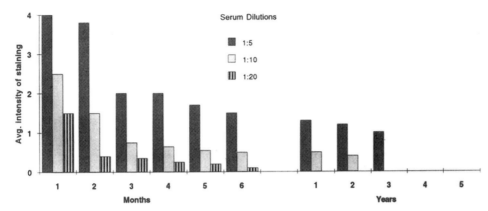

**FIG. 36.3.** Serial heart-reactive antibody titers in 40 patients with documented acute rheumatic fever. Note: the slow decline of these titers during the first 2 years after the initial episode and the absence of these antibodies 5 years after the initial attack.

phocytes obtained from experimental animals sensitized to cell membranes but not cell walls are specifically cytotoxic for syngeneic embryonic cardiac myofibers *in vitro* (63). In humans, normal mononuclear cells primed *in vitro* by M-protein molecules from an RF-associated strain are also cytotoxic for myofibers, but specificity solely for cardiac cells was lacking in the human studies (64). Similar studies have not been performed yet using lymphocytes from active ARF patients.

## CLINICAL FEATURES OF ACUTE DISEASE

The clinical presentation of ARF is variable, and the lack of a single pathognomonic feature has resulted in the development of the revised Jones criteria (Table 36.3), which are used to establish a diagnosis (65,66). These criteria were established only as guidelines for the diagnosis and were never intended to be unchanging. Thus, depending on the

age, geographic location, or ethnic population, emphasis on one criterion for the diagnosis of ARF may be more important than consideration of others. Manifestations of rheumatic fever that are not clearly expressed pose a dilemma because of the importance of identifying a first rheumatic attack clearly to establish the need for prophylaxis of recurrences (see later). Some of the isolated manifestations, particularly polyarthritis, may be difficult or impossible to distinguish from other diseases, especially at their onset. The diagnosis can be made, however, when "pure" chorea is the sole manifestation because of the rarity with which this syndrome has any other cause.

## ARTHRITIS

In the classic, untreated case, the arthritis of rheumatic fever affects several joints in quick succession, each for a short time. The legs are usually affected first and later the arms.

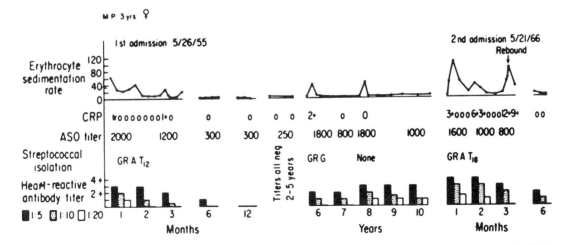

**FIG. 36.4.** Heart-reactive antibody titers and laboratory data obtained from a patient with rheumatic fever who had two well-documented acute attacks 11 years apart. Note the absence of the heart-reactive antibody during years 2 to 5 and its reappearance during years 6 to 10 after evidence of two intercurrent streptococcal infections secondary to breaks in penicillin prophylaxis (see anti–streptolysin O [*ASO*] titers). High titers of heart-reactive antibody appeared with the second attack. *CRP*, C-reactive protein.

**TABLE 36.3.** *Revised Jones criteria for diagnosis of acute rheumatic fever*

Major manifestations
  Carditis
  Polyarthritis
  Chorea
  Erythema marginatum
  Subcutaneous nodules
Minor manifestations
  Fever
  Arthralgia
  Previous rheumatic fever or rheumatic heart disease
Laboratory findings
  Elevated acute-phase reactants
    C-reactive protein
    Erythrocyte sedimentation rate
  Prolonged PR interval rate
Supporting evidence of preceding streptococcal infection
  Increased ASO or other streptococcal antibodies
  Positive throat culture for group A hemolytic streptococci
  Recent scarlet fever

ASO, anti-streptolysin O
From Special Writing Group of the Committee on Rheumatic Fever, Endocarditis, and Kawasaki Disease of the Council on Cardiovascular Disease in the Young of the American Heart Association. Guidelines for the diagnosis of rheumatic fever. Jones criteria, 1992 update [published erratum appears in *JAMA* 1993;269:476 [see comments]. *JAMA* 1992;268:2069–2073, with permission.

The terms *migrating* and *migratory* are often used to describe the polyarthritis of RF, but these designations are not meant to signify that the inflammation necessarily disappears in one joint when it appears in another. Rather, the various locations usually overlap in time, and the onset, as opposed to the full course of the arthritis, "migrates" from joint to joint.

Joint involvement is more common and also more severe in teenagers and young adults than in children. This involvement occurs early in the rheumatic illness and is usually the earliest symptomatic manifestation of the disease, although asymptomatic carditis may precede it. Rheumatic polyarthritis may be excruciatingly painful but is almost always transient. The pain is usually more prominent than the objective signs of inflammation.

When the disease is allowed to express itself fully, unchecked by antiinflammatory treatment, more than half of patients studied show a true polyarthritis, with inflammation in anywhere from 6 to 16 joints. Classically, each joint is maximally inflamed for only a few days or a week at the most. The inflammation decreases, perhaps lingering for another week or so, and then disappears completely. Radiographs at this point may show a slight effusion but most likely will be unremarkable.

In routine practice, however, many patients with arthritis or arthralgias are treated empirically with salicylates or other nonsteroidal antiinflammatory drugs. Accordingly, arthritis subsides quickly in the joints already affected and does not migrate to new joints. Thus, therapy may deprive the diagnostician of a useful sign. In a large series of patients with rheumatic fever and associated arthritis, most of whom had been treated, involvement of only a single large joint was common (25%). One or both knees were affected in 76% of patients and 1 or both ankles in 50%. Elbows, wrists, hips, or small joints of the feet were involved in 12% to 15% of patients, and shoulder or small joints of the head were affected in 7% to 8%. Joints rarely affected were the lumbosacral (2%), cervical (1%), sternoclavicular (0.5%), and temporomandibular (0.5%). Involvement of the small joints of the hands or feet alone occurred in only 1% of these patients.

Analysis of the synovial fluid in well-documented cases of rheumatic fever with arthritis generally reveals a sterile, inflammatory fluid. There may be a decrease of the complement components C1q, C3, and C4 and the presence of immunoglobulins indicating their consumption by immune complexes in the joint fluid (59).

## POSTSTREPTOCOCCAL REACTIVE ARTHRITIS

A number of investigators (67,68) have raised the question of whether poststreptococcal migratory arthritis (in adults and children) in the absence of carditis might be a distinct entity from ARF, for the following reasons:

1. The latent period between the antecedent streptococcal infection and the onset of ARF is shorter (1 to 2 weeks) than the 3 to 4 weeks usually seen in classic ARF.
2. The response of the arthritis to aspirin and other nonsteroidal medications is poor in comparison to the dramatic response seen in classic ARF.
3. Evidence of carditis is not usually seen in these patients; further, the severity of the arthritis is marked.
4. Extraarticular manifestations (such as tenosynovitis and renal abnormalities) are often seen in these patients.

Although these features may be seen (admittedly rarely), migratory arthritis without evidence of other major Jones criteria, if supported by two minor manifestations (Table 36.3), must still be considered ARF, especially in children. Variations in the response to aspirin in these children are often not documented with serum salicylate levels, and an unusual clinical course is not sufficient to exclude the diagnosis of ARF. Thus, appropriate prophylactic measures should be taken (69). Support for this concept may be found in the work of Crea (70). In this series of patients with ARF, 50% of the children who presented solely with signs of migratory arthritis went on to develop significant valvular damage.

RF in adults also occurs. Although migratory arthritis is a common presenting symptom, a recent outbreak in the San Diego Naval Training Camp (71) revealed a 30% incidence of valvular damage in these patients. The lower attack rate of ARF in adults has usually been attributed to the fact that in patients older than 18 to 20 years of age, the incidence of streptococcal infection declines, mainly as a result of a broad-based immunity to the organism. As the likelihood of getting a streptococcal infection diminishes, the incidence of ARF would be lower in adults.

In our opinion, reactive arthritis after a streptococcal infection should be considered an rheumatic fever variant, and secondary prophylactic treatment should be instituted. We disagree with the contention of some investigators that poststreptococcal reactive arthritis is a benign condition without need for prophylaxis. These patients by and large do fulfill the Jones criteria (one major, two minor). Thus, they should be considered as having rheumatic fever and treated as such.

## CARDITIS

Cardiac valvular and muscle damage can manifest in a variety of signs or symptoms. These manifestations include organic heart murmurs, cardiomegaly, congestive heart failure (CHF), or pericarditis. Mild to moderate chest discomfort, pleuritic chest pain, and a pericardial friction rub can be indications of pericarditis. On clinical examination, the patient may have new or changing organic murmurs, most commonly mitral regurgitant murmurs, and occasionally aortic regurgitant murmurs or systolic ejection murmurs caused by acute valvular inflammation and deformity. Rarely, a Carey–Coombs mid-diastolic murmur caused by rapid flow over the mitral valve is heard. If the valvular damage is severe and there is concurrent cardiac dysfunction, CHF can occur. CHF is the most life-threatening clinical syndrome of ARF and must be treated aggressively and early with a combination of antiinflammatory drugs, diuretics, and, occasionally, steroids to decrease cardiac inflammation acutely. Electrocardiographic abnormalities may include all degrees of heart block, including atrioventricular dissociation, but first-degree heart block is not associated with a poor prognosis. Second- or third-degree heart block can occasionally be symptomatic. If heart block is associated with CHF, temporary pacemaker placement may be required. The most common manifestation of carditis is cardiomegaly, as seen on radiograph.

In the patient population reviewed from the Rockefeller University Hospital who were diagnosed with ARF between 1950 and 1970 with an average of 20 years of follow-up, 90% had evidence of carditis at diagnosis. In Bland and Jones' (72) classic review of 1000 patients, only 65% of the patients were diagnosed with carditis. When Doppler ultrasonography was employed in the clinical evaluation of patients during the Utah outbreak, however, 91% of patients had carditis (1), indicating that with more sensitive measurements of cardiac dysfunction, almost all ARF patients have signs of acute carditis.

## RHEUMATIC HEART DISEASE

Rheumatic heart disease (RHD) is the most severe complication of ARF. Usually occurring 10 to 20 years after the original attack, it is the major cause of acquired valvular disease in the world. The mitral valve is mainly involved, and aortic valve involvement occurs less often. Mitral stenosis is a classic RHD finding and can manifest as a combination of mitral insufficiency and stenosis, secondary to severe calcification of the mitral valve. When symptoms of left atrial enlargement are present, mitral valve replacement may become necessary.

In various studies, the incidence of RHD in patients with a history of ARF has varied. In Bland and Jones' classic study (72), after 20 years, one third of patients had no murmur, another one third died, and the remaining one third were alive with RHD (72). Most of the patients who died had RHD. Although the classic dogma is that patients with RHD invariably had more than one attack of ARF, an analysis of the authors' patients at the Rockefeller University Hospital disproved this notion. The population studied was 87 patients who had only one documented attack of ARF without any evidence (clinical or laboratory) of a recurrence during a 20-year follow-up under close supervision. More than 80% had carditis at admission, and about 50% now have organic murmurs. Thus, valvular damage manifesting as organic murmurs later in life is still likely to occur in 50% of patients, particularly if they presented with evidence of carditis at initial diagnosis. All of the patients in this who ended up with RHD had carditis at diagnosis.

## CHOREA

Sydenham's chorea, chorea minor, or "St. Vitus dance," is a neurologic disorder consisting of abrupt, purposeless, non-rhythmic involuntary movements, muscular weakness, and emotional disturbances. These symptoms disappear during sleep but may occur at rest and may interfere with voluntary activity. Initially, it may be possible to suppress these movements, which may affect all voluntary muscles, with the hands and face usually the most obvious. Grimaces and inappropriate smiles are common. Handwriting usually becomes clumsy and provides a convenient way of following the patient's course. Speech is often slurred. The movements are commonly more marked on one side and are occasionally completely unilateral (hemichorea).

Chorea may follow streptococcal infections after a latent period, which is longer on the average than the latent period of other rheumatic manifestations. Some patients with chorea have no other symptoms, but other patients develop chorea weeks or months after arthritis. In both cases, examination of the heart may reveal murmurs.

A new and potentially interesting chapter is unfolding concerning this manifestation of RF. It has been known for years that the early symptoms of chorea often present as emotional or behavioral changes in the patient, and that only later do the choreiform motor symptoms appear (73). It was also noted that some chorea patients, years after the choreiform symptoms had subsided, would present with behavioral disorders, such as tics or obsessive compulsive disorder (OCD).

These earlier observations, coupled with the known presence of antibrain antibodies in the sera of Sydenham's chorea patients (31), raised the question of whether a prior streptococcal infection (or infection with other microbes) might induce antibodies cross-reactive with brain antigen involved in neural pathways associated with obsessive behaviors but not with classic Sydenham's chorea. Two papers (74,75) indicated there is a strong association of the D8/17 B-cell marker (described previously in children with OCD). Although Swedo et al. (75) selected patients on the basis of a strong history of prior streptococcal infections, Murphy et al. (74) noted a strong association of the marker with OCD patients without a history of streptococcal infections. These patients also exhibit antibrain antibodies in the sera, and the pattern appears to be different from the antibrain antibodies seen in classic chorea.

These preliminary studies suggest that streptococci and probably other microbes may induce antibodies that functionally disrupt the basal ganglia pathways, leading not only to classic chorea but also to disorders more behavioral in nature. It is our belief that the type of antibrain antibody produced is different in each group, which would account for the different clinical manifestations of each disease group.

## SUBCUTANEOUS NODULES

The subcutaneous nodules of rheumatic fever are firm and painless. The overlying skin is not inflamed and can usually be moved over the nodules. The diameter of these round lesions varies from a few millimeters to 1 or even 2 cm. They are located over a bony surface or prominences or near tendons; their number varies from a single nodule to a few dozen and averages three or four. When numerous, they are usually symmetric. These nodules are present for 1 week or longer but rarely for more than 1 month. They are smaller and more short lived than the nodules of RA. Although in both diseases, the elbows are most frequently involved, the rheumatic nodules are more common on the olecranon, and the rheumatoid nodules are usually found 3 or 4 cm distal to it. Rheumatic subcutaneous nodules generally appear only after the first few weeks of illness, usually only in patients with carditis.

## ERYTHEMA MARGINATUM

Erythema marginatum is an evanescent, nonpruritic skin rash, pink or faintly red, affecting usually the trunk and sometimes the proximal parts or the limbs but not the face. This lesion extends centrifugally, whereas the skin in the center returns gradually to normal; hence, the name *erythema marginatum*. The outer edge of the lesion is sharp, whereas the inner edge is diffuse. Because the margin of the lesion is usually continuous, making a ring, it is also known as *erythema annulare*.

The individual lesions may appear and disappear in a matter of hours, usually to return. A hot bath or shower may make them more evident or may even reveal them for the first time.

Erythema marginatum usually occurs in the early phase of the disease. It often persists or recurs, even when all other manifestations of the disease have disappeared. Occasionally, the lesions appear for the first time or, more likely, are noticed for the first time, late in the course of the illness or even during convalescence. This disorder usually occurs only in patients with carditis.

## MINOR MANIFESTATIONS

### Fever

Temperature is increased in almost all rheumatic attacks and ranges from 38.4° to 40°C. Temperature usually decreases in about 1 week without antipyretic treatment and may become low grade for another 1 or 2 weeks. Fever rarely lasts for more than 3 to 4 weeks.

### Abdominal Pain

The abdominal pain of rheumatic fever resembles that of other conditions associated with acute microvascular mesenteric inflammation and is nonspecific. It usually occurs at or near the onset of the rheumatic attack, so that other manifestations may not be present yet to clarify the diagnosis. In many cases, it may mimic acute appendicitis.

### Epistaxis

In the past, epistaxis occurred most prominently and severely in patients with severe and protracted rheumatic carditis. Early clinical studies reported a frequency as high as 48%, but it probably occurs even less frequently now (Table 36.3). Although epistaxis has been correlated in the past with the severity of rheumatic inflammation, it is difficult to assess retrospectively the possible thrombasthenic effect of large doses of salicylates administered for prolonged periods in protracted attacks.

### Rheumatic Pneumonia

Rheumatic pneumonia may appear during the course of severe rheumatic carditis. This inflammatory process is difficult or impossible to distinguish from pulmonary edema or the alveolitis associated with respiratory distress syndromes caused by a variety of pathophysiologic states.

## LABORATORY FINDINGS

The diagnosis of rheumatic fever cannot readily be established by laboratory tests. Nevertheless, these may be helpful in two ways: first, in demonstrating that an antecedent streptococcal infection has occurred; and second, in documenting the presence or persistence of an inflammatory process. Serial chest radiographs may be helpful in following the course of carditis, and the electrocardiogram may reflect the inflammatory process on the conduction system.

Throat cultures are usually negative by the time rheumatic fever appears, but an attempt should be made to isolate the organism. It is our practice to take three throat cultures during the first 24 hours before administration of antibiotics. Streptococcal antibodies are more useful because (a) they reach a peak titer at about the time of onset of RF, (b) they indicate true infection rather than transient carriage, and (c) by performing several tests for different antibodies, any significant recent streptococcal infection can be detected. To demonstrate a rising titer, it is useful to take a serum specimen when the patient is first seen and another one 2 weeks later for comparison.

The specific antibody tests that have been used to diagnosis streptococcal infections most frequently are those directed against extracellular products. They include anti–streptolysin O, anti–DNAse B, antihyaluronidase, anti-NADase (anti-DPNase), and antistreptokinase. Anti–streptolysin O has been the most widely used test and is generally available in hospitals in the United States.

Streptococcal antibodies, when increased, support but do not make the diagnosis of ARF, nor are they a measure of rheumatic activity. Even in the absence of intercurrent streptococcal infection, titers decline during the rheumatic attack despite the persistence or severity of rheumatic activity.

### Acute-Phase Reactants

Acute-phase reactants are elevated during ARF, just as they are during other inflammatory conditions. The C-reactive protein and erythrocyte sedimentation rate (ESR) are almost invariably abnormal during the active rheumatic process, if it is not suppressed by antirheumatic drugs. These may be normal, however, during episodes of pure chorea or persistent erythema marginatum. Particularly when treatment has been discontinued or is being tapered, the C-reactive protein and ESR are useful in monitoring rebounds of rheumatic inflammation, which indicate that the rheumatic process is still active. If either the C-reactive protein or ESR remains normal a few weeks after discontinuing antirheumatic therapy, the attack may be considered ended unless chorea appears. Even then, there is usually no exacerbation of the systemic inflammation, and chorea is present as an isolated manifestation.

### Other Supporting Tests

As noted in Fig. 36.3 and Table 36.2, two other tests have, in our experience, been helpful in confirming the diagnosis of ARF, especially when the diagnosis is in doubt. First, elevated titers of heart-reactive antibodies to sarcolemmal antigens can be detected in most ARF patients. In our experience, antibodies to cardiac tropomyosin were most elevated in these patients and could be detected by enzyme-linked immunosorbent assay (58).

Second, the use of the D8/17 monoclonal antibody mentioned previously has proved helpful in the differential diagnosis of ARF from other disorders. In our experience, all rheumatic fever patients expressed abnormal levels of D8/17-positive B cells, especially during the acute attack. In those cases in which the diagnosis of ARF has been in doubt, the presence of elevated levels of D8/17-positive B cells has been helpful in establishing the correct diagnosis (49).

## CLINICAL COURSE AND TREATMENT OF ACUTE DISEASE

Since the late 1800s, the mainstay of treatment of ARF has always been antiinflammatory agents, most commonly aspirin. In 1876, Maclagan (76) suggested willow bark ingestion as a primary treatment of RF. He reasoned that plants that arise from "conditions analogous to those under which the rheumatic miasm" occurred would contain a likely therapeutic agent. The salicylates as a class of agents were popularized by Lees three decades later (77). Dramatic improvement in symptoms is seen in most patients after the start of therapy. Usually, 80 to 100 mg/kg/day in children and 4 to 8 g/day in adults is required for an effect to be seen. Aspirin levels can be measured, and 20 to 30 mg/dL is the therapeutic range. The duration of antiinflammatory therapy can vary, but treatment needs to be maintained until all symptoms are absent and laboratory values are normal.

The primary treatment of ARF is antiinflammatory. The accepted treatment of the rheumatic carditis with corticosteroids has remained predominantly unchanged since the controlled trials of the drug in the 1950s. There is little clear evidence of the benefit of corticosteroids over salicylates, however, because of the limited number of studies and the fact that more than 80% of rheumatic carditis cases heal completely without treatment. In addition, mild changes in mitral valve function are difficult to define and standardize with echocardiography (78,79). If severe carditis is also present (as indicated by significant cardiomegaly, CHF, or third-degree heart block), steroid therapy should be instituted. The usual dosage is 2 mg/kg/day of oral prednisone during the first 1 to 2 weeks. Depending on clinical and laboratory improvement, the dosage is then tapered over the next 2 weeks, and during the last week, aspirin may be added in the dosage recommended previously, sufficient to achieve the 20 to 30 mg/dL level.

Whether or not signs of pharyngitis are present at the time of diagnosis, antibiotic therapy with penicillin should be started and maintained for at least 10 days, given in doses recommended for the eradication of a streptococcal pharyngitis. In addition, all family contacts should be cultured and, if positive, treated for streptococcal infection. If compliance is an issue, depot penicillins, that is, benzathine penicillin G, 600,000 U in children or 1.2 million U in adults, should be given. Recurrences of ARF are most common within 2 years of the original attack but can occur at any time. The risk for recurrence decreases with age. Recurrence rates have been decreasing from 20% to between 2% and 4% in recent outbreaks.

## PROPHYLAXIS

Antibiotic prophylaxis with penicillin should be started immediately after resolution of the acute episode. The optimal regimen consists of oral penicillin VK, 250,000 U twice a day, or by injecting penicillin G, 1.2 million U given intramuscularly every 4 weeks. Data suggest, however, that injections given every 3 weeks are more effective than those given every 4 weeks in preventing ARF recurrences. If the patient is allergic to penicillin, oral erythromycin, 250 mg twice daily, can be substituted.

The end point of prophylaxis is unclear; most believe it should continue at least until the patient is a young adult, which is usually 10 years from an acute attack with no recurrence. In our opinion, patients with documented evidence of rheumatic heart disease should be on continuous prophylaxis indefinitely because we have seen recurrences even in the fifth or sixth decades. Another potential problem for ARF recurrences is young children in the household who could transmit new group A streptococcal infections to RF-susceptible people.

## VACCINATION

The alternative to long-term prophylaxis in individuals who are susceptible to ARF will be the introduction of streptococcal vaccines designed not only to prevent recurrent infections but also to prevent streptococcal disease in general. Although it is not within the scope of this paper to discuss the prospects of these vaccines, at least a few words should be written regarding prospects. Immunization of mice with either M-protein C repeat peptides or a cloned M protein in a vaccinia virus vector protected them against intranasal infection of homologous or heterologous strains of group A streptococci. Whether these antigens or vectors are protective in humans is under investigation. Additional promising work on a group A carbohydrate vaccine (80) and multivalent M-protein–based vaccines (81) is also taking place. One of the major problems with all these candidates will be to avoid using the parts of the molecule that cross-react with mammalian tissue.

## CONCLUSIONS

Despite its disappearance in many areas of the world, rheumatic fever continues to be a serious problem in those geographic areas where two thirds of the population live. Even in developed countries with full access to medical care, better nutrition, and better housing, the recent resurgence of the disease in these areas emphasizes the need for continued vigilance of physicians and other health officials in diagnosing and treating RF. Whether this resurgence represents a change in the virulence of the organism or failure to recognize the importance and adequate treatment of an antecedent streptococcal infection remains an area of intense debate and will therefore require careful and controlled epidemiologic surveillance. The importance of early diagnosis and therapy cannot be overemphasized. Although the joint manifestations are transient and self-limiting, the cardiac sequelae are chronic and life-threatening.

Nevertheless, rheumatic fever remains one of the few autoimmune disorders known to occur as a result of infection with a specific organism. The confirmed observation of an increased frequency of a B-cell alloantigen in several populations of rheumatic patients suggests that it might be possible to identify RF-susceptible people at birth. If so, then from a public health standpoint, (a) these people would be prime candidates for immunization with any streptococcal vaccine that might be developed in the future; (b) careful monitoring of streptococcal disease in the susceptible population could lead to early and effective antibiotic strategies, resulting in disease prevention; and (c) in people previously infected, who later present with subtle or nonspecific manifestations of the disease, the presence or absence of the marker could be of value in arriving at a diagnosis.

The continued study of rheumatic fever as a prime example of microbe–host interactions also has important implications for the study of autoimmune diseases in general and rheumatic diseases in particular. Further insights into this intriguing host–parasite relationship may shed additional light onto those diseases in which the infection is presumed but has not yet been identified.

## REFERENCES

1. Veasy LG, Wiedmeier SE, Orsmond GS, et al. Resurgence of acute rheumatic fever in the intermountain area of the United States. *N Engl J Med* 1987;316:421–427.
2. Gordis L. The virtual disappearance of rheumatic fever in the United States: lessons in the rise and fall of disease. T. Duckett Jones memorial lecture. *Circulation* 1985;72:1155–1162.
3. Pope RM. Rheumatic fever in the 1980s. *Bull Rheum Dis* 1989;38:1–8.
4. Markowitz M, Gordis L. Rheumatic fever. *Major Probl Clin Pediatr* 1972;11:1–309.
5. Kaplan EL, Johnson DR, Cleary PP. Group A streptococcal serotypes isolated from patients and sibling contacts during the resurgence of rheumatic fever in the United States in the mid-1980s. *J Infect Dis* 1989;159:101–103.
6. Whitnack E, Bisno AL. Rheumatic fever and other immunologically mediated cardiac diseases. In: Parker C, ed. *Clinical immunology*. Philadelphia: WB Saunders, 1980:894–929.
7. Stollerman GH. *Rheumatic fever and streptococcal infection*. Boston: Grune & Stratton, 1975.
8. Denny FW, Wannamaker LW, Brink WR. Prevention of rheumatic fever: treatment of the preceding streptococcal infection. *JAMA* 1950; 143:151–153.
9. Markowitz M, Gerber MA. Rheumatic fever: recent outbreaks of an old disease. *Conn Med* 1987;51:229–233.
10. Stollerman GH, Schultz AJ. Relationship of the immune response to group A streptococci to the cause of the acute, chronic and recurrent rheumatic fever. *Am J Med* 1956;20:163–169.
11. Potter EV, Svartman M, Mohammed I, et al. Tropical acute rheumatic fever and associated streptococcal infections compared with concurrent acute glomerulonephritis. *J Pediatr* 1978;92:325–333.
12. Carapetis JR, Currie BJ. Group A streptococcus, pyoderma, and rheumatic fever [Letter; Comment]. *Lancet* 1996;347:1271–1272.
13. Kendall F, Heidelberger M, Dawson M. A serologically inactive polysaccharide elaborated by mucoid strains of group A hemolytic streptococcus. *J Biol Chem* 1937;118:61–82.
14. Quinn RW, Singh KP. Antigenicity of hyaluronic acid. *Biochem J* 1957; 95:290–301.
15. Seastone CV. The virulence of group C hemolytic streptococci of animal origin. *J Exp Med* 1939;70:361–378.
16. Fillit HM, McCarty M, Blake M. Induction of antibodies to hyaluronic acid by immunization of rabbits with encapsulated streptococci. *J Exp Med* 1986;164:762–776.

17. Fischetti VA. Streptococcal M protein: molecular design and biological behavior. *Clin Microbiol Rev* 1989;2:285–314.

18. Dale JB, Beachey EH. Multiple, heart-cross-reactive epitopes of streptococcal M proteins. *J Exp Med* 1985;161:113–122.

19. Sargent SJ, Beachey EH, Corbett CE, et al. Sequence of protective epitopes of streptococcal M proteins shared with cardiac sarcolemmal membranes. *J Immunol* 1987;139:1285–1290.

20. Cunningham MW, McCormack JM, Talaber LR, et al. Human monoclonal antibodies reactive with antigens of the group A streptococcus and human heart. *J Immunol* 1988;141:2760–2766.

21. McCarty M. The streptococcal cell wall. *Harvey Lect* 1970;65:73–96.

22. Goldstein I, Caravano R. Determination of anti group A streptococcal polysaccharide antibodies in human sera by an hemagglutination technique. *Proc Soc Exp Biol Med* 1967;124:1209–1212.

23. Salvadori LG, Blake MS, McCarty M, et al. Group A streptococcus-liposome ELISA antibody titers to group A polysaccharide and opsonophagocytic capabilities of the antibodies. *J Infect Dis* 1995;171:593–600.

24. Chetty C, Schwab JH, Chemistry of endotoxins. In: Rietschel-Elsenier ET, ed. *Handbook of endotoxin*. Hamburg, Germany: Science Publishers, 1984:376–410.

25. Cromartie WJ, Craddock JG, Schwab JH, et al. Arthritis in rats after systemic injection of streptococcal cells or cell walls. *J Exp Med* 1977;146:1585–1602.

26. Cromartie WJ, Craddock JG. Rheumatic-like cardiac lesions in mice. *Science* 1966;154:285–287.

27. Heymer B, Schleifer KH, Read S, et al. Detection of antibodies to bacterial cell wall peptidoglycan in human sera. *J Immunol* 1976;117:23–26.

28. Dziarski R, Tapping RI, Tobias PS. Binding of bacterial peptidoglycan to CD14. *J Biol Chem* 1998;273:8680–8690.

29. Hattor Y, Kasai K, Akimoto K, et al. Induction of NO synthesis by lipoteichoic acid from Staphylococcus aureus in J774 macrophages: involvement of a CD14-dependent pathway. *Biochem Biophys Res Commun* 1997;233:375–379.

30. Kingston D, Glynn LE. A cross-reaction between Str. pyogenes and human fibroblasts, endothelial cells and astrocytes. *Immunology* 1971;21:1003–1016.

31. Husby G, van de Rijn I, Zabriskie JB, et al. Antibodies reacting with cytoplasm of subthalamic and caudate nuclei neurons in chorea and acute rheumatic fever. *J Exp Med* 1976;144:1094–1110.

32. Froude J, Gibofsky A, Buskirk DR, et al. Cross-reactivity between streptococcus and human tissue: a model of molecular mimicry and autoimmunity. *Curr Top Microbiol Immunol* 1989;145:5–26.

33. Zabriskie JB. Rheumatic fever: the interplay between host, genetics, and microbe. Lewis A. Conner Memorial Lecture. *Circulation* 1985;71:1077–1086.

34. Tomai M, Kotb M, Majumdar G, et al. Superantigenicity of streptococcal M protein. *J Exp Med* 1990;172:359–362.

35. Fleischer B, Schmidt KH, Gerlach D, et al. Separation of T-cell-stimulating activity from streptococcal M protein. *Infect Immunol* 1992;60:1767–1770.

36. Schmidt KH, Gerlach D, Wollweber L, et al. Mitogenicity of M5 protein extracted from Streptococcus pyogenes cells is due to streptococcal pyrogenic exotoxin C and mitogenic factor MF. *Infect Immunol* 1995;63:4569–4575.

37. Read SE, Reid HF, Fischetti VA, et al. Serial studies on the cellular immune response to streptococcal antigens in acute and convalescent rheumatic fever patients in Trinidad. *J Clin Immunol* 1986;6:433–441.

38. Guilherme L, Cunha-Neto E, Coelho V, et al. Human heart-infiltrating T-cell clones from rheumatic heart disease patients recognize both streptococcal and cardiac proteins. *Circulation* 1995;92:415–420.

39. Dziarski R. Peptidoglycan and lipopolysaccharide bind to the same binding site on lymphocytes. *J Biol Chem* 1991;266:4719–4725.

40. Herman A, Labrecque N, Thibodeau J, et al. Identification of the staphylococcal enterotoxin A superantigen binding site in the beta 1 domain of the human histocompatibility antigen HLA-DR. *Proc Natl Acad Sci U S A* 1991;88:9954–9958.

41. Marrack P, Kappler J. The staphylococcal enterotoxins and their relatives [published erratum appears in *Science* 1990;248:1066; see Comments]. *Science* 1990;248:705–711.

42. White J, Herman A, Pullen AM, et al. The V beta-specific superantigen staphylococcal enterotoxin B: stimulation of mature T cells and clonal deletion in neonatal mice. *Cell* 1989;56:27–35.

43. Paliard X, West SG, Lafferty JA, et al. Evidence for the effects of a superantigen in rheumatoid arthritis. *Science* 1991;253:325–329.

44. Cheadle WB. Harvean Lectures on the various manifestations of the rheumatic state as exemplified in childhood and early life. *Lancet* 1889;1:821–832.

45. Wilson MG. The familial epidemiology of rheumatic fever. *J Pediatr* 1943;22:468–442.

46. Taranta A, Torosdag S, Metrakos JD. Rheumatic fever in monozygotic and dizygotic twins. *Circulation* 1959;20:778–792.

47. Glynn LE, Halborrow EJ. Relationship between blood groups, secretion status and susceptibility to rheumatic fever. *Arthritis Rheum* 1961;4:203.

48. Patarroyo ME, Winchester RJ, Vejerano A, et al. Association of a B-cell alloantigen with susceptibility to rheumatic fever. *Nature* 1979;278:173–174.

49. Khanna AK, Buskirk DR, Williams RC Jr, et al. Presence of a non-HLA B cell antigen in rheumatic fever patients and their families as defined by a monoclonal antibody. *J Clin Invest* 1989;83:1710–1716.

50. Ayoub EM, Barrett DJ, Maclaren NK, et al. Association of class II human histocompatibility leukocyte antigens with rheumatic fever. *J Clin Invest* 1986;77:2019–2026.

51. Maharaj B, Hammond MG, Appadoo B, et al. HLA-A, B, DR, and DQ antigens in black patients with severe chronic rheumatic heart disease. *Circulation* 1987;76:259–261.

52. Guilherme L, Weidebach W, Kiss MH, et al. Association of human leukocyte class II antigens with rheumatic fever or rheumatic heart disease in a Brazilian population. *Circulation* 1991;83:1995–1998.

53. Watson RF, Hirst GK, Lancefield RC. Bacteriological studies of cardiac tissues obtained at autopsy from eleven patients dying with rheumatic fever. *Arthritis Rheum* 1961;4:74–85.

54. Halbert SP, Bircher R, Dahle E. The analysis of streptococcal infections. V. Cardiotoxicity of streptolysin O for rabbits in vivo. *J Exp Med* 1961;113:759–784.

55. Wagner BM. Studies in rheumatic fever. III. Histochemical reactivity of the Aschoff body. *Ann N Y Acad Sci* 1960;86:992–1008.

56. Zabriskie JB, Hsu KC, Seegal BC. Heart-reactive antibody associated with rheumatic fever: characterization and diagnostic significance. *Clin Exp Immunol* 1970;7:147–159.

57. Schlievert PM, Johnson LP, Tomai MA. Characterization and genetics of group A streptococcal pyrogenic exotoxins. In: Ferreti J, Curtis R, ed. *Streptococcal genetics*. Washington DC: ASM, 1987:136–142.

58. Khanna AK, Nomura Y, Fischetti VA, et al. Antibodies in the sera of acute rheumatic fever patients bind to human cardiac tropomyosin. *J Autoimmunol* 1997;10:99–106.

59. Svartman M, Potter EV, Poon-King T, et al. Immunoglobulins and complement components in synovial fluid of patients with acute rheumatic fever. *J Clin Invest* 1975;56:111–117.

60. van de Rijn I, Fillit H, Brandeis WE, et al. Serial studies on circulating immune complexes in post-streptococcal sequelae. *Clin Exp Immunol* 1978;34:318–325.

61. Kemeny E, Grieve T, Marcus R, et al. Identification of mononuclear cells and T cell subsets in rheumatic valvulitis. *Clin Immunol Immunopathol* 1989;52:225–237.

62. Amoils B, Morrison RC, Wadee AA, et al. Aberrant expression of HLA-DR antigen on valvular fibroblasts from patients with active rheumatic carditis. *Clin Exp Immunol* 1986;66:88–94.

63. Yang LC, Soprey PR, Wittner MK, et al. Streptococcal-induced cell-mediated-immune destruction of cardiac myofibers in vitro. *J Exp Med* 1977;146:344–360.

64. Dale JB, Beachey EH. Human cytotoxic T lymphocytes evoked by group A streptococcal M proteins. *J Exp Med* 1987;166:1825–1835.

65. Special Writing Group of the Committee on Rheumatic Fever, Endocarditis, and Kawasaki Disease of the Council on Cardiovascular Disease in the Young of the American Heart Association. Guidelines for the diagnosis of rheumatic fever. Jones Criteria: 1992 update [published erratum appears in *JAMA;*269:476; see Comments]. *JAMA* 1992;268:2069–2073.

66. Stollerman GH, Markowitz M, Taranta A. Jones criteria (revised) for guidance in the diagnosis of rheumatic fever. *Circulation* 1965;32:664–668.

67. Arnold MH, Tyndall A. Poststreptococcal reactive arthritis [see Comments]. *Ann Rheum Dis* 1989;48:686–688.

68. Fink CW. The role of the streptococcus in poststreptococcal reactive arthritis and childhood polyarteritis nodosa. *J Rheumatol Suppl* 1991;29:14–20.

69. Gibofsky A, Zabriskie JB. Rheumatic fever: new insights into an old disease. *Bull Rheum Dis* 1993;42:5–7.
70. Crea MA. The nature of scarlatinal arthritis. *Pediatrics* 1959;23: 879–884.
71. Wallace MR, Garst PD, Papadimos TJ, et al. The return of acute rheumatic fever in young adults [see Comments]. *JAMA* 1989;262: 2557–2561.
72. Bland EF, Jones TD. Rheumatic fever and rheumatic heart disease: a twenty year report on 1,000 patients followed since childhood. *Circulation* 1951;4:836–843.
73. Osler W. *On chorea and choreioform movements.* Baltimore: HK Lewis, 1894.
74. Murphy TK, Goodman WK, Fudge MW, et al. B lymphocyte antigen D8/17: a peripheral marker for childhood-onset obsessive-compulsive disorder and Tourette's syndrome? *Am J Psychiatry* 1997;154:402–407.
75. Swedo SE, Leonard HL, Mittleman BB, et al. Identification of children with pediatric autoimmune neuropsychiatric disorders associated with streptococcal infections by a marker associated with rheumatic fever [see Comments]. *Am J Psychiatry* 1997;154:110–112.
76. Maclagan T. The treatment of acute rheumatic fever by salicin. *Lancet* 1876;1:342–343.
77. Lees DB. The treatment of some acute visceral inflammations: acute rheumatic carditis and pericarditis. *Br Med J* 1903;2:1318–1322.
78. Stollerman GH. Rheumatic carditis. *Lancet* 1995;346:390–392.
79. Albert DA, Harel L, Karrison T. The treatment of rheumatic carditis: a review and meta-analysis. *Medicine* (Baltimore) 1995;74:1–12.
80. Zabriskie JB, Poon-King T, Blake MS, et al. Phagocytic, serological, and protective properties of streptococcal group A carbohydrate antibodies. *Adv Exp Med Biol* 1997;418:917–919.
81. Dale JB. Group A streptococcal vaccines [In Process Citation]. *Infect Dis Clin North Am* 1999;13:227–243, viii.

*Textbook of the Autoimmune Diseases,*
Edited by R. G. Lahita, N. Chiorazzi, and W. H. Reeves,
Lippincott Williams & Wilkins, Philadelphia © 2000.

# CHAPTER 37

# Postinfectious Autoimmunity

Stanley J. Naides

Infectious agents are attractive etiologic candidates for various diseases of unknown cause. Speculation and hypotheses proposing specific microbial triggers for idiopathic autoimmune disease are fueled by the description of autoimmune or autoimmune-like responses to known infections. Potential mechanisms of initiation and perpetuation of autoimmunity by pathogens are discussed in Section I of this text. Animal models showing autoimmunity after infection by intact pathogens or exposure to microbial components further pique interest in the role of viruses, bacteria, and fungi as triggers of autoimmunity. Features of autoimmune diseases, such as rheumatoid arthritis, include arthralgia and frank arthritis, often prominent features of acute viral infection. Togaviruses are known to cause epidemics of acute febrile arthritis affecting thousands of people. Some affected patients may continue to have symptoms for months. Bacterial infections may have immune-mediated manifestations, such as the immune complex tenosynovitis associated with gonorrhea. Poststreptococcal infection sequelae are well recognized (see Chapter 36). Similarly, individual responses to mycobacterial or fungal infection may have autoimmune features. Demonstration of latency in microbial infections suggests the possibility that the triggering infectious agent may not always be cleared from the host after initiating the autoimmune process. Rather, its presence, even in amounts undetectable by standard assays, may be required to perpetuate the autoimmune response. Describing the mechanisms by which specific infectious agents cause symptoms and signs associated with autoimmunity may offer insights into the pathogenic mechanisms of idiopathic disease and identify specific etiologic agents for subsets of idiopathic autoimmune disease.

The definition of *autoimmunity* in the context of infectious disease agents needs further elaboration. Many idiopathic processes in which arthritis is a prominent feature are considered autoimmune. The first cases of Lyme disease identi-

fied in children in Connecticut were diagnosed as juvenile rheumatoid arthritis and carried that label until the specific etiologic agent, *Borrelia burgdorferi,* was identified and the epidemiology and pathogenesis delineated. Many infectious agents cause acute and chronic syndromes with clinical features that are mediated by activation of the immune system. In many instances, it is not yet known whether the activation of the immune response is initially induced by the pathogen itself or its antigens, or whether the pathogen alters the immune system's ability to control response to self antigens. Initial immune response to a specific pathogen's antigens may broaden to target self antigen through epitope spreading. Alternatively, virus may interact with host cell regulatory genes to increase cell growth or eliminate the host cell through cytopathic effects or induction of apoptosis. Selective enhancement or elimination of target populations could lead to dysregulation of immune homeostasis. To decide whether postchlamydial infection reactive arthritis, for example, represents an immune response to persistent chlamydia or chlamydial antigens or instead is an autoimmune response to cross-reactive self antigens is academic in the absence of a clear understanding of the mechanisms by which a particular pathogen causes disease. Targeted immune responses to specific pathogens may cause more nonspecific immune-mediated destruction of host tissues. For many of the pathogens discussed in this chapter, the determination of whether the disease they cause is immune or autoimmune awaits elucidation of the mechanisms by which they induce disease.

## VIRUSES

### Parvovirus B19

Human parvovirus B19 was first discovered in sera from normal blood donors in 1975 (1). B19 is a member of the virus family Parvoviridae, subfamily Parvovirinae, genus *Erythrovirus.* B19 is a nonenveloped, icosahedral, single-stranded DNA virus that replicates in erythroid precursors.

S. J. Naides: Department of Medicine, Section of Rheumatology, Pennsylvania State Univesity College of Medicine, Milton S. Hershey Medical Center, Hershey, Pennsylvania 17033.

Infection in nonerythroid tissues may occur but is less efficient. Numerous mammalian parvoviruses (e.g., canine parvovirus) are known, but parvoviruses do not cross species. Many of the syndromes associated with B19 infection have been well known, but the recognition of B19 as the etiologic agent has led to its designation as an emerging virus (2).

### Incidence and Epidemiology

Parvovirus B19 infection is a common worldwide community-acquired infection transmitted through respiratory secretions. Up to 70% of children in community outbreaks do not develop symptoms. Children often present to pediatricians with undiagnosed nonspecific viral symptoms (3). Up to 60% of adults have serologic evidence of past B19 infection (4). Outbreaks are reported throughout the year but occur most frequently in late winter and spring when indoor crowding is most common. Outbreaks tend to occur in 3- to 5-year cycles within a community, representing the time necessary to accumulate a new cohort of susceptible children in the schools (2). Workers in occupations with increased exposure to children, such as school teachers, day care workers, and hospital personnel, are at increased risk for infection (5). In nonepidemic periods, the risk to susceptible adults is less than 1%. With multiple classroom exposures during an outbreak, the risk for infection in susceptible teachers may be as high as 50% (6). Sporadic cases occur during nonepidemic periods.

The incubation period is 7 to 18 days after natural infection. Human volunteer studies demonstrated an influenza-like illness associated with viremia, viral shedding in nasal secretions, and areticulocytosis that occurs 7 days after nasal inoculation of virus. Specific immunoglobulin M (IgM) appears 4 to 6 days after onset viremia and was associated with resolution of viremia and viral shedding and with reticulocyte rebound. Onset of specific IgG occurs almost concurrently with the IgM response (7).

### Clinical Features

An influenza-like illness characterized by fever, malaise and myalgia is associated with viremia (2). Areticulocytosis occurs during the viremia as viral replication causes maturation arrest at the giant pronormoblast stage of erythrocyte development (8). A second phase of clinical illness, consisting of rash, arthralgia, and arthritis, occurs concomitant with the onset of IgM response (7,9–12).

Parvovirus B19 causes transient aplastic crisis in the setting of chronic hemolytic anemia (2). Failure to maintain reticulocytosis in the face of chronic hemolysis causes marked anemia lasting 7 to 10 days and usually requires transfusion support (13,14). In normal children, erythema infectiosum, or fifth disease, is the most common manifestation. This common rash illness in children is characterized by bright red "slapped cheeks" and a macular or maculopapular rash on the torso and extremities (Fig. 37.1) (15,16). Rash recurs after initial clearing in about half of children. Sore

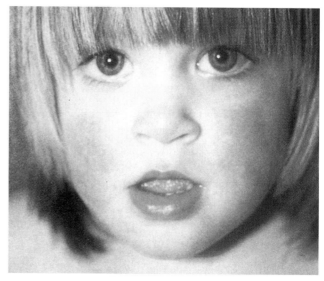

**FIG. 37.1.** Classic "slapped cheeks" of a child with erythema infectiosum, or fifth disease, caused by parvovirus B19. A lacy macular erythematous eruption is also present on the trunk but is not in focus. (From Feder HM Jr. Fifth disease. *N Engl J Med* 1994;331:1062, with permission.) See color plate 29.

throat, headache, fever, cough, anorexia, vomiting, diarrhea, and arthralgia may occur but are often absent (17). In adults, the rash tends to be subtler or absent (12). Uncommon dermatologic manifestations include vesiculopustular eruption, purpura with or without thrombocytopenia, Henoch–Schönlein purpura, and an acral erythema in a "socks-and-gloves" distribution (16,18–25). B19 infection may be associated with peripheral neuropathies, including distal paresthesias and arm weakness (26–28). Nerve conduction may be slowed and motor and sensory potential amplitudes decreased (26,29). Aseptic meningitis occurs rarely (30–32).

Parvovirus B19 may be transmitted transplacentally at a rate of about 30% of infected mothers. Of infected fetuses, about 9% develop hydrops fetalis as a result of high-output cardiac failure from anemia (33,34). Rarely, fetuses develop viral cardiomyopathy (35). In fetuses, children, and adults, B19 may cause pancytopenia or isolated anemia, thrombocytopenia, leukopenia, myocarditis, or hepatitis (36–39). B19 viremia has been reported in a few cases of idiopathic thrombocytopenic purpura, self-limited benign acute lymphadenopathy, or hemophagocytic syndrome (39–44). Hemophagocytic syndrome in association with lymphadenopathy resembling necrotizing lymphadenitis (Kikuchi's disease) has also been reported (45). B19 infection may occur in association with cutaneous vasculitis, polyarteritis nodosa or Wegener's granulomatosis (46–50). Screening large series of patients with polyarteritis nodosa or Wegener's granulomatosis for evidence of B19 infection, however, failed to demonstrate a significant prevalence of B19 infection (51,52).

B19 infection may be persistent in patients with congenital or acquired immune deficiencies, including prior chemotherapy for lymphoproliferative disorders, immunosuppressive therapy for transplantation, or human acquired immunodeficiency syndrome (AIDS) (53–65). Infection manifests as chronic or recurrent anemia, thrombocytopenia, or leukopenia. B19 infection is the leading cause of pure red blood cell aplasia in patients with AIDS (66).

In an outbreak study in which infection was defined by the presence of rash, about 5% and 3% of children under 10 years of age had arthralgia and joint swelling, respectively. In adolescents, joint pain and swelling occurred in 12% and 5%, respectively. In adults 20 years of age or older, joint pain and swelling occurred in 77% and 60%, respectively (67). In adults, B19 infection is often characterized by sudden onset of severe polyarthralgia (68). Joint swelling is prominent. An associated severe influenza-like illness may occur, but alternatively, joint symptoms may also occur in the absence of a viral prodrome (12). Joint involvement is rheumatoid in distribution with symmetric involvement of the metacarpophalangeal, finger proximal interphalangeal, wrist, knee, and ankle joints. Joint symptoms may initially be limited to a few joints but, within 24 to 48 hours, spreads to include the wrists, ankles, feet, elbows, and shoulders. Axial joints are usually not involved. Joint symptoms are usually self-limited in adults, but symptoms are prolonged in a minority. Two thirds of chronic B19 arthropathy patients have continuous symptoms of morning stiffness and arthralgias between intermittent flares, whereas the remaining one third are symptom free between flares (9). Morning stiffness and arthralgia are prominent during flares (9–11,69,70). Rheumatoid factor may be present in low to moderate titer during the acute phase of infection but usually resolves (71). Low to moderate titer anti-DNA, antilymphocyte, antinuclear antibodies and antiphospholipid antibodies may be detected (72–74). Chronic arthropathy may last for up to 9 years, the longest follow-up to date. About 12% of patients presenting with "early synovitis," most of whom are women, have B19-induced rheumatoid-like arthropathy (12).

The distribution and symmetry of B19 arthropathy may suggest a diagnosis of rheumatoid arthritis (9–12). Half of all patients with chronic B19 arthropathy meet American Rheumatism Association diagnostic criteria for rheumatoid arthritis: morning stiffness lasting an hour or more, symmetric joint involvement, involvement of at least three joints, and involvement of the metacarpophalangeal and proximal interphalangeal joints (12,75,76). Joint erosions and rheumatoid nodules are absent in B19 arthropathy. Synovial thickening is absent, and arthroscopy fails to identify evidence of inflammation. Although an initial report suggested that chronic B19 arthropathy was associated with HLA-DR4, subsequent studies by the same group demonstrated no increased association with DR4 (2,77). The absence of rheumatoid nodules or joint destruction aids in the differential diagnosis of B19 arthropathy from classic, erosive rheumatoid arthritis (78).

Acute B19 infection may be confused with onset of systemic lupus erythematosus based on the presence of rash, arthralgia, arthritis, cytopenias, neuropathy, constitutional symptoms, and autoantibodies (79–81).

## Diagnostic Testing

Detection of B19 viremia by polymerase chain reaction or DNA hybridization technologies may confirm the diagnosis of chronic or early acute B19 infection. Diagnostic testing is usually not sought during the viremic phase and influenza-like prodrome accompanying erythema infectiosum or arthropathy. Patients with rash, arthralgia, or arthritis have usually developed anti-B19 IgM by the time of presentation, and B19 DNA may no longer be detectable, depending on the sensitivity of the DNA assay. Both radioimmunoassay and enzyme-linked immunoabsorbent assay have been used to detect B19 antigen and antibody to B19 capsid (2,12). The anti-B19 IgM response usually lasts for 2 months and then wanes. Specific IgM may be detectable for 6 months or longer (4). Anti-B19 IgG is usually present when anti-B19 IgM is detectable. Anti-B19 IgG antibody in the absence of anti-B19 IgM is usually not diagnostically helpful because of the high seroprevalence of anti-B19 IgG in the adult population. B19 infection should be considered in all patients presenting with sudden onset of symmetric polyarthralgia or polyarthritis. Failure to obtain serologic testing at presentation misses anti-B19 IgM, which is necessary for diagnosis in patients who develop chronic arthropathy. Fetuses infected early in development may not develop an anti-IgM antibody response detectable in cord blood. Anti-B19 IgG, when detected, may be of maternal origin; follow-up serology in surviving neonates at 9 months of age is required to differentiate endogenous IgG antibodies from passively acquired maternal IgG (2,82).

## Pathophysiology

The mechanisms by which B19 induces arthritis remain obscure. The onset of arthralgia, arthritis, and rash is associated temporally with the onset of anti-B19 IgM antibody response (7). This temporal association suggests that the acute phase of B19 arthritis is mediated by immune complexes. Indeed, the common clinical observation that B19 arthritis is worse for the first 2 weeks of symptoms and then ameliorates or resolves is consistent with an initial phase in which immune complexes circulate (9); however, there is little evidence of circulating virus in patients who have chronic symptoms (83).

Evidence is accumulating suggesting that B19 is a virus that persists even in patients with asymptomatic disease. B19 DNA may be found in the bone marrow and synovium of patients with chronic B19 arthropathy (78,84). In otherwise healthy people undergoing arthroscopy for trauma, B19 DNA has been found in synovium using sensitive nested polymerase chain reaction techniques (85). Finding evidence of persistence of a DNA virus such as B19, however, is insufficient in itself to explain disease. Many DNA viruses are known to remain latent without necessarily causing disease. Some patients with chronic B19 arthropathy reportedly have antibodies to the NS1 nonstructural protein (86). Because these antibodies have not been consistently identified in chronic B19 arthropathy patients, it is more likely that the presence of anti-NS1 antibody reflects an immune response to either NS1 on the surface of B19 virions or that NS1 spilled during cell death, rather than the antibodies themselves playing a pathogenic role. NS1 protein, however, may play a pathogenic role in perpetuating chronic B19 arthropathy through its interaction with cellular genes. NS1 has been shown to upregulate transcription of the interleukin-6 promotor and the human immunodeficiency virus long terminal repeat (LTR) in the presence of tat and an intact *tar* element (87,88).

Of interest, a study reported B19 DNA and proteins with a high prevalence in rheumatoid arthritis synovium and concluded that B19 was responsible for upregulation of interleukin-6 and tumor necrosis factor (89). These findings remain controversial. NS1 may also induce apoptosis through NS1 production in liver-derived cells nonpermissive for B19 replication (90). Similar mechanisms in synoviocyte subpopulations may induce autoimmunity by disrupting normal patterns of cell interactions and intercellular regulation. In chronic B19 arthropathy patients, IgG antibody to the N-terminus of the minor capsid protein, known to encode neutralizing epitopes, is absent, which may allow quantitatively greater B19 persistence (91).

### Treatment

No specific treatment or vaccine has been successful in the treatment of B19 infection; therefore, treatment is symptomatic. Patients with aplastic crisis usually require transfusion support during the areticulocytosis. Fetuses may require transfusion support *in utero* for anemia or digitalis therapy for cardiomyopathy (35,92). Arthropathy is treated symptomatically with nonsteroidal antiinflammatory drugs (NSAIDs). Immunocompromised patients with bone marrow suppression from persistent B19 infection may be treated with intravenous immunoglobulin 0.4 g/kg daily for 5 days (55,56).

## TOGAVIRUSES

### Rubella Virus

Rubella virus is the sole member of the genus *Rubivirus* in the Togaviridae family of enveloped single-stranded RNA viruses (93).

### Incidence and Epidemiology

Wild-type rubella virus infection in childhood is uncommon in the developed world because of a successful program of early childhood vaccination. After rubella vaccination campaigns, the incidence of rubella fell sharply. From 1969 to 1989, the number of rubella cases reported annually in the United States fell 99.6%, and the number of congenital rubella cases fell 97.4% (94). Similarly, the at-risk population in England and Wales has decreased (95). Select populations that have eschewed vaccination remain at increased risk (96).

Rubella is transmitted by nasopharyngeal secretions. Susceptible patients in close quarters, such as military recruits and cruise ship crews, are at increased risk for infection (97,98). Local outbreaks have occurred in high school and college students whose immunity since childhood vaccination had waned, suggesting that with widespread vaccination, the age profile has shifted toward young adults (99). Peak incidence is during late winter and early spring. The incubation period before rash appears is 14 to 21 days. Viral shedding in nasopharyngeal secretions is detectable from 7 days before and until 14 days after onset of rash but is maximal just before eruption until 5 to 7 days after eruption (100,101).

### Clinical Features

Infection in children and adults may be asymptomatic. In some cases, the rash is only a transient blush. The classic presentation consists of rash, low-grade fever, malaise, coryza, and prominent posterior cervical, postauricular, and occipital lymphadenopathy. Constitutional symptoms may precede rash by 5 days. A morbilliform facial rash spreads to the torso and upper then lower extremities over a 2- to 3-day period (Fig. 37.2).

Joint symptoms are common in women, occurring 1 week before or after onset of the rash (102). Symmetric or migratory arthralgias, and less commonly frank arthritis, usually resolve within 2 weeks. Stiffness is prominent during this time. Proximal interphalangeal, metacarpophalangeal, wrist, elbow, ankle, and knee joints are most frequently involved.

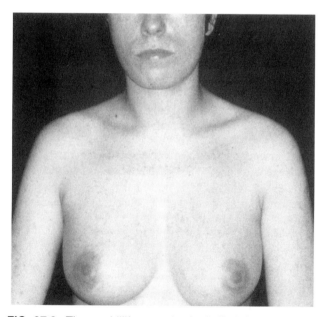

**FIG. 37.2.** The morbilliform rash of rubella infection. (From Naides SJ. Viral arthritis. In: Klippel JH, Dieppe PA, eds. *Rheumatology.* 2nd ed. London: CV Mosby, 1998:6.6.3.) See color plate 30.

Periarthritis, tenosynovitis, and carpal tunnel syndrome may occur (102). In a subset of patients, joint symptoms may be prolonged (103–106).

Rubella vaccines use live attenuated virus and have a high frequency of postvaccination arthralgia, myalgia, arthritis, and paresthesias (107–113). Arthrogenicity of early vaccine strains (e.g., HPV77/DK12, HPV77/DE5, and Cendehill) has led to use of the vaccine strain RA27/3. RA27/3, however, may also cause postvaccination joint symptoms, which have been reported to occur in 15% or more of recipients (114). In adults, joint involvement similar to natural infection occurs 2 weeks after inoculation and usually lasts less than a week. In some patients, however, symptoms may persist for more than a year (115).

Two neuropathic syndromes have been reported in children after natural infection or vaccination (116). In the arm syndrome, brachial radiculopathy causes arm and hand pain. Dysesthesias worsen at night. The "catcher's crouch" syndrome is a lumbar radiculopathy characterized by popliteal fossa pain on arising in the morning, which gradually subsides through the day. Pain is exacerbated by knee extension and minimized in a catcher's crouch position. Both syndromes appear 1 to 2 months after vaccination. The initial episode lasts up to 2 months. Recurrences up to 1 year are shorter in duration. The neuropathy eventually resolves without permanent sequelae (117).

### Diagnostic Testing

Rubella is readily cultured from tissues and body fluids, including throat swabs. Antirubella IgM positivity or anti-IgG seroconversion is diagnostic. Antirubella IgM and IgG are usually present at the onset of joint symptoms. IgM antibody peaks 8 to 21 days after symptom onset and is undetectable in most patients after 5 weeks. Specific IgG levels rise over 7 to 21 days after symptom onset; this high IgG level is long lived. A diagnosis of rubella infection by IgG serology requires paired acute and convalescent sera. A positive IgG screen on an isolated serum sample documents only immunity (101,118).

### Pathophysiology

Synoviocytes and chondrocytes can be persistently infected with rubella virus *in vitro* (119). Antirubella antibody concentrations are higher in synovial fluid than in serum, and synoviocytes *in vitro* spontaneously secrete antirubella antibody (120,121), suggesting that there is an *in situ* immune response to rubella infection in the joint.

### Treatment

Treatment of rubella infection is supportive. NSAIDs may be used for joint symptoms. Low to moderate doses of steroids have been reported to control symptoms and viremia, particularly in patients with a chronic course (113).

## Alphaviruses

### Incidence and Epidemiology

The alphaviruses are members of the Togaviridae family and include viruses responsible for large epidemics of febrile polyarthritis (Table 37.1). All alphaviruses use mosquitoes as vectors (122–128). The geographic distribution of transmitting vector and animal reservoir for each virus determine geographic distribution of disease. The importance of recognizing these infections lies in their presentation far from the location of endemic infection because of the rapidity of patient travel. The spread of mosquito vector and animal host ranges raises the specter that these infections may emerge in new geographic areas. *Aedes aegypti* has reinfested and *Aedes albopictus* has been reintroduced into the Western hemisphere. Mayaro virus has been isolated from a bird in Louisiana (129).

**TABLE 37.1.** *Viral arthritis*

| Virus | Pattern | Symptom duration | Associated symptoms | Geographic distribution | Mode of transmission |
|---|---|---|---|---|---|
| Erythrovirus Parvovirus B19 | Symmetric polyarthralgia and polyarthritis in a rheumatoid pattern | Days to weeks; in 12%, months to years | Fever, malaise, slapped-cheek, reticular, morbilliform rash | Worldwide | Respiratory secretions |
| Togaviruses Rubella virus | Symmetric or migratory polyarthritis of PIPs. MCPs, wrists, elbows, ankles, knees; arm syndrome; "catcher's crouch" syndrome | Days to months | Morbilliform rash, fever, malaise, coryza, lymphadenopathy | Worldwide | Respiratory secretions |

continued

**TABLE 37.1.** *Continued.*

| Virus | Pattern | Symptom duration | Associated symptoms | Geographic distribution | Mode of transmission |
|---|---|---|---|---|---|
| Chikungunya virus | Polyarthralgia and polyarthritis, small joints more than large joints | 10% up to 1 year | Explosive-onset fever, macular and maculopapular rash, petechiae, mucosal hemorrhage, headache, photophobia, pharyngitis, anorexia, nausea, vomiting | Africa, Asia | *Aedes* species, *Mansonia africana* |
| O'nyong-nyong virus | Polyarthralgia and polyarthritis | Days to weeks | Fever, rash, post-cervical lymphadenopathy | Uganda, central Africa | *Anopheles funestus, Anopheles gambiae* |
| Igbo Ora virus | Arthralgia | | Fever, rash, myalgia | Ivory Coast | *Anopheles funestus, Anopheles gambiae* |
| Ross River virus (epidemic polyarthritis) | Asymmetric or migratory severe polyarthralgia of DIPs, PIPs, MCPs, wrists, knees, ankles, shoulders, elbows; one third with synovitis | 4 weeks; a few up to 3 years | Fever, headache, nausea, myalgia, rash | Australia, New Zealand, New Guinea and the Pacific islands | *Aedes vigilax, Aedes camptorhynchus, Culex annulirostris, Mansonia uniformus, Aedes polynesiensis, Aedes aegypti* |
| Barmah Forest virus | Polyarthritis similar to Ross River virus | Clinically indistinguishable from Ross River virus | Fever, rash | Australia | |
| Sindbis virus | Polyarthritis of small joints of hands and feet, wrists, elbows, ankles, knees | Acute symptoms days to weeks; minority lasts 2 or more years | Fever, headache, malaise, fatigue, nausea, vomiting, pharyngitis; macular rash evolves to vesicles on pressure points that may become hemorrhagic | Sweden, Finland, and the Karelian isthmus of Russia | *Aedes* species, *Culex* species, *Culista* species |
| Mayaro virus | Arthralgias of wrist, fingers, ankles, toes; 20% with joint swelling | Days to weeks; few with arthralgias at 3 months | Fever, headache, dizziness, chills, rash | Rain forests of Brazil, Bolivia, and Peru | *Haemogogus* species |
| Hepadnavirus Hepatitis B virus | Symmetric or migratory and additive small and large joint arthritis | Preicteric prodrome up to 1 month | Preicteric fever, malaise, anorexia, nausea, myalgia, arthritis and urticarial rash; followed by icterus | Worldwide | Bloodborne, sexual contact |
| Flavivirus Hepatitis C virus | Acute polyarthritis in acute infection (see Chapter 35) | 80% of cases asymptomatic acutely | Cryoglobulinemia in chronic infection | Worldwide | Bloodborne |
| Retroviruses Human T-lymphocytic leukemia virus type 1 | Oligoarthritis | | Nodular rash and association with abnormal cellular infiltrates | Endemic in southern | Bloodborne |

DIP, distal interphalangeal joint; MCP, metacarpophalangeal joint; PIP, proximal interphalangeal joint.

Chikungunya ("that which twists or bends up") virus was isolated during an epidemic of febrile arthritis in Tanzania in 1952 to 1953. In a 1964 epidemic in Bangkok, Thailand, an estimated 40,000 patients out of an urban area of 2 million were infected (130). The seroconversion rate was 31%. O'ny-ong-nyong ("joint breaker") virus was first described in an outbreak in the Acholi province of northwestern Uganda in February, 1959. Within 2 years, 2 million people in Uganda and the surrounding region were infected. Serologically determined attack rates ranged from 50% to 60%, with 9% to 78% of infected patients developing symptoms (131–134). Disease spread at a rate of 2 to 3 kilometers daily. After the epidemic, the virus was not detected again until it was isolated from *Anopheles funestus* mosquitoes in Kenya in 1978. A new outbreak began in 1996 (135).

Ross River virus is responsible for annual outbreaks of febrile polyarthritis observed in Australia since 1928 (136–141). Weber's line is a hypothetical demarcation separating the Australian geographic zone from the Asiatic zone. West of Weber's line, antibodies to Ross River virus are absent. Antibodies to Ross River virus are found in endogenous populations in Papua New Guinea, West New Guinea, the Bismarck Archipelago, Rossel Island, and the Solomon Islands (142–146). In Australia, both endemic cases and epidemics occur in tropical and temperate regions (147). High rain fall, which increases mosquito populations, usually precedes epidemic periods. Cases occur from spring through autumn. Infection rates in Australia range from 0.2% to 3.5% per year. Although male and female infection rates are similar, there is a predominance of women in presenting cases. A major epidemic of febrile polyarthritis occurred in the Fiji Islands from 1979 to 1980, affecting more than 40,000 people.

Infection with Sindbis virus, named for the Egyptian village where it was first isolated from local mosquitoes in 1952, presents as Okelbo disease, Pogosta disease, or Karelian fever in Sweden, Finland, and the neighboring Karelian isthmus of Russia, respectively (148,149). Cases are confined to forested areas where vector mosquitoes live and where people involved in outdoor activities or occupations are at risk. Sindbis virus infection has also been reported as sporadic cases or small outbreaks from Uganda, South Africa, Zimbabwe, Central Africa, and Australia (136).

Mayaro virus was first recognized in Trinidad in 1954 and has caused outbreaks in Bolivia, Brazil, and Peru (150). In an outbreak in Belterra, Brazil in 1988, 800 of 4000 exposed latex gatherers were infected, a clinical attack rate of 80%. Travelers to endemic areas have returned to the United States with illness (150).

### Clinical Features

The clinical features of alphavirus infections are similar in that patients characteristically have explosive onset of fever, rash, and severe polyarthritis. Chikungunya virus incubation period is usually 2 to 3 days but ranges from 1 to 12 days (149,151). Intense viremia occurs within 48 hours after mos-

quito bite but begins to wane by about day 3 of illness. Body temperature elevations of up to 39° to 40°C, associated with rigors, last 1 to 7 days. Facial and neck flushing is followed by macular or maculopapular rash on the torso, extremities, and occasionally the face, palms, and soles. The rash may be pruritic. Typically, the rash occurs on days 2 through 5 of the illness and is associated with defervescence. The rash may recur with fever. Suffusion of the conjunctiva is prominent. Isolated petechiae and mucosal bleeding may occur. In some patients, involved skin desquamates. Sore throat, pharyngitis, headache, photophobia, retroorbital pain, anorexia, nausea, vomiting, and abdominal pain may accompany the acute illness. Lymph nodes may be tender but are usually not markedly enlarged. Diffuse myalgia with back and shoulder pain is common (152,153). Migratory polyarthralgia, stiffness, and swelling predominantly affect the small joints of the hands, wrists, feet, and ankles. Large joints are less severely affected. Previously injured joints may be disproportionately affected. Large effusions are uncommon.

In some cases, symptoms persist for months before resolution. About 10% of patients have joint symptoms 1 year after infection (152). A destructive arthropathy may occur in a few adult patients with chronic symptoms (154). Low-titer rheumatoid factor may be found in those with long-standing symptoms. Symptoms in children tend to be milder; nausea and vomiting, pharyngitis, and facial flushing are prominent features in affected children, but arthralgia, arthritis, and rash are uncommon and, when present, are milder and briefer in duration (155–158).

O'nyong-nyong fever is clinically similar to Chikungunya fever (136,159). The incubation period lasts at least 8 days and is followed by sudden onset of polyarthralgia or polyarthritis. Rash, which tends to be uniform, typically begins 4 days later as the joints improve and lasts 4 to 7 days before fading. Fever is less prominent than in Chikungunya fever, but postcervical lymphadenopathy may be marked. Although residual joint pain may persist, there appear to be no long-term sequelae.

Igbo Ora ("the disease that breaks your wings") virus is in the serologic group of Chikungunya and O'nyong-nyong viruses (160). A single patient with fever, sore throat, and arthritis was initially identified. In 1984, an epidemic of fever, myalgias, arthralgias, and rash occurred in four villages on the Ivory Coast.

Polyarthralgia ("febrile polyarthritis')' caused by Ross River virus occurs abruptly after a 7- to 11-day incubation period (161). Macular, papular, or maculopapular rash, which may be pruritic, typically follows onset of arthralgia by 1 to 2 days but may precede or follow joint symptoms by 11 or 15 days, respectively. Vesicles, papules or petechia are typically found on the trunk and extremities. Involvement of the palms, soles, and face may occur. The rash resolves by fading to a brownish discoloration or by desquamation. Despite its name, only half of affected patients have fever, which may be only modest and last 1 to 3 days. Nausea, headache, and myalgia are common. Respiratory symptoms, mild photophobia, and lymphadenopathy may occur. Arthralgia is severe and incapacitating in most patients. Joint distribution is often migratory and asymmetric, with metacarpophalangeal and finger interphalangeal joint, wrist, knee, and ankle involvement. Shoulders, elbows, and toes may also be involved. Axial, hip, and temporomandibular involvement occasionally occurs. Arthralgias are worse in the morning and after periods of inactivity. Mild exercise tends to improve joint symptoms. One third of patients have frank synovitis. Polyarticular swelling and tenosynovitis are common. Up to one third have paresthesias and palm or sole pain. Half of all patients are able to resume their daily activities within 4 weeks, although residual polyarthralgia may be present. Joint symptoms may recur. Episodes of relapse gradually resolve. A few patients continue to have joint symptoms for up to 3 years (147,162–164). Barmah Forest virus, another alphavirus recently described in Australia, may present in a fashion similar to epidemic febrile polyarthritis (165).

Rash and arthralgia are the presenting symptoms in Sindbis virus infection, although one may precede the other by a few days. A low-grade fever may be present. Constitutional symptoms are usually mild and include headache, fatigue, malaise, nausea, vomiting, pharyngitis, and paresthesias. A macular rash typically begins on the torso and then spreads to the arms and legs, palms, soles, and occasionally head. Macules evolve to form papules, which tend to vesiculate. Vesiculation is prominent on pressure points, including the palms and soles. As the rash fades, a brownish discoloration is left. Vesicles on the palms and soles may become hemorrhagic. The rash may recur during convalescence (166). Arthralgia and arthritis involve the small joints of the hands and feet, wrists, elbows, ankles, and knees. The axial skeleton is involved occasionally. Tendonitis is common, often involving the extensor tendons of the hand and the Achilles tendon. Nonerosive chronic arthropathy is common, with up to one third of patients having arthropathy 2 or more years after onset. A smaller number have symptoms for as long as 5 to 6 years (167).

Mayaro virus infection symptoms invariably include fever and headache. Myalgia, eye pain, chills, and arthralgia occur in most patients. Rash occurs in about one third of patients. Nausea, cough, sore throat, vomiting, abdominal pain, nasal congestion, diarrhea, photophobia, and gum bleeding may occur (150). About 20% of patients have joint swelling. Unilateral inguinal lymphadenopathy may be seen in some patients. Leukopenia is common. Fever lasts 2 to 5 days, then a maculopapular rash on the trunk and extremities appears, lasting about 3 days. Some patients with Mayaro virus infection still have persistent arthralgias at 2 months' follow-up (168–170).

### Diagnosis

The possibility of alphavirus infection should be entertained in any febrile patient residing in or returning from an endemic area. A history of a recent outbreak is helpful but not necessary. Diagnosis requires laboratory confirmation. Virus may be isolated from serum early in illness (151). Hemagglutination inhibition or complement fixation tests may be used to detect antibody (131,136). Chikungunya, O'nyong-nyong, and Igbo Ora viruses are closely related serologically. Specific hemagglutination inhibition, neutralizing antibody, and plaque reduction tests help differentiate the viruses (150,171). Specific IgM antibodies are helpful in making the diagnosis in patients dwelling in endemic areas (136). IgG seroconversion in patients returning from brief visits to endemic areas is helpful. Anti-Sindbis virus IgM may persist for years, raising the possibility that Sindbis virus arthritis is associated with viral persistence (167).

### Pathophysiology

Little is known about the pathophysiology of alphavirus-induced arthritis for those viruses most prevalent in medically underserved developing geographic areas. In Chikungunya rash, lymphocytic perivascular cuffing and erythrocyte extravasation occur at superficial capillaries (158). In a single case, arthroscopy revealed an atrophic-appearing synovium, but histology was normal. In another case, atypical, destructive arthritis was associated with pannus formation and synovial germinal centers (152). The pathogenesis of O'nyong-nyong and Sindbis virus arthritides is unknown. In the latter, the evidence argues against immune complex involvement (172). Prolonged persistence of IgM antibodies to Sindbis virus for 3 to 4 years after initial infection suggests failure of the immune response to mature and possibly persistence of virus (167).

More is known about Ross River virus pathogenesis. In mice, selective tissue targets of infection include periosteum, perichondrium, and muscle. Viral replication in muscle results in myositis. Certain strains may cause myocarditis in mice (173). In affected joints in humans, Ross River virus antigen, but not virus, can be detected. Synovial fluids have elevated numbers of lymphocytes, monocytes, and vacuolated macrophages (162,174,175). In synoviocytes *in vitro*, Ross River virus induces transient and partial cytopathologic effects, killing 25% to 75% of the cell layer with partial regeneration (176). The immune response to alphavirus or viral antigens localized to synovium could explain the acute arthritis. In some patients, anti–Ross River virus IgM antibody response and arthritis may be prolonged (162,177).

About 10% of patients with Chikungunya virus arthritis have joint symptoms 1 year after initial infection (142). Whether chronic arthritis represents ongoing immune response to local persistent viral antigen or virus or development of an autoimmune response to self antigens remains to be determined. The major histocompatibility antigens DR7 and possibly B12 confer increased susceptibility to Ross River virus arthritis (162,178).

### Treatment

Treatment is supportive. During the acute attack, range-of-motion exercises decrease stiffness. NSAIDs are useful.

Chloroquine phosphate (250 mg/day) has been used in Chikungunya fever when NSAIDs fail (179).

Vaccines to the alphaviruses are under development but are yet not available for widespread human use. An inactivated Ross River virus vaccine elicits neutralizing antibodies in mice (181). An attenuated live virus vaccine for Chikungunya fever virus has been found safe in initial human testing (182–185).

## Hepatitis B Virus

Hepatitis B virus (HBV), a member of the family Hepadnaviridae, genus *Orthohepadnavirus,* is an enveloped double-stranded DNA icosahedral virus (186,187).

### Incidence and Epidemiology

HBV infection occurs worldwide, but the prevalence is higher in Asia, the Middle East, and sub-Sahara Africa. The prevalence in China may be as high as 10%, compared with 0.01% in the United States. In a serosurvey of patients seen for emergency treatment at 10 California hospitals chosen to reflect geographic and demographic diversity, HBV seroprevalence was 2.6% (57 of 2209 patients) (188). HBV is transmitted by parenteral and sexual routes. Most acute infections in endemic regions occur at an early age, with many acquired perinatally. Early HBV infection is usually asymptomatic. The annual incidence of infection in endemic areas in children may be as high as 5%. The rate of HBV carriage and specific antibody declines with age. HBV is a common cause of chronic liver disease and a leading cause of hepatocellular carcinoma in endemic regions (189). In Western countries, most infections are acquired during adulthood through sexual or needle exposures, and HBV is more often associated with acute hepatitis. Of patients with acute hepatitis, 5% to 10% develop persistent infection (186).

### Clinical Features

The incubation period in HBV infection is usually 45 to 120 days. A preicteric prodromal period lasts several days to 1 month and may be associated with fever, myalgia, malaise, anorexia, nausea, and vomiting. Significant viremia occurs early in infection. Soluble immune complexes with circulating hepatitis B surface antigen (HBsAg) form as antibodies (HBsAb) to HBsAg are produced. An immune complex–mediated arthritis is usually sudden in onset and often severe. Joint involvement is usually symmetric, with simultaneous involvement of several joints at onset, but arthritis may be migratory or additive (190). Hand and knee joints are most often affected, but wrists, ankles, elbows, shoulders, and other large joints may be involved as well. Fusiform swelling may be seen in the small joints of the hand. Morning stiffness is common. Urticaria may accompany arthritis, and both may precede jaundice by days or weeks and may persist several weeks after jaundice. Arthritis and urticaria usually subside soon after onset of clinical jaundice. Patients who develop chronic active hepatitis or chronic HBV viremia may have recurrent polyarthralgia or polyarthritis. Polyarteritis nodosa may be associated with chronic hepatitis B viremia (191,192).

### Diagnosis

Urticaria in the presence of polyarthritis should raise the possibility of HBV infection. Acute hepatitis may be asymptomatic, but elevated bilirubin and transaminases are usually present when the arthritis appears. At the time of arthritis onset, peak levels of serum HBsAg are detectable. Virions, viral DNA, viral polymerase, and hepatitis B e antigen may be detectable in serum. IgM to hepatitis B core antigen is present and indicates acute HBV infection as opposed to past or chronic infection (193,194).

### Treatment

HBV urticaria and arthritis are self-limited. Treatment is symptomatic. Patients with persistent viremia and chronic active hepatitis may require antiviral therapy.

## OTHER VIRUSES

Apart from specific viral infections described previously in which arthralgia and arthritis are typically prominent manifestations, a host of commonly encountered viral syndromes present with signs typically seen in autoimmune processes. Adenovirus and coxsackieviruses A9, B2, B3, B4, and B6 infections have been associated with recurrent polyarthritis, pleuritis, myalgia, rash, pharyngitis, myocarditis, and leukocytosis. Echovirus 9 infection rarely causes polyarthritis, fever, or myalgias. Hepatitis C virus infection is commonly associated with cryoglobulinemia and rheumatoid factor positivity and is discussed in Chapter 35.

## BACTERIAL INFECTIONS

### Reiter's Syndrome and Reactive Arthritis

#### Incidence and Prevalence

Enteric infection with *Salmonella, Shigella,* or *Campylobacter* species and urogenital infections with *Chlamydia trachomatis* or *Ureaplasma urealyticum* have all been implicated as triggers of Reiter's syndrome, a triad of urethritis, arthritis, and uveitis (195). *C. trachomatis* DNA, RNA, and proteins are found in the synovium of patients with Reiter's disease (196–199). Similar arthritis in the absence of the complete triad following infection has been labeled *reactive arthritis* (200). *Yersinia enterocolitica, Yersinia pseudotuberculosis, Chlamydia pneumoniae, Vibrio parahemolyticus, Clostridium difficile,* and *Gardnerella vaginalis* infections have all been implicated as potential triggers of reactive arthritis (201,202).

Patients with Reiter's syndrome and reactive arthritis have a high prevalence of HLA-B27 positivity, about 75% of cases (203). The incidence of Reiter's syndrome and reactive arthritis reflects the prevalence of HLA-B27 in the population (204). The age-adjusted annual incidence of Reiter's syndrome for male patients younger than 50 years old in an upper Midwest, predominantly white, community-based population was 3.5 per 100,000, or 0.0035%. No female cases were identified. In 63% of the patients, either a prolonged or relapsing disease course occurred (205). In contrast, Chukotka natives of Siberia have a frequency of HLA-B27 positivity as high as 40%, and spondyloarthropathies are present in up to 2%, including Reiter's syndrome (4 of 86 patients, or 4.7%) (206).

Increased use of condoms and more conservative sexual practices resulting from concern about acquired immunodeficiency syndrome (AIDS) may have had a positive effect on the incidence of Reiter's syndrome and reactive arthritis in non-AIDS populations (207). In AIDS populations, the incidence of Reiter's syndrome and reactive arthritis may be increased as a result of increased exposure to triggering organisms.

### Clinical Features

Enthesitis, inflammation at the site of tendon and ligament insertion into bone, is a characteristic feature of Reiter's syndrome and reactive arthritis. Patients may present with peripheral arthritis in an asymmetric, oligoarticular pattern. Heel pain and Achilles tendonitis may be prominent features.

Complaints of low-back pain are common. Prolonged morning stiffness lasting at least 1 hour is common. Dactylitis may be present (208). Urethritis may manifest as urethral discharge and pain or may be minimally symptomatic, with the patient reporting only undergarment soiling on close questioning. Uveitis, particularly iridocyclitis, may present as photophobia, blurred vision, or eye pain. Syncytia formation representing adhesions between the iris and the posterior aspect of the cornea, resulting from inflammation in the anterior chamber of the eye, may distort the pupil and further impair visual acuity. Reiter's syndrome is predominantly a disease of males, perhaps in part because of the difficulty of identifying urethritis in women; however, cervical mucositis or salpingitis may be found in women instead of urethritis (209,210).

Cutaneous manifestations aid in the diagnosis. Small, shallow ulcers may be present on the glans of the penis (balanitis circinata). In uncircumcised men, they may be moist, whereas in circumcised men, they may become encrusted and painful. The ulcers may coalesce (Fig. 37.3). Similar ulcerations may be found on the oral mucosa. The nails may become hyperkeratotic with onycholysis. Plaquelike or papular hyperkeratosis of the palms and soles may be found (keratoderma blennorrhagica) (Fig. 37.4). Diarrhea and urethritis may recur over time despite failure to isolate a triggering organism. Radiographic findings include sacroiliitis, spondylitis with syndesmophyte formation, and peripheral joint erosive disease (211–215).

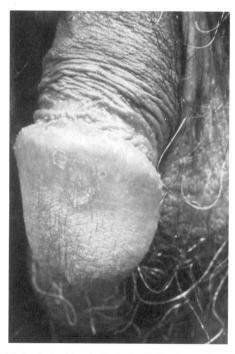 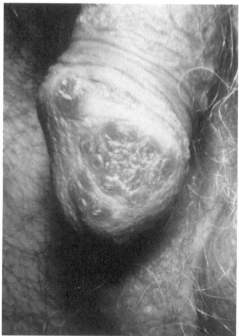

**FIG. 37.3.** Balanitis circinata in Reiter's syndrome. **Left:** Early discrete moist superficial ulcer on the glans. **Right:** Multiple coalesced lesions with crust. (Courtesy of the Arthritis Foundation Slide Collection, Atlanta, GA, U.S.A.)

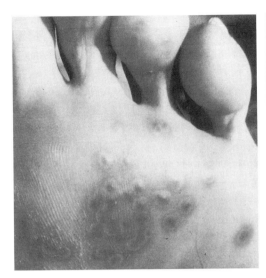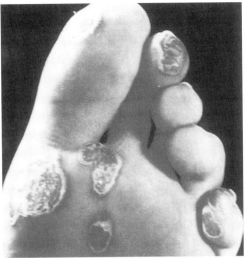

**FIG. 37.4.** Keratoderma blennorrhagica in Reiter's syndrome. **Left:** Early pustules and vesicles on the sole. **Right:** More advanced discrete plaque-like lesions. (Courtesy of the Arthritis Foundation Slide Collection, Atlanta, GA, U.S.A.)

### Diagnosis

The diagnosis is based on clinical findings with radiographic confirmation. Synovial fluid is inflammatory. Although useful as a research tool, determination of HLA-B27 has no role in the clinical diagnosis of spondyloarthropathies.

### Treatment

Long-term management uses multiple modalities to decrease inflammation and avoid long term disability. Antibiotics are appropriate if a triggering organism is isolated. Antibiotic treatment after the onset of synovitis cannot, however, cure the arthritis. Tetracycline has been used for several months after onset of arthritis by some practitioners. Patients may show some benefit from a 3-month course of tetracycline in the setting of acute chlamydial arthritis (216). Lymecycline given for the first 3 months appears to accelerate recovery from chlamydial arthritis (217,218). The mechanism by which tetracyclines may ameliorate reactive arthritis may not be caused by antimicrobial effects. Rather, tetracyclines, including minocycline and lymecycline, appear to have an anti-inflammatory effect through inhibition of metalloproteinases, such as collagenase (218,219). Long-term antibiotic therapy in reactive arthritis has not been shown to be of benefit (220). There has not been the kind of lay interest and demand for long-term therapy as has surrounded the treatment of chronic Lyme arthritis, for which popular fervor has sought practitioners willing to treat an array of symptoms attributed to Lyme disease with chronic long-term antibiotics.

Medical treatment includes NSAIDs for arthritis. Prednisone has a role as an adjunct in the treatment of arthritis and ocular inflammation. Sulfasalazine has proved helpful in controlling chronic disease (221). Instruction in posture and a low-impact program of stretching exercises are helpful in maintaining patient function. Orthotics and fitted shoes may be helpful in maintaining ambulation and preventing disability when heel involvement is severe.

### Erythema nodosum

#### Incidence and Prevalence

Erythema nodosum most commonly occurs in young adults between 18 and 34 years of age (222). In a retrospective study of 157 patients with a diagnosis of erythema nodosum, the mean age was 34 years, with a female-to-male ratio of 5:1. Streptococcal infection was found in 28% and chlamydial infection in 1.5% of patients, and one case each was found of *Mycoplasma* species, *Yersinia* species, HBV, and tuberculosis infection (223–225). In other studies, the incidence of tuberculosis is higher (226). In children, the incidence of *Yersinia* species infection may be as high as 20% of cases (227). Erythema nodosum may be the only sign of brucellosis (228). It may be seen in active tuberculosis, coccidioidomycosis, histoplasmosis, and blastomycosis (229,230). Most cases of erythema nodosum, however, do not have an identifiable trigger (83).

#### Clinical Features

Erythematous, often exquisitely tender nodules appear predominantly on the lower extremities on the extensor surfaces, although lesions may be seen elsewhere on the legs and arms and occasionally on the torso. Nodules may recur in crops. It is often common to see nodules resolving as others appear. Erythema nodosum is often self-limited, with resolution in 1 to 2 months, but chronic forms do occur. Löfgren's syndrome (the triad of erythema nodosum, bilateral hilar lym-

**TABLE 37.2.** *Infections associated with erythema nodosum*

Viral
  Epstein–Barr virus
  Hepatitis B virus
  Paravaccinia virus
Bacterial
  β-Hemolytic streptococci
  Brucellosis
  Cat scratch fever (*Bartonella henslae*)
  *Chlamydia psittaci*
  *Chlamydia trachomatis*
  *Moraxella catarrhalis*[235]
  *Mycobacterium leprae*
  *Mycobacterium tuberculosis*
  *Mycoplasma pneumoniae*
  Q fever (*Coxiella burnettii*)[236]
  *Salmonella enteritidis*[237]
  Tularemia (*Francisella tularensis*)
  *Yersinia enterocolitica*[238]
Fungal
  Blastomyces
  *Coccidiodes immitis*
  *Histoplasma capsulatum*
  *Trichophyton mentagrophytes*

phadenopathy, and periarthritis, particularly of the ankles) may be seen with infection as well as sarcoidosis (231).

### Diagnosis

Full-thickness biopsy of an erythema nodosum lesion demonstrates inflammation and thickening of the septa of fat lobules. Evaluation for triggering organisms should include anti–streptolysin O titer, throat culture, chest radiographs, and skin testing for tuberculosis. Consideration should be given to serology or skin testing for coccidioidomycosis, histoplasmosis, and blastomycosis (232). *Yersinia* species titers may be helpful (Table 37.2) (233).

### Treatment

NSAIDs are helpful. Oral steroids may be necessary to control inflammation. Potassium iodide has been used in refractory cases in the setting of Crohn's disease (234).

### REFERENCES

1. Pattison JR. The discovery of human parvovirus. In: Pattison JR, ed. *Parvoviruses and human disease.* Boca Raton, FL: CRC Press, 1988: 1–4.
2. Naides SJ. Parvoviruses. In: Specter S, Lancz G, ed. *Clinical virology manual.* 2nd ed. Essex, England: Elsevier Science Publishers, 1992:547–569.
3. Mosley JW. Should measures be taken to reduce the risk of human parvovirus (B19) infection by transfusion of blood components and clotting factor concentrates. *Transfusion* 1994;34:744–746.
4. Anderson LJ, Tsou RA, Chorba TL, et al. Detection of antibodies and antigens of human parvovirus B19 by enzyme-linked immunosorbent assay. *J Clin Microbiol* 1986;24:522–526.
5. Bell LM, Naides SJ, Stoffman P, et al. Human parvovirus B19 infection among hospital staff members after contact with infected patients. *N Engl J Med* 1989;321:485–491.
6. Gillespie SM, Cartter ML, Asch S, et al. Occupational risk of human parvovirus B19 infection for school and day-care personnel during an outbreak of erythema infectiosum. *JAMA* 1990;263:2061–2065.
7. Anderson MJ, Higgins PG, Davis LR, et al. Experimental parvoviral infection in humans. *J Infect Dis* 1985;152:257–265.
8. Young N, Ozawa K. Studies of the B19 virus in bone marrow cell culture. In: Pattison JR, ed. *Parvoviruses and human disease.* Boca Raton, FL: CRC Press, 1988:117–132.
9. White DG, Woolf AD, Mortimer PP, et al. Human parvovirus arthropathy. *Lancet* 1985;1:419–421.
10. Reid DM, Reid TM, Brown T, et al. Human parvovirus-associated arthritis: a clinical and laboratory description. *Lancet* 1985;1:422–425.
11. Woolf AD, Campion GV, Chishick A, et al. Clinical manifestations of human parvovirus B19 in adults. *Arch Intern Med* 1989;149: 1153–1156.
12. Naides SJ, Scharosch LL, Foto F, Howard EJ. Rheumatologic manifestations of human parvovirus B19 infection in adults: initial two-year clinical experience. *Arthritis Rheum* 1990;33:1297–1309.
13. Serjeant GR, Goldstein AR. B19 virus infection and the aplastic crisis. In: Pattison JR, ed. *Parvoviruses and human diseases.* Boca Raton, FL: CRC Press, 1988:85–92.
14. Rao SP, Miller ST, Cohen BJ. Transient aplastic crisis in patients with sickle cell disease: B19 parvovirus studies during a 7-year period. *Am J Dis Child* 1992;146:1328–1330.
15. Anderson MJ, Jones SE, Fisher Hoch SP, et al. Human parvovirus, the cause of erythema infectiosum (fifth disease)? *Lancet* 1983;1:1378.
16. Etienne A, Harms M. Cutaneous manifestations of parvovirus B19 infection. *Presse Med* 1996;25:1162–1165.
17. Anderson MJ, Lewis E, Kidd IM, et al. An outbreak of erythema infectiosum associated with human parvovirus infection. *J Hyg (Lond)* 1984;93:85–93.
18. Naides SJ, Piette W, Veach LA, et al. Human parvovirus B19-induced vesiculopustular skin eruption. *Am J Med* 1988;84:968–972.
19. Lefrere JJ, Courouce AM, Muller JY, et al. Human parvovirus and purpura. *Lancet* 1985;1:730.
20. Mortimer PP, Cohen BJ, Rossiter MA, et al. Human parvovirus and purpura. *Lancet* 1985;1:730–731.
21. Shiraishi H, Umetsu K, Yamamoto H, et al. Human parvovirus (HPV/B19) infection with purpura. *Microbiol Immunol* 1989;33: 369–372.
22. Kilbourne ED, Cerini CP, Khan MW, et al. Immunologic response to the influenza virus neuraminidase is influenced by prior experience with the associated viral hemagglutinin. *J Immunol* 1987;138: 3010–3013.
23. Lefrere JJ, Courouce AM, Kaplan C. Parvovirus and idiopathic thrombocytopenic purpura. *Lancet* 1989;1:279.
24. Anderson MJ. Rash illness due to B19 virus. In: Pattison JR, ed. *Parvoviruses and human diseases.* Boca Raton, FL: CRC Press, 1988: 93–104.
25. Lefrere JJ, Courouce AM, Soulier JP, et al. Henoch-Schonlein purpura and human parvovirus infection. *Pediatrics* 1986;78:183–184.
26. Faden H, Gary GW Jr, Korman M. Numbness and tingling of fingers associated with parvovirus B19 infection. *J Infect Dis* 1990;161: 354–355.
27. Faden H, Gary GW Jr, Anderson LJ. Chronic parvovirus infection in a presumably immunologically healthy woman. *Clin Infect Dis* 1992;15: 595–597.
28. Denning DW, Amos A, Rudge P, et al. Neuralgic amyotrophy due to parvovirus infection. *J Neurol Neurosurg Psychiatry* 1987;50: 641–642.
29. Walsh KJ, Armstrong RD, Turner AM. Brachial plexus neuropathy associated with human parvovirus infection. *Br Med J* 1988;296:896.
30. Okumura A, Ichikawa T. Aseptic meningitis caused by human parvovirus B19. *Arch Dis Child* 1993;68:784–785.
31. Koduri PR, Naides SJ. Aseptic meningitis caused by parvovirus B19. *Clin Infect Dis* 1995;21:1053.
32. Tribe GW, Fleming MP. Parvovirus vaccination. *Vet Rec* 1984; 115:284.
33. Anonymous. Prospective study of human parvovirus (B19) infection in pregnancy. Public Health Laboratory Service Working Party on Fifth Disease. *Br Med J* 1990;300:1166–1170.

34. Gray ES, Davidson RJ, Anand A. Human parvovirus and fetal anaemia. *Lancet* 1987;1:1144.

35. Naides SJ, Weiner CP. Antenatal diagnosis and palliative treatment of non-immune hydrops fetalis secondary to fetal parvovirus B19 infection. *Prenat Diagn* 1989;9:105–114.

36. Naides SJ, Cuthbertson G, Murray JC, et al. Neonatal sequelae of parvovirus B19 infection in utero. *28th Interscience Conference on Antimicrobial Agents and Chemotherapy Proceedings.* 1988:199(abst).

37. Metzman R, Anand A, DeGiulio PA, et al. Hepatic disease associated with intrauterine parvovirus B19 infection in a newborn premature infant. *J Pediatr Gastroenterol Nutr* 1989;9:112–114.

38. Anderson MJ, Cohen BJ. Human parvovirus B19 infections in United Kingdom 1984-86. *Lancet* 1987;1:738–739.

39. Van Elsacker-Niele AMW, Weiland HT, Kroes ACM, et al. Parvovirus B19 infection and idiopathic thrombocytopenic purpura. *Ann Hematol* 1996;72:141–144.

40. Tsuda H, Maeda Y, Nakagawa K. Parvovirus B19-related lymphadenopathy. *Br J Haematol* 1993;85:631–632.

41. Boruchoff SE, Woda BA, Pihan GA, et al. Parvovirus B19-associated hemophagocytic syndrome. *Arch Intern Med* 1990;150:897–899.

42. Muir K, Todd WTA, Watson WH, et al. Viral-associated haemophagocytosis with parvovirus-B19-related pancytopenia. *Lancet* 1992;339: 1139–1140.

43. Watanabe M, Shimamoto Y, Yamaguchi M, et al. Viral-associated haemophagocytosis and elevated serum TNF-α with parvovirus-B19-related pancytopenia in patients with hereditary spherocytosis. *Clin Lab Haematol* 1994;16:179–182.

44. Shirono K, Tsuda H. Parvovirus B19-associated haemophagocytic syndrome in healthy adults. *Br J Haematol* 1995;89:923–926.

45. Yufu Y, Matsumoto M, Miyamura T, et al. Parvovirus B19-associated haemophagocytic syndrome with lymphadenopathy resembling histiocytic necrotizing lymphadenitis (Kikuchi's disease). *Br J Haematol* 1997;96:868–871.

46. Andres E, Grunenberger F, Schlienger JL, et al. Cutaneous vasculitis disclosing parvovirus B19 infection [Letter]. *Ann Med Interne* 1997; 148:107–108.

47. Finkel TH, Torok TJ, Ferguson PJ, et al. Chronic parvovirus B19 infection and systemic necrotizing vasculitis: opportunistic infection or aetiological agent? *Lancet* 1994;343:1255–1258.

48. Corman LC, Dolson DJ. Polyarteritis nodosa and parvovirus B19 infection. *Lancet* 1992;339:491.

49. Corman LC, Staud R. Association of Wegener's granulomatosis with parvovirus B19 infection: comment on the concise communication by Nikkari et al [Letter; Comment]. *Arthritis Rheum* 1995;38:1174–1175.

50. Nikkari S, Mertsola J, Korvenranta H, et al. Wegener's granulomatosis and parvovirus B19 infection [see Comments]. *Arthritis Rheum* 1994;37:1707–1708.

51. Leruez-Ville M, Lauge A, Morinet F, et al. Polyarteritis nodosa and parvovirus B19 [Letter; Comment]. *Lancet* 1994;344:263–264.

52. Nikkari S, Vainionpaa R, Toivanen P, et al. Association of Wegener's granulomatosis with parvovirus B19 infection [comment on the concise communication by Nikkari et al.; Reply]. *Arthritis Rheum* 1997; 38:1175.

53. Cooling LLW, Koerner TAW, Naides SJ. Multiple glycosphingolipids determine the tissue tropism of parvovirus B19. *J Infect Dis* 1995; 172:1198–1205.

54. Naides SJ, Howard EJ, Swack NS, et al. Parvovirus B19 as a cause of anemia in human immunodeficiency virus-infected patients [Reply]. *J Infect Dis* 1994;169:939–940.

55. Kurtzman GJ, Ozawa K, Cohen B, et al. Chronic bone marrow failure due to persistent B19 parvovirus infection. *N Engl J Med* 1987; 317:287–294.

56. Kurtzman GJ, Cohen B, Meyers P, et al. Persistent B19 parvovirus infection as a cause of severe chronic anaemia in children with acute lymphocytic leukaemia. *Lancet* 1988;2:1159–1162.

57. Kurtzman G, Frickhofen N, Kimball J, et al. Pure red-cell aplasia of 10 years' duration due to persistent parvovirus B19 infection and its cure with immunoglobulin therapy. *N Engl J Med* 1989;321:519–523.

58. Graeve JL, de Alarcon PA, Naides SJ. Parvovirus B19 infection in patients receiving cancer chemotherapy: the expanding spectrum of disease. *Am J Pediatr Hematol Oncol* 1989;11:441–444.

59. Young NS, Baranski B, Kurtzman G. The immune system as mediator of virus-associated bone marrow failure: B19 parvovirus and Epstein-Barr virus. *Ann N Y Acad Sci* 1989;554:75–80.

60. Frickhofen N, Young NS. Persistent parvovirus B19 infections in humans. *Microb Pathog* 1989;7:319–327.

61. de Mayolo JA, Temple JD. Pure red cell aplasia due to parvovirus B19 infection in a man with HIV infection. *South Med J* 1990;83: 1480–1481.

62. Chrystie IL, Almeida JD, Welch J. Electron microscopic detection of human parvovirus (B19) in a patient with HIV infection. *J Med Virol* 1990;30:249–252.

63. Rao SP, Miller ST, Cohen BJ. Severe anemia due to B19 parvovirus infection in children with acute leukemia in remission. *Am J Pediatr Hematol Oncol* 1990;12:194–197.

64. Frickhofen N, Young NS. Polymerase chain reaction for detection of parvovirus B19 in immunodeficient patients with anemia. *Behring Inst Mitt* 1990;85:46–54.

65. Naides SJ, Howard EJ, Swack NS, et al. Parvovirus B19 infection in HIV-1 infected individuals failing or intolerant to zidovudine therapy. *J Infect Dis* 1993;168:101–105.

66. Frickhofen N, Abkowitz JL, Safford M, et al. Persistent B19 parvovirus infection in patients infected with human immunodeficiency virus type 1 (HIV-1): a treatable cause of anemia in AIDS. *Ann Intern Med* 1990;113:926–933.

67. Ager EA, Chin TDY, Poland JD. Epidemic erythema infectiosum. *N Engl J Med* 1966;275:1326–1331.

68. Naides SJ. Rheumatic manifestations of parvovirus B19 infection. *Rheum Dis Clin North Am* 1998;24:375–401.

69. Smith CA, Woolf AD, Lenci M. Parvoviruses: infections and arthropathies. *Rheum Dis Clin North Am* 1987;13:249–263.

70. Stoll T, Brühlmann P, Brunner U, et al. Parvovirus-B19-induced arthritis/arthropathy and its importance in differential diagnosis of rheumatoid arthritis. *Schweiz Med Wochenschr* 1995;125:347–354.

71. Naides SJ, Field EH. Transient rheumatoid factor positivity in acute human parvovirus B19 infection. *Arch Intern Med* 1988;148: 2587–2589.

72. Sasaki T, Takahashi Y, Yoshinaga K, et al. An association between human parvovirus B-19 infection and autoantibody production. *J Rheumatol* 1989;16:708–709.

73. Solonika CA, Anderson MJ, Laskin CA. Anti-DNA and antilymphocyte antibodies during acute infection with parvovirus B19. *J Rheumatol* 1989;16:777–781.

74. Kerr JR, Boyd N. Autoantibodies following parvovirus B19 infection. *J Infect* 1996;32:41–47.

75. Arnett FC, Edworthy SM, Bloch DA, et al. The American Rheumatism Association 1987 revised criteria for the classification of rheumatoid arthritis. *Arthritis Rheum* 1988;31:315–324.

76. Silman AJ. The 1987 revised American Rheumatism Association criteria for rheumatoid arthritis [Editorial]. *Br J Rheumatol* 1988;27: 341–343.

77. Klouda PT, Corbin SA, Bradley BA, et al. HLA and acute arthritis following human parvovirus infection. *Tissue Antigens* 1986;28: 318–319.

78. Naides SJ, Foto F, Marsh JL, et al. Synovial tissue analysis in patients with chronic parvovirus B19 arthropathy. *Clin Res* 1991;39:733(abst).

79. Vigeant P, Ménard H-A, Boire G. Chronic modulation of the autoimmune response following parvovirus B19 infection. *J Rheumatol* 1994;21:1165–1167.

80. Fawaz-Estrup F. Human parvovirus infection: rheumatic manifestations, angioedema, C1 esterase inhibitor deficiency, ANA positivity, and possible onset of systemic lupus erythematosus. *J Rheumatol* 1996;23:1180–1185.

81. Loizou S, Cazabon JK, Walport MJ, et al. Similarities of specificity and cofactor dependence in serum antiphospholipid antibodies from patients with human parvovirus B19 infection and from those with systemic lupus erythematosus. *Arthritis Rheum* 1997;40:103–108.

82. Karetnyi YV, Naides SJ. Parvovirus B19. In: Rose NR, Conway de Macario E, Folds JD, et al., eds. *Manual of clinical laboratory immunology.* 5th ed. Washington DC: American Society of Microbiology, 1997:667–672.

83. White JW Jr, Winkelmann RK. Weber-Christian panniculitis: a review of 30 cases with this diagnosis. *J Am Acad Dermatol* 1998;39:56–62.

84. Foto F, Saag KG, Scharosch LL, et al. Parvovirus B19-specific DNA in bone marrow from B19 arthropathy patients: evidence for B19 viral persistence. *J Infect Dis* 1993;167:744–748.

85. Söderlund M, von Essen R, Haapasaari J, et al. Persistence of parvovirus B19 DNA in synovial membranes of young patients with and without chronic arthropathy. *Lancet* 1997;349:1063.

86. Von Poblotzki A, Gigler A, Lang B, et al. Antibodies to parvovirus B19 NS-1 protein in infected individuals. *J Gen Virol* 1995;76: 519–527.

87. Moffatt S, Tanaka N, Tada K, et al. A cytotoxic nonstructural protein, NS1, of human parvovirus B19 induces activation of interleukin-6 gene expression. *J Virol* 1996;70:8485–8491.

88. Sol N, Morinet F, Alizon M, et al. Trans-activation of the long terminal repeat of human immunodeficiency virus type 1 by the parvovirus B19 NS1 gene product. *J Gen Virol* 1993;74:2011–2014.

89. Takahashi Y, Murai C, Shibata S, et al. Human parvovirus B19 as a causative agent for rheumatoid arthritis. *Proc Nat Acad Sci U S A* 1998;95:8227–8232.

90. Karetnyi YV, Beck PR, Markin RS, et al. Human parvovirus B19 infection in acute fulminant liver failure. *Arch Virol* 1999;144: 1713–1724.

91. Naides SJ, Scharosch LL, Hays-Goldsmith S, et al. Defective parvovirus B19 capsid protein epitope recognition in B19 arthropathy. *Arthritis Rheum* 1999;35:S36.

92. Sahakian V, Weiner CP, Naides SJ, et al. Intrauterine transfusion treatment of nonimmune hydrops fetalis secondary to human parvovirus B19 infection. *Am J Obstet Gynecol* 1991;164:1090–1091.

93. Frey TK. Molecular biology of rubella virus. *Adv Virus Res* 1994; 44:69–160.

94. Anonymous. Rubella and congenital rubella syndrome—United States, 1994-1997. *MMWR Morb Mortal Wkly Rep* 1997;46:350–354.

95. Miller E, Waight P, Gay N, et al. The epidemiology of rubella in England and Wales before and after the 1994 measles and rubella vaccination campaign: fourth joint report from the PHLS and the National Congenital Rubella Surveillance Programme. *Communicable Dis Rep CDR Rev* 1997;7:R26–32.

96. Briss PA, Fehrs LJ, Hutcheson RH, et al. Rubella among the Amish: resurgent disease in a highly susceptible community. *Pediatr Infect Dis J* 1992;11:955–959.

97. Hoey J. Rubella outbreaks on cruise ships. *CMAJ* 1998;158:516–517.

98. Anonymous. Rubella among crew members of commercial cruise ships—Florida, 1997. *MMWR Morb Mortality Wkly Rep* 1998;46: 1247–1250.

99. Centers for Disease and Prevention. Increase in rubella and congenital rubella syndrome—United States, 1988–1990. *MMWR Morb Mortal Wkly Rep* 1991;40:93–99.

100. Anonymous. Rubella. In: Peter G, ed. *Report of the Committee on Infectious Diseases.* 21st ed. Elk Grove Village, IL: American Academy of Pediatrics, 1988:362–370.

101. Wolinsky JS. Rubella. In: Fields BN, Knipe DM, Chanock RM, et al., eds. *Fields virology.* 2nd ed. New York: Raven Press, 1990:815–838.

102. Bayer AS. Arthritis related to rubella: a complication of natural rubella and rubella immunization. *Postgrad Med* 1980;67:131–134.

103. Smith CA, Petty RE, Tingle AJ. Rubella virus and arthritis [Review]. *Rheum Dis Clin North Am* 1987;13:265–274.

104. Ueno Y. Rubella arthritis: an outbreak in Kyoto. *J Rheumatol* 1994; 21:874–876.

105. Chantler JK, Tingle AJ, Petty RE. Persistent rubella virus infection associated with chronic arthritis in children. *N Engl J Med* 1985; 313:1117–1123.

106. Tingle AJ, Allen M, Petty RE, et al. Rubella-associated arthritis. I. Comparative study of joint manifestations associated with natural rubella infection and RA 27/3 rubella immunisation. *Ann Rheum Dis* 1986;45:110–114.

107. Chin J, Werner SB. Neuritis and arthritis following rubella immunization. *JAMA* 1971;215:485–486.

108. Cooper LZ, Ziring PR, Weiss HJ, et al. Transient arthritis after rubella vaccination. *Am J Dis Child* 1969;118:218–225.

109. Gold JA. Arthritis after rubella vaccination of women. *N Engl J Med* 1969;281:109.

110. Howson CP, Katz M, Johnston RB Jr, et al. Chronic arthritis after rubella vaccination. *Clin Infect Dis* 1992;15:307–312.

111. Weibel RE, Benor DE. Chronic arthropathy and musculoskeletal symptoms associated with rubella vaccines: a review of 124 claims submitted to the National Vaccine Injury Compensation Program. *Arthritis Rheum* 1996;39:1529–1534.

112. Mitchell LA, Tingle AJ, Shukin R, et al. Chronic rubella vaccine-associated arthropathy. *Arch Intern Med* 1993;153:2268–2274.

113. Chin J, Werner SB, Kusumoto HH, Lennette EH. Complications of rubella immunization in children. *California Med* 1971;114:7–12.

114. Polk BF, Modlin JF, White JA, et al. A controlled comparison of joint reactions among women receiving one of two rubella vaccines. *Am J Epidemiol* 1982;115:19–25.

115. Tingle AJ, Chantler JK, Pot KH, et al. Postpartum rubella immunization: association with development of prolonged arthritis, neurological sequelae, and chronic rubella viremia. *J Infect Dis* 1985;152:606–612.

116. Deinard AS, Hoban TW, Venters HD. Clinical reactions in children after rubella vaccination. *Health Services Reports* 1973;88:457–462.

117. Kilroy AW, Schaffner W, Fleet WF Jr, et al. Two syndromes following rubella immunization. *JAMA* 1970;214:2287–2292.

118. Meurman OH. Persistence of immunoglobulin G and immunoglobulin M antibodies after postnatal rubella infection determined by solid-phase radioimmunoassay. *J Clin Microbiol* 1978;7:34–38.

119. Miki NPH, Chantler JK. Differential ability of wild-type and vaccine strains of rubella virus to replicate and persist in human joint tissue. *Clin Exp Rheumatol* 1992;10:3–12.

120. Mims CA, Stokes A, Grahame R. Synthesis of antibodies, including antiviral antibodies, in the knee joints of patients with arthritis. *Ann Rheum Dis* 1985;44:734–737.

121. Chattopadhyay H, Chattopadhyay C, Natvig JB, et al. Demonstration of anti-rubella antibody-secreting cells in rheumatoid arthritis patients. *Scand J Immunol* 1979;10:47–54.

122. Turell MJ, Beaman JR, Tammariello RF. Susceptibility of selected strains of Aedes aegypti and Aedes albopictus (Diptera: Culicidae) to chikungunya virus. *J Med Entomol* 1992;29:49–53.

123. Jupp PG, McIntosh BM. Aedes furcifer and other mosquitoes as vectors of chikungunya virus at Mica, northeastern Transvaal, South Africa. *J Am Mosquito Control Assoc* 1990;6:415–420.

124. Gard G, Marshall ID, Woodroofe GM. Annually recurrent epidemic polyarthritis and Ross River virus activity in a coastal area of New South Wales. II. Mosquitoes, viruses, and wildlife. *Am J Tropical Med Hygiene* 1973;22:551–560.

125. Doherty RL. Arthropod-borne viruses in Australia, 1973–1976. *Aust J Exp Biol Med Sci* 1977;55:103–130.

126. Gubler DJ. Transmission of Ross River virus by Aedes polynesiensis and Aedes aegypti. *Am J Tropical Med Hygiene* 1981;30:1303–1306.

127. Rosen L, Gubler DJ, Bennett PH. Epidemic polyarthritis (Ross River) virus infection in the Cook Islands. *Am J Trop Med Hyg* 1981;30: 1294–1302.

128. Niklasson B, Espmark A, LeDuc JW, et al. Association of a Sindbis-like virus with Ockelbo disease in Sweden. *Am J Trop Med Hyg* 1984;33:1212–1217.

129. Calisher CH, Gutierrez E, Maness KS, et al. Isolation of Mayaro virus from a migrating bird captured in Louisiana in 1967. *Bull Pan Am Health Org* 1974;8:243–248.

130. Halstead SB, Nimmannitya S, Margiotta MR. Dengue and chikungunya virus infection in man in Thailand, 1962–1964. II. Observations on disease in outpatients. *Am J Trop Med Hyg* 1969;18:972–983.

131. Williams MC, Woodall JP, Porterfield JS. O'Nyong-nyong fever: an epidemic virus disease in east africa. V. Human antibody studies by plaque inhibition and other serological tests. *Trans R Soc Trop Med Hyg* 1962;56:166–172.

132. Williams MC, Woodall JP, Porterfield JS. O'nyong-nyong fever: an epidemic virus disease in East Africa. *Trans R Soc Trop Med Hyg* 1962;56:166–172.

133. Williams MC, Woodall JP, Corbet PS, et al. O'nyong-nyong fever: an epidemic in east Africa. VIII. Virus isolations from Anopheles mosquitoes. *Trans R Soc Trop Med Hyg* 1965;59:300–306.

134. Williams MC, Woodall JP, Gillett JD. O'nyong-nyong fever: an epidemic in East Africa. VII. Virus isolations from man and serological studies up to July 1961. *Trans R Soc Trop Med Hyg* 1965;59:186–197.

135. Rwaguma EB, Lutwama JJ, Sempala SD, et al. Emergence of epidemic O'nyong-nyong fever in southwestern Uganda, after an absence of 35 years [Letter]. *Emerg Infect Dis* 1997;3 (online: cdc.gov/ncidod/eid/vol3nol/rwaguma.htm)

136. Peters CJ, Dalrymple JM. Alphaviruses. In: Fields BN, Knipe DM, Chanock RM, et al., eds. *Fields virology.* 2nd ed. New York: Raven Press, 1990:713–761.

137. Halliday JH, Horan JP. An epidemic of polyarthritis in the Northern Territory. *Med J Aust* 1943;2:293–295.

138. Sibree EW. Acute polyarthritis in Queensland. *Med J Aust* 1944;2: 565–567.

139. Anderson SG, French EL. An epidemic exanthem associated with polyarthritis in Murray Valley, 1956. *Med J Aust* 1957;2:113–117.

140. Aaskov JG, Ross PV, Harper JJ, et al. Isolation of Ross River virus from epidemic polyarthritis patients in Australia. *Aust J Exp Biol Med Sci* 1985;63:587–597.

141. Marshall ID, Woodroofe GM, Gard GP. Arboviruses of coastal south-eastern Australia. *Aust J Exp Biol Med Sci* 1980;58:91–102.

142. Schuchmann L, Neumann Haefelin D. Persistent (chronic active) Epstein-Barr virus infection and arthritis in childhood [German]. *Monatsschrift Kinderheilkunde* 1985;133:845–847.

143. Clarke JA, Marshall ID, Gard G. Annually recurrent epidemic polyarthritis and Ross river virus activity in a coastal area of New South Wales. I. Occurrence of the disease. *Am J Trop Med Hyg* 1973;22:543–550.

144. Tesh RB, Gajdusek DC, Garruto RM, et al. The distribution and prevalence of group A arbovirus neutralizing antibodies among human populations in Southeast Asia and the Pacific islands. *Am J Trop Med Hyg* 1975;24:664–675.

145. Scrimgeour EM, Aaskov JG, Matz LR. Ross River virus arthritis in Papua New Guinea. *Trans R Soc Trop Med Hyg* 1987;81:833–834.

146. Scrimgeour EM, Matz LR, Aaskov JG. A study of arthritis in Papua New Guinea. *Aust N Z J Med* 1987;17:51–54.

147. Mudge PR, Aaskov JG. Epidemic polyarthritis in Australia, 1980-1981. *Med J Aust* 1983;2:269–273.

148. Skogh M, Espmark A. Ockelbo disease: epidemic arthritis-exanthema syndrome in Sweden caused by Sindbis-virus like agent. *Lancet* 1982;1:795–796.

149. Tesh RB. Arthritides caused by mosquito-borne viruses. *Ann Rev Med* 1982;33:31–40.

150. Tesh RB, Watts DM, Russell KL, et al. Mayaro virus disease: an emerging mosquito-borne zoonosis in tropical South America. *Clin Infect Dis* 1999;28:67–73.

151. Nimmannitya S, Halstead SB, Cohen SN, et al. Dengue and chikungunya virus infection in man in Thailand, 1962–1964. I. Observations on hospitalized patients with hemorrhagic fever. *Am J Trop Med Hyg* 1969;18:954–971.

152. Brighton SW, Prozesky OW, De la Harpe AL. Chikungunya virus infection: a retrospective study of 107 cases. *S Afr Med J* 1983;63:313–315.

153. Kennedy AC, Fleming J, Solomon L. Chikungunya viral arthropathy: a clinical description. *J Rheumatol* 1980;7:231–236.

154. Brighton SW, Simson IW. A destructive arthropathy following Chikungunya virus arthritis: a possible association. *Clin Rheumatol* 1984;3:253–258.

155. Tomori O, Fagbami A, Fabiyi A. The 1974 epidemic of Chikungunya fever in children in Ibadan. *Trop Geographical Med* 1975;27:413–417.

156. Halstead SB, Scanlon JE, Umpaivit P, et al. Dengue and chikungunya virus infection in man in Thailand, 1962–1964. IV. Epidemiologic studies in the Bangkok metropolitan area. *Am J Trop Med Hyg* 1969;18:997–1021.

157. Halstead SB, Udomsakdi S, Scanlon JE, et al. Dengue and chikungunya virus infection in man in Thailand, 1962–1964. V. Epidemiologic observations outside Bangkok. *Am J Trop Med Hyg* 1969;18:1022–1033.

158. Fourie ED, Morrison JG. Rheumatoid arthritic syndrome after Chikungunya fever. *S Afr Med J* 1979;56:130–132.

159. Shore H. O'Nyong-nyong fever: an epidemic virus disease in east africa. III. Some clinical and epidemiological observations in the northern province. *Trans R Soc Trop Med Hyg* 1961;55:361–373.

160. Moore DL, Causey OR, Carey DE, et al. Arthropod-borne viral infections of man in Nigeria, 1964–1970. *Ann Trop Med Parasitol* 1975;69:49–64.

161. Nimmo JR. An unusual epidemic. *Med J Aust* 1928;1:549–550.

162. Fraser JRE. Epidemic polyarthritis and Ross River virus disease. *Clin Rheum Dis* 1986;12:369–388.

163. Hawkes RA, Boughton CR, Naim HM, et al. A major outbreak of epidemic polyarthritis in New South Wales during the summer of 1983/1984. *Med J Aust* 1985;143:330–333.

164. Fraser JR, Cunningham AL. Incubation time of epidemic polyarthritis. *Med J Aust* 1980;1:550–551.

165. Lindsay MDA, Johansen CA, Broom AK, et al. Emergence of Barmah Forest virus in western Australia. *Emerg Infect Dis* (online) 1995;1:1–6.

166. Tesh RB. Arthritides caused by mosquito-borne viruses. *Annu Rev Med* 1982;33:31–40.

167. Niklasson B, Espmark A, Lundstrom J. Occurrence of arthralgia and specific IgM antibodies three to four years after Ockelbo disease. *J Infect Dis* 1988;157:832–835.

168. Pinheiro FP, Freitas RB, Travassos da Rosa JF, et al. An outbreak of Mayaro virus disease in Belterra, Brazil. I. Clinical and virological findings. *Am J Trop Med Hyg* 1981;30:674–681.

169. LeDuc JW, Pinheiro FP, Travassos da Rosa AP. An outbreak of Mayaro virus disease in Belterra, Brazil. II. Epidemiology. *Am J Trop Med Hyg* 1981;30:682–688.

170. Hoch AL, Peterson NE, LeDuc JW, et al. An outbreak of Mayaro virus disease in Belterra, Brazil. III. Entomological and ecological studies. *Am J Trop Med Hyg* 1981;30:689–698.

171. Aaskov JG, Mataika JU, Lawrence GW, et al. An epidemic of Ross River virus infection in Fiji, 1979. *Am J Trop Med Hyg* 1981;30:1053–1059.

172. Julkunen I, Brummer-Korvenkontio M, Hautanen A, et al. Elevated serum immune complex levels in Pogosta disease, an acute alphavirus infection with rash and arthritis. *J Clin Lab Immunol* 1986;21:77–82.

173. Murphy FA, Taylor WP, Mims CA, et al. Pathogenesis of Ross River virus infection in mice. II. Muscle, heart, and brown fat lesions. *J Infect Dis* 1973;127:129–138.

174. Fraser JRE, Cunningham AL, Clarris BJ, et al. Cytology of synovial effusions in epidemic polyarthritis. *Aust N Z J Med* 1981;11:168–173.

175. Hazelton RA, Hughes C, Aaskov JG. The inflammatory response in the synovium of a patient with Ross River arbovirus infection. *Aust N Z J Med* 1985;15:336–339.

176. Cunningham AL, Fraser JR. Ross River virus infection of human synovial cells in vitro. *Aust J Exp Biol Med Sci* 1985;63:197–204.

177. Carter IW, Smythe LD, Fraser JR, et al. Detection of Ross River virus immunoglobulin M antibodies by enzyme-linked immunosorbent assay using antibody class capture and comparison with other methods. *Pathology* 1985;17:503–508.

178. Fraser JR, Tait B, Aaskov JG, Cunningham AL. Possible genetic determinants in epidemic polyarthritis caused by Ross River virus infection. *Aust N Z J Med* 1980;10:597–603.

179. Brighton SW. Chloroquine phosphate treatment of chronic Chikungunya arthritis: an open pilot study. *S Afr Med J* 1984;66:217–218.

180. Reference deleted.

181. Yu S, Aaskov JG. Development of a candidate vaccine against Ross River virus infection. *Vaccine* 1994;12:1118–1124.

182. Levitt NH, Ramsburg HH, Hasty SE, et al. Development of an attenuated strain of Chikungunya virus for use in vaccine production. *Vaccine* 1986;4:157–162.

183. Turrell MJ, Malinoski FJ. Limited potential for mosquito transmission of a live, attenuated chikungunya virus vaccine. *Am J Trop Med Hyg* 1992;47:98–103.

184. McClain DJ, Lewis TE, Ramsburg H, et al. Evaluation of the immunogenicity and reactogenicity of a live, attenuated Chikungunya vaccine (abst). *Am Soc Virol* 1993;A1.

185. McClain DJ, Pitman PR, Ramsburg HH, et al. Immunologic interference from sequential administration of live attenuated alphavirus vaccines. *J Infect Dis* 1998;177:634–641.

186. Hollinger FB. Hepatitis B. In: Fields BN, Knipe DM, Chanock RM, et al., eds. *Fields virology*. 2nd ed. New York: Raven Press, 1990:2171–2236.

187. Seeger C. Hepatitis B viruses: molecular biology (human). In: Webster RG, Granoff A, eds. *Encyclopedia of virology*. San Diego: Academic Press, 1994:560–564.

188. Rhee KJ, Albertson TE, Kizer KW, et al. A comparison of HIV-1, HBV, and HTLV-I/II seroprevalence rates of injured patients admitted through California emergency departments. *Ann Emerg Med* 1992;21:397–401.

189. Robinson WS. Hepatitis B viruses: general features (human). In: Webster RG, Granoff A, eds. *Encyclopedia of virology*. San Diego: Academic Press, 1994:554–559.

190. Alarcon GS, Townes AS. Arthritis in viral hepatitis: report of two cases and review of the literature. *Johns Hopkins Med J* 1973;132:1–15.

191. Calabro JJ, Londino AV Jr. Infectious vasculitis: viral and rickettsial diseases. In: Hicks RV, ed. *Vasculopathies of childhood*. Littleton, MA: PSG Publishing, 1988:285–296.

192. Guillevin L, Lhote F, Cohen P, et al. Polyarteritis nodosa related to hepatitis B virus: a prospective study with long-term observation of 41 patients. *Medicine* (Baltimore) 1995;74:238–253.

193. Cohen BJ. The IgM antibody responses to the core antigen of hepatitis B virus. *J Med Virol* 1970;3:141–149.

194. Hoofnagle JH. Serologic markers of hepatitis B virus infection. *Annu Rev Med* 1981;32:1–11.

195. Gladman DD. Clinical aspects of the spondyloarthropathies. *Am J Med Sci* 1998;316:234–238.
196. Beutler AM, Schumacher HR Jr, Whittum-Hudson JA, et al. Case report: in situ hybridization for detection of inapparent infection with Chlamydia trachomatis in synovial tissue of a patient with Reiter's syndrome. *Am J Med Sci* 1995;310:206–213.
197. Branigan PJ, Gerard HC, Hudson AP, et al. Comparison of synovial tissue and synovial fluid as the source of nucleic acids for detection of Chlamydia trachomatis by polymerase chain reaction [errata in *Arthritis Rheum* 1997;40:387 and 1997;40:782]. *Arthritis Rheum* 1996;39:1740–1746.
198. Gerard HC, Branigan PJ, Schumacher HR Jr, et al. Synovial Chlamydia trachomatis in patients with reactive arthritis/Reiter's syndrome are viable but show aberrant gene expression. *J Rheumatol* 1998;25:734–742.
199. Nanagara R, Li F, Beutler A, et al. Alteration of Chlamydia trachomatis biologic behavior in synovial membranes: suppression of surface antigen production in reactive arthritis and Reiter's syndrome. *Arthritis Rheum* 1995;38:1410–1417.
200. Kirchner JT. Reiter's syndrome: a possibility in patients with reactive arthritis [Review] [35 refs]. *Postgrad Med* 1995;97:111–112.
201. Stolk-Engelaar VM, Hoogkamp-Korstanje JA. Clinical presentation and diagnosis of gastrointestinal infections by Yersinia enterocolitica in 261 Dutch patients. *Scand J Infect Dis* 1996;28:571–575.
202. Toussirot E, Plesiat P, Wendling D. Reiter's syndrome induced by Gardnerella vaginalis. *Scand J Rheumatol* 1998;27:316–317.
203. Arnett FC. Reactive arthritis (Reiter's syndrome) and enteropathic arthritis. In: Klippel JH, Weyand CM, Wortmann RL, eds. *Primer on the rheumatic diseases.* 11th ed. Atlanta: Arthritis Foundation, 1997:184–188.
204. Reveille JD. HLA-B27 and the seronegative spondyloarthropathies. *Am J Med Sci* 1998;316:239–249.
205. Michet CJ, Machado EB, Ballard DJ, et al. Epidemiology of Reiter's syndrome in Rochester, Minnesota: 1950–1980. *Arthritis Rheum* 1988;31:428–431.
206. Krylov MY, Reveille JD, Alexeeva LI, et al. HLA-B27 subtypes among the Chukotka Native groups. *Arch Immunol Ther Exp* 1995;43:135–138.
207. Iliopoulos A, Karras D, Ioakimidis D, et al. Change in the epidemiology of Reiter's syndrome (reactive arthritis) in the post-AIDS era? An analysis of cases appearing in the Greek Army. *J Rheumatol* 1995;22:252–254.
208. Rothschild BM, Pingitore C, Eaton M. Dactylitis: implications for clinical practice. *Semin Arthritis Rheum* 1998;28:41–47.
209. Yli-Kerttula UI, Kataja MJ, Vilppula AH. Urogenital involvements and rheumatic disorders in females: an interview study. *Clin Rheumatol* 1985;4:170–175.
210. Wolf P, Smolle J. Reiter syndrome in an 82-year-old female [German]. *Hautarzt* 1990;41:277–279.
211. Kettering JM, Towers JD, Rubin DA. The seronegative spondyloarthropathies. *Semin Roentgenol* 1996;31:220–228.
212. Secundini R, Scheines EJ, Gusis SE, et al. Clinico-radiological correlation of enthesitis in seronegative spondyloarthropathies (SNSA). *Clin Rheumatol* 1997;16:129–132.
213. Fan PT, Yu DTY. Reiter's syndrome. In: Kelly WN, Ruddy S, Harris ED Jr, et al., eds. *Textbook of Rheumatology.* 5th ed. Philadelphia: WB Saunders, 1997:983–997.
214. Toivanen A. Reactive arthritis and Reiter's syndrome: history and clinical features. In: Klippel JH, Dieppe PA, eds. *Rheumatology.* 2nd ed. London: CV Mosby, 1998:1–8.
215. Calin A. Reactive arthropathy, Reiter's syndrome, and enteric arthropathy in adults. In: Maddison PJ, Isenberg DA, Woo P, et al., eds. *Oxford textbook of rheumatology.* 2nd ed. Oxford, England: Oxford Medical Publications, 1998:1084–1097.
216. Leirisalo-Repo M. Therapeutic aspects of spondyloarthropathies: a review. *Scand J Rheumatol* 1998;27:323–328.
217. Lauhio A, Leirisalo-Repo M, Lähdevirta J, et al. Double-blind, placebo controlled study of three-month treatment with lymecycline in reactive arthritis, with special reference to Chlamydia arthritis. *Arthritis Rheum* 1991;34:6–14.
218. Toussirot E, Depaux J, Wendling D. Do minocycline and other tetracyclines have a place in rheumatology? *Rev Rhum Engl Ed* 1997; 64:474–480.
219. Lauhio A, Konttinen YT, Salo T, et al. The in vivo effect of doxycycline treatment on matrix metalloproteinases in reactive arthritis. *Ann N Y Acad Sci* 1994;732:431–432.
220. Schumacher HR Jr. Reactive arthritis. *Rheum Dis Clin North Am* 1998; 24:261–273.
221. Clegg DO, Reda DJ, Weisman MH, et al. Comparison of sulfasalazine and placebo in the treatment of reactive arthritis (Reiter's syndrome). A Department of Veterans Affairs Cooperative Study. *Arthritis Rheum* 1996;39:2021–2027.
222. Bohn S, Buchner S, Itin P. Erythema nodosum: 112 cases. Epidemiology, clinical aspects and histopathology [German]. *Schweiz Med Wochenschrift* 1997;127:1168–1176.
223. Cribier B, Caille A, Heid E, et al. Erythema nodosum and associated diseases: a study of 129 cases. *Int J Dermatol* 1998;37:667–672.
224. Hassink RI, Pasquinelli-Egli CE, Jacomella V, et al. Conditions currently associated with erythema nodosum in Swiss children. *Eur J Pediatr* 1997;156:851–853.
225. Bottone EJ. Yersinia enterocolitica: the charisma continues. *Clin Microbiol Rev* 1997;10:257–276.
226. Puavilai S, Sakuntabhai A, Sriprachaya-Anunt S, et al. Etiology of erythema nodosum. *J Med Assoc Thai* 1995;78:72–75.
227. Labbe L, Perel Y, Maleville J, et al. Erythema nodosum in children: a study of 27 patients. *Pediatr Dermatol* 1996;13:447–450.
228. Alpanez S, Carrasco I, Pons M, et al. Lesions of erythema nodosum type as the only manifestation of brucellosis [Spanish]. *Enferm Infecc Microbiol Clin* 1998;16:43–44.
229. Boonchai W, Suthipinittharm P, Mahaisavariya P. Panniculitis in tuberculosis: a clinicopathologic study of nodular panniculitis associated with tuberculosis. *Int J Dermatol* 1998;37:361–363.
230. Chao D, Steier KJ, Gomila R. Update and review of blastomycosis. *J Am Osteopath Assoc* 1997;97:525–532.
231. Werth VP. Miscellaneous syndromes involving skin and joints. In: Klippel JH, Weyand CM, Wortmann RL, eds. *Primer on the rheumatic diseases.* 11th ed. Atlanta: Arthritis Foundation, 1997:365–369.
232. Soderstrom RM, Krull EA. Erythema nodosum: a review. *Cutis* 1978;21:806–810.
233. Hoogkamp-Korstanje JA, Stolk-Engelaar VM. Yersinia enterocolitica infection in children. *Pediatr Infect Dis J* 1995;14:771–775.
234. Marshall JK, Irvine EJ. Successful therapy of refractory erythema nodosum associated with Crohn's disease using potassium iodide. *Can J Gastroenterol* 1997;11:501–502.
235. Periyakoil V, Krasner C. Moraxella catarrhalis bacteremia as a cause of erythema nodosum. *Clin Infect Dis* 1996;23:650–651.
236. Vazquez-Lopez F, Rippe ML, Soler T, et al. Erythema nodosum and acute Q fever: report of a case with granulomatous hepatitis and immunological abnormalities. *Acta Derm Venereol* 1997;77:73–74.
237. Villirillo A, Balsano L, Quinti S, et al. Erythema nodosum associated with Salmonella enteritidis infection. *Pediatr Infect Dis J* 1995;14: 919–920.
238. Martinez-Roig A, Llorens-Terol J, Torres JM. Erythema nodosum and kerion of the scalp. *Am J Dis Child* 1982;136:440–442.
239. Hicks JH. Erythema nodosum in patients with tinea pedis and onychomycosis. *South Med J* 1977;70:27–28.

*Textbook of the Autoimmune Diseases,*
Edited by R. G. Lahita, N. Chiorazzi, and W. H. Reeves,
Lippincott Williams & Wilkins, Philadelphia © 2000.

# CHAPTER 38

# Fibromyalgia

Robert M. Bennett

Fibromyalgia is not an autoimmune disease, not even a questionable one. The relevance of its inclusion in a textbook on autoimmune diseases is that it that it is often associated with the classic autoimmune connective tissue diseases (CTDs). This association has relevance for several reasons. The symptoms of fibromyalgia may be mistaken for those of the underlying CTDs. Fibromyalgia symptoms often further impair the quality of life of CTD patients. The association may provide clues to unravel the conundrum of fibromyalgia pathogenesis. During the last 5 years, important insights into the generation of fibromyalgia symptoms have been provided by neuroscience researchers investigating the anatomic and molecular basis for "central sensitization." An awareness of this paradigm shift in understanding fibromyalgia is relevant to clinicians and researchers interested in the classic autoimmune CTDs.

*Fibromyalgia* is the name given to a common syndrome of widespread musculoskeletal pain. It cannot be considered a discrete disease entity but is instead a process involving sensory amplification at the level of the dorsal horn and subcortical nuclei.

## DIAGNOSIS

In 1990, the American College of Rheumatology (ACR) offered guidelines for diagnosing fibromyalgia (1): a history of widespread pain of 3 months or more, with *widespread* is defined as pain in an axial distribution plus pain of left and right sides of the body and pain above and below the waist. A patient with axial pain plus pain in three body segments would qualify. The diagnosis requires pain in 11 or more of 18 specified tender point sites on digital palpation with an approximate force of 4 kg (i.e., the amount of pressure required to blanch a thumbnail) (Fig. 38.1).

R. M. Bennett: Department of Medicine, Division of Arthritis and Rheumatic Diseases, Oregon Health Sciences University, Portland, Oregon, 97201.

The recommended number of tender points ($\geq 11$) was originally derived from a receiver operating curve and relates to the number producing the best sensitivity and specificity. In clinical practice, the diagnosis of fibromyalgia can be entertained when fewer than 11 tender points are identified. In such cases, it is useful to palpate other areas that are commonly tender, including the infraspinatus, the upper portion of the latissimus dorsi, the scapular insertion of the levator scapulae, the humeral insertion of the deltoid, the interossei muscles in the first web space of the hand, the junction of the tensor fascia lata and the iliotibial tract, the junction of the soleus and Achilles' tendon, and the origin of the foot flexor muscles from the medial aspect of the calcaneum. In general, designated tender points are more tender than control areas (i.e., distal dorsal third of forearm, thumbnail, and mid-foot of the midpoint of the dorsal third metatarsal), but it is now appreciated that such a differentiation cannot be used to exclude fibromyalgia or indicate malingering.

Although it is semi-subjective, the tender point examination has been shown to be reproducible among different observers (2,3) and difficult to fake (4). The 1990 criteria suggested abolishing the distinction between primary and secondary fibromyalgia. This notion is important, because some fibromyalgia patients get extensive workups to exclude another diagnosis.

## EPIDEMIOLOGY

Chronic musculoskeletal pain is commonly encountered in the general population. Patients with this symptom often have areas of hyperalgesia in muscles and nearby structures–the so-called tender points or trigger points. In a postal survey of 2034 adults in the north of England, Croft reported prevalence rates of 11.2% for chronic widespread pain, 43% for regional pain, and 44% for no pain (5). When subjects with widespread pain were examined, 21.5% had 11 or more tender points, 63.8% had between 1 and 10 tender points, and 14.7% had no tender points (6). In general, there was a positive correlation between the finding of a tender point and a history of pain in that location.

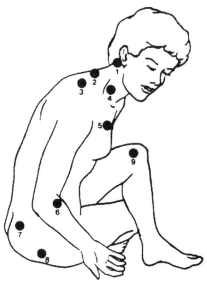

**FIG. 38.1.** American College of Rheumatology 1990 Fibromyalgia Criteria, indicating the recommended tender point locations. A total of 11 or more tender points in conjunction with a history of widespread pain is characteristic of the fibromyalgia syndrome. *1,* Insertion of the nuchal muscles into the occiput. *2,* Upper border of the trapezius (midportion). *3,* Muscle attachments to the upper medial border of the scapula. *4,* Anterior aspects of the C5 to C7 intertransverse spaces. *5,* Second rib space, which is about 3 cm lateral to the sternal border. *6,* Muscle attachments to the lateral epicondyle. *7,* Upper outer quadrant of the gluteal muscles. *8,* Muscle attachments just posterior to the greater trochanter. *9,* Medial fat pad of the knee proximal to the joint line.

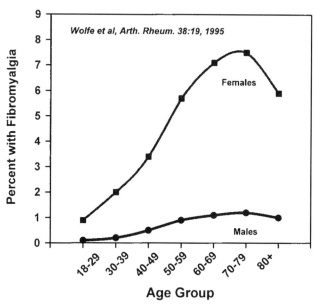

**FIG. 38.2.** Prevalence of fibromyalgia in the general population. (Data from Wolfe F, Ross K, Anderson J, et al. The prevalence and characteristics of fibromyalgia in the general population. *Arthritis Rheum* 1995;38:19–28.)

Wolf conducted a similar study in Wichita, Kansas (7). It was found that the prevalence of chronic widespread musculoskeletal pain was more common in women and increased progressively from ages 18 to 70, with 23% prevalence in the seventh decade. Chronic regional pain had a similar prevalence in men and women and displayed an almost linear increase with age, approaching 30% by the eighth decade. When Wolfe examined patients with a history of widespread pain, 25.2% of women and 6.8% of men had 11 or more tender points. The overall (male and female) prevalence of fibromyalgia in the Wichita population was 2%, with a prevalence of 3.4% for women and 0.5% for men. There was an almost linear increase in the prevalence of fibromyalgia, affecting nearly 8% of women in their eighth decade (Fig. 38.2). The results of Croft's and Wolfe's studies indicate that a history of chronic widespread pain is more prevalent than the strictly defined diagnosis of fibromyalgia. The concept is emerging that fibromyalgia is at one end of a continuous spectrum of chronic pain.

## CLINICAL FEATURES

The defining symptom of the fibromyalgia syndrome is chronic, widespread pain (1). Fibromyalgia pain typically waxes and wanes in intensity; flares are associated with unaccustomed exertion, soft tissue injuries, lack of sleep, cold exposure, and psychologic stressors. Fibromyalgia pain is predominantly axial in distribution, but pain in the hands and feet is not uncommon and may lead a misdiagnosis of "early" rheumatoid arthritis (8). Although most patients have widespread body pain, there are typically one or two locations that are the major foci. These pain centers often shift to other locations, often in response to new biomechanical stresses or trauma. Many patients describe a feeling of swelling in their soft tissues; this is often localized to the area of joints, leading to self-diagnosis of arthritis. Stiffness, a prominent feature of most fibromyalgia patients, can further reinforce the impression of early arthritis. Most patients with this array of pain symptoms have multiple tender points (9).

Fibromyalgia is more than a muscle pain syndrome; most patients have an array of other somatic complaints (10). Nearly all fibromyalgia patients have severe fatigue, poor sleep, and postexertional pain (1). Other symptoms include tension type headaches, cold intolerance, sicca symptoms, unexplained bruising, fluid retention, chest pain, jaw pain, dyspnea, dizziness, abdominal pain, paresthesia, and low-grade depression and anxiety (11–17). Some symptoms are related to specific syndromes whose prevalence appears to be increased; these include irritable bowel syndrome, migraine, premenstrual syndrome, Raynaud's phenomenon, female urethral syndrome, and restless leg syndrome (18–21).

## ASSOCIATIONS WITH AUTOIMMUNE DISORDERS

### Lupus and Fibromyalgia

Lupus patients often have a concurrent fibromyalgia syn.drome. Wallace reported a 22% prevalence among 464 lupus patients (22); Middleton reported a 22% prevalence of fibromyalgia meeting the ACR criteria, with another 23% having probable fibromyalgia (23); and Morand reported a 25% prevalence of fibromyalgia in a cohort of 87 lupus patients (24). The latter investigators observed that having concurrent fibromyalgia interfered with the rating of lupus activity using the SLAM assessment questionnaire. Gladman compared the Systemic Lupus Erythematosus Disease Activity Index (SLEDAI) and Systemic Lupus International Coordinating Committee/American College of Rheumatology (SLICC/ACR) Damage Index with Short Form 36 quality of life index (SF-36) for 119 SLE patients (25). Fibromyalgia occurred in 21% of the lupus patients. However, the presence of fibromyalgia was not related to the overall scores or any of the components of SLEDAI or Damage Index, but it was highly correlated with all eight domains of the SF-36. Fibromyalgia in a lupus patient is a major determinant in a reduced quality of life.

Middleton reported that lupus patients with fibromyalgia were much more likely to have the following symptoms compared with lupus patients without fibromyalgia: widespread pain, myalgias, nonrestorative sleep, depression, abdominal pain or bloating, dysmenorrhea, and sensitivity to light and noise. The fibromyalgia patients were less likely to be able to perform daily activities or be employed. Lupus activity was the same in the two groups (using SLAM) after the data were corrected for subjective fibromyalgia symptoms. Wysenbeek evaluated 77 lupus patients using factor analysis to identify distinctive subgroups (26). Six factors accounted for 64% of the variance. They were, in descending order of each feature, skin disease, renal involvement, thrombotic disease, lymphopenia, fibromyalgia, and abnormal serology. The individual components of the fibromyalgia group were myalgias, arthralgias, muscle tenderness, headaches, and nervousness. These studies indicate fibromyalgia is a common accompaniment of lupus and that it has a considerable impact on morbidity.

Lupus is not alone in having an association with fibromyalgia; about 25% of patients with rheumatoid arthritis (27) and about 50% of Sjögren's have been reported to have concurrent fibromyalgia. In some patients with mild primary Sjögren's syndrome, fibromyalgia may be the presenting problem (28).

## Misdiagnosis of Systemic Lupus Erythematosus

Wallace has commented on the adverse effects of incorrectly labeling a patient as having lupus (29). The misdiagnosis of fibromyalgia for lupus is not uncommon. A study from the University of Alabama analyzed 230 patients being followed for a presumptive diagnosis of lupus (30). It turned out that only 39% fulfilled the 1982 ACR criteria for lupus. The remaining 61% were readily divisible into three groups: 16% had probable SLE (i.e., classic organ involvement but not fulfilling four or more criteria); 26% had fibromyalgia; and 58% could not be classified or had cutaneous lupus (n=8) or a nonlupus antiphospholipid antibody syndrome (n=3). The

fibromyalgia group had predominantly arthralgias or myalgias, self-reported skin problems, fatigue, and a positive antinuclear antibody (ANA) result. This was a different clinical profile from that of the definite and probable lupus groups, who most often presented with clinically evident arthritis, serositis, renal disease, and observable skin findings.

There are two major reasons for mistaking fibromyalgia for lupus. First, fibromyalgia patients have a high prevalence of lupus-like symptoms (1,10). All have musculoskeletal pain, which in about 25% of fibromyalgia patients has a peripheral distribution (8) and is often described as coming from their joints (1). However, fibromyalgia patients are negative on radioactive joint scans (31). About 40% of fibromyalgia patients have cold-induced vasospasm (32), but this is not caused by digital vessel pathology as seen in cases of secondary Raynaud's (20). Some fibromyalgia patients have IgG deposits at the dermal-epidermal junction (33). However, this finding can be differentiated from a classic lupus band test by the absence of other immunoglobulins and complement components (34). Sicca symptoms are common in fibromyalgia patients (1,15); this appears to be a primary feature in many but may also be caused by anticholinergic medications (e.g., tricyclic antidepressants). It may also be a clue to an association with primary Sjögren's syndrome (28). One study found a 50% prevalence of fibromyalgia in patients with primary Sjögren's syndrome (35). Cognitive dysfunction and fatigue are common complaints in both conditions (1,36); the extent to which a concurrent fibromyalgia contributes to these symptoms in lupus has not been evaluated. Fibromyalgia has been linked to at least three infectious diseases that may develop clinical and serologic features suggesting a diagnosis of lupus. They are hepatitis C (37,38), human immunodeficiency virus infection (HIV) (39,40), and Lyme disease (41,42). All three diseases have increased immune reactivity with a tendency to autoantibody production (38,43,44). Hepatitis C in particular may develop a low-grade synovitis and an associated Sjögren's syndrome (45). Patients with these infections and concurrent fibromyalgia may be misdiagnosed as having lupus.

Second, fibromyalgia is not a popular diagnosis with many physicians. Repeated ANA testing may eventually disclose a weakly positive ANA result. Several careful studies have not found an increased prevalence of positive ANA results for fibromyalgia patients (46,47). Wallace describes 44 patients seen over a 3-month period for a "rule out lupus" consultation (29). All patients had tested ANA positive on at least one occasion. After retesting, using multiple substrates, 20% had a true-negative ANA result. At the 6-month follow-up, the diagnoses were lupus (43%), fibromyalgia (32%), rheumatoid arthritis (9%), and myasthenia gravis (2%), and 15% were undiagnosed.

Long-term follow-up studies of fibromyalgia patients have never shown an increased predilection for the development of any another rheumatic disorder (48–50). It is important not to misdiagnose lupus in fibromyalgia patients, because its treatment with steroids and cytotoxic drugs puts patients at an increased risk for iatrogenic disease. Steroid withdrawal may mimic fibromyalgia symptoms (51) and make fibromyalgia worse. One controlled study of steroids in fibromyalgia showed no therapeutic efficacy (52). Although there are no effective medications for treating fibromyalgia patients, a conservative approach stressing lifestyle modification and gentle exercise is very different that the usual approach to treating lupus (53,54).

## PATHOGENESIS OF FIBROMYALGIA

Fibromyalgia is a chronic pain syndrome. About 30 years ago, Melzack and Wall proposed that pain is a complex integration of noxious stimuli, affective traits, and cognitive factors (55). In other words, the emotional aspects of having a chronic pain state and one's rationalization of the problem may influence the final experience of pain. The International Association for the Study of Pain (IASP) (56) defines pain an unpleasant sensory and emotional experience associated with actual or potential tissue damage or described in terms of such damage.

This definition explicitly affirms that pain has a sensory and an affective or evaluative component and furthermore acknowledges that it may occur in the absence of obvious peripheral or visceral pathology. To fully understand chronic pain one must integrate the sensory and affective or evaluative elements of the pain experience. It is equally misguided to focus exclusively on the psychologic aspects of pain, as it is to address only the sensory component and ignore the affective dimensions. For the sake of clarity, these two constitutive elements are considered separately.

### Sensory Component

Pain is generally envisaged as the perceptual result of a cascade of impulses that originate from nociceptors in somatic or visceral tissues. The impulses travel in peripheral nerves with a first synapse in the dorsal horn, a second synapse in the thalamus, and end up in the cerebral cortex and other supraspinal structures. This results in an experience of pain and the activation of reflex and later reflective behaviors. These reflex and reflective behaviors are aimed at eliminating further pain. The expectation is that nociceptor-driven pain can be successfully abolished, allowing healing and a return to a pain-free state. The problem with chronic pain is that the linear relationship between nociception and pain experience is inappropriate or even absent, and the expected recovery does not occur.

In 1965, Mendell and Wall provided the first experimental evidence that the nervous system was not hard wired (57). They observed that repetitive stimulation of a peripheral nerve, at sufficient intensity to activate C fibers, resulted a progressive buildup of the magnitude of the electrical response recorded in the second order dorsal horn neurons (57). If the system had been hard wired, each stimulus should have elicited the same response in the second order neuron.

**TABLE 38.1.** *Central sensitization*

| |
|---|
| Definition |
|    Increased excitability of neurones in spinal cord |
| Pathophysiology |
|    Reduction in pain threshold |
|    Increased size of receptive fields |
|    Recruitment of input from type A fibers |
| Clinical manifestations |
|    Heightened sensitivity (hyperalgesia) |
|    Spatial spread (secondary hyperalgesia) |
|    Pain on light touch (allodynia) |

They called this phenomenon *wind-up*. The phenomenon of wind-up is crucial to understanding the problem of chronic pain. The biochemical basis for this phenomenon is being unraveled in terms of increased activation of $N$-methyl-D-aspartate (NMDA) receptors by their cognate ligand, glutamate (58). Amplification of normally mildly painful (hyperalgesia) or even nonpainful (nonnociceptive) impulses is a cardinal feature of many chronic pain states in which a peripheral cause for pain is not apparent; this is referred to as *central sensitization* (Table 38.1).

Central sensitization refers to an increased excitability of second-order neurons in the spinal cord resulting from injury or inflammation-induced activation of peripheral nociceptors. Sensory input from muscle, as opposed to skin, is a much more potent effector of central sensitization (59). This may be the clue to the role of muscle pain in the total spectrum of the fibromyalgia syndrome. It has been hypothesized that muscle microtrauma, a normal occurrence after unaccustomed exertion, is a potent stimulus to perpetuation of central sensitization in fibromyalgia patients (60). Growth hormone deficiency in a subset of fibromyalgia patients (61,62) may impair the healing of muscle microtrauma (60); treatment of these patients with recombinant growth hormone leads to a worthwhile clinical improvement (63).

The two types of second-order spinal neurons involved in central sensitization are nociceptive-specific neurons, which respond only to nociceptive stimuli, and wide-dynamic-range neurons, which respond to nociceptive and nonnociceptive afferent stimuli. Both may be sensitized by noxious stimuli, but wide-dynamic-range neurons are generally more intensely sensitized than nociceptive-specific neurons. Nociceptive and nonnociceptive afferents often converge onto the same wide-dynamic-range neuron (Fig. 38.3). Once sensitized by ongoing nociceptive impulses from peripheral nerves, wide-dynamic-range neurons respond to nonnoxious stimuli just as intensely as they had to some noxious stimuli before sensitization. This results in sensations such as light touch being experienced as pain (i.e., allodynia). Sensitization of wide-dynamic-range neurons by prior noxious stimuli provides the pathophysiologic foundation for nonnociceptive pain.

The central nervous system of subjects who have ongoing pain (e.g., arthritis) or have had previous pain experiences

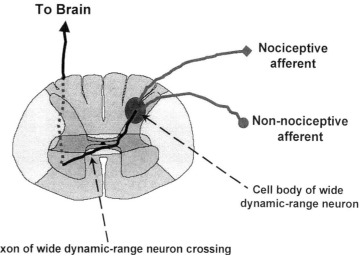

**FIG. 38.3.** Convergence of nociceptive and nonnociceptive afferent nerves onto a wide-dynamic-range neuron in the dorsal horn of the spinal cord.

(e.g., postinjury pain) may be permanently altered because of changes that can now be understood at the physiologic, molecular and structural levels (64). At a clinical level, persistent pain in survivors of serious illnesses who experienced high levels of pain during hospitalization (65), persistent pain after breast surgery (66), or the occurrence of fibromyalgia after automobile accidents (67) may reflect ongoing central sensitization that remains even after healing of peripheral injury. The reason why the phenomenon of central sensitization only occurs in a minority of individuals is unknown. A genetic susceptibility is one possibility. This has gained some support from the impressive familial occurrence in female relatives of fibromyalgia patients (68,69).

At a molecular level, there are many studies demonstrating the important role of excitatory amino acids such as glutamate and neuropeptides such as substance P in the generation of central sensitization (70–73) (Fig. 38.4). One study has shown that activation of NMDA receptors in the spinal cord causes a release of substance P and dramatic structural changes in the dendrites of neurons having substance P receptors (74). Substance P, unlike the excitatory amino acids, can diffuse long distances in the spinal cord and sensitize dorsal horn neurons in spinal segments above and below the input segment, potentially resulting the generation of nonnociceptive pain from afferent input to several segments of the spinal cord. Clinically, this would appear as an expansion of receptive fields, such as the perception of pain in apparently uninjured locations after an automobile accident. The common association of lupus and other CTDs with fibromyalgia may be a result of persistent stimulation of pain pathways by arthritis and the subsequent development of central sensitization. Another potential mechanism for this association

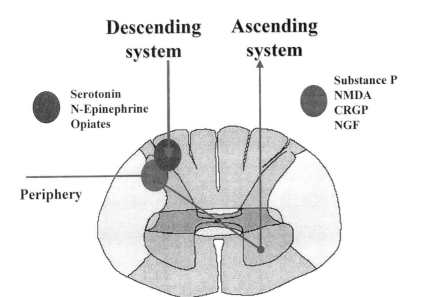

**FIG. 38.4.** Neurotransmitters involved in the ascending and descending transmission and modulation of pain impulses.

is the activation of neural circuits by proinflammatory cytokines (75).

## Psychologic Component

Chronic pain can occur in the absence of ongoing tissue damage; this is an example of the *sensory* component of pain. Subcortical areas of the brain contain several discrete nuclei (e.g., the thalamus, cingulate gyrus, hippocampus, amygdala, and locus ceruleus) that interact to form a functional unit called the *limbic system*. This is the part of the brain that serves many reflex phenomena, including the association of sensory input with specific mood states (e.g., pleasure, fear, aversion). These facts form the physiologic basis for considering the *emotional* aspect of pain.

Electrical stimulation of the brain during neurosurgical procedures does not induce pain sensations in pain-free subjects. However, in past pain patients, it often reawakens previous pain experiences (76,73). It is surmised that such stimulation reactivates cortical and subcortical pain circuits that were previously dormant. It is not known whether there is a single cortical structure that serves pain memory. Currently, it appears that different cortical and subcortical structures are involved in different aspects of the pain experience. For instance removal of the somatosensory cortex does not abolish chronic pain, but excision or lesions of the anterior cingulate cortex reduces the unpleasantness of pain (77). The anterior cingulate cortex is involved in the integration of affect, cognition, and motor response aspects of pain (78) and exhibits increased activity on positron emission tomography (PET) studies of pain patients (79). Other structures involved in cortical pain processing include the prefrontal cortex (i.e., activation of avoidance strategies, diversion of attention and motor inhibition), the insula (i.e., alerting mechanisms and integration of other relevant sensations), the amygdala (i.e., emotional significance and activation of hypervigilance), and the locus ceruleus (i.e., activation of the fight or flight response) (80). All these structures are linked to the medial thalamus, whereas the lateral thalamus is linked to the somatosensory cortex (i.e., pain localization). One example of limbic system activation is the hypervigilance that accompanies many chronic pain states, including fibromyalgia (81).

The emotional component of pain is multifactorial and includes past experiences, genetic factors, general state of health, the presence of depression and other psychologic diagnoses, coping mechanisms, and beliefs and fears surrounding the pain diagnosis. Thoughts and other sensations can influence the sensory pain input to consciousness and the emotional coloring of the pain sensation. The term given for this modulation of pain impulses is the *gate control theory of pain*. Thoughts (e.g., beliefs, fears, depression, anxiety, anger, helplessness) and peripherally generated sensations can dampen or amplify pain. There are important consequences of having pain that does not go away (as is the expected experience for most pain in most people). The unsettling realization that the problem may well be lifelong

generates a varied mix of emotions and behaviors that are often counterproductive to coping with a chronic problem. Many of these changes (which are partly reflex in origin) would be appropriate for dealing with acute self-healing pain events but become a liability when dealing with chronic pain. The end result of chronic pain is often depressive illness, marital discord, vocational difficulties, chemical dependency, social withdrawal, sleep disorders, increasing fatigue, and inappropriate beliefs. Various degrees of functional disability are a common accompaniment of chronic pain states. The reasons for dysfunction are multiple and vary from individual to individual. Pain often monopolizes attention (causing lack of focus on the task at hand). It is usually associated with poor sleep (causing emotional fatigue). Movements may aggravate pain (causing a reluctance to engage in activity). Fear of activity often leads to deconditioning (which predisposes to muscle and tendon injuries and reduced stamina). Pain causes stress, which may result in anxiety, depression, and inappropriate behavior (causing disability because of secondary psychologic distress). The modern era of psychologic imaging is providing an important new framework for understanding these "emotional" responses.

## Central Sensitization

There are several lines of evidence to suggest that the pain experience of fibromyalgia patients is in part the result of central sensitization leading to nonnociceptive pain.

### Qualitative Differences in Pain

An objective measure of applied force to a tender point can be obtained by dolorimetry (9). Various instruments have been used, most commonly, a spring-loaded balance or an electric palpometer (82). One study using the latter instrument recorded the subject's assessment of pain intensity on a 0- to 10-cm visual analogue scale (VAS) at various levels of applied force (83). Distinctly different response curves were obtained for controls and fibromyalgia patients. Similar abnormalities of pain processing in fibromyalgia patients have also been reported for heat and cold (84). When a muscle is isometrically contracted, there is normally an increase in the pain threshold to palpation (85). In fibromyalgia patients, there is a decrease in the pain threshold (86). It has been hypothesized that this is a result of sensitization of mechanoreceptors in fibromyalgia or dysfunction of afferent inhibition activated by muscle contraction (as posited by the gate control theory of pain) (86). Whatever the mechanism, it provides a partial explanation for the increased pain experienced by fibromyalgia patients on exertion.

### Hyperresponsive Somatosensory-Induced Potentials

Somatosensory induced potentials refer to the electroencephalographic (EEG) fluctuations that can be measured by skull electrodes in response to peripheral sensory stimulation.

Lorenz et al. (87) reported increased amplitude of the N170 and P390 brain somatosensory potentials in fibromyalgia compared with controls evoked by laser stimulation of the skin. They observed a spreading of the brain impulse to the other side of the cerebral cortex; in controls, the somatosensory potential was strictly localized to one side of the brain. Gibson et al. reported an increased late nociceptive ($CO_2$ laser stimulation of skin) evoked somatosensory response in 10 fibromyalgia patients compared with 10 matched controls (88). These two studies provide objective evidence that fibromyalgia patients have an altered processing of nociceptive stimuli in comparison to pain-free controls.

### Abnormalities on Single-Photon Emission Computed Tomography Imaging

Pain related functional central nervous system changes can be demonstrated by imaging techniques. For instance, several PET studies have shown increased activity in the anterior cingulate gyrus in response to pain (79). Mountz et al. reported that fibromyalgia patients, characterized by low pain thresholds, had a decreased regional blood flow compared with healthy controls on single-photon emission computed tomography (SPECT) imaging (89). The decreased perfusion was particularly prominent in the thalamic and caudate nuclei (structures involved in the processing of nociceptive stimuli). A similar finding has been reported in patients with unilateral chronic neuropathic pain, using $^{15}O$ PET (90). Functional imaging studies are also supportive of an altered processing of sensory input in fibromyalgia patients.

### Elevated Levels of Substance P in the Cerebrospinal Fluid

Substance P and calcitonin gene–related peptide are important nociceptive neurotransmitters. They lower the threshold of synaptic excitability, permitting the unmasking of normally silent interspinal synapses and the sensitization of second-order spinal neurons (91–93). Substance P can diffuse long distances in the spinal cord and sensitize dorsal horn neurons at some distance from the initial input level. This results in an expansion of receptive fields and the activation of wide-dynamic-range neurons by nonnociceptive afferent impulses. An increased production of neurotransmitters within the spinal cord may be detected as increased levels in cerebrospinal fluid (CSF) (94). Two definitive studies have shown a threefold increase of substance P in the CSF of fibromyalgia patients compared with controls (95,96). The relevance of this finding has been highlighted by a animal model of central sensitization that implicated substance P as a major etiologic factor (97). The finding of elevated levels of substance P in fibromyalgia patients is in accord with the notion that central sensitization is germane to its pathogenesis.

### Beneficial Response to an NMDA Receptor Antagonist

Previous evidence has been offered to support the role of the excitatory amino acid glutamine and NMDA receptors in the generation of nonnociceptive pain. If this were relevant to pain in fibromyalgia, the NMDA receptor antagonists would be expected to have a beneficial therapeutic effect. Two studies from Sweden reported that intravenous ketamine (an NMDA receptor antagonist) attenuates pain and pain threshold and improves muscle endurance in fibromyalgia patients (98,99). In some patients, a single intravenous infusion over a course of 10 minutes (0.3 mg/kg) resulted in a significant reduction in pain that persisted for up to 7 days. Ketamine, at this subanesthetic dose, was more potent than intravenous morphine (10 mg) and intravenous lidocaine (5 mg/kg). This is a therapeutic example of altered pain processing in fibromyalgia patients at the molecular level of glutamate-NMDA receptor interaction.

## TREATMENT

Pain is the primary overriding problem for most fibromyalgia patients. Many of the other problems they experience are largely a secondary consequence of having chronic pain. When pain is even partly relieved, fibromyalgia patients experience a significant improvement in psychologic distress, cognitive abilities, sleep, and functional capacity. A total elimination of pain is currently not possible in most fibromyalgia patients. However, worthwhile improvements can nearly always be achieved by a careful systematic analysis of the pain complaints. Fibromyalgia-related pain can be divided into general pain (i.e., the chronic background pain experience) and focal pain (i.e., the intensification of pain in a specific region, usually aggravated by movement). The latter is probably a potent driving force in the generation of central sensitization.

### Generalized Pain

The use of nonsteroidal antiinflammatory drugs in fibromyalgia is usually disappointing; it is unusual for fibromyalgia patients to experience more than a 20% relief of their pain, but many consider this to be worthwhile. Narcotics (i.e., propoxyphene, codeine, and oxycodone) often provide a worthwhile relief of pain. In most patients, concerns about addiction, dependency, and tolerance are ill founded. Tramadol (Ultram, Ortho-McNeil Pharmaceutical, Raritan, NJ, U.S.A.), a recently introduced analgesic, has been shown to be beneficial in managing fibromyalgia pain in a placebo-controlled trial (100). It has advantages of having a low abuse potential and is not a prostaglandin inhibitor; it does reduce the epileptogenic threshold and should be used cautiously with antidepressants. Looking to the future, it appears logical to use drugs that modulate the neurotransmitters involved in pain transmission and inhibition (Fig. 38.4). Experimental studies have reported the effectiveness of NMDA inhibitors (98,99). The severity of pain and the location of "hot spots" typically varies from month to month, and the judicious use of myofascial trigger point injections and spray and stretch is worthwhile in selected patients. These modalities should be viewed as an aid to active participation in a regular stretching and aerobic exercise program. Evaluation by an occupational and physical therapist often provides worthwhile advice on improved ergonomics, biomechanical imbalance, and the formulation of a regular stretching program. Hands-on physical therapy treatment with heat modalities is reserved for major flares of pain, because there is no evidence that long-term therapy alters the course of the disorder. The same comments can be made for acupuncture, trans-cutaneous electrical nerve stimulation (TENS) units, manipulation, and various massage techniques.

### Local Pain

Although fibromyalgia patients complain of widespread body pain—a manifestation of central sensitization—they also have multiple areas of tenderness in muscles called myofascial trigger points. I think these focal pain sites are a potent cause for the persistence of central sensitization; their elimination, when possible, should be of general benefit. The essential prerequisites of myofascial therapy are as follows:

1. Accurate identification of the trigger point
2. Identification and elimination of aggravating factors
3. Passive stretching of the involved muscle after the local anesthetic has taken effect; this is often aided by spraying the overlying skin with Fluori-Methane spray before passive stretching
4. Precise injection of the myofascial trigger points with 1% procaine (101)

In most patients, this treatment regimen needs to be repeated over a period of several weeks and occasionally over several months. Recalcitrant cases are usually caused by a failure to eliminate an aggravating factor, imprecise injection of the trigger point, or failure to inject satellite trigger points.

### Recognition and Treatment of Psychologic Distress

Patients with chronic pain often develop secondary psychologic disturbances, such as depression, anger, fear, withdrawal, and anxiety. When "an event" is associated with the onset of the fibromyalgia, they may adopt the role of a victim. Sometimes, these secondary reactions become the "major problem," but it is a common mistake to attribute all of the patients symptoms to an aberrant psyche. The prompt diagnosis and treatment of these secondary features is essential to effective overall management of fibromyalgia patients. Some patients develop a reduced functional ability and have difficulty being competitively employed. In such cases, the treating physician needs to act as an advocate in sanctioning a reduced or modified load at work and at home. Unless the patient has an obvious psychiatric illness, referral to psychiatrists is usually nonproductive. Psychologic counseling, particularly the use of techniques such as cognitive restructuring and biofeedback, may benefit some patients who are having difficulties coping with the realities of living with their pain and associated problems.

### Exercise

A gentle program of stretching and aerobic exercise is essential to counteract the tendency for deconditioning that leads to progressive dysfunction in fibromyalgia patients. Before stretching, muscles should be warmed actively by gentle exercise or passively by a heating pad, warm bath, or hot tub. Stretching aids the release of tightened muscle bands and, when properly performed, provides pain relief. The amount of the stretch is important. Stretching to point of resistance and then holding the stretch allows the Golgi tendon apparatus to signal the muscle fibers to relax. Stretching to the point of increased pain precipitates a contraction of additional fibers and has a deleterious effect. The stretch should be gentle and sustained for 60 seconds. Patients often must work up to this amount of time and start with 10 to 15 seconds on and then 10 to 15 seconds off. There is evidence that fibromyalgia patients benefit from increased aerobic conditioning (102,103), but many are reluctant to exercise on account of increased pain and fatigue. However, most patients, can be motivated to increase their level of fitness if they are provided realistic guidelines for exercise and have regular follow-up. Exercise prescription should emphasize non–impact-loading exercise such as use of walking, stationary exercycles, and water therapy. The aim is to exercise three to four times each week at 60% to 70% of the maximal heart rate for 20 to 30 minutes. Many patients cannot start out at this level but need to establish a regular pattern of exercise. An acceptable initiation for most patients is to start with two or three daily exercise sessions of only 3 to 5 minutes each. The duration should then be increased until they are doing three 10-minute sessions, then two 15-minute sessions, and one 20- to 30-minute session performed 3 times per week (104).

## REFERENCES

1. Wolfe F, Smythe HA, Yunus MB, et al. The American College of Rheumatology 1990 criteria for the classification of fibromyalgia: report of the Multicenter Criteria Committee. *Arthritis Rheum* 1990; 33:160–172.
2. Jacobs JW, Geenen R, van der Heide A, et al. Are tender point scores assessed by manual palpation in fibromyalgia reliable? An investigation into the variance of tender point scores. *Scand J Rheumatol* 1995; 24:243–247.
3. Tunks E, McCain GA, Hart LE, et al. The reliability of examination for tenderness in patients with myofascial pain, chronic fibromyalgia and controls. *J Rheumatol* 1995;22:944–952.
4. Smythe HA, Gladman A, Mader R, et al. Strategies for assessing pain and pain exaggeration: controlled studies. *J Rheumatol* 1997;24: 1622–1629.
5. Croft P, Rigby AS, Boswell R, et al. The prevalence of chronic widespread pain in the general population. *J Rheumatol* 1993;20: 710–713.
6. Croft P, Schollum J, Silman A. Population study of tender point counts and pain as evidence of fibromyalgia. *BMJ* 1994;309:696–699.
7. Wolfe F, Ross K, Anderson J, et al. The prevalence and characteristics of fibromyalgia in the general population. *Arthritis Rheum* 1995;38: 19–28.
8. Reilly PA, Littlejohn GO. Peripheral arthralgic presentation of fibrositis/fibromyalgia syndrome. *J Rheumatol* 1992;19:281–283.
9. Campbell SM, Clark S, Tindall EA, et al. Clinical characteristics of fibrositis. I. A blinded, controlled study of symptoms and tender points. *Arthritis Rheum* 1983;26:817–824.

10. Bennett RM. Confounding features of the fibromyalgia syndrome: a current perspective of differential diagnosis. *J Rheumatol* 1989; 16[Suppl 19]:58–61.
11. Deodhar AA, Fisher RA, Blacker CVR, Woolf AD. Fluid retention syndrome and fibromyalgia. *Br J Rheumatol* 1994;33:576–582.
12. Pellegrino MJ. Atypical chest pain as an initial presentation of primary fibromyalgia. *Arch Phys Med Rehabil* 1990;71:526–528.
13. Caidahl K, Lurie M, Bake B, et al. Dyspnoea in chronic primary fibromyalgia. *J Intern Med* 1989;226:265–270.
14. Blasberg B, Chalmers A. Temporomandibular pain and dysfunction syndrome associated with generalized musculoskeletal pain: a retrospective study. *J Rheumatol Suppl* 1989;19:87–90.
15. Dinerman H, Goldenberg DL, Felson DT. A prospective evaluation of 118 patients with the fibromyalgia syndrome: prevalence of Raynaud's phenomenon, sicca symptoms, ANA, low complement, and Ig deposition at the dermal-epidermal junction. *J Rheumatol* 1986;13:368–373.
16. Gerster JC, Hadj Djilani A. Hearing and vestibular abnormalities in primary fibrositis syndrome. *J Rheumatol* 1984;11:678–680.
17. Burckhardt CS, O'Reilly CA, Wiens AN, et al. Assessing depression in fibromyalgia patients. *Arthritis Care Res* 1994;7:35–39.
18. Yunus M, Masi AT, Calabro JJ, et al. Primary fibromyalgia (fibrositis): clinical study of 50 patients with matched normal controls. *Semin Arthritis Rheum* 1981;11:151–171.
19. Wallace DJ. Genitourinary manifestations of fibrositis: an increased association with the female urethral syndrome. *J Rheumatol* 1990;17: 238–239.
20. Bennett RM, Clark SR, Campbell SM, et al. Symptoms of Raynaud's syndrome in patients with fibromyalgia: a study utilizing the Nielsen test, digital photoplethysmography, and measurements of platelet alpha 2-adrenergic receptors. *Arthritis Rheum* 1991;34:264–269.
21. Veale D, Kavanagh G, Fielding JF, Fitzgerald O. Primary fibromyalgia and the irritable bowel syndrome: different expressions of a common pathogenetic process. *Br J Rheumatol* 1991;30:220–222.
22. Sigal LH. Illness behavior and the biomedical model. *Bull Rheum Dis* 1997;46:1–4.
23. Middleton GD, McFarlin JE, Lipsky PE. The prevalence and clinical impact of fibromyalgia in systemic lupus erythematosus [see comments]. *Arthritis Rheum* 1994;37:1181–1188.
24. Morand EF, Miller MH, Whittingham S, Littlejohn GO. Fibromyalgia syndrome and disease activity in systemic lupus erythematosus. *Lupus* 1994;3:187–191.
25. Shadick NA, Phillips CB, Logigian EL, et al. The long-term clinical outcomes of Lyme disease—a population-based retrospective cohort study. *Ann Intern Med* 1994;121:560–567.
26. Wysenbeek AJ, Leibovici L, Amit M, Weinberger A. Disease patterns of patients with systemic lupus erythematosus as shown by application of factor analysis. *J Rheumatol* 1992;19:1096–1099.
27. Wolfe F, Cathey MA, Kleinheksel SM. Fibrositis (fibromyalgia) in rheumatoid arthritis. *J Rheumatol* 1984;11:814–818.
28. Bonafede RP, Downey DC, Bennett RM. An association of fibromyalgia with primary Sjögren's syndrome: a prospective study of 72 patients. *J Rheumatol* 1995;22:133–136.
29. Wallace DJ, Schwartz E, Chi-Lin H, Peter JB. The "rule out lupus" rheumatology consultation: clinical outcomes and perspectives. *J Clin Rheumatol* 1995;1:158–164.
30. Calvo-Alen J, Bastian HM, Straaton KV, et al. Identification of patient subsets among those presumptively diagnosed with, referred, and/or followed up for systemic lupus erythematosus at a large tertiary care center. *Arthritis Rheum* 1995;38:1475–1484.
31. Yunus MB, Berg BC, Masi AT. Multiphase skeletal scintigraphy in primary fibromyalgia syndrome: a blinded study. *J Rheumatol* 1989;16:1466–1468.
32. Bengtsson A, Henriksson KG, Jorfeldt L, et al. Primary fibromyalgia: a clinical and laboratory study of 55 patients. *Scand J Rheumatol* 1986;15:340–347.
33. Caro XJ. Immunofluorescent detection of IgG at the dermal-epidermal junction in patients with apparent primary fibrositis syndrome. *Arthritis Rheum* 1984;27:1174–1179.
34. Caro XJ, Wolfe F, Johnston WH, Smith AL. A controlled and blinded study of immunoreactant deposition at the dermal-epidermal junction of patients with primary fibrositis syndrome. *J Rheumatol* 1986;13: 1086–1092.
35. Vitali C, Tavoni A, Neri R, et al. Fibromyalgia features in patients with primary Sjögren's syndrome: evidence of a relationship with psychological depression. *Scand J Rheumatol* 1989;18:21–27.
36. Petri M. Clinical features of systemic lupus erythematosus. *Curr Opin Rheumatol* 1995;7:395–401.
37. Barkhuizen A, Schoeplin GS, Bennett RM. Fibromyalgia: a prominent feature in patients with musculoskeletal problems in chronic hepatitis C: a report of 12 patients. *J Clin Rheumatol* 1996;2:180–184.
38. Lovy MR, Starkebaum G, Uberoi S. Hepatitis C infection presenting with rheumatic manifestations: a mimic of rheumatoid arthritis. *J Rheumatol* 1996;23:979–983.
39. Simms RW, Zerbini CA, Ferrante N, et al. Fibromyalgia syndrome in patients infected with human immunodeficiency virus. *Am J Med* 1992;92:368–374.
40. Buskila D, Gladman DD, Langevitz P, et al. Fibromyalgia in human immunodeficiency virus infection. *J Rheumatol* 1990;17:1202–1206.
41. Sigal LH. Persisting complaints attributed to chronic Lyme disease: possible mechanisms and implications for management. *Am J Med* 1994;96:365–373.
42. Steere AC, Taylor E, McHugh GL, Logigian EL. The overdiagnosis of Lyme disease. *JAMA* 1993;269:1812–1816.
43. Savige JA, Chang L, Horn S, Crowe SM. Anti-nuclear, anti-neutrophil cytoplasmic and anti-glomerular basement membrane antibodies in HIV-infected individuals. *Autoimmunity* 1994;18:205–211.
44. Schned ES, Williams DN. Special concerns in Lyme disease: seropositivity with vague symptoms and development of fibrositis. *Postgrad Med* 1992;91:65–68, 70.
45. Mariette X, Zerbib M, Jaccard A, et al. Hepatitis C virus and Sjögren's syndrome. *Arthritis Rheum* 1993;36:280–281.
46. Yunus MB, Hussey FX, Aldag JC. Antinuclear antibodies and connective disease features in fibromyalgia syndrome: a controlled study. *J Rheumatol* 1993;20:1557–1560.
47. Bengtsson A, Ernerudh J, Vrethem M, Skogh T. Absence of autoantibodies in primary fibromyalgia. *J Rheumatol* 1990;17:1682–1683.
48. Bengtsson A, Backman E, Lindblom B, Skogh T. Long-term follow-up of fibromyalgia patients: clinical symptoms, muscular function, laboratory tests—an eight year comparison study. *J Musculoskel Pain* 1994;2:67–80.
49. Kennedy M, Felson DT. A prospective long-term study of fibromyalgia syndrome. *Arthritis Rheum* 1996;39:682–685.
50. Ledingham J, Doherty S, Doherty M. Primary fibromyalgia syndrome—an outcome study. *Br J Rheumatol* 1993;32:139–142.
51. Dixon RP, Christy NP. On the various forms of corticosteroid withdrawal syndrome. *Am J Med* 1980;68:224–229.
52. Clark S, Tindall E, Bennett RM. A double blind crossover trial of prednisone versus placebo in the treatment of fibrositis. *J Rheumatol* 1985; 12:980–983.
53. Bennett RM, Campbell S, Burckhardt C, et al. A multidisciplinary approach to fibromyalgia treatment. *J Musculoskel Med* 1991;8:21–32.
54. McCain GA, Boissevain MD. Comment on "Toward an integrated understanding of fibromyalgia syndrome. I. Medical and pathophysiological aspects" by Boissevain and McCain in *Pain* 1991;45:227–238. Response. *Pain* 1991;47:370.
55. Melzack R, Wall PD. Pain mechanisms: a new theory. *Science* 1965; 150:971–979.
56. Merskey H, Bogduk N. *Classification of chronic pain: descriptions of chronic pain syndromes and definitions of pain terms.* 2nd ed. Seattle: IASP Press, 1994.
57. Mendell LM, Wall PD. Response of single dorsal cord cells to peripheral cutaneous unmyelinated fibers. *Nature* 1965;206:97–99.
58. Woolf CJ. Central mechanisms of acute pain. *Pain* 1990;5:218.
59. Wall PD, Woolf CJ. Muscle but not cutaneous C-afferent input produces prolonged increases in the excitability of the flexion reflex in the rat. *J Physiol* 1984;356:443–458.
60. Bennett RM. The contribution of muscle to the generation of fibromyalgia symptomatology. *J Musculoskel Pain* 1996;4:35–59.
61. Bennett RM, Clark SR, Campbell SM, Burckhardt CS. Low levels of somatomedin C in patients with the fibromyalgia syndrome: a possible link between sleep and muscle pain. *Arthritis Rheum* 1992;35: 1113–1116.
62. Bennett RM, Cook DM, Clark SR, et al. Hypothalamic-pituitary-insulin–like growth factor-I axis dysfunction in patients with fibromyalgia. *J Rheumatol* 1997;24:1384–1389.
63. Bennett RM. A randomized, double-blind, placebo-controlled study of growth hormone in the treatment of fibromyalgia. *Am J Med* 1998; 104:227–231.

64. Dubner R, Ruda MA. Activity-dependent neuronal plasticity following tissue injury and inflammation. *Trends Neurol Sci* 1992;15:96–103.

65. Desbien NA, Wu AW, Alzola MS, et al. Pain during hospitalization is associated with continued pain six months later in survivors of serious illness. *Am J Med* 1997;103:269–276.

66. Wallace MS. Pain after breast surgery: a survey of 282 women. *Pain* 1996;66:195–205.

67. Buskila D, Neumann L, Vaisberg G, et al. Increased rates of fibromyalgia following cervical spine injury: a controlled study of 161 cases of traumatic injury. *Arthritis Rheum* 1997;40:446–452.

68. Buskila D, Neumann L, Hazanov I, Carmi R. Familial aggregation in the fibromyalgia syndrome. *Semin Arthritis Rheum* 1996;26:605–611.

69. Buskila D, Neumann L. Fibromyalgia syndrome (FM) and nonarticular tenderness in relatives of patients with FM. *J Rheumatol* 1997;24:941–944.

70. Dubner R. Hyperalgesia and expanded receptive fields. *Pain* 1992;48:3–4.

71. Dickenson AH, Sullivan AF. NMDA receptors and central hyperalgesic states. *Pain* 1991;46:344–345.

72. Woolf CJ, Thompson SW. The induction and maintenance of central sensitization is dependent on *N*-methyl-D-aspartic acid receptor activation; implications for the treatment of post-injury pain hypersensitivity states. *Pain* 1991;44:293–299.

73. Basbaum AI. Memories of pain. *Science and Medicine* 1996;1:22–31.

74. Liu H, Mantyh CR, Basbaum AI. NMDA-receptor regulation of substance P release from primary afferent nociceptors. *Nature* 1997;386:721–724.

75. Watkins LR, Maier SF, Goehler LE. Immune activation: the role of pro-inflammatory cytokines in inflammation, illness responses and pathological pain states. *Pain* 1995;63:289–302.

76. Lenz FA. Thalamic stimulation reproduces previously experienced pain. *Nat Med* 1995;1:910–913.

77. Folz EL, White LEJ. Pain relief form frontal cingulotomy. *Neurosurgery* 1962;19:89–100.

78. Devinsky O, Morrell MJ, Vogt BA. Contributions of the anterior cingulate to behaviour. *Brain* 1995;118:279–306.

79. Hsieh JC, Belfrage M, Stone-Elander S, et al. Central representation of chronic ongoing neuropathic pain studied by positron emission tomography. *Pain* 1995;63:225–236.

80. Jones AKP. Pain, its perception, and imaging. *IASP Newslett* 1997;May/June:3–5.

81. McDermid AJ, Rollman GB, McCain GA. Generalized hypervigilance in fibromyalgia: evidence of perceptual amplification. *Pain* 1996;66:133–144.

82. Atkins CJ, Zielinski A, Makosinski A. Palpometry: a novel concept in pain measurement. *Nat Med* 1995;1:1138–1139.

83. Bendtsen L, Norregaard J, Jensen R, Olesen J. Evidence of qualitatively altered nociception in patients with fibromyalgia. *Arthritis Rheum* 1997;40:98–102.

84. Kosek E, Ekholm J, Hansson P. Sensory dysfunction in fibromyalgia patients with implications for pathogenic mechanisms. *Pain* 1996;68:375–383.

85. Pertovaara A, Kemppainen P. Lowered cutaneous sensitivity to nonpainful electrical stimulation during isometric exercise in humans. *Exp Brain Res* 1992;89:447–452.

86. Kosek E, Ekholm J, Hansson P. Modulation of pressure pain thresholds during and following isometric contraction in patients with fibromyalgia and in healthy controls. *Pain* 1996;64:415–423.

87. Lorenz J, Grasedyck K, Bromm B. Middle and long latency somatosensory evoked potentials after painful laser stimulation in patients with fibromyalgia syndrome. *Electroencephalogr Clin Neurophysiol* 1996;100:165–168.

88. Gibson SJ, Littlejohn GO, Gorman MM, et al. Altered heat pain thresholds and cerebral event-related potentials following painful $CO_2$ laser stimulation in subjects with fibromyalgia syndrome. *Pain* 1994;58:185–193.

89. Mountz JM, Bradley LA, Modell JG, et al. Fibromyalgia in women: abnormalities of regional cerebral blood flow in the thalamus and the caudate nucleus are associated with low pain threshold levels. *Arthritis Rheum* 1995;38:926–938.

90. Iadarola MJ, Max MB, Berman KF. Unilateral decrease in thalamic activity observed in positron emission tomography in patients with chronic neuropathic pain. *Pain* 1995;63:55–64.

91. Arnetz BB, Fjellner B. Psychological predictors of neuroendocrine responses to mental stress. *J Psychosom Res* 1986;30:297–305.

92. Sastry BR. Substance P effects on spinal nociceptive neurones. *Life Sci* 1979;24:2169–2178.

93. Coderre TJ, Katz J, Vaccarino AL, Melzack R. Contribution of central neuroplasticity to pathological pain: review of clinical and experimental evidence. *Pain* 1993;52:259–285.

94. Tsigos C, Diemel LT, White A, et al. Cerebrospinal fluid levels of substance P and calcitonin-gene–related peptide: correlation with sural nerve levels and neuropathic signs in sensory diabetic polyneuropathy. *Clin Sci* 1993;84:305–311.

95. Vaeroy H, Helle R, Forre O, et al. Elevated CSF levels of substance P and high incidence of Raynaud phenomenon in patients with fibromyalgia: new features for diagnosis. *Pain* 1988;32:21–26.

96. Russell IJ, Orr MD, Littman B, et al. Elevated cerebrospinal fluid levels of substance P in patients with the fibromyalgia syndrome. *Arthritis Rheum* 1994;37:1593–1601.

97. Watkins LR. Illness-induced hyperalgesia is mediated by spinal neuropeptides and excitatory amino acids. *Brain Res Bull* 1994;664:17–24.

98. Sorensen J, Bengtsson A, Backman E, et al. Pain analysis in patients with fibromyalgia: effects of intravenous morphine, lidocaine and ketamine. *Scand J Rheumatol* 1995;24:360–365.

99. Sorensen J, Bengtsson A, Ahlner J, et al. Fibromyalgia—are there different mechanisms in the processing of pain? A double blind crossover comparison of analgesic drugs. *J Rheumatol* 1997;24:1615–1621.

100. Russell IJ. Efficacy of Ultram™ [tramadol HCL] treatment of fibromyalgia syndrome: preliminary analysis of a multi-center, randomized, placebo-controlled study. *Arthritis Rheum* 1997;40:S214.

101. Bennett RM. Bursitis, tendinitis, myofascial pain and fibromyalgia. In: Rakel RE, ed. *Current therapy*. Philadelphia: WB Saunders, 1998:990–995.

102. Wigers SH, Stiles TC, Vogel PA. Effects of aerobic exercise versus stress management treatment in fibromyalgia: a 4.5 year prospective study. *Scand J Rheumatol* 1996;25:77–86.

103. McCain GA, Bell DA, Mai FM, Halliday PD. A controlled study of the effects of a supervised cardiovascular fitness training program on the manifestations of primary fibromyalgia. *Arthritis Rheum* 1988;31:1135–1141.

104. Clark SR. Prescribing exercise for fibromyalgia patients. *Arthritis Care Res* 1994;7:221–225.

*Textbook of the Autoimmune Diseases,*
Edited by R. G. Lahita, N. Chiorazzi, and W. H. Reeves,
Lippincott Williams & Wilkins, Philadelphia © 2000.

# CHAPTER 39

# Diseases Associated With Silicone Implants

Luis R. Espinoza and Marta Lucia Cuellar

The term *silicone* refers to a family of chemically related organosilicon compounds, prepared by reducing silica, $SiO_2$, to elemental silicon and then reacting it with methyl chloride. Silicon is an element not found in its simplest form, is the second most abundant element after oxygen, and constitutes 28% of the earth's crust (1).

Silicone polymers are extensively used in medicine since their introduction in the 1940s. Almost every field in clinical medicine uses these synthetic materials. One of their most frequent uses, however, is in breast cosmetic and reconstructive surgery.

The first indication that the use of these synthetic polymeric materials may be associated with connective tissue disorders appeared in the Japanese medical literature in 1964, when it was reported the presence of hypergammaglobulinemia in association with augmentation mammaplasty. During the ensuing years, a variety of connective tissue disorders were reported in association with the presence of foreign material, including paraffin and injections of free silicone. In 1973, Miyoshi et al. (2) introduced the term human adjuvant disease (HAD) to describe the clinical and laboratory characteristics presented by patients who had a mammaplasty with a foreign substance followed by the development of a variety of connective tissue disorders, including scleroderma, systemic lupus erythematosus (SLE), rheumatoid arthritis, and other nonspecific rheumatic disorders (Table 39.1). It is difficult to assess the nature of this association because of the complexity of the material used for mammaplasty. This consisted of a mixture of compounds, all not well characterized.

In 1962, silicone gel prostheses were introduced in the United States, and approximately 1 million women have since received these prostheses. There are several types,

including tissue expanders, silicone gel implant textured silicone coating, double-lumen implants, biocompatible gel implants, polyurethane-coated implants, and saline implants. The reasons for this variety are many and include efforts to decrease the rate of silicone gel bleed and to diminish the rate of local complication or encapsulation.

In 1982, van Nunen et al. (3) first described the association of connective tissue disorders with silicone gel breast implants. They described three women, who developed SLE, mixed connective tissue disease, and rheumatoid arthritis complicated by Sjögren's syndrome after cosmetic surgery with silicone breast implants. After this report, over the ensuing years numerous case reports were published describing the association of autoimmune abnormalities, connective tissue disorders, or both types of disorders with silicone breast implants (4–6). In the past several years, series with larger number of patients began to appear describing the possible association of silicone breast implants and underlying connective tissue disease (7–13).

## EPIDEMIOLOGIC CONSIDERATIONS

In general, epidemiologic studies have failed to demonstrate a significant association between distinct connective tissue disorders and silicone breast implants. However, later studies have shown a small but significant increase with breast and nonbreast silicone implants (14–24). In the past 10 years, several attempts to establish the frequency of distinct connective tissue disorders, particularly progressive systemic sclerosis, have been attempted. However, results obtained suggest no significant increase in the risk for progressive systemic sclerosis or other distinct connective tissue disease in women with silicone breast implants. However, no study has been designed to specifically address atypical connective tissue disease, and there are some studies that suggest that women with silicone breast implants may have an unusually high frequency of complaints suggestive of atypical connective tissue disorder.

L. R. Espinoza: Department of Medicine, Section of Rheumatology, Louisiana State University School of Medicine, New Orleans, Louisiana 70112-2822.

M. L. Cuellar: Department of Medicine, Section of Rheumatology, Tulane University Medical Center, New Orleans, Louisiana 70112; Department of Medicine, Tulane University Hospital and Clinic, New Orleans, Louisiana 70112.

**TABLE 39.1.** *Characteristics of human adjuvant disease*

- Autoimmune disease–like symptoms years after foreign substance implantation
- Recipient of paraffin, silicone, or substances that may have adjuvant effect
- Formation of foreign-body granulomas
- Serologic abnormality such as autoantibodies
- Symptoms of some patients improve after removal of foreign substance
- No concomitant infection or malignancy

These studies, however, without exception have had major flaws that severely hampered their interpretation. For example, Gabriel et al. (14), in their study of patients followed at Mayo Clinic in Olmsted County, Minnesota, found no increased risk for defined connective tissue disorders. However, increased morning stiffness among breast implant women (relative risk (RR): 1.8; confidence interval (CI), 1.1 to 3.0) was present. The sample size in this study was inadequate to detect rare outcomes, and the design of the study would not allow the detection of atypical syndromes or symptom complexes not recorded in the medical record.

Similarly, Sanchez-Guerrero et al. (15) also failed to demonstrate an increased risk for defined connective tissue disease in silicone implant recipients. However, history of connective tissue disease was sought only in participants reporting diagnosed rheumatologic, musculoskeletal, or connective tissue disease. Duration of silicone exposure was short in some silicone recipients.

Hochberg el al. (16), in the case-control telephone interviews and self-administered questionnaires of 896 patients with scleroderma at several medical centers, found no association between scleroderma and silicone breast implants. Flaws in this study include lack of specification of response rates for controls and type of implant used, and also differences in the duration of exposure to silicone between case patients and controls.

Surveys of silicone breast women attending rheumatology clinics have produced conflicting data. Weisman et al. (17) were one of the first groups to search for distinct connective tissue disorders, and they found no cases of inflammatory systemic rheumatic disease in 278 silicone breast implant women. There was, however, no control group. Goldman et al. (18), in their cross-sectional, retrospective record analysis of a rheumatology or primary care practice, also found no association between distinct connective tissue diseases, including rheumatoid arthritis and silicone breast implants. This study did not consider atypical connective tissue disease, but Giltay et al. (19), in a cohort, mailed questionnaire survey of 287 silicone breast implant patients compared with 287 patients who had cosmetic surgery without silicone exposure matched by age and year of surgery, also found no difference in risk for distinct connective tissue disorders. In contrast, implant patients had an increased risk for rheumatic symptoms (odds ratio (OR): 2.3; CI: 1.5 to 3.5), painful joints (OR: 2.6; CI: 1.5 to 4.7), burning eyes (OR: 2.4; CI: 1.3 to 4.6), and skin abnormalities (OR: 5.1; CI: 1.7 to 15.0).

In the past 5 years, an increasing number of cross-sectional, retrospective, and prospective studies of women with silicone breast implants attending rheumatology clinics have failed to demonstrate an association with distinct connective tissue disorders but have demonstrated an unusually high prevalence of atypical connective tissue disease. Large numbers of patients were included, but lack of a control group hampered the interpretation of data (7–13).

A large epidemiologic study (20) showed an association between silicone breast implants and connective tissue disorders. The design was a retrospective cohort study of 395,543 female health professionals who completed mailed questionnaires for potential inclusion in the Women's Health Study. The RR of the combined end point of any connective tissue disease among women with implants was 1.24 (CI: 95% 1.08 to 1.41, $P = 0.0015$). With respect to the individual diseases, the finding for other connective tissue diseases was statistically significant ($P = 0.017$), the findings for rheumatoid arthritis, Sjögren's syndrome, dermatomyositis or polymyositis, and scleroderma were of borderline statistical significance ($0.05 < P < 0.10$), and the finding for SLE was not statistically significant ($P = 0.44$). Atypical connective tissue disorders were not investigated. Coleman et al. (21) found similar findings in a telephone survey of 820 women with implants.

Intriguing and of great interest are the finding of Greenland and Findle (22) in patients with prosthetic nonbreast implants, including penile, testicular, and articular implants. They found an association between this type of implants and certain connective tissue disorders, including vasculitis and ankylosing spondylitis, and neurologic disorders.

There is a need for epidemiologic studies involving large numbers of patients, appropriate controls, and sufficient duration of silicone exposure to ascertain the presence of distinct, but rare, connective tissue diseases and atypical connective tissue disorders (23). The evidence accumulated, however, seems to indicate the presence of an increased frequency of atypical or undifferentiated connective tissue diseases in women with silicone breast implants (24).

## PATHOGENIC CONSIDERATIONS

Increasing data support a role for silicone in the development of the clinical manifestations associated with silicone breast implants (Table 39.2). These include adjuvant activity of silicone in animals, the formation of a capsular synovial-like membrane reaction around the implant, the detection of autoantibodies in the sera of patients with silicone breast implants, T-cell stimulatory responses induced by silicone *in vitro,* and numerous reports of autoimmune (typical and atypical) disorders in patients with silicone breast implants with improvement or remission after explantation.

Naim et al. (25) clearly demonstrated the adjuvant effect of silicone gel from mammary implants on antibody formation in rats. Their study compared the immune potentiation effects of silicone gel with that of Freund's adjuvant, using

**TABLE 39.2.** *Pathogenic mechanisms that may participate in silicone breast implant–associated connective tissue disease*

1. Adjuvant effect of silicone
    Potent adjuvant effect for antibody production against multiple antigens
    Mediates collagen-induced arthritis
2. Formation of a capsular synovial-like membrane reaction
3. Induction of multiple autoantibodies in sera
4. Cell-mediated immune responses
    Presence of specific T-cell responses
    Decreased NK-cell activity
5. HLA-mediated genetic predisposition (DR53)
6. Association with autoimmune-like disorders and improvement and/or remission after explanation

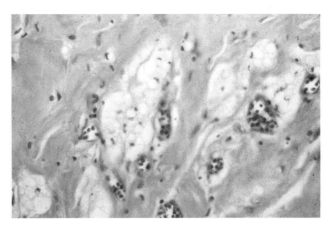

**FIG. 39.1.** Histologic appearance of a capsule, showing a mononuclear cell infiltrate, fibrous tissue, vacuolar cells, and increased vascularization (hematoxylin and eosin stain; original magnification, ×160).

bovine serum albumin (BSA) as the test antigen in rats. The results indicate that silicone gel is a potent immunologic adjuvant compared with complete and incomplete Freund's adjuvant. They further demonstrated that the humoral adjuvancy of silicone oil appears to depend on its molecular weight. Others also have confirmed and extended these observations. Nicholson et al. (26) showed other components present in silicone implants in addition to silicone gel such as octamethylcycoltetrasiloxane (D4) are potent adjuvants for antibody production against bovine serum albumin.

Naim et al. (27) also demonstrated that silicone gel is capable of eliciting autoantibodies to rat thyroglobulin and bovine collagen II. However, this immune response did not produce any histologic evidence of thyroiditis or arthritis. The same group also showed that silicone gel taken from a commercial breast implant can serve as an effective adjuvant in collagen-induced arthritis in rats (28). However, silicone gel alone does not appear to be arthritogenic. Narini et al. (29) showed that silicone gel may induce an antigen-specific lymphocyte-mediated response comparable to complete Freund's adjuvant. It appears that silicone gel can enhance immune responses, humoral and cell-mediated, which suggests that this material is bioactive.

The most common histologic reaction to the implant is the formation of mature scar tissue with mononuclear cells, histiocytes, neovascularization, vacuoles containing a highly refractile, nonpolarizable material consistent with silicone, and foreign-body giant cells (30,31) (Fig. 39.1). Occasionally, the tissue reaction is exuberant and resembles a villous papillary hyperplasia with a striking histologic appearance to proliferative synovitis (30,31). The formation of this periprosthetic tissue is a dynamic process subject to ongoing restructuring. This reaction differs in thickness and cellular composition from patient to patient. This tissue has been shown to stain with concanavalin A and peanut agglutinin and for vimentin and cytokeratin. In this regard, it behaves in identical manner in the staining pattern to that for dendritic synovitis and normal synovium. Under certain circumstances, local immune responses induced by silicone involve activation of macrophages, B and T lymphocytes, and selected T-cell receptor use (31).

Katzin et al. (32) showed that 89% of the implant-associated lymphocytes were T cells. Twenty-five percent of the CD3$^+$ T cells coexpressed HLA-DR, compared with 7.9% of matched peripheral blood lymphocytes. Sixty-eight percent of the implant-associated T cells coexpressed CD4 and CD29, but only 3% of the T cells coexpressed CD4 and CD45RO. The expression of HLA-DR and the predominance of CD29$^+$ CD4$^+$ T cells indicate the presence of immune activation with the potential for stimulating antigen-specific antibody production.

The presence of a variety of autoantibodies has been recognized in the sera of women with silicone breast implants (Table 39.3). Hypergammaglobulinemia and rheumatoid factor were reported early on (2). Antinuclear antibodies (ANAs) have been found in approximately one half of women with silicone breast implants (33–36). However, some of these studies lack adequate controls. Claman et al. (35) performed a cross-sectional analysis of 150 women, of whom 131 had implants. Four groups were studied. Group 0 consisted of 19 healthy volunteer women without breast implants, group 1 had 38 healthy volunteer women with silicone breast implants, group 2 had 82 women with implants

**TABLE 39.3.** *Autoantibodies associated with silicone breast implants*

- Antinuclear antibodies
- Rheumatoid factor
- Anticentromere antibodies
- Anti-SS-A (Ro), SS-B (La) antibodies
- Anti–double stranded DNA antibodies
- Antimitochondrial, Scl-70, RNP antibodies
- Anticollagen antibodies
- Antibodies to silicone surface–associated antigens
- Anti-nuclear envelope antibodies
- Anti-GM$_1$ and anti-MAG antibodies
- B-cell antibodies
- Antipolymer antibodies
- Antibodies to silicone

who had various symptoms, and group 3 had 11 women who had autoimmune disease, including scleroderma in 6. They found ANA positivity in 0% of group 0, 18% of group 1 ($P < 0.05$ versus group 0), 26% of group 2, and 64% of group 3. Cuellar et al. (34) confirmed and expanded these ANA studies in a larger number of patients with silicone breast implants. Their data indicated a higher prevalence of ANA in individuals with silicone breast implants regardless of the clinical presentation. Of relevance was the finding of a high incidence of antinucleolar and anticentromere antibodies, highly specific for the scleroderma group disorders, including silica-associated disorders. There are some studies reporting a lower incidence of ANA in silicone breast implant patients. These studies, however, differ from the others in patient selection, smaller numbers of patients, and a high incidence of ANAs in the control population.

Specific ANA systems, including anti-SS-A (Ro), SS-B (La), RNP, and Sm, have been reported, particularly in women with longer exposure to silicone implants (37). Antibodies to collagen types I and II have also been significantly increased in sera of women with silicone breast implants (38). The epitope specificity of the autoantibodies differed markedly. Sera from women with silicone implants reacted strongly in an individually specific manner with multiple peptides of type I collagen, whereas sera from women with SLE and rheumatoid arthritis reacted only weakly with a restricted range of peptides of type I collagen. Sera from women with rheumatoid arthritis reacted strongly with multiple peptides of type II, whereas sera from women with silicone implants or SLE reacted only weakly (38). Data suggest that silicone or its biodegradation products can act as adjuvants *in situ* to enhance the immunogenicity of type I collagen or protein-silicone conjugates.

Kossovsky et al. (13) first demonstrated the immunogenicity of silicone-protein complexes. In their model, they suggest that protein-silicone complexes in animals can evoke an inflammatory reaction consistent with a delayed hypersensitivity response.

Cell-mediated immunity appears to play a role in the development of abnormal immune reactions associated with silicone. Ojo-Amaize et al. (39) demonstrated that silicone-specific T-cell responses were present in twice as many symptomatic as asymptomatic women exposed to silicone breast implants. $CD4^+$ T cells were the target cells for silicon or silicone. T cells also proliferate on stimulation with silicone dioxide (silica). A human leukocyte antigen (HLA)–mediated genetic predisposition for the development of autoimmune-like disorders in women with silicone breast implants is suggested by the finding of an increased frequencies of HLA-DR53, -DR7, and -DQ2 in symptomatic women with implants (40).

Forty-two percent of symptomatic patients with implants formed autoantibodies to their own B cells, and of these, 81% were DR53 positive. These data suggest that symptomatic patients with implants share important genetic characteristics (primarily HLA-DR53 positivity) that differentiate them

**TABLE 39.4.** *Distinct and ill-defined autoimmune disorders associated with silicone breast implants*

- Progressive systemic sclerosis
- Systemic lupus erythematosus
- Rheumatoid arthritis
- Polymyositis
- Sjögren's syndrome
- Primary biliary cirrhosis
- Multiple sclerosis–like syndrome
- Peripheral neuropathy
- Undifferentiated or atypical connective tissue disease
- Chronic fatigue syndrome
- Raynaud's disease
- Fibromyalgia

from their asymptomatic counterparts. DR53 may be a marker of women who are predisposed by their HLA genotype to become symptomatic after exposure to silicone breast implant (40). Suppressed natural killer (NK) cell activity in women with silicone breast implants may contribute to some of the B-cell abnormalities seen, particularly hypergammaglobulinemia and autoantibodies (41).

The association of silicone breast implants with typical and atypical connective tissue disorders is well-recognized, and a large variety of connective tissue disorders in women with implants have been reported (3–13) (Table 39.4). An increasing number of reports have stressed improvement or disease remission after explantation (4,9,12,42).

A working hypothesis of disease induction in women with silicone breast implants has been postulated. A silicone gel prosthesis is implanted into breast tissue, and this is followed in the ensuing weeks, months, and years by bleeding of the low-molecular-weight polymer into the surrounding tissue, triggering a local inflammatory and immune response, with infiltration of immune cells, $CD4^+$ T cells, macrophages, histiocytes, fibroblasts, and neovascularization (i.e., capsule formation). Silicone-protein complexes are formed and, in combination with the adjuvant effect of silicone and suppressed NK-cell activity, give rise to the formation of multiple autoantibodies and to specific T-cell responses. Interaction of these humoral and cell-mediated immune responses with joints, muscles, nerves, and other tissues, results in inflammation, epitope spreading, and cytokine production.

## CLINICAL MANIFESTATIONS

Clinical manifestations associated with silicone breast implants can be subdivided into local and systemic types.

### Local Clinical Manifestations

Local clinical manifestations are related to symptoms and signs of encapsulation or contracture and to silicone gel migration. They include pain, tenderness, hardening, change in the size or shape, burning and numb feeling, asymmetry, and disfigurement. Diagnosis and measurement of the severity of contracture are subjective and range from 1 (i.e., breast with a soft and natural appearance) to 4 (i.e., hard breast with spherical distortion) on the Baker scale. Contractures occur more frequently with silicone gel implants but can also occur with saline implants and may have an incidence as low as 1% and as high as 100%. Higher incidence is seen with implants of longer duration.

Several other local complications may occur, including breast pain, axillary lymph node enlargement, infection, delayed wound healing, hematoma, seratoma, numbness in breast or nipples, galactorrhea, shifting, displacement, extrusion of the implant, unsatisfactory cosmetic results, and rupture (43,44). The latter is the most serious complication, may be asymptomatic, but more often is accompanied by severe pain, swelling, decreased breast size, and disfigurement. The rate of implant rupture increases with age of implant and has been described in 35.7% of implants after 1 to 9 years to 95.7% of implants after 10 to 17 years (44).

Physical examination is not sensitive for diagnosing implant rupture. Ultrasonography and magnetic resonance imaging are more sensitive than physical examination in the detection of rupture implants, but their true sensitivity and specificity are unknown. Confirmation of ruptured implant is best determined by explantation and inspection of the implant.

### Systemic Clinical Manifestations

The clinical spectrum exhibited by women with silicone breast implants is quite diverse and ranges from asymptomatic with or without breast encapsulation to undifferentiated or atypical connective tissue disease to well-defined or distinct connective tissue disorders such as scleroderma (3–13).

In an analysis of 300 patients with breast implants seen at Louisiana State University Medical Center in 1991, a wide spectrum of clinical manifestation was found (12). Two hundred seventy-six patients had silicone gel implants, and the remaining 24 had saline-filled implants. Augmentation mammaplasty was performed in 209 (69.6%) individuals and reconstructive mammaplasty after mastectomy for cancer or fibrocystic disease in 91 (30.4%). Clinical evidence of encapsulation was seen in 75.6%, and implant rupture or leakage in 26.3%. Most women with implants exhibited ill-defined or poorly characterized rheumatic complaints, and most complained of fatigue, arthralgia, alopecia, sicca symptoms,

myalgia, or rash. Only 2% of patients had frank arthritis. Distinct connective tissue disorders such as scleroderma, SLE, or rheumatoid arthritis were diagnosed in 13.2% of the patients. Two hundred fifty (83.3%) of the 300 patients had clinical manifestations suggesting some connective tissue disease. Among these 250 patients, fatigue was the predominant complaint in 170 (68%). When these 170 patients were further analyzed, 46 (27%) of 170 fulfilled diagnostic criteria for chronic fatigue syndrome and 79 (43.4%) of 170 fulfilled criteria for fibromyalgia.

By comparing large series, the conclusion can be reached that women with silicone breast implants tend to be in the fourth decade of life and exhibit a clinical picture characterized by fatigue, myalgia, cognitive dysfunction, and sicca symptoms as their main complaints (Table 39.5). Even studies aimed at determining whether the frequency of distinct connective tissue disorders is increased in this population have shown an increased frequency of these atypical manifestations.

### LABORATORY FINDINGS

Most laboratory findings seen in women with silicone breast implants are nonspecific. ANA positivity is the hallmark of autoimmunity and is found in almost one half of symptomatic patients. Positive ANA findings in this population are often misinterpreted by physicians not experienced with this type of patient. Specific ANA systems, including Ro, La, Sm, and DNA, are seldom present. Mild elevation of the erythrocyte sedimentation rate may be seen in 20% to 30% of patients. Special consideration should be given to the antipolymer antibody (APA). APAs bind or recognize a complex of synthetic polymers immobilized on nitrocellulose using an assay similar in general format to western immunoblotting (46). The frequency of APA was found significantly increased in women with silicone breast implants, particularly in symptomatic ones (46). Elevation of IgG, IgM, and IgA levels can be found, but this usually occurs in less than one half of patients and is of mild degree. Monoclonal gammopathy of indeterminate significance, frank multiple myeloma, and antisilicone antibodies have been described, but their exact frequency and significance remain to be determined (46–48). Other autoantibodies including rheumatoid factor, antimicrosomal, and antimitochondrial antibodies, may occasionally be seen.

**TABLE 39.5.** *Clinical manifestations associated with silicone breast implants*

| Manifestation | Vasey et al. (25) | Borenstein (24) | Solomon (26) | Cuellar (28) |
|---|---|---|---|---|
| No. of patients | 50 | 100 | 176 | 300 |
| Age (years) | 44 | 44.2 | 45.1 | 44.4 |
| Fatigue | 84% | 91% | 77% | 68% |
| Myalgia | 84% | 62% | 42% | 66% |
| Arthralgia | 60% | 69% | 56% | 65% |
| Cognitive dysfunction | N.A. | 13% | 65% | 30% |
| Sicca symptoms | 10% | 26% | 50% | 12.6% |
| Hair loss | 12% | 35% | 40% | 24.1% |
| Raynaud's | 14% | 8% | 24% | 43% |

Mammography is not very sensitive nor specific in diagnosing contractures or implant rupture. Ultrasound and magnetic resonance imaging are more sensitive tests. Migration and biodegradation of free silicone from silicone and gel-filled implants have been detected with more sensitive techniques including proton nuclear magnetic resonance localized spectroscopy, but further studies are needed to confirm their usefulness (49).

## DIAGNOSIS

Preliminary diagnostic criteria have been proposed for women with silicone implants. They have a sensitivity and specificity of approximately 77%. There is a need for further validation of these criteria by other groups and with larger number of patients (50).

## THERAPEUTIC MANAGEMENT

### Local Complications

Management of the local complications depend on their severity and whether the implant has ruptured. Symptomatic therapy with analgesics, nonsteroidal antiinflammatory drugs (NSAIDs), local heat and cold packs, and gentle massage may provide relief for most patients. Closed capsulotomy should never be performed because of the increased likelihood of implant rupture or extrusion of silicone from the implant. The presence of severe encapsulation (Baker III or IV) may require explantation, but implant rupture is an absolute indication for explantation.

Asymptomatic women with breast implants or mildly symptomatic women do not necessarily need to have the implants removed. These women should be followed periodically and for long period, keeping in mind that the average life span of an implant is approximately 8 to 10 years and that the frequency of encapsulation or contracture and implant rupture increases with time.

### Systemic Complications

Most patients with systemic complaints can be managed symptomatically with a combination of analgesics, NSAIDs, tricyclics, exercise, and counseling. Patients exhibiting rapidly progressive distinct connective tissue disorders such as scleroderma or who are incapacitated by their systemic atypical complaints, including fatigue, cognitive dysfunction, and myalgias, should have their implants removed, even in the absence of severe encapsulation or rupture. For these patients, the capsule should also be removed. Patients with specific connective tissue disease such as polymyositis, rheumatoid arthritis, or SLE should be treated like patients with the idiopathic forms in addition to explantation. These disorders, fortunately, occur infrequently.

## REFERENCES

1. Lane TH, Burns SA. Silica, silicon and silicones . . . unraveling the mystery. *Curr Top Microbiol Immunol* 1996;210:3–12.
2. Miyoshi K, Shiragami H, Yoshida K. Adjuvant disease of man. *Clin Immunol* 1973;5:785–794.
3. Van Nunen S, Gatemby P, Basten A. Post-mammaplasty connective tissue disease. *Arthritis Rheum* 1982;25:694–697.
4. Brozema SJ, Fenske NA, Cruse W, et al. Human adjuvant disease following augmentation mammaplasty. *Arch Dermatol* 1988;124:1383–1386.
5. Spiera H, Kerr LD. Scleroderma following silicone implantation: accumulative experience of 11 cases. *J Rheumatol* 1993;20:958–961.
6. Gutierrez FJ, Espinoza LR. Progressive systemic sclerosis complicated by severe hypertension: Reversal after silicone implant removal. *Am J Med* 1990;89:390–392.
7. Bridges AJ, Conley C, Wang G, et al. A clinical and immunological evaluation of women with silicone breast implants and symptoms of rheumatic disease. *Ann Intern Med* 1993;118:929–936.
8. Borenstein D. Siliconosis: a spectrum of illness. *Semin Arthritis Rheum* 1994;24[Suppl 1]:1–7.
9. Vasey FB, Havice DL, Bocanegra TS, et al. Clinical findings in symptomatic women with silicone breast implants. *Semin Arthritis Rheum* 1994;24[Suppl 1]:22–28.
10. Solomon G. A clinical and laboratory profile of symptomatic women with silicone breast implants. *Semin Arthritis Rheum* 1994;24 [Suppl 1]:29–37.
11. Freundlich B, Altman C, Sandorfi N, et al. A profile of symptomatic patients with silicone breast implants: a Sjögren's like syndrome. *Semin Arthritis Rheum* 1994;24[Suppl 1]:44–53.
12. Cuellar ML, Gluck O, Molina JF, et al. Silicone breast implant-associated musculoskeletal manifestations. *Clin Rheumatol* 1995;14:667–672.
13. Kossovsky N, Gornbein JA, Zeidler M, et al. Self-reported signs and symptoms in breast implant patients with novel antibodies to silicone surface associated antigens [anti-SSAA(x)]. *J Appl Biometer* 1995;6:153–160.
14. Gabriel SE, O'Fallon WM, Kurland LT, et al. Risk of connective tissue diseases and other disorders after breast implantation. *N Engl J Med* 1994;330:1697–1702.
15. Sanchez-Guerrero J, Colditz GA, Karlson EW, et al. Silicone breast implants and the risk of connective tissue diseases and symptoms. *N Engl J Med* 1995;332:1666–1670.
16. Hochberg MC, Perlmutter DL, White B, et al. The association of augmentation mammaplasty with systemic sclerosis: results from a multicenter case-control study. *Arthritis Rheum* 1994;37[Suppl]:S369(abst).
17. Weisman MH, Vecchione TR, Albert D, et al. Connective tissue disease following breast augmentation: a preliminary test of the human adjuvant disease hypothesis. *Plast Reconstr Surg* 1988;82:626–630.
18. Goldman JA, Grenblatt J, Joines R, et al. Breast implants, rheumatoid arthritis, and connective tissue diseases in a clinical practice. *J Clin Epidemiol* 1995;48:571–582.
19. Giltay EJ, Bernelot Moens HJ, Riley AH, Tan RG. Silicone breast prostheses and rheumatic symptoms: a retrospective follow-up study. *Ann Rheum Dis* 1994;53:194–196.
20. Hennekens CH, Lee I-M, Cook NR, et al. Self-reported breast implants and connective-tissue disease in female health professionals: a retrospective cohort study. *JAMA* 1996;275:616–621.
21. Coleman EA, Lemon SJ, Rudick J, et al. Rheumatic disease among 1167 women reporting local implant and systemic problems after breast implant surgery. *J Women Health* 1994;3:165–177.
22. Greenland S, Finkle WD. A case-control study of prosthetic implants and selected chronic disease. *Ann Epidemiol* 1996;6:530–540.
23. Silverman BG, Brown SL, Bright RA, et al. Reported complications of silicone gel breast implants: an epidemiologic review. *Ann Intern Med* 1996;124:744–756.
24. Laing TJ, Guillespie BW, Lacey JV, et al. The association between silicone exposure and undifferentiated connective tissue disease among women in Michigan and Ohio. *Arthritis Rheum* 1996;39:S150.
25. Naim JO, Lanzafame RJ, van Oss CJ. The adjuvant effect of silicone gel on antibody formation in rats. *Immunol Invest* 1993;22:151–161.
26. Nicholson JJ III, Wong GE, Frondoza CG, et al. Silicone gel and Octamethylcyclotetrasiloxane potentiate antibody production to bovine serum albumin in mice. *Curr Top Microbiol Immunol* 1996;210:139–144.

27. Naim JO, Lanzafame RJ, van Oss CJ. The effect of silicone gel on the immune response. *J Biometer Sci Polymer Edu* 1995;7:123–132.
28. Naim JO, Ippolito KML, Lanzafame RJ, van Oss CJ. Induction of type II collagen arthritis in the DA rat using silicone gel as adjuvant. *Curr Top Microbiol Immunol* 1996;210:103–111.
29. Narini PP, Semple JL, Hay JB. Repeated exposure to silicone gel can induce delayed hypersensitivity. *Plast Reconstr Surg* 1995;96:371–380.
30. Hameed MR, Erlandson R, Rosen PP. Capsular synovial-like hyperplasia around mammary implants similar to dendritic synovitis. *Am J Surg Pathol* 1995;19:433–438.
31. O'Hanlon TP, Okada S, Love LA, et al. Immunohistopathology and T cell receptor gene expression in capsules surrounding silicone breast implants. *Curr Top Microbiol Immunol* 1996;210:237–242.
32. Katzin WE, Feng L-J, Abbuhl M, Klein MA. Phenotype of lymphocyte associated with the inflammatory reaction to silicone gel breast implants. *Clin Diagn Lab Immunol* 1996;3:156–161.
33. Press RI, Peebles CL, Kumagai Y, et al. Antinuclear autoantibodies in women with silicone breast implants. *Lancet* 1992;340:1304–1307.
34. Cuellar ML, Scopelitis E, Tenenbaum SA, et al. Serum antinuclear antibodies in women with silicone breast implants. *J Rheumatol* 1995;22:236–240.
35. Claman HN, Robertson AD. Antinuclear antibodies and breast implants. *West J Med* 1994;160:225–228.
36. Tan EM, Ochs RL, Kumagai Y, et al. Re-evaluation of autoantibodies and clinical overview of silicone-related disorders. *Curr Top Microbiol Immunol* 1996;210:291–298.
37. Zandman-Goddard G, Blank M, Ehrenfeld M, et al. A comparison of autoantibody production in asymptomatic and symptomatic women with silicone breast implants. *Arthritis Rheum* 1996;39:S51.
38. Rowley MJ, Cook AD, Reuber SS, Gershwin ME. Antibodies to collagen: comparative epitopes mapping in women with silicone breast implants, systemic lupus erythematosus and rheumatoid arthritis. *J Autoimmun* 1994;7:775–789.
39. Ojo-Amaize EA, Conte V, Lin H-C, Brucker RF, et al. Silicone-specific blood lymphocyte response in women with silicone breast implants. *Clin Diagn Lab Immunol* 1994;1:689–695.
40. Young VL, Nemecek JR, Schwartz BD, et al. HLA typing in women with breast implants. *Plast Reconstr Surg* 1995;96:1497–1519.
41. Wilson SD, Munson AE. Silicone-induced modulation of natural killer cell activity. *Curr Top Microbiol* 1996;210:199–208.
42. Kaiser W, Biesenbach G, Stuby U, et al. Human adjuvant disease: remission of silicone induced autoimmune disease after explantation of breast augmentation. *Ann Rheum Dis* 1990;49:937–938.
43. Truong LD, Cartwright J, Goodman MD, Woznicki D. Silicone lymphadenopathy associated with augmentation mammaplasty. Morphologic features of nine cases. *Am J Surg Pathol* 1988;12:484–491.
44. De Camara DL, Sheridan JM, Kammer BA. Rupture and aging of silicone gel breast implants. *Plast Reconstr Surg* 1993;91:828–834.
45. Edworthy SM, Maztin L, Barr SG, et al. A clinical study of the relationship between silicone breast implants and CTD. *J Rheumatol* 1998;25:254–260.
46. Tennenbaum SA, Rice JC, Espinoza LR, et al. Use of antipolymer antibody assay in recipients of silicone breast implants. *Lancet* 1997;349:449–454.
47. Silverman S, Vescio R, Silver D, et al. Silicone gel implants and monoclonal gammopathies: three cases of multiple myeloma and monoclonal gammopathy of undetermined significance. *Curr Top Microbiol Immunol* 1996;210:367–374.
48. Wolf LE, Lappé M, Peterson RD, Ezrailson EG. Human immune response to polydimethylsiloxane (silicone): screening studies in a breast implant population. *FASEB J* 1993;7:1265–1268.
49. Pfleiderer B, Garrido L. Migration and accumulation of silicone in the liver of women with silicone gel-filled breast implants. *Magn Res Imaging* 1995;33:8–17.
50. Silverman S, Borenstein D, Solomon G, et al. Preliminary operational criteria for systemic silicone related disease (SSRD). *Arthritis Rheum* 1996;39:S51.

Textbook of the Autoimmune Diseases,
Edited by R. G. Lahita, N. Chiorazzi, and W. H. Reeves,
Lippincott Williams & Wilkins, Philadelphia © 2000.

# CHAPTER 40

# How to Interpret Autoimmune Tests

Peter H. Schur

The interpretation of autoimmune tests follows the traditional interpretation methods of any laboratory test. The test results help in the diagnosis of a particular disease, and sometimes they may be helpful in monitoring the activity of disease. Critical in the interpretation of any autoimmune test is determining its sensitivity (i.e., proportion of patients with the target disorder who have a positive test), specificity (i.e., proportion of patients who are free of the target disorder and have negative or normal test results), and the positive and negative predictive values, which allow a calculation of how useful a positive test is in facilitating or negating a diagnosis (Fig. 40.1).

A nomogram based on pretest probability and likelihood ratios can be used to interpret diagnostic test results (1,2). Contingent on making these calculations are data from the study of an adequate number of patients and controls (with related and unrelated diseases and with normal subjects), using standardized, reproducible tests. Unfortunately, adequate information is often lacking (3). This chapter reviews available information regarding a number of serologic tests that are used in the diagnosis and evaluation of patients with autoimmune, rheumatic, and related disorders.

## ANTINUCLEAR ANTIBODIES

Antinuclear antibodies (ANAs) were initially discovered in the 1940s using the lupus erythematosus (LE) cell test (4). This test is no longer performed because of the lack of sensitivity, specificity, and predictive value and because of the difficulty of performance. It has been replaced by immunofluorescent techniques for the detection of ANAs in general and solid-phase immunoassays, such as enzyme-linked immunosorbent assays (ELISAs), for the detection of specific ANAs, although immunodiffusion, immunoblotting, and radioimmunoassays are occasionally performed.

P. H. Schur: Department of Medicine, Harvard Medical School, Boston, Massachusetts 02115; Department of Medicine, Division of Rheumatology, Immunology, and Allergy, Brigham and Women's Hospital, Boston, Massachusetts 02115.

The most commonly performed autoimmune test is the immunofluorescent ANA test. This test is especially useful for screening for the diagnosis of systemic lupus erythematosus (SLE), but it is also useful for the evaluation of patients with related rheumatic conditions.

## Diseases Associated with Antinuclear Antibody Positivity

ANA positivity can be seen with systemic autoimmune diseases, organ-specific autoimmune diseases, and a variety of infections. The presence of ANAs does not mandate the presence of illness, because they can also be found in normal, healthy individuals.

A positive ANA result is an essential component of the definition of some systemic autoimmune disorders, such as SLE. A positive serologic finding can also be associated with many autoimmune disorders that are not defined by these antibodies. As a result, the sensitivity of a positive ANA for a particular autoimmune disease can widely vary :

- SLE sensitivity: 95% to 100%
- Scleroderma: 60% to 80%
- Mixed connective tissue disease: 100%
- Polymyositis/dermatomyositis (5): 61%
- Rheumatoid arthritis: 52%
- Rheumatoid vasculitis: 30% to 50%
- Sjögren's syndrome: 40% to 70%
- Drug-induced lupus: 100%
- Discoid lupus: 15%
- Pauciarticular juvenile chronic arthritis (6): 71%
- Drug-induced lupus: 100%

Positive ANA results are occasionally observed for patients with autoimmune diseases that are limited to a specific organ such as the thyroid gland, liver, or lung. The following sensitivities have been reported for these disorders:

- Hashimoto's thyroiditis (7): 46%
- Graves' disease (7): 50%
- Autoimmune hepatitis (8): 100%

Target Disorders

|  |  | Present | Absent |
|---|---|:---:|:---:|
| Diagnostic | Positive | a | b |
| Test | Negative | c | d |

Sensitivity = a/(a+c)

Specificity = d/(b+d)

Pos likelihood ratio = sensitivity/(1-specificity)

Neg likelihood ratio = (1-sensitivity)/specificity

Pos predictive value = a/(a+b)

Neg predictive value = d/(c+d)

Prevalence = pretest probability = (a+c)/(a+b+c+d)

**FIG. 40.1.** Bayes' theorem is applied to calculate sensitivity, specificity, and predictive values.

- Primary autoimmune cholangitis (9): 100%
- Primary pulmonary hypertension (10): 40%

Other well-recognized disorders associated with a positive ANA titer include chronic infectious diseases, such as mononucleosis (11), subacute bacterial endocarditis, and tuberculosis, and some lymphoproliferative diseases (12,13). ANAs have also been identified in up to 90% of patients taking certain drugs; however, most of these patients do not develop drug-induced lupus.

False-positive ANAs (i.e., ANAs in the absence of autoimmune disease or known antigenic stimuli) are more commonly seen in normal women and in elderly patients. They are usually found in low titer.

## Performance of the Assay

The titer and specificity of antinuclear antigens vary depending on the antigen substrate used for the assay. Most laboratories use Hep2 cells (Human epithelial cell tumor line), which provide certain advantages over the frozen sections of murine (rat or mouse) liver or kidney. Hep2 cells offer a standardized substrate with larger nucleoli. They also provide better sensitivity for antibodies to nuclear antigens during cell division, such as the centromere antigens. ANA titers are almost always higher when measured on Hep2 cells. One study, for example, found that the ANA titer was higher when measured on Hep2 cells than on rat livers in 78 of 79 patients (14). However, the increased sensitivity of using Hep2 cells is offset by its decreased specificity (and predictive value) for SLE.

The assay is performed by first incubating Hep2 cells or cut sections of murine organs with the patient's serum and then overlaying this combination with fluorescein-tagged antihuman γ-globulin. When viewed through a fluorescent microscope, antibodies bound to nuclear antigens produce an apple green nuclear pattern. The pattern of fluorescence and the dilution at which nuclear fluorescence disappears (i.e., titer) are observed. Differences in titer of one tube dilution commonly occur when a test is repeated on the same specimen but are without clinical significance.

The different types of ANAs are defined by their target antigen, including single-stranded DNA (ssDNA) and double-stranded DNA (dsDNA), individual nuclear histones, nonhistone nuclear proteins, and RNA-protein complexes. Some of these antibodies are relatively specific for a particular disease or for specific clinical manifestations in patients with lupus.

Certain antibody specificities, such as that for the anticentromere antibody, can be read directly from the ANA test performed on Hep2 cells. However, further testing must be performed for other antibody determinations. The following are examples:

- Anti-Sm, RNP, Ro (SSA), La (SSB), Scl-70, and Jo-1 antibodies are detected by immunoblotting, ELISA, and occasionally immunodiffusion.
- Antibodies to dsDNA may be measured by ELISA or immunofluorescence.
- Antibodies to histones are generally detected by ELISA.

In the past, the tremendous interlaboratory variability of ANA results led to much confusion. However, current ANA testing is reliable and reproducible because most laboratories use commercially available tissue culture cell substrates and participate in proficiency testing. The ability to accurately perform an ANA assay is extremely important. This test is the cornerstone of the laboratory investigation of systemic connective tissue and often is of critical diagnostic significance.

### Interpretation of the Staining Pattern

A variety of nuclear staining patterns can result from antibodies directed against different nuclear antigens. The accurate interpretation of these patterns requires considerable experience and evaluation of the patient. When used properly, an accurate ANA with titer, in combination with a full history and physical examination, can be extremely useful in the diagnosis and exclusion of connective tissue diseases.

ANAs produce a wide range of different staining patterns. A positive ANA result can therefore reflect the presence of antibodies to one or a combination of nuclear proteins. The nuclear staining pattern has been recognized to have a relatively low sensitivity and specificity for different autoimmune disorders, although it was commonly used in the past to detect specific antibody and antigen specificity. Several specific tests have largely supplanted the use of these patterns:

- The homogeneous or diffuse pattern represents antibodies to the DNA-histone complex, also called deoxyribonucleoprotein or nucleosome. It is believed that these anti-bodies are responsible for the LE phenomenon.

- The peripheral or rim pattern is produced by antibodies to DNA.
- The speckled pattern is produced by antibodies to Sm, RNP, Ro/SSA, La/SSB, Scl-70, RNA polymerase II and III, and other antigens.
- The nucleolar pattern is produced by antibodies to nucleolar RNA.
- The centromeric pattern is produced by antibodies to centromeres.

Despite these general observations, it is increasingly clear that accurate interpretation of different nuclear patterns is confounded by several difficulties. The recognition of specific patterns is operator dependent, and does not produce a permanent record. The fluorescence fades in 1 or 2 days, so that one cannot compare a result with other samples without photographing each test result.

Different serum dilutions can produce varying nuclear patterns. One nuclear pattern may obscure and prevent the recognition of another pattern if several antibodies are present simultaneously. Certain specificities are visible only on specific substrates. Anti-Ro antibodies and anticentromere antibodies, for example, are not detected with murine organs, but can be found using HEp2 cells. Nuclear patterns are neither sensitive nor specific. As a result, no single pattern denotes a single disease, and conversely, several diseases may produce a particular ANA pattern.

Because of these difficulties, specific nuclear pattern recognition is not as useful as previously thought. Pattern recognition has been progressively supplanted by assays that detect specific antibodies to an ever increasing array of nuclear antigens and to antigens not normally found in the nucleus (e.g., Jo-1 in dermatomyositis/polymyositis).

### Usefulness of the Antinuclear Antibody Titer

Unlike nuclear pattern recognition, the determination of the titer of ANAs still provides clinically relevant information. As an example, a patient with no objective clinical evidence of an autoimmune disorder but with an extremely high ANA titer should be followed expectantly for the possible emergence of an illness. However, ANA titers are less helpful or important in patients with unmistakable clinical evidence of a systemic connective tissue disease.

The presence of very high concentrations of antibody (titer of more than 1:640) should arouse suspicion of an autoimmune disorder. However, its presence alone is not diagnostic of disease. If no initial diagnosis can be made, it is our practice to watch the patient carefully over time and to exclude ANA associated diseases.

The combination of very low titers of antibody (<1:80), and no or few signs or symptoms of disease portend a much smaller likelihood of an autoimmune disease. These patients need to be reevaluated far less frequently than those with extremely high antibody titers.

### False-Positive Results

Positive ANA results are commonly found for the normal population. When Hep2 cells are used as a substrate, one study of 125 normal individuals found an ANA titer above 1:40 in 32%, above 1:80 in 13%, and above 1:320 in 3% (15). No patient had anti-dsDNA antibodies.

Antibody titers in healthy individuals usually remain relatively constant over time, a finding that can also be seen in patients with known disease. My colleagues and I feel strongly that the very low specificity of a positive ANA in the absence of clinical findings of an autoimmune disorder precludes its use as a screening test for disease in the general healthy population.

### False-Negative Results

Certain ANAs can be detected at high titer using certain methods and techniques, but they are only found at low titer or may be absent when assayed using other techniques. These confounding findings result from a number of technical and physical nuances, including the method of substrate fixation, the solubility of the antigen (e.g., Ro, La, PCNA, Ku), and the localization of the antigen outside the nucleus (e.g., Jo-1, ssDNA). Because of this limitation, a patient with a negative ANA finding and strong clinical evidence of a systemic autoimmune disorder may require specific antibody assays to accurately diagnosis a rheumatic disease.

### Antibodies to DNA

Autoantibodies to DNA were first described in the late 1950s (16). These are the best recognized autoantibodies found in patients with SLE. Antibodies to DNA can be primarily divided into two groups: those reactive with denatured (single-stranded) DNA and those recognizing native (double-stranded) DNA. Some anti-dsDNA antibodies also react with Z-DNA (17).

Anti-ssDNA antibodies that identify denatured DNA are probably reacting with the purine and pyrimidine bases that are accessible on ssDNA but are buried within the β helix of dsDNA. Antidenatured DNA antibodies do not cross-react with native DNA.

Antibodies to ssDNA have several properties. They have been eluted from the kidneys of patients with proliferative nephritis and may therefore be of pathogenic significance (18). They are much less specific for SLE than antibodies to dsDNA. For example, anti-ssDNA antibodies have been reported for persons with rheumatoid arthritis, those with drug-related lupus, healthy relatives of patients with SLE (19), and less commonly, in patients with other rheumatic diseases (Table 40.1). Anti-ssDNA has limited usefulness for the diagnosis of SLE. They do not correlate well with disease activity and are therefore not useful for disease management.

Anti-dsDNA antibodies have received a significant amount of attention during the past 35 to 40 years. They are relatively specific (95%) and 70% to 75% sensitive for SLE,

**TABLE 40.1.** *Sensitivity, specificity, and predictive value of different antinuclear antibodies*

| Disease[a] | Antibody | | | | | | | |
|---|---|---|---|---|---|---|---|---|
| | dsDNA | ssDNA | Histone | Nucleoprotein | Sm | RNP | Ro | La |
| **SLE** | | | | | | | | |
| Sen | 70% | 80 | 30–80 | 58 | 25–30 | 50 | 25–35 | 15 |
| Spec | 95% | 50 | Mod | Mod | 99 | 87–94 | | |
| Pre | 95% | 50 | Mod | Mod | 97 | 46–85 | | |
| **Drug LE** | | | | | | | | |
| Sen | | 80 | 95 | 50 | 1% | | Low | Low |
| Spec | 1–5% | 50 | High | Mod | | | | |
| Pre | 1–5% | 50 | High | Mod | | | | |
| **RA** | | | | | | | | |
| Sen | | Mod | Low | 25 | 1% | 47 | Low | Low |
| Spec | 1% | Mod | | Low | | | | |
| Pre | 1% | Mod | | Low | | | | |
| **Scleroderma** | | | | | | | | |
| Sen | | | <1% | <1% | <1% | 20 | | |
| Spec | <1% | Low | | | | | | |
| Pre | <1% | Low | | | | | | |
| **PM/DM** | | | | | | | | |
| Sen | | | <1% | <1% | <1% | | Low | |
| Spec | <1% | Low | | | | | | |
| Pre | <1% | Low | | | | | | |
| **Sjögren's** | | | | | | | | |
| Sen | | Mod | Low | Mod | 1–5% | 5–60 | 8–70 | 14–60 |
| Spec | 1–5% | Mod | Low | Mod | | | 87 | 94 |
| Pre | 1–5% | Mod | Low | Mod | | | 5–48 | 26–41 |

Drug LE, drug-induced lupus; PM/DM, polymyositis/dermatomyositis; Pre, predictive value; RA, rheumatoid arthritis; Sen, sensitivity; SLE, systemic lupus erythematosus; Spec, specificity.

[a] Other associations, RNP with mixed connective tissue disease; Ro with subacute cutaneous lupus, first-degree biliary cirrhosis, vasculitis, chronic hepatitis B.

making them very useful for diagnosis (20) (Table 40.1). They are occasionally found in other conditions, including rheumatoid arthritis, juvenile arthritis, drug-induced lupus, autoimmune hepatitis, and even normal, healthy persons. Titers of anti-dsDNA antibodies often fluctuate with disease activity and are therefore useful for following the course of SLE in many patients (21–23). There is a well-recognized association of high anti-dsDNA titers with active glomerulonephritis (23–25); there also appear to be highly enriched amounts of anti-dsDNA antibodies in the glomerular deposits of immune complexes found in patients with lupus nephritis. These observations have led many investigators to believe that anti-dsDNA antibodies are of primary importance in the pathogenesis of lupus nephritis (23,26).

### Measurement of Anti–Double-Stranded DNA Antibodies

Three methods are used by most clinical laboratories to quantitate anti-dsDNA antibodies. Most of these tests measure high- and low-avidity antibodies.

The Farr assay is based on the precipitation of radiolabeled DNA–anti-DNA antibody complexes in 50% saturated ammonium sulfate. This assay detects primarily high-avidity IgG antibodies. Approximately 50% to 78% of all patients with SLE have elevated titers of anti-DNA antibodies measured by this method; the titers appear to correlate closely with disease activity, especially with active proliferative nephritis (20,27). Because the test requires radioactivity and because some of the DNA tends to become denatured (i.e., single stranded during labeling and during the performance of the assay), it is used much less commonly today and has been largely been replaced by the methods subsequently described.

The *Crithidia luciliae* assay is an indirect immunofluorescent assay that makes use of the fact that the basal body of this unicellular flagellate contains circular DNA that is "entirely" dsDNA (28). The test is performed as serial dilutions. This method, although of comparable sensitivity to the Farr assay, is more cumbersome to quantitate, and the antibodies detected correlate less closely with active nephritis (29,30).

The third method in routine use uses the ELISA technique (31,32). The dsDNA adherent to polystyrene microwells is treated to increase adhesiveness and serves as antigen to capture antibodies. These antibodies are then quantitated using a second antiserum to human immunoglobulin conjugated to a detector enzyme. This method is positive in approximately 70% of patients with SLE. The IgG antibody titers correlate moderately well with active nephritis, and in our experience, there is a good correlation with disease activity in general.

### Properties of Anti–Double-Stranded DNA Antibodies

Anti-dsDNA antibodies can demonstrate different properties based on avidity that affect their usefulness as a diagnostic tool. As an example, high-affinity IgG anti-dsDNA antibodies can be demonstrated in 70% to 80% of patients with SLE when their disease is active (24). In contrast, some patients with SLE have predominantly IgM or low-avidity IgG antibodies to dsDNA. These antibodies are less useful diagnostically, because they can be found in association with drug-induced lupus, rheumatoid arthritis, Sjögren's syndrome, other connective tissue diseases, chronic infection, chronic liver disease, and normal aging (20); in these instances, the antibodies have no clinical significance. Lower-avidity antibodies may be reacting with ssDNA fragments in the DNA preparations used as antigenic substrates.

A number of properties of anti-dsDNA antibodies other than avidity also affect their pathogenicity, including the isoelectric point, isotype, idiotype, and ability to activate mediators of inflammation such as complement (20). Light microscopic and electron microscopic studies have shown that the degree of renal damage in SLE is proportional to the quantity of IgG anti-DNA deposited in the subendothelial region of the glomerular basement membrane (33). A specific group of anti-DNA antibodies, which are IgG, cationic, and bind with high affinity, correlate best with renal activity.

The antigen-binding region may be another determinant of the likelihood of renal disease. In addition to binding to dsDNA, the antibody may bind to *in situ* antigens at different sites in the glomerular capillary wall, thereby leading to different histologic and clinical manifestations (34,35).

The IgG subclass also may be a determinant of the inflammatory response that is induced by immune complex deposition. IgG1 and IgG3 fix complement, but IgG2 and IgG4 do not (36). The latter two subclasses should lead to less inflammation.

These antibody properties may vary among individuals, over time in the same individual, or with disease activity, even in the face of a stable antibody titer. Some patients with SLE have persistent anti-dsDNA antibody activity despite improvement in disease activity. Similarly, a small but significant minority of patients have active nephritis without elevations of anti-dsDNA antibody titer. These findings may be related in part to differences in the anti-DNA antibodies over time. Anti-DNA antibodies manifesting in some patients during periods of active nephritis may differ idiotypically from the anti-DNA antibodies in the same patient during periods of inactive disease (37).

### Antibody Titer and Correlation with Activity

Titers of anti-dsDNA antibodies are important in the management of some patients with SLE. Titers rise when disease is active and usually fall (generally into the normal range) when the flare subsides. Early studies reported a tight correlation between high titer anti-dsDNA antibodies and nephritic activity (23,25), particularly in the setting of hypocomplementemia (23,38). Later studies reported exceptions to this correlation of titers and disease activity (e.g., some patients have elevated titers of anti-dsDNA antibodies in the setting of inactive or minimally active lupus) (39).

This phenomenon may be attributable to sensitive assays that are more likely to detect low-avidity antibodies that previously would have been missed. Clinical correlations that hold about high-avidity antibodies appear not to be applicable to those of lower avidity, and current assays are unable to distinguish between high- and low-avidity (i.e., pathogenic and nonpathogenic) antibodies. Although the correlation between antibody titer and disease activity holds for most patients with SLE, this assay has limited clinical utility for some patients.

The association between anti-DNA antibodies and other disease manifestations of SLE is far less clear. As an example, there is no relationship between antibody titer and disease activity of neuropsychiatric SLE (40).

Distinguishing active lupus from infectious complications (e.g., secondary to treatment with immunosuppressive agents), from the toxic effects of drugs, and from unrelated disease is always a challenge. Anti-DNA antibodies may be helpful in some patients in making this distinction. Although there is clear variability among patients, the test becomes useful after a given patient is shown to follow the characteristic pattern of rising DNA and falling complement in the setting of a flare. After a patient shows a disassociation between his or her anti-DNA antibody titer and clinical evidence of nephritis, future changes in anti-DNA antibody activity are unlikely to accurately reflect disease activity. In this setting, therapeutic decisions must be guided by the clinical picture and perhaps by other serologic findings such as complement levels.

## Anti-Smith Antibodies and Antiribonucleoprotein Antibodies

The anti-Smith (anti-Sm) and antiribonucleoprotein (anti-RNP) systems are considered together, because they coexist in many patients with SLE and bind to related but distinct antigens (16).

### Anti-Smith Antibodies

The Smith antigen is a nuclear nonhistone protein that was characterized in 1966 and was the first nuclear protein autoantigen to be described in SLE (41). The antigen to which anti-Sm antibodies bind consists of a series of proteins (B, B′, D, E, F, and G) that are complexed with small nuclear RNAs (U1, U2, U4-6, and U5) that can be characterized by Western and Northern blots. These complexes of nuclear proteins and RNAs are called small nuclear ribonucleoprotein particles (snRNPs). They are important in the splicing of precursor messenger RNA (42), an integral step in the processing of RNA transcribed from DNA.

The anti-Sm immune reaction consists of multiple antibodies binding to multiple protein antigens. Although we speak of the anti-Sm antibody, it is better described as an antibody system. Anti-Sm antibodies are found in only 18% to 30% (depending on the assay used) of patients with SLE but infrequently in patients with other conditions (43–45) (Table 40.1). Measurement of anti-Sm titers may be useful diagnostically, particularly at a time when DNA antibodies are undetectable.

## Antiribonucleoprotein Antibodies

The anti-RNP system binds to antigens that are different from but related to Sm antigens. These antibodies bind to proteins (especially to a 68- to 70-kd protein) containing only U1-RNA. The U1-RNP particle is involved in splicing heterogenous nuclear RNA into messenger RNA.

### Methods and Usefulness of Antibody Measurement

Although anti-Sm antibodies and anti-RNP antibodies can be detected by immunodiffusion or counterimmunoelectrophoresis in agarose gels, these methods are relatively insensitive and difficult to quantitate (28,46). Most clinical laboratories now employ ELISA to detect these antibodies (47).

Anti-Sm antibodies occur more frequently in African Americans and Asians than in Caucasians with SLE. As an example, one series reported a prevalence rate of 25% in blacks and 10% in whites (by immunodiffusion) (48). The prevalence of anti-Sm antibodies in SLE using the ELISA depends on whether Sm is measured alone or in combination with RNP. Generally accepted rates of anti-Sm antibody positivity in SLE are in the range of 10% to 30% in Caucasians and 30% to 40% in Asians and African Americans (48).

Antibody titers may fluctuate somewhat over time, although this is a controversial issue. Levels occasionally drift into the negative range when the immunodiffusion technique is used, but this should not occur when the more sensitive ELISA method is employed.

Many studies have tried to correlate anti-Sm antibody with disease activity in general and with specific disease manifestations. These investigations have often yielded conflicting results. Several investigators have reported an association between anti-Sm antibodies and a low frequency of progression to end-stage renal disease (i.e., milder renal disease) (49–51). However, others have found that the severity of renal disease is similar in patients who do and do not make antibodies to Sm (52). One report concluded that the presence of anti-Sm antibodies in the absence of antibodies to DNA was associated with an increased incidence of serositis and a decrease in the incidence of hematologic abnormalities (53). Another study found an association between anti-Sm antibodies and the presence of central nervous system (CNS) disease occurring as an isolated clinical finding (40). These often contradictory results may be explained by the use of different methods of antibody assay by different investigators and by the application of inappropriate statistical methods.

There is no evidence that anti-Sm antibodies can be useful for following or predicting disease activity in the way that we use anti-dsDNA antibodies. Antibodies to Sm do function as an important diagnostic marker for SLE. As an example, the presence of antibodies to the Sm antigen system in a patient in whom we suspect the diagnosis of SLE strongly supports the diagnosis. Similarly, in a patient with a less convincing clinical picture, the presence of these antibodies suggests that even a nonspecific symptom complex is likely to progress to SLE. Given their relatively low prevalence, however, a negative value in no way excludes a presumptive diagnosis of SLE.

Anti-RNP antibodies are found in about 40% to 60% of patients with SLE but are not specific for SLE, because they are a defining feature in the related syndrome, mixed connective tissue disease (Table 40.1). The antibody is present in lower titers and lower frequencies in several other rheumatic diseases, including rheumatoid arthritis and scleroderma.

## Anti-Ro/SSA and Anti-La/SSB Antibodies

Anti-Ro/SSA and anti-La/SSB are specific ANAs that have been detected in high frequency in patients with Sjögren's syndrome and in SLE (54). Antibodies to Ro are detected clinically by immunodiffusion, ELISA, or Western blot. Most but not all sera react in all three assays. ELISA and Western blots are the most sensitive in detecting low titer antibodies.

### Anti-Ro/Anti-SSA Antibodies

The anti-Ro/anti-SSA antibodies are ANAs that recognize cellular proteins with molecular weights of approximately 52 and 60 kd. The 60-kd protein is complexed with the hY1-5 species of small nuclear RNAs (42).

In 1969, Reichlin et al. described the presence of antibodies in the sera of some patients with SLE that reacted with ribonucleoprotein antigens present in saline extracts of rabbit and human spleen (55). When purified preparations of this antibody were incubated with a human epithelial cell line (i.e., Hep2), the nuclei and the cytoplasm were stained in a speckled pattern. These investigators named the antibody anti-Ro after the original patient in whom the antibodies were identified.

Subsequently, Alspaugh and Tan found antibody activity in sera from many patients with Sjögren's syndrome that gave the same immunofluorescent staining pattern as that reported for anti-Ro antibodies (56). These workers referred to this antibody as anti-SSA. It was soon shown that these two antibody systems (Ro and SSA) produced a line of identity on immunodiffusion, indicating that they were reacting with the same nuclear RNA protein (57). Subsequent research found that anti-Ro antibodies in SLE and anti-SSA antibodies in primary Sjögren's syndrome react with different epitopes on the same 60-kd particle (58).

Anti-Ro/SSA antibodies are primarily found in patients with SLE and Sjögren's syndrome but are also found in patients with photosensitive dermatitis. They are infrequently seen in other connective tissue diseases such as scleroderma, polymyositis, mixed connective tissue disease, and rheumatoid arthritis. There is a strong linkage between the production of anti-Ro antibodies and a genetic deficiency in the production of the C4 complement component and the HLA-DR3 genotype (59).

### Clinical Significance in Systemic Lupus Erythematosus

Anti-Ro/SSA antibodies are found in approximately 50% of patients with SLE (Table 40.1). They have been associated with photosensitivity, a rash known as subacute cutaneous lupus, cutaneous vasculitis (i.e., palpable purpura), interstitial lung disease, neonatal lupus, and congenital heart block (60–65).

Several observations have been made about the associations with neonatal lupus and congenital heart block. The Ro/SSA antibody has been found in almost all newborns who have neonatal lupus manifested by the combination of rash and heart block. In women who have had children with congenital heart block, approximately 15% of subsequent pregnancies will result in an infant who has heart block (66). The incidence of congenital complete heart block appears to be even more common in offspring of women with high titers of anti-Ro/SSA and anti-La/SSB (66). The anti-Ro and anti-La antibodies may induce autoimmune injury that prevents normal development of the conduction fibers (65). Many women who give birth to children with congenital complete heart block show no evidence of SLE or other connective tissue disease, although they uniformly test positive for anti-Ro/SSA and anti-La/SSB antibodies. On follow-up, most of these women have not developed SLE or Sjögren's syndrome (67).

### Clinical Significance in Sjögren's Syndrome

Anti-Ro/SSA antibodies are found in approximately 75% of patients with primary Sjögren's syndrome (Table 40.1), and high titers of these antibodies are associated with a greater incidence of extraglandular features, especially purpura and vasculitis (68). In contrast, Ro/SSA antibodies are present in only 10% to 15% of patients with secondary Sjögren's syndrome associated with rheumatoid arthritis. The presence of Ro/SSA or anti-La/SSB antibodies in patients with suspected primary Sjögren's syndrome strongly supports the diagnosis. A sicca syndrome can also occur in association with other autoimmune diseases (e.g., secondary Sjögren's syndrome), and the anti-Ro/SSA antibodies may be directed against different epitopes than in primary Sjögren's syndrome.

Anti-Ro/SSA antibodies recognize at least two proteins: a 52-kd, 475–amino acid protein and a 60-kd, 525–amino acid protein. Anti-52-kd antibodies are found more frequently in primary Sjögren's syndrome, and anti-60-kd antibodies are more prevalent in Sjögren's syndrome associated with SLE

(69). The anti-Ro/SSA antibodies in the sicca syndrome associated with primary biliary cirrhosis appear to be directed against a smaller epitope on the 52-kd protein than in Sjögren's syndrome (70).

### Association of Anti-Ro Antibodies with Other Disorders

Anti-Ro/SSA antibodies occasionally are observed in patients with rheumatoid arthritis, progressive systemic sclerosis, cutaneous vasculitis, dermatomyositis/polymyositis, undifferentiated connective tissue disease, mixed connective tissue disease, juvenile rheumatoid arthritis, chronic active hepatitis, or homozygous C2 or C4 deficiency (61). They are also found in 0.1% to 0.5% of normal subjects; such individuals may have an enhanced sensitivity to ultraviolet light.

In the 1970s, there were several reports of patients who met the American College of Rheumatology criteria for SLE but were persistently negative for ANA (71). Although not recognized at the time, this consistently negative finding occurred because sera were tested using mouse rather than human tissue as substrate (61). By comparison, anti-Ro/SSA antibodies were found in most of these patients because a human cell line extract was used as the substrate to detect Ro. Substitution of Hep2 cells (a human cell line) for mouse tissue sections in the ANA test resulted in only a small number of patients who test persistently negative for ANA (72). Nevertheless, on rare occasions, the anti-Ro/SSA antibody test may be useful in establishing a diagnosis of systemic autoimmune disease in the face of a negative ANA.

### Anti-La/SSB Antibodies

Approximately 50% of sera from patients with SLE who have anti-Ro antibody activity also contain antibody to La, a closely related RNA-protein antigen. Similarly, most sera from patients with Sjögren's syndrome that demonstrate anti-SSA activity also contain a second anti-RNA-protein antibody, anti-SSB. La is identical to SSB.

The antigen is a nuclear phosphoprotein with a molecular weight of 46 kd; this antigen is complexed with pre-5S RNA and pretransfer RNA, suggesting that it may be involved in the maturation and transport of RNA. The La protein is involved with all RNA polymerase III transcripts and acts as a transcription and termination factor (42).

### Clinical Associations of Anti-La Antibodies

Anti-La/SSB antibodies are found in several circumstances. It is unusual to encounter sera that contain anti-La/SSB activity without demonstrable antibodies to Ro/SSA in patients with SLE or Sjögren's syndrome. Isolated anti-La/SSB antibody activity has been seen in some patients with primary biliary cirrhosis and autoimmune hepatitis. Antibodies to the La/SSB antigen are present in 40% to 50% of patients with primary Sjögren's syndrome and in 15% of patients with SLE, but they are rarely seen in other connective tissue diseases.

### Indications for Anti-Ro/SSA and Anti-La/SSB Testing

There are several indications for ordering an anti-Ro/SSA and anti-La/SSB antibody test:

- Women with SLE who have become pregnant
- Women who have a history of giving birth to a child with heart block or myocarditis
- Patients with a history of unexplained photosensitive skin eruptions
- Patients suspected of having a systemic connective tissue disease including in those in whom the screening ANA test is negative
- Patients with symptoms of xerostomia, keratoconjunctivitis sicca or salivary and lacrimal gland enlargement
- Patients with unexplained small vessel vasculitis

### Anticentromere Antibodies

Anticentromere antibodies (ACAs) are found almost exclusively in patients with limited cutaneous systemic sclerosis, especially those with CREST syndrome (calcinosis, Raynaud's phenomenon, esophageal hypomotility, sclerodactyly, telangiectasias) (73). ACAs have been observed in 32% to 57% of patients with CREST (74) but have also been identified in patients with other conditions, including in some patients with Raynaud's phenomenon (75). ACAs are typically detected by the characteristic immunofluorescent pattern on Hep2 cells.

### Anti-Scl-70 Antibodies

Approximately 15% to 20% of patients with scleroderma have antibodies to a 70-kd protein, topoisomerase-1, a nucleoplasmic and nucleolar enzyme subsequently named Scl-70 (74). The usual method for detection was immunodiffusion, but most laboratories now detect it by ELISA (76). Scl-70 is important diagnostic marker for systemic sclerosis, and its presence appears to increase the risk for pulmonary fibrosis in patients with scleroderma.

### Antikeratin and Antiperinuclear Factor Antibodies

Antikeratin antibodies (AKA) and antiperinuclear factor antibody (APF) have a similar antigenic specificity, recognizing filaggrin and profilaggrin related proteins of buccal epithelial cells (76); they are thought to be the same or closely related antibodies (77).

AKAs are primarily detected by indirect immunofluorescence of cryosections of rat esophagus (78). The staining pattern of AKA specific for rheumatoid arthritis is linear laminated and is localized to the stratum corneum of the epithelium.

AKAs have also been detected by immunoblotting, but the results often differ from those obtained with immunofluorescence (79,80); this method of detection is therefore not frequently used. Only IgG (not IgM) AKAs react with stratum corneum of rat esophagus and are specific for rheumatoid arthritis.

A pathogenetic role for AKAs in rheumatoid arthritis has not been established. However, the study of AKAs and APFs may eventually provide insight into the pathogenesis of early rheumatoid arthritis, because they may be detected at the time of polyarthritis but before there are sufficient be symptoms and signs to establish a diagnosis of rheumatoid arthritis (81).

Although the sensitivity of AKA in rheumatoid arthritis is only 40% to 55% (82,83), the specificity is extremely high, ranging from 95% to 99% (84). The sensitivity of APF varies between 50% and 90%, and the specificity is similar to that seen with AKA (85).

AKA and APF may play an important role in the differential diagnosis of patients presenting with symptoms and signs suggestive of a connective tissue disorder. They are rarely found in patients with nonrheumatoid arthritis, inflammatory arthritides, or other autoimmune diseases. Their expression is also independent of rheumatoid factor; AKA and APF antibodies have been detected in up to one third of patients with seronegative rheumatoid arthritis (86,87). There are no consistently observed clinical associations between AKA and APF and any specific manifestations of rheumatoid arthritis.

### Nucleosome-Specific Autoantibodies

The first autoantibody described in SLE, the "LE factor," was a nucleosome specific autoantibody (76). These antibodies are now called nucleosome-restricted antibodies because they bind to the complex of DNA and histones but not to the individual components—and are the same as what used to be called nucleoprotein. Several reports suggest that nucleosomes might be critical antigens in the eventual generation of ANAs in SLE.

Detection of antinucleosome-specific antibodies remains problematic because the nucleosomal material used as substrate also binds anti-dsDNA and antihistone antibodies. The traditional method of circumventing this problem, absorption techniques, is cumbersome and difficult to perform. An epitope recognized only by nucleosome specific antibodies has not been identified.

Because of the difficulties in detection, there is a paucity of data concerning the incidence and accuracy of antinucleosome-specific autoantibodies. A prevalence of 48% to more than 80% has been observed among patients with SLE (80) (Table 40.1). They usually are associated with anti-dsDNA and antihistone antibodies (88). The specificity of these antibodies remains a source of controversy. Some series have found a weak but significant association with clinical manifestations (89), but others have not (90).

### Anti–Heterogeneous Nuclear Ribonuclear Protein Antibodies

The spliceosome refers to a complex of nuclear RNA binding proteins that processes pre-mRNA into spliced mature mRNA (76). Among the subunits of the spliceosome are a group of 30 structurally related proteins known as heterogeneous nuclear ribonuclear proteins (hnRNPs) (91).

Autoantibodies specific for the RNA binding regions of two of the hnRNP proteins, A2 (also called RA33) and A1, produce a finely speckled pattern of staining in the nucleoplasm on indirect immunofluorescence microscopy. Their presence must be confirmed by immunoblotting or dot blot assays (92).

Anti-hnRNP antibodies against the A1 and A2 proteins have been reported with the following frequencies (93,94):

- Rheumatoid arthritis: 50% for the A1 protein and 35% for the A2 protein.
- SLE: 22% to 38% for A1 and 23% for A2
- Mixed connective tissue disease: 40% for A1 and 38% for A2
- Scleroderma, myositis, Sjögren's syndrome: less than 5% for A2
- No connective tissue disease: less than 7% for A1 and A2

The presence of these antibodies does not appear to correlate with any of the clinical features of rheumatoid arthritis or SLE, although their presence in patients with SLE is strongly associated with anti-U1 RNP and anti-Sm antibodies.

The clinical utility of anti-hnRNP antibodies is limited because they cross-react with multiple antigens, and antibodies not directed against A1 and A2 may be found in different autoimmune disorders. As an example, one study found that sera from 22 of 40 patients with scleroderma contained antibodies reactive with a structurally and immunologically distinct component of the spliceosome, named hnRNP I (95). In a case report, antibodies to the C1 and C2 core proteins of hnRNP were found in a patient with scleroderma and psoriatic arthritis but not in patients with scleroderma alone or those with SLE or rheumatoid arthritis (96). Patients with psoriatic arthritis alone were not evaluated.

### Anti–Proliferating Cell Nuclear Antigen Antibodies

A number of proteins accumulate in the nucleoplasm of cells during the $G_1$/S phase of the cell cycle, which corresponds to the period of DNA synthesis (76). Approximately 2% to 10% of sera from patients with SLE sera contain antibodies that react with one such protein, the proliferating cell nuclear antigen (PCNA) (97).

PCNA has a molecular weight of approximately 33 kd and can be induced in resting cells by several growth factors; the protein binds to at least two nuclear enzymes, uracil-DNA glycosylase and DNA-(cytosine-5) methyltransferase, which are involved in the nucleotide excision, repair, and mismatch repair aspects of DNA synthesis (98).

Anti-PCNA antibodies can be detected by indirect immunofluorescence as a finely granular nuclear staining pattern on rapidly dividing cells (99). An ELISA is used for the detection of these antibodies. The dominant epitope of PCNA is an area of 14 contiguous amino acids (100).

Anti-PCNA antibodies appear to be specific (>95%) but not sensitive (3% to 5%), for SLE; they have not been found in sera from patients with other diseases (97). The incidence of this antibody varies because its production is rapidly inhibited by the administration of corticosteroids and immunosuppressive drugs. The presence of anti-PCNA antibodies in patients with SLE is not associated with any particular clinical manifestation other than arthritis.

### Anti-Hu Antibodies

Antibodies reactive with neuron specific RNA-binding nuclear proteins have been detected in most patients with the paraneoplastic syndromes of sensory neuropathy, encephalomyelitis, and opsoclonus or myoclonus (76,101). The proteins, which have molecular weights of 33 to 35 kd, function in the terminal differentiation of the neuron; they are named HuD, HuC, Hel-N1, and Hel-N2. Autoantibodies that react with a cross-reacting epitope on all of these proteins have been referred to as anti-Hu antibodies or as type 1 antineuron and nuclear antibodies (anti-ANNA-1 antibodies) (102).

The anti-Hu antibodies have been classically detected by indirect immunofluorescence on brain tissue sections; they produce a finely speckled staining of the neuronal nuclei but do not stain glial cell nuclei (103). An ELISA has been described for these antibodies (104).

Because undifferentiated tumor cells may express the Hu antigens, anti-Hu antibodies have been found most frequently in patients with small cell carcinoma of the lung. They have been associated with a paraneoplastic neurologic syndrome, including certain gastrointestinal disorders (such as achalasia or chronic intestinal pseudo-obstruction) (105–107). Patients with sensory neuropathy and anti-Hu antibodies have also been reported in association with primary Sjögren's syndrome (108).

### Miscellaneous Antinuclear Antibodies

Other autoantibodies reactive with nuclear and perinuclear antigens have been associated with connective tissue diseases (76):

- Anti-RNA polymerase I, II, and III: scleroderma (109)
- Antifibrillarin (U3 nucleolar RNP): scleroderma (110)
- Antinucleolus organizer region (NOR 90): possibly with scleroderma (111)
- Antinucleolar RNA helicase (Gu): scleroderma, SLE, watermelon stomach (112)
- Anti-DNA associated acidic protein (Ku): scleroderma and polymyositis overlap (113)
- Anti-Mi-2: dermatomyositis (114)
- Antinucleosomal high mobility group proteins (HMG): juvenile rheumatoid arthritis (115)
- Antimajor nucleolar phosphoprotein (B23): antiphospholipid antibody syndrome (116)
- Antiannexin XI (56K): most connective tissue diseases (117)

These antibodies have less clinical significance than others, because they are not routinely assayed in clinical laboratories and appear to have more limited specificity and sensitivity than other ANAs.

## ANTIRIBOSOMAL P PROTEIN ANTIBODIES

### Characterization

Serum from patients with SLE had been previously recognized to have precipitating antibodies to ribosomes (118,119). The targets of these antibodies were three phosphoproteins (P proteins) located on the 60S subunit of ribosomes (120,121). The proteins were designated P0, P1, and P2, with molecular weights of 35, 19, and 17 kd, respectively. They were thought to be involved in protein synthesis; specifically, in the interaction of EF-1α and EF-2 with ribosomes.

P proteins were initially identified on ribosomes in the cytoplasm of cells. Two papers, however, documented epitopes recognized by anti-P protein antibodies on the surface of neuronal and other non-CNS cells (122). The binding of these proteins to cell surfaces is hypothesized to be of pathogenic significance.

### Clinical Associations

All published studies agree on the specificity of antiribosomal P protein antibodies for SLE (123,124). These antibodies have not been found using conventional assays in normal controls (124,125), or in patients with other autoimmune diseases (e.g., rheumatoid arthritis, scleroderma, and myositis) (126).

Alternative tests, however, may defect antiribosomal P protein antibodies in healthy individuals. One study of 88 normal children, for example, found that an affinity assay "unmasked" these antibodies in 79 (127). The existence of an idiotypic antibody in normals may "mask" the presence of these antiribosomal antibodies (which disappear with increasing age) to detection through conventional assays. These observations suggest that pathogenic antiribosomal P antibodies, such as in patients with SLE, may be caused by a dysregulation of idiotypic networks.

The reported incidence of antiribosomal P protein antibodies among patients with SLE is variable. They were initially detected in 10% to 20% of patients with SLE (123,124,128); however, several investigators (particularly those studying Asian populations) have reported incidence rates as high as 40% to 50% (126,129).

The presence of ribosomal P protein antibodies may be highly specific for lupus manifested by psychosis (125). Using Western Blot and radioimmunoassay, for example, one study found that these antibodies were detected in the serum of 18 of 20 patients with lupus-related psychosis compared with three of 20 who had non-CNS manifestations of lupus and none of the nonlupus patients with psychosis (125). Another study found ribosomal P protein antibodies by ELISA in 13 of 29 lupus patients with psychosis (45%), 7 of

8 lupus patients with severe depression (88%), and only 4 of 45 patients without neuropsychiatric manifestations of lupus (9%) (124). A third report detected antiribosomal P protein antibodies in 37 of 89 (42%) patients with active lupus versus only four of 49 (8%) patients with inactive disease (126). Although there was no significant increase in frequency among patients with SLE-induced psychosis, there was an apparent association of the presence of antiribosomal P protein antibodies with depression (5 of 5 patients).

However, not all studies have found a strong correlation between the incidence of antiribosomal antibodies and neuropsychiatric lupus (128,130). Some investigators have therefore concluded that there is no association between these antibodies and neuropsychiatric manifestations. One confounding factor is that correlation studies are based on a relatively small number of patients. Only the results of a prospective study of large numbers of patients can properly determine whether there is a correlation between active SLE and antiribosomal antibodies. Data on the correlation of antiribosomal P antibody with activity of neuropsychiatric manifestations of SLE are scant and conflicting. Antiribosomal P protein antibodies have also been occasionally found in SLE patients with hepatic or renal involvement (131,132).

## ANTIHISTONE ANTIBODIES

### Association with Drug-Induced Lupus

One important immunologic characteristic of drug-induced lupus is the presence of antihistone antibodies (133). These antibodies are present in more than 95% of cases (Table 40.1), particularly those taking procainamide, hydralazine, chlorpromazine, and quinidine; other autoantibodies are uncommon in this disorder (134). Antihistone antibodies are also seen in up to 80% of patients with idiopathic lupus (134); however, patients with SLE also form a variety of other autoantibodies, including those directed against DNA and small ribonucleoproteins.

The autoantibodies in drug-induced lupus are primarily formed against a complex of the histone dimer H2A-H2B and DNA (135) and, with hydralazine, to the H1 and H3-H4 complex (134). DNA is required to stabilize the complex or perhaps to contribute part of the antigenic epitope (135). Although the drugs that can cause drug-induced lupus are markedly heterogeneous, there may be a common pathway for disease induction because the autoantibodies produced are in most, but not all (136), cases nearly identical (135). In contrast, the antihistone antibodies in idiopathic lupus are primarily directed against the H1 and H2B histone subunits (134).

The development of IgG antibodies to the complex of H2A-H2B and DNA soon after starting procainamide is associated with a high risk of developing drug-induced lupus; by comparison, autoantibodies to ssDNA or histones alone do not distinguish between symptomatic or asymptomatic individuals (137). It is unknown whether these observations apply to other causes of drug-induced lupus.

It remains unclear, however, what the particular characteristic is of those drugs that induce autoantibody formation. One possibility, which has been demonstrated *in vitro,* is that the offending drugs are capable of serving as substrates for myeloperoxidase in activated neutrophils (138). This interaction results in the formation of reactive drug metabolites that may directly affect lymphocyte function.

An alternative hypothesis is that drugs such as procainamide and hydralazine decrease T cell DNA methylation, leading to overexpression of lymphocyte function–associated antigen-1 (134). These T cells may then become autoreactive, leading to autoantibody formation. It is also possible that genetic differences in cytochrome P450 enzymes, which facilitate the metabolism of many medications, results in the generation of toxic metabolites that facilitate the development of autoimmunity (139).

### Associated Drugs

A variety of drugs have been identified as being definite, probable, or possible causes of drug-induced lupus (139a). Among the definite agents are procainamide, hydralazine, diltiazem, minocycline, penicillamine, isoniazid (INH), methyldopa, chlorpromazine, and practolol. INH induces ANAs in approximately 15% of patients but symptomatic lupus is rare. Diltiazem may result in the induction of subacute cutaneous lupus (140). Minocycline can induce lupus in some patients with acne (141). (As a result, my colleagues and I recommend that minocycline not be used for the treatment of acne in patients with SLE.)

Possible agents causing drug-induced lupus are anticonvulsants (e.g., phenytoin, mephenytoin, trimethadione, ethosuximide), quinidine, antithyroid drugs, sulfonamides, lithium, β blockers, nitrofurantoin, para-aminosalicylate, captopril, interferon-alfa, hydrochlorothiazide, glyburide, carbamazepine, sulfasalazine, rifampin and hydrazine. A component of alfalfa sprouts, L-canavanine, induces a lupus-like syndrome in monkeys. There is, however, no definite evidence that this occurs in humans.

Drugs unlikely to cause drug-induced lupus are gold salts, penicillin, tetracycline, reserpine, valproate, lovastatin, simvastatin, griseofulvin, gemfibrozil, valproate, and ophthalmic timolol.

The drugs associated with the highest risk of inducing lupus in an individual patient are procainamide, hydralazine, and penicillamine. A lupus-like syndrome is most commonly seen with procainamide, which may be mediated by the reactive metabolite procainamide hydroxylamine. A positive ANA titer occurs in almost all patients, particularly slow acetylators (142). Symptoms, however, develop in only 15% to 20% of patients; the determining factors for susceptibility to symptomatic disease are not known (136,142). Risk factors include HLA-DR6Y but not DR4 or DR3 (143).

In contrast to this high risk, there is little or no ANA formation or symptomatic lupus after the administration of *N*-acetylprocainamide (NAPA), the major active metabolite

of procainamide (144). Remission of procainamide-induced lupus can be achieved by switching to NAPA (145). These observations suggest an important pathogenetic role for the aromatic amino group on procainamide.

The incidence of clinical disease is generally lower with drugs other than procainamide, averaging 5% to 10% with hydralazine, being infrequent with quinidine, and rarely occurring with chlorpromazine (137,146). With hydralazine, for example, a number of risk factors have been identified, including drug dose, female sex, slow hepatic acetylation, the HLA-DR4 genotype, and the null gene for the fourth component of complement, C4 (137,148). In one study, lupus developed in 19% of women taking 200 mg of hydralazine per day, compared with 13 of 13 who also had the HLA-DR4 genotype (147). It is possible that slow acetylation increases free drug levels while low levels of C4 might prevent clearance of any immune complexes that are formed (1140). Even low doses may not be safe as clinical disease can develop in up to 5% of slow acetylators taking 100 mg per day (139).

The presence of drug-induced lupus should be suspected when a lupus-like syndrome develops in a patient taking one or more of the previously described drugs. Confirming the diagnosis is difficult, however, because of the clinical overlap with the more common idiopathic disease. If available, the finding of antihistone antibodies in the absence of other autoantibodies strongly suggests that a drug is responsible (146). The gold standard is spontaneous resolution of the disease within 1 to 7 months after the offending drug has been discontinued.

## ANTIBODIES IN AUTOIMMUNE HEPATITIS

### Type 1 Autoimmune Hepatitis

Type 1 or classic autoimmune hepatitis is characterized by ANA or antibodies to smooth muscle (ASMA); the latter are thought to reflect more specific antiactin antibodies (AAA) (Table 40.2). AAA is not generally measured in most clinical laboratories, but ASMA with titers of 1:320 or greater almost always reflect the presence of AAA (149). Antibodies to soluble liver antigens (SLA) occur in approximately 10% of patients with type 1 autoimmune hepatitis (150).

Other antibodies described in type 1 autoimmune hepatitis include those directed against DNA (including dsDNA), a liver-pancreas protein, a plasma-membrane sulfatide, the nuclear envelope proteins lamins A and C, and a number of cytoskeleton antigens. Antineutrophil cytoplasmic antibodies (ANCA), which characterize primary sclerosing cholangitis, are commonly present in type 1 but not type 2 autoimmune hepatitis; they appear to occur in association with AAA and have a P-ANCA pattern on immunofluorescence (151).

Circulating antibodies against the liver-specific asialoglycoprotein receptor are found in a large percentage of European, Asian, and North American patients with autoimmune hepatitis. These antibodies serve primarily as a research tool (152).

Occasionally, antimitochondrial antibodies (AMA), which are generally seen in primary biliary cirrhosis, accompany ANA, SLA, or ASMA in autoimmune hepatitis (153). In contrast, the isolated presence of AMA almost always signifies primary biliary cirrhosis, except in those rare instances in which an overlap syndrome occurs (153).

### Type 2 Autoimmune Hepatitis

Type 2 autoimmune hepatitis is defined by the presence of antibodies to liver/kidney microsomes (ALKM-1), which are directed at an epitope of CYP2D6 (cytochrome P450IID6) (154), or antibodies to a liver cytosol antigen (ALC-1) (155) (Table 40.2). On occasion, type 2 autoimmune hepatitis may be marked exclusively by ALC-1. ALKM-2 antibodies, seen in ticrynafen-induced hepatitis, and ALKM-3 antibodies, seen in chronic delta hepatitis, are not characteristic of type 2 autoimmune hepatitis (156,157).

### Overlap Syndromes

There are two conditions in which features of autoimmune hepatitis and primary biliary cirrhosis occur, obscuring the classic boundaries between these two putative autoimmune liver disorders.

In the so-called overlap syndrome (153), the histologic findings of autoimmune hepatitis are accompanied by serologic findings of primary biliary cirrhosis, i.e., isolated AMA (directed toward enzymes in the 2-oxo-acid dehydrogenase family).

In autoimmune cholangiopathy (i.e., autoimmune cholangitis, immune cholangiopathy, and immunocholangitis), the histologic features of primary biliary cirrhosis occur in the absence of circulating AMA but with circulating ANA or ASMA (158). Some investigators refer to this syndrome as AMA-negative primary biliary cirrhosis. Antibodies to a form of carbonic anhydrase (anti CA-II) present in biliary duct epithelium have been reported in this syndrome (159), but their specificity is unknown because they also occur in other ductopenic disorders, such as primary biliary cirrhosis and primary sclerosing cholangitis.

**TABLE 40.2.** *Classification of autoantibodies in autoimmune hepatitis*

| Type | Autoantibodies |
|---|---|
| 1 (classic) | Antinuclear |
| | Antismooth muscle |
| | Anti-actin |
| | Antisoluble liver antigen |
| | ANCA |
| 2 | Anti-LKM-1 |
| | Antiliver cytosol-1 |
| Overlap syndrome | Antimitochondrial |
| Autoimmune cholangiopathy | Antinuclear |
| | Antismooth muscle |
| | Anticarbonic anhydrase II |

Overlap syndromes in which features of autoimmune hepatitis and primary sclerosing cholangitis coexist have also been proposed in children and adults, but criteria are not clearly established (160,161).

## ANTINEUTROPHIL CYTOPLASMIC ANTIBODIES

Two immunofluorescence patterns can be seen when the patient's serum is incubated with ethanol-fixed, normal human neutrophils (162). In the first group, cytoplasmic antineutrophil cytoplasmic antibodies (C-ANCA) that stain the cytoplasm diffusely. These antibodies are usually directed against a serine protease called proteinase 3 (PR3) (163). In the second, perinuclear antineutrophil cytoplasmic antibodies (P-ANCA) are usually directed against myeloperoxidase (MPO). The P-ANCA fluorescence pattern represents an artifact of ethanol fixation; with ethanol, positively charged granule constituents rearrange around and on the negatively charged nuclear membrane (164).

P-ANCA identified by indirect immunofluorescence techniques using ethanol-fixed neutrophils must be distinguished from ANAs. This can be accomplished by the use of cross-linking fixatives, such as formalin. Unlike ethanol, cross-linking fixatives prevent the rearrangement of charged cellular components. Serum containing P-ANCA in ethanol-fixed neutrophils produce diffuse granular cytoplasmic staining with formalin-fixed polymorphonuclear cells, allowing distinction from ANAs (165). The concurrent use of formalin- and ethanol-fixed polymorphonuclear cells permits P-ANCA and ANA to be distinguished from each other in serum containing both antibodies.

Immunoblotting techniques or ELISAs are more accurate than immunofluorescence studies, and enable the identification of the target antigens associated with these autoantibodies. The identification of anti-MPO antibodies is particularly important, because P-ANCA directed against non-MPO molecules, such as elastase, cathepsin G, lactoferrin, lysozyme, and azurocidin, may occur in a variety of nonvasculitic disorders (165).

ANCA are primarily associated with Wegener's granulomatosis, microscopic polyangiitis, idiopathic necrotizing glomerulonephritis (pauci-immune glomerulonephritis), and Churg-Strauss syndrome. They may also be seen in a variety of gastrointestinal and other rheumatic disorders and after the administration of certain drugs.

C-ANCA, that is antiproteinase 3 (PR3) is found primarily in patients with Wegener's granulomatosis and microscopic polyarteritis, and occasionally or rarely in other diseases (163,166–172) (Table 40.3).

P-ANCA, which is directed primarily against myeloperoxidase (MPO) but also to lactoferrin, elastase, cathepsin G, lysozyme, and enolase, has been described in patients with a variety of rheumatic autoimmune diseases (Tables 40.4 and 40.5) and in patients with polymyositis and dermatomyositis, juvenile chronic arthritis, reactive arthritis, relapsing polychondritis, scleroderma, and antiphospholipid antibody syndrome (164,166–169,173–182). ANCA testing had a speci-

**TABLE 40.3.** *Significance of cANA*

| PR3 | Frequency |
| --- | --- |
| Wegener's granulomatosis | 90% |
| Microscopic polyarteritis | 50% |
| Hypersensitivity vasculitis | Rare |
| Henoch–Schönlein purpura | Rare |
| IgA nephropathy | Rare |
| Postinfectious glomerulonephritis | Rare |
| Systemic lupus erythematosus | Rare |
| Kawasaki disease | + |
| Controls | ± |

+, reported to be present; ±, occasionally present.

ficity for vasculitis of 99.5% among patients with connective tissue disease. Although patients with rheumatic autoimmune diseases have an increased frequency of vasculitis, data suggesting that ANCA positivity enhances the risk of vasculitis are contradictory (165). Nonvasculitic aspects of rheumatic disease activity, severity, and chronicity also fail to consistently correlate with ANCA status. As a result, there is little clinical utility for ANCA testing in patients with rheumatic autoimmune diseases in whom the presence of an ANCA-associated systemic vasculitis is not suspected on clinical grounds.

### Clinical Associations

#### *Autoimmune Gastrointestinal Disorders*

ANCA positivity is seen in 60% to 80% of patients with ulcerative colitis and the related disorder primary sclerosing cholangitis but in only 10% to 27% of patients with Crohn's disease (in whom only low titers are present) (183) (Table 40.5). The P-ANCA in these conditions is directed against a variety of proteins. The most common are lactoferrin, cathepsin G, elastase, lysozyme, and antigens not characterized; antibodies that recognize MPO may also be seen (166,183,184).

The pathogenetic significance of these antibodies is unclear because the ANCA titer does not seem to vary with the activity or severity of the disease and, in ulcerative coli-

**TABLE 40.4.** *Significance of pANCA against myeloperoxidase*

| Disease | Frequency |
| --- | --- |
| Microscopic polyarteritis | 50–70% |
| Idiopathic necrotizing glomerulonephritis | 50–85% |
| Churg–Strauss syndrome | 70–85% |
| Goodpasture's (anti-GBM) | 10–30 |
| Polyarteritis nodosa | + |
| Polyangiitis overlap | + |
| Systemic lupus erythematosus | + |
| Hydralazine-induced crescenteric glomerulonephritis | + |
| Kawasaki disease | + |
| Ill children | + |

+, reported to be present.

**TABLE 40.5.** *Significance of pANCA against lactoferrin, cathepsin G, elastase, and lysozyme*

| Disease | Frequency |
| --- | --- |
| Giant cell arteritis | + |
| Rheumatoid arthritis | + |
| Systemic lupus erythematosus | 25% |
| Sjögren's | + |
| Inflammatory bowel disease | + |
| Ulcerative colitis | + |
| Crohn's disease | 10–27% |
| Primary sclerosing cholangitis | + |
| Unaffected relatives of patients with ulcerative colitis or primary sclerosing cholangitis | 25–30% |
| Chronic active hepatitis | + |
| Primary biliary cirrhosis | + |

+, reported to be present.

tis, does not fall after colectomy. The observation that P-ANCA can be demonstrated in 25% to 30% of unaffected relatives of patients with ulcerative colitis or primary sclerosing cholangitis has led to the suggestion that ANCA may be a genetic marker for susceptibility to these diseases. Similar considerations may apply to the frequent presence of P-ANCA in type 1 autoimmune hepatitis.

#### *Drug-Associated Antineutrophil Cytoplasmic Antibodies*

The administration of certain drugs has been reported to induce ANCA reactivity in association with various symptoms. These include the following:

- Hydralazine-induced lupus with anti-MPO and antielastase antibodies.
- Hydralazine-associated vasculitis and anti-MPO and anti-lactoferrin antibodies(185).
- Minocycline-induced arthritis, fever, and livedo reticularis and anti-MPO antibodies(186)
- Propylthiouracil-induced vasculitis, and positive ANCA specificities to several different target antigens, including PR3, MPO, and elastase (187).

#### *Antiglomerular Basement Membrane Antibody Disease*

Another disorder in which ANCA may be seen is antiglomerular basement membrane (GBM) antibody disease, which has similar renal and pulmonary manifestations to Wegener's granulomatosis and which seems to be associated with ANCA in 10 to as many as 38% of cases (188).

The clinical significance of combined ANCA and anti-GBM antibodies is uncertain. It has been suggested that most of these patients have low titers of ANCA and no clinical manifestations of vasculitis. There are, however, some patients with findings that are uncommon in anti-GBM antibody disease alone and that suggest that there is a concurrent systemic vasculitis. These include purpuric rash, arthralgias, granulomas in the kidney, and a more favorable renal prognosis.

## Clinical Applications

There are a variety of clinical issues that must be addressed in patients who are ANCA-positive. Perhaps the most common is whether ANCA alone can establish the diagnosis without tissue biopsy.

### Diagnostic Utility

Can ANCA alone establish the diagnosis? The diagnostic accuracy of ANCA was evaluated in a large multicenter European collaborative study that compared 169 newly diagnosed and 189 historic patients with idiopathic systemic vasculitis or rapidly progressive glomerulonephritis with 184 disease controls (including those with other vasculitides, such as giant cell or Takayasu arteritis, or nonvasculitic glomerulonephritides) and 740 healthy controls (189). Indirect immunofluorescence testing and the anti-PR3 and anti-MPO ELISAs were evaluated.

In Wegener's granulomatosis, the sensitivity of C-ANCA, P-ANCA, anti-PR3, and anti-MPO, was 64%, 21%, 66%, and 24%, respectively. In microscopic polyarteritis, the sensitivities were 23%, 58%, 26%, and 58%, respectively. These results confirm other studies showing a relative association of anti-PR3 with Wegener's granulomatosis and anti-MPO with microscopic polyarteritis. In idiopathic rapidly progressive glomerulonephritis, the sensitivities were 36%, 45%, 50%, and 64%, respectively.

Compared with the results in disease controls, the specificity of C-ANCA, P-ANCA, anti-PR3, and anti-MPO was 95%, 81%, 87%, and 91%, respectively. The combination of indirect and ELISA testing resulted in increased sensitivity and specificity. The sensitivity of C-ANCA plus anti-PR3 or P-ANCA plus anti-MPO was 73%, 67%, and 82% for Wegener's granulomatosis, microscopic polyangiitis, and rapidly progressive glomerulonephritis, respectively. Specificity was 99% for both combinations.

Combination testing consisting of C-ANCA immunofluorescence plus anti-PR3 ELISA, and P-ANCA immunofluorescence plus anti-MPO ELISA was therefore much more accurate than immunofluorescence or ELISA alone.

The predictive value of ANCA testing also depends on the clinical presentation of the patient in whom the test is performed. As an example, the finding of an elevated ANCA titer in a patient presenting with acute or rapidly progressive glomerulonephritis predicts the presence of Wegener's granulomatosis, microscopic polyarteritis, or idiopathic necrotizing glomerulonephritis with an accuracy that can reach 98% (190,191). C-ANCA is much more specific than P-ANCA; it is therefore recommended that a positive P-ANCA be followed by an antigen-specific assay to document the presence of anti-MPO antibodies (165,168).

However, the specificity of ANCA, even C-ANCA, is substantially less in patients referred for evaluation for the possible diagnosis of vasculitis and in those presenting with sinusitis alone.

One study, which evaluated 346 patients with possible vasculitis, found a sensitivity and positive predictive value of C-ANCA for the presence of Wegener's granulomatosis of 28% and 50% (192). Similar findings were reported in a meta-analysis of published studies in which the pooled sensitivity and specificity in all patients was 66% and 98%, respectively (190). The values increased to 91% and 99% when only patients with active disease were included.

Among those presenting with sinusitis alone, a positive C-ANCA in one analysis had a posttest probability of accurately predicting Wegener's granulomatosis of only 7% to 16% (193).

Although controversial, some investigators feel that treatment may be instituted among such patients based on a presumptive diagnosis of systemic vasculitis without the traditional reliance on invasive biopsy procedures to confirm the diagnosis. In this setting, the diagnosis must be reconsidered if there is a poor response to appropriate treatment. However, others feel that confirmation of the diagnosis by biopsy of an affected tissue is still indicated despite the presence of strong circumstantial evidence of an underlying ANCA-associated vasculitis because the available therapies are extremely toxic.

### Antineutrophil Cytoplasmic Antibodies and Renal Disease

To more adequately assess the diagnostic predictive value of ANCA serology among patients with evidence of renal involvement at clinical presentation, data from the European collaborative study was combined with that from nearly 4200 consecutive patients from the University of North Carolina group (191). The predictive value of serologic testing was assessed based on a sensitivity and specificity of 72.5% and 98.4%, respectively (values similar to those obtained with combined indirect immunofluorescence and ELISA testing). The predictive value of ANCA varied markedly depending on the age and degree of renal disease at presentation.

Among those with a positive serology and a clinical presentation of rapidly progressive glomerulonephritis, the positive predictive value of finding a pauci-immune crescentic glomerulonephritis on renal biopsy was at least 98% in all age groups.

By comparison, among adults with hematuria, proteinuria, and a serum creatinine of less than 1.5 mg/dL (133 µmol/L), the positive predictive value of a positive ANCA was only 47%; as a result, one half of all such patients with a positive serology do not have a pauci-immune crescentic glomerulonephritis by renal biopsy. However, a negative serology in this setting has a predictive value of 99% of not uncovering a pauci-immune glomerulonephritis with renal biopsy.

Despite the usefulness of ANCA serologies, a biopsy, when clinically indicated, is still required to document the presence or absence of a pauci-immune crescentic glomerulonephritis. Many available assays are not sufficiently accurate and the potential toxicity of present therapies for ANCA-positive diseases is too great to rely on serology alone.

A related question is whether the monitoring of ANCA titers over time has a role in treatment decisions. Persistent high titers or rising titers of ANCA (anti-MPO or anti-PR3) are often associated with relapse from remission in patients with microscopic polyangiitis or Wegener's granulomatosis. However, this association may not occur in one third or more of those with such ANCA profiles during one or more years of follow-up (166,194).

The use of an elevation in ANCA titer as the sole parameter to justify immunosuppressive therapy cannot be endorsed because its prognostic value is imperfect and, if used, places approximately one third of patients at risk for unnecessary toxicity. Therapy should only be instituted based on unequivocal evidence of relapse.

What role sequential ANCA studies should play in patient care, after the diagnosis is established, is still unclear. If titers are sequentially followed and an increase is seen in an asymptomatic patient, surveillance should be increased to help detect a possible relapse. It is currently unknown whether it is cost effective or prudent to sequentially follow ANCA titers.

## RHEUMATOID FACTORS

Rheumatoid factors are antibodies directed against the Fc portion of IgG (195). The rheumatoid factor (RF) was initially described by Waaler and Rose in 1940 and is measured in clinical practice is an IgM RF, although other immunoglobulin types, including IgG and IgA, have been described.

The presence of RF can be detected by a variety of techniques such as agglutination of IgG-sensitized sheep red cells or bentonite or latex particles coated with human IgG, radioimmunoassay, ELISA, or nephelometry (196–199). Measurement of RF is not standardized in many laboratories (leading to problems with false-positive results) and no one technique has clear advantage over others. Testing for RF is primarily used for the diagnosis of rheumatoid arthritis; however, RF may also be present in other rheumatic diseases and chronic infections.

### Clinical Associations

A positive RF test result can be found in rheumatic disorders, nonrheumatic disorders, and healthy subjects (200).

### *Rheumatic Disorders*

Patients may have detectable serum RF in a variety of rheumatic disorders, many of which share similar features, such as symmetric polyarthritis and constitutional symptoms. These include (200) the following examples:

- Rheumatoid arthritis: 26% to 90%
- Sjögren's syndrome: 75% to 95%
- Mixed connective tissue disease: 50% to 60%
- Mixed cryoglobulinemia (types II and III): 40% to 100%
- Systemic lupus erythematosus: 15% to 35%
- Polymyositis/dermatomyositis: 5% to 10%

The reported sensitivity of the RF test in rheumatoid arthritis has been as high as 90%. However, population-based studies, which include patients with mild disease, have found much lower rates of RF-positive rheumatoid arthritis (26% to 60%) (201–204). This difference may reflect classification criteria that lead published series of patients with rheumatoid arthritis to be biased toward more severe (and more seropositive) disease, thereby overestimating the sensitivity of RF in rheumatoid arthritis.

### *Nonrheumatic Disorders*

Nonrheumatic disorders characterized by chronic antigenic stimulation (especially with circulating immune complexes or polyclonal B lymphocyte activation) commonly induce RF production (Table 40.6). Included in this group are (200):

Indolent or chronic infection, as with SBE or hepatitis B or C virus infection. An an example, studies have demonstrated that hepatitis C infection, especially when accompanied by cryoglobulinemia, is associated with a RF positivity in 70% to 76% of cases (205). RF production typically ceases with resolution of the infection in these disorders: inflammatory or fibrosing pulmonary disorders, such as sarcoidosis; malignancy; and primary biliary cirrhosis.

### *Healthy Individuals*

RFs have been found in up to 5% of young, healthy individuals. The reported incidence may be higher in elderly subjects without rheumatic disease, ranging from 3% to 25% (206). Part of this wide range may be explained by a higher incidence of RF among the chronically ill elderly as compared with healthy older patients (206). RF is typically present in low to moderate titer (1:40 to 1:160) in individuals with no demonstrable rheumatic or inflammatory disease.

**TABLE 40.6.** *Rheumatoid factors in nonrheumatoid diseases*

| Condition | Frequency of rheumatoid factors (%) |
|---|---|
| Aging (age >60) | 5–25 |
| Infection | |
|   Bacterial endocarditis | 25–50 |
|   Hepatitis B or hepatitis C | 20–75 |
|   Tuberculosis | 8 |
|   Syphilis | ≤13 |
|   Parasitic diseases | 20–90 |
|   Leprosy | 5–58 |
|   Viral infection | 15–65 |
| Pulmonary disease | |
|   Sarcoidosis | 3–33 |
|   Interstitial pulmonary fibrosis | 10–50 |
|   Silicosis | 30–50 |
|   Asbestosis | 30 |
| Miscellaneous diseases | |
|   Primary biliary cirrhosis | 45–70 |
|   Malignancy | 5–25 |
|   After multiple immunizations | 10–15 |

## Measurement of Rheumatoid Factor

Population-based studies have shown that some healthy people with a positive RF develop rheumatoid arthritis over time. However, most of these subjects do not progress to rheumatoid arthritis; as a result, measurement of RF is a poor screening test for future rheumatic disease.

The predictive value of RF testing has not been widely studied. The sensitivity of RF in rheumatoid arthritis has ranged from 26% to 90%. The specificity is reported as high as 95%, but the positive predictive value for rheumatoid arthritis has been only 24%, and the value has been 34% for any rheumatic disease (207). A negative test result had a negative predictive value for rheumatoid arthritis and for any rheumatic disease of 89% and 85%, respectively.

The RF titer should be considered when analyzing its utility. The higher the titer, the greater the likelihood that the patient has rheumatic disease. There are, however, frequent exceptions to this rule, particularly among patients with one of the chronic inflammatory disorders previously described. The use of a higher titer for diagnosis decreases the sensitivity of the test at the same time as it increases the specificity (by decreasing the incidence of false-positive results). In one study, for example, an RF titer of 1:40 or greater was 28% sensitive and 87% specific for rheumatoid arthritis; in comparison, a titer of 1:640 or greater increased the specificity to 99% (i.e., almost no false-positive results) but reduced the sensitivity to 8% (207).

RF-positive patients with rheumatoid arthritis may experience more aggressive and erosive joint disease and extraarticular manifestations than those who are RF negative (208). Similar prognostic associations have been found for juvenile rheumatoid arthritis. These general observations, however, are of limited utility in an individual patient because of wide interpatient variability. In this setting, accurate prediction of the disease course is not possible from the RF alone.

## ANTIPHOSPHOLIPID ANTIBODIES

Antiphospholipid antibodies (APLs) are antibodies directed against phospholipids or plasma proteins bound to anionic phospholipids (209). Patients with these patients may have a variety of clinical manifestations including venous and arterial thrombosis, recurrent fetal losses, and thrombocytopenia. Patients with these antibodies have the primary antiphospholipid antibody syndrome (APS) when it occurs alone, the secondary APS when it is seen in association with SLE, or other rheumatic or autoimmune disorders.

## Clinical Associations

Four major types of antiphospholipid antibodies have been characterized: false-positive serologic test for syphilis (STS), lupus anticoagulants, anticardiolipin antibodies, and anti-β₂-glycoprotein-1 antibodies.

### False-Positive Serologic Test for Syphilis

Some patients with SLE have a false-positive serologic test for syphilis. Such patients have fewer successful pregnancies, an increased number of thrombotic events, livedo reticularis, and migraine headaches.

When patient sera contain anticardiolipin antibodies, the false-positive STS occurs because the syphilis antigen used in the test is embedded in cardiolipin. As a result, a reaction against this molecule is incorrectly interpreted as being directed against the treponemal antigen. The STS should not be used to screen for APL because it has a low sensitivity and specificity (210).

### Lupus Anticoagulants

Lupus anticoagulants (LA) are antibodies directed against plasma proteins bound to anionic phospholipids (211). The LA blocks the *in vitro* assembly of the prothrombinase complex, resulting in a prolongation of *in vitro* clotting assays such as the activated partial thromboplastin time (aPTT), the dilute Russell viper venom time (RVTT), the kaolin clotting time, and rarely the prothrombin time. These abnormalities are not reversed when the patient's plasma is diluted 1:1 with normal platelet-free plasma, a procedure that corrects clotting disorders due to deficient clotting factors (212). The abnormal clotting test results can be largely reversed by incubation with a hexagonal phase phospholipid that neutralizes the inhibitor (212). Although these changes suggest impaired coagulation, patients with a LA have a paradoxical increase in frequency of arterial and venous thrombotic events (213).

### Anticardiolipin Antibodies

Anticardiolipin antibodies (aCL) react with phospholipids such as cardiolipin and phosphatidylserine. There is an approximate 85% concordance between the presence of a LA and aCL. In many cases, the LA is a separate population of antibodies from aCL (212,214). Testing should be performed for LA and aCL when APS is clinically suspected. LA positivity incurs a somewhat greater risk for thrombosis than aCL.

Different immunoglobulin isotypes and subclasses are associated with aCL, including IgG, IgA, IgM, and IgG subclasses 1 to 4. Elevated levels of IgG aCL (particularly IgG2) incur a greater risk of thrombosis than do other immunoglobulin isotypes (215).

### Anti-β₂-Glycoprotein 1 Antibodies

Antibodies to β₂-glycoprotein 1, a phospholipid-binding inhibitor of coagulation, are found in a large percentage of patients with primary or secondary APS (216). Although antibodies to β₂-glycoprotein 1 are commonly found in those with other antiphospholipid antibodies, they are the sole antiphospholipid antibody found in approximately 11% of patients with APS (216).

The antigens against which the antiphospholipid antibodies are directed are incompletely understood. Rather than binding directly to anionic phospholipids, antiphospholipid antibodies appear to be directed against epitopes on plasma proteins that are uncovered or generated by the binding of these proteins to phospholipids (212).

Antiphospholipid antibodies may be largely directed against neoepitopes generated by the oxidation of phospholipids or by the adduct resulting from a combination of the breakdown products of oxidized phospholipids and different proteins. One study of antibodies from patients with APS found that the antibodies bound to cardiolipin in increasing amounts as the phospholipid became progressively oxidized on exposure to atmosphere (217). In contrast, affinity purified antiphospholipid antibodies did not bind a nonoxidized cardiolipin analog.

Different coagulation proteins may be involved in binding to phospholipids, which may explain the predisposition to thrombosis. Examples include $\beta_2$-glycoprotein 1, prothrombin, protein C, and protein S (212,218–220).

### $\beta_2$-*Glycoprotein 1*

$\beta_2$-Glycoprotein 1 (apolipoprotein H) is a naturally occurring phospholipid-binding (especially phosphatidylserine and phosphatidylinositol) inhibitor of coagulation and platelet aggregation. The importance of $\beta_2$-glycoprotein I as a pathogenic cofactor in at least some patients with aCL and LA has been demonstrated by the several observations. Antiphospholipid antibodies prolong the PTT if added to normal plasma but not to plasma depleted of $\beta_2$-glycoprotein 1 (218).

In one group of patients with SLE, antibodies directed against free $\beta_2$-glycoprotein 1 were found in 35 of 39 patients with symptoms of the APS versus only two of 55 without such symptoms (219,220). Patients with syphilis and other infections (e.g., malaria, human immunodeficiency virus infection, Q fever) (221) do not form anti-$\beta_2$-glycoprotein 1 antibodies, which may explain why they are not hypercoagulable even though they may have anticardiolipin antibodies (219,220).

Antibodies to $\beta_2$-glycoprotein 1 correlate better with symptoms of APS than do antibodies to cardiolipin alone. (212,219,220,222). $\beta_2$-Glycoprotein I avidly binds negatively charged phospholipids (223), and inhibits contact activation of the clotting cascade (213) and prothrombin-thrombin conversion (224). The $\beta_2$-glycoprotein 1 may be a natural plasma anticoagulant (225), which could explain why neutralizing antibodies directed against this protein may promote thrombosis. Two studies have described patients with antibodies to $\beta_2$-glycoprotein I antigen but without LA or aCL who displayed clinical features of APS, including venous or arterial thromboses (216,226).

### Prevalence of Antiphospholipid Antibodies

Although antiphospholipid antibodies are associated with a propensity for thrombosis and with various autoimmune disorders, they can sometimes be found in normal, asymptomatic individuals. Normal individuals occasionally have elevated levels of IgG or IgM aCL (227,228). In one study, for example, the prevalence was 5% on a first test but only 2% on retesting (228). Increased levels of IgG or IgM aCL have been observed in 12 to 52% of the elderly (227,229). One study found that 40 of 499 normal blood donors had a positive LA test (frequently young women); however, only three had elevated levels of aCL (230).

Antiphospholipid antibody levels are increased in patients with SLE. Approximately 31% of patients have a LA, and 40% to 47% have an aCL (231). Roughly 50% of patients with a LA have SLE (214,231). Antiphospholipid antibodies also occur with increased frequency (5% to 10%) in women with greater than three spontaneous recurrent abortions (232).

LA and aCL have also been found in patients with a variety of autoimmune and rheumatic diseases (231):

- Hemolytic anemia
- Idiopathic thrombocytopenic purpura: up to 30%
- Juvenile arthritis
- Rheumatoid arthritis: 7% to 50%
- Psoriatic arthritis: 28%
- Scleroderma, especially with severe disease (233): 25%
- Behçet's syndrome: 20%
- Sjögren's syndrome: 25% to 42%
- Mixed connective tissue disease: 22%
- Polymyositis and dermatomyositis
- Polymyalgia rheumatica (234): 20%
- Osteoarthritis: less than 14%
- Occasionally in gout and in multiple sclerosis
- Chronic discoid LE (235)
- Eosinophilia myalgia and toxic oil syndrome (236)
- Raynaud's phenomenon (237)

Antiphospholipid antibodies have been found in patients with infections and after the administration of certain drugs. These are usually IgM aCL antibodies, which rarely result in thrombotic events (231). The antibodies do not appear to have anti-$\beta_2$-glycoprotein 1 antibody activity (238). The infections that have been associated with these antibodies include hepatitis A, mumps, bacterial septicemia, HIV infection, syphilis, HTLV-I, malaria, *Pneumocystis carinii*, infectious mononucleosis, and rubella. Among the drugs that have been implicated are phenothiazines (chlorpromazine), phenytoin, hydralazine, procainamide, quinidine, quinine, valproate, amoxicillin, propranolol, cocaine, sulfadoxine, pyrimethamine, and streptomycin (239,240).

## ANTITHYROID ANTIBODIES

Nearly all patients with Hashimoto's thyroiditis have high titers of autoantibodies to one or more thyroid antigens (241,242), which include thyroglobulin (Tg), thyroid peroxidase (TPO) (formerly known as the microsomal antigen), the thyrotropin (TSH) receptor, and the iodine transporter.

## Antibodies Thyroglobulin and Thyroid Peroxidase

Nearly all patients with Hashimoto's thyroiditis have high serum concentrations of antibodies to Tg and TPO (243). These antibodies are also found, although usually in lower concentration, in patients with other thyroid diseases and in some subjects, especially older women, with no clinical or biochemical evidence of thyroid disease (Table 40.7).

Most patients with Graves' disease have circulating autoantibodies to Tg and TPO. Neither the frequency of positive tests for these antibodies nor the titers are as high in patients with Graves' hyperthyroidism as they are in patients with chronic autoimmune thyroiditis.

## Antibodies to the Thyrotropin Receptor

TSH receptor antibodies were first identified by their prolonged thyroid-stimulating activity when serum from patients with Graves' hyperthyroidism; this activity was originally called the long-acting thyroid stimulator (LATS) (243,244). Subsequently, IgG fractions of serum from these patients were found to have thyroid-stimulating actions qualitatively similar to those of TSH in many bioassays and to block binding of radiolabeled TSH to thyroid membranes; in other words the IgG fraction contained TSH receptor antibodies that acted as TSH agonists.

Later, with the use of binding assays, TSH receptor antibodies were detected in the serum of patients with Hashimoto's thyroiditis (244). However, these antibodies, which are usually polyclonal, block the action of TSH rather than activating thyroid tissue. Stimulating and blocking antibodies may bind to different regions of the extracellular domain of the TSH receptor; some evidence suggests that the binding sites for the blocking antibodies are fewer in number and more often located in the region of the ectodomain near the plasma membrane.

TSH receptor antibodies are, therefore, specific for Graves' and Hashimoto's diseases, in contrast to Tg and TPO antibodies, which are found in patients with many other thyroid diseases, and many normal subjects. Patients who had Hashimoto's thyroiditis and Graves' hyperthyroidism at different times have also been well described; at the appropriate times their serum contained TSH receptor-blocking antibodies and TSH receptor-stimulating antibodies.

## Antibodies to the Iodide Transporter

In addition to its role in thyroid iodide transport, this symporter may be an autoantigen. Serum from patients with autoimmune thyroiditis binds to symporter peptides and inhibits TSH-stimulated radioiodine uptake in cultured thyroid follicular cells and in transfected CHO cells expressing the symporter (29). Antibodies to this protein have been identified in the serum of 12% to 20% of patients with Hashimoto's thyroiditis (248).

The titers of TSHR antibody tend to decline in patients treated with an antithyroid drug; if high titers persist, the patient is likely to become hyperthyroid again when the drug is discontinued (245). Whether monitoring TSHR antibody titers in these patients is clinically useful is debated (246). We do measure TSHR antibody titers at the time of cessation of drug therapy because of the association of higher titers with recurrence (245).

In patients treated with radioactive iodine, the titers of TSHR antibody tend to rise, reaching a peak 3 to 5 months after treatment, and then gradually decline (247). In contrast, the titers decline progressively after thyroidectomy, often being undetectable 1 year later. The initial increase in antibody titers may explain why, in some patients, Graves' ophthalmopathy or infiltrative dermopathy are transiently exacerbated by or first appear after radioiodine therapy.

Not all TSHR antibodies are stimulatory. Some, usually found in the serum of patients with chronic autoimmune thyroiditis, block not only the binding but also the action of TSH, and therefore can cause hypothyroidism.

## ANTIGLOMERULAR BASEMENT MEMBRANE ANTIBODY

Antibodies to the GBM are discussed in Chapter 32.

## ISLET CELL ANTIBODIES

Islet cell antibodies (ICAs) were first detected in serum from patients with autoimmune polyendocrine deficiency; they have subsequently been identified in 70% to 80% of patients with newly diagnosed type 1 diabetes and in prediabetic subjects (249,250). Detection of serum ICAs is important clinically because it is the major screening test used to identify patients at risk for the development of clinical diabetes.

**TABLE 40.7.** *Estimated prevalence of antithyroid antibodies*

| Group | Anti-TSHR Ab (%) | Anti-Tg Ab (%) | Anti-TPO Ab (%) |
|---|---|---|---|
| General population | 0 | 5–20 | 8–27 |
| Graves' disease | 80–95 | 50–70 | 50–80 |
| Autoimmune (Hashimoto's thyroiditis) | 10–20 | 80–90 | 90–100 |
| Relatives of patients | 0 | 30–50 | 30–50 |
| Type 1 diabetes | 0 | 30–40 | 30–40 |
| Pregnant women | 0 | ~14 | ~14 |

Anti-TSHR Ab, antithyroid stimulating hormone receptor antibodies; Anti-Tg Ab, antithyroglobulin antibodies; Anti-TPO AB, antithyroid peroxidase antibodies.

An ongoing search has identified several autoantigens within the pancreatic β cells that may play important roles in the initiation or progression of autoimmune islet injury (251). It is not clear, however, which of these autoantigens is involved in the initiation of islet injury and which are secondary, being released only after the injury.

One of the first and most important autoantigens against which antibodies are detected is the enzyme glutamic acid decarboxylase (GAD), which is found in the islets, central nervous system, and testes (252). Antibodies to GAD (a 65-kd protein) are found in about 70% of patients with recent-onset type 1 diabetes. Other antibodies that appear early in the course of the disease include antibodies against a 40-kd fragment of tyrosine phosphatase (IA2) (253) and a 38-kd membrane glycoprotein called glima 38 (254). Antibodies have also been detected against insulin, islet cells, and carboxypeptide H (255).

Prediabetic subjects with a high GAD antibody response but low GAD-T cell response are less likely to develop overt type 1 diabetes (256). It must be emphasized, however, that the pathogenetic importance of GAD is still unproven (257). In prospective studies of offspring of mothers with type 1 diabetes, antiinsulin antibodies are often detected before anti-GAD antibodies (258).

Another autoantigen is a neuroendocrine protein called insulinoma-associated protein 2 (IA-2), which is a tyrosine phosphatase. Antibodies to this antigen have been found in the serum of 58% of patients with newly diagnosed type 1 diabetes (259). The pathophysiologic importance of autoantibodies to this protein is not clear. However, in contrast to the other autoantibodies found in type 1 diabetes, the presence of antibodies to this protein is highly correlated with cellular immune responses triggered by this antigen. The cellular immune response to IA-2 may be a good marker for the disease in as yet unaffected persons and may be involved in the destruction of the pancreatic β cells.

Patients with type 1 diabetes may also have antibodies to 21-hydroxylase, a common autoantigen in primary adrenal insufficiency (260), and to endomysial antigens (such as found in patients with celiac disease)—but without GI symptoms (261).

## ANTIADRENAL ANTIBODIES

Serum antibodies that react with all three zones of the adrenal cortex are present in the serum of 60% to 75% of patients with primary adrenal insufficiency caused by autoimmune adrenalitis; in contrast, these antibodies are rarely found in patients with other causes of adrenal insufficiency, in first-degree relatives of patients with autoimmune primary adrenal insufficiency, or in normal subjects (262–266). Antiadrenal antibodies are more common in women, particularly those with the polyglandular autoimmune syndrome.

Some patients with other autoimmune endocrine diseases who do not have adrenal insufficiency have antiadrenal anti-

**TABLE 40.8.** *Incidence of antiadrenal antibodies in patients with autoimmune disease of other endocrine glands*

| Autoimmune endocrine disease | Incidence of antiadrenal antibodies (%) |
|---|---|
| Hypoparathyroidism | 16 |
| Goitrous autoimmune thyroiditis | 1.9 |
| Atrophic autoimmune thyroiditis | 1.7 |
| Hyperthyroidism | 1.9 |
| Diabetes mellitus | 1.2 |
| Pernicious anemia | <1 |

bodies (Table 40.8). These patients develop adrenal insufficiency at a rate of up to 19% per year (267,268).

Antiadrenal antibodies target the steroidogenic enzymes P450scc (CYP11A1, side-chain cleavage enzyme), P450c17 (CYP17, 17α-hydroxylase), and P450c21 (CYP21A2, 21-hydroxylase) (269,270). The presence of adrenal antibodies may be a stronger risk factor for developing adrenal insufficiency in children than adults (271). Approximately 60% of patients with adrenal insufficiency have antithyroid peroxidase (microsomal) antibodies (272), and almost one half of these patients have overt hypothyroidism. Many other patients have subclinical hypothyroidism (i.e., increased serum thyrotropin (TSH) and normal serum thyroxine concentrations) and are at risk for developing overt hypothyroidism (263).

Some patients with adrenal insufficiency and antiadrenal antibodies also have gastric parietal cell, intrinsic factor, and gonadal antibodies, which correlates with the presence of atrophic gastritis, pernicious anemia, and premature ovarian failure, respectively (Table 40.9). Antigonadal antibodies are much less common in men, as is testicular failure.

## ANTI–TYPE II COLLAGEN ANTIBODIES

It has long been recognized that patients with relapsing polychondritis (RPC) may have humoral or cell-mediated immune responses to extracellular matrix components of cartilage (273). Although their pathophysiologic significance is not completely understood, antibodies to native and denatured type II collagen and proteoglycans have largely been regarded as epiphenomena, emanating from tissue destruction, that lack disease specificity (274). Anti-type II collagen antibodies have been identified in other diseases including rheumatoid arthritis, the seronegative spondyloarthropathies, hip and knee osteoarthritis, and connective tissue disorders such as systemic sclerosis, lupus, and Sjögren's syndrome (275).

Anti–type II collagen antibodies are found in less than one half of patients with RPC, occurring more frequently in the early active phase of disease (274). Their usefulness in monitoring disease activity and the response to therapy requires further analysis.

Later studies found differences in the epitope specificity of the anti-type II collagen antibody appearing in RPC compared with that in rheumatoid arthritis (276). The spectrum of

**TABLE 40.9.** *Incidence of antiadrenal and other autoantibodies in patients with autoimmune adrenal insufficiency*

| Tissue | Incidence of antibodies (%) |
| --- | --- |
| Adrenal | 60–70 |
| Thyroid peroxidase | 50 |
| Parathyroid | 26 |
| Islet cell | 8 |
| Gonad | |
| Ovary | 22 |
| Testes | 5 |
| Stomach | |
| Parietal cell | 30 |
| Intrinsic factor | 9 |

anticollagen response has also been extended. Antibodies to native and denatured type IX and denatured type XI collagen have been identified using immunoblotting and ELISAs (277,278). These antibodies also lack specificity.

## ACKNOWLEDGMENTS

I am indebted to the work of many authors of *Uptodate in Medicine,* whose work provided a useful framework for the development of this chapter.

## REFERENCES

1. Griner PF, Mayewski RJ, Mushlin AI, Greenland P. Selection and interpretation of diagnostic tests and procedures: principles and applications. *Ann Intern Med* 1981;94:553.
2. Sackett DL, Strauss S. On some clinically useful measures of the accuracy of diagnostic tests. *ACP J Club* 1998;129:A17.
3. Kavanuagh A. Personal communications.
4. Barland P, Wachs J. Measurement and clinical significance of antinuclear antibodies. In: Rose B, Schur PH, eds. *Uptodate in Medicine.* Wellesley, MA: UpToDate, Inc., 1998.
5. Reichlin M, Arnett FC Jr. Multiplicity of antibodies in myositis sera. *Arthritis Rheum* 1984;27:1150.
6. Rosenberg AM. Clinical associations of antinuclear antibodies in juvenile rheumatoid arthritis. *Clin Immunol Pathol* 1988;49:19.
7. Petri M, Karlson EW, Cooper DS, Ladenson PW. Autoantibody tests in autoimmune thyroid disease: a case-control study. *J Rheumatol* 1991;18:1529.
8. Czaja AJ, Nishioka M, Morshed SA, Hachiya T. Patterns of nuclear immunofluorescence and reactivities to recombinant nuclear antigens in autoimmune hepatitis. *Gastroenterology* 1994;107:200.
9. Taylor SL, Dean PJ, Riely CA. Primary autoimmune cholangitis: an alternative to anti-mitochondrial antibody-negative primary biliary cirrhosis. *Am J Surg Pathol* 1994;18:91.
10. Rich S, Kieras K, Hart K, et al. Antinuclear antibodies in primary pulmonary hypertension. *J Am Coll Cardiol* 1986;8:1307.
11. Kaplan M, Tan E. Antinuclear antibodies in infectious mononucleosis. *Lancet* 1968;1:561.
12. Burnham T. Antinuclear antibodies in patients with malignancies. *Lancet* 1972;2:436.
13. Seiner M, Klein E, Klein G. Antinuclear reactivity or sera in patients with leukemia and other neoplastic diseases. *Clin Immunol Pathol* 1975;4:374.
14. Miller MH, Littlejohn GO, Jones BW, Strand H. Clinical comparison of cultured human epithelial cells and rat liver as substrates for the fluorescent antinuclear antibody test. *J Rheumatol* 1985;12:265.
15. Tan EM, Feltkamp TE, Smolen JS, et al. Range of antinuclear antibodies in "healthy" individuals. *Arthritis Rheum* 1997;40:1601.
16. Wachs J, Barland P. Antibodies to DNA, SM, and RNP in systemic lupus erythematosus. In: Rose B, Schur PH, eds. *Uptodate in Medicine.* Wellesley, MA: UpToDate, Inc., 1998.
17. Lafer EM, Valle RPC, Moller A, et al. Z-DNA–specific antibodies in human systemic lupus erythematosus. *J Clin Invest* 1983;71:314.
18. Koffler D, Schur PH, Kunkel HG. Immunological studies concerning nephritis of systemic lupus erythematosus. *J Exp Med* 1967;126:607.
19. Karlson EW, Hankinson SE, Liang MH, et al. Association of silicone breast implants with immunologic abnormalities: a prospective study. *Am J Med* 1999;106:11.
20. Hahn BH. Antibodies to DNA. *N Engl J Med* 1998;338:1359.
21. Swaak AJ, Groenwold J, Bronsveld W. Predictive value of complement profiles and dsDNA in systemic lupus erythematosus. *Ann Rheum Dis* 1986;5:359.
22. ter Borg EJ, Horst G, Hummel EJ, et al. Measurement of increases in anti-double-stranded DNA antibody levels as a predictor of disease exacerbation in systemic lupus erythematosus. *Arthritis Rheum* 1990;33:634.
23. Schur PH, Sandson J. Immunologic factors and clinical activity in systemic lupus erythematosus. *N Engl J Med* 1968;278:553.
24. Cervera R, Kharmasta M, Font J, et al. Systemic lupus erythematosus: clinical and immunological patterns of disease expression in a cohort of 1,000 patients. *Medicine (Baltimore)* 1993;72:113.
25. Rothfield NF, Stollar BD. The relation of immunoglobulin class, pattern of antinuclear antibody, and complement-fixing antibodies to DNA in sera from patients with systemic lupus erythematosus. *J Clin Invest* 1967;46:1785.
26. Tan EM, Schur PH, Carr RI, Hunkel HG. DNA and antibodies to DNA in the serum of patients with systemic lupus erythematosus. *J Clin Invest* 1966;45:1732.
27. Hughes GRV, Cohen SA, Christian CL. Anti-DNA activity in systemic lupus erythematosus. *Ann Rheum Dis* 1971;30:259.
28. Arden LA, deGroot ER, Feltkamp TEW. Immunology of DNA III. *Crithidia luciliae:* a simple substrate for the determination of anti-dsDNA with the immunofluorescence technique. *Ann N Y Acad Sci* 1975;254:505.
29. Smeenk R, Lily G, Aarden L. Avidity of antibodies to dsDNA: comparison of IFT on *Crithidia luciliae,* Farr assay and PEG assay. *J Immunol* 1982;128:73.
30. Crowe W, Kushner I, Clough JD. Comparison of the Crithidia luciliae, millipore filter, Farr and hemagglutination methods for detection of antibodies to DNA. *Arthritis Rheum* 1978;21:390.
31. Miller TE, Lahita RG, Zarro VJ, et al. Clinical significance of anti-double stranded DNA antibodies detected by a solid phase immunoassay. *Arthritis Rheum* 1981;24:602.
32. Avina-Zubieta JA, Galindo-Rodriguez G, Kwar-Yeung L, et al. Clinical evaluation of various selected ELISA kits for the detection of anti-DNA antibodies. *Lupus* 1995;4:370.
33. Coobick A, Southerson B, Williams J, Ziff M. An appraisal of tests for native DNA antibodies in connective tissue diseases. *Ann Intern Med* 1978;89:186.
34. Vlahakos DV, Foster MH, Adams S, et al. Anti-DNA antibodies form immune deposits at distinct glomerular and vascular sites. *Kidney Int* 1992;41:1690.
35. D'Andrea DM, Coupaye-Gerard B, Kleyman TR, et al. Lupus autoantibodies interact directly with distinct glomerular and vascular cell surface antigens. *Kidney Int* 1996;49:1214.
36. Schur PH, Monroe M, Rothfield N. The gamma G subclass of antinuclear and antinucleic acid antibodies. *Arthritis Rheum* 1972;15:174.
37. Ronsuke S, Evans M, Abdou N. Idiotypic and immunochemical differences of anti-DNA antibodies of lupus patients during active and inactive disease. *Clin Immunol Immunopathol* 1991;61:320.
38. Lloyd W, Schur P. Immune complexes, complement and anti-DNA in exacerbations of systemic lupus erythematosus (SLE). *Medicine (Baltimore)* 1981;60:208.
39. Gladman DD, Urowitz MB, Keystone EC. Serologicially active clinically quiescent systemic lupus erythematosus. *Am J Med* 1979;66:210.
40. Winfield J, Brunner C, Koffler D. Serologic studies in patients with systemic lupus erythematosus and central nervous system dysfunction. *Arthritis Rheum* 1978;21:289.
41. Tan EM, Kunkel HG. Characteristics of a soluble nuclear antigen precipitating with sera of patients with systemic lupus erythematosus. *J Immunol* 1966;96:464.

42. Bush H, Reddy R, Ruthblum L, Choy YC. SnRNAs, SnRNPs, and RNA processing. *Annu Rev Biochem* 1982;51:617.
43. Barad FA Jr, Andrews BS, Davis JS, Taylor RP. Antibodies to Sm in patients with systemic lupus erythematosus: correlation of Sm antibody titers with disease activity and other laboratory parameters. *Arthritis Rheum* 1981;24:1236.
44. Beaufils M, Kouki F, Mignon F, et al. Clinical significance of anti-Sm antibodies in systemic lupus erythematosus. *Am J Med* 1983;74:201.
45. Munves EF, Schur PH. Antibodies to Sm and RNP: prognosticators of disease involvement. *Arthritis Rheum* 1983;26:848.
46. Karata N, Tan EM. Identification of antibodies to nuclear acid antigens by counterimmunoelectrophoresis. *Arthritis Rheum* 1976;19:574.
47. Houtman PM, Kallenberg CGM, Lumburg PC, et al. Quantitation of antibodies to nucleoribonucleoprotein by ELISA: relations between antibody levels and disease activity in patients with connective tissue disease. *Clin Exp Immunol* 1985;62:696.
48. Arnett FC, Hamilton RG, Roebber MG, et al. Increased frequencies of Sm and nRNP autoantibodies in American blacks compared to whites with systemic lupus erythematosus. *J Rheumatol* 1988;15:1773.
49. Homma M, Mimori T, Takeda Y, et al. Autoantibodies to the Sm antigen: immunological approach to clinical aspects of systemic lupus erythematosus. *J Rheumatol* 1987;14[Suppl 13]:188.
50. Takeda Y, Wang G, Wang R, et al. Enzyme-linked immunosorbent assay using isolated (U) small nuclear ribonucleoprotein polypeptides as antigens to investigate the clinical significance of autoantibodies to these polypeptides. *Clin Immunol Immunopathol* 1989;50:213.
51. Winn D, Wolfe J, Lindberg D, et al. Identification of a clinical subset of systemic lupus erythematosus by antibodies to the Sm antigen. *Arthritis Rheum* 1979;22:1334.
52. Reinitz E, Grayzel A, Barland P. Specificity of Smith antibodies. *Arthritis Rheum* 1977;20:693.
53. Janwityanuchit S, Verasertniyom O, Vanichapuntu M, Vatanasuk M. Anti-Sm: its predictive value in systemic lupus erythematosus. *Clin Rheumatol* 1993;12:350.
54. Barland P, Wachs J. Clinical significance of anti-Ro/SSA and anti-La/SSB antibodies. In: Rose B, Schur PH, eds. *Uptodate in Medicine.* Wellesley, MA: UpToDate, Inc., 1998.
55. Clark G, Reichlin M, Tomeri T. Characterization of a soluble cytoplasmic antigen reactive with sera from patients with systemic lupus erythematosus. *J Immunol* 1969;102:117.
56. Alspaugh MA, Tan EM. Antibodies to cellular antigens in Sjögren's syndrome. *J Clin Invest* 1975;55:1067.
57. Alspaugh M, Maddison P. Resolution of the identity of certain antigen-antibody systems in systemic lupus erythematosus and Sjögren's syndrome: an interlaboratory collaboration. *Arthritis Rheum* 1979;22:796.
58. Barakat S, Meyer G, Torterotot F, et al. IgG antibodies from patients with primary Sjögren's syndrome and systemic lupus erythematosus recognize different epitopes in 60-Kd-A/Ro protein. *Clin Exp Immunol* 1992;89:38.
59. Wilson RW, Provost TT, Bias WB, et al. Sjögren's syndrome: influence of multiple HLA-D region alloantigens on clinical and serologic expression. *Arthritis Rheum* 1984;27:1245.
60. Sanchez-Guerrero J, Lew RA, Fossel AH, Schur PH. Utility of anti-Sm, anti-RNP, anti-Ro/SS-A, and anti-La/SS-B (extractable nuclear antigens) detected by enzyme-linked immunosorbent assay for the diagnosis of systemic lupus erythematosus. *Arthritis Rheum* 1996; 39:1055.
61. Provost TT, Watson R, Simmons-O'Brien E. Significance of the anti-Ro (SS-A) antibody in the evaluation of patients with cutaneous manifestations of a connective tissue disease. *J Am Acad Dermatol* 1996; 35:147.
62. Maddison P, Mogavero H, Provost TT, et al. The clinical significance of autoantibodies to a soluble cytoplasmic antigen in systemic lupus erythematosus and other connective tissue diseases. *J Rheumatol* 1979; 6:189.
63. Lockshin MD, Bonja E, Elkon K, Druzen ML. Neonatal lupus risk to newborns of mothers with systemic lupus erythematosus. *Arthritis Rheum* 1988;31:697.
64. Buyon JP, Ben-Chetrit E, Karp S, et al. Acquired congenital heart block: pattern of maternal antibody response to biochemically defined antigens of the SSA/Ro-SSB/La system in neonatal lupus. *J Clin Invest* 1989;84:627.
65. Garcia S, Nascimento JH, Bonfa E, et al. Cellular mechanism of the conduction abnormalities induced by serum from anti-Ro/SSA positive patients in rabbit heart. *J Clin Invest* 1994;93:718.
66. Buyon JP, Hiebert R, Copel J, et al. Autoimmune associated congenital heart block: demographics, mortality, morbidity and recurrence rates obtained from a national neonatal lupus registry. *J Am Coll Cardiol* 1998;31:1658.
67. Brucato A, Francechini F, Buyon JP. Neonatal lupus: long-term outcomes of mothers and children and recurrence rate. *Clin Exp Rheumatol* 1997;15:467.
68. Harley JB, Alexander EL, Bias WB, et al. Anti-Ro (SSA) and anti-La (SSB) in patients with Sjögren's syndrome. *Arthritis Rheum* 1986; 29:196.
69. St Clair EW, Burch J, Saitta M. Specificity of autoantibodies for recombinant 60-kd and 52-kD Ro autoantigens. *Arthritis Rheum* 1994; 37:1373.
70. Dorner T, Feist E, Held C, et al. Differential recognition of the 52-kd Ro (SS-A) antigen by sera from patients with primary biliary cirrhosis and primary Sjögren's syndrome. *Hepatology* 1996;24:1404.
71. Maddison P, Provost T, Reichlin M. Serological findings in patients with "ANA-negative" systemic lupus erythematosus. *Medicine (Baltimore)* 1981;60:87.
72. Harmon C, Deng J, Peebles C, et al. The importance of tissue substrate in the SS-A/Ro antigen-antibody system. *Arthritis Rheum* 1984; 27:166.
73. Denton CP, Black CM. Classification of scleroderma. In: Rose B, Schur PH, eds. *Uptodate in Medicine.* Wellesley, MA: UpToDate, Inc., 1998.
74. Black CM. The aetiopathogenesis of systemic sclerosis: thick skin-thin hypotheses. The Parkes Weber Lecture, 1994. *J R Coll Physicians Lond* 1995;29:119.
75. Wade JP, Sack B, Schur PH. Anticentromere antibodies—clinical correlates. *J Rheumatol* 1988;15:1759.
76. Wachs, Barland P. Miscellaneous antinuclear antibodies. In: Rose B, Schur PH, eds. *Uptodate in Medicine.* Wellesley, MA: UpToDate, Inc., 1998.
77. Sebbag M, Simon M, Vincent C, et al. The antiperinuclear factor and the so-called antikeratin antibodies are the same rheumatoid arthritis-specific autoantibodies. *J Clin Invest* 1995;95:2672.
78. Young BJ, Mallya RK, Leslie RD, et al. Antikeratin antibodies in rheumatoid arthritis. *Br Med J* 1979;1:97.
79. Simon M, Girbal E, Sebbag M, et al. The cytokeratin filament-aggregating protein filaggrin is the target of the so-called "antikeratin antibodies" in rheumatoid arthritis. *J Clin Invest* 1993;92:1387.
80. Gomes-Daudrix V, Sebbag M, Girbal E, et al. Immunoblotting detection of so-called "antikeratin antibodies": A new assay for the diagnosis of rheumatoid arthritis. *Ann Rheum Dis* 1994;53:735.
81. Berthelot JM, Maugars Y, Castagne A, et al. Antiperinuclear factors are present in polyarthritis before ACR criteria for rheumatoid arthritis are fulfilled. *Ann Rheum Dis* 1997;56:123.
82. Paimela L, Gripenberg M, Kurki P, Leirisalo-Repo M. Antikeratin antibodies: diagnostic and prognostic markers for early rheumatoid arthritis. *Ann Rheum Dis* 1992;51:743.
83. Boki KA, Kurki P, Holthofer H, et al. Prevalence of antikeratin antibodies in Greek patients with rheumatoid arthritis: a clinical, serologic and immunogenetic study. *J Rheumatol* 1995;22:2046.
84. Adebajo AO, Hazleman BL, Williams DG, Maini RN. Diagnostic role of antikeratin antibodies in rheumatoid arthritis [Letter]. *Ann Rheum Dis* 1992;51:1264.
85. Le Goff P, Saraux P, Yauinou P. New autoantibodies in rheumatoid arthritis. *Rev Rheum Engl Ed* 1997;64:638.
86. Serre G, Vincent C. Filaggrin (keratin) autoantibodies. In: Peter JB, Schoenfeld Y, eds. *Autoantibodies.* Amsterdam: Elsevier Science, 1996:271.
87. Hoet R, Van Venraij WJ. The antiperinuclear factor (APF) and antikeratin antibodies (AKA) in rheumatoid arthritis. In: Smolen JS, Kalden JR, Maini RN, eds. *Rheumatoid arthritis.* Berlin: Springer-Verlag, 1992:299.
88. Chabre H, Amoura Z, Piette J, et al. Presence of nucleosome-restricted antibodies in patients with systemic lupus erythematosus. *Arthritis Rheum* 1995;38:1485.
89. Tupchong M, Wither J, Hallett D, Gladman D. Anti-nucleosome antibodies as markers for renal disease in lupus nephritis. *Arthritis Rheum* 1997;40:304.
90. Massa M, de Benedetti F, Pignatti P. Anti-double-stranded DNA, anti-histone and antinucleosome IgG reactivities in children with systemic lupus erythematosus. *Clin Exp Rheumatol* 1994;12:219.

91. Dreyfus G, Matunes MJ, Pinol-Roma S, Bard CG. Hn RNP proteins and the biogenesis of mRNA. *Annu Rev Biochem* 1993;62:289.

92. Montecucco C, Caporali R, Negri C, et al. Antibodies from patients with rheumatoid arthritis and systemic lupus erythematosus recognize different epitopes of a single heterogeneous nuclear RNP core protein. *Arthritis Rheum* 1990;33:180.

93. Hassfeld W, Steiner G, Sludnicka-Benke A, et al. Autoimmune response to the spliceosome: an immunologic link between rheumatoid arthritis, mixed connective tissue disease, and systemic lupus erythematosus *Arthritis Rheum* 1995;38:777.

94. Biamonti G, Ghigna C, Caporali R, Montecucco C. Heterogeneous nuclear ribonucleoproteins (hnRNPs): an emerging family of autoantigens in rheumatic diseases. *Clin Exp Rheumatol* 1998;16:317.

95. Montecucco C, Caporali R, Cobianchi F, Biamonte G. Identification of autoantibodies to the I protein of the heterogeneous nuclear ribonucleoprotein complex in patients with systemic sclerosis. *Arthritis Rheum* 1996;39:1669.

96. Stanek D, Vencovsky J, Kafkova J, Raska I. Heterogeneous nuclear RNP C1 and C2 core proteins are targets for an autoantibody found in the serum of a patient with systemic sclerosis and psoriatic arthritis. *Arthritis Rheum* 1997;40:2172.

97. Fritzler MJ, McCarty GA, Ryan JP, Kinsella TD. Clinical features of patients with antibodies directed against proliferating cell nuclear antigen. *Arthritis Rheum* 1983;26:140.

98. Muller-Weeks SJ, Caradonna S. Specific association of cyclin-like uracil-DNA glycosylase with the proliferating cell nuclear antigen. *Exp Cell Res* 1996;226:346.

99. Miyachi K, Fritzler MJ, Tan EM. Autoantibody to a nuclear antigen in proliferating cells. *J Immunol* 1978;121:2228.

100. Roos G, Landberg G, Huff JP, et al. Analysis of the epitopes of proliferating cell nuclear antigen recognized by monoclonal antibodies. *Lab Invest* 1993;68:204.

101. Furneaux HM, Reich L, Posner JB. Central nervous system synthesis of autoantibodies in paraneoplastic syndromes. *Neurology* 1990;40:1085.

102. Furneaux HM. Neuronal nuclear autoantibodies, type 1 (Hu). In: Peter JB, Schoenfeld Y, eds. *Autoantibodies*. Amsterdam: Elsevier Science, 1996:551.

103. Graus F, Elkon KB, Cordon-Cardo C, Posner JB. Sensory neuropathy and small cell lung cancer: antineuronal antibody that also reacts with the tumor. *Am J Med* 1986;80:45.

104. Dropcho EJ, King PH. Autoantibodies against the Hcl-N1 RNA-binding protein among patients with lung carcinoma: an association with type I antineuronal antibodies. *Ann Neurol* 1994;36:200.

105. Alamowitch S, Graus F, Uchuya M, et al. Limbic encephalitis and small cell lung cancer: clinical and Immunological features. *Brain* 1997;120:923.

106. Darnell RB, De Angelis LM. Regression of small-cell lung carcinoma in patients with paraneoplastic neuronal antibodies. *Lancet* 1993;341:21.

107. Lennon VA, Sas DF, Busk MF, et al. Enteric neuronal autoantibodies in pseudoobstruction with small-cell lung carcinoma. *Gastroenterology* 1991;100:137.

108. Griffin JW, Cornblath DR, Alexander E. Sensory ganglionitis associated with connective tissue disorders. *Neurology* 1988;38:243(abst).

109. Hirakata M, Okano Y, Pati U, et al. Identification of autoantibodies to RNA polymerase II: occurrence in systemic sclerosis and association with autoantibodies to RNA polymerase I and III. *J Clin Invest* 1993;91:2665.

110. Okano Y, Steen VD, Medsger TA Jr. Autoantibody to U3 nucleolar ribonucleoprotein (fibrillarin) in patients with systemic sclerosis. *Arthritis Rheum* 1992;35:95.

111. Dick T, Mierau R, Steinfeld R, et al. Clinical relevance and HLA association of autoantibodies against the nucleolus organizer region (NOR-90). *J Rheumatol* 1995;22:67.

112. Arnett FC, Reveille JD, Benigno VC. Autoantibodies to a nucleolar RNA helicase protein in patients with connective tissue diseases. *Arthritis Rheum* 1997;40:1487.

113. Mimori T, Akizuki M, Yamagata H, et al. Characterization of a high molecular weight acidic nuclear protein recognized by autoantibodies in sera from patients with polymyositis-scleroderma overlap. *J Clin Invest* 1981;68:611.

114. Love LA, Leff RL, Fraser DD, et al. A new approach to the classification of idiopathic inflammatory myopathy: myositis-specific auto-

antibodies define useful homogeneous patient groups. *Medicine (Baltimore)* 1991;70:360.

115. Jung F, Neuer G, Bautz FA. Antibodies against a peptide sequence located in the linker region of the HMG-1/2 box domains in sera from patients with juvenile rheumatoid arthritis. *Arthritis Rheum* 1997;40:1803.

116. Li X, McNeilage J, Whittingham S. Autoantibodies to the major nucleolar phosphoprotein B23 define a novel subset of patients with anti-cardiolipin antibodies. *Arthritis Rheum* 1989;32:1165.

117. Misaki Y, Van Venrooij WJ, Pruijn GJ. Prevalence and characteristics of anti-56K/annexin XI autoantibodies in systemic autoimmune diseases. *J Rheumatol* 1995;22:97.

118. Wachs J, Barland P. Antiribosomal P protein antibodies. In: Rose B, Schur PH, eds. *Uptodate in Medicine*. Wellesley, MA: UpToDate, Inc., 1998.

119. Schur PH, Moroz L, Kunkel HG. Precipitating antibodies to a ribosomal antigen in the serum of patients with systemic lupus erythematosus. *Immunochemistry* 1967;4:447.

120. Elkon KB, Parnassa AP, Foster CL. Lupus autoantibodies target ribosomal P proteins. *J Exp Med* 1985;162:459.

121. Francour AM, Peebles CL, Heckman KJ, et al. Identification of ribosomal protein autoantigens. *J Immunol* 1985;135:2878.

122. Koren E, Reichlin MW, Koscec M, et al. Autoantibodies to the ribosomal P proteins react with a plasma membrane related target on human cells. *J Clin Invest* 1992;89:1236.

123. Bonfa E, Elkon KB. Clinical and serologic associations of the antiribosomal P protein antibody. *Arthritis Rheum* 1986;29:981.

124. Schneebaum AB, Singleton JD, West SG, Blodgett JK. Association of psychiatric manifestations with antibodies to ribosomal P proteins in systemic lupus erythematosus. *Am J Med* 1991;90:54.

125. Bonfa E, Golombek S, Kaufman L, et al. Association between lupus psychosis and antiribosomal P protein antibodies. *N Engl J Med* 1987;317:265.

126. Sato T, Uchiumi T, Ozawa T, et al. Autoantibodies against ribosomal proteins found with high frequency in patients with systemic lupus erythematosus with active disease. *J Rheumatol* 1991;18:1681.

127. Anderson CJ, Neas BR, Pan Z, et al. The presence of masked antiribosomal P autoantibodies in healthy children. *Arthritis Rheum* 1998;41:33.

128. Van Dam A, Nossent H, de Jong J, et al. Diagnostic value of antibodies against ribosomal phosphoproteins: a cross sectional and longitudinal study. *J Rheumatol* 1991;18:1026.

129. Nojima Y, Minota S, Yamada A, et al. Correlation of antibodies to ribosomal P protein with psychosis in patients with systemic lupus erythematosus. *Ann Rheum Dis* 1992;51:1053.

130. Teh L, Bedwell A, Isenberg D, et al. Antibodies to protein P in systemic lupus erythematosus. *Ann Rheum Dis* 1992;51:489.

131. Arnett FC, Reichlin M. Lupus hepatitis: an under-recognized disease feature associated with autoantibodies to ribosomal P. *Am J Med* 1995;99:465.

132. Martin AL, Reichlin M. Fluctuations of antibody to ribosomal P proteins correlate with appearance and remission of nephritis in SLE. *Lupus* 1996;5:22.

133. Schur PH, Rose BD. Drug-induced lupus. In: Rose B, Schur PH, eds. *Uptodate in Medicine*. Wellesley, MA: UpToDate, Inc., 1998.

134. Yung RL, Johnson KJ, Richardson BC. New concepts in the pathogenesis of drug-induced lupus. *Lab Invest* 1995;73:746.

136. Burlingame RW, Rubin RL. Drug-induced anti-histone autoantibodies display two patterns of reactivity with substructures of chromatin. *J Clin Invest* 1991;88:680.

135. Rubin RL, Bell SA, Burlingame RW. Autoantibodies associated with lupus induced by diverse drugs target a similar epitope in the (H2A-H2B)-DNA complex. *J Clin Invest* 1992;90:165.

137. Rubin RL, Burlingame RW, Arnett JL, et al. IgG but not other classes of anti-(H2A-H2B)-DNA) is an early sign of procainamide induced lupus. *J Immunol* 1995;154:2403.

138. Jiang X, Khursigara G, Rubin RL. Transformation of lupus-inducing drugs to cytotoxic products by activated neutrophils. *Science* 1994;266:810.

139. McKinnon RA, Nebert DW. Possible role of cytochrome P450 in lupus erythematosus and related disorders. *Lupus* 1994;3:473.

139a Fritzler MJ. Drugs recently associated with lupus syndromes. *Lupus* 1994;3:455.

140. Crowson AN, Magro CM. Diltiazem and subacute cutaneous lupus erythematosus-like lesions [Letter]. *N Engl J Med* 1995;333:1429.

141. Gough A, Chapman S, Wagstaff K, et al. Minocycline induced auto-immune hepatitis and systemic lupus erythematosus-like syndrome. *BMJ* 1996;312:169.
142. Totoritis MC, Tan EM, McNally EM, Rubin RL. Association of anti-body to histone complex H2A-H2B with symptomatic procainamide-induced lupus. *N Engl J Med* 1988;318:1431.
143. Adams LE, Mongey A-B. Role of genetic factors in drug-related autoimmunity. *Lupus* 1994;3:443.
144. Reidenberg MM, Drayer DE. Procainamide, *N*-acetylprocainamide, antinuclear antibody and systemic lupus erythematosus. *Angiology* 1986;37:968.
145. Stec GP, Lertora JJ, Atkinson AJ Jr, et al. Remission of procainamide-induced lupus with *N*-acetylprocainamide therapy. *Ann Intern Med* 1979;90:799.
146. Hess E. Drug-induced lupus. *N Engl J Med* 1988;318:1460.
147. Batchelor JR, Welsh KI, Tinoco RM, et al. Hydralazine-induced systemic lupus erythematosus: influence of HLA-DR and sex on sus-ceptibility. *Lancet* 1980;1:1107.
148. Speirs C, Fielder AH, Chapel H, et al. Complement system protein C4 and susceptibility to hydralazine-induced systemic lupus erythemato-sus. *Lancet* 1989;1:922.
149. Krawitt EL. Classification of autoimmune hepatitis. In: Rose B, Schur PH, eds. *Uptodate in Medicine*. Wellesley, MA: UpToDate, Inc., 1998.
150. Czaja AJ, Carpenter HA, Manns MP. Antibodies to soluble liver anti-gen P450IID6, and mitochondrial complexes in chronic hepatitis. *Gas-troenterology* 1993;105:1522.
151. Zauli D, Ghetti S, Grassi A, et al. Anti-neutrophil cytoplasmic antibodies in type 1 and 2 autoimmune hepatitis. *Hepatology* 1997;25:1105.
152. Treichel U, McFarlane BM, Seki T, et al. Demographics of anti-asialoglycoprotein receptor autoantibodies in autoimmune hepatitis. *Gastroenterology* 1994;107:799.
153. Davis PA, Leung P, Manns M, et al. M4 and M9 antibodies in the over-lap syndrome of primary biliary cirrhosis and chronic active hepatitis: epitopes or epiphenomena? *Hepatology* 1992;16:1128.
154. Lohr HF, Schlaak JF, Lohse AW, et al. Autoreactive CD4+ LKM-specific and anticlonotypic T-cell responses in LKM-1 antibody-positive autoimmune hepatitis. *Hepatology* 1996;24:1416.
155. Homberg J-C, Abuaf N, Bernard O, et al. Chronic active hepatitis asso-ciated with antiliver/kidney microsome antibody type 1: a second type of "autoimmune" hepatitis. *Hepatology* 1987;7:1333.
156. Robin MA, Maratrat M, Le Roy M, et al. Antigenic targets in tienilic acid hepatitis: both cytochrome P450 2C11 and 2C11-tienilic acid adducts are transported to the plasma membrane of rat hepatocytes and recognized by human sera. *J Clin Invest* 1996;98:1471.
157. Philipp T, Durazzo M, Trautwein C, et al. Recognition of uridine diphosphate glucuronosyl transferases by LKM-3 antibodies in chronic hepatitis D. *Lancet* 1994;344:578.
158. Sherlock S. Autoimmune cholangitis: a unique entity? *Mayo Clin Proc* 1998;73:184.
159. Gordon SC, Quattrociocchi-Longe TM, Khan BA, et al. Antibodies to carbonic anhydrase in patients with immune cholangiopathies. *Gas-troenterology* 1995;108:1802.
160. Gohlke F, Lohse AW, Dienes HP, et al. Evidence for an overlap syn-drome of autoimmune hepatitis and primary sclerosing cholangitis. *J Hepatol* 1996;24:699.
161. Boberg KM, Fausa O, Haaland T, et al. Features of autoimmune hepatitis in primary sclerosing cholangitis: an evaluation of 114 pri-mary sclerosing cholangitis patients according to a scoring system for the diagnosis of autoimmune hepatitis. *Hepatology* 1996;23:1369.
162. Rose BD, Hoffman GS. Clinical spectrum of antineutrophil cytoplas-mic antibodies. In: Rose B, Schur PH, eds. *Uptodate in Medicine*. Wellesley, MA: UpToDate, Inc., 1998.
163. Jennette JC, Hoidal JR, Falk RJ. Specificity of anti-neutrophil cyto-plasmic autoantibodies for proteinase 3. *Blood* 1990;75:2263.
164. Falk RJ, Jennette JC. Anti-neutrophil cytoplasmic autoantibodies with specificity for myeloperoxidase in patients with systemic vasculitis and idiopathic necrotizing and crescentic glomerulonephritis. *N Engl J Med* 1988;25:1651.
165. Hagen EC, Andrassy K, Csernok E, et al. Development and standard-ization of solid phase assays for the detection of anti-neutrophil cyto-plasmic antibodies (ANCA): a report on the second phase of an inter-national cooperative study on the standardization of ANCA assays. *J Immunol Methods* 1996;196:1.
166. Hoffman GS, Specks U. Antineutrophil cytoplasmic antibodies (ANCA). *Arthritis Rheum* 1998;41:1521.
167. Merkel PA, Polisson RP, Chang Y, et al. Prevalence of antineutrophil cytoplasmic antibodies in a large inception cohort of patients with con-nective tissue disease. *Ann Intern Med* 1997;126:866.
168. Kallenberg CG, Brouwer E, Weening JJ, Cohen Tervaert JW. Anti-neutrophil cytoplasmic antibodies: current diagnostic and pathophysi-ological potential. *Kidney Int* 1994;46:1.
169. Specks U, Homburger HA. Anti-neutrophil cytoplasmic antibodies. *Mayo Clin Proc* 1994;69:1197.
170. Ronda N, Esnault VLM, Layward L, et al. Antineutrophil cytoplasm antibodies (ANCA) of IgA isotype in adult Henoch-Schönlein purpura. *Clin Exp Immunol* 1994;95:49.
171. Robson WL, Leung AK, Woodman RC. The absence of antineutrophil cytoplasmic antibodies in patients with Henoch-Schönlein purpura. *Pediatr Nephrol* 1994;8:295.
172. Nash MC, Shah V, Reader JA, Dillon MJ. Anti-neutrophil cytoplasmic antibodies and anti-endothelial cell antibodies are not increased in Kawasaki disease. *Br J Rheumatol* 1995;34:882.
173. Hauschild S, Csernok E, Schmitt WH, Gross WL. Antineutrophil cyto-plasmic antibodies in systemic polyarteritis nodosa with and without hepatitis B virus infection and Churg-Strauss syndrome—62 patients. *J Rheumatol* 1994;21:1173.
174. Baranger TA, Audrain MA, Castagne A, et al. Absence of antineu-trophil cytoplasmic antibodies in giant cell arteritis. *J Rheumatol* 1994;21:871.
175. Eichhorn J, Sima D, Thiele B, et al. Anti-endothelial cell antibodies in Takayasu arteritis. *Circulation* 1996;94:2396.
176. Braun MG, Csernok E, Schmitt WH, Gross WL. Incidence, target anti-gens, and clinical implications of antineutrophil cytoplasmic antibodies in rheumatoid arthritis. *J Rheumatol* 1996;23:826.
177. Schnabel A, Csernok E, Isenberg DA, et al. Antineutrophil cytoplasmic antibodies in systemic lupus erythematosus. *Arthritis Rheum* 1995;38:633.
178. Guillevin L, Lhote F. Distinguishing polyarteritis nodosa from micro-scopic polyangiitis and implications for treatment. *Curr Opin Rheumatol* 1995;7:20.
179. Mulder L, van Rossum M, Hosrst G, et al. Antineutrophil cytoplasmic antibodies in juvenile chronic arthritis. *J Rheumatol* 1997;24:568.
180. Locht H, Peen E, Skogh T. Antineutrophil cytoplasmic antibodies in reactive arthritis. *J Rheumatol* 1995;22:2304.
181. Papo T, Piette JC, Du LTH, et al. Antineutrophil cytoplasmic antibod-ies in polychondritis. *Ann Rheum Dis* 1993;52:384.
182. Locke IC, Worrall JG, Leaker B, et al. Autoantibodies to myeloperox-idase in systemic sclerosis. *J Rheumatol* 1997;24:86.
183. Seibold F, Slametschka D, Gregor M, Weber P. Neutrophil antibodies in primary sclerosing cholangitis and ulcerative colitis. *Gastroenterol-ogy* 1994;107:532.
184. Mulder AH, Horst G, Haagsma EB, et al. Prevalence and characteri-zation of neutrophil cytoplasmic antibodies in autoimmune liver dis-eases. *Hepatology* 1993;17:411.
185. Short AK, Lockwood CM. Antigen specificity in hydralazine associ-ated ANCA positive systemic vasculitis. *Q J Med* 1995;88:775.
186. Elkayam O, Yaron M, Caspi D. Minocycline induced arthritis associ-ated with fever, livedo reticularis, and pANCA. *Ann Rheum Dis* 1996;55:769.
187. Kitahara T, Hiromura K, Maezawa A, et al. Case of propylthiouracil-induced vasculitis associated with anti-neutrophil cytoplasmic anti-body (ANCA): review of literature. *Clin Nephrol* 1997;47:336.
188. Hellmark T, Niles JL, Collins AB, et al. Comparison of anti-GBM anti-bodies in sera with to without ANCA. *J Am Soc Nephrol* 1997;8:376.
189. Hagen EC, Daha MR, Hermans J, et al for the EC/BCR project for ANCA assay standardization. Diagnostic value of standardized assays for anti-neutrophil cytoplasmic antibodies in idiopathic systemic vas-culitis. *Kidney Int* 1998;53:743.
190. Rao JK, Weinberger M, Oddone EZ, et al. The role of antineutrophil cytoplasmic antibody (c-ANCA) testing in the diagnosis of Wegener's granulomatosis: a literature review and meta-analysis. *Ann Intern Med* 1995;123:925.
191. Jennette JC, Wilkman AS, Falk RJ. Diagnostic predictive value of ANCA serology. *Kidney Int* 1998;53:796.
192. Rao JK, Allen NB, Feussner JR, Weinberger M. A prospective study of antineutrophil cytoplasmic antibody (c-ANCA) and clinical criteria in diagnosing Wegener's granulomatosis. *Lancet* 1995;346:926.

193. Langford CA. The diagnostic utility of c-ANCA in Wegener's granulomatosis. *Cleve Clin J Med* 1998;65:135.
194. Jayne DRW, Gaskin G, Pusey CD, Lockwood CM. ANCA and predicting relapse in systemic vasculitis. *Q J Med* 1995;88:127.
195. Shmerling RH. Origin and utility of measurement of rheumatoid factors. In: Rose B, Schur PH, eds. *Uptodate in Medicine*. Wellesley, MA: UpToDate, Inc., 1998.
196. Waaler E. On the occurrence of a factor in human serum activating the specific agglutination of sheep blood corpuscles. *Acta Pathol Microbiol Scand* 1940;17:172.
197. Singer JM, Plotz CM. The latex fixation test. *Am J Med* 1956;21:888.
198. Panush RS, Bianco NE, Schur PH. Serum and synovial fluid IgG, IgA, and IgM antigammaglobulins in rheumatoid arthritis. *Arthritis Rheum* 1971;14:737.
199. Wolfe F. A comparison of IgM rheumatoid factor by nephelometry and latex methods: clinical and laboratory significance. *Arthritis Care Res* 1998;11:89.
200. Shmerling RH, Delbanco TL. The rheumatoid factor: an analysis of clinical utility. *Am J Med* 1991;91:528.
201. Lichtenstein MJ, Pincus T. Rheumatoid arthritis identified in population-based cross sectional studies: low prevalence of rheumatoid factor. *J Rheumatol* 1991;18:989.
202. Mikkelsen WM, Dodge HJ, Duff IF, Kato H. Estimates of the prevalence of rheumatic diseases in the population of Tecumseh, Michigan, 1959. *J Chron Dis* 1967;20:351.
203. Cathcart ES, O'Sullivan JB. Rheumatoid arthritis in a New England town: a prevalence study in Sudbury, Massachusetts. *N Engl J Med* 1970;282:421.
204. Kellgren JH. Epidemiology of rheumatoid arthritis. *Arthritis Rheum* 1966;9:658.
205. Clifford BD, Donahue D, Smith L, et al. High prevalence of serological markers of autoimmunity in patients with chronic hepatitis C. *Hepatology* 1995;21:613.
206. Juby AG, Davis P, McElhaney JE, Gravenstein S. Prevalence of selected autoantibodies in different elderly subpopulations. *Br J Rheumatol* 1994;33:1121.
207. Shmerling RH, Delbanco TL. How useful is the rheumatoid factor? An analysis of sensitivity, specificity, and predictive value. *Arch Intern Med* 1992;152:2417.
208. van der Heijde DM, van Riel PL, van Rijswijk MH, van de Putte LB. Influence of prognostic features on the final outcome in rheumatoid arthritis: a review of the literature. *Semin Arthritis Rheum* 1988;17:284.
209. Bermas BL, Schur PH, Rose BD. Clinical manifestations and diagnosis of the antiphospholipid antibody syndrome. In: Rose B, Schur PH, eds. *Uptodate in Medicine*. Wellesley, MA: UpToDate, Inc., 1998.
210. Sammaritano LR, Gharavi AE, Lockshin MD. Antiphospholipid antibody syndrome: immunologic and clinical aspects. *Semin Arthritis Rheum* 1990;20:81.
211. Santoro SA. Antiphospholipid antibodies and thrombotic predisposition: underlying pathogenetic mechanisms. *Blood* 1994;83:2389.
212. Roubey RA. Immunology of the antiphospholipid antibody syndrome. *Arthritis Rheum* 1996;39:1444.
213. Asherson RA, Khamashta MA, Ordi-Ros J, et al. The "primary" antiphospholipid syndrome: major clinical and serological features. *Medicine (Baltimore)* 1989;68:366.
214. Triplett DA, Brandt JT, Musgrave KA. Relationship between lupus anticoagulants and antibodies to phospholipids. *JAMA* 1988;259:550.
215. Sammaritano LR, Ng S, Sobel R, et al. Anticardiolipin IgG subclasses: association of IgG2 with arterial and/or venous thrombosis. *Arthritis Rheum* 1997;40:1998.
216. Day HM, Thiagarajan P, Ahn C, et al. Autoantibodies to beta(2)-glycoprotein I in systemic lupus erythematosus and primary antiphospholipid antibody syndrome: clinical correlations in comparison with other antiphospholipid antibody tests. *J Rheumatol* 1998;5:667.
217. Hörkkö S, Miller E, Dudl E, et al. Antiphospholipid antibodies are directed against epitopes of oxidized phospholipid. *J Clin Invest* 1996;98:815.
218. Roubey RA, Pratt CW, Buyon JP, Winfield JB. Lupus anticoagulant activity of autoimmune antiphospholipid antibodies is dependent upon β2-glycoprotein I. *J Clin Invest* 1992;90:1100.
219. Cabral AR, Cabiedes J, Alarcon-Segovia D. Antibodies to phospholipid-free beta 2-glycoprotein-I in patients with primary antiphospholipid syndrome. *J Rheumatol* 1995;22:1894.
220. Cabiedes J, Cabral AR, Alarcon-Segovia D. Clinical manifestations of the antiphospholipid syndrome in patients with systemic lupus erythematosus associate more strongly with anti-beta 2-glycoprotein-I than with antiphospholipid antibodies. *J Rheumatol* 1995;22:1899.
221. Shapiro SS. The lupus anticoagulant/antiphospholipid syndrome. *Annu Rev Med* 1996;47:533.
222. Roubey RA, Maldonado MA, Byrd SN. Comparison of an enzyme-linked immunosorbent assay for antibodies to beta2-glycoprotein I and a conventional anticardiolipin immunoassay. *Arthritis Rheum* 1996;39:1606.
223. Schousboe I. Beta-2 glycoprotein 1: a plasma inhibitor of the contact activation of the intrinsic blood coagulation pathway. *Blood* 1985;66:1086.
224. Nimpf J, Bevers EM, Bomans PH, Till U. Prothrombinase activity of human platelets is influenced by beta-2-glycoprotein 1. *Biochim Biophys Acta* 1986;884:142.
225. Harris EN, Gharavi A, Asherson RA, et al. Antiphospholipid antibodies—middle aged but robust. *J Rheumatol* 1994;21:6.
226. Cabral AR, Amigo C, Cabiedes J, Alarcon-Segovia D. The antiphospholipid/cofactor syndromes: a primary variant with antibodies to beta 2-glycoprotein-I but no antibodies detectable in standard antiphospholipid assays. *Am J Med* 1996;101:472.
227. Fields RA, Toubbeh H, Searles RP, Bankhurst AD. The prevalence of anticardiolipin antibodies in a healthy elderly population and its association with antinuclear antibodies. *J Rheumatol* 1989;16:623.
228. Vila P, Hernandez MC, Lopez-Fernandez MF, Battle J. Prevalence, follow-up and clinical significance of the anticardiolipin antibodies in normal subjects. *Thromb Haemost* 1994;72:20.
229. Manoussakis MN, Tzioufas AG, Silis MP, et al. High prevalence of anti-cardiolipin and other autoantibodies in a healthy elderly population. *Clin Exp Immunol* 1987;68:557.
230. Shi W, Krilis SA, Chong BH, et al. Prevalence of lupus anticoagulant in a healthy population: lack of correlation with anticardiolipin antibodies. *Aust N Z J Med* 1990;20:231.
231. McNeil HP, Chesterman CN, Krilis SA. Immunology and clinical importance of antiphospholipid antibodies. *Adv Immunol* 1991;49:193.
232. Melk A, Mueller Eckhardt G, Polten B, et al. Diagnostic and prognostic significance of anticardiolipin antibodies in patients with recurrent spontaneous abortions. *Am J Reprod Immunol* 1995;33:228.
233. Picillo U, Migliaresi S, Marcialis MR, et al. Clinical significance of anticardiolipin antibodies in patients with systemic sclerosis. *Autoimmunity* 1995;20:1.
234. Chakravarty K, Pountain G, Merry P, et al. A longitudinal study of anticardiolipin antibody in polymyalgia rheumatica and giant cell arteritis. *J Rheumatol* 1995;22:1694.
235. Ruffatti A, Veller-Fornasa C, Patrassi GM, et al. Anticardiolipin antibodies and antiphospholipid syndrome in chronic discoid lupus erythematosus. *Clin Rheumatol* 1995;14:402.
236. Carreira PE, Montalvo MG, Kaufman LD, et al. Antiphospholipid antibodies in patients with eosinophilia myalgia and toxic oil syndrome. *J Rheumatol* 1997;24:69.
237. Vayssairat M, Abuaf N, Baudot N, et al. Abnormal IgG cardiolipin antibody titers in patients with Raynaud's phenomenon and/or related disorders: prevalence and clinical significance. *J Am Acad Dermatol* 1998;38:555.
238. McNally T, Purdy G, Mackie IJ, et al. The use of anti-beta 2-glycoprotein-I assay for discrimination between anticardiolipin antibodies associated with infection and increased risk of thrombosis. *Br J Haematol* 1995;91:471.
239. Merrill JT, Shen C, Gugnani M, et al. High prevalence of antiphospholipid antibodies in patients taking procainamide. *J Rheumatol* 1997;24:1083.
240. Devine DV, Brigden ML. The anti-phospholipid antibody syndrome. *Postgrad Med* 1996;99:105.
241. Davies TF. Pathogenesis of Hashimoto's thyroiditis (chronic autoimmune thyroiditis). In: Rose B, Schur PH, eds. *Uptodate in Medicine*. Wellesley, MA: UpToDate, Inc., 1998.
242. Davies TF. Pathogenesis of Graves' disease. In: Rose B, Schur PH, eds. *Uptodate in Medicine*. Wellesley, MA: UpToDate, Inc., 1998.
243. Nagayama Y, Rapoport B. The thyrotropin receptor 25 years after its discovery: new insight after its molecular cloning. *Mol Endocrinol* 1992;6:145.
244. Kraiem Z, Lahat N, Glaser B, et al. Thyrotropin receptor blocking antibodies: incidence, characterization and in vitro synthesis. *Clin Endocrinol* 1987;27:409.

245. Wilson R, McKillop JH, Henderson N, et al. The ability of the serum TSH receptor antibody index and HLA status to predict long-term remission of thyrotoxicosis following medical therapy for Graves' disease. *Clin Endocrinol* 1986;25:151.

246. Feldt-Rasmussen U, Schleusner H, Carayon P. Meta-analysis evaluation of the impact of thyrotropin receptor antibodies on long term remission after medical therapy of Graves' disease. *J Clin Endocrinol Metab* 1994;78:98.

247. Aizawa Y, Yoshida K, Kaise N, et al. Long-term effects of radioiodine on thyrotrophin receptor antibodies in Graves' disease. *Clin Endocrinol (Oxf)* 1995;42:517.

248. Morris JC, Bergert ER, Bryant WP. Binding of immunoglobulin G from patients with autoimmune thyroid disease to rat sodium-iodide symporter peptides: evidence for the iodide transporter as an autoantigen. *Thyroid* 1997;7:527.

249. McCulloch DK. Pathogenesis of type 1 (insulin-dependent) diabetes mellitus. In: Rose B, Schur PH, eds. *Uptodate in Medicine*. Wellesley, MA: UpToDate, Inc., 1998.

250. Atkinson MA, Maclaren NK. Mechanisms of disease: the pathogenesis of insulin-dependent diabetes mellitus. *N Engl J Med* 1994;331:1428.

251. Tisch R, McDevitt H. Insulin-dependent diabetes mellitus. *Cell* 1996;85:291.

252. Aanstoot HJ, Kang SM, Kim J, et al. Identification and characterization of glima 38, a glycosylated islet cell membrane antigen, which together with GAD65 and IA2 marks the early phases of autoimmune response in type 1 diabetes. *J Clin Invest* 1996;97:2772.

253. Hawa M, Rowe R, Lan MS, et al. Value of antibodies to islet protein tyrosine phosphatase-like molecule in predicting type 1 diabetes. *Diabetes* 1997;46:1270.

254. Kaufman DL, Clare-Salzler M, Tian J, et al. Spontaneous loss of T-cell tolerance to glutamic acid decarboxylase in murine insulin-dependent diabetes. *Nature* 1993;366:69.

255. Khalil I, d'Auriol L, Gobet M, et al. A combination of HLA-DQb Asp[57]-negative and HLA DQa Arg[52] confers susceptibility to insulin-dependent diabetes mellitus. *J Clin Invest* 1990;85:1315.

256. Eisenbarth GS. Mouse or man: is GAD the cause of type I diabetes? *Diabetes Care* 1994;17:605.

257. Ziegler AG, Hillebrand B, Rabl W, et al. On the appearance of islet associated autoimmunity in offspring of diabetic mothers: a prospective study from birth. *Diabetologia* 1993;36:402.

258. Ko IY, Jun HS, Kim GS, Yoon JW. Studies on autoimmunity for initiation of beta-cell destruction. X. Delayed expression of a membrane-bound islet cell-specific 38 kDa autoantigen that precedes insulitis and diabetes in the diabetes-prone BB rat. *Diabetologia* 1994;37:460.

259. Ellis TM, Schatz DA, Ottendorfer EW, et al. The relationship between humoral and cellular immunity to IA-2 in IDDM. *Diabetes* 1998;47:566.

260. Brewer KW, Parziale VS, Eisenbarth GS. Screening patients with insulin-dependent diabetes mellitus for adrenal insufficiency [Letter]. *N Engl J Med* 1997;337:202.

261. Cronin CC, Shanahan F. Insulin-dependent diabetes mellitus and coeliac disease. Lancet 1997;349:1096.

262. Orth DN. Pathogenesis of autoimmune adrenal insufficiency. In: Rose B, Schur PH, eds. *Uptodate in Medicine*. Wellesley, MA: UpToDate, Inc., 1998.

263. Blizzard RM, Chee D, Davis W. The incidence of adrenal and other antibodies in the sera of patients with idiopathic adrenal insufficiency (Addison's disease). *Clin Exp Immunol* 1967;2:19.

264. Irvine WJ, Barnes EW. Addison's disease, ovarian failure and hypoparathyroidism. *Clin Endocrinol Metab* 1975;4:379.

265. Colls J, Betterle C, Volpato M, et al. Immunoprecipitation assay for autoantibodies to steroid 21-hydroxylase in autoimmune adrenal diseases. *Clin Chem* 1995;41:375.

266. Falorni A, Nikoshkov A, Laureti S, et al. High diagnostic accuracy for idiopathic Addison's disease with a sensitive radiobinding assay for autoantibodies against recombinant human 21-hydroxylase. *J Clin Endocrinol Metab* 1995;80:2752.

267. Ahonen P, Miettinen A, Perheentupa J. Adrenal and steroidal cell antibodies in patients with autoimmune polyglandular disease type I and risk of adrenocortical and ovarian failure. *J Clin Endocrinol Metab* 1987;64:494.

268. Betterle C, Scalici C, Presotto F, et al. The natural history of adrenal function in autoimmune patients with adrenal autoantibodies. *J Endocrinol* 1988;117:467.

269. Boscaro M, Betterle C, Sonino N, et al. Early adrenal hypofunction in patients with organ-specific autoantibodies and no clinical adrenal insufficiency. *J Clin Endocrinol Metab* 1994;79:452.

270. Song YH, Connor EL, Muir A, et al. Autoantibody epitope mapping of the 21-hydroxylase antigen in autoimmune Addison's disease. *J Clin Endocrinol Metab* 1994;78:1108.

271. Betterle C, Volpato M, Rees Smith B, et al. II. Adrenal cortex and steroid 21-hydroxylase autoantibodies in children with organ-specific autoimmune diseases: markers of high progression to clinical Addison's disease. *J Clin Endocrinol Metab* 1997;82:939.

272. Zelissen PM, Bast EJ, Croughs RJ. Associated autoimmunity in Addison's disease. *J Autoimmun* 1995;8:121.

273. Herman JH. Diagnostic evaluation of relapsing polychondritis. In: Rose B, Schur PH, eds. *Uptodate in Medicine*. Wellesley, MA: UpToDate, Inc., 1998.

274. Ebinger R, Rook G, Swana GT, et al. Antibodies to cartilage and type II collagen in relapsing polychondritis and other rheumatic diseases. *Ann Rheum Dis* 1981;40:473.

275. Charriere J, Hartman DJ, Vignon E, et al. Antibodies to types I, II, IX, and XI collagen in the serum of patients with rheumatic diseases. *Arthritis Rheum* 1988;31:325.

276. Terato K, Shimozuru Y, Katayama K, et al. Specificity of antibodies to type II collagen in rheumatoid arthritis. *Arthritis Rheum* 1990;33:1493.

277. Yang CL, Brinckmann J, Rui HF, et al. Autoantibodies to cartilage collagens in relapsing polychondritis. *Arch Dermatol Res* 1993; 285:245.

278. Alsalameh S, Mollenhauer J, Scheuplein F, et al. Preferential cellular and humoral immune reactivities to native and denatured collagen types IX and XI in a patient with fatal relapsing polychondritis. *J Rheumatol* 1993;20:1419.

*Textbook of the Autoimmune Diseases,*
Edited by R. G. Lahita, N. Chiorazzi, and W. H. Reeves,
Lippincott Williams & Wilkins, Philadelphia © 2000.

# CHAPTER 41

# Autoimmunity Induced by Metals

Pierluigi E. Bigazzi

Clinical reports and experimental investigations have demonstrated that chronic exposure of human subjects and laboratory animals to xenobiotics can affect the immune system and cause immunosuppression or allergic and autoimmune reactions (1–8). Xenobiotics are foreign substances of synthetic, natural, or biologic origin that may be present in the environment or are administered for therapeutic reasons. They comprise industrial chemicals, drugs, and cytokines. In particular, many metals can cause a decrease or enhancement of immune responses. For each metal discussed in this chapter, I first provide a summary of its effects on the cellular components of the immune system and its possible allergic activity. I then examine its reported autoimmune effects.

The demonstration that some metals act on the immune system does not necessarily imply that they have autoimmune consequences. From this point of view, it is important to distinguish different groups of metals. The first group, comprising arsenic, beryllium, nickel, vanadium, and iron, has recognized immunotoxic activity but is characterized by the lack of well-documented reports of autoimmune responses or autoimmune disease (9). It is difficult to explain why nickel, generally considered as the most common cause of human cutaneous allergy (10), does not also induce autoimmunity. A second group, including zinc, copper, chromium, lead, cadmium, platinum, and silver, is capable of affecting the immune system but has been only occasionally associated with autoimmune responses in human subjects or experimental animals. Overall, these metals do not seem to be potent inducers of autoimmunity, despite their recognized immunotoxic effects. Exposure to lithium, gold, and mercury has been clearly linked with autoimmune responses and autoimmune disease. These activities are discussed because they have theoretical and practical interest. Some of the animal models caused by administration of metals may provide information applicable to the much wider areas of xenobiotic-induced autoimmunity and on "idiopathic" autoimmune disease (11).

## METALS OCCASIONALLY ASSOCIATED WITH AUTOIMMUNITY

In this group are several metals (i.e., zinc, copper, chromium, lead, cadmium, platinum, and silver) and a metalloid (silicon) that have *in vitro* and *in vivo* effects on the immune system (9). However, their autoimmune effects have been reported only occasionally and are still uncertain (Table 41.1).

### Silicon

Crystalline silicon is a nonmetallic, light element whose dioxide is silica. It is included in this review as a xenobiotic close to metals (i.e., metalloid) that has been associated with autoimmune manifestations (12,13).

#### *Effects of Silicon on Cells of the Immune System*

A review of the literature revealed no published studies of silicon effects on lymphocytes, macrophages, and other cells of the immune system. Such a lack of experimental data is surprising, considering its reported autoimmune effects and the hypothesized links with the activity of high molecular weight polymeric siloxanes (14).

#### *Silicon-Induced Allergy*

I have found no reports of allergic reactions induced by silicon, even though this element is known to accumulate in dialysis patients (15).

#### *Autoimmune Effects of Silicon*

##### *Human Autoimmune Disease*

The inhalation of silicon dusts, which results in the occupational disease called *silicosis*, stimulates the production of antinuclear antibodies (ANAs) and rheumatoid factors. Some patients experience a systemic lupus erythematosus–like or scleroderma-like syndrome, with deposition of immune

P. E. Bigazzi: Department of Pathology, University of Connecticut School of Medicine, Farmington, Connecticut 06030.

**TABLE 41.1.** *Metals associated with autoimmunity*

| Metal | Autoimmune responses (human and/or animal) | Human autoimmune disease | Animal autoimmune disease |
|---|---|---|---|
| Cadmium | Autoantibodies to laminin 1 | None reported | None reported |
| Chromium | Antinuclear antibodies | SLE-like syndrome, pemphigus | None reported |
| Copper | Autoantibodies to red cells | None reported | None reported |
| Gold | Anti-Ro autoantibodies, antiplatelet autoantibodies, ANA | Autoimmune kidney disease, autoimmune thrombocytopenia, SLE-like syndrome, pemphigus | Autoimmune kidney disease |
| Lead | IgM autoantibodies to NF160 and MBP IgG autoantibodies to NF-68 and GFAP | None reported | None reported |
| Lithium | Autoantibodies to thyroglobulin, autoantibodies to thyroid peroxidase, ANA, autoantibodies to gastric parietal cells | Autoimmune thyroid disease, SLE-like syndrome | Autoimmune thyroid disease |
| Mercury | Autoantibodies to fibrillarin, autoantibodies to laminin 1, autoantibodies to DNA, autoantibodies to thyroglobulin | Autoimmune kidney disease, lichen planus, scleroderma-like disease | Autoimmune kidney disease, GvH-like disease, arthritis, vasculitis |
| Platinum | ANA | None reported | None reported |
| Silicon (silica) | ANA | Scleroderma-like syndrome | None reported |
| Silver | Autoantibodies to fibrillarin | None reported | None reported |
| Zinc | None reported to date | Multiple sclerosis cluster (?) | None reported |

ANA, antinuclear antibodies; GvH, graft-versus-host; SLE, systemic lupus erythematosus.

complexes in the glomeruli and focal renal glomerulosclerosis (16). Patients with silicosis have higher levels of antibodies to type I and type III collagen (17). A fulminant form of silicosis known as *silicoproteinosis* is characterized by elevated levels of ANA and rapidly progressive crescentic glomerulonephritis (16).

### *Autoimmune Disease in Experimental Animals*

In experimental animals, silicon has strong adjuvant activity in the induction of experimental allergic encephalomyelitis (EAE) when mixed with spinal cord homogenate (18). Pretreatment of LEW rats with silicon accelerates the onset and increases the incidence and severity of EAE (19). Rats with silicosis have higher cell numbers in thoracic lymph nodes, with increases in T cells, B cells, natural killer (NK) cells, and macrophages (20). A significantly higher percentage of activated CD8+ and CD4+ T cells was present in their lymph nodes.

### Zinc

Zinc is a trace element critical for a variety of cellular activities. It is essential as a cofactor for many enzymes. Deficiencies or excesses of this metal may have important pathophysiologic consequences.

### *Effects of Zinc on Cells of the Immune System*

Zinc has a major role in the induction of immune responses, because specific and nonspecific immunity are conditioned by adequate levels of this metal (21). Antibody responses are

significantly suppressed in humans and experimental animals with zinc deficiencies. Development and maintenance of cellular immunity also depend on this metal.

### *Zinc-Induced Allergy*

Despite its stimulatory effects on the immune system, zinc is a rare cause of allergic reactions. A case of allergic dermatitis to a shampoo containing zinc pirithione has been reported (22).

### *Autoimmune Effects of Zinc*

Zinc's involvement in autoimmune responses is rather hypothetical and is related to its consideration as a possible risk factor for multiple sclerosis (MS) (23–26).

### *Human Autoimmune Disease*

Areas with high MS prevalence rates have significantly higher concentrations of soluble zinc in the soil compared with control areas with a lower MS prevalence rate. Zinc levels are significantly elevated in erythrocytes from patients with MS and vary with disease activity (27). A cluster of MS with high zinc levels has also been reported (23). Eleven cases of MS were diagnosed within a 10-year period in a zinc-related manufacturing plant, an incidence greater than expected from population data. The MS patients and controls working in that plant had higher serum zinc levels than subjects (MS and controls) not working there. Because immunologic studies of this cluster of MS patients were not performed, the connection between zinc and autoimmune mechanisms in MS is still hypothetical. I also found no published reports of zinc's association with other autoimmune diseases, which suggests that this metal does not have autoimmune effects.

### Autoimmune Disease in Experimental Animals

To obtain experimental evidence supporting the hypothesis that zinc may be involved in the pathogenesis of MS, dietary supplements of this metal were administered to SJL/J mice (24–26). Zinc appeared to affect the incidence and severity of EAE induced by immunization with syngeneic spinal cord homogenate. EAE was observed in 17% of mice on a control diet, 25% of mice on a high-zinc diet, and 5% of mice on a high-nickel diet. The severity of inflammation and demyelination was also higher in zinc-treated mice than in the other groups. However, these differences were not statistically significant. In conclusion, studies of experimental animals have provided some clues but not a convincing demonstration that zinc can induce or modulate EAE or MS.

## Copper

Copper is an essential element, a constituent of every natural food product (28). The major route of host exposure is by ingestion. Deficiencies or excesses of this metal may have important pathophysiologic consequences.

### Effects of Copper on Cells of the Immune System

Adequate levels of copper are required for normal immune response to occur (28). Overall, the experimental evidence available suggests that specific and nonspecific immunity are more sensitive to deficiencies than excesses of copper.

### Copper-Induced Allergy

Contact dermatitis is one of the major immunologic consequences of exposure to copper compounds (28).

### Autoimmune Effects of Copper

*Human Autoimmune Disease*

I have found no published reports of autoimmune responses induced by copper in humans.

*Autoimmune Disease in Experimental Animals*

Mice exposed to copper in their drinking water show an increased production of autoantibodies to red cells, an increase that is not modified by augmenting their zinc supply (29).

## Chromium

Chromium has numerous industrial uses in metallurgy and in the manufacture of paints, preservatives, and other products.

Despite its pathogenic potential as a frequent cause of contact hypersensitivity, it is usually not associated with autoimmunity (28).

### Effects of Chromium on Cells of the Immune System

The effects of chromium on the various cellular components of the immune system have not received much attention. However, this metal seems to have suppressive rather than stimulatory activity on T and B lymphocytes (9). One study of chromium exposed workers has detected significant reductions of $CD4^+$ T lymphocytes, B lymphocytes, and NK cells (30). A reduced production of interleukin-6 (IL-6) was observed in individuals from Hudson County, New Jersey, an area contaminated with chromium (31). These results are difficult to understand, considering the recognized allergic potential of chromium.

### Chromium-Induced Allergy

Chromium metal is insoluble and seems to have scarce potential to sensitize (10,32). However, its salts are a common cause of contact dermatitis and occupational asthma (10).

### Autoimmune Effects of Chromium

As for the other metals discussed above, there are only sparse reports of autoimmunity related to chromium.

*Human Autoimmune Disease*

Long-term low-dose exposure to inorganic chromium and other chemicals in contaminated well water has been associated with increased symptoms and signs of SLE (33). One case of pemphigus developing after occupational contact with basochrom (basic chromium sulfate) was reported in 1990 (34). Immune-mediated renal disease has not been observed after industrial exposure to chromium (16).

*Autoimmune Disease in Experimental Animals*

A literature search revealed no reports of chromium-induced autoimmunity in experimental animals. An investigation of delayed-type hypersensitivity to chromium in various strains of mice revealed genetic control influenced by the I-A region of H-2 (35).

## Lead

The toxic and immunotoxic activity of lead is well known (36). It is still employed in the production of storage batteries, but its use in gasoline, paints, solders, and plumbing supplies has decreased considerably in recent years.

### Effects of Lead on Cells of the Immune System

The immune system appears to be an excellent target for low-dose lead toxicity (37,38). Lead, like silver, copper, cadmium, and mercury, has high affinity for thiol groups, which are essential for the functional performance of immune cells (39). Not surprisingly, early investigations of the immunomodulatory effects of lead demonstrated that *in vitro* exposure of lymphocytes to this metal resulted in enhanced responsiveness to mitogens and increased B-cell differentiation and T-cell proliferation (40). The same group reported that lead and mercury stimulated *in vitro* IL-4 production by a murine $T_H2$ clone and inhibited interferon-$\gamma$ (IFN-$\gamma$) production by a murine $T_H1$ clone (41). The same investigators detected higher IL-4 and lower IFN-$\gamma$ levels in plasma of BALB/c mice exposed to $PbCl_2$ or $HgCl_2$. When spleen T cells from *in vivo* lead-treated mice were stimulated *in vitro* with anti-CD3, there was an increase in IL-4 and a decrease in IFN-$\gamma$ production (41).

### Lead-Induced Allergy

Despite its well-demonstrated effects on cells of the immune system and the suggestion that lead can stimulate type 2 cytokine production, there are no published reports of allergic disease caused by this metal.

### Autoimmune Effects of Lead

Considering that lead has immunostimulatory effects similar to those of mercury, it was logical to expect that it could also induce autoimmune responses and disease (40,42). However, early suggestions that lead can cause an immune-mediated nephropathy have not been confirmed (16,43,44). One study has found no evidence of marked immunotoxic effects of lead in occupationally exposed workers (45).

#### Human Autoimmune Disease

Three clinical forms of lead-induced kidney disease are recognized. Brief but massive lead absorption causes an acute lead nephropathy, with a transient Fanconi syndrome (i.e., aminoaciduria, glycosuria, phosphaturia, and hypercalciuria). Cumulative excessive lead absorption, often without symptomatic acute lead poisoning, results in a chronic slowly progressive interstitial nephritis. One half of the patients with this type of lead nephropathy also exhibit gout. The kidney shows the characteristic signs of relatively acellular tubulointerstitial nephritis. The third form is observed in low-level exposure to environmental lead and is characterized by hypertension arising in the absence of symptomatic lead intoxication and before the clinical appearance of renal failure. None of these nephropathies have indications suggesting autoimmunity.

More exciting are reports that autoantibodies against neuroproteins (e.g., neurofilament triplet proteins) predominated in cohorts of lead-exposed workers (46). Titers of autoantibodies to NF-68, NF-160, NF-200, GFAP, and MBP were determined by enzyme-linked immunosorbent assay (ELISA). Higher levels of IgM autoantibodies against NF-160 and

MBP, as well as IgG autoantibodies against GFAP, were detected in these subjects. Hopefully, these observations will be pursued and confirmed by additional detailed studies. In that case, lead may join lithium, gold, and mercury in the group of metals with autoimmune activity.

#### Autoimmune Disease in Experimental Animals

In a literature search, we found only one report of autoimmunity induced in experimental animals by treatment with lead. Male Fischer rats exposed to 50 or 450 ppm lead acetate in drinking water developed IgM and IgG autoantibodies to neuroproteins (46). In another study, the plasma of BALB/c mice treated with $PbCl_2$ had increased IL-4 and lower IFN-$\gamma$ levels (41). However, there was no mention of autoimmune responses, which suggests that they were not detected in those mice.

### Cadmium

Cadmium is used for many industrial purposes (e.g., manufacturing of batteries, pigments, metal coatings), but the largest potential sources of exposure for humans are food and cigarette smoke (47).

### Effects of Cadmium on Cells of the Immune System

This heavy metal has well-demonstrated immunotoxic properties (9). Suppression or potentiation of antibody responses and cellular immunity has been observed *in vitro* and *in vivo* after exposure to cadmium.

### Cadmium-Induced Allergy

A survey of the literature has not revealed published reports of allergic disease caused by cadmium. Immediate hypersensitivity reactions caused by cadmium must be very rare or nonexistent, which contrasts with the well-demonstrated immunotoxic activities of this metal and is reminiscent of the situation previously discussed for lead.

### Autoimmune Effects of Cadmium

It would not be surprising if cadmium had autoimmune effects in humans. However, the published literature does not support this suggestion.

#### Human Autoimmune Disease

Workers exposed to cadmium may develop low-molecular-weight proteinuria, tubulointerstitial nephritis, and occasionally glomerular damage (16). However, there is no solid evidence demonstrating that their renal pathology is caused by immune mechanisms. Similarly, reports that occupational exposure to cadmium induced the production of autoantibodies to laminin or other autoimmune responses have not been confirmed (48).

*Autoimmune Disease in Experimental Animals*

The oral administration of cadmium to outbred Sprague–Dawley rats induced a diffuse membranous glomerulonephritis after 30 weeks of exposure (49). Electron microscopy revealed irregular thickening of the glomerular basement membrane (GBM) and electron-opaque deposits within mesangial cells. Granular IgG deposits were observed within most glomeruli. It has also been reported that rats treated with cadmium have circulating antilaminin antibodies (50). Sprague–Dawley and Brown Norway (BN) rats were chronically exposed to cadmium administered in their drinking water or by intraperitoneal injection. Antibodies to laminin were transiently detected in the sera of Sprague–Dawley rats but not BN rats. Circulating antibodies to type IV collagen and linear deposits of immunoglobulins in the kidneys were not present in either group of rats. After 13 months of exposure to cadmium, granular renal deposits of immunoglobulins were observed in 25% of animals, a prevalence not significantly different from that observed in control rats. Renal immune deposits were not detected in C57BL/6 mice exposed to cadmium in their drinking water (51). ICR mice treated with cadmium for a period of 10 weeks developed ANAs (52). BALB/c mice were less susceptible than ICR mice to the autoimmune effects of cadmium, which occurred only after the administration of higher doses of this metal. Mice chronically treated with cadmium develop T cells against stress protein HSP70 and show renal tubular damage followed by peritubular inflammation and interstitial fibrosis (53). These studies of rats and mice suggest that cadmium may induce autoimmunity but only in certain genetically predisposed individuals.

## Platinum

Platinum has a variety of industrial and therapeutic uses (54). It also has diverse effects on the immune system, with the potential to induce allergic and autoimmune reactions.

### *Effects of Platinum on Cells of the Immune System*

Few studies have examined the immunotoxic effects of compounds containing platinum (54). However, some chemotherapeutic agents that contain this metal (e.g., cisplatin) may stimulate or inhibit immune responses of human and murine lymphocytes.

### *Platinum-Induced Allergy*

Investigations of workers with occupational exposure to complex platinum salts have detected a variety of allergic responses, mediated by immediate and delayed hypersensitivity reactions (54). There are occasional reports of contact stomatitis due to sensitization to platinum, alone or combined with palladium (55).

### *Autoimmune Effects of Platinum*

A survey of the literature revealed only a few publications on the autoimmune effects of platinum compounds.

### *Human Autoimmune Disease*

An occasional case of scleroderma has been associated with cisplatin treatment, but there are no detailed reports of autoimmune responses or autoimmune disease in humans exposed to platinum (6,56).

### *Autoimmune Disease in Experimental Animals*

Experimental animal studies have failed to demonstrate allergic reactions but have shown specific immune responses to platinum-containing compounds (54). In particular, a selective production of type 2 cytokines has been observed *in vitro* using cultures of lymph node cells from mice exposed to platinum salts (57). Investigations of laboratory animals injected with this metal have revealed T-cell–dependent popliteal lymph node reactions and the induction of autoimmunity (58,59). Mice of the C57/BL6 strain produce ANAs after 14 weeks of treatment (subcutaneous injections of 0.4 or 2.0 µg three times per week) with $Na_2PtCl_6$. Similarly treated B10.S mice did not experience autoimmune responses.

## Silver

Exposure to silver can occur as a result of industrial activities (an occurrence that is relatively rare) or the use of certain medical and dental products (60). In the past, this metal was administered orally as silver nitrate for the treatment of peptic ulcers or applied to mucous membranes in the form of colloidal silver compounds. Currently, silver is used as a component of certain antibacterial drugs for the treatment of burns (silver sulfadiazine), dietary supplements, catheters, acupuncture needles, iontophoretic devices, and dental amalgam. Silver has traditionally been classified in the "minor toxic metals" category and usually receives scarce attention in toxicology textbooks (61). Chronic exposure to this metal may result in argyria (or argyrosis), characterized by a slate blue-gray discoloration of the skin. A similar pigmentation of the conjunctiva may be caused by long-term instillation of drops containing soluble silver preparations or after occupational exposure to silver compounds in dry form or in solution, in circumstances that allow their inhalation or ingestion over long periods (62). These patients may have silver in lymph nodes, spleen, and lungs. Effects on the nervous system have been rarely reported, but a review of metal toxicity on the choroid plexus mentions a 72-year-old patient, who developed argyria after 2 to 5 years of using nose drops containing a silver preparation and had deposits of this metal at the level of the epithelial basal lamina of the choroid plexus (63).

### Effects of Silver on Cells of the Immune System

Immunotoxicology studies of silver are scarce. Some reviews of the immunotoxicology of drugs and chemicals do not even include silver (9). A study published in 1920 found *in vitro* enhancement or inhibition of guinea pig complement activity by different concentrations of silver (42). Later investigations demonstrated that, as previously observed for other metals, silver has a variety of immunotoxic effects that depend on its concentration (64). *In vitro* studies have shown that silver inhibits the respiratory burst activity of human lymphocytes and neutrophils, increases superoxide production by human neutrophils and has cytotoxic effects on human lymphocytes, including T and B cells. Lipid peroxidation of mouse peritoneal macrophages is increased by exposure to silver. These various activities are not surprising, considering that silver, like copper, cadmium, lead, and mercury, has a high affinity for thiol groups, which are essential components for the functional performance of immune cells (39).

### Silver-Induced Allergy

A survey of the literature revealed one report suggesting that silver may have allergenic potential (65). In comparative patch testing of various dental alloys, reactions to silver nitrate ranked at an intermediate level, below those to nickel sulfate, potassium dichromate, and cobalt nitrate, and above responses to copper sulfate, palladium chloride, and platinum chloride.

### Autoimmune Effects of Silver

Despite its reported effects on various components of the immune system, silver does not seem to be a common cause of allergic or autoimmune disease. However, it is capable of inducing autoimmune responses in experimental animals.

#### Human Autoimmune Disease

I have found no published reports of silver-induced autoimmune disease in humans. Studies in mice suggest that it may induce autoimmune responses that do not result in disease.

#### Autoimmune Disease in Experimental Animals

It is to the credit of Hultman et al. to have discovered the autoimmune effects of silver on mice of various strains (66–68). The peritoneal implantation of alloy (the non–mercury-containing component of dental fillings) in SJL mice was followed by the development of circulating autoantibodies to nucleolar antigens (66). This observation was pursued in a follow-up study, in which SJL/N mice treated with silver nitrate in their drinking water (0.05% or 0.01% for 5 to 10 weeks) were found to develop IgG antinucleolar autoantibodies after 5 weeks (67). High titers of these autoantibodies

were detected during the following 5 weeks. The clumpy nucleolar staining observed by indirect immunofluorescence was similar to that observed in mercury-treated mice with circulating autoantibodies to the nucleolar protein fibrillarin. In additional studies, Hultman et al. observed that antinucleolar autoantibodies developed in all silver nitrate-treated SJL/N, A.SW, A.TH, and B10.G mice; in 60% of B10.S mice; and 22% of B10.S(9R) mice (68). Similarly treated A.TL, B6, and DBA mice did not develop any antinucleolar autoantibodies. Immunoblotting showed that sera from mice with antinucleolar autoantibodies detected by indirect immunofluorescence reacted with a 34-kd nucleolar protein (i.e., fibrillarin). The development of these autoantibodies depends on susceptibility genes in the H-2A locus and on non-H-2 background genes. Mice with circulating antinucleolar autoantibodies had no significant immune deposits in their kidneys.

## METALS THAT FACILITATE OR INDUCE AUTOIMMUNITY

This group of elements comprises a light metal (lithium) and two heavy metals (gold and mercury) that, in addition to their *in vitro* and *in vivo* activities on the immune system, have been clearly associated with autoimmune responses and autoimmune disease in humans and experimental animals (9) (Table 41.1).

### Lithium

Lithium is a light metal used in the treatment of manic-depressive patients. In addition to its recognized psychiatric effects, it may influence the immune system (69).

### Effects of Lithium on Cells of the Immune System

Lithium has stimulatory effects on T and B lymphocytes, NK cells, macrophages, mast cells, and polymorphonuclear leukocytes (69–71). Most of the investigations on the immunotoxic activity of lithium were performed in the 1980s, at a time when the functional significance of T lymphocyte subsets was not well understood. Little information is available on the effects of this chemical on cytokine profiles.

### Lithium-Induced Allergy

Early reports of lithium allergy have been attributed to hypersensitivity to nonlithium ingredients in commercial preparations (69). The lack of publications on allergic disease caused by lithium suggests that immediate hypersensitivity reactions caused by this metal are rare or still undiscovered. This is surprising, considering lithium's demonstrated immunotoxic effects and in particular its facilitating activity on autoimmune responses.

## Autoimmune Effects of Lithium

### Human Autoimmune Disease

Early reports described lithium-induced adverse effects on thyroid function (6,72–74). Patients treated with lithium for periods up to 2 years develop goiters with a frequency that varies from 4% to 60%, depending on the study and duration of treatment. Overt or subclinical hypothyroidism occurs in 2% to 15% of patients after lithium treatment. These patients show a higher incidence of autoantibodies to thyroglobulin, thyroid peroxidase, or both. Lithium is also associated with the production of antibodies against gastric parietal cells and ANAs.

Investigations of manic-depressive patients tested before and after lithium therapy have shown that only patients who had detectable serum levels of autoantibodies to thyroid antigens before therapy showed an increase in autoantibody titers and hypothyroidism after lithium treatment. This evidence has been interpreted as suggesting that lithium facilitates autoimmunity in patients with a predisposition to autoimmune thyroid disease (72). Lithium has also been associated with a relatively small number of cases of hyperthyroidism with exophthalmos (74). Some have occurred on discontinuation of lithium, while others were observed during lithium therapy. The presence of circulating autoantibodies to the thyroid-stimulating hormone (TSH) receptor was not reported. It is not clear whether lithium treatment can cause autoimmune Graves' disease. Similarly unexplained is the association with exacerbations of myasthenia gravis or the development of a nephrotic syndrome (NS) with minimal change disease (70,71). Lithium does not cause relapses of MS, another disease with a putative autoimmune pathogenesis (70,71).

### Autoimmune Disease in Experimental Animals

Initial research of lithium effects on experimentally induced autoimmune disease showed that this metal had inhibitory activity on Arthus and delayed-type hypersensitivity reactions to thyroglobulin (72). It also decreased the production of autoantibodies to thyroglobulin as well as thyroiditis. Later investigators found that lithium increased the production of autoantibodies to thyroglobulin during the initial stages of autoimmune thyroiditis experimentally induced in rats of the August strain (75). Autoantibody levels decreased if lithium was administered at later stages, when thyroiditis was spontaneously resolving. Treatment with lithium had no effects on the degree of lymphocytic infiltration of the thyroid or on serum TSH. It did not induce production of autoantibodies to thyroglobulin in a group of normal, not immunized rats. These experimental results favor the suggestion (derived from clinical studies) that lithium may have an immunomodulatory effect on existing autoimmune disease but cannot induce autoimmune thyroid disease *de novo*.

## Gold

Gold was traditionally used for the treatment of pruritus, tuberculosis, and syphilis (76). Such practice has been discontinued, but gold compounds are still employed widely for the treatment of rheumatoid arthritis (RA) (77). This metal was considered relatively inert and incapable of adversely affecting the immune system, but its presence in jewelry and its administration to patients with RA have been frequently associated with allergic or autoimmune reactions.

### Effects of Gold on Cells of the Immune System

Gold can modulate metabolic events in phorbol ester-stimulated polymorphonuclear leukocytes and B lymphocytes (78). It is also capable of inhibiting T-cell activation by mitogens and IL-2 production by peptide-specific murine CD4$^+$ T-cell clones (79). Mononuclear phagocytes exposed to Au(I) *in vitro* generate the reactive metabolite Au(III), a possible explanation of the diverse immune responses stimulated by gold-containing compounds (80).

### Gold-Induced Allergy

The main source of skin contact with gold is jewelry, a primary cause of allergic contact dermatitis (10,32). Gold has become one of the most common allergens. In some countries, it is only second to nickel as a cause of cutaneous hypersensitivity reactions (81).

### Autoimmune Effects of Gold

### Human Autoimmune Disease

Preparations containing gold salts are widely used in the treatment of RA and are associated with a variety of autoimmune responses, including case reports of drug-related lupus (82). Gold therapy has been linked with the development of circulating anti-Ro autoantibodies or antidextran antibodies in patients with RA (83). Gold-specific T cells have been detected in RA patients treated with this metal (84). In the period from the late 1960s to the late 1970s, numerous reports described a NS and immune complex-mediated glomerulonephropathy induced by administration of gold (62,83, 85–91). Treatment of RA with gold salts resulted in mild proteinuria in approximately 10% and massive proteinuria in 1% of patients. The NS usually disappeared after gold therapy was discontinued. The relative risk of proteinuria during gold treatment of RA was found to be increased 32 times in HLA-DR3–positive patients, suggesting an immunogenetic influence. Gold directly binds to the HLA-DR molecule (84). Kidney biopsies examined by immunofluorescence showed diffuse granular deposits of IgG and C3 along the glomerular capillary walls (92). IgM and IgA were observed less frequently. Gold was detected in tubular and glomerular tuft epithelial cells but not in the electron-opaque immune deposits (92). Light and electron microscopy revealed a variety of histopathologic changes, including membranous glomerulonephropathy, mesangial glomerulonephritis, or minimal change nephropathy.

Autoimmune thrombocytopenia (ATP) is another complication observed in 1% to 3% of patients receiving gold therapy (93). ATP usually developed after the patient had been treated with gold for several weeks or months. Platelet counts returned to normal within 5 to 7 days after cessation of therapy. However, there are published reports of ATP persisting for longer than 30 days. Drug-dependent antibodies to platelets (i.e., antibodies binding to platelets in the presence of the drug or metabolites of the drug) were detected in the circulation of these patients. An association with HLA-DR3 was reported. Other autoimmune responses or diseases have also been associated with gold treatment, as shown by the occurrence of pemphigus in a RA patient who had previously developed myasthenia gravis after penicillamine treatment (94). It has been suggested that pulmonary fibrosis, a rare complication of gold treatment, might have an autoimmune pathogenesis (95).

### Autoimmune Disease in Experimental Animals

Studies in experimental animals have clarified the autoimmune effects of gold. In initial studies, outbred Wistar rats injected with sodium aurothiomalate developed proteinuria as well as histopathologic and immunohistopathologic lesions similar to those observed in gold-treated patients (96). An immune complex nephropathy was obtained in rabbits fed a preparation of gold oxide, used in India as an oral tonic (97). Guinea pigs injected with sodium aurothiomalate produced autoantibodies to renal tubular antigens, autoimmune tubulointerstitial nephritis, or immune complex nephropathy (98). When exposed to gold salts, BN rats develop autoimmune responses and a membranous glomerulonephropathy mediated by antibodies to the renal GBM (99,100). After treatment with gold, mercury, or penicillamine, mice that bear the H-2$^s$ haplotype exhibit similar autoimmune responses to nucleolar antigens (101). The autoimmune activity of different gold compounds, including some thiol-containing salts, has been examined in rats and mice (99,102). Sulfur-containing groups do not seem to induce autoimmune responses but may potentiate gold's autoimmune effects.

### Mercury

The inorganic and organic forms of mercury have immunotoxic effects (9). Suppression or potentiation of cellular immunity and antibody responses have been observed *in vitro* and *in vivo*. There is also solid evidence that mercury can induce autoimmunity in humans and experimental animals (5,6,8,103). Mercury is widely present in the environment, and its levels are increasing as a consequence of discharges from various industries, medical and scientific waste, and the processing of raw ores. Mercury vapor released from dental amalgam fillings may be a major source of inorganic mercury in humans; its potential health risks are still a source of controversy (104–108).

### Effects of Mercury on Cells of the Immune System

The adverse effects of mercury on various components of the immune system have been reviewed (103). Low concentrations of mercury can depress or stimulate the immune system and even induce autoimmune disease in various animal species through mechanisms that are still incompletely understood. Immunotoxicity studies have found that experimental animals exposed to mercury have a decreased resistance to certain viruses (e.g., pseudorabies, encephalomyocarditis, herpes simplex virus type 2) (109). Mercury may affect early, nonspecific defense mechanisms, interfere with the production of cytokines by macrophages, and change the function of various other components of the immune system. Investigations of its effects on lymphocytes, macrophages, and other immune cells are relevant to human health because they may elucidate the cellular and molecular basis of immunotoxicity induced by mercury and other xenobiotics.

### T Lymphocytes

Old studies using human and animal lymphocytes demonstrated a stimulatory or a inhibitory effect of mercury on T-lymphocyte function (110,111). Early experiments with lymphocytes from BALB/c mice demonstrated that mercury induces mitogenesis, cell-mediated cytotoxicity, and interferon production (112,113). Purified human T cells treated *in vitro* with $HgCl_2$ or MeHgCl have shown a monocyte-dependent inhibition of PHA- and PMA-induced cell proliferation and a decreased production of IL-2 (114). *In vivo* exposure to mercury increases T-lymphocyte responses in BALB/c mice and decreases them in Swiss and (B6×C3)F$_1$ hybrid mice (115). A very low (10 µM) *in vitro* concentration of $HgCl_2$ has been reported to increase the rate of DNA synthesis in murine lymphocytes, with the most significant increase in spleen cells from A.SW and BALB/c mice, strains that experience *in vivo* autoimmune responses to mercury (116). Both CD4$^+$ and CD8$^+$ T cells were activated by mercury in responder mice, whereas only CD8$^+$ T cells were affected in nonresponder (DBA/2) mice. Accessory cells were required for this effect, as suggested by lack of response when adherent cells were removed. CD4$^+$ T cells are crucial for $HgCl_2$-induced activation, because cell proliferation after exposure to mercury was completely inhibited by the administration of monoclonal antibodies to CD4. Higher IL-4 and lower IFN-γ levels were detected in plasma of BALB/c mice exposed to $HgCl_2$ (41). However, a later study reported that a single injection of $HgCl_2$ enhanced mixed type 1 and type 2 cytokine responses in mice of this strain (117). Exposure to mercury also induces time- and dose-dependent cell death of various T-cell lines, with typical features of apoptosis and necrosis (118). Inorganic mercury has also been reported to protect Jurkat T cells against CD95-mediated apoptosis (119). Rats of the BN strain injected with a low dose of $HgCl_2$ show a marked decrease in the ConA-induced generation of

IFN-γ–producing cells from splenocyte cultures prepared 1 hour after mercury administration (120). The inhibition of IFN-γ production by spleen cells of mercuric chloride-injected BN rats is likely caused by nitric oxide (121). No inhibitory effects on splenic IFN-γ production is observed in Lewis (LEW) rats after exposure to mercury.

*B Lymphocytes*

Inhibition or stimulation of B cells by mercury was reported in early studies (122). Later treatment of purified human B cells with HgCl₂ or MeHgCl resulted in a dose-dependent inhibition of B-cell proliferation and in IgM and IgG production (123). *In vitro* treatment of resting murine B cells with mercury inhibits RNA and DNA synthesis and has significant inhibitory effects on immunoglobulin isotype (especially IgG3) expression (124). Early reports of *in vivo* effects of methylmercury also showed suppressed antibody responses to influenza virus and sheep red blood cells in rabbits and mice but increased activity of lipopolysaccharide-stimulated B lymphocytes from BALB/c mice (122). Mercury treatment of mice from certain strains (A.SW and C57BL/6J) and BN rats results in increased serum IgE levels (125). IgM, IgG1, IgG2b, IgG2c, and IgA are also increased in BN rats injected with mercury (126). Mercury-treated LEW rats do not have such an increase in IgE or other immunoglobulins.

*Macrophages*

Most studies of mercury effects on macrophages have reported inhibitory effects on superoxide and free radicals production and phagocytosis (127). Depending on its *in vitro* concentration, HgCl₂ stimulates H₂O₂ release from LEW but not BN macrophages and inhibits phagocytosis in LEW and BN "resident" peritoneal macrophages (128). Treatment with HgCl₂ induces IL-1 production by murine macrophages (129) and higher gene expression of IL-12 in spleen cells of LEW rats (130).

*Polymorphonuclear Leukocytes*

Early studies of mercury effects on human polymorphonuclear leukocytes (PMNs) showed that HgCl₂ inhibited adherence, polarization, chemotaxis, and erythrophagocytosis (131). Low concentrations of HgCl₂ significantly increased chemoluminescence and stimulated H₂O₂ production. Other studies of human PMNs have reported inhibition of microbicidal activities and respiratory burst (132) and decreased superoxide anion formation and chemotaxis after exposure to methyl mercury, mercuric chloride and silver lactate (133). In my laboratory, my colleagues and I examined the *in vitro* effects of mercury on peritoneal PMNs from inbred rats and found that HgCl₂ stimulates *in vitro* H₂O₂ release from LEW, but not BN, cells (128).

*Mast Cells*

HgCl₂ increases the sensitivity of peritoneal mast cells from BN rats to degranulation by a monoclonal antibody to IgE (134). In contrast, mast cells from rats of the LEW strain exhibit very little degranulation by anti-IgE and no enhancement by HgCl₂. The same group also demonstrated that HgCl₂ inhibits cell proliferation and expression of mRNA for IL-8, tumor necrosis factor-α (TNF-α), and IL-4 in cells of a human leukemic mast cell line (HMC-1) (135).

*Natural Killer Cells*

NK cells have an early and important role in host resistance and the control of the initiation of the adaptive immune response (136). This subpopulation of large granular lymphocytes that do not express the T-cell receptor or immunoglobulin surface molecules has attracted considerable attention because of their ability to recognize and lyse certain virally infected or neoplastic cells without prior sensitization and in a manner that is not restricted by classic major histocompatibility complex (MHC) gene products (137). NK cells produce IFN-γ, TNF-α, and various colony-stimulating factors (e.g., granulocyte colony-stimulating colony, granulocyte-macrophage colony-stimulating factor, IL-3). They regulate the expression of costimulatory activities on antigen-presenting cells and instruct the adaptive immune system to develop a particular effector response by releasing effector cytokines. There have been few studies of immunotoxic effects of mercury on NK cells. A 44% reduction of NK-cell activity has been observed in BALB/c mice treated with methylmercury (138). Splenic NK-cell activity was also suppressed in 15-day-old rats after exposure to methylmercury *in utero* and during lactation (138). One study has detected a similar decrease in NK-cell activity in 12-week-old Sprague–Dawley rats exposed to mercury during gestation and nursing (139).

**Mercury-Induced Allergy**

Allergic reactions are the best known immunologic alteration induced in humans by exposure to inorganic mercury and in particular thimerosal (used as an antiseptic and preservative) (32). Allergy to mercury can occur as an anaphylactic reaction or as a delayed-type hypersensitivity response (e.g., contact dermatitis). Lichenoid contact dermatitis in red tattoos (obtained with mercuric sulfide) or adjacent to amalgam fillings has also been reported (140). The onset of allergic reactions to mercury depends on individual susceptibility traits that are still unrecognized.

**Autoimmune Effects of Mercury**

*Human Autoimmune Disease*

Autoimmune disease induced in humans by exposure to mercury is rare. For example, one review article does not include mercury among the causes of the NS (141). However, autoimmune disease did occur in the past after treatment with drugs containing mercury, a practice that has since been discontinued. Fillastre et al. documented several instances of mercury-associated NS (142). About 20 cases of NS were reported between 1947 and 1968 after treatment with organomercurial diuretics for congestive heart failure. In France, NS was observed in seven patients after the ingestion of mercury-containing laxatives. Similarly, the protracted use of ammoniated mercury in skin ointments for the treatment of psoriasis resulted in 10 cases of NS. Mercury-containing skin-lightening creams were associated with several cases of NS observed in East Africa (143). Kidney biopsies from these patients have shown binding of IgG and complement at the level of the renal GBM, with linear staining (reminiscent of that observed in Goodpasture's syndrome) in some cases, granular staining (as seen in deposition of antigen-antibody complexes) in others, and mixed linear-granular patterns in other cases (144,145).

Autoimmune responses from occupational exposure may still occur, but the evidence available is scarce and inconclusive (146). Circulating antilaminin antibodies were detected in workers exposed to mercury vapors, but this finding was not confirmed by later studies. Later investigations have not revealed significant autoimmune responses to renal autoantigens in two different cohorts of workers exposed to mercury (106,147). However, a slight increase in antibodies against DNA has been detected in workers of one cohort (148). Similarly, development of ANAs and systemic autoimmune disease have been observed in a few patients with long-standing exposure to mercury (140).

In conclusion, mercury absorbed through the skin, respiratory tract, or gastrointestinal system may cause autoimmune responses and disease in humans. However, studies of this environmental hazard are usually quite difficult because low doses of mercury may be absorbed over a long period and escape notice. Once the autoimmune disease develops, a retrospective study may not reveal the etiologic agent or establish a cause-effect relationship. By contrast, investigations using experimental animals have provided excellent evidence that administration of mercury causes autoimmunity in rabbits, rats, and mice (149,150).

### Autoimmune Disease in Experimental Animals

*Rabbits.* An early study by Andres' group showed that mercury treatment of outbred New Zealand White rabbits results in the formation of immune deposits in kidneys and other organs, a process that in this species is characterized by two-stage kinetics (151). During the first stage (the first 3 to 4 weeks of injections with HgCl$_2$), linear deposits of rabbit IgG were detected at the level of the GBM and tubular basement membrane (TBM). Deposits of C3 were not detectable. Eluates from the IgG deposits reacted with antigens of the extracellular matrix (152). In this initial stage, there was normal renal histology and only slight proteinuria. In the second

stage (the next 5 to 7 weeks of HgCl$_2$ treatment), granular deposits of IgG as well as C3 were present in GBM and TBM. Eluates from these IgG deposits also reacted with extracellular matrix components (152). A membranous nephropathy developed in this stage; light microscopy showed a slight thickening of the glomerular capillary wall in 60% of the rabbits and electron microscopy revealed focal electron-opaque subepithelial deposits. The number and size of subepithelial deposits increased in rabbits sacrificed after 8 to 12 weeks of mercury treatment. A continuous granular layer of deposits, occasionally surrounded by a newly formed layer of basement membrane, was observed in rabbits sacrificed at later dates. These animals had heavy proteinuria. Similar deposits were observed in a variety of other organs, including hepatic and adrenal sinusoids, lung, choroid plexus, sarcolemma of striated muscles, red pulp and vessels of the spleen, and tunica propria of ileum and colon. No histopathologic or functional damage was consistently observed in those tissues.

Exposure of outbred rabbits to mercury likely resulted in autoimmune responses to epitopes of the extracellular matrix. In these animals, the kidney glomerulus was the major target for *in situ* formation of immune complexes followed by morphologic and functional damage. Other organs and tissues, despite the presence of immune deposits, showed minor effects or appeared normal.

This would be a useful model to revisit. Unfortunately, it has not been pursued further because of the lack of inbred rabbit strains and reagents to characterize lymphocyte subpopulations and cytokine production. However, the early results obtained in this species are still of value and show that an outbred population of animals may experience autoimmune responses to antigens of the extracellular matrix and an immune complex-mediated NS after exposure to mercury. These findings may be extrapolated to primates, including humans.

*Rats.* Numerous studies of mercury-induced cell injury and acute renal failure had been performed in the past using experimental animals of various species. However, it is to the credit of Bariety et al. to have initiated and established a rat model for immunopathologic investigations of autoimmunity caused by mercury (153). Outbred Wistar rats divided in several groups were injected subcutaneously 3 times each week with doses of HgCl$_2$ that varied from 0.25 to 0.05 mg/100 g body weight. Approximately 28% of animals injected with 0.15 mg, and 33% of those injected with 0.25 mg HgCl$_2$ developed a membranous glomerulonephropathy. Significant proteinuria was observed in three rats. Light microscopy showed that these animals had diffuse thickening of glomerular capillary walls, with diffuse subepithelial deposits visible by electron microscopy. Granular deposits of immunoglobulins and complement were detected by direct immunofluorescence. Segmental and focal glomerulonephropathy was observed in four rats that did not show proteinuria. Their kidneys looked mostly normal by light microscopy, but electron microscopy revealed scattered and small opaque subepithelial deposits. Direct immunofluorescence showed granular immunoglobulin and complement deposits in some glomeruli.

As a follow-up of these observations, Druet's group developed a similar model in inbred BN rats (154). In the past 20 years, studies of this rat model have provided exciting data that may be applicable to autoimmune responses induced by other xenobiotics.

*Autoimmune responses.* Initial studies showed that mercury-treated BN, MAXX, and Dorus Zadel Black (DZB) rats have high levels of circulating autoantibodies to antigens of the renal GBM (155–163). Autoantibody levels usually start increasing on day 9 or 10 of mercury treatment and reach a peak on days 14 or 15 (Fig. 41.1). A decrease is seen by day 18 and levels continue to decrease in the following days. As shown in Fig. 41.1, there is considerable variability in serum levels of anti-GBM autoantibodies in MAXX rats. These autoantibodies do not bind rat complement *in vitro* (158). Autoimmune responses of mercury-treated BN and MAXX rats have a self-limiting course somewhat similar to that observed in rats with "monophasic" experimental allergic encephalomyelitis. BN rats that have recovered from mercury-induced autoimmunity are subsequently resistant to additional treatment with this metal.

In the initial studies, the target autoantigen for assays of circulating autoantibodies was a rather crude preparation of rat GBM, solubilized by treatment with bacterial collagenase.

However, it was soon observed that ELISAs using mouse laminin provided an easier and reliable determination of mercury-induced autoimmune responses to rat GBM (156, 157,159–161,163,164). Laminins, a superfamily of large trimeric proteins, are structural components of basement membranes and have numerous biologic functions in cell differentiation, adhesion, migration, and proliferation (165). There are more than 10 different isoforms of laminins, one of which, now defined as laminin 1, was originally derived from the Engelbreth-Holm-Swarm (EHS) mouse tumor and is considered the prototype of this family (166). Because laminin 1 is remarkably conserved across mammalian species (167), the finding of serum antibodies reacting with mouse laminin 1 suggested that mercury-treated BN rats produce autoantibodies to rat laminin 1. A formal proof of the autoantibody nature of these antilaminin antibodies was still needed, because antigenic differences between mouse and rat laminin 1 have been previously observed (167). This proof has been provided by examination of monoclonal antibodies prepared from lymph node cells of mercury-treated DZB rats with circulating autoantibodies to laminin 1 (160). These monoclonal antibodies react by ELISA with mouse and rat laminin 1 (164). I also observed that 100% of sera from BN rats injected with HgCl$_2$ react with mouse and rat laminin 1 (i.e., contain autoantibodies to laminin 1) (163). Serum autoantibodies against laminin 1 are also present in BB rats with insulin-

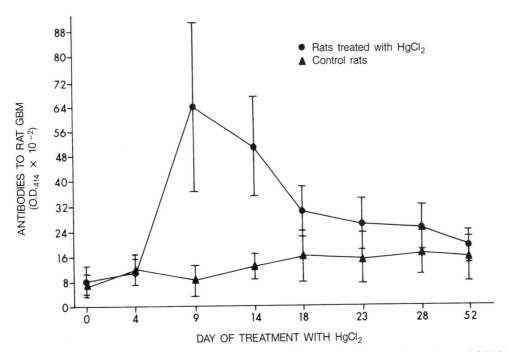

**FIG. 41.1.** Kinetics of circulating autoantibodies to renal glomerular basement membrane (*GBM*) in MAXX rats injected with HgCl$_2$. Values observed on days 0 and 4 of treatment were similar to those of controls treated with acidified distilled water. Autoantibody levels increased to a peak on days 9 and 14, then decreased on day 18, and continued decreasing to near baseline values in the following days. (From Henry GA, Jarnot BM, Steinhoff MM, Bigazzi PE. Mercury-induced renal autoimmunity in the MAXX rat. *Clin Immunol Immunopathol* 1988;49:187–203, with permission.)

dependent diabetes mellitus (IDDM), and exposure to mercury increases autoantibody levels and percentage of positive BB rats (168).

The autoantibodies to laminin 1 detected in $HgCl_2$-treated BN rats belong mostly to the IgG1 and IgG2a isotypes. Highly significant increases of IgG1 and IgG2a autoantibodies to laminin 1 were observed on day 11 of mercury treatment (Fig. 41.2.). Only the levels of IgG1 autoantibodies to laminin 1 were still significantly elevated on day 15. Diabetes-prone BB rats not treated with mercury have circulating autoantibodies to laminin 1 of the IgG2a (56%), IgG1 (11%), and IgG2c (11%) isotypes (168). After mercury treatment of diabetes-prone BB rats, autoantibodies to laminin 1 are detected in all IgG isotypes (i.e., IgG2a in 92%, IgG1 in 67%, IgG2b in 67% and IgG2c in 25% of diabetes-prone rats) (168).

Autoantibodies to other autoantigens (e.g., thyroglobulin, type IV collagen, heparan sulfate proteoglycan, entactin) have also been detected in BN rats after exposure to mercury, but they are present in lower concentrations and for shorter periods. They do not appear to be associated with functional or morphologic alterations of the thyroid or other organs. High levels of IgE are produced by mercury-treated BN rats, but the target antigens of this immune response are still unknown (125). Rats of the PVG strain develop autoantibodies to nuclear antigens after mercury treatment (169–171). No antibodies to laminin 1 or other autoantibodies have been detected in these animals.

*Immunopathology.* Mercury treatment of BN and MAXX rats results in renal immune deposits with two-stage kinetics that are morphologically similar but temporally not identical to those observed in similarly treated outbred rabbits. The first stage peaks at approximately day 15 and is characterized by linear deposits of IgG at the level of GBM (Fig. 41.3) and TBM (Fig. 41.4). The immunoglobulins present in these linear deposits belong mostly to the IgG2a and IgG1 isotypes and contain autoantibodies to laminin 1 (156,157,159–161, 164,172). Complement components (e.g., C3) are not usually present in these deposits (173). In addition to the renal immunoglobulin deposits, linear binding of IgG is observed at the level of the basement membranes in various organs, such as reticulum and wall of central arteries in splenic white pulp, portal spaces, and posthepatic vein of the liver, adrenal vessels, and capillaries and arteries of the heart (174). Oral administration of $HgCl_2$ to BN rats induces linear deposits of IgA and of IgG in the basement membranes of the ileum (175). In $HgCl_2$-injected rats we have observed a similar linear IgG pattern in various tissues, particularly striking in the basement membranes of the intestine (Fig. 41.5). The second stage of immune deposition occurs after 15 to 20 days and shows granular IgG in renal GBM and TBM. These deposits also contain autoantibodies that react most strongly with laminin 1 (157).

Kidneys of DZB rats injected with $HgCl_2$ show faint linear deposition of IgG along the GBM on days 6 to 10 but later

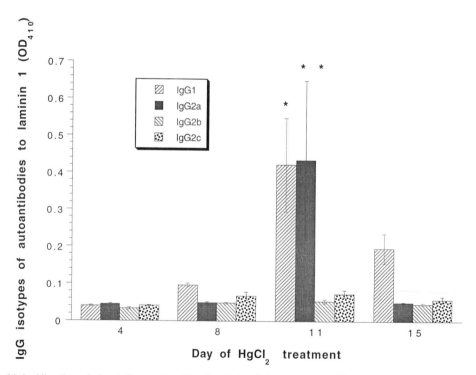

**FIG. 41.2.** Kinetics of circulating autoantibodies to laminin 1 in Brown Norway rats injected with $HgCl_2$. Highly significant increases of IgG1 (*$P < 0.0001$ vs. D4 and $P = 0.0004$ vs. D8) and IgG2a (**$P = 0.0031$ vs. D4 and $= 0.0034$ vs. D8) autoantibodies were observed on D11. IgG1 autoantibodies to laminin 1 were still increased on D15 ($P = 0.0324$), whereas IgG2 autoantibody levels were not significantly changed ($P = 0.9587$). (From Kosuda LL, Whalen B, Greiner DL, Bigazzi PE. Mercury-induced autoimmunity in Brown Norway rats: kinetics of changes in RT6⁺ T lymphocytes correlated with IgG isotypes of circulating autoantibodies to laminin 1. *Toxicology* 1998;125:215–231, with permission.)

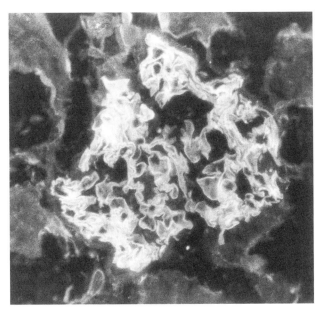

**FIG. 41.3.** Linear staining of rat IgG on glomerular capillary walls of kidney from HgCl₂-treated MAXX rat (direct immuno-fluorescence on cryostat sections of rat kidney incubated with FITC-conjugated rabbit antibodies to rat IgG; original magnification ×128). (From Henry GA, Jarnot BM, Steinhoff MM, Bigazzi PE. Mercury-induced renal autoimmunity in the MAXX rat. *Clin Immunol Immunopathol* 1988;49:187–203, with permission.)

have strong granular IgG deposits (160). Only a granular IgG pattern (not preceded by linear deposits) is observed in the GBM of similarly treated PVG rats (171). BB rats with circulating autoantibodies to laminin 1 show no immunoglobulin binding to renal or other structures (168).

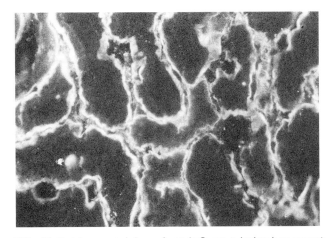

**FIG. 41.4.** Linear staining of rat IgG on tubular basement membranes of kidney from HgCl₂-treated MAXX rat (direct immunofluorescence on cryostat sections of rat kidney incubated with FITC-conjugated rabbit antibodies to rat IgG; original magnification, ×128). (From Henry GA, Jarnot BM, Steinhoff MM, Bigazzi PE. Mercury-induced renal autoimmunity in the MAXX rat. *Clin Immunol Immunopathol* 1988;49:187–203, with permission.)

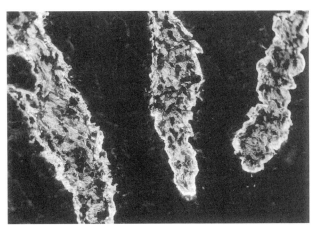

**FIG. 41.5.** Linear staining of rat IgG in the intestinal mucosa of HgCl₂-treated Brown Norway rat. IgG is deposited in a linear fashion at the level of the basement membrane of the villi, with some staining of the stroma. The epithelial cells lining the villi are completely negative and barely visible (direct immunofluorescence on cryostat sections of rat intestine incubated with FITC-conjugated affinity purified F(ab′)₂ fragment of goat antibodies to rat IgG; original magnification ×80).

*Histopathology and functional alterations.* All rat models of mercury autoimmunity are characterized histopathologically by a membranous glomerulonephropathy (176). Light and electron microscopy studies performed on animals perfused *in vivo* with fixatives before obtaining kidneys and other tissues have revealed only minor alterations (158). Kidneys from MAXX rats treated with HgCl₂ for 9 days showed some sloughing of tubular epithelial cells in renal proximal tubules and mild changes in glomeruli, with focal separation of endothelial cells from the GBM. There was a moderate increase in the amount of mesangial matrix. Kidneys obtained after 32 days showed mild increases in cellularity, increased mesangial matrix and cells, and accumulation of electron-opaque material between endothelial cells and GBM.

Proteinuria is a functional alteration that has been observed after exposure to mercury in BN, MAXX, and DZB rats (158,160,177). As shown in Fig. 41.6, MAXX rats exhibit significant proteinuria with peak levels on days 14 to 16 of mercury treatment, followed by a decrease to levels still higher than baseline on day 32. The absence of notable inflammatory reactions at the renal level and the presence of kidney immunoglobulin deposits correlated with proteinuria indicate that mercury causes a membranous glomerulonephropathy (MGP) in rats of susceptible strains.

Other effects of mercury include splenomegaly, lymph node hyperplasia and thymic atrophy in BN rats (178). Light microscopy studies of thymuses from BN rats have revealed extensive disorganization within 14 days after HgCl₂ treatment, with loss of demarcation between cortex and medulla but without any detectable increase in apoptotic cells. The numbers of thymus cells were significantly decreased in BN and (BN×LEW)F₁ hybrid rats injected with HgCl₂. Single- and two-color FCM showed significant increases in percent-

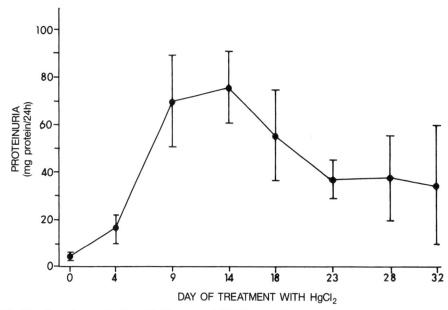

**FIG. 41.6.** Kinetics of proteinuria in HgCl$_2$-treated MAXX rats. Peak levels of proteinuria were observed on days 9 and 14 of mercury treatment. (From Henry GA, Jarnot BM, Steinhoff MM, Bigazzi PE. Mercury-induced renal autoimmunity in the MAXX rat. *Clin Immunol Immunopathol* 1988;49:187–203, with permission.)

ages of single-positive CD8$^+$ or CD4$^+$ and double-negative CD8$^-$CD4$^-$ thymocytes compared with H$_2$O-treated controls ($P = 0.0001$, $= 0.0003$, and $= 0.0016$, respectively). In contrast, the percentage of CD8$^+$CD4$^+$ double positive thymocytes was significantly decreased ($P = 0.0004$). Total numbers of CD4$^+$ single-positive thymocytes were significantly increased ($P = 0.0007$), whereas the total numbers of double-positive CD8$^+$CD4$^+$ thymocytes were decreased ($P = 0.0041$). Mercury-treated LEW rats had no changes in thymus architecture or significant decreases in cell numbers. Thus, exposure to low doses of HgCl$_2$ causes changes in thymocyte subpopulations of "mercury-susceptible" but not of "mercury-resistant" rats.

Changes in peripheral lymphocyte subpopulations of mercury-treated rats have also been detected. I have observed that HgCl$_2$-treated BN rats have a decrease of RT6$^+$ T cells, inversely correlated with autoimmune responses to laminin 1 (163,179,180). Figure 41.7 shows a kinetic analysis of the decrease in RT6.2$^+$ T cells in cervical lymph nodes of HgCl$_2$-injected BN rats, demonstrating a significant percentage decrease on days 8, 11, and 15 of treatment. I have also observed by two-color flow cytometry that BN rats sacrificed on day 15 of mercury treatment experience a significant decrease in percentages of RT6.2$^+$CD4$^+$ and RT6.2$^+$CD8$^+$ T lymphocytes (Fig. 41.8).

Lesions in other tissues were not usually reported (160). However, publications from some laboratories have described inflammatory processes in various organs and tissues of mercury-treated BN rats. In particular, Mathieson's group has reported that HgCl$_2$-treated BN rats develop inflammation and ulceration of the skin, hepatic periportal

mononuclear cell infiltrates, and hemorrhagic lesions of the gut, with intense submucosa inflammation and leukocytoclastic vasculitis (181). These rats may produce antibodies to myeloperoxidase and develop a CD8$^+$ T lymphocyte-mediated inflammatory polyarthritis (182–184). Other investigators have demonstrated a focal inflammatory process in the parotid, submandibular, lachrymal, and thyroid glands of HgCl$_2$-treated BN rats (185). These inflammatory reactions, similar to those occurring in BN rats injected neonatally with (BN×LEW)F$_1$ hybrid spleen cells, have suggested the possibility that a common mechanism may be responsible for allogeneic reactions and the effects of certain xenobiotics (150). Because previous publications never mentioned the occurrence of inflammatory reactions in HgCl$_2$-treated BN rats, we carefully reexamined a variety of tissues from BN rats injected with mercury. I have found no inflammatory changes in thyroid, pancreas, intestine, skin, liver, parotid, and lung (Bigazzi et al., unpublished data). The discrepancy between our observations and the descriptions of polyarthritis and dermatitis by other groups is still unexplained.

*Cytokine profiles.* A deficiency in IL-2 production (186) and a marked decrease in the ConA-induced generation of IFN-$\gamma$ (120) have been observed in BN rats after mercury treatment. Cytokine profiles obtained using quantitative and semiquantitative polymerase chain reaction methods have shown an increase in type 2 cytokines, suggesting that an imbalance between T$_H$1 and T$_H$2 cells may be the basis of mercury-induced autoimmunity (187,188). Another approach to assess the *in vivo* functional effects of cytokines relies on the determination of immunoglobulin isotypes of autoantibodies (189). Relatively scarce information is presently available on the reg-

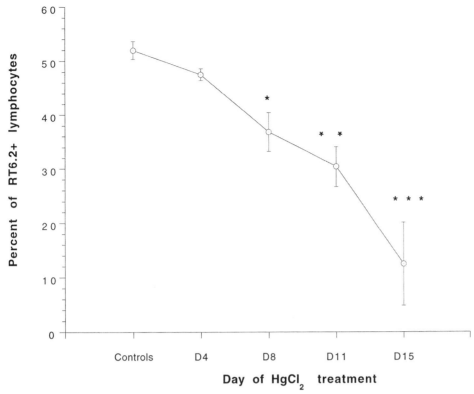

**FIG. 41.7.** Flow cytometry kinetic analysis of changes in the percentage of RT6.2⁺ T cells in cervical lymph nodes of HgCl₂-treated Brown Norway rats. Significant decreases were present on D8 of treatment (*$P = 0.0012$ vs. controls and = 0.0332 vs. mercury-treated rats sacrificed on D4), D11 (**$P < 0.0001$). and D15 (***$P < 0.0001$). (From Kosuda LL, Whalen B, Greiner DL, Bigazzi PE. Mercury-induced autoimmunity in Brown Norway rats: kinetics of changes in RT6⁺ T lymphocytes correlated with IgG isotypes of circulating autoantibodies to laminin 1. *Toxicology* 1998;125:215–231, with permission.)

ulation of IgG isotype expression in rats, but rat IgG1 and IgG2a may be induced by IL-4 similarly to what occurs for mouse IgG1 (190). Autoantibodies to laminin 1 detected in HgCl₂-treated BN rats are of the IgG1 and IgG2a isotypes, confirming the suggestion of a polarized, type 2 cytokine profile in these animals (163). After exposure to mercury, BB rats develop autoantibodies to laminin 1 of all IgG isotypes, including those that probably depend on type 1 cytokines (168). Thus, mercury is not only "the God of T_H2 cells" (191) but may affect various cellular components of the immune system.

*Immunogenetics.* BN and MAXX rats (RT-1ⁿ haplotype) have autoimmune responses to laminin 1 after mercury administration. Early immunogenetic studies showed that rats from 17 other strains, with the Lewis (LEW) strain (RT-1ˡ haplotype) as the prototype, are resistant to these autoimmune effects (155). Susceptibility to the first autoimmune phase (linear deposition of IgG in kidneys) was shown to depend on several genes, one of which is RT-1–linked, whereas the second phase (renal granular deposits of IgG) is associated with one major RT-1–linked gene or cluster of genes, with other non-RT-1–linked genes controlling the magnitude of the response. Later investigations, showing that rats from other strains (i.e., DZB and August, both of the

RT-1ᵘ haplotype) respond to mercury, have confirmed the role of MHC genes but have also stressed the importance of non-MHC genes (192). Particularly relevant in this regard are the findings in mercury-treated congenic BN.1L and LEW.1N rats (Table 41.2), which do not show autoimmune responses to laminin, renal immune deposits or proteinuria (192). Circulating autoantibodies to laminin and IgG deposits in renal GBM can be induced by exposure to mercury in BN → LEW.1N chimeras (193) (Table 41.2).

*Pathogenesis.* The pathogenesis of mercury-induced autoimmune disease in rats is not completely clear. The major target organ is the kidney, which exhibits MGP. Other organs and tissues show minor effects or seem to be spared. Circulating autoantibodies against laminin 1 in BN (as well as MAXX and DZB) rats may have a pathogenic role, as demonstrated by their correlation with proteinuria. BN and MAXX rats with autoantibodies to laminin 1 but no C3 deposited in their kidneys may experience proteinuria as a direct consequence of autoantibody binding to the GBM. Glomerular injury and proteinuria caused by antibodies alone, in the absence of complement, neutrophils, or other known secondary mediators, are a well-documented phenomenon (194). Activation of the complement cascade in

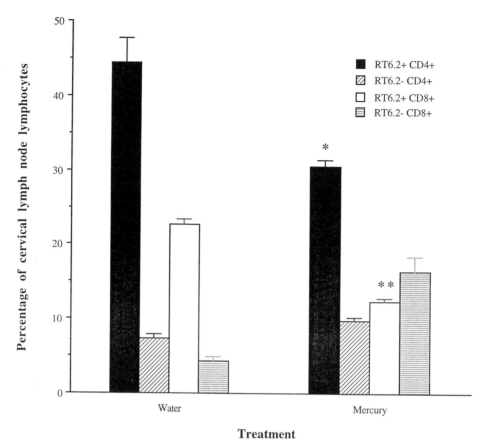

**FIG. 41.8.** Two-color flow cytometry analysis demonstrates a significant decrease in the percentage of RT6.2$^+$CD4$^+$ T lymphocytes (*$P$ = 0.0041) and RT6.2$^+$CD8$^+$ T lymphocytes (**$P$ = 0.0003) in the cervical lymph nodes of HgCl$_2$-treated Brown Norway rats sacrificed on day 15. (From Kosuda LL, Whalen B, Greiner DL, Bigazzi PE. Mercury-induced autoimmunity in Brown Norway rats: kinetics of changes in RT6$^+$ T lymphocytes correlated with IgG isotypes of circulating autoantibodies to laminin 1. *Toxicology* 1998;125:215–231, with permission.)

**TABLE 41.2.** *Autoimmune effects of mercury in congenic and chimeric rats*

| Rat strain | Pretreatment | Treatment | Rats with IgG deposits in renal GBM (%)[a] | Percent of rats with serum autoantibodies to laminin 1[b] |
|---|---|---|---|---|
| LEW.1N | None | HgCl$_2$ | 0 | 0 |
| LEW.1N | None | H$_2$O | 0 | 0 |
| BN.1L | None | HgCl$_2$ | 0 | 0 |
| BN.1L | None | H$_2$O | 0 | 0 |
| BN→LEW.1N | 600 rad[c] + 80 × 10$^6$ L[d] | HgCl$_2$ | 20 | 20 |
| BN→LEW.1N | 600 rad[c] + 80 × 10$^6$ L[d] | H$_2$O | 0 | 0 |
| BN→LEW.1N | 700 rad[c] + 80 × 10$^6$ L[d] | HgCl$_2$ | 62.5 | 62.5 |
| BN→LEW.1N | 700 rad[c] + 80 × 10$^6$ L[d] | H$_2$O | 0 | 0 |

[a] Determined by direct immunofluorescence of kidneys obtained on day 16 of mercury treatment.

[b] Determined by ELISA of sera obtained on day 16 of mercury treatment.

[c] Gamma irradiation.

[d] L, adoptively transferred spleen lymphocytes from untreated BN rats.

Adapted from Kosuda LL, Greiner DL, Bigazzi PE. Mercury-induced renal autoimmunity in BN→LEW.1N chimeric rats. *Cell Immunol* 1994;155:77–94.

DZB rats with renal deposits of autoantibodies to laminin 1 and complement components is a possible cause of proteinuria. PVG rats with circulating autoantibodies to nuclear antigens may experience proteinuria through a similar mechanism (i.e., the renal deposition of immune complexes and complement activation). Lymphocytes and macrophages, often present in the renal interstitium, may be an additional damaging factor, but direct proof of their pathogenic involvement is still lacking.

*Etiology.* The administration of various forms of mercury by the oral, respiratory, subcutaneous, or intraperitoneal routes is the initial cause of autoimmune responses and disease in rats of various strains. Less clear are the immune mechanisms involved in the induction of autoimmunity by mercury. T lymphocytes play a central role, as shown by the absence of mercury-induced effects in T-cell deprived animals. Less successful have been experiments attempting to identify T lymphocytes with immunoregulatory activity. Depletion of CD8+ T lymphocytes obtained in BN rats by a combination of thymectomy and treatment with a monoclonal antibody against rat CD8 (195) did not affect the initial induction and spontaneous regression of renal autoimmune response after exposure to mercury. Similarly negative were the results obtained in LEW rats, which are "resistant" to the autoimmune effects of mercury (i.e., they do not produce autoantibodies to laminin or develop renal immune complexes). It was suggested that CD8+ T lymphocytes might be responsible for this lack of response to mercury (196). However, LEW rats depleted of their CD8+ T lymphocytes did not develop the autoimmune abnormalities observed after mercury treatment in BN rats. As described above, the RT6+ subset of T cells (which have a regulatory role in other rat models of autoimmune disease) decreases in mercury-treated BN rats.

Mercury may activate B lymphocytes directly or indirectly through IL-4 production by T cells. The presence of hyper-IgE has suggested that IL-4 could be an important mediator of T-cell–dependent B-cell activation. Some investigators have suggested that HgCl₂ induces autoimmunity by the stimulation of $T_H2$ cells (197). Investigations of $HgCl_2$-treated BN rats have shown increases in IL-4 mRNA and decreased IFN-γ production in their spleen, leading to the conclusion that mercury is a stimulator of $T_H2$ cell functions (188,191,198,199). However, this effect may be limited to some rat strains, because my colleagues and I demonstrated that HgCl₂ can stimulate in BB rats the production of autoantibodies that belong to rat IgG isotypes regulated by $T_H1$ and $T_H2$ lymphocytes (168). Another effect of mercury is an increased expression of MHC class II molecules on B cells, which can be detected as early as 3 days after the first injection of the metal.

The $\alpha_4\beta_1$ integrin, which has essential functions in leukocyte migration, is also involved in autoimmunity caused by HgCl₂. BN rats treated with monoclonal antibodies to this integrin had decreased levels of autoantibodies to the renal GBM, did not show immunoglobulins bound to the kidney *in vivo*, and had a drastic reduction in proteinuria (200).

*Mercury-induced immunosuppression in rats.* Administration of mercury may result in immunosuppression of autoimmune disease (201–203). Protective effects were first observed in LEW rats treated with mercury and immunized with renal brush border antigen gp330 in complete Freund's adjuvant (CFA) to obtain Heymann's nephritis (202). These animals had low antibody responses to gp330 and no renal autoimmune disease. Mercury also attenuated or prevented the clinical manifestations of EAE in LEW rats and inhibited myelin basic protein (MBP)–induced proliferative responses of T cells as well as antibody responses to MBP. This activity of HgCl₂ has been explained as resulting from a non–antigen-specific immunosuppression mediated by an increase in the number of CD8+ (suppressor/cytotoxic) T lymphocytes (201). High levels of CD8+ suppressor T cells and at least 10-fold less frequent MBP-specific helper T cells were detected in mercury-treated LEW rats, together with a third cell type (i.e., contrasuppressor cells) that allows proliferative responses of helper T cells despite the presence of suppressor T cells (204). HgCl₂ reportedly induces in BN and LEW rats autoreactive anti–class II CD4+ T cells. T-cell lines derived from LEW CD4+ T cells of this type proliferated in the presence of normal class II–bearing cells, secreted IL-2, and did not induce B cells to produce immunoglobulins. Transfer of one of these lines into normal LEW rats led to the appearance of CD8+ T cells responsible for a non–antigen-specific immunosuppression that induced complete protection from EAE. Later studies have questioned the regulatory role of CD8+ T cells, because CD4+ (not CD8+) T cells directly prevent autoimmunity in IDDM of diabetes-prone BB rats and irradiated thymectomized PVG rats (205,206). Similarly, mercury-treated (BN×LEW)F₁ hybrid rats are protected against the development of experimental autoimmune uveitis (EAU) independently of the presence of CD8+ T cells (207). The protection effect was interpreted as resulting from activation of CD4+ $T_H2$ cells, in line with the suggestion that the $T_H1/T_H2$ cell balance has a prominent role in autoimmune disease (208–210). The LEW T-cell lines with inhibitory activity against autoimmunity induced by mercury produce IL-2, IFN-γ, and transforming growth factor-β (TGF-β) (211). Their protective effects may depend on TGF-β, because it is abrogated by treatment with antibodies to this cytokine (211).

Immunosuppressive activity of mercury has been observed only in experimentally induced autoimmune diseases (e.g., Heymann's nephritis, EAE, EAU) and only in one strain of rats (LEW or the F₁ hybrids between LEW and BN rats). No reports of protection in other rat strains against naturally occurring (i.e., spontaneous) autoimmune disease have been published. My colleagues and I investigated possible immunosuppressive effects of HgCl₂ on IDDM and thyroiditis of BB rats (168). Autoimmune disease of BB rats is likely determined by the relative balance of autoreactive effector T cells and regulatory T cells with a possible predominance of $T_H1$-type lymphocytes (212). We showed that exposure to mercury had no inhibitory effects on the development and progression of IDDM and thyroiditis in diabetes-prone BB rats (168). Thus, the immunosuppressive effects of HgCl$_2$ may be a unique characteristic of the LEW rat strain. This possibility is not surprising, because the autoimmune effects of mercury vary with inbred strain of rats and are associated with certain MHC and non-MHC genes.

*Mice.* Murine models have proven extremely useful in dissecting the various components of mercury-induced autoimmunity. In particular, the availability of transgenic and knockout mice has provided the opportunity for elegant and insightful experiments, resulting in information that may be relevant to autoimmunity in general (213).

*Autoimmune responses.* The parenteral or oral administration of HgCl$_2$ to mice of various inbred strains (i.e., A/J, A.SW, B10.S, and SJL/J) or outbred ICR mice stimulates the production of anti-nucleolar and antinuclear autoantibodies (214–221) (Fig. 41.9). Antinucleolar autoantibodies detected in mercury-treated mice react with a 34-kd nucleolar protein (i.e., fibrillarin or U3 RNP protein) and occasionally with other nucleolar proteins of 60 to 70 kd and 10 to 15 kd. They seem to recognize nucleolar epitopes similar to those reacting with autoantibodies from certain patients with scleroderma (222) (Fig. 41.9). Autoantibodies to fibrillarin belong to all IgG subclasses, but there is a predominance of IgG1 and IgG2a isotypes (216). Their production gradually develops after 3 to 5 weeks of mercury exposure, is characterized by high concentrations of autoantibodies, and lasts for 10 to 12 weeks or longer (216). One investigation showed two patterns of persistence of autoantibody production after cessation of treatment (223). In one group, comprising mice of SJL and A.SW strains, antinucleolar autoantibodies were detectable until the end of the study, 12 months after mercury treatment was terminated. However, mice of the B10.S strain had lower titers of autoantibodies or became negative 6 to 9 months after treatment (223).

Mercury toxicokinetics differ significantly among inbred mouse strains, are regulated by non-H-2 genes and correlate with autoimmune responses in genetically susceptible strains (224). Dose-response studies have shown that autoantibodies to fibrillarin are detected in susceptible mice given at least

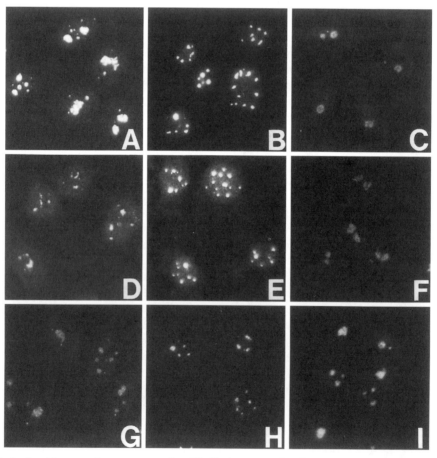

**FIG. 41.9.** Indirect immunofluorescence of antifibrillarin autoantibodies using human HEp-2 **(A, D, G)**, mouse 3T3 **(B, E, H)**, and *Xenopus* XlK-2 **(C, F, I)** cells as substrates. The reactivity of human scleroderma serum is shown in **A, B,** and **C**; HgCl$_2$-treated mouse serum in **D, E,** and **F**; and antifibrillarin monoclonal 72B9 in **G, H,** and **I**. (From Takeuchi J, Turley SJ, Tan EM, Pollard KM. Analysis of the autoantibody response to fibrillarin in human disease and murine models of autoimmunity. *J Immunol* 1995;154:961–971, with permission.)

1.225 ppm of $HgCl_2$ in their drinking water for 10 weeks, a dose resulting in a mercury body burden similar to that observed in some occupationally exposed human subjects (220). The lowest concentration of mercury vapor causing autoimmune effects in SJL/N mice was found to be 170 µg of Hg/kg per week, corresponding to a renal mercury concentrations of 4.0 to 0.76 µg of Hg/g of wet weight (225). The investigators compared this body burden with that observed in occupationally exposed humans and concluded that the safety margin may be narrow for genetically susceptible individuals (225).

The antinuclear autoantibodies stimulated by exposure to mercury occur in a smaller percentage of mice and are directed against epitopes of chromatin and/or histones (216). The administration of $HgCl_2$ to New Zealand Black × New Zealand White (NZB×NZW)$F_1$ mice stimulates a polyclonal B-cell activation, with high levels of IgG1, IgG3, and IgE immunoglobulins, an intense antibody production against double-stranded DNA, IgG, collagen, phosphatidylethanolamine, and the hapten trinitrophenol (226). However, an early report of mercury-induced development of antilaminin antibodies has not been confirmed. Significant levels of autoantibodies to tissue-specific antigens of kidney, thyroid, and skin do not seem to be present in the circulation of $HgCl_2$-treated mice (227).

*Immunopathology and histopathology.* Immune deposits are detected in the kidneys of inbred (SJL, ASW, BALB/c) and outbred (ICR) mice exposed to mercury (214,220,228–230). The pattern of immune complex deposition is granular, with a predominant localization in the glomerular mesangium and the walls of interlobular arterioles and arteries (Fig. 41.10).

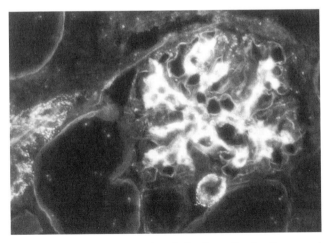

**FIG. 41.10.** Heavy granular IgG deposits in the renal glomerular mesangium and in the arteriolar wall of a H-2s (SJL) mouse treated with subcutaneous injection of 1.0 mg of $HgCl_2$/kg body weight every third day for 6 weeks (direct immunofluorescence on kidney cryostat sections incubated with FITC-conjugated goat anti-mouse IgG; original magnification ×900). (Photograph courtesy of Dr. Per Hultman, Division of Molecular and Immunological Pathology, Department of Health and Environment, Linköping University, Linköping, Sweden.)

Direct immunofluorescence does not detect linear staining of the renal GBM or TBM. Kidney immune deposits associated with mercury treatment of SJL and A.SW mice contain IgG and C3. Eluates from these deposits contain autoantibodies to fibrillarin. Renal immune deposits from $HgCl_2$-treated BALB/c mice (that do not have circulating autoantibodies to fibrillarin) do not contain autoantibodies to nucleolar antigens (215). In a dose-response study, kidneys from all SJL mice showed granular mesangial IgG staining irrespective of treatment (220). However, mice given 5.0 ppm of $HgCl_2$ in their drinking water had higher levels of renal mesangial and vascular immune deposits than controls. Granular IgG deposits were also found in the vessel walls of arteries and arterioles of the spleen and intramyocardial arteries. In contrast, after exposure to mercury A.CA, DBA, and P mice develop serum antinucleolar autoantibodies but do not have renal immune deposits (230).

Mercury-treated mice with circulating antifibrillarin autoantibodies and renal immune deposits develop a mesangial glomerulopathy, with minimal histopathologic findings that comprise widening of glomerular mesangial areas, electron-opaque deposits and a moderate increase of endocapillary cells (215,220,229). Popliteal lymph node hyperplasia has also been observed in mice injected in a footpad with $HgCl_2$ or $CH_3HgCl$ (231). Functional alterations (i.e., effects seen in mercury-treated rats such as proteinuria, graft-versus-host–like syndrome or immunosuppression) have not been reported.

*Immunogenetics.* Mice of various strains are susceptible to the autoimmune effects of mercury, with autoimmune responses that are in large part determined by the MHC (7). In particular, H-2$^s$ strains (e.g., A.SW, B10.S, SJL/J) produce antinucleolar and antinuclear autoantibodies. Responsiveness has been mapped to H-2A, with H-2E acting as an "immune suppression" locus (232). Resistance to mercury, found in H-2$^d$ strains, was attributed to IFN-γ–mediated effects (233). It has been suggested that resistance may be an intrinsic property of B cells (234,235). Tissue concentrations of mercury in the spleen are higher in susceptible strains and lower in resistant strains (236). Inbred mouse strains show significant differences in the toxicokinetics of mercury, which are regulated by non-H-2 genes and correlate with autoimmune responses in genetically susceptible animals (224).

*Pathogenesis.* The pathogenesis of mercury-induced autoimmune disease in mice seems rather straightforward. As in the rat model, the major target organ is the kidney, affected by a mesangial glomerulopathy. Other organs and tissues appear normal. Activation of the complement cascade in mice with renal deposits of autoantibodies to fibrillarin and complement components might cause proteinuria. The role of lymphocytes and macrophages as additional damaging factors to kidney structures is still uncertain.

*Etiology.* The administration of mercury in various forms and routes is the initial cause of autoimmunity in susceptible mice. Investigations have shown that the metal induces molecular and antigenic modifications of a nucleolar component, fibrillarin (237) (Fig. 41.11). Very low doses of mercury have been found effective in SJL/J mice, but exposure needs to be more prolonged than in rats. Athymic SJL/J mice treated with mercury do not produce antinucleolar antibodies and do not experience systemic immune complex deposition (238). A similar lack of mercury-induced autoimmune responses was observed in euthymic SJL/J mice depleted of CD4$^+$ T lymphocytes before exposure to the metal. The SJL/J mice treated with mercury and then injected with monoclonal antibodies against CD4$^+$ T cells showed no decline in antinucleolar antibody levels despite a severe reduction of CD4$^+$ cells (238). Induction of autoimmunity by mercury strictly depends on the presence of T cells, but after autoimmunity is well established, it is no longer susceptible to CD4$^+$ T-cell depletion. Lymphocyte costimulatory pathways are also an essential factor of mercury-induced autoimmune responses (239).

Mercury strongly activates CD4$^+$ T cells from responder but not from nonresponder mice (240). In contrast, CD8$^+$ T cells were activated by mercury in all strains, regardless of their responder or nonresponder status (240). These observations indirectly confirm previous evidence that had suggested IL-4 as an important mediator of T-cell–dependent B-cell activation. Increased levels of IL-4 mRNA have been detected within CD4$^+$ T cells of mercury-treated H-2$^s$ mice and treatment with antimouse IL-4 monoclonal antibody reportedly caused a switch in the immunoglobulin subclass of antifibrillarin antibodies (197). At least in H-2$^s$ mice, T$_H$2

cells secreting IL-4 may be responsible for B-cell stimulation. T$_H$2 hyperactivity may be associated with decreased T$_H$1 functions (i.e., impaired ability to produce IL-2 and IFN-$\gamma$ *in vitro*). Highly susceptible strains such as A.SW, SJL, and B10.S (H-2$^s$ haplotype) do not develop contact dermatitis in an ear swelling test (a form of delayed-type hypersensitivity reaction). The H-2$^d$ mice, which are resistant or low responders, develop contact dermatitis. On the basis of these observations, it has been suggested that mercury induces a T$_H$1/T$_H$2 imbalance, as hypothesized for the rat model (150).

Investigations of gene-targeted mice have provided intriguing results that contradict the hypothesis of a mercury-induced lack of balance between T$_H$1 and T$_H$2 cells (213). HgCl$_2$-injected IL-4–deficient mice develop serum autoantibodies to fibrillarin and immune complex deposits in their kidneys, showing that IL-4 is not essential for their development (Fig. 41.12). Conversely, similarly treated IFN-$\gamma$–deficient mice have very low serum autoantibody levels and no disease (Fig. 41.12). Autoantibodies to fibrillarin of all isotypes (not just those thought to depend on IFN-$\gamma$) are lacking in these animals.

## QUESTIONS ABOUT METAL-INDUCED AUTOIMMUNITY

The data summarized in this chapter provide answers to some questions often asked about autoimmunity associated with exposure to metals.

### Can Metals Induce Autoimmunity?

As observed in humans after therapeutic or occupational exposure and in animals after experimental administration, various metals can cause autoimmune responses. The preceding sections reviewed the well-demonstrated consequences of gold and mercury administration. Other metals (e.g., lithium, silver) may also be responsible for inducing or favoring autoimmunity. Studies of experimental animals have provided a clear-cut correlation between exposure to certain metals and onset of autoimmune responses. It is usually difficult to reproduce in animals the metal-induced autoimmune consequences observed in humans. However, use of the appropriate animal species and/or inbred strain may result in parallel, albeit not analogous, models of human autoimmunity.

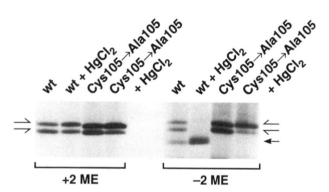

**FIG. 41.11.** Mercury-induced modification of fibrillarin requires two cysteines. The 35S-labeled wild type (*wt*) and fibrillarin with Cys$^{105}$ → Ala$^{105}$ mutation (*Cys105→Ala105*) were incubated in the presence and absence of 40 μM HgCl$_2$ before fractionation by SDS-PAGE in the presence and absence of mercaptoethanol (*2ME*). In the presence of 2ME wild type fibrillarin migrated as a doublet at 34 and 36 kd, in the presence and absence of HgCl$_2$ (*half arrows*). In the absence of 2ME, a 32-kd band appeared (*arrow*). Addition of HgCl$_2$ resulted in an accumulation of material at 32 kd. Migration of mutated fibrillarin (*Cys105→Ala105*) as the 34- and 36-kd doublet (*half arrows*) was unchanged in the presence of 2ME or by addition of HgCl$_2$. (Photograph courtesy of Dr. K. Michael Pollard, Keck Autoimmune Disease Center, The Scripps Research Institute, La Jolla, CA, U.S.A. New figure based on data from Pollard KM, Lee DK, Casiano CA, et al. The autoimmunity-inducing xenobiotic mercury interacts with the autoantigen fibrillarin and modifies its molecular and antigenic properties. *J Immunol* 1997;158:3521–3528.)

### Do Metals Cause Only Autoimmune Responses or Are They Capable of Inducing Autoimmune Disease?

Metal-induced autoimmune responses may be relatively harmless or result in autoimmune disease. The circumstances controlling such an outcome are still unknown. This is not surprising, because autoimmune responses are often observed in apparently healthy, normal individuals. Circulating autoantibodies in a normal subject do not necessarily suggest immediate or future pathologic consequences.

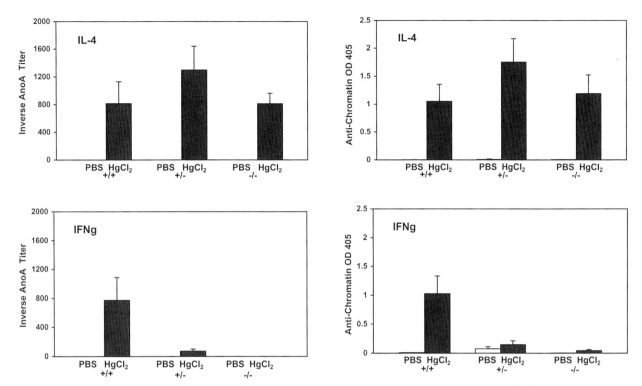

**FIG. 41.12.** Mercury-induced autoantibody responses in mice depend on interferon-γ (*IFN-γ*). Antinucleolar (*AnoA*) and antichromatin antibody responses of HgCl₂- or saline- (*PBS*) treated wild-type (+/+) H-2s mice are compared with those of H-2s mice heterozygous (+/−) or homozygous (−/−) for lack of expression of interleukin-4 (*IL-4*) or IFN-γ. HgCl₂-treated mice lacking wild-type expression of IFN-γ produce little or no autoantibody, whereas disruption of IL-4 has no effect on HgCl₂-induced autoantibody production. (Courtesy of Deborah L. Pearson and Dr. K. Michael Pollard, Keck Autoimmune Disease Center, The Scripps Research Institute, La Jolla, CA, U.S.A. New figure adapted from data from Kono DH, Balomenos D, Pearson DL, et al. The prototypic Th2 autoimmunity induced by mercury is dependent on IFN-γ and not Th1/Th2 imbalance. *J Immunol* 1998;161:234–240.)

However, autoantibodies can be associated with disease. Some metals (e.g., silver) stimulate the production of autoantibodies without causing tissue-specific or systemic autoimmune disorders. The gold- and mercury-induced autoantibody responses can cause tissue damage. T cells specific for gold or mercury have been detected in mice and humans exposed to these metals, and damaging cytotoxic effects or release of proinflammatory cytokines are therefore possible.

### Is Metal-Induced Autoimmune Disease Analogous to Idiopathic Autoimmune Disease?

Autoimmunity associated with xenobiotics is often different from idiopathic or spontaneously occurring autoimmunity. Good examples are the toxic oil syndrome and the eosinophilia-myalgia syndrome, disorders that had a variety of autoimmune manifestations but did not reproduce completely any well-characterized systemic autoimmune disease. Similarly, target antigens, autoimmune responses, and the course of the disease in drug-related lupus do not usually match those of SLE. However, penicillamine-induced autoimmune diseases (i.e., SLE, pemphigus, and myasthenia

gravis) appear identical or very similar to the corresponding idiopathic disorders. In the case of metal-induced MGP, the linear or granular deposition of immunoglobulins observed in the kidneys of some subjects after exposure to gold or mercury is not different from that observed in similar pathology of an idiopathic nature or from other causes. There are also no major discrepancies between gold-associated ATP and other spontaneously occurring forms of this condition. Autoimmune thyroiditis facilitated or induced by lithium does not seem to differ from Hashimoto's disease.

The target autoantigens responsible for the MGP caused in humans by gold and mercury are unknown. Are they laminins, collagens, DNA or fibrillarin? Animal models have provided some answers, showing that laminin 1, fibrillarin, and nuclear histones are involved in metal-induced autoimmunity, depending on species and strain. Human subjects with different immunogenetic and ecogenetic phenotypes may respond to one or the other of these autoantigens after exposure to gold or mercury.

Most animal models of metal-induced autoimmunity are parallel but not necessarily analogous to the human situations. It is often incorrectly stated that the systemic autoimmune responses induced by mercury in rats and mice are similar or equivalent to human SLE. Patients with SLE exhibit autoimmune responses to autoantigens present in various tissues, but the most relevant autoantibodies may be directed against double-stranded DNA. The most pronounced autoimmune responses observed in BN rats exposed to mercury are directed against laminin 1. Similarly, mercury-treated SJL mice produce autoantibodies to a nucleolar antigen, fibrillarin, that also induces autoimmune responses in a subset of scleroderma patients but not in human subjects with SLE. BN rats injected with mercury have linear immunoglobulin deposits in their kidneys, an immunopathology that is reminiscent of Goodpasture's syndrome, not SLE. However, the rat autoantibodies binding to basement membranes in a linear fashion are directed against epitopes of laminin 1 and not $\alpha_3$ type IV collagen, as occurs in Goodpasture's patients. The granular immunoglobulin deposits observed in mercury-treated SJL mice are mostly localized in the mesangium, without major involvement of the GBM, in contrast to the more diffuse involvement in SLE. Renal histopathology in rats and mice shows scarce alterations and no major inflammatory reactions. In conclusion, the systemic disease caused by mercury in animals does not resemble SLE but at best may reproduce the pathology induced by this metal in human subjects.

## Is Metal-Induced Autoimmunity Permanent or Does It Disappear When the Affected Individuals Are No Longer Exposed to the Xenobiotic Involved?

The pathology and autoimmune responses caused in humans by gold or mercury usually disappear after withdrawal of the metal. Mercury-induced autoimmunity in BN and MAXX rats is a short-term process that spontaneously terminates within a month even if the administration of the metal is continued. The situation is slightly different in susceptible mice, which require a much longer exposure to mercury before the appearance of autoimmune responses and immunopathology. In this case, production of autoantibodies to fibrillarin continues for several months after mercury treatment is interrupted. Other examples of xenobiotic-induced autoimmunity are even longer-lasting. Autoimmune disease may persist after the interruption of exposure in a few subjects treated with penicillamine, a drug with autoimmune-inducing activity similar to gold and mercury. The possibility that dietary iodine may be responsible for the reported increase of human autoimmune thyroiditis also suggests that the effects of some xenobiotics may become permanent.

## Which Individuals Are Susceptible to Metal-Induced Autoimmunity?

Clinical studies suggest that only a limited percentage of human subjects exposed to similar levels of metals develop autoimmunity. The rat and mouse models of mercury-induced autoimmunity are induced by exposure to relatively low doses of the metal in inbred animals with the appropriate

MHC and non-MHC genes. They show that a genetically controlled predisposition is indispensable for the expression of autoimmune disease induced by metals. I have repeatedly stressed the possible role of immunogenetic and pharmacogenetic (ecogenetic) factors (6). The importance of immunogenetics in idiopathic or naturally occurring autoimmune disease is well known. Unfortunately, there is only preliminary immunogenetic information of patients with autoimmunity caused by xenobiotics. For example, we know that certain MHC (e.g., HLA-DR3) and complement C4 null haplotypes are associated with gold-induced autoimmune disease. The role of pharmacogenetics and ecogenetics in abnormal and untoward drug reactions is also well known. Susceptibility to autoimmune effects caused by exposure to xenobiotics may be influenced by various phenotypes (e.g., metallothionein, sulfoxidizer, acetylator, aromatic hydrocarbon receptor, cytochrome P450). Metallothioneins (241) may be involved in the autoimmune effects of various metals, but we know nothing about this possibility or the involvement of other ecogenetic phenotypes.

## Do Metals Cause Autoimmunity *De Novo*, or Do They Facilitate Its Appearance in Individuals Predisposed To It and Who Would Eventually Become Autoimmune?

It is difficult to distinguish between facilitated and *de novo* induced autoimmunity (6). Facilitation of an underlying disease may be suggested by a relatively short period of exposure to the metal, whereas a longer period may imply *de novo* induction of autoimmunity. On the basis of the published evidence, lithium is likely to facilitate rather than induce autoimmune responses. Mercury's effects are more complex, because treatment with this metal increases autoantibody production in mice susceptible to murine lupus and diabetes-prone BB rats. Mercury is also capable of inducing autoimmune disease *de novo* in rat and mouse strains that otherwise do not spontaneously respond to autoantigens. Exposure to gold also causes *de novo* autoimmune disease in animals without a genetic predisposition to naturally occurring autoimmunity.

## Are Particular Structure–Activity Relationships Involved in Metal-Induced Autoimmunity?

A possible role of interaction with thiols was initially suggested by studies with gold compounds. Mercury and silver also have high affinity for thiol groups and are capable of inducing autoimmune responses. The formation of disulfide bonds between -SH groups and thiols of self-proteins may change the structure of autoantigens, render them foreign, or expose hidden epitopes. Alternatively, disulfide bonds may be formed with surface structures of immune cells, causing their stimulation. However, aurothiomalate and aurothioglucose contain a sulfur atom, not as sulfhydryl or disulfide, and still have similar autoimmune effects (99). It is difficult to understand why lead, copper, and cadmium, which also have high affinity for thiol groups, do not usually induce autoimmunity. Finally, the adjuvant capacity of certain metals does not seem to correlate with their autoimmune effects. A good example is provided by aluminum, which is used in a number of vaccines for its powerful adjuvant activity but which is not associated with autoimmune disease.

## Which Immunologic Effector Mechanisms Are Involved in the Pathogenesis of Autoimmune Disease Caused by Metals?

The immunologic and pathologic profile of autoimmune disease induced by exposure to gold or mercury is similar to that observed in idiopathic or naturally occurring autoimmune disease (5,6,8,103). The pathogenesis of metal-induced ATP involves cytotoxic autoantibodies that destroy platelets. Renal binding of autoantibodies against components of the renal GBM (e.g., laminin 1) present in gold- or mercury-treated human subjects, BN rats, and outbred NZW rabbits, may have a pathogenetic role, causing proteinuria through activation of the complement cascade or direct autoantibody effects. Renal deposition of immune complexes containing autoantibodies to nuclear and nucleolar antigens and complement activation in human patients, PVG rats, and SJL mice exposed to gold or mercury may also result in proteinuria. Cytotoxic T lymphocytes and cytokine-producing T lymphocytes and macrophages may have a similar pathogenetic role, but we have no direct evidence of their involvement in human autoimmunity induced by metals.

## Which Etiologic Mechanisms Are Responsible for the Induction of Autoimmune Responses and Disease by Metals?

The cause of metal-induced autoimmune disease is obvious in experimental animal models, where we know the initial time and dose of exposure to mercury or gold. In humans it is more difficult to determine whether the autoimmune process is initiated by exposure to an environmental metal, especially when the exposure to the metal does not occur in the workplace or when multiple xenobiotics are involved. However, there are clear-cut examples of human autoimmune responses and disease induced by gold and mercury. Less understood are the molecular, biochemical, and cellular events occurring in the immune system after administration of metals and leading to autoimmunity (242).

Metals may cause autoimmunity by their indirect or direct effects on the immune system. The first possibility occurs when metals, acting on tissues and organs of the body, induce modifications of autoantigen structure, exposing new or cryptic epitopes. Some CD4$^+$ T-cell hybridomas obtained from HgCl$_2$-treated mice specifically respond to fibrillarin bound to mercury, whereas other react against untreated fibrillarin (243). Elegant studies have shown that mercury interacts with the autoantigen fibrillarin and modifies its molecular and antigenic properties (237). Mercury can also generate the expression of stress proteins (i.e., heat shock proteins) that

may have a role in autoimmunity (244–248). Stress proteins are also induced by arsenic, cadmium, copper, zinc, lead, iron, and gold (249), but only cadmium has been associated with a T-cell response to heat shock proteins (53). Metals may release cellular or extracellular matrix components, normally present at very low levels or completely absent in the circulation. Even though the possibility is remote and not yet demonstrated, there may be molecular mimicry between epitopes of gold or mercury and host autoantigens.

Metals can directly stimulate the immune system by a variety of mechanisms (242). The first is independent of antigen and may be similar to the activity of conventional mitogens. Early studies showed that oxidation or reduction of thiol or disulfide groups modulates murine T-cell proliferation (39). Mercury may dimerize the thiol group–bearing proteins on the cell membrane and induce tyrosine phosphorylation and cell death (250). *In vitro* treatment with HgCl$_2$ of spleen cells or thymocytes from C57BL/6 mice results in aggregation of transmembrane CD4, CD3, CD45, Thy-1, and protein tyrosine kinase p56lck (251). Methylmercury causes a rapid increase in intracellular free Ca$^{2+}$ levels in rat splenocytes, whereas HgCl$_2$ increases Ca$^{2+}$ influx from extracellular sources (252). Direct effects of metals can occur when they act as immunogens or haptens (253). The induction of mercury-specific helper T cells, reacting with mercury or a mercury-protein complex stored in macrophages, has been detected in mice (254). Gold-specific T cells are present in patients with RA treated with this metal (84). Mercury may sequentially activate helper T and regulatory lymphocytes (150). B lymphocytes may be stimulated by mercury directly or indirectly through cytokine (e.g., IL-4) production by T cells (150). Lymphocyte costimulatory pathways and adhesion molecules are also involved in mercury-induced autoimmunity (239). Macrophages and other antigen-presenting cells may be induced by metals to become more active in epitope presentation and production of cytokines (e.g., IL-1).

The end result of the interactions between heavy metals and cells of the immune system probably is a change in the cytokine network and a loss of immune tolerance to autoantigens. The presence of hyper-IgE and hyper-IgG1 in mercury-treated rats and mice has suggested that IL-4 could be an important mediator of T-cell–dependent B-cell activation. T$_H$2 hyperactivity may be associated with decreased T$_H$1 functions (e.g., impaired ability to produce IL-2 *in vitro*). Mercury may induce an imbalance between T$_H$1 and T$_H$2 cells (150). However, experiments using cytokine-knockout mice treated with mercury contradict this hypothesis (213). Metals may also have diverse effects on immunoregulatory (suppressor?) T cells and cause their inhibition or activation. Mercury-induced suppressor T cells producing TGF-β have been detected in LEW rats (211). The percentage of RT6$^+$ T lymphocytes that have an immunoregulatory role in various rat models of autoimmune disease decreases in mercury-treated BN rats, a change correlated with the appearance of autoimmunity (163,179,180,255). Alterations of the idiotype-antiidiotype network may occur through an "internal image" phenomenon, but there is no solid evidence that such a mechanism has an initiating role in metal-induced autoimmunity (159).

## CONCLUSIONS

Because of changes in therapeutics, there have been few recent reports of human autoimmune disease induced by mercury. Similarly, initial medical attention to the possible side effects of gold compounds may have decreased the incidence of autoimmunity caused by this metal. Occupational exposure to mercury and gold seldom results in persistent immunologic consequences (256). The paucity of metal-induced human pathology may therefore be caused by lack of sufficient exposure or the bias of individual susceptibility traits. However, the occasional patients with gold- or mercury-induced autoimmune responses or disease should not be discounted. The huge amount of evidence obtained from experimental animal studies shows the diverse and polymorphic pathologic consequences of gold and mercury exposure. It is clear that these metals can act on the immune system and cause autoimmunity in humans, rabbits, mice, and rats.

Apart from the obvious conclusion that occupational or therapeutic exposure to mercury and gold should be avoided as much as possible, there are positive consequences from studies of the immunotoxic effects of these metals. An example of the progress that can be achieved through such investigations is provided by data on the cytokine network in mercury-treated mice. The $T_H1/T_H2$ paradigm has been used as an explanation for the pathogenesis of autoimmune disease and a rationale for therapeutic strategies (208,209,257). However, in vivo studies have led to the realization that it may not fully explain the mechanisms involved in autoimmunity, allergy, and transplantation (258–260). Blocking IFN-$\gamma$ with soluble IFN-$\gamma$ receptor (IFN-$\gamma$R) inhibits murine lupus in (NZB$\times$NZW)F$_1$ hybrid (BW) mice (261). IFN-$\gamma$R–knockout MRL mice do not develop murine lupus, possibly because of an inhibition of autoantibody production (262). Murine lupus is also inhibited in IFN-$\gamma$R–knockout BW mice (263). In this case, the effects of genetic targeting of IFN-$\gamma$R on autoantibody production were not limited to an inhibition of IFN-$\gamma$-dependent mouse IgG isotypes (IgG2a and IgG3) but also involved IgG1 and IgM isotypes. IFN-$\gamma$-knockout mice immunized with acetylcholine receptor (AChR) in CFA do not develop experimental autoimmune myasthenia gravis, a disease mediated by autoantibodies to AChR (264). The resistance of these mice was associated with greatly reduced levels of circulating autoantibodies to AchR, a dramatic decrease involving autoantibodies to AChR of IgG isotypes that are $T_H1$-cytokine–dependent (IgG2a, IgG3) and isotypes that are $T_H2$-dependent (IgG1, IgG2b). Immunization of IFN-$\gamma$-knockout mice apparently failed to elicit significant amounts of autoantibodies to AChR in any IgG subclass.

As summarized for the mercury-induced mouse model, similar results have been obtained from elegant studies of

mercury-treated gene-targeted mice (213). Those investigations have revealed that IFN-$\gamma$ is essential, whereas IL-4 is not required for the development of autoantibodies to fibrillarin in HgCl$_2$-injected mice. In contrast, other experimental models of autoimmune disease that are T-cell mediated, such as EAE, collagen-induced arthritis, and EAU, have been produced in IFN-$\gamma$ knockout mice by immunization with high doses of antigen and CFA (265). These findings suggest that IFN-$\gamma$ is essential in the early stages of induction of spontaneous and experimental models of autoimmunity that are mediated by autoantibodies. IFN-$\gamma$ may be required to activate adaptive immune responses to self-antigens, possibly through the induction of costimulatory factors (e.g., B7.2) or increased MHC class II and class I expression that favor epitope presentation (266). These responses, depending on cytokine levels, costimulatory molecules and other environmental factors may eventually differentiate in autoantibody production driven by type 2 and/or type 1 cytokines (267). Experiments in IFN-$\gamma$–knockout mice and evidence from rat models lead to similar conclusions (i.e., the early role of IFN-$\gamma$ in some autoimmune responses mediated by autoantibodies). However, IFN-$\gamma$ may not be absolutely necessary for the early induction of cell-mediated models of autoimmunity where other cytokines (e.g., IL-1, lymphotoxin, migration inhibition factor, TNF-$\alpha$), together with or independently of IFN-$\gamma$, may be responsible for activating effector functions (268).

Another research topic that may be clarified by investigations of animal models is the difference between metals capable of inducing autoimmune responses and those that do not. For example, there are no published reports of autoimmune disease induced by aluminum, a metal with good adjuvant capabilities. Exposure to various other metals (e.g., arsenic, cobalt) that affect lymphocytes and macrophages might also result in autoimmune responses, but they have not been detected. In particular, lead has well-known immunotoxic properties, but there are no confirmed observations of its autoimmune effects. Beryllium can induce chronic beryllium disease by means of an immune pathogenesis, but early suggestions of its association with autoimmune disease have not been corroborated. It is possible that many metals have immunotoxic effects but cannot cause autoimmune responses and disease. Alternatively, if they act at very low environmental levels with extremely long periods of exposure we may have difficulties in associating them with autoimmunity. This is an interesting area that has been mostly ignored but deserves additional studies.

Synergism between metals and microorganisms may increase the autoimmune-inducing potential of these agents. Metals can induce autoimmunity. Similarly, numerous bacteria and viruses can generate autoimmune responses and disease (269–278). An intriguing graft-versus-host–like syndrome with a variety of autoimmune responses and tissue lesions may develop in BN rats treated with mercury (181). This syndrome disappears after antibiotic treatment, suggesting a possible role of microorganisms. It would be of interest to know whether it is caused by synergistic effects of mercury and bacteria on the immune system.

Considering the variety of environmental metals and other xenobiotics, the complexity of the immune system, and the diversity of immunogenetic and ecogenetic phenotypes, a single mechanism is unlikely to be responsible for the induction of autoimmune responses and disease by metals. Understanding the sequence of these complex events may require in depth studies of diverse animal models in which some of the variables are more easily controlled. On the basis of its range of immunotoxic properties, I have suggested that the pleiotropic effects of mercury should be considered a paradigm of metal-induced autoimmunity (11). *In vitro* and *in vivo* research of autoimmune disease caused by mercury, gold, and other metals has already yielded extremely valuable information and answered a number of important questions. At the same time, it has raised various issues connected to the possible mechanisms of xenobiotic activity, whether they suppress or stimulate the various components of the immune system. Investigations of metal-induced autoimmunity have the potential to produce new knowledge with relevance to autoimmune disease caused by other xenobiotics and idiopathic autoimmunity.

## ACKNOWLEDGMENTS

I wish to thank Dr. K. Michael Pollard (W. M. Keck Autoimmune Disease Center, Department of Molecular and Experimental Medicine, The Scripps Research Institute, La Jolla, CA) and Professor Per Hultman (Division of Molecular and Immunological Pathology, Department of Health and Environment, Linköping University, Linköping, Sweden) for kindly providing illustrations and data from their work on mercury-induced autoimmunity in mice. I am also grateful for their comments on this manuscript. Our studies of xenobiotic-induced autoimmunity are supported by grant ES03230 from USPHS.

## REFERENCES

1. Bigazzi PE. Autoimmunity induced by chemicals. *J Toxicol Clin Toxicol* 1988;26:125–156.
2. Druet P, Pelletier L, Rossert J, et al. Autoimmune reactions induced by metals. In: Kammüller ME, Bloksma N, Seinen W, eds. *Autoimmunity and toxicology.* Amsterdam: Elsevier, 1989:347–361.
3. Hess EV. The role of drugs and environmental agents in lupus syndromes. *Curr Opin Rheumatol* 1992;4:688–692.
4. Yoshida S, Gershwin ME. Autoimmunity and selected environmental factors of disease induction. *Semin Arthritis Rheum* 1993;22, 399–419.
5. Bigazzi PE. Autoimmunity induced by metals. In: Chang LW, ed. *Toxicology of metals.* Boca Raton, FL: CRC Lewis Publishers, 1996:835–852.
6. Kosuda LL, Bigazzi PE. Chemical-induced autoimmunity. In: Smialowicz RJ, Holsapple MP, eds. *Experimental immunotoxicology.* Boca Raton, FL: CRC Press, 1996:419–465.
7. Pollard KM, Hultman P. Effects of mercury on the immune system. In: Sigel A, Sigel H, eds. *Metal ions in biological systems.* New York: Marcel Dekker, 1997:421–440.
8. Bigazzi PE. Autoimmunity caused by xenobiotics. *Toxicology* 1997;119:1–21.
9. Descotes J. *Immunotoxicology of drugs and chemicals.* New York: Elsevier, 1986.
10. Kimber I. Chemical-induced hypersensitivity. In: Smialowicz RJ, Holsapple MP, eds. *Experimental immunotoxicology.* Boca Raton, FL: CRC Press, 1996:391–417.
11. Bigazzi PE. Mercury, In: Zelikoff J, Thomas P, eds. *Immunotoxicology of environmental and occupational metals.* London: Taylor & Francis, 1998:131–161.
12. Bolton WK, Suratt PM, Sturgill BC. Rapidly progressive silicon nephropathy. *Am J Med* 1081;71:823–828.
13. Hauglustaine D, Van Damme B, Daenens P, Michielsen P. Silicon nephropathy: a possible occupational hazard. *Nephron* 1980;26:219–224.
14. Brawer AE. Silicon and matrix macromolecules: new research opportunities for old diseases from analysis of potential mechanisms of breast implant toxicity. *Med Hypotheses* 1998;51:27–35.
15. van Landeghem GF, de Broe ME, D'Haese PC. Al and Si: their speciation, distribution, and toxicity. *Clin Biochem* 1998;31:385–397.
16. Wedeen RP. Heavy metals and the kidney. In: Cameron S, Davison AM, Grunfeld J-P, et al, eds. *Oxford textbook of clinical nephrology.* Oxford: Oxford University Press, 1992:837–848.
17. Nagaoka T, Tabata M, Kobayashi K, Okada A. Studies on production of anticollagen antibodies in silicosis. *Environ Res* 1993;60:12–29.
18. Levine S, Sowinski R. Experimental allergic encephalomyelitis: inhibition of clinical signs and paradoxical enhancement of lesions in second attacks. *Am J Pathol* 1980;101:375–385.
19. Levine S, Sowinski R. Enhancement of allergic encephalomyelitis by particulate adjuvants inoculated long before antigen. *Am J Pathol* 1980;99:291–304.
20. Garn H, Friedetzky A, Davis GS, et al. T-lymphocyte activation in the enlarged thoracic lymph nodes of rats with silicosis. *Am J Respir Cell Mol Biol* 1997;16:309–316.
21. Omara FO, Brousseau P, Blakley BR, Fournier M. Iron, zinc, and copper. In: Zelikoff J, Thomas P, eds. *Immunotoxicology of environmental and occupational metals.* London: Taylor & Francis, 1998:231–262.
22. Nielsen NH, Menne T. Allergic contact dermatitis caused by zinc pyrithione associated with pustular psoriasis. *Am J Contact Dermatol* 1997;8:170–171.
23. Stein EC, Schiffer RB, Hall WJ, Young N. Multiple sclerosis and the workplace: report of an industry-based cluster. *Neurology* 1987;37:1672–1677.
24. Schiffer RB, Herndon RM, Stabrowski A. Effects of dietary trace metals on experimental allergic encephalomyelitis in SJL mice. *Ann Neurol* 1988;24:141.
25. Schiffer RB, Herndon RM, Eskin T. Effects of altered dietary trace metals upon experimental allergic encephalomyelitis. *Neurotoxicology* 1990;11:443–450.
26. Schiffer RB, Sunderman FWJ, Baggs RB, Moynihan JA. The effects of exposure to dietary nickel and zinc upon humoral and cellular immunity in SJL mice. *J Neuroimmunol* 1991;34:229–239.
27. Ho S-Y, Catalanotto FA, Lisak RP, Dore-Duffy P. Zinc in multiple sclerosis. II: Correlation with disease activity and elevated plasma membrane-bound zinc in erythrocytes from patients with multiple sclerosis. *Ann Neurol* 1986;20:712–715.
28. Zelikoff JT, Cohen MD. Immunotoxicology of inorganic metal compounds. In: Smialowicz RJ, Holsapple MP, eds. *Experimental immunotoxicology.* Boca Raton, FL: CRC Press, 1996:189–228.
29. Pocino M, Malavé I, Baute L. Zinc administration restores the impaired immune response observed in mice receiving excess copper by oral route. *Immunopharmacol Immunotoxicol* 1990;12:697–713.
30. Boscolo P, DiGioacchino M, Bavazzano P, et al. Effects of chromium on lymphocyte subsets and immunoglobulins from normal populations and exposed workers. *Life Sci* 1997;60:1319–1325.
31. Snyder CA, Udasin I, Waterman SJ, et al. Reduced IL-6 levels among individuals in Hudson County, New Jersey, an area contaminated with chromium. *Arch Environ Health* 1996;51:26–28.
32. Kimber I, Basketter DA. Contact hypersensitivity to metals. In: Chang LW, ed. *Toxicology of metals.* Boca Raton, FL: CRC Lewis Publishers, 1996:827–833.
33. Kilburn KH, Warshaw RH. Prevalence of symptoms of systemic lupus erythematosus (SLE) and of fluorescent antinuclear antibodies associated with chronic exposure to trichloroethylene and other chemicals in well water. *Environ Res* 1992;57:1–9.
34. Tsankov N, Stransky L, Kostowa M, et al. Induced pemphigus caused by occupational contact with Basochrom. *Occup Environ Dermatol* 1990;38:91–93.

35. Ishii N, Takahashi K, Kawaguchi H, et al. Genetic control of delayed-type hypersensitivity to chromium chloride. *Int Arch Allergy Immunol* 1993;100:333–337.

36. McCabe MJJ. Lead. In: Zelikoff J, Thomas P, eds. *Immunotoxicology of environmental and occupational metals.* London: Taylor & Francis, 1998:111–130.

37. McCabe MJ, Lawrence DA. The heavy metal lead exhibits B cell-stimulatory factor activity by enhancing B cell Ia expression and differentiation. *J Immunol* 1990;145:671–677.

38. McCabe MJ, Lawrence DA. Lead, a major environmental pollutant, is immunomodulatory by Its differential effects on CD4⁺ T cell subsets. *Toxicol Appl Pharmacol* 1991;111:13–23.

39. Noelle RJ, Lawrence DA. Modulation of T-cell function. II. Chemical basis for the involvement of cell-surface thiol-reactive sites in control of T-cell proliferation. *Cell Immunol* 1981;60:453–469.

40. Lawrence DA, McCabe MJ Jr. Immune modulation by toxic metals. In: Goyer RA, Klaassen CD, Waalkes, MP, eds. *Metal toxicology.* San Diego: Academic Press, 1995:305–337.

41. Heo Y, Parsons PJ, Lawrence DA. Lead differentially modifies cytokine production in vitro and in vivo. *Toxicol Appl Pharmacol* 1996;138:149–157.

42. Lawrence DA. Immunotoxicity of heavy metals. In: Dean J, Luster MI, Munson AE, Amos H, eds. *Immunotoxicology and immunopharmacology.* New York: Raven Press, 1985:341–353.

43. Wedeen RP, Mallik DK, Batuman V. Detection and treatment of occupational lead nephropathy. *Arch Intern Med* 1979;139:53–57.

44. Wedeen RP. Lead nephrotoxicity. In: Porter GA, ed. *Nephrotoxic mechanisms of drugs and environmental toxins.* New York: Plenum Medical Books, 1982:255–265.

45. Pinkerton LE, Biagini RE, Ward EM, et al. Immunologic findings among lead-exposed workers. *Am J Ind Med* 1998:33:400–408.

46. El-Fawal HAN. Concepts of immunological biomarkers of metal toxicity. In: Chang LW, ed. *Toxicology of metals.* Boca Raton, FL: CRC Lewis Publishers, 1996:45–59.

47. Jarup L, Berglund M, Elinder CG, et al. Health effects of cadmium exposure—a review of the literature and a risk estimate. *Scand J Work Environ Health* 1998;24[Suppl 1]:1–51.

48. Bernard AM, Roels HR, Foidart JM, Lauwerys RL. Search for anti-laminin antibodies in the serum of workers exposed to cadmium, mercury vapour or lead. *Int Arch Occup Environ Health* 1987;59:303–309.

49. Joshi BC. Immune complex nephritis in rats induced by long-term oral exposure to cadmium. *J Comp Pathol* 1981;91:11–15.

50. Bernard A, Lauwerys R, Gengoux P, et al. Anti-laminin antibodies in Sprague–Dawley and Brown Norway rats chronically exposed to cadmium. *Toxicology* 1984;31:307–313.

51. Chowdhury BA, Friel JK, Chandra RK. Cadmium-induced immunopathology is prevented by zinc administration in mice. *J Nutr* 1987; 117:1788–1794.

52. Ohsawa M, Takahashi K, Otsuka F. Induction of anti-nuclear antibodies in mice orally exposed to cadmium at low concentrations. *Clin Exp Immunol* 1988;73:98–102.

53. Weiss RA, Madaio MP, Tomaszewski JE, Kelly CJ. T cells reactive to an inducible heat shock protein induce disease in toxin-induced interstitial nephritis. *J Exp Med* 1994;180:2239–2250.

54. Rodgers K, Platinum. In: Zelikoff J, Thomas P, eds. *Immunotoxicology of environmental and occupational metals.* London: Taylor & Francis, 1998:195–206.

55. Koch P, Baum HP. Contact stomatitis due to palladium and platinum in dental alloys. *Contact Dermatitis* 1996;34:253–257.

56. Schuppe H-C, Ronnau AC, von Schmiederberg S, et al. Immunomodulation by heavy metal compounds. *Clin Dermatol* 1998;16:149–157.

57. Dearman RJ, Basketter DA, Kimber I. Selective induction of type 2 cytokines following topical exposure of mice to platinum salts. *Food Chem Toxicol* 1998;36:199–207.

58. Schuppe H-C, Haas-Raida D, Kulig J, et al. T-cell–dependent popliteal lymph node reactions to platinum compounds in mice. *Int Arch Allergy Immunol* 1992;97:308–314.

59. Schuppe H-C, Haas-Raida D, Kulig J, et al. Platinum compounds induce pathological immune reactions in mice. *Immunobiology* 1990; 181:238.

60. Fung MC, Bowen DL. Silver products for medical indications: risk-benefit assessment. *J Toxicol Clin Toxicol* 1996;34:119–126.

61. Klaassen CD, ed. *Casarett and Doull's toxicology.* New York: McGraw-Hill, 1996.

62. Goyer RA. Toxic effects of metals. In: Klaassen CD, ed. *Casarett and Doull's toxicology.* New York: Pergamon Press, 1996:691–736.

63. Zheng W. Choroid plexus and metal toxicity. In: Chang LW, ed. *Toxicology of metals.* Boca Raton, FL: CRC Lewis Publishers, 1996: 609–626.

64. Hollinger MA. Toxicological aspects of topical silver pharmaceuticals. *Crit Rev Toxicol* 1996;26:255–260.

65. Kansu G, Aydin AK. Evaluation of the biocompatibility of various dental alloys: Part 2. Allergenical potentials. *Eur J Prosthodont Restor Dent* 1996;4:155–161.

66. Hultman P, Johansson U, Turley SJ, et al. Adverse immunological effects and autoimmunity induced by dental amalgam and alloy in mice. *FASEB J* 1994;8:1183–1190.

67. Hultman P, Eneström S, Turley SJ, Pollard KM. Selective induction of anti-fibrillarin autoantibodies by silver nitrate in mice. *Clin Exp Immunol* 1994;96:285–291.

68. Hultman P, Ganowiak K, Turley SJ, Pollard KM. Genetic susceptibility to silver-induced anti-fibrillarin autoantibodies in mice. *Clin Immunol Immunopathol* 1995;77:291–297.

69. Hart DA. Modulation of the immune system elements by lithium. In: Bach RO, Gallicchio VS, eds. *Lithium and cell physiology.* New York: Springer–Verlag, 1990:58–81.

70. Hart DA. Lithium, lymphocyte stimulation and the neuroimmune interface. *Lithium Ther Monogr* 1991;4:46–67.

71. Hart DA. Immunoregulation in patients treated with lithium for affective disorders. *Lithium Ther Monogr* 1991;4:68–78.

72. Hassman RA, McGregor AM. Lithium and autoimmune thyroid disease. *Lithium Ther Monogr* 1988;2, 134–146.

73. Hassman RA, McGregor AM. Lithium and autoimmune thyroid disease. In: Johnson FN, ed. *Lithium and the endocrine system.* Basel: Karger, 1988:134–146.

74. Kushner JP, Wartofsky L. Lithium-thyroid interactions: an overview. *Lithium Ther Monogr* 1988;2:74–98.

75. Hassman R, Solic N, Jasani B, et al. Immunological events leading to destructive thyroiditis in the AUG rat. *Clin Exp Immunol* 1988;73: 410–416.

76. Insel PA. Analgesic-antipyretic and anti-inflammatory agents and drugs employed in the treatment of gout. In: Hardman JG, Limbird LE, Molinoff PB, Ruddon RW, eds. *Goodman and Gilman's the pharmacological basis of therapeutics.* New York: McGraw–Hill 1996: 644–646.

77. Jones G, Brooks PM. Injectable gold compounds: an overview. *Br J Rheumatol* 1996;35:1154–1158.

78. Ward PA, Goldschmidt P, Greene ND. Suppressive effects of metal salts on leukocyte and fibroblastic functions. *J Reticuloendoth Soc* 1975;18:313–321.

79. Griem P, Takahashi K, Kalbacher H, Gleichmann E. The antirheumatic drug disodium aurothiomalate inhibits CD4⁺ T cell recognition of peptides containing two or more cysteine residues. *J Immunol* 1995;155:1575–1587.

80. Goebel C, Kubicka-Muranyi M, Tonn T, et al. Phagocytes render chemicals immunogenic: oxidation of gold(I) to the T cell-sensitizing gold(III) metabolite generated by mononuclear phagocytes. *Arch Toxicol* 1995;69:450–459.

81. Hostynek JJ. Gold: an allergen of growing significance. *Food Chem Toxicol* 1997;35:839–844.

82. Adams LE, Hess EV. Drug-related lupus: incidence, mechanisms and clinical implications. *Drug Safety* 1991;6:431–449.

83. Palosuo T, Milgrom F. Gold-induced autoimmune reactions. In: Porter GA, ed. *Nephrotoxic mechanisms of drugs and environmental toxins.* New York: Plenum Medical Books, 1982:409–412.

84. Romagnoli P, Spinas GA, Sinigaglia F. Gold-specific T cells in rheumatoid arthritis patients treated with gold. *J Clin Invest* 1992; 89:254–258.

85. Lee JC, Dushkin M, Eyring EJ, et al. Renal lesions associated with gold therapy: light and electron microscopic studies. *Arthritis Rheum* 1965;8:1–13.

86. Katz A, Little AH. Gold nephropathy. *Arch Pathol* 1973;96:133–136.

87. Törnroth T, Skrifvars B. Gold nephropathy prototype of membranous glomerulonephritis. *Am J Pathol* 1974;75:573–586.

88. Watanabe I, Whittier FC, Moore J, Cuppage FE. Gold nephropathy. *Arch Pathol Lab Med* 1976;100:632–635.

89. Hall CL. Gold nephropathy. *Nephron* 1988;50:265–272.

90. Hall CL. The natural course of gold and penicillamine nephropathy: a long-term study of 54 patients. *Adv Exp Med Biol* 1989;252:247–256.

91. Fillastre JP, Godin M. Drug-induced nephropathies. In: Cameron S, Davison AM, Grünfeld, et al, eds. *Oxford textbook of clinical nephrology.* Oxford: Oxford University Press, 1992:159–175.

92. Heptinstall RH. Polyarteritis (periarteritis) nodosa and rheumatoid arthritis. In: Heptinstall RH, ed. *Pathology of the kidney.* Boston: Little, Brown, 1983:828–832.

93. Kosty MP, Hench PK, Tani P, McMillan R. Thrombocytopenia associated with auronofin therapy: evidence for a gold-dependent immunologic mechanism. *Am J Hematol* 1989;30:236–239.

94. Ciompi ML, Marchetti G, Bazzichi L, et al. D-Penicillamine and gold salt treatments were complicated by myasthenia and pemphigus, respectively, in the same patient with rheumatoid arthritis. *Rheumatol Int* 1995;15:95–97.

95. Smith W, Ball GV. Lung injury due to gold treatment. *Arthritis Rheum* 1980;23:351–354.

96. Nagi AH, Alexander F, Barabas AZ. Gold nephropathy in rats: light and electron microscopic studies. *Exp Mol Pathol* 1971;15:354–362.

97. Nagi AH, Khan AH. Gold nephropathy in rabbits using an indigenous preparation: a morphological study. *Int Urol Nephrol* 1984;16:49–59.

98. Ueda S, Wakashin M, Wakashin Y, et al. Experimental gold nephropathy in guinea pigs: detection of autoantibodies to renal tubular antigens. *Kidney Int* 1986;29:539–548.

99. Tournade H, Guery JC, Pasquier R, et al. Effect of the thiol group on experimental gold-induced autoimmunity. *Arthritis Rheum* 1991;34:1594–1599.

100. Tournade H, Guery J-C, Pasquier R, et al. Experimental gold-induced autoimmunity. *Nephrol Dial Transplant* 1991;6:621–630.

101. Goter-Robinson CJ, Balasz T, Egorov IK. Mercuric chloride, gold sodium thiomalate, and D-penicillamine induced antinucleolar antibodies in mice. *Toxicol Appl Pharmacol* 1986;86:159–169.

102. Schuhmann D, Kubicka-Muranyi M, Mirtschewa J, et al. Adverse immune reactions to gold. I. Chronic treatment with an Au(I) drug sensitizes mouse T cells not to Au(I), but to Au(III) and induces autoantibody formation. *J Immunol* 1990;145, 2132–2139.

103. Bigazzi PE. Autoimmunity and heavy metals. *Lupus* 1994;3:449–453.

104. Eley BM, Cox SW. The release, absorption and possible health effects of mercury from dental amalgam: a review of recent findings, *Br Dent J* 1993;175:355–362.

105. Jokstad A, Thomassen Y, Bye E, et al. Dental amalgam and mercury. *Pharmacol Toxicol* 1992;70, 308–313.

106. Langworth S, Elinder CG, Sundquist KG. Minor effects of low exposure to inorganic mercury on the human immune system. *Scand J Work Environ Health* 1993;19:405–413.

107. Molin C. Amalgam—fact and fiction. *Scand J Dent Res* 1992;100:66–73.

108. Olsson S, Bergman M. Daily dose calculations from measurements of intra-oral mercury vapor. *J Dent Res* 1992;71:414–423.

109. Christensen MM, Ellermann-Eriksen S, Rungby J, Mogensen SC. Influence of mercuric chloride on resistance to generalized infection with herpes simplex virus type 2 in mice. *Toxicology* 1996;114:57–66.

110. Schopf E, Schulz KH, Gromm M. Transformationen und Mitosen von Lymphozyten in vitro durch Quecksilber(II)-chlorid. *Naturwissenschaften* 1967;54:568–569.

111. Schopf E, Schulz KH, Isensee I. Investigations on lymphocyte transformation in mercury sensitivity: nonspecific transformation due to mercury compounds. *Arch Klin Exp Dermatol* 1969;234:420–433.

112. Reardon CL, Lucas DO. $Zn^{2+}$ and $Hg^{2+}$-mediated induction of mitogenesis, cell-mediated cytotoxicity, and interferon production in murine lymphocytes. In: Parker JW, O'Brien RL, eds. *Intercellular communication in leukocyte function.* New York: J Wiley & Sons, 1983:449–452.

113. Reardon CL, Lucas DO. Heavy metal mitogenesis: $Zn^{2+}$ and $Hg^{2+}$ induce cellular cytotoxicity and interferon production in murine T lymphocytes. *Immunobiology* 1987;175:455.

114. Shenker BJ, Rooney C, Vitale L, Shapiro IM. Immunotoxic effects of mercuric compounds on human lymphocytes and monocytes. I. Suppression of T cell activation. *Immunopharmacol Immunotoxicol* 1992;14:539–553.

115. Sharma RP, Dugyala RR. Effects of metals on cell-mediated immunity and biological response modulators. In: Chang LW, ed. *Toxicology of metals.* Boca Raton, FL: CRC Lewis Publishers, 1996:785–796.

116. Jiang Y, Möller G. *In vitro* effects of $HgCl_2$ on murine lymphocytes. I. Preferable activation of $CD4^+$ T cells in a responder strain. *J Immunol* 1995;154:3138–3146.

117. Albers R, de Heer C, Bol M, et al. Selective immunomodulation by the autoimmunity-inducing xenobiotics streptozotocin and $HgCl_2$. *Eur J Immunol* 1998;28:1233–1242.

118. Aten J, Prigent P, Poncet P, et al. Mercuric chloride-induced programmed cell death of a murine hybridoma. I. Effect of the proto-oncogene Bcl-2. *Cell Immunol* 1995;161:98–106.

119. Whitekus MJ, Santini RP, Rosenspire AJ, McCabe MJJ. Protection against CD95-mediated apoptosis by inorganic mercury in Jurkat T cells. *J Immunol* 1999;162:7162–7170.

120. van der Meide PH, de Labie MCDC, Botman CAD, et al. Mercuric chloride down-regulates T cell interferon-γ production in brown Norway but not in Lewis rats; role of glutathione. *Eur J Immunol* 1993;23:675–681.

121. van der Meide PH, de Labie MCDC, Botman CAD, et al. Nitric oxide suppresses IFN-γ production in the spleen of mercuric chloride-exposed Brown Norway rats. *Cell Immunol* 1995;161:195–206.

122. Exon JH, South EH, Hendrix K. Effects of metals on the humoral immune response. In: Change LW, ed. *Toxicology of metals.* Boca Raton, FL: CRC Lewis Publishers, 1996:797–810.

123. Shenker BJ, Berthold P, Rooney C, et al. Immunotoxic effects of mercuric compounds on human lymphocytes and monocytes. III. Alterations in B-cell function and viability. *Immunopharmacol Immunotoxicol* 1993;15:87–112.

124. Daum JR, Shepherd DM, Noelle RJ. Immunotoxicology of cadmium and mercury on B-lymphocytes. I. Effects on lymphocyte function. *Int J Immunopharmacol* 1993;15:383–394.

125. Prouvost-Danon A, Abadie A, Sapin C, et al. Induction of IgE synthesis and potentiation of anti-ovalbumin IgE antibody response by $HgCl_2$ in the rat. *J Immunol* 1981;126:699–702.

126. Pelletier L, Pasquier R, Guettier C, et al. $HgCl_2$ induces T and B cells to proliferate and differentiate in BN rats. *Clin Exp Immunol* 1988;71:336–342.

127. Zelikoff JT, Smialowicz RJ. Metal-induced alterations in innate immunity. In: Chang LW, ed. *Toxicology of metals.* Boca Raton, FL: CRC Press, 1996:811–826.

128. Contrino J, Kosuda LL, Marucha P, et al. The in vitro effects of mercury on peritoneal leukocytes (PMN and macrophages) from inbred Brown Norway and Lewis rats. *Int J Immunopharmacol* 1992;14:1051–1059.

129. Zdolsek JM, Soder O, Hultman P. Mercury induces in vivo and in vitro secretion of interleukin-1 in mice. *Immunopharmacology* 1994;28, 201–208.

130. Mathieson PW, Gillespie KM. Cloning of a partial cDNA for rat interleukin-12 (IL-12) and analysis of IL-12 expression in vivo. *Scand J Immunol* 1996;44:11–14.

131. Contrino J, Marucha P, Ribaudo R, et al. Effects of mercury on human polymorphonuclear leukocyte function in vitro. *Am J Pathol* 1988;132:110–118.

132. Baginski B. Effect of mercuric chloride on microbicidal activities of human polymorphonuclear leukocytes. *Toxicology* 1988;50:247–256.

133. Obel N, Hansen B, Christensen MM, et al. Methyl mercury, mercuric chloride, and silver lactate decrease superoxide anion formation and chemotaxis in human polymorphonuclear leucocytes. *Hum Exp Toxicol* 1993;12:361–364.

134. Oliveira DBG, Wolfreys K, Coleman JW. Compounds that induce Th2-driven autoimmunity in Brown Norway rats sensitize their mast cells in vitro. *Hum Exp Toxicol* 1994;13:615.

135. Warbrick EV, Thomas AL, Coleman JW. The effects of mercuric chloride on growth, cytokine and MHC class II gene expression in a human leukemic mast cell line. *Toxicology* 1995;104:179–186.

136. Medzhitov R, Janeway CAJ. Innate immunity: impact on the adaptive immune response. *Curr Opin Immunol* 1997;9:4–9.

137. Moretta A, Bottino C, Vitale M, et al. Receptors for HLA class-I molecules in human natural killer cells. *Annu Rev Immunol* 1996;14:619–648.

138. Ilback NG, Sundberg J, Oskarsson A. Methyl mercury exposure via placenta and milk impairs natural killer (NK) cell function in newborn rats. *Toxicol Lett* 1991;58:149–158.

139. Wild LG, Ortega HG, Lopez M, Salvaggio JE. Immune system alteration in the rat after indirect exposure to methyl mercury chloride or methyl mercury sulfide. *Environ Res* 1997;74:34–42.

140. Schrallhammer-Benkler K, Ring J, Przybilla B, Landthaler M. Acute mercury intoxication with lichenoid drug eruption followed by mercury contact allergy and development of antinuclear antibodies. *Acta Dermatol Venereol (Stockh)* 1992;72:294–296.

141. Orth SR, Ritz E. The nephrotic syndrome. *N Engl J Med* 1998; 338:1202–1211.

142. Fillastre J-P, Druet P, Mery J-P. Proteinuric nephropathies associated with drugs and substances of abuse. In: Cameron JS, Glassock RJ, eds. *The nephrotic syndrome*. New York: Marcel Dekker, 1988:697–744.

143. Barr RD, Rees PH, Cordy PE, et al. Nephrotic syndrome in adult Africans in Nairobi. *Br Med J* 1972;2:131–134.

144. Lindqvist KJ, Makene WJ, Shaba JK, Nantulya V. Immunofluorescence and electron microscopic studies of kidney biopsies from patients with nephrotic syndrome, possibly induced by skin lightening creams containing mercury. *E Afr Med J* 1974;51:168–169.

145. Charpentier B, Moullot P, Faux N, et al. Fonctions lymphocytaires T au cours d'une glomérulonéphrite extramembraneuse induite par une intoxication chronique au mercure. *Nephrologie* 1981;2:153–157.

146. Tubbs RR, Gephardt GN, McMahon JT, et al. Membranous glomerulonephritis associated with industrial mercury exposure. *Am J Clin Pathol* 1982;77:409–413.

147. Langworth S, Elinder CG, Sundquist KG, Vesterberg O. Renal and immunological effects of occupational exposure to inorganic mercury. *Br J Ind Med* 1992;49:394–401.

148. Cardenas A, Roels HR, Bernard AM, et al. Markers of early renal changes induced by industrial pollutants. I. Application to workers exposed to mercury vapour. *Br J Ind Med* 1993;50:17–27.

149. Bigazzi PE. Lessons from animal models: the scope of mercury-induced autoimmunity. *Clin Immunol Immunopathol* 1992;65:81–84.

150. Goldman M, Druet P, Gleichmann E. $T_H2$ cells in systemic autoimmunity: insights from allogeneic diseases and chemically induced autoimmunity. *Immunol Today* 1991;12:223–227.

151. Roman-Franco AA, Turiello M, Albini B, et al. Anti-basement membrane antibodies and antigen-antibody complexes in rabbits injected with mercuric chloride. *Clin Immunol Immunopathol* 1978;9:464–481.

152. Albini B, Andres GA. Autoimmune disease induced in rabbits by administration of mercuric chloride: evidence suggesting a role for antigens of the connective tissue matrix. In: Cummings NB, Michael AF, Wilson CB, eds. *Immune mechanisms in renal disease*. New York: Plenum Medical Books, 1983:249–260.

153. Bariety J, Druet P, Laliberte F, Sapin C. Glomerulonephritis with γ- and β1c-globulin deposits induced in rats by mercuric chloride. *Am J Pathol* 1971;65:293–300.

154. Sapin C, Druet E, Druet P. Induction of anti-glomerular basement membrane antibodies in the Brown Norway rat by mercuric chloride. *Clin Exp Immunol* 1977;28:173–179.

155. Druet E, Sapin C, Günther E, et al. Mercuric chloride-induced anti-glomerular basement membrane antibodies in the rat: genetic control. *Eur J Immunol* 1977;7:348–351.

156. Bellon B, Verroust P, Mandet C, Druet P. Spontaneous circulating immune complex like material in Brown Norway rats: role of environmental factors. *J Clin Lab Immunol* 1982;8:133–136.

157. Fukatsu A, Brentjens JR, Killen PD, et al. Studies on the formation of glomerular immune deposits in Brown Norway rats injected with mercuric chloride. *Clin Immunol Immunopathol* 1987;45:35–47.

158. Henry GA, Jarnot BM, Steinhoff MM, Bigazzi PE. Mercury-induced renal autoimmunity in the MAXX rat. *Clin Immunol Immunopathol* 1988;49:187–203.

159. Bigazzi PE, Michaelson JH, Potter NT. Epibodies in autoimmunity: antisera against autoantibodies to the renal glomerular basement membrane react with idiotypes as well as with autoantigens. *Autoimmunity* 1989;5:3–16.

160. Aten J, Veninga A, Bruijn JA, et al. Antigenic specificities of glomerular-bound autoantibodies in membranous glomerulopathy induced by mercuric chloride. *Clin Immunol Immunopathol* 1992;63:89–102.

161. Icard P, Pelletier L, Vial M-C, et al. Evidence for a role of antilaminin-producing B cell clones that escape tolerance in the pathogenesis of $HgCl_2$-induced membranous glomerulopathy. *Nephrol Dial Transplant* 1993;8:122–127.

162. Druet E, Guery J-C, Ayed K, et al. Characteristics of polyreactive and monospecific IgG anti-laminin autoantibodies in the rat mercury model. *Immunology* 1994;83:489–494.

163. Kosuda LL, Whalen B, Greiner DL, Bigazzi PE. Mercury-induced autoimmunity in Brown Norway rats: kinetics of changes in RT6+ T lymphocytes correlated with IgG isotypes of circulating autoantibodies to laminin 1. *Toxicology* 1998;125:215–231.

164. Aten J, Veninga A, Coers W, et al. Autoantibodies to the laminin P1 fragment in $HgCl_2$-induced membranous glomerulopathy. *Am J Pathol* 1995;146:1467–1480.

165. Timpl R. Macromolecular organization of basement membranes. *Curr Opin Cell Biol* 1996;8:618–624.

166. Burgeson RE, Chiquet M, Deutzmann R, et al. A new nomenclature for the laminins. *Matrix Biol* 1994;14:209–211.

167. Engvall E, Krusius T, Wewer U, Ruoslahti E. Laminin from rat yolk sac tumor: isolation, partial characterization, and comparison with mouse laminin. *Arch Biochem* 1983;222:649–656.

168. Kosuda LL, Greiner DL, Bigazzi PE. Effects of $HgCl_2$ on the expression of autoimmune responses and disease in diabetes-prone (DP) BB rats. *Autoimmunity* 1997;26:173–187.

169. Weening JJ, Fleuren GJ, Hoedemaeker PJ. Demonstration of antinuclear antibodies in mercuric chloride-induced glomerulopathy in the rat. *Lab Invest* 1978;39:405–411.

170. Weening JJ, Grond J, Van der Top D, Hoedemaeker PJ. Identification of the nuclear antigen involved in mercury-induced glomerulopathy in the rat. *Invest Cell Pathol* 1980;3:129–134.

171. Weening JJ, Hoedemaeker PJ, Bakker WW. Immunoregulation and anti-nuclear antibodies in mercury-induced glomerulopathy in the rat. *Clin Exp Immunol* 1981;45:64–71.

172. Aten J, Bosman CB, Rozing J, et al. Mercuric chloride-induced autoimmunity in the Brown Norway rat. *Am J Pathol* 1988;133:127–138.

173. Capron M, Ayed K, Druet E, et al. Complement studies in BN rats with mercuric chloride-induced immune glomerulonephritis. *Ann Immunol* 1980;131D:43–55.

174. Bernaudin JF, Druet E, Belair MF, et al. Extrarenal immune complex type deposits induced by mercuric chloride in the Brown Norway rat. *Clin Exp Immunol* 1979;38:265–273.

175. Andres P. IgA-IgG disease in the intestine of Brown Norway rats ingesting mercuric chloride. *Clin Immunol Immunopathol* 1984;30:488–494.

176. Hinglais N, Druet P, Grossetete J, et al. Ultrastructural study of nephritis induced in Brown Norway rats by mercuric chloride. *Lab Invest* 1979;41:150–159.

177. Druet P, Druet E, Potdevin F, Sapin C. Immune type glomerulonephritis induced by $HgCl_2$ in the Brown Norway rat. *Ann Immunol* 1978;129C:777–792.

178. Kosuda LL, Hannigan MO, Bigazzi PE, et al. Thymus atrophy and changes in thymocyte subpopulations of BN rats with mercury-induced renal autoimmune disease. *Autoimmunity* 1996;23:77–89.

179. Kosuda LL, Wayne A, Nahounou M, et al. Reduction of the RT6.2+ subset of T lymphocytes in Brown Norway rats with mercury-induced renal autoimmunity. *Cell Immunol* 1991;135:154–167.

180. Kosuda LL, Greiner DL, Bigazzi PE. Mercury-induced renal autoimmunity: changes in RT6+ T lymphocytes of "susceptible" and "resistant" rats. *Environ Health Persp* 1993;101:178–185.

181. Mathieson PW, Thiru S, Oliveira DBG. Mercuric chloride-treated Brown Norway rats develop widespread tissue injury including necrotizing vasculitis. *Lab Invest* 1992;67:121–129.

182. Kiely PDW, Thiru S, Oliveira DBG. Inflammatory polyarthritis induced by mercuric chloride in the Brown Norway rat. *Lab Invest* 1995;73, 284–293.

183. Kiely PDW, Gillespie KM, Oliveira DBG. Oxpentifylline inhibits tumor necrosis factor-α mRNA transcription and protects against arthritis in mercuric chloride-treated Brown Norway rats. *Eur J Immunol* 1995;25:2899–2906.

184. Kiely PDW, O'Brien D, Oliveira DBG. Anti-CD8 treatment reduces the severity of inflammatory arthritis, but not vasculitis, in mercuric chloride-induced autoimmunity. *Clin Exp Immunol* 1996:106:280–285.

185. Peszkowski MJ, Warfvinge G, Larsson Å. $HgCl_2$-induced glandular pathosis in the Brown Norway rat. *Clin Immunol Immunopathol* 1993;69:272–277.

186. Baran D, Lantz O, Dosquet P, et al. Interleukin-2 production in Brown Norway rats with $HgCl_2$-induced autoimmune disease: paradoxical in vivo versus in vitro findings. *Clin Exp Immunol* 1988;73:401–405.

187. Gillespie K, Qasim F, Tibbatts L, et al. Interleukin-4 gene expression in mercury-induced autoimmunity, *Scand J Immunol* 1995;41:268–272.

188. Gillespie KM, Saoudi A, Kuhn J, et al. Th1/Th2 cytokine gene expression after mercuric chloride in susceptible and resistant rat strains. *Eur J Immunol* 1996;26:2388–2392.

189. Finkelman FD, Holmes J, Katona IM, et al. Lymphokine control of in vivo immunoglobulin isotype selection. *Annu Rev Immunol* 1990;8:303–333.

190. Benbenou N, Matsiota-Bernard P, Guenounou M. Antisense oligonu-cleotides to interleukin-4 regulate IgE and IgG2a production by spleen cells from *Nippostrongylus brasiliensis*-infected rats. *Eur J Immunol* 1993;23:659–663.

191. Mathieson PW. Mercury: god of Th2 cells? *Clin Exp Immunol* 1995;102, 229–230.

192. Aten J, Veninga A, DeHeer E, et al. Susceptibility to the induction of either autoimmunity or immunosuppression by mercuric chloride is related to the major histocompatibility complex class II haplotype. *Eur J Immunol* 1991;21:611–616.

193. Kosuda LL, Greiner DL, Bigazzi PE. Mercury-induced renal autoim-munity in BN → LEW.1N chimeric rats. *Cell Immunol* 1994; 155:77–94.

194. Salant DJ, Natori Y, Shimizu F. Glomerular injury due to antibody alone. In: Neilson EG, Couser WG, eds. *Immunologic renal disease*. Philadelphia: Lippincott-Raven Publishers, 1997:359–375.

195. Mathieson PW, Stapleton KJ, Oliveira DBG, Lockwood CM. Immunoregulation of mercuric chloride-induced autoimmunity in Brown Norway rats: a role for CD8+ T cells revealed by in vivo deple-tion studies. *Eur J Immunol* 1991;21:2105–2109.

196. Pelletier L, Rossert J, Pasquier R, et al. Role of CD8+ T cells in mer-cury-induced autoimmunity or immunosuppression in the rat. *Scand J Immunol* 1990;31:65–74.

197. Ochel M, Vohr HW, Pfeiffer C, Gleichmann E. IL-4 is required for the IgE and IgG1 increase and IgG1 autoantibody formation in mice treated with mercuric chloride. *J Immunol* 1991;146:3006–3011.

198. Druet P, Sheela R, Pelletier L. T$_H$1 and T$_H$2 lymphocytes in autoim-munity. *Adv Nephrol* 1996;25:217–241.

199. Druet P, Sheela R, Pelletier L. Th1 and Th2 cells in autoimmunity. *Chem Immunol* 1996;63:158–170.

200. Molina A, Sánchez-Madrid F, Bricio T, et al. Prevention of mercuric chloride-induced nephritis in the Brown Norway rat by treatment with antibodies against the $\alpha_4$ integrin. *J Immunol* 1995;153:2313–2320.

201. Pelletier L, Pasquier R, Rossert J, Druet P. HgCl$_2$ induces nonspecific immunosuppression in Lewis rats. *Eur J Immunol* 1987;17:49–54.

202. Pelletier L, Galceran M, Pasquier R, et al. Down modulation of Hey-mann's nephritis by mercuric chloride. *Kidney Int* 1987;32:227–232.

203. Pelletier L, Rossert J, Pasquier R, et al. Effect of HgCl$_2$ on experimen-tal allergic encephalomyelitis in Lewis rats: HgCl$_2$-induced down-modulation of the disease. *Eur J Immunol* 1988;18:243–247.

204. Rossert J, Pelletier L, Pasquier R, et al. HgCl$_2$-induced perturbation of the T cell network in experimental allergic encephalomyelitis. I. In vitro characterization of T cells involved. *Cell Immunol* 1991; 137:367–378.

205. Mordes JP, Gallina DL, Handler ES, et al. Transfusions enriched for W3/25+ helper/inducer T lymphocytes prevent spontaneous diabetes in the BB/W rat. *Diabetologia* 1987;30:22–26.

206. Crisá L, Mordes JP, Rossini AA. Autoimmune diabetes mellitus in the BB rat. *Diabetes Metabol Rev* 1992;8:9–37.

207. Saoudi A, Bellon B, De Kozak Y, et al. Prevention of experimental autoimmune uveoretinitis and experimental autoimmune pinealitis in (Lewis × Brown Norway) F$_1$ rats by HgCl$_2$ injections. *Immunology* 1991;74:348–354.

208. Liblau RS, Singer SM, McDevitt HO. Th1 and Th2 CD4+ T cells in the pathogenesis of organ-specific autoimmune diseases. *Immunol Today* 1995;16:34–38.

209. Adorini L, Guéry J-C, Trembleau S. Manipulation of the Th1/Th2 cell balance: an approach to treat human autoimmune diseases? *Autoim-munity* 1996;23:53–68.

210. Nicholson LB, Kuchroo VK. Manipulation of the Th1/Th2 balance in autoimmune disease. *Curr Opin Immunol* 1996;8:837–842.

211. Bridoux F, Badou A, Saoudi A, et al. Transforming growth factor beta (TGF-beta)–dependent inhibition of T helper cell 2 (Th2)–induced autoimmunity by self-major histocompatibility complex (MHC) class II-specific regulatory CD4(+) T cell lines. *J Exp Med* 1997;185: 1769–1775.

212. Rossini AA, Greiner DL, Friedman HP, Mordes JP. Immunopatho-genesis of diabetes mellitus. *Diabetes Rev* 1993;1:43–75.

213. Kono DH, Balomenos D, Pearson DL, et al. The prototypic Th2 autoimmunity induced by mercury is dependent on IFN-γ and not Th1/Th2 imbalance. *J Immunol* 1998;161:234–240.

214. Goter Robinson CJ, Abraham AA, Balasz T. Induction of anti-nuclear antibodies by mercuric chloride in mice. *Clin Exp Immunol* 1984;58: 300–306.

215. Hultman P, Enestrom S. Mercury induced antinuclear antibodies in mice: characterization and correlation with renal immune complex deposits. *Clin Exp Immunol* 1988;71:269–274.

216. Hultman P, Enestrom S, Pollard KM, Tan EM. Anti-fibrillarin autoan-tibodies in mercury-treated mice. *Clin Exp Immunol* 1989;78:470–477.

217. Reuter R, Tessars G, Vohr H-W, et al. Mercuric chloride induces autoantibodies to small nuclear ribonucleoprotein in susceptible mice. *Proc Natl Acad Sci USA* 1989;86:237–241.

218. Hultman P, Enestrom S. Mercury induced B-cell activation and anti-nuclear antibodies in mice. *J Clin Lab Immunol* 1989;28:143.

219. Saegusa J, Yamamoto S, Iwai H, Ueda K. Antinucleolar autoantibody induced in mice by mercuric chloride. *Ind Health* 1990;28:21–30.

220. Hultman P, Enestrom S. Dose-response studies in murine mercury-induced autoimmunity and immune-complex disease. *Toxicol Appl Pharmacol* 1992;113:199–208.

221. Monestier M, Losman MJ, Novick KE, Aris JP. Molecular analysis of mercury-induced antinucleolar antibodies in H-2s mice. *J Immunol* 1994;152:667–675.

222. Reimer G. Autoantibodies against nuclear, nucleolar, and mitochon-drial antigens in systemic sclerosis (scleroderma). *Rheum Dis Clin North Am* 1990;16:169–183.

223. Hultman P, Turley SJ, Enestrom S, et al. Murine genotype influences the specificity, magnitude and persistence of murine mercury-induced autoimmunity. *J Autoimmun* 1996;9:139–149.

224. Hultman P, Nielsen JB. The effects of toxicokinetics on murine mer-cury-induced autoimmunity. *Environ Res* 1998;77[Suppl A]:141–148.

225. Warfvinge K, Hansson H, Hultman P. Systemic autoimmunity due to mercury vapor exposure in genetically susceptible mice: dose-response studies. *Toxicol Appl Pharmacol* 1995;132:299–309.

226. Al-Balaghi S, Möller E, Möller G, Abedi-Valugerdi M. Mercury induces polyclonal B-cell activation, autoantibody production and renal immune complex deposits in young (NZB × NZW) F$_1$ hybrids. *Eur J Immunol* 1996;26:1519–1526.

227. Hultman P, Bell LJ, Enestrom S, Pollard KM. Murine susceptibility to mercury. I. Autoantibody profiles and systemic immune deposits in inbred, congenic and intra-H-2 recombinant strains. *Clin Immunol Immunopathol* 1992;65:98–109.

228. Enestrøm S, Hultman P. Immune-mediated glomerulonephritis induced by mercuric chloride in mice. *Experientia* 1984;40:1234–1240.

229. Hultman P, Enestrøm S. The induction of immune complex deposits in mice by peroral and parenteral administration of mercuric chloride: strain dependent susceptibility. *Clin Exp Immunol* 1987;67:283–292.

230. Goter-Robinson CJ, White HJ, Rose NR. Murine strain differences in response to mercuric chloride: antinucleolar antibodies production does not correlate with renal immune complex deposition. *Clin Immunol Immunopathol* 1997;83:127–138.

231. Stiller-Winkler R, Radaskiewicz T, Gleichmann E. Immunopatholog-ical signs in mice treated with mercury compounds. I. Identification by the popliteal lymph node assay of responder and nonresponder strains. *Int J Immunopharmacol* 1988;10:475–484.

232. Mirtcheva J, Pfeiffer C, De Bruijn JA, et al. Immunological alterations inducible by mercury compounds. III. H-2A acts as an immune response and H-2E as an immune "suppression" locus for HgCl$_2$-induced antinucleolar autoantibodies. *Eur J Immunol* 1989;19: 2257–2261.

233. Doth M, Fricke M, Nicoletti F, et al. Genetic differences in immune reactivity to mercuric chloride (HgCl$_2$): immunosuppression of H-2d mice is mediated by interferon-gamma (IFN-γ). *Clin Exp Immunol* 1997;109:149–156.

234. Hanley GA, Schiffenbauer J, Sobel ES. Class II haplotype differen-tially regulates immune response in HgCl$_2$-treated mice. *Clin Immunol Immunopathol* 1997;84, 328–337.

235. Hanley GA, Schiffenbauer J, Sobel ES. Resistance to HgCl$_2$-induced autoimmunity in haplotype-heterozygous mice is an intrinsic property of B cells. *J Immunol* 1998;161:1778–1785.

236. Griem P, Scholz E, Turfeld M, et al. Strain differences in tissue con-centrations of mercury in inbred mice treated with mercuric chloride. *Toxicol Appl Pharmacol* 1997;144:163–170.

237. Pollard KM, Lee DK, Casiano CA, et al. The autoimmunity-inducing xenobiotic mercury interacts with the autoantigen fibrillarin and mod-ifies its molecular and antigenic properties. *J Immunol* 1997;158: 3521–3528.

238. Hultman P, Johansson U, Dagnaes-Hansen F. Murine mercury-induced autoimmunity: the role of T-helper cells. *J Autoimmun* 1995;8: 809–823.

239. Biancone L, Andres G, Ahn H, et al. Distinct regulatory roles of lymphocyte costimulatory pathways on T helper type 2-mediated autoimmune disease. *J Exp Med* 1996;183:1473–1481.

240. Jiang Y, Möller G. Unresponsiveness of CD4⁺ T cells from a nonresponder strain to HgCl₂ is not due to CD8⁺-mediated immunosuppression: an analysis of the very early activation antigen CD69. *Scand J Immunol* 1996;44:565–570.

241. Kägi JHR. Overview of metallothionein. *Methods Enzymol* 1991;205: 613–626.

242. Griem P, Gleichmann E. Metal ion induced autoimmunity. *Curr Opin Immunol* 1995;7:831–838.

243. Kubicka-Muranyi M, Griem P, Lübben B, et al. Mercuric chloride-induced autoimmunity in mice involves an upregulated presentation of altered and unaltered nucleolar self antigen. *Int Arch Allergy Immunol* 1995;108:1–10.

244. Levinson W. Metal-binding drugs induce synthesis of four proteins in normal cells. *Biol Trace Element Res* 1979;1:15–23.

245. Levinson W. Transition series metals induce the synthesis of four proteins in eukaryotic cells. *Biochim Biophys Acta* 1980;606:170–180.

246. Levinson W, Oppermann H, Jackson J. Transition series metals and sulfhydryl reagents induce the synthesis of four proteins in eukaryotic cells. *Biochim Biophys Acta* 1980;606:170–180.

247. Goering PL, Fisher BR, Chaudhary PP, Dick CA. Relationship between stress protein induction in rat kidney by mercuric chloride and nephrotoxicity. *Toxicol Appl Pharmacol* 1992;113:184–191.

248. Cohen IR. Autoimmunity to HSP65 and the immunologic paradigm. *Adv Intern Med* 1992;37:295–311.

249. Goering PL, Fisher BR. Stress protein. In: Goyer RA, Cherian MG, eds. *Toxicology of metals: biochemical aspects.* Berlin: Springer–Verlag, 1995:229–266.

250. Rahman SMJ, Pu M, Hamaguchi M, et al. Redox-linked ligand-independent cell surface triggering for extensive protein tyrosine phosphorylation. *FEBS Lett* 1993;317:35–38.

251. Nakashima I, Pu M, Nishizaki A, et al. Redox mechanism as alternative to ligand binding for receptor activation delivering disregulated cellular signals. *J Immunol* 1994;152, 1064–1071.

252. Tan X, Tang C, Castoldi AF, et al. Effects of inorganic and organic mercury on intracellular calcium levels in rat T lymphocytes. *J Toxicol Environ Health* 1993;38:159–170.

253. Wylie DE, Lu D, Carlson LD, et al. Monoclonal antibodies specific for mercuric ions. *Proc Natl Acad Sci USA* 1992;89:4104–4108.

254. Kubicka-Muranyi M, Behmer O, Uhrberg M, et al. Murine systemic autoimmune disease induced by mercuric chloride (HgCl₂): Hg-specific helper T cells react to antigen stored in macrophages. *Int J Immunopharmacol* 1993;15:151–161.

255. Kosuda LL, Hosseinzadeh H, Greiner DL, Bigazzi PE. The role of RT6⁺ T lymphocytes in mercury-induced renal autoimmunity: experimental manipulations of "susceptible" and "resistant" rats. *J Toxicol Environ Health* 1994;42:303–321.

256. Ellingsen DG, Gaarder PI, Kjuus H. An immunological study of chloralkali workers previously exposed to mercury vapour. *Acta Pathol Microbiol Immunol Scand* 1994;102:170–176.

257. Röcken M, Racke M, Shevach EM. IL-4–induced immune deviation as antigen-specific therapy for inflammatory autoimmune disease. *Immunol Today* 1996;17:225–231.

258. Kelso A. Th1 and Th2 subsets: paradigms lost? *Immunol Today* 1995;16:374–379.

259. Nickerson P, Steurer W, Steiger J, et al. Cytokines and the Th1/Th2 paradigm in transplantation. *Curr Opin Immunol* 1994;6:757–764.

260. Aebischer I, Stadler BM. T$_H$1-T$_H$2 cells in allergic responses: at the limits of a concept. *Adv Immunol* 1996;61:341–403.

261. Ozmen L, Roman D, Fountoulakis M, et al. Experimental therapy of systemic lupus erythematosus: the treatment of NZB/W mice with soluble interferon-γ receptor inhibits the onset of glomerulonephritis. *Eur J Immunol* 1995;25:6–12.

262. Haas C, Ryffel B, Le Hir M. IFN-γ is essential for the development of autoimmune glomerulonephritis in MRL/lpr mice. *J Immunol* 1997; 158:5484–5491.

263. Haas C, Ryffel B, Le Hir M. IFN-γ receptor deletion prevents autoantibody production and glomerulonephritis in lupus-prone (NZB × NZW)F₁ mice. *J Immunol* 1998;160:3713–3718.

264. Balasa B, Deng C, Lee J, et al. Interferon γ (IFN-γ) is necessary for the genesis of acetylcholine receptor-induced clinical experimental autoimmune Myasthenia gravis in mice. *J Exp Med* 1997;186: 385–391.

265. Ferber IA, Brocke S, Taylor-Edwards C, et al. Mice with a disrupted IFN-γ gene are susceptible to the induction of experimental autoimmune encephalomyelitis (EAE). *J Immunol* 1996;156:5–7.

266. Lenschow DJ, Walunas TL, Bluestone JA. CD28/B7 system of T cell costimulation. *Annu Rev Immunol* 1996;14:233–258.

267. Carter L, Dutton RW. Type 1 and type 2: a fundamental dichotomy for all T-cell subsets. *Curr Opin Immunol* 1996;8:336–342.

268. Durum SK, Schmidt JA, Oppenheim JJ. Interleukin 1: an immunological perspective. *Annu Rev Immunol* 1985;3:263–287.

269. Baughn RE. Triggering of autoimmune antibody responses in syphilis. In: Friedman H, Rose NR, Bendinelli M, eds. *Microorganisms and autoimmune diseases.* New York: Plenum Press, 1996:79–103.

270. Cunningham MW. Streptococci and rheumatic fever. In: Friedman H, Rose NR, Bendinelli M, eds. *Microorganisms and autoimmune diseases.* New York: Plenum Press, 1996:13–66.

271. Dyrberg T, Mackay P, Michelsen B, et al. Viruses and diabetes mellitus. In: Friedman H, Rose NR, Bendinelli M, eds. *Microorganisms and autoimmune diseases.* New York: Plenum Press, 1996:105–127.

272. Garzelli C. Epstein-Barr virus and autoimmunity. In: Friedman H, Rose NR, Bendinelli M, eds. *Microorganisms and autoimmune diseases.* New York: Plenum Press, 1996:197–218.

273. Rose NR. Infection as a precursor to autoimmunity. In: Friedman H, Rose NR, Bendinelli M, eds. *Microorganisms and autoimmune diseases.* New York: Plenum Press, 1996:277–284.

274. Teixeira ARL, Ripoll CM, Santos-Buch CA. Autoimmunity in Chagas disease. In: Friedman H, Rose NR, Bendinelli M, eds. *Microorganisms and autoimmune diseases.* New York: Plenum Press, 1996:233–255.

275. Ugen KE, Fernandes L, Schumacher HR, et al. Retroviruses and autoimmunity. In: Friedman H, Rose NR, Bendinelli M, eds. *Microorganisms and autoimmune diseases.* New York: Plenum Press, 1996:219–231.

276. van Eden W, Anderton SM, Prakken ABJ, Van der Zee R. Bacterial heat-shock proteins and autoimmune disease. In: Friedman H, Rose NR, Bendinelli M, eds. *Microorganisms and autoimmune diseases.* New York: Plenum Press, 1996:1–12.

277. Welsh CT, Fujinami RS. Neuropathic viruses and autoimmunity. In: Friedman H, Rose NR, Bendinelli M, eds. *Microorganisms and autoimmune diseases.* New York: Plenum Press, 1996:159–180.

278. Yoon JW, Kominek H. The role of Coxsackie B viruses in the pathogenesis of Type I diabetes. In: Friedman H, Rose NR, Bendinelli M, eds. *Microorganisms and autoimmune diseases.* New York: Plenum Press, 1996:129–158.

*Textbook of the Autoimmune Diseases,*
Edited by R. G. Lahita, N. Chiorazzi, and W. H. Reeves,
Lippincott Williams & Wilkins, Philadelphia © 2000.

# CHAPTER 42

# Drug-Induced Autoimmunity

Jan H. Vaile and Anthony S. Russell

## MECHANISMS OF DRUG-INDUCED AUTOIMMUNITY

The concept of autoimmune disease should include two components: first, the disease features are caused by a response of the body's own immune system (i.e., an autoaggressive response); second, the antigens against which the response is directed are host antigens. This second criterion remains difficult to demonstrate in many cases of drug induced immune-mediated disease. Thus, autoimmune disease can be further defined as follows:

1. Allergic responses may cause widespread or focal damage (e.g., by histamine release or complement-induced lysis), but the antibody remains directed against the drug or a metabolite.
2. Responses termed autoaggressive generally show histologic features of an immune-mediated attack, but with no notion of the antigens involved.
3. True autoimmune responses would be directed against normal antigen (e.g., histone, acetyl choline receptor, rhesus antigen), and one or more of these antigenic specificities should be known. Ideally, this response should be in part responsible for features of damage, but this requirement is often waived. Autoimmune responses (e.g., antinuclear antibodies [ANAs]) are still much more common, whether or not they are drug induced, than is an associated disease. This is in contrast to those situations (e.g., anti–acetyl choline receptor antibody) in which the antibody is usually both necessary and sufficient for disease. A response directed against a neoantigen caused by drug or protein binding would not correctly be designated as autoimmune unless it was associated with broadening of the response to include normal adjacent epitopes.

J. H. Vaile: Department of Medicine, University of Sydney, Sydney, Australia 2006; Department of Rheumatology, Royal Prince Alfred Hospital, Camperdown, Australia 2050.

A. S. Russell: Department of Medicine, University of Alberta, Edmonton, Alberta, Canada T6G 2S2.

Self recognition, such as that of major histocompatibility complex (MHC) determinants, is part of normal immune regulation, but no active response directed against these determinants ensues, except under *in vitro* conditions (e.g., the autologous mixed lymphocyte culture). Such a widespread T-cell activation does, however, occur *in vivo* in, for example, a graft-versus-host response, and may then be associated with a variety of autoimmune responses (1). It is possible that the autoimmune responses seen in association with defects of the Fas ligand system may be on a similar basis (2). As yet, no drugs have been reported to interfere in this area.

Peripheral T-cell tolerance mechanisms exist, suggesting that not all such cells reacting with self antigen have been permanently eliminated (3). Furthermore, such cells may develop in rats after prolonged cyclosporine treatment is discontinued, suggesting that intrathymic class II antigen presentation may have been affected (4), but this mechanism of drug-induced autoimmunity has not been reported in humans.

Many mechanisms have been suggested for drug-induced autoimmunity, but rarely is the specific mechanism clear for any given clinical situation. Unfortunately, these disorders are not usually experienced in animals, thus removing one potential experimental approach. Self antigen responsive B cells do exist normally, and if T-cell help can be provided, such as by "T-cell bypass," a humoral autoimmune response develops (5). T-cell help may occur nonspecifically in the presence of superantigens or with graft-versus-host disease, as mentioned previously.

In some cases, drug (hapten) or protein binding may occur, but the antibody response is to the hapten only (e.g., as in penicillin-induced hemolytic anemia), and the process is not autoimmune and is immediately abrogated once the drug is metabolized or excreted.

An intriguing mechanism for true autoimmunity, described by Richardson and colleagues (6–9), relates to hypomethylation of DNA, leading to abnormal gene regulation and overexpression of lymphocyte function–associated antigen 1 (LFA-1). T cells treated with inhibitors of DNA methyltransferase may thus be activated by antigen-presenting cells alone in the absence of a specific antigen (8,10,11). Furthermore, procainamide, hydralazine, and 5-azacytidine (5-AZA) all inhibit DNA methylation *in vitro* and induce autoreactivity (12,13). Acetyl procainamide, known not to induce systemic lupus erythematosus (SLE) *in vivo,* is nonreactive in this system (13).

Mice transfected to overexpress LFA-1 also develop SLE-like disease (8). Furthermore, in rats, an adoptive transfer of T cells made autoreactive by agents that inhibit methylation of DNA induces an SLE-like disease in unirradiated syngeneic recipients, and in this circumstance, autoreactivity correlates with overexpression of LFA-1 (14). Stably transfecting a clonal murine T-cell line with a c-DNA construct that increases LFA-1 also gives rise to autoreactivity, particularly against self Ia-bearing macrophages (15,16). These cells induced an SLE-like disease *in vivo,* perhaps akin to a graft-versus-host response (8). This transfection has nothing to do directly with hypomethylation but shows the importance of the overexpression of LFA-1 (10).

A change in cytokine profile, perhaps by a decrease in apoptosis, may also induce autoimmune responses. Thus, the use of anti–tumor necrosis factor-α (anti–TNF-α) antisera has been associated with the development of positive ANAs and even with antibodies to native DNA with SLE-like disease (17). Therapy with TNF receptors bound to a fusion protein for longer half-life, which also downregulate the production of TNF-α, has similar effects (18).

Other cytokine changes have been noted in mouse and rat models in which autoimmune or autoaggressive syndromes are produced by mercury, gold, and D-penicillamine (19) and are associated with overexpression of $T_H2$ cells secreting interleukin-4 (IL-4) and with a decreased activity of IL-2 secreting subset 1 helper T ($T_H1$) cells (19).

Other theories involve polyclonal activation of B cells, possibly by inhibition of suppressor T-cell function (20) or modification of MHC class II molecules (21). Activation of an SLE diathesis or of latent viral infection has also been suggested as an alternative to production of SLE *de novo,* and molecular mimicry may be important (14).

## MAJOR DRUGS THAT INDUCE SYSTEMIC LUPUS ERYTHEMATOSUS–LIKE DISEASE

### Hydralazine

Hydralazine modifies the pyrimidine bases of DNA and may thereby increase its immunogenicity (22). It has been suggested that alteration of T-cell DNA may be responsible for hydralazine-mediated induction of autoimmunity (23). Hydralazine has structural similarities to the nucleic acid adenosine, and cross-reaction of antibodies to hydralazine may be a mechanism associated with development of autoimmunity (24). Hydralazine, like procainamide, isoniazid, and penicillamine, can also induce the transformation of DNA from the right-handed B from to the more immunogenic left-handed Z conformation (24). Despite this, hydralazine-

associated SLE is not characterized by antibodies to double-stranded DNA (ds-DNA).

### Methyldopa

Methyldopa is associated with positive direct Coombs' tests, occasionally with hemolysis, and rarely with aspects of SLE.

### Procainamide

Procainamide contains an amine group linked to an aromatic ring. Oxidation of the nitro moiety can result in a reactive intermediary that may be important in the production of autoimmunity. Acetylation of procainamide prevents oxidation, and acetylated procainamide is not associated with clinical autoimmunity (7,15). Slow acetylators of procainamide develop features of autoimmunity more rapidly and at lower doses than fast acetylators (25,26). Procainamide binds and reversibly inhibits methyltransferase (11,27) and is thus associated with DNA hypomethylation, a phenomenon associated with development of autoimmunity (see later).

### Sulfasalazine

Sulfasalazine has been associated with development of an SLE-like disease, with some features unusual for drug-induced lupus (DIL), including production of antibodies to ds-DNA, hypocomplementemia, cutaneous vasculitis, nephropathy, and months to resolution after discontinuation of drug (28).

### Penicillamine

A wide range of autoimmune syndromes are associated with penicillamine, including SLE, autoimmune thyroiditis, Goodpasture's syndrome, myasthenia gravis (MG), pemphigus, membranous glomerulopathy, polymyositis, and Sjögren's syndrome (29). Rheumatoid arthritis patients appear to be at increased risk for adverse reactions from penicillamine if they possess HLA-DR3 or are poor sulfoxidizers (30).

### Chlorpromazine

Chlorpromazine is associated with ANA positivity, DIL, and circulating anticoagulants (31).

### Cytokines and Monoclonal Antibodies

Interferon-α (IFN-α) has been associated with autoimmune thyroid disease, SLE, pernicious anemia, hemolytic anemia, thrombocytopenia, vasculitis, and a number of autoimmune skin conditions (32–34). Human leukocyte and recombinant forms have been implicated (32). Other cytokines have been associated with skin conditions, including psoriasis, eosinophilic fasciitis, linear immunoglobulin A (IgA) bullous dermatitis, and vitiligo, possibly by stimulation of T and B lymphocytes. IL-2 has been associated with autoimmune thyroid disease, pemphigus, vitiligo, vasculitis, and development of autoantibodies (34). Antibodies to TNF-α in patients with rheumatoid arthritis have also been shown to induce ANA, and in at least one patient with features of typical SLE and antibodies to ds-DNA (17). ANAs were also seen in association with TNF receptor therapy (18).

## Quinidine and Quinine

Quinidine has been associated with ANA positivity, DIL, polymyalgia–rheumatica–like illness, hemolytic anemia, and thrombocytopenia (35).

## Anticonvulsants

SLE may be induced by phenytoin, mephenytoin, ethosuximide, trimethadione, carbamazepine, valproate, and primidone (36,37). Valproate has been associated with development of immune thrombocytopenia (34). Phenytoin, carbamazepine (unusually), and trimethadione have been associated with vasculitis (36,37). Phenytoin may be associated with autoimmune thyroiditis, and phenytoin and trimethadione have been suggested as possible causes of MG. Anticonvulsants do not appear to exacerbate idiopathic SLE (24).

## Minocycline

Minocycline is a recent addition to the DIL list, and one of particular interest to rheumatologists. SLE and a hepatitis with autoimmune serology have both been described in more than 100 patients taking minocycline. Minocycline-associated SLE appears to be reversible, at least in the early stages (38).

## CLINICAL PRESENTATION OF DRUG-INDUCED AUTOIMMUNE DISEASES

### Systemic Lupus Erythematosus

#### Mechanisms

The large number of drugs implicated in the production of DIL suggests more than a single mechanism (21,24,34). It is not clear to what extent mechanisms overlap with those of idiopathic SLE, and the failure of most drugs that induce SLE to exacerbate preexisting idiopathic SLE suggests that different mechanisms may be relevant (21,24). Most of the research associated with the pathogenesis of drug-induced SLE concerns the prototypical agents, procainamide and hydralazine.

Procainamide appears to exert different immunologic effects depending on dose, with lower doses enhancing and higher doses inhibiting peripheral lymphocyte mitogenic responses (25). Procainamide may inhibit suppressor T-cell function and therefore increase immunoglobulin function (25). A number of drugs, including procainamide, hydralazine,

and 5-AZA appear to interfere with DNA methylation, which is important in the regulation of gene expression (10,16,25). Procainamide appears to do this by reversible inhibition of DNA methyltransferase (10,11). 5-AZA is incorporated into newly synthesized DNA and binds DNA methyltransferase (7,10). Procainamide and hydralazine also appear to facilitate a conformational change in DNA, which may enhance immunogenicity (39). Hydralazine, isoniazid, penicillamine, and a metabolite of procainamide all bind to the active site of C4 and thereby inhibit binding, possibly inhibiting clearance of immune complexes (24).

#### Prevalence and Epidemiology

Up to 10% of cases of SLE are drug related (22,24,25,40,41), and it is likely that mild cases are overlooked. More than 70 medications have been reported to cause DIL; the most clearly established of these include procainamide, hydralazine, isoniazid, phenytoin, chlorpromazine, penicillamine, methyldopa, quinidine, and sulfasalazine (25,34,40). To establish a clear-cut relationship between a drug and the subsequent development of SLE, ideally one has to show remission with withdrawal and relapse with reexposure. Although this has been done occasionally (e.g., with procainamide), it is clearly unusual, and remission on withdrawal may be all that has been shown (42,43). With some drugs, such as D-penicillamine, remission does not occur with withdrawal; therefore, one has to rely on the demonstration of an increased prevalence of SLE developing in patients taking the drug, compared with patients not taking the drug (44). If the manifestations are characteristic, as in the autoimmunity after methyldopa administration, this too may be acceptable. For many of the drugs cited in the lower part of Table 42.1, the association remains relatively anecdotal (25,33, 34,40,43,45,46). In children, the most common association is with anticonvulsants (45).

Many more patients develop positive ANAs than clinical disease. ANAs appear in most patients receiving long-term procainamide therapy, with clinical lupus developing in 15% to 35% (25,26,47). ANA appears in about 40% of patients taking hydralazine for 3 years, with 2% to 21% likely to develop clinical lupus (25,40,48). The risk appears to be dose related (40,48). Of patients taking chlorpromazine, 16% to 52% develop positive ANAs, but less than 1% develop DIL (25,40). About one fourth of patients taking isoniazid develop positive ANAs, with less than 1% developing disease (25,40). ANAs may develop in up to 67% of rheumatoid patients using penicillamine, with up to 2% of these patients developing disease (25). About one fourth of patients taking isoniazid and methyldopa develop positive ANAs (40). IFN therapy may be associated with positive ANAs in up to 72% of patients, and although a DIL syndrome occurs, its frequency is not clear (25). Regarding the anticonvulsants, positive ANAs may develop in up to 60% of patients taking long-term phenytoin, primidone, and carbamazepine (24).

**TABLE 42.1.** *Drugs associated with systemic lupus erythematosus*

*Most clearly established*
  Hydralazine
  Methyldopa
  Penicillamine
  Chlorpromazine
  Quinidine
  Isoniazid
  Sulfasalazine
  Minocycline
*Others*
  β-Blockers: timolol, practolol
  Lithium
  Interferon-α
  Interferon-γ
  Ethosuximide
  Propylthiouracil
  Valproate
  Captopril
  Carbamazepine
  Hydrochlorothiazide
  Interleukin-2
  Leuprolide acetate
  Mesalazine
  Simvastatin
  Lovastatin
  Clobazam
  Phenytoin
  Mephenytoin
  Diphenyl hydantoin
  Trimethadione
  Carbimazole
  Oral contraceptive pill
  Sulphonamides
  Griseofulvin

Most studies indicate that patients who are slow acetylators using procainamide, hydralazine, and sulfasalazine develop ANA positivity more quickly and in higher titer and appear more likely to develop DIL (23,24,47,49–51), although the influence of acetylator status on eventual development of ANA positivity has been questioned in other studies (48). The role of acetylator status in anticonvulsant-induced SLE is unclear (36). Acetylator status does not appear to be important in idiopathic SLE (24).

The role of HLA status in influencing susceptibility to DIL is unclear (24). An increased frequency of HLA-DR4 in hydralazine-induced SLE has been suggested but not confirmed (48,50,52). No definite HLA associations with SLE induced by procainamide, chlorpromazine, or penicillamine have been established (25,47). The presence of a C4 null allele may predispose to some forms of DIL, with complement deficiencies known to increase the risk for idiopathic SLE (24).

It has been suggested that viral infection may act in conjunction with drug agents to influence the development of autoimmunity (53).

The epidemiology of DIL differs in a number of respects from that of idiopathic SLE. Patients with DIL are generally 50 to 70 years of age, compared with an average age of 20 to 50 years in patients with idiopathic SLE; patients in the older age group are more likely to be taking those medications that can induce SLE. An exception to this pattern is the occurrence of DIL in children using anticonvulsants (25,45). The female preponderance seen in idiopathic SLE is not usually evident in DIL (24,25,40,54), except that female patients may be more likely to develop hydralazine-associated SLE (48,50,52). White patients appear more likely to develop DIL and to have more severe disease than African-American patients, in contrast to the pattern seen in idiopathic SLE (24,25).

### Clinical Presentation

Distinct diagnostic criteria for DIL have not been established, and patients may fail to meet criteria for idiopathic SLE (26,41,55). Generally, DIL should be considered in previously unaffected patients who develop both a positive ANA and at least one feature of SLE while taking a suspicious drug, and most particularly, if these resolve after cessation of the drug (25).

In general, DIL is a milder disease with fewer manifestations than idiopathic SLE (24,54). Clinical features may develop weeks to years after commencing the drug, often abruptly, and resolve days to weeks, but occasionally months, after cessation (40,54). Arthralgia or arthritis, usually affecting multiple joints in a symmetric fashion, occurs in more than 75% of patients in both DIL and idiopathic SLE (24). It may be migratory, most commonly affects small joints, and characteristically, is not destructive (24,25). Arthritis in addition to arthralgia may be more common in hydralazine-associated disease than in that associated with other drugs (25). Diffuse myalgia may be severe in up to half of patients; myopathy and weakness are rare (24,25).

Pulmonary infiltrates may be equally common in idiopathic SLE and procainamide-induced disease but are uncommon in other forms of DIL (40). Fever, frequently present in idiopathic SLE, occurs in less than half of patients with DIL, but body temperature in these patients may be high, and weight loss may be prominent. Malaise may also be a feature (24,25). Rash is present in less than one fourth of patients with DIL but may be present in up to half of patients with quinidine-induced disease (40). The patterns of skin involvement are similar to those in idiopathic disease (25), but malar rash, photosensitivity, and alopecia are less common (36,54). Mucocutaneous involvement is rare in DIL (54).

Serositis is present in 25% to 56% of DIL patients and is more common with procainamide-induced disease (24,25). Pleural involvement with effusions is particularly likely. Pericardial involvement is far less common than pleural disease but may be severe. It is most commonly associated with procainamide (25).

Renal involvement, present in up to 75% of idiopathic SLE patients, rarely occurs in patients with DIL but may be seen in hydralazine-induced disease, possibly as a result of the preexisting medical conditions in patients using hydralazine (26,40), and may be seen in sulfasalazine-induced disease (42). Renal involvement, however, is characteristic of D-penicillamine–induced SLE and fails to remit when the medication is discontinued, thus providing an exception to the usual experience (44). Renal involvement appears rarely with minocycline use, although anti-DNA antibodies have been described along with others, such as perinuclear antineutrophil cytoplasmic antibody (p-ANCA) (56).

Central and peripheral nervous system involvement is similarly rare in DIL but may occur in 20% to 50% of patients with idiopathic disease (25,40). Raynaud's phenomenon is less common in DIL (5%) than in idiopathic SLE (30%) (24,26,54). Lymphadenopathy, present in up to half of patients with idiopathic, is present in a minority of DIL patients, and hepatomegaly and splenomegaly may be less common than in idiopathic SLE (25,40,54). Renal, retinal, and systemic vasculitis may occur but are uncommon (24).

*Diagnostic Testing*

Mild thrombocytopenia, leukopenia, and normocytic, normochromic anemia may occur in DIL, but are seen less commonly than in idiopathic disease, and severe hematologic abnormalities are uncommon (24,40). Thrombocytopenia is more common with quinidine-induced disease than with disease associated with other drugs (35). The erythrocyte sedimentation rate is usually elevated, as in idiopathic disease, and usually normalizes as symptoms subside (54).

ANAs, usually in a homogeneous pattern, are present in essentially all cases but are also present in patients exposed to a number of implicated drugs in the absence of disease (15,25,40). ANA shows more restricted specificity in DIL than in idiopathic disease (25). Antibodies to individual histones and complexes of histones, components of chromatin, are often considered a hallmark of DIL, with most studies indicating a prevalence of 60% to 75% (24,40,57). Antihistone antibodies are also seen in 30% to 50% of patients taking the relevant drugs who do not have clinical disease (25). The reported incidence of antihistone antibodies in idiopathic SLE varies greatly (0% to 75%) and may correlate with disease activity (26,57,58). Antibodies to histones may also appear in rheumatoid arthritis, juvenile rheumatoid arthritis, Felty's syndrome, and undifferentiated connective tissue disease (25).

In DIL, different drugs may be associated with different histone antibodies, with hydralazine-associated disease showing principally H2A and H2B and procainamide associated disease showing predominantly H3 and H4 antibodies (24–26,36,47,59). The pattern and frequency of antihistone antibodies may differ between patients with symptoms and those without symptoms (26,47,60). In addition, the pattern of antihistone antibodies may be different in idiopathic SLE, in which specificity appears mostly to trypsin-sensitive areas, than in DIL, in which antibodies may be less restricted (59). Anti-Sm and anti–ds-DNA are uncommon

in DIL (24–26,36,61), except that anti–ds-DNA may be present in many patients with sulfasalazine-induced SLE (42) and in many cases of DIL related to D-penicillamine (44).

Autoantibodies generally predate clinical symptoms and may persist for months after resolution of clinical features (40).

Rheumatoid factor is positive in a minority of patients with DIL, as in idiopathic SLE (62). A positive Coombs' test may occur as in idiopathic disease, particularly with procainamide, chlorpromazine, or methyldopa use (24, 25,54).

Anticardiolipin antibodies may be present, particularly with chlorpromazine and procainamide, but do not appear to be associated with thrombotic syndromes (24,25). Lymphocytotoxic antibodies have been reported with procainamide, hydralazine, and some anticonvulsants, and in idiopathic SLE (25). Specific antibodies have been identified against hydralazine and procainamide but are not considered to be responsible for disease manifestations (25,63). Antineutrophil cytoplasmic or antimyeloperoxidase antibodies of uncertain significance have occasionally been reported (25,64).

Hypocomplementemia is rarely a feature of DIL, except in quinidine-associated disease, although it is often present in idiopathic SLE. Hypergammaglobulinemia is less frequent than in idiopathic disease (54).

Synovial fluid may be inflammatory or noninflammatory, with predominance of lymphocytes or neutrophils, and does not appear different from that seen in idiopathic SLE (65).

*Treatment*

Resolution of clinical features characteristically accompanies cessation of the drug (especially with procainamide and hydralazine), although this is not always the case (40); with D-penicillamine SLE, it occurs rarely (44). Symptomatic treatment, such as use of nonsteroidal antiinflammatory drugs (NSAIDs) for joint complaints, may be required. Occasionally, corticosteroids may be required for severe symptoms or visceral involvement. Serositis may respond to NSAIDs or corticosteroids. Renal involvement is treated along the same lines as idiopathic disease (54). Corticosteroids or immunosuppression may be required for the rare occurrence of vasculitis.

It is not necessary to follow ANAs in patients taking drugs capable of inducing DIL because most patients who develop positive ANAs do not develop overt disease. Thus, the drug need not be discontinued on the basis of a positive ANA alone; instead, vigilance for development of clinical features should be maintained. Determination of acetylator status is rarely used in clinical practice (54).

Rechallenge usually results in recurrence, often after a shorter period of use, and should be avoided if possible (25,36,62). Development of DIL with one anticonvulsant may increase risk for the syndrome with other classes of anticonvulsants (37).

## Hematologic Disorders

### General

A number of immune mechanisms have been proposed for drug-induced blood cell dyscrasias. Such reactions may require ongoing presence of the drug or a metabolite (drug-dependent antibodies) or may persist in the absence of drug (drug-independent autoantibodies) (66). Antibodies may or may not bind complement. The principal theories proposed to explain drug-induced cytopenias include involvement of hapten, neoantigens, immune complexes, and autoimmune mechanisms. Only the autoimmune mechanisms are reviewed in detail here.

The true incidence of immunologically mediated cytopenias is unknown, in part because of the difficulty in distinguishing such reactions from other toxic reactions or from idiopathic disease, the frequent coadministration of other drugs, and failure to recognize a potentially drug-related effect. Most frequently, a single cell line is affected, but antibodies against other lines may also be produced (66). Most reactions occur in adults, and in some specific cases, a female or male prevalence has been suggested (67,68).

Normally, a period of at least 6 days is required after initial administration of a drug before an immune-mediated reaction may occur (66), but in the case of methyldopa, it is 3 to 6 months. The onset may be much faster after subsequent administration, even years after the initial event. The risk for second reactions is poorly quantified, although it is known that antibodies may persist for months to years after resolution of the clinical toxicity (66).

### Anemia

#### Mechanisms

A drug may induce anemia by hemolysis or, less commonly, aplasia. Many drugs may give rise to positive direct Coombs' tests and sometimes hemolysis because of antidrug antibodies (e.g., against penicillin) reacting with a drug absorbed on the surface of the red blood cell. The presence of immune complexes absorbed on the surface of red blood cells may have an equivalent effect (stibophen). Methyldopa (and L-dopa) fall into an entirely different category because they induce an autoimmune hemolysis. The antibodies are true autoantibodies, usually with specificities related to rhesus antigens (e.g., c or e, or core antigens), as in spontaneous autoimmune hemolytic anemia (69). ANA may also develop in relation to this drug, but this appears to be independent of the direct Coombs' test results, arguing against the suggested mechanism of an alteration in suppressor T-cell function (20). Mefenamic acid, now rarely used, may also be associated with similar antibodies.

Ranitidine has been associated with hemolytic anemia and thrombocytopenia, possibly as a result of an inhibiting autoimmune process at the histamine receptor on mature and immature erythrocytes, also present in other progenitor cell lines and on mature neutrophils (70).

Up to half of cases of aplastic anemia are drug related. Possible roles for chloramphenicol and quinidine acting as haptens in binding with stem cells and a possible immunologically mediated mechanism for cimetidine in illnesses of this type have been proposed (71). However, the relative contribution of immunologic causes in most drug-related cases of aplastic anemia remains controversial, with only occasional identification of antibodies to drugs or cells (72,73). Postulated mechanisms of drug-induced isolated red blood cell aplasia include IgG-mediated destruction in the presence of the drug as a hapten, a direct effect on DNA synthesis, and true autoantibody formation (67).

### Prevalence and Epidemiology

Autoantibodies to one or more specific rhesus antigens appear in up to 20% of patients using methyldopa for longer than 4 months, but AHA occurs in less than 1% (74). Other drugs that have been associated with an antibody-mediated hemolysis include penicillins, cephalosporin, quinine, quinidine, hydantoins, methysergide, and chlorpromazine (69).

Drug-induced pure red blood cell aplasia, with specific absence of red blood cell precursors from the bone marrow, is rare, and even with the most strongly implicated drug, phenytoin, the mechanism appears to involve antibodies reacting with drug bound to erythrocyte precursors, that is, not an autoantibody.

### Clinical Presentation

The hemolytic anemia associated with methyldopa is clinically indistinguishable from idiopathic warm autoimmune hemolytic anemia (69), with gradual onset followed by a gradual recovery after cessation of the drug.

### Diagnostic Testing

In hemolytic anemia associated with penicillins and cephalosporin, the direct antiglobulin test is usually strongly positive for IgG but negative for complement, and it becomes negative with withdrawal of the drug (66). In some cases, the direct antiglobulin test is positive only with C3b, and causative antibodies may be detected in the presence of drug (66). Red blood cell autoantibodies induced by methyldopa are IgG and usually rhesus specific (69,74), and if the direct antiglobulin test if positive, it is usually only to IgG, although a reaction to complement has been reported (69). The direct test may remain positive for years after cessation. Risk for overt hemolysis appears to be directly related to the antibody titer (69). In some cases (e.g., quinidine-induced hemolysis), drug-dependent, but also drug-independent, antibodies occur. The drug-independent antibodies may react with homologous cells and appear to be true autoantibodies (66).

## Thrombocytopenia

### Mechanism

The mechanisms of drug-induced thrombocytopenia may be as varied as those of drug-induced hemolysis (75). Possibilities include binding of drug to the platelet surface with production of antibodies against the drug or the ensuing complex, or formation of drug–antibody complexes, with subsequent "innocent" binding by Fc receptors on the platelet surface (75). In addition, both drug-dependent and drug-independent antibodies probably play a role, sometimes for the same drug. The latter mechanisms appear to be relevant in patients with thrombocytopenia induced by quinidine, phenazopyridine, acetaminophen, thioguanine, dexamyl, phenytoin, ampicillin, and sulfamethoxazole (75). Heparin-induced thrombocytopenia results from increased destruction of platelets. The onset is delayed, although more rapid for second courses (76,77). The existence of an IgG, heparin-dependent, antiplatelet antibody suggests that heparin-induced thrombocytopenia may be autoimmune (76).

### Prevalence and Epidemiology

More than 50 drugs have been reported to cause autoimmune thrombocytopenia; the more common of these are quinine, quinidine, heparin, gold, penicillin, cephalosporin, penicillamine, alprenolol, cocaine, co-trimoxazole, digoxin, phenytoin, IFN-α, levodopa, oxprenolol, rifampicin, and sulfonamides (74). Gold-induced thrombocytopenia appears to be related to the presence of HLA-DR3 (78), but other drug-related blood dyscrasias do not appear to have a genetic predisposition (66,68). Gold-induced thrombocytopenia is usually reported in rheumatoid arthritis patients who are at risk for autoimmune thrombocytopenia independent of gold. With most drugs, the mechanism, and whether the thrombocytopenia is truly autoimmune, remains unknown.

### Clinical Presentation

It may be difficult to distinguish thrombocytopenia resulting from drug-induced antibodies from idiopathic disease because the presentation of this variant may not be dramatic. Drug-dependent antibodies, however, may result in a severe and abrupt clinical picture. Accompanying involvement of red blood cells or leukocytes may occur. Petechiae, ecchymoses, and mucosal bleeding are common.

### Diagnostic Testing

The marrow in gold-induced thrombocytopenia is normal, suggesting peripheral destruction as in idiopathic thrombocytopenic purpura, and up to 70% of patients may have antiplatelet antibodies detectable in serum (78). With quinine and quinidine, most patients have multiple drug-dependent antibodies (74).

### Treatment

In most cases, platelet counts recover within less than a week after drug withdrawal (74). Platelet destruction may persist for weeks or months when there is autoantibody formation, and supportive therapy, such as immunoglobulin or corticosteroids, may be required (66). Drug-dependent antibody-related thrombocytopenia, although more severe, tends to resolve within days. Substantial supportive therapy, however, such as immunoglobulin, corticosteroids, plasmapheresis, and platelet transfusions, may be required in the interim.

Gold-induced thrombocytopenia usually responds quickly to corticosteroids, splenectomy, or both (78).

## Neutropenia

An immune mechanism has been proposed to explain the role of a number of drugs in inducing neutropenia (79). Aminopyrine, sulfonamides, quinidine, propylthiouracil, procainamide, gold thiomalate, and penicillins may be associated with production of antineutrophil antibodies capable of opsonizing normal neutrophils (21,79). The drug may combine with protein and result in immune complex formation, with attachment to the neutrophil and subsequent clearing. Alternatively, the drug may incite an immune response by attaching to the cell directly and acting as a hapten. There is also evidence that aminopyrine acts by this mechanism rather than by an autoimmune mechanism (21). Clozapine appears to affect marrow precursors, although the evidence for the importance of antibody formation in this reaction is not strong (21). Ibuprofen may induce an autoimmune destruction of myeloid progenitors (80).

## Marrow Aplasia and Pancytopenia

It has been suggested that marrow aplasia associated with quinidine may be mediated by a destructive immune process directed at precursor cells (81), with altered antigenicity as cells mature accounting for lack of effect on more mature cells. Quinidine may be associated with other manifestations in some cases, in association with hypercellular marrow, implying more than a single mechanism (81). Pancytopenia has been associated with cimetidine and chloramphenicol (71,82). There is little evidence to support an autoimmune basis for chloramphenicol-induced pancytopenia (82), but immune mechanisms are suspected in the case of cimetidine (71).

## Phospholipid Syndromes

Antiphospholipid antibodies are induced by the same drugs that induce SLE-like syndromes, particularly chlorpromazine and other phenothiazines and quinidine (24,59,83–85). The clinical syndrome occurring with autoimmune antiphospholipid antibodies tends not to occur with drug-induced antiphospholipid antibodies (24,83–85). Drug-induced antiphospholipid antibodies are predominantly IgM, as opposed to the usual IgG type of the autoimmune form (83,85). Antiphospholipid antibodies generally require no specific treatment.

## Skin Disorders

### Pemphigus

#### Mechanism

Pemphigus is characterized by autoantibodies against epidermal and epithelial cell surfaces, resulting in acantholysis and blistering of the skin (86). A number of drugs can induce pemphigus, with evidence for both direct drug effects on epidermis and indirect effects by immune modification. In the cases of penicillamine and captopril, interaction with cell adhesion molecules, perhaps by the active sulfhydryl group of both drugs, may render them antigenic (86–88); however, the diseases do not rapidly remit with drug discontinuation. Penicillamine, β-blockers, progesterone, and rifampin may all impair suppressor T-cell function, perhaps allowing production of autoantibodies against epidermal cell surface antigens (86,88).

#### Prevalence and Epidemiology

Drug-induced pemphigus accounts for a small proportion of all cases. Drugs reported to be associated with production of pemphigus include thiols (penicillamine, captopril, pyritinol, thiopronine, piroxicam, thiamazole, golf thiomalate), antibiotics (penicillins, ampicillin, carbenicillin, rifampicin, cephalexin), pyrazolon derivatives (phenylbutazone, aminophenazone, azapropazone, oxyphenylbutazone), β-blockers, progesterone, heroin, levodopa, lysine acetylsalicylate, phenobarbital, α-mercaptopropionylglycine, enalapril, optalidon, pentachlorophenol, phosphamide, IFN-α and IFN-β, IL-2, and hydantoins (hydantoin and barbitone) (86–91). A link with HLA-B15 has been suggested (86).

#### Clinical Presentation

The clinical features of drug-induced pemphigus may differ from those of idiopathic disease, with a prodromal widespread erythema or eruption frequent in drug-induced disease. Typical pemphigus lesions may then appear after a variable period. Lesions are often similar to those seen in pemphigus foliaceus, with erythema, scaly patches, and superficial blisters. Seborrheic lesions in a butterfly distribution may predominate (88). Groups of small vesicular lesions that spread with a serpiginous edge are common (88). The typical large bullae on otherwise normal-looking skin that are typical of pemphigus vulgaris are uncommon in drug-induced disease (86,88). The disease can be severe, and fatalities have been reported (91).

#### Diagnostic Testing

Direct immunofluorescence shows IgG antibodies at the cell surface in 90% of patients with drug-induced pemphigus, with complement deposition frequent. Antibodies to cell-surface antigens are detected in 70%, but titer correlates poorly with extent and severity of disease (88). Penicillamine induces antibodies to intercellular cement substance with the same specificities as those found in idiopathic forms of pemphigus (87,92). With this drug, other autoantibodies may exist, including ANAs and antibodies to smooth muscle, striated muscle, thyroid, glomerular basement membrane, and gastric mucosa (44,86).

#### Treatment

Cessation of the offending agent does not guarantee resolution of drug-induced pemphigus, and topical or systemic immunosuppressive therapy similar to that used in idiopathic disease may be required (86,88). Resolution appears more likely in the minority of patients with no circulating or tissue-bound antibodies (86,87). Surveillance for recurrence of antibodies has been advocated for early detection of relapse (88).

### Bullous Pemphigoid

#### Mechanism

The postulated mechanisms of drug-induced bullous pemphigoid are similar to those of drug-induced pemphigus, namely drug acting as hapten, altered immunogenicity of skin components, and direct effect on the immune system (88). Whether the antigenic sites are the same as those of idiopathic disease is controversial. The presence of sulfhydryl groups in many drugs causing bullous pemphigoid appears to be important and may be responsible for cleavage of epidermal intercellular cement substance, resulting in the production of antibodies (93).

#### Incidence and Epidemiology

Furosemide is the most commonly implicated drug in bullous pemphigoid; others include penicillamine, penicillin derivatives, sulfasalazine, salicylosulfapyridine, phenacetin, captopril, enalapril, ibuprofen, and topical fluorouracil (88,93–97).

Patients tend to be younger than those with idiopathic disease, except in the case of furosemide (97). No definite HLA association for drug-induced bullous pemphigoid has been established (88,92).

#### Clinical Presentation

Blisters may appear abruptly after a single dose of inciting drug or may appear after years of therapy (94). Two patterns are evident: an acute self-limited form, often requiring no systemic therapy; and a more persistent form, which may not resolve entirely and appears to evolve into a condition indistinguishable from the idiopathic form (93). Clinical features may be classic or atypical, and mild or severe (88). One third of cases have oral mucosal involvement, but involvement of other mucosal surfaces is rare (95). Recurrence has occurred after rechallenge (97).

*Diagnostic Testing*

Detectable antibodies may include anti–basement membrane zone, intercellular, and antiepidermal cytoplasmic antibodies (92). Both circulating and bound antibodies are found. Disappearance of the antibodies accompanies clinical resolution. Immunofluorescence shows IgG and C3 deposits.

*Treatment*

A proportion of cases resolve after cessation of drug, possibly after steroid therapy, but some cases appear to evolve into a form indistinguishable from the idiopathic form. Immunosuppression with methotrexate or azathioprine in conjunction with steroids may be required (94).

*Psoriasis*

The cytokines IFN-α and IFN-β, granulocyte-macrophage colony-stimulating factor, and IL-2 have been associated with appearance *de novo* or exacerbation of psoriasis (91). Exacerbations may be generalized or occur predominantly at the injection site. The mechanism has been linked to mimicking of the $T_H1$ profile of idiopathic psoriasis (91). It has been hypothesized that β-blocker–induced psoriasis is mediated by binding of drug to β receptors in the skin, rendering them more immunogenic. Subsequent antibody formation against the receptors results in impaired function and development of psoriasis (98).

**Gastrointestinal Disease**

*Liver Disease*

*Mechanisms*

More than 600 drugs have been associated with liver abnormalities, but in only a small proportion of cases has an immune mechanism been considered the primary pathology. Halothane, enflurane, isaxonine, erythromycin, amineptine, phenytoin, sulfonamides, tienilic acid, amitryptyline, imipramine, allopurinol, amodiaquine, iproniazid, phenindione, phenylbutazone, quinidine, ranitidine, sulindac, carbamazepine, cimetidine, clometacin, dextropropoxyphene, hydralazine dihydralazine, and α-methyldopa have all been implicated in acute allergic hepatitis (99). A number of mechanisms have been proposed for drug-induced hepatic immunotoxicity. Inhibition of suppressor T-cell activity or polyclonal B-cell activation may play a role (100). A number of drugs, including α-methyldopa, iproniazid, minocycline, tienilic acid, nitrofurantoin, dihydralazine, oxyphenisatin, nitrofurantoin, clometacin, halothane, and the herbal medicine dai-saiko-to may induce hepatitis in association with

production of organ-nonspecific autoantibodies (99–102). Tienilic acid appears to be metabolized to a reactive metabolite by P450, with subsequent binding of the metabolite to the enzyme and generation of specific anti-P450 antibodies, and a similar mechanism has been postulated for dihydralazine (103). Even viral hepatitis may be associated with antibodies to a P450 enzyme (CYP.2C9), which is an example of an autoimmune response, but whether this underlies progressive damage is unclear (21).

The liver may be a particularly likely site for drug-induced immune reactions because it is the main site for metabolism and is exposed to possibly immunotoxic metabolites (100). Metabolism may also result in generation of new antigens on hepatic plasma membranes, either formed there directly or formed in the endoplasmic reticulum and then transported to the membrane (99). Liver damage as a result of this new antigen presentation has been termed *allergic hepatitis*. Thus, halothane is metabolized to trifluoroacetyl chloride, which may interact with amino groups on lysine residues. Patients who develop hepatic necrosis have antibodies that react with these trifluoroacetyl chloride hepatic proteins, for example, on the endoplasmic reticulum where they are formed (104,105). Some antibodies, however, recognize native proteins and are therefore autoantibodies (21). Their role is unclear, but they could be a marker of a T-cell autoimmune response.

As many as 60 drugs are known to be associated with the development of hepatic granulomas, in which a drug or metabolite presumably acts as a hapten to stimulate specific T cells (106). Phenylbutazone, penicillins, and sulfonamides, in particular, are recognized as causing disease (106).

Specific mechanisms resulting in chronic active hepatitis (CAH) have not been elucidated. It has been suggested that some drugs may unmask idiopathic CAH rather than cause it *de novo* (100), but as with chronic viral hepatitis, autoantibodies may be seen. Whether they may reflect a T-cell mediated autoimmune attack is unclear. They generally remit when the drug is discontinued.

Patients with alcoholic liver disease have increased frequency of a number of autoantibodies: ANAs, anti–smooth muscle antibodies, and antibodies to liver-specific lipoprotein complex and liver membrane antigen, although these may also be found in CAH and in viral hepatitis (100,107). Alcohol may also result in alteration of liver cell membrane antigens, and antibodies to these altered antigens have been described. Until we understand the mechanisms better, the term "autoimmune hepatitis" is best avoided, and a descriptive term may be used, such as *drug-induced hepatitis with autoantibodies*.

*Prevalence and Epidemiology*

Specific risk factors for immunologically mediated liver damage have not been ascertained in most circumstances, but malnutrition, use of drugs inducing microsomal enzymes, and coexistent liver disease may increase the risk for adverse hepatic reactions to drugs (99).

Halothane hepatitis is more common in women. A suggestion that HLA-DR2 may confer increased risk for halothane hepatitis has been disputed (100). In virtually all studies, previous exposure to halothane has been documented, and the risk increases after multiple exposures (105).

α-Methyldopa, nitrofurantoin, oxyphenisatin, isoniazid, sulfonamides, dantrolene, hydralazine, phenylbutazone, and ethanol have all been reported to cause CAH (99,108). Reported incidence rates range from 3% to 60% (100). HLA-B8 may be overrepresented in some cases, as in the idiopathic form (100,108).

### Clinical Presentation

Drug-induced hepatic disease may mimic many other kinds of liver disease (99). Allergic hepatitis may be manifest as hepatocellular, cholestatic, or mixed picture and may have accompanying features of hypersensitivity, such as fever and eosinophilia, and less commonly rash, interstitial nephritis, serum sickness, lymphadenopathy, hemolytic anemia, immune neutropenia, leukopenia, or thrombocytopenia (99,101,103). Clinical features of the illness otherwise are similar to those of other causes of fulminant hepatitis and CAH. Rapid recurrence after rechallenge is characteristic of allergic hepatitis (99).

Halothane may result in a mild hepatitis in about 20% of patients, with a moderate transaminase increase, or in a severe and sometimes fatal form in less than 1% of patients. The more severe form appears more commonly after multiple exposures. Fever and eosinophilia are frequently associated (100).

In most circumstances, if damage is not already severe, recovery quickly follows removal of the inciting agent, although hepatitis associated with iproniazid and tienilic acid (often with autoantibodies present) may continue to worsen after drug withdrawal (99).

Hepatic granulomas may be asymptomatic or may manifest as acute icteric hepatitis (106). Withdrawal of the drug is generally followed by improvement.

### Diagnostic Testing

ANAs and smooth muscle antibodies, respectively, may be found in 69% and 34% of cases of drug-induced CAH and in 32% and 49% of patients with alcoholic liver cirrhosis (107–109). Antimitochondrial antibodies and antibodies against liver cell membranes may also be more prevalent in patients with alcoholic cirrhosis (107). An antibody against altered hepatocytes has been identified in patients with halothane hepatitis but not in patients exposed to halothane without developing hepatitis (104). Analogous antibodies have been demonstrated in patients with hepatic reactions to α-methyldopa and rifampicin (100,105). Autoantibodies, particularly to liver–kidney microsomes, appear in up to one third of halothane hepatitis patients (101,105). Tienilic acid hepatitis is usually associated with autoantibodies directed against an isoenzyme of cytochrome P450 and against liver–kidney microsomes (99,101). An antimitochondrial antibody is produced in iproniazid hepatitis (99,101). Methyldopa may be associated with a positive Coombs' test.

A search for alternative explanations for liver disease by viral serology and imaging may be helpful.

### Treatment

Treatment of drug-induced liver disease is similar to that of idiopathic disease, after cessation of the drug.

### Colitis

Although a number of drugs, including gold, oral contraceptives, NSAIDs, and chemotherapeutic agents, have been associated with colitis resembling Crohn's disease or ulcerative colitis, immune mechanisms have not been definitely implicated in these conditions (109,111,112). A possible autoimmune basis for the colitis rarely associated with α-methyldopa has been suggested in view of the accompanying fever, rash, and eosinophilia in some cases (109).

### Pernicious Anemia

Autoimmune gastritis is a $CD4^+$-mediated disorder with similarities to pernicious anemia associated with antibodies to gastric $H^+/K^+$-ATPase. In murine studies, autoimmune gastritis can be induced in neonates by thymectomy or treatment with cyclosporine; in adult mice, thymectomy and cyclophosphamide can induce autoimmune gastritis. Administration of antibody to the $T_H1$ cytokine IFN-γ prevents development of autoimmunity. It has been suggested that transient lymphopenia and lack of thymic regulation produced by these means can induce autoimmunity by expansion and activation of "resting" autoreactive peripheral T cells. It is not known whether these mechanisms are relevant in human pernicious anemia, and these drugs are not known to produce the condition in humans (113,114).

### Primary Biliary Cirrhosis

Primary biliary cirrhosis is an autoimmune condition characterized by intrahepatic bile destruction in association with antibodies against mitochondria. Although we are not aware of therapeutic drugs producing a similar clinical picture, mercury is known to damage mitochondria and is excreted by the biliary route. It has been hypothesized that mercury may bind to microsomal enzymes and alter immunogenicity to produce autoimmune destructive disease (19,115).

### Vasculitis

Drug-induced vasculitis usually involves small vessels, and most identified drug-related small vessel vasculitis has been confined to the skin, with drugs accounting for 10% of cases (116). Drugs that appear to be associated with skin vasculitis include propylthiouracil, hydralazine, penicillins, aminopenicillins, sulfonamides, allopurinol, thiazides, pyrazolon, retinoids, quinolones, hydantoins, streptokinase, cytokines, and monoclonal antibodies (116–119). Induction of ANCA appears to be an important aspect with propylthiouracil and hydralazine, whereas immune complex formation and deposition appears to be a more common mechanism in general (116). In the case of anticonvulsants, the mechanism is unknown but may involve binding of the drug to macromolecules to act as a hapten (36).

Localized vasculitis syndromes of the kidney have also been described (36,117). In the case of skin disease (characteristically leukocytoclastic angiitis), a single episode lasting weeks to months is common (116). The reaction may occur after days, after long-term use, or after discontinuation (36).

Hydralazine, propylthiouracil, phenytoin, and penicillamine have been associated with renal vasculitis (110, 117,120). The systemic vasculitis associated with propylthiouracil and carbamazepine may be accompanied by ANCA autoantibodies, the titer of which parallels clinical improvement when the drug is ceased (119).

Skin biopsy typically shows lesions of similar age, in contrast to the varied ages of lesions in idiopathic disease (36). Deposits of complement and immunoglobulin, most commonly IgM, in the vessel wall are usual. In anticonvulsant-induced disease, involvement of venules with inflammatory infiltrate is characteristic, and leukocytoclasia may be present (36).

Implicated drugs should be stopped. Treatment is symptomatic, with oral corticosteroids sometimes required in severe disease.

## Myasthenia Gravis

### Incidence and Epidemiology

MG may be aggravated or unmasked by a large number of drugs, but the list of drugs inducing the disease is much shorter, and penicillamine is the best established (121,122). Antibodies to the acetylcholine receptor characteristic of idiopathic disease are present and appear to be sufficient to induce disease, in contrast to the relationship of ANAs and drug-induced SLE (123,124). Trimethadione and diphenylhydantoin have also been reported to be associated with MG syndromes in small numbers of patients (125,126). For penicillamine, no relationship has been established between cumulative dose and severity of symptoms (122).

The age of onset of penicillamine-induced MG is older than for idiopathic disease. The female preponderance may be explained by the common use of penicillamine in rheumatoid arthritis. The association with HLA-A1 and HLA-B6 seen in idiopathic MG may be less evident in penicillamine-induced disease, but HLA-DR1 and Bw35 may be overrepresented (122). Polymorphism of the acetylcholine receptor and immunoglobulin genes may also be important (123).

### Clinical Presentation

The treatment duration before onset of MG symptoms ranges from days to years, with a median of about 8 months. Penicillamine-induced disease may be clinically indistinguishable from idiopathic disease, may be localized or generalized, and tends to be mild (122). Usually, the extraocular muscles are the first affected in penicillamine-induced disease, as in the idiopathic form (121).

### Diagnostic Testing

Edrophonium or neostigmine tests appear to be positive in all patients with penicillamine-induced disease, with abnormal decremental tests less common (122). Elevated levels of antibodies to the acetylcholine receptor are present in at least 80%, and declining levels appear to parallel clinical improvement after removal of the drug (121,122,124).

### Treatment

The disease and its associated antibody usually resolve after cessation of the drug, although this may take months, and a small proportion of patients have persisting disease (122,124). Treatment with anticholinesterases may be required for some weeks (121).

## Polymyositis and Dermatomyositis

Penicillamine has been implicated as a causative agent in a number of reports of dermatomyositis and polymyositis (121,127,128). Penicillin, levodopa, cromoglycate, cimetidine, propylthiouracil, and bacille Calmette-Guérin vaccination have also been reported to induce this disease, and myositis may occur as part of DIL (121,129,130). Zidovudine results in a polymyositis-like syndrome in up to 20% of patients with human immunodeficiency virus treated with the drug; this syndrome appears to be dose-related and usually appears after months of therapy (131,132). It may be difficult to distinguish this complication from the myopathy accompanying the disease. HLA associations with Bw35, DR1, or DR2 may exist with penicillamine-induced disease, as opposed to the idiopathic associations with B8 and DR3 (29,92). The disease appears to remit over months on cessation of therapy in most cases, although fatalities have been reported (130).

## Thyroid Disease

### Mechanism

Autoimmune lymphocytic thyroiditis may be induced by anticonvulsants and sulfonamides in a syndrome characterized by hypersensitivity reactions, overt hypothyroidism, and antithyroid antibodies (133–135). This may be mediated by metabolism of sulfonamides and phenytoin by thyroid peroxidases to produce reactive metabolites, which may then interact with the peroxidase or with other cell macromolecules to produce antimicrosomal antibodies against the peroxidase complex (133). Binding of the reactive metabolites to other cell molecules may result in neoantigen formation. In one series of five patients, onset was acute in all, none had a goiter, and all recovered (133). Hypothyroidism was preceded by a hypersensitivity phase characterized by fever, rash, and involvement of liver, kidney, bone marrow, lung, heart and central nervous system, occurring over days to weeks. Resolution with withdrawal of the drug is thought to be related to absence of the metabolite and generation of new peroxidase.

It has been shown that alimemazine (a phenothiazine) and IFN-γ can increase MHC class II antigen expression on thyroid cells (136). This phenomenon also occurs in idiopathic thyroid autoimmune disorders and is thought to contribute to the development and persistence of autoimmunity. It is also possible that such drugs upregulate class II expression on APCs and thereby stimulate CD4 responses, or that upregulation unmasks latent thyroid autoimmunity (136).

Iodine has been implicated in the production of autoimmune thyroid disease in genetically susceptible patients (3). Hypothesized mechanisms of this include overiodination of thyroglobulin, rendering it more immunogenetic, and binding of a reactive intermediary to enzymes, interfering with intracellular signaling (3).

The mechanism of amiodarone-induced thyroid disease is not entirely clear, but changes such as antibodies to thyroglobulin, thyroid peroxidase, thyroid-stimulating receptor, and T-cell subset changes have been reported and suggest an immunologic influence (74). The hypothyroidism in up to 15% of patients treated with lithium may also be associated with increased titer of antibodies to thyroglobulin or thyroid peroxidase in patients with antibodies previously detectable, suggesting unmasking rather than *de novo* occurrence of autoimmunity (74).

### Renal Disease

Drugs associated with development of autoimmune renal disease include gold, mercury, cadmium, captopril, propylthiouracil, IFN-α, α-mercaptopropionylglycine, lithium, organic solvents, paraquat, penicillamine, and perchlorethylene; membranous glomerulopathy is the most common histopathology (74).

The mechanism of drug-induced acute interstitial nephritis is not always clear, and autoimmunity is one possible factor (137). Both cell-mediated damage and antibody-mediated damage have been proposed as mechanisms (137). Penicillin derivatives are associated with the production of antibodies to tubular basement membrane, and the presence of fever, rash, arthralgia, and eosinophilia in conjunction with tubulointerstitial disease suggests an immune mechanism (137). Cimetidine-induced immunomodulation has been suggested as a mechanism of cimetidine nephritis (138). Drug-induced interstitial nephritis usually presents as renal failure (110).

The glomerulonephritis associated with hydralazine may resemble vasculitis more closely than SLE nephritis (117), and it may occur as an isolated manifestation (139). Most patients are hypertensive and present with rapidly progressive renal impairment (140). This may present as a rapidly progressive glomerulonephritis, with focal and segmental necrosis and crescents, in association with ANAs and anti-histone antibodies (139–141). Circulating antibodies to myeloperoxidase and elastase appear in most cases and are not found in hydralazine-treated patients without this effect (64). A similar condition may arise with the use of thiazides (141).

Penicillamine and gold may produce proliferative or membranous glomerulonephritis mediated by immune complex disease arising as a result of drug-induced tubular injury, release of tubular protein, and subsequent antibody formation (110,120,142). This may be more common in patients with HLA-B8 and HLA-DR3. Penicillamine has been reported to cause proteinuria in up to 24% of patients (142). It may also be associated with a condition resembling Goodpasture's syndrome in which glomerulonephritis is accompanied by pulmonary hemorrhage (110,143,144). The immunofluorescence pattern seen in this syndrome, however, is not always concordant with the linear deposition of complement and IgG on the glomerular basement membrane seen in idiopathic Goodpasture's syndrome, and circulating anti–basement membrane antibodies are not present (143,144).

Phenytoin-induced renal disease usually manifests as interstitial nephritis or vasculitis and, although uncommon, may be fatal (110,145). It may be accompanied by rash. Circulating and bound IgG antibodies to tubular basement membrane may be present (146). Methicillin has been associated with a similar picture (146).

Propylthiouracil has been associated with vasculitis, manifesting as rapidly progressive renal impairment in a number of reports (147,148). Clinical presentation may include a preceding influenza-like illness, proteinuria, hematuria, and anemia in conjunction with deteriorating renal function. ANCA is frequently positive, with specificity for myeloperoxidase, proteinase-3, or both (148). Biopsy usually shows crescentic disease. Chlorpropramide has been reported as the cause of proliferative glomerulonephritis and nephrotic syndrome with a suspected immunologic basis (149).

ANCAs have been demonstrated in glomerulonephritis associated with hydralazine, propylthiouracil, and carbamazepine (117,147); in these patients, ANA was not always detected.

In isolated hydralazine-associated renal impairment, recovery of renal function appears to accompany cessation of the drug, although in some cases, immunosuppression may be required (139,140). Cessation of propylthiouracil does not always result in resolution of renal abnormalities (148).

### Autoimmune Eye Disease

Sulfonamides have been implicated in a number of cases of bilateral anterior uveitis, and although an immune mechanism is suspected, the exact pathophysiology remains unclear (150).

## Breast Implant Problems

Both specific autoimmune conditions, such as systemic sclerosis, inflammatory arthritis, and adult-onset Still's disease, and atypical syndromes have been proposed as possible associations of silicone breast implants, but epidemiologic evidence does not support this. Large population studies have failed to confirm a relationship between implants and subsequent development of connective tissue disease (151–154), but the issue remains controversial (155). The significance of local complications, such as rupture, in determination of adverse outcome remains poorly defined.

## Pulmonary Disease

More than 75 drugs are known to cause adverse pulmonary reactions, and alterations in the immune system have been implicated in many cases (156). Most cases postulated to involve autoimmune mechanisms, however, involve penicillamine or those drugs producing manifestations of SLE described previously (157). Most patients with DIL have some pleuropulmonary features. Penicillamine, gold, and sulfasalazine have been reported to be associated with bronchiolitis obliterans, but the mechanisms are not well understood (156,158). Penicillamine is also associated with alveolitis and with pulmonary renal syndrome, with similarities to Goodpasture's syndrome, which may have a fulminant onset and is frequently fatal (156). The pathogenesis of methotrexate pneumonitis probably involves an immune mechanism, although induction of autoimmunity does not appear to be an issue (159). Amiodarone pneumonitis may be associated with antibodies to the drug, and the possibility of amiodarone acting as a hapten linked to pulmonary tissue with subsequent lung damage has been raised (158).

## CONCLUSIONS

The interest in drug-induced autoimmune disease stems from the obvious possibility that if the association is recognized and the drug discontinued, the disease may well be cured, although clearly this is not always so. The other issue relates to the understanding of spontaneous disease that it may provide. Thus, it is possible that the decrease in apoptosis seen with a reduction in TNF-$\alpha$ production may be an important aspect in the development of ANAs and SLE, and this is supported by the suppressive effects of TNF-$\alpha$ in spontaneous disease of B/W mice. The role of hydralazine and procainamide in increasing LFA-1 expression—a feature that may also be found in spontaneous SLE—is fascinating, but still does not explain why this form of DIL syndrome is particularly characterized by the absence of anti-DNA antibodies. We have a great deal to learn, and although they are hardly "experiments of nature," how these puzzling phenomena can be induced, often by simple chemicals, surely provides a model worthy of further study.

## REFERENCES

1. Rozendaal L, Pals ST, Gleichmann E, et al. Persistence of allospecific helper T cells is required for maintaining autoantibody formation in lupus-like graft versus host disease. *Clin Exp Immunol* 1990;82:527–532.
2. Mountz JD, Wu J, Cheng J, et al. Autoimmune disease: a problem of defective apoptosis. *Arthritis Rheum* 1994;37:1415–1420.
3. Yoshida S, Gershwin ME. Autoimmunity and selected environmental factors of disease induction. *Semin Arthritis Rheum* 1993;22:399–419.
4. Sorokin R, Kimura H, Schroder K, et al. Cyclosporine-induced autoimmunity. *J Exp Med* 1986;164:1615–1625.
5. Allison AC, Denman AM, Barnes RD. Cooperating and controlling functions of thymus derived lymphocytes in relation to autoimmunity. *Lancet* 1971;2:135–140.
6. Richardson B, Scheinbart L, Strahler J, et al. Evidence for impaired T cell DNA methylation in systemic lupus erythematosus and rheumatoid arthritis. *Arthritis Rheum* 1990;33:1665–1673.
7. Richardson B. Effect of an inhibitor of DNA methylation on T cells. II. 5-Azacytidine induces self-reactivity in antigen-specific T4$^+$ cells. *Human Immun* 1986:17;456–470.
8. Yung R, Powers D, Johnson K, et al. Mechanisms of drug-induced lupus. II. T cells overexpressing lymphocyte function-associated antigen 1 become autoreactive and cause a lupuslike disease in syngeneic mice. *J Clin Invest* 1996:97;2866–2871.
9. Richardson BC, Strahler JR, Pivirotto TS, et al. Phenotypic and functional similarities between 5 azacytidine-treated T cells and a T cell subset in patients with active systemic lupus erythematosus. *Arthritis Rheum* 1992;35;647–662.
10. Richardson B, Powers D, Hooper F, et al. Lymphocyte function-associated antigen 1 overexpression and cell autoreactivity. *Arthritis Rheum* 1994;37;1363–1372.
11. Scheinbart LS, Johnson MA, Gross LA, et al. Procainamide inhibits DNA methyltransferase in a human T cell line. *J Rheumatol* 1991;18:530–534.
12. Yung R, Chang S, Hemati N, et al. Mechanisms of drug-induced lupus. IV. Comparison of procainamide and hydralazine with analogs in vitro and in vivo. *Arthritis Rheum* 1997;40;1436–1443.
13. Yung RL, Quddus J, Chrisp CE, et al. Mechanisms of drug-induced lupus. I. Cloned H2 cells modified with DNA methylation inhibitors in vitro cause autoimmunity in vivo. *J Immunol* 1995;154;3025–3035.
14. Quddus J, Johnson KJ, Gavalchin J, et al. Treating activated CD4$^+$ T cells with either of two distinct DNA methyltransferase inhibitors, 5-azacytidine or procainamide, is sufficient to cause a lupus-like disease in syngeneic mice. *J Clin Invest* 1993;92:38–53.
15. Richardson BC, Buckmaster T, Keren DF, et al. Evidence that macrophages are programmed to die after activating autologous, cloned, antigen-specific, CD4$^+$ T cells. *Eur J Immunol* 1993:23;1450–1455.
16. Yung R, Williams R, Johnson K, et al. Mechanisms of drug-induced lupus. IV. Comparison of procainamide and hydralazine with analogs in vitro and in vivo. *Arthritis Rheum* 1997;40;1334–1343.
17. Feldmann M, Elliott MJ, Woody JN, et al. Anti tumor necrosis factor alpha therapy of rheumatoid arthritis. *Adv Immunol* 1997;64:283–350.
18. Moreland LW, Baumgartner SW, Schiff MH, et al. Treatment of rheumatoid arthritis with a recombinant human tumor necrosis factor receptor (p75)-Fc fusion protein. *N Engl J Med* 1997;337:141–147.
19. Goldman M, Druet P, Gleichmann E. Th2 cells in systemic autoimmunity: insights from allogeneic diseases and chemically-induced autoimmunity. *Immunol Today* 1991;12:223–227.
20. Kirtland HH, Mohler DN, Horwitz DA. Methyldopa inhibition of suppressor lymphocyte function. *N Engl J Med* 1980;302:825–832.
21. Uetrecht JP. Current trends in drug-induced autoimmunity. *Toxicology* 1997;119:37–43.
22. Dubroff LM, Reid RJ. HydralazIne-pyrimidine interactions may explain hydralazine-induced lupus erythematosus. *Science* 1980;208:4046.
23. Litwin A, Adams LE, Zimmer H, et al. Immunologic effects of hydralazine in hypertensive patients. *Arthritis Rheum* 1981;24:1074–1077.

24. Price EJ, Venables PJW. Drug-induced lupus. *Drug Safety* 1995;12: 283–290.

25. Yung RL, Richardson BC. Drug-induced lupus. *Rheum Dis Clin North Am* 1994;20:61–86.

26. Tan EM, Rubin RL. Autoallergic reactions induced by procainamide. *J Allergy Clin Immunol* 1984;74:631–634.

27. Cornacchia E, Golbus J, Maybaum J, et al. Hydralazine and procainamide inhibit T cell DNA methylation and induce autoreactivity. *Immunology* 1988;140:2197–2200.

28. Laversuch CJ, Collins DA, Charles PJ, et al. Sulphasalazine-induced autoimmune abnormalities in patients with rheumatic disease. *Br J Rheumatol* 1995;34:435–439.

29. Balint G, Gergely P. Clinical immunotoxicity of antirheumatic drugs. *Inflamm Res* 1996;45:S91–S95.

30. Emery P, Panayi GS, Huston G, et al. D-penicillamine induced toxicity in rheumatoid arthritis: the role of sulphoxidation status and HLA-DR3. *J Rheumatol* 1984;11:626–632.

31. Zarrabi MH, Zucker S, Miller F, et al. Immunologic and coagulation disorders in chlorpromazine disorders in chlorpromazine-treated patients. *Ann Intern Med* 1979;91:194–199.

32. Ronnblom LE, Alm GV, Oberg KE. Autoimmunity after alpha-interferon therapy for malignant carcinoid tumours. *Ann Intern Med* 1991;115:178–183.

33. Tolaymat A, Lenethal B, Sakarcan A, et al. Systemic lupus erythematosus in a child receiving long-term interferon therapy. *J Pediatr* 1992;120:429–432.

34. Fritzler MJ. Drugs recently associated with lupus syndromes. *Lupus* 1994;3:455–459.

35. Alloway JA, Salate MP. Quinidine-induced rheumatic syndromes. *Semin Arthritis Rheum* 1995;24:315–322.

36. Totoritis MC, Rubin RL. Drug-induced lupus. *Postgrad Med* 1985; 78:149–160.

37. Drory VE, Korczyn AD. Hypersensitivity vasculitis and systemic lupus erythematosus induced by anticonvulsants. *Clin Neuropharmacol* 1993;1:19–29.

38. Emery P, Gough A, Griffiths B. Minocycline related lupus. *J Rheumatol* 1997;24:1850.

39. Thomas TJ, Messner RP. Effects of lupus-inducing drugs on the B to Z transition of synthetic DNA. *Arthritis Rheum* 1986;29:638–645.

40. Rich MW. Drug-induced lupus. *Postgrad Med* 1996;100:299–308.

41. Hess E. Drug-related lupus. *N Engl J Med* 1988;318:1460–1462.

42. Gunnarsson I, Kanerud L, Pettersson E, et al.: Predisposing factors in sulphasalazine induced systemic lupus erythematosus. *Br J Rheumatol* 1997;36:1089–1094.

43. Gunnarsson I, Pettersson E, Lindblad S, et al. Olsalazine-induced lupus syndrome. *Scand J Rheumatol* 1997;26:65–66.

44. Chalmers A, Thompson D, Stein HE, et al. Systemic lupus erythematosus during penicillamine therapy for rheumatoid arthritis. *Ann Intern Med* 1982;97:659–663.

45. Ansell BM. Drug-induced systemic lupus erythematosus in childhood. *Lupus* 1993;2:139–140.

46. Graninger WB, Hassfeld W, Pesau BB, et al. Induction of systemic lupus erythematosus by interferon gamma in a patient with rheumatoid arthritis. *J Rheumatol* 1991;18:1621–1622.

47. Totoritis MC, Tan EM, McNally EM, et al. Association of antibody to histone complex H2A-2B with symptomatic procainamide-induced lupus. *N Engl J Med* 1988;318:1431–1436.

48. Hughes GRV, Rynes RI, Gharavi A, et al. The heterogeneity of serologic findings and predisposing host factors in drug-induced lupus erythematosus. *Arthritis Rheum* 1981;24:1070–1073.

49. Perry HM, Tan EM, Carmody S, et al. Relationship of actual transferase activity to antinuclear antibodies and toxic symptoms in hypertensive patients treated with hydralazine. *J Lab Clin Med* 1970;76: 114–125.

50. Batchelor JR, Welsh KI, Tinoco RM, et al. Hydralazine-induced systemic lupus erythematosus: influence of HLA-DR and sex on susceptibility. *Lancet* 1980;1:1107–1109.

51. Woosley RL, Drayer DE, Reidenberg MM, et al. Effect of acetylator phenotype on the rate at which procainamide induces antinuclear antibodies and the lupus syndrome. *N Engl J Med* 1978;298:1157–1159.

52. Brand C, Davidson A, Littlejohn G, et al. Hydralazine-induced lupus: no association with HLA-DR4. *Lancet* 1984;1:462.

53. Schattner A, Sthoeger Z, Geltner D. Effect of acute cytomegalovirus infection on drug-induced SLE. *Postgrad Med J* 1994;70:738–740.

54. Solinger AM. Drug-related lupus. *Rheum Dis Clin North Am* 1988;14: 187–202.

55. Tan EM, Cohen AS, Fries JF, et al. The 1982 revised criteria for the classification of systemic lupus erythematosus. *Arthritis Rheum* 1982; 25:1271–1277.

56. Masson C, Laine P, Audran M. Minocycline related lupus. *J Rheumatol* 1997;24:1851.

57. Gioud M, Ait Kaci M, Monier JC. Histone antibodies in systemic lupus erythematosus. *Arthritis Rheum* 1982;25:407–413.

58. Reeves WH, Satoh M, Wang J, et al. Systemic lupus erythematosus. Antibodies to DNA, DNA-binding proteins, and histones. *Rheum Dis Clin North Am* 1994;1–28.

59. Portanova JP, Arndt RE, Tan RE, et al. Anti-histone antibodies in idiopathic and drug-induced lupus recognize intrahistone regions. *J Immunol* 1987;138:446–451.

60. Epstein A, Barland P. The diagnostic value of antihistone antibodies in drug-induced lupus erythematosus. *Arthritis Rheum* 1985;28:158–163.

61. West SG, McMahon M, Portanova JP. Quinidine-induced lupus erythematosus. *Ann Intern Med* 1984;100:840–842.

62. Blomgren SE. Drug-induced lupus erythematosus. *Semin Hematol* 1973;10:345–349.

63. Russell AS, Ziff M. Natural antibodies to procainamide. *Clin Exp Immunol* 1968;3:901–909.

64. Nassberger L, Johansson AC, Bjorck S, et al. Antibodies to neutrophil granulocyte myeloperoxidase and elastase: autoimmune responses in glomerulonephritis due to hydralazine treatment. *J Int Med* 1991; 229:261–265.

65. Vivino FB, Schumacher HR. Synovial fluid characteristics and the lupus erythematosus cell phenomenon in drug-induced lupus. *Arthritis Rheum* 1989;32:560–568.

66. Salama A, Mueller-Eckhardt C. Immune mediated blood cell dyscrasias related to drugs. *Semin Hematol* 1992;29:54–63.

67. Thompson DF, Gales MA. Drug-induced pure red cell aplasia. *Pharmacotherapy* 1996:16;1002–1008.

68. Mueller-Eckhardt G, Giers G, Salama A, et al. Major histocompatibility complex markers in patients with nomifensene-induced immune hemolytic anemia. *Vox Sang* 1988;54:59–61.

69. Worlledge SM. Immune drug-induced hemolytic anemias. *Semin Hematol* 1973;10:327–344.

70. Pixley JS, MacKintosh FR, Sahr E, et al. Mechanisms of ranitidine associated anemia. *Am J Med Sci* 1989;297:369–371.

71. Nagler A, Rozenbaum H, Enat R, et al. Immune basis for cimetidine-induced pancytopenia. *Am J Gastroenterol* 1987;82:359–361.

72. Malkin D, Koren G, Saunders EF. Drug-induced aplastic anemia: pathogenesis and clinical aspects. *Am J Pediatr Hematol Oncol* 1990; 12:402–410.

73. Young NS, Maciejewski J. The pathophysiology of acquired aplastic anaemia. *N Engl J Med* 1997;336:1365–1372.

74. Bigazzi PE. Autoimmunity caused by xenobiotics. *Toxicology* 1997; 119:1–21.

75. Lerner W, Caruso R, Faig D, et al. Drug-dependent and non-drug-dependent antiplatelet antibody in drug-induced immunologic thrombocytopenic purpura. *Blood* 1985;2:306–311.

76. Kelton JG. Heparin-induced thrombocytopenia. *Haemostasis* 1986;16: 173–186.

77. Schmitt BP, Adelman B. Heparin-associated thrombocytopenia: a critical review and pooled analysis. *Am J Med Sci* 1993;305:208–215.

78. von dem Borne AEGR, Pegels JG, van der Stadt RJ, et al. Thrombocytopenia associated with gold therapy: a drug-induced autoimmune disease? *Br J Haematol* 1986;63:509–516.

79. Boxer LA. Immune neutropenias: clinical and biological implications. *Am J Pediatr Hematol Oncol* 1981;3:89–96.

80. Mamus SW, Burton JD, Groat JD, et al. Ibuprofen-associated pure white-cell aplasia. *N Engl J Med* 1986;314:624–625.

81. Kelton JG, Huang AT, Mold N, et al. The use of in vitro technics to study drug-induced pancytopenia. *N Engl J Med* 1979;301:621–624.

82. Best WR. Chloramphenicol-associated blood dyscrasias. *JAMA* 1967;201:99–106.

83. Lockshin MD. Antiphospholipid antibody syndrome. *Rheum Dis Clin North Am* 1994;20:45–59.

84. Lillicrap DP, Pinto M, Benford K, et al. Heterogeneity of laboratory test results for antiphospholipid antibodies treated with chlorpromazine and other phenothiazines. *Am J Clin Pathol* 1990;93:771–775.

85. Canosa RT, de Oliveira RM. Chlorpromazine-induced anticardiolipin antibodies and lupus anticoagulant: absence of thrombosis. *Am J Hematol* 1988;27:272–275.

86. Mutasim DF, Pelc NJ, Anhalt GJ. Drug-induced pemphigus. *Dermatol Clin* 1993;3:463–471.

87. Korman NJ, Eyre RW, Zone J, et al. Drug-induced pemphigus: autoantibodies directed against the pemphigus antigen complexes are present in penicillamine and captopril-induced pemphigus. *J Invest Dermatol* 1991;96:273–276.

88. Ruocco V, Sacerdoti G. Pemphigus and bullous pemphigoid due to drugs. *Int J Dermatol* 1991;30:307–312.

89. Magro CM, Crowson AN. Drug-induced immune dysregulation as a cause of atypical cutaneous lymphoid infiltrates. *Human Pathol* 1996;27:125–132.

90. Fellner MJ, Moshell A, Mont MA. Pemphigus vulgaris and drug reactions. *Int J Dermatol* 1981;20:115–118.

91. Asnis LA, Gaspari AA. Cutaneous reactions to recombinant cytokine therapy. *J Am Acad Dermatol* 1995;33:393–410.

92. Mobini N, Ahmed AR. Immunogenetics of drug-induced bullous diseases. *Clin Dermatol* 1993;11;449–460.

93. Smith EP, Taylor TB, Meyer LJ, et al. Antigen identification in drug-induced bullous pemphigoid. *J Am Acad Dermatol* 1993;29;879–882.

94. Koch CA, Mazzafem EL, Larry JA, et al. Bullous pemphigoid after treatment with furosemide. *Cutis* 1996;58:341–344.

95. Alcalay J, David M, Ingber A, et al. Bullous pemphigoid mimicking bullous erythema multiforme: an untoward side effect of penicillins. *J Am Acad Dermatol* 1988;18:345–349.

96. Hodak E, Ben-Sehtrit A, Ingber A, et al. Bullous pemphigoid: an adverse effect of penicillin. *Clin Exp Dermatol* 1990;15:50–52.

97. Fellner MJ. Drug-induced bullous pemphigoid. *Clin Dermatol* 1993;11:515–520.

98. Wolf R. A new concept in the pathogenesis of drug-induced psoriasis. *Med Hypotheses* 1986;21:277–279.

99. Pessayre D, Larrey D. Acute and chronic drug-induced hepatitis. *Baillieres Clin Gastroenterol* 1988;2:385–422.

100. Neuberger J, Williams R. Immunology of drug and alcohol-induced liver disease. *Baillieres Clin Gastroenterol* 1987;1:707–722.

101. Beaune PH, Bourdi M. Autoantibodies against cytochromes P-450 in drug-induced autoimmune hepatitis. *Ann N Y Acad Sci* 1993;685:641–645.

102. Kamiyama T, Nouchi T, Kpojima S, et al. Autoimmune hepatitis triggered by administration of a herbal medicine. *Am J Gastroenterol* 1997;92:703–704.

103. Lecoeur S, Gautier J-C, Belloc C, et al. Use of heterologous expression systems to study autoimmune drug-induced hepatitis. *Methods Enzymol* 1996;272:76–85.

104. Vergani D, Mieli-Vergani G, Alberti A, et al. Antibodies to the surface of halothane altered rabbit hepatocytes in patients with severe halothane associated hepatitis. *N Engl J Med* 1980;303:66–71.

105. Neuberger J, Kenna JG. Halothane hepatitis: a model of immune mediated drug hepatotoxicity. *Clin Sci* 1987;72:263–270.

106. Ishak KG, Zimmerman HJ. Drug-induced and toxic granulomatous hepatitis. *Baillieres Clin Gastroenterol* 1988;2:463–480.

107. Gluud C, Tage-Jensen U, Bahnsen M, et al. Autoantibodies, HLA and testosterone in males with alcoholic liver disease. *Clin Exp Immunol* 1981;44:31–37.

108. Lindberg J, Lindholm A, Lundin P, et al. Trigger factors and HLA antigens in chronic acute hepatitis. *Br Med J* 1975;4:77–79.

109. Fortson WC, Tedesco FJ. Drug-induced colitis: a review. *Am J Gastroenterol* 1984;79:878–883.

110. Swainson CP, Thomson D, Short AIK, et al. Plasma exchange in the successful treatment of drug-indcued renal disease. *Nephron* 1982;30:244–249.

111. Tedesco FJ, Volpicelli NA, Moore FS. Estrogen- and progesterone-associated colitis: a disorder with clinical and endoscopic features mimicking Crohn's colitis. *Gastrointest Endosc* 1982;28:247–249.

112. Aabakken L, Osnes M. Non-steroidal anti-inflammatory drug-induced disease in the distal ileum and large bowel. *Scand J Gastroenterol* 1989;163[Suppl]:48–55.

113. Toh B-H, van Driel IR, Gleeson PA. Pernicious anaemia. *N Engl J Med* 1997;338:1441–1448.

114. Barrett SP, Toh B-H, Alderuccio F, et al. Organ-specific autoimmunity induced by adult thymectomy and cyclophosphamide-induced lymphopenia. *Eur J Immunol* 1995;25:238–244.

115. Strubelt O, Kremer J, Tilse A, et al. Comparative studies on the toxicity of mercury, cadmium, and copper toward the isolated, perfused rat liver. *J Toxicol Environ Health* 1996;47:267–283.

116. Jennette JC, Falk RJ. Small-vessel vasculitis. *N Engl J Med* 1997;337:1512–1523.

117. Cambridge G, Wallace H, Bernstein RM, et al. Autoantibodies to myeloperoxidase in idiopathic and drug-induced systemic lupus erythematosus and vasculitis. *Br J Rheumatol* 1994;33:109–114.

118. Bernstein RM, Egerton-Vernon J, Webster J. Hydralazine-induced cutaneous vasculitis. *Br Med J* 1980;280:156–157.

119. Dolman KM, Gans ROB, Vervaat TJ, et al. Vasculitis and antineutrophil cytoplasmic autoantibodies associated with propylthiouracil therapy. *Lancet* 1993;342:651–652.

120. Banfi G, Imbasciatti E, Guerra L, et al. Extracapillary glomerulonephritis with necrotizing vasculitis in D-penicillamine-treated rheumatoid arthritis. *Nephron* 1983;33:56–60.

121. Lane RJM, Routledge PA. Drug-induced neurological disorders. *Drugs* 1983;26:124–147.

122. Kaeser HE. Drug-induced myasthenic syndromes. *Acta Neurol Scand* 1984;70:39–46.

123. Dawkins RL, Kay PH, Garlepp MJ, et al. Immunogenetics of spontaneous, drug-induced, and experimental myasthenia gravis. *Ann N Y Acad Sci* 1987;505:398–406.

124. Russell AS, Lindstrom JM. Penicillamine-induced myasthenia gravis associated with antibodies to acetylcholine receptor. *Neurology* 1978;28:847–849.

125. Booker HE, Chun RWM, Sanguino M. Myasthenia gravis syndrome associated with trimethadione. *JAMA* 1970;212:2262–2263.

126. Peterson HD. Association of trimethadione therapy and myasthenia gravis. *N Engl J Med* 1966;274:506–507.

127. Lund HI, Nielsen M. Penicillamine-induced dermatomyositis. *Scand J Rheumatol* 1983;12:350–352.

128. Fernandes L, Swinson DR, Hamilton EBD. Dermatomyositis complicating penicillamine treatment. *Ann Rheum Dis* 1977;36:94–95.

129. Shergy WJ, Caldwell DS. Polymyositis after propylthiouracil treatment for hyperthyroidism. *Ann Rheum Dis* 1988;47:340–343.

130. Watson AJS, Dalbow MH, Stachura I, et al. Cimetidine and polymyositis. *N Engl J Med* 1983;309:188.

131. Zuckner J. Drug-related myopathies. *Rheum Dis Clin North Am* 1994;20:1017–1032.

132. Bessen LJ, Greene JB, Louie E, et al. Severe polymyositis-like syndrome associated with zidovudine therapy of AIDS and ARD. *N Engl J Med* 1988;318:708.

133. Gupta A, Eggo MC, Uetrecht JP, et al. Drug-induced hypothyroidism: the thyroid as a targe organ in hypersensitivity reactions to anticonvulsants and sulfonamides. *Clin Pharmacol Ther* 1992;51:56–67.

134. Kuiper JJ. Lymphocytic thyroiditis possibly induced by diphenylhydantoin. *JAMA* 1969;210:2370–2372.

135. Nishimaya S, Matsukura M, Fujimoto S, et al. Reports of two cases of autoimmune thyroiditis while receiving anticonvulsant therapy. *Eur J Pediatr* 1983;140:116–117.

136. Takorabet L, Ropars A, Raby C, et al. Phenothiazine induces de novo MHC class ll antigen expression on thyroid epithelial cells. *J Immunol* 1995;154:3593–3602.

137. McCluskey RT, Bhan AK. Cell-mediated mechanisms in renal diseases. *Kidney Int* 1982;21:S6–S12.

138. Watson AJS, Dalbow MH, Stachura I, et al. Immunologic studies in cimetidine-induced nephropathy and polymyositis. *N Engl J Med* 1983;308:142–145.

139. Bjorck S, Svalander C, Westberg G. Hydralazine-associated glomerulonephritis. *Acta Med Scand* 1985;218:261–269.

140. Mason PD, Lockwood CM. Rapidly progressive nephritis in patients taking hydralazine. *J Clin Lab Immunol* 1986;20:151–153.

141. Nassberger L. Granulocyte autoantibodies: markers for drug-induced autoimmune adverse effects. *Clin Nephrol* 1992;39:288.

142. Jaffe IA, Treser G, Suzuki Y, et al. Nephropathy induced by D-penicillamine. *Ann Intern Med* 1968;69:549–556.

143. Gibson T, Burry HC, Ogg C. Goodpasture syndrome and D-penicillamine. *Ann Intern Med* 1976;84:100.

144. Sternlieb I, Bennett B, Scheinberg IH. D-penicillamine induced Goodpasture's syndrome in Wilson's disease. *Ann Intern Med* 1975;82:673–676.

145. Agarwal BN, Cabebe FG, Hoffman BI. Diphenylhydantoin-induced acute renal failure. *Nephron* 1977;18:249–251.

146. Hyman LR, Ballow M, Knieser MR. Diphenylhydantoin interstitial nephritis: roles of cellular and humoral immunologic injury. *J Pediatr* 1978;92:915–920.

147. D'Cruz D, Chesser AMS, Lightowler C, et al. Antineutrophil cytoplasmic antibody-positive crescentic glomerulonephritis associated with anti-thyroid drug treatment. *Br J Rheumatol* 1995;34:1090–1091.

148. Tanemoto M, Miyakawa H, Hanai J, et al. Myeloperoxidasantineutrophil cytoplasmic antibody-positive crescentic glomerulonephritis complicating the course of Graves' disease: report of three adult cases. *Am J Kidney Dis* 1995;26:774–780.

149. Appel GB, D'Agati V, Bergman M, et al. Nephrotic syndrome and immune complex glomerulonephritis associated with chlorpropamide therapy. *Am J Med* 1983;74:337–342.

150. Tilden ME, Rosenbaum JT, Fraunfelder FT. Systemic sulfonamides as a cause of bilateral, anterior uveitis. *Arch Ophthalmol* 1991;109:67–69.

151. Williams HJ, Weisman MH, Berry CC. Breast implants in patients with differentiated and undifferentiated connective tissue disease. *Arthritis Rheum* 1997;40:437–440.

152. Goldman JA, Greenblatt J, Joines R, et al. Breast implants, rheumatoid arthritis and connective tissue diseases in a clinical practice. *J Clin Epidemiol* 1995;48:571–582.

153. Nyren O, Yin L, Josefsson S, et al. Risk of connective tissue disease and related disorders among women and breast implants: a nationwide retrospective cohort study in Sweden. *Br Med J* 1998;316:417–422.

154. Edelman DA, Grant S, van Os WAA. Autoimmune disease following the use of silicone gel-filled breast implants: a review of the clinical literature. *Semin Arthritis Rheum* 1994;24:183–189.

155. Angell M. Do breast implants cause systemic disease? *N Engl J Med* 1994;320:1748–1749.

156. Allen J, Cooper D, White DA, et al. Drug-induced pulmonary disease. *Am Rev Respir Dis* 1986;133:488–505.

157. Rosenow EC. Drug-induced bronchopulmonary pleural disease. *J Allergy Clin Immunol* 1987;80:780–787.

158. Israel-Biet D, Labrune S, Huchon GJ. Drug-induced lung disease: 1990 review. *Eur Respir J* 1991;4:465–478.

159. White DA, Rankin JA, Stover DE, et al. Methotrexate pneumonitis: bronchoalveolar lavage findings suggest an immunologic disorder. *Am Rev Respir Dis* 1989;139:18–21.

*Textbook of the Autoimmune Diseases,*
Edited by R. G. Lahita, N. Chiorazzi, and W. H. Reeves,
Lippincott Williams & Wilkins, Philadelphia © 2000.

# CHAPTER 43

# Experimental Autoimmune Encephalomyelitis

Rhonda R. Voskuhl

Experimental autoimmune encephalomyelitis (EAE) is a demyelinating disease of the central nervous system (CNS) mediated by CD4$^+$ major histocompatibility complex (MHC) class II restricted T lymphocytes specific for myelin proteins. It serves as a useful animal model for the study of autoantigen-specific T-lymphocyte responses in the human demyelinating disease multiple sclerosis (MS) (1). EAE has been induced in many mammalian species, including mice, rats, guinea pigs, rabbits, and monkeys.

The two methods of EAE induction are passive and active (2). Passive EAE is the adoptive transfer method whereby the animal with EAE has *passively* received T lymphocytes specific for a given encephalitogenic myelin protein epitope. These T lymphocytes have been generated by immunization of a separate group of animals with a myelin protein emulsified in complete Freund's adjuvant. This group of mice is sacrificed, and cell suspensions containing myelin protein–specific T lymphocytes are made from draining lymph nodes. After *in vitro* stimulation with myelin protein, these T lymphocytes are adoptively transferred into a second group of animals, which subsequently develop EAE. This method thereby separates the induction phase (immunization) from the effector phase (disease development), with each phase taking place in separate groups of animals.

In the active EAE model, the mouse with EAE has *actively* generated its own T lymphocytes specific for the encephalitogenic myelin epitope. A single group of animals is immunized with myelin protein emulsified in complete Freund's adjuvant. Pertussis is injected during the 1 to 2 days that follow and is thought to affect blood-brain barrier permeability. Within a few weeks, these mice develop clinical signs of EAE. This method thereby combines the induction phase and the effector phase, with both phases taking place in the same animal.

Although both the passive and active methods of EAE induction have been extensively used, the passive EAE method is considered a "cleaner" system than the active EAE method because disease is induced by the transfer of only antigen-specific T lymphocytes in the absence of antigen or antibody. In addition, the mouse with passive EAE has not received complete Freund's adjuvant or pertussis, which may artificially alter immune responsiveness and the blood-brain barrier, respectively.

EAE was originally induced using spinal cord homogenate, then with purified myelin basic protein (MBP) (3). Proteolipid protein (PLP) (4) and myelin oligodendrocyte glycoprotein (5) were later shown to be encephalitogenic, as were epitopes within myelin proteins expressed during remyelination (6). Interestingly, a nonmyelin protein, S-100-β, a calcium-binding protein in astroglia, has also been shown to cause panencephalomyelitis accompanied by uveoretinitis (7). Thus, multiple CNS proteins have been shown to be encephalitogenic.

Animals vary in their susceptibility to EAE induction (3). Some inbred strains are highly susceptible, whereas others are relatively resistant. Outbred animals demonstrate variability in susceptibility. Disease susceptibility has been clearly linked to MHC background (8,9). Because there are examples of MHC congenic mice that differ in EAE susceptibility, however, non-MHC genes also appear to contribute to susceptibility. The precise identification of these non-MHC genes and their role in disease susceptibility remains to be elucidated. Linkage analysis has been performed on mice derived from back-crosses between MHC congenic mice with high and low levels of susceptibility. Multiple non-MHC loci have been identified as being associated with susceptibility using this approach; however, the loci identified vary depending on which MHC congenic pairs are examined (10–12). Thus, in addition to MHC genes, multiple non-MHC genes appear to contribute to susceptibility to EAE. Unlike diabetes and lupus, there is no spontaneous model for MS in nontransgenic mice. Perhaps when the full array of genes that contribute to EAE susceptibility is characterized, a mouse that contains these combined susceptibility loci will develop EAE spontaneously.

R. R. Voskuhl: Department of Neurology, University of California at Los Angeles, Los Angeles, California 90095.

MHC background is important not only in determining the level of susceptibility of a given strain but also in determining which region within a myelin protein will be encephalitogenic. For example, the encephalitogenic epitope for H-2$^s$ mice lies within the 83–102 region of MBP (13) and the 139–151 region of PLP (4), whereas the encephalitogenic epitope for H-2$^u$ mice lies within the 1–9 region of MBP (14) and the 43–64 region of PLP (15). Thus, the immunodominant region for each protein differs for each strain, and immunodominance correlates with encephalitogenicity. Subdominant epitopes of myelin proteins can also induce disease if the frequency of T cells for this epitope reaches a given threshold.

The importance of the EAE model is demonstrated by its extensive use for the study of immune mechanisms in MS and other cell-mediated autoimmune diseases. Immune mechanisms in this model are discussed in this chapter, including adhesion molecules, cytokines, T-cell–receptor (TCR) use, epitope spreading, and gender differences in susceptibility.

## ADHESION MOLECULES

For T lymphocytes to be encephalitogenic, they must not only be specific for a protein expressed within the CNS, they must also be activated. This is best demonstrated by the fact that myelin protein–specific T lymphocytes that are not activated *in vitro* before adoptive transfer do not induce disease. This activation step is thought to be crucial for two reasons. Activation increases expression of adhesion molecules essential for homing to the CNS, and it induces the production of cytokines central to disease immunopathogenesis.

Although several adhesion molecules may play a role in migration of T lymphocytes into the CNS, the clearest role has been demonstrated for a molecule within the integrin family. Surface expression of $\alpha_4$ integrins (very late antigen 4, VLA-4) have been shown to correlate with the ability of cloned myelin protein–specific T cells to induce disease upon transfer (16,17). Moreover, antibodies to $\alpha_4$ integrin or its ligand, vascular cell adhesion molecule 1 (VCAM-1), on endothelial cells has been shown to reduce pathogenicity of myelin protein–specific cells *in vivo* (16,18). These reports demonstrate that VLA-4 expression on activated T lymphocytes is crucial to their ability to leave the blood and enter the CNS.

The importance of the specificity of these T lymphocytes has also been shown. Although all activated T lymphocytes, regardless of specificity, can enter the CNS, only T lymphocytes that are specific for an antigen expressed within the CNS remain and induce disease (19).

## CYTOKINES

In addition to inducing adhesion molecule expression, activation of myelin protein–specific T lymphocytes before adoptive transfer is also important in inducing the production of cytokines that are proinflammatory for disease. It has been shown that the ability of myelin protein–specific T lymphocytes to induce disease correlates with their ability to produce cytokines of the helper T-cell subset 1 ($T_H1$) type (17,20,21), specifically tumor necrosis factor (TNF) and interferon-$\gamma$ (IFN-$\gamma$). Such cytokines have been shown to cause increased expression of VCAM on CNS endothelial cells, thereby promoting the binding of VLA-4 expressing T lymphocytes to endothelium and also causing upregulated expression of MHC class II molecules on antigen-presenting cells (APCs) within the CNS.

$T_H1$ cytokine mRNA expression has been demonstrated within the CNS of mice during the peak of disease, with levels dropping to background during remission (22). Further, MBP-specific T-cell lines derived from mouse strains expressing identical k haplotype-derived MHC class II molecules, B10.A and B10.BR, have demonstrated important differences in encephalitogenicity. B10.BR T-cell lines, which produced high levels of TNF-$\alpha$ were highly encephalitogenic, whereas B10.A T-cell lines that produced low levels of TNF-$\alpha$ were weakly encephalitogenic (23). These data underscore the importance of $T_H1$ cytokines in EAE pathogenesis and also suggest that non-MHC genes that influence disease susceptibility may affect $T_H1$ cytokine production.

It was hoped that the use of cytokine gene knockout mice would be an informative approach in examining the role of a given cytokine in EAE; however, such approaches have yielded conflicting results. In two studies, mice with either a single knockout of TNF-$\alpha$ or a double knockout of TNF-$\alpha$ and TNF-$\beta$ (lymphotoxin) were not resistant to EAE as anticipated, thereby providing evidence against a pathogenic role for TNF in EAE (24,25). In another study, however, TNF-$\beta$ knockout mice were protected from disease (26). In yet another study, TNF-$\alpha$ knockout mice demonstrated a delayed onset of disease with reduced perivascular cuff formation, as compared with wild-type litter mates. Severe EAE ensued, however, with widespread inflammation and demyelination, suggesting that TNF-$\alpha$ may play a role in initial leukocyte movement into the CNS but may have little influence on demyelination (27).

Unexpected results have been obtained with IFN-$\gamma$ knockout mice as well. These mice demonstrated either worse disease or no difference in disease compared with wild-type litter mates, suggesting that IFN-$\gamma$ may also not be involved in EAE pathogenesis (28,29). Transgenic mice expressing $T_H1$ cytokine genes within the CNS have, on the other hand, demonstrated a pathogenic role for $T_H1$ cytokines in CNS inflammation. Transgenic mice that constitutively expressed a murine TNF-$\alpha$ transgene in their CNS spontaneously developed a chronic inflammatory demyelinating disease (30). Also, transgenic mice expressing IFN-$\gamma$ in the CNS through an oligodendrocyte-specific promoter demonstrated primary demyelination, upregulation of MHC molecules, and lymphocytic infiltration. The expression of the IFN-$\gamma$ transgene occurred after 8 weeks of age, a time when the murine immune and nervous systems were fully developed (31).

Together, these conflicting data suggest that factors such as the location and timing of expression of a cytokine gene are important in determining the ultimate effect on disease.

Conditional knockout and transgenic approaches are clearly advantageous over conventional approaches. In conventional knockout or transgenic approaches, one observes the effect of the absence or presence of gene expression, respectively, on the developing immune and nervous systems as well as on the adult immune and nervous systems. In contrast, conditional knockout or transgenic approaches create the desired effect only on the adult immune or nervous systems. Alterations in gene expression only in adulthood are theoretically not complicated by an extensive network of redundancy pathways, as compared with alterations in gene expression beginning neonatally, because plasticity decreases with age. Thus, the role of TNF-$\alpha$ and IFN-$\gamma$ on EAE pathogenesis using knockout and transgenic mice awaits further study with conditional approaches.

An alternative approach in studying the role of cytokines in EAE pathogenesis involves altering cytokine function at the protein level and examining the effects on EAE. Rolipram, a selective type IV phosphodiesterase inhibitor, suppresses the production of TNF, lymphotoxin and to a lesser extent IFN-$\gamma$ in autoreactive T lymphocytes resulting in an amelioration of EAE (32). In addition, treatments with antibody to TNF and with soluble TNF receptor have been shown to cause clinical improvement in EAE (33–35). In contrast, antibodies to IFN-$\gamma$ unexpectedly exacerbated EAE (36). Interleukin-12 (IL-12) is a potent inducer of IFN-$\gamma$ and is widely considered to be the principal cytokine that regulates the generation of $T_H1$-type effector cells. Thus, the findings that IL-12 treatment exacerbates EAE and antibody to IL-12 ameliorates disease are consistent with the hypothesis that $T_H1$ cytokines are central to the pathogenesis of EAE (37,38).

Because $T_H2$ cytokines are known to downregulate $T_H1$ responses, $T_H2$ cytokines have been administered to mice with EAE. Treatments with IL-4 and IL-10 have been shown to ameliorate MBP-induced EAE when administered systemically (39–41). In addition, IL-4 has been delivered to the CNS by retrovirally transduced myelin protein–specific T lymphocytes (42), and IL-10 has been delivered to the CNS by genetically modified myelin protein–specific T lymphocytes (43). Each resulted in EAE amelioration. In contrast, one report has demonstrated that MBP-specific $T_H2$ cells induced CNS pathology when transferred to immunodeficient mice. In this case, the pathologic picture resembled an atypical allergic process, which is a process that does not occur in mice with an intact immune system, as demonstrated by a study in which the same $T_H2$ cells were transferred to normal mice, but no pathology developed (44). Together, these data demonstrate the protective effect of $T_H2$ cytokines, such as IL-4 and IL-10, on the pathogenesis of EAE in the setting of a normal immune system.

In EAE induced by MBP or PLP, numerous successful therapeutic approaches have been designed that shift MBP- or PLP-specific responses away from $T_H1$ and toward $T_H2$.

Oral tolerance using low doses of myelin has been shown to be effective in ameliorating EAE by inducing a favorable shift in cytokine production. T cells from rodents fed with MBP have demonstrated decreased IL-2 and IFN-$\gamma$ with increased IL-4, IL-10, and transforming growth factor $\beta$ production (45,46). Thus, EAE induced with PLP can be suppressed by feeding MBP through bystander suppression. Oral tolerance using higher doses of myelin works through an alternative deletional mechanism. Myelin antigen–coupled splenocytes have also been shown to ameliorate EAE by reducing IL-2 and IFN-$\gamma$ production while concomitantly increasing IL-4 production (47).

Another therapeutic approach in EAE that involves alteration in the balance between $T_H1$ and $T_H2$ cytokine production includes the use of altered peptide ligands of encephalitogenic myelin protein epitopes. An amino acid substitution at a crucial TCR contact residue within the MBP 87–99 epitope was shown to antagonize in vitro responses of T lymphocytes to native ligand and to result in an amelioration of EAE with an associated reduced production of the $T_H$ cytokines TNF-$\alpha$ and IFN-$\gamma$ (48). Similarly, an altered peptide ligand involving an amino acid substitution at a crucial TCR contact point within the PLP 139–151 epitope was shown to inhibit the development of EAE induced by native peptide. The altered peptide ligand was shown to inhibit EAE through the generation of T cells that secreted the $T_H2$ cytokines IL-4 and IL-10 (49).

Thus, alteration in the balance between $T_H1$ and $T_H2$ has been shown to affect EAE pathogenesis, with improvement occurring with shifts away from $T_H1$ and toward $T_H2$. The timing and anatomic location of this shift, however, appear to be important. Although $T_H1$ cells clearly cause EAE and $T_H2$ cells clearly do not, highly polarized $T_H2$ cells have been shown to be unable to suppress EAE caused by $T_H1$ cells (50). It was hypothesized that highly polarized $T_H2$ cells may be inefficient at crossing the blood-brain barrier, thereby limiting their suppressive potential. In contrast, incompletely skewed T-cell populations that produce both $T_H1$ and $T_H2$ cytokines have been weakly encephalitogenic, thereby suggesting that disease inhibition with $T_H2$ cytokines may occur at early time points during disease development, at times preceding the development of polarized $T_H1$ cells (50).

Coadministration of myelin protein–specific $T_H1$ and $T_H2$ cells to immunodeficient mice has confirmed the observation that $T_H2$ cells cannot alter disease induction by $T_H1$ cells after transfer (44). It has been shown, however, that $T_H2$ cells specific for an exogenous, nonself antigen, keyhole limpet hemocyanin (KLH), could shift the cytokine profile of encephalitogenic T cells from an inflammatory $T_H1$ toward a protective $T_H2$ type by releasing IL-4 in the lymphoid microenvironment. Mice were preimmunized with KLH and incomplete Freund's adjuvant to generate KLH-specific $T_H2$ cells. Later, when mice were immunized with MBP and complete Freund's adjuvant, EAE occurred in mice that were not rechallenged with KLH, whereas it did not occur in mice that were rechallenged with KLH. It was shown that KLH-specific memory T cells secreted IL-4 upon KLH rechallenge, resulting in a shift in cytokine profile of MBP-specific T cells away from $T_H1$ and toward $T_H2$. These data demonstrate that $T_H2$ cytokines in the lymphoid microenvironment early during the time when autoreactive T lymphocytes are being generated can result in protection from the development of $T_H1$-mediated disease (51).

## COSTIMULATORY MOLECULES

T lymphocytes require two signals for full activation. The first signal is provided by TCR recognition of antigenic peptides within MHC complexes on APCs. The second signal is provided by other receptors on T cells that bind to their respective ligands on APCs. Interactions that produce this second signal are known as *costimulatory*. B7-2 is constitutively expressed on APCs, whereas both B7-2 and B7-1 are upregulated after activation. CD28 is constitutively expressed on T lymphocytes, whereas CTLA-4 is expressed only during T-cell activation (52). Interactions of B7-1 and B7-2 ligands on APCs with CD28 and CTLA-4 receptors on T lymphocytes have been shown to play a role in the pathogenesis of EAE. Initial studies used CTLA-4Ig, a fusion protein ligand capable of blocking both B7-1 and B7-2, to address the role of costimulation in EAE. CTLA-4Ig administered *in vivo* during active EAE ameliorated disease (53). In the passive EAE model, in which the induction of the encephalitogenic response and the effector phase of disease are separate, it was shown that *in vivo* treatment of donor mice during immunization reduced the encephalitogenicity of the T cells generated, whereas treatment of recipients had no effect (54). In addition, if myelin protein–specific T cells were treated *in vitro* with CTLA-4Ig before adoptive transfer, it reduced their encephalitogenicity. Further, if APCs were treated *in vitro* with CTLA-4Ig during stimulation with peptide, injection of these APCs could protect against active EAE induction (55). Together, these data suggest that costimulation by B7-1 or B7-2 on APCs is important in the generation of encephalitogenic T cells.

B7-1 and B7-2 costimulation was then addressed more extensively during in the effector phase of disease. B7-1 expression was shown to be increased on immune cells in spleen during the effector phase of EAE. Therefore, antibodies specific for B7-1 (Fab fragments) were administered *in vivo* during the effector phase. Disease was ameliorated, and myelin protein–specific responses were decreased (56). In another study, antibodies to B7-1 again ameliorated disease, but in this case, amelioration was associated with a shift in the myelin protein–specific response toward the $T_H2$ type (57). Experiments addressing the role of B7-2 during the effector phase of disease have yielded conflicting results. Antibodies to B7-2 had no effect on EAE in one study (56), whereas disease was of increased severity in another (57). Thus, although these results have demonstrated that B7-1 is an important costimulatory molecule in the perpetuation of

the effector phase of EAE, the role of B7-2 during the effector phase of disease has remained unclear.

Because B7-1 and B7-2 could theoretically interact with either CD28 or CTLA-4 on T lymphocytes, mice with EAE were treated *in vivo* with an anti–CTLA-4 antibody (or their Fab fragment) to observe effects when only the CTLA-4 receptor on T lymphocytes was blocked. Surprisingly, this treatment resulted in an exacerbation of EAE with an increase in TNF-$\alpha$, IFN-$\gamma$ and IL-2 production (58,59). Thus, CTLA-4–receptor ligation clearly delivers a negative signal with regard to the production of proinflammatory cytokines and encephalitogenicity.

To address whether B7-1 or B7-2 might be binding to the CTLA-4 receptor to deliver the downregulatory signal, experiments were designed using a mutant form of CTLA-4Ig, CTLA-4IGY100F, which would bind only to B7-1. Effects on EAE were compared using CTLA-4Ig, which binds to both B7-1 and B7-2, or the mutant form of CTLA-4Ig, CTLA-4IGY100F, which binds only to B7-1. In contrast to the disease protection observed when CTLA-4Ig was given *in vivo*, there was no protection or disease worsening when CTLA-4IGY100F was given. These data indicate that either B7-2 plays a role in the generation of myelin protein–specific T lymphocyte responses or that interactions of B7-1 with CTLA-4 are important in downregulating EAE (60).

These data concerning disease worsening using CTLA-4IGY100F to block B7-1 are in contrast to previous data of disease amelioration when B7-1 was blocked with antibodies (Fab fragments) specific for B7-1 (56,57). Differences between results may be related to partial agonistic effects of CTLA-4IGY100F or B7-1 antibodies. Alternatively, differences in results may suggest immunopathogenic differences between EAE in Lewis rats, as compared with EAE in SJL mice, because Lewis rats were used when B7-1 was blocked with with CTLA-4IGY100F, whereas SJL mice were used when B7-1 was blocked with anti B7-1 antibodies. Thus, although there is clear evidence that B7-1 and B7-2 costimulation plays a major role in EAE, the details of this role appear to be complex and need further study. It can be said, however, that the combined reports demonstrate that stimulation of CD28 on T lymphocytes is important in the generation of myelin protein–specific T lymphocyte responses, whereas stimulation of CTLA-4 on T lymphocytes is important in downregulating myelin protein–specific T-lymphocyte responses (61).

## T-CELL RECEPTOR USE

T lymphocytes specific for MBP Ac1–9, which are responsible for EAE in B10.PL and (SJL $\times$ B10.PL)F1 mice, as well as T lymphocytes specific for MBP 72–89, which induce EAE in Lewis rats, have restricted TCR use, predominantly using the TCR V$\beta$8.2 gene segment. The disease course in each is monophasic, and most animals recover permanently from the disease. Remission of the disease has been attributed to a regulatory circuitry of T lymphocytes that is expanded spontaneously during disease, which recognizes a determinant within framework region 3 of the Vβ8.2 chain (62). The importance of this regulatory circuitry has been demonstrated by protection from disease when regulatory T cells were primed *in vivo* through three vaccination approaches: with a peptide containing the Vβ8.2 TCR determinant, with recombinant single-chain TCRs containing appropriate Vβ domains, or with naked DNA encoding the Vβ8.2 TCR (63–65). Conversely, an increase in disease severity and duration with the appearance of relapses occurred when this regulatory circuitry was blocked (66,67). These observations indicate an important role for a regulatory TCR-specific network in strains of mice and rats that demonstrate restricted TCR use by encephalitogenic T cells and a monophasic disease course.

In contrast to the above models of EAE, the disease in SJL mice is not monophasic. The disease course is characterized by spontaneous remissions and relapses, with myelin protein–specific TCR use that is less restricted (68). Further, strains of mice and rats with a monophasic disease course have been shown to be resistant to reinduction of disease, whereas SJL mice remain susceptible after recovery (69). These observations demonstrate that SJL mice have a defect in immunoregulation, which may be due at least in part to their lack of restricted TCR use during initial disease induction and subsequent inadequate priming of regulatory TCR-specific circuitry.

## AUTOREACTIVE T LYMPHOCYTES

The observation that SJL mice remain susceptible to reinduction of disease after recovery, with reinduced disease occurring earlier than initial disease, indicates not only the absence of regulatory mechanisms but also the persistence of autoreactive T lymphocytes that can subsequently be reactivated outside the CNS by stimulation with the appropriate antigen and adjuvant. If the initial episode of EAE is elicited using a synthetic peptide of PLP, for example, reinjection of the same PLP peptide can reinduce disease. These data have indicated that T cells specific for the disease inciting autoantigen persist after the initial episode of disease for at least 20 weeks after initial disease induction. Such autoantigen-specific T lymphocytes can also be reactivated by other means because mice in conventional housing facilities relapsed spontaneously, whereas mice in specific pathogen-free facilities did not (69). These data regarding the persistence of T lymphocytes specific for the disease inciting autoantigen in mice with relapsing EAE are consistent with data from other reports, which have demonstrated either a persistence or an increase in the frequency of T cells specific for the disease inciting autoantigen in lymph node, spleen, and thymus for up to 18 weeks after disease induction (70–74).

In addition to an increase in T lymphocytes specific for an epitope within the disease inciting autoantigen, there is an increase in T lymphocytes specific for other epitopes within the same or different autoantigens during relapsing EAE (75–78). These events have been termed *intramolecular epitope spreading* when the new reactivity is directed toward an epitope within the same autoantigen and as *intermolecular epitope spreading* when the new reactivity is directed toward an epitope within a different autoantigen. These "spreading" responses have been detected in lymph node and spleen during the relapsing phase of disease. The importance of each of these T lymphocyte responses has been demonstrated by observations that treatments that downregulate or eliminate either T lymphocytes specific for spreading epitopes or T lymphocytes specific for epitopes within the disease inciting autoantigen each ameliorate disease.

A central question in the immunopathogenesis of relapsing EAE concerns the mechanisms that underlie the perpetuation and generation of myelin protein–specific T-lymphocyte responses *in vivo* during disease. One hypothesis is that myelin protein breakdown within EAE lesions in the CNS leads to the presentation of epitopes therein, thereby resulting in the chronic *in vivo* stimulation of T lymphocytes specific for myelin proteins. Chemokines, such as macrophage inflammatory protein-1, monocyte chemotactic protein-1, and neurotactin, have each been shown to be expressed in an upregulated fashion in EAE lesions (79–82). They are thought to play a role in the chemotaxis of T lymphocytes, macrophages, and other immune cells to the lesion. Myelin proteins within lesions may be presented to T lymphocytes by infiltrating macrophages, resident microglia, or astrocytes (83,84). The detection of spreading T-lymphocyte responses in lymph node and spleen would imply that T lymphocytes stimulated within the CNS exit and recirculate in the periphery.

The discovery that MBP and PLP are not sequestered behind the blood-brain barrier but are expressed at the mRNA and protein levels within lymph node, thymus, and spleen (85–89) has led to an alternative hypothesis regarding the mechanisms through which T lymphocytes are chronically stimulated *in vivo* during relapsing EAE. The site of T-lymphocyte stimulation *in vivo* may be within lymphoid tissues. Not only has myelin protein expression been demonstrated in lymphoid tissues, the expression of myelin proteins has also been shown to be upregulated during the relapsing phase of EAE (89). Lymph node cells, thymocytes, and splenocytes have been shown to present endogenous myelin proteins in a manner that is stimulatory to T lymphocytes specific for immunodominant and subdominant MBP and PLP epitopes (88–90).

These observations, combined with the observation that costimulatory molecule expression is upregulated within immune tissues during EAE (56), suggest a mechanism for the break in the peripheral tolerance of myelin protein–specific T lymphocytes during relapsing EAE. This activation of myelin protein–specific T lymphocytes in the peripheral immune compartment would allow their entry into the CNS for relapses. The hypothesis that myelin protein–specific T lymphocytes are activated *in vivo* within lymphoid tissues is consistent with numerous reports in which antibodies that target either the trimolecular complex or costimulatory interactions result in amelioration of relapsing EAE when administered systemically. It is also consistent with the observation that KLH-specific memory T lymphocytes that secrete IL-4 in the lymphoid microenvironment can induce a shift in the cytokine profile of MBP-specific T cells from $T_H1$ toward $T_H2$ and result in disease protection (51).

## GENDER-RELATED DIFFERENCES IN EXPERIMENTAL AUTOIMMUNE ENCEPHALITIS

An enhanced female susceptibility, as compared with male susceptibility, has characterized a variety of autoimmune diseases, including spontaneous diabetes in nonobese diabetic (NOD) mice, lupus in New Zealand black (NZB) and New Zealand white (NZW) mice, and most recently, EAE in SJL mice (91,92). Using the adoptive EAE model, it has been shown that there is a gender difference in both the ability to generate encephalitogenic T-lymphocyte responses (induction phase) and the ability of encephalitogenic T lymphocytes to cause disease (effector phase). Mechanisms underlying decreased disease expression in male subjects appear to involve a protective effect of testosterone because castration of male subjects increases disease severity and testosterone treatment of female subjects reduces severity (93,94). Further, it has been shown that male subjects and testosterone-treated females subjects have a relatively higher level of $T_H2$ cytokine production when lymph node cells or splenocytes are stimulated with myelin proteins (92,93,95).

It is not yet known whether sex hormones interact directly with receptors on myelin protein–specific T lymphocytes to affect cytokine gene expression or whether sex hormones act more indirectly by interacting with receptors on APCs. Previous studies have demonstrated an effect of sex hormones on T lymphocytes, B lymphocytes, and macrophages (96–99). A defect in the ability of male subjects to generate $CD4^+$ $T_H1$ delayed-type hypersensitivity responses and EAE effector T cells after immunization has been attributed to a defect in macrophage function in male SJL mice (100). Further characterization of the expression of androgen receptors and estrogen receptors $\alpha$ and $\beta$ on immune cells and the functional consequences of ligand binding *in vivo* are needed.

Gender-related differences in EAE susceptibility may also be related to gender differences in stimulation of the hypothalamic pituitary axis during stress (101,102). The ramifications of gender-related differences in stimulation of this axis may be complex because releasing factors and pituitary hormones can directly affect immune responses (103–106). For example, corticotropin-releasing factor not only may increase cortisol production to ameliorate EAE but also may act more directly because it has been shown to suppress EAE in adrenalectomized rats (107).

In summary, the effects of sex hormones on EAE may influence myelin protein–specific T lymphocytes or APCs. Additional effects may be mediated through the hypothalamic-pituitary axis. Finally, the effects of sex hormones on sus-

ceptibility of the target organ, the CNS, to autoimmune attack remain to be determined.

## CONCLUSIONS

The EAE model has yielded insight into several cell-mediated autoimmune disease processes. Adhesion molecule interactions have been identified that are crucial for homing of T lymphocytes to the target organ, and treatment strategies to block these interactions have been successful in amelioration of disease. In addition, the importance of specific cytokines in immunopathogenesis has been appreciated, and multiple therapeutic approaches have been designed that have successfully shifted the autoantigen-specific immune response away from the production of proinflammatory cytokines and toward the production antiinflammatory cytokines. Costimulatory molecule expression on APCs *in vivo* during the disease is being investigated, and the binding of these molecules to receptors on autoantigen-specific T lymphocytes during EAE have generated important but complex results with positive and negative effects. Further, it has been established that myelin protein–specific T lymphocytes specific for the disease inciting autoantigen, as well as T lymphocytes specific for other autoantigens through spreading, are stimulated *in vivo* in chronic relapsing EAE. Whether the site of this T-lymphocyte stimulation *in vivo* is within the CNS or within lymphoid tissues remains to be determined. Finally, gender differences in susceptibility to EAE have been demonstrated that result at least in part from a protective effect of testosterone. This protective effect on disease appears to involve a favorable shift in cytokine production. How sex hormones bias cytokine production mechanistically remains to be determined. Thus, although major strides have been made in understanding the immunopathogenesis of EAE and other cell-mediated autoimmune diseases, these answers have led to yet more questions in the path ahead.

## REFERENCES

1. Martin R, McFarland HF, McFarlin DE. Immunological aspects of demyelinating diseases. *Ann Rev Immunol* 1992;10:153–187.
2. Pettinelli CB, McFarlin DE. Adoptive transfer of experimental allergic encephalomyelitis in SJL/J mice after in vitro activation of lymph node cells by myelin basic protein: requirement for Lyt 1+2− T lymphocytes. *J Immunol* 1981;127:1420–1423.
3. Fritz RB, McFarlin DE. Encephalitogenic epitopes of myelin basic protein. *Chem Immunol* 1989;46:101–125.
4. Tuohy VK, Lu Z, Sobel RA, et al. Identification of an encephalitogenic determinant of myelin proteolipid protein for SJL mice. *J Immunol* 1989;142:1523–1527.
5. Johns TG, Kerlero de Rosbo N, Menon KK, et al. Myelin oligodendrocyte glycoprotein induces a demyelinating encephalomyelitis resembling multiple sclerosis. *J Immunol* 1995;154:5536–5541.
6. Segal BM, Raine CS, McFarlin DE, et al. Experimental allergic encephalomyelitis induced by the peptide encoded by exon 2 of the MBP gene, a peptide implicated in remyelination. *J Neuroimmunol* 1994;51:7–19.
7. Kojima K, Berger T, Lassmann H, et al. Experimental autoimmune panencephalitis and uveoretinitis transferred to the Lewis rat by T lymphocytes specific for the S100 beta molecule, a calcium binding protein of astroglia. *J Exp Med* 1994;180:817–829.

8. Raine CS, Barnett LB, Brown A, et al. Neuropathology of experimental allergic encephalomyelitis in inbred strains of mice. *Lab Invest* 1980;43:150–157.

9. Fritz RB, Skeen MJ, Chou CH, et al. Major histocompatibility complex-linked control of the murine immune response to myelin basic protein. *J Immunol* 1985;134:2328–2332.

10. Baker D, Rosenwasser OA, O'Neill JK, et al. Genetic analysis of experimental allergic encephalomyelitis in mice. *J Immunol* 1995;155:4046–4051.

11. Sundvall M, Jirholt J, Yang HT, et al. Identification of murine loci associated with susceptibility to chronic experimental autoimmune encephalomyelitis. *Nat Genet* 1995;10:313–317.

12. Encinas JA, Lees MB, Sobel RA. Genetic analysis of susceptibility to experimental autoimmune encephalomyelitis in a cross between SJL/J and B10.S mice. *J Immunol* 1996;157:2186–2192.

13. Kono DH, Urban JL, Horvath SJ, et al. Two minor determinants of myelin basic protein induce experimental allergic encephalomyelitis in SJL/J mice. *J Exp Med* 1988;168:213–227.

14. Zamvil SS, Mitchell DJ, Moore AC, et al. T-cell epitope of the autoantigen myelin basic protein that induces encephalomyelitis. *Nature* 1986;324:258–260.

15. Whitham RH, Jones RE, Hashim GA, et al. Location of a new encephalitogenic epitope (residues 43 to 64) in proteolipid protein that induces relapsing experimental autoimmune encephalomyelitis in PL/J and (SJL × PL)F1 mice. *J Immunol* 1991;147:3803–3808.

16. Baron JL, Madri JA, Ruddle NH, et al. Surface expression of alpha 4 integrin by CD4 T cells is required for their entry into brain parenchyma. *J Exp Med* 1993;177:57–68.

17. Kuchroo VK, Martin CA, Greer JM, et al. Cytokines and adhesion molecules contribute to the ability of myelin proteolipid protein-specific T cell clones to mediate experimental allergic encephalomyelitis. *J Immunol* 1993;151:4371–4382.

18. Yednock TA, Cannon C, Fritz LC, et al. Prevention of experimental autoimmune encephalomyelitis by antibodies against alpha 4 beta 1 integrin. *Nature* 1992;356:63–66.

19. Hickey WF, Hsu BL, Kimura H. T-lymphocyte entry into the central nervous system. *J Neurosci Res* 1991;28:254–260.

20. Ando DG, Clayton J, Kono D, et al. Encephalitogenic T cells in the B10.PL model of experimental allergic encephalomyelitis (EAE) are of the Th-1 lymphokine subtype. *Cell Immunol* 1989;124:132–143.

21. Powell MB, Mitchell D, Lederman J, et al. Lymphotoxin and tumor necrosis factor-alpha production by myelin basic protein-specific T cell clones correlates with encephalitogenicity. *Int Immunol* 1990;2:539–544.

22. Renno T, Krakowski M, Piccirillo C, et al. TNF-alpha expression by resident microglia and infiltrating leukocytes in the central nervous system of mice with experimental allergic encephalomyelitis: regulation by Th1 cytokines. *J Immunol* 1995;154:944–953.

23. Conboy IM, DeKruyff RH, Tate KM, et al. Novel genetic regulation of T helper 1 (Th1)/Th2 cytokine production and encephalitogenicity in inbred mouse strains. *J Exp Med* 1997;185:439–451.

24. Frei K, Eugster HP, Bopst M, et al. Tumor necrosis factor alpha and lymphotoxin alpha are not required for induction of acute experimental autoimmune encephalomyelitis. *J Exp Med* 1997;185:2177–2182.

25. Liu J, Marino MW, Wong G, et al. TNF is a potent anti-inflammatory cytokine in autoimmune-mediated demyelination. *Nat Med* 1998;4:78–83.

26. Suen WE, Bergman CM, Hjelmstrom P, et al. A critical role for lymphotoxin in experimental allergic encephalomyelitis. *J Exp Med* 1997;186:1233–1240.

27. Korner H, Riminton DS, Strickland DH, et al. Critical points of tumor necrosis factor action in central nervous system autoimmune inflammation defined by gene targeting. *J Exp Med* 1997;186:1585–1590.

28. Ferber IA, Brocke S, Taylor-Edwards C, et al. Mice with a disrupted IFN-gamma gene are susceptible to the induction of experimental autoimmune encephalomyelitis (EAE). *J Immunol* 1996;156:5–7.

29. Krakowski M, Owens T. Interferon-gamma confers resistance to experimental allergic encephalomyelitis. *Eur J Immunol* 1996;26:1641–1646.

30. Probert L, Akassoglou K, Pasparakis M, et al. Spontaneous inflammatory demyelinating disease in transgenic mice showing central nervous system-specific expression of tumor necrosis factor alpha. *Proc Natl Acad Sci U S A* 1995;92:11294–11298.

31. Horwitz MS, Evans CF, McGavern DB, et al. Primary demyelination in transgenic mice expressing interferon-gamma. *Nat Med* 1997;3:1037–1041.

32. Sommer N, Loschmann PA, Northoff GH, et al. The antidepressant rolipram suppresses cytokine production and prevents autoimmune encephalomyelitis. *Nat Med* 1995;1:244–248.

33. Ruddle NH, Bergman CM, McGrath KM, et al. An antibody to lymphotoxin and tumor necrosis factor prevents transfer of experimental allergic encephalomyelitis. *J Exp Med* 1990;172:1193–200.

34. Selmaj K, Raine CS, Cross AH. Anti-tumor necrosis factor therapy abrogates autoimmune demyelination. *Ann Neurol* 1991;30:694–700.

35. Selmaj K, Papierz W, Glabinski A, et al. Prevention of chronic relapsing experimental autoimmune encephalomyelitis by soluble tumor necrosis factor receptor I. *J Neuroimmunol* 1995;56:135–141.

36. Duong TT, St. Louis J, Gilbert JJ, et al. Effect of anti-interferon-gamma and anti-interleukin-2 monoclonal antibody treatment on the development of actively and passively induced experimental allergic encephalomyelitis in the SJL/J mouse. *J Neuroimmunol* 1992;36:105–115.

37. Leonard JP, Waldburger KE, Goldman SJ. Prevention of experimental autoimmune encephalomyelitis by antibodies against interleukin 12. *J Exp Med* 1995;181:381–386.

38. Segal BM, Shevach EM. IL-12 unmasks latent autoimmune disease in resistant mice. *J Exp Med* 1996;184:771–775.

39. Racke MK, Bonomo A, Scott DE, et al. Cytokine-induced immune deviation as a therapy for inflammatory autoimmune disease. *J Exp Med* 1994;180:1961–1966.

40. Rott O, Fleischer B, Cash E. Interleukin-10 prevents experimental allergic encephalomyelitis in rats. *Eur J Immunol* 1994;24:1434–1440.

41. Crisi GM, Santambrogio L, Hochwald GM, et al. Staphylococcal enterotoxin B and tumor-necrosis factor-alpha-induced relapses of experimental allergic encephalomyelitis: protection by transforming growth factor-beta and interleukin-10. *Eur J Immunol* 1995;25:3035–3040.

42. Shaw MK, Lorens JB, Dhawan A, et al. Local delivery of interleukin 4 by retrovirus-transduced T lymphocytes ameliorates experimental autoimmune encephalomyelitis. *J Exp Med* 1997;185:1711–1714.

43. Mathisen PM, Yu M, Johnson JM, et al. Treatment of experimental autoimmune encephalomyelitis with genetically modified memory T cells. *J Exp Med* 1997;186:159–164.

44. Lafaille JJ, Keere FV, Hsu AL, et al. Myelin basic protein-specific T helper 2 (Th2) cells cause experimental autoimmune encephalomyelitis in immunodeficient hosts rather than protect them from the disease. *J Exp Med* 1997;186:307–3112.

45. Chen Y, Inobe J, Weiner HL. Induction of oral tolerance to myelin basic protein in CD8-depleted mice: both CD4+ and CD8+ cells mediate active suppression. *J Immunol* 1995;155:910–916.

46. Meyer AL, Benson JM, Gienapp IE, et al. Suppression of murine chronic relapsing experimental autoimmune encephalomyelitis by the oral administration of myelin basic protein. *J Immunol* 1996;157:4230–4238.

47. Kennedy KJ, Smith WS, Miller SD, et al. Induction of antigen-specific tolerance for the treatment of ongoing, relapsing autoimmune encephalomyelitis: a comparison between oral and peripheral tolerance. *J Immunol* 1997;159:1036–1044.

48. Karin N, Mitchell DJ, Brocke S, et al. Reversal of experimental autoimmune encephalomyelitis by a soluble peptide variant of a myelin basic protein epitope: T cell receptor antagonism and reduction of interferon gamma and tumor necrosis factor alpha production. *J Exp Med* 1994;180:2227–2237.

49. Nicholson LB, Greer JM, Sobel RA, et al. An altered peptide ligand mediates immune deviation and prevents autoimmune encephalomyelitis. *Immunity* 1995;3:397–405.

50. Khoruts A, Miller SD, Jenkins MK. Neuroantigen-specific Th2 cells are inefficient suppressors of experimental autoimmune encephalomyelitis induced by effector Th1 cells. *J Immunol* 1995;155:5011–5017.

51. Falcone M, Bloom BR. A T helper cell 2 (Th2) immune response against non-self antigens modifies the cytokine profile of autoimmune T cells and protects against experimental allergic encephalomyelitis. *J Exp Med* 1997;185:901–907.

52. Bluestone JA. New perspectives of CD28-B7-mediated T cell cost imulation. *Immunity* 1995;2:555–559.

53. Khoury SJ, Akalin E, Chandraker A, et al. CD28-B7 costimulatory blockade by CTLA4Ig prevents actively induced experimental autoimmune encephalomyelitis and inhibits Th1 but spares Th2 cytokines in the central nervous system. *J Immunol* 1995;155:4521–4524.

54. Perrin PJ, Scott D, Quigley L, et al. Role of B7:CD28/CTLA-4 in the induction of chronic relapsing experimental allergic encephalomyelitis. *J Immunol* 1995;154:1481–1490.

55. Khoury SJ, Gallon L, Verburg RR, et al. Ex vivo treatment of antigen-presenting cells with CTLA4Ig and encephalitogenic peptide prevents experimental autoimmune encephalomyelitis in the Lewis rat. *J Immunol* 1996;157:3700–3705.

56. Miller SD, Vanderlugt CL, Lenschow DJ, et al. Blockade of CD28/B7-1 interaction prevents epitope spreading and clinical relapses of murine EAE. *Immunity* 1995;3:739–745.

57. Kuchroo VK, Das MP, Brown JA, et al. B7-1 and B7-2 costimulatory molecules activate differentially the Th1/Th2 developmental pathways: application to autoimmune disease therapy. *Cell* 1995;80:707–718.

58. Karandikar NJ, Vanderlugt CL, Walunas TL, et al. CTLA-4: a negative regulator of autoimmune disease. *J Exp Med* 1996;184:783–788.

59. Perrin PJ, Maldonado JH, Davis TA, et al. CTLA-4 blockade enhances clinical disease and cytokine production during experimental allergic encephalomyelitis. *J Immunol* 1996;157:1333–1336.

60. Gallon L, Chandraker A, Issazadeh S, et al. Differential effects of B7-1 blockade in the rat experimental autoimmune encephalomyelitis model. *J Immunol* 1997;159:4212–4216.

61. Bluestone JA. Is CTLA-4 a master switch for peripheral T cell tolerance? *J Immunol* 1997;158:1989–1993.

62. Kumar V, Tabibiazar R, Geysen HM, et al. Immunodominant framework region 3 peptide from TCR V beta 8.2 chain controls murine experimental autoimmune encephalomyelitis. *J Immunol* 1995;154:1941–1950.

63. Kumar V, Coulsell E, Ober B, et al. Recombinant T cell receptor molecules can prevent and reverse experimental autoimmune encephalomyelitis: dose effects and involvement of both CD4 and CD8 T cells. *J Immunol* 1997;159:5150–5156.

64. Waisman A, Ruiz PJ, Hirschberg DL, et al. Suppressive vaccination with DNA encoding a variable region gene of the T-cell receptor prevents autoimmune encephalomyelitis and activates Th2 immunity. *Nat Med* 1996;2:899–905.

65. Offner H, Hashim GA, Vandenbark AA. T cell receptor peptide therapy triggers autoregulation of experimental encephalomyelitis. *Science* 1991;251:430–432.

66. Kumar V, Stellrecht K, Sercarz E. Inactivation of T cell receptor peptide-specific CD4 regulatory T cells induces chronic experimental autoimmune encephalomyelitis (EAE). *J Exp Med* 1996;184:1609–1617.

67. Offner H, Malotky MK, Pope L, et al. Increased severity of experimental autoimmune encephalomyelitis in rats tolerized as adults but not neonatally to a protective TCR V beta 8 CDR2 idiotope. *J Immunol* 1995;154:928–935.

68. Su XM, Sriram S. Analysis of TCR V beta gene usage and encephalitogenicity of myelin basic protein peptide p91-103 reactive T cell clones in SJL mice: lack of evidence for V gene hypothesis. *Cell Immunol* 1992;141:485–495.

69. Lindsey JW, Pappolla M, Steinman L. Reinduction of experimental autoimmune encephalomyelitis in mice. *Cell Immunol* 1995;162:235–240.

70. Fallis RJ, Powers ML, Sy M, et al. Adoptive transfer of murine chronic-relapsing autoimmune encephalomyelitis: analysis of basic protein-reactive cells in lymphoid organs and the nervous system of donor and recipient animals. *J Neuroimmunol* 1987;14:205.

71. Sakai K, Tabira T, Endoh M, et al. Ia expression in chronic relapsing experimental allergic encephalomyelitis induced by long-term cultured T cell lines in mice. *Lab Invest* 1986;54:345.

72. Voskuhl, RR, Farris RW, Nagasato K, et al. Epitope spreading occurs in active but not passive EAE induced by myelin basic protein. *J Neuroimmunol* 1996;70:103.

73. Naparstek Y, Holoshitz J, Eisenstein S, et al. Effector T lymphocyte line cells migrate to the thymus and persist there. *Nature* 1982;300:262.

74. Naparstek Y, Ben-Nun A, Holoshitz J, et al. T lymphocyte lines producing or vaccinating against autoimmune encephalomyelitis (EAE): functional activation induces peanut agglutinin receptors and accumulation in the brain and thymus of cell lines. *Eur J Immunol* 1983;13:418.

75. Lehmann PV, Forsthuber T, Miller A, et al. Spreading of T-cell autoimmunity to cryptic determinants of an autoantigen. *Nature* 1992;358:155.

76. Cross AH, Tuohy VK, Raine CS. Development of reactivity to new myelin antigens during chronic relapsing autoimmune demyelination. *Cell Immunol* 1993;146:261.

77. Yu M, Johnson JM, Tuohy VK. A predictable sequential determinant spreading cascade invariably accompanies progression of experimental autoimmune encephalomyelitis: a basis for peptide-specific therapy after onset of clinical disease. *J Exp Med* 1996;183:1777.

78. McRae BL, Vanderlugt CL, Del Canto MC, et al. Functional evidence for epitope spreading in the relapsing pathology of experimental autoimmune encephalomyelitis. *J Exp Med* 1995;182:75.

79. Karpus WJ, Lukacs NW, McRae BL, et al. An important role for the chemokine macrophage inflammatory protein-1 alpha in the pathogenesis of the T cell-mediated autoimmune disease, experimental autoimmune encephalomyelitis. *J Immunol* 1995;155:5003–5010.

80. Glabinski AR, Balasingam V, Tani M, et al. Chemokine monocyte chemoattractant protein-1 is expressed by astrocytes after mechanical injury to the brain. *J Immunol* 1996;156:4363–4368.

81. Berman JW, Guida MP, Warren J, et al. Localization of monocyte chemoattractant peptide-1 expression in the central nervous system in experimental autoimmune encephalomyelitis and trauma in the rat. *J Immunol* 1996;156:3017–3023.

82. Pan Y, Lloyd C, Zhou H, et al. Neurotactin, a membrane-anchored chemokine upregulated in brain inflammation. *Nature* 1997;387:611–617.

83. Ford AL, Goodsall AL, Hickey WF, et al. Normal adult ramified microglia separated from other central nervous system macrophages by flow cytometric sorting: phenotypic differences defined and direct ex vivo antigen presentation to myelin basic protein-reactive CD4+ T cells compared. *J Immunol* 1995;154:4309–4321.

84. Nikcevich KM, Gordon KB, Tan L, et al. IFN-gamma-activated primary murine astrocytes express B7 costimulatory molecules and prime naive antigen-specific T cells. *J Immunol* 1997;158:614–621.

85. Pribyl TM, Campagnoni CW, Kampf K, et al. The human myelin basic protein gene is included within a 179-kilobase transcription unit: Expression in immune and central nervous systems. *Proc Natl Acad Sci U S A* 1993;90:10695.

86. Zelenika D, Grima B, Pessac B. A new family of transcripts of the myelin basic protein gene: expression in the brain and immune system. *J Neurochem* 1993;60:1574.

87. Pribyl TM, Campagnoni CW, Kampf K, et al. Expression of myelin proteolipid protein gene in the human fetal thymus. *J Neuroimmunol* 1996;67:125.

88. Fritz RB, Zhao ML. Thymic expression of myelin basic protein (MBP). Activation of MBP-specific T cells by thymic cells in the absence of exogenous MBP. *J Immunol* 1996;157:5249–5253.

89. MacKenzie-Graham A, Pribyl TM, Kim S, et al. Myelin protein expression is increased in lymph nodes of mice with relapsing experimental autoimmune encephalomyelitis. *J Immunol* 1997;159:4602.

90. Voskuhl RR. Myelin protein expression in lymphoid tissues: implications for peripheral tolerance. *Immunol Rev* 1998;164:81–92.

91. Voskuhl RR, Pitchekian-Halabi H, MacKenzie-Graham A, et al. Gender differences in autoimmune demyelination in the mouse: implications for multiple sclerosis. *Ann Neurol* 1996;39:724–733.

92. Cua DJ, Hinton DR, Stohlman SA. Self-antigen-induced Th2 responses in experimental allergic encephalomyelitis (EAE)-resistant mice: Th2-mediated suppression of autoimmune disease. *J Immunol* 1995;155:4052–4059.

93. Dalal M, Kim S, Voskuhl RR. Testosterone therapy ameliorates experimental autoimmune encephalomyelitis and induces a T helper 2 bias in the autoantigen-specific T lymphocyte response. *J Immunol* 1997;159:3–6.

94. Bebo BF Jr, Zelinka-Vincent E, Adamus G, et al. Gonadal hormones influence the immune response to PLP 193-151 and the clinical course of relapsing experimental autoimmune encephalomyelitis. *J Neuroimmunol* 1998;84:122–130.

95. Bebo BF Jr, Vandenbark AA, Offner H. Male SJL mice do not relapse after induction of EAE with PLP 139-151. *J Neurosci Res* 1996;45:680–689.

96. Gilmore W, Weiner LP, Correale J. Effect of estradiol on cytokine secretion by proteolipid protein-specific T cell clones isolated from multiple sclerosis patients and normal control subjects. *J Immunol* 1997;158:446–451.

97. Piccinni MP, Giudizi MG, Biagiotti R, et al. Progesterone favors the development of human T helper cells producing Th2-type cytokines

and promotes both IL-4 production and membrane CD30 expression in established Th1 cell clones. *J Immunol* 1995;155:128–133.

98. Medina KL, Kincade PW. Pregnancy-related steroids are potential negative regulators of B lymphopoiesis. *Proc Natl Acad Sci U S A* 1994;91:5382–5386.

99. Chao TC, Van Alten PJ, Grager JA, et al. Steroid sex hormones regulate the release of tumor necrosis factor by macrophages. *Cell Immunol* 1995;160:43–49.

100. Cua DJ, Hinton DR, Kirkman L, et al. Macrophages regulate induction of delayed-type hypersensitivity and experimental allergic encephalomyelitis in SJL mice. *Eur J Immunol* 1995;25:2318–2324.

101. Griffin AC, Lo WD, Wolny AC, et al. Suppression of experimental autoimmune encephalomyelitis by restraint stress: sex differences. *J Neuroimmunol* 1993;44:103–116.

102. Grewal IS, Heilig M, Miller A, et al. Environmental regulation of T-cell function in mice: group housing of males affects accessory cell function. *Immunology* 1997;90:165–168.

103. Jacobson JD, Nisula BC, Steinberg AD. Modulation of the expression of murine lupus by gonadotropin-releasing hormone analogs. *Endocrinology* 1994;134:2516–2523.

104. Athreya BH, Pletcher J, Zulian F, et al. Subset-specific effects of sex hormones and pituitary gonadotropins on human lymphocyte proliferation in vitro. *Clin Immunol Immunopathol* 1993;66:201–211.

105. Batticane N, Morale MC, Gallo F, et al. Luteinizing hormone-releasing hormone signaling at the lymphocyte involves stimulation of interleukin-2 receptor expression. *Endocrinology* 1991;129:277–286.

106. Mann DR, Ansari AA, Akinbami MA, et al. Neonatal treatment with luteinizing hormone-releasing hormone analogs alters peripheral lymphocyte subsets and cellular and humorally mediated immune responses in juvenile and adult male monkeys. *J Clin Endocrinol Metab* 1994;78:292–298.

107. Poliak S, Mor F, Conlon P, et al. Stress and autoimmunity: the neuropeptides corticotropin-releasing factor and urocortin suppress encephalomyelitis via effects on both the hypothalamic-pituitary-adrenal axis and the immune system. *J Immunol* 1997;158:5751–5756.

*Textbook of the Autoimmune Diseases,*
Edited by R. G. Lahita, N. Chiorazzi, and W. H. Reeves,
Lippincott Williams & Wilkins, Philadelphia © 2000.

# CHAPTER 44

# Experimental Autoimmune Disease of the Testis and the Ovary

Kenneth S. K. Tung

## OVERVIEW

### The Clinical Diseases

Autoimmune diseases of the testis and its efferent ducts are responsible for spontaneous infertility in animals and may cause similar diseases in humans (Table 44.1). Immunologic infertility in male patients can occur as a result of sperm antibodies binding to the ejaculated sperm, and in these patients, there is no associated orchitis. Antibodies that develop after vasectomy may cause infertility in patients after vasovasostomy. A second form of male immunologic infertility is associated with testicular immunopathology that mirrors the two testicular changes in the spontaneously infertile dark mink: granulomatous orchitis and loss of germ cells with or without peritubular immune complexes. In addition, some patients with epididymal granulomas of noninfectious origin may have an autoimmune basis (1).

Autoimmune oophoritis is responsible for infertility in a subset of women with premature ovarian failure (see Chap. 23). Ovarian inflammation (oophoritis), dominated by lymphocytic or eosinophilic infiltrates early in disease, is reported in some patients (1,2). Of the autoantibodies detected, some react with antigens of steroid-producing cells common to ovaries, placenta, adrenal gland, and testis, including the P450 side-chain cleavage enzyme, the 17α-hydroxyl enzyme, and the zona pellucida (ZP). As additional evidence for an autoimmune basis, both human testicular and ovarian diseases can occur in patients with the autoimmune multiendocrinopathy syndromes.

### Experimental Testicular and Ovarian Autoimmune Diseases and the Nature of the Self Antigens

In contrast to clinical studies, extensive literature exists on the experimental models of autoimmune disease that affects

the gonads, and detailed protocols for their induction are available (3). These studies have contributed to the elucidation of the principles governing tolerance and autoimmunity (4), and in this chapter, I describe the models and emphasize their contributions to autoimmunity in general.

Experimental autoimmune orchitis (EAO) and autoimmune ovarian disease (AOD) can be elicited by two experimental approaches (Table 44.1). Immunization with testis or ovarian antigen or peptide in adjuvant is the classic approach. Severe diseases also occur after deliberate perturbation of T-cell compositions of the common laboratory mice and rats, such as thymectomy, at a narrow time window of days 1 to 4 but usually on day 3 (D3TX) after birth, or the transfer of defined T-cell populations from normal laboratory inbred mice to syngeneic athymic nu/nu mice recipients (5,6) (Table 44.1). Because these treatments also lead to autoimmune disease of the thyroid, prostate, salivary, and lachrymal glands and the eye and pancreatic islets, the research on this model will likely elucidate the fundamental mechanisms of self tolerance or unresponsiveness, relevant to the physiologic control against pathogenic autoimmune responses.

Pathogenic testicular autoimmune responses are directed to haploid germ cells, including spermatozoa. An EAO-inducing testis protein of known function has been identified as PH20, the testicular isoform of hyaluronidase (7). EAO and reversible male infertility are induced in guinea pigs with guinea pig PH20. PH20, expressed in male haploid germ cells of species including human and mouse, is located on both the plasma membrane of the intact spermatozoa and the inner acrosomal membrane of the acrosome-reacted spermatozoa. In addition to its potent hyaluronidase activity, PH20 is required for sperm penetration of the ZP in fertilization (8).

Experimental murine AOD is induced by immunization with a peptide from murine ZP3, in complete Freund's adjuvant or incomplete Freund's adjuvant (Fig. 44.1) (9). ZP3 is the sperm receptor and a component of the ZP. The ZP is the

K. S. K. Tung: Department of Pathology, University of Virginia, Charlottesville, Virginia 22908.

**TABLE 44.1.** *Experimental autoimmune diseases of testis and ovary*

---

*Experimental autoimmune (allergic) orchitis (EAO) and experimental autoimmune oophoritis that result from immunization with tissue antigen*

    Classic EAO induced by immunization with testis antigen with adjuvant

    EAO induced by immunization with testis antigen without adjuvant

    Autoimmune oophoritis induced by immunization with a peptide from murine ZP3 (Table 44.2)

*Autoimmune diseases of ovary, testis, or other organs that result from manipulations of the normal immune system*

    Thymectomize mice on days 1 to 4 (D3TX) after birth.

    Transfer adult murine CD5$^{low}$ or CD25-negative spleen T cells to athymic mice, to mice without T cells, or to SCID mice.

    Treat neonatal mice with cyclosporine.

    Engraft fetal rat thymus in athymic mice.

    Engraft neonatal mouse thymus in athymic mice.

    Inject normal murine T cells from adult or neonatal thymus, or neonatal spleen in athymic mice.

    Mice with a transgenic V protein of the T-cell receptor

    Inject RT6-depleted rat spleen T cells in athymic rats

    Inject OX22$^{high}$ (or CD45RC$^{high}$) rat spleen T cells in athymic rats.

*Other models of autoimmune orchitis*

    Spontaneous autoimmune orchitis in dog, mink, rat, and humans

    Postvasectomy autoimmune orchitis

    Orchitis in rats with the transgenic HLA-B27 molecule

---

acellular matrix that surrounds developing and ovulated oocytes and that exists as degraded proteins within the atretic follicles. The murine *zp3* gene encodes a polypeptide of 424 amino acids (10). Its peptide, pZP3 (amino acids 330–342; ZP3[330–342]), has well-defined native B-cell and T-cell epitopes that enable the independent analysis of T-cell and B-cell effector mechanisms (Table 44.2). The shortest oophoritogenic T-cell epitope is the 8-mer sequence, ZP3(330–337). These mice developed ZP3-specific T-cell responses and produced antibodies to ZP3 detectable in serum and bound to the ovarian ZP. The pZP3 peptide is unique in being both a tissue-specific and gender-specific antigen. The investigation of pZP3 permits the comparison of immune responses to self and foreign antigen in female and male animals with an ovarian graft. The versatility of this AOD model is illustrated by a study on neonatal tolerance to pZP3, wherein male mice were shown to be tolerant to the neonatal injection of the foreign pZP3 antigen, whereas female mice responded to neonatal injection of self pZP3 (11). The gender difference in the response was dependent on the presence of the ovaries in the neonatal female mice.

In this chapter, I review systemic and regional mechanisms that normally prevent the occurrence of gonadal autoimmune diseases, events that might overcome these control mechanisms, and pathogenetic pathways that amplify the disease processes. When appropriate, findings in the testes and the ovaries are compared. Finally, the location of some of

the genetic loci that regulate gonadal autoimmunity are reviewed.

## SYSTEMIC MECHANISMS THAT PREVENT GONADAL AUTOIMMUNE DISEASES

### Phenotype of T Cells in Normal Mice With Capacity to Induce and Prevent Autoimmune Ovarian and Testicular Diseases

The existence of pathogenic T cells in normal subjects and their regulation by other normal T cells are documented in the following series of experiments. When CD4$^+$, CD8$^-$ thymocyte from normal female adults or neonatal BALB/c mice are transferred to athymic BALB/c mice, about 75% of the recipients develop significant oophoritis or autoimmune gastritis within 2 months (12). This is associated with detectable serum autoantibody to the oocytes and the gastric autoantigen, H$^+$/K$^+$-ATPase, respectively. Because the CD4$^+$, CD8$^-$ subset represents mature thymocytes beyond deletion of self-reactive T cells, pathogenic self-reactive T cells for gonadal and other self antigens are not deleted in the normal thymus. This conclusion is supported by a study on mice with the transgenic expression of the gastric H$^+$/K$^+$-ATPase β chain in the thymus; their thymocytes no longer elicit gastritis but continue to transfer oophoritis in athymic recipients (13).

Oophoritis and gastritis develop in athymic syngeneic recipients that receive neonatal but not adult splenic T cells. Therefore, tolerance to self antigens, including those relevant to AOD, is ontogenetically regulated. The neonatal repertoire is enriched in self-reactive T cells, which do not require regulation. That thymectomy soon after birth limits the T-cell repertoire to that of the neonate, and skews it to one enriched in self-reactive T cells, could explain in part autoimmune diseases in the D3TX mice (14).

Although adult spleen T cells do not transfer oophoritis and gastritis to athymic recipients, a fraction of adult splenic CD4$^+$ T cells can do so (15–17). The phenotype of these pathogenic T cells has been defined to bear the following markers: CD5$^{low}$, CD45RB$^{high}$, CD25$^{low}$, and in rats, RT6$^-$. Studies have established the existence of potentially pathogenic T cells within the peripheral T cells of normal adult mice. In normal rats, these pathogenic CD4$^+$ T cells produced interleukin-2 (IL-2), but not IL-4, upon activation, consistent with the T$_H$1, CD4$^+$ inflammatory T-cell subset (18).

The existence of regulatory T cells with the capacity to suppress oophoritogenic T cells has also been demonstrated. When adult splenic T cells and neonatal T cells are co-injected into athymic recipients, oophoritis and gastritis do not develop. The nature of the regulatory T cells in these models have phenotypes that are reciprocal to those of the pathogenic T cells: CD5$^{high}$, CD45RB$^{low}$, CD25$^{high}$; and in rats, RT6$^+$ (16–19). These findings suggest that the regulatory T-cell population shares the phenotype of activated or memory T cells.

This series of experiments emphasizes the physiologic role of regulatory T cells in rendering oophoritogenic T cells non-

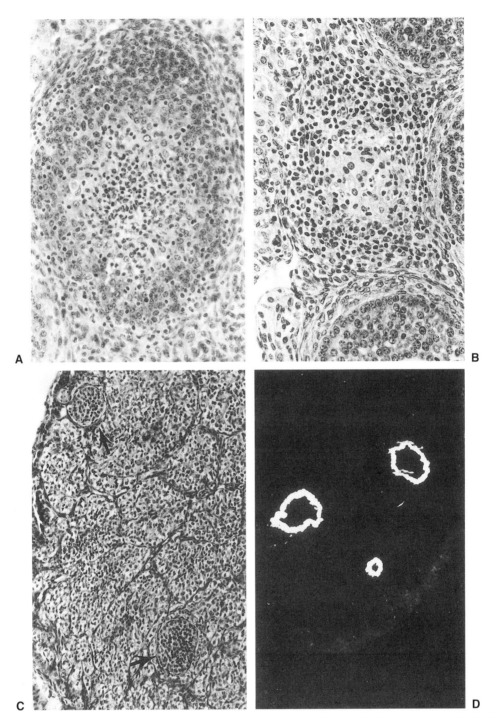

**FIG. 44.1.** Histopathology of experimental autoimmune oophoritis induced by immunization with the ZP3 (330–342) peptide in complete Freund's adjuvant **(A, B, C)**. **A:** Inflammatory cells have replaced the oocytes in the center of a graafian follicle; many lymphoid cells can be seen amid granulosa cells (original magnification, ×100). **B:** A granuloma is found in the interestitial region (original magnification, ×200). **C:** In severe oophoritis, all oocytes disappear; inflammation is not present, and the ovary is atrophic (original magnification, ×100). **D:** Ovaries with autoimmune oophoritis show *in vivo* binding of immunoglobulin G antibody to the zona pellucida, as demonstrated by direct immunofluorescence (original magnification, ×100). (From Rhim SH, Millar SE, Robey F, et al. Autoimmune diseases of the ovary induced by a ZP3 peptide from the mouse zona pellucida. *J Clin Invest* 1992;89:28–35, with permission.)

**TABLE 44.2.** *Functional domains of the murine ZP3 self peptide and their modified forms*

| Peptide | Amino acid sequence | Biologic function |
| --- | --- | --- |
| ZP3 (330–342) | NSSSSQFQIHGPR | Pathogenic T-cell epitopes and native B-cell epitope |
| ZP3 (330–340) | NSSSSQFQIHG | Pathogenic T-cell epitopes without native B-cell epitope, but containing a peptidic B-cell epitope |
| ZP3 (330–337) | NSSSSQFQ | Minimum T-cell and pathogenic epitope |
| ZP3 (335–342) | QFQIHGPR | Native B-cell epitope |
| Polyalanine with the crucial T-cell epitope residues | NAAAAQFQA | Pathogenic T-cell epitope |
| Chimeric peptide | NCAYKTTQANK-QAQIHGPR | Modified native B-cell epitope linked to a foreign T-cell peptide of bovine ribonuclease (94–104) |

pathogenic in normal rodents. However, the antigen specificity of disease suppression in this model remains unclear. The mechanism of regulation is under active investigation and may involve cytokines or contact between T cells and antigen-presenting cells (APCs).

### Regulatory T Cells for Testis Antigen Demonstrable in the Experimental Autoimmune Orchitis Model

Classic murine EAO is elicited by immunization with testis antigen in complete Freund's adjuvant and *Bordetella pertussis* toxin (20). Adjuvant independent EAO can also be induced in the C3H/He mice by multiple subcutaneous injections of viable testicular cells (21). The pathology is transferable to normal mice by CD4[+] T-cell lines derived from the mice with EAO (21). Antigen-specific tolerance is induced by intravenous injections of deaggregated, soluble testis antigens, and mice so treated develop long-lasting resistance to EAO induction (22). CD8[+] splenic T cells from mice that receive intravenous soluble testis antigen transfer EAO resistance to normal mice. In addition, a CD4[+] T-cell line with the capacity to suppress the EAO has been derived from the spleens of C3H/He mice injected with testis cells (23). Regulatory T cells have also been demonstrated in the classic murine EAO model induced by testis homogenate in adjuvants. Sublines of the BALB/c mice differ in EAO susceptibility (24); BALB/cBy are susceptible, whereas BALB/cJ are highly resistant. When CD4[+] spleen cells from the resistant BALB/cJ line, immunized with testis antigen in adjuvant, are transferred to BALB/cBy mice, the recipients become resistant to EAO induction (25,26).

### REGIONAL IMMUNOREGULATION IN THE TESTIS AND OVARY

#### Testis Self Antigens of Late Ontogeny Are Incompletely Sequestered, Whereas Ovarian Self Antigens Are Fully Accessible to the Immune System

Testicular isoforms of somatic antigens, expressed on haploid germ cells, develop after puberty and are not available to interact with lymphocytes early in life. Because immunologic tolerance might require the interaction between self antigens and developing lymphocytes long before puberty, it has been

speculated that tolerance to male germ cell antigens might not exist. Instead, testis antigen might be protected by a complete immunologic blood-testis barrier. A structural barrier consists of the peritubular myoid cells, and the junctional complexes between adjacent Sertoli's cells effectively separate circulating antibodies and lymphocytes from the intratubular haploid germ cells and limit the access of germ cell antigens to the APCs outside the seminiferous tubules.

Several findings indicate that tissue barrier and antigen sequestration are important, but not sufficient, to protect male germ cell antigens or to prevent EAO. Antibody can enter the rete testis to bind to spermatozoa (27), and immunogenic autoantigens are detected on the diploid, preleptotene spermatocytes located outside the blood-testis barrier (28). In cell transfer experiments, pathology occurs in a unique location, suggesting that target peptides may be presented to T cells outside the blood-testis barrier along the straight tubules linking the seminiferous tubules to the rete testis (29). Indeed, this is the precise location where peptides from ovalbumin microinjected into the seminiferous tubules are recognized by ovalbumin-specific T cells (30).

There is also evidence for local immunoregulation against autoimmune response to testis antigens. The testicular interstitial space may be immunologically privileged and function as an immunochemical barrier. Accordingly, the testicular autoantigens are likely protected by the confinement of most of the germ cell antigens by a strong but regionally incomplete anatomic barrier, whereas systemic and regional mechanisms prevent activation of autoreactive lymphocytes.

The situation for the ovarian autoantigens is quite different. Normal ovaries are endowed with a fixed number of primordial oocytes. In cycling female mice, a cohort of 30 to 40 oocytes develop and mature in every ovarian cycle that lasts for 4 to 5 days. Most of the oocytes degenerate and undergo a process of atresia wherein oocyte antigens, including the ZP, are phagocytosed by major histocompatibility complex (MHC) class II positive macrophages. Thus, a potential source of ovarian peptides is presented by activated macrophages located in ovarian interstitial space. Indeed, ZP3 peptide-specific T-cell clones can transfer, within 2 days, granulomatous inflammation that targets the atretic follicles in normal recipients. Antigens of the ZP in normal ovarian follicles and within atretic follicles are accessible to circulating antibody of immunoglobulin G (IgG) class and to circulating immune complexes (9,31,32). As described later, there is evidence that oocyte antigens can leave normal ovaries to reach lymphoid tissues. Thus, compared with the testis, ovarian autoantigens turn over continuously in cycling female mice, and they are fully accessible to the immune system.

## Suppressor Factors Within Testicular Local Environment

Parathyroid and pancreatic islet allografts, placed under the renal capsule, would be rapidly rejected, but they survive for prolonged periods when engrafted inside the testis (33). T-cell response elicited by mitogen or antibody to the T-cell receptor is suppressed by proteins in fluid obtained from the testicular interstitial space and in the supernatant of cultured testicular interstitial cells. Thus, factors exist within the testicular interstitial space that are responsible for immunosuppression.

Activated lymphocytes that express FAS undergo apoptosis upon interaction with cells bearing the FAS ligand (34). FAS ligand has been detected in Sertoli's cells of the rodent testis (35). Its possible role in immunoprotection is suggested by the finding that seminiferous tubules of normal mice survived under kidney capsule of an allogeneic host for a longer period than did seminiferous tubules from the gld mutant mice that lack a functional FAS ligand (35).

## Altered Ovarian Environment in Postrecovery Resistance in ZP3-Induced Ovarian Autoimmune Disease

In both EAO and AOD induced by the ZP3 peptide, the inflammatory infiltrates eventually regress (7,36). Recovery from ovarian pathology is associated with resistance of the animals to reinduction of AOD. Oophoritis resistance is not explicable by the immunosuppressive effect of adjuvant priming, nor by the suppression of pathogenic T cells. Moreover, the recovered mice produce ZP3 antibodies of IgG class when challenged with the ZP3 peptide. Ovarian disease resistance is also not a result of the limitation of accessible target antigens; when mated, the recovered mice produce normal litters. Moreover, pathogenic ZP3-specific T cells elicit oophoritis when transferred to recovered mice.

The oophoritis resistance state has been ascribed to an altered target organ (36). Thus, the recovered mice immunized with the ZP3 peptide develop oophoritis in normal ovaries implanted under the renal capsule, whereas their endogenous ovaries are spared.

## EVENTS THAT OVERCOME THE IMMUNOREGULATORY MECHANISMS AND LEAD TO GONADAL AUTOIMMUNE DISEASES

The studies described earlier on autoimmune disease induction by normal murine T cells indicate that pathogenic self-reactive T cells exist in normal mice and that they are controlled by regulatory T cells. This is consistent with the concept of tolerance based on the balance of T-cell subpopulations. It follows that if the balance is tipped in favor of effector T-cell activation, autoimmune diseases might occur. This scenario has been substantiated in AOD, in which disease occurs under the following circumstances: the depletion of regulatory cells by D3TX or other manipulations of the normal immune system, or the activation of oophoritogenic T cells by nonovarian peptides that mimic an oophoritogenic T-cell peptide.

## Depletion of Regulatory T Cells

Important models of autoimmune endocrinopathy that feature oophoritis and orchitis were described by Nishizuka and Sakakura (5) and later by Penhale et al. (37). Excellent reviews on these autoimmune models, summarized in Table 44.1, have been published (3,38,39).

(C57BL/6 × A/J)F1 mice with D3TX develop AOD spontaneously by 4 to 6 weeks, and the disease is transferred to young recipients by CD4+ (but not CD8+) T cells from the diseased mice (Fig. 44.1) (16,40). Of particular significance is the observation that the autoimmune disease is prevented by T cells from normal adult mice, given to D3TX recipients that are less than 10 days of age (16,41). Both adult thymocytes and adult spleen cells contain effective regulatory T cells. They express CD4 and high levels of CD5 (16); more recently, these regulatory T cells have been identified within the fraction of CD4+ T cells (less than 10%) that express CD25, the IL-2 α chain (17,42,43).

Disease suppression by normal T cells in D3TX mice indicates that autoimmune diseases in D3TX mice have resulted from deprivation of physiologically relevant regulatory T cells. This conclusion is corroborated by the finding that the same T-cell subpopulation also suppresses all of the autoimmune models based on the perturbation of the normal immune system (Table 44.1). Therefore, two mechanisms are invoked for the pathogenesis of D3TX oophoritis and orchitis: the maintenance and expansion of the self-reactive, neonatal T-cell repertoire, as discussed earlier, and the preferential deprivation of regulatory T cells that exit the thymus after the pathogenic T cells. Additional factors that influence autoimmune disease induction are thymic abnormality, which influences the thymic-hypothalamic-pituitary axis (44), and lymphopenia (39); both factors have been described in the manipulated mice with autoimmune diseases. Because selective reduction of CD25 T cells by *in vivo* antibody treatment of normal euthymic mice also results in autoimmune disease, however, the loss of the regulatory T cells appears to be the single most crucial factor responsible for the autoimmune state (42).

## Activation of Pathogenic T Cells Through Molecular Mimicry

Autoimmune oophoritis also develops when the host is immunized with peptides that mimic the self T-cell peptide, as in AOD induced by immunization with pZP3. A peptide from the δ chain of murine acetylcholine receptor (AcCRδ) is recognized by ZP3-specific T-cell clones and induces AOD (45). Of the nine amino acids in the ZP3 and AcCRδ peptides, four are shared between the peptides, and three of these four residues are crucial for induction of AOD. Direct evidence for molecular mimicry based on sharing of the crucial residues is obtained by induction of oophoritis and ZP3-specific T-cell response by nanomer polyalanine peptides, into which selected residues of the ZP3 or the AcCRδ peptides are inserted. The study provides one of the first pieces of evidence for molecular mimicry at the level of T-cell peptides that results in autoimmune disease (4).

The phenomenon of molecular mimicry also applies to foreign peptides, and the occurrence can be frequent. Of 16 randomly-selected, nonovarian peptides that share partial sequence homology with the crucial residue motif as ZP3(330–338), 7 (44%) induced AOD and autoantibody responses (46).

### Ovarian Endogenous Antigens Drive a Rapid Autoantibody Response After T-Cell Activation

It has been shown that induction of T-cell response to a self peptide can lead to the spontaneous development of autoantibodies to the peptide-bearing antigen. Thus, mice injected with a ZP3 T-cell peptide lacking a native B epitope (Table 44.2) spontaneously produce autoantibodies to the native ZP3 protein (47,48). Similar antibody response is also induced in mice by nonovarian peptides that cross-react with the ZP3 T-cell peptide, and even by polyalanine peptides that contain the crucial residues of the ZP3 peptide (47,48). This T-cell to B-cell epitope spreading phenomenon was confirmed by reaction of the antibodies to non–cross-reactive ZP3 B-cell epitopes outside the ZP3-immunizing T-cell peptide (48). Endogenous ovarian antigens are responsible for induction of ZP autoantibodies; antibodies are not detected in mice ovariectomized 2 days before immunization. However, ovarian pathology is not required for antibody induction because ovariectomy 2 days after immunization fails to abrogate antibody response (48). The antibodies are therefore not merely a secondary response to antigens released from diseased ovaries. Importantly, the antibody response occurs rapidly and has been detected 2 days after T-cell response, concordant with the onset of ovarian inflammation. This series of studies support the conclusion that ovarian antigens normally reach regional lymphoid tissues.

The phenomenon of autoantibody induction by T-cell peptide is explicable as follows. In normal mice, ovarian antigenic macromolecules or macromolecular complexes that include ZP3 normally reach the regional lymph nodes, where they encounter ZP3-specific B cells. ZP3 is internalized and processed, and its T-cell peptides are presented on MHC class II molecules. In normal mice, the series of events ends here because such B cells normally undergo apoptotic cell death. In mice immunized with T-cell peptide, however, the

ZP3-specific T cells can recognize and be activated by the peptide–MHC complexes on the ZP3-specific B cells. In turn, the T cells stimulate the B cells to produce antibodies. Importantly, the antibody specificity would match that of the antigen receptor on B cells that initially capture the ovarian antigen. An implication is that self-reactive B cells in normal female mice can respond to ovarian self antigen; therefore, they are not intrinsically tolerized. In addition, the occurrence of amplified autoantibodies indicates that serum autoantibodies need not mirror the immunogens that initiate an autoimmune disease; therefore, investigation of molecular mimicry in autoimmunity using autoantibodies as reagents can be misleading.

The phenomenon of autoantibody production by epitope spreading has also been described in other models of autoimmunity (reviewed in 4), including, for example, immune response to a peptide from murine myelin basic protein in experimental allergic encephalomyelitis (EAE), antibody response to murine gastric parietal cell $K^+/H^+$-dependent ATPase in autoimmune gastritis of the D3TX mice, and antibody response to the pancreatic islet β-cell autoantigen, glutamic acid decarboxylase, in the nonobese diabetic (NOD) mice. Even more importantly, epitope spreading from one antigen to another within nuclear macromolecular complexes has been reported and provides a potential mechanism for autoantibody induction in systemic autoimmunity, such as systemic lupus erythematosus.

### Loss of Physical Barrier

Vasectomy, a common male contraceptive approach, results in the production of autoantibody response to sperm antigens of all subjects and in T-cell response to testicular antigens in guinea pigs (49). In addition, postvasectomy autoimmune orchitis has been documented in vasectomized rabbits, guinea pigs, and monkeys.

## PATHOGENETIC MECHANISMS OF AUTOIMMUNE TESTICULAR AND OVARIAN DISEASES

### Pathogenetic Role of Inflammatory $T_H1$, CD4$^+$T Cells

The importance of the T-cell–mediated mechanism is established by experiments involving disease transfer by lymphocytes of known function and antigen specificity. T cells that have been activated *in vitro* transfer severe orchitis and vasitis to syngeneic euthymic mice (22,23,50). Similarly, T cells from mice immunized with oophoritogenic pZP3 rapidly transfer AOD to syngeneic recipients (9). In both cases, CD4$^+$ T cells are responsible for disease transfer. The importance of CD4$^+$ T cells in disease transfer is substantiated by studies using CD4$^+$ T-cell lines and clones (9,23,51).

A study based on T-cell clones has further defined the pathogenetic mechanism of EAO (51). Despite the use of crude testis antigens, both T-cell lines and all of 16 independent T-cell clones transfer EAO to normal syngeneic mice with pathology that affects the testis, epididymis, or vas deferens. Thus, orchitogenic peptides are likely to be immunodominant among peptides in the crude testis antigenic preparation. Although testis antigen–derived T-cell clones respond preferentially to testis antigen and sperm antigen–derived clones respond more to sperm antigens, each of the 16 clones responded to both antigens. Thus, common and unique orchitogenic antigens exist in the germ cell populations, and their quantity may differ in distribution. The fact that sperm-specific T-cell clones elicit disease indicates that male germ cell antigens alone can elicit EAO. All orchitogenic T-cell clones express CD4, and when activated, they produced IL-2 and interferon-γ (IFN-γ), but not IL-4. They are therefore typical of the $T_H1$, CD4$^+$ T cells responsible for the delayed-type immunologic reaction that includes granulomatous inflammation. Importantly, disease transfer is significantly and reproducibly attenuated when recipients are given neutralizing antibody to tumor necrosis factor (TNF), but not neutralizing antibody to IFN-γ. Hence, TNF is a cytokine important in the pathogenesis of this autoimmune disease.

Based on the unique distribution of testicular pathology in recipients of activated orchitogenic T-cell lines or T-cell clones, a main location of accessible testis peptides to the CD4$^+$ T cells has been defined (Fig. 44.2) (29,51). The predominant testicular inflammation affects the straight tubules. CD4$^+$ T cells recognize peptides in association with MHC class II molecules, and in normal mouse testis, MHC class II–positive macrophages are sparse but form a dense cuff around the straight tubules. These are the likely APCs that present the germ cell peptides to orchitogenic T cells to initiate EAO (29). The inflammatory infiltrate then blocks the passage of tubular spermatozoa and fluids to cause dilation of the proximal seminiferous tubules. Severe orchitis spreads centripetally to involve peripheral seminiferous tubules, and eventually testicular atrophy and necrosis ensue.

CD4$^+$ T-cell clones against the ZP3 peptide that produce IL-2 and IFN-γ, but not IL-4, are also responsible for oophoritis transfer, and disease transfer is also blocked by antibody to TNF (Bagavant H, Luo AM, and Tung KSK, unpublished observations). The target antigenic structure in the ovaries is the atretic follicles. In contrast, the growing follicles, antral follicles, and corpus luteum are not involved (9).

## Costimulation Requirements in Clonal Expansion and Functional Acquisition of Ovarian Antigen–Specific T Cells

Naive T-cell activation by self peptides requires costimulation between ligands on the T cells with the corresponding receptors on the APCs. The role of two costimulation pathways in AOD induction have been analyzed: CD28 on T cells with CD80/CD86 (or B7) on the APCs, and CD40 ligand on activated T cells with CD40 on the APCs (52). Blockage of the CD40 pathway by CD40 ligand antibody results in failure to induce AOD and autoantibodies. Inhibition of ligand

binding to the CD28 receptors by the fusion protein, murine CTLA4Ig (which blocks CD80/CD86), likewise results in the failure to generate antibody to ZP and significantly reduces disease severity and prevalence. The frequencies of antigen-specific T cells in CD40 ligand antibody–treated mice, CTLA4Ig-treated mice, and mice given control reagents are equivalent, however, as determined by limiting dilution analysis (1:5000). These T cells, which produce comparable amounts of cytokines *in vitro* but fail to cause ovarian inflammation in the original hosts, can transfer oophoritis to normal recipients. When CD40 ligand antibody and CTLA4Ig are given together, the effect is additive; the frequency of pZP3-specific T cells is reduced to 1:190,000, and disease and antibody responses are absent. Thus, oophoritis and ZP3 antibody production can be inhibited by blocking either of the costimulatory pathways, whereas inhibition of clonal expansion of the pathogenic T-cell population requires blockade of both pathways. This *in vivo* study has effectively dissociated two sequential activation steps of autoreactive ZP3-specific T cells.

## Pathogenic Role of Antibodies

### Experimental Autoimmune Orchitis

As indicated earlier, autoimmunogenic germ cells have been identified outside the blood-testis barrier that react with circulating autoantibodies *in vivo* (28). In mice immunized with testis antigens in adjuvant, intense deposits of IgG are detected on the surface of cells of the seminiferous tubules outside the blood-testis barrier (Fig. 44.3). This is detected as early as day 7 after immunization, 5 to 6 days before the onset of orchitis. The IgG deposits, transferred by serum to normal mice, were defined as antibodies to the preleptotene spermatocytes that are located outside the Sertoli's cell barrier.

Testis IgG deposits are also elicited by immunization with testis homogenate in incomplete Freund's adjuvant, which does not elicit EAO. Thus, the immune deposits are not sufficient to cause EAO. The lack of pathogenicity may be related to the unique immunoglobulin subclass of the IgG deposits because only antibodies of the IgG1 and IgG3 subclasses are detected, without complement components. However, the immune complexes may provide a source of peptides for effector T-cell activation, outside the anatomic blood-testis barrier, to initiate EAO. The inflammatory process then alters the blood-testis barrier and allows inflammatory cells to enter the seminiferous tubules.

In EAO, antibodies have also been detected as granular immune complexes in basal lamina around aspermatogenic tubules that are free of orchitis. Although deposits of immune complexes occur only focally in EAO of rabbits (53) and mice (20,21), massive immune complexes surrounding the aspermatogenic tubules are detected in spontaneous EAO of the dark mink, the aging brown Norway rat, and vasectomized rabbits (54).

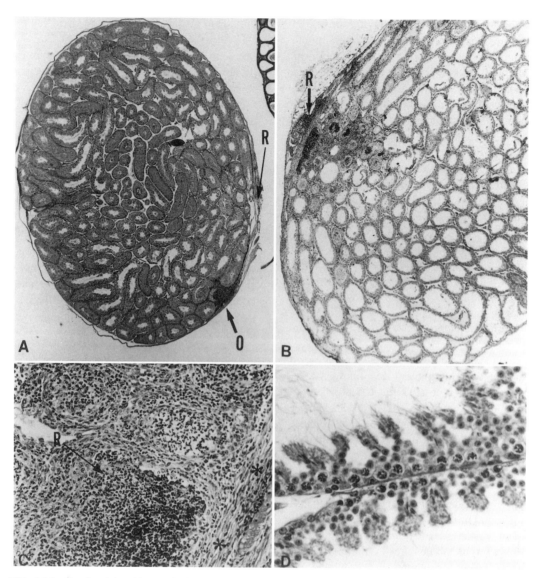

**FIG. 44.2.** Predominant histopathologic lesions in active and passive experimental autoimmune orchitis (EAO) **(A, B)**. **A:** A common lesion in active EAO is found under the testicular capsule (*arrow*), away from the rete testis (*R*) *O*, orchitis. (original magnification, ×50) **B:** In passive EAO, inflammation in the regions of straight tubules, adjacent to the rete testis (*R*), is common, and this leads to severe dilation of the seminiferous tubules (original magnification, ×50). **C:** In passive EAO, inflammation in the rete regions (*R*) is severe and obstructs the lumen (original magnification, ×200). **D:** In passive EAO, dilated seminiferous tubules have attenuated but intact germinal epithelium, without evidence of orchitis (original magnification, ×400). (From Tung KSK, Yule TD, Mahi-Brown CA, et al. Distribution of histopathology and Ia positive cells in actively-induced and adoptively-transferred experimental autoimmune orchitis. *J Immunol* 1987;138:752–759, with permission.)

### ZP3-Induced Autoimmune Ovarian Disease

Immune complexes have been detected in the ZP in two experimental conditions without concomitant autoimmune oophoritis. Female mice with experimental systemic lupus erythematosus, including the (NZBXW)F1, MRL/1, and BXSB strains, spontaneously accumulate antigen–antibody complexes in the ovarian ZP (31). Rabbits injected with antibody to angiotensin-converting enzyme, an antigen expressed on the plasmalemma of oocytes, also form abundant immune complexes in the ZP (32).

The role of antibody has been investigated in more detail in AOD, based on a chimeric peptide of ZP3 that induces antibody without concomitant T-cell response (55). The chimeric peptide is made up of a promiscuous foreign T-cell peptide capable of eliciting $T_H$ cell response and a native B-cell peptide of ZP3 that has been modified by substitution of residue crucial for T-cell, but not for B-cell, response to ZP3 (Table 44.2). Mice immunized with the chimeric peptide produce antibodies to native ZP but are free of oophoritis. Thus, antibody *per se*, without concomitant T-cell response, is not

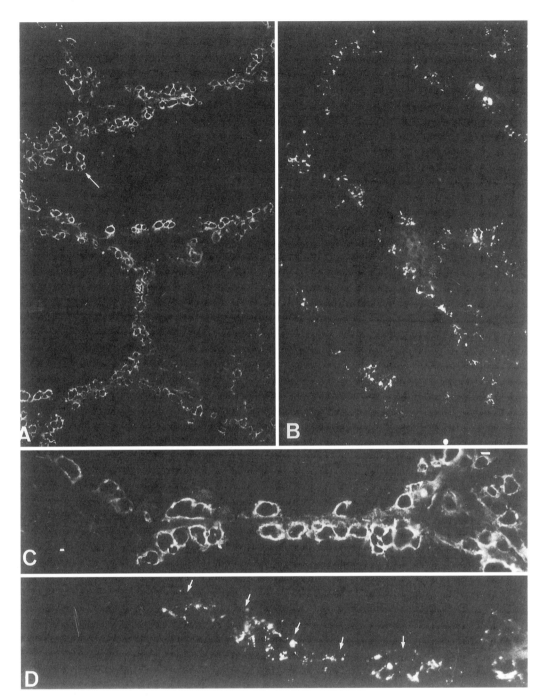

**FIG. 44.3. A:** Immunofluorescence localization of *in vivo* binding of immunoglobulin G antibody on preleptotene spermatocytes at the periphery of seminiferous tubules; these cells are located outside the blood-testis barrier (original magnification, ×100). **B:** In some testes, the deposits appear granular (original magnification, ×100). **C, D:** Immune deposits seen in parts **A** and **B** are shown at higher magnification (original magnification, ×400). (From Yule TD, Montoya GD, Russell LD, et al. Autoantigenic germ cells exist outside the blood testis barrier. *J Immunol* 1988;141:1161–1167, with permission.)

sufficient to induce AOD. ZP3 autoantibody, however, can inhibit fertility *in vivo* and fertilization *in vitro* (10,55).

Although ZP3 antibodies do not cause oophoritis, their reaction to the target tissue strongly influences the distribution of oophoritis mediated by T cells. As described earlier, ZP3-specific T cells transfer pathology confined to the atretic fol-

licles and spare the growing and antral follicles. When mice also receive ZP3 antibodies, which bind to the ZP of growing and antral follicles, the T-cell–mediated inflammation is retargeted to those ovarian follicles (56). This is the first demonstration that autoantibody binding to a tissue antigen can modify the distribution of a T-cell–mediated inflammation.

## IMMUNOGENETIC APPROACH TO AUTOIMMUNE DISEASE OF TESTIS AND OVARY

Several testicular and ovarian autoimmune disease susceptibility and resistance gene loci have been mapped by the microsatellite approach.

### Major Histocompatibility Complex Class III Locus for Experimental Autoimmune Orchitis Susceptibility

Studies based on intra-MHC recombinant inbred mice indicate that *Orch-1* is an orchitis-susceptibility gene mapped within the *H-2S/H-2D* interval (57), between the *IR* gene controlling antibody responsiveness to trinitrophenol-Ficoll (TNP-Ficoll) and the locus encoding TNF (26). This has established the gene order in the region as follows: *H-2S*, *TNP-Ficoll, Orch-1, Tnf, H-2D*. Recent molecular analysis has further mapped *Orch-1* within a 50- to 60-kb segment from *Hsp70.1* to a region proximal to *G7* that encompasses the *Hsp70.1, Hsp70.3, Hsc70t, G7b,* and *G7a/Bat6* genes (58).

### An Experimental Autoimmune Orchitis Resistance Gene Locus

Genes located outside the MHC strongly influence EAO susceptibility. DBA/2J (*H-2^d*) mice are resistant to EAO, BALB/cByJ (*H-2^d* mice are susceptible to EAO, whereas (BALB/cByJ × DBA/2J)F1 (CD2F1) mice are resistant (57). Among a (BALB/cBy × DBA/2J)F1 × BALB/cByJ (BC1) population (n = 172), 54% of the animals are resistant, whereas 46% are susceptible. Using DNA isolated from the phenotyped BC1 population and previously mapped microsatellite markers distinguishing DBA/2J and BALB/ cByJ, an orchitis-resistant gene locus, *Orch-3*, was mapped to *D11Mit8* (59). The *Orch-3* gene is of particular interest because it is located in a region of chromosome 11 encoding a variety of immune modulatory genes of intense research interest, including important interleukins, chemokines, and Tpm1, a locus controlling the differential induction of $T_H1$- and $T_H2$-type responses to murine *Leishmania* species infection (60).

### Independent Genetic Regulation of Three Lesions of Experimental Autoimmune Orchitis: Orchitis, Epididymitis, and Vasitis

A study investigated 109 back-cross mice between B10.S and (B10.S × SJL)F1 for linkage analysis of gene loci with orchitis, epididymitis, and vasitis (61). Linkage with orchitis was mapped to a gene locus in chromosome 8 *(Orch-6)*, epididymitis to chromosome 16 *(Epd-1)*, and vasitis to chromosome 1 *(Vas-1)*. Thus, in EAO, the inflammation affecting three different anatomic sites is under separate genetic control.

### A Common Immunoregulatory Locus Controls Susceptibility of Experimental Autoimmune Orchitis and Experimental Allergic Encephalomyelitis in BALB/c Mice

The BALB/cByJ substrain is highly susceptible to EAO and EAE, whereas the BALB/cJ substrain is highly resistant to both diseases. Segregation analysis of 11 second-generation back-cross lines demonstrated that 6 were responders and 5 were nonresponders, and a perfect concordance was found in disease susceptibility and resistance between EAO and EAE (62). This study also provided data to indicate that disease resistance is dependent on a regulatory T-cell population; however, environmental factors also influence disease susceptibility.

### Two Genetic Loci Govern Distinct Pathologic Expression of Autoimmune Ovarian Disease Induced by D3TX

*H-2*-linked genes play little, if any, role in determining disease outcome in the D3TX mice. This is corroborated by a study on autoimmune oophoritis and other polyendocrinopathy that developed in mice with the transgenic T-cell receptor Vα protein; the organ distribution of pathology is strictly controlled by the genetic background of the mice that carry the transgene (63).

Studies have mapped two gene loci that control susceptibility to D3TX-induced AOD. One hundred and forty-four D3TX (C57BL/6J × A/J)F1 × C57BL/6J back-cross mice were cross-bred between the disease susceptible A/J strain (90% disease incidence), (C57BL/6J × A/J)F1 hybrid (100% disease incidence), and the disease-resistant C57BL/6J (8% disease incidence). On histologic analysis of the ovaries at 60 days of age, 77 exhibited oophoritis and oocytic autoimmunity, whereas 67 were resistant. The ratio of 1.15 between susceptible and resistant animals is consistent with that expected for a single locus. Microsatellites have been employed to generate a genomic exclusion map that localizes the autoimmune oophoritis and autoantibody susceptibility gene *(Aod-1)* to chromosome 16, linked to *D16Mit4*. Several candidate genes of immunologic relevance reside on chromosome 16, including *Ly-7, Ifgt, Ifrc, Igl-1, Mls-3,* and *VpreB* (64).

In AOD of the D3TX mice, an independent genetic locus strongly influences the development of ovarian atrophy of this disease (65). This gene *(Aod-3)* has been mapped to chromosome 3, within the interval between *D3Mit21* and *D3Mit154*. This interval contains the *il2* gene and also the basic fibroblast growth factor *(bgfb)* gene. The latter is known to regulate cell growth and differentiated functions of ovarian cells, including granulosa cells.

## CONCLUSIONS

This chapter has presented current knowledge concerning the tolerance mechanisms that prevent gonadal autoimmunity and the potential events that can overcome such mechanisms to trigger autoimmune diseases. It has also summarized our understanding of the mechanisms responsible for the immunopathology of these diseases.

The local testicular immunoregulatory environment, provided by the strong blood-testis barrier and perhaps intratesticular humoral factors, partially impedes autoimmune responses to testis antigens of late ontogeny. Although ovarian self antigens are fully accessible to the immune system, the ovaries become resistant to disease induction in animals that have recovered from AOD and that is based on mechanism other than loss of self antigens.

In addition, systemic tolerance mechanisms regulate autoreactive T cells that recognize testicular and ovarian antigen. These studies indicate that pathogenic T cells capable of eliciting autoimmune diseases in the gonads develop in both the neonatal and adult thymus, and they persist in the normal peripheral immune system. The function of the pathogenic T cells in adult mice, however, is normally under the control of regulatory T cells, which maintain peripheral tolerance, and important phenotypic differences are being defined between these two functional CD4$^+$ T-cell subsets. When the clonal balance of these T-cell subsets is tipped in favor of pathogenic T cells, autoimmune diseases of the gonads could ensue. Because these findings also apply to autoimmune disease affecting many other organs, they should be of general significance in the pathogenesis of the autoimmune state.

The loss of regulatory T cells may occur through aberrant T-cell development. This has been documented in several novel models of autoimmune oophoritis and orchitis caused by deliberate perturbation of the normal immune system, including D3TX. On the other hand, oophoritogenic T cells can be activated through stimulation by nonovarian peptides that cross-react with self peptides. This novel form of antigen mimicry can occur frequently and is dependent in part on partial sharing, between unrelated peptides, of the crucial amino acids required for activation of pathogenic T cells.

The inflammatory (T$_H$1) CD4$^+$ T-cell mechanism has been established as a crucial pathogenetic pathway for autoimmune orchitis and autoimmune oophoritis. In both diseases, the pathogenic T-cell clones secrete IL-2, IFN-γ, and TNF; moreover, neutralizing TNF *in vivo* markedly reduces disease severity transferred by pathogenic T-cell clones. The tissue locations wherein pathogenic T cells encounter testicular and ovarian target antigens have been surmised by the rather precise localization of histopathology that follows the adoptive transfer of the pathogenic T-cell clones. Activation of the pathogenic CD4$^+$ oophoritogenic T cells has been shown to depend on the integrity of CD28 and gp39 costimulation pathways. Inhibition of either of the pathways does not inhibit clonal proliferation, but the pathogenicity of the expanded T cells is blocked.

Antibodies can access both testicular and ovarian target antigens during the development of autoimmune orchitis and autoimmune oophoritis. Studies indicates that antibody is not sufficient to cause oophoritis; however, antibody to ZP has been shown to retarget the location of T-cell–mediated pathology in the ovary.

In the case of ovarian disease, a novel mechanism of autoantibody induction has been uncovered. Immunization of female mice with a pure T-cell peptide from ZP3 can lead to the production of antibodies against ZP3 domains outside the immunogenic ZP3 peptide. Evidently, endogenous antigens from normal and pathologic ovaries may reach peripheral immune tissues and provide the antigenic stimulus to trigger an autoantibody response. This occurs at the same time as activation of ZP3-specific T cells is detected and is therefore not a consequence of tissue injury. Importantly, similar autoantibody induction has been produced against lupus antigens, and the mechanism is potentially important in systemic autoimmune disease pathogenesis.

Finally, progress has been made based on gene linkage analysis of inbred mice that helps to map genetic loci responsible for the susceptibility and resistance to autoimmune diseases of the testis and ovary. This approach can potentially elucidate new and unanticipated mechanisms that underlie the complex gonadal and other autoimmune diseases. Some of the genetic loci are the same as those associated with EAE and NOD mice, and as such, they may code for functional molecules involved in autoimmune disease pathogenesis in general.

Contemporary research on experimental testicular and ovarian autoimmune diseases has led to rapid accumulation of new information on self tolerance and autoimmune disease pathogenesis. The findings have emphasized the similarities between these two organs as well as their similarities with autoimmune diseases affecting other organs. Research based on the unique models of gonadal autoimmune diseases and the well-defined self antigens can be expected to clarify further the human autoimmune diseases of the gonads as well as the autoimmune process in general.

## ACKNOWLEDGMENTS

I wish to thank Drs. Cory Teuscher, Cherri Mahi-Brown, Teresita Yule, Hedy Smith, An-Ming Luo, Yahuan Lou, and Nathan Griggs and Ms. Kristine Garza for their conceptual and experimental contributions to our studies described in this chapter. I also thank Ms. Marianne Volpe for her excellent editorial skills and manuscript preparation. The studies are supported by National Institutes of Health grants AI-41236 and HD-29099.

## REFERENCES

1. Tung KSK, Lu CY. Immunologic basis of reproductive failure. In: Kraus FT, Damjanov I, Kaufman, N, eds. *Pathology of reproductive failure.* New York: Williams & Wilkins, 1991:308–333.
2. Lewis J. Eosinophilic perifolliculitis: a variant of autoimmune oophoritis? *Int J Gynecol Pathol* 1993;12:360.
3. Tung KSK, Taguchi O, Teuscher C. Testicular and ovarian autoimmune diseases. In: Cohen, IR, Millers, A, eds. *Guidebook to animal models for autoimmune diseases.* New York: Academic Press, 1994:267–290.
4. Tung KSK, Lou YH, Garza KM, et al. Autoimmune ovarian disease: mechanism of disease induction and prevention. *Curr Opin Immunol* 1997;9:839–845.

5. Nishizuka Y, Sakakura T. Thymus and reproduction: sex linked dysgenesis of the gonad after neonatal thymectomy. *Science* 1969;166: 753–755.

6. Taguchi O, Nishizuka Y. Experimental autoimmune orchitis after neonatal thymectomy in the mouse. *Clin Exp Immunol* 1981;46: 425–434.

7. Tung KSK, Primakoff P, Woolman-Gamer L, et al. Mechanism of infertility in male guinea pigs immunized with sperm PH-20. *Biol Reprod* 1997;56:1133–1141.

8. Primakoff P, Hyatt H, Myles DG. A role for the migrating sperm surface antigen, PH-20, in guinea pig sperm binding to the egg zona pellucida. *J Cell Biol* 1985;101:2239–2244.

9. Rhim SH, Millar SE, Robey F, et al. Autoimmune diseases of the ovary induced by a ZP3 peptide from the mouse zona pellucida. *J Clin Invest* 1992;89:28–35.

10. Dean J. Biology of mammalian fertilization: role of the zona pellucida. *J Clin Invest* 1992;89:1055–1059.

11. Garza K, Griggs ND, Tung KSK. Neonatal injection of an ovarian peptide induces autoimmune ovarian disease in female mice: requirement of endogenous neonatal ovaries. *Immunity* 1997;6:89–96.

12. Smith H, Lou, YH, Lacy P, et al. Tolerance mechanism in ovarian and gastric autoimmune disease. *J Immunol* 1992;149:2212–2218.

13. Alderuccio F, Toh BH, Tan SS, et al. An autoimmune disease with multiple molecular targets abrogated by the transgenic expression of a single autoantigen in the thymus. *J Exp Med* 1993;178:419–426.

14. Smith H, Chen IM, Kubo R, et al. Neonatal thymectomy results in a repertoire enriched in T cells deleted in adult thymus. *Science* 1989;245:749–752.

15. Sakaguchi SK, Fukuma K, Kuribayashi, et al. Organ-specific autoimmune diseases induced in mice by elimination of T cell subset. I. Evidence for the active participation of T cells in natural self-tolerance. Deficit of a T cell subset as a possible cause of autoimmune disease. *J Exp Med* 1985;161:72–87.

16. Smith H, Sakamoto Y, Kasai L, et al. Effector and regulatory cells in autoimmune oophoritis elicited by neonatal thymectomy. *J Immunol* 1991;147:2928–2933.

17. Sakaguchi S, Sakaguchi N, Asano M, et al. Immunologic self-tolerance maintained by activated T cells expressing IL-2 receptor α-chains (CD25). *J Immunol* 1995;155:1151–1164.

18. Fowell K, McKnight AJ, Powrie F, et al. Subsets of CD4 T cells and their roles in the induction and prevention of autoimmunity. *Immunol Rev* 1991;123:37–64.

19. McKeever U, Mordes, JP, Greiner DL, et al. Adoptive transfer of autoimmune diabetes and thyroiditis to athymic rats. *Proc Natl Acad Sci U S A* 1990;87:7618–7622.

20. Kohno S, Munoz JA, Williams TM, et al. Immunopathology of murine experimental allergic orchitis. *J Immunol* 1983;130:2675–2582.

21. Itoh M, Mukasa A, Tokunaga Y, et al. New experimental model for adoptive transfer of murine autoimmune orchitis. *Andrologia* 1991;23: 415–420.

22. Mukasa A, Itoh M, Tokunaga Y, et al. Inhibition of a novel model of murine experimental autoimmune orchitis by intravenous administration with a soluble testicular antigen: participation of CD8⁺ regulatory T cells. *Clin Immunol Immunopathol* 1992;62:210–219.

23. Itoh M, Hiramine C, Mukasa A, et al. Establishment of an experimental model of autoimmune epididymo-orchitis induced by the transfer of a T-cell line in mice. *Int J Androl* 1992;15:170–181.

24. Teuscher C, Smith SM, Tung KSK. Experimental allergic orchitis in mice. III. Differential susceptibility in BALB/c sublines. *J Reprod Immunol* 1987;10:219–230.

25. Mahi-Brown CA, Tung KSK. Transfer of susceptibility to experimental autoimmune orchitis from responder to non-responder substrains of BALB/C mice. *J Reprod Immunol* 1990;18:247–257.

26. Teuscher C, Gasser DL, Woodward SR, et al. Experimental allergic orchitis in mice. VI. Recombinations within the H-2S/H-2D interval define the map position of the H-2 associated locus controlling disease susceptibility. *Immunogenetics* 1990;32:237–344.

27. Tung KSK, Unanue ER, Dixon FJ. Pathogenesis of experimental allergic orchitis. II. The role of antibody. *J Immunol* 1971;106:1463–1472.

28. Yule TD, Montoya GD, Russell LD, et al. Autoantigenic germ cells exist outside the blood testis barrier. *J Immunol* 1988;141:1161–1167.

29. Tung KSK, Yule TD, Mahi-Brown CA, et al. Distribution of histopathology and Ia positive cells in actively-induced and adoptively-transferred experimental autoimmune orchitis. *J Immunol* 1987;138: 752–759.

30. Grafer C, Maddocks S, Miller D, et al. Micro-surgical injection of surrogate testis antigen provides a versatile experimental model of murine immunologic orchitis. *J Reprod Immunol* 1997;34:37–38.

31. Accinni L, Albini B, Andres G, et al. Deposition of immune complexes in ovarian follicles of mice with lupus-like syndrome. *Am J Pathol* 1980;99:589–596.

32. Matsuo B, Caldwell PRB, Brentjens JR, et al. In vitro interaction of antibodies with cell surface antigens: a mechanism responsible for in vivo formation of immune deposits in the zona pellucida of rabbit oocytes. *J Clin Invest* 1985;75:1369–1380.

33. Head JR, Neaves WB, Billingham RE. Immune privilege in the testis. I. Basic parameters of allograft survival. *Transplantation* 1983;36: 423–431.

34. Nagata S, Golstein P. The Fas death factor. *Science* 1995;267: 1449–1456.

35. Bellgrau D, Gold D, Selawry H, et al. A role for CD95 ligand in preventing graft rejection. *Nature* 1995;377:630–632.

36. Lou YH, McElveen F, Adams S, et al. Altered target organ: a mechanism of postrecovery resistance to murine autoimmune oophoritis. *J Immunol* 1995;155:3667–3673.

37. Penhale WJ, Farmer A, McKenna RP, et al. Spontaneous thyroiditis in thymectomized and irradiated wistar rats. *Clin Exp Immunol* 1973; 15:225–236.

38. Sakaguchi S, Sakaguchi N. Thymus, T cells, and autoimmunity: various causes but a common mechanism of autoimmune disease. In: Coutinho A, Kazatchkine M, eds. *Autoimmunity: physiology and disease.* New York: Wiley-Liss, 1994:203–227.

39. Gleeson PA, Toh BH, van Driel IR. Organ-specific autoimmunity induced by lymphopenia. *Immunol Rev* 1996;149:97–125.

40. Sakaguchi S, Sakaguchi N. Thymus and autoimmunity: capacity of the normal thymus to produce self-reactive T cells and conditions required for their induction of autoimmune disease. *J Exp Med* 1990;172: 537–545.

41. Sakaguchi S, Takahashi T, Nishizuka Y. Study on cellular events in post-thymectomy autoimmune oophoritis in mice. II. Requirement of Lyt-1 cells in normal female mice for the prevention of oophoritis. *J Exp Med* 1982;156:1577–1586.

42. Taguchi O, Takahashi T. Administration of anti-interleukin 2 receptor alpha antibody in vivo induces localized autoimmune disease. *Eur J Immunol* 1996;26:1608–1612.

43. Suri-Payer E, Kehn PJ, Cheever AW, et al. Pathogenesis of post-thymectomy autoimmune gastritis: identification of anti-H/K adenosine triphosphatase-reactive T cells. *J Immunol* 1996;157:1799–1805.

44. Michael SD, Taguchi O, Nishizuka Y. Effect of neonatal thymectomy on ovarian development and plasma LH, FSH, GH and PRL in the mouse. *Biol Reprod* 1980;22:343–350.

45. Luo AM, Garza KM, Hunt D, et al. Antigen mimicry in autoimmune disease: sharing of amino acid residues critical for pathogenic T cell activation. *J Clin Invest* 1993;92:2117–2123.

46. Garza K, Tung KSK. Frequency of T cell peptide crossreaction determined by experimental autoimmune disease and autoantibody induction. *J Immunol* 1995;155:5444–5448.

47. Lou YH, Tung KSK. T cell peptide of a self protein elicits autoantibody to the protein antigen: Implications for specificity and pathogenetic role of antibody in autoimmunity. *J Immunol* 1993;151:5790–5799.

48. Lou YH, McElveen F, Garza K, et al. Rapid induction of autoantibodies by endogenous ovarian antigens and activated T cells: implication in autoimmunity pathogenesis and B cell tolerance. *J Immunol* 1996; 156:3535–3540.

49. Meng AL, Tung KSK. Cell-mediated and humoral immune responses to aspermatogenic antigen in experimental allergic orchitis in guinea pig. *J Reprod Fertil* 1983;69:279–288.

50. Mahi-Brown CA, Tung KSK. Activation requirements of donor T cells and host T cell recruitment in adoptive transfer of murine experimental autoimmune orchitis (EAO). *Cell Immunol* 1989;124:368–379.

51. Yule TD, Tung KSK. Experimental autoimmune orchitis induced by testis and sperm antigen-specific T cell clones: an important pathogenic cytokine is tumor necrosis factor. *Endocrinology* 1993;133:1098–1107.

52. Griggs ND, Agersborg SS, Noelle RJ, et al. The relative contribution of the CD28 and GP39 costimulatory pathways in the clonal expansion and pathogenic acquisition of self reactive T cells. *J Exp Med* 1996;183: 801–810.

53. Tung KSK, Woodroffe A. Immunopathology of experimental allergic orchitis in the rabbit. *J Immunol* 1978;120:320–328.

54. Tung KSK, Ellis L, Teuscher C, et al. The black mink (mustela vison): a natural model of immunologic male infertility. *J Exp Med* 1981; 154:1016–1032.

55. Lou YH, Ang J, Thai H, et al. A ZP3 peptide vaccine induces antibody and reversible infertility without ovarian pathology. *J Immunol* 1995; 155:2715–2720.

56. Lou YH, Park KK, Tung KSK. Binding of autoantibody to the tissue antigen directs targeting of T cell-mediated autoimmune inflammation. Keystone Symposia on Lymphocyte Activation. Hilton Head, South Carolina, Abst. 2051, 1996.

57. Teuscher C, Smith SM, Goldberg EH, et al. Experimental allergic orchitis in mice. I. Genetic control of susceptibility and resistance to induction of autoimmune orchitis. *Immunogenetics* 1985;22:323–333.

58. Snoek M, Jansen M, Olavessen MG, et al. The Hsp7-genes are located in the Cr-H-2D region: possible candidates for the Orch-1 locus. *Genomics* 1993;15:350–356.

59. Meeker ND, Hickey WF, Korngold R, et al. Multiple loci govern the bone marrow-derived immunoregulatory mechanism controlling dominant resistance to autoimmune orchitis. *Proc Natl Acad Sci U S A* 1995;92:5684–5688.

60. Gorham JD, Guler ML, Steen RG, et al. Genetic mapping of a murine locus controlling development of T helper 1/T helper 2 type responses. *Proc Natl Acad Sci U S A* 1997;93:12467–12472.

61. Roper RJ, Doerge RW, Stanford BC, et al. Autoimmune orchitis, epididymitis, and vasitis are immunogenetically distinct lesions. *Am J Pathol* 1998;152:1337–1345.

62. Teuscher C, Hickey WF, Grafer CM, et al. A common immunoregulatory locus controls susceptibility to actively induced experimental allergic encephalomyelitis and experimental allergic orchitis in BALB/c mice. *J Immunol* 1998;160:2725–2756.

63. Sakaguchi S, Ermak TH, Toda M, et al. Induction of autoimmune disease in mice by germline alteration of the T cell receptor gene expression. *J Immunol* 1994;152:1471–1484.

64. Wardell BB, Michael SD, Tung KSK, et al. Multiple genes regulate neonatal thymectomy-induced autoimmune ovarian dysgenesis (AOD) with linkage of ovarian atrophy to Idd-3. *Proc Natl Acad Sci U S A* 1995;92:4758–4762.

65. Teuscher C, Wardell BB, Lunceford JK, et al. Aod2, the locus controlling development of atrophy in neonatal thymectomy-induced autoimmune ovarian dysgenesis of atrophy, is linked to IL2, Fgfb, and Idd3. *J Exp Med* 1996;183:631–637.

*Textbook of the Autoimmune Diseases,*
Edited by R. G. Lahita, N. Chiorazzi, and W. H. Reeves,
Lippincott Williams & Wilkins, Philadelphia © 2000.

# CHAPTER 45

# Collagen Arthritis

David E. Trentham

The aim of this chapter is to describe collagen arthritis (CA) as an experimentally inducible animal model of rheumatoid arthritis (RA) and, in particular, to review important new information that has been obtained in the past 5 years regarding this system. This chapter does not duplicate material contained in previous reviews (1–8).

## INDUCTION AND IMMUNOPATHOGENESIS

CA is induced in susceptible strains of rats, mice, or monkeys by immunization with native cartilage- or ocular-derived type II collagen (CII) (9–12). Homologous and heterologous CII, derived from a variety of species, including chickens, cows, pigs, deer, or humans, are equivalently arthritogenic. Interestingly, rabbits, which react only to nonhelical epitopes on CII, are resistant to the disease. Also intriguing is the adequacy of incomplete Freund's adjuvant, emulsified with CII, to induce CA efficiently in rats (9). This contrasts markedly to all other host-antigen adjuvant–incited disease, in which use of complete Freund's, which consists of adjuvant oil and mycobacterial products, is obligatory.

CA appears to be created by T-cell sensitization to CII, leading to the release of $T_H1$ proinflammatory cytokines and the generation of help for B cells to produce synovitic immunoglobulin G (IgG) antibodies to collagen (13). In the highly susceptible DBA/1 mouse strain, the immunodominant epitope of CII has been localized to the 260– to 267–amino acid region of the molecule (14). Additive evidence for this being the governing region are both the induction and suppression of CA by analog peptides of CII 260–267 (14,15).

CII continues to be an attractive candidate autoantigen in RA. About 30% of patients with RA have demonstrable antibody (16) and T cell (17) responses to CII, although the frequency of intraarticular responses appears to be much higher (18). Further evidence for a role for CII in the pathogenesis of RA has derived from the results of oral tolerance trials using native chicken CII (16,19). Although these positive outcomes could be attributable to oral tolerance–triggered $T_H2$ inhibitory cytokines (i.e., bystander suppression), it is equally plausible that disease-relevant CII-specific cells are anergized or eliminated by the ingestion of appropriate quantities of CII (20).

New molecular genetics techniques have helped to identify hereditary influences on autoimmune disease (21). It is now clear that gene polymorphisms within the HLA class II loci play a predisposing role for T-cell–mediated autoimmune disease in mice and humans. Crystallography has shown that major histocompatibility complex (MHC) molecules have a peptide-binding cleft that contains the variable region of the molecule. Genetic polymorphism at the MHC thereby determines the specificity and affinity of peptide binding by the antigen-presenting cell and subsequent T-cell recognition.

RA is strongly associated with alleles of the DRB1 locus (21). Animals bearing transgenes for HLA have been used to explore this association. A "humanized" transgenic mouse was created with class II molecules similar to those associated with RA (22). Specifically, this involved creation of a mouse in which the class II molecules were encoded solely by *HLA-DQ8,* a gene known to occur in linkage with RA associated DR molecules. Immunization of these *HLA-DQ8* mice with CII created severe CA (23). This experiment identified for the first time that a specific human MHC class II molecule could be associated as a pathogen with an autoimmune disease. It further suggested that the HLA-DQ molecule might be pivotal in governing susceptibility to RA. The mechanism could involve the class II molecule functioning in the antigen presentation of CII to pathogenic T cells.

CA has also been used to scrutinize the potential contributory roles of other pathways in RA. Sometimes, the findings have been quite unexpected. For example, knockout techniques can be used to create mice that are deficient in one specific trait. The knockout strain can then be compared with the normal wild-type counterpart to probe, in a heretofore

D. E. Trentham: Department of Medicine, Harvard Medical School, Boston, Massachusetts 02215; Department of Medicine, Beth Israel Deaconess Medical Center, Boston, Massachusetts 02215.

unprecedented way, the role of the deficient pathway in a disease. Stromelysin-1 (SLN1) is a major member of the matrix metalloproteinase-3 family, which has been implicated in the destruction of cartilage matrix components in inflammatory arthritis (24,25). SLN1 has been detected in cartilage and synovial tissue of patients with RA or osteoarthritis as well as CA (26). Inhibitors of metalloproteinase have suppressed CA in mice (27), further favoring an important role for SLN1 in tissue degradation during arthritis. In one analysis, however, SLN1 knockout mice were just as susceptible to CA as were their wild-type counterparts (26). Meticulous histologic assessments confirmed the authors' clinical conclusion. This startling outcome throws into question whether inhibitors of metalloproteinase would be truly beneficial drugs for the treatment of arthritis.

## CLINICAL PRESENTATION

CA has many features that closely parallel RA (2). These include fairly symmetric involvement of the peripheral large and small joints of the extremities as well as sparing of the axial skeleton; synovial pannus formation with contiguous cartilage and subchondral bone erosion; and infiltration of the synovial tissue and joint space by inflammatory cells. Contrasting with these physical resemblances, production of antibodies with rheumatoid factor activity does not occur at any stage of disease (2).

The time of onset of CA differs in rats and mice. In rats, CA begins between 9 and 18 days after primary immunization, whereas it is delayed in mice. To induce CA in mice, it is generally required to administer a booster dose of CII, conventionally given 21 days after primary immunization; the disease then begins to be clinically apparent 35 to 60 days after primary exposure to CII. In both species, the onset to CA is abrupt, and the inceptual phase is severe. Considerable joint redness and swelling are found, and radiographic appraisal shows that abundant bone damage occurs during the first week of disease. Animals continue to eat and imbibe water, but ambulation is markedly impaired. Avoidance of weight-bearing is characteristic. For ethical reasons, animals are typically sacrificed just as soon as the required outcome data are acquired. For drug or biologic testing, experiments in rats are generally terminated between days 21 and 25.

There is a gradual defervescence in arthritis after the initial 2 weeks or so of clinical disease. Nonetheless, rats and mice are left with permanent joint deformity. Histologic evidence of persistent joint inflammation can be found for more than 100 days after primary immunization. A prompt and severe relapse of CA occurs if the animals are reimmunized during this period. The disease is largely monophasic in rats and mice, with a prompt peak and gradual subsidence over time. In susceptible strains of monkeys, such as the rhesus or squirrel, CA is decidedly fluctuant (11,12). Also contrasting to the situation in rodents, monkeys frequently refuse to eat, act quite ill, and rapidly succumb to the process. The basis for

this extreme systemic effect in primates, almost resembling a toxicity, is unknown.

Serial microscopic analyses in rats, including electron (28) and immunocytochemical (29) techniques, have shown morphologic changes in the synovial membrane beginning about 3 days after immunization. Initially, there is dense fibrin deposition on the surface of the synovium, and synoviocytes round up and dislodge themselves from abutting cells and the underlying subsynovial fat. Polymorphonuclear leukocytes and cells appearing to be of monocyte-macrophage lineage appear within the synovial tissue. Shortly thereafter, pannus production begins and progresses. By immunocytochemistry, T cells are encountered in the inflamed synovium by day 5 and constantly increase in numbers (29). Between days 5 and 10, before the emergence of macroscopically evident arthritis, the predominant cell type is $CD4^+$. Thereafter, appreciable numbers of $CD8^+$ cells emerge.

In rodents, extraarticular manifestations of CA can be found on occasion. These lesions characteristically occur in other CII-containing tissue, such as the ear and eye. Infrequently, Sprague–Dawley rats, which are a highly susceptible strain, develop auricular chondritis late in the course of CA (30,31). As in relapsing polychondritis (32), the auricular lesion in rats is highly inflammatory in nature and can destroy the integrity of the elastic cartilage supporting the ear. Initially, polymorphonuclear and mononuclear inflammatory cells, along with rare eosinophils, invade the margin of the cartilaginous plate and adjacent soft tissue. Chondrocyte death and cartilage matrix dissolution then ensue, along with expansion of the mixed inflammatory cell nest in the soft tissue contiguous to the diseased cartilage. Later, multinucleated giant cells can be found in the granulation tissue. True granuloma formation does not occur. Gradually, the cartilage begins a partial attempt at repair, and occasionally nodular sites of elastic cartilage overgrowth can be found. In the early lesion, dense deposits of complement (C3), immunoglobulin, and fibrin can be detected by immunofluorescence. All these features exemplify the histopathologic changes of relapsing polychondritis. As in the animal model, autoantibodies to CII have been found in the human disease (33). Thus, autoimmunity to CII could have relevance for relapsing polychondritis, a disease like RA in its association with HLA-DR4 (32).

In a collaborative effort involving Drs. Joan O'Brien, Henry Adler, and Daniel Albert of the Massachusetts Eye and Ear Institute, as well as myself, a CII hyperimmunization schedule was shown to create, as a composite, an animal model of juvenile rheumatoid arthritis (JRA) (34). Unlike adult RA, anterior uveitis is a characteristic feature of JRA. Sprague–Dawley rats received varying antigenic doses of CII. Although all doses induced CA, greater antigenic exposure was significantly ($p < 0.005$) associated with increasing degrees of anterior uveitis, as measured by histopathologic assessments of the ocular globe. Similar to the ocular lesion in JRA, CII-induced eye inflammation had a pattern that included loss of epithelium in the corneas with stromal disruption by inflammatory infiltrate and vascularization and scarring; anterior and posterior synechiae with angle closure; uveal inflammation, predominantly involving the iris; confinement of choroidal inflammation to anterior regions; and essentially normal sclera, retina, and posterior choroid.

The uveitogenic, as well as the arthritogenic, properties of native CII are consistent with the physically restricted presence of the protein as a major structural component of both cartilage and the vitreous of the eye (35), but not elsewhere in the body. By inference, these observations support the concept that autoimmunity to CII plays a role in the pathogenesis of JRA, a disease with distinctly different serologic and immunogenetic features from RA.

## LABORATORY TESTING

In contrast to the other experimentally inducible animal models of inflammatory polyarthritis, such as adjuvant arthritis and streptococcal cell wall arthritis in rats and pristane-induced arthritis in mice, CA readily affords a multitude of surrogate markers of autoimmunity to be measured and followed. Therefore, a protocol that suppresses clinical disease activity in CA can be easily scrutinized for immunosuppressive properties. B-cell responses to collagen can be easily quantified by enzyme-linked immunosorbent assay (ELISA) measurement of isotype-specific antibodies to native CII (7). Likewise, T-cell responses to CII can be analyzed *in vivo* by delayed-type hypersensitivity reactions, assessed by microcaliper measurement of ear swelling after antigen challenge or by a radiometric ear assay (7). *In vitro,* T-cell reactivity to CII can be graded by thymidine incorporation or $T_H1$ cytokine release (7).

In animals, measurement of acute-phase reactants has been difficult to standardize. On the other hand, tissue injury can be easily and objectively assessed by light microscopic appraisal (7). Plain radiographs of hind limbs, disarticulated after sacrifice and mounted on cardboard, accurately quantifies bone damage in CA (7). Radioscintigraphy, using indium-111, is an additional, albeit expensive, way to quantify joint inflammation in rats with CA (36).

Synovial tissue–derived fibroblasts from rats with CA grow readily in culture and release appreciable quantities of collagenase and prostaglandin $E_2$ ($PGE_2$) (37). Production of both mediators can be suppressed in rats given effective antirheumatic treatment (37).

T-cell numbers and subset type can be analyzed by immunophenotyping in synovial, splenic, or lymph node tissue (7). To monitor for toxicity in drug trials, food or water consumption can be measured and weight gain (a normal occurrence throughout young adulthood in rats and mice) noted.

Despite their sophistication and objectivity, there is no better way to evaluate disease severity of CA than by enumerating the incidence of CA in experimental groups and grading the severity of arthritis in individual rats by a macroscopic arthritic index, whereby paw involvement is graded in inte-

gers from 0 to 4, resulting in a maximum score per animal of 16 (7). Similarly, a way to assess globally the immune response to collagen immunization that is preferable to the ELISA antibody assay has not been found.

## TREATMENT

The chief contribution of the CA model to the field of autoimmune disease is the identification of a potential role of CII autoimmunity in RA, relapsing polychondritis, or JRA. On the utilitarian level, however, its major significance is probably an ongoing ability to screen predictably compounds for possible antirheumatic activity.

CA, like RA, is readily responsive to steroidal or nonsteroidal antiinflammatory compounds. A major justification for the use of total lymphoid irradiation in the treatment of RA was its successful application to CA. More recently, cyclophosphamide, cyclosporine, and FK-506 have efficiently suppressed CA and have also shown activity in RA. The drug development of the novel and nontoxic synthetic hexose sugar, amiprilose hydrochloride, was fostered in large part by preclinical screening in CA (37). A large study has validated its efficacy in RA. The rationale for the 200-patient, minocycline in RA (MIRA) trial (38) was in part based on antirheumatic actions observed in CA (39). Increasingly, minocycline, which has potent antiinflammatory, enzyme-inhibitory, and T-cell–immunosuppressive properties in animals, is gaining a niche as an excellently tolerated and effective drug for treating patients with RA (40).

CA has advanced biologic therapy for RA as well. Early work used polyclonal antithymocyte globulin or anti-CD4 monoclonal antibodies to suppress CA. Subsequent trials showed that anti–tumor necrosis factor-α (anti–TNF-α) strategies were effective, helping to foster the current interest in this therapy for RA.

Antigen-specific suppression of autoimmune disease has been achieved in CA. Initially, intravenous injection of spleen or red blood cells coupled to CII was used (41). Later, intravenous injection of large quantities of solubilized CII (42) and the instillation of CII-specific T-line cells (43) were successful. Most recently, the saga of oral tolerance has emerged (20). It was first shown in rats (44) or mice (45) that oral delivery of CII abrogated CA. Outcomes in RA have been positive as well (16,19); intriguingly, they have shown an inverse dose relationship of CII ingestion with disease suppression in both CA and RA.

Lately, additional immunointerventions have delineated novel preclinical findings in CA that could, in the future, be applied to RA. The following paragraphs outline some of this work.

As discussed earlier, stimulation of T cells involves recognition of peptide bound to MHC proteins by the antigen-specific T-cell receptor (TCR). This T-cell response to a cognate peptide–MHC molecule can be governed by a finite set of TCR V-region gene segments. Thus, similar V regions on oligoclonal T-cell populations could provide a target whereby antigen-specific immunosuppression would be accomplished (46). Attempts to use Vβ domains to reach this goal have met with limited success, in part because of technical factors, such as a limited supply of material. Recently, however, a recombinant Vα domain of a disease-relevant TCR was used to downregulate CA in mice (47). This Vα domain was highly immunogenic, and vaccinated mice proved to be resistant to CA. They also displayed attenuated antibody and cellular responses to CII. This is the first demonstration that recombinant TCR vaccines may be applied to RA, assuming that restricted TCR usage is a feature shared by the human disease. At this time, the latter aspect remains one of the most controversial topics in cellular immunology.

Paralleling the largely frustrating attempts to employ TCR vaccination as a treatment for autoimmune disease has been the use of anti-CD4 monoclonal antibodies. Apart from problems such as the immunogenicity of these nonhumanized molecules has been the occasional discordance of immunologic and clinical outcomes. For example, administering some products induced a protracted acquired immunodeficiency syndrome–like immunodeficiency state in humans but failed to modify the patients' RA. In contrast, one fairly current effort has been remarkably successful in murine CA (48). In the first step, a highly complex series of back-cross matings of CA-susceptible and CA-resistant mouse strains finally resulted in a transgenic model that exhibited a much slower onset but elongated chronic stage of CA. To the investigators, both aspects more closely resembled RA than the more self-limited disease in the wild counterparts. The chronicity of CA in the transgenic animals also permitted experiments during the later stage of CA to be more readily performed. Using a nondepleting anti-CD4 monoclonal antibody, it was next shown that the induction of this new model could be blocked (48). Moreover, the molecule was also therapeutic because the chronic stage of the established disease could be suppressed as well. The mechanism for this antirheumatic action appeared to be the induction of CII-specific T-cell anergy. This state was defined by the lack of proliferation, a $T_H1$ response, by CII stimulation *in vitro* (48). Collagen antibody production in treated mice was also attenuated. In summary, a nondepleting anti-CD4 monoclonal antibody was shown to suppress CA by specific inhibition of the $T_H1$ subset. These outcomes argue that similar agents may yet be found for RA.

Interleukin-4 (IL-4) is of considerable interest as a cytokine that could be used to modify autoimmune disease. It is a pleiotropic molecule derived from T cells and mast cells that exerts multiple biologic actions on B and T cells as well as macrophages, endothelial cells, and fibroblasts. Expression of IL-4 is characteristic of $T_H2$ responses, such as those involved in IgE production in allergy and parasitic infections. Conceivably, IL-4 could downplay the $T_H1$ drive in autoimmune disease. Supporting this possibility is the sharp increase in the $T_H1$ attributable IFN-γ production at the onset of CA but absence of the $T_H2$ cytokines, IL-4 and IL-10, by cultured

lymph node cells (49). In contrast, the $T_H2$ cytokines dominate during the later improvement stage of CA. In additional experiments, continuous IL-4 infusion for 28 days suppressed the induction of CA in mice (50). The most striking immunologic effect was a 1000-fold reduction in TNF-α production by synovial cells from IL-4 treated animals.

Further evidence for an inhibitory role of IL-4 in CA has been reported (51). A standard oral tolerization protocol was used to abrogate the onset of CA in mice. However, when mice fed CII also received an anti–IL-4 monoclonal antibody, which eliminated IL-4–mediated bioactivity, this suppressive effect on CA disappeared. The neutralization of IL-4 activity also abolished the suppression of IgG antibody and proliferation response to CII that was encountered in the fed but not treated control group.

Yet another cytokine-based treatment of autoimmune disease has emerged using the CA model (52). IL-12 is another pleiotropic cytokine. It promotes the growth of activated T cells and NK cells. IL-12 also selectively acts to foster $T_H1$ development from naive T cells and augments the release of IFN-γ by differentiated $T_H1$ cells. Production of TNF-α can also be upregulated by IL-12. IL-12 may be a major protector during bacterial infections. Intriguingly, it could also function in the putative role of bacterial infections in the induction of $T_H1$-triggered autoimmune disease. In addition, IL-12 is a potent stimulus for IL-10 production by $T_H2$ cells, a pathway that could limit tissue injury during inflammatory or infectious states. A report suggests that IL-12 is an inducer of IL-10 generation by T cells and macrophages; this process could culminate in a negative-feedback loop to curtail excessive immunologic activity and resultant tissue injury.

Accordingly, interesting dichotomous findings emerged when IL-12 was studied in the early and late stages of the murine CA model (52). When IL-12 was administered intraperitoneally at the time of arthritis onset, a more explosive onset and pronounced acceleration in the severity of arthritis were noted. Both exacerbating features could be dampened by the coadministration of a monoclonal antibody directed against IL-12. These outcomes provide combinatorial evidence that IL-12 participates in the induction stage of CA. A complex outcome was encountered when anti–IL-12 treatment was applied to established murine CA. Here, exaggerated disease expression was observed. There was also an abnormal expression of TNF-α mRNA in the synovial tissue.

To analyze further the dual role of IL-12 in early and late CA, mice with established CA were treated with recombinant IL-12 (52). A marked suppression of arthritis was noted. Sera of recombinant IL-12–treated mice showed a 10-fold increase in the level of IL-10, and upregulated release of IL-10, IFN-γ, and IL-12 was detected in synovial tissue. In addition, the antagonistic effect of IL-12 on established CA could be blocked by coadministration of anti–IL-10 antibodies. In concert, this multiplicity of experiments has provided evidence of pivotal roles for IL-12, as well as IL-10, in the control of CA. By inference, intuitive reasoning would conclude that because of biologic harmony, immunoregulatory cytokines, both at a proactive and antiexertional level, like-wise influence human autoimmune arthritic disease.

These IL-12 outcomes have just been validated by an additional assessment (53). This involved insertion of a gene regulating transient IL-12 expression and subsequent analysis of its effect on CA. In this system, there was clear-cut exacerbation of disease, as defined by enhanced disease progression and severity. Enhancement of IFN-γ release accompanied these outcomes. In further appraisals, neutralization of IL-12 aborted these clinical and IFN-γ augmentations. Considered as a whole, these independent results (52,53) strongly implicate IL-12 as an important mediator in CA and suggest that inflammatory arthritis in humans is a complex byproduct of multiple cytokine and, perhaps, antibody-mediated orchestrations.

## INSIGHTS DERIVED FROM PRIMATE TYPE II COLLAGEN

In rodents, susceptibility to CA is crucially dependent on MHC haplotypes. In inbred strains of mice, particular regions on the CII molecule play dominant roles in both arthritogenicity and immunogenicity. These regions vary in different strains. For example, the cyanogen bromide cleavage peptide CB11 (amino residues 147 to 403) of both chicken and bovine CII is the dominant peptide in DBA/1 mice, whereas B10.RIII mice respond to CB8 rather than CB11 (12).

In general, nonhuman primates are highly susceptible to CA. Squirrel (11), rhesus, and cynomolgus (12) monkeys are susceptible, but cebus (11) monkeys are not. These findings have been refined and extended in a recent study (12). Outbred cynomolgus monkeys were found to be highly susceptible to both heterologous and homologous CII. Multiple regions on CII (i.e., CB12, CB11, and CB10) were capable of inducing high titers of antibodies to CII, and arthritis generally developed as well. Many of these experimentally induced antibodies reacted to autologous CII, clearly indicating that an autoimmune reactivity had been created. In these outbred animals, in contrast to inbred strains, epitope switching occurred. For example, early after immunization with denatured CB11 or CB12, antibodies reacted better to denatured CII than to the native molecule. In contrast, at later stages, when severe arthritis had been present for some time, a broader cascade of reactivities, including reactions dominantly directed to native CII, were encountered. As a composite, this latter pattern resembled CII autoantibody profiles frequently encountered in different patients with RA. The data also support a complex and multifactorial role for MHC molecules in the immunorecognition of CII epitopes in RA.

## CONCLUSIONS

No animal model of autoimmune disease, with the probable exception of the experimental myasthenia gravis analog, has proved persuasively to delineate the etiology of its human counterpart. Nonetheless, CA joins experimental autoim-

mune encephalomyelitis in exemplifying the utility of model systems to identify pathogenic pathways that are highly probable to operate in human disease. This chapter has provided a selected update of insights into immunopathologic processes acquired by means of CA. As a whole, this knowledge strongly infers that cytokines accelerate and dampen autoimmune disease. What remains unanswered, although suggested (54), is whether T-cell products can actually initiate an autoimmune process. Therapeutically, what appears to be most important is whether cytokine limbs can be harnessed to ameliorate these disorders. Materials delivered to counteract deleterious cytokines, such as TNF-α, or to promote the bioactivity of desirable species, such as IL-4 or IL-10, may provide major novel approaches to the future treatment of autoimmunity. By helping study these feasibilities, CA has already served an invaluable function. Of course, these potential benefits for the treatment of human disease have to be counterbalanced against the harm and suffering inflicted on the experimental animals. After 25 years of working with CA, I remain insecure about the bioethics of animal experimentation.

## REFERENCES

1. Trentham DE. Autoimmunity to collagen as a disease mechanism. In: Weissman JG, ed. *Advances in inflammation research.* Vol. 2. New York: Raven Press, 1981:149–164.
2. Trentham DE. Collagen arthritis as a relevant model for rheumatoid arthritis: evidence pro and con. *Arthritis Rheum* 1982;25:911–916.
3. Trentham DE. Immunity to collagen in rheumatoid and experimental arthritis. In: Franklin EC, ed. *Clinical immunology update.* New York: North Holland/American Elsevier, 1983:37–55.
4. Trentham DE. Immune response to collagen. In: Gupta S, Talal N, eds. *Immunology of rheumatic diseases.* New York: Plenum, 1985:301–323.
5. Trentham DE. Clues provided by animal models of arthritis. *Rheum Dis Clin North Am* 1987;13:307–318.
6. Breedveld FC, Trentham DE. Progress in the understanding of inducible models of chronic arthritis. *Rheum Dis Clin North Am* 1987;13:532–544.
7. Trentham DE, Dynesius-Trentham RA. Type II collagen-induced arthritis in the rat. In: Chang JY, Lewis AJ, eds. *Pharmacological methods in the control of inflammation.* New York: Alan R Liss, 1989:395–414.
8. Trentham DE, Dynesius-Trentham RA. Collagen-induced arthritis. In: Henderson B, Edwards JCW, Pettipher ER, eds. *Mechanisms and models in rheumatoid arthritis.* London: Academic Press, 1995:447–456.
9. Trentham DE, Townes AS, Kang AH. Autoimmunity to type II collagen: an experimental model of arthritis. *J Exp Med* 1977;146:857–868.
10. Courtenay JS, Dallman MJ, Dayan AD, et al. Immunisation against heterologous type II collagen induces arthritis in mice. *Nature* 1980;283:666–668.
11. Cathcart ES, Hayes KC, Gonnerman WA, et al. Experimental arthritis in a nonhuman primate. I. Induction by bovine type II collagen. *Lab Invest* 1986;54:26–31.
12. Shimozuru Y, Yamane S, Fujimoto K, et al. Collagen-induced arthritis in nonhuman primates: multiple epitopes of type II collagen can induce autoimmune-mediated arthritis in outbred cynomolgus monkeys. *Arthritis Rheum* 1998;41:507–514.
13. Seki N, Sudo T, Yoshioka S, et al. Type II collagen-induced murine arthritis. I. Induction and perpetuation of arthritis require synergy between humoral and cell-mediated immunity. *J Immunol* 1988;140:1477–1484.
14. Brand DD, Myers LK, Terato K, et al. Characterization of the T cell determinants in the induction of autoimmune arthritis by bovine α 1(II)-CB11 in H-2q mice. *J Immunol* 1994;152:3088–3097.
15. Tang B, Myers LK, Rosloniec EF, et al. Characterization of signal transduction through the TCR-δ chain following T cell stimulation with

analogue peptides of type II collagen 260-267. *J Immunol* 1998;160:3135–3142.

16. Barnett ML, Kremer JM, St Clair EW, et al. Treatment of rheumatoid arthritis with oral type II collagen: results of a multicenter, double-blind, placebo-controlled trial. *Arthritis Rheum* 1998;41:290–297.

17. Snowden N, Reynolds I, Morgan K, et al. T cell responses to human type II collagen in patients with rheumatoid arthritis and healthy controls. *Arthritis Rheum* 1997;40:1210–1218.

18. Tarkowski A, Klareskog L, Carlsten H, et al. Secretion of antibodies to types I and II collagen by synovial tissue cells in patients with rheumatoid arthritis. *Arthritis Rheum* 1989;32:1087–1092.

19. Trentham DE, Dynesius-Trentham RA, Orav EJ, et al. Effects of oral administration of type II collagen on rheumatoid arthritis. *Science* 1993;261:1727–1730.

20. Trentham DE. Oral tolerization as a treatment for rheumatoid arthritis. *Rheum Dis Clin North Am* 1998;24:525–536.

21. Taneja V, David CS. HLA transgenic mice as humanized mouse models of disease and immunity. *J Clin Invest* 1998;101:921–926.

22. Cheng S, Baisch J, Krco C, et al. Expression and function of HLA-DQ8 (DQA1*0301/DQB1*0302) genes in transgenic mice. *Eur J Immunogenet* 1996;23:15–20.

23. Nabozny GH, Baisch JM, Cheng D, et al. HLA-DQ8 transgenic mice are highly susceptible to collagen-induced arthritis: a novel model for human polyarthritis. *J Exp Med* 1996;183:27–37.

24. Matrisian LM. Metalloproteinases and their inhibitors in matrix remodeling. *Trends Genet* 1990;6:121–125.

25. Brinckerhoff CR. Joint destruction in arthritis: metalloproteinases in the spotlight. *Arthritis Rheum* 1991;34:1073–1075.

26. Mudgett JS, Hutchinson NI, Chartrain NA, et al. Susceptibility of stromelysin 1-deficient mice to collagen-induced arthritis and cartilage destruction. *Arthritis Rheum* 1998;41:110–121.

27. Carmichael DF, Stricklin GP, Stuart JM. Systemic administration of TIMP in the treatment of collagen-induced arthritis in mice. *Agents Actions* 1989;27:378–379.

28. Caulfield JP, Hein A, Dynesius-Trentham RA, et al. Morphological demonstration of two stages in the development of type II collagen-induced arthritis. *Lab Invest* 1982;46:321–343.

29. Breedveld FC, Dynesius-Trentham RA, deSousa M, et al. Collagen arthritis in the rat is initiated by CD4+ T cells and can be amplified by iron. *Cell Immunol* 1989;121:1–12.

30. Cremer MA, Pitcock JA, Stuart JM, et al. Auricular chondritis in rats: an experimental model of relapsing polychondritis induced with type II collagen. *J Exp Med* 1981;154:535–540.

31. McCune WJ, Schiller AL, Dynesius-Trentham RA, et al. Type II collagen-induced auricular arthritis. *Arthritis Rheum* 1982;25:266–273.

32. Trentham DE, Le CH. Relapsing polychondritis. *Ann Intern Med* 1998;129:114–122.

33. Foidart JM, Abe S, Martin GR, et al. Antibodies to type II collagen in relapsing polychondritis. *N Engl J Med* 1978;299:1203–1207.

34. O'Brien JM, Adler HJ, Albert DM, et al. Induction of ocular and joint inflammation by type II collagen simulating juvenile rheumatoid arthritis. *Arthritis Rheum* 1989;32:S89(abst).

35. Bornstein P. Structurally distinct collagen types. *Am Rev Biochem* 1980;49:957–1003.

36. deSousa M, Lima Bastos A, Dynesius-Trentham RA, et al. Potential of indium-111 to measure inflammatory arthritis. *J Rheumatol* 1986;13:1108–1116.

37. Kieval RI, Young CT, Prohazka D, et al. Evaluation of a modified hexose sugar, amiprilose hydrochloride, in experimental models of synovitis. *J Rheumatol* 1989;16:67–74.

38. Tilley BC, Alarcón GS, Heyse SP, et al. Minocycline in rheumatoid arthritis: a 48 week double-blind, placebo-controlled trial. *Ann Intern Med* 1995;122:81–89.

39. Sewell KL, Breedveld F, Furrie E, et al. The effect of minocycline in rat models of inflammatory arthritis: correlation of arthritis suppression with enhanced T cell calcium flux. *Cell Immunol* 1996;167:195–204.

40. Trentham DE, Dynesius-Trentham RA. Antibiotic therapy for rheumatoid arthritis: scientific and anecdotal appraisals. *Rheum Dis Clin North Am* 1995;21:817–834.

41. Schoen RT, Greene MI, Trentham DE. Antigen-specific suppression of type II collagen-induced arthritis by collagen-coupled spleen cells. *J Immunol* 1982;128:717–719.

42. Cremer MA, Hernandez AD, Townes AS, et al. Collagen-induced arthritis in rats: antigen-specific suppression of arthritis and immunity by intravenously injected native type II collagen. *J Immunol* 1983;131:2995–3000.

43. Brahn E, Trentham DE. Attenuation of collagen arthritis and modulation of delayed-type hypersensitivity by type II collagen reactive T cell lines. *Cell Immunol* 1987;109:139–147.

44. Thompson HSG, Staines NA. Gastric administration of type II collagen delays the onset and severity of collagen-induced arthritis in rats. *Clin Exp Immunol* 1985;64:581–586.

45. Nagler-Anderson C, Bober LA, Robinson ME, et al. Suppression of type II collagen-induced arthritis by intragastric administration of soluble type II collagen. *Proc Natl Acad Sci U S A* 1986;83:7443–7446.

46. Acha-Orbea H, Mitchell DJ, Timmerman L, et al. Limited heterogeneity of T cell receptors from lymphocytes mediating autoimmune encephalomyelitis allows specific immune intervention. *Cell* 1988;54:263–273.

47. Rosloniec EF, Brand DD, Whittington KB, et al. Vaccination with recombinant Vα domain of a TCR prevents the development of collagen-induced arthritis. *J Immunol* 1995;155:4504–4511.

48. Mauri C, Chu C-QQ, Woodrow D, et al. Treatment of a newly established transgenic model of chronic arthritis with nondepleting anti-CD4 monoclonal antibody. *J Immunol* 1997;159:5032–5041.

49. Mauri C, Williams R, Walmsley M, et al. Relationship between Th1/Th2 cytokine patterns and the arthritogenic response in collagen-induced arthritis. *Eur J Immunol* 1996;26:1511–1518.

50. Horsfall AC, Butler DM, Marinova L, et al. Suppression of collagen-induced arthritis by continuous administration of IL-4. *J Immunol* 1997;159:5687–5696.

51. Yoshino S. Treatment with an anti-IL-4 monoclonal antibody blocks suppression of collagen-induced arthritis in mice by oral administration of type II collagen. *J Immunol* 1998;160:3067–3071.

52. Joosten LAB, Lubberts E, Helsen MMA, et al. Dual role of IL-12 in early and late stages of murine collagen type II arthritis. *J Immunol* 1997;159:4094–4102.

53. Parks E, Strieter RM, Lukacs NW, et al. Transient gene transfer of IL-12 regulates chemokine expression and disease severity in experimental arthritis. *J Immunol* 1998;160:4615–4619.

54. Brahn E, Trentham DE. Experimental synovitis induced by collagen-specific T cell lines. *Cell Immunol* 1989;118:491–503.

Textbook of the Autoimmune Diseases,
Edited by R. G. Lahita, N. Chiorazzi, and W. H. Reeves,
Lippincott Williams & Wilkins, Philadelphia © 2000.

# CHAPTER 46

# Inbred Murine Models of Autoimmunity

## David I. Daikh and David Wofsy

Several strains of mice spontaneously develop autoimmune diseases that closely resemble diseases that occur in humans. Since the 1970s, these murine models have been extremely important in clarifying the genetic, cellular, and molecular mechanisms that lead to autoimmunity. These advances have in turn led to the development of new strategies for the prevention and treatment of autoimmune diseases, with the murine models serving as important testing grounds for these ideas. Some of the therapeutic strategies that have been developed in this way have already found their place in the routine treatment of humans, and many more are undergoing clinical investigation.

## SYSTEMIC LUPUS ERYTHEMATOSUS

Several strains of mice serve as models for systemic lupus erythematosus (SLE) (1,2). These strains include NZB/NZW F1 (B/W) mice, MRL-*lpr/lpr* (MRL/*lpr*) mice, and BXSB mice. These mice all produce antibodies to double-stranded DNA (anti-dsDNA) and develop immune complex glomerulonephritis, but the B/W model most closely resembles SLE in humans with respect to disease manifestations and the predilection for more severe illness in female than in male subjects (1,2).

### New Zealand Mice (NZB and NZB/NZW)

In 1959, in the process of generating new inbred strains of mice to study at the University of Otago Medical School in New Zealand, Dr. Marianne Bielschowsky noted that mice in one of the strains, New Zealand black (NZB) mice, died at an early age with anemia, jaundice, and splenomegaly (3). Sub-

sequent evaluation of these mice established that the cause of their illness was an autoimmune hemolytic anemia. This was the first spontaneous autoimmune disease described in animal models, and its discovery led to a series of back-crosses with apparently healthy strains of mice that were performed in an effort to determine the genetic basis for the new autoimmune disease. The most interesting of these back-crosses involved New Zealand white (NZW) mice. This cross produced F1 offspring (B/W mice) that were found to have clinical and serologic features that bore a strong similarity to SLE in humans (4). Since that time, these mice have served as the principal model for SLE.

### Clinical and Serologic Manifestations

NZB mice develop autoimmune hemolytic anemia early in life (5). Antibodies to erythrocytes first appear at about 3 months of age, followed by progressive anemia, reticulocytosis, jaundice, and splenomegaly later in life. Other autoantibodies are found in some NZB mice, including antinuclear antibodies (ANAs), but these tend to be present in low titer. During the second year of life, most NZB mice develop B-cell lymphomas that resemble the lymphomas that occur in people with Sjögren's syndrome (6). The median life expectancy is about 16 months for female NZB mice and 17 months for male NZB mice, compared with about 2 years for most strains of healthy mice (1).

B/W mice develop an autoimmune disease that is different and considerably more aggressive than the disease that occurs in NZB mice (5). B/W mice develop LE cells, high ANA titers, anti-dsDNA antibodies, and severe immune complex glomerulonephritis. Female mice are more severely affected than are male mice. Clinical evidence of nephritis is evident in female mice by 5 to 6 months of age, and death from lupus nephritis follows relatively shortly thereafter. Examination of the glomeruli reveals deposition of DNA-containing immune complexes and complement (7). Median life expectancy for B/W female mice is 8 months, whereas male B/W mice do not succumb from their disease until about 15 months of age (Table 46.1).

D. I. Daikh: Department of Medicine, University of California at San Francisco, San Francisco, California 94143; Department of Medicine, Rheumatology Section, Veterans Administration Medical Center, San Francisco, California 94121.

D. Wofsy: Departments of Medicine and Microbiology/Immunology, University of California, San Francisco, San Francisco, California 94121; Department of Medicine, Rheumatology Section, Veterans Administration Medical Center, San Francisco, California 94121.

**TABLE 46.1.** *Life expectancy in murine models for systemic lupus erythematosus*

| Strain | Sex | 50% Mortality rate (mos of age) | 90% Mortality rate (mos of age) |
|---|---|---|---|
| NZB/NZW F$_1$ | Female | 8 | 13 |
| | Male | 15 | 19 |
| MRL/*lpr* | Female | 5 | 7 |
| | Male | 6 | 9 |
| MRL/+ | Female | 17 | 23 |
| | Male | 23 | 27 |
| BXSB | Female | 15 | 24 |
| | Male | 5 | 8 |

Adapted from Andrews BS, Eisenberg RS, Theofilopoulos AN, et al. Spontaneous murine lupus-like syndromes: clinical and immunopathological manifestations in several strains. *J Exp Med* 1978;148:1198, by copyright permission of the Rockefeller University Press.

Although renal disease is the most prominent manifestation of SLE in B/W mice, it is accompanied by other abnormalities that are also seen in humans with SLE. These include generalized lymphadenopathy and sialadenitis resembling Sjögren's syndrome (Table 46.2) (8). Serologic and immunologic abnormalities also parallel the abnormalities that are characteristic of SLE in humans, including the presence of LE cells, hypergammaglobulinemia, anti-dsDNA antibodies, antilymphocyte antibodies, and hypocomplementemia, (1,2).

### Role of B Cells

The development of hypergammaglobulinemia, the production of autoantibodies, and the glomerular deposition of immune complexes and complement strongly suggest a role for B cells in the pathophysiology of murine lupus in B/W mice. Consistent with this hypothesis, several abnormalities in B-cell function have been identified in NZB and B/W mice. B cells from both NZB and B/W mice spontaneously proliferate and secrete antibodies *in vitro* (9). In addition, B cells from B/W mice are hyperresponsive to T-cell–derived cytokines, such as interleukin-5 (IL-5) and IL-6 (10,11).

Several lines of investigation have focused attention on a distinct subset of B cells, designated B1. In B/W mice, there is an early expansion of the B1 subset, and elimination of B1 cells reduces autoantibody production and substantially prolongs life (12). These findings establish that B1 cells play an important role in the development of autoimmunity in B/W mice. However, the mechanism by which B1 cells contribute to murine lupus and the role of these cells in humans with SLE have yet to be determined. For example, in other murine lupus models and in humans, expansion of B1 cells is not required for the development of SLE. Although B1 cells are the source of low-affinity immunoglobulin M (IgM) autoantibodies, they do not appear to be the source of the high-affinity pathogenic IgG autoantibodies. Thus, autoantibody production may not be the mechanism by which B1 cells promote autoimmunity. Studies have shown that B1 cells augment presentation of autoantigens to pathogenic T cells (13). This finding suggests an alternative mechanism by which B1 cells might contribute to autoimmunity.

### Role of T Cells

The demonstration of B-cell abnormalities in B/W mice initially suggested that murine lupus might reflect a primary B-cell defect. Extensive work, however, has also implicated T cells in the pathogenesis of disease in these mice. First, genetic variants of B/W mice that lack B1 cells are protected from murine lupus, but they nonetheless manifest T-cell abnormalities that may contribute to autoimmunity. These abnormalities include resistance to tolerance induction and impaired production of, and response to, cytokines (12,14). Second, the isotype and specificity of the autoantibodies in B/W mice suggest that they are under T-cell control (15). Third, lupus nephritis does not occur in athymic B/W mice (16). Finally, monoclonal antibodies (MAb) against CD4$^+$ T cells can prevent murine lupus in B/W mice (17). These findings establish that T cells are required for the development of autoimmune disease in B/W mice.

### Role of Sex Hormones

The female-predominant pattern of disease among B/W mice has made this an attractive model for studies designed to gain insight into the mechanisms responsible for the female pre-

**TABLE 46.2.** *Key characteristics of murine models for systemic lupus erythematosus*

| Strain | Characteristic features | | | |
|---|---|---|---|---|
| | Genes | Sex | Lymphoproliferation | Clinical features |
| B/W | Multiple genes from each parent | Female predominance (androgens protect; estrogens augment) | Generalized hyperplasia | Glomerulonephritis Sjögren's syndrome |
| MRL/*lpr* | *Fas* defect (and multiple background genes) | Both sexes affected (modest protection by androgens) | Marked increase in CD4$^-$/CD8$^-$ T cells | Lymphadenopathy; glomerulonephritis; arthritis, vasculitis |
| BXSB | Y chromosome (and multiple background genes) | Male predominance (unrelated to sex hormones) | Increase in B cells and monocytes | Glomerulonephritis |

disposition to autoimmune diseases in humans. In B/W mice, the female predisposition to SLE can be explained almost entirely by the effects of sex hormones. For example, castration of male B/W mice early in life (i.e., before puberty) produces a female pattern of disease with enhanced autoantibody production and markedly accelerated mortality relative to control male B/W mice (18). Prepubertal castration of females did not alter the course of the disease (19). When these mice were treated with androgenic hormones, however, autoimmune disease was retarded; when these mice were treated with estrogenic hormones, autoimmune disease was accelerated (19). These findings provide strong evidence that androgens exert a protective effect in B/W mice, whereas estrogens exert a detrimental effect.

The mechanism by which sex hormones influence the expression of autoimmune disease in B/W mice remains uncertain. Experiments designed to identify primary abnormalities in sex hormone metabolism in B/W mice have generally produced negative results (20). Therefore, it has been speculated that the influence of sex hormones in the setting of autoimmunity may simply be a manifestation of the effects of sex hormones on immune function generally. For example, in nonautoimmune mice, estrogens enhance immune responses and interfere with tolerance induction, whereas androgens inhibit immune responses (21–23). The precise molecular mechanisms through which sex hormones exert these effects has not been established, but evidence suggests that effects on cytokine gene expression may play a role (24).

The profound effects of sex hormone manipulation in B/W mice have led to some new ideas regarding the treatment of SLE. Roubinian et al. (25) showed that androgen administration retards lupus nephritis and prolongs life even in the advanced stages of disease in B/W female mice. Based on this observation, Petri et al. (26) tested a relatively nonvirilizing androgen, dehydroepiandrosterone (DHEA), in humans with SLE. Preliminary results of this work have demonstrated a modest benefit. The full potential of hormone manipulation as a therapeutic strategy remains to be determined.

### Role of Viruses

There has long been interest in the possible role of endogenous retroviruses in B/W mice, just as there has been continuing speculation that a yet undiscovered virus may contribute to SLE in people. Initially, studies of the role of viruses in murine lupus focused on an endogenous retroviral envelope protein designated gp70. All mouse strains express gp70, but nonautoimmune strains are tolerant to this antigen. In contrast, B/W mice produce large amounts of anti-gp70 antibody and have been shown to have circulating and intrarenal immune complexes that contain gp70 (27). These observations suggested that gp70 might be an important inciting antigen in murine lupus. Subsequent analyses of NZB backcrosses, however, cast doubt on this hypothesis. In particular, virus-negative offspring from these crosses develop other autoantibodies, and the development of glomerulonephritis

in the offspring does not correlate with viral expression (28,29). Studies using oligonucleotide probes have confirmed these observations by demonstrating that the levels of viral transcripts do not correlate with disease expression (30,31).

Another endogenous retroviral product has been implicated in murine lupus. This product is derived from a polytropic, or Mink cell focus–forming (MCF), retrovirus. It is abundantly expressed as a full-length transcript in thymic RNA from all lupus-prone strains of mice, whereas it is expressed only in small quantities in nonautoimmune strains (30,31). Studies are in progress to determine the significance of this retroviral sequence in the pathogenesis of murine lupus.

### Genetic Basis of Autoimmune Disease in B/W Mice

The genetics of autoimmunity in B/W mice are complex. Both the NZB and the NZW parents provide multiple genes that contribute to the development of autoimmune disease. The key contribution from the NZW parent resides on chromosome 17 and appears to involve the major histocompatibility complex (MHC) genes of the $H\text{-}2^z$ genotype (32,33). Heterozygosity for $H\text{-}2^{d/z}$ confers maximum susceptibility, thus implicating an MHC-linked contribution by the NZB parent as well (32–34). Another gene within the H-2 complex may also contribute to murine lupus. This gene codes for tumor necrosis factor-α (TNF-α). A polymorphism in the TNF-α gene in NZW mice causes a deficiency of TNF-α activity (35). Correction of this deficiency by administration of TNF-α ameliorates lupus nephritis in B/W mice, suggesting that this genetic polymorphism may contribute to autoimmunity.

Genome-wide linkage studies in mice derived from the NZB and NZW strains have mapped the position of at least 12 non-MHC loci that can enhance disease susceptibility and influence disease expression in B/W mice (reviewed in 32). In addition, there appear to be other loci that can diminish the effects of the disease-susceptibility genes. Among the non-MHC disease susceptibility loci, three regions have received particular attention. Sle1 on chromosome 1, Sle2 on chromosome 4, and Sle3 on chromosome 7 all strongly contribute to lupus susceptibility in B/W mice. Genetic studies designed to dissect the contribution of each of these loci have shown that they have different effects (32,36). Sle1 is associated with selective loss of tolerance to distinct subnucleosomal antigens and the development of mild nephritis. Sle2 is associated with expansion of B1 cells and polyclonal increases in IgM, but not with IgG autoantibody production or nephritis. Sle3 is associated with the production of ANAs and the development of mild nephritis. Thus, individual susceptibility genes appear to contribute some, but not all, of the abnormalities characteristic of SLE (32,37–39). Thus far, only the MHC region has been linked to all three of the cardinal features of murine lupus, including autoantibody production, severe glomerulonephritis, and mortality (37).

### Treatment of B/W Mice

The similarities between murine lupus in B/W mice and SLE in humans have suggested that therapeutic strategies that prove to be effective in B/W mice may also be effective in people with SLE. Consistent with this expectation, corticosteroids ameliorate autoimmune disease in B/W mice (5), and pulse cyclophosphamide was shown to be effective in B/W mice (40) before it became established as an important therapeutic option for humans with lupus nephritis (41).

The B/W model has been used to test a host of new therapeutic strategies that are based on the rapid progress that has occurred in our understanding of the molecular biology of the immune system. Some of these strategies are designed to interfere with distinct cell-surface molecules that are required for T-cell recognition of antigen (42,43). Other strategies are designed to prevent the production of pathogenic autoantibodies by modulating the B-cell repertoire (44). Still others are designed to block distinct cytokines that promote autoimmunity (45–47) or to augment cytokines that may inhibit autoimmunity (35). Considerable attention is focused on the use of agents that block T-cell costimulation. Specifically, blockade of either the B7/CD28 pathway of T-cell costimulation or the CD40/CD40-ligand pathway of T-cell costimulation dramatically retards lupus nephritis in B/W mice (48–50). Moreover, brief simultaneous blockade of both of these pathways produces long-lasting clinical benefit in B/W mice without causing sustained generalized immune suppression (Fig. 46.1). These strategies are the subject of clinical trials that are designed to determine whether the promising results in B/W mice will herald a new era of improved treatments for humans with SLE.

### MRL/*lpr* and Other FAS-Defective Mice

The MRL/*lpr* mouse has been a particularly informative model of autoimmunity because it has led to the identification and characterization of a single gene, *lpr*, that dramatically accelerates murine lupus. The parent MRL strain was established from crosses of several standard mouse strains. During these crosses, a mutant with lymphadenopathy and splenomegaly, as well as marked systemic autoimmunity, was discovered and designated *lpr*, for lymphoproliferation (51). This autosomal recessive *lpr* mutation was then localized to chromosome 19 (52). Subsequently, a second, phenotypically similar autosomal recessive mutation was described in the inbred C3H/HeJ strain and localized to chromosome 1 (53,54). This mutation was designated *gld*, for generalized lymphoproliferative disease. Homozygosity of either mutation results in lymphoproliferation and autoimmunity. F1 mice derived by crossing *lpr/lpr* mice with *gld/gld* mice are phenotypically normal, however, indicating that these two mutations are not complementary. To determine the relationship between these mutations, Allen et al. (55) performed a series of bone marrow transplantations between wild-type MRL mice and *lpr* and *gld* mutant mice. These studies established

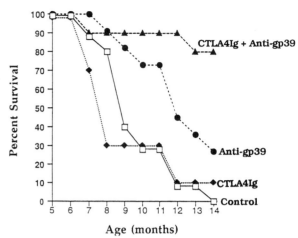

**FIG. 46.1.** Female B/W mice were treated for 2 weeks at age 5 months with either CTLA4Ig alone (*closed diamond*), hamster monoclonal antibody (MAb) to gp39 alone (*closed circle*), a combination of both CTLA4Ig and mAb to gp39 (*closed triangle*), or a combination of a control mAb and purified hamster immunoglobulin G (*open square*). CTLA4Ig blocks CD28-mediated T-cell costimulation, and anti-gp39 blocks CD40-ligand–mediated T-cell costimulation. This experiment demonstrates that brief simultaneous blockade of both costimulation pathways significantly prolongs survival in B/W mice. (From Daikh DI, Finck BK, Linsley PS, et al. Long-term inhibition of murine lupus by brief simultaneous blockade of the B7/CD28 and CD40/gp39 costimulation pathways. *J Immunol* 1997;159:3104–3108, with permission Copyright 1997 by The American Association of Immunologists.)

that the *lpr* and *gld* mutations represent a receptor–ligand pair of molecules. Another similar, but clinically less severe mutation, which is allelic to *lpr*, was subsequently discovered in CBA/KlJms mice. This mutation was designated *lprcg* because it complements the *gld* mutation (56).

### Molecular Basis of the lpr and gld Defects

The *lpr* and *gld* defects represent mutations in the genes encoding the FAS protein and its ligand (FASL), respectively (57,58). FAS is a 45-kd protein that was originally identified as the target of an MAb that could induce a stereotypical process of programmed cell death, or apoptosis, in lymphocytes (59). FAS is a type I membrane protein and is a member of the TNF receptor family. This gene is expressed in activated T lymphocytes as well as the thymus, liver, lung, heart, and ovary (60). Antibodies against FAS are cytotoxic; in particular, anti–human FAS antibody induces apoptosis in murine cells that express human FAS, implying that FAS is able to transduce an apoptotic signal (61). The ligand for FAS was isolated from a cytotoxic T-lymphocyte (CTL) cell line that was able to kill FAS$^+$, but not FAS$^-$, cells. FASL is a 40-kd type II membrane protein with significant homology to the TNF family in its extracellular domain (62,63). The role of this receptor–ligand pair in apoptosis was proved by the demonstration that Cos cells expressing recombinant FASL can induce apoptosis of FAS-expressing cells (64).

When the chromosomal localization of the *fas* gene was determined, it mapped to the same region as the *lpr* mutation on chromosome 19 (60). Northern analysis indicated that little FAS is expressed in MRL/*lpr* tissues. Analysis of the structure of the *fas* gene cloned from MRL/*lpr* mice demonstrated that it contains an early transposable element within the second intron, resulting in premature termination and abnormal splicing of the primary FAS transcript (65). Although a few full-length FAS transcripts are produced, their level is a fraction of that observed in wild-type mice (57). In contrast, the *lprcg* mutant has normal levels of FAS mRNA. In this mutant, however, there is a T-to-A transversion, resulting in replacement of an isoleucine with asparagine within the cytoplasmic domain of FAS, which renders it unable to transduce an apoptotic signal (57). Formal demonstration of the role of FAS in MRL/*lpr* mice was provided by an experiment in which normal FAS protein expressed by a transgene prevented disease (66). The *gld* mutation is a T-to-C transition that replaces a phenylalanine near the C terminus of FASL with leucine, which destroys its ability to bind FAS (58).

### Clinical and Serologic Features

MRL/*lpr* mice develop massive nonmalignant lymphoproliferation as well as many manifestations of autoimmunity, including autoantibody production, glomerulonephritis, vasculitis, and arthritis (1,51). Female mice are affected slightly more severely than male mice and have a mean life expectancy of 5 months, compared with 6 months in male mice (Table 46.1). At the time of death, there is massive lymphadenopathy, with lymph node enlargement up to 100 times normal, and frequent lymph node medullary necrosis. Lymphocytic infiltration of other organs, such as the spleen and salivary glands, also occurs (67,68). This lymphoproliferation, which is begins to appear at about age 6 weeks, is the result of the accumulation of large numbers of an unusual T-lymphocyte subpopulation that is not seen in normal adult mice. Like other T-cell subpopulations, these cells undergo polyclonal rearrangement of the T-cell receptor (TCR); however, the expression of cell-surface TCR is low (69–71). These cells also display a number of other T-cell markers, including CD3 and Thy1, but they are CD4 and CD8 negative (72,73). These so-called double-negative (DN) T cells also express the B-cell marker B220 (74). These cells can be distinguished from the normal population of DN thymic T cells in the normal developing thymus on the basis of differences in surface markers and function (75). Although there is expansion of these abnormal cell populations in *lpr/lpr* mice, these cells do not proliferate in culture at baseline, nor in response to anti-CD3 or IL-2, which may in part result from a decrease in IL-2 receptor levels (76). Thus, the accumulation of DN T cells in the periphery does not appear to be the result of abnormal proliferation, but rather of the loss of normal programmed cell death (77).

Although profound lymphoproliferation is a distinguishing feature of MRL/*lpr* mice, these mice also develop a number of clinical features that are similar to those seen in other lupus-prone mouse strains and in humans with SLE (Table 46.2). These include proliferative glomerulonephritis with immune complex and complement deposition (78); necrotizing vasculitis involving medium-sized arteries, especially in the renal, mesenteric, and coronary vasculature (79); lupus-like inflammation at the dermoepidermal junction (80); interstitial pneumonitis or pulmonary vasculitis (81); and production of autoantibodies (1). The clinical features in *lpr/lpr* mice and the range of autoantibodies that they produce are critically dependent on background genes. Thus, MRL/*lpr* mice develop severe nephritis and produce antibodies to nuclear antigens and chromatin, dsDNA, Sm, Su, and the ribosomal P antigen, whereas B6/*lpr* mice have much milder nephritis and produce only antichromatin autoantibodies (1,82–84). MRL/*lpr* mice also demonstrate some features that are suggestive of rheumatoid arthritis (RA), including the production of IgM rheumatoid factor and the development of an inflammatory, proliferative synovitis (1,85,86). High levels of circulating IgG3 results in cryoglobulins in some mice (87,88). The clinical manifestations in *gld* mice are remarkably similar to those in *lpr* mice, including clinical autoimmunity and lymphoproliferation with large numbers of DN T cells (53,73).

### Immunological Features

The *lpr* and *gld* mice display many abnormalities of immune function. Nonspecific polyclonal B-cell activation occurs, resulting in extremely high levels of circulating IgG and a wide range of autoantibodies (89). MHC class II expression is also increased (90). Moreover, B cells from MRL/*lpr* mice are relatively resistant to tolerance induction compared those from with wild-type mice (91). B-cell responses to specific antigens and polyclonal B-cell activators are diminished, however (92,93).

The function of the T-cell compartment is also aberrant in these mice. In addition to the abnormalities involving DN T cells, there are abnormalities among the phenotypically normal CD4$^+$ T cells. CD4$^+$ T cells in these mice have decreased IL-2 production and decreased proliferation in response to mitogen stimulation (94). CD4$^+$ T cells are also resistant to activation-induced cell death by anti-CD3 or anti-TCR antibodies (95). Autoreactive CD4$^+$ T cells are present before the onset of clinical lymphadenopathy, and their numbers are increased compared with wild-type mice (96). These autoreactive cells are capable of proliferating in response to IL-2 *in vitro* (97). Evidence that autoimmunity in *lpr* mice is dependent on autoreactive CD4$^+$ T cells comes from studies demonstrating that treatment with MAb to CD4 can retard, and in some cases prevent, autoimmunity (98,99). This conclusion is also supported by studies indicating that MHC class II–deficient or CD4-deficient MRL/*lpr* mice do not develop autoimmunity (100,101).

### Relationship Between Lymphoproliferation and Autoimmunity

Although elimination of CD4$^+$ T cells prevents autoimmunity, it does not reduce lymphoproliferation (100,101). Conversely, elimination of CD8$^+$ T cells prevents lymphoproliferation but has little effect on autoantibody production (102,103). Other interventions, such as treatment with cyclosporine (104) or anti–interferon-γ (IFN-γ) antibody (105), have also been shown to reduce lymphoproliferation but not autoimmunity. These findings imply that the accumulation of DN T cells is not directly responsible for the development of autoimmunity. This conclusion is consistent with the observation that the levels of total IgG, or of specific autoantibodies, do not correlate with the absolute numbers of DN T cells in MRL/lpr mice (105).

Examination of the effects of the lpr and gld mutations on diverse genetic backgrounds has also revealed a dissociation between lymphoproliferation and autoimmunity. Although lymphoproliferation is invariably present in mouse strains that bear the lpr or gld mutations, autoimmune phenomena are variable (106). Antinuclear, antichromatin, and anti-dsDNA antibodies are found in most lpr strains, but anti-Sm, anti-Su, and anti–ribosomal-P autoantibodies are found only in the MRL background (82). On the other hand, IgM rheumatoid factor is produced in the highest levels in C57BL/6-lpr mice (107). Unlike MRL/lpr mice, most lpr strains do not develop nephritis or arthritis (106). Interestingly, wild-type MRL mice develop low autoantibody titers late in life, even when they lack lpr. Taken together, these findings imply that the development of autoimmunity is dependent on the action of various background genes and is greatly accentuated by the lpr and gld mutations.

### BXSB Mice

Like B/W and MRL/lpr mice, BXSB mice spontaneously produce anti-dsDNA antibodies and develop immune complex glomerulonephritis suggestive of SLE in humans (1,108). BXSB mice are unique among murine models for SLE, however, in that male BXSB mice are more severely affected than female BXSB mice (Table 46.1) (108). Acceleration of disease in the male mice is not a result of hormonal influences, but rather reflects genetic factors residing on the Y chromosome (108,109). Interestingly, when BXSB male mice are crossed with other lupus-prone mice, the F1 male offspring develop a lupus-like illness that resembles murine lupus in BXSB males (110). When BXSB male mice are crossed with mice from normal strains, however, the male offspring do not develop autoimmunity (111). These findings indicate that the Y chromosome provides an accelerating factor for autoimmunity but that predisposing background genes are also required for the development of lupus.

The mechanism of autoimmune disease in BXSB mice is poorly understood. The lymphoid abnormalities that occur in BXSB male mice differ somewhat from the lymphoid abnor-

malities in other lupus-prone mice in that BXSB male mice develop B-cell hyperplasia (112) and marked monocytosis (113). The importance of B cells in the development of autoimmunity in this model has been confirmed by the demonstration that the xid mutation protects BXSB mice against lupus nephritis. Like murine lupus in B/W mice, however, murine lupus in BXSB mice is also dependent on T cells. Male BXSB mice exhibit marked shifts from naive to memory CD4$^+$ T cells early in life (114), and their disease can be suppressed by treatment with MAb to CD4 (115) or by blockade of T-cell costimulation (116).

Although the male-predominant pattern of disease in BXSB mice suggests fundamental differences between lupus in this strain and lupus in humans, it is possible that the mechanisms that promote autoimmunity in BSXB mice may contribute to autoimmunity in at least a subset of humans. In this respect, it is interesting that a pattern of father-to-son inheritance of SLE has been described in some human families (117).

## AUTOIMMUNE DIABETES MELLITUS

### Nonobese Diabetic Mice

The nonobese diabetic mouse (NOD) is a spontaneous model of organ-specific autoimmune diabetes that shares many features with autoimmune diabetes in humans. The NOD mouse was derived in Japan from a diabetic female mouse discovered among a group of outbred Jcl-ICR mice being used to derive a spontaneous cataract model. Inbreeding of diabetes-prone sublines from the original founder resulted in the NOD mouse (118). The frequency of insulin-dependent diabetes mellitus (IDDM) varies among different NOD colonies, with an incidence ranging from 20% to 100% in 30-week-old female mice (119). Because NOD colonies all represent the same highly inbred strain, the differences in disease incidence are most likely a result of incompletely defined environmental factors rather than genetic differences between colonies (120). The presence of microbial agents may be one of the environmental factors because the incidence of disease in a given colony is higher when the mice are kept in a pathogen-free environment (121). In this respect, NOD mice differ from other autoimmune murine models, including B/W mice, in which disease severity is typically reduced by maintaining the colony in a pathogen-free environment.

### Clinical and Pathologic Characteristics

In typical high-incidence colonies, 80% to 90% of female mice and 45% to 50% of male mice become insulin-dependent between 3 and 7 months of age (119). The pathologic basis for IDDM in NOD mice, and in humans, is destruction of β cells in the pancreatic islets. The progression of this β-cell destruction in NOD mice is well characterized. The earliest pathologic abnormality is the development of an insulitis, beginning at 3 to 4 weeks of age (122). This inflammatory islet cell infiltration is seen in all NOD mice and consists of dendritic cells, macrophages, B cells, and large numbers of T cells (123). While virtually all NOD mice develop insulitis, some do not progress to insulin dependence, suggesting that multiple factors contribute to the full expression of disease.

### Role of T Cells

A number of lines of evidence point to T cells as the primary mediator of β-cell destruction. First, athymic *(nu/nu)* NOD mice do not develop diabetes (124). Second, adoptive transfer of T cells from diabetic NOD mice transfers insulitis and diabetes to adult NOD-*scid* mice (125) or to healthy neonatal NOD mice (126). Third, treatment with anti–T-cell MAb blocks the development of disease (127).

Both CD4$^+$ and CD8$^+$ T cells have been implicated in the β-cell destruction in NOD mice (125,126,128,129). CD8$^+$ T cells, along with monocytes, are the first cells to appear in the insulitic lesion (130); CD4$^+$ T cells appear later. In addition, the NOD-β$_2$-microglobulin knockout mouse, which has very few CD8$^+$ T cells, does not develop significant insulitis or diabetes (131,132). These results indicate that CD8$^+$ T cells function as effector cells in IDDM in the NOD mouse. It is clear, however, that a subset of CD4$^+$ T cells also constitutes important effector cells in NOD mice. In particular, T$_H$1-type T cells are much more numerous among islet-infiltrating T cells (133–136). These cells secrete high levels of IFN-γ and TNF-α. As a result, there is an increased IFN-γ–to–IL-4 ratio in pancreatic islets of female NOD mice with insulitis, beginning around age 4 weeks (132,136). These female mice have a high rate of progression to IDDM. On the other hand, male mice with insulitis, but a much lower rate of diabetes, have a high IL-4–to–IFN-γ ratio, reflecting a predominance of T$_H$2 cells.

The importance of T$_H$1 cells in autoimmune diabetes is also supported by studies demonstrating that treatment with IL-12, which promotes differentiation of T$_H$1 cells and induces expression of IFN-γ, results in the rapid induction of IDDM (137). Thus, islet cell destruction in NOD mice is associated with a skewing of the helper T-cell population toward a T$_H$1 phenotype, implying that the balance of T$_H$1 versus T$_H$2 T cells within the pancreatic islet is a crucial factor in determining whether there will be β-cell destruction and subsequent diabetes. This hypothesis is also supported by studies in CD28-deficient or CTLA4Ig transgenic NOD mice (138). In the absence of T-cell costimulation by CD28, the autoreactive T cells that develop in these mice produce increased levels of T$_H$1 cytokines and decreased levels of T$_H$2 cytokines, a factor that is associated with the development of an accelerated pattern of disease.

Although both CD4$^+$ and CD8$^+$ T cells contribute to the development of diabetes in NOD mice, there is also evidence that some T cells may exert a regulatory effect that protects against β-cell destruction. For example, a subset of CD4$^+$ T cells from prediabetic NOD mice was able to prevent transfer of diabetes by splenic cells from diabetic mice (139). The

existence of protective regulatory T cells is also postulated to explain the seemingly paradoxical observation that the lymphotoxic alkylating agent cyclophosphamide rapidly induces diabetes in mice with preexisting insulitis, presumably by preferentially killing regulatory cells that inhibit islet cell destruction (140–142). These observations are consistent with the postulate that some CD4$^+$ T cells (T$_H$1 cells) promote diabetes in NOD mice, whereas other CD4$^+$ T cells (T$_H$2 cells) may inhibit diabetes.

T-cell lines from NOD mice have also been helpful in confirming the role of T$_H$1 and T$_H$2 cells in the development of β-cell destruction. Katz et al. (143) produced T$_H$1 and T$_H$2 cell lines that expressed identical diabetogenic TCRs. Cells from both of these lines caused insulitis when injected into neonatal NOD mice, but only the T$_H$1 line caused diabetes.

### Role of Autoantigens

A major unanswered question about the pathogenesis of both insulitis and β-cell destruction in the NOD mouse, and in humans, is whether T cells initially recognize a single autoantigen, or whether the disease is the result of autoreactivity toward multiple islet antigens. Several possible targets of autoreactive T cells have been identified in NOD mice, including insulin, proinsulin, glutamic acid decarboxylase (GAD), and heat shock protein 60 (hsp60). Identification of a long-recognized 65-kd autoantigen as GAD, and the observation that T-cell reactivity toward GAD65 is present in 3-week-old NOD mice, suggested that this could be the primary antigen in autoimmune diabetes (144–146). Consistent with this hypothesis, tolerization of neonatal NOD mice with GAD65 prevents the development of insulitis and diabetes (147). However, tolerization with insulin β chain, insulin, proinsulin, or a fragment of hsp70 also prevents IDDM (148–152). In addition, among the various diabetogenic antigens that have been proposed, only insulin is specific to the β-cell, and insulin-reactive T cells are present very early in NOD mice (153,154). Nevertheless, active immunization with insulin, or with any of the other candidate autoantigens, does not induce insulitis in NOD mice (121).

Identification of the putative initiating autoantigens is further complicated by the phenomenon of epitope spreading, which has been demonstrated in islet-specific T cells from NOD mice (146,155). It is not possible, therefore, to implicate with certainty any single antigen as the inciting or primary autoantigen in the NOD model of autoimmune diabetes.

Other efforts to identify relevant autoantigens in the NOD mouse have taken an indirect approach by looking for restricted TCR repertoires. Islet cell–reactive T-cell clones isolated from infiltrated islets and from the periphery of NOD mice have been studied by several groups. In almost all cases, there has been heterogeneity of TCR expression (156–160). T cells expressing a single Vβ gene product, however, were isolated from preinsulitic 2-week-old NOD mice (161), suggesting that insulitis may be initiated by a single autoantigen.

Simone et al. (160) studied TCR gene use among T-cell clones isolated from early (prediabetic) islet lesions and found that, although there was no restriction in Vβ-chain use, a single Vα chain was expressed. These clones were reactive with a peptide from the insulin β chain and could adoptively transfer IDDM to prediabetic NOD mice (160). In addition, CD8+ T-cell clones isolated from islets of diabetic NOD mice were found to have highly homologous Vα and Vβ gene sequences (162), also suggesting that CD8+ T cells may be recognizing a single or limited number of islet autoantigens.

### Role of Viruses

An alternate theory for the pathogenesis of IDDM in humans and in NOD mice is that the initial diabetogenic antigen is a viral antigen and that much of the abnormal T-cell reactivity observed is the result of molecular mimicry. Interestingly, there is significant structural homology between a GAD65 epitope and a protein from coxsackievirus B4 (163), a virus that has been epidemiologically linked to the development of IDDM in humans (164). The role of viral infection in NOD mice is not clear. Lymphocytic infiltrates occur in NOD mice in organs other than the endocrine pancreas, such as lacrimal and salivary glands, suggesting at least the possibility that this may represent a response to a chronic endogenous viral infection (165).

### Genetic Basis of Autoimmune Disease in NOD Mice

Our understanding of the genetic control of autoimmunity has been advanced significantly by genetic studies in NOD mice. Crosses of NOD mice with nondiabetic strains indicate that diabetes is a polygenic trait (166). At least 14 genetic loci have been linked to the development of IDDM; however, genetic back-crosses demonstrating a high incidence of insulitis without IDDM have suggested that the development of insulitis is controlled by one or only a few genes (120). The first locus identified, *Idd1,* maps to the MHC locus on chromosome 17 (167–169). Susceptibility to diabetes is associated with several genes within the MHC complex. In particular, a number of abnormalities of specific MHC class II alleles correlate highly with disease onset and severity (120). NOD mice ($K^d$, I-A$^{g7}$, I-E$^{null}$, D$^b$) lack I-E expression because of a deletion in the Ea promoter (167). The I-Aβ$^{g7}$ of NOD mice contains serine at residue 57 rather than aspartic acid, which is present at this position in other strains. Serine, alanine, or valine in position 57 of the homologous locus in humans (HLA-DQβ) correlates with susceptibility to IDDM, whereas aspartic acid in this position is associated with resistance to IDDM (170). These similarities between the NOD mouse and humans with IDDM strongly implicate this MHC class II allele in autoimmune diabetes and further support the value of the NOD strain as a model for IDDM in humans.

Although the expression of native I-A$^{g7}$ is necessary for the development of diabetes, mutation of amino acid 57 to aspartic acid does not prevent the development of insulitis (171).

Thus, the expression of I-A$^{g7}$ does not prevent the development of autoreactive T cells. The function of aspartic acid in position 57 of the Aβ (DQ) chain has not been established, but by analogy with other class II structures, this residue likely affects peptide binding by the MHC class II molecule (172). Thus, I-A$^{g7}$ molecules may present antigen inefficiently to autoreactive T cells, resulting in persistence, rather than deletion, of these clones during selection of the T-cell repertoire (173,174). In addition to I-A$^{g7}$ and other MHC-linked genes, a number of non-MHC genes are required for the development of IDDM in NOD mice (120). The eventual mapping of these loci will ultimately lead to the identification of these genes and the determination of their function. These discoveries can be expected to provide not only a better understanding of the pathogenesis of autoimmune diabetes but also provide insight into the development of polygenic autoimmune diseases in general.

## MURINE MODELS FOR OTHER AUTOIMMUNE DISEASES

### Motheaten Mice

Severe systemic autoimmunity and immunodeficiency occur in mice that have an autosomal recessive mutation, designated motheaten (*me*), on chromosome 6 (175). These mice have severe defects in hematopoiesis, including developmental and structural abnormalities in T cells, B cells, natural killer cells, macrophages, and granulocytes (176). One of the earliest clinical abnormalities in these mice is the development at age 3 to 4 days of patchy loss of pigment from the skin, followed shortly thereafter by patchy thinning or absence of hair, resulting in the motheaten appearance from which this model gets its name (175). The skin changes are associated with the development of skin abscesses, with marked accumulations of neutrophils. These cutaneous manifestations are followed by severe pneumonitis with infiltration by lymphocytes and macrophages. Motheaten mice also develop immune complex glomerulonephritis, associated with hypergammaglobulinemia and production of anti-dsDNA antibodies (175,176). They die at a mean age of only 3 weeks. A variant of the motheaten mutation, designated motheaten viable (*me^v/me^v*), produces a slightly more protracted course of illness with a mean life expectancy of 9 weeks (177).

The basic defect in motheaten mice appears to reside in hematopoietic progenitor cells in the bone marrow. Thus, bone marrow from *me/me* (or *mev/mev*) mice can transfer the disease into irradiated recipients; conversely, reconstitution of motheaten mice with bone marrow from normal mice can protect them against the disease (176). The precise defect in hematopoietic cells has been elucidated by the discovery that the *me* mutation involves a gene that encodes the SHP-1 protein tyrosine phosphatase, previously termed hematopoietic cell phosphatase (*Hcph*) (178). This phosphatase is an important negative regulator of signal transduction in hematopoietic cells. In particular, it associates with CD22 on B cells and produces dephosphorylation of the B-cell–receptor complex (179). These findings imply that failure to provide down-regulation of B cells may be the mechanism by which the SHP-1 defect causes autoimmunity in motheaten mice. This postulate is supported by the observation that similar auto-immune syndromes develop in knockout mice that lack either Lyn or CD22, two other molecules that contribute to B-cell–receptor signaling (179,180).

## Tight Skin Mice

Two strains of mice that have tight skin (Tsk1 and Tsk2 mice) have been used as models for scleroderma (181,182). These mice overproduce collagen and develop thickened skin that is bound down to the subcutaneous tissue and underlying muscle. In each strain, the pathology can be traced to an autosomal dominant gene. In Tsk1 mice, the disease is caused by a gene on chromosome 2; in Tsk2 mice, the disease is caused by a gene on chromosome 1. The precise nature of these genes remains to be determined. Although the cutaneous abnormalities in Tsk mice bear a resemblance to scleroderma in humans, other abnormalities are quite distinct from scleroderma. For example, Tsk1 mice develop pulmonary emphysema rather than pulmonary fibrosis (183). It is not clear whether autoimmunity is the basis for the pathology in Tsk mice.

## Transgenic and Knockout Mice

Advances in molecular biology have made it possible to insert, or delete, selected genes in inbred strains of mice. This strategy has made it possible to create many new murine models in which to study the role of distinct genes and gene products in the pathogenesis of autoimmunity.

The insertion of distinct genes creates new models that are referred to as *transgenic*. The development of transgenic models is accomplished by injecting a gene, in the form of a DNA fragment, into a fertilized egg (184). The animal that subsequently arises from that egg expresses the gene and can be used to breed a colony of animals, all of which express the transgene. This approach has already been used to clarify the role of numerous genes and their products in the development of autoimmunity. For example, the *HLA-B27* gene has been transferred into mice and rats, where its expression produces a murine model for seronegative arthritis and inflammatory bowel disease (185). The TNF-α gene has also been expressed in transgenic mice, where it causes a chronic inflammatory arthritis with features of RA (186). This model has received particular attention lately in light of clinical trials indicating that selective blockade of TNF-α reduces inflammation in humans with RA (187,188). Other cytokines, including IFN-γ, IL-10, and transforming growth factor-β, have all been studied in transgenic models to determine their role in the pathogenesis of autoimmune diabetes (189). Transgenic models have also been used to examine the effects of costimulatory cell-surface molecules, such as B7-1, in promoting the development of diabetes (190).

The deletion of distinct genes by targeted mutagenesis has created other models that are useful in determining the functions of individual genes *in vivo*. In these models, gene deletion (or "knockout") is accomplished by homologous recombination of a specific gene in embryonic stem cells (184). After the gene has been inactivated by this technique, the stem cells are transferred into blastocyst embryos, which then develop into animals that can be used to breed a colony of mice with the selected gene knockout. Like transgenic technology, this technology has been used to examine the role of distinct cytokines (191–197) and cell-surface molecules (198–201) in the pathogenesis of autoimmunity. Together, these twin technologies hold the promise of countless new inbred murine models that will help to clarify our understanding of the mechanisms of autoimmunity in humans.

## REFERENCES

1. Andrews BS, Eisenberg RS, Theofilopoulos AN, et al. Spontaneous murine lupus-like syndromes: clinical and immunopathological manifestations in several strains. *J Exp Med* 1978;148:1198–1215.
2. Steinberg AD, Raveché ES, Laskin CA, et al. Systemic lupus erythematosus: insights from animal models. *Ann Intern Med* 1984;100: 714–727.
3. Bielschowsky M, Helyer BJ, Howie JB. Spontaneous anemia in mice of the NZB/Bl strain. *Proc Univ Otago Med School* 1961;39:3–4.
4. Helyer BJ, Howie JB. Renal disease associated with positive lupus erythematosus in cross-bred strains of mice. *Nature* 1963;197:197.
5. Howie JB, Helyer BJ. The immunology and pathology of NZB mice. *Adv Immunol* 1968;9:215–266.
6. Talal N. Autoimmunity and lymphoid malignancy in New Zealand black mice. *Prog Clin Immunol* 1974;2:101–120.
7. Lambert PH, Dixon FS. Pathogenesis of the glomerulonephritis of NZB/NZW mice. *J Exp Med* 1968;127:507–522.
8. Jonsson R, Tarkowski A, Bäckman K, et al. Immunohistochemical characterization of sialadenitis in NZB × NZW F1 mice. *Clin Immunol Immunopathol* 1987;42:93–101.
9. Yoshida S, Castles JJ, Gershwin ME. The pathogenesis of autoimmunity in New Zealand mice. *Semin Arthritis Rheum* 1990;19:224–242.
10. Herron LR, Coffman RL, Bond MW, et al. Increased autoantibody production by NZB/NZW B cells in response to IL-5. *J Immunol* 1988; 141:842–848.
11. Alarcon-Riguelme ME, Moller G, Fernandez C. Age-dependent responsiveness of interleukin-6 in B lymphocytes from systemic lupus erythematosus-prone (NZB × NZW) F1 hybrid. *Clin Immunol Immunopathol* 1992;62:264–269.
12. Steinberg B, Smathers P, Frederiksen K, et al. Ability of the *xid* gene to prevent autoimmunity in (NZB x NZW) F1 mice during the course of their natural history, after polyclonal stimulation, or following immunization with DNA. *J Clin Invest* 1982;70:587–597.
13. Mohan C, Morel L, Yang P, et al. Accumulation of splenic B1a cells with potent antigen-presenting capability in NZM2410 lupus-prone mice. *Arthritis Rheum* 1998;41:1652–1662.
14. Taurog J, Raveché E, Smathers P, et al. T cell abnormalities in NZB mice occur independently of autoantibody production. *J Exp Med* 1981;153:221–234.
15. Datta SK, Patel H, Berry D. Induction of a cationic shift in IgG anti-DNA autoantibodies: role of T helper cells with classical and novel phenotypes in three murine models of lupus nephritis. *J Exp Med* 1987; 165:1252–1268.
16. Mihara M, Ohsugi Y, Saito K, et al. Immunologic abnormality in NZB/NZW F1 mice: thymus-independent occurrence of B cell abnormality and requirement for T cells in the development of autoimmune disease, as evidenced by an analysis of the athymic nude individuals. *J Immunol* 1988;141:85–90.

17. Wofsy D, Seaman WE. Successful treatment of autoimmunity in NZB/NZW F1 mice with monoclonal antibody to L3T4. *J Exp Med* 1985;161:378–391.

18. Roubinian JR, Papoian R, Talal N. Androgenic hormones modulate autoantibody responses and improve survival in murine lupus. *J Clin Invest* 1977;59:1066–1070.

19. Roubinian JR, Talal N, Greenspan JS, et al. Effect of castration and sex hormone treatment on survival, anti-nucleic acid antibodies, and glomerulonephritis in NZB/NZW F1 mice. *J Exp Med* 1978;147:1568–1583.

20. Baer AN, Green FA. Estrogen metabolism in the (New Zealand black × New Zealand white)F1 murine model of systemic lupus erythematosus. *Arthritis Rheum* 1990;33:107–112.

21. Terres G, Morrison SL, Habicht. A quantitative difference in the immune response response between male and female mice. *Proc Soc Exp Biol Med* 1968;127:664–667.

22. Eidinger D, Garrett TJ. Studies of the regulatory effects of the sex hormones on antibody formation and stem cell differentiation. *J Exp Med* 1972;136:1098–1116.

23. Fujii H, Yakibumi N, Tsuchiya H, et al. Effect of a single administration of testosterone on the immune response of lymphoid tissues in mice. *Cell Immunol* 1975;20:315–326.

24. Fox HS, Bond B, Parslow TG. Estrogen regulates the IFN-gamma promoter. *J Immunol* 1991;146:4362–4367.

25. Roubinian JR, Talal N, Greenspan JS, et al. Delayed androgen treatment prolongs survival in murine lupus. *J Clin Invest* 1979;63:902–911.

26. Petri M, Lahita R, McGuire J, et al. Results of the GL701 (DHEA) multicenter steroid-sparing SLE study (abst.). *Arthritis Rheum* 1997;40:S327.

27. Izui S, McConahey PJ, Theofilopoulos AN, et al. Association of circulating retroviral gp70-anti-gp70 immune complexes with murine systemic lupus erythematosus. *J Exp Med* 1979;149:1099–1116.

28. Datta SK, Manny N, Andrzejewski C, et al. Genetic studies of autoimmunity and retrovirus expression in crosses of New Zealand black mice. I. Xenotropic virus. *J Exp Med* 1978;147:854–871.

29. Datta SK, McConahey PJ, Manny N, et al. Genetic studies of autoimmunity and retrovirus expression in crosses of New Zealand black mice. II. The viral envelope glycoprotein gp70. *J Exp Med* 1978;147:872–881.

30. Krieg AM, Steinberg AD, Kahn AS. Increased expression of novel full-length endogenous mink cell focus-forming (MCF)-related transcripts in autoimmune mouse strains. *Virology* 1988;162:274–276.

31. Krieg AM, Kahn AS, Steinberg AD. Expression of an endogenous retroviral transcript is associated with murine lupus. *Arthritis Rheum* 1989;32:322–329.

32. Vyse TJ, Kotzin BL. Genetic susceptibility to systemic lupus erythematosus. *Annu Rev Immunol* 1998;16:261–292.

33. Chiang BL, Bearer E, Ansari A, et al. The BM12 mutation and autoantibodies to dsDNA in NZB.H-2bm12 mice. *J Immunol* 1990;145:94–101.

34. Hirose S, Ueda G, Noguchi K, et al. Requirement of H-2 heterozygosity for autoimmunity in (NZB × NZW) F1 hybrid mice. *Eur J Immunol* 1986;16:1631–1633.

35. Jacob CO, McDevitt HO. Tumor necrosis factor-α in murine autoimmune 'lupus' nephritis. *Nature* 1988;331:356–358.

36. Mohan C, Morel L, Yang P, et al. Genetic dissection of systemic lupus erythematosus pathogenesis. *J Immunol* 1997;159:454–465.

37. Kono DH, Burlingame RW, Owens DG, et al. Lupus susceptibility loci in New Zealand mice. *Proc Natl Acad Sci U S A* 1994;91:10168–10172.

38. Morel L, Rudofsky UH, Longmate JA, et al. Polygenic control of susceptibility to murine systemic lupus erythematosus. *Immunity* 1994;1:219–229.

39. Drake CG, Rozzo SJ, Hirschfeld HF, et al. Analysis of the New Zealand black contribution to lupus-like renal disease: multiple genes that operate in a threshold manner. *J Immunol* 1995;154:2441–2447.

40. Hahn BH, Knotts L, Ng M, et al. Influence of cyclophosphamide and other immunosuppressive drugs on immune disorders and neoplasia in NZB/NZW mice. *Arthritis Rheum* 1976;18:145–152.

41. Austin HA III, Klippel JH, Balow JE, et al. Therapy of lupus nephritis: controlled trial of prednisone and cytotoxic drugs. *N Engl J Med* 1986;314:614–619.

42. Wofsy D, Seaman WE. Reversal of advanced murine lupus in NZB/NZW F1 mice by treatment with monoclonal antibody to L3T4. *J Immunol* 1987;138:3247–3253.

43. Adelman NE, Watling DL, McDevitt HO. Treatment of (NZB × NZW)F1 disease with anti-I-A monoclonal antibodies. *J Exp Med* 1983;158:1350–1355.

44. Hahn BH, Ebling FM. Suppression of NZB/NZW murine nephritis by administration of a syngeneic monoclonal antibody to DNA: possible role of anti-idiotypic antibodies. *J Clin Invest* 1983;71:1728–1736.

45. Jacob CO, van der Meide PH, McDevitt HO. In vivo treatment of (NZB × NZW)F1 lupus-like nephritis with monoclonal antibody to gamma interferon. *J Exp Med* 1987;166:798–803.

46. Finck BK, Chan B, Wofsy D. Interleukin 6 promotes murine lupus in NZB/NZW F1 mice. *J Clin Invest* 1994;94:585–591.

47. Ishida H, Muchamuel T, Sakaguchi S, et al. Continuous administration of anti-interleukin 10 antibodies delays the onset of autoimmunity in NZB/W F1 mice. *J Exp Med* 1994;179:305–310.

48. Finck BK, Linsley PS, Wofsy D. Treatment of murine lupus with CTLA4Ig. *Science* 1994;265:1225–1227.

49. Mohan C, Shi Y, Laman JD, et al. Interaction between CD40 and its ligand gp39 in the development of murine lupus nephritis. *J Immunol* 1995;154:1470–1480.

50. Daikh DI, Finck BK, Linsley PS, et al. Long-term inhibition of murine lupus by brief simultaneous blockade of the B7/CD28 and CD40/gp39 costimulation pathways. *J Immunol* 1997;159:3104–3108.

51. Murphy ED, Roths JB. New inbred strains. *Mouse News Letter* 1978;58:51.

52. Watanabe T, Sakai Y, Miyawaki S, et al. A molecular genetic linkage map of mouse chromosome 19, including the lpr, Ly-44, and Tdt genes. *Biochem Genet* 1991;29:325–335.

53. Roths JB, Murphy ED, Eicher EM. A new mutation, gld, that produces lymphoproliferation and autoimmunity in C3H/HeJ mice. *J Exp Med* 1984;159:1–20.

54. Seldin MF, Morse HC, Reeves JP, et al. Genetic analysis of autoimmune gld mice. I. Identification of a restriction fragment length polymorphism closely linked to the gld mutation within a conserved linkage group. *J Exp Med* 1988;167:688–693.

55. Allen RD, Marshall JD, Roths JB, et al. Differences defined by bone marrow transplantation suggest that lpr and gld are mutations of genes encoding an interacting pair of molecules. *J Exp Med* 1990;172:1367–1375.

56. Matsuzawa A, Moriyama T, Kaneko T, et al. A new allele of the lpr locus, lpr-cg, that complements the gld gene in induction of lymphadenopathy in the mouse. *J Exp Med* 1990;171:519–531.

57. Watanabe-Fukunaga R, Brannan CI, Copeland NG, et al. Lymphoproliferative disorder in mice explained by defects in fas antigen that mediates apoptosis. *Nature* 1992;356:314–317.

58. Takahashi T, Tanaka M, Brannan CI, et al. Generalized lymphoproliferative disease in mice caused by a point mutation in the Fas ligand. *Cell* 1994;76:969–976.

59. Yonehara S, Ishii A, Yonehara M. A cell-killing monoclonal antibody (anti-Fas) to a cell surface antigen co-downregulated with the receptor of tumor necrosis factor. *J Exp Med* 1989;169:1747–1756.

60. Watanabe-Fukunaga R, Brannan CI, Itoh N, et al. The cDNA structure, expression and chromosomal assignment of the mouse Fas antigen. *J Immunol* 1992;148:1274–1279.

61. Itoh N, Yonehara S, Ishii A, et al. The polypeptide encoded by the cDNA for human surface antigen fas can mediate apoptosis. *Cell* 1992;66:233–243.

62. Rouvier E, Luciani M-F, Golstein P. Fas involvement in Ca$^{2+}$-independent T cell-mediated cytotoxicity. *J Exp Med* 1993;177:195–200.

63. Suda T, Nagata S. Purification and characterization of the Fas-ligand that induces apoptosis. *J Exp Med* 1994;179:873–879.

64. Suda T, Takahashi T, Golstein P, et al. Molecular cloning and expression of the Fas ligand, a novel member of the tumor necrosis family. *Cell* 1993;75:1169–1175.

65. Adachi M, Watanabe-Fukunaga R, Nagata S. Aberrant transcription caused by the insertion of an early transposable element in the intron of the Fas antigen gene of lpr mice. *Proc Natl Acad Sci U S A* 1993;90:1756–1760.

66. Wu J, Zhou T, Zhang J, et al. Correction of accelerated autoimmune disease by early replacement of the mutated lpr gene with the normal Fas apoptosis gene in the T cells of transgenic MRL-lpr/lpr mice. *Proc Natl Acad Sci U S A* 1994;91:2344–2348.

67. Hoffman RW, Alspaugh MA, Waggie KS, et al. Sjögren's syndrome in MRL/l and MRL/n mice. *Arthritis Rheum* 1984;27:157–165.

68. Jabs DA, Pendergast RA. Reactive lymphocytes in lacrimal gland and vasculitic renal lesions of autoimmune MRL/lpr mice express L3T4. *J Exp Med* 1987;166:1198–1203.

69. Nemanzee DA, Studer S, Steinmetz M, et al. The lymphoproliferating cells of MRL-lpr/lpr mice are a polyclonal population that bear the T lymphocyte receptor for antigen. *Eur J Immunol* 1985;15:760–764.

70. Mountz JD, Huppi KE, Seldin MF, et al. T cell receptor gene expression in autoimmune mice. *J Immunol* 1986;137:1029–1036.

71. Croghan TW, Evans J, Davignon JL, et al. Diminished expression of the T cell receptor on the expanded lymphocyte population in MRL/Mp-lpr/lpr mice. *Autoimmunity* 1990;2:97–111.

72. Wofsy D, Hardy RR, Seaman WE. The proliferating cells in autoimmune MRL/lpr mice lack L3T4, an antigen on "helper" T cells that is involved in the response to class II major histocompatibility antigens. *J Immunol* 1984;132:2686–2689.

73. Davidson WF, Dumont FJ, Bedigian HG, et al. Phenotypic, functional, and molecular genetic comparisons of abnormal lymphoid cells of CH3-lpr/lpr and CH3-gld/gld mice. *J Immunol* 1986;136:4075–4084.

74. Kato K, Ohzawa N, Nakayama K, et al. Effects of ulinastatin on experimental arthritis. *Nippon Yakurigaku Zasshi* 1988;91:29–40.

75. Katagiri K, Katagiri T, Eisenberg RA, et al. Interleukin 2 responses of lpr and normal L3T4-/Lyt-2-T cells induced by TPA plus A23187. *J Immunol* 1987;138:149–156.

76. Rosenberg YJ, Nurse F, Begley C. IL-2 receptor expression in autoimmune MRL-lpr/lpr mice: the expanded L3T4-, Lyt-2- population does not express p75 and cannot generate functional high-affinity IL-2 receptor. *J Immunol* 1989;143:2216–2222.

77. Singer GG, Carrera AC, Marshak-Rothstein A, et al. Apoptois, FAS and systemic autoimmunity: the MRL-lpr/lpr model. *Curr Opin Immunol* 1994;6:913–920.

78. Theofilopoulos AN, Dixon FJ. Murine models of systemic lupus erythematosus. *Adv Immunol* 1985;37:269–290.

79. Berden JH, Hang L, McConahey PJ, et al. Analysis of vascular lesions in murine SLE. I. Association with serologic abnormalities. *J Immunol* 1983;130:1699–1705.

80. Ansel JC, Mountz JD, Steinberg AD, et al. Effects of UV radiation on autoimmune strains of mice: increased mortality and accelerated autoimmunity in BXSB male mice. *J Invest Dermatol* 1985;85:181–186.

81. Sunderrajan EV, McKenzie WN, Lieske TR, et al. Pulmonary inflammation in autoimmune MRL/Mp-lpr/lpr mice: histopathology and bronchoalveolar lavage evaluation. *Am J Pathol* 1986;124:353–362.

82. Cohen PL, Eisenberg RA. lpr And gld: single gene models of systemic autoimmunity and lymphoproliferative disease. *Annu Rev Immunol* 1991;9:243–269.

83. Eisenberg RA, Tan EM, Dixon FJ. Presence of anti-Sm reactivity in autoimmune mouse strains. *J Exp Med* 1978;147:582–587.

84. Bonfa E, Marshak-Rothstein A, Weissbach H, et al. Frequency and epitope recognition of anti-ribosome P antibodies from humans with systemic lupus erythematosus and MRL/lpr mice are similar. *J Immunol* 1989;140:3434–3437.

85. Hang L, Theofilopoulos AN, Dixon FJ. A spontaneous rheumatoid arthritis-like disease in MRL/l mice. *J Exp Med* 1982;155:1690–1701.

86. Koopman WJ, Gay S. The MRL-lpr/lpr mouse: a model for the study of rheumatoid arthritis. *Scand J Rheumatol Suppl* 1988;75:284–289.

87. Gyotoku Y, Abdelmoula M, Spertini F, et al. Cryoglobulinemia induced by monoclonal immunoglobulin G rheumatoid factors derived from autoimmune MRL/MpJ-lpr/lpr mice. *J Immunol* 1987;138:3785–3792.

88. Abdelmoula M, Spertini F, Shibata T, et al. IgG3a is the major source of cryoglobulins in mice. *J Immunol* 1989;143:526–532.

89. Klinman DM, Steinberg AD. Systemic autoimmune disease arises from polyclonal B cell activation. *J Exp Med* 1987;165:1755–1760.

90. Monroe JG, Cambier SA, Moody EA, et al. Hyper-Ia antigen expression on B cells from B6-lpr/lpr mice correlates with manifestations of the autoimmune state. *Clin Immunol Immunopathol* 1985;34:124–129.

91. Amagi T, Cinader B. Resistance of MRL/Mp-lpr/lpr mice to tolerance induction. *Eur J Immunol* 1989;11:923–926.

92. Creighton D, Katz DH, Dixon FJ. Antigen-specific immunocompetency, B cell function, and regulatory helper and suppressor T cell activities in spontaneously autoimmune mice. *J Immunol* 1979;126:2627–2636.

93. Dziarski R. Comparison of in vitro and in vivo mitogenic and polyclonal antibody and autoantibody responses to peptidoglycan, LPS, protein A, PWM, PHA and Con A in normal and autoimmune mice. *J Clin Lab Immunol* 1985;16:93–109.

94. Asano T, Tomooka S, Serushago BA, et al. A new T cell subset expressing B220 and CD4 in lpr mice: defects in the response to mitogens and in the production of IL-2. *Clin Exp Immunol* 1988;74:36–40.

95. Bossu P, Singer GG, Andres P, et al. Mature CD4+ T lymphocytes from MRL/lpr mice are resistant to receptor-mediated tolerance and apoptosis. *J Immunol* 1993;151:7233–7239.

96. Weston KM, Ju ST, Lu CY, et al. Autoreactive T cells in MRL/Mp-lpr/lpr mice: characterization of the lymphokines produced and analysis of antigen-presenting cells required. *J Immunol* 1988;141:1941–1948.

97. Cohen PL, Rapoport R, Eisenberg RA. Characterization of functional T-cell lines derived from MRL mice. *Clin Immunol Immunopathol* 1986;40:485–496.

98. Santoro TJ, Portanova JP, Kotzin BL. The contribution of L3T4+ T cells to lymphoproliferation and autoantibody production in MRL-lpr/lpr mice. *J Exp Med* 1988;167:1713–1718.

99. Jabs DA, Kuppers RC, Saboori AM, et al. Effects of early and late treatment with anti-CD4 monoclonal antibody on autoimmune disease in MRL/Mp-lpr/lpr mice. *Cell Immunol* 1994;154:66–76.

100. Jevnikar AM, Grusby MJ, Glimcher LH. Prevention of nephritis in MHC class-II-deficient MRL-lpr mice. *J Exp Med* 1994;179:1137–1143.

101. Chesnutt MS, Finck BK, Killeen N, et al. Enhanced lymphoproliferation and diminished autoimmunity in CD4-deficient MRL/lpr mice. *Clin Immunol Immunopathol* 1998;87:23–32.

102. Giese T, Davidson WF. Chronic treatment of C3H-lpr/lpr and C3H-gld/gld mice with anti-CD8 monoclonal antibody prevents the accumulation of double negative T cells but not autoantibody production. *J Immunol* 1994;152:2000–2010.

103. Koh DR, Ho A, Rahemtulla A, et al. Murine lupus in MRL/lpr mice lacking CD4 or CD8 T cells. *Eur J Immunol* 1995;25:2558–2562.

104. Mountz JD, Smith HR, Wilder RL, et al. CS-A therapy in MRL-lpr/lpr mice: amelioration of immunopathology despite autoantibody production. *J Immunol* 1987;138:157–163.

105. Cohen PL, Rapoport RG, Eisenberg RA, et al. Effects of anti-IFN-gamma on MRL-Mp-lpr/lpr mice (abst.). *Arthritis Rheum* 1989;32:S52.

106. Izui S, Kelly VE, Masuda K, et al. Induction of various autoantibodies by mutant gene lpr in several strains of mice. *J Immunol* 1984;133:227–233.

107. Warren RW, Roths JB, Murphy ED, et al. Mechanisms of polyclonal B-cell activation in autoimmune B6-lpr/lpr mice. *Cell Immunol* 1984;84:22–31.

108. Murphy ED, Roths JB. Autoimmunity and lymphoproliferation: induction by mutant gene lpr and acceleration by a male-associated factor in strain BXSB mice. In: Rose NR, Bigazzi PE, Warner NL, eds. *Genetic control of autoimmune disease.* New York: Elsevier–North Holland, 1979:207–221.

109. Kastner D, Steinberg A. Determinants of B cell hyperactivity in murine lupus. *Concepts Immunopathol* 1988;6:22–31.

110. Theofilopoulos AN, Dixon FJ. Etiopathogenesis of murine SLE. *Immunol Rev* 1981;55:179–216.

111. Izui S, Higaki M, Morrow D, et al. The Y chromosome from autoimmune BXSB/MpJ mice induces a lupus-like syndrome in (NZB × NZW)F₁ male mice, but not in C57BL/6 male mice. *Eur J Immunol* 1988;18:911–915.

112. Theofilopoulos AN, Eisenberg RA, Bourdon M, et al. Distribution of lymphocytes identified by surface markers in murine strains with systemic lupus erythematosus-like syndromes. *J Exp Med* 1979;149:516–534.

113. Wofsy D, Kerger CD, Seaman WE. Monocytosis in the BXSB model for systemic lupus erythematosus. *J Exp Med* 1984;159:629–634.

114. Chu EB, Ernst DN, Hobbs MV, et al. Maturational changes in CD4+ cell subsets and lymphokine production in BXSB mice. *J Immunol* 1994;152:4129–4138.

115. Wofsy D. Administration of monoclonal anti-T cell antibodies retards murine lupus in BXSB mice. *J Immunol* 1986;136:4554–4560.

116. Chu EB, Hobbs MV, Wilson CB, et al. Intervention of CD4+ cell subset shifts and autoimmunity in the BXSB mouse by murine CTLA4Ig. *J Immunol* 1996;156:1262–1268.

117. Lahita RG, Chiorazzi N, Gibofsky A, et al. Familial systemic lupus erythematosus in males. *Arthritis Rheum* 1983;26:39–44.

118. Makino S, Kunimoto K, Maraoka Y, et al. Breeding of a non-obese diabetic strain of mice. *Exp Anim* 1980;29:1–13.

119. Pozilli P, Signore A, Williams AJK, et al. NOD mouse colonies around the world: recent facts and figures. *Immunol Today* 1993;14:193–196.

120. Wicker LS, Todd JA, Peterson LB. Genetic control of autoimmune diabetes in the NOD mouse. *Annu Rev Immunol* 1995;13:179–200.

121. Delovitch TL, Singh B. The nonobese diabetic mouse as a model of autoimmune diabetes: immune dysregulation gets the NOD. *Immunity* 1997;7:727–738.

122. Fujita T, Yui R, Kusumoto Y, et al. Lymphocytic insulitis in a 'non-obese diabetic (NOD)' strain of mice: an immunohistochemical and electron microscope investigation. *Biomed Res* 1982;3:429–443.

123. Lo D, Reilly CR, Scott B, et al. Antigen-presenting cells in adoptively transferred and spontaneous autoimmune diabetes. *Eur J Immunol* 1993;23:1693–1698.

124. Yagi H, Matsumoto M, Kunimoto K, et al. Analysis of the roles of CD4+ and CD8+ T cells in autoimmune diabetes of NOD mice using transfer to NOD athymic nude mice. *Eur J Immunol* 1992;22:2387–2393.

125. Christianson SW, Shultz LD, Leiter EH. Adoptive transfer of diabetes into immunodeficient NOD-scid/scid mice: relative contributions of CD4+ and CD8+ T-cells from diabetic versus prediabetic NOD.NON-Thy-1a donors. *Diabetes* 1993;42:44–55.

126. Bendelac A, Carnaud C, Boitard C, et al. Syngeneic transfer of autoimmune diabetes from diabetic NOD mice to healthy neonates: requirements for both L3T4+ and Lyt-2+ T cells. *J Exp Med* 1987;166:823–832.

127. Chatenoud L, Thervet E, Primo J, et al. Anti-CD3 antibody induces long-term remission of overt autoimmunity in nonobese diabetic mice. *Proc Natl Acad Sci U S A* 1993;91:123–127.

128. Miller BJ, Appel MC, O'Neil JJ, et al. Both the Lyt-2+ and L3T4+ T cell subsets are required for the transfer of diabetes in nonobese diabetic mice. *J Immunol* 1988;140:52–58.

129. Haskins K, McDuffie M. Acceleration of diabetes in young NOD mice with a CD4+ islet-specific T cell clone. *Science* 1990;24:1433–1436.

130. Jarpe AJ, Hickman MR, Anderson JT, et al. Flow cytometric enumeration of mononuclear cell populations infiltrating the islets of Langerhans in prediabetic NOD mice: development of a model of autoimmune insulitis for type I diabetes. *Reg Immunol* 1991;3:305–317.

131. Serreze DV, Leiter EH, Christianson GJ, et al. Major histocompatibility comples class I-deficient NOD-β2m$_{null}$ mice are diabetes and insulitis resistant. Diabetes 1994;43:505–509.

132. Wicker LS, Leiter EH, Todd JA, et al. β²-Microglobulin-deficient NOD mice do not develop insulitis or diabetes. *Diabetes* 1994;45:500–504.

133. Rabinovitch A. Immunoregulatory and cytokine imbalances in the pathogenesis of IDDM: therapeutic intervention by immunostimulation? *Diabetes* 1994;43:613–621.

134. Katz JD, Benoist C, Mathis D. T helper cell subsets in insulin-dependent diabetes. *Science* 1995;268:1185–1188.

135. Shimada A, Rohane P, Fathman CG, et al. Pathogenic and protective roles of CD45RB(low) CD4+ cells correlate with cytokine profiles in the spontaneously autoimmune diabetic mouse. *Diabetes* 1996;45:71–78.

136. Fox CJ, Danska JS. IL-4 expression at the onset of islet inflammation predicts nondestructive insulitis in nonobese diabetic mice. *J Immunol* 1997;158:2414–2424.

137. Trembleau S, Penn G, Bosi E, et al. Interleukin 12 administration induces T helper type 1 cells and accelerates autoimmune diabetes in NOD mice. *J Exp Med* 1995;181:817–821.

138. Lenschow DJ, Herold KC, Rhee L, et al. CD28/B7 regulation of Th1 and Th2 subsets in the development of autoimmune diabetes. *Immunity* 1996;5:285–293.

139. Boitard C, Yasunami R, Dardenne M, et al. T cell-mediated inhibition of the transfer of autoimmune diabetes in NOD mice. *J Autoimmun* 1989;169:1669-1680.

140. Harada M, Makino S. Promotion of spontaneous diabetes in nonobese diabetes-prone mice by cyclophosphamide. *Diabetologia* 1984;27:604–606.

141. Yasunami R, Bach J-F. Anti-suppressor effect of cyclophosphamide on the development of spontaneous diabetes in NOD mice. *Eur J Immunol* 1988;18:481–484.

142. Healey DG, Burt J, Shevket M, et al. Variation in CD4 TH1/TH2 phenotypes prior to cyclophosphamide induced diabetes in the NOD mouse. *Autoimmunity* 1993;15[Suppl]:45–52.

143. Katz JD, Benoist C, Mathis D. T helper cell subsets in insulin-dependent diabetes. *Science* 1995;268:1185–1189.

144. Baekkeskov S, Aanstoot HJ, Christgau S, et al. Identification of the 64K autoantigen in insulin-dependent diabetes as GABA-synthesizing enzyme glutamic acid. *Nature* 1990;347:151–156.

145. Tisch R, Yang XD, Singer SM, et al. Immune response to glutamic acid decarboxylase correlates with insulitis non-obese diabetic mice. *Nature* 1993;366:72–75.

146. Kaufman D, Clare-Salzler M, Tian J, et al. Spontaneous loss of T-cell tolerance to glutamic acid decarboxylase in murine insulin-dependent diabetes. *Nature* 1993;366:69–72.

147. Tian J, Atkinson MA, Clare-Salzler, et al. Nasal administration of glutamate decarboxylase (GAD65) peptides induces Th2 responses and prevents murine insulin-dependent diabetes. *J Exp Med* 1996;183:1561–1567.

148. Zhang ZL, Davidson L, Eisenbarth G, et al. Suppression of diabetes in nonobese diabetic mice by oral administration porcine insulin. *Proc Natl Acad Sci U S A* 1991;88:10252–1110256.

149. Bergerot I, Fabien N, Maguer V, et al. Oral administration of human insulin to NOD mice generates CD4+ T cells that suppress adoptive transfer of diabetes. *J Autoimmun* 1994;7:655–663.

150. Muir A, Peck A, Clare-Salzler M, et al. Insulin immunization of nonobese diabetic mice induces a protective insulitis characterized by diminished intraislet interferon-gamma transcription. *J Clin Invest* 1995;95:628–634.

151. Harrison LC, Demsey-Collier M, Kramer DR, et al. Aerosol insulin induces regulatory CD8 gamma delta T cells that prevents murine insulin-dependent diabetes. *J Exp Med* 1996;184:2167–2174.

152. Elias D, Marcus H, Reshef T, et al. Induction of diabetes in standard mice by immunization with the p277 of a 60-kDa heat shock protein. *Eur J Immunol* 1995;25:2851–2857.

153. Daniel D, Gill RG, Schloot N, et al. Epitope specificity, cytokine production profile and diabetogenic activity of insulin-specific T cell clones isolated from NOD mice. *Eur J Immunol* 1994;25:1056–1062.

154. Eisenbarth GS. Mouse or man: is GAD the cause of type I diabetes? *Diabetes Care* 1994;17:605–607.

155. Tian J, Lehmann PV, Kaufman DL. Determinant spreading of T helper cell 2 (Th2) responses to pancreatic islet autoantigens. *J Exp Med* 1997;186:2039–2043.

156. Haskins K, Portas M, Bradley B, et al. T-lymphocyte clone specific for pancreatic islet antigen. *Diabetes* 1988;37:1444–1448.

157. Nakano N, Kikutani H, Nishimoto H, et al. T cell receptor V gene usage of islet beta cell-reactive T cells is not restricted in non-obese diabetic mice. *J Exp Med* 1991;173:1091–1097.

158. Waters SH, O'Neil JJ, Melican DT, et al. Multiple TCR V beta usage by infiltrates of young NOD mouse islets of Langerhans: a polymerase chain reaction analysis. *Diabetes* 1992;41:308–312.

159. Galley KA, Danska JS. Peri-islet infiltrates of young non-obese diabetic mice display TCR beta-chain diversity. *J Immunol* 1995;154:2969–22222982.

160. Simone E, Daniel D, Schloot N, et al. T cell receptor restriction of diabetogenic autoimmune NOD T cells. *Proc Natl Acad Sci U S A* 1997;94:2518–2521.

161. Yang Y, Charlton B, Shimada A, et al. Monoclonal T cells identified in early NOD islet infiltrates. *Immunity* 1996;4:189–194.

162. Santamaria P, Utsugi T, Park B-J, et al. Beta-cell-cytotoxic CD8+ T cells from nonobese diabetic mice use highly homologous T cell receptor alpha-chain CDR3 sequences. *J Immunol* 1995;154:2494–2503.

163. Tian J, Lehmann PV, Kaufman DL. T cell cross-reactivity between coxsackievirus and glutamate decarboxylase associated with a murine diabetes susceptibility allele. *J Exp Med* 1994;180:1979–1984.

164. Gamble DR, Taylor KW, Cumming H. Coxsackie viruses and diabetes mellitus. *Br Med J* 1973;4:260–262.

165. Bach JF. Insulin-dependent diabetes mellitus as an autoimmune disease. *Endocr Rev* 1994;15:516–542.

166. Ikegami H, Makino S. Genetic susceptibility to insulin-dependent diabetes mellitus: from NOD mice to humans. In: Shafrir E, ed. *Lessons from animal diabetes.* London: Smith-Gordon, 1993:39–50.

167. Hattori M, Buse JB, Jackson RA, et al. The NOD mouse: recessive diabetogenic gene in the major histocompatibility complex. *Science* 1986;231:733–735.

168. Wicker LS, Miller BJ, Coker LZ. Genetic control of diabetes and insulitis in the nonobese diabetic (NOD) mouse. *J Exp Med* 1987;165:1639–1654.

169. Prochazka M, Leiter EH, Serreze, et al. Three successive loci required for insulin-dependent diabetes in NOD mice. *Science* 1987;237: 286–289.

170. Todd JA, Bell JI, McDevitt HO. HLA-DQβ gene contributes to susceptibility and resistance to insulin-dependent diabetes mellitus. *Nature* 1987;329:599–604.

171. Lund TM, O'Reilly L, Hutchings P, et al. Prevention of insulin-dependent diabetes mellitus in non-obese diabetic mice by transgenes encoding modified I-A beta-chain or normal I-E alpha-chain. *Nature* 1990;345: 727–729.

172. Brown JH, Jardetzky TS, Gorga JC, et al. The three-dimensional structure of the human class II histocompatibility antigen HLA-DR1. *Nature* 1993;364:33–39.

173. Serreze DV. Autoimmune diabetes results from genetic defects manifest by antigen presenting cells. *FASEB J* 1993;7:1092–1096.

174. Carrasco-Marin E, Shimizu J, Kanagawa O, et al. The class II MHC I-A$^{g7}$ molecules from non-obese diabetic mice are poor peptide binders. *J Immunol* 1996;156:450–458.

175. Green MC, Schultz LD. Motheaten, an immunodeficient mutant of the mouse. I. Genetics and pathology. *J Hered* 1975;66:250–258.

176. Schultz LD. Pleiotropic effects of deleterious alleles at the "motheaten" locus. *Curr Top Microbiol Immunol* 1988;137:216–222.

177. Shultz LD, Coman DR, Bailey CL, et al. "Viable motheaten": a new allele at the motheaten locus. I. Pathology. *Am J Pathol* 1984;116: 179–192.

178. Schultz LD, Schweitzer PA, Rajan TV, et al. Mutations at the murine motheaten locus are within the hematopoietic cell protein-tyrosine phosphatase *(Hcph)* gene. *Cell* 1993;73:1445–1154.

179. Hibbs ML, Tarlington DM, Armes J, et al. Multiple defects in the immune system of *Lyn*-deficient mice, culminating in autoimmune disease. *Cell* 1995;83:301–311.

180. Tedder TF, Tuscano J, Sato S, et al. CD22, a B lymphocyte-specific adhesion molecule that regulates antigen receptor signaling. *Annu Rev Immunol* 1997;15:481–504.

181. Jimenez S, Bashey R, Williams C, et al. The tight skin (TSK) mouse as an experimental model of scleroderma. In: Greenwald R, Diamond H, eds. *CRC handbook of animal models for the rheumatic diseases.* Boca Raton, FL: CRC Press, 1988:169–193.

182. Christner PJ, Peters J, Hawkins D, et al. The tight skin 2 mouse: an animal model of scleroderma displaying cutaneous fibrosis and mononuclear cell infiltration. *Arthritis Rheum* 1995;38:1791–1798.

183. Szapiel S, Fulmer J, Hunninghake, et al. Hereditary emphysema in the tight-skin (TSK/+) mouse. *Am Rev Respir Dis* 1981;123:680–685.

184. Westphal H. Transgenic mammals and biotechnology. *FASEB J* 1989; 3:117–120.

185. Hammer RE, Maika SD, Richardson JA, et al. Spontaneous inflammatory disease in transgenic rats expressing HLA-B27 and human β2-m: an animal model of the HLA-B27-associated human disorders. *Cell* 1990;63:1099–1112.

186. Keffer J, Probert L, Cazlaris H, et al. Transgenic mice expressing human tumor necrosis factor: a predictive genetic model of arthritis. *EMBO J* 1991;10:4025–031.

187. Elliott MJ, Maini RN, Feldman M, et al. Randomised double-blind comparison of chimeric monoclonal antibody to tumour necrosis factor α (cA2) versus placebo in rheumatoid arthritis. *Lancet* 1994;344: 1105–1110.

188. Moreland LW, Baumgartner SW, Schiff MH, et al. Treatment of rheumatoid arthritis with a recombinant human tumor necrosis factor (p75)-Fc fusion protein. *N Engl J Med* 1997;337:141–147.

189. Lee M-S, Sarvetnick N. Cytokine transgenic mice and autoimmunity. In: Abbas AK, Flavell RA, eds. *Genetic models of immune and inflammatory diseases.* New York: Springer–Verlag, 1996:121–128.

190. Guerder S, Picarella DE, Linsley PS, et al. Costimulator B7-1 confers antigen-presenting-cell function to parenchymal tissue and in conjunction with tumour necrosis factor-α leads to autoimmunity in transgenic mice. *Proc Natl Acad Sci U S A* 1994;91:5138–5142.

191. Shull MM, Ormsby I, Kier AB, et al. Targeted disruption of the mouse transforming growth factor-β1 gene results in multifocal inflammatory disease. *Nature* 1992;359:693–699.

192. Yaswen L, Kulkarni AB, Fredrickson T, et al. Autoimmune manifestations in the transforming growth factor-β1 knockout mouse. *Blood* 1996;86:1439–1445.

193. Kühn R, Löhler J, Rennick D, et al. Interleukin-10-deficient mice develop chronic enterocolitis. *Cell* 1993;75:263–274.

194. Strober W, Lúdviksson BR, Fuss IJ. The pathogenesis of mucosal inflammation in murine models of inflammatory bowel disease and Crohn disease. *Ann Intern Med* 1998;128:848–856.

195. Peng SL, Moslehi J, Craft J. Roles of interferon-γ and interleukin-4 in murine lupus. *J Clin Invest* 1997;99:1936–1946.

196. Ferber IA, Brocke S, Taylor-Edwards C, et al. Mice with a disrupted IFN-γ gene are susceptible to the induction of experimental autoimmune encephalomyelitis (EAE). *J Immunol* 1996;156:5–7.

196. Alonzi T, Fattori E, Lazzaro D, et al. Interleukin 6 is required for the development of collagen-induced arthritis. *J Exp Med* 1998;187: 461–468.

198. Chen S-Y, Takeoka Y, Ansari AA, et al. The natural history of disease expression in CD4 and CD8 gene-deleted New Zealand black (NZB) mice. *J Immunol* 1996;157:2676–2684.

199. Lenschow DJ, Herold KC, Rhee L, et al. CD28/B7 regulation of Th1 and Th2 subsets in the development of autoimmune diabetes. *Immunity* 1996;5:285–293.

200. Jevnikar AM, Grusby MJ, Glimcher LH. Prevention of nephritis in major histocompatibility complex class II-deficient MRL-*lpr* mice. *J Exp Med* 1994;179:1137–1143.

201. Maldonado MA, Eisenberg RA, Roper E, et al. Greatly reduced lymphoproliferation in *lpr* mice lacking major histocompatibility complex class I. *J Exp Med* 1995;181:641–648.

*Textbook of the Autoimmune Diseases,*
Edited by R. G. Lahita, N. Chiorazzi, and W. H. Reeves,
Lippincott Williams & Wilkins, Philadelphia © 2000.

# CHAPTER 47

# Experimental Therapies of Autoimmune Disease

Noel R. Rose

*Autoimmunity* is defined as the immune response of the body to the tissues of the body, regardless of whether it is induced by a foreign antigen or a self antigen. The pathologic consequence of the autoimmune response is autoimmune disease. The autoimmune diseases can affect any site in the body, including connective tissue, brain, skin, heart, blood, lungs, kidney, liver, gastrointestinal tract, and endocrine system. Because the organ system affected varies widely in different diseases, autoimmune diseases are traditionally treated by different clinical specialists. Diseases affecting the connective tissues come to the attention of the rheumatologist; those involving the brain, like multiple sclerosis (MS), are seen by neurologists; skin diseases, like pemphigus, are treated by dermatologists; and type 1 diabetes is the province of the endocrinologist.

Approaches to therapy differ greatly among these specialized clinicians. In general, however, they have two goals. If the autoimmune disorder increases or decreases the function of the target organ, the therapeutic approach is to correct the malfunction. In diabetes, insulin remedies the deficiency in islet cell production, whereas thyroxine compensates for the hypothyroidism of thyroiditis. Propylthiouracil and methimazole ameliorate the thyrotoxicosis of Graves' disease by decreasing thyroid hormone secretion. To treat the more generalized autoimmune diseases, a general reduction of the inflammatory and immune responses is sometimes necessary. Lupus and severe rheumatoid arthritis can be managed by cautious use of immunosuppressive and antiinflammatory drugs, such as antimetabolites and steroids.

None of these treatments is curative because none corrects the basic cause of the autoimmune dysfunction. As our understanding of the pathogenesis of autoimmune disease has increased, it has become clear that many pathogenetic mechanisms are involved. The differing underlying mechanisms

suggest different opportunities for therapy. The promise of the future is to develop novel therapies that will arrest the autoimmune responses producing the injury, thereby leading to long-lasting remission and possibly even cure. Ultimately, measures should be devised to prevent autoimmune disease before irreversible tissue damage has occurred.

The goals of this chapter are to assess the fundamental, common mechanisms underlying the immunopathogenesis of autoimmune disease and to point out steps at which therapeutic intervention may interrupt the disease-producing process. Stress is placed on novel approaches to treatment using biologic agents.

## IMMUNOPATHOGENESIS OF AUTOIMMUNE DISEASE

A highly simplified scheme for visualizing the immunopathogenesis of autoimmune disease is presented in Fig. 47.1. It emphasizes, first, the many ways in which the autoimmune process may emerge. Second, it indicates the multiple consequences of the immune response that can lead to disease. One factor common to virtually all autoimmune diseases is the central role played by self-reactive CD4 helper T ($T_H$) cells. For that reason, many of the newer therapies for treating autoimmune disease are aimed at inactivating the self-reactive T cell.

With respect to inductive mechanisms, the five given in Fig. 47.1 are illustrative of the large number of possibilities. One of the most attractive ideas is molecular mimicry (1). It suggests that an encounter with a cross-reacting antigen from an external source, such as an invading microorganism, initiates a response that affects a structurally similar self antigen. Appealing as this idea is, there are no clear-cut examples of molecular mimicry as a cause of a human autoimmune disease. The association of β-hemolytic streptococcal infection with rheumatic heart disease is based primarily on an epidemiologic association. Cross-reactions between streptococcal M-protein, enteroviruses, and cardiac myosin have been demonstrated on the antibody level, but the streptococcal

N. R. Rose: Departments of Pathology and Molecular Microbiology and Immunology, The Johns Hopkins Medical Institutions, Baltimore, Maryland 21205; Department of Medicine, The Johns Hopkins Hospital, Baltimore, Maryland 21205.

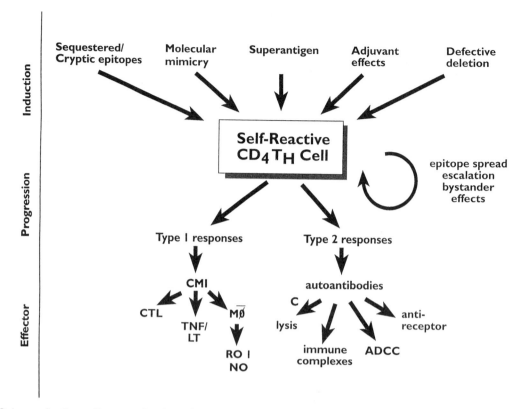

**FIG. 47.1.** Scheme for the pathogenesis of autoimmune disease. ADCC, antibody-dependent cell-mediated cytotoxicity; C, complement; $CD_4T_{h1}$, type 1 helper (CD4+) T cell; CMI, cell-mediated immunity; CTL, cytotoxic lymphocyte; MØ, macrophage; ROI, reactive oxygen intermediate; TNF/LT, tumor necrosi factor/lymphotoxin.

antigens actually responsible for the damaging autoimmune response have not yet been delineated (2).

As an alternative to molecular mimicry, infectious agents may instigate an autoimmune response if they produce superantigens (3). These substances bind to the T-cell receptor (TCR) β chain outside the antigen-binding site and stimulate a subpopulation of T cells based on their shared β chains. Included in this population may be some self-reactive T cells, which proliferate and generate an autoimmune response.

Cryptic epitopes are poorly presented by antigen-presenting cells and consequently have limited immunogenic capability. These same epitopes avoid the induction of tolerance in the thymus. They are, therefore, the epitopes that are most likely to encounter self-reactive T cells and to induce a pathogenic autoimmune response (4,5). The concept of cryptic epitopes has a certain parallel to the older idea of sequestered antigens. Located in "privileged" sites, such as the lens and the testes, these substances do not normally contact the immune system and, therefore, fail to generate normal self-tolerance. It is relatively easy to induce autoimmune responses to these antigens. Research suggests that privileged sites are less a result of anatomic isolation and more an expression of FAS ligand (FASL) or other apoptosis-inducing signals that prevent the local proliferation of T cells (6).

The process of clonal deletion of self-reactive T cells is often incomplete. Either the self antigen is not expressed in the thymus at all or its expression is limited and inefficient (7). The result is that T cells, especially low-affinity T cells,

reactive with many self antigens, escape intrathymic deletion. When such T cells encounter the corresponding self-antigen, particularly when given with a powerful immunopotentiating agent, like Freund's complete adjuvant, in experimental animals, they initiate an autoimmune response. In human autoimmune disease, infection may provide adjuvant-like activity. Thus, infection may initiate, or enhance, autoimmunization as a result of the production of proinflammatory cytokines, upregulation of costimulatory signs, expression of major histocompatibility complex (MHC) products class II, and the mobilization of immunologically active cells.

Based on the abundance of mechanisms that can instigate an autoimmune response, we might expect that autoimmunity is rather common. Indeed, experience has shown it to be so. Nevertheless, autoimmune disease is a relatively unusual outcome of an autoimmune response. It depends on the availability and accessibility of the appropriate self antigen as well as the appearance of the appropriate effector mechanism. If the self antigen is not accessible to the autoimmune response, a long-lasting state of immunologic ignorance may prevail; self-reactive T cells are present but ignore the cellular antigen (8). The state of clonal indifference may be terminated when the antigen becomes accessible through contact with an infectious agent bearing the appropriate antigenic determinant.

In considering effector mechanisms, it is convenient to distinguish helper T-cell subtype 1 ($T_H1$) from subtype 2 ($T_H2$) responses (9). The distinction between $T_H1$ and $T_H2$ T cells is based primarily on studies of leishmaniasis in experimental animals. The dichotomy has never been as clear-cut in autoimmune disease in humans, in which type 1 and type 2 responses are mixed. Nevertheless, there is heuristic value in dealing separately with type 1 responses that result primarily in cell-mediated immunity and type 2 responses associated with antibody production. It must be emphasized, however, that type 1 responses include certain isotypes of antibody and that type 2 responses encompass cell-mediated effects, especially those associated with eosinophils and mast cells.

Among the autoimmune diseases, our firmest understanding of pathogenetic mechanisms stems from the study of antibody-mediated disorders. The antibody, of course, must have access to the antigen. Antibody to blood cells is responsible for the hemolytic anemias and thrombocytopenias, either through enhanced phagocytosis or complement-mediated lysis. Antibodies to receptors also produce the symptoms of myasthenia gravis and Graves' disease. Pemphigus vulgaris and bullous pemphigoid are associated with antibodies to extracellular antigens of the skin. In lupus, the major antigens are found within cells but are released when cells die. The deposition of immune complexes in the kidneys and other tissues is the main pathogenetic process. Finally, antibody-dependent, cell-mediated cytotoxicity has been demonstrated *in vitro* in a number of autoimmune diseases, although its relevance to the process *in vivo* has not been established.

In most of the autoimmune diseases, $T_H1$ responses dominate the effector mechanisms. Cytotoxic T cells are prominent in diseases such as multiple sclerosis and type 1 diabetes, although direct evidence for their effect in the body is still lacking. The cytokine products of T cells are important intermediates in a number of autoimmune diseases. Finally, the role of activated macrophages must be emphasized. These cells supply a number of potentially damaging mediators, including interleukin-1 (IL-1), tumor necrosis factor (TNF), nitric oxide, and reactive oxygen intermediates.

With the possible exception of some forms of hemolytic anemia mediated by cold-reactive immunoglobulin M (IgM) autoantibodies, the progression of the autoimmune response from initiation to pathologic effect requires mobilization of self-reactive T cells. It makes them a logical target for therapeutic intervention because the ultimate goal is to affect the pathogenic immune response specifically. There are, however, problems in developing therapies at the T-cell level. In most, if not all, autoimmune diseases, multiple epitopes on the initiating antigenic molecule are recognized. Unlike inbred mice, humans are genetically heterogeneous, and the peptides of even a single antigen molecule presented in individual patients are dissimilar. This initial complexity is augmented as the autoimmune response progresses and additional epitopes are recruited through the phenomenon of epitope spread (10). By the time a patient is considered for therapy, therefore, multiple T cells with varying specificities are involved. Probably because of the elaboration locally of proinflammatory cytokines, T cells that recognize additional antigens of the affected organ become involved (11). Termed *immunologic escalation,* this phenomenon was first described in autoimmune thyroiditis in nonhuman primates (12). Based on the observation that virtually all autoimmune diseases are characterized by multiple autoantibodies, it appears that immune escalation is a common phenomenon. This complexity of the autoimmune response complicates efforts to develop specific therapies based on inactivating self-reactive T cells.

## THERAPEUTIC APPROACHES AT THE INDUCTIVE LEVEL

Despite the wide variety of mechanisms for inducing an autoimmune response, a number of novel therapies can be envisioned. The first prospective treatment considers errors in central tolerance as a result of faulty deletion. One possible strategy is to provide the patient's T cells with a "second chance" to distinguish self from nonself properly. It is accomplished by destroying the bone marrow, thereby completely ablating the existing faulty immune system, followed by reconstitution with hematopoietic stem cells from a histocompatible donor (13). Such bone marrow transplantation has become accepted therapy for a number of malignancies and, in experienced hands, can be carried out with minimal risk. Patients are treated by irradiation or cytotoxic drugs and reconstituted with histocompatible bone marrow cells. Infection is always a risk during the reconstitution phase, but reconstitution is significantly hastened by administration of colony-stimulating factors.

A hazard of this approach is the possibility of graft-versus-host disease. To eliminate this risk, some investigators have employed autologous rather than allogeneic bone marrow transplantation (14). Surprisingly, the reconstituted lymphoid system that follows transplantation of the patient's own hematopoietic stem cells does not lead to a recurrence of autoimmune disease. The stem cells reconstituting the immune system are capable of distinguishing self from nonself antigens.

Bone marrow transplantation, allogeneic or autologous, has been applied in a limited way in instances of life-threatening autoimmune disease, such as severe type 1 diabetes, rheumatoid arthritis, or systemic lupus erythematosus (15).

Based on the evidence that reconstituted bone marrow stem cells restore the ability of the immune system to distinguish self from nonself, another experimental therapy is focused on administration of pulsed, high-dose cyclophosphamide. This drug depletes bone marrow of most of its cells but spares the hemopoietic stem cell, which produces high levels of an aldehyde dehydrogenase that inactivates the drug. Patients are treated with a short-term regimen of cyclophosphamide followed by rescue, using colony-stimulating factors. Although this form of therapy has not yet been tested on a large scale, a number of remissions from severe autoimmune disease have been reported (16).

A second experimental therapy aimed at the inductive level is based on peripheral regulatory mechanisms. A promising procedure to protect an organ from autoimmune damage is local production of Fas ligand L (FasL); this appears to be the mechanism used at privileged sites (17). An artificial privileged site is produced in the targeted organ by engineering antigen-presenting cells to produce FasL. This procedure has been suggested as a method for ensuring the survival of transplanted pancreas islets (17). This approach may be broadly applicable to autoimmune disorders involving immune-mediated destruction of a solid organ (18).

If infection plays an important role in initiating autoimmune diseases, an effective strategy of prevention is prompt treatment of the infection. Antimicrobial treatment of streptococcal pharyngitis has been used with great success in preventing rheumatic heart disease. Because the disease is associated with repeated infections by β-hemolytic streptococci, children who have had rheumatic fever are treated perennially with long-acting penicillins. These drugs prevent colonization by the streptococcus and, therefore, avoid any possibility of infection-induced autoimmunity. This procedure may be responsible for the virtual elimination of rheumatic heart disease from most North American and West European countries.

Generalizing from the experience with rheumatic fever, many episodes of autoimmune disease occur in patients who are genetically predisposed and then come into contact with some environmental trigger, be it biologic, chemical, or physical. The identification of the environmental agent responsible for the initiation of the autoimmune response may be, in the long run, the most effective and least costly approach to the prevention of autoimmune disease. Considerable circumstantial evidence, for example, indicates that ingestion of excessive doses of iodine can intensify thyroid autoimmunity and lead to the development of thyroiditis (19). If further research supports this view, it may be possible to control the rising incidence of autoimmune thyroid disease by reducing dietary iodine.

## THERAPEUTIC APPROACHES AT THE LEVEL OF THE EFFECTOR CELL

As explained previously, a number of autoimmune diseases result from the direct or indirect action of antibodies. In these instances, removal of the pathogenic antibody may produce remission. The most direct means of accomplishing antibody removal is through plasmapheresis. For short-term improvement, such as in Guillain–Barré syndrome, replacement of the patient's plasma can be life-saving. Even for chronic diseases, such as myasthenia gravis, plasmapheresis can provide temporary benefit and offer a window of opportunity to establish longer-lasting treatments (20).

A great deal of attention has been devoted to the use of large pools of immunoglobulin administered intravenously (IVIg). These immunoglobulin preparations have been modified to prevent aggregation, so that they can safely be administered intravenously. In addition to treatment of immunodeficiency, IVIg is being used in the management of Kawasaki's disease and idiopathic thrombocytopenia (21). IVIg has also been widely used in other autoimmune diseases, and there is anecdotal evidence for its value in some cases. The mechanism of action of IVIg is unknown at this time. Several investigators, however, have presented evidence indicating that IVIg contains antiidiotypes to many common autoantibodies. If confirmed, this may explain the mechanism by which this material prevents autoantibody synthesis. It would, moreover, clear the path for deliberate production of antiidiotypes for the treatment of particular autoimmune diseases in which an autoantibody is the paramount effector. Unfortunately, the history of treating autoimmune disease with antiidiotypes has been disappointing.

In a number of autoimmune diseases, such as lupus, a major mechanism of tissue damage is the deposition of immune complexes. The damaging effect of the immune complex depends on activation of complement and the resultant phlogistic response. This observation suggests that blocking the complement cascade might be a useful treatment, particularly during flare-ups of the disease. Because complement activation also plays a crucial role in the early rejection of tissue xenografts, active research is being carried out on possible maneuvers to reduce or prevent complement activation. Similar mechanisms may be applicable to those autoimmune disorders in which complement-mediated damage is paramount. Receptors for the Fc portion of IgG (FcγRs) play a significant role in diseases mediated by immune complexes. FcγRs bind the Fc portion of IgG in the immune complexes and aid in their removal from the circulation by cells of the monocyte phagocytic system. Soluble forms of these receptors bind to the IgG in complexes and enhance their clearance. They may be useful therapeutic agents in diseases like lupus (22).

The inflammatory organ-localized autoimmune diseases are mainly attributable to cell-mediated immunity and to the production of proinflammatory cytokines and related mediators. For treatment of these diseases, a number of novel strategies suggest themselves. One approach is to employ methods to interfere with the cytokine responsible for tissue damage. IL-1, for example, is a macrophage product that may initiate the inflammatory process. In this case, one can make therapeutic use of a naturally occurring peptide, IL-1 receptor antagonist, which acts as a competitive inhibitor of proinflammatory IL-1 (23). Because the peptide is of small molecular weight, it is rapidly excreted, but its half-life can be prolonged by coupling to a carrier protein.

A similar approach can be envisioned for the cytokine TNF-α. Monoclonal antibodies can be produced to this molecule. Because these antibodies are foreign proteins, however, they evoke an immune response. Therefore, the effort was made to engineer genetically ("humanize") the monoclonal antibody, so that its half-life can be prolonged. This material has already been shown to have a remarkable effect in rheumatoid arthritis and some forms of vasculitis (24). A related approach has been to use soluble TNF receptor as a competitive inhibitor. Soluble dimeric TNF-R55 coupled to human immunoglobulin has been tested in a number of autoimmune diseases (25). Drugs are known to serve as pharmacologic inhibitors of TNF synthesis. Thalidomide, for instance, has already been subjected to preliminary clinical trial and has shown some promise (26).

Other cytokines are important in progression of autoimmune diseases. For example, administration of interferon-γ (IFN-γ) produced a sharp increase in exacerbations of multiple sclerosis. Because IFN-β and IFN-α generally have opposite effects from IFN-γ, they were tried as therapeutic agents and found to be effective in reducing exacerbations of multiple sclerosis (27).

The more distal mediators of cell-mediated immunity may also be suitable targets for therapeutic intervention. A number of drugs are available that block the synthesis of macrophage-derived inducible nitric oxide. These compounds have relatively little effect on the constitutive or endothelial form of nitric oxide synthase (NOS). In those autoimmune diseases in which nitric oxide is a major mediator of tissue injury, such agents may be efficacious. A potential drawback, however, is that inducible NOS may play an important role in resistance to infection (28). Similar cautions pertain to agents that interfere with the synthesis of reactive oxygen intermediates.

## THERAPEUTIC APPROACHES AT THE LEVEL OF THE SELF-REACTIVE T CELL

The central role of the self-reactive T cell in the progression from an autoimmune response to autoimmune disease was emphasized previously. Early attempts to employ biologic agents to treat autoimmune disease by depleting the entire cell population or the CD4$^+$ T cells were generally unsuccessful in producing a significant or sustained clinical response (29). This approach, moreover, has the potential drawback of producing general immunosuppression. More recent efforts have been directed at devising immune-based therapies that specifically inactivate the "pathogenic" T cell.

The trimolecular complex of TCR, antigenic peptide, and MHC molecule is required for the generation of an autoimmune response. This trimolecular complex, therefore, may be considered to be the optimal target for antigen-specific, highly selective therapies. Each component of the trimolecular complex can be inactivated by multiple means, singly or in concert.

Many autoimmune diseases are associated with particular MHC alleles, providing the rationale for therapies targeting disease-associated MHC molecules. Two approaches may be considered. In the first, antibody to a particular MHC allele product is used (30). Although such methods may be applicable to inbred experimental animals, humans are genetically heterogeneous. One would require, therefore, a series of anti-MHC reagents, and an individual panel would be required for each patient. A second approach is to immunize with the portion of the MHC involved in antigen binding, such as peptides from MHC class II β-chain hypervariable region (31).

Whether such a method would be useful for the heterogeneous response of human patients is still to be ascertained. Moreover, a single MHC binds a number of peptides, so that the response to the vaccine would not be strictly specific for the pathogenic peptide.

If the peptide responsible for induction of disease can be identified, it is another logical target for immune intervention. One possible therapeutic approach is to develop a blocking peptide that binds the contact sites on the MHC but offers different amino acids to the TCR (32). Copolymer-1, a synthetic, basic random polymer of L-alanine, L-glutamic acid, L-lysine and L-tyrosine, has been used successfully for the treatment of relapsing–remitting multiple sclerosis. It was discovered in a study of basic copolymers in an attempt to simulate the action of myelin basic protein in inducing experimental autoimmune encephalomyelitis (EAE) but was found to suppress the disease. It is believed to act by competing with myelin basic protein for binding to the MHC class II molecules expressed on antigen-presenting cells. As more of the binding pockets of the MHC are defined in the future, synthesis of such peptides will become more feasible. It is important, however, to determine that the deviant peptides act as antagonists rather than agonists of the pathogenic autoimmune response. In initiating T-cell proliferation, they must have great affinity for the MHC, so that they will not be displaced by the natural self peptide. In addition, the effect of such peptide analogs must be defined in terms of their effect on the various T-cell populations. T-cell unresponsiveness may be temporary, requiring continued contact with the altered peptide, or long-lasting, a result of elimination of corresponding T cells or generation of specific regulatory cells.

In applying this strategy to human autoimmune disease, a major limitation is the lack of knowledge of the antigen initiating the pathogenic autoimmune response. There are relatively few autoimmune diseases in which the responsible antigen has been identified. Equally important, the particular epitope responsible for initiation of the immune response needs to be delineated. The issues of epitope spread and immune escalation represent potential limitations to this approach to therapy of autoimmune disease.

Logic would dictate that the most specific point of attack for an immune-based therapy for autoimmune disease is the receptor of the self-reactive T cell itself. This concept requires a specific immune response against potentially self-reactive T-cell clones. The theoretical basis for this approach was laid in the 1970s when we demonstrated that it is possible to induce an immune response to the recognition structure of T cells and, thereby, abrogate a graft-versus-host reaction (33). The next conceptual step was taken by Ben-Nun and Cohen (34), who showed that it is possible to harvest T cells from a mouse undergoing an autoimmune response, attenuate the cells, and immunize a syngeneic recipient with these cells. T-cell vaccination protected the recipient against the induction of the particular autoimmune disease or even arrested the progression of active disease.

The original concept of T-cell vaccination required the isolation of self-reactive T-cell clones and their cultivation and expansion, inactivation or attenuation *in vitro*, and reinjection into a syngeneic recipient. In terms of a human therapy, a more effective approach has been to isolate the antigen-specific TCR of the autoreactive T cells, rather than employing the whole cell. The most variable portion of the TCR is the CDR-3 region. Going one step further, a peptide representing the CDR-3 can be prepared, combined with an appropriate adjuvant, and administered as a preventive or therapeutic vaccine (35).

Several successful applications of T-cell vaccination against autoimmune disease have been reported, using experimental models of human diseases, such as encephalomyelitis (36) and myasthenia gravis (37). The method has been to isolate a T-cell line capable of transferring the disease and to inactivate it by irradiation, hyperbaric pressure, or fixation with cross-linking agents, such as glutaraldehyde. Administration of such attenuated T cells protects animals against actively induced disease.

The mechanism of protection conferred by T-cell vaccines is unclear, but it is possible that vaccination leads to the proliferation of CD8$^+$ regulatory T cells that act directly to inactivate self-reactive CD4 T cells or act as regulatory T cells by production of soluble factors. In experimental models, such as allergic encephalomyelitis, the success of this approach may depend on the fact that this disease in animals is genetically highly restricted. Most encephalitogenic T-cell clones use the TCR β chain Vβ8.2. It is not clear, however, that the ultimate immune response is Vβ8.2 specific. There is evidence that regulatory T cells induced by immunization with the Vβ peptide produce soluble factors that inhibit not only the stimulating Vβ8.2 T cells but also T cells expressing different Vβ genes (38). This observation would make the method more attractive for human application because it is unlikely that any human disease is genetically so narrowly restricted as is allergic encephalomyelitis in mice.

An innovation has been to employ DNA vaccine rather than the Vβ peptides for immunization (35). Intramuscular administration of "naked DNA" is capable of inducing an effective immune response to a number of antigens. The advantage of this procedure is that it eliminates the need for repeated injections and the use of an adjuvant.

In addition to the trimolecular complex of an antigen-specific TCR and an antigenic peptide bound to the MHC molecule, an effective immune response requires the participation of costimulatory signals. The absence of such secondary signals leads to inactivation or anergy of the T cell. Another therapeutic approach is to block these costimulatory pathways. A major advantage of this strategy is that the antigen responsible for initiating the autoimmune process need not be known. Activated T cells actually undergoing an immune response are anergized, whereas most resting T cells are not influenced. One promising procedure is to block the CD28$^-$ B7 pathway. The experimental therapy may use either an anti-B7 monoclonal antibody or a CTLA4Ig fusion protein (39,40). Administration of anti-B7.1 may either prevent an immune response by blocking the necessary costimulatory pathway or shift the response from a $T_H1$ to a $T_H2$ pattern. CTLA4Ig, representing an alternative, high-affinity ligand for B7, also effectively blocks the response. With its Ig fusion partner, it remains in the circulation for the required period of time. An attractive feature of this approach is that it may lead to long-term anergy after a short course of treatment.

A second costimulatory pathway is represented by CD40 and its ligand CD40L, or CD154 (gp39). Although originally thought of as stimulatory for B cells, it is now apparent that there is also a profound effect on cell-mediated immune responses. Antibodies to CD40 have already shown promise for use in mice in autoimmune disease (41). A combination of CTLA4Ig and anti-CD154 may be more effective than either reagent alone (42).

Another therapeutic maneuver that has shown promise in experimental models has been the inhibition of intercellular adhesion molecules. Monoclonal antibodies to adhesion molecules may interrupt the association of the self-reactive T cell with its antigen-presenting cell or may impair the localization of effector cells at the target organ site. Either of these effects would arrest the progression of the autoimmune process. Monoclonal antibody to the intercellular adhesion molecule 1 (ICAM-1) has already been shown to suppress EAE in actively immunized rats (43). It had little effect on the adoptive T-cell transfer model, however, indicating that the monoclonal antibody to ICAM-1 acted mainly at the inductive phase of the immune response, rather than on T-cell localization. On the other hand, recombinant soluble ICAM-1 inhibited lymphocyte attachment to cultured cerebral endothelial cells, indicating that the soluble molecule might impede lymphocyte localization. Because adhesion molecules play an important role in the inflammatory process, it is possible that these reagents interfere with the inflammatory reaction as well as with the autoimmune process.

As T cells undergo immune activation, they express a number of markers on their surface. These surface molecules provide attractive targets for immune-based therapies. An example of such an activation marker is the IL-2 receptor. Monoclonal antibodies to the IL-2 receptor or IL-2 itself can be conjugated to toxin, such as the A chain of ricin (46) or the enzymatically active portion of diphtheria toxin (44). Antibody to IL-2 receptor or IL-2 guides the toxic molecule to the activated T cells, which would, thereby, be killed. The use of activation markers as targets is not antigen specific because T cells activated at the time of treatment by other antigens would also serve as target for the immunotoxin. It may be an advantage in instances in which the "pathogenic" antigen is unknown.

A considerable amount of research has been expended on the production of monoclonal antibodies against T-cell differentiation molecules. Antibody to CD4, for example, is useful for the control of transplantation rejection. In several murine models of lupus, anti-CD4 was effective in delaying the onset of disease or even in arresting the progress of ongoing disease. Both depleting and nondepleting forms of the antibody have been used in experimental models (45). The humanized form of anti-CD4 autoantibody has been tested in a number of autoimmune diseases, such as rheumatoid arthritis and multiple sclerosis (46). Although the administration of anti-CD4 caused depletion of circulating CD4$^+$ T cells, there was little appreciable effect on the progression of the human diseases. Similar studies were carried out with antibody against CD52, a marker that is expressed on all lymphocytes and some monocytes. In one study of multiple sclerosis, infusion of this antibody was accompanied by exacerbation of the disease, possibly resulting from increased production of proinflammatory cytokines (47). This type of treatment, therefore, would have to be employed with great caution.

Depending on the conditions of activation, as well as the genetic background of the host, activation of self-reactive T cells may lead primarily to a $T_H1$ or a $T_H2$ response. In mice, $T_H1$ cells secrete IL-2, IFN-$\gamma$, and lymphotoxin, whereas $T_H2$ cells produce IL-4, IL-5, IL-9, IL-10, and IL-13. In humans, the distinction between these two types of T cells is blurred. There is some evidence that the $T_H1$ cytokines are primarily responsible for a number of the organ-specific autoimmune diseases (48). A plausible therapeutic approach, therefore, is to shift the spectrum of cytokines produced during the immune response by immune deviation. Because the cytokine products of $T_H1$ and $T_H2$ cells are mutually inhibitory for the differentiation in effector functions of the reciprocal type, there are several ways to produce such deviation. For example, IFN-$\gamma$ selectively inhibits the proliferation of $T_H2$ cells, whereas IL-10 inhibits cytokine synthesis by $T_H1$ cells (49).

Therapeutic use of cytokine administration is fraught with hazards because the dosage and timing of the cytokine often determine its effect. Although IL-12 is known primarily for its ability to favor $T_H1$ responses, administration of this cytokine later in the course of an autoimmune response may actually diminish autoimmune thyroiditis (50). Clearly, a great deal more needs to be learned about the intricacies of the cytokine network before safe and effective interventions involving cytokines can be devised.

The application of oral tolerance to the treatment of autoimmune diseases is based on old observations that administration of antigen through the gastrointestinal tract results in antigen-specific hyporesponsiveness. It apparently uses a physiologic mechanism to prevent unwanted immune responses to ingested proteins. Animals fed bovine serum albumin (BSA), for example, and then immunized with BSA, subsequently show a reduced immune response against the fed antigen but not against other antigens (51). Depending on the dose of antigen administered, orally administered antigens can either lead to the deletion of antigen-specific T cells or inhibit antigen-specific T cells by the induction of clonal anergy (52). Moreover, antigens that pass through the intestine preferentially induce the $T_H2$ type of T cells. Such T cells migrate from the gut to the organs containing the fed antigen. These $T_H2$ cells are then locally stimulated to release regulatory cytokines. Thus, oral tolerization results in the production of regulatory T cells that are triggered in an antigen-specific manner but suppress in an antigen-nonspecific fashion. The regulatory cytokines TGF-$\beta$, IL-10, and IL-4, produced by cells from an animal fed a tissue-specific antigen, may mediate "bystander suppression" when the T cells encounter the autoantigen at the target organ (53). Therefore, oral tolerance as a therapy may have the advantage that the antigen directly responsible for causing the pathologic consequences of the autoimmune response need not be identified.

Oral tolerance has proved to be effective in suppressing several experimental autoimmune diseases, including EAE (54), experimental uveitis (55), and collagen-induced arthritis (56). In some models, intranasal application of the antigen has proved to be even more effective than oral administration (57). Early studies were inconclusive, and the value of oral or nasal tolerance in human autoimmune disease needs to be tested in large-scale clinical trials. Under some conditions, oral administration of autoantigen can induce or exacerbate autoimmune disease (58).

## CONCLUSIONS

The past decade has seen a marked change in the approach to the treatment of autoimmune disease. Rather than depending on correction of a particular organ function or global immunosuppression, attention has turned to more specific strategies for arresting the development of the autoimmune response and the progression from benign to pathogenic autoimmunity (59). The efforts to develop more directed therapies have been enhanced by greater understanding of the etiology of the autoimmune diseases at the induction level, greater knowledge of the effector mechanisms responsible for the cellular and tissue injury, and more awareness of the intricacies of T-cell activation. Many different approaches are being actively pursued because each entails certain risks as well as advantages. It may well be that no single approach will be appropriate for all autoimmune diseases. Nevertheless, this research has emphasized the common threads that unite all of the autoimmune disorders. The importance of strengthening cross-specialty collaboration, however, has become increasingly obvious as the same modality of treatment finds application in diverse autoimmune diseases.

It is not too daring to suggest that the treatment of autoimmune diseases is at a point in time similar to the late 1940s and 1950s in the study of infectious diseases. Before that time, there were few specific remedies, and most treatments of infectious disease were symptomatic and supportive. The introduction of antibiotics for the first time opened the possibility of a cure for many of the infectious diseases. It required a much enhanced ability to diagnose these diseases early and to identify the causative agent. In the case of the autoimmune diseases, early intervention would appear to be equally important. A great opportunity has been created by studies of genetic predisposition to identify people at an inordinate risk for developing an autoimmune disorder. If an intervention is sufficiently harmless, it may well be possible to administer a treatment before there are any clinical manifestations of disease. Similarly, the identification of environmental triggers of autoimmune disease may permit people at increased risk to avoid the incriminated infectious or chemical agent. Based on the fundamental knowledge obtained and on progress made during the recent past, it is likely that the first decade of the 21st century will see a dramatic change in the approach to therapy and prevention of the autoimmune diseases.

## ACKNOWLEDGMENT

This chapter was supported by National Institutes of Health research grant #HL33878.

## REFERENCES

1. Oldstone MBA. Molecular mimicry and immune-mediated diseases. *Ocular Immunol* 1998;12:1255–1265.
2. Cunningham MW, Antone SM, Gulizia JM, et al. Cytotoxic and viral neutralizing antibodies crossreact with streptococcal M protein, enteroviruses, and human cardiac myosin. *Proc Natl Acad Sci U S A* 1992;89:1320–1324.
3. Schiffenbauer J, Soos J, Johnson H. The possible role of bacterial superantigens in the pathogenesis of autoimmune disorders. *Immunol Today* 1998;19:117–120.
4. Lehmann PV, Forsthuber T, Miller A, et al. Spreading of T cell autoimmunity to cryptic determinants of an autoantigen. *Nature (London)* 1992;358:155–157.
5. Moudgil KD, Sercarz EE. Antigenic determinants involved in induction and propagation of autoimmunity. In: Rose NR, Mackay IR, eds. *The autoimmune diseases.* 3rd ed. San Diego: Academic Press, 1998:45–58.
6. Griffith TS, Brunner T, Fletcher SM, et al. Fas ligand-induced apoptosis as a mechanism of immune privilege. *Science* 1995;270:1189–1197.
7. Ada GL, Rose NR. The initiation and early development of autoimmune diseases. *Clin Immunol Immunopathol* 1988;47:3–9.
8. Miller JFAP, Heath WR, Allison J, et al. T cell tolerance and autoimmunity. In: *The molecular basis of defence.* Melbourne, Australia: Ciba Foundation Symposium, 1997:159–168.
9. Romagnani S. T-cell subsets (Th1, Th2) and cytokines in autoimmunity. In: Rose NR, Mackay IR, eds. *The autoimmune diseases.* 3rd ed. San Diego: Academic Press, 1998:163–191.
10. Vandenbark AA, Chou JK, Whitham R, et al. Effects of vaccination with T cell receptor peptides: epitope switching to a possible disease-protective determinant of myelin basic protein that is cross-reactive with a TCR BV peptide. *Immunol Cell Biol* 1998;76:83–90.
11. Wong S, Guerder S, Visintin I, et al. Expression of the co-stimulator molecule B7-1 in pancreatic E1-cells accelerates diabetes in the NOD mouse. *Diabetes* 1995;44:326–329.
12. Rose NR, Skelton FR, Kite JH Jr, et al. Experimental thyroiditis in the rhesus monkey. III. Course of the disease. *Clin Exp Immunol* 1966;1:171–188.
13. Nelson JL, Torrez R, Louie FM, et al. Pre-existing autoimmune disease in patients with long-term survival after allogenic bone marrow transplantation. *J Rheumatol Suppl* 1997;48:23–29.
14. van Bekkum DW. New opportunities for the treatment of severe autoimmune diseases: bone marrow transplantation. *Clin Immunol Immunopathol* 1998;89:1–10.
15. Marmont AM. Immune ablation followed by allogeneic or autologous bone marrow transplantation: a new treatment for severe autoimmune disease? *Stem Cells* 1994;12:125–135.
16. Brodsky A, Petri M, Smith BD, et al. Immunoablative high-dose cyclophosphamide without stem cell rescue for refractory, severe autoimmune disease. *Ann Intern Med* 1998;129:1031–1035.
17. Lau HT, Yu M, Fontana A, et al. Prevention of islet allograft rejection with engineered myoblasts expressing FasL in mice. *Science* 1996;273:109–112.
18. Revillard J-P, Adorini L, Goldman M, et al. Apoptosis: potential for disease therapies. *Immunol Today* 1998;19:292–293.
19. Rose NR, Rasooly L, Saboori AM, Burek CL. Linking iodine with autoimmune thyroiditis. *Environ Health Perspect* 1999;107:749–752.
20. Keesey J, Buffkin D, Kebo D, et al. Plasma exchange as therapy for myasthenia gravis. *Ann N Y Acad Sci* 1981;377:729–743.
21. Strand V, Lee ML. Intravenous immunoglobulin (IVIg) in the treatment of autoimmune diseases. In: Strand V, Scott DL, Simon LS, eds. *Novel therapeutic agents for the treatment of autoimmune diseases.* New York: Marcel Dekker, 1997:235–256.
22. Watanabe H, Sherris D, Gilkeson GS. Soluble D16 in the treatment of murine lupus nephritis. *Clin Immunol Immunopathol* 1998;88:91–95.
23. Arend WP. Interleukin 1 receptor antagonist: a new member of the interleukin 1 family. *J Clin Invest* 1991;88:1445–1451.
24. Choy EHS, Panayi GS. Engineered human anti-tumor necrosis factor-alpha (TNFα) antibody, CDP571, in rheumatoid arthritis. In: Stramd V, Scott DL, Simon LS, eds. *Novel therapeutic agents for the treatment of autoimmune diseases.* New York: Marcel Dekker, 1997:121–129.
25. Heaney ML, Golde DW. Soluble cytokine receptors. *Blood* 1996;87:847–857.
26. Hamuruydan V, Mat C, Saip S, et al. Thalidomide in the treatment of the mucocutaneous lesions of the Behçet syndrome. *Ann Intern Med* 1998;128:443–450.
27. Bashir K, Whitaker JN. Current immunotherapy in multiple sclerosis. *Immunol Cell Biol* 1998;76:55–64.
28. Lowenstein CJ, Hill SL, Lafond-Walker A, et al. Nitric oxide inhibits viral replication in murine myocarditis. *J Clin Invest* 1996;97:1837–1843.
29. Moreland LW, Koopman WJ. Chimeric anti-CD4 antibody as a potential therapeutic agent for rheumatoid arthritis. In: Strand V, Scott DL, Simon LS, eds. *Novel therapeutic agents for the treatment of autoimmune diseases.* New York: Marcel Dekker, 1997:41–53.
30. Steinman L, Rosenbaum JT, Sriram S, et al. In vivo protective effects of antibodies to immune response gene products: prevention of experimental allergic encephalomyelitis. *Proc Natl Acad Sci U S A* 1981;78:7111–7114.
31. Bright JJ, Topham DJ, Nag B, et al. Vaccination with peptides from MHC class II beta chain hypervariable region causes allele-specific suppression of EAE. *J Neuroimmunol* 1996;67:119–124.
32. Arnon R. The development of Cop-1 (Copaxone), an innovative drug for the treatment of multiple sclerosis. *Immunol Lett* 1996;50:1–15.
33. Rose NR. Modification of hybrid responsiveness in the local graft-versus-host reaction by injection of parental lymphocytes. *Transplantation* 1975;20:248–254.
34. Ben-Nun A, Cohen IR. Vaccination against autoimmune encephalomyelitis (EAE): attenuated autoimmune T lymphocytes confer resistance to induction of active EAE but not to EAE mediated by the intact T lymphocyte line. *Eur J Immunol* 1981;11:949–952.
35. Bona CA, Casares S, Brumeanu T-D. Towards development of T-cell vaccines. *Immunol Today* 1998;19:126–133.
36. VandenBark AA, Hashim G, Offner H. Immunization with a synthetic T-cell receptor V-region peptide protects against experimental autoimmune encephalomyelitis. *Nature* 1989;341:541–544.
37. Kahn CR, McIntosh KR, Drachman DB. T-cell vaccination in experimental myasthenia gravis: a double-edged sword. *J Autoimmun* 1990;3:659–669.
38. Offner H, Hashim GA, Vandenbark AA. T cell receptor peptide therapy triggers autoregulation of experimental encephalomyelitis. *Science* 1991;251:430–432.
39. Bluestone JA. New perspectives of CD28-B7-mediated T cell costimulation. *Immunity* 1995;2:555–559.
40. Linsley PS, Wallace PM, Johnson J, et al. Immunosuppression in vivo by a soluble form of the CTLA-4 T cell activation molecule. *Science* 1992;257:792–795.
41. Early GS, Zhao W, Burns CM. Anti-CD40 ligand antibody treatment prevents the development of lupus-like nephritis in a subset of New Zealand black × New Zealand white mice. *J Immunol* 1996;157:3159–3164.
42. Griggs ND, Agersborg SS, Noelle RJ, et al. The relative contribution of the CD28 and gp39 costimulatory pathways in the clonal expression and pathogenic acquisition of self reactive T cells. *J Exp Med* 1996;183:801–810.

43. Archelos JJ, Jung S, Mäurer M, et al. Inhibition of experimental autoimmune encephalomyelitis by an antibody to the intercellular adhesion molecule ICAM-1. *Ann Neurol* 1993;34:145–154.

44. Woodworth TG, Parker K. Early clinical studies of IL-2 fusion toxin in patients with severe rheumatoid arthritis, recent-onset insulin-dependent diabetes mellitus, and psoriasis. In: Strand V, Scott DL, Simon LS, eds. *Novel therapeutic agents for the treatment of autoimmune diseases.* New York: Marcel Dekker, 1997:25–39.

45. Carteron NL. Schimenti CL, Wofsy D. Treatment of murine lupus with F(ab′)$_2$ fragments of monoclonal antibody to L3T4: suppression of autoimmunity does not depend on T helper cell depletion. *J Immunol* 1989;142:1470–1475.

46. Levy R, Weisman M, Wiesenhutter C, et al. Results of a placebo-controlled, multicenter trial using a primatized non-depleting, anti-CD4 monoclonal antibody in the treatment of rheumatoid arthritis. *Arthritis Rheum* 1996;39:S122.

47. Moreau T, Coles A, Wing M, et al. Transient increase in symptoms associated with cytokine in patients with multiple sclerosis. *Brain* 1996;119:225–237.

48. Adorini L. Guéry J-C, Trembleau S. Manipulation of the Th1/Th2 cell balance: an approach to treat human autoimmune diseases? *Autoimmunity* 1996;23:53–68.

49. Romagnani S, Maggi M. Th1 versus Th2 responses in AIDS. *Curr Opin Immunol* 1994;6:616–622.

50. Stafford EA, Hill SL, Rose NR. IL12 treatment increases or decreases the severity of autoimmune thyroiditis in mice, depending on timing and strain. *FASEB J Part II* 1998;A1084:6276(abst).

51. Weiner HL, Friedman A, Miller A, et al. Oral tolerance: immunologic mechanisms and treatment of animal and human organ-specific autoimmune diseases by oral administration of autoantigens. *Annu Rev Immunol* 1994;12:809–837.

52. Melamed D, Fredman A. *In vivo* tolerization of Th1 lymphocytes following a single feeding with ovalbumin: anergy in the absence of suppression. *Eur J Immunol* 1994;24:1974–1981.

53. Chen Y, Kuchroo VK, Inobe J-I, et al. Regulatory T cell clones induced by oral tolerance: suppression of autoimmune encephalomyelitis. *Science* 1994;265:1237–1240.

54. Al-Sabbagh A, Miller A, Santos LMB, et al. Antigen-driven tissue-specific suppression following oral tolerance: orally administered myelin-basic protein suppresses proteolipid protein-induced experimental autoimmune encephalomyelitis in the SJL mouse. *Eur J Immunol* 1994;24:2105–2109.

55. Thurau SR, Diedrichs-Möhring, Fricke H, et al. Molecular mimicry as a therapeutic approach for an autoimmune disease: oral treatment of uveitis-patients with an MHC-peptide crossreactive with autoantigen—first results. *Immunol Lett* 1997;57:193–201.

56. Sieper J, Kary S, Sorensen H, et al. Oral type II collagen treatment in early rheumatoid arthritis: a double-blind, placebo-controlled, randomized trial. *Arthritis Rheum* 1996;39:41–51.

57. Shi F-D, Bai X-F, Huang Y-M, et al. Nasal tolerance in experimental autoimmune myasthenia gravis (EAMG): induction of protective tolerance in primed animals. *Clin Exp Immunol* 1998;111:506–512.

58. Blanas E, Carbone FR, Allison J, et al. Induction of autoimmune diabetes by oral administration of autoantigen. *Science* 1996;274:1707–1709.

59. Willenborg DO, Staykova MA. Approaches to the treatment of central nervous system autoimmune disease using specific neuroantigen. *Immunol Cell Biol* 1998;76:91–103.

# Subject Index

# Subject Index

in systemic lupus erythematosus, 538
tests for, 727–736
for anticentromere antibodies, 734
false-positive/false-negative results,
728, 729
in fibromyalgia, 711
Antiovarian antibodies, 489, 492–493
Antioxidants, 307
Antiperinuclear factor antibodies
as rheumatoid arthritis marker, 586
tests for, 734
Antiphospholipid antibodies, 203–204,
538, 641–642, 742–743
tests for, 656–657, 742–743
Antiphospholipid antibody syndromes, 8,
203–204, 641–668
catastrophic, 654, 655, 658
clinical manifestations of, 643–656
adrenal, 650–651
cardiac, 647–649
dermatologic, 653–654
digestive, 652
hematologic, 654
hepatic, 651–652
large-vessel, 643–644
microangiopathic syndromes, 655
neurologic, 644–647
obstetric, 652–653
pulmonary, 649
renal, 649–650
drug-induced, 789–790
hepatitis C virus infection–associated,
670–671, 674
incidence and epidemiology of, 641–643
thrombotic, 204, 205
Antiplatelet drugs, as immunoglobulin A
nephropathy therapy, 327
Anti-proliferating cell nuclear antigen antibodies, tests for, 735
Anti-ribonucleoprotein antibodies, tests for,
732
Antiribosomal P protein antibody, tests for,
736
Anti-Ro (SSA) antibodies
Sjögren's syndrome–associated, 569,
570, 571
tests for, 732–733, 734
Anti-Scl-70 antibodies, tests for, 734
Anti-Smith antibodies, tests for, 731–732
Antisperm antibodies, in orchitis, 484, 485,
486, 487, 488, 489
Antisynthetase autoantibody syndrome, 89
Antithyroid antibodies
Hashimoto's thyroiditis–associated,
384–385
tests for, 743–744
Antithyroid drugs, 381
Anti-type II collagen antibody tests, 745–746
APECED syndrome, 398–399
Aplasia
drug-induced, 788, 789

marrow, 789
pure red cell, 192
acquired, 194–195
in immunocompromised patients, 208
Apolipoprotein E, 454
Apoptosis
autoantibody production during, 95
of B cells, 17
CD95-mediated, 760
definition of, 71–72
Fas/FasL in, 383
in T-cell negative selection, 71–72
of T cells, 4, 7
Appendectomy, 243
Appetite suppressants, as scleroderma
cause, 558
Arachidonic acid metabolites, 8, 49, 307
Arbovirus, as myocarditis cause, 275
Arenavirus (Lassa fever), as myocarditis
cause, 275
Argyria, silver-associated, 757
Aromatase, in endometriosis, 481
Arrhythmia, myocarditis-associated,
279–280, 283
Arterial disease, as Raynaud's phenomenon
cause, 559
Arteritis
giant cell, 291, 549, 550, 551–552
Takayasu's, 291, 505, 549, 550, 551
temporal, 549, 550
Arthralgia
antiphospholipid syndromes–associated,
653
hepatitis C virus infection–associated,
671–672
silicone breast implant–associated, 723
Arthritides, infection-associated, 581
Arthritis. See also Rheumatoid arthritis
acute rheumatic fever–associated,
288–289
antiphospholipid syndromes–associated,
653
collagen-induced, 577, 823–828
autoimmune costimulation in, 180, 182
hepatitis B–associated, 701
infectious, 581
inflammatory, scleromyositis-associated,
453
juvenile
antiphospholipid antibodies associated
with, 743
pauciarticular chronic, 727
parvovirus-associated, 695, 697
peripheral, inflammatory bowel disease–
associated, 253
poststreptococcal reactive, 685–687
psoriatic, antiphospholipid antibodies
associated with, 642, 743
reactive, 701–703
rheumatic fever–associated, 685–686

systemic lupus erythematosus–associated,
538, 540, 541–542
togavirus-associated, 697
viral, 697–701
Arthus reaction, 86
Asbestosis, 304, 314–315, 316, 741
Aschoff's lesions, 682, 684
Aspartate aminotransferase, as idiopathic
inflammatory myopathy marker,
430–431, 437
Aspartate transaminase, as juvenile
dermatomyositis marker, 448
*Aspergillus*, as myocarditis cause, 275
Aspirin
as antiphospholipid syndrome prophylaxis, 658
as rheumatic carditis therapy, 288
Asthma, 308–312, 511
bronchial, 8
late-phase, 304–305
Astrocytes, in multiple sclerosis, 598
Ataxia
cerebellar, 646
paraneoplastic, 361
Atlantoaxial joint, rheumatoid arthritis of,
581, 586
Atopy, 8
Atrophy, idiopathic adrenal, 387
Auranofin, as rheumatoid arthritis therapy,
590
Austin–Dyck syndrome, 354
Autoantibodies, 81–100
classification of, 81, 82
conventional, 91–92
detection techniques for, 81–83
in disease pathogenesis
antibody-mediated cytotoxic hypersensitivity mechanism, 83, 84–86
immune complex–mediated hypersensitivity mechanism, 83, 86–87
genetic determination of, 93–94
as markers of disease processes, 87–90
natural, 91
origins of, 90–93
production of, 94–95
environmental triggers of, 93–94
genetic determination of, 93–94
Autoantibody-mediated cytolytic
syndromes, 197–203
Autoantibody responses, memory cells in, 7
Autoimmune disease
definition of, 783
differentiated from autoimmunity, 83
immunopathogenesis of, 843–845
superantigen-related exacerbation of, 30
Autoimmunity
definition of, 843
differentiated from autoimmune disease,
83
immune system suppression of, 515
origin of term, 81